KT-509-296

Meyler's Side Effects of Drugs

The International Encyclopedia of Adverse Drug Reactions and Interactions

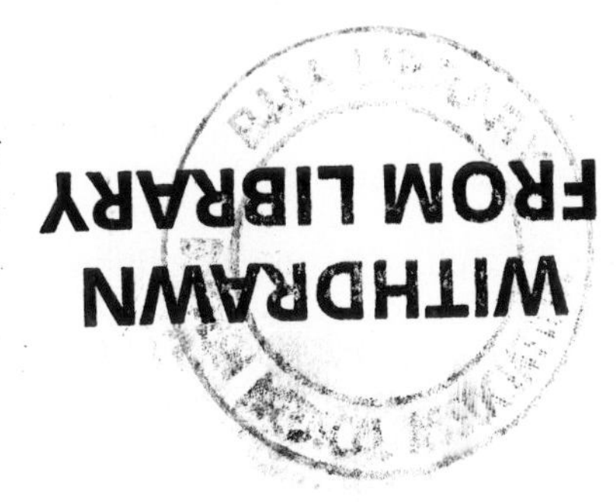

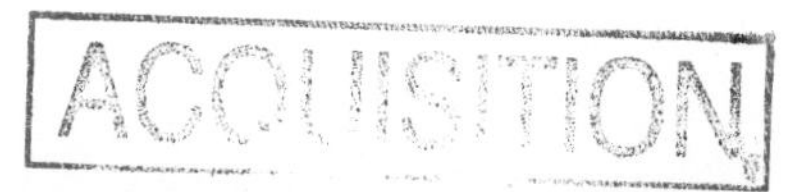

Complementary to this volume

Side Effects of Drugs Annuals 24–29 (1999–2006)
Edited by Jeffrey K. Aronson (Earlier annuals are no longer available in print)

Drugs During Pregnancy and Lactation, Second edition (2006)
Edited by Christof Schaefer et al.

The Law and Ethics of the Pharmaceutical Industry (2005)
By Graham Dukes

Introduction to Clinical Pharmacology, Fifth edition (2006)
By Marilyn Edmunds

Principles of Clinical Pharmacology, Second edition (2006)
Edited by Arthur Atkinson et al.

Writing Clinical Research Protocols (2006)
By E. De Renzo

A Pharmacology Primer (2003)
By Terry Kenakin

Publishing history of *Meyler's Side Effects of Drugs*

*Volume**	*Date of publication*	*Editors*
First published in Dutch	1951	L Meyler
First published in English	1952	L Meyler
First updating volume	1957	L Meyler
Second volume	1958	L Meyler
Third volume	1960	L Meyler
Fourth volume	1964	L Meyler
Fifth volume	1966	L Meyler, C Dalderup, W Van Dijl, and HGG Bouma
Sixth volume	1968	L Meyler and A Herxheimer
Seventh volume	1972	L Meyler and A Herxheimer
Eighth volume	1975	MNG Dukes
Ninth edition	1980	MNG Dukes
Tenth edition	1984	MNG Dukes
Eleventh edition	1988	MNG Dukes
Twelfth edition	1992	MNG Dukes
Thirteenth edition	1996	MNG Dukes
Fourteenth edition	2000	MNG Dukes & JK Aronson
Fifteenth edition	2006	JK Aronson

*The first eight volumes were updates; the ninth edition was the first encyclopedic version and updating continued with the Side Effects of Drugs Annual (SEDA) series.

At various times, full or shortened editions of volumes in the Side Effects series have appeared in French, Russian, Dutch, German, and Japanese.
The website of *Meyler's Side Effects of Drugs* can be viewed at:
http://www.elsevier.com/locate/Meyler.

Meyler's Side Effects of Drugs

The International Encyclopedia of Adverse Drug Reactions and Interactions

Fifteenth edition

Editor

JK Aronson, MA, DPhil, MBChB, FRCP, FBPharmacol S
Oxford, United Kingdom

Honorary Editor

MNG Dukes, MA, DPhil, MB, FRCP
Oslo, Norway

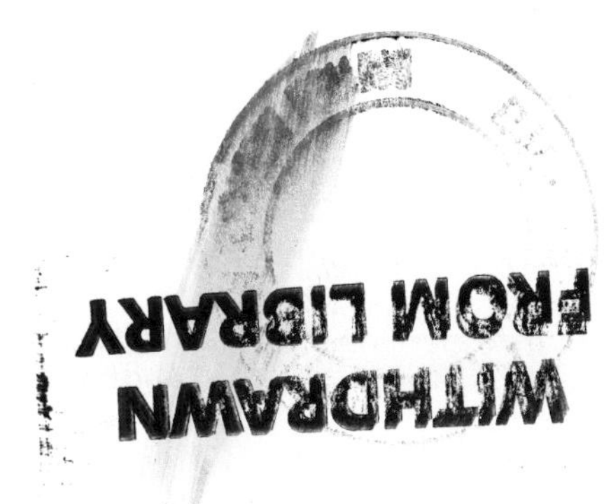

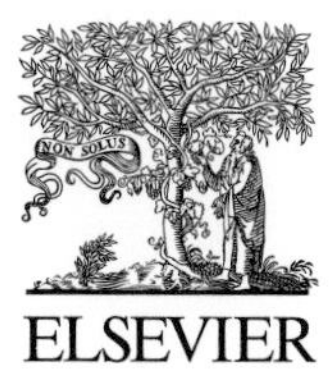

AMSTERDAM • BOSTON • HEIDELBERG • LONDON • NEW YORK • OXFORD
PARIS • SAN DIEGO • SAN FRANCISCO • SINGAPORE • SYDNEY • TOKYO

Elsevier
Radarweg 29, PO Box 211, 1000 AE Amsterdam, The Netherlands

Fifteenth edition 2006
Reprinted 2007

British Library Cataloguing in Publication Data
A catalogue record for this book is available from the British Library

Library of Congress Cataloging-in-Publication Data
A catalog record for this book is available from the Library of Congress

ISBN: 978-0-444-50998-7 (Set)
ISBN: 978-0-444-52251-1 (Volume 1)
ISBN: 978-0-444-52252-8 (Volume 2)
ISBN: 978-0-444-52253-5 (Volume 3)
ISBN: 978-0-444-52254-2 (Volume 4)
ISBN: 978-0-444-52255-9 (Volume 5)
ISBN: 978-0-444-52256-6 (Volume 6)

For information on all Elsevier publications visit our website at books.elsevier.com

Printed and bound in *Great Britain*

07 08 09 10 10 9 8 7 6 5 4 3 2

Contents

Contributors

In this list the main contributors to the Encyclopedia are identified according to the original chapter material to which they made the most contribution. Most have contributed the relevant chapters in one or more editions of the *Side Effects of Drugs Annuals* 23-27 and/or the 14th edition of *Meyler's Side Effects of Drugs*. A few have contributed individual monographs to this edition.

M. Allwood
Derby, United Kingdom
Intravenous infusions—solutions and emulsions

M. Andersen
Odense, Denmark
Antihistamines

M. Andrejak
Amiens, France
Drugs affecting blood coagulation, fibrinolysis, and hemostasis

J.K. Aronson
Oxford, United Kingdom
Antiepileptic drugs
Antiviral drugs
Positive inotropic drugs and drugs used in dysrhythmias

S. Arroyo
Milwaukee, Wisconsin, USA
Antiepileptic drugs

I. Aursnes
Oslo, Norway
Drugs that affect lipid metabolism

H. Bagheri
Toulouse, France
Radiological contrast agents

A.M. Baldacchino
London, United Kingdom
Opioid analgesics and narcotic antagonists

D. Battino
Milan, Italy
Antiepileptic drugs

Z. Baudoin
Zagreb, Croatia
General anesthetics and therapeutic gases

A.G.C. Bauer
Rotterdam, The Netherlands
Antihelminthic drugs
Dermatological drugs, topical agents, and cosmetics

M. Behrend
Deggendorf, Germany
Drugs acting on the immune system

T. Bicanic
London, United Kingdom
Antiprotozoal drugs

L. Biscarini
Perugia, Italy
Anti-inflammatory and antipyretic analgesics and drugs used in gout

J. Blaser
Zurich, Switzerland
Various antibacterial drugs

C. Bokemeyer
Tübingen, Germany
Cytostatic drugs

S. Borg
Stockholm, Sweden
Antidepressant drugs

J. Bousquet
Montpellier, France
Antihistamines

P.J. Bown
Redhill, Surrey, United Kingdom
Opioid analgesics and narcotic antagonists

C.N. Bradfield
Auckland, New Zealand
General anesthetics and therapeutic gases

C.C.E. Brodie-Meijer
Amstelveen, The Netherlands
Metal antagonists

P.W.G. Brown
Sheffield, United Kingdom
Radiological contrast agents

A. Buitenhuis
Amsterdam, The Netherlands
Sex hormones and related compounds, including hormonal contraceptives

H. Cardwell
Auckland, New Zealand
Local anesthetics

A. Carvajal
Valladolid, Spain
Antipsychotic drugs

R. Cathomas
Zurich, Switzerland
Drugs acting on the respiratory tract

A. Cerny
Zurich, Switzerland
Various antibacterial drugs

G. Chevrel
Lyon, France
Drugs acting on the immune system

C.C. Chiou
Bethesda, Maryland, USA
Antifungal drugs

N.H. Choulis
Attika, Greece
Metals
Miscellaneous drugs and materials, medical devices, and techniques not dealt with in other chapters

L.G. Cleland
Adelaide, Australia
Corticotrophins, corticosteroids, and prostaglandins

P. Coates
Adelaide, Australia
Miscellaneous hormones

J. Costa
Badalona, Spain
Corticotrophins, corticosteroids, and prostaglandins

P. Cottagnoud
Bern, Switzerland
Various antibacterial drugs

P.C. Cowen
Oxford, United Kingdom
Antidepressant drugs

S. Curran
Huddersfield, United Kingdom
Hypnosedatives and anxiolytics

H.C.S. Daly
Perth, Western Australia
Local anesthetics

A.C. De Groot
Hertogenbosch, The Netherlands
Dermatological drugs, topical agents, and cosmetics

M.D. De Jong
Amsterdam, The Netherlands
Antiviral drugs

A. Del Favero
Perugia, Italy
Anti-inflammatory and antipyretic analgesics and drugs used in gout

P. Demoly
Montpellier, France
Antihistamines

J. Descotes
Lyon, France
Drugs acting on the immune system

A.J. De Silva
Ragama, Sri Lanka
Snakebite antivenom

H.J. De Silva
Ragama, Sri Lanka
Gastrointestinal drugs

F.A. De Wolff
Leiden, The Netherlands
Metals

S. Dittmann
Berlin, Germany
Vaccines

M.N.G. Dukes
Oslo, Norway
Antiepileptic drugs
Antiviral drugs
Metals
Sex hormones and related compounds, including hormonal contraceptives

H.W. Eijkhout
Amsterdam, The Netherlands
Blood, blood components, plasma, and plasma products

E.H. Ellinwood
Durham, North Carolina, USA
Central nervous system stimulants and drugs that suppress appetite

C.J. Ellis
Birmingham, United Kingdom
Drugs used in tuberculosis and leprosy

P. Elsner
Jena, Germany
Dermatological drugs, topical agents, and cosmetics

T. Erikkson
Lund, Sweden
Thalidomide

E. Ernst
Exeter, United Kingdom
Treatments used in complementary and alternative medicine

M. Farré
Barcelona, Spain
Corticotrophins, corticosteroids, and prostaglandins

P.I. Folb
Cape Town, South Africa
Cytostatic drugs
Intravenous infusions—solutions and emulsions

J.A. Franklyn
Birmingham, United Kingdom
Thyroid hormones and antithyroid drugs

M.G. Franzosi
Milan, Italy
Beta-adrenoceptor antagonists and antianginal drugs

J. Fraser
Glasgow, Scotland
Cytostatic drugs

H.M.P. Freie
Maastricht, The Netherlands
Antipyretic analgesics

C. Fux
Bern, Switzerland
Various antibacterial drugs

P.J. Geerlings
Amsterdam, The Netherlands
Drugs of abuse

A.H. Ghodse
London, United Kingdom
Opioid analgesics and narcotic antagonists

P.L.F. Giangrande
Oxford, United Kingdom
Drugs affecting blood coagulation, fibrinolysis, and hemostasis

G. Gillespie
Perth, Australia
Local anaesthetics

G. Girish
Sheffield, United Kingdom
Radiological contrast agents

V. Gras-Champel
Amiens, France
Drugs affecting blood coagulation, fibrinolysis, and hemostasis

A.I. Green
Boston, Massachusetts, USA
Drugs of abuse

A.H. Groll
Münster, Germany
Antifungal drugs

H. Haak
Leiden, The Netherlands
Miscellaneous drugs and materials, medical devices, and techniques not dealt with in other chapters

F. Hackenberger
Bonn, Germany
Antiseptic drugs and disinfectants

J.T. Hartmann
Tübingen, Germany
Cytostatic drugs

K. Hartmann
Bern, Switzerland
Drugs acting on the respiratory tract

A. Havryk
Sydney, Australia
Drugs acting on the respiratory tract

E. Hedayati
Auckland, New Zealand
General anesthetics and therapeutic gases

E. Helsing
Oslo, Norway
Vitamins

R. Hoigné
Wabern, Switzerland
Various antibacterial drugs

A. Imhof
Seattle, Washington, USA
Various antibacterial drugs

L.L. Iversen
Oxford, United Kingdom
Cannbinoids

J. W. Jefferson
Madison, Wisconsin, USA
Lithium

D.J. Jeffries
London, United Kingdom
Antiviral drugs

M. Joerger
St Gallen, Switzerland
Drugs acting on the respiratory tract

G.D. Johnston
Belfast, Northern Ireland
Positive inotropic drugs and drugs used in dysrhythmias

P. Joubert
Pretoria, South Africa
Antihypertensive drugs

A.A.M. Kaddu
Entebbe, Uganda
Antihelminthic drugs

C. Koch
Copenhagen, Denmark
Blood, blood components, plasma, and plasma products

H. Kolve
Münster, Germany
Antifungal drugs

H.M.J. Krans
Hoogmade, The Netherlands
Insulin, glucagon, and oral hypoglycemic drugs

M. Krause
Scherzingen, Switzerland
Various antibacterial drugs

S. Krishna
London, United Kingdom
Antiprotozoal drugs

M. Kuhn
Chur, Switzerland
Drugs acting on the respiratory tract

R. Latini
Milan, Italy
Beta-adrenoceptor antagonists and antianginal drugs

T.H. Lee
Durham, North Carolina, USA
Central nervous system stimulants and drugs that suppress appetite

P. Leuenberger
Lausanne, Switzerland
Drugs used in tuberculosis and leprosy

M. Leuwer
Liverpool, United Kingdom
Neuromuscular blocking agents and skeletal muscle relaxants

G. Liceaga Cundin
Guipuzcoa, Spain
Drugs that affect autonomic functions or the extrapyramidal system

P.O. Lim
Dundee, Scotland
Beta-adrenoceptor antagonists and antianginal drugs

H.-P. Lipp
Tübingen, Germany
Cytostatic drugs

C. Ludwig
Freiburg, Germany
Drugs acting on the immune system

T.M. MacDonald
Dundee, Scotland
Beta-adrenoceptor antagonists and antianginal drugs

G.T. McInnes
Glasgow, Scotland
Diuretics

I.R. McNicholl
San Francisco, California, USA
Antiviral drugs

P. Magee
Coventry, United Kingdom
Antiseptic drugs and disinfectants

A.P. Maggioni
Firenze, Italy
Beta-adrenoceptor antagonists and antianginal drugs

J.F. Martí Massó
Guipuzcoa, Spain
Drugs that affect autonomic functions or the extrapyramidal system

L.H. Martín Arias
Valladolid, Spain
Antipsychotic drugs

M.M.H.M. Meinardi
Amsterdam, The Netherlands
Dermatological drugs, topical agents, and cosmetics

D.B. Menkes
Wrexham, United Kingdom
Hypnosedatives and anxiolytics

R.H.B. Meyboom
Utrecht, The Netherlands
Metal antagonists

T. Midtvedt
Stockholm, Sweden
Various antibacterial drugs

G. Mignot
Saint Paul, France
Gastrointestinal drugs

S.K. Morcos
Sheffield, United Kingdom
Radiological contrast agents

W.M.C. Mulder
Amsterdam, The Netherlands
Dermatological drugs, topical agents, and cosmetics

S. Musa
Wakefield, United Kingdom
Hypnosedatives and anxiolytics

K.A. Neftel
Bern, Switzerland
Various antibacterial drugs

A.N. Nicholson
Petersfield, United Kingdom
Antihistamines

L. Nicholson
Auckland, New Zealand
General anesthetics and therapeutic gases

I. Öhman
Stockholm, Sweden
Antidepressant drugs

H. Olsen
Oslo, Norway
Opioid analgesics and narcotic antagonists

I. Palmlund
London, United Kingdom
Diethylstilbestrol

J.N. Pande
New Delhi, India
Drugs used in tuberculosis and leprosy

J.K. Patel
Boston, Massachusetts, USA
Drugs of abuse

J.W. Paterson
Perth, Australia
Drugs acting on the respiratory tract

K. Peerlinck
Leuven, Belgium
Drugs affection blood coagulation, fibrinolysis, and hemostasis

E. Perucca
Pavia, Italy
Antiepileptic drugs

E.H. Pi
Los Angeles, California, USA
Antipsychotic drugs

T. Planche
London, United Kingdom
Antiprotozoal drugs

B.C.P. Polak
Amsterdam, The Netherlands
Drugs used in ocular treatment

T.E. Ralston
Worcester, Massachusetts, USA
Drugs of abuse

P. Reiss
Amsterdam, The Netherlands
Antiviral drugs

H.D. Reuter
Köln, Germany
Vitamins

I. Ribeiro
London, United Kingdom
Antiprotozoal drugs

T.D. Robinson
Sydney, Australia
Drugs acting on the respiratory tract

Ch. Ruef
Zurich, Switzerland
Various antibacterial drugs

M. Schachter
London, United Kingdom
Drugs that affect autonomic functions or the extrapyramidal system

A. Schaffner
Zurich, Switzerland
Various antibacterial drugs
Antifungal drugs

S. Schliemann-Willers
Jena, Germany
Dermatological drugs, topical agents, and cosmetics

M. Schneemann
Zürich, Switzerland
Antiprotozoal drugs

S.A. Schug
Perth, Australia
Local anesthetics

G. Screaton
Oxford, United Kingdom
Drugs acting on the immune system

J.P. Seale
Sydney, Australia
Drugs acting on the respiratory tract

R.P. Sequeira
Manama, Bahrain
Central nervous system stimulants and drugs that suppress appetite

T.G. Short
Auckland, New Zealand
General anesthetics and therapeutic gases

D.A. Sica
Richmond, Virginia, USA
Diuretics

G.M. Simpson
Los Angeles, California, USA
Antipsychotic drugs

J.J. Sramek
Beverly Hills, California, USA
Antipsychotic drugs

A. Stanley
Birmingham, United Kingdom
Cytostatic drugs

K.J.D. Stannard
Perth, Australia
Local anesthetics

B. Sundaram
Sheffield, United Kingdom
Radiological contrast agents

J.A.M. Tafani
Toulouse, France
Radiological contrast agents

M.C. Thornton
Auckland, New Zealand
Local anesthetics

B.S. True
Campbelltown, South Australia
Corticotrophins, corticosteroids, and prostaglandins

C. Twelves
Glasgow, Scotland
Cytostatic drugs

W.G. Van Aken
Amsterdam, The Netherlands
Blood, blood components, plasma, and plasma products

C.J. Van Boxtel
Amsterdam, The Netherlands
Sex hormones and related compounds, including hormonal contraceptives

G.B. Van der Voet
Leiden, The Netherlands
Metals

P.J.J. Van Genderen
Rotterdam, The Netherlands
Antihelminthic drugs

R. Verhaeghe
Leuven, Belgium
Drugs acting on the cerebral and peripheral circulations

J. Vermylen
Leuven, Belgium
Drugs affecting blood coagulation, fibrinolysis, and hemostasis

P. Vernazza
St Gallen, Switzerland
Antiviral drugs

T. Vial
Lyon, France
Drugs acting on the immune system

P. Vossebeld
Amsterdam, The Netherlands
Blood, blood components, plasma, and plasma products

G.M. Walsh
Aberdeen, United Kingdom
Antihistamines

T.J. Walsh
Bethesda, Maryland, USA
Antifungal drugs

R. Walter
Zurich, Switzerland
Antifungal drugs

D. Watson
Auckland, New Zealand
Local anesthetics

J. Weeke
Aarhus, Denmark
Thyroid hormones and antithyroid drugs

C.J.M. Whitty
London, United Kingdom
Antiprotozoal drugs

E.J. Wong
Boston, Massachusetts, USA
Drugs of abuse

C. Woodrow
London, United Kingdom
Antiprotozoal drugs

Y. Young
Auckland, New Zealand
General anesthetics and therapeutic gases

F. Zannad
Nancy, France
Antihypertensive drugs

J.-P. Zellweger
Lausanne, Switzerland
Drugs used in tuberculosis and leprosy

A. Zinkernagel
Zürich, Switzerland
Antiprotozoal drugs

M. Zoppi
Bern, Switzerland
Various antibacterial drugs

O. Zuzan
Hannover, Germany
Neuromuscular blocking agents and skeletal muscle relaxants

Foreword

My doctor is
A good doctor
He made me no
Iller than I was

Willem Hussem (The Netherlands) 1900–1974
Translation: Peter Raven

"*Primum non nocere*"—in the first place, do no harm—is often cited as one of the foundation stones of sound medical care, yet its origin is uncertain. Hippocrates? There are some who will tell you so;[1] but the phrase is not a part of the Hippocratic Oath, and the Father of Medicine wrote in any case in his native Greek.[2] It could be that the Latin phrase is from the Roman physician Galenius, while others attribute it to Scribonius Largus, physician to one of the later Caesars,[3] and there is a lot of reason to believe that it actually originated in 19th century England.[4] Hippocrates himself, in the first volume of his *Epidemics*, put it at all events better in context: "When dealing with diseases have two precepts in mind: to procure benefit and not to harm."[5] One must not become overly obsessed by the safety issue, but it is a necessary element in good medical care.

The ability to do good with the help of medicines has developed immensely within the last century, but with it has come the need to keep a watchful eye on the possibility of inflicting harm on the way. The challenge is to recognize at the earliest possible stage the adverse effects that a valuable drug may induce, and to find ways of containing them, so that risk never becomes disproportionate to benefit. The process of drug development will sometimes result in methods of treatment that are more specific to their purpose than were their predecessors and hence less likely to produce unwanted complications; yet the more novel a therapeutic advance the greater the possibility of its eliciting adverse effects of a type so unfamiliar that they are not specifically looked for and long remained unrecognized when they do occur. The entire process of keeping medicines safe today involves all those concerned with them, whether as researchers, manufacturers, regulators, prescribers, dispensers, or users, and it demands an effective and honest flow of information and thought between them.

For several decennia, concerned by its own errors in the past, the science of therapeutics put unbounded faith in the ability of well-planned clinical trials to arrive at the truth about the properties of medicines. Insofar as efficacy was concerned that was and remains a sound move, closing the door to charlatanism as well as to well-meant amateurism. Therapeutic trials with a new medicine were also able to delineate those adverse effects that occurred in a fair proportion of users. If serious, they would bar the drug from entry to the market altogether, while if transient and reasonably tolerable they would form the basis for warnings and precautions as well as the occasional contraindication. The problem lay with those adverse drug reactions that occurred rather less commonly or not at all in populations recruited for therapeutic trials, yet which could soon arise in the much broader spectrum of patients exposed to the drug once it was marketed across the world. The influence of race or climate might explain some of them; others might reflect interactions with foods, alcohol, or other drugs; yet others could only be explained, if at all, in terms of the particular susceptibility of certain individuals. Scattered across the globe, these effects might readily be overlooked, regarded as coincidental, or at worst dismissed contemptuously as "merely anecdotal".

The seriousness of the adverse effects issue became very apparent even as the reputation of controlled trials deservedly grew, and it touched on both newer and older drugs. The thalidomide calamity, involving several thousand cases of drug-induced phocomelia, was fortunately recognized by Widukind Lenz and others in the light of individual case reports within two years of the introduction of the product. On the other hand, generations elapsed between the patenting of aspirin in 1899 and the realization in 1965 that it might induce Reye's syndrome when used to treat fever in children. Such events, and many less spectacular, showed that, however vital well-controlled studies had become, there was good reason to remain alert for signals emerging from individual cases. Unanticipated events occurring during drug treatment might indeed reflect mere coincidence, but again they might not; and for many of the patients who suffered in consequence there was nothing in the least anecdotal about them.

Fortunately, the 1950s and 1960s of the 20th century saw the first positive reactions to the adverse reaction issue. Effective drug regulation emerged in one country after another. In 1952, Prof. Leo Meyler of The Netherlands produced his first "Side Effect of Drugs" to pull together data from the world literature. A number of national adverse reaction monitoring bureaux were established to gather data from the field and examine carefully reports of suspected side effects of medicines, creating the basis for the World Health Organization to establish its global reporting system. The pharmaceutical industry has increasingly realized its duty to collect and pass on the information that comes into its possession through its wide contacts with the health professions. Later years have seen the emergence, notably in Sweden and in Britain, of systems through which patients themselves can report possible adverse effects to the medicines they have taken. All these processes fit together in what the French language so appropriately terms "pharmacovigilance", with vigilance as the watchword for all concerned.

In this continuing development, the medical literature provides a resource with vast potential. The world is believed to have some 20 000 medical journals, of which a nuclear group of a thousand or so can be relied upon to publish reports and analyses of adverse effects—not only in the framework of formal investigations but also in letters, editorials, and reports of meetings large and small. Much of that information comprises not so much firm facts as emergent knowledge, based directly on experience in the field and calling urgently for attention. The book that Leo Meyler created has, in the course of fifteen editions and with the support of an ever-larger team of professionals, provided the means by which that attention can be mobilized. It has become the world's principal tool in bringing together, encyclopedically but critically, the evidence on the basis of which adverse drug effects and interactions can be recognized, discussed, and accommodated into medical practice. Together with its massive database and its complementary *Side Effects of Drugs Annuals*, it has evolved into a vital instrument in ensuring that drugs are used wisely and well and with due caution, in the light of all that is known about them. There is nothing else like it, nor need there be; across the world, *Meyler* has become a pillar of responsible medical care.

M.N. Graham Dukes
Honorary Editor, *Meyler's Side Effects of Drugs*
Oslo, Norway

Notes

1. Lichtenhaeler C. Histoire de la Médicine, Fayard, Paris, 1978:117.
2. Smith CM. Origin and uses of *Primum non nocere*. J Clin Pharmacol 2005;45:371–7.
3. Albrecht H. Primum nil nocere. Die Zeit, 6 April, 2005.
4. Notably in a book by Inman T. *Foundation for a New Theory and Practice of Medicine*. London, 1860.
5. I am indebted to Jeffrey Aronson for his own translation of the Greek original from Hippocrates *Epidemics*, Book I, Section XI, which seems to convey the meaning of the original [ἀσκεῖν περὶ τὰ νοσημάτα δῦο, ὠφελειν ἤ μὴ βλάπτειν] rather better than the published translations of his work.

Preface

This is a completely new edition of what has become the standard reference text in the field of adverse drug reactions and interactions since Leopold Meyler published his first review of the subject 55 years ago. Although we have retained the old title, *Meyler's Side Effects of Drugs*, the subtitle of this edition, *The Encyclopedia of Adverse Drug Reactions and Interactions*, reflects both modern terminology and the scope of the review. The structure of the book may have changed, but the *Encyclopedia* remains the most comprehensive reference source on adverse drug reactions and interactions and a major source of informed discussion about them.

Scope

The scope of the *Encyclopedia* remains wide. It covers not only the vast majority of prescription drugs, old and new, but also non-prescribed substances (such as anesthetics, antiseptics, lifestyle compounds, and drugs of abuse), herbal medicines, devices (such as blood glucose meters), and methods in alternative and complementary medicine. For this edition, entries on some substances that were regarded as obsolete, such as thalidomide and smallpox vaccine, have been rewritten and restored. Other compounds, such as diethylstilbestrol, although no longer in use, continue to cast their shadow and are included. Yet others, currently regarded as obsolete, have been retained, both for historical reasons and because one can never be sure when an old compound may once more become relevant or provide useful information in relation to another compound. Some drugs have been withdrawn from the market in some countries since the last edition of *Meyler* was published; rofecoxib, cisapride, phenylpropanolamine, and kava (see Piperaceae) are examples. Nevertheless, detailed monographs have been included on these substances because of the lessons that they can teach us and in some cases because of their relevance to other compounds in their classes that are still available; it is also not possible to predict whether these compounds will eventually reappear in some other form or for some new indication.

In the last 15 years there has been increasing emphasis on the use of high-quality evidence in therapeutic practice, principally as obtained from large, randomized clinical trials and from systematic reviews of the results of many such trials. However, while it has been possible to obtain useful information about the beneficial effects of interventions in this way, evidence about harms, including adverse drug reactions, has been more difficult to obtain. Even trials that yield good estimates of benefits are poor at providing evidence about harms for several reasons:

- benefits are usually single, whereas harms are usually multiple;
- the chance of any single form of harm is usually smaller than the chance of benefit and therefore more difficult to detect; however, multiple harms can accumulate and affect the benefit-to-harm balance;
- benefits are identifiable in advance, whereas harms are not or not always;
- the likely time-course of benefits can generally be predicted, while the time-course of harms often cannot and may be much delayed by comparison with the duration of a trial.

For all these reasons, larger and sometimes longer studies are needed to detect harms. In recent years attempts have been made to conduct systematic reviews of adverse reactions, but these have also been limited by several problems:

- harms are in general poorly collected in randomized trials and trials may not last long enough to detect them all;
- even when they are well collected, as is increasingly happening, they are often poorly reported;
- even when they are well reported in the body of a report, they may not be mentioned in titles and abstracts;
- even when they are well reported in the body of a report, they may be poorly indexed in large databases.

All this means that it is difficult to collect information on adverse drug reactions from randomized, controlled trials for systematic review. This can be seen from the evidence provided in Table 1, which shows the proportion of different types of information that have been used in the preparation of two volumes of the *Side Effects of Drugs Annual*, proportions that are likely be the same in this *Encyclopedia*.

Wherever possible, emphasis in this *Encyclopedia* has been placed on information that has come from systematic reviews and clinical trials of all kinds; this is reflected in new headings under which trial results are reported (observational studies, randomized studies, placebo-controlled studies). However, because many reports of adverse drug reactions (about 30%) are anecdotal, with evidence from one or just a few cases, many individual case studies (see below) have also been included. We need better methods to make use of the information that this large body of anecdotes provides.

Structure

The first major change that readers will notice is that the chapter structure of previous editions has given way to a monographic structure. That is because some of the information about individual drugs has previously been scattered over different chapters in the book; for example ciclosporin was previously covered in Chapter 37 and in scattered sections throughout Chapter 45; it is now dealt with in a single monograph. The monographs are arranged in alphabetical order, with cross-referencing as required. For example, if you turn to the monograph on cetirizine, you will be referred to the complementary general monograph on antihistamines, where much information that is relevant to cetirizine is given; the monograph on cetirizine itself contains information that is relevant only to cetirizine and not to other antihistamines. Within each monograph the material is arranged in the same way as in the *Side Effects of Drugs Annuals* (see "How to use this book").

Case Reports

A new feature, recognizable from the Annuals, but not incorporated into previous editions, is the inclusion of case reports of adverse effects. This feature reflects the fact that about 30% of all the literature that is reported and discussed in the Annuals derives from such reports (see Table 1). In some cases the only information about an adverse effect is contained in an anecdotal report; in other cases the report illustrates a variant form of the reaction. A case report also gives more immediacy to an adverse reaction, allowing the reader to appreciate more precisely the exact nature of the reported event.

Classification of Adverse Drug Reactions

Another new feature of this edition is the introduction of the DoTS method of classifying adverse drug reactions, based on the **Dose** at which they occur relative to the beneficial dose, the **Time-course** of the reaction, and individual **Susceptibility factors** (see "How to use this book"). This has been done for selected adverse effects, and I hope that as volumes of SEDA continue to be published and the *Encyclopedia's* electronic database is expanded, it will be possible to classify increasing numbers of adverse reactions in this way.

References

Because all the primary and secondary literature is thoroughly surveyed in the Annuals, the *Encyclopedia* has become increasingly compact relative to the amount of information available (even though it has increased in absolute size), with many unreferenced statements and cross-references to the Annuals, on the assumption that all the information would be readily available to the reader, although that may not always be the case. To restore all the reference material on which the *Encyclopedia* has been based as it has evolved over so many years would be a gargantuan task, but in this edition a major start has been made. Many references to original material have been restored, and there is now hardly a statement that is not backed up by at least one reference to primary literature. In addition, almost all of the material that was published in Annuals 23 to 27 (SEDA-23 to SEDA-27) has been included, complete with citations. This has resulted in the inclusion of more than 40 000 references in this edition. Readers will still have to refer to earlier editions of the Annual (SEDA-1 to SEDA-22) and occasionally to earlier editions of *Meyler's Side Effects of Drugs* for more detailed descriptions, but now that the *Encyclopedia* is available electronically this will be repaired in future editions.

Methods and Contributors

I initially prepared the text of the *Encyclopedia* by combining text from the 14th edition of *Meyler's Side Effects of Drugs* and the five most recent annuals (SEDA-23 to SEDA-27). [Later literature is covered in SEDA-28 and the forthcoming SEDA-29.] I next restored missing references to the material and extended it where important information had not been included. The resulting monographs were then sent to experts for review, and their comments were incorporated into the finished monographs. I am grateful to all those, both authors of chapters in previous editions and Annuals and those who have reviewed the monographs for this edition, for their hard work and for making their expertise available.

Acknowledgements

This 15th edition of *Meyler's Side Effects of Drugs* was initiated and carefully planned with Joke Jaarsma at Elsevier, who has provided unstinting support during the production of several previous editions of *Meyler's Side Effects of Drugs* and the *Side Effects of Drugs Annuals*. Early discussions with Dieke van Wijnen at Elsevier about the structure of the text were invaluable. Professor Leufkens from the Faculty of Pharmacy at the University of Utrecht was instrumental in helping us to assemble the preliminary content for this edition; pharmacy students in his department entered the text

Table 1 Types of articles on adverse drug reactions published in 6576 papers in the world literature during 1999 and 2003 (as reviewed in SEDA-24 and SEDA-28)

Type of article	Number of descriptions* (%)
An anecdote or set of anecdotes (that is reported case histories)	2084 (29.9)
A major, randomized, controlled trial or observational study	1956 (28.1)
A minor, randomized, controlled trial or observational study or a non-randomized study (including case series)	1099 (15.8)
A major review, including non-systematic statistical analyses of published studies	951 (13.7)
A brief commentary (for example an editorial or a letter)	362 (5.19)
An experimental study (animal or in vitro)	263 (3.77)
A meta-analysis or other form of systematic review	172 (2.47)
Official statements (for example by Governmental organizations, the WHO, or manufacturers)	75 (1.07)
Total no. of descriptions*	6962
Total no. of articles	6576

* Some articles are described in more than one way

electronically into templates under the guidance of Joke Zwetsloot from Elsevier. Christine Ayorinde provided excellent assistance while I expanded and edited the material. The International Non-proprietary Names were checked by Renée Aronson. At Elsevier the references were then checked and collated by Liz Perill, who also copyedited the material, with Ed Stolting, and shepherded it through conversion to different electronic formats. Bill Todd created the indexes. Stephanie Diment oversaw the project and coordinated everyone's efforts.

The History of Meyler

The history of *Meyler's Side Effects of Drugs* goes back 55 years; a full account can be found at http://www.elsevier.-com/locate/Meyler and the various volumes are listed before the title page of this set. When Leopold Meyler, a physician, experienced unwanted effects of drugs that were used to treat his tuberculosis, he discovered that there was no single text to which medical practitioners could turn for information about the adverse effects of drug therapy; Louis Lewin's text *Die Nebenwirkungen der Arzneimittel* ("The Untoward Effects of Drugs") of 1881 had long been out of print (SEDA-27, xxv–xxix). Meyler therefore surveyed the current literature, initially in Dutch as *Schadelijke Nevenwerkingen van Geneesmiddelen* (Van Gorcum, 1951), and then in English as *Side Effects of Drugs* (Elsevier, 1952). He followed up with what he called surveys of unwanted effects of drugs. Each survey covered a period of two to four years and culminated in Volume VIII (1976), edited by Graham Dukes (SEDA-23, xxiii-xxvi), Meyler having died in 1973. By then the published literature was too extensive to be comfortably encompassed in a four-yearly cycle, and an annual cycle was started instead; the first *Side Effects of Drugs Annual* (SEDA-1) was published in 1977. The four-yearly review was replaced by a complementary critical encyclopaedic survey of the entire field; the first encyclopaedic edition of *Meyler's Side Effects of Drugs*, which appeared in 1980, was labeled the ninth edition.

Since then, *Meyler's Side Effects of Drugs* has been published every four years, providing an encyclopaedic survey of the entire field. Had the cycle been adhered to, the 15th edition would have been published in 2004, but over successive editions the quantity and nature of the information available in the text has changed. In the new millennium it was clear that for this edition a revolutionary approach was needed, and that has taken a little longer to achieve, with a great deal of effort from many different individuals.

We have come a long way since Meyler published his first account in a book of 192 pages. I think that he would have approved of this new *Encyclopedia*.

J. K. Aronson
Oxford, October 2005

How to use this book

In a departure from its previous structure, this edition of *Meyler's Side Effects of Drugs* is presented as individual drug monographs in alphabetical order. In many cases a general monograph (for example Antihistamines) is complemented by monographs about specific drugs (for example acrivastine, antazoline, etc.); in that case a cross-reference is given from the latter to the former.

Monograph Structure

Within each monograph the information is presented in sections as follows:

GENERAL INFORMATION

Includes, when necessary, notes on nomenclature, information about the results of observational studies, comparative studies, and placebo-controlled studies in relation to reports of adverse drug reactions, and a general summary of the major adverse effects.

ORGANS AND SYSTEMS

- Cardiovascular (includes heart and blood vessels)
- Respiratory
- Ear, nose, throat
- Nervous system (includes central and peripheral nervous systems)
- Neuromuscular function
- Sensory systems (includes eyes, ears, taste)
- Psychological, psychiatric
- Endocrine (includes hypothalamus, pituitary, thyroid, parathyroid, adrenal, pancreas, sex hormones)
- Metabolism
- Nutrition (includes effects on amino acids, essential fatty acids, vitamins, micronutrients)
- Electrolyte balance (includes sodium, potassium)
- Mineral balance (includes calcium, phosphate)
- Metal metabolism (includes copper, iron, magnesium, zinc)
- Acid–base balance
- Fluid balance
- Hematologic (includes blood, spleen, and lymphatics)
- Mouth and teeth
- Salivary glands
- Gastrointestinal (includes esophagus, stomach, small bowel, large bowel)
- Liver
- Biliary tract
- Pancreas
- Urinary tract (includes kidneys, ureters, bladder, urethra)
- Skin
- Hair
- Nails
- Sweat glands
- Serosae (includes pleura, pericardium, peritoneum)
- Musculoskeletal (includes muscles, bones, joints)
- Sexual function
- Reproductive system (includes uterus, ovaries, breasts)
- Immunologic (includes effects on the immune system and hypersensitivity reactions)
- Autacoids
- Infection risk
- Body temperature
- Multiorgan failure
- Trauma
- Death

LONG-TERM EFFECTS

- Drug abuse
- Drug misuse
- Drug tolerance
- Drug resistance
- Drug dependence
- Drug withdrawal
- Genotoxicity
- Mutagenicity
- Tumorigenicity

SECOND-GENERATION EFFECTS

- Fertility
- Pregnancy
- Teratogenicity
- Fetotoxicity
- Lactation

SUSCEPTIBILITY FACTORS (relates to features of the patient)

- Genetic factors
- Age
- Sex
- Physiological factors
- Cardiac disease
- Renal disease
- Hepatic disease
- Thyroid disease
- Other features of the patient

DRUG ADMINISTRATION

- Drug formulations
- Drug additives
- Drug contamination (includes infective agents)
- Drug adulteration
- Drug dosage regimens (includes frequency and duration of administration)
- Drug administration route
- Drug overdose

DRUG–DRUG INTERACTIONS

FOOD–DRUG INTERACTIONS

SMOKING

OTHER ENVIRONMENTAL INTERACTIONS

INTERFERENCE WITH DIAGNOSTIC TESTS

DIAGNOSIS OF ADVERSE DRUG REACTIONS

MANAGEMENT OF ADVERSE DRUG REACTIONS

MONITORING THERAPY

Classification of Adverse Drug Reactions

Selected major reactions are classified according to the DoTS system (BMJ 2003;327:1222–5). In this system adverse reactions are classified according to the **Dose** at which they usually occur relative to the beneficial dose, the **Time-course** over which they occur, and the **Susceptibility factors** that make them more likely, as follows:

1 **Relation to dose**
- *Toxic reactions* (reactions that occur at supratherapeutic doses)
- *Collateral reactions* (reactions that occur at standard therapeutic doses)
- *Hypersusceptibility reactions* (reactions that occur at subtherapeutic doses in susceptible patients)

2 **Time-course**
- *Time-independent reactions* (reactions that occur at any time during a course of therapy)
- *Time-dependent reactions*
  - Immediate reactions (reactions that occur only when a drug is administered too rapidly)
  - First-dose reactions (reactions that occur after the first dose of a course of treatment and not necessarily thereafter)
  - Early reactions (reactions that occur early in treatment then abate with continuing treatment)
  - Intermediate reactions (reactions that occur after some delay but with less risk during longer- term therapy, owing to the "healthy survivor" effect)
  - Late reactions (reactions the risk of which increases with continued or repeated exposure), including withdrawal reactions (reactions that occur when, after prolonged treatment, a drug is withdrawn or its effective dose is reduced)
  - Delayed reactions (reactions that occur some time after exposure, even if the drug is withdrawn before the reaction appears)

3 **Susceptibility factors**
- *Genetic*
- *Age*
- *Sex*
- *Physiological variation*
- *Exogenous factors* (for example drug–drug or food–drug interactions, smoking)
- *Diseases*

Drug Names And Spelling

Drugs are usually designated by their recommended or proposed International Non-proprietary Names (rINN or pINN); when these are not available, chemical names have been used. If a fixed combination has a generic combination name (for example co-trimoxazole for trimethoprim + sulfamethoxazole) that name has been used; in some cases brand names have been used.

Spelling

Where necessary, for indexing purposes, American spelling has been used, for example anemia rather than anaemia, estrogen rather than oestrogen.

Cross-references

The various editions of *Meyler's Side Effects of Drugs* are cited in the text as SED-13, SED-14, etc.; the *Side Effects of Drugs Annuals* 1-22 are cited as SEDA-1, SEDA-2, etc. This edition includes most of the contents of SEDA-23 to SEDA-27. SEDA-28 and SEDA-29 are separate publications, which were prepared in parallel with the preparation of this edition.

Indexes

Index of drug names
An index of drug names provides a complete listing of all references to a drug for which adverse effects and/or drug interactions are described. The monograph on herbal medicines contains tabulated cross-indexes to the plants that are covered in separate monographs.

Index of adverse effects
This index is necessarily selective, since a particular adverse effect may be caused by very large numbers of compounds; the index is therefore mainly directed to adverse effects that are particularly serious or frequent, or are discussed in special detail; before assuming that a given drug does not have a particular adverse effect, consult the relevant monograph.

Alphabetical list of drug monographs

The number in parentheses after each heading is the number of the corresponding chapter in the Side Effects of Drug Annuals (SEDA-28 and later) in which the item is usually covered.

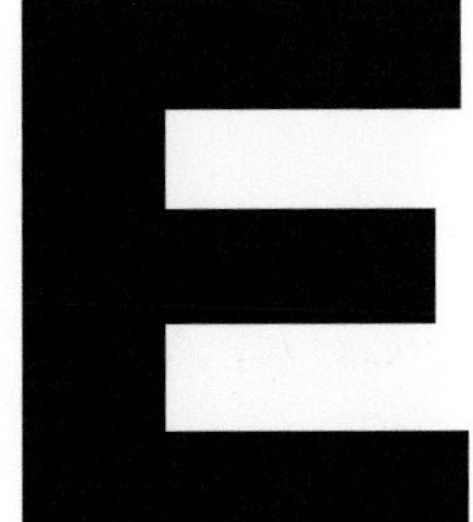

Ebastine

See also Antihistamines

General Information

Ebastine is a second-generation antihistamine with proven efficacy in the treatment of allergic disease (1). It is rapidly absorbed after oral administration, and undergoes extensive first-pass metabolism by CYP3A4 to its active carboxylic acid metabolite, carebastine.

Organs and Systems

Cardiovascular

Cardiac effects were reported from early experimental work using very high doses of ebastine, but they are not believed to be clinically relevant in normal use. In one study serial electrocardiograms showed no changes with doses up to the maximum used (30 mg). Ebastine in doses up to five times the recommended therapeutic dose did not cause clinically relevant changes in QT_c interval in healthy subjects (2). Co-administration of ebastine with ketoconazole or erythromycin did not lead to significant changes in the QT_c interval (3,4).

Psychological, psychiatric

The effects of ebastine 10 mg on cognitive impairment have been assessed in 20 healthy volunteers who performed six types of attention-demanding cognitive tasks, together with objective measurements of reaction times and accuracy (5). Ebastine was compared with placebo and a positive control, chlorphenamine 2 mg and 6 mg. Compared with placebo, ebastine had no effect on any objective cognitive test nor any effect on subjective sleepiness. In contrast, chlorphenamine significantly increased reaction times, reduced accuracy in cognitive tasks, and increased subjective sleepiness. The effect of chlorphenamine increased with plasma concentration.

Susceptibility Factors

Age

The effect of age on the pharmacokinetics of ebastine and carebastine has been studied (6). Ebastine can be safely given to elderly subjects and there are no clinically important age-related differences in the pharmacokinetics of ebastine/carebastine.

Sex

The effect of sex on the pharmacokinetics of ebastine and carebastine has been studied (6). There were no clinically important sex-related differences in the pharmacokinetics of ebastine/carebastine.

Food–Drug Interactions

Like other antihistamines that rely on activation by metabolism, the systemic availability of ebastine can be affected by food. In a double-blind, placebo-controlled, parallel-group study, 215 patients with seasonal allergic rhinitis took ebastine with solid food (immediately after breakfast), while 218 took it 1–2 hours after breakfast (7). Food taken at the time of dosing did not alter the therapeutic or adverse effects of ebastine for 2 weeks in seasonal allergic rhinitis. Although carebastine steady-state concentrations were 15% higher when ebastine was taken with food this was not considered clinically important.

References

1. Wiseman LR, Faulds D. Ebastine. a review of its pharmacological properties and clinical efficacy in the treatment of allergic disorders. Drugs 1996;51(2):260–77.
2. Gillen MS, Miller B, Chaikin P, Morganroth J. Effects of supratherapeutic doses of ebastine and terfenadine on the QT interval. Br J Clin Pharmacol 2001;52(2):201–4.
3. Moss AJ, Chaikin P, Garcia JD, Gillen M, Roberts DJ, Morganroth J. A review of the cardiac systemic side-effects of antihistamines: ebastine. Clin Exp Allergy 1999;29(Suppl 3):200–5.
4. Moss AJ, Morganroth J. Cardiac effects of ebastine and other antihistamines in humans. Drug Saf 1999;21(Suppl 1):69–80 discussion 81–7.
5. Tagawa M, Kano M, Okamura N, Higuchi M, Matsuda M, Mizuki Y, Arai H, Fujii T, Komemushi S, Itoh M, Sasaki H, Watanabe T, Yanai K. Differential cognitive effects of ebastine and (+)-chlorpheniramine in healthy subjects: correlation between cognitive impairment and plasma drug concentration. Br J Clin Pharmacol 2002;53(3):296–304.
6. Rohatagi S, Gillen M, Aubeneau M, Jan C, Pandit B, Jensen BK, Rhodes G. Effect of age and gender on the pharmacokinetics of ebastine after single and repeated dosing in healthy subjects. Int J Clin Pharmacol Ther 2001;39(3):126–34.
7. Frank H Jr, Gillen M, Rohatagi SS, Lim J, George G; Ebastine Study Group. A double-blind, placebo-controlled study of the efficacy and safety of ebastine 20 mg once daily given with and without food in the treatment of seasonal allergic rhinitis J Clin Pharmacol 2002;42(10): 1097–104.

Echinocandins

General Information

The echinocandins are a class of semisynthetic antifungal lipopeptides that are structurally characterized by a cyclic hexapeptide core linked to a variably configured lipid side chain. The echinocandins act by non-competitive inhibition of the synthesis of 1,3-α-D-glucan, a major polysaccharide component of the cell wall of many pathogenic fungi, which plays a key role in cell division and cell growth and is absent from mammalian cells. In concert with chitin, the rope-like glucan fibrils are important in maintaining the osmotic integrity of the fungal cell and play a key role in cell division and cell growth.

The currently available echinocandins are anidulafungin (rINN; Versicor Inc, Freemont, CA), caspofungin (rINN) (Merck & Co, Inc, Rahway, NJ), and micafungin (rINN; Fujisawa Inc, Deerfield, IL). They have relatively similar pharmacological properties. All three have potent and broad-spectrum antifungal activity against *Candida* species and *Aspergillus* species without cross-resistance to existing agents. They have prolonged post-antifungal effects and fungicidal activity against *Candida* and they cause severe damage to *Aspergillus* at the sites of hyphal growth. Their efficacy against these organisms in vivo has been demonstrated in animals (1,2). Their activity against other fungal pathogens in vitro is variable (3).

Pharmacokinetics

The echinocandins are currently available only for intravenous administration. They have dose-proportional plasma pharmacokinetics, with half-lives of 10–15 hours, which allows once-daily dosing. All echinocandins are highly protein-bound (over 95%) and distribute into all major tissues, including the brain; concentrations in non-inflammatory CSF are low. The echinocandins are eliminated by degradation and/or hepatic metabolism, and are slowly excreted as inactive metabolites in the urine and feces; only small fractions are excreted unchanged in the urine. As a class they are generally well tolerated and lack significant potential for drug interactions mediated by CYP450 isozymes (1–4). In vitro biotransformation studies of caspofungin have shown that it is not a substrate of P-glycoprotein and is a poor substrate and a weak inhibitor of cytochrome P450 enzymes (5). However, other in vitro studies have shown that it may inhibit CYP3A4 (6).

Observational studies

The clinical efficacy of anidulafungin, caspofungin, and micafungin against *Candida* species has been documented in phase II or phase III studies in immunocompromised patients with esophageal candidiasis. All achieved therapeutic efficacy at least comparable with standard agents. Phase III efficacy studies of caspofungin for esophageal candidiasis, invasive candidiasis, and empirical antifungal therapy in persistently febrile neutropenic patients have been completed. Caspofungin had no serious adverse effects and had therapeutic efficacy that was at least as good as standard agents (7–9). It is approved in the USA and the EU for second-line therapy of definite or probable invasive aspergillosis and for primary therapy in non-neutropenic patients with invasive *Candida* infections (3,5).

Caspofungin has been studied in a multicenter, open, non-comparative phase II trial in 83 patients with definite or probable invasive aspergillosis refractory to or intolerant of standard therapies (10,11). Common underlying conditions included hematological malignancies (48%), allogeneic blood and marrow transplantation (25%), and solid organ transplantation (11%). Caspofungin was administered in a dose of 70 mg on day 1, followed by 50 mg/day for a mean duration of 34 (range 1–162) days. There was a favorable response to caspofungin in 37 patients, including 32 of 64 with pulmonary aspergillosis and 3 of 13 with disseminated aspergillosis. Caspofungin was generally well tolerated. One serious adverse event was reported as possibly drug-related. Infusion-related reactions, nephrotoxicity, and hepatotoxicity were uncommon. Two patients discontinued caspofungin because of adverse effects.

The safety and tolerability of caspofungin have been studied in 623 patients, including 295 who received at least 50 mg/day for at least 1 week in clinical studies. In 263 patients who received caspofungin in randomized, double-blind, active-control trials, there were no serious clinical or laboratory drug-related adverse events; caspofungin was withdrawn in 2% of these patients because of drug-related adverse effects (12).

Comparative studies

Amphotericin

Caspofungin (Cancidas; 50 and 70 mg/day for 14 days; $n = 74$) has been compared with conventional amphotericin (0.5 mg/kg/day for 14 days; $n = 54$) in the treatment of esophageal candidiasis in a randomized, double-blind, multicenter trial in South America (13). Most of the patients (over 75%) were HIV-infected and about half of them had CD4+ lymphocyte counts of under 50×10^6/l. Caspofungin was well tolerated: eight patients in the amphotericin group and one patient in the combined caspofungin group developed a raised serum creatinine of over 176 μmol/l (2 mg/dl) during treatment. Of the patients who received caspofungin, 4.1% withdrew prematurely owing to drug-associated adverse effects, compared with 22% in the amphotericin arm. There was a clinical response (symptoms plus endoscopy) in 85% of the patients in the combined caspofungin group versus 67% in the amphotericin group.

Caspofungin has been compared with amphotericin in a multicenter, double-blind, randomized trial in 128 adults with endoscopically documented symptomatic *Candida* esophagitis (7). There was endoscopically verified clinical success in 74 and 89% of the patients who received caspofungin 50 and 70 mg/day respectively, and in 63% of patients given amphotericin deoxycholate 0.5 mg/kg/day. Therapy was withdrawn because of drug-related adverse events in 24% of the patients who were given amphotericin and in 4 and 7% of those who were given caspofungin 50 and 70 mg/day respectively. The most frequent adverse events with caspofungin were fever, phlebitis, headache, and rash. Fewer patients who received caspofungin had drug-related fever, chills, or nausea than those who received amphotericin. More patients who received amphotericin (91%) than caspofungin (61 and 32%) developed drug-related laboratory abnormalities, the most common in the caspofungin groups being hypoalbuminemia and increased serum activities of alkaline phosphatase and transaminases. There were drug-related increases in blood urea nitrogen concentrations in 15% of the patients who received amphotericin but in none of those who received caspofungin. Likewise, serum creatinine concentrations increased in 16 patients who received amphotericin but in only one who received caspofungin. In summary, caspofungin was as effective as amphotericin but better tolerated in the treatment of esophageal candidiasis.

In a double-blind, randomized trial, caspofungin was compared with amphotericin deoxycholate for the primary treatment of invasive candidiasis (9). Patients who had clinical evidence of infection and a positive culture for *Candida* species from blood or another site were enrolled. They were stratified according to the severity of disease, as indicated by the presence or absence of neutropenia and the Acute Physiology and Chronic Health Evaluation (APACHE II) score, and were randomly assigned to receive either caspofungin (50 mg/day with a loading dose of 70 mg on day 1) or amphotericin (0.6–0.7 mg/kg/day or 0.7–1.0 mg/kg/day for patients with neutropenia). Of the 239 patients enrolled, 224 were included in the modified intention-to-treat analysis. Baseline characteristics, including the percentage of patients with neutropenia and the mean APACHE II score, were similar in the two treatment groups. The efficacy of caspofungin was similar to that of amphotericin, with successful outcomes in 73% of the patients treated with caspofungin and in 62% of those treated with amphotericin. There were significantly fewer drug-related adverse events associated with caspofungin: fever, chills, and infusion-related events were less frequent with caspofungin. Caspofungin caused less nephrotoxicity (as defined by an increase in serum creatinine of at least twice the baseline value or an increase of at least 88.4 μmol/l: 8.4 versus 25%). Only 2.6% of those who were given caspofungin were withdrawn because of adverse events, compared with 23% of those who were given amphotericin. Thus, caspofungin was at least as effective as amphotericin for the treatment of mostly non-neutropenic patients with invasive candidiasis but significantly better tolerated.

The safety, tolerability, and efficacy of caspofungin in patients with oropharyngeal and/or esophageal candidiasis have been investigated in a phase II dose-ranging study (14). The patients were randomized, double-blind to either caspofungin acetate (35, 50, or 70 mg) or amphotericin (0.5 mg/kg intravenously) once daily for 7–14 days. Of 140 patients, 63% had esophageal involvement and 98% were infected with HIV. Response rates with caspofungin groups were 74–91%, and 63% with amphotericin. Fewer patients receiving any dose of caspofungin had drug-related adverse effects (fever, chills, nausea, vomiting). Two patients who took caspofungin 35 mg and one who was given amphotericin withdrew because of adverse effects. Drug-related laboratory abnormalities were also more common in patients who received amphotericin. The most common drug-related laboratory abnormalities in patients who received caspofungin were raised alanine transaminase, aspartate transaminase, and alkaline phosphatase, which were typically less than five times the upper limit of normal and resolved despite continued treatment. None of the patients receiving caspofungin and nine of those who received amphotericin developed drug-related increases in serum creatinine concentrations. No patient withdrew because of drug-related laboratory adverse effects.

Antifungal azoles

Caspofungin and fluconazole have been compared in adults with *Candida* esophagitis in a double-blind, randomized trial (8). Eligible patients had symptoms compatible with esophagitis, endoscopic mucosal plaques, and microscopic *Candida*. They were randomized to receive caspofungin (50 mg) or fluconazole (200 mg) intravenously once a day for 7–21 days. Most of them (154/177) had HIV infection, with a median CD4 count of 30×10^6/l. Favorable response rates were achieved in 66 of the 81 patients in the caspofungin arm and in 80 of the 94 patients in the fluconazole arm; symptoms had resolved in over 50% of the patients in both groups by the fifth day of treatment. Drug-related adverse effects were reported in 41% of patients given caspofungin and 32% of those given fluconazole; the most common events in both groups were phlebitis, headache, fever, nausea, diarrhea, abdominal pain, and rashes. Drug-related laboratory abnormalities developed in 29% of patients given caspofungin and in 34% of those given fluconazole. The most frequent laboratory abnormalities included reduced white blood cell count, hemoglobin concentration, and serum albumin concentration, and increased alkaline phosphatase and transaminases. No patient given caspofungin developed a serious drug-related adverse effect; therapy was withdrawn in only one patient (who was receiving fluconazole), because of an unspecified adverse effect.

Drug–Drug Interactions

Amphotericin

There were no pharmacokinetic interactions of caspofungin with amphotericin deoxycholate in healthy volunteers (5).

Antifungal azoles

In rats, caspofungin did not alter the plasma pharmacokinetics of ketoconazole, a potent inhibitor of CYP3A4 (5). Co-administration of caspofungin 50 mg/day and itraconazole 200 mg/day to healthy subjects for 14 days did not alter the pharmacokinetics of either drug (15).

Ciclosporin

Ciclosporin increased the AUC of caspofungin by about 35%, but caspofungin did not increase the plasma concentrations of ciclosporin. Because of transient rises in hepatic transaminases not exceeding 2–3 times the upper limit of the reference range in single-dose interaction studies, concomitant use of caspofungin with ciclosporin should be undertaken with care (5), although limited experience in patients studied by the manufacturers suggests that it may be safe.

Enzyme inducers

Regression analysis of pharmacokinetic data from patients has suggested that co-administration of caspofungin with inducers of drug metabolism and mixed inducer/inhibitors, namely carbamazepine, dexamethasone, efavirenz, nelfinavir, nevirapine, phenytoin, and rifampicin, can cause clinically important reductions in caspofungin concentrations. However, no data are currently available from formal interaction studies, and it is not known which clearance mechanisms of caspofungin are inducible. The manufacturer currently recommends considering an increase in the daily dose of caspofungin to 70 mg in patients who are taking these drugs concurrently and who are not responding (5).

Indinavir

In rats, caspofungin did not alter the plasma pharmacokinetics of indinavir, a substrate and competitive inhibitor of CYP3A2 (5).

Tacrolimus

While tacrolimus had no effect on the plasma pharmacokinetics of caspofungin, chronic caspofungin reduced the AUC of tacrolimus by about 20% (5).

References

1. Kurtz MB, Douglas CM. Lipopeptide inhibitors of fungal glucan synthase. J Med Vet Mycol 1997;35(2):79–86.
2. Georgopapadakou NH. Update on antifungals targeted to the cell wall: focus on beta-1,3-glucan synthase inhibitors. Expert Opin Investig Drugs 2001;10(2):269–80.
3. Groll AH, Walsh TJ. Antifungal chemotherapy: advances and perspectives. Swiss Med Wkly 2002;132(23–24):303–11.
4. Groll AH, Gea-Banacloche JC, Glasmacher A, Just-Nuebling G, Maschmeyer G, Walsh TJ. Clinical pharmacology of antifungal compounds. Infect Dis Clin North Am 2003;17(1):159–91.
5. Groll AH, Walsh TJ. Caspofungin: pharmacology, safety and therapeutic potential in superficial and invasive fungal infections. Expert Opin Investig Drugs 2001;10(8): 1545–58.
6. Colburn DE, Giles FJ, Oladovich D, Smith JA. In vitro evaluation of cytochrome P450-mediated drug interactions between cytarabine, idarubicin, itraconazole and caspofungin. Hematology 2004;9(3):217–21.
7. Villanueva A, Arathoon EG, Gotuzzo E, Berman RS, DiNubile MJ, Sable CA. A randomized double-blind study of caspofungin versus amphotericin for the treatment of candidal esophagitis. Clin Infect Dis 2001;33(9):1529–35.
8. Villanueva A, Gotuzzo E, Arathoon EG, Noriega LM, Kartsonis NA, Lupinacci RJ, Smietana JM, DiNubile MJ, Sable CA. A randomized double-blind study of caspofungin versus fluconazole for the treatment of esophageal candidiasis. Am J Med 2002;113(4):294–9.
9. Mora-Duarte J, Betts R, Rotstein C, Colombo AL, Thompson-Moya L, Smietana J, Lupinacci R, Sable C, Kartsonis N, Perfect J; Caspofungin Invasive Candidiasis Study Group. Comparison of caspofungin and amphotericin B for invasive candidiasis. N Engl J Med 2002;347(25):2020–9.
10. Maertens J, Raad I, Sable CA, Ngui A, Berman R, Patterson TF, Denning D, Walsh TJ. Multicenter, noncomparative study to evaluate safety and efficacy of caspofungin in adults with invasive aspergillosis refractory or intolerant to amphotericin B, amphotericin B lipid formulations, or azoles. Abstracts of the 40th International Conference on Antimicrobial Agents and Chemotherapy, 2000;1103.
11. Maertens J, Raad I, Petrikkos G, Boogaerts M, Selleslag D, Petersen FB, Sable CA, Kartsonis NA, Ngai A, Taylor A, Patterson TF, Denning DW, Walsh TJ; Caspofungin Salvage Aspergillosis Study Group. Efficacy and safety of caspofungin for treatment of invasive aspergillosis in patients refractory to or intolerant of conventional antifungal therapy. Clin Infect Dis 2004;39(11):1563–71.
12. Sable CA, Nguyen BY, Chodakewitz JA, DiNubile MJ. Safety and tolerability of caspofungin acetate in the treatment of fungal infections. Transpl Infect Dis 2002; 4(1):25–30.
13. Sable CA, Villanueva A, Arathon E, Gotuzzo E, Turcato G, Uip D, Noriega L, Rivera C, Rojas E, Taylor V, Berman R, Calandra GB, Chodakewitz J. A randomized, double-blind, multicenter trial of MK-991 (L-743,872) vs. amphotericin B (AMB) in the treatment of *Candida* esophagitis in adults. Abstracts of the 37th Interscience Conference on Antimicrobial Agents and Chemotherapy, 1997;LB-33.
14. Arathoon EG, Gotuzzo E, Noriega LM, Berman RS, DiNubile MJ, Sable CA. Randomized, double-blind, multicenter study of caspofungin versus amphotericin B for treatment of oropharyngeal and esophageal candidiases. Antimicrob Agents Chemother 2002;46(2):451–7.
15. Stone JA, McCrea J, Wickersham P, Holland S, Deutsch P, Bi S, Cicero T, Greenberg H, Waldman SA. Phase I study of caspofungin evaluating the potential for drug interactions with itraconazole, the effect of gender and the use of a loading dose. Abstracts of the 40th Interscience Conference on Antimicrobial Agents and Chemotherapy, 2000;854.

Edetic acid and its salts

General Information

Edetic acid is a metal chelator. The effect of an intravenous dose of 1 g of calcium disodium edetate on the urinary excretion on the elements aluminium, boron, barium, calcium, copper, iron, lead, magnesium, manganese, phosphorus, potassium, silicon, sodium, strontium, sulphur, and zinc was measured in healthy volunteers. The ratio of the increase of urinary elimination was about two for iron, five for aluminium, lead, and manganese, and 15 for zinc (1).

Salts of edetic acid are still used in intravenous "chelation therapy" as an alternative treatment for atherosclerotic disease in several countries (SEDA-10, 225) (2–7). Many of the data on their adverse effects are derived from older studies. There is some evidence of efficacy, although the dangers are obvious (SED-14, 722) (8,9).

Urea edetate (with methylhexyl ether) has been used for the dissolution of calcified gallbladder stones, without adverse effects (10).

Adverse effects of disodium edetate include hypocalcemia, tetany, convulsions, cardiac dysrhythmias, respiratory arrest, and renal insufficiency. Other possible symptoms include nausea, vomiting, diarrhea, fever, headache, and urinary urgency. Pain and phlebitis at the site of injection can occur (11). The sodium load in "chelation therapy" can precipitate heart failure. Renal tubular necrosis can occur (2).

Sodium calcium edetate can cause the same adverse effects as the disodium salt, with the exception of hypocalcemia.

In children receiving disodium ethylenediaminetetraacetate by intravenous infusion, an influenza-like syndrome developed, characterized by lacrimation, rhinorrhea, sneezing, and cough (12). Other symptoms included malaise, fatigue, nausea, and vomiting; one patient had a fever of 39.2°C.

Five patients became ill shortly after chelation therapy at an out-patients clinic, where they had received an infusion of Na_2EDTA 3 g, MgCl 2 g, vitamin B_1 100 mg, vitamin B complex 1 ml, and vitamin C 15 g in sterile water at a rate of 180 ml/hour (13). One patient also received 10 ml of 50% dimethylsulfoxide. All initially had gastrointestinal and musculoskeletal symptoms (trembling, muscle spasms) and complained of dry mouth or excessive thirst. All had fever and hypotension, four had tachycardia and sweating. Laboratory data were collected in four patients, all of whom had varying degrees of thrombocytopenia, leukopenia, and lymphocytopenia, reflecting transient bone marrow suppression. Subsequent measurements showed leukocytosis with early cell forms. Urinalysis showed transient proteinuria (in four), microscopic hematuria (in three), hyaline casts (in two), and ketonuria (in four). Three had mild transient rises in serum urea and creatinine concentrations. Three had hypocalcemia, requiring supplementation in one (probably accounting for the muscular symptoms). In these patients, acute edetate toxicity appeared to be related to errors in dosage or the rate at which the formulation was administered.

Organs and Systems

Respiratory

Additives to drug for inhalation, such as disodium edetate or benzalkonium chloride, can cause bronchoconstriction (14). This can lead to reduced therapeutic effectiveness of bronchodilators, for example salbutamol or ipratropium. Some products do and others do not contain these additives and an unexpected reduction in response to a bronchodilator may be the result of a casual change of product.

- In one case, paradoxical bronchoconstriction and laryngospasm necessitated emergency admission after the use of salbutamol in a metered-dose inhaler, which also contained edetate disodium as a preservative (15). Although there was prompt relapse on re-exposure, there were no positive findings demonstrating the role of edetate disodium.

Sensory systems

In two patients with atypical band keratopathy, the combined use of the preservatives sodium edetate, boric acid, and benzalkonium chloride in eye-drops for glaucoma treatment was identified as the cause (16).

Metal metabolism

Salts of edetic acid have been reported to cause symptomatic zinc deficiency, with abnormalities of the skin, including crusted lesions of the mouth and eyelids, leukokeratosis of the tongue, stomatitis, and a papular, pustular, erosive rash of the face and perianally, alopecia, and white bands on the nails (17,18).

Hematologic

For pseudothrombocytopenia, pseudoneutropenia, and pseudoleukocytosis caused by the use of edetic acid as an in vitro anticoagulant, see the section on "Interference with diagnostic tests" in this monograph.

Urinary tract

Intravenous administration of disodium edetate can cause renal insufficiency and acute tubular necrosis (2). In children with subclinical lead poisoning, the administration of sodium calcium edetate and dimercaprol together was associated with mild and transient biochemical evidence of renal damage in 13% of patients, whereas another 3% had acute renal insufficiency (19).

Edetate-induced renal damage is associated with vacuolization of the proximal tubules, loss of the brush border, and eventually degeneration of the proximal tubular cells. A possible mechanism underlying this renal toxicity is an interaction between edetate and endogenous metals in the proximal tubule (13).

Skin

Disodium edetate can cause contact dermatitis, for instance when used in local anesthetics (20).

Immunologic

Derivatives of edetic acid are allergenic and can cause allergic reactions, with rashes, fever, edema, and arthralgia. There can be cross-allergy to ethylenediamine, which is a constituent of various drug formulations (for example aminophylline, some ointments) (SED-8, 538). In addition, disodium edetate is found in small amounts in certain drugs, as a result of the removal of trace quantities of heavy metals. However, ethylenediaminetetraacetate was administered for lead poisoning without ill effects to a child with a proven allergy to ethylenediamine hydrochloride (21).

Second-Generation Effects

Teratogenicity

Salts of edetic acid are teratogenic in animals, probably by causing zinc deficiency (22,23). However, there is no evidence of teratogenicity in humans.

Drug–Drug Interactions

Phenylmercuric preservatives

The activity of phenylmercuric preservatives can be reduced by interaction with disodium edetate (24).

Warfarin

Reduced anticoagulation has been reported in a patient taking warfarin when he was given chelation therapy (25).

- A 64-year-old man with coronary artery disease taking atenolol, lisinopril, atorvastatin, glyceryl trinitrate, triamterene, hydrochlorothiazide, omeprazole, nizatidine, enteric-coated aspirin, and a liquid multivitamin formulation containing spinach and broccoli extracts was given warfarin for bilateral pulmonary embolism. About 3 weeks later he received chelation therapy with a cocktail including sodium edetate 3 g and heparin 2500 units. The next day his INR had fallen from 2.6 to 1.6. He denied having missed a dose of warfarin, having taken other drugs, or having made dietary changes. The dose of warfarin was increased and the INR reached the target range.

The authors did not propose a mechanism for this interaction, although the rapidity of the effect suggests protein binding displacement of warfarin; nor did they comment on the possible role of the extract of broccoli, which contains vitamin K.

Interference with Diagnostic Tests

Cell counters

A major unwanted effect of edetic acid, related to its use as an in vitro anticoagulant in blood samples, is the phenomenon of pseudothrombocytopenia by interference with electronic cell counters, which occurs in 0.1–2.0% of blood samples (26–36). It is assumed that about 15–30 minutes after collecting blood, edetic acid, presumably by extraction of calcium, causes changes in the platelet membrane, exposing a hidden glycoprotein antigen (28). An already circulating immunoglobulin — mostly IgG, but sometimes IgM or IgA — behaves as a drug-dependent antibody and reacts with glycoproteins in the cell membrane, resulting in the agglutination of platelets and falsely low platelet counts (26,30,35). It is more frequent in hospital patients with significant concurrent illnesses, suggesting that the antibody involved is acquired. A variety of disorders, including viral infections, neoplastic diseases, autoimmune disorders, liver disease, trauma, atherosclerosis, and thrombotic disorders, are thought to be risk factors (26). Sometimes the use of a medicine, for example mexiletine (37), is involved in the development of edetic acid-induced pseudothrombocytopenia. Pseudothrombocytopenia is more likely to occur when there is a delay between taking and testing the blood samples. The agglutinin crosses the placenta and can cause transient pseudothrombocytopenia in neonatal blood samples (26).

The clinical importance of edetic acid as a cause of pseudothrombocytopenia can be illustrated by the following findings. In a retrospective study, 15% of patients thought to have true thrombocytopenia were found to be cases of edetic acid-induced pseudothrombocytopenia (28). In another study, there were eight cases of pseudothrombocytopenia, compared with only three patients with Werlhof's disease (idiopathic thrombocytopenic purpura) during the same period (26). Among pregnant women with isolated thrombocytopenia, 7% had edetic acid-mediated pseudothrombocytopenia (38). Although it is rarer, pseudothrombocytopenia can also occur in connection with other anticoagulants, such as citrate or heparin. Sometimes different anticoagulants cause pseudothrombocytopenia in one and the same patient (26). Moreover, similar antibodies can occur that are not edetate dependent (39). Obviously, pseudothrombocytopenia deserves a place in the differential diagnosis of thrombocytopenia.

Failure to recognize pseudothrombocytopenia can lead to diagnostic errors, unnecessary invasive procedures (for example bone marrow puncture), delayed surgery, and wrong treatments (for example unnecessary withdrawal of wrongly suspected drugs, unnecessary transfusions, the use of potentially harmful drugs, splenectomy). Confusion can arise when pseudothrombocytopenia develops during hospitalization, especially in patients with pre-existing or expected (true) thrombocytopenia.

Artefactual pseudothrombocytopenia is typically an error of automated cell counters. When platelet clumps are mistaken for leukocytes this can result in pseudoleukocytosis (30,36). Edetic acid can also cause agglutination of granulocytes, and confusing findings such as combined pseudothrombocytopenia, pseudoneutropenia, and pseudolymphocytosis can occur (28).

Whenever pseudothrombocytopenia is suspected, for example in the case of unexpected thrombocytopenia without signs of bleeding, the diagnosis can be confirmed by finding normal platelet counts immediately after drawing the blood specimen or by examination of a blood smear. When serial counts are made, the number of platelets falls linearly with time. Pseudothrombocytopenia is usually associated with a normal mean platelet volume, whereas true thrombocytopenia is associated with a reduced mean platelet volume (28).

A case report from Germany has underlined the clinical importance of early recognition of edetate-induced pseudothrombocytopenia (SEDA-21, 250) (40). In this case, artefactual thrombocytopenia led to a bone marrow puncture and treatment with high doses of glucocorticoids, with severe Cushing's syndrome as a result. In such patients, concomitant bleeding disorders (without true thrombocytopenia), for example menorrhagia due to an intrauterine contraceptive device, can add to the confusion.

References

1. Allain P, Mauras Y, Premel-Cabic A, Islam S, Herve JP, Cledes J. Effects of an EDTA infusion on the urinary elimination of several elements in healthy subjects. Br J Clin Pharmacol 1991;31(3):347–9.
2. Magee R. Chelation treatment of atherosclerosis. Med J Aust 1985;142(9):514–15.
3. McGillem MJ, Mancini GB. Inefficacy of EDTA chelation therapy for coronary atherosclerosis. N Engl J Med 1988;318(24):1618–19.
4. Scott J. Chelation therapy—evolution or devolution of a nostrum? NZ Med J 1988;101(841):109–10.
5. Sloth-Nielsen J, Guldager B, Mouritzen C, Lund EB, Egeblad M, Norregaard O, Jorgensen SJ, Jelnes R. Arteriographic findings in EDTA chelation therapy on peripheral arteriosclerosis. Am J Surg 1991;162(2):122–5.
6. Anonymous. EDTA-chelatie behandeling. Ned Tijdschr Geneeskd 1991;135:2296.
7. Guldager B, Jelnes R, Jorgensen SJ, Nielsen JS, Klaerke A, Mogensen K, Larsen KE, Reimer E, Holm J, Ottesen S.

EDTA treatment of intermittent claudication—a double-blind, placebo-controlled study. J Intern Med 1992;231(3):261–7.
8. Ogata K, Nakajima H, Ikeda M, Yamamoto Y, Amagai M, Hashimoto T, Kodama H. Drug-induced pemphigus foliaceus with features of pemphigus vulgaris. Br J Dermatol 2001;144(2):421–2.
9. Frishman WH. Chelation therapy for coronary artery disease: panacea or quackery? Am J Med 2001;111(9):729–30.
10. Swobodnik W, Baumgaertel H, Janowitz P, Fuchs S, Ditschuneit H. Dissolution of calcified gallbladder stones by treatment with methyl-hexyl ether and urea-EDTA. Lancet 1988;2(8604):216.
11. Christensen K, Theilade D. EDTA chelation therapy: an ethical problem. Med Hypotheses 1999;53(1):69–70.
12. Ramirez JA, Goodman WG, Menezes C, Segre GV, Salusky IB. Disodium ethylenediaminetetraacetate: adverse effects in dialyzed children. Pediatr Nephrol 1993;7(2):182–4.
13. Morgan BW, Kori S, Thomas JD. Adverse effects in 5 patients receiving EDTA at an outpatient chelation clinic. Vet Hum Toxicol 2002;44(5):274–6.
14. Beasley R, Fishwick D, Miles JF, Hendeles L. Preservatives in nebulizer solutions: risks without benefit. Pharmacotherapy 1998;18(1):130–9.
15. Mutlu GM, Moonjelly E, Chan L, Olopade CO. Laryngospasm and paradoxical bronchoconstriction after repeated doses of beta 2-agonists containing edetate disodium. Mayo Clin Proc 2000;75(3):285–7.
16. Kremer I, Fink-Cohen S, Zer I. Atypical band keratopathy associated with antiglaucoma therapy. Ann Ophthalmol Glaucoma 1996;28:164–7.
17. Ridley CM. Zinc deficiency developing in treatment for thalassaemia. J R Soc Med 1982;75(1):38–9.
18. Vicari A, Banfi G, Bonini PA. EDTA-dependent pseudothrombocytopaenia: a 12-month epidemiological study. Scand J Clin Lab Invest 1988;48(6):537–42.
19. Moel DI, Kumar K. Reversible nephrotoxic reactions to a combined 2,3-dimercapto-1-propanol and calcium disodium ethylenediaminetetraacetic acid regimen in asymptomatic children with elevated blood lead levels. Pediatrics 1982;70(2):259–62.
20. Bhushan M, Beck MH. Allergic contact dermatitis from disodium ethylenediamine tetra-acetic acid (EDTA) in a local anaesthetic. Contact Dermatitis 1998;38(3):183.
21. Fisher AA. Safety of ethylenediamine tetraacetate in the treatment of lead poisoning in persons sensitive to ethylenediamine hydrochloride. Cutis 1991;48(2):105–6.
22. Marsh L, Fraser FC. Letter: Chelating agents and teratogenesis. Lancet 1973;2(7833):846.
23. Swenerton H, Hurley LS. Teratogenic effects of a chelating agent and their prevention by zinc. Science 1971;173(991):62–4.
24. Parkin JE, Duffy MB, Loo CN. The chemical degradation of phenylmercuric nitrate by disodium edetate during heat sterilization at pH values commonly encountered in ophthalmic products. J Clin Pharm Ther 1992;17(5):307–14.
25. Grebe HB, Gregory PJ. Inhibition of warfarin anticoagulation associated with chelation therapy. Pharmacotherapy 2002;22(8):1067–9.
26. Radaelli A, Reiner M, Balestra B. Die Antikoagulantien-bedingte Pseudothrombozytopenie: ein wichtiges Laborartefakt. [Anticoagulant-induced pseudothrombocytopenia: an important laboratory artifact.] Schweiz Rundsch Med Prax 1996;85(48):1550–2.
27. Maniscalchi T, Corbo A, Figliola G, Vaccaro S, Cicatello C, Di Rosa S. EDTA-induced pseudothrombocytopenia. Policlin Sez Med 1996;103:7–12.
28. Allerheiligen D, Houston R, Vermedahl B. EDTA-induced pseudothrombocytopenia. J Am Board Fam Pract 1996;9(3):212–14.
29. Lippi U, Schinella M, Nicoli M, Modena N, Lippi G. EDTA-induced platelet aggregation can be avoided by a new anticoagulant also suitable for automated complete blood count. Haematologica 1990;75(1):38–41.
30. Lavender RC, Salmon JS, Golden WE. Pseudothrombocytopenia in an elderly preoperative patient. Anesth Analg 1989;69(3):396–7.
31. Lombarts AJ, de Kieviet W. Recognition and prevention of pseudothrombocytopenia and concomitant pseudoleukocytosis. Am J Clin Pathol 1988;89(5):634–9.
32. Perrier JF, Nace L, Mariot J, et al. Pseudothrombopénie en présense d'ETDA évoquant une thrombopénie à l'héparine. Reanim Soins Intens Med Urg 1988;4:313–15.
33. Berkman N, Michaeli Y, Or R, Eldor A. EDTA-dependent pseudothrombocytopenia: a clinical study of 18 patients and a review of the literature. Am J Hematol 1991;36(3): 195–201.
34. Foresti V, Parisio E, Tronci M, Casati O, Zubani R, Pedretti D. Pseudothrombocitopenia da EDTA. [EDTA-induced pseudothrombocytopenia.] Recenti Prog Med 1990;81(10):661–2.
35. Pestana D, Marcote C, de Castro MF. EDTA-dependent pseudothrombocytopenia in a preoperative patient. Acta Anaesthesiol Scand 1992;36(4):328–30.
36. D'Angelo G, Calvano D, Mattaini R, Cosini I, Giardini C. Platelet aggregation in presence of anticoagulants dependent pseudothrombocytopenia. Minerva Med 1993; 84(7–8):399–402.
37. Gutensohn K, Cassens U, Riggert J, Kuehnl P. Effect of storage conditions on the CD34+ counts in flow cytometric analysis after anticoagulation of samples with EDTA. Transfus Sci 1996;17(4):591–4.
38. Altes A, Muniz-Diaz E, Pujol-Moix N, Mateo J, Fontcuberta J, Parra J, Brunet S, Madoz P. Trombocitopenia aislada en el curso de la gestación. Estudio etiopatogénico y actitud terapéutica en 60 pacientes. [Isolated thrombocytopenia in pregnancy. Etiopathogenic study and therapeutic approach in 60 patients.] Med Clin (Barc) 1996;107(19):721–5.
39. Hoyt RH, Durie BG. Pseudothrombocytopenia induced by a monoclonal IgM kappa platelet agglutinin. Am J Hematol 1989;31(1):50–2.
40. Germing U, Giagounidis A, Sohngen D, Schneider W. EDTA-induced pseudothrombocytopenia: a case report. Z Allgmed 1998;740:891–4.

Edrecolomab

See also Monoclonal antibodies

General Information

Edrecolomab (17-1A antibody), a mouse monoclonal antibody, has been used in the adjuvant treatment of colorectal cancer.

Organs and Systems

Immunologic

Severe exacerbation of Wegener's granulomatosis with multiorgan involvement has been reported after the first infusion of edrecolomab (500 mg over 2 hours) in a 64-year-old man (1).

Hypersensitivity and anaphylactic reactions have been noted, and urticaria prolonged over a 4-month period was reported in one patient (2).

References

1. Franz A, Bewersdorf H, Hartung G, Dencausse Y, Queisser W. Exacerbation of Wegener's granulomatosis following single administration of monoclonal antibody 17-1A (Panorex®) during adjuvant immunotherapy of colon cancer. Onkologie 2000;23(5):472–4.
2. Sizmann N, Korting HC. Prolonged urticaria with 17-1A antibody. BMJ 1998;317(7173):1631.

Efavirenz

See also Non-nucleoside reverse transcriptase inhibitors (NNRTIs)

General Information

Efavirenz is a non-nucleoside reverse transcriptase inhibitor with excellent inhibitory activity against HIV-1. Its most frequent adverse effects involve the central nervous system and the skin (1). At the start of therapy, dizziness, insomnia, or fatigue is observed in most patients, and headache and even psychotic reactions have also been observed. A maculopapular rash is seen in about 10%. These adverse effects usually vanish within the first 2–4 weeks of therapy (2). About 1–2% of individuals stop taking efavirenz because of neurological or dermatological adverse events. Administration of efavirenz at bedtime reduces the incidence of severe adverse effects, and the rash can be managed by short-term antihistamines or topical corticosteroids (1). Nausea and vomiting are less often observed than in patients treated with zidovudine, lamivudine, or indinavir.

There is other evidence that efavirenz is in some respects better tolerated than certain of the alternatives used in HIV infection. However, comparisons are difficult, since efavirenz will generally be used with drugs of other types in order to avoid the rapid development of resistance. Combined efavirenz with nucleoside analogues reduces toxicity (3). Efavirenz-induced adverse effects often begin on the first day of therapy and resolve within 14–28 (median 13) days (4).

Because efavirenz is metabolized by cytochrome P450, several clinically significant interactions have been described. Efavirenz induces CYP3A4 (5); there was 55% mean induction at a dose of 400 mg/day and 33% at 200 mg/day. However, no significant interaction was noted with co-administration of nelfinavir, zidovudine, lamivudine, fluconazole, or azithromycin (2).

Observational studies

In 77 HIV-positive subjects randomized to switch from protease inhibitors to nevirapine or efavirenz or to continue taking protease inhibitors, quality of life significantly improved among those who switched (6). In those who took efavirenz there was an increase in gamma-glutamyltransferase activity and three patients interrupted treatment because of central nervous system symptoms. Eight patients withdrew because of adverse events: rashes ($n = 3$), dizziness ($n = 2$), irritability and depression ($n = 1$), depression ($n = 1$), or hepatotoxicity ($n = 1$).

Comparative studies

In an open comparison of efavirenz and indinavir (plus two nucleoside analogues) in predominantly treatment-naive patients efavirenz-based triple therapy provided at least similar antiviral effects over 48 weeks (7). Furthermore, fewer patients discontinued efavirenz-based triple therapy than indinavir-based therapy because of adverse events. Adverse effects associated with efavirenz included a maculopapular rash and central nervous system disturbances (dizziness, vivid dreams, poor concentration, sleep disturbances), which generally occurred (but later resolved) within the first weeks of therapy.

Organs and Systems

Nervous system

In a randomized comparison of an efavirenz-containing regimen and a protease inhibitor-containing regimen, nervous system adverse effects were specifically sought (8). Patients were randomized to two NRTIs plus efavirenz ($n = 51$) or two NRTIs plus one or more protease inhibitors ($n = 49$). The patients who took efavirenz reported the following at week 4: dizziness (66%), abnormal dreaming (48%), light-headedness (37%), and difficulty in sleeping (35%). At week 24, dizziness (13%), abnormal dreaming (18%), light-headedness (13%), difficulty in sleeping (7%), and nervousness (13%) were significantly less common. Irritability, abnormal dreaming, and nervousness persisted at week 48 in 13%, 10%, and 8% respectively.

Psychological, psychiatric

Efavirenz has been associated with psychiatric problems, such as anxiety, depression, and confusion (9,10). In a retrospective study of 1897 patients, dementia and depression were significantly associated with efavirenz compared with other drugs; the respective odds ratios were 4.0 (95% CI = 1.2, 14) and 1.7 (1.0, 3.0) (11). However, those who were given efavirenz were perhaps more ill than those who were not, judging by CD4 counts and opportunistic infections.

Most clinicians tend to avoid efavirenz in patients with a psychiatric history. However, it is important to remember that efavirenz can precipitate sudden and severe psychiatric symptoms in patients with no such history. Three patients developed sudden irritability; excitability with anxiety; and insomnia, confusion, and amnesia (12).

The psychiatric adverse effects of efavirenz correlate with its plasma concentrations. In 130 HIV-infected patients, toxicity was three times more common in patients who had an efavirenz concentration over 4000 ng/ml (13).

Metabolism

In a randomized, double blind study of 327 patients, cholesterol and triglycerides were raised in patients taking efavirenz, although this did not reach statistical significance (4).

Liver

In a prospective study of the incidence of severe hepatotoxicity among 312 patients taking efavirenz, hepatitis C and hepatitis B viruses were detected in 7.7% of the patients (14). There was severe hepatotoxicity in 8.0%, but only 50% of the episodes were detected during the first 12 weeks of therapy. The risk was significantly greater among those with chronic viral hepatitis (69% of cases) and those taking concurrent protease inhibitors (82% of cases). However, 84% of patients with chronic hepatitis C or hepatitis B did not have severe hepatotoxicity.

Skin

Efavirenz has been associated with UV photosensitivity, which recurred after skin challenge with efavirenz powder (15).

Reproductive system

Gynecomastia and breast hypertrophy have been reported in at least three patients. All had had indinavir replaced by efavirenz. No other medications were changed, and gynecomastia was not present before substitution (16). The breast enlargement was generally asymmetrical and painful. Needle biopsy was consistent with gynecomastia. Six other reports have confirmed painful breast hypertrophy in patients taking efavirenz (17).

However, gynecomastia has also been reported in 15 patients taking a variety of antiretroviral drugs (18). The authors suggested that it was due to increased cytokine concentrations following immune restoration and this adverse effect may therefore not be unique to efavirenz among drugs used to treat HIV infection.

Immunologic

The incidence of allergic reactions to efavirenz is 10–34%. They usually cause an erythematous maculopapular rash, with or without fever, 1–3 weeks after the start of therapy. Desensitization has been reported (19).

- A 37-year-old HIV-positive white man was given efavirenz, amprenavir, stavudine, lamivudine, and didanosine after failure of a previous regimen. After 8 days he developed a generalized pruritic rash and all the drugs were withdrawn. Two weeks later he was given efavirenz, stavudine, didanosine, lamivudine, and lopinavir, but developed red itchy skin within a day. All the drugs were withdrawn. He was then successfully restarted on stavudine, didanosine, lamivudine, lopinavir, and amprenavir. Desensitization to efavirenz was undertaken, but on day 12 he again developed a rash on the trunk and limbs, which was treated with a topical steroid and diphenhydramine 45 minutes before each dose of efavirenz. The desensitization protocol was continued for another 4 days, and 16 months later he was taking full-dose efavirenz in combination with the other antiretroviral drugs.

Efavirenz can cause an allergic syndrome called the DRESS syndrome (Drug Rash with Eosinophilia and Systemic Symptoms). It is a life-threatening reaction that typically includes a rash, fever, lymphadenopathy, hepatitis, interstitial nephritis, pneumonia, myocarditis, and hematological abnormalities, particularly eosinophilia and a mononucleosis-like atypical lymphocytosis. The DRESS syndrome has been described in an HIV-infected woman taking efavirenz (20).

- A 44-year-old HIV-1 infected woman from the Ivory Coast, who was taking stavudine, lamivudine, efavirenz, and pyrimethamine plus sulfadiazine for *Toxoplasma* encephalitis, developed a maculopapular rash on both arms. The sulfadiazine was withdrawn and clindamycin was added. Ten days later her condition had worsened. Her temperature was 40°C, pulse rate 137/minute, and respiratory rate 26/minute. She had a generalized maculopapular rash without mucosal involvement, moderate abdominal tenderness, hepatomegaly, jaundice, and bilateral crackles. Her white cell count was 16×10^9/l with 9% eosinophils and 51% lymphocytes. A chest X-ray showed moderate bilateral interstitial pneumonitis. All drugs were withdrawn and she was given intravenous methylprednisolone. The skin rash and all systemic manifestations resolved within 1 week and HIV treatment was restarted uneventfully with lamivudine, stavudine, and nelfinavir.

Although this syndrome has been described with sulfonamides (which the patient had taken), the fact that her condition worsened after withdrawal of sulfadiazine, and the characteristic timing of the syndrome (2–6 weeks after starting a drug), suggested efavirenz as the cause.

- In a 39-year-old man efavirenz caused a confluent maculopapular rash, and pulmonary interstitial infiltrates without lymphadenopathy (21). The symptoms resolved when efavirenz was withdrawn while other antiretroviral drugs were continued. The patient was rechallenged, and the rash and fever reappeared; however, recurrence of the pulmonary infiltrates was not addressed.

A leukocytoclastic vasculitis has been attributed to efavirenz (22).

- A 44-year-old man, having taken various antiretroviral drugs, started to take efavirenz; 5 days later he developed palpable purpura on both legs, with pruritus. His white cell count was 14.4×10^9/l and a skin biopsy showed a leukocytoclastic vasculitis. Efavirenz was withdrawn and he was given prednisolone for 3 days; the lesions disappeared, leaving only minimal hyperpigmentation.

Second-Generation Effects

Teratogenicity

- A boy, born at full term to a woman who had taken efavirenz, stavudine, and zidovudine before pregnancy and for the first 24 weeks, had a myelomeningocele (23). The baby was HIV-positive.

The authors suggested that the efavirenz had been responsible, based on previous studies in monkeys.

Drug–Drug Interactions

Ciclosporin

Efavirenz causes increased requirements of ciclosporin by inducing CYP3A4.

- A 39-year-old man took ciclosporin 200 mg bd after a kidney transplant (24). The blood ciclosporin concentration was 307 ng/ml. The co-administration of prednisone caused the blood ciclosporin concentration to rise to 372 ng/ml, but it fell to 203 ng/ml when the dose was reduced to 175 mg bd. Efavirenz 600 mg/day, zidovudine 300 mg bd, and lamivudine 150 mg bd were added, and 7 days later the blood ciclosporin concentration fell to 80 ng/ml and later to 50 ng/ml.

HIV protease inhibitors

The effect of multiple-dose efavirenz 600 mg/day on the steady-state pharmacokinetics of the combination of indinavir (800 mg) + low-dose ritonavir (100 mg) bd, in which ritonavir is used to increase indinavir plasma concentrations, has been investigated in 14 healthy men (25). Efavirenz significantly reduced indinavir AUC (25%), C_{max} (17%), and C_{min} (50%). Ritonavir AUC, C_{max}, and C_{min} were reduced by 36%, 34%, and 39% respectively. The authors proposed that efavirenz had induced the activity of CYP3A and concluded that the dose of indinavir or ritonavir may need to be increased to maintain similar indinavir drug concentrations after the addition of efavirenz.

Indinavir

Increased dosage of indinavir is recommended if efavirenz is co-administered (25).

Methadone

Following a report of withdrawal symptoms in three patients taking methadone maintenance therapy, serum methadone concentrations were measured before and after starting efavirenz in one patient (26). Serum methadone concentrations were as follows: (*R*)-methadone (the active enantiomer) 168 ng/ml and 90 ng/ml before and after efavirenz. The corresponding (*S*)-methadone concentrations were 100 and 28 ng/ml. The dosage of methadone was increased from 100 to 180 mg/day before the patient's withdrawal symptoms resolved.

- Three patients taking methadone were given efavirenz-containing regimens and started to complain of opioid withdrawal symptoms 3–7 days later (27). In one case the plasma methadone concentration fell from about 170 ng/ml to about 50 ng/ml over 6 days.

Since methadone is partly metabolized by CYP3A4, the interaction of efavirenz with methadone has been investigated prospectively in 11 patients taking stable methadone maintenance therapy (28). Efavirenz reduced the steady-state methadone AUC by 50%. However, patients generally only needed a 22% increase in their methadone dose to eliminate the symptoms of methadone withdrawal, and the full basis of the interaction is not understood.

Rifamycins

Rifampicin induces the metabolism of efavirenz. In 24 patients (21 men, 3 women; mean age 37 years) with HIV infection and tuberculosis the C_{max}, C_{min}, and AUC of efavirenz interval fell by 24%, 25%, and 22% respectively in the presence of rifampicin (29).

References

1. Morales-Ramirez J, Tashima K, Hardy D, et al. A phase II, multi-center randomized, open label study to compare the antiretroviral activity and tolerability of efavirenz (EFV) + indinavir (IDV), versus EFV + zidovudine (ZDV) + lamivudine (3TC), versus IDV + 3TC at >36 weeks (DMP 266-006). 38th ICAAC, San Diego, 24–27 September 1998: Abstract 103.
2. Adkins JC, Noble S. Efavirenz. Drugs 1998;56(6):1055–64.
3. Gazzard BG. Efavirenz in the management of HIV infection. Int J Clin Pract 1999;53(1):60–4.
4. Haas DW, Fessel WJ, Delapenha RA, Kessler H, Seekins D, Kaplan M, Ruiz NM, Ploughman LM, Labriola DF, Manion DJ. Therapy with efavirenz plus indinavir in patients with extensive prior nucleoside reverse-transcriptase inhibitor experience: a randomized, double-blind, placebo-controlled trial. J Infect Dis 2001;183(3):392–400.
5. Mouly S, Lown KS, Kornhauser D, Joseph JL, Fiske WD, Benedek IH, Watkins PB. Hepatic but not intestinal CYP3A4 displays dose-dependent induction by efavirenz in humans. Clin Pharmacol Ther 2002;72(1):1–9.
6. Negredo E, Cruz L, Paredes R, Ruiz L, Fumaz CR, Bonjoch A, Gel S, Tuldra A, Balague M, Johnston S, Arno A, Jou A, Tural C, Sirera G, Romeu J, Clotet B. Virological, immunological, and clinical impact of switching from protease inhibitors to nevirapine or to efavirenz in patients with human immunodeficiency virus infection and long-lasting viral suppression. Clin Infect Dis 2002;34(4):504–10.
7. Moyle GJ. Efavirenz: shifting the HAART paradigm in adult HIV-1 infection. Expert Opin Investig Drugs 1999;8(4):473–86.
8. Fumaz CR, Tuldra A, Ferrer MJ, Paredes R, Bonjoch A, Jou T, Negredo E, Romeu J, Sirera G, Tural C, Clotet B. Quality of life, emotional status, and adherence of HIV-1-infected patients treated with efavirenz versus protease inhibitor-containing regimens. J Acquir Immune Defic Syndr 2002;29(3):244–53.
9. Morales-Ramirez J, Tashima K, Hardy D, et al. A phase III, multicenter randomized open-label study to compare the antiretroviral activity and tolerability of efavirenz (EFV) + indinavir (IDV), versus EFV + zidovudine (ZDV) + lamivudine (3TC), versus IDV + ZDV + 3TC at 36 weeks (DMP 266-006). 38th Interscience Conference on Antimicrobial Agents and Chemotherapy (San Diego). Washington DC: American Society for Microbiology, 1998:I-103.
10. Mayers D, Jemesk J, Eyster E, et al. A double-blind, placebo-controlled study to assess the safety, tolerability and antiretroviral activity of efavirenz (EFV DMP 266) in combination with open-label zidovudine (ZDV) and lamivudine (3TC) in HIV infected patients (DMP 266–004). 38th Interscience Conference on Antimicrobial Agents and Chemotherapy (San Diego). Washington DC: American Society for Microbiology, 1998:22340.
11. Welch KJ, Morse A. Association between efavirenz and selected psychiatric and neurological conditions. J Infect Dis 2002;185(2):268–9.

12. Peyriere H, Mauboussin JM, Rouanet I, Fabre J, Reynes J, Hillaire-Buys D. Management of sudden psychiatric disorders related to efavirenz. AIDS 2001;15(10):1323–4.
13. Marzolini C, Telenti A, Decosterd LA, Greub G, Biollaz J, Buclin T. Efavirenz plasma levels can predict treatment failure and central nervous system side effects in HIV-1-infected patients. AIDS 2001;15(1):71–5.
14. Sulkowski MS, Thomas DL, Mehta SH, Chaisson RE, Moore RD. Hepatotoxicity associated with nevirapine or efavirenz-containing antiretroviral therapy: role of hepatitis C and B infections. Hepatology 2002;35(1):182–9.
15. Treudler R, Husak R, Raisova M, Orfanos CE, Tebbe B. Efavirenz-induced photoallergic dermatitis in HIV. AIDS 2001;15(8):1085–6.
16. Caso JA, Prieto Jde M, Casas E, Sanz J. Gynecomastia without lipodystrophy syndrome in HIV-infected men treated with efavirenz. AIDS 2001;15(11):1447–8.
17. Mercie P, Viallard JF, Thiebaut R, Faure I, Rispal P, Leng B, Pellegrin JL. Efavirenz-associated breast hypertrophy in HIV-infection patients. AIDS 2001; 15(1):126–9.
18. Qazi NA, Morlese JF, King DM, Ahmad RS, Gazzard BG, Nelson MR. Gynaecomastia without lipodystrophy in HIV-1-seropositive patients on efavirenz: an alternative hypothesis. AIDS 2002;16(3):506–7.
19. Phillips EJ, Kuriakose B, Knowles SR. Efavirenz-induced skin eruption and successful desensitization. Ann Pharmacother 2002;36(3):430–2.
20. Bossi P, Colin D, Bricaire F, Caumes E. Hypersensitivity syndrome associated with efavirenz therapy. Clin Infect Dis 2000;30(1):227–8.
21. Behrens GM, Stoll M, Schmidt RE. Pulmonary hypersensitivity reaction induced by efavirenz. Lancet 2001;357(9267):1503–4.
22. Domingo P, Barcelo M. Efavirenz-induced leukocytoclastic vasculitis. Arch Intern Med 2002;162(3):355–6.
23. Fundaro C, Genovese O, Rendeli C, Tamburrini E, Salvaggio E. Myelomeningocele in a child with intrauterine exposure to efavirenz. AIDS 2002;16(2):299–300.
24. Tseng A, Nguyen ME, Cardella C, Humar A, Conly J. Probable interaction between efavirenz and cyclosporine. AIDS 2002;16(3):505–6.
25. Aarnoutse RE, Grintjes KJ, Telgt DS, Stek M Jr, Hugen PW, Reiss P, Koopmans PP, Hekster YA, Burger DM. The influence of efavirenz on the pharmacokinetics of a twice-daily combination of indinavir and low-dose ritonavir in healthy volunteers. Clin Pharmacol Ther 2002;71(1):57–67.
26. Marzolini C, Troillet N, Telenti A, Baumann P, Decosterd LA, Eap CB. Efavirenz decreases methadone blood concentrations. AIDS 2000;14(9):1291–2.
27. Boffito M, Rossati A, Reynolds HE, Hoggard PG, Back DJ, Di Perri G. Undefined duration of opiate withdrawal induced by efavirenz in drug users with HIV infection and undergoing chronic methadone treatment. AIDS Res Hum Retroviruses 2002;18(5):341–2.
28. Clarke SM, Mulcahy FM, Tjia J, Reynolds HE, Gibbons SE, Barry MG, Back DJ. The pharmacokinetics of methadone in HIV-positive patients receiving the non-nucleoside reverse transcriptase inhibitor efavirenz. Br J Clin Pharmacol 2001;51(3):213–17.
29. Lopez-Cortes LF, Ruiz-Valderas R, Viciana P, Alarcon-Gonzalez A, Gomez-Mateos J, Leon-Jimenez E, Sarasanacenta M, Lopez-Pua Y, Pachon J. Pharmacokinetic interactions between efavirenz and rifampicin in HIV-infected patients with tuberculosis. Clin Pharmacokinet 2002;41(9):681–90.

Eflornithine

General Information

Eflornithine is a specific irreversible inhibitor of ornithine decarboxylase, the enzyme involved in the first step of mammalian polyamine biosynthesis (1). Decarboxylation of ornithine is an obligatory and rate-limiting step in the biosynthesis of polyamines, such as putrescine, spermidine, and spermine. These low molecular weight polyamines play an essential role in the growth, differentiation, and replication of the cell by participating in nucleic acid and protein synthesis, and are needed in the process of decoding genetic messages. In vitro studies of different types of cell lines (including human malignant cells) exposed to eflornithine demonstrated inhibition of growth. Eflornithine added to human erythrocytes infected with *Plasmodium falciparum* reduced parasite growth and intracellular polyamine content. Polyamines play an important role in the cellular metabolism of trypanosomatids (SED-12, 708) (2,3). Eflornithine can arrest viral replication.

Eflornithine hydrochloride can be given intravenously and orally. Absorption after oral administration is adequate. After intravenous administration, 80% is excreted unchanged in the urine within 14 hours. It penetrates the nervous system, and cerebrospinal fluid concentrations are 10–45% of serum concentrations.

Eflornithine has been used in the chemotherapy and chemoprevention of some tumors, including glioblastoma and colorectal carcinoma in the presence of polyposis coli (4). It has been used in the treatment of malaria tropica, in AIDS, and in *Pneumocystis jiroveci* infections, with varied success. It has also been approved for use in *Trypanosoma gambiense* (SED-12, 708) (5,6).

The most important adverse effect of eflornithine is a natural consequence of its mode of action, myelosuppression, which is frequent and sometimes treatment-limiting. Gastrointestinal toxicity is also common, and is more marked with oral administration. Seizures, hearing loss, alterations in liver function tests, and rash have been described in the treatment of *P. jiroveci* infections in patients with AIDS (SED-13, 835). In 31 patients with AIDS and *P. jiroveci* pneumonia, intolerant of and/or unresponsive to co-trimoxazole or pentamidine, about 50% reacted favorably to eflornithine. The adverse effects were no different from those seen in patients without AIDS, but the frequency of adverse effects was higher. The most common effects in this group were myelosuppression, thrombocytopenia being the most serious, with hepatitis (3%) and hearing loss (9%) among the others (SEDA-17, 332).

Eflornithine in trypanosomiasis

Melarsoprol (an arsenical compound) is still the most effective compound against stage II (nervous system) disease in both East and West African trypanosomiasis. However, it is toxic and causes death in about 2–8% of subjects treated. Eflornithine is an alternative to melarsoprol for West African trypanosomiasis (both early and late). However, it is very expensive, and its usefulness in endemic areas may therefore be limited. The standard regimen is 100 mg/kg intravenously 6-hourly for 14 days.

There have been some anecdotal reports that a shorter 7-day course may be equally effective, with obvious cost-saving advantages.

There has been a multicenter, randomized, open comparison of treatment with eflornithine for 7 or 14 days ($n = 321$) (7). The subjects were divided into new cases and relapses. The 14-day course of eflornithine was superior to the 7-day course for the new cases, but there was no difference in the relapsing cases. However, the numbers of patients who relapsed were small ($n = 47$) and this may not have allowed the detection of a small difference between the groups. The most common adverse events associated with eflornithine were convulsions, altered consciousness, diarrhea, vomiting, nausea, abdominal pain, and secondary infections. Diarrhea and secondary infection were more common in subjects who took the 14-day course.

In 42 patients with late-stage *Trypanosoma brucei gambiense* trypanosomiasis, who relapsed after initial treatment with melarsoprol, a sequential combination of intravenous eflornithine (100 mg/kg every 6 hours for 4 days) followed by three daily injections of melarsoprol (3.6 mg/kg, up to 180 mg) was used (8). They were followed for 24 months. In one case, the administration of eflornithine had to be interrupted for 48 hours because of convulsions, but treatment was then resumed without recurrence. Other adverse effects during treatment were abdominal pain or vomiting ($n = 4$ each), diarrhea ($n = 1$), and loss of hearing ($n = 1$). Two patients died during treatment:

- A 37-year-old man died of an acute cholera-like syndrome, with severe diarrhea, vomiting, and dehydration, after the last dose of eflornithine but before receiving his first dose of melarsoprol.
- A 34-year-old man died of an unknown cause after having received all 16 doses of eflornithine as well as the first injection of melarsoprol.

Organs and Systems

Nervous system

The frequency of seizures in patients with trypanosomiasis taking eflornithine is about 7% (SEDA-16, 316) (9).

Sensory systems

Hearing loss is the dose-limiting toxic effect for eflornithine in patients taking over 2 g/m^2/day (10) (SEDA-11, 394). In one study, it was found in 48% of patients. In some cases the hearing loss was characterized audiographically as bilateral, sensorineural, primarily high frequency, with a median loss of 25–30 dB. All patients recovered within 1–3 months of withdrawal of therapy. There was no clear association between the total dose of eflornithine and the degree of hearing loss (11). Tinnitus has been reported in some patients taking eflornithine (12).

Hearing loss due to eflornithine is usually reversible, but irreversible hearing loss has also been described.

- A patient in a Barrett's esophagus chemoprevention trial developed a hearing deficit of 15 dB at frequencies of 250, 2000, and 3000 Hz in the right ear and a deficit of 20 dB or more at 4000–6000 Hz in the left ear after taking eflornithine 0.5 g/m^2/day for about 13 weeks (cumulative dose 45 g/m^2); clinical hearing was not affected, but the threshold shifts persisted 7 months after eflornithine was withdrawn (13).

In a placebo-controlled study in 123 patients with colorectal polyps and normal hearing at frequencies of 250–2000 Hz, eflornithine 0.075–0.4 g/m^2/day for 12 months had no effect on auditory pure-tone thresholds or distortion product otoacoustic emission (14). There was no hearing loss, in contrast to studies with higher dosages.

In 58 patients with metastatic malignant melanoma, 179 sequential audiograms were obtained from patients treated with eflornithine 2–12 g/m^2/day alone ($n = 16$) or in combination with interferon alfa-2b ($n = 42$) for 2–50 weeks (15). Total doses of 60–1390 g/m^2 correlated with clinical effects and pure-tone audiometric changes at multiple frequencies (500, 1000, 2000, 4000, and 8000 Hz). Patients with normal baseline audiography had more hearing loss than those with abnormal baseline audiography at the higher frequencies. Of the patients with normal prestudy hearing thresholds 10% or less developed a demonstrable hearing deficit at cumulative doses below 150 g/m^2. Conversely, up to 75% of the patients who received more than 250 g/m^2 developed hearing loss. Other factors that adversely affected hearing included age, male sex, and the concomitant use of interferon alfa-2b.

Hematologic

Myelosuppression, as evidenced by anemia, leukopenia, and thrombocytopenia, is common in patients taking eflornithine. The manufacturers quote respective incidence rates of 55, 37, and 14%. However, other reports have suggested that thrombocytopenia is the most frequent problem; it is dose-dependent and occurred in 90% of patients with cancer on a dose of 6–8 g/m^2 with eflornithine concentrations over 400 mmol/l (SED-12, 709) (16).

- A 32-year-old Haitian man with AIDS developed complications of *Isospora belli* enteritis (17). He was given intravenous eflornithine and developed severe thrombocytopenia, nausea, and vomiting, which recurred on rechallenge with low-dose oral eflornithine.

There is an impression that patients with AIDS have a higher incidence of adverse effects. The myelosuppression is reversible on withdrawal (SED-12, 708) (SEDA-16, 316).

Gastrointestinal

Nausea, vomiting, abdominal pain, and diarrhea, mild or severe, are seen with parenteral and oral administration, but more markedly after oral administration (SED-12, 708) (18).

Hair

Alopecia has been reported in 5–10% of patients with trypanosomiasis taking eflornithine (9).

Second-Generation Effects

Teratogenicity

Animal studies have shown arrest of the growth of malignant cells and decrease in tumor size, but as one might expect, there was also an arrest of embryonic growth if eflornithine was given in the first days of pregnancy (SED-12, 708). On theoretical grounds, one would expect an effect on the development of the fast-growing embryo; whether or not this could lead to defects and/or deformities is not known.

References

1. Pasic TR, Heisey D, Love RR. Alpha-difluoromethylornithine ototoxicity. Chemoprevention clinical trial results. Arch Otolaryngol Head Neck Surg 1997;123(12):1281–6.
2. Anonymous. d,l-alpha-Difluoromethyl ornithine. DFMO. Eflornithine. Drugs Future 1985;10:242.
3. Anonymous. DFMO. Ann Drug Data Rep 1982;71.
4. Courtney ED, Melville DM, Leicester RJ. Review article: chemoprevention of colorectal cancer. Aliment Pharmacol Ther 2004;19(1):1–24.
5. Notification. New drug for trypanosomiasis. Lancet 1991;337(8732):42.
6. Anonymous. Sleeping sickness. Wake-up call. Economist 1990;Dec 12:110.
7. Pepin J, Khonde N, Maiso F, Doua F, Jaffar S, Ngampo S, Mpia B, Mbulamberi D, Kuzoe F. Short-course eflornithine in Gambian trypanosomiasis: a multicentre randomized controlled trial. Bull World Health Organ 2000;78(11):1284–95.
8. Mpia B, Pepin J. Combination of eflornithine and melarsoprol for melarsoprol-resistant Gambian trypanosomiasis. Trop Med Int Health 2002;7(9):775–9.
9. Burri C, Brun R. Eflornithine for the treatment of human African trypanosomiasis. Parasitol Res 2003;90(Suppl 1): S49–52.
10. van der Velden JW, van Putten WL, Guinee VF, Pfeiffer R, van Leeuwen FE, van der Linden EA, Vardomskaya I, Lane W, Durand M, Lagarde C, et al. Subsequent development of acute non-lymphocytic leukemia in patients treated for Hodgkin's disease. Int J Cancer 1988;42(2):252–5.
11. Meyskens FL, Kingsley EM, Glattke T, Loescher L, Booth A. A phase II study of alpha-difluoromethylornithine (DFMO) for the treatment of metastatic melanoma. Invest New Drugs 1986;4(3):257–62.
12. Levin VA, Chamberlain MC, Prados MD, Choucair AK, Berger MS, Silver P, Seager M, Gutin PH, Davis RL, Wilson CB. Phase I-II study of eflornithine and mitoguazone combined in the treatment of recurrent primary brain tumors. Cancer Treat Rep 1987;71(5):459–64.
13. Lao CD, Backoff P, Shotland LI, McCarty D, Eaton T, Ondrey FG, Viner JL, Spechler SJ, Hawk ET, Brenner DE. Irreversible ototoxicity associated with difluoromethylornithine. Cancer Epidemiol Biomarkers Prev 2004;13(7):1250–2.
14. Doyle KJ, McLaren CE, Shanks JE, Galus CM, Meyskens FL. Effects of difluoromethylornithine chemoprevention on audiometry thresholds and otoacoustic emissions. Arch Otolaryngol Head Neck Surg 2001;127(5):553–8.
15. Croghan MK, Aickin MG, Meyskens FL. Dose-related alpha-difluoromethylornithine ototoxicity. Am J Clin Oncol 1991;14(4):331–5.
16. Ajani JA, Ota DM, Grossie VB Jr, Levin B, Nishioka K. Alterations in polyamine metabolism during continuous intravenous infusion of alpha-difluoromethylornithine showing correlation of thrombocytopenia with alpha-difluoromethylornithine plasma levels. Cancer Res 1989;49(20):5761–5.
17. Tietze KJ, Gaska JA, Cosgrove EM. Thrombocytopenia and vomiting due to difluoromethylornithine. Drug Intell Clin Pharm 1987;21(7–8):627–30.
18. Anonymous. Eflornithine hydrochloride. d,l-alpha-Difluoromethyl ornithine. DFMO. Drugs Future 1986;11:220.

Emedastine

See also Antihistamines

General Information

Emedastine is a potent second-generation antihistamine with proven efficacy in allergic conjunctivitis (1).

Organs and Systems

Nervous system

The potential sedative effects of single and repeated doses of emedastine 2 mg and 4 mg bd on actual driving performance have been assessed in healthy volunteers (9 men and 10 women, aged 21–45 years) (2). The study was a four-period, double-blind, crossover design, and driving performance was measured in a standardized test at 3–4 hours after administration of the morning dose on days 1, 4, and 5. Emedastine significantly impaired driving in every test at both doses and the authors concluded that the drug could constitute a traffic hazard and that its users should be warned accordingly.

Drug–Drug Interactions

Ketoconazole

In a study of the interaction of emedastine difumarate 4 mg bd with ketoconazole 200 mg bd in 12 subjects there was a moderate but statistically significant interaction; however, there was no increase in the QT_c interval during concomitant therapy (3). The authors concluded that these findings are consistent with the multiple metabolic pathways that supplement the metabolism of emedastine by different enzymatic isoforms of CYP450, and that concomitant treatment with emedastine and ketoconazole in people with normal QT intervals can be undertaken without special precautions. However, it is difficult to determine the precise cardiac risk, if any, posed by the administration of emedastine eye-drops (4).

References

1. Verin P, Easty DL, Secchi A, Ciprandi G, Partouche P, Nemeth-Wasmer G, Brancato R, Harrisberg CJ, Estivin-Ebrardt C, Coster DJ, Apel AJ, Coroneo MT, Knorr M,

Carmichael TR, Kent-Smith BT, Abrantes P, Leonardi A, Cerqueti PM, Modorati G, Martinez M. Clinical evaluation of twice-daily emedastine 0.05% eye drops (Emadine eye drops) versus levocabastine 0.05% eye drops in patients with allergic conjunctivitis. Am J Ophthalmol 2001;131(6):691–8.
2. Vermeeren A, Ramaekers JG, O'Hanlon JF. Effects of emedastine and cetirizine, alone and with alcohol, on actual driving of males and females. J Psychopharmacol 2002;16(1):57–64.
3. Herranz U, Rusca A, Assandri A. Emedastine–ketoconazole: pharmacokinetic and pharmacodynamic interactions in healthy volunteers. Int J Clin Pharmacol Ther 2001;39(3):102–9.
4. Anonymous. Emedastine and allergic conjunctivitis: new preparation. Poor assessment. Prescrire Int 2001;10(52): 39–40.

Emepronium bromide

See also Anticholinergic drugs

General Information

Emepronium bromide is an anticholinergic drug. Doses of 200 mg tds (sometimes with a double dose in the evenings) are useful in relieving urinary frequency. It causes the expected milder anticholinergic adverse effects.

Organs and Systems

Gastrointestinal

Emepronium has repeatedly been shown to cause ulceration of the mouth and esophagus and widespread esophagitis (1–3). The buccal irritation is particularly marked if the tablets are retained in the mouth instead of being swallowed, and the problem as a whole is greater if the drug is not taken with sufficient fluid.

- Two women taking emepronium bromide developed extended ulcers of the esophageal mucosa. They had taken the tablets late in the evening with only a little fluid (4).

Drug Administration

Drug overdose

Central effects of emepronium are only serious in gross overdosage. In one case of attempted suicide with 100 tablets, there was severe confusion and derangement of breathing (due to neuromuscular paralysis) demanding mechanical ventilation (SED-12, 330).

References

1. Puhakka HJ. Drug-induced corrosive injury of the oesophagus. J Laryngol Otol 1978;92(10):927–31.
2. Pilbrant A. Ulceration due to emepronium bromide tablets. Lancet 1977;1(8014):749.

3. Leonard RC, Adams PC, Parker S, Adams DM. Oesophageal injury associated with emepronium bromide (Cetiprin). Br J Clin Pract 1984;38(11-12):429–30.
4. Berges W, Rohner HG, Wienbeck W. Osophagusulkus nach Einnahme von Emeproniumbromid. [Ulcer of the esophagus after intake of emeproniumbromide.] Leber Magen Darm 1980;10(1):37–40.

Emorfazone

General Information

Emorfazone is a pyridazinone NSAID that was developed in Japan. Sleepiness, dry mouth, rash, and various gastrointestinal disturbances are its most important adverse effects (1).

Reference

1. Anonymous. Emorfazone. Drugs Today 1985;21:63.

Enadoline

General Information

Enadoline is an opioid agonist at OP_2 (κ) receptors and has no effects attributable to OP_3 (μ) receptor actions, such as respiratory depression. However, enadoline does not offer any benefits over other currently available opioids (1).

Reference

1. Pande AC, Pyke RE, Greiner M, Wideman GL, Benjamin R, Pierce MW. Analgesic efficacy of enadoline versus placebo or morphine in postsurgical pain. Clin Neuropharmacol 1996;19(5):451–6.

Enalapril

See also Angiotensin converting enzyme inhibitors

General Information

Enalapril is an ACE inhibitor used in the treatment of hypertension and heart failure and prophylactically in patients with asymptomatic left ventricular dysfunction.

Organs and Systems

Cardiovascular

Of all studies of the effects of ACE inhibitors on mortality in acute myocardial infarction, only the CONSENSUS II trial did not show a positive effect. In this trial enalaprilat was infused within 24 hours after the onset of symptoms, followed by oral enalapril. The reasons for the negative result of CONSENSUS II remain unresolved, but hypotension linked to a poorer prognosis has been suggested as an explanation. In a small substudy of this large trial, 60 patients were investigated for residual ischemia before discharge, with exercise testing and Holter monitoring (1). Episodes of hypotension and predischarge ischemia were more common with enalapril than with placebo. The authors suggested that enalapril induced a proischemic effect in hypotension-prone patients, mediated through exacerbation of the hemodynamic response, since the initial blood pressure fall after myocardial infarction is related to residual ischemia and recurrent acute ischemic syndromes. This conclusion seems very speculative. The data were derived from a small substudy with multiple subanalyses and cannot support a cause-and-effect relation between the acute hemodynamic effect and the predischarge ischemic conditions. ACE inhibitors should still be used in acute myocardial infarction with cautious dose titration.

Neuromuscular function

Muscular weakness has been reported in a patient with mild renal impairment taking enalapril (2).

- A 78-year-old man, taking enalapril (10 mg/day), furosemide, and digoxin for cardiac failure due to ischemic heart disease, suddenly developed generalized muscle weakness. He had grade 3/5 weakness of all four limbs, his cranial nerves were intact, and there was no sensory impairment. His tendon reflexes were reduced and he had flexor plantar reflexes. The initial diagnosis was Guillain–Barré syndrome. Further investigation showed peaked T waves on his electrocardiogram, with a serum potassium of 9.4 mmol/l and a creatinine of 266 μmol/l. He was treated with glucose plus insulin, calcium gluconate, and sodium bicarbonate. Enalapril was withdrawn. His potassium concentration normalized.

Hyperkalemic muscle paralysis has been reported in renal insufficiency and trauma and in patients taking spironolactone and amiloride plus hydrochlorothiazide (co-amilozide). ACE inhibitors inhibit the release of aldosterone, reducing renal potassium loss, which can be enhanced by potassium-sparing diuretics or pre-existing renal insufficiency.

Endocrine

A single case of the syndrome of inappropriate secretion of antidiuretic hormone has been reported with enalapril (3).

Hematologic

Thrombocytopenia has been reported with enalapril in two elderly sisters (4). Both had the same HLA phenotype (B8DR3), which the authors postulated may reflect a genetic predisposition to this reaction. However, no further cases have been reported.

Enalapril-induced anemia has been reported in hemodialysis patients and in kidney transplant recipients. The anemia is usually normocytic, normochromic, and non-regenerative. Deficient bone-marrow erythropoiesis has occasionally been described. The anemia is reversible after withdrawal. Although the hypothesized mechanism of a reduction in erythropoietin blood concentrations by enalapril is controversial, in a prospective controlled study enalapril increased recombinant human erythropoietin requirements to maintain hemoglobin concentrations (5).

Enalapril-induced anemia has been reported in a child (6).

- A 7-year-old girl with segmental glomerulosclerosis and nephrotic syndrome failed to respond to prednisolone and cyclophosphamide, which were withdrawn. While her renal function was deteriorating she was given enalapril 2.5 mg bd. After 3 months, the enalapril was withdrawn because her hemoglobin fell from 12.7 to 6.2 g/dl. Ferritin, folate, and vitamin B_{12} were normal. Recovery was incomplete. Only 10 weeks after enalapril withdrawal her hemoglobin rose to 8.5 g/dl and remained unchanged thereafter.

The incomplete resolution of anemia in this case suggests that factors other than the speculated enalapril-related inhibition of erythropoietin may have contributed to the initial anemia (worsening renal function, frequent blood sampling, withdrawal of prednisolone).

An equivocal case of neutropenia has been ascribed to enalapril (7).

- A 52-year-old male renal transplant recipient on stable therapy (4.5 months) with ciclosporin, mycophenolate mofetil, and co-trimoxazole developed erythrocytosis and hypertension. His leukocyte count fell 19 days after he started to take enalapril. Enalapril was withdrawn, the dose of co-trimoxazole was halved, and the dose of mycophenolate was first reduced and then withdrawn on day 25. On day 28 the leukocyte and neutrophil counts were so low that granulocyte-stimulating factor had to be used. The leukocyte count normalized during continued treatment with ciclosporin and co-trimoxazole. CMV tests were negative.

The authors suggested a synergistic effect between enalapril and mycophenolate. As leukopenia is the commonest clinically significant adverse effect of mycophenolate, the evidence in this case is inadequate to support this hypothesis, particularly in the absence of information on mycophenolate blood concentrations.

Liver

Hepatitis has been attributed to enalapril.

- A 45-year-old man who had taken enalapril (dose not reported) for more than 2 years presented with hepatitis with negative viral serology (8). Biopsy showed necrosis and cholestasis. He recovered fully after drug withdrawal (timing not reported).
- A 46-year-old man had taken enalapril for hypertension for 3 years before he presented with jaundice and progressive liver failure (9). He was taking no other drugs and had a moderate daily consumption

of alcohol. All known causes of acute liver failure were excluded by careful and extensive investigation. Analysis of liver biopsies showed a pathological pattern comparable to that observed in severe halothane hepatitis. Serological studies, including T cell stimulation with enalapril and a broad spectrum of tests for autoimmunity, were negative. The hepatitis persisted despite enalapril withdrawal and finally led to orthotopic liver transplantation and subsequently to death.

The mechanism of enalapril-induced liver injury in this case was obscure. The causal relation was unconvincing.

Skin

Adult Henoch-Schönlein purpura has been attributed to enalapril (10).

- A 41-year-old man with a history of hypertension and a recent stroke was admitted 10 days after starting to take enalapril (dose not reported). He complained of severe abdominal pain, myalgia, arthralgia, paresthesia, and Raynaud's phenomenon, and had a high erythrocyte sedimentation rate, but no leukocytosis or thrombocytopenia. He developed purpura-like cutaneous lesions with acute renal insufficiency, severe hematuria, and proteinuria. Liver tests became altered. There was a polyclonal rise in IgA concentrations. Skin biopsy suggested leukocytoclastic vasculitis, with deposition of IgA and complement. Other diagnostic procedures were negative. Enalapril was withdrawn and he was given glucocorticoids, after which he fully recovered (timing not reported).

The acantholytic potential of enalapril has been shown in vitro in skin cultures and in vivo acantholysis without pemphigus has been reported.

- A 66-year-old man, who had taken enalapril 10 mg/day for 1 year, had a basal cell carcinoma removed surgically (11). Histology showed suprabasal acantholytic clefts in the perilesional epidermis. Direct immunofluorescence did not show intracellular deposits of IgG, IgA, IgM, or C3. Indirect immunofluorescence showed serum anticellular antibodies (titer 1:80). He stopped taking enalapril, and 3 months later his anticellular antibody titer was 1:320. A further biopsy of apparently healthy skin on the back showed new foci of acantholysis. Another biopsy in the same location 2 months later showed no acantholytic changes. Direct immunofluorescence was negative and the anticellular antibody titer was 1:80. HLA typing showed pemphigus-predisposing antigens (DR14, DQ1), which has previously been reported as a predisposing factor for acantholytic changes in the epidermis exposed to enalapril.

As pemphigus vulgaris has been attributed to ACE inhibitors, it is not surprising that giving an ACE inhibitor to a patient with pemphigus could worsen the disease. Aggravation of pre-existing childhood pemphigus by enalapril has been reported (12).

- A 12-year-old boy with pemphigus vulgaris was treated with intravenous dexamethasone and prednisolone. He developed severe hypertension, which was unresponsive to atenolol, and he was given enalapril 2.5 mg bd. Although the blood pressure responded, the pemphigus deteriorated markedly over the next 2 weeks. Additional dexamethasone did not produce improvement. Enalapril was replaced by amlodipine, and the disease resolved over 3 weeks.

The evidence to date suggests that ACE inhibitors should be avoided in patients with pre-existing pemphigus.

Immunologic

Eosinophilic gastroenteritis after enalapril has been described (13). The authors briefly reviewed this rare condition, which is diagnosed on the basis of the presence of gastrointestinal symptoms, eosinophilic infiltration of the gastrointestinal tract, and the absence of parasitic or extra-intestinal disease. It has also been reported after clofazimine and naproxen.

- A 63-year-old hypertensive woman, who had a carcinoma of the distal esophagus resected 19 months earlier, developed chronic diarrhea. *Clostridium difficile* toxin was identified in her stools and the diarrhea resolved after treatment with metronidazole. Enalapril was added to her antihypertensive treatment, and 3 months later the diarrhea recurred. Stool examination was negative and there was no *Clostridium difficile* toxin. Her condition worsened and she lost 5 kg in weight. She had marked eosinophilia (2.4×10^9/l), and a small bowel biopsy showed mild chronic inflammation and edema, partial villous atrophy, and large clusters of eosinophils in the lamina propria with some focal infiltration of the epithelium. She stopped taking enalapril and her diarrhea promptly abated and the eosinophil count fell to 0.5×10^9/l at 3 weeks and 0.1×10^9/l at 2 months.

Body temperature

Fever has been attributed to enalapril (14).

- A 50-year-old man with heart failure and a valve prosthesis, taking digoxin, furosemide, and spironolactone, was given enalapril 5 mg/day. Two days later, after increasing the dose to 10 mg, he developed a fever with cough and clear sputum, with a normal chest X-ray. Enalapril was withdrawn and 24 hours later the fever resolved. It recurred immediately after rechallenge.

Drug Administration

Drug overdose

A single case of overdose of enalapril has been reported (15).

References

1. Sogaard P, Thygesen K. Potential proischemic effect of early enalapril in hypotension-prone patients with acute myocardial infarction. The CONSENSUS II Holter Substudy Group. Cardiology 1997;88(3):285–91.
2. Dutta D, Fischler M, McClung A. Angiotensin converting enzyme inhibitor induced hyperkalaemic paralysis. Postgrad Med J 2001;77(904):114–15.

3. Castrillon JL, Mediavilla A, Mendez MA, Cavada E, Carrascosa M, Valle R. Syndrome of inappropriate antidiuretic hormone secretion (SIADH) and enalapril. J Intern Med 1993;233(1):89–91.
4. Grosbois B, Milton D, Beneton C, Jacomy D. Thrombocytopenia induced by angiotensin converting enzyme inhibitors. BMJ 1989;298(6667):189–90.
5. Albitar S, Genin R, Fen-Chong M, Serveaux MO, Bourgeon B. High dose enalapril impairs the response to erythropoietin treatment in haemodialysis patients. Nephrol Dial Transplant 1998;13(5):1206–10.
6. Sackey AH. Anaemia after enalapril in a child with nephrotic syndrome. Lancet 1998;352(9124):285–6.
7. Donadio C, Lucchesi A. Neutropenia after treatment of posttransplantation erythrocytosis with enalapril. Transplantation 2001;72(3):553–4.
8. Quilez C, Palazon JM, Chulia T, Cordoba YC. Hepatatoxicided por enalapril. [Hepatoxicity by enalapril.] Gastroenterol Hepatol 1999;22(2):113–14.
9. Jeserich M, Ihling C, Allgaier HP, Berg PA, Heilmann C. Acute liver failure due to enalapril. Herz 2000;25(7):689–93.
10. Goncalves R, Cortez Pinto H, Serejo F, Ramalho F. Adult Schönlein–Henoch purpura after enalapril. J Intern Med 1998;244(4):356–7.
11. Lo Schiavo A, Guerrera V, Cozzani E, Aurilia A, Ruocco E, Pinto F. In vivo enalapril-induced acantholysis. Dermatology 1999;198(4):391–3.
12. Thami GP, Kaur S, Kanwar AJ. Severe childhood pemphigus vulgaris aggravated by enalapril. Dermatology 2001;202(4):341.
13. Barak N, Hart J, Sitrin MD. Enalapril-induced eosinophilic gastroenteritis. J Clin Gastroenterol 2001;33(2):157–8.
14. Lorente L, Falguera M, Jover A, Rubio M. Fiebra secundaria a la administracion de enalapril. [Fever secondary to enalapril administration.] Med Clin (Barc) 1999;112(16):638–9.
15. Newby DE, Lee MR, Gray AJ, Boon NA. Enalapril overdose and the corrective effect of intravenous angiotensin II. Br J Clin Pharmacol 1995;40(1):103–4.

Encainide

See also Antidysrhythmic drugs

General Information

Encainide is a class I antidysrhythmic drug. Reviews of its clinical pharmacology, clinical use, efficacy, and adverse effects have appeared (1–6).

Organs and Systems

Cardiovascular

In the wake of the preliminary and final reports of the Cardiac Arrhythmia Suppression Trial (CAST) (7,8), which showed that there was an increased risk of death among patients who took encainide and flecainide after myocardial infarction, there have been many publications in which the implications of these findings have been thoroughly discussed (9–13). The relative risk of death or cardiac arrest due to dysrhythmias in the treated patients was 2.6 and the relative risk due to all causes was 2.38. The risk of non-fatal cardiac adverse effects was no different in treated patients from that in those taking placebo and there was no difference between the groups in the use of other drugs.

Although there is a consensus that encainide and flecainide were associated with an increase in the rate of mortality in CAST, there are still some open questions. First, all the patients recruited to CAST had asymptomatic ventricular dysrhythmias after myocardial infarction, and it is not clear whether the results can be extrapolated to other patients. Secondly, the reasons for the increased mortality in the treated patients are not clear: ventricular dysrhythmias and worsening of left ventricular function are both possible. Thirdly, it is not clear whether the results of CAST in patients with asymptomatic ventricular dysrhythmias after myocardial infarction can also be applied to other Class I antidysrhythmic drugs.

Separate studies have confirmed the prodysrhythmic actions of encainide (14–17). The incidence of prodysrhythmias is much higher in patients being treated for ventricular dysrhythmias than in those being treated for supraventricular dysrhythmias (18).

Encainide has been reported to cause sinus node arrest in association with prolonged sinus node recovery time (19). It also raises the pacing threshold in patients with chronic implanted pacemakers (20), although this has not been reported to increase the failure rate of pacemakers.

Encainide has a negative inotropic effect on the heart and can cause hypotension (21) or worsen heart failure (22).

Nervous system

The most common non-cardiac effects of encainide are on the central nervous system, and include abnormal or blurred vision (11%), dizziness (7.3%), headaches (6.0%), nausea (4.3%), vertigo (2.3%), insomnia, and fatigue. The figures in parentheses are taken from a review of 349 patients with supraventricular dysrhythmias treated with encainide (14). These effects are common during long-term therapy, but may also occur transiently during intravenous administration and appear to be dose-related (23,24).

A case of encephalopathy has been attributed to encainide (25).

Sensory systems

There have been reports of a metallic taste in the mouth after intravenous administration of encainide (24).

Endocrine

Encainide can cause hyperglycemia (26), perhaps due to insulin resistance.

Gastrointestinal

Nausea can occur during long-term therapy with encainide, probably due to a central nervous effect (27).

Skin

Skin rashes have been reported occasionally during long-term therapy with encainide (27).

Musculoskeletal

There have been reports of leg cramps after intravenous administration of encainide (24).

Susceptibility Factors

Genetic factors

Encainide is metabolized, at least partly, by oxidation to *O*-desmethylencainide, 3-methoxy-*O*-desmethylencainide, *N*-desmethylencainide, and *N*,*O*-didesmethylencainide. Of 112 healthy Caucasians 9 (8%) were defective in their ability to 4-hydroxylate debrisoquine (28). The cumulative frequency distribution of the 8-hour urinary recovery ratio of encainide/*O*-desmethylencainide indicated two distinct populations, an extensive metabolizer (EM) phenotype and a poor metabolizer (PM) phenotype. There was no 3-methoxy-*O*-desmethylencainide in the urine of the poor metabolizers. As *O*-desmethylencainide is a more potent antidysrhythmic drug than encainide and 3-methoxy-*O*-desmethylencainide is at least equipotent, these metabolites contribute significantly to the overall antidysrhythmic effect in extensive metabolizers. The low plasma concentrations of *O*-desmethylencainide and 3-methoxy-*O*-desmethylencainide in poor metabolizers would be expected to result in ineffective therapy when usual doses of encainide are given. However, in such individuals, chronic oral therapy results in accumulation of unmetabolized encainide to far higher concentrations than in extensive metabolizers, and as encainide itself has antidysrhythmic activity at these concentrations, this generally results in the desired response. It is possible that poor hydroxylators are at greater risk of adverse effects than extensive hydroxylators.

In 110 healthy subjects the changes in atrioventricular (PR) and intraventricular (QRS) conduction times produced by encainide were different in extensive and poor metabolizers and correlated with CYP2D6 activity, although the electrocardiographic response was never 100% specific and sensitive for the identification of either phenotype (29). Moreover, genotypic identification of heterozygous and homozygous extensive metabolizer subjects did not predict CYP2D6 activity, as determined by encainide metabolic ratios or encainide responses, as determined by intraventricular and atrioventricular changes.

Age

Children under the age of 6 months may be more liable to the prodysrhythmic effects of encainide than older children (30).

References

1. Keefe DL, Kates RE, Harrison DC. New antiarrhythmic drugs: their place in therapy. Drugs 1981;22(5):363–400.
2. Harrison DC, Winkle R, Sami M, Mason J. Encainide: a new and potent antiarrhythmic agent. Am Heart J 1980;100(6 Pt 2):1046–54.
3. Lynch JJ, Lucchesi BR. New antiarrhythmic agents. II. The pharmacology and clinical use of encainide. Pract Cardiol 1984;10:109–32.
4. Roden DM, Woosley RL. Clinical pharmacology of the new antiarrhythmic encainide. Clin Progr Pacing Electrophysiol 1984;2:112–19.
5. Rinkenberger RL, Naccarelli GV, Dougherty AH. New antiarrhythmic agents. X. Safety and efficacy of encainide in the treatment of ventricular arrhythmias. Pract Cardiol 1987;13:110–32.
6. Naccarelli GV, et al. A symposium: The use of encainide in supraventricular tachycardias. June 3 and 4, 1988, Bermuda. Proceedings. Am J Cardiol 1988;62(19):1L–84L.
7. The Cardiac Arrhythmia Suppression Trial (CAST) Investigators. Preliminary report: effect of encainide and flecainide on mortality in a randomized trial of arrhythmia suppression after myocardial infarction. N Engl J Med 1989;321(6):406–12.
8. Echt DS, Liebson PR, Mitchell LB, Peters RW, Obias-Manno D, Barker AH, Arensberg D, Baker A, Friedman L, Greene HL, et al. Mortality and morbidity in patients receiving encainide, flecainide, or placebo. The Cardiac Arrhythmia Suppression Trial. N Engl J Med 1991;324(12):781–8.
9. Gottlieb SS. The use of antiarrhythmic agents in heart failure: implications of CAST. Am Heart J 1989;118(5 Pt 1):1074–7.
10. Podrid PJ, Marcus FI. Lessons to be learned from the Cardiac Arrhythmia Suppression Trial. Am J Cardiol 1989;64(18):1189–91.
11. Bigger JT Jr. The events surrounding the removal of encainide and flecainide from the Cardiac Arrhythmia Suppression Trial (CAST) and why CAST is continuing with moricizine. J Am Coll Cardiol 1990;15(1):243–5.
12. Akhtar M, Breithardt G, Camm AJ, Coumel P, Janse MJ, Lazzara R, Myerburg RJ, Schwartz PJ, Waldo AL, Wellens HJ, et al. CAST and beyond. Implications of the Cardiac Arrhythmia Suppression Trial. Task Force of the Working Group on Arrhythmias of the European Society of Cardiology. Circulation 1990;81(3):1123–7.
13. Thomis JA. Encainide—an updated safety profile. Cardiovasc Drugs Ther 1990;4(Suppl 3):585–94.
14. Soyka LF. Safety considerations and dosing guidelines for encainide in supraventricular arrhythmias. Am J Cardiol 1988;62(19):L63–8.
15. Miles WM, Zipes DP, Rinkenberger RL, Markel ML, Prystowsky EN, Dougherty AH, Heger JJ, Naccarelli GV. Encainide for treatment of atrioventricular reciprocating tachycardia in the Wolff–Parkinson–White syndrome. Am J Cardiol 1988;62(19):L20–5.
16. Rinkenberger RL, Naccarelli GV, Miles WM, Markel ML, Dougherty AH, Prystowsky EN, Heger JJ, Zipes DP. Encainide for atrial fibrillation associated with Wolff–Parkinson–White syndrome. Am J Cardiol 1988;62(19): L26–30.
17. Naccarelli GV, Jackman WM, Akhtar M, Rinkenberger RL, Friday KJ, Dougherty AH, Tchou P, Yeung-Lai-Wah JA. Efficacy and electrophysiologic effects of encainide for atrioventricular nodal reentrant tachycardia. Am J Cardiol 1988;62(19):L31–6.
18. The Encainide-Ventricular Tachycardia Study Group. Treatment of life-threatening ventricular tachycardia with encainide hydrochloride in patients with left ventricular dysfunction. Am J Cardiol 1988;62(9):571–5.
19. Lemery R, Talajic M, Nattel S, Theroux P, Roy D. Sinus node dysfunction and sudden cardiac death following treatment with encainide. Pacing Clin Electrophysiol 1989;12(10):1607–12.
20. Salel AF, Seagren SC, Pool PE. Effects of encainide on the function of implanted pacemakers. Pacing Clin Electrophysiol 1989;12(9):1439–44.

21. Rinkenberger RL, Prystowsky EN, Jackman WM, Naccarelli GV, Heger JJ, Zipes DP. Drug conversion of nonsustained ventricular tachycardia to sustained ventricular tachycardia during serial electrophysiologic studies: identification of drugs that exacerbate tachycardia and potential mechanisms. Am Heart J 1982;103(2):177–84.
22. DiBianco R, Fletcher RD, Cohen AI, Gottdiener JS, Singh SN, Katz RJ, Bates HR, Sauerbrunn B. Treatment of frequent ventricular arrhythmia with encainide: assessment using serial ambulatory electrocardiograms, intracardiac electrophysiologic studies, treadmill exercise tests, and radionuclide cineangiographic studies. Circulation 1982;65(6):1134–47.
23. Kesteloot H, Stroobandt R. Clinical experience of encainide (MJ 9067): a new anti-arrhythmic drug. Eur J Clin Pharmacol 1979;16(5):323–6.
24. Sami M, Mason JW, Peters F, Harrison DC. Clinical electrophysiologic effects of encainide, a newly developed antiarrhythmic agent. Am J Cardiol 1979;44(3):526–32.
25. Tartini A, Kesselbrenner M. Encainide-induced encephalopathy in a patient with chronic renal failure. Am J Kidney Dis 1990;15(2):178–9.
26. Winter WE, Funahashi M, Koons J. Encainide-induced diabetes: analysis of islet cell function. Res Commun Chem Pathol Pharmacol 1992;76(3):259–68.
27. Sami M, Harrison DC, Kraemer H, Houston N, Shimasaki C, DeBusk RF. Antiarrhythmic efficacy of encainide and quinidine: validation of a model for drug assessment. Am J Cardiol 1981;48(1):147–56.
28. McAllister CB, Wolfenden HT, Aslanian WS, Woosley RL, Wilkinson GR. Oxidative metabolism of encainide: polymorphism, pharmacokinetics and clinical considerations. Xenobiotica 1986;16(5):483–90.
29. Funck-Brentano C, Thomas G, Jacqz-Aigrain E, Poirier JM, Simon T, Bereziat G, Jaillon P. Polymorphism of dextromethorphan metabolism: relationships between phenotype, genotype and response to the administration of encainide in humans. J Pharmacol Exp Ther 1992;263(2):780–6.
30. Strasburger JF, Smith RT Jr, Moak JP, Gothing C, Garson A Jr. Encainide for resistant supraventricular tachycardia in children: follow-up report. Am J Cardiol 1988;62(19):L50–4.

Endothelin receptor antagonists

See also Individual agents

General Information

It is disappointing that mechanistically novel antihypertensive drugs have not emerged during the last decade or two. The only real novelty was the addition of angiotensin II receptor antagonists as a refinement of the approach introduced with ACE inhibitors. The expectations for direct renin antagonists have not been realized. Some of the cornerstone classes of antihypertensive drugs, such as the diuretics, beta-adrenoceptor antagonists, calcium channel blockers, and direct vasodilators, have been around for several decades. Advances have predominantly been made in the pharmacokinetic properties and pharmacodynamic specificities of compounds in existing antihypertensive drug classes.

With the emergence of knowledge about endothelial factors such as nitric oxide and endothelin, there was much expectation that endothelin antagonists would become useful in the management of hypertension. Endothelin was discovered in 1988 (1) and is the most potent vasoconstrictor known. In terms of pathophysiology, endothelin receptor antagonists could play a role in a variety of diseases associated with vasoconstriction, such as hypertension, renal disease, occlusive vascular disease, pulmonary hypertension, and congestive heart failure (2). Apart from vasoconstriction, endothelin is also involved in the structural changes associated with these diseases, and it is now recognized that there is a wider target in hypertension treatment than lowering blood pressure. Vascular and myocardial remodelling may be key issues in determining long-term outcome (3) and effects on myocardial fibrosis and vascular compliance may be as important as lowering blood pressure. ACE inhibitor treatment can produce regression of hypertensive myocardial fibrosis in animal models (4) and in hypertensive patients (5).

Trials of the effects of endothelin receptor antagonists in patients with heart failure, coronary artery disease, arterial hypertension, and pulmonary hypertension have been reviewed (6), as have their uses in treating cancers (7) and cerebral vasospasm (8), and their potential uses in atherosclerosis, re-stenosis, myocarditis, shock, and portal hypertension (9)

As far as hypertension is concerned, there is a substantial body of preclinical evidence of the potential efficacy of endothelin antagonists in hypertension, and this has been extensively reviewed (10). Circulating endothelin concentrations are not increased in hypertension, but it is postulated that there is an imbalance between the vasodilatory effects of nitric oxide and the vasoconstrictor effects of endothelin at a local vascular level, resulting in increased endothelin vasoconstrictor tone and endothelin-mediated end-organ damage (11,12).

References

1. Yanagisawa M, Kurihara H, Kimura S, Tomobe Y, Kobayashi M, Mitsui Y, Yazaki Y, Goto K, Masaki T. A novel potent vasoconstrictor peptide produced by vascular endothelial cells. Nature 1988;332(6163):411–15.
2. Luscher TF, Barton M. Endothelins and endothelin receptor antagonists: therapeutic considerations for a novel class of cardiovascular drugs. Circulation 2000;102(19):2434–40.
3. Weber KT. Cardioreparation in hypertensive heart disease. Hypertension 2001;38(3 Pt 2):588–91.
4. Brilla CG, Matsubara L, Weber KT. Advanced hypertensive heart disease in spontaneously hypertensive rats. Lisinopril-mediated regression of myocardial fibrosis. Hypertension 1996;28(2):269–75.
5. Brilla CG, Funck RC, Rupp H. Lisinopril-mediated regression of myocardial fibrosis in patients with hypertensive heart disease. Circulation 2000;102(12):1388–93.
6. Neunteufl T, Berger R, Pacher R. Endothelin receptor antagonists in cardiology clinical trials. Expert Opin Investig Drugs 2002;11(3):431–43.
7. Wu-Wong JR. Endothelin receptor antagonists as therapeutic agents for cancer. Curr Opin Investig Drugs 2002;3(8):1234–9.
8. Chow M, Dumont AS, Kassell NF, Seifert V, Zimmermann M, Elliott JP, Awad IA, Dempsey RJ,

Hodge CJ Jr. Endothelin receptor antagonists and cerebral vasospasm: an update. Neurosurgery 2002;51(6):1333–42.
9. Doggrell SA. The therapeutic potential of endothelin-1 receptor antagonists and endothelin-converting enzyme inhibitors on the cardiovascular system. Expert Opin Investig Drugs 2002;11(11):1537–52.
10. Moreau P. Endothelin in hypertension: a role for receptor antagonists? Cardiovasc Res 1998;39(3):534–42.
11. Taddei S, Virdis A, Ghiadoni L, Sudano I, Magagna A, Salvetti A. Role of endothelin in the control of peripheral vascular tone in human hypertension. Heart Fail Rev 2001;6(4):277–85.
12. Donckier JE. Therapeutic role of bosentan in hypertension: lessons from the model of perinephritic hypertension. Heart Fail Rev 2001;6(4):253–64.

Enflurane

See also General anesthetics

General Information

Enflurane is a non-explosive halogenated volatile anesthetic that was first marketed in 1966. It was developed in the search for agents safer than halothane and methoxyflurane (1). However, the list of its halothane-like adverse effects has continued to grow.

Organs and Systems

Cardiovascular

Despite conflicting results, enflurane is generally considered to have little effect on the cardiovascular system. Cardiac output was mildly influenced in healthy men and the negative inotropic effects of enflurane (2) were more pronounced in patients with congestive heart failure (3). Myocardial damage was suggested to be an unlikely complication of enflurane anesthesia, even in patients with ischemic heart disease (4).

Cardiac dysrhythmias are generally considered to be less frequent, or at least less severe, with enflurane than with halothane (5,6). However, caution in the use of adrenaline is advisable, especially in patients with cardiac disease or hyperthyroidism. Isorhythmic atrioventricular dissociation was seen in 16 of 105 patients after the use of 1.0–1.5% enflurane (7).

Respiratory

Enflurane is usually not irritant to the respiratory tract, although bronchospasm has been reported (8). However, it is generally considered to be a bronchodilator. It causes respiratory depression at concentrations over 2%.

Nervous system

Cerebral irritability is a potential consequence of enflurane anesthesia, as evidenced by electroencephalographic recordings and by reported cases of convulsions (SED-11, 208) (9). Enflurane should be used with care (although it is probably not absolutely contraindicated) in patients with epileptiform tendencies, especially if they are deeply anesthetized and hyperventilated. There are reports of delayed convulsions after light general anesthesia not involving hyperventilation. A patient had a convulsion in a car after being discharged from a day-care anesthetic involving enflurane (9).

Motor neuron disease has been attributed to enflurane (10). The authors proposed that enflurane-induced release of glutamate may have caused changes in the spinal cord motor neurons. It is not clear what role alcohol abuse had in this case.

Neuromuscular function

Enflurane increased the sensitivity of the neuromuscular junction to d-tubocurarine in man (11).

Psychological, psychiatric

There was a reduced capacity for learning and decision-making in healthy volunteers after exposure to subanesthetic concentrations of enflurane (12,13).

Endocrine

The endocrine effects of enflurane anesthesia are minimal and clinically insignificant (14).

Metabolism

The effect of enflurane on heme metabolism has been tested in mice (15); the authors suggested that enflurane be added to the list of drugs that can precipitate acute attacks of porphyria.

Liver

One of the main advantages of enflurane over halothane is a reduced rate of liver damage, although such damage can occur (about one in 800 000 exposures) (16,17). With increasing use since 1980 there has been an increasing number of reports of enflurane-induced hepatitis (SED-11, 209), some in patients previously affected by halothane (18), and with some evidence that the risk may be higher in obese middle-aged women (19); some deaths have occurred. All the same, its hepatotoxic potential, although not entirely defined, is probably low, as evidenced by prospective studies of liver function during repeated enflurane anesthesia (20). Indeed, in May 1982 the FDA decided against incorporating a warning of hepatotoxicity on the drug's American labelling, and this policy has been maintained since.

Two patients with hepatic failure after enflurane anesthesia were reported from a hepatic transplant unit in France; both died while waiting for a liver transplant (21). In common with halothane, hepatic failure after enflurane is thought to be caused by the metabolite trifluoroacetic acid.

Urinary tract

Nephrotoxicity leading to renal insufficiency, particularly after prolonged anesthesia, is a potential consequence of general anesthesia with enflurane (22). Several cases of renal insufficiency have been described (SED-11, 209) (23,24), and the mechanism studied. On experimental grounds, it has been suspected that the inorganic fluoride ions to which enflurane is transformed may play a role. Despite evidence that enflurane can cause a significant reduction in maximum urinary osmolarity (tested using vasopressin administration) and in creatinine clearance in healthy volunteers (25), further investigations are warranted. Superimposition of nephrotoxic factors, for example drugs or underlying disease, should be avoided (1).

Musculoskeletal

Myoglobinuria, developing immediately after enflurane anesthesia, has been reported (26).

Second-Generation Effects

Teratogenicity

Experimental evidence is against a teratogenic role of enflurane (1).

Susceptibility Factors

Renal disease

It has been thought that patients with chronically impaired renal function might be at increased risk of nephrotoxicity due to enflurane, because of an increased fluoride load due to reduced excretion. However, this was not confirmed in 41 patients undergoing elective surgery with a stable increased preoperative serum creatinine concentration who were randomly allocated to receive sevoflurane ($n = 21$) or enflurane ($n = 20$) at a fresh gas inflow rate of 4 l/minute for maintenance of anesthesia (27). Peak serum inorganic fluoride concentrations were significantly higher after sevoflurane than after enflurane anesthesia. Laboratory measures of renal function remained stable throughout the postoperative period in both groups. No patient had permanent deterioration of pre-existing renal insufficiency and none required dialysis.

Drug–Drug Interactions

Amitriptyline

Amitriptyline may potentiate enflurane-induced cerebral irritability (19).

References

1. Black GW. Enflurane. Br J Anaesth 1979;51(7):627–40.
2. Shimosato S, Iwatsuki N, Carter JG. Cardio-circulatory effects of enflurane anesthesia in health and disease. Acta Anaesthesiol Scand Suppl 1979;71:69–70.
3. Rifat K. Effets cardiovasculaires de l'enflurane. Med Hyg 1979;37:3602.
4. Reves JG, Samuelson PN, Lell WA, McDaniel HG, Kouchoukos NT, Rogers WJ, Smith LR, Carter MR. Myocardial damage in coronary artery bypass surgical patients anaesthetized with two anaesthetic techniques: a random comparison of halothane and enflurane. Can Anaesth Soc J 1980;27(3):238–45.

5. Saarnivaara L. Comparison of halothane and enflurane anaesthesia for tonsillectomy in adults. Acta Anaesthesiol Scand 1984;28(3):319–24.
6. Willatts DG, Harrison AR, Groom JF, Crowther A. Cardiac arrhythmias during outpatient dental anaesthesia: comparison of halothane with enflurane. Br J Anaesth 1983;55(5):399–403.
7. Chander S. Isorhythmic atrioventricular dissociation during enflurane anesthesia. South Med J 1982;75(8):945–50.
8. Lowry CJ, Fielden BP. Bronchospasm associated with enflurane exposure—three case reports. Anaesth Intensive Care 1976;4(3):254–8.
9. Fahy LT. Delayed convulsions after day case anaesthesia with enflurane. Anaesthesia 1987;42(12):1327–8.
10. Schnorf H, Landis T. Motor neuron disease after enflurane/propofol anaesthesia in patient with alcohol abuse. Lancet 1995;346(8978):850–1.
11. Stanski DR, Ham J, Miller RD, Sheiner LB. Time-dependent increase in sensitivity to d-tubocurarine during enflurane anesthesia in man. Anesthesiology 1980;52(6):483–7.
12. Bentin S, Collins GI, Adam N. Decision-making behaviour during inhalation of subanaesthetic concentrations of enflurane. Br J Anaesth 1978;50(12):1173–8.
13. Bentin S, Collins GI, Adam N. Effects of low concentrations of enflurane on probability learning. Br J Anaesth 1978;50(12):1179–83.
14. Oyama T, Taniguchi K, Ishihara H, Matsuki A, Maeda A, Murakawa T, Kudo T. Effects of enflurane anaesthesia and surgery on endocrine function in man. Br J Anaesth 1979;51(2):141–8.
15. Buzaleh AM, Enriquez de Salamanca R, Batlle AM. Porphyrinogenic properties of the anesthetic enflurane. Gen Pharmacol 1992;23(4):665–9.
16. Holt C, Csete M, Martin P. Hepatotoxicity of anesthetics and other central nervous system drugs. Gastroenterol Clin North Am 1995;24(4):853–74.
17. Kenna JG, Jones RM. The organ toxicity of inhaled anesthetics. Anesth Analg 1995;81(Suppl 6):S51–66.
18. Sigurdsson J, Hreidarsson AB, Thjodleifsson B. Enflurane hepatitis. A report of a case with a previous history of halothane hepatitis. Acta Anaesthesiol Scand 1985;29(5):495–6.
19. Paull JD, Fortune DW. Hepatotoxicity and death following two enflurane anaesthetics. Anaesthesia 1987;42(11):1191–6.
20. Fee JP, Black GW, Dundee JW, McIlroy PD, Johnston HM, Johnston SB, Black IH, McNeill HG, Neill DW, Doggart JR, Merrett JD, McDonald JR, Bradley DS, Haire M, McMillan SA. A prospective study of liver enzyme and other changes following repeat administration of halothane and enflurane. Br J Anaesth 1979;51(12):1133–41.
21. Lo SK, Wendon J, Mieli-Vergani G, Williams R. Halothane-induced acute liver failure: continuing occurrence and use of liver transplantation. Eur J Gastroenterol Hepatol 1998;10(8):635–9.
22. Motuz DJ, Watson WA, Barlow JC, Velasquez NV, Schentag JJ. The increase in urinary alanine aminopeptidase excretion associated with enflurane anesthesia is increased further by aminoglycosides. Anesth Analg 1988;67(8):770–4.
23. Eichhorn JH, Hedley-Whyte J, Steinman TI, Kaufmann JM, Laasbert LH. Renal failure following enflurane anesthesia. Anesthesiology 1976;45(5):557–60.
24. Delhumeau A, Cocaud J, Bourganneau MC, Cavellat M. La toxicité rénale de l'enflurane: hypothése ou certitude? Anesth Analg Reanim 1981;38:549.
25. Mazze RI, Calverley RK, Smith NT. Inorganic fluoride nephrotoxicity: prolonged enflurane and halothane anesthesia in volunteers. Anesthesiology 1977;46(4):265–71.

26. Miyagishima T, Takagi N, Oka N, et al. Myoglobinuria associated with enflurane anesthesia. Hiroshima J Anesth 1981;16:122.
27. Conzen PF, Nuscheler M, Melotte A, Verhaegen M, Leupolt T, Van Aken H, Peter K. Renal function and serum fluoride concentrations in patients with stable renal insufficiency after anesthesia with sevoflurane or enflurane. Anesth Analg 1995;81(3):569–75.

Enoximone

See also Phosphodiesterase type III, selective inhibitors of

General Information

Enoximone is an inhibitor of phosphodiesterase type III, and has a positive inotropic effect. Its most common adverse effects are gastrointestinal and cardiac. The gastrointestinal effects include anorexia, nausea, vomiting, and diarrhea (1,2).

Other rarely reported adverse effects include thrombocytopenia, leukocytosis, increased appetite, increased serum activity of alanine transaminase, hyperglycemia, headache, lethargy, anxiety, dyspnea, and skin rashes (2–6).

Organs and Systems

Cardiovascular

The cardiac effects of enoximone include hypotension, transient atrial fibrillation, and bradycardia (3). Ventricular tachydysrhythmias have been reported in about 4% of patients (2) and myocardial ischemia can also occur (4,7).

Musculoskeletal

Enoximone has been reported to cause increased contraction in skeletal muscle in vitro in patients with a predisposition to malignant hyperthermia (8,9).

- Vastus lateralis muscle from a 48-year-old man with rhabdomyolysis had an increased in vitro response to increasing concentrations of enoximone above 0.6 mmol/l (10). He also had a heterozygous mutation in his ryanodine receptor gene, with substitution of arginine for glycine in position 2433, a mutation that is associated with malignant hyperthermia.

Phosphodiesterase inhibitors, such as enoximone, increase the release of calcium from the sarcoplasmic reticulum by activating ryanodine receptors, and the authors suggested that this may have been the mechanism whereby enoximone precipitated rhabdomyolysis in this case.

Death

Long-term treatment with inhibitors of phosphodiesterase type III is associated with increased mortality in congestive heart failure (SEDA-17, 217).

In 102 patients taking digoxin and diuretics the addition of enoximone did not confer any therapeutic advantage and there was a significantly higher dropout rate and a significantly higher mortality rate in those taking enoximone (11).

The use of a lower dose of enoximone in 105 patients with heart failure (New York Heart Association classes 2 or 3) has been studied over 12 weeks (12). Enoximone 25–50 mg tds improved exercise capacity and reduced dyspnea. There was no evidence of a dysrhythmic effect. The rates of adverse events were similar with enoximone and placebo, and there were fewer cases of dizziness, vertigo, or hypotension in those who took enoximone. There were two deaths in the 70 patients who took enoximone compared with four of the 35 who took placebo. However, this small short-term study does not rule out the possibility that even this small dose of enoximone can cause increased mortality during long-term administration or in patients with more severe cardiac failure.

References

1. Shah PK, Amin DK, Hulse S, Shellock F, Swan HJ. Inotropic therapy for refractory congestive heart failure with oral fenoximone (MDL-17,043): poor long-term results despite early hemodynamic and clinical improvement. Circulation 1985;71(2):326–31.
2. Kereiakes D, Chatterjee K, Parmley WW, Atherton B, Curran D, Kereiakes A, Spangenberg R. Intravenous and oral MDL 17043 (a new inotrope–vasodilator agent) in congestive heart failure: hemodynamic and clinical evaluation in 38 patients. J Am Coll Cardiol 1984;4(5):884–9.
3. Leeman M, Lejeune P, Melot C, Naeije R. Reduction in pulmonary hypertension and in airway resistances by enoximone (MDL 17,043) in decompensated COPD. Chest 1987;91(5):662–6.
4. Martin JL, Likoff MJ, Janicki JS, Laskey WK, Hirshfeld JW Jr, Weber KT. Myocardial energetics and clinical response to the cardiotonic agent MDL 17043 in advanced heart failure. J Am Coll Cardiol 1984;4(5):875–83.
5. Rubin SA, Tabak L. MDL 17,043: short- and long-term cardiopulmonary and clinical effects in patients with heart failure. J Am Coll Cardiol 1985;5(6):1422–7.
6. Uretsky BF, Generalovich T, Verbalis JG, Valdes AM, Reddy PS. MDL 17,043 therapy in severe congestive heart failure: characterization of the early and late hemodynamic, pharmacokinetic, hormonal and clinical response. J Am Coll Cardiol 1985;5(6):1414–21.
7. Amin DK, Shah PK, Hulse S, Shellock FG, Swan HJ. Myocardial metabolic and hemodynamic effects of intravenous MDL-17,043, a new cardiotonic drug, in patients with chronic severe heart failure. Am Heart J 1984;108(5):1285–92.
8. Fiege M, Wappler F, Scholz J, von Richthofen V, Brinken B, Schulte am Esch J. Diagnostik der Disposition zur malignen Hyperthermie durch einen in vitro Kontrakturtest mit dem Phosphodiesterase-III-Hemmstoff Enoximon. [Diagnosis of susceptibility to malignant hyperthermia with an in vitro contracture test with the phosphodiesterase iii inhibitor enoximone.] Anasthesiol Intensivmed Notfallmed Schmerzther 1998;33(9):557–63.
9. Fiege M, Wappler F, Scholz J, Weisshorn R, von Richthofen V, Schulte am Esch J. Effects of the phosphodiesterase-III inhibitor enoximone on skeletal muscle specimens from malignant hyperthermia susceptible patients. J Clin Anesth 2000;12(2):123–8.
10. Riess FC, Fiege M, Moshar S, Bergmann H, Bleese N, Kormann J, Weisshorn R, Wappler F. Rhabdomyolysis

following cardiopulmonary bypass and treatment with enoximone in a patient susceptible to malignant hyperthermia. Anesthesiology 2001;94(2):355–7.

11. Uretsky BF, Jessup M, Konstam MA, Dec GW, Leier CV, Benotti J, Murali S, Herrmann HC, Sandberg JA. Multicenter trial of oral enoximone in patients with moderate to moderately severe congestive heart failure. Lack of benefit compared with placebo. Enoximone Multicenter Trial Group. Circulation 1990;82(3):774–80.
12. Lowes BD, Higginbotham M, Petrovich L, DeWood MA, Greenberg MA, Rahko PS, Dec GW, LeJemtel TH, Roden RL, Schleman MM, Robertson AD, Gorczynski RJ, Bristow MR. Low-dose enoximone improves exercise capacity in chronic heart failure. Enoximone Study Group. J Am Coll Cardiol 2000;36(2):501–8.

Enprofylline

General Information

Enprofylline (3-propylxanthine) is a xanthine derivative that has some actions in common with theophylline but has a negligible antagonistic effect at most adenosine receptor subtypes (1,2). Enprofylline is a more potent smooth muscle relaxant and antiasthmatic drug than theophylline but does not produce, for example diuresis, stimulant behavioral effects (restlessness and seizures) in the nervous system, gastric secretory effects, or free fatty acid release. Selectivity for the A_{2B} adenosine receptor subtype may underlie this lack of typical adverse effects associated with other theophylline-related drugs (3). Enprofylline has a short half-life (about 2 hours). The target plasma concentration is about 3 μg/ml. Its efficacy and tolerability have been briefly reported (4).

The most severe adverse effects of theophylline, namely seizures, are claimed to be absent even at high doses of enprofylline, although there are other disadvantages, such as cardiovascular effects, nausea, vomiting, and headache. Much more information is needed before claims of greater safety can be taken seriously.

The possibility of obtaining a steady-state plasma enprofylline concentration of 5 μg/ml by two constant rate infusions was examined in six asthmatic patients (5). The resulting adverse effects and bronchodilatation were compared with those obtained with theophylline at a steady-state concentration of 15 μg/ml. Headache, nausea, and vomiting became pronounced in two patients in whom the plasma enprofylline concentration was about 6 μg/ml. The authors concluded that by varying the infusion rate the plasma concentration of enprofylline can be controlled like that of theophylline, but they stressed the need for further studies of efficacy versus adverse effects.

References

1. Persson CG. The profile of action of enprofylline, or why adenosine antagonism seems less desirable with xanthine antiasthmatics. Agents Actions Suppl. 1983;13:115–29.
2. Persson CG, Andersson KE, Kjellin G. Effects of enprofylline and theophylline may show the role of adenosine. Life Sci 1986;38(12):1057–72.
3. Linden J, Auchampach JA, Jin X, Figler RA. The structure and function of A1 and A2B adenosine receptors. Life Sci 1998;62(17–18):1519–24.
4. Pauwels R. Enprofylline, a new bronchodilating xanthine derivative. Eur J Respir Dis 1983;64(5):331–2.
5. Laursen LC, Johannesson N, Fagerstrom PO, Weeke B. Intravenous administration of enprofylline to asthmatic patients. Eur J Clin Pharmacol 1983;24(3):323–7.

Enprostil

See also Prostaglandins

General Information

Enprostil is a synthetic analogue of PGE_2.

Organs and Systems

Gastrointestinal

Even in doses insufficient to control ulcer symptoms, enprostil has a higher incidence of adverse effects than the H_2-receptor antagonists. In a randomized, double-blind, endoscopically controlled study, 98 patients with gastric ulcers were treated with either enprostil 70 micrograms bd or ranitidine 150 mg bd (1). The healing rates at 4, 8, and 12 weeks were similar. After ulcer healing, half the patients were followed for 1 year without treatment and the others were given enprostil 70 micrograms/day. Diarrhea was a common adverse effect of enprostil, and seven patients withdrew because of diarrhea or abdominal pain.

Reference

1. Morgan AG, Pacsoo C, Taylor P, McAdam WA. A comparison between enprostil and ranitidine in the management of gastric ulceration. Aliment Pharmacol Ther 1990;4(6): 635–41.

Entacapone

General Information

Entacapone is an inhibitor of catechol-*O*-methyltransferase, which catalyses a relatively minor pathway of dopamine metabolism. It therefore enhances the action of dopamine.

The safety of entacapone has been specifically addressed in a Finnish study in 326 patients (mean age 62 years, 217 men) taking levodopa plus a decarboxylase inhibitor (1). Two-thirds were randomized to take entacapone 200 mg/day and the remainder to take placebo. The withdrawal rate due to adverse events was 14% with entacapone compared to 11% with placebo. Dyskinesias were greatly increased in the former (29 versus 11%) and entacapone was also associated with increased incidences of diarrhea (9.2 versus 1.9%), dry mouth (6.0% versus 0), and discolored urine (6.9% versus 0). However, there was no evidence of liver toxicity with entacapone.

Placebo-controlled studies

In a placebo-controlled study in Germany and Austria, 301 patients with Parkinson's disease were randomized to receive placebo or entacapone 200 mg with each dose of levodopa, together with their other usual therapy (2). The mean age was 61 years and 40% of the entacapone group and 48% of the placebo group were men; the groups were also unequal in size (197 versus 104), for reasons that were not clearly defined. Entacapone reduced the Unified Parkinson's Disease Rating Scale score, increased "on" periods, and reduced "off" periods. In the patients who took entacapone there was more frequent dyskinesia (34 versus 26%), nausea (10 versus 4.8%), and diarrhea (8.1 versus 3.8%). All of these findings are consistent with enhanced dopaminergic activity. There was no evidence of hepatotoxicity in any of the patients.

Comparative studies

In 40 patients (mean age 64 years, 22 men) who took tolcapone for 3–7 months and were given entacapone in dosages titrated to 800–2000 mg/day after a transition period of 3–6 months with co-beneldopa, the improvements in "on" and "off" times were less impressive than they had been with tolcapone and there were more adverse effects (3). One patient had diarrhea and orthostatic hypertension with both drugs, but another six patients had increased dyskinesias and hallucinations and one developed myoclonus. There was no evidence of liver toxicity with either drug. The authors pointed out that entacapone, unlike tolcapone, not only increases the half-life of levodopa but also its peak concentration, causing significantly enhanced levodopa-related adverse effects. There is therefore a paradox: entacapone appears to be safer but overall causes more adverse effects.

Organs and Systems

Nervous system

Fatigue and light-headedness or dizziness have occurred relatively frequently during oral entacapone administration in small studies (up to 60% of patients) (4). Other less frequent central nervous system effects include confusion, anxiety, syncope (related to postural hypotension), and insomnia (5,6). Mood elevation has been observed occasionally (5). The inclusion of entacapone in levodopa therapy for Parkinson's disease increases the risk of dyskinesias, possibly through enhanced brain penetration of levodopa (4,5,7). This can be adjusted by reducing the dose of levodopa.

Gastrointestinal

Gastrointestinal adverse effects have been reported in up to 50% of patients taking oral entacapone, and include epigastric pain, abdominal pain, nausea, anorexia, and loose stools or diarrhea (4–6,8). These effects have generally been mild and not dose-limiting.

Liver

Whether entacapone is hepatotoxic is debatable.

- A 76-year-old Australian woman complained of nausea, anorexia, and malaise 2 weeks after starting to take entacapone 200 mg five times a day (9). A week later her bilirubin, alanine transaminase, alkaline phosphatase, and gamma-glutamyl transpeptidase were all raised (2–8 times higher than the upper limits of the reference ranges). Clotting was normal. Over the next 3 days her liver function tests deteriorated and the entacapone was withdrawn. All the laboratory data improved within 2 days, but not all were fully normal 4 weeks later. She refused a rechallenge.

The authors noted that two other patients in the Australian adverse reactions database also appeared to have had hepatotoxicity related to entacapone. In response, representatives of the manufacturers (Novartis) strongly contested the conclusion that any of the three reported cases demonstrated entacapone-induced hepatotoxicity, and concluded that two of the three patients had cholestasis, which is unlikely to be related to entacapone, while the third had no real evidence of hepatic dysfunction (10). These arguments were in turn rebutted by the original authors, and the possible hepatotoxicity of entacapone remains a matter of debate, although there can be no doubt that it is safer than tolcapone.

References

1. Myllyla VV, Kultalahti ER, Haapaniemi H, Leinonen M; FILOMEN Study Group. Twelve-month safety of entacapone in patients with Parkinson's disease. Eur J Neurol 2001;8(1):53–60.
2. Poewe WH, Deuschl G, Gordin A, Kultalahti ER, Leinonen M; Celomen Study Group. Efficacy and safety of entacapone in Parkinson's disease patients with suboptimal levodopa response: a 6-month randomized placebo-controlled double-blind study in Germany and Austria (Celomen study). Acta Neurol Scand 2002;105(4):245–55.
3. Onofrj M, Thomas A, Iacono D, Di Iorio A, Bonanni L. Switch-over from tolcapone to entacapone in severe Parkinson's disease patients. Eur Neurol 2001;46(1):11–16.
4. Kaakkola S, Teravainen H, Ahtila S, Rita H, Gordin A. Effect of entacapone, a COMT inhibitor, on clinical disability and levodopa metabolism in parkinsonian patients. Neurology 1994;44(1):77–80.
5. Ruottinen HM, Rinne UK. Effect of one month's treatment with peripherally acting catechol-O-methyltransferase inhibitor, entacapone, on pharmacokinetics and motor response to levodopa in advanced parkinsonian patients. Clin Neuropharmacol 1996;19(3):222–33.
6. Ruottinen HM, Rinne UK. Entacapone prolongs levodopa response in a one month double blind study in parkinsonian patients with levodopa related fluctuations. J Neurol Neurosurg Psychiatry 1996;60(1):36–40.
7. Merello M, Lees AJ, Webster R, Bovingdon M, Gordin A. Effect of entacapone, a peripherally acting catechol-O-methyltransferase inhibitor, on the motor response to acute treatment with levodopa in patients with Parkinson's disease. J Neurol Neurosurg Psychiatry 1994;57(2):186–9.
8. Illi A, Sundberg S, Koulu M, Scheinin M, Heinavaara S, Gordin A. COMT inhibition by high-dose entacapone does not affect hemodynamics but changes catecholamine

metabolism in healthy volunteers at rest and during exercise. Int J Clin Pharmacol Ther 1994;32(11):582–8.
9. Fisher A, Croft-Baker J, Davis M, Purcell P, McLean AJ. Entacapone-induced hepatotoxicity and hepatic dysfunction. Mov Disord 2002;17(6):1362–5.
10. Beck S, Hubble J, Reinikainen K. Entacapone-induced hepatotoxicity and hepatic dysfunction. Mov Disord 2002;17:1397–400.

Enteral nutrition

General Information

Enteral nutrition refers to any method of feeding that involves instillation of food into the gastrointestinal tract, such as normal feeding, feeding by nasogastric or nasoenteric tube, or feeding into a gastrostomy or enterostomy (for example a so-called PEG, a percutaneous endoscopic gastrostomy). Enteral nutrition should be tailored to the needs of the individual, but on average should provide about 30–40 kcal/kg/day.

Organs and Systems

Gastrointestinal

There is a risk of gastroesophageal reflux during nasogastric feeding, especially in mechanically ventilated and sedated patients (1).

- A 77-year-old man had a ruptured abdominal aortic aneurysm repaired and developed acute renal, respiratory, and heart failure. Six days postoperatively, enteral feeding was started with a standard formulation. This was well tolerated and the volume was increased to 2 l/day continuously. After 9 days, the nasogastric tube was accidentally dislodged. Reinsertion was attempted but failed owing to apparent obstruction at 25 cm. Until this, the patient had been nursed supine. Esophagoscopy showed impacted enteral feed obstructing the esophagus almost completely.

Gastroesophageal reflux during enteral nutrition is caused by a number of factors, including the presence of the nasogastric tube, the supine position, leakage from the tube at the teeth, and the administration of sucralfate. While the cause in this case was not entirely clear, it does show that mechanical obstruction of the esophagus due to reflux can occur without any obvious symptoms.

Reference

1. Paling A, Girbes ARJ. Esophageal obstruction: an unusual complication of enteral nutrition. Care Crit Ill 2000;16: 224–5.

Ephedra, ephedrine, and pseudoephedrine

General Information

Ephedra consists of a mixture of different members of the Ephedraceae family (*E. sinica*, *E. equisetina*, and *E. gerardiana*). Its actions are due to the presence of ephedrine and pseudoephedrine.

Ephedrine is a sympathomimetic drug prepared from members of the *Ephedra* family, such as *Ephedra vulgaris*, also called the sea grape. It is available as ordinary pharmaceutical formulations of ephedrine, but also in herbal formulations of *Ephedra*, including a Chinese herbal medicine called Ma huang, which has been used since ancient times as a stimulant and in the treatment of asthma, and in formulations combined with caffeine. It is used to treat asthma, nasal congestion, fever, obesity, and anhidrosis. It is also abused as a recreational drug. Of 140 reports of adverse events related to *Ephedra* supplements submitted to the FDA between June 1997 and March 1999, 31% were definitely or probably causally related to *Ephedra* (1). In 47% of the cases, there were cardiovascular symptoms and in 18% central nervous system effects; 10 patients died.

Pseudoephedrine is a stereoisomer of ephedrine, in which two of three chiral centers are different.

"Herbal ecstasy" is a term used for many different herbal formulations, none of which contains ecstasy. Some of the names for these herbs (which can be sold in stores) include "The Bomb," "Reds," and "Sublime." In New Zealand analysis of "The Bomb" showed substantial amounts of ephedrine and the Ministry of Health removed it from the market. Some symptoms associated with herbal ecstasy include headache, dizziness, palpitation, tachycardia, and raised blood pressure. Thus, in countries where the term "herbal ecstasy" is commonly used, it is important that those who see patients who have taken Herbal Ecstasy should not confuse it with ecstasy, as toxicity and medical management may be quite different (2).

Ephedrine is longer-acting than adrenaline and can exert any type of adrenergic effect, including metabolic changes and dysuria. It has a somewhat smaller effect on the cardiovascular system than adrenaline but a relatively larger effect on the central nervous system; even low doses can, in sensitive patients, cause tremor, insomnia, and anxiety, and such problems are much more marked if ephedrine is given together with caffeine, as it sometimes is for appetite control (SEDA-17, 161). In children, ephedrine sometimes paradoxically induces sedation. Psychosis has resulted from excessive self-medication (3).

Both ephedrine and pseudoephedrine remain worryingly popular (4) and are widely available without prescription. Based on increasing evidence of the risks of *Ephedra* self-medication, various national regulatory authorities are currently considering recalling *Ephedra* products from over-the-counter sales. Oral doses of ephedrine 25–30 mg are often prescribed, for example for orthostatic hypotension. Lower oral doses, present in some "cold remedies" in tablet form, are unlikely to be efficacious, although they are risky where the drug is contraindicated, for example in patients with cardiac disease. Ephedrine used in nasal sprays and drops can have systemic effects in the doses normally used. Such products are widely available over the counter in many countries. In Texas some 500 cases of adverse reactions were reported between 1993 and 1995 (SEDA-21, 153). Three of these cases have been highlighted because of their serious nature: one patient died from myocardial infarction, one had a series of generalized absence seizures, and a third had a fatal subarachnoid hemorrhage as the result of taking an unsuitable dose (SEDA-21, 153).

Organs and Systems

Cardiovascular

Cardiologists and pharmacologists from Boston have reviewed cases of possible cardiovascular toxicity associated with the use of Ma huang. Among over 900 cases of possible toxicity reported to the Food and Drug Administration, they identified 37 patients (23 women) in whom stroke ($n = 16$), myocardial infarction ($n = 10$), and sudden death ($n = 11$) appeared to be temporally related to consumption of Ma huang. The authors noted that in all but one of these cases the doses used were within the range recommended by the manufacturers. In the seven patients on whom autopsies were performed, coronary artery disease was found in three and cardiomyopathy in another three, with features suggesting sympathomimetic toxicity. The authors emphasized the toxicity of Ma huang in relatively young individuals—the mean age of the 37 patients was about 43 years—even though the relevant pathogenic mechanisms remain to be fully defined.

Hypertension

The cardiovascular effects, subjective effects, and abuse potential of single intranasal doses of ephedrine 5 and 10 mg have been compared with oral doses of (−)ephedrine 50 mg in 16 healthy Caucasian men with no drug/alcohol/nicotine abuse or dependence (5). Intranasal ephedrine caused an increase in blood pressure but associated orthostatic hypotension.

Pseudoephedrine is a component of some non-prescription basal decongestants given by mouth; even quite ordinary doses of such products (for example 120 mg) can cause a hypertensive reaction in sensitive subjects, such as those with a pheochromocytoma and those with at least a family history of hypertension (SEDA-17, 162).

- A 21-year-old man presented with hypertension (blood pressure 220/110 mmHg) and ventricular dysrhythmias after taking four capsules of herbal ecstasy (6). He was treated with lidocaine and sodium nitroprusside and his symptoms resolved within 9 hours.

Severe hypertension has been attributed to pseudoephedrine abuse (7).

- A 36-year-old man with hypertension taking no less than seven antihypertensive drugs had outpatient systolic pressures of over 190 mmHg. Investigations for primary causes of hypertension were negative and there was increasing suspicion of treatment non-compliance or factitious hypertension. Urine screening showed the presence of pseudoephedrine, which the patient could not explain. When he was given his normal antihypertensive drugs under close supervision his systolic blood pressure fell to 70 mmHg and his serum creatinine doubled. His blood pressure became normal when his medication was briefly suspended but he continued to deny any deliberate attempt to alter his blood pressure and discharged himself soon afterwards.

The authors concluded that this represented factitious hypertension due to pseudoephedrine, the first such case reported and a very unusual example of Munchausen's syndrome.

Cardiac dysrhythmias

Cardiac dysrhythmias have been attributed to ephedrine both in therapeutic doses (8) and when used as a drug of abuse (6).

- A 25-year-old woman became hypotensive after the administration of epidural anesthesia for an elective cesarean section. She was given intravenous ephedrine 9 mg, after which she complained of nausea. For an unexplained reason this was taken as an indication to give a further 9 mg of ephedrine. She immediately developed sinus tachycardia with atrial and multifocal ventricular extra beats, followed by short runs of ventricular tachycardia. She remained asymptomatic and recovered after about 5 minutes.

One must have some concerns about the high dose used here for a relatively modest level of hypotension with a systolic blood pressure of 100 mmHg.

- A 21-year-old Canadian man presented with severe headache, nausea and vomiting, hypertension (220/120 mmHg), and a sinus tachycardia of about 120/minute with frequent multifocal ventricular extra beats. He was treated with intravenous sodium nitroprusside and lidocaine and recovered fully within 24 hours.

The authors concluded that ephedrine was very largely responsible for the cardiovascular toxicity.

Myocardial ischemia

Myocardial infarction has been attributed to *Ephedra* (9).

- A previously healthy 19-year-old man took tablets containing a total of 24 mg of Ephedra alkaloids and 100 mg of caffeine, and 15 minutes later developed severe chest pain radiating down the left arm. An electrocardiogram showed an inferolateral myocardial infarct, confirmed by creatine kinase and troponin I measurements. He made a full recovery, and coronary angiography showed only minimal atherosclerotic disease of the left anterior descending artery.

The authors emphasized the dangers of *Ephedra*-containing over-the-counter formulations, even in fit young people.

Ephedrine is sometimes used to treat vasovagal episodes and has been reported to cause coronary artery spasm and myocardial infarction in these circumstances (10).

- Two apparently healthy women, aged 26 and 34 years, who were given spinal anesthesia for pelvic or hip surgery, both developed hypotension and bradycardia and were given intravenous ephedrine in divided doses, in one case a total of 20 mg and in the other 30 mg. In both cases this resulted in ventricular tachycardia and raised troponin I concentrations and creatine kinase activity, but Q waves did not follow. Coronary angiography showed normal arteries in both cases and the women recovered, apparently fully.

The authors rightly pointed out that atropine is a safer and more appropriate intervention in circumstances such as these.

Arteritis

Arteritis has been attributed to ephedrine (11).

- A 44-year-old French woman was given intravenous ephedrine during anesthesia and developed hypertension (systolic pressure 180 mmHg) with nausea, vomiting, and progressive drowsiness. She had a history of migraine, antiphospholipid antibodies, mitral valve prolapse, and atrial fibrillation treated with propranolol. Immediately after anesthesia she developed headache, vomiting, and drowsiness. CT scanning showed frontal and parietal hemorrhagic infarcts, and cerebral angiography showed multiple segments of constriction and dilatation consistent with arteritis. She was left with residual visual and memory deficits.

This is the first case of this kind associated with ephedrine, and it seems plausible that the patient's previous history indicated a genetic predisposition to vascular disease.

Others

A form of toxic shock syndrome on more than one occasion occurred in one patient who used pseudoephedrine (SEDA-18, 158).

Nervous system

In a consecutive stroke registry since 1988, 22 patients (10 men and 12 women) had strokes associated with over-the-counter sympathomimetic drugs (12). There was intracerebral hemorrhage in 17, subarachnoid hemorrhage in four, and ischemic stroke in one. Stroke was associated with the use of pseudoephedrine (60–300 mg) in four cases.

The largest manufacturer of *Ephedra*-containing supplements is Metabolife. The firm has repeatedly insisted that it was not aware of adverse events associated with its products, and claimed that they were "absolutely safe" (13). An investigation by the US Justice Department into the truth of these statements showed that between 1997 and 2002 the company had received over 13 000 reports of suspected adverse drug reactions; they included nearly 2000 reports of significant adverse reactions.

- A 33-year-old man had a stroke while taking a herbal remedy (Thermadrene) containing *Ephedra* alkaloids and guaraná for "boosting his energy" (14). He was immediately treated with alteplase and was referred for rehabilitation 9 days later. At follow-up 5 months later he still had a minor neurological deficit.

Psychological, psychiatric

Ma huang can cause psychiatric complications, which can last several weeks. These have been reviewed in the context of two cases of psychotic reactions (15).

- A 27-year-old US Marine presented with depressed affect, irritability, and poor concentration and eventually admitted 2 years self-medication with Ma huang to improve workout performance.
- A 27-year-old US Marine developed a frank psychosis with ideas of reference and some paranoid ideation. He had been taking two preparations containing Ma huang, although the duration of use was unclear.

After discontinuing the drug both made a full recovery. The authors emphasized the importance of recognizing possible abuse of such "natural" medications, widely perceived to be harmless despite warnings and attempted restrictions by regulatory authorities. Treatment is supportive while awaiting spontaneous recovery after drug withdrawal.

Pseudoephedrine is often used by scuba divers to avoid ear barotrauma. The psychometric and cardiac effects of pseudoephedrine have been evaluated at 1 atmosphere (100 kPa, sea level) and 3 atmospheres (30 kPa, 20 m) in a double-blind, placebo-controlled, crossover study in 30 active divers in a hyperbaric chamber (16). Pseudoephedrine did not cause significant alterations in psychometric performance at 3 atmospheres.

A young child suffered from visual hallucinations caused by high doses of pseudoephedrine (17).

Endocrine

One patient with Graves' disease who used pseudoephedrine developed a thyroid storm, suggesting that hyperthyroidism is a susceptibility factor (18).

Gastrointestinal

The vasoconstrictor action of pseudoephedrine can predispose susceptible patients to ischemic colitis, particularly in the watershed area of the splenic flexure. Perimenopausal women may be more susceptible (19). A group from Yale have described four patients, women aged 35–50 years, who developed ischemic colitis while taking pseudoephedrine (19). Three of them had taken the drug for about 1 week, the fourth for 6 months. In all cases there was ischemic colitis affecting predominantly the splenic flexure, and there was full recovery after drug withdrawal.

- A 33-year-old man took pseudoephedrine 240 mg/day for 5 days (20). His mesenteric vasculature was normal on subsequent magnetic resonance angiography and no other abnormalities were found, leading to the presumption that the drug had caused mesenteric vasoconstriction. He made a full recovery.
- A 51-year-old woman presented for the second time in 4 months with abdominal pain (21). On this as on the previous occasion, emergency laparotomy was needed and she was found to have patchy infarction of the terminal ileum and the ascending colon. It emerged that she had been taking pseudoephedrine for 2 years, because she found that it relieved her headaches. In fact she had often noticed abdominal pain and distension, with occasional bloody diarrhea, after taking

pseudoephedrine. Before each of her two admissions she had been taking a remarkably high dose of 900 mg/day, and on many other occasions had taken as much as 600 mg/day. She made a good recovery and was said to have stopped taking pseudoephedrine.

The authors quoted seven other published cases of pseudoephedrine-related ischemic colitis, all occurring at much lower dosages, at most 240 mg/day.

Urinary tract

Seven patients (four men, three women, aged 21–52 years) taking large doses of over-the-counter formulations containing ephedrine and guaifenesin developed urinary stones (22). These largely contained guaifenesin metabolites, but presumably dependence on ephedrine was the reason for abuse of these formulations.

Skin

Non-pigmenting fixed drug eruptions proven by oral rechallenge have been reported with pseudoephedrine; in each of these cases the erythematous lesions spontaneously remitted without residual pigmentation (23–25).

- A 10-year-old boy given pseudoephedrine 60 mg/day developed a solitary eruption in the groin; rechallenge was positive (24).

Generalized skin reactions are even less frequent. A group of allergy specialists in Madrid have described two cases of generalized dermatitis with dissimilar histological findings in men aged 64 and 73 years (26). In one case there was severe eczema, in the other vacuolar interface dermatitis, which is rarer. Both patients had taken a proprietary formulation containing codeine and chlorphenamine as well as pseudoephedrine. Oral challenges with the former two drugs was negative in both cases, but was positive for pseudoephedrine in one patient; the other was not rechallenged, because of the severity of the original reaction.

- A hypersensitivity reaction was confirmed by patch testing in a 73-year-old woman who had taken a single (unspecified) dose of a compound formulation containing pseudoephedrine (27). This caused the memorably named baboon syndrome, a widespread symmetrical erythematous rash with papules and pustules.

Immunologic

Pseudoephedrine can cause hypersensitivity, as in three cases reported by allergy specialists from Spain (28).

- A 33-year-old man developed anaphylaxis on a second exposure to pseudoephedrine, having developed urticaria after a first exposure.
- A 24-year-old woman developed severe urticaria and fever, but no other systemic reaction, after a single dose of pseudoephedrine.
- A 67-year-old woman developed urticaria and angioedema of the eyelids after a single dose of pseudoephedrine.

In all three cases skin testing was performed; it was positive in the first two instances but not the third. The authors noted that such cases are reportedly uncommon and that cross-sensitivity is to be expected between pseudoephedrine and ephedrine.

Body temperature

Pseudoephedrine may have played a role in an episode of hyperthermia (29).

- A 21-year-old American military recruit, moderately obese, collapsed during a 3-mile run and was asystolic and hyperthermic (rectal temperature 42.2°C); he could not be resuscitated. Only 75 minutes earlier he had received vaccinations against typhoid and Japanese encephalitis and he was taking over-the-counter pseudoephedrine to promote weight loss.

The authors noted that this was only one of the factors predisposing to hyperthermia; one might also wonder whether it was wise to undertake such a run so soon after the vaccinations.

Death

Ephedra was implicated in the deaths of eight patients, and although it was pointed out that several had pre-existing conditions such as chest pain and hypertension (30), the authors justifiably responded that these were contraindications to the use of *Ephedra* in the first place, and they cast doubt on the adequacy of the warnings provided (31).

Susceptibility Factors

In patients with ischemic heart disease, ephedrine can cause myocardial infarction and potentially fatal dysrhythmias (31). Caution is needed in patients with any form of cardiac disease. At one time an attempt was made to use high doses of ephedrine for the early treatment of ventricular fibrillation, but its pharmacological effects militated against its use, since the immediate survival rate actually fell.

Thyrotoxic patients are unduly sensitive to the effects of ephedrine (SEDA-14, 179).

Drug Administration

Drug overdose

- In a suicide attempt, a 32-year-old woman took 60 tablets of a weight-loss supplement containing Ephedra (32). She was delivered to hospital comatose. Her symptoms resolved over the next 5 days without treatment. At follow-up 5 months later she was euthymic, had no suicidal ideation, and was not taking any psychotropic medications.

Drug–Drug Interactions

Amfebutamone

Acute coronary syndrome has been attributed to a combination of pseudoephedrine with amfebutamone (bupropion) (33).

- A 21-year-old man developed acute myocardial ischemia. Smoking was the only risk factor for coronary artery disease and he denied using cocaine. Angiography showed normal coronary arteries. He had recently started to take amfebutamone for smoking cessation and pseudoephedrine as a non-prescription influenza remedy.

The authors postulated that the combination of two sympathomimetics had caused acute coronary artery vasospasm. This is the first report linking amfebutamone to acute coronary syndrome, and one of a few cases associated with pseudoephedrine. It is also possible that erythromycin, which this patient was also taking, could have impaired the hepatic metabolism of amfebutamone.

Antihypertensive drugs

In patients taking antihypertensive drugs, self-medication with ephedrine-containing remedies can cause an increase in blood pressure (31).

Barbiturates

In intravenous solutions, ephedrine is physically incompatible with several barbiturates (34).

Cocaine

Chronic cocaine use sensitizes coronary arterial alpha-adrenoceptors up to agonists (SEDA-22, 154).

Dextromethorphan

Combinations of pseudoephedrine with dextromethorphan are often used in over-the-counter formulations. Although they are generally considered safe, two reports have emphasized the potential adverse effect of these cold and cough formulations (35,36).

- A 2-year-old child developed hyperirritability, psychosis, and ataxia after being overmedicated with a cough formulation containing pseudoephedrine and dextromethorphan. The child made an uneventful recovery after an observation period of 4 hours in the emergency department.
- Three adolescent girls developed acute psychoses associated with the use of similar over-the-counter formulations. They required several days of hospitalization, extensive invasive medical evaluation, and consultations with neurologists, infectious disease specialists, toxicologists, and psychiatrists. They were treated with risperidone.

It is not clear which was the primary causative drug in these cases or whether there was some degree of synergy or at least additive toxicity.

Entacapone

An interaction of ephedrine with entacapone, a specific, reversible, peripherally acting inhibitor of catechol-*O*-methyl transferase, has been reported (37).

- A 76-year-old woman with Parkinson's disease and closed-angle glaucoma was scheduled for eye surgery. She had severe choreoathetoid movements, and 3 weeks before surgery began to take entacapone 200 mg/day, in addition to her five daily doses of co-careldopa. General anesthesia was induced with intravenous propofol 80 mg and fentanyl 25 mg, and maintained with nitrous oxide–oxygen (2:1) and sevoflurane 1–1.5%. After 30 minutes her blood pressure fell from 145/85 to 85/35 mmHg. She was given an intravenous bolus of ephedrine 3 mg and her blood pressure immediately rose to 225/125 mmHg; it remained high despite an increase in the dose of sevoflurane, but was controlled by repeated doses of hydralazine 2 mg.

The effect of ephedrine, which is both a direct and indirect sympathomimetic, may have been enhanced by its not being metabolized by catechol-*O*-methyl transferase, because of the action of entacapone.

Halothane

Halothane and some other anesthetics sensitize patients to the risk of ephedrine-induced ventricular dysrhythmias and acute pulmonary edema, especially if hypoxia is present (31).

Hydrocortisone

In intravenous solutions, ephedrine is physically incompatible with hydrocortisone (34).

Monoamine oxidase inhibitors

Monoamine oxidase inhibitors can dangerously potentiate the hypertensive effects of ephedrine (38).

Propofol

An interaction of propofol with ephedrine has been described (11).

- A 44-year-old woman was given ephedrine intravenously, to manage hypotension during spinal anesthesia. She developed intracranial hypertension and focal cerebral deficits related to multiple hemorrhagic cerebral infarcts. Angiography showed reversible beading, consistent with cerebral arteritis.

Owing to the risk of tachycardia, resulting in myocardial ischemia, the combination of propofol with ephedrine in elderly patients undergoing genitourinary surgery is not recommended (39). These reports should alert physicians to the potential hazards associated with the use of ephedrine during anesthesia.

SSRIs

- A 37-year-old New Zealand woman took a total of 480 mg of pseudoephedrine in various cold remedies over 4 days (40). She had also been taking fluoxetine 20 mg/day for seasonal affective disorder. She developed rapidly swinging mood changes, alternating between laughing and crying, and was sweating and shaking violently. Although her pulse rate was only 70/minute her blood pressure was 220/130 mmHg. She recovered within 4 hours and had no recurrence of her behavioral disturbance.

Although pseudoephedrine toxicity was a possible diagnosis, the authors concluded that serotonin syndrome was more likely, from an interaction of pseudoephedrine with fluoxetine. Patients should be warned about the hazards of taking selective serotonin re-uptake blockers and then self-medicating with ephedrine or pseudoephedrine.

Tricyclic antidepressants

Tricyclic antidepressants inhibit the uptake of catecholamines, such as ephedrine, into sympathetic neurons and can enhance their cardiovascular effects (41).

- A 61-year-old woman taking amitriptyline 25 mg/day underwent oophorectomy for ovarian cancer under combined general and epidural lumbar anesthesia. After the administration of the local anesthetic she developed hypotension refractory to high doses of ephedrine and dopaminergic drugs. Control was achieved with noradrenaline 200 μg.

The authors suggested that even the small amounts of ephedrine present as additives in some local anesthetics can have a marked effect on the cardiovascular system.

Vaccines

Hyperthermia occurred shortly after immunization with typhoid and Japanese encephalitis vaccines in a service member using an over-the-counter formulation of pseudoephedrine (29).

- While exercising in mild weather the patient collapsed 75 minutes after vaccination. He presented with asystole, with a core temperature of 42.2°C, and there was no evidence of urticaria or angioedema.

References

1. Haller CA, Benowitz NL. Adverse cardiovascular and central nervous system events associated with dietary supplements containing ephedra alkaloids. N Engl J Med 2000;343(25):1833–8.
2. Yates KM, O'Connor A, Horsley CA. "Herbal Ecstasy": a case series of adverse reactions. NZ Med J 2000;113(1114):315–17.
3. Herridge CF, a'Brook MF. Ephedrine psychosis. BMJ 1968;2(598):160.
4. Samenuk D, Link MS, Homoud MK, Contreras R, Theoharides TC, Wang PJ, Estes NA 3rd. Adverse cardiovascular events temporally associated with ma huang, an herbal source of ephedrine. Mayo Clin Proc 2002;77(1): 12–16.
5. Berlin I, Warot D, Aymard G, Acquaviva E, Legrand M, Labarthe B, Peyron I, Diquet B, Lechat P. Pharmacodynamics and pharmacokinetics of single nasal (5 mg and 10 mg) and oral (50 mg) doses of ephedrine in healthy subjects. Eur J Clin Pharmacol 2001;57(6–7):447–55.
6. Zahn KA, Li RL, Purssell RA. Cardiovascular toxicity after ingestion of "herbal ecstacy". J Emerg Med 1999;17(2):289–91.
7. Jacobs KM, Hirsch KA. Psychiatric complications of Ma-huang. Psychosomatics 2000;41(1):58–62.
8. Kluger MT. Ephedrine may predispose to arrhythmias in obstetric anaesthesia. Anaesth Intensive Care 2000;28(3):336.
9. Traub SJ, Hoyek W, Hoffman RS. Dietary supplements containing ephedra alkaloids. N Engl J Med 2001;344(14):1096.
10. Wahl A, Eberli FR, Thomson DA, Luginbuhl M. Coronary artery spasm and non-Q-wave myocardial infarction following intravenous ephedrine in two healthy women under spinal anaesthesia. Br J Anaesth 2002;89(3):519–23.
11. Mourand I, Ducrocq X, Lacour JC, Taillandier L, Anxionnat R, Weber M. Acute reversible cerebral arteritis associated with parenteral ephedrine use. Cerebrovasc Dis 1999;9(6):355–7.
12. Cantu C, Arauz A, Murillo-Bonilla LM, Lopez M, Barinagarrementeria F. Stroke associated with sympathomimetics contained in over-the-counter cough and cold drugs. Stroke 2003;34(7):1667–72.
13. Durbin RJ, Waxman HA, Davis SA. Adverse event reports from Metabolife. House Committee on Government Reform, Oct 2002.
14. Kaberi-Otarod J, Conetta R, Kundo KK, Farkash A. Ischemic stroke in a user of thermadrene: a case study in alternative medicine. Clin Pharmacol Ther 2002;72(3):343–6.
15. Jacobs KM, Kirsch KA. Psychiatric complications of Ma-huang. Psychosomatics 2000;41:58–62.
16. Taylor D, O'Toole K, Auble T, Ryan C, Sherman D. The psychometric and cardiac effects of pseudoephedrine and antihistamine in the hyperbaric environment. S Pac Underw Med Soc J 2001;31:50–7.
17. Sauder KL, Brady WJ Jr, Hennes H. Visual hallucinations in a toddler: accidental ingestion of a sympathomimetic over-the-counter nasal decongestant. Am J Emerg Med 1997;15(5):521–6.
18. Wilson BE, Hobbs WN. Case report: pseudoephedrine-associated thyroid storm: thyroid hormone—catecholamine interactions. Am J Med Sci 1993;306(5):317–9.
19. Dowd J, Bailey D, Moussa K, Nair S, Doyle R, Culpepper-Morgan JA. Ischemic colitis associated with pseudoephedrine: four cases. Am J Gastroenterol 1999;94(9):2430–4.
20. Lichtenstein GR, Yee NS. Ischemic colitis associated with decongestant use. Ann Intern Med 2000;132(8):682.
21. Klestov A, Kubler P, Meulet J. Recurrent ischaemic colitis associated with pseudoephedrine use. Intern Med J 2001;31(3):195–6.
22. Assimos DG, Langenstroer P, Leinbach RF, Mandel NS, Stern JM, Holmes RP. Guaifenesin- and ephedrine-induced stones. J Endourol 1999;13(9):665–7.
23. Anibarro B, Seoane FJ. Nonpigmenting fixed exanthema induced by pseudoephedrine. Allergy 1998;53(9):902–3.
24. Hindioglu U, Sahin S. Nonpigmenting solitary fixed drug eruption caused by pseudoephedrine hydrochloride. J Am Acad Dermatol 1998;38(3):499–500.
25. Vidal C, Prieto A, Perez-Carral C, Armisen M. Nonpigmenting fixed drug eruption due to pseudoephedrine. Ann Allergy Asthma Immunol 1998;80(4):309–10.
26. Vega F, Rosales MJ, Esteve P, Morcillo R, Panizo C, Rodriguez M. Histopathology of dermatitis due to pseudoephedrine. Allergy 1998;53(2):218–20.
27. Sanchez TS, Sanchez-Perez J, Aragues M, Garcia-Diaz A. Flare-up reaction of pseudoephedrine baboon syndrome after positive patch test. Contact Dermatitis 2000;42(5): 312–13.
28. Venturini M, Lezaun A, Abos T, Fraj J, Monzon S, Colas C, Duce F. Immediate hypersensitivity due to pseudoephedrine. Allergy 2002;57(1):52–3.
29. Franklin QJ. Sudden death after typhoid and Japanese encephalitis vaccination in a young male taking pseudoephedrine. Mil Med 1999;164(2):157–9.
30. Hutchins GM. Dietary supplements containing ephedra alkaloids. N Engl J Med 2001;344(14):1095–6.
31. Haller CA, Benowitz NL. Dietary supplements containing Ephedra alkaloids. New Engl J Med 2001;344:1096–7.
32. Traboulsi AS, Viswanathan R, Coplan J. Suicide attempt after use of herbal diet pill. Am J Psychiatry 2002;159(2):318–19.
33. Pederson KJ, Kuntz DH, Garbe GJ. Acute myocardial ischemia associated with ingestion of bupropion and pseudoephedrine in a 21-year-old man. Can J Cardiol 2001;17(5):599–601.
34. Griffin JP, D'Arcy PF. A Manual of Adverse Drug Reactions. Bristol: John Wright and Sons Ltd, 1979.
35. Roberge RJ, Hirani KH, Rowland PL 3rd, Berkeley R, Krenzelok EP. Dextromethorphan- and pseudoephedrine-induced agitated psychosis and ataxia: case report. J Emerg Med 1999;17(2):285–8.

36. Soutullo CA, Cottingham EM, Keck PE Jr. Psychosis associated with pseudoephedrine and dextromethorphan. J Am Acad Child Adolesc Psychiatry 1999;38(12):1471–2.
37. Renfrew C, Dickson R, Schwab C. Severe hypertension following ephedrine administration in a patient receiving entacapone. Anesthesiology 2000;93(6):1562.
38. Elis J, Laurence DR, Mattie H, Prichard BN. Modification by monoamine oxidase inhibitors of the effect of some sympathomimetics on blood pressure. BMJ 1967;2(544): 75–8.
39. Gamlin F, Freeman J, Winslow L, Berridge J, Vucevic M. The haemodynamic effects of propofol in combination with ephedrine in elderly patients (ASA groups 3 and 4). Anaesth Intensive Care 1999;27(5):477–80.
40. Wilson H, Woods D. Pseudoephedrine causing mania-like symptoms. NZ Med J 2002;115(1148):86.
41. Boada S, Solsona B, Papaceit J, Saludes J, Rull M. Hipotension por bloqueo simpatico refractaria a efedrina en una paciente en tratamiento cronico con antidepresivos triciclicos. [Hypotension refractory to ephedrine after sympathetic blockade in a patient on long-term therapy with tricyclic antidepressants.] Rev Esp Anestesiol Reanim 1999;46(8):364–6.

Eplerenone

See also Diuretics

General Information

Eplerenone is a potassium-sparing diuretic. It is similar to spironolactone as an aldosterone antagonist, but has less affinity for androgen and progesterone receptors and may therefore have fewer adverse effects (1).

Eplerenone is metabolized by CYP3A4 (2) and should not be given with inhibitors of CYP3A4 because of the risk of hyperkalemia (3).

Eplerenone has been compared with spironolactone in patients with heart failure (NYHA classes II–IV). In a dose-finding study, 321 patients maintained on ACE inhibitors and diuretics, with or without digoxin, were randomized to receive eplerenone 25–100 mg/day, spironolactone 25 mg/day, or placebo (4). After 12 weeks there was no improvement in heart failure in patients taking either eplerenone or spironolactone. Increases in plasma testosterone were significantly greater in men taking spironolactone than in those taking eplerenone. However, hyperkalemia was more frequent in patients taking eplerenone 100 mg/day (12%) than in those taking spironolactone 25 mg/day (8.7%). The potency of eplerenone relative to spironolactone remains to be established in patients with heart failure.

Organs and Systems

Electrolyte balance

In the Eplerenone Post-Acute Myocardial Infarction Heart Failure Efficacy and Survival Study (EPHESUS), the addition of eplerenone 25–50 mg/day to optimal medical therapy in patients with an acute myocardial infarction complicated by left ventricular dysfunction and heart failure significantly reduced all-cause and cardiovascular mortality (5). Patients with a serum potassium concentration over 5.0 mmol/l at baseline were excluded. The incidence of hypokalemia was significantly lower with eplerenone. However, there was serious hyperkalemia (serum potassium 6.0 mmol/l or more) in 5.5% of those who took eplerenone compared with 3.9% of those who took placebo.

Reproductive system

Eplerenone has been reported to produce less gynecomastia than spironolactone (6,7). In patients with gynecomastia from spironolactone, eplerenone can be substituted and gynecomastia status reassessed.

Drug–Drug Interactions

ACE inhibitors

Co-administration of potassium-sparing diuretics with ACE inhibitors can cause severe hyperkalemia (SED-14, 674).

NSAIDs

The interaction between potassium-sparing diuretics and NSAIDs is well documented (SED-14, 674). The major complications are deterioration of renal function and hyperkalemia. The risk associated with the non-selective COX-2 inhibitors is unknown. However, three patients had hyperkalemia (8.5, 5.4, and 5.1 mmol/l) after developing acute renal insufficiency while taking these drugs (8).

References

1. Zillich AJ, Carter BL. Eplerenone—a novel selective aldosterone blocker. Ann Pharmacother 2002;36(10):1567–76.
2. Cook CS, Berry LM, Kim DH, Burton EG, Hribar JD, Zhang L. Involvement of CYP3A in the metabolism of eplerenone in humans and dogs: differential metabolism by CYP3A4 and CYP3A5. Drug Metab Dispos 2002;30(12):1344–51.
3. Moore TD, Nawarskas JJ, Anderson JR. Eplerenone: a selective aldosterone receptor antagonist for hypertension and heart failure. Heart Dis 2003;5(5):354–63.
4. Pitt B, Roniker B. Eplerenone a novel selective aldosterone receptor antagonist (SARA): dose finding study in patients with heart failure. J Am Coll Cardiol 1999;33(Suppl A):A188–9.
5. Keating GM, Plosker GL. Eplerenone : a review of its use in left ventricular systolic dysfunction and heart failure after acute myocardial infarction. Drugs 2004;64(23):2689–707.
6. Burgess ED, Lacourciere Y, Ruilope-Urioste LM, Oparil S, Kleiman JH, Krause S, Roniker B, Maurath C. Long-term safety and efficacy of the selective aldosterone blocker eplerenone in patients with essential hypertension. Clin Ther 2003;25(9):2388–404.
7. Hollenberg NK, Williams GH, Anderson R, Akhras KS, Bittman RM, Krause SL. Symptoms and the distress they cause: comparison of an aldosterone antagonist and a calcium channel blocking agent in patients with systolic hypertension. Arch Intern Med 2003;163(13):1543–8.
8. Perazella MA, Eras J. Are selective COX-2 inhibitors nephrotoxic? Am J Kidney Dis 2000;35(5):937–40.

Epoprostenol

See also Prostaglandins

General Information

Epoprostenol is PGI_2 available for exogenous administration. It has become the preferred long-term treatment for patients with primary pulmonary hypertension who continue to have symptoms in spite of conventional therapy. However, tolerance, which always occurs, has made dosing uncertain. The effectiveness of epoprostenol given according to an aggressive dosing strategy for longer than 1 year has been investigated in these patients (1). The dose of epoprostenol was increased by 2.4 nanograms/kg/minute each month to the maximum tolerated dose. Adverse effects were common and included diarrhea, jaw pain, headaches, and flushing in all patients.

Organs and Systems

Respiratory

Pulmonary veno-occlusive disease is a rare form of pulmonary hypertension associated with fibrotic occlusion of the smaller pulmonary veins. Although vasodilator therapy is effective in many patients with primary pulmonary hypertension, the role of vasodilators in veno-occlusive disease is unclear, because of concerns about precipitating pulmonary edema. There have been reports of successful therapy with oral vasodilators or intravenous prostacyclin. In contrast, there has been a description of a patient who developed acute pulmonary edema and respiratory failure 15 minutes after the start of a low-dose prostacyclin infusion 2 nanograms/kg/minute, leading to death an hour later (2). This case has several important implications for the management of patients with pulmonary hypertension. Although previous reports suggested that prostacyclin may be safe in patients with pulmonary veno-occlusive disease, the experience reported here suggests that even in very low doses prostacyclin can produce acute decompensation. Thus, consideration must be given to the diagnosis of pulmonary veno-occlusive disease in all patients with suspected primary pulmonary hypertension.

Further cases of pulmonary edema have been reported during continuous intravenous epoprostenol in patients with severe pulmonary hypertension and pulmonary capillary hemangiomatosis, a rare condition characterized by proliferation of thin-walled microvessels in the alveolar walls (3). This report suggests that epoprostenol should not be used in such patients.

- A 66-year-old woman with scleroderma and severe pulmonary hypertension was given continuous intravenous epoprostenol 2 and then 4 nanograms/kg/minute (total duration 48 hours) (4). Two weeks later her dyspnea had improved, but her leg was swollen and her oxygen saturation had fallen. Her dosage of epoprostenol was increased to 5 nanograms/kg/minute. One month later she developed increasing dyspnea, a non-productive cough, severe edema of her legs, and severe hypoxemia. She had gained 5 kg in weight and there were new bibasal lung crackles. A chest X-ray showed bilateral air-space opacities and bilateral effusions. Her PaO_2 was 5.7 kPa, $PaCO_2$ 3.9 kPa, and the arterial pH 7.51. Pulmonary veno-occlusive disease was diagnosed and the infusion of epoprostenol was gradually tapered over the next 48 hours. She died 6 days later with right-sided heart failure. At autopsy, histological examination showed thickening of the alveolar septa by proliferation of dilated capillaries on both sides of the alveolar walls, consistent with pulmonary capillary hemangiomatosis.
- A 61-year-old woman developed pulmonary edema during treatment with epoprostenol for severe pulmonary hypertension associated with limited scleroderma (5). She received an infusion of epoprostenol 1 nanogram/kg/minute, and the dosage was increased by 1–2 nanograms/kg/minute every 15 minutes. At a dosage of 6 nanograms/kg/minute, her pulmonary vascular resistance had fallen by 60% and her cardiac output had increased by 55%. However, at this dosage, she became acutely dyspneic. Epoprostenol was withdrawn, she was treated with furosemide and high-flow oxygen, and her symptoms resolved. Because no other therapy was available, she agreed to restart epoprostenol therapy the next day, 1 nanogram/kg/minute, increasing by 1 nanogram/kg/minute every 24 hours to 3 nanograms/kg/minute at discharge. Over the next 6 months, the dosage of epoprostenol was gradually increased to 20 nanograms/kg/minute. She had a significant improvement in her exercise tolerance and there was no evidence of pulmonary edema. However, after about 7 months of marked clinical improvement, she developed right ventricular decompensation. Increased doses of epoprostenol were ineffective and she died. Autopsy showed severe obliterative and plexogenic pulmonary arteriopathy.

This is the first case in which epoprostenol has been successfully restarted. The authors commented that pulmonary edema during acute infusion of epoprostenol is considered a contraindication to its further use. They theorized that the pulmonary edema could have occurred secondary to the dramatic increase in pulmonary perfusion at 6 nanograms/kg/minute of epoprostenol and subsequent rapid shifts in vascular hydrostatic pressure. The slow increase in dosage during reinstitution may have averted the dramatic increase in pulmonary perfusion.

Hematologic

Patients with end-stage liver failure, portal hypertension, and associated pulmonary artery hypertension (portopulmonary hypertension) have a high mortality when undergoing liver transplantation. Successful transplantation in these patients may depend on efforts to reduce pulmonary artery pressure. To this end, some centers are using a continuous intravenous infusion of epoprostenol, which has been shown to improve symptoms, extend life span, and reduce pulmonary artery pressure in patients with primary pulmonary hypertension. There have been four cases in which treatment of portopulmonary hypertension with continuous intravenous epoprostenol was followed by the development of progressive splenomegaly, with worsening thrombocytopenia and leukopenia (6). This finding may limit the usefulness of epoprostenol in portopulmonary hypertension and influence the timing of transplantation in such patients.

References

1. McLaughlin VV, Genthner DE, Panella MM, Rich S. Reduction in pulmonary vascular resistance with long-term epoprostenol (prostacyclin) therapy in primary pulmonary hypertension. N Engl J Med 1998;338(5):273–7.
2. Palmer SM, Robinson LJ, Wang A, Gossage JR, Bashore T, Tapson VF. Massive pulmonary edema and death after prostacyclin infusion in a patient with pulmonary veno-occlusive disease. Chest 1998;113(1):237–40.
3. Humbert M, Maitre S, Capron F, Rain B, Musset D, Simonneau G. Pulmonary edema complicating continuous intravenous prostacyclin in pulmonary capillary hemangiomatosis. Am J Respir Crit Care Med 1998;157(5 Pt 1):1681–5.
4. Gugnani MK, Pierson C, Vanderheide R, Girgis RE. Pulmonary edema complicating prostacyclin therapy in pulmonary hypertension associated with scleroderma: a case of pulmonary capillary hemangiomatosis. Arthritis Rheum 2000;43(3):699–703.
5. Farber HW, Graven KK, Kokolski G, Korn JH. Pulmonary edema during acute infusion of epoprostenol in a patient with pulmonary hypertension and limited scleroderma. J Rheumatol 1999;26(5):1195–6.
6. Findlay JY, Plevak DJ, Krowka MJ, Sack EM, Porayko MK. Progressive splenomegaly after epoprostenol therapy in portopulmonary hypertension. Liver Transpl Surg 1999; 5(5):362–5.

Eprazinone

General Information

Eprazinone hydrochloride is a cough suppressant that is also reported to have expectorant properties.

Drug Administration

Drug overdose

In a retrospective study of 199 cases of accidental or intentional acute poisoning with eprazinone, eprozinol, and zipeprol, collected at the Poison Control Center in Paris from 1975 to 1982, there were seven cases of seizures, all after ingestion of eight times the therapeutic dose. They resolved rapidly and without recurrence with symptomatic treatment (1).

Reference

1. Merigot P, Garnier R, Efthymiou ML. Les convulsions avec trois antitussifs dérivés substitués de la pipérazine (zipeprol, eprazinone, eprozinol). [Convulsions with 3 antitussive substituted derivatives of piperazine (zipeprol, eprazinone, eprozinol).] Ann Pediatr 1985;32(6):504–6.

Eprosartan

See also Angiotensin II receptor antagonists

General Information

Eprosartan is a non-biphenyl, non-tetrazole competitive antagonist at angiotensin II type 1 (AT_1) receptors that is chemically distinct from other angiotensin II receptor antagonists (1). It causes dual blockade of AT_1 receptors both presynaptically and postsynaptically, reducing sympathetic nerve activity significantly more than other receptor antagonists.

Organs and Systems

Respiratory

In a multicenter controlled study in patients with hypertension and a history of ACE inhibitor-induced cough, eprosartan significantly reduced the risk of cough by 88% compared with enalapril (2).

References

1. Puig JG, Lopez MA, Bueso TS, Bernardino JI, Jimenez RT; Grupo MAPA-MADRID Investigators. Clinical profile of eprosartan. Cardiovasc Drugs Ther 2002;16(6):543–9.
2. Oparil S. Eprosartan versus enalapril in hypertensive patients with angiotensin-converting enzyme inhibitor-induced cough. Curr Ther Res Clin Exp 1999;60:1–4.

Eprozinol

General Information

Eprozinol hydrochloride inhibits bronchoconstriction and has been used in the treatment of asthma and bronchitis.

Drug Administration

Drug overdose

In a retrospective study of 199 cases of accidental or intentional acute poisoning with eprozinol, eprazinone, and zipeprol, collected at the Poison Control Center in Paris from 1975 to 1982, there were seven cases of seizures, all after ingestion of eight times the therapeutic dose. They resolved rapidly and without recurrence with symptomatic treatment (1).

Reference

1. Merigot P, Garnier R, Efthymiou ML. Les convulsions avec trois antitussifs dérivés substitués de la pipérazine (zipeprol, eprazinone, eprozinol). [Convulsions with 3 antitussive substituted derivatives of piperazine (zipeprol, eprazinone, eprozinol).] Ann Pediatr 1985;32(6):504–6.

Ergot derivatives

General Information

Ergot derivatives include ergotamine tartrate (rINNM), dihydroergotamine (BAN, USAN), ergometrine (rINNM, also called ergonovine), and methylergotamine (rINNM). They are potent alpha$_1$-adrenoceptor and 5-HT receptor antagonists, and have been used to treat migraine (ergotamine, dihydroergotamine) and to stimulate uterine contraction (ergometrine, methylergotamine).

Ergotamine and dihydroergotamine

Ergotamine and dihydroergotamine have been used in preventing migraine attacks and dihydroergotamine in the treatment of hypotension (either orthostatic or caused by spinal or epidural anesthesia). When dihydroergotamine was given intravenously after coronary bypass surgery, despite increased filling pressure there was no rise in cardiac output, and despite increased cardiac work the bypass flow fell significantly. The significant decrease in regional myocardial vascular resistance found after the administration of dihydroergotamine may explain the absence of the expected increase in cardiac output and coronary bypass flow.

The combination of heparin with dihydroergotamine has been used in the prevention of thromboembolic complications. It was claimed that these two components act synergistically, allowing a lower dosage of heparin to be used. However, the lower risk of hemorrhagic complications is certainly not counterbalanced by a lowered risk of ergotism (SEDA-8, 147). Vasospastic reactions after giving heparin with dihydroergotamine seem to occur particularly in traumatized patients or when a limb is injured. Since the risk of vasospasm increases with treatment time, the Swedish Adverse Reactions Committee recommended that the duration of treatment with dihydroergotamine with heparin should not exceed 7 days (SEDA-15, 135).

With daily use of dihydroergotamine by injection, there is an ill-defined frequency of nausea, vomiting, abdominal pain, and diarrhea, but also a high incidence of muscle cramps and some cases of lethargy and peripheral edema (SEDA-17, 171).

An expert European group has re-evaluated the preclinical and clinical data on ergotamine as they relate to treatment of migraine and have tried to reach a consensus on how to use it prudently (1).

Ergometrine

Ergometrine is used in obstetrics, since its oxytocic effects are relatively more marked than its vascular effects. Nausea and vomiting can occur if it is given orally. Slight bradycardia is common, but tachycardia occurs in some patients, and there can be changes in intracardiac conduction and pacemaker function. Very rarely, hypertensive reactions and cardiac arrest have been described and there are two reports of myocardial infarction in healthy women who were smokers (SEDA-18, 160). A newborn infant inadvertently injected with ergometrine and oxytocin developed depression of respiration and convulsions (2).

The "ergonovine provocation test" has been used in the diagnosis of angina pectoris (by producing vasospasm during angiography) but it can cause myocardial infarction and even death (SED-12, 324) (3).

Co-dergocrine

Co-dergocrine mesylate (Hydergine) is a mixture of the methane sulfonates of the dihydrogenated derivatives of the three alkaloids of ergotoxin (dihydroergocornine, dihydroergocristine, and dihydroergocryptine). Dihydrogenation eliminates the vasoconstrictor effects of ergotoxin and enhances its alpha-adrenoceptor antagonist and 5-HT receptor antagonist properties. Co-dergocrine has other pharmacological effects, including inhibition of brain-specific phosphodiesterases, several of which are still poorly described.

Co-dergocrine is claimed to have some effect in brain ageing and has also been promoted as a "metabolic enhancer," mainly because it protects against metabolic alterations induced by hypothermia and ischemia in animals (4).

Many double-blind, controlled trials have been conducted with co-dergocrine in senile dementia, and almost all have reported improvements in scores on at least one psychomotor test scale. However, despite this evidence of short-term efficacy, many skeptical clinicians still consider it to be no better than placebo, and find support from a double-blind, placebo-controlled trial in which a group treated with the recommended dosage of 1 mg tds for 24 weeks did not perform better after treatment than did the placebo-treated group (5). The clinical value of co-dergocrine in patients with claudication and rest pain is poorly documented.

Although the recommended dosage has been tripled over the years (from 0.5 to 1.5 mg tds), significant unwanted effects are rare. Vomiting, blurred vision, skin rashes, nasal stuffiness, bad taste, postural hypotension, and vasospastic reactions are all uncommon (SED-12, 472). Diffuse fibrotic processes (for example retroperitoneal fibrosis), repeatedly reported with other ergot derivatives, such as methysergide and dihydroergotamine, have not been observed with co-dergocrine. In elderly people, co-dergocrine only occasionally causes diarrhea, nausea, gastric pain, orthostatic hypotension, and headache. In 40 children, nasal stuffiness and anorexia were most common adverse effects of co-dergocrine (6).

Organs and Systems

Cardiovascular

Ergot derivatives are powerful vasoconstrictors. The extremities become pale and cold, and arterial spasm in the arms and legs has been demonstrated; even the face can be affected. The condition can develop acutely even after brief use of the drug, and there is real risk of gangrene; if given early, intra-arterial infusion of prostaglandin E$_1$ can reverse the spasms. Protracted coronary spasm has also been reported in some cases (SEDA-14, 122). Renal arterial spasm has occurred after a dose of ergotamine of 10 mg in the form of suppositories given over 60 hours (SED-8, 308) (7), and bilateral papillitis with ischemia of the periaxial fibers has resulted from 2 weeks of maximum-dose treatment. High doses have also led on occasion to mesenteric vascular constriction, ischemic bowel disease, and partial necrosis of the tongue. Arterial stenosis can even result in aneurysm formation (8). The absence of symptoms does not mean that there is no adverse effect; in 30 patients who had taken ergotamine 1–5 mg/day for a year all had lowered systolic blood pressures in the foot.

Arterial spasm induced by ergotamine can be due to overdose, but some patients have an exaggerated response to a therapeutic dose. Interaction with other drugs, leading to potentiation, is a third mechanism. Four patients developed extreme limb ischemia after a therapeutic dose of ergotamine: one even took only a single dose of 1 mg. The symptoms responded to vasodilator therapy after withdrawal of ergotamine, but one needed a minor amputation. All patients were taking antiviral treatment for HIV infection, and ritonavir and indinavir may have potentiated the effect of ergotamine by inhibiting its metabolism (9–12).

Treatment of migraine can lead to subclinical ergotism for a prolonged period, and thence to occlusive peripheral vascular disease; peripheral systolic pressure (and liver function tests) should be monitored in patients taking regular ergotamine (SEDA-15, 135). Tolerance to these vasoconstrictive effects varies widely among individuals; such symptoms as cyanosis of the limbs, syncope, hypotension, and paresthesia have been seen in sensitive subjects after doses of up to 8 mg taken over as little as 10 days. The Swedish drug authorities have recommended that treatment should not be continued for more than 7 days (SEDA-13, 113).

- A 78-year-old woman developed gangrene in three fingertips on the right hand and two on the left after being given dihydroergotamine 10 mg/day as migraine prophylaxis (13). She had had Raynaud's syndrome for at least the previous 5 years and was thought to have a relatively mild form of systemic sclerosis.
- A 44-year-old woman developed claudication and rest pain after gross overuse of ergotamine 100 mg suppositories (up to 6 times a day) for chronic headaches over a period of several years (14). Angiography showed occlusion of both femoral arteries. Intra-arterial prostaglandin E (presumably E_1) followed by chemical sympathectomy normalized the circulation in both the legs.
- A 63-year-old Canadian woman who had been taking ergotamine (dosage unspecified) for migraine for 20 years developed acute ischemia of the right arm, with no palpable pulses below the axilla (15). Angiography showed multiple filling defects in upper limb arteries, partially reversible with intravenous phentolamine. She was given prazosin 2 mg/day and became pain-free after 5 days. Treatment was continued for 3 months and during this time attacks of migraine were treated with sumatriptan without adverse effects. Her pulses were entirely normal after 3 months, as was angiography.

Myocardial infarction has been reported.

- A 27-year-old woman with familial hypercholesterolemia already treated with lipid-lowering drugs developed acute chest pain after a prophylactic intramuscular injection of 0.5 mg ergometrine, given during the late stages of labor (16). Angiography showed three-vessel atherosclerotic disease and occlusion of the left anterior descending coronary artery. Angioplasty with stenting was successful and she made an excellent recovery.
- A 34-year-old woman had a myocardial infarction after being given ergonovine for an atonic uterus after cesarean section (17). Within minutes she became unresponsive, with bradycardia and then asystole followed by ventricular fibrillation during cardiopulmonary resuscitation. An electrocardiogram showed an acute anterior infarct and coronary angiography showed diffuse spasm of the circumflex and left anterior descending arteries, with subtotal occlusion of the latter. The spasm was reversed with intracoronary glyceryl trinitrate but she required ventilation for another 2 days and was eventually discharged 11 days after the infarct, with a borderline left ventricular ejection fraction of 45%.

The authors commented that the latter patient was of Asian origin and that such individuals are thought to have increased susceptibility to the vasoconstrictor effects of ergot derivatives.

The role of arterial spasm as a cause of angina after angioplasty has been studied in two men, aged 45 and 58 years, who had emergency angioplasties for acute coronary thrombosis (18). Although the primary procedures were successful in both cases, ischemic chest pain returned after 4 and 6 months respectively. Perhaps a little surprisingly, in both cases intravenous ergonovine (0.4 mg) was given during coronary angiography, causing severe arterial spasm, which resolved with intravenous isosorbide dinitrate. There was no evidence of restenosis. The authors noted that recurrence of angina does not necessarily imply restenosis, although it is not clear how many cardiologists will repeat this procedure with their own patients.

- A 48-year-old woman developed a cold pulseless right leg and no measurable blood pressure at the right ankle (19). She was a migraine sufferer and had been taking over-the-counter medications, some of which contained ergot derivatives, although the nature and quantity were not specified. Arteriography showed severe stenosis of the superficial femoral artery, with no identifiable tibial vessels. There was an initial improvement with intra-arterial glyceryl trinitrate infusion, and sustained normalization of the circulation in the leg after administration of sodium nitroprusside, nifedipine, prazosin, and heparin. She made a full recovery.

The authors reviewed the pharmacology of the ergot alkaloids and the acute and subclinical ischemic syndromes that they can produce. They pointed out that in some countries, notably in Latin America, ergot-containing formulations are freely available without a prescription.

Acute hypertensive encephalopathy has occurred in a patient given methylergotamine (SEDA-3, 121).

Diverticulum formation in the internal carotid artery occurred in a patient who had taken ergotamine for

4 years (SEDA-10, 119). Rupture of a splenic artery aneurysm in a 46-year-old woman was ascribed to excessive ergotamine ingestion for migraine (20). The authors thought that significant vasospasm may have led to damage and weakening of the vessel wall and consequently to the development of a false aneurysm. It should be noted that splanchnic aneurysms are occasionally discovered in otherwise healthy people and carry a 5% risk of spontaneous rupture.

Long-term abuse of ergotamine can occasionally cause fibrosis of the cardiac valves (SEDA-18, 160).

Ear, nose, throat

During intranasal administration for migraine, nasal congestion, irritation, and sneezing can occur (21).

Nervous system

The cerebral vasculature can also be vulnerable to ergot-induced vasoconstriction.

- A 54-year-old woman with a 20-year history of migraine used a nasal ergotamine spray one evening during an episode of migraine (22). She used a second dose at 4 p.m. the next day since the migraine had persisted. The following morning she was given subcutaneous sumatriptan 6 mg. Some 30–45 minutes later she developed the symptoms of global amnesia, which resolved by the following morning. Magnetic resonance imaging showed a small infarct in the right thalamus.

It seems likely that the co-administration of two cerebral vasoconstrictors increased the likelihood of such an event.

- A 36-year-old woman developed a "cerebral angiopathy" within 36 hours after starting to take oral metergoline, an ergot derivative prescribed after delivery to suppress lactation (23). This angiopathy was apparently due to severe narrowing of small and medium cerebral arteries; its main features were sudden hypertension, seizures, and variable reversible neurological deficits.

Transient cortical blindness, with severe headache and hallucinations, has been associated with the intravenous injection of methylergometrine 0.2 mg in a postpartum patient reference.

The role of ergotamine and sumatriptan in drug-induced headache has been surveyed in over 2000 patients at a regional headache clinic (24). About 600 had taken ergot derivatives previously and a similar number had used sumatriptan, while nearly 250 had experience of both. Drug overuse was defined as the use of at least one dose of either drug on 18 or more days every month for at least 3 months. By these criteria the rates of ergotamine and sumatriptan overuse were estimated at 14 and 3.5% respectively. Drug-induced headache was much more common among ergotamine overusers than sumatriptan overusers (68 versus 32%).

Sensory systems

Bilateral ischemic optic neuropathy can develop secondary to acute ergotism after administration of ergotamine tartrate (25).

Psychological, psychiatric

Unlike the dopamine-mimetic ergolines, ergotamine is not usually regarded as a drug with major effects on the brain. However, this may not always be true.

- A 75-year-old woman in Arizona developed progressive confusion, auditory hallucinations, and aggressive behavior (26). Her systolic pressure was raised (194 mmHg). She had a history of migraine and many other problems, including hypertension. Her headaches had become more severe over the weeks before admission and she had been gradually increasing her intake of a formulation containing ergotamine 1 mg and caffeine 100 mg: just before the emergence of her psychiatric symptoms she was taking 14 tablets per week. After withdrawal of the ergotamine/caffeine, her mental state and blood pressure returned to normal, without antihypertensive medication, and remained so 12 months later.

Although there has been extensive discussion of the phenomenon of ergotism in medieval and early modern times, its features do not closely resemble this case, perhaps because of the co-administration of caffeine. However, regardless of that, there does seem to be a strong case for a drug effect here.

A syndrome resembling reversible dementia has been described in chronic ergotamine intoxication (SEDA-3, 121).

Gastrointestinal

Nausea and vomiting are common problems with effective doses of ergotamine. Rectal stenosis demanding treatment has several times been described after prolonged use or overuse (27). This pattern of use can also rarely cause reversible gastrointestinal ischemia, presenting as lower abdominal pain (SEDA-17, 146).

- A 50-year-old woman developed ischemic necrosis of the stomach wall after taking up to 5 mg/day of ergotamine tablets for 10 years because of daily headaches (28). The necrosis was seen on the greater curvature and was about 10 cm in diameter. She required laparotomy because of peritonitis and there was a 4 cm area of full-thickness necrosis within the ischemic area. She made a full recovery.
- A necrotic small intestine was resected in a 65-year-old man with ergotamine abuse (29). Histological examination showed hypertrophy of the smooth muscle of the mesenteric arteries resulting from chronic vasospasm. The patient developed postoperatively limb ischemia and tongue gangrene before he died.

Liver

Portal hypertension, presumably due to vasoconstriction, has been reported (SEDA-11, 131).

Skin

Anocutaneous ergotism (characterized by anal ulceration) has been observed in one case after excessive use of ergot suppositories (SEDA-10, 119).

Serosae

Retroperitoneal fibrosis, as produced classically by methysergide, has been reported after the administration of ergotamine (SEDA-8, 147) and dihydroergotamine (SEDA-17, 170).

Other fibrotic reactions have been reported in patients taking ergot derivatives.

- A 67-year-old man in Germany with Parkinson's disease took co-careldopa and (somewhat unusually) alpha-dihydroergocryptine 45 mg/day, the latter in order to regulate fluctuations on motor function (30). After 2 years he developed a dry cough with dyspnea. Chest X-rays showed severe thickening of the pleura bilaterally with associated effusions. Biopsy confirmed fibrosis. The ergot drug was immediately replaced with pramipexole, eventually at a dose of 3 mg/day. Respiratory symptoms improved markedly within weeks, but there was little change radiologically.

Although this is the first description of such a reaction to this particular drug, it has been well documented with several other dopaminergic ergot derivatives.

Long-Term Effects

Drug dependence

If ergotamine tartrate is used chronically, which is in any case undesirable because of its vascular effects, a vicious cycle can arise, withdrawal headaches leading to the use of ever-increasing doses (SEDA-13, 113). Tolerance can develop to the point at which the doses being used exceed those that are normally regarded as safe. The only possible treatment is to withdraw the drug; the withdrawal symptoms tend to be poorly responsive to other drugs, but they usually abate within 72 hours, after which the patient can be treated with other antimigraine drugs. The best means of preventing ergotamine dependence is to limit the use of ergotamine tartrate to no more than 2 days per week and to ensure that the drug is not used unnecessarily for plain headaches, which have been labeled as migrainous.

Second-Generation Effects

Teratogenicity

Microcephaly occurred in a child whose mother had used ergotamine and caffeine (during the first trimester) and propranolol (during the second) for the relief of migraine (SEDA-13, 114). Although this suggests the possibility of teratogenicity, data in animals are not consistent. However, ergotamine should in any case not be used in pregnancy in view of its oxytocic effects (SEDA-8, 147), which can lead to fetal stress requiring cesarean section (31).

Lactation

Ergotamine does not affect the amount of milk secreted during lactation (32). It has been said that if ergotamine is used during lactation, the infant may have gastrointestinal upsets, cardiovascular instability, and even convulsions, but there is little documented evidence of this.

Susceptibility Factors

Hepatic disease

There are special risks in giving ergotamine in liver disease, since most of the drug is metabolized by the liver. Ergotamine also reduces liver blood flow by vasoconstriction and therefore reduces its own first-pass metabolism.

Other features of the patient

Women taking oral contraceptives and pregnant women are more susceptible to the vasospastic effects of the ergot alkaloids, as are patients in shock, with sepsis, and with Raynaud's disease or Buerger's disease. The risk of severe vascular reactions is increased in the presence of peripheral vascular disease or when sympathomimetic agents are given at the same time.

Drug Administration

Drug overdose

The signs of ergot poisoning initially include dizziness, frontal headache, depression, and leg and low back pain; more severe poisoning results in formication, severe cyanosis of the extremities, muscular twitching, tonic spasms, convulsions, delirium, and ultimately death (33).

Drug–Drug Interactions

Clarithromycin

Clarithromycin has been reported to potentiate the effects of ergotamine.

- A 41-year-old woman presented with pain and pallor in the leg and a sensation of coolness exacerbated by exercise (34). For many years she had been taking a formulation containing ergotamine 1 mg plus caffeine 100 mg, at a dose of one or two tablets daily, for both prophylaxis and treatment of migraine. For 7 days she had also taken clarithromycin (dose is not stated) for a chest infection. Her legs were cool and cyanosed, with no palpable popliteal or foot pulses and an ankle–brachial index of only 0.6 (normal >0.8).

The authors concluded that her symptoms had been precipitated by the introduction of clarithromycin, an inhibitor of CYP isozymes like the other macrolide antibiotics. However, she was also taking omeprazole, another inhibitor, which may have contributed to the problem. All drugs were withdrawn and nifedipine was given, with full recovery within a couple of days.

Ritonavir

Ritonavir has been reported to potentiate the effects of ergotamine.

- A 28-year-old woman was taking triple therapy for HIV infection, including the protease inhibitor ritonavir (35).

She had also started to take a combined formulation containing ergotamine (0.6 mg/day), phenobarbital (40 mg/day), and belladonna extract (0.4 mg/day). Four days later she noted pain in both legs and all her extremities were cold, pale, and pulseless. She had diffuse arterial spasm in the aorta and all four limbs. Despite intensive vasodilator therapy, she developed bilateral gangrene of the toes, requiring transmetatarsal amputations.

- A 37-year-old woman with AIDS who had been taking ritonavir developed acute dysphasia and right-sided weakness having taken a total of 10 mg of ergotamine in suppository form for severe headaches that were presumed to be migraine (36). Transcranial Doppler and angiography showed multiple stenoses in vessels in the circle of Willis, and an MRI scan showed watershed infarcts in the right and left hemispheres. It was presumed that she had had ergotamine-induced vasospasm due to inhibition of ergotamine metabolism by ritonavir. She was treated with "hemodilution, hypertension and hypervolemia"; the cerebral flow velocities normalized over the next 18 days and the angiographic appearances by day 90. She was left with a slight right expressive dysphasia and weakness in the right leg.

Ritonavir is a very potent inhibitor of CYP3A4, which is responsible for the metabolism of ergotamine, and this interaction obviously led to toxic plasma concentrations of the alkaloid.

Sumatriptan

The combination of ergotamine with sumatriptan has been associated with vasospasm in the cerebral arteries (37).

- A 20-year-old woman developed a severe headache 24 hours after a spontaneous normal delivery. She was given sumatriptan 6 mg subcutaneously followed 24 hours later by three tablets of ergotamine. Shortly after this she had a secondarily generalized tonic-clonic seizure, starting in the left arm, and became hemiplegic. A CT scan showed cerebral edema and angiography showed multiple narrowings of the right vertebrobasilar and middle cerebral arteries. After several further seizures she gradually improved and was clinically normal after 10 days. An MRI angiogram was normal two days later.

The danger of combining two cerebral and coronary vasoconstrictors needs no emphasis.

References

1. Renfrew C, Dickson R, Schwab C. Severe hypertension following ephedrine administration in a patient receiving entacapone. Anesthesiology 2000;93(6):1562.
2. Kenna AP. Accidental administration of syntometrine to a newborn infant. J Obstet Gynaecol Br Commonw 1972;79(8):764–6.
3. Hays JT, Hamill RD, DeFelice CA, Raizner AE. Coronary artery spasm culminating in thrombosis following ergonovine stimulation. Cathet Cardiovasc Diagn 1993;28(3):221–4.
4. Hollister LE, Yesavage J. Ergoloid mesylates for senile dementias: unanswered questions. Ann Intern Med 1984;100(6):894–8.
5. Thompson TL 2nd, Filley CM, Mitchell WD, Culig KM, LoVerde M, Byyny RL. Lack of efficacy of hydergine in patients with Alzheimer's disease. N Engl J Med 1990;323(7):445–8.
6. Tareen KI, Bashir A, Saeed K, Hussain T. Clinical efficacy of codergocrine mesylate in children with learning difficulties. J Int Med Res 1988;16(3):204–9.
7. Fedotin MS, Hartman C. Ergotamine poisoning producing renal arterial spasm. N Engl J Med 1970;283(10):518–20.
8. Pajewski M, Modai D, Wisgarten J, Freund E, Manor A, Starinski R. Iatrogenic arterial aneurysm associated with ergotamine therapy. Lancet 1981;2(8252):934–5.
9. Lambert DH. Transient neurologic symptoms when phenylephrine is added to tetracaine spinal anesthesia—an alternative. Anesthesiology 1998;89(1):273.
10. Poldermans D, Rambaldi R, Bax JJ, Cornel JH, Thomson IR, Valkema R, Boersma E, Fioretti PM, Breburda CS, Roelandt JR. Safety and utility of atropine addition during dobutamine stress echocardiography for the assessment of viable myocardium in patients with severe left ventricular dysfunction. Eur Heart J 1998;19(11):1712–18.
11. Elhendy A, Valkema R, van Domburg RT, Bax JJ, Nierop PR, Cornel JH, Geleijnse ML, Reijs AE, Krenning EP, Roelandt JR. Safety of dobutamine-atropine stress myocardial perfusion scintigraphy. J Nucl Med 1998;39(10):1662–6.
12. Lin SS, Roger VL, Pascoe R, Seward JB, Pellikka PA. Dobutamine stress Doppler hemodynamics in patients with aortic stenosis: feasibility, safety, and surgical correlations. Am Heart J 1998;136(6):1010–16.
13. Hahne T, Balda BR. Fingerkuppennekrosen nach Dihydroergotaminmedikation bei limitierter systemischer Sklerodermie. [Finger tip necroses after dihydroergotamine medication in limited systemic scleroderma.] Hautarzt 1998;49(9):722–4.
14. Rommel JD, Klee P, Burkard A, Ratthey KP. Normalisierung des Gefäßbildes durch Sympathikusblockade bei schwerer arterieller Durchblutungsstörung durch Ergotismus. [Normalization of the vascular picture with sympathetic block in severe arterial ischemia from ergotism.] Anästhesiol Intensivmed Notfallmed Schmerzther 1999;34(9):578–81.
15. Safar HA, Alanezi KH, Cina CS. Successful treatment of threatening limb loss ischemia of the upper limb caused by ergotamine. A case report and review of the literature. J Cardiovasc Surg (Torino) 2002;43(2):245–9.
16. Mousa HA, McKinley CA, Thong J. Acute postpartum myocardial infarction after ergometrine administration in a woman with familial hypercholesterolaemia. BJOG 2000;107(7):939–40.
17. Tsui BC, Stewart B, Fitzmaurice A, Williams R. Cardiac arrest and myocardial infarction induced by postpartum intravenous ergonovine administration. Anesthesiology 2001;94(2):363–4.
18. Yoshitomi Y, Kojima S, Sugi T, Matsumoto Y, Yano M, Kuramochi M. Coronary artery spasm induced by ergonovine in an infarct related coronary artery late after primary angioplasty. J Interv Cardiol 2000;13:31–4.
19. Zavaleta EG, Fernandez BB, Grove MK, Kaye MD. St. Anthony's fire (ergotamine induced leg ischemia)—a case report and review of the literature. Angiology 2001;52(5):349–56.
20. Kernan WN, Viscoli CM, Brass LM, Broderick JP, Brott T, Feldmann E, Morgenstern LB, Wilterdink JL, Horwitz RI. Phenylpropanolamine and the risk of hemorrhagic stroke. N Engl J Med 2000;343(25):1826–32.

21. Scott AK. Dihydroergotamine: a review of its use in the treatment of migraine and other headaches. Clin Neuropharmacol 1992;15(4):289–96.
22. Pradalier A, Lutz G, Vincent D. Transient global amnesia, migraine, thalamic infarct, dihydroergotamine, and sumatriptan. Headache 2000;40(4):324–7.
23. Crippa G, Sverzellati E, Pancotti D, Carrara GC. Severe postpartum hypertension and reversible cerebral angiopathy associated with ergot derivative (methergoline) administration. Ann Ital Med Int 2000;15(4):303–5.
24. Smith MA, Ross MB. Oral 5-HT_1 receptor agonists for migraine: comparative considerations. Formulary 1999;34:324–8.
25. Sommer S, Delemazure B, Wagner M, Xenard L, Rozot P. Neuropathie optique ischémique bilateral sécondaire à un ergotisme aigu. [Bilateral ischemic optic neuropathy secondary to acute ergotism.] J Fr Ophtalmol 1998;21(2):123–5.
26. Gulbranson SH, Mock RE, Wolfrey JD. Possible ergotamine–caffeine-associated delirium. Pharmacotherapy 2002;22(1):126–9.
27. Gordon RD, Ballantine DM, Bachmann AW. Effects of repeated doses of pseudoephedrine on blood pressure and plasma catecholamines in normal subjects and in patients with phaeochromocytoma. Clin Exp Pharmacol Physiol 1992;19(5):287–90.
28. Papalampros EL, Salakou SG, Felekouras ES, Scopa C, Tsamandas AC, Bastounis E. Ischemic necrosis of gastric wall after long-term ergotamine pill abuse: case report and review of the literature. Dig Dis Sci 2001;46(5):981–4.
29. Hamilton RS, Sharieff G. Phenylpropanolamine-associated intracranial hemorrhage in an infant. Am J Emerg Med 2000;18(3):343–5.
30. Oechsner M, Groenke L, Mueller D. Pleural fibrosis associated with dihydroergocryptine treatment. Acta Neurol Scand 2000;101(4):283–5.
31. de Groot AN, van Dongen PW, van Roosmalen J, Eskes TK. Ergotamine-induced fetal stress: review of side effects of ergot alkaloids during pregnancy. Eur J Obstet Gynecol Reprod Biol 1993;51(1):73–7.
32. Jolivet A, Robyn C, Huraux-Rendu C, Gautray JP. Effêt de derives des alcaloïdes de l'ergot de seigle sur la secretion lactée dans le post-partum immediat. [Effect of ergot alkaloid derivatives on milk secretion in the immediate postpartum period.] J Gynecol Obstet Biol Reprod (Paris) 1978;7(1):129–34.
33. Loew DM, Van Deusen EB, Meier-Ruge W. Effect on the central nervous system. In: Berde B, Schild HO, editors. Handbook of Experimental Pharmacology. Vol. 49. Ergot Alkaloids and Related Compounds. Berlin-Heidelberg-New York: Springer-Verlag, 1978;79:421.
34. Ausband SC, Goodman PE. An unusual case of clarithromycin associated ergotism. J Emerg Med 2001;21(4): 411–13.
35. Liaudet L, Buclin T, Jaccard C, Eckert P. Drug points: severe ergotism associated with interaction between ritonavir and ergotamine. BMJ 1999;318(7186):771.
36. Spiegel M, Schmidauer C, Kampfl A, Sarcletti M, Poewe W. Cerebral ergotism under treatment with ergotamine and ritonavir. Neurology 2001;57(4):743–4.
37. Granier I, Garcia E, Geissler A, Boespflug MD, Durand-Gasselin J. Postpartum cerebral angiopathy associated with the administration of sumatriptan and dihydroergotamine—a case report Intensive Care Med 1999; 25(5): 532–4.

Ericaceae

See also Herbal medicines

General Information

The genera in the family of Ericaceae (Table 1) include heather, huckleberry, and rhododendron.

Arctostaphylos uva-ursi

Arctostaphylos uva-ursi (bearberry) contains a steroid, sitosterol, and triterpenoids, such as amyrin, betulinic acid, lupeol, oleanolic acid, taraxenol, ursolic acid, and uvaol. The main constituent is a glucoside called arbutin. Other constituents are methylarbutin, ericolin, ursone, gallic acid, and ellagic acid.

Its reputed antibacterial activity is ascribed to the urinary metabolite hydroquinone, which is excreted in the form of inactive conjugates and needs an alkaline urine to be liberated. As the urine of people who consume a Western non-vegetarian diet is usually acidic, it is sometimes suggested that one should alkalinize the urine of bearberry users with sodium bicarbonate. However, as the dosage recommended for this purpose is usually high, this carries well-known risks such as a high sodium load and interference with the renal clearance of certain other drugs.

Table 1 The genera of Ericaceae

Agarista (Florida hobblebush)
Andromeda (bog rosemary)
Arbutus (madrone)
Arctostaphylos (manzanita)
Befaria (befaria)
Calluna (heather)
Cassiope (mountain heather)
Chamaedaphne (leather leaf)
Comarostaphylis (summer holly)
Elliottia (elliottia)
Epigaea (trailing arbutus)
Erica (heath)
Gaultheria (snowberry)
Gaylussacia (huckleberry)
Gonocalyx (brittle leaf)
Harrimanella (harrimanella)
Kalmia (laurel)
Kalmiopsis (kalmiopsis)
Ledum (Labrador tea)
Leiophyllum (leiophyllum)
Leucothoe (dog hobble)
Loiseleuria (loiseleuria)
Lyonia (stagger bush)
Menziesia (menziesia)
Ornithostaphylos (ornithostaphylos)
Oxydendrum (swamp cranberry)
Phyllodoce (mountain heath)
Pieris (fetter bush)
Rhododendron (rhododendron)
Symphysia (symphysia)
Vaccinium (blueberry)
Xylococcus (mission manzanita)
Zenobia (honeycup)

Adverse effects

The urine of patients taking bearberry can darken on standing.

Toxic reactions to bearberry have not been reported, except for an anomalous case of dyspnea, cyanosis, and skin reactions after the consumption of an aqueous decoction (1).

- A 56-year-old woman who had taken *uva ursi* for 3 years developed reduced visual acuity (2). She had a typical bull's-eye maculopathy bilaterally.

The authors suggested that the effect was due to impaired melanin synthesis.

Reports of carcinogenicity of hydroquinone after prolonged administration of high doses to rats or mice raise a question about the long-term safety of *A. uva-ursi* and other medicinal herbs that contain substantial amounts of arbutin (3).

Gaultheria procumbens

The volatile oil of *Gaultheria procumbens* (wintergreen) leaves consists largely of methyl salicylate (more than 95%).

Adverse effects

Salicylism has been attributed to the use of oil of wintergreen as part of an herbal skin cream for the treatment of psoriasis (4).

- A 40-year-old man became acutely unwell after receiving oil of wintergreen from an unregistered naturopath. Transcutaneous absorption of the methyl salicylate was enhanced in this case owing to the abnormal areas of skin that were covered and the use of an occlusive dressing. The patient developed tinnitus, vomiting, tachypnea, and the typical acid/base disturbance of salicylate toxicity. Decontamination of the skin followed by rehydration and establishment of good urine flow was successful.

Laryngeal edema has been attributed to oil of wintergreen (5).

Methyl salicylate in topical analgesic preparations can cause irritant or allergic contact dermatitis and anaphylactic reactions (6).

In a retrospective study 80 subjects who had taken aspirin tablets ($n = 42$) or topical oil of wintergreen ($n = 38$) were compared (7). The admission plasma salicylate concentrations were generally higher in those who had taken aspirin tablets, but the two highest readings (4.3 and 3.5 mmol/l) belonged to two of the subjects who had taken oil of wintergreen.

Oil of wintergreen in the form of candy flavoring was ingested by a 21-month-old boy who developed vomiting, lethargy, and hyperpnea but recovered rapidly with parenteral fluids and sodium bicarbonate (8).

Methylsalicylate is also an important constituent of the Red Flower Oil formulations that are popular herbal analgesics for topical application in Southeast Asia. Some users take small amounts of the oil orally to enhance its analgesic effects. There are many different brands, which provide variable amounts of declared or undeclared methylsalicylate (up to 0.78 g/ml of oil). A suicide attempt by deliberate ingestion of about 100 ml resulted in severe salicylate poisoning (9).

Ledum palustre

The essential oil of *Ledum palustre* (marsh Labrador tea), which contains flavones, monoterpenoids, and sesquiterpenoids, is a potent irritant of the gastrointestinal tract, kidneys, and urinary tract; other toxic effects include abortion.

Vaccinium macrocarpon

Vaccinium macrocarpon (cranberry, marsh apple) has been used to prevent and treat urinary tract infections, although it is not useful in established infections (10,11). It is supposed to act by preventing adhesion of bacteria to the bladder wall. It may also reduce the risk of formation of some types of urinary stone (12,13).

Adverse effects

Hematologic

Cranberry juice may contain small amounts of quinine, which can cause immune thrombocytopenia.

- After transurethral resection of his prostate, a 68-year-old man developed immune thrombocytopenic purpura (platelet count 1×10^9/l) (14). He had self-medicated with cranberry juice for 10 days before the operation and had also taken amlodipine and aspirin. He had oral petechiae, bleeding gums, hematuria, and bruises. He recovered within 3 days of being given human immunoglobulin and oral prednisolone, and 18 months later his platelet count was still normal.

Drug interactions

Cranberry juice has been reported to enhance the action of warfarin (15)

- After a chest infection a man in his 70s had a poor appetite for 2 weeks and ate next to nothing, taking only cranberry juice as well as his regular drugs (digoxin, phenytoin, and warfarin) (16). Six weeks later his international normalized ratio was over 50, having previously been stable. He died of gastrointestinal and pericardial haemorrhage. He had not taken any over the counter preparations or herbal medicines, and he had been taking his drugs correctly.

The Committee on Safety of Medicines has received several other reports through the yellow card-reporting scheme about a possible interaction between warfarin and cranberry juice.

In one case this effect was suggested to have been due to contamination with salicylic acid, which displaces warfarin from protein binding sites (17).

References

1. Meijers FS. Idio-synkrasie voor folia uvae ursi. Ned Tijdschr Geneeskd 1902;46:1226–8.
2. Wang L, Del Priore LV. Bull's-eye maculopathy secondary to herbal toxicity from uva ursi. Am J Ophthalmol 2004;137(6):1135–7.

3. De Smet PA. Health risks of herbal remedies. Drug Saf 1995;13(2):81–93.
4. Bell AJ, Duggin G. Acute methyl salicylate toxicity complicating herbal skin treatment for psoriasis. Emerg Med (Fremantle) 2002;14(2):188–90.
5. Botma M, Colquhoun-Flannery W, Leighton S. Laryngeal oedema caused by accidental ingestion of oil of wintergreen. Int J Pediatr Otorhinolaryngol 2001;58(3):229–32.
6. Chan TY. Potential dangers from topical preparations containing methyl salicylate. Hum Exp Toxicol 1996;15(9): 747–50.
7. Chan TY. The risk of severe salicylate poisoning following the ingestion of topical medicaments or aspirin. Postgrad Med J 1996;72(844):109–12.
8. Howrie DL, Moriarty R, Breit R. Candy flavoring as a source of salicylate poisoning. Pediatrics 1985;75(5): 869–71.
9. Chan TH, Wong KC, Chan JC. Severe salicylate poisoning associated with the intake of Chinese medicinal oil ("red flower oil"). Aust NZ J Med 1995;25(1):57.
10. Raz R, Chazan B, Dan M. Cranberry juice and urinary tract infection. Clin Infect Dis 2004;38(10):1413–19.
11. Jepson RG, Mihaljevic L, Craig J. Cranberries for preventing urinary tract infections. Cochrane Database Syst Rev 2004;(2):CD001321.
12. Kessler T, Jansen B, Hesse A. Effect of blackcurrant-, cranberry- and plum juice consumption on risk factors associated with kidney stone formation. Eur J Clin Nutr 2002;56(10):1020–3.
13. McHarg T, Rodgers A, Charlton K. Influence of cranberry juice on the urinary risk factors for calcium oxalate kidney stone formation. BJU Int 2003;92(7):765–8.
14. Davies JK, Ahktar N, Ranasinge E. A juicy problem. Lancet 2001;358(9299):2126.
15. Grant P. Warfarin and cranberry juice: an interaction? J Heart Valve Dis 2004;13(1):25–6.
16. Suvarna R, Pirmohamed M, Henderson L. Possible interaction between warfarin and cranberry juice. BMJ 2003; 327(7429):1454.
17. Isele H. Todliche Blutung unter Warfarin plus Preiselbeersaft. Liegt's an der Salizylsäaure. [Fatal bleeding under warfarin plus cranberry juice. Is it due to salicylic acid?] MMW Fortschr Med 2004;146(11):13.

Erythromycin

See also Macrolide antibiotics

General Information

For some decades erythromycin was the only macrolide antibiotic available, but with the development of new macrolides with remarkable pharmacokinetic and safety features (1), it has met fierce competition and has, at least in some health-care systems, lost its place as the most important macrolide.

Comparative studies

In a direct comparison of clarithromycin with erythromycin stearate, the rate of adverse events was 19% in 96 patients taking clarithromycin and 35% in 112 patients taking erythromycin (2). Most of the adverse events associated with clarithromycin affect the gastrointestinal tract (7%).

In a prospective, single-blind, randomized study of a 7-day course of clarithromycin (7.5 mg/kg bd) and a 14-day course of erythromycin (13.3 mg/kg tds) in 153 children with pertussis, the incidence of treatment-emergent drug-related adverse events was significantly higher with erythromycin than with clarithromycin (62 versus 45%) (3). Three subjects given erythromycin withdrew prematurely because of adverse events: one because of a rash; one with vomiting and diarrhea; and one with vomiting, abdominal pain, and rash.

In a double-blind, randomized, multicenter trial in 302 children, a 10-day course of erythromycin estolate (40 mg/kg/day in two doses) was as safe and effective as amoxicillin (50 mg/kg/day in two doses) in acute otitis media. Treatment-related adverse events occurred in 5.3% of patients given erythromycin and in 7.3% of patients given amoxicillin (4).

General adverse effects

Erythromycin is relatively well tolerated, with the exception of gastrointestinal adverse effects. Cholestasis resulting from the use of all forms of erythromycin is virtually the only serious effect. However, local irritation (affecting the gastrointestinal system, the muscles, or the veins, depending on the route of administration) is common. Erythromycin can increase serum theophylline concentrations and occasionally causes theophylline toxicity. Hypersensitivity reactions are rare, unless cholestasis is to be regarded as allergic. They probably have clinical effects in under 0.5% of treated patients, and consist mainly of maculopapular rashes, pruritus, urticaria, and angioedema; anaphylaxis and acute respiratory distress have also been reported. Fixed drug eruptions, urticaria, and Stevens–Johnson syndrome have also been reported.

Organs and Systems

Cardiovascular

Erythromycin has antidysrhythmic properties similar to those of Class IA antidysrhythmic drugs, and causes an increase in atrial and ventricular refractory periods. This is only likely to be a problem in patients with heart disease or in those who are receiving drugs that delay ventricular repolarization (5). High-doses intravenously have caused ventricular fibrillation and torsade de pointes (6). Each episode of dysrhythmia, QT interval prolongation, and myocardial dysfunction occurred 1–1.5 hours after erythromycin infusion and resolved after withdrawal.

In an FDA database analysis, 346 cases of cardiac dysrhythmias associated with erythromycin were identified. There was a preponderance of women, as there was among those with life-threatening ventricular dysrhythmias and deaths after intravenous erythromycin lactobionate. A sex difference in cardiac repolarization response to erythromycin is a potential contributing factor, since in an in vitro experiment on rabbit hearts, erythromycin caused significantly greater QT prolongation in female than in male hearts (7).

In 35 women and 28 men erythromycin caused QT interval prolongation after the first few doses of erythromycin (8). Similarly, in a prospective, comparative study in 19 patients with uncomplicated community-acquired pneumonia, a single dose of intravenous erythromycin 500 mg increased the heart rate and prolonged the QT interval. These effects were seen after 15 minutes of infusion and disappeared 5 minutes after the infusion had been stopped (9).

Owing to prolongation of the QT interval, a newborn with congenital AV block developed ventricular extra beats and non-sustained ventricular tachycardia after intravenous erythromycin; the QT interval normalized after withdrawal (10).

- Intravenous erythromycin (1 g 6-hourly by intravenous infusion over 30 minutes) resulted in QT interval prolongation, ventricular fibrillation, and torsade de pointes in a 32-year-old woman (6).

Intravenous administration of erythromycin into peripheral veins relatively commonly causes thrombophlebitis, although the lactobionate form of erythromycin may be less irritating to veins than other parenteral forms (11,12). In a prospective study of 550 patients with 1386 peripheral venous catheters, the incidence of phlebitis was 19% with antibiotics and 8.8% without; erythromycin was associated with an increased risk (13).

Respiratory

Adverse effects involving the respiratory system were reported in 2% of patients taking erythromycin stearate (2).

A beneficial effect of erythromycin on sputum volume has been reported in a patient with severe airways obstruction due to bronchorrhea (14).

Nervous system

In patients without neuromuscular disease erythromycin caused subclinical loss of motor unit contractions, which improved with intravenous edrophonium or neostigmine (15).

Sensory systems

Ototoxicity, resulting in hearing loss, and usually reversible, has been reported in patients treated with erythromycin lactobionate 4 g/day or more or large oral doses of erythromycin estolate (16). Ototoxic reactions have also been seen after the use of esters of erythromycin, such as the ethylsuccinate, stearate, and propionate (17). High parenteral doses of erythromycin have resulted in transient perceptive deafness (18–21). Since renal and hepatic disease was a prominent feature in these patients, ototoxicity was thought to result from high blood concentrations (22). Recovery occurred within a few days after withdrawal. The phenomenon differs from the permanent type of ototoxicity caused by aminoglycosides. Erythromycin should not be given together with other potentially ototoxic drugs and hearing acuity should be monitored during erythromycin therapy, especially in the elderly. Acute psychotic reactions have been related to ototoxicity and high-dose erythromycin therapy (23).

Psychological, psychiatric

Erythromycin has been associated with complications such as confusion, paranoia, visual hallucinations, fear, lack of control, and nightmares. These suspected psychiatric adverse effects were seen within 12–48 hours of starting therapy with conventional doses. Such complications may even be under-reported (23–26).

Gastrointestinal

Erythromycin is a motilin receptor agonist (27–29). This mechanism may be at least partly responsible for the gastrointestinal adverse effects of macrolides.

Pylorospasm and hypertrophic pyloric stenosis is associated with early postnatal erythromycin exposure and has been observed in neonates after 1–2 days of oral erythromycin therapy (30). The prominent gastrokinetic properties of erythromycin have been postulated as the mechanism (31).

- Pyloric stenosis has also been reported in a boy born at 23 weeks gestation, weight 690 g, after treatment of the child with three doses of oral erythromycin 10 mg/kg/day (32).

The use of erythromycin in postexposure prophylaxis for pertussis in 200 infants was followed by an increased number of cases of infantile hypertrophic pyloric stenosis, and all seven cases had taken erythromycin prophylactically (33). A case review and cohort study supported these preliminary findings (34). In a retrospective study in 314 029 children, very early exposure to erythromycin (at 3–13 days of life) was associated with a nearly eightfold increased risk of pyloric stenosis (35). There was no increased risk in infants exposed to erythromycin after 13 days of life or in infants exposed to antibiotics other than erythromycin.

Intravenous erythromycin should be restricted to as few patients as possible. It can cause severe abdominal cramps, probably by a direct action on smooth muscle (36–38).

Liver

Erythromycin can cause two different types of liver damage (39,40). Administration of erythromycin as base or salt can be followed in 0–10% of cases by apparently benign increases in serum transaminases, which may or may not recur on rechallenge. In children, raised transaminases were noted at dosages of 40 mg/kg/day but not 20 mg/kg/day.

Cholestatic hepatitis, which is associated primarily with erythromycin estolate, can be caused by all forms of erythromycin, including the base, estolate, ethylsuccinate, propionate, and stearate (39,41). Although it was originally speculated that a hypersensitivity reaction to the estolate ester rather than to the erythromycin itself was responsible for this adverse reaction (42), erythromycin does inhibit bile flow (43). Most probably the differences in hepatotoxicity between the various erythromycin derivatives are of a quantitative rather than a qualitative nature (44,45), perhaps because of better intestinal absorption of the estolate. Potentially severe but rare cholestatic liver injury occurs in perhaps up to 2–4% of treated patients. Erythromycin-induced cholestasis is rare in children under the age of 12 years, but has occurred in infants at 6 weeks of age, in whom it can mimic acute cholecystitis, biliary atresia, or neonatal hepatitis (46).

- A young woman developed severe cholestasis and jaundice after taking erythromycin stearate (47). A second severe episode of jaundice and malaise occurred after treatment with erythromycin succinate 2 years later pointing to erythromycin itself as the culprit.

The syndrome generally starts 10–14 days after the start of therapy, but earlier after re-exposure, sometimes within 12–24 hours (48). At all ages it often begins with abdominal pain, nausea, vomiting, pyrexia, pruritus, and jaundice; fever, rash, leukocytosis, raised serum transaminases, and eosinophilia can also occur. However, it can be ushered in with severe acute upper abdominal pain or right subcostal tenderness, simulating an acute abdomen, or it can resemble obstructive jaundice. Serum bilirubin, alkaline phosphatase, and transaminases are raised. Histological examination typically shows intrahepatic cholestasis and periportal inflammatory infiltration, with lymphocytes, neutrophils, and disproportionate numbers of eosinophils (49). These histological findings could be interpreted as reflecting a hypersensitivity reaction, but this hypothesis has been rejected (43). If erythromycin is promptly withdrawn, the clinical signs often improve rapidly, although prolonged jaundice has been reported.

Urinary tract

Acute renal insufficiency has been observed in a patient with Henoch–Schönlein syndrome (50). Another case presented as interstitial nephritis with acute renal insufficiency (51).

Skin

Topical erythromycin in benzoylperoxide, marketed for acne treatment, must be compounded by a pharmacist and requires subsequent refrigeration, warranting the development of alternative formulations. In a double-blind, parallel-group, multicenter study in 327 patients, a single-use erythromycin in benzoylperoxide combination package was compared with the vehicle alone and the original, reconstituted formulation packaged in a jar. Dry skin was the most frequently reported skin-related adverse event; it occurred in 3.2% of patients who used the preformulated erythromycin in benzoylperoxide and 5.0% of those who used the reconstituted erythromycin in benzoylperoxide (52).

A fixed drug eruption due to erythromycin has been observed (53). In another case skin tests with erythromycin were positive for the immediate and or delayed types of hypersensitivity (54).

- A 27-year-old woman developed urticaria 30 minutes after taking a single dose of erythromycin (55). An identical episode had occurred three years before. Erythromycin-specific IgE was detected in her serum by radioimmunoassay.
- Stevens–Johnson syndrome developed in a 64-year-old man who took erythromycin stearate for non-specific upper respiratory tract symptoms (56). After four doses of 250 mg, he developed a fever and typical lesions in the mouth and conjunctivae and on the lips. He was treated with prednisolone and recovered rapidly.

Second-Generation Effects

Teratogenicity

In a retrospective study there was no evidence of an increased risk of pyloric stenosis among infants born to mothers exposed to erythromycin during pregnancy (57).

Drug–Drug Interactions

Antihistamines

The association of ventricular dysrhythmias with co-administration of erythromycin and terfenadine (58) is thought to be due to inhibition of CYP3A4 by erythromycin. This combination should be avoided.

Erythromycin increases concentrations of astemizole (59). This combination should be avoided.

A double-blind, crossover study of the potential interaction between erythromycin and loratadine in 24 healthy volunteers showed that the AUCs of loratadine and its metabolite descarboethoxyloratadine were increased 40% and 46% respectively by erythromycin, but with no discernible effect on the QT interval (60).

Combined desloratadine 7.5 mg/day plus erythromycin 500 mg qds in 24 healthy volunteers was well tolerated and had no clinically important electrocardiographic effects (61). Although co-administration of erythromycin slightly increased plasma concentrations of desloratadine, this change did not correlate with prolongation of the QT interval, and there was no toxicity.

Benzodiazepines

Erythromycin can increase concentrations of midazolam and triazolam by inhibition of CYP3A4, and dosage reductions of 50% have been proposed if concomitant therapy is unavoidable (59).

Buspirone

Co-administration of erythromycin with the anxiolytic drug buspirone increased the plasma concentration of buspirone (62).

Carbamazepine

Erythromycin can cause acute carbamazepine intoxication, probably by inhibiting its hepatic metabolism (63). Erythromycin may also directly inhibit the conversion of carbamazepine to its epoxide. In a controlled study of the effects of erythromycin on carbamazepine pharmacokinetics in healthy volunteers, the clearance of a single dose of carbamazepine was reduced by 19% during erythromycin treatment (64). In contrast, the single-dose pharmacokinetics of phenytoin were not affected by erythromycin (65,66). After withdrawal of the macrolide, carbamazepine concentrations quickly return to normal (67). If co-administration of erythromycin and carbamazepine cannot be avoided, a dosage reduction of carbamazepine of around 25% should be considered, with careful monitoring of serum concentrations (59).

Cilostazol

When erythromycin was given to 16 healthy non-smoking male volunteers taking cilostazol, the C_{max} and AUC of cilostazol increased significantly by 47 and 73% respectively, and the unbound clearance of the major metabolite of cilostazol, OPC-13015, fell by about 50% (68).

Cisapride

- QT interval prolongation and torsade de pointes occurred after co-administration of cisapride and erythromycin 500 mg qds for 1 week in a 47-year-old woman (69).

Digoxin

The interaction of erythromycin with digoxin (70,71) is probably due to inhibition of its presystemic metabolism by inhibition of the growth of *Eubacterium glenum.*

Disopyramide

Disopyramide altered protein binding of erythromycin and this resulted in increased plasma erythromycin concentrations in vitro (72). The interaction between erythromycin and disopyramide was potentially fatal in two cases (73).

Ergot alkaloids

The interaction of erythromycin with ergotamine or dihydroergotamine can cause ergotism, sometimes leading to gangrene, by inhibition of the metabolism of the ergopeptides (74).

Felbamate

Erythromycin (333 mg tds for 10 days) had no effect on the pharmacokinetics of felbamate (3.0 or 3.6 g/d) used as monotherapy in epilepsy (75).

Halofantrine

Erythromycin inhibited halofantrine metabolism in vitro, suggesting that increased cardiotoxicity might be clinically important (76).

Lidocaine

Erythromycin can increase the plasma concentration and toxicity of oral lidocaine, as shown in a crossover study in nine volunteers who took erythromycin orally (500 mg tds) for 4 days and 1 mg/kg of oral lidocaine on day 4 (77).

Oral anticoagulants

Erythromycin can interact with warfarin, resulting in a modest increase in blood concentrations and a rise in the prothrombin time of around 8% (78).

Erythromycin may potentiate acenocoumarol anticoagulant treatment, as reported in a 68-year-old man on stable anticoagulation with acenocoumarol 3 mg/day who took erythromycin ethylsuccinate 1.5 g/day (79).

Quinidine

Erythromycin reduced the total clearance of quinidine, reduced its partial clearance by 3-hydroxylation, and increased its maximal serum concentration in an open study in 30 healthy young volunteers (80).

Quinine

Erythromycin is a competitive in vitro inhibitor of quinine 3-hydroxylation and may therefore interact with quinine (81).

Selective serotonin re-uptake inhibitors (SSRIs)

- A 12-year-old boy developed the serotonin syndrome, which is normally associated with the interaction of two or more serotonergic agents, after the co-administration of erythromycin and sertraline.

This could have been due to erythromycin-induced inhibition of sertraline metabolism by CYP3A (82).

Statins

It has been proposed that the risk of myotoxicity increases when statins are prescribed concurrently with erythromycin (83). There are no data for any pharmacokinetic interaction with fluvastatin or pravastatin, but as in the case of simvastatin the major route of metabolism of these drugs is by CYP3A4 and there is potential for an adverse interaction.

Atorvastatin

When erythromycin was co-administered with atorvastatin, the mean C_{max} and AUC of atorvastatin increased by more than 30% (5,84).

Lovastatin

Rhabdomyolysis with or without renal impairment has been reported in patients taking both erythromycin and lovastatin (85). The exact mechanism is unknown, but lovastatin is extensively metabolized by CYP3A4 and its metabolism may therefore be inhibited by erythromycin. The manufacturers have advised that careful monitoring is required when these two drugs are given together.

Simvastatin

A case-control analysis of 7405 cases and 28 327 controls suggested that concomitant use of simvastatin and erythromycin is associated with an increased risk of cataract (86). Studies in dogs have shown that some statins are associated with cataract when given in excessive doses (87).

Theophylline and other xanthines

Erythromycin can increase the serum concentrations of theophylline by 20–25%. However, patients with an average serum concentration of theophylline under 15 μg/ml will probably only experience a small increase in their serum theophylline concentration during erythromycin therapy, whereas patients with steady-state concentrations above 15 μg/ml deserve careful monitoring and close observation for symptoms of theophylline toxicity during treatment with erythromycin (88,89).

Tiagabine

Both tiagabine and erythromycin are metabolized by cytochrome P450. In an open, crossover study in 13 healthy volunteers, tiagabine (4 mg bd) and erythromycin (500 mg bd) were co-administered for 4 days (90). Maximum plasma concentration, AUC, and half-life of tiagabine were comparable when tiagabine was administered alone or in combination with erythromycin. The t_{max} was prolonged after administration with erythromycin in women; this effect may be due to a differential effect of erythromycin on gastric emptying. The interpretation of these findings is limited by the rather low doses of tiagabine used in the study and the short time of co-administration.

References

1. Schlossberg D. Azithromycin and clarithromycin. Med Clin North Am 1995;79(4):803–15.
2. Anderson G, Esmonde TS, Coles S, Macklin J, Carnegie C. A comparative safety and efficacy study of clarithromycin and erythromycin stearate in community-acquired pneumonia. J Antimicrob Chemother 1991;27(Suppl A):117–24.
3. Lebel MH, Mehra S. Efficacy and safety of clarithromycin versus erythromycin for the treatment of pertussis: a prospective, randomized, single blind trial. Pediatr Infect Dis J 2001;20(12):1149–54.
4. Scholz H, Noack R. Multicenter, randomized, double-blind comparison of erythromycin estolate versus amoxicillin for the treatment of acute otitis media in children. AOM Study Group. Eur J Clin Microbiol Infect Dis 1998;17(7):470–8.
5. Rubinstein E. Comparative safety of the different macrolides. Int J Antimicrob Agents 2001;18(Suppl 1):S71–6.
6. Orban Z, MacDonald LL, Peters MA, Guslits B. Erythromycin-induced cardiac toxicity. Am J Cardiol 1995;75(12):859–61.
7. Drici MD, Knollmann BC, Wang WX, Woosley RL. Cardiac actions of erythromycin: influence of female sex. JAMA 1998;280(20):1774–6.
8. Kdesh A, McPherson CA, Yaylali Y, Yasick D, Bradley K, Manthous CA. Effect of erythromycin on myocardial repolarization in patients with community-acquired pneumonia. South Med J 1999;92(12):1178–82.
9. Mishra A, Friedman HS, Sinha AK. The effects of erythromycin on the electrocardiogram. Chest 1999;115(4):983–6.
10. Brixius B, Lindinger A, Baghai A, Limbach HG, Hoffmann W. Ventrikuläre Tachykardie nach Erythromycin-Gabe bei einem Neugeborenen mit angeborenem AV-Block. [Ventricular tachycardia after erythromycin administration in a newborn with congenital AV-block.] Klin Padiatr 1999;211(6):465–8.
11. Washington JA 2nd, Wilson WR. Erythromycin: a microbial and clinical perspective after 30 years of clinical use (1). Mayo Clin Proc 1985;60(3):189–203.
12. Washington JA 2nd, Wilson WR. Erythromycin: a microbial and clinical perspective after 30 years of clinical use (2). Mayo Clin Proc 1985;60(4):271–8.
13. Lanbeck P, Odenholt I, Paulsen O. Antibiotics differ in their tendency to cause infusion phlebitis: a prospective observational study. Scand J Infect Dis 2002;34(7):512–19.
14. Marom ZM, Goswami SK. Respiratory mucus hypersecretion (bronchorrhea): a case discussion—possible mechanisms(s) and treatment. J Allergy Clin Immunol 1991;87(6):1050–5.
15. Herishanu Y, Taustein I. The electromyographic changes by antibiotics. A preliminary study. Confin Neurol 1971;33(1): 41–5.
16. Eckman MR, Johnson T, Riess R. Partial deafness after erythromycin. N Engl J Med 1975;292(12):649.
17. Schweitzer VG, Olson NR. Ototoxic effect of erythromycin therapy. Arch Otolaryngol 1984;110(4):258–60.
18. Brummett RE, Fox KE. Vancomycin- and erythromycin-induced hearing loss in humans. Antimicrob Agents Chemother 1989;33(6):791–6.
19. Haydon RC, Thelin JW, Davis WE. Erythromycin ototoxicity: analysis and conclusions based on 22 case reports. Otolaryngol Head Neck Surg 1984;92(6):678–84.
20. Huang MY, Schacht J. Drug-induced ototoxicity. Pathogenesis and prevention. Med Toxicol Adverse Drug Exp 1989;4(6):452–67.
21. Agusti C, Ferran F, Gea J, Picado C. Ototoxic reaction to erythromycin. Arch Intern Med 1991;151(2):380.
22. Quinnan GV Jr, McCabe WR. Ototoxicity of erythromycin. Lancet 1978;1(8074):1160–1.
23. Umstead GS, Neumann KH. Erythromycin ototoxicity and acute psychotic reaction in cancer patients with hepatic dysfunction. Arch Intern Med 1986;146(5):897–9.
24. Black RJ, Dawson TA. Erythromycin and nightmares. BMJ (Clin Res Ed) 1988;296(6628):1070.
25. Williams NR. Erythromycin: a case of nightmares. BMJ (Clin Res Ed) 1988;296(6616):214.
26. Murdoch J. Psychiatric complications of erythromycin and clindamycin. Can J Hosp Pharm 1988;41:277.
27. Lin HC, Sanders SL, Gu YG, Doty JE. Erythromycin accelerates solid emptying at the expense of gastric sieving. Dig Dis Sci 1994;39(1):124–8.
28. Hasler WL, Heldsinger A, Chung OY. Erythromycin contracts rabbit colon myocytes via occupation of motilin receptors. Am J Physiol 1992;262(1 Pt 1):G50–5.
29. Kaufman HS, Ahrendt SA, Pitt HA, Lillemoe KD. The effect of erythromycin on motility of the duodenum, sphincter of Oddi, and gallbladder in the prairie dog. Surgery 1993;114(3):543–8.
30. SanFilippo A. Infantile hypertrophic pyloric stenosis related to ingestion of erythromycine estolate: A report of five cases. J Pediatr Surg 1976;11(2):177–80.
31. Hauben M, Amsden GW. The association of erythromycin and infantile hypertrophic pyloric stenosis: causal or coincidental? Drug Saf. 2002;25(13):929–42.
32. Shiima Y, Tsukahara H, Kobata R, Hayakawa K, Hiraoka M, Mayumi M. Erythromycin in ELBW infants. J Pediatr 2002;141(2):297–8.
33. Centers for Disease Control and Prevention (CDC). Hypertrophic pyloric stenosis in infants following pertussis prophylaxis with erythromycin—Knoxville, Tennessee, 1999. MMWR Morb Mortal Wkly Rep 1999;48(49): 1117–20.
34. Honein MA, Paulozzi LJ, Himelright IM, Lee B, Cragan JD, Patterson L, Correa A, Hall S, Erickson JD. Infantile hypertrophic pyloric stenosis after pertussis prophylaxis with erythromcyin: a case review and cohort study. Lancet 1999;354(9196):2101–5.
35. Cooper WO, Griffin MR, Arbogast P, Hickson GB, Gautam S, Ray WA. Very early exposure to erythromycin and infantile hypertrophic pyloric stenosis. Arch Pediatr Adolesc Med 2002;156(7):647–50.
36. Tomomasa T, Kuroume T, Arai H, Wakabayashi K, Itoh Z. Erythromycin induces migrating motor complex in human gastrointestinal tract. Dig Dis Sci 1986;31(2): 157–61.
37. Omura S, Tsuzuki K, Sunazuka T, Marui S, Toyoda H, Inatomi N, Itoh Z. Macrolides with gastrointestinal motor stimulating activity. J Med Chem 1987;30(11):1941–3.
38. Lehtola J, Jauhonen P, Kesaniemi A, Wikberg R, Gordin A. Effect of erythromycin on the oro-caecal transit time in man. Eur J Clin Pharmacol 1990;39(6):555–8.

39. Braun P. Hepatotoxicity of erythromycin. J Infect Dis 1969;119(3):300–6.
40. Ginsburg CM, Eichenwald HF. Erythromycin: a review of its uses in pediatric practice. J Pediatr 1976;89(6): 872–84.
41. Ginsburg CM. A prospective study on the incidence of liver function abnormalities in children receiving erythromycin estolate, erythromycin ethylsuccinate or penicillin V for treatment of pneumonia. Pediatr Infect Dis 1986;5(1):151–3.
42. Tolman KG, Sannella JJ, Freston JW. Chemical structure of erythromycin and hepatotoxicity. Ann Intern Med 1974;81(1):58–60.
43. Lee WM. Drug-induced hepatotoxicity. N Engl J Med 1995;333(17):1118–27.
44. Funck-Brentano C, Pessayre D, Benhamou JP. Hepatites dues à divers derivés de l'érythromycine. [Hepatitis caused by various derivatives of erythromycin.] Gastroenterol Clin Biol 1983;7(4):362–9.
45. Inman WH, Rawson NS. Erythromycin estolate and jaundice. BMJ (Clin Res Ed) 1983;286(6382):1954–5.
46. Krowchuk D, Seashore JH. Complete biliary obstruction due to erythromycin estolate administration in an infant. Pediatrics 1979;64(6):956–8.
47. Horn S, Aglas F, Horina JH. Cholestasis and liver cell damage due to hypersensitivity to erythromycin stearate—recurrence following therapy with erythromycin succinate. Wien Klin Wochenschr 1999;111(2):76–7.
48. Eichenwald HF. Adverse reactions to erythromycin. Pediatr Infect Dis 1986;5(1):147–50.
49. Lunzer MR, Huang SN, Ward KM, Sherlock S. Jaundice due to erythromycin estolate. Gastroenterology 1975;68(5 Pt 1):1284–91.
50. Handa SP. The Schönlein-Henoch syndrome: Glomerulonephritis following erythromycin. Sth Med J (Bgham Ala) 1972;65:917.
51. Rosenfeld J, Gura V, Boner G, Ben-Bassat M, Livni E. Interstitial nephritis with acute renal failure after erythromycin. BMJ (Clin Res Ed) 1983;286(6369):938–9.
52. Thiboutot D, Jarratt M, Rich P, Rist T, Rodriguez D, Levy S. A randomized, parallel, vehicle-controlled comparison of two erythromycin/benzoyl peroxide preparations for acne vulgaris. Clin Ther 2002;24(5):773–85.
53. Pigatto PD, Riboldi A, Riva F, Altomare GF. Fixed drug eruption to erythromycin. Acta Dermatol Venereol 1984;64(3):272–3.
54. van Ketel WG. Immediate- and delayed-type allergy to erythromycin. Contact Dermatitis 1976;2(6):363–4.
55. Pascual C, Crespo JF, Quiralte J, Lopez C, Wheeler G, Martin-Esteban M. In vitro detection of specific IgE antibodies to erythromycin. J Allergy Clin Immunol 1995;95(3):668–71.
56. Pandha HS, Dunn PJ. Stevens–Johnson syndrome associated with erythromycin therapy. NZ Med J 1995;108(992):13.
57. Hussain N, Herson VC. Erythromycin use during pregnancy in relation to pyloric stenosis. Am J Obstet Gynecol 2002;187(3):821–2; author reply 822.
58. Wynn RL. Erythromycin and ketoconazole (Nizoral) associated with terfenadine (Seldane)-induced ventricular arrhythmias. Gen Dent 1993;41(1):27–9.
59. Amsden GW. Macrolides versus azalides: a drug interaction update. Ann Pharmacother 1995;29(9):906–17.
60. Brannan MD, Reidenberg P, Radwanski E, Shneyer L, Lin CC, Cayen MN, Affrime MB. Loratadine administered concomitantly with erythromycin: pharmacokinetic and electrocardiographic evaluations. Clin Pharmacol Ther 1995;58(3):269–78.
61. Banfield C, Hunt T, Reyderman L, Statkevich P, Padhi D, Affrime M. Lack of clinically relevant interaction between desloratadine and erythromycin. Clin Pharmacokinet 2002;41(Suppl 1):29–35.
62. Mahmood I, Sahajwalla C. Clinical pharmacokinetics and pharmacodynamics of buspirone, an anxiolytic drug. Clin Pharmacokinet 1999;36(4):277–87.
63. Hedrick R, Williams F, Morin R, Lamb WA, Cate JC 4th. Carbamazepine–erythromycin interaction leading to carbamazepine toxicity in four epileptic children. Ther Drug Monit 1983;5(4):405–7.
64. Wong YY, Ludden TM, Bell RD. Effect of erythromycin on carbamazepine kinetics. Clin Pharmacol Ther 1983;33(4):460–4.
65. Bachmann K, Schwartz JI, Forney RB Jr, Jauregui L. Single dose phenytoin clearance during erythromycin treatment. Res Commun Chem Pathol Pharmacol 1984;46(2):207–17.
66. Milne RW, Coulthard K, Nation RL, Penna AC, Roberts G, Sansom LN. Lack of effect of erythromycin on the pharmacokinetics of single oral doses of phenytoin. Br J Clin Pharmacol 1988;26(3):330–3.
67. Wroblewski BA, Singer WD, Whyte J. Carbamazepine–erythromycin interaction. Case studies and clinical significance. JAMA 1986;255(9):1165–7.
68. Suri A, Forbes WP, Bramer SL. Effects of CYP3A inhibition on the metabolism of cilostazol. Clin Pharmacokinet 1999;37(Suppl 2):61–8.
69. Kyrmizakis DE, Chimona TS, Kanoupakis EM, Papadakis CE, Velegrakis GA, Helidonis ES. QT prolongation and torsades de pointes associated with concurrent use of cisapride and erythromycin. Am J Otolaryngol 2002;23(5):303–7.
70. Lindenbaum J, Rund DG, Butler VP Jr, Tse-Eng D, Saha JR. Inactivation of digoxin by the gut flora: reversal by antibiotic therapy. N Engl J Med 1981;305(14):789–94.
71. Morton MR, Cooper JW. Erythromycin-induced digoxin toxicity. DICP 1989;23(9):668–70.
72. Zini R, Fournet MP, Barre J, Tremblay D, Tillement JP. In vitro study of roxithromycin binding to serum proteins and erythrocytes in man. Br J Clin Pract 1987;42(Suppl 5):54.
73. Ragosta M, Weihl AC, Rosenfeld LE. Potentially fatal interaction between erythromycin and disopyramide. Am J Med 1989;86(4):465–6.
74. Eadie MJ. Clinically significant drug interactions with agents specific for migraine attacks. CNS Drugs 2001;15(2):105–18.
75. Sachdeo RC, Narang-Sachdeo S, Montgomery PA, Shumaker RC, Perhach JL, Lyness WH, Rosenberg A. Evaluation of the potential interaction between felbamate and erythromycin in patients with epilepsy. J Clin Pharmacol 1998;38(2):184–90.
76. Baune B, Flinois JP, Furlan V, Gimenez F, Taburet AM, Becquemont L, Farinotti R. Halofantrine metabolism in microsomes in man: major role of CYP 3A4 and CYP 3A5. J Pharm Pharmacol 1999;51(4):419–26.
77. Isohanni MH, Neuvonen PJ, Olkkola KT. Effect of erythromycin and itraconazole on the pharmacokinetics of oral lignocaine. Pharmacol Toxicol 1999;84(3):143–6.
78. Bachmann K, Schwartz JI, Forney R Jr, Frogameni A, Jauregui LE. The effect of erythromycin on the disposition kinetics of warfarin. Pharmacology 1984;28(3):171–6.
79. Grau E, Real E, Pastor E. Macrolides and oral anticoagulants: a dangerous association. Acta Haematol 1999;102(2):113–4.
80. Damkier P, Hansen LL, Brosen K. Effect of diclofenac, disulfiram, itraconazole, grapefruit juice and erythromycin on the pharmacokinetics of quinidine. Br J Clin Pharmacol 1999;48(6):829–38.
81. Zhao XJ, Ishizaki T. A further interaction study of quinine with clinically important drugs by human liver

microsomes: determinations of inhibition constant (Ki) and type of inhibition. Eur J Drug Metab Pharmacokinet 1999;24(3):272–8.
82. Lee DO, Lee CD. Serotonin syndrome in a child associated with erythromycin and sertraline. Pharmacotherapy 1999;19(7):894–6.
83. Prieto JC. El perfil de seguridad de las estatinas. [Safety profile of statins.] Rev Med Chil 2001;129(11):1237–40.
84. Williams D, Feely J. Pharmacokinetic–pharmacodynamic drug interactions with HMG-CoA reductase inhibitors. Clin Pharmacokinet 2002;41(5):343–70.
85. Garnett WR. Interactions with hydroxymethylglutaryl-coenzyme: a reductase inhibitors. Am J Health Syst Pharm 1995;52(15):1639–45.
86. Schlienger RG, Haefeli WE, Jick H, Meier CR. Risk of cataract in patients treated with statins. Arch Intern Med 2001;161(16):2021–6.
87. Bernini F, Poli A, Paoletti R. Safety of HMG-CoA reductase inhibitors: focus on atorvastatin. Cardiovasc Drugs Ther 2001;15(3):211–8.
88. Zarowitz BJ, Szefler SJ, Lasezkay GM. Effect of erythromycin base on theophylline kinetics. Clin Pharmacol Ther 1981;29(5):601–5.
89. Paulsen O, Hoglund P, Nilsson LG, Bengtsson HI. The interaction of erythromycin with theophylline. Eur J Clin Pharmacol 1987;32(5):493–8.
90. Thomsen MS, Groes L, Agerso H, Kruse T. Lack of pharmacokinetic interaction between tiagabine and erythromycin. J Clin Pharmacol 1998;38(11):1051–6.

Erythropoietin, epoetin alfa, epoetin beta, epoetin gamma, and darbepoetin

General Information

Erythropoietin is an endogenous glycosylated protein hormone that is produced mainly in the kidneys and stimulates the production of members of the erythroid series of blood cells. Epoetin is the name that has been given to recombinant forms, of which there are four: epoetin alfa, epoetin beta, epoetin omega, and darbepoetin alfa. Darbepoetin alfa is a supersialylated form of erythropoietin with a longer half-life.

Uses

Recombinant human erythropoietin (epoetin and darbepoetin) provides effective therapy with a very favorable risk–benefit ratio in hemodialysis patients with end-stage chronic renal insufficiency, and in patients with progressive renal insufficiency who are not yet being dialysed (1). It improves cognitive function and the quality of life of patients with chronic uremia (2–5) and is very effective in children with chronic renal graft rejection and anemia (6). It also offers new opportunities for treating anemia in non-uremic patients. In patients with chemotherapy-induced anemia, epoetin increases hemoglobin concentration, reduces transfusion requirements, and improves quality of life (7,8). The response rate to epoetin in patients with multiple myeloma and anemia, which is 55–85% (9), increases when GM-CSF or G-CSF is co-administered (10). Epoetin is also approved for indications such as anemia induced by zidovudine in HIV-infected patients, the prevention of anemia in surgical patients, and anemia of prematurity (10,11). Treatment with epoetin results in a substantial improvement in the rehabilitation and quality of life of patients with cancer, AIDS, and rheumatoid arthritis (12).

Anemia due to prematurity can also be treated with epoetin. However, there are still questions to be answered about its efficacy, dosage regimen, and route of administration (subcutaneously or intravenously) (13,14). A comparison of the efficacy of daily versus less frequent dosing schedules in preterm infants showed that dosage regimens that achieve lower peak serum concentrations over a more prolonged period of time may be more efficacious (14). Although growth retardation in children with renal insufficiency does not improve (15,16), well-being, energy, appetite, and cardiac function are enhanced, and by obviating the need for regular blood transfusions, iron overload, allo-immunization to cellular antigens, and transfusion-transmitted viral infections are avoided (17).

Patients with cancer often develop anemia, and several studies have shown that recombinant human epoetin is a useful alternative to blood transfusion in such patients (18). Response rates of up to about 80% have been reported in patients with cancer-related anemia, especially in patients treated with platinum-based chemotherapy (18). Whether epoetin will improve tumor control after radiotherapy is being investigated (19). Epoetin corrects low hemoglobin concentrations, resulting in a better quality of life and probably improving cure rates in cancer patients undergoing radiotherapy (19). It also relieves symptoms of fatigue in patients with cancer (20,21), increasing hemoglobin and reducing transfusion requirements (22). No acceleration of tumor growth by epoetin has been observed (23). Epoetin has also been used in combination with G-CSF and amifostine or G-CSF and IL-3 as adjunctive treatment for cytopenias complicating myelodysplastic syndrome (24,25). Although these combinations are well tolerated, they promote hemopoiesis only in a subgroup of these patients.

Epoetin combined with parenteral iron is effective and safe for moderate and severe iron deficiency anemia during pregnancy (26), and iron supplementation is often required (27). The use of epoetin in combination with intravenous iron makes collection of larger numbers of autologous erythrocyte units feasible. However, epoetin does not synergize with G-CSF for the mobilization of peripheral blood progenitor cells in healthy donors (28).

Epoetin has been used to reduce allogeneic transfusion needs by increasing the efficacy of autologous transfusion for elective surgery (29). The combination of autologous predonation and epoetin treatment reduces blood requirements during and after orthopedic and cardiac surgery (30). In elective open-heart surgery, 26 of 30 patients who received only iron preoperatively needed blood transfusions compared with one of 30 patients who received iron plus epoetin (30).

While epoetin is not of benefit after autologous bone marrow transplantation, in patients receiving allogeneic bone marrow transplantation epoetin accelerates erythroid engraftment, increases hemoglobin concentrations, reduces requirements for erythrocyte transfusions, and shortens the time to transfusion independence (31).

The main limiting factor in obtaining an optimal response to epoetin is the adequacy of the patient's iron stores (32,33); the response is abated in the presence of iron deficiency, occult blood loss, hemolysis, and other hematological diseases (34,35). Other causes of an inadequate response to epoetin include concurrent infection or inflammatory disease (1), aluminium toxicity, vitamin deficiencies, secondary hyperparathyroidism (36,37), and osteitis fibrosa (38,39).

Pharmacokinetics

Subcutaneous epoetin in patients undergoing hemodialysis can maintain the hematocrit at a desired target range using an average weekly dose lower than with intravenous administration (40). Intravenous administration leads to higher initial epoetin concentrations compared with subcutaneous administration. However, after intravenous administration the half-life is only 4–5 hours, compared with 19–22 hours after subcutaneous administration (41).

Observational studies

In a prospective trial in 3012 patients, the clinical benefits and adverse events profiles were similar with once-weekly epoetin compared with historical experience with thrice-weekly dosing (42).

In 194 patients a low dose of epoetin beta before elective surgery was well tolerated and reduced the need for transfusions (43).

Effective epoetin treatment has been reported in a transfusion-dependent beta-thalassemia major patient: there were no adverse effects (44).

In four patients with chronic diffuse gastrointestinal bleeding that was difficult to control, epoetin was successfully used as a hemostatic agent (45).

Placebo-controlled studies

In a double-blind, randomized, placebo-controlled, multicenter study in 80 critically ill patients, epoetin led to a 45% reduction in the number of erythrocyte units transfused. There were no epoetin-related adverse effects (46).

General adverse effects

Both epoetin alfa and beta and darbepoetin alfa are quite well tolerated (47). Common adverse effects are infection, hypertension, hypotension, shunt thrombosis, myalgia, nausea, headache, and chest pain (34,48). After the first few doses of epoetin, flu-like symptoms occur transiently, with an incidence of 5.4–18% (34,49). These can be avoided by injecting epoetin subcutaneously rather than intravenously (31,33,50,51). It has also been suggested that such symptoms can be avoided by dose escalation, starting with an ultra-low dose (49). Subcutaneous injection can cause local reactions, probably due to allergy (52).

Darbepoetin

Darbepoetin alfa is a long-acting form of erythropoietin, with additional sialic acid residues, and does not require such frequent administration as epoetin; its long half-life allows administration once every 1 or 2 weeks (53).

The safety profiles of epoetin and darbepoetin are similar. Adverse effects of darbepoetin include hypertension, injection site pain (generally mild and transient) in the case of subcutaneous administration, cardiovascular events, headache, vascular disorders (vascular access thrombosis), flu-like symptoms, and skin rashes (20,53,54). Adverse effects such as hypertension and thrombophlebitis are observed in uremic patients requiring dialysis but not in patients with hematological malignancies (55).

Organs and Systems

Cardiovascular

In a randomized study of 180 patients with anemia due to hormone-refractory prostate cancer, who were treated with epoetin beta 1000 IU or 5000 IU subcutaneously 3 times a week for 12 weeks, cardiovascular events were more frequent with the higher dosage. Four patients had deep vein thrombosis and two had myocardial infarctions; all were taking the higher dosage. However, only one of the patients with deep vein thrombosis had a high hemoglobin concentration (21).

Hypertension

Epoetin causes or aggravates hypertension in about 20–35% of dialysis patients (56–60). It can be accompanied by encephalopathy or seizures (61). In 44 children with chronic renal insufficiency treated with epoetin 150 U/kg/week, hypertension was mostly observed in patients on hemodialysis (66%) compared with peritoneal dialysis (33%) and predialysis patients (16%) (62).

Several factors contribute to the development of hypertension. One is the loss of the hypoxic vasodilatory response, leading to an increase in peripheral vascular resistance (63), but more important is the rise in blood viscosity, which increases with the hematocrit in both normotensive and hypertensive individuals (64). It is still being debated whether hypertension occurs only in patients with pre-existing hypertension or in normotensive patients as well, but about 30% of all patients require increased or de novo antihypertensive therapy as they respond to erythropoietin treatment (65).

Hypertension after epoetin has mostly been seen in uremic patients (66). However, in two of 44 cancer patients treated with epoetin during cisplatin-containing chemotherapy, epoetin was withdrawn owing to hypertension (diastolic pressure over 100 mmHg) (67).

Hypertensive encephalopathy can arise in connection with the sudden and extreme rises in blood pressure that occur in some patients given epoetin (52,68).

- A 14-year-old child developed hypertensive encephalopathy, a known rare adverse effect of erythropoietin, after 2 months (69).

During an open, uncontrolled study in 22 patients with end-stage renal disease treated with epoetin omega there was one case of hypertensive encephalopathy (70).

Susceptibility factors

It is not clear why certain patients develop hypertension and hypertensive encephalopathy and others do not, but transfusion-dependent anemic patients with a low hematocrit (<20%) are particularly susceptible, as are those with previous hypertension and seizures. Careful control of blood pressure at the start of epoetin treatment and the use of low doses are therefore advised in patients at high risk.

If epoetin is given preoperatively without autologous predonation, there is an increased risk of hypertension, an increased risk of graft thrombosis and myocardial infarction in cardiac surgery, and an increased risk of venous thromboembolism in orthopedic patients (71).

Because of an increase in cardiac-related deaths, it has been recommended that in patients with congestive heart failure or ischemic heart disease the hematocrit should not be raised above 42% (3).

Mechanisms

One of the possible mechanisms of epoetin-induced hypertension is an imbalance of local endothelial factors, such as endothelium-derived relaxation factor and endothelin (61), a potent vasoactive peptide produced by endothelial cells (13), increased concentrations of which have been observed in adults with an increase in mean blood pressure of more than 10 mmHg. In contrast, in preterm infants receiving epoetin there were no acute effects of epoetin on endothelin-1 concentrations or mean blood pressure (13). When intravenous and subcutaneous epoetin were compared, only intravenous epoetin was accompanied by hypertension (57,61). Plasma concentrations of proendothelin-1 and endothelin-1 increased after infusion of epoetin only in patients with hypertension. In addition the molar ratio of endothelin-1 to proendothelin-1 was significantly higher in patients with hypertension than in patients without (61). The authors suggested that endothelin-1 converting enzyme may play a role in the pathogenesis of epoetin-induced hypertension (61). Studies in rats have confirmed that epoetin stimulates endothelin release and synthesis of vascular tissue (72). There is a relation between the dose of epoetin and post-dialysis blood pressure, but not predialysis blood pressure (57). Risk factors for the development or worsening of hypertension are pre-existing hypertension, the presence of native kidney, a rapid increase in hematocrit, a low baseline hematocrit, high dosages of epoetin, and intravenous administration (57).

Epoetin has vascular effects that can cause an imbalance between vasoconstrictor-proproliferative-proatherogenic factors (angiotensin, endothelin, thromboxane) and vasodilator-antiproliferative-antiatherogenic factors (nitric oxide, prostacyclin). These changes may be related to the occurrence or aggravation of pre-existing hypertension in humans and can cause vascular hypertrophy and potentially accelerate the development of atherosclerosis (66).

Adrenomedullin, an endocrine peptide with vasodilatory and natriuretic actions, is increased in patients with hypertension and chronic renal insufficiency. In 54 patients with renal anemia, treated with epoetin 6000 IU once a week, there was a correlation between the progression of renal disease and circulating adrenomedullin; however, there was no relation between adrenomedullin and epoetin-induced hypertension (73).

The induction of hypertension by epoetin has been attributed to increased blood viscosity after a rapid increase in hematocrit and a loss of hypoxia-induced vasodilatation (59). Another pathogenic mechanism for the induction of hypertension by epoetin is enhanced endothelin production by endothelial cells (59).

In 10 normotensive hemodialysis patients with severe anemia treated with epoetin there was increased adrenergic activity (74).

Epoetin-induced hypertension may be associated with an angiotensinogen gene polymorphism; the incidence of hypertension was increased in patients carrying a homozygous T on position 235 of the angiotensinogen gene (75). The authors speculated that erythropoietin causes a rise in blood pressure via the T allele, which influences components of the renin–angiotensin system, thereby stimulating production of angiotensinogen, which leads to hypertension.

Management

Blood pressure should be monitored during treatment (18).

Erythropoietin-induced hypertension can easily be treated by initiating or increasing antihypertensive medication (76). For example, two of 26 pregnant women treated with epoetin for iron deficiency anemia had worsening of mild hypertension, which was managed effectively with methyldopa 250 mg tds (26).

Antiplatelet therapy reduces the incidence of epoetin-induced hypertension in predialysis patients (60).

Vascular disease

There is an increased incidence of peripheral vascular diseases in diabetic patients who receive peritoneal dialysis and epoetin (4). In these patients the time to a first vascular incident is shorter, the number of vascular events is increased, and more hospital days associated with vascular disease have been reported compared with patients receiving peritoneal dialysis without epoetin (4). Significant risk factors for the development of peripheral vascular disease are epoetin therapy, epoetin dose, and smoking (4). Peripheral vascular disease may be related to increased blood viscosity or other changes in blood rheology (4).

Thrombotic events related to epoetin include vascular access thrombosis, renal and temporal vein thrombosis, transient ischemic attacks, and myocardial infarction (66).

Vascular access thrombosis has been reported in up to 26% of patients treated with epoetin alfa (3,34,38). Most of the failures occurred in polytetrafluoroethylene grafts. There was no comparison with patients not treated with epoetin. It has been suggested that the increased risk of extracorporeal circuit clotting and the higher heparin requirements during hemodialysis may not be due to a hypercoagulable state, but rather to an increase in erythrocyte mass and consequently in whole blood viscosity (66).

- A patient with end-stage renal disease treated with epoetin-alfa developed a dural sinus thrombosis (5).

It was postulated that it was caused by polycythemia, because the hematocrit more than doubled in under 2 months, reaching 0.55 (5).

Nervous system

Several neurological complications of epoetin, such as headache, seizures, visual hallucinations, transient myalgia, and hypertensive leukoencephalopathy, have been described (5,77).

Headache, probably due to intracranial hypertension, has been reported in 15% of patients with renal insufficiency treated with epoetin (23). Analysis of the safety of epoetin in cancer patients is often hampered by toxicity of the concomitant chemotherapy. In a prospective open study, three of 183 anemic cancer patients who did not receive chemotherapy complained of headache, possibly or probably related to epoetin (22). Complaints of dizziness and headache, possible due to epoetin, occurred in two of 44 cancer patients during cisplatin-containing chemotherapy (67).

Seizures have been reported in 2–17% of dialysis patients treated with epoetin (38,78). The mechanism is not known, but is most likely multifactorial, including increased peripheral vascular resistance, reversal of hypoxic vasodilatation, and a direct pressor effect of epoetin mediated by enhanced production of serum endothelin-1 (78). Seizures occur most often during the correction of anemia and are associated with a rapid increase in hemoglobin concentration and poor control of hypertension (38).

Reversible posterior leukoencephalopathy syndrome, in which imaging abnormalities are present in the parieto-occipital regions of the brain, is reversible after blood pressure control and withdrawal of epoetin (59,79). Monitoring of the blood pressure is indicated and the hematocrit should be increased slowly, with a target of not more than 30%. If hypertension and seizures are under control, epoetin therapy can be resumed (59).

Psychological, psychiatric

Visual hallucinations have been reported in patients receiving epoetin (59).

Endocrine

In two patients with non-insulin-dependent diabetes and uremia, glucose control deteriorated after the introduction of epoetin, requiring insulin therapy (80).

Hematologic

Iron deficiency is a common adverse effect (30%) in children with chronic renal insufficiency treated with epoetin, even with iron supplementation (62). In premature infants given enteral epoetin, there was a significant fall in ferritin concentrations despite iron supplementation (81), and there were increased numbers of hypochromic erythrocytes and soluble transferrin receptors (14). This implies that active erythropoiesis in premature infants causes increased iron requirements.

Erythrocytes

Worldwide, 112 cases of pure red cell aplasia have been reported after subcutaneous administration of epoetin alfa (especially Eprex) in patients with chronic renal insufficiency. In these patients, neutralizing anti-erythropoietin antibodies were detected (82–84); these antibodies cross-react with all other erythropoietin products. This adverse effect was probably restricted to patients with renal insufficiency because these patients had used subcutaneous erythropoietin for many years. The incidence was calculated as one in 10 000 patients after 1 year of use of erythropoietin.

In other reports from Canada and the UK, patients typically developed sudden worsening of anemia unresponsive to increasing doses of epoetin alfa or any other form of erythropoietin and became transfusion dependent (85). In patients who develop sudden lack of efficacy or worsening of anemia, typical causes of non-response (for example deficiencies of iron, folate, and vitamin B_{12}, infection or inflammation, blood loss, hemolysis, and aluminium intoxication) should be investigated. If pure red cell aplasia is suspected and no cause can be identified, erythropoietin antibodies should be sought.

The Australian Adverse Drug Reactions Advisory Committee has also received 12 reports of pure red cell aplasia associated with the use of epoetin alfa (Eprex) in patients with renal insufficiency (86). The patients were aged 28–76 years and the duration of epoetin alfa use, when known, was 4–13 months.

Janssen-Ortho Inc, in association with Health Canada, have issued a "Dear Health Professional" letter about the addition of a boxed section to the product monograph of epoetin-alfa (Eprex). The addition recommends that epoetin alfa should be administered intravenously rather than subcutaneously in patients with chronic renal insufficiency. This advice is based on the fact that most of the worldwide reports of pure red cell aplasia in patients treated with epoetin alfa have been associated with subcutaneous administration.

The suggested mechanism for these cases of pure red cell aplasia is an immune reaction that is probably induced by repeated, subcutaneous administration of a foreign protein, a biotechnologically processed erythropoietin. However, no antibodies toward darbepoetin alfa were detected in over 1534 patients treated for 2 years (87).

- A 70-year-old woman with a history of diabetes mellitus and renal insufficiency rapidly developed a severe anemia (with a hemoglobin concentration of 3.5 mmol/l). She had been treated with recombinant erythropoietin (4000 IU/week) for 6 months with an initial favorable response (hemoglobin concentration between 6.8 and 7.5 mmol/l) (82). Her bone marrow showed pure red cell aplasia with early termination of maturation. The dose of recombinant erythropoietin was increased to 8000 IU/week. She required 3 units of packed red cells per month.

This patient had developed antibodies against recombinant erythropoietin. After recombinant erythropoietin was withdrawn, the concentration of antibodies fell slightly. Because of persistent transfusion requirements, she received prednisone (1 mg/kg/day) for 6 months. At that time, antibodies against erythropoietin could not be detected anymore and the hemoglobin concentration was around 5.6 mmol/l.

Leukocytes

In neonates neutropenia has been described after treatment with high doses of epoetin. Neutrophil counts increased in these neonates after withdrawal of epoetin (88). Lymphopenia has been described (89), but the fall in lymphocyte count in patients with renal insufficiency is less significant. Pretreatment with imidazole-2-hydroxybenzoate, which inhibits the synthesis of prostaglandins, causes a less marked and delayed reduction of lymphocytes (89). However, neutropenia has not been noted in recent studies (14).

Thrombotic events have been reported in patients given epoetin (90,91), but there have been contradictory results on its effects on blood coagulation and fibrinolysis. There is currently no definitive evidence that epoetin further enhances hypercoagulability in uremic patients (66). In a prospective controlled study, epoetin for elective hip surgery did not activate coagulation and fibrinolysis (92). In 26 patients the effect of epoetin on hemostasis was minimal, with only a clinically insignificant fall in the total amount of protein S (93). In contrast to earlier studies, this study did not show changes in the number of platelets or platelet function. Regular epoetin treatment in 39 hemodialysis patients with anemia did not result in adversely high blood viscosity, and in an overview of data from 3000 patients there was no increase in shunt or fistula occlusion (94).

In a placebo-controlled study of severely anemic patients with low-grade non-Hodgkin's lymphoma, chronic lymphocytic leukemia, or multiple myeloma, a fatal case of pulmonary embolism was thought to have been related to treatment with epoetin beta (95). Thrombotic events, such as vascular access thrombosis, venous thrombosis, and pulmonary embolism, have occurred after treatment with epoetin or darbepoetin alfa (96). It is therefore recommended that a rapid rise in the hemoglobin concentration be avoided and that care should be taken that the hemoglobin concentration does not exceed 12.1 g/dl (7.5 mmol/l) (97).

In 173 renal patients with anemia, in which once-weekly administration of subcutaneous epoetin beta was compared with thrice-weekly administration, there were seven serious adverse events, possible related to epoetin beta (98). There were two cases of arteriovenous fistula thrombosis in the once-weekly group and three in the thrice-weekly group. A transient ischemic attack and a hypertensive crisis occurred in one patient in the once-weekly group.

Treatment of patients with sickle cell anemia has led to disastrous sickling crises (99), and there are at present no clinical data to support the use of erythropoietin in sickle cell disease (100).

Gastrointestinal

Of 183 anemic cancer patients who did not receive chemotherapy in a prospective open study, seven complained of nausea, possibly or probably related to epoetin (22).

Urinary tract

Because the erythrocyte volume increases under the influence of erythropoietin, the clearance achieved by the dialyser can fall, with a consequent increase in creatinine, potassium, and phosphate (101). However, earlier fears that the renal function of predialysis patients receiving epoetin might deteriorate prematurely have not been realized (65).

The use of darbepoetin alfa is associated with an increase in erythrocytes and a reduction in plasma volume, which can lead to reduced efficacy of dialysis (48).

Skin

Generalized skin rash and local swelling at the injection site have been reported after subcutaneous epoetin (8,20), as have urticaria and other skin rashes (48,102). Of 61 patients with malignancies of the oral cavity and oropharynx who were treated with epoetin before perioperative chemoradiation, one had a mild transient skin rash related to epoetin (103).

- Strawberry hemangiomas developed in a premature infant after 1 week of treatment with epoetin (104).

Strawberry hemangiomas are congenital vascular lesions characterized by endothelial hyperplasia during the proliferative phase. The development and proliferation of capillary endothelium requires the presence of angiogenic factors, such as vascular endothelial growth factor. Epoetin has a proliferative effect on endothelial cells and can induce angiogenesis (104,105).

- A rare case of generalized exfoliative dermatitis secondary to epoetin has been described (38). Epoetin was withdrawn and the lesions disappeared spontaneously after 20 days.

Hair

- At the start of treatment with epoetin alpha for anemia, a 60-year-old man with nephrotic syndrome developed reversible total alopecia (106).

Sexual function

- Veno-occlusive priapism occurred in a 25-year-old man with chronic renal insufficiency treated with epoetin. The episodes resolved after the epoetin dosage was reduced (107).

The exact mechanism of this adverse effect is not known. Several cases of priapism have been reported, and it has been hypothesized that androgen therapy probably contributes (107).

Immunologic

Occasionally low-titer antibodies have been reported in patients treated with epoetin (38,108). Neutralizing anti-erythropoietin antibodies have been found in patients with chronic renal insufficiency who develop pure red cell aplasia after subcutaneous administration of epoetin alfa (especially Eprex). This adverse effect was probably restricted to patients with renal insufficiency because they had used subcutaneous erythropoietin for many years. The incidence was calculated as one in 10 000 patients after 1 year of use of erythropoietin (82–84).

There is no evidence of antibody formation to darbepoetin alfa, probably in part owing to the fact that carbohydrate chains are rarely immunogenic (54,109,110). No antibodies to darbepoetin alfa were detected in over 1534 patients treated for 2 years (87).

An allergic reaction led to early termination of epoetin treatment in one of 26 pregnant women treated with epoetin for iron deficiency anemia (26).

Anaphylaxis has been observed after the administration of epoetin that contained bovine gelatine as a stabilizer (2). Antibovine gelatine IgE antibodies were found. No anaphylactic reaction was observed after the administration of epoetin that contained human serum albumin as a stabilizer in the same patient.

Body temperature

Of 183 anemic cancer patients who did not receive chemotherapy in a prospective, open study, four had fever, possibly or probably related to the use of epoetin (22).

Long-Term Effects

Drug abuse

Epoetin has been abused by athletes, increasing the risk of hypertension and disseminated intravascular coagulopathy (10). In athletes epoetin causes increased blood viscosity, which will further increase during dehydration, leading to risks of myocardial infarction, cerebrovascular accident, or encephalopathy (10). Epoetin induces accelerated fibrinolysis, and so epoetin doping can be detected by analysis of fibrin degradation products in urine (10). In addition, hypochromic macrocytes are increased (10).

Susceptibility Factors

Age

The adverse effects of erythropoietin in neonates are minimal compared with adults. There were no hypertensive effects reported and no effect on development and growth measured at 18–22 months (111). In a multicenter, randomized, double-blind trial in 21 anemic HIV-infected children, who were concomitantly treated with antiretroviral drugs, epoetin was effective and safe (112).

In 30 preterm infants epoetin 300 μg/kg three times a week for 4 weeks reduced transfusion requirements without problems with tolerability (113).

High doses of epoetin in children undergoing long-term hemodialysis is associated with increased heparin requirements during hemodialysis, suggesting that careful monitoring of thrombotic events, especially in small children who need catheters for hemodialysis access, is warranted (114).

Drug Administration

Drug formulations

In the past, subcutaneous epoetin alfa resulted in more pain than epoetin beta, owing to citrate buffer in the product. Although the formulation of epoetin alfa has been changed to a phosphate buffer, discomfort after epoetin alfa is still greater than after epoetin beta (115,116).

Drug administration route

Epoetin can be administered in four ways: intravenously, subcutaneously, orally, and intraperitoneally (37). The subcutaneous route is preferred in patients undergoing dialysis, because subcutaneous epoetin provides better long-term utilization and maintains the same hematocrit with 20% lower dosages than intravenous administration. After intraperitoneal administration the absorption time is prolonged and only 5–10% of the dose is utilized (37). Local reactions occur at the site of injection when epoetin is given subcutaneously (117), and local pain has been reported after the administration of citrate- or phosphate-buffered epoetin (117,118).

After subcutaneous administration the systemic availability of epoetin is not complete (20%) and lower plasma concentrations are observed than after intravenous administration. However, the apparent half-life of epoetin is prolonged after subcutaneous injection, and this allows the use of lower doses to obtain an equivalent hemoglobin concentration (38). Subcutaneous injections are more effective when given thrice weekly rather than once weekly (38).

Patients with a skin-fold thickness of less than 20 mm at the injection site have a mean reduction in the maintenance dose of 36% when treatment is changed from two injections a week to daily injections (119). In patients with a thin layer of subcutaneous fat, the diffusion distance of epoetin to bloodstream is shorter than in patients with a thicker layer of subcutaneous fat. Therefore, the diffusion time in lean patients is shorter and the increase in plasma epoetin concentration is more pronounced but of shorter duration after each injection. More frequent injections of reduced amounts of epoetin creates an absorption curve whose area is more congruent with the area of the therapeutic plasma concentration.

Epoetin can also be given orally in premature infants, resulting in a significant increase in plasma epoetin concentration, increased peak reticulocyte counts, and reduced blood transfusion requirements (62,81).

In children undergoing peritoneal dialysis, epoetin is usually given intraperitoneally, resulting in similar systemic availability and dosages compared with subcutaneous administration. A follow-up study is required to determine if the risk of peritonitis is increased by intraperitoneal epoetin (120).

Drug–Drug Interactions

ACE inhibitors

During treatment of renal hypertension or heart failure with ACE inhibitors the response to epoetin therapy is reduced; this can be avoided by the use of angiotensin-II receptor antagonists instead (39).

Moxifloxacin

Possible synergy between erythropoietin and moxifloxacin was observed in a patient with myelodysplastic syndrome who did not respond to erythropoietin alone (121).

References

1. Adamson JW, Eschbach JW. The use of recombinant human erythropoietin (rHuEpo) in humans. Cancer Surv 1990;9(1):157–67.
2. Sakaguchi M, Kaneda H, Inouye S. A case of anaphylaxis to gelatin included in erythropoietin products. J Allergy Clin Immunol 1999;103(2 Pt 1):349–50.
3. Mingoli A, Sapienza P, Puggioni A, Modini C, Cavallaro A. A possible side-effect of human erythropoietin therapy: thrombosis of peripheral arterial reconstruction. Eur J Vasc Endovasc Surg 1999;18(3): 273–4.
4. Wakeen M, Zimmerman SW. Association between human recombinant EPO and peripheral vascular disease in diabetic patients receiving peritoneal dialysis. Am J Kidney Dis 1998;32(3):488–93.
5. Finelli PF, Carley MD. Cerebral venous thrombosis associated with epoetin alfa therapy. Arch Neurol 2000;57(2):260–2.
6. Aufricht C, Marik JL, Ettenger RB. Subcutaneous recombinant human erythropoietin in chronic renal allograft dysfunction. Pediatr Nephrol 1998;12(1):10–13.
7. Barosi G, Marchetti M, Liberato NL. Cost-effectiveness of recombinant human erythropoietin in the prevention of chemotherapy-induced anaemia. Br J Cancer 1998;78(6):781–7.
8. Csaki C, Ferencz T, Schuler D, Borsi JD. Recombinant human erythropoietin in the prevention of chemotherapy-induced anaemia in children with malignant solid tumours. Eur J Cancer 1998;34(3):364–7.
9. Dalton WS. Anemia in multiple myeloma and its management. Cancer Control 1998;5(2 Suppl 1):46–50.
10. Veys N. Use and abuse of erythropoietin. Tijdschr Geneeskd 1998;54:1315–22.
11. Cazzola M. How and when to use erythropoietin. Curr Opin Hematol 1998;5(2):103–8.
12. Foa P. Erythropoietin: clinical applications. Acta Haematol 1991;86(3):162–8.
13. Cogar AA, Hartenberger CH, Ohls RK. Endothelin concentrations in preterm infants treated with human recombinant erythropoietin. Biol Neonate 2000;77(2):105–8.
14. Ohls RK. The use of erythropoietin in neonates. Clin Perinatol 2000;27(3):681–96.
15. Fischback M, Simeoni U, Mengus L, et al. Le génie génétique au service de l'anémi rénale. J Med Strasbourg 1990;21:433.
16. Watson AJ. Adverse effects of therapy for the correction of anemia in hemodialysis patients. Semin Nephrol 1989;9(1 Suppl 1):30–4.
17. Offner G, Hoyer PF, Latta K, Winkler L, Brodehl J, Scigalla P. One year's experience with recombinant erythropoietin in children undergoing continuous ambulatory or cycling peritoneal dialysis. Pediatr Nephrol 1990;4(5):498–500.
18. Engert A. Recombinant human erythropoietin as an alternative to blood transfusion in cancer-related anaemia. Dis Manage Heath Outcomes 2000;8:259–72.
19. Henke M, Guttenberger R. Erythropoietin in radiation oncology—a review. 1st International Conference, Freiburg, June 11–12, 1999. Oncology 2000;58(2):175–82.
20. Turner R, Anglin P, Burkes R, Couture F, Evans W, Goss G, Grimshaw R, Melosky B, Paterson A, Quirt I; Canadian Cancer and Anemia Guidelines Development Group. Epoetin alfa in cancer patients: evidence-based guidelines. J Pain Symptom Manage 2001;22(5):954–65.
21. Johansson JE, Wersall P, Brandberg Y, Andersson SO, Nordstrom L; EPO-Study Group. Efficacy of epoetin beta on hemoglobin, quality of life, and transfusion needs in patients with anemia due to hormone-refractory prostate cancer—a randomized study. Scand J Urol Nephrol 2001;35(4):288–94.
22. Quirt I, Robeson C, Lau CY, Kovacs M, Burdette-Radoux S, Dolan S, Tang SC, McKenzie M, Couture F; Canadian Eprex Oncology Study Group. Epoetin alfa therapy increases hemoglobin levels and improves quality of life in patients with cancer-related anemia who are not receiving chemotherapy and patients with anemia who are receiving chemotherapy. J Clin Oncol 2001;19(21):4126–34.
23. Beguin Y. A risk-benefit assessment of epoetin in the management of anaemia associated with cancer. Drug Saf 1998;19(4):269–82.
24. Musto P, Sanpaolo G, D'Arena G, Scalzulli PR, Matera R, Falcone A, Bodenizza C, Perla G, Carotenuto M. Adding growth factors or interleukin-3 to erythropoietin has limited effects on anemia of transfusion-dependent patients with myelodysplastic syndromes unresponsive to erythropoietin alone. Haematologica 2001;86(1):44–51.
25. Neumeister P, Jaeger G, Eibl M, Sormann S, Zinke W, Linkesch W. Amifostine in combination with erythropoietin and G-CSF promotes multilineage hematopoiesis in patients with myelodysplastic syndrome. Leuk Lymphoma 2001;40(3–4):345–9.
26. Sifakis S, Angelakis E, Vardaki E, Koumantaki Y, Matalliotakis I, Koumantakis E. Erythropoietin in the treatment of iron deficiency anemia during pregnancy. Gynecol Obstet Invest 2001;51(3):150–6.
27. Kaufman JS, Reda DJ, Fye CL, Goldfarb DS, Henderson WG, Kleinman JG, Vaamonde CA; Department of Veterans Affairs Cooperative Study Group on Erythropoietin in Hemodialysis Patients. Diagnostic value of iron indices in hemodialysis patients receiving epoetin. Kidney Int 2001;60(1):300–8.
28. Sautois B, Baudoux E, Salmon JP, Michaux S, Schaaf-Lafontaine N, Pereira M, Paulus JM, Fillet G, Beguin Y. Administration of erythopoietin and granulocyte colony-stimulating factor in donor/recipient pairs to collect peripheral blood progenitor cells (PBPC) and red blood cell units for use in the recipient after allogeneic PBPC transplantation. Haematologica 2001;86(11):1209–18.
29. Shapiro GS, Boachie-Adjei O, Dhawlikar SH, Maier LS. The use of epoetin alfa in complex spine deformity surgery. Spine 2002;27(18):2067–71.
30. Podesta A, Carmagnini E, Parodi E, Dottori V, Crivellari R, Barberis L, Audo A, Lijoi A, Passerone G. Elective coronary and valve surgery without blood transfusion in patients treated with recombinant human erythropoietin (epoetin-alpha). Minerva Cardioangiol 2000;48(11):341–7.
31. Klaesson S. Clinical use of rHuEPO in bone marrow transplantation. Med Oncol 1999;16(1):2–7.
32. Fischer JW, Bonner J, Eschback J, et al. Statement on the clinical use of recombinant erythropoietin in anemia of end-stage renal disease. Ad Hoc Committee for the National Kidney Foundation. Am J Kidney Dis 1989;14(3):163–9.
33. McMahon LP, Dawborn JK. Experience with low dose intravenous and subcutaneous administration of recombinant human erythropoietin. Am J Nephrol 1990;10(5):404–8.
34. MacKinnon GE, Singla D. Epoetin alfa in chronic renal failure. P&T 1998;23:437–46.
35. Jain AK, Bastani B. Safety profile of a high dose ferric gluconate in patients with severe chronic renal insufficiency. J Nephrol 2002;15(6):681–3.
36. Eschbach JW, Adamson JW. Anemia of end-stage renal disease (ESRD). Kidney Int 1985;28(1):1–5.
37. Morris AT, Ronco C. Erythropoietin therapy in peritoneal dialysis patients. Perit Dial Int 2000;20(Suppl 2):S178–82.

38. Cameron JS, Barany P, Barbas J, Carrera F, Chanard J. European best practice guidelines for the management of anaemia in patients with chronic renal failure. Working Party for European Best Practice Guidelines for the Management of Anaemia in Patients with Chronic Renal Failure. Nephrol Dial Transplant 1999;14(Suppl 5):1–50.
39. Schiffl H, Bergner A. Angiotensin-II, renal anemia and hyporesponsiveness to recombinant human erythropoietin. Int J Artif Organs 1999;22(10):672–5.
40. Kaufman JS, Reda DJ, Fye CL, Goldfarb DS, Henderson WG, Kleinman JG, Vaamonde CA. Subcutaneous compared with intravenous epoetin in patients receiving hemodialysis. Department of Veterans Affairs Cooperative Study Group on Erythropoietin in Hemodialysis Patients. N Engl J Med 1998;339(9):578–83.
41. Goodnough LT. Guidelines for the treatment of preoperative anaemia with epoetin. Biodrugs 1998;10:183–91.
42. Gabrilove JL, Cleeland CS, Livingston RB, Sarokhan B, Winer E, Einhorn LH. Clinical evaluation of once-weekly dosing of epoetin alfa in chemotherapy patients: improvements in hemoglobin and quality of life are similar to three-times-weekly dosing. J Clin Oncol 2001;19(11):2875–82.
43. Wurnig C, Schatz K, Noske H, Hemon Y, Dahlberg G, Josefsson G, Milbrink J, Hamard C; Collaborative Study Group. Subcutaneous low-dose epoetin beta for the avoidance of transfusion in patients scheduled for elective surgery not eligible for autologous blood donation. Eur Surg Res 2001;33(5–6):303–10.
44. Makis AC, Chaliasos N, Hatzimichael EC, Bourantas KL. Recombinant human erythropoietin therapy in a transfusion-dependent beta-thalassemia major patient. Ann Hematol 2001;80(8):492–5.
45. Zaharia-Czeizler V. Erythropoietin stops chronic diffuse transfusion-dependent gastrointestinal bleeding. Ann Intern Med 2001;135(10):933.
46. Corwin HL, Gettinger A, Rodriguez RM, Pearl RG, Gubler KD, Enny C, Colton T, Corwin MJ. Efficacy of recombinant human erythropoietin in the critically ill patient: a randomized, double-blind, placebo-controlled trial. Crit Care Med 1999;27(11):2346–50.
47. Nissenson AR, Swan SK, Lindberg JS, Soroka SD, Beatey R, Wang C, Picarello N, McDermott-Vitak A, Maroni BJ. Randomized, controlled trial of darbepoetin alfa for the treatment of anemia in hemodialysis patients. Am J Kidney Dis 2002;40(1):110–18.
48. Cada DJ, Levien T, Baker DE. Darbepoetin alfa. Hosp Pharm 2002;37:46–57.
49. Ohira N, Takasugi K, Takasugi N, Yorioka N, Ito T, Kushihata S, Takemasa A. Dose escalation induces tolerance to side-effects of erythropoietin in a patient with dialysis anaemia: case report. J Int Med Res 1998;26(2):102–5.
50. Freuken LAM, Koene RPA. Recombinant human erythropoietin and the effects of different routes of administration. Nephrologia 1990;10:33.
51. Winearls CG, Oliver DO, Pippard MJ, Reid C, Downing MR, Cotes PM. Effect of human erythropoietin derived from recombinant DNA on the anaemia of patients maintained by chronic haemodialysis, Lancet 1986;2(8517):1175–8.
52. Macdougall IC. Adverse reactions profile 4. Erythropoietin in chronic renal failure, 1992.
53. Ibbotson T, Goa KL. Darbepoetin alfa. Drugs 2001;61(14):2097–104.
54. Locatelli F, Vecchio LD. Darbepoetin alfa. Amgen. Curr Opin Investig Drugs 2001;2(8):1097–104.
55. Kasper C. Recombinant human erythropoietin in the treatment of anemic patients with hematological malignancies. Ann Hematol 2001;80(6):319–29.
56. Frei U, Nonnast-Daniel B, Koch KM. Erythropoietin und Hypertonie. [Erythropoietin and hypertension.] Klin Wochenschr 1988;66(18):914–19.
57. Ifudu O, Dawood M, Homel P. Erythropoietin-induced elevation in blood pressure is immediate and dose dependent. Nephron 1998;79(4):486–7.
58. Buemi M, Allegra A, Aloisi C, Corica F, Frisina N. Hemodynamic effects of recombinant human erythropoietin. Nephron 1999;81(1):1–4.
59. van den Bent MJ, Bos GM, Sillevis Smitt PA, Cornelissen JJ. Erythropoietin induced visual hallucinations after bone marrow transplantation. J Neurol 1999;246(7):614–16.
60. Kuriyama S, Tomonari H, Hosoya T. Antiplatelet therapy decreases the incidence of erythropoietin-induced hypertension in predialysis patients. Clin Exp Hypertens 1999;21(3):213–22.
61. Kang DH, Yoon KI, Han DS. Acute effects of recombinant human erythropoietin on plasma levels of proendothelin-1 and endothelin-1 in haemodialysis patients. Nephrol Dial Transplant 1998;13(11):2877–83.
62. Brandt JR, Avner ED, Hickman RO, Watkins SL. Safety and efficacy of erythropoietin in children with chronic renal failure. Pediatr Nephrol 1999;13(2):143–7.
63. Raine AE. Seizures and hypertension events. Semin Nephrol 1990;10(2 Suppl 1):40–50.
64. Levin N. Management of blood pressure changes during recombinant human erythropoietin therapy. Semin Nephrol 1989;9(1 Suppl 2):16–20.
65. Eschbach JW, Kelly MR, Haley NR, Abels RI, Adamson JW. Treatment of the anemia of progressive renal failure with recombinant human erythropoietin. N Engl J Med 1989;321(3):158–63.
66. Cases A. Recombinant human erythropoietin treatment in chronic renal failure: effects on hemostasis and vasculature. Drugs Today (Barc) 2000;36(8):541–56.
67. Savonije JH, Spanier BW, van Groeningen CJ, Giaccone G, Pinedo HM. Afname van de transfusiebehoefte bij oncologiepatienten door het gebruik van epoetine tijdens cisplatinebevattende chemotherapie. [Decline in the need for blood transfusions in cancer patients due to the use of epoietin alfa during cisplatin based chemotherapy.] Ned Tijdschr Geneeskd 2001;145(18):878–81.
68. Tomson CRV, Venning MC, Ward MK. Blood pressure and erythropoietin. Lancet 1988;1(8581):351–2.
69. Taylor J, Pahl M, Rajpoot D. Erythropoietin-induced hypertensive encephalopathy in a child: possible mechanisms. Dial Transplant 2002;31:170–88.
70. Sikole A, Spasovski G, Zafirov D, Polenakovic M. Epoetin omega for treatment of anemia in maintenance hemodialysis patients. Clin Nephrol 2002;57(3):237–45.
71. Faught C, Wells P, Fergusson D, Laupacis A. Adverse effects of methods for minimizing perioperative allogeneic transfusion: a critical review of the literature. Transfus Med Rev 1998;12(3):206–25.
72. Tsukahara H, Hori C, Tsuchida S, Hiraoka M, Fujisawa K, Mayumi M. Role of endothelin in erythropoietin-induced hypertension in rats. Nephron 1998;79(4):499–500.
73. Kuriyama S, Kobayashi H, Tomonari H, Tokudome G, Hayashi F, Kaguchi Y, Horiguchi M, Ishikawa M, Hosoya T. Circulating adrenomedullin in erythropoietin-induced hypertension. Hypertens Res 2000;23(5):427–32.
74. Ksiazek A, Zaluska WT, Ksiazek P. Effect of recombinant human erythropoietin on adrenergic activity in normotensive hemodialysis patients. Clin Nephrol 2001;56(2):104–10.
75. Kuriyama S, Tomonari H, Tokudome G, Kaguchi Y, Hayashi H, Kobayashi H, Horiguchi M, Ishikawa M, Hara Y, Hosoya T. Association of angiotensinogen gene polymorphism with erythropoietin-induced hypertension: a preliminary report. Hypertens Res 2001;24(5): 501–5.

76. Tong EM, Nissenson AR. Erythropoietin and anemia. Semin Nephrol 2001;21(2):190–203.
77. Anonymous. Erythropoietin (Procrit; Epogen) revisited. Med Lett Drugs Ther 2001;43(1104):40–1.
78. Beccari M. Erythropoietin-induced epilepsy in hemodialysis patients? Nephron 1998;78(3):354.
79. Rodrigo E, San Millan JCR, Heras M, Pinera C, Fresnedo F, Sanz De Castro S, Martin De Francisco YM, Arias AL. Posterior leukoencephalopathy in erythropoietin induced hypertensive encephalopathy. Neurologica 1999;19:360–4.
80. Rigalleau V, Blanchetier V, Aparicio M, Baillet L, Sneed J, Dabadie H, Gin H. Erythropoietin can deteriorate glucose control in uraemic non-insulin-dependent diabetic patients. Diabetes Metab 1998;24(1):62–5.
81. Ballin A, Bilker-Reich A, Arbel E, Davidovitz Y, Kohelet D. Erythropoietin, given enterally, stimulates erythropoiesis in premature infants. Lancet 1999;353(9167):1849.
82. Mercadal L, Sutton L, Casadevall N, Bagnis C, Jacobs C. Immunological reaction against erythropoietin causing red-cell aplasia. Nephrol Dial Transplant 2002;17(5):943.
83. Gershon SK, Luksenburg H, Cote TR, Braun MM. Pure red-cell aplasia and recombinant erythropoietin. N Engl J Med 2002;346(20):1584–6.
84. Casadevall N, Nataf J, Viron B, Kolta A, Kiladjian JJ, Martin-Dupont P, Michaud P, Papo T, Ugo V, Teyssandier I, Varet B, Mayeux P. Pure red-cell aplasia and antierythropoietin antibodies in patients treated with recombinant erythropoietin. N Engl J Med 2002;346(7):469–75.
85. Anonymous. Epoetin alpha. Reports of pure red blood cell aplasia. WHO Pharmaceuticals Newslett 2002;1:7.
86. Anonymous. Epoetin alpha. Pure red cell aplasia. WHO Pharmaceuticals Newslett 2002;4:7.
87. Anonymous. Darbepoetin alfa: profile report. Drugs Ther Perspect 2002;18:4–5.
88. Latini G, Rosati E. Transient neutropenia may be a risk of treating preterm neonates with high doses of recombinant erythropoietin. Eur J Pediatr 1998;157(5):443–4.
89. Buemi M, Allegra A, Corica F, Cavallaro G, Aloisi C, Pettinato G, Frisina N. Rapid and transient lymphocytopenia after i.v. administration of high doses of human recombinant erythropoietin. Hematopathol Mol Hematol 1997–98;11(1):13–17.
90. Koppensteiner R, Stockenhuber F, Jahn C, Balcke P, Minar E, Ehringer H. Changes in determinants of blood rheology during treatment with haemodialysis and recombinant human erythropoietin. BMJ 1990;300(6740):1626–7.
91. Macdougall IC, Hutton RD, Cavill I, Coles GA, Williams JD. Treating renal anaemia with recombinant human erythropoietin: practical guidelines and a clinical algorithm. BMJ 1990;300(6725):655–9.
92. Hasegawa Y, Takamatsu J, Iwase T, Iwasada S, Kitamura S, Iwata H. Effects of recombinant human erythropoietin on thrombosis and fibrinolysis in autologous transfusion for hip surgery. Arch Orthop Trauma Surg 1999;119(7–8):384–7.
93. Christensson AG, Danielson BG, Lethagen SR. Normalization of haemoglobin concentration with recombinant erythropoietin has minimal effect on blood haemostasis. Nephrol Dial Transplant 2001;16(2):313–19.
94. Silberberg J. Total correction of renal anaemia does not lead to adversely high blood viscosity. Erythropoiesis New Dimens Treat Anaemia 2001;11:25–6.
95. Osterborg A, Brandberg Y, Molostova V, Iosava G, Abdulkadyrov K, Hedenus M, Messinger D; Epoetin Beta Hematology Study Group. Randomized, double-blind, placebo-controlled trial of recombinant human erythropoietin, epoetin Beta, in hematologic malignancies. J Clin Oncol 2002;20(10):2486–94.
96. Hudson JQ, Sameri RM. Darbepoetin alfa, a new therapy for the management of anemia of chronic kidney disease. Pharmacotherapy 2002;22(9 Pt 2):S141–9.
97. Overbay DK, Manley HJ. Darbepoetin-alpha: a review of the literature. Pharmacotherapy 2002;22(7):889–97.
98. Locatelli F, Baldamus CA, Villa G, Ganea A, Martin de Francisco AL. Once-weekly compared with three-times-weekly subcutaneous epoetin beta: results from a randomized, multicenter, therapeutic-equivalence study. Am J Kidney Dis 2002;40(1):119–25.
99. Barber WH. Fetal hemoglobin and erythropoietin. N Engl J Med 1987;318:449.
100. Williamson PJ. Erythropoietin. Transfus Sci 1991;12:15.
101. Zehnder C. Erythropoietin treatment: influence of hemoglobin concentration on dialyser creatinine clearance in haemodialysed patients. 1996.
102. Terpos E, Mougiou A, Kouraklis A, Chatzivassili A, Michalis E, Giannakoulas N, Manioudaki E, Lazaridou A, Bakaloudi V, Protopappa M, Liapi D, Grouzi E, Parharidou A, Symeonidis A, Kokkini G, Laoutaris NP, Vaipoulos G, Anagnostopoulos NI, Christakis JI, Meletis J, Bourantas KL, Zoumbos NC, Yataganas X, Viniou NA; For The Greek MDS Study Group. Prolonged administration of erythropoietin increases erythroid response rate in myelodysplastic syndromes: a phase II trial in 281 patients. Br J Haematol 2002;118(1):174–80.
103. Glaser CM, Millesi W, Kornek GV, Lang S, Schull B, Watzinger F, Selzer E, Lavey RS. Impact of hemoglobin level and use of recombinant erythropoietin on efficacy of preoperative chemoradiation therapy for squamous cell carcinoma of the oral cavity and oropharynx. Int J Radiat Oncol Biol Phys 2001;50(3):705–15.
104. Leung SP. Multiple strawberry haemangiomas—side effect of rhuEpo? Acta Paediatr 2000;89(7):890.
105. Fabb SA, Dickson JG. Technology evaluation: AAV factor IX gene therapy, Avigen Inc. Curr Opin Mol Ther 2000;2(5):601–6.
106. Reddy V, Turney JH. Epoietin-alpha-associated total alopecia. Nephrol Dial Transplant 2001;16(7):1525.
107. Brown JA, Nehra A. Erythropoietin-induced recurrent veno-occlusive priapism associated with end-stage renal disease. Urology 1998;52(2):328–30.
108. Leikis MJ, Forbes IK, McMahon LP, Becker GJ. Resolution of pure red cell aplasia with continued production of low titer anti-epoetin antibodies. Clin Nephrol 2004;62(6):481–2.
109. Smith RE Jr, Jaiyesimi IA, Meza LA, Tchekmedyian NS, Chan D, Griffith H, Brosman S, Bukowski R, Murdoch M, Rarick M, Saven A, Colowick AB, Fleishman A, Gayko U, Glaspy J. Novel erythropoiesis stimulating protein (NESP) for the treatment of anaemia of chronic disease associated with cancer. Br J Cancer 2001;84(Suppl 1):24–30.
110. Heatherington AC, Schuller J, Mercer AJ. Pharmacokinetics of novel erythropoiesis stimulating protein (NESP) in cancer patients: preliminary report. Br J Cancer 2001;84(Suppl 1):11–16.
111. Ohls RK. Erythropoietin treatment in extremely low birth weight infants: blood in versus blood out. J Pediatr 2002;141(1):3–6.
112. Rendo P, Freigeiro D, Barboni G, Donato H, Drelichman G, Gonzalez F. A multicenter, randomized, double-blind trial with recombinant human erythropoietin (rhuEPO) in anemic HIV-infected children treated with antiretrovirals. Int J Pediatr Hematol Oncol 2001;7:235–9.
113. Bader D, Kugelman A, Maor-Rogin N, Weinger-Abend M, Hershkowitz S, Tamir A, Lanir A, Attias D, Barak M. The role of high-dose oral iron supplementation

during erythropoietin therapy for anemia of prematurity. J Perinatol 2001;21(4):215–20.
114. Seeherunvong W, Rubio L, Abitbol CL, Montane B, Strauss J, Diaz R, Zilleruelo G. Identification of poor responders to erythropoietin among children undergoing hemodialysis. J Pediatr 2001;138(5):710–14.
115. Cumming MN, Sharkey IM, Sharp J, Plant ND, Coulthard MG. Subcutaneous erythropoietin alpha (Eprex) is more painful than erythropoietin beta (Recormon). Nephrol Dial Transplant 1998;13(3):817.
116. Veys N, Dhondt A, Lameire N. Pain at the injection site of subcutaneously administered erythropoietin: phosphate-buffered epoetin alpha compared to citrate-buffered epoetin alpha and epoetin beta. Clin Nephrol 1998;49(1):41–4.
117. Raftery MJ, Auinger M, Hertlova M. Safety and tolerability of a multidose formulation of epoetin beta in dialysis patients. Collaborative Study Group. Clin Nephrol 2000;54(3):240–5.
118. Ruiz PG, Balcke P, Martinez JM, Harris K. Tolerability of the epoetin-beta multidose formulation (Reco-Pen) in patients with renal anaemia. Clin Drug Invest 2000;20:151–8.
119. Brahm M. Subcutaneous treatment with recombinant human erythropoietin—the influence of injection frequency and skin-fold thickness. Scand J Urol Nephrol 1999;33(3):192–6.
120. Kausz AT, Watkins SL, Hansen C, Godwin DA, Palmer RB, Brandt JR. Intraperitoneal erythropoietin in children on peritoneal dialysis: A study of pharmacokinetics and efficacy. Am J Kidney Dis 1999;34(4):651–6.
121. Fragasso A, Mannarella C, Sacco A. Response to erythropoietin and moxifloxacin in a patient with myelodysplastic syndrome non-respondent to erythropoietin alone. Eur J Intern Med 2002;13(8):521–3.

Esmolol

See also Beta-adrenoceptor antagonists

General Information

Esmolol is a beta$_1$-selective adrenoceptor antagonist with an extremely short half-life (about 10 minutes), because of extensive metabolism by esterases in blood, liver, and other tissues.

Organs and Systems

Cardiovascular

Esmolol causes hypotension, sometimes symptomatic, in up to 44% of patients (1–3).

Drug Administration

Drug administration route

Irritation at the infusion site occurs in up to 9% of patients and depends on the duration of the infusion (4).

Drug–Drug Interactions

Digoxin

Esmolol increased digoxin concentrations by 10–20% in healthy volunteers (5).

Morphine

Co-administration of esmolol with morphine resulted in increased steady-state concentrations of esmolol (5).

References

1. Benfield P, Sorkin EM. Esmolol. A preliminary review of its pharmacodynamic and pharmacokinetic properties, and therapeutic efficacy. Drugs 1987;33(4):392–412.
2. Gray RJ, Bateman TM, Czer LS, Conklin CM, Matloff JM. Esmolol: a new ultrashort-acting beta-adrenergic blocking agent for rapid control of heart rate in postoperative supraventricular tachyarrhythmias. J Am Coll Cardiol 1985;5(6):1451–6.
3. Morganroth J, Horowitz LN, Anderson J, Turlapaty P. Comparative efficacy and tolerance of esmolol to propranolol for control of supraventricular tachyarrhythmia. Am J Cardiol 1985;56(11):F33–9.
4. Angaran DM, Schultz NJ, Tschida VH. Esmolol hydrochloride: an ultrashort-acting, beta-adrenergic blocking agent. Clin Pharm 1986;5(4):288–303.
5. Lowenthal DT, Porter RS, Saris SD, Bies CM, Slegowski MB, Staudacher A. Clinical pharmacology, pharmacodynamics and interactions with esmolol. Am J Cardiol 1985;56(11):F14–18.

Esomeprazole

See also Proton pump inhibitors

General Information

Esomeprazole is the *S*-isomer of omeprazole. The pharmacology, pharmacokinetics, efficacy, and safety of esomeprazole have been reviewed (1). Esomeprazole produces acid control comparable to that of currently available proton pump inhibitors. It undergoes less hepatic metabolism than omeprazole, has an oral availability of 89% at a dose of 40 mg, and a half-life of 1.5 hours. Esomeprazole is well tolerated; its common adverse effects are diarrhea, headache, nausea, abdominal pain, respiratory infection, and sinusitis.

To assess symptom control, esomeprazole 20 mg on demand has been compared with placebo on demand (maximum of one dose a day) for 6 months in a multicenter, double-blind study in 342 endoscopy-negative patients with gastro-esophageal reflux disease (2). There was complete resolution of heartburn after 4 weeks of daily esomeprazole therapy. On-demand therapy with esomeprazole was significantly more effective than placebo in controlling symptoms. The frequencies of adverse effects and laboratory profiles were similar in the two groups when adjusted for the time spent in the study.

To examine the pharmacokinetics and pharmacodynamics of esomeprazole, 12 healthy men took once-daily esomeprazole 5, 10, or 20 mg, or omeprazole 20 mg for 5 days in a crossover study (3). The pharmacokinetics of esomeprazole were time- and dose-dependent. There was greater acid inhibition with esomeprazole than with omeprazole.

References

1. Kale-Pradhan PB, Landry HK, Sypula WT, Mena R, Perreault MM. Esomeprazole for acid peptic disorders. Ann Pharmacother 2002;36(4):655–63.
2. Talley NJ, Lauritsen K, Tunturi-Hihnala H, Lind T, Moum B, Bang C, Schulz T, Omland TM, Delle M, Junghard O. Esomeprazole 20 mg maintains symptom control in endoscopy-negative gastro-oesophageal reflux disease: a controlled trial of "on-demand" therapy for 6 months. Aliment Pharmacol Ther 2001;15(3):347–54.
3. Andersson T, Rohss K, Bredberg E, Hassan-Alin M. Pharmacokinetics and pharmacodynamics of esomeprazole, the S-isomer of omeprazole. Aliment Pharmacol Ther 2001;15(10):1563–9.

Estrogens

See also Individual agents

General Information

For a complete account of the adverse effects of estrogens, readers should consult the following monographs as well as this one:

- Diethylstilbestrol
- Hormonal contraceptives—emergency contraception
- Hormonal contraceptives—oral
- Hormone replacement therapy—estrogens
- Hormone replacement therapy—estrogens + androgens
- Hormone replacement therapy—estrogens + progestogens.

The physiological secretion of endogenous estrogens rises and falls during the monthly cycle; it is much lower before the menarche and after the menopause than during the period of fertility. Any use of estrogens that deviates from this pattern is therefore unphysiological.

Types of estrogen

The primary estrogen in premenopausal women is 17-β-estradiol (E2), which is synthesized by developing ovarian follicles. Estradiol is oxidized to estrone (E1) and then to estriol (E3). Estrone is also produced in peripheral tissues by aromatization of androstenedione, an androgen precursor that is produced by both the ovaries and the adrenal glands; after the menopause, estrone produced in this way becomes the predominant estrogen. All of the estrogens are sulfated and glucuronidated before excretion.

Natural 17-β-estradiol undergoes first-pass metabolism when given by mouth, and other compounds have therefore been preferred for therapeutic purposes. For the estrogen component of the oral contraceptives, mestranol (ethinylestradiol-3-methyl ether) was originally used, but since it was suspected of adverse effects it was by 1969 largely replaced by unesterified ethinylestradiol. 17-α-estradiol has also been synthesized (or extracted from pomegranates) and studied, but it binds much more weakly than the 17-α congener to estrogen receptors. 17-β-estradiol in micronized form, to improve systemic availability, has also been used in various products, especially in Scandinavia.

For estrogen replacement therapy, the less potent estrogens, estrone and estriol, have been widely used, as well as the semi-synthetic compound epimestrol.

In North America, much publicity has for many years been devoted to the supposed merits of "equine estrogens," also known as "conjugated estrogens" (Premarin), described as comprising a natural product extracted from the urine of pregnant mares. However, since pregnant mares were an inadequate source of starting material, these preparations have for a long time apparently been based primarily on synthetic substances (estrone with some equilin), although in some products a small amount of natural material may be present. The Food and Drug Administration in the USA long took the view that sodium estrone sulfate and sodium equilin sulfate were the sole active ingredients of the original product, but this was challenged by the manufacturers, who adduced evidence that dehydroestrone sulfate, and perhaps other components, could play a role. Overall, however, the view seems to be that the effects of Premarin are similar to those of other weak estrogens, whether given singly or in combination.

For injectable formulations used in estrogenic hormone replacement therapy, various esters of beta-estradiol have been most widely used.

Estradiol (E2) (rINN)

As noted above, 17-β-estradiol has hardly been used by the oral route, except in micronized form. The micronized product is also available in the form of an intranasal spray for the treatment of menopausal symptoms; this can give rise to mild irritation, leading to sneezing (1).

Estriol (E3) (rINN) and estrone (E1) (rINN)

Estriol is a very weak estrogen, usually given in oral doses of 1–2 mg/day, which has effects similar to those of ethinylestradiol at about 1/100th of this dosage: that is the vulva and vagina respond, but there is little effect on the endometrium. Similar considerations apply to estrone and to conjugated equine estrogens; most of the activity in the latter is in fact due to the presence of sodium estrone, which appears to be added to most formulations, in view of the limited supply of genuine equine estrogens.

Epimestrol (rINN)

The adverse effects of epimestrol (3-methoxy-17-epiestriol), a very weak estrogen with some ovulation-inducing effects, are largely as one would expect. In one series, hot flushes, insomnia, anorexia, nausea, and vomiting were reported in 1.5%, headache in 3%, and uterine bleeding in 38% (2). Ovarian hyperstimulation is rare but not unknown. As is usual with such treatment, the incidence of the adverse effects reported varies greatly, no doubt reflecting differences in the motivation of the patients and the schemes of administration used.

Ethinylestradiol (rINN)
Ethinylestradiol is discussed under hormonal contraceptives.

Fosfestrol (rINN)
Fosfestrol is an unusual agent used in Japan for the treatment of prostatic carcinoma but not accepted by experts in Europe. Described as an estrogen, in European studies it had a high incidence of complications, including fluid retention (16%), myocardial infarction (10%), and thromboembolism (6.3%). A case of adrenocortical insufficiency has now been documented in Japan, involving a 59-year-old man who had taken the drug for 10 years (3).

Quinestrol (rINN)
Quinestrol is an ether of ethinylestradiol. It is stored in body fat and hence acts for weeks or months after a single oral dose; in the event of adverse reactions, this makes prompt termination of exposure impossible.

Non-steroidal estrogens
The non-steroidal estrogens diethylstilbestrol (rINN) and cyclofenine (rINN) are covered in separate monographs.

Uses

Estrogens are used principally for:

- relief of the symptoms of the menopause
- treatment of postmenopausal vaginal atrophy
- contraception, in combination with a progestogen
- hormone replacement therapy, alone or in combination with a progestogen, an androgen, or both.

Hormone replacement therapy should be distinguished from the short-term therapeutic use of estrogen (or hormonal combinations) around the time of the climacteric for the relief of acute (primarily vasomotor) symptoms; such treatment can generally be limited to some 6–12 months although if it is then withdrawn the symptoms may recur (4). Confusion between these two forms of treatment has led to a series of misunderstandings regarding the adverse effects of true hormone replacement therapy.

Oral contraception and hormone replacement therapy are dealt with specifically in separate monographs. Here the general adverse effects of estrogens for any indication are reviewed.

"Equine estrogens" (Premarin)

The controversy regarding the composition of Premarin and what are regarded as its generic equivalents has been outlined above. While still in use for hormone replacement therapy, these products have also been used as a means of reducing unwanted bleeding, for example in uremia (5,6), although their efficacy has been challenged. Estrogens have also been used in the treatment of bleeding in hereditary hemorrhagic telangiectasia (7,8).

General adverse effects

Salt and water retention due to estrogens can cause weight gain and a rise in blood pressure. Changes in liver function tests can occur and jaundice is sometimes seen. Mild gastrointestinal upsets are not unusual. Unwanted endocrine effects include uncomfortable stimulation of the breasts and endometrial bleeding. In men, estrogens produce gynecomastia. Hypersensitivity reactions are rare and include urticaria, edema, and bronchospasm.

Estrogens can be associated with endometrial carcinoma, liver tumors, and breast tumors; they can also promote the further growth of pre-existing estrogen-dependent tumors.

When conjugated estrogens are used to control bleeding they are generally given only in short courses and are therefore well tolerated. As recommendations for control of bleeding involve administration of Premarin on a limited number of occasions (no more than five or seven doses) the usual hormonal problems associated with estrogens will be avoided. Gross hepatic disease is regarded as a contraindication. Headache, flushing, and nausea have been observed after intravenous injections and slow injection is therefore recommended.

Men taking estrogens generally do so in the course of palliative treatment for malignancies (prostatic carcinoma), for which high doses have sometimes been used. Estrogen therapy in men with prostate cancer may be superior to castration in terms of efficacy, but orally administered estrogens are associated with adverse effects: gynecomastia, loss of sexual function, and unacceptable cardiovascular toxicity (9). Low-dose estrogens in combination with anti-androgens or antithrombotic agents may be better tolerated.

Estrogenic effects of non-estrogens

Over the last 50 years, it has been realized that environmental chemicals, such as pesticides and industrial chemicals, can have hormone-like effects in wildlife and humans (10). These chemicals may:

- mimic the effect of endogenous hormones
- antagonize the effect of endogenous hormones
- alter the synthesis and metabolism of endogenous hormones
- alter the synthesis and metabolism of hormone receptors.

There have been reports that aviation crop dusters handling DDT had reduced sperm counts and workers at a plant producing the insecticide kepone had reduced libido, became impotent, and had low sperm counts. Subsequently, animal experiments showed that these pesticides have estrogen-like activity. Man-made compounds used in the manufacture of plastics interfered with experiments on natural estrogens. Some detergents and antioxidants are not themselves estrogenic, but on degradation during sewage treatment can release estrogenic alkyl phenols, such as bisphenol-A, nonylphenol, and phenylphenols. Polycarbonate flasks release bisphenol-A, which can also contaminate the contents of canned food in which polycarbonate coatings are used; bisphenol-A is also used in dental sealants and composites and can leach from teeth into saliva. Polystyrene tubes can release nonylphenol. The surfactant nonoxynol is used as intravaginal spermicide and condom lubricant; in animals it is metabolized to free nonylphenol. Other xeno-estrogens include the plasticizers benzylbutylphthalate and dibutylphthalate, the antioxidant butylhydroxyanisole, the rubber additive *para*-phenylphenol, and the disinfectant *ortho*-phenylphenol.

Organs and Systems

Cardiovascular

Estrogens have both wanted and unwanted effects on the cardiovascular system, depending on the manner in which they are used. Hormone replacement therapy is used in the hope of reducing the risk of ischemic heart disease after the menopause. The reduction in risk may be as much as 50% and is attributed variously to vasodilatation mediated by the endothelial production of prostaglandin I_2 (prostacyclin), effects on coagulation factors and endothelial function, and improvements in serum lipids (increased concentrations of HDL cholesterol and reduced concentrations of LDL and total cholesterol) (11), but variable effects on triglycerides. However, estrogens (especially as used in contraception but also postmenopausally) can have a marked effect on clotting factors and renin substrate, increasing the risk of thromboembolism.

The Coronary Drug Project in men taking different doses of estrogens showed a dose-related increase in myocardial infarction and thromboembolic diseases (12).

Respiratory

Allergic bronchospasm occurs very rarely with estrogens (13), but has been reported several times in women with an existing allergic tendency or a history of asthma; some asthmatic women have worse symptoms during the luteal phase of the menstrual cycle. In affected cases, the link with estrogens can be demonstrated by rechallenge.

Nervous system

Various types of headache can occur; in patients with migraine, attacks can be precipitated, usually with prominent visual phenomena.

- In a woman with history of chorea in the distant past, a vaginal cream containing estrogens precipitated an attack.

In a randomized, double-blind, placebo-controlled arm of the Women's Health Initiative, 10 739 postmenopausal women, aged 50–79 years, with prior hysterectomies, were randomly assigned to receive either conjugated equine estrogen 0.625 mg/day or placebo. There was an increased risk of stroke (RR = 1.39; 95% CI = 1.10, 1.77).

Sensory systems

Retinal vein occlusion (14–17), retinal artery occlusion (18), and optic neuritis (19,20) have been described in women taking estrogens.

In older women, estrogens cause a slight rise in intraocular pressure (SED-12, 1031) (21).

Psychological, psychiatric

The effects of estrogens on mood tend to be positive, and improved performance in intellectual tests has been described (SEDA-20, 382) (22); this is in parallel with the known effects of endogenous estrogens. During the menopause some women become depressed and irritable, and the ability of estrogens to correct this has been delineated in various studies, including work with estradiol given transdermally (23). Some workers also claim increased vigilance, and have concluded that this is reflected in encephalographic changes. There is even some evidence of an improvement in mental balance and self-control when estrogens are given to demented and aggressive old people of both sexes (24). However, all of these effects of estrogens on mood or mental performance are only likely to last for as long as the treatment does, and the effects on mood may occur only at the start of treatment; altered mood can follow acute withdrawal.

Endocrine

In postmenopausal women taking long-term mestranol there was a fall in the serum concentration of unbound (free) thyroxine, but it was not associated with hypothyroidism; the serum concentration of thyroid-stimulating hormone was unchanged (25).

Metabolism

Conflicting data concerning the effects of oral contraceptives on carbohydrate metabolism have been presented; the effects are probably clinically insignificant. However, estrogen hormone replacement therapy with a sequential-type product containing mestranol and norethisterone caused significantly impaired glucose tolerance (26).

There is no doubt that with appropriate treatment regimens, altered lipid metabolism due to estrogens can improve (27). In women with familial hypertriglyceridemia or increased triglycerides from other causes, oral estrogens can increase triglyceride concentrations. However, transdermal estrogens can lower triglycerides and generally produce smaller changes in lipoproteins than oral therapy, although it may be that whatever differences are observed merely reflect differing degrees of absorption.

Porphyria can be precipitated by estrogens, and familial porphyria cutanea tarda can become manifest (28).

Metal metabolism

Estrogens increase serum copper concentrations (SED-12, 1030) (29).

Fluid balance

Retention of water and salt and consequent weight gain are common during estrogen therapy. Fluid retention can cause a feeling of abdominal pressure, sensations resembling the premenstrual syndrome, breast tenderness, bloating, and edema. These symptoms can largely be relieved by a mild diuretic, but it is only practicable to use this approach if the estrogen treatment is cyclical and the symptoms thus intermittent, since it is undesirable to give diuretics continuously to healthy women over a long period of time.

Hematologic

There is a risk of thrombosis with estrogens, discussed in detail in the monograph on Hormonal contraception. Both superficial and deep complications can occur in either sex. Effects on clotting factors and renin are involved: in one small study, men taking estrogens had increased concentrations of factor VII, factor VIII, and fibrinogen, pointing to a hypercoagulable state and platelet activation (30).

In hormone replacement therapy, the risk of deep vein thrombosis is increased by a factor of 2–4 (31–33). The absolute increase in the treated population as a whole is low, with about one case of venous thromboembolism in 5000 women-years of use of hormone replacement therapy. However, in the subgroup with pre-existing risk factors, such as obesity, varicose veins, smoking, and a prior history of venous thromboembolism or superficial thrombophlebitis, the increase in risk from hormone replacement therapy can be substantial; among these women are those with a genetic predisposition to thrombosis, generally due to some form of thrombophilia, such as deficiency of the coagulation inhibitors protein S, protein C, or antithrombin III. In any of these subjects thrombosis can occur early in hormone replacement therapy. However, this tendency to early occurrence of deep vein thrombosis also seems to be present in all those who take hormone replacement therapy.

The mechanisms of thrombotic complications are multiple. Fibrinolytic activity falls in postmenopausal women when a high dose (250 micrograms/day) of ethinylestradiol is given for 10 days in preparation for prolapse operation (34). On the other hand, long-term administration of mestranol 80 micrograms/day to postmenopausal women for 1 year or longer increased the concentrations of fibrinogen and l-trypsin inhibitor and reduced plasminogen (SED-12, 1030) (35). There is also evidence that even low doses of oral estrogens increase the amount of thrombin generated in vivo.

It has been suggested, on the basis of a case of multiple systemic arterial thrombi in a patient with a prosthetic heart valve, that if estrogens are needed in such individuals they should be combined with anticoagulants. One would be inclined to extend the warning: any woman with a pre-existing risk of thrombosis should be examined very carefully before deciding to give estrogens at all.

The hypercoagulability that can occur with conjugated estrogens has been reported to be less pronounced than with oral contraceptives, but it is not clear that it is less than that seen with other types of estrogen used in hormone replacement therapy (36). The hematological effects of different estrogens are additive; various reports have demonstrated this for ethinylestradiol and diethylstilbestrol (37), which would mean that nothing would be gained by using several estrogens in parallel at reduced doses.

Some work suggests that when estrogens are given parenterally or transdermally rather than orally, the unwanted effects on the clotting process are reduced (38). The most important pharmacokinetic difference is that first-pass metabolism in the liver is avoided in all forms of non-oral therapy, which in the case of estrogens includes percutaneous gels, implants into the abdominal wall or buttocks, transdermal patches, and vaginal tablets, rings, and creams. It may therefore be prudent to use transdermal estrogens or another form of parenteral therapy when seeking to prevent osteoporosis in women with a tendency to thrombosis or hypertension.

For reasons that are not clear, other facets of the blood system are also affected by estrogens. After 6-months treatment with low doses of conjugated estrogens, hemoglobin concentration and mean erythrocyte counts were significantly reduced (39); on the other hand, the hematocrit was significantly increased by high-dose estrogen + androgen at 6 months, while the mean white blood cell count was significantly increased by low-dose estrogen + androgen at 12 months (39).

Mesenteric venous thrombosis has been reported in men taking estrogen therapy for carcinoma of the prostate (SED-12, 1032) (40).

Gastrointestinal

Estrogens can cause dose-related nausea, which is not reduced by using enteric-coated tablets. It has been claimed that there is a significantly lower incidence of nausea with estrogen + androgen than with conjugated estrogens.

Intestinal ischemia has occasionally been attributed to conjugated estrogens (22,41).

There is some reason to distinguish this from the ischemia that can be caused by oral contraceptives, in that it is restricted to the colon, can have a chronic or remitting course, can present with non-specific abdominal and colonic symptoms, can be reversible despite continued use of estrogen, and does not require surgical treatment. The symptoms of intestinal ischemia resolve within days to weeks after withdrawal of the estrogen. However, oral contraceptives have also been reported to cause ischemic colitis.

- A 19-year-old woman developed abdominal cramps, nausea, vomiting, diarrhea, and rectal bleeding (42). She was taking no medications other than Norinyl-2 (norethindrone 2 mg and mestranol 1 mg), which she had taken for 6 months. Just before the onset of the symptoms she had taken dimenhydrinate 100 mg and two ExLax tablets (90 mg of phenolphthalein) for constipation. Colonic X-rays showed impaired mesenteric circulation and bowel ischemia. Her symptoms subsided within 96 hours of withdrawing the oral contraceptive and giving supportive therapy (including intravenous fluid infusion, nasogastric suction, analgesics, and antiemetics). Further radiology showed that the ischemia had resolved.

Estrogens can cause or aggravate constipation (43), but when it occurs it is more likely to be due to the calcium carbonate that many women take as a daily supplement in postmenopausal treatment.

Liver

Changes in liver function tests can occur during estrogen treatment (44). In one comparative study, ethinylestradiol had an unfavorable effect on liver protein synthesis (SED-12, 1030) (45).

Cholestatic jaundice has often been reported with oral estrogens and is probably related to an effect on the permeability of the canalicular membrane (SEDA-20, 381). Cholestatic jaundice induced by a subcutaneous estrogen implant has also been reported in the absence of any other cause of liver disease (SEDA-20, 381). After removal of the implant the patient's symptoms resolved. The authors' explanation was that fragmentation of the implant had led to release of excessive amounts of estradiol.

The effects of estrogens on liver function differ with the type of estrogen used, problems being particularly associated with 17-substituted steroids. Significant reductions in transaminases, lactate dehydrogenase, and alkaline phosphatase have been found at 6 and 12 months with various forms of estrogen therapy. A reduction in mean bilirubin concentration has been described at 6 months with high-dose conjugated estrogens, and a significant increase in mean bilirubin concentration with low-dose estrogen + androgen at 12 months.

In some studies, women taking estradiol or conjugated estrogens for hormone replacement therapy had no cholestasis or hepatotoxicity, as assessed by rises in serum alkaline phosphatase, bilirubin, or transaminases, whereas these effects did occur with ethinylestradiol.

Pancreas

There is a small but significant risk of acute pancreatitis at 2–78 weeks after the start of hormone replacement therapy; the pain usually abates within 10 days of withdrawal (46).

Urinary tract

In the past, hypernephroma was thought to result from estrogen treatment. However, there is no clear evidence that this is so. There is evidence that older women with an intact uterus become more susceptible to urinary tract infections by taking estrogens (47). This is surprising, since some other studies, admittedly in selected patients, have shown a reduction in such infections when hormone replacement therapy is used. In another study, hormone replacement therapy improved urinary incontinence and nocturia after 6 months in postmenopausal women, without affecting bacteriuria (48).

Skin

Diffuse prickly erythema has been attributed to ethinylestradiol in various oral contraceptive formulations.

- A woman taking an oral contraceptive (Marvelon, ethinylestradiol 30 micrograms + desogestrel 150 micrograms) developed diffuse prickly erythema in an exposed site less than 20 minutes after sun exposure (49). Phototesting showed photosensitivity in the UVB and UVA ranges, but routine patch and photopatch tests with Marvelon were negative. All abnormal findings reversed 4 months after withdrawal of the oral contraceptive, but reappeared when she started using another oral contraceptive (Microgynon 30, ethinylestradiol 30 micrograms + levonorgestrel 150 micrograms). Phototesting was again abnormal. Her symptoms disappeared after withdrawal of the oral contraceptive. Porphyrin production was normal.

Although the estrogen and progestogen were not tested separately in this patient, the photosensitivity was most probably due to the estrogen, because the oral contraceptives that she used contained ethinylestradiol 30 micrograms with different progestogens, and photosensitivity has been described with estrogens (50).

- A 47-year-old postmenopausal woman developed eczematous lesions at the sites of application of an estradiol transdermal system and subsequently at the sites of application of an estradiol gel (51). She was therefore given oral estrogen instead, but this promptly elicited a systemic pruritic rash. The causal link was in all instances confirmed by patch-testing.

Estrogens can cause chloasma (52).

Papillomatous melanocytic nevi can be induced by estrogens (53), and melanocytic lesions can contain large numbers of estrogen and progestogen receptors (54).

When transdermal estrogens are used there can be problems with poor adhesion and skin irritation. The latter occurs more often in hot humid weather and can rarely proceed to edema, induration, a vesicular rash, residual pigmentation, itching, and erythema (55).

Three patients developed erythema nodosum during estrogen replacement therapy (56).

Topical estrogens can reduce skin aging (57), for example with reduced wrinkling and increased firmness in the dermis of perimenopausal women, although it is not clear that the effect is more marked than with oral treatment. Certainly, estrogens augment dermal water content by increasing hyaluronic acid and mucopolysaccharides, improving the structure of elastic fibers, and increase vascularization.

Sexual function

Libido, sexual activity (including masturbation), and orgasm increase in women taking the combination of an estrogen with an androgen, but it is not clear that estrogens alone have any such effect (58,59). Reduced libido and reduced sexual activity are to be expected in men treated with estrogens.

Reproductive system

All estrogens, even less potent ones, can cause endometrial hypertrophy and bleeding in a proportion of users after the menopause; in high doses the complication is common (60). With continuous estrogen therapy, the bleeding is irregular and unpredictable, whereas cyclical use of a combination with a progestogen is likely to produce something resembling normal menstruation, although it generally abates as treatment continues (60).

Estrogens can cause painful tingling and swelling of the breasts, sometimes requiring withdrawal of treatment. Frank gynecomastia can occur in men by exposure to estrogens in a factory environment and has even been described in an elderly man whose wife used an estrogen-containing vaginal lubricant (SEDA-6, 350).

In men, estrogens cause pigmentation of the areola followed by gynecomastia, both during oral treatment and local application (61). Estrogen-induced gynecomastia can be prevented in men with prostatic carcinoma by irradiating the breast region before starting therapy.

Immunologic

Estrogens can have adverse immunological effects, which could predispose to infections (62).

The immunological effects of two contraceptive combinations, namely Valette (dienogest 2.0 mg + ethinylestradiol 0.03 mg) and Lovelle (desogestrel 0.15 mg + ethinylestradiol 0.02 mg), have been examined during one treatment cycle (63). Lovelle significantly increased the numbers of lymphocytes, monocytes, and granulocytes. Valette reduced the CD4 lymphocyte count after 10 days and Lovelle did the opposite. Lovelle increased CD19 and CD23 cell counts after 21 days. Phagocytic activity was unaffected by either formulation. After 10 days both contraceptives reduced serum IgA, IgG, and IgM concentrations, which remained low at day 21 with Lovelle but returned to baseline with Valette. Secretory IgA was unaffected by either contraceptive. Neither treatment affected concentrations of interleukins, except for a significant difference between the treatment groups in interleukin-6 after 10 days, which resolved after 21 days. Concentrations of non-immunoglobulin serum components fluctuated; macroglobulin was increased by Valette. However, total protein and albumin concentrations were reduced more by Lovelle than Valette. Complement factors also fluctuated. There was no evidence of sustained immunosuppression with either Valette or Lovelle.

A severe anaphylactic reaction occurred in one patient who was given an intravenous formulation of conjugated estrogens (SED-12, 1033) (64). Some formulations of conjugated estrogens contain foreign (equine) material.

Long-Term Effects

Tumorigenicity

For the sake of simplicity the carcinogenic effects of estrogens in all formulations, including the combined oral contraceptives, are included here.

Knowledge of tumor induction by sex steroids is largely based on interpretation of epidemiological data, with careful exclusion of possible confounding elements. Hepatic tumors have given rise to most concerns, but some evidence also indicates an increased incidence of various other malignancies, including carcinomas of the breast, endometrium, and prostate (65).

The overall incidence of reproductive cancers attributable to oral contraceptive use has been estimated in a modeling analysis (66). The authors assumed a 50% reduction in ovarian and endometrial cancers associated with 5 years or more of tablet use, and used two alternative scenarios for breast and cervical cancer effects. If oral contraceptive use produces a 20% increase in breast cancer before age 50 and the same increase in cervical cancer, then for every 100 000 tablet users there would be 44 fewer reproductive cancers and these users would gain one more day free of cancer. If instead the increase in risk of early breast cancer and of cervical cancer is 50%, oral contraceptive users would have 11 fewer cancer-free days.

Liver tumors

In dealing with liver tumors, it is essential to consider all the various types of sex steroids in a single review since they seem to resemble one another closely in their long-term effects on this organ. The nomenclature used in the literature is unfortunately confusing: most reports differentiate between "hepatic adenoma" and "focal nodular hyperplasia," but the latter term is also sometimes used to cover the whole range. Other terms that have been used are "focal cirrhosis," "regenerative hyperplasia," "hamartoma," "mixed adenoma," and "benign hepatoma," while "peliosis" may constitute a precancerous state.

Androgens and anabolic steroids

There is no essential difference between androgens and so-called anabolic steroids. High doses of either, such as can be used in refractory anemias, have been associated with the induction of benign liver tumors and primary hepatocellular carcinoma. The fact that primary hepatoma, liver adenoma, and peliosis are uncommon conditions and that there is a considerable overlap between the patients concerned and the tiny fraction of the population taking high-dose androgens strongly suggests that the association of both events is more than coincidental (67). Some animal studies and in vitro studies have also pointed to a hepatic carcinogenic effect of anabolic steroids. No cases seem to have been described in sportsmen who have used high-dose androgens or in girls suffering from precocious puberty, but the former at least often use these drugs for relatively short periods; furthermore, such use is likely to be surreptitious and thus poorly documented. Most of the widely used compounds in this class, including methyltestosterone, have been reported to induce liver tumors. The apparent exceptions are the nortestosterone derivatives without 17-alpha substitution. Whether these drugs are indeed safer or whether they have merely been used less often in high doses is not known.

The incidence of liver tumors following the use of androgens and anabolic steroids still cannot be calculated. What is clear is that if these products are used in high doses or over long periods of time (and there is now much doubt about whether they are more than marginally effective in such conditions as osteoporosis and aplastic anemia), techniques such as CT scanning and ultrasonography should be used routinely to ensure early detection of liver lesions.

Oral contraceptives, estrogens, and benign liver tumors

The effects of oral contraceptives on the liver include not only benign liver tumors (focal nodular hyperplasia, hepatic adenoma, and hemangioma) (68) and hepatocellular carcinoma, but also peliosis hepatis (69), sinusoid dilatation (70), and such probably unrelated shorter-term complications as jaundice and gallstones.

However, the causal association between oral contraceptives and certain benign liver tumors has been well documented in humans, and the same association arises with conjugated estrogens (71), diethylstilbestrol, and probably antiestrogens. The evidence for the link is based on many case reports, reviewed in SEDA, and on some case-control studies, which first appeared in 1976 and 1981, pointing to a correlation (SED-14, 1450). The relative risk of benign liver tumors in users of conjugated estrogens or oral contraceptives compared with non-users may be about 40:1, although the figure is still low in absolute terms. Animal studies suggest in fact that estrogens, taken alone or in combination with progestogens, can increase the size of pre-existing liver tumors, but do not initiate tumor formation themselves; however, whether these formulations actually induce tumors or promote a latent tendency to tumor development is not of essential importance. Although there is some evidence that liver cell adenomas can regress after oral contraceptives are withdrawn (72), they do not always do so (73).

It is clear that any woman with "pill"-associated liver lesions should avoid all further use of hormonal contraceptives and related products.

Oral contraceptives and malignant liver cancer

Malignant cancer of the liver is still a very rare disease in young women, but case-control studies are possible. Evidence from both sides of the Atlantic suggested from 1987 onwards that there might be a significant relation between oral contraceptives and hepatocellular carcinoma (74–76). However, even the best of these studies had some limitations, for example incomplete data as regards a history of hepatitis or the extent of contraceptive use. One authoritative attempt to estimate the degree of risk was made by the World Health Organization in 1989, matching 122 newly diagnosed cases of primary liver cancer to 802 controls; the relative risk of liver cancer in women who had at any time used combined oral contraceptives was estimated at 0.71; there was no consistent link with months of use or time since first or last use (77). A major examination of the issue appeared in 1992, when it was concluded that the relative risk for sometime users of oral contraceptives was 1.6, rising to 2.0 in those who used the products for more than 10 years (78).

In a review of the earliest studies of hepatocellular carcinoma, it was concluded that oral contraceptives may not interact with other hepatic carcinogens, and that if they do not interact they may not measurably enhance the risk of liver cancer in parts of the world where hepatitis B virus is endemic and hepatocellular carcinoma is common (79). Others have since suggested a positive association between parity or gravidity and hepatocellular carcinoma, which needs to be further explored (80).

Conjugated estrogens

The same association with benign liver tumors arises with conjugated estrogens (71), diethylstilbestrol (q.v.), and probably antiestrogens. The evidence for the link is based on very numerous case reports from the field, reviewed in the Annuals in this series, but also on some case-control investigations. Studies of the latter type first appeared in 1976 and 1981, and both pointed to a correlation (SED-12, 1024). The relative risk of benign liver tumors in users of conjugated estrogens or oral contraceptives compared with non-users may be about 40:1, although the figure is still low in absolute terms.

Uterine tumors

The extent to which tumors of the reproductive tract are associated with hormonal treatment varies greatly with the type of tumor and the type of treatment involved.

Hormonal replacement therapy and endometrial carcinoma

In untreated women, the main risk factors for endometrial carcinoma are age, obesity, nulliparity, late menopause (and possibly early menarche), the Stein–Leventhal syndrome, exposure to exogenous estrogens, radiation, and certain systemic diseases, including diabetes mellitus, hypertension, hypothyroidism, and arthritis (SED-14, 1451) (81). Certain of these risk factors indicate that an altered endocrine state with increased estrogen stimulation is a predisposing cause, and one might thus in theory expect estrogen treatment (and notably hormonal replacement therapy) to increase the risk (SEDA-22, 466).

In women with an intact uterus, the risk of endometrial hyperplasia and cancer increases with increasing dose and duration of estrogen use. Adding a progestogen to estrogen-only therapy for at least 12 days a month greatly reduces this risk. However, it is not clear why the complication develops only in certain users. The risk of developing endometrial cancer during HRT seems to vary individually, perhaps because of genetic rather than exogenous factors. In women with endometrial cancer, women who reported ever taking HRT were more than twice as likely to develop endometrial cancer as women who had never taken it (OR = 2.24; 95% CI = 1.19, 4.23) and among these women the risk of endometrial cancer was higher for women homozygous for the CYP17 T-allele (OR = 4.10; 95% CI = 1.64, 10.3), but not for women with the C-allele. These preliminary findings suggest that CYP17 or other variants in estrogen biosynthesis or metabolism pathways may be markers of susceptibility to endometrial cancer among users of estrogen replacement therapy (82).

Two epidemiological studies published in 1975 first suggested that the use of estrogens during and after the menopause increased the risk of endometrial cancer, and in 1986 the authors of an authoritative review (83) endorsed these findings, concluding that there was an increase in risk among users, relative to non-users, of 4–9 times; the risk increased with both the strength of the medication and the duration of use. A 1990 review of data up to that time suggested that estrogen replacement therapy, continued for over 2 years without concurrent progesterone therapy, was associated with an approximately three-fold increase in the risk of both localized and extrauterine cancer; this risk increased with duration of use and persisted for over 6 years after withdrawal of therapy (84). These studies have been criticized from a methodological point of view, particularly since there is evidence of a detection bias that arises from the increased diagnostic attention received by women with uterine bleeding after estrogen exposure and perhaps also from a greater tendency of women to bleed from a pre-existing tumor when estrogens are given (85). It could be that the magnitude of the association between estrogens and endometrial cancer has been greatly overestimated for such reasons, and that the real odds ratio is less than estimated, but it seems unlikely that the risk can be disproved. There is, for example, some older evidence that even when the above-mentioned bias has largely been eliminated, there is still a correlation between the use of estrogens and endometrial carcinoma, the evidence being strongest for the first-generation oral contraceptive products, which contained large amounts of estrogen. One such study still found a six-fold risk among estrogen users compared with non-users (86); long-term users (over 5 years) had a 15-fold risk; there were excess risks for both diethylstilbestrol and conjugated estrogens. Another well-controlled study, from 1986, similarly found increased risks with conjugated estrogens, the greatest increases in risk being associated with a dosage of 0.625 mg/day or greater and duration of use of 10 years or more (87). Although according to this study the risk remained high even among women who had stopped using conjugated estrogens 5 or more years before, one cannot ignore an earlier finding, based on evidence from a large group practice, that a sharp downward trend in the incidence of endometrial cancer occurred in parallel with a substantial reduction in prescriptions for replacement estrogens (88).

Among the many papers that have since then incriminated estrogens, particularly the conjugated estrogens so widely used in North America, some have presented more subtle conclusions. One paper specifically incriminated estrone (89), but this is of course a major component of conjugated estrogens. A case-control study from Buffalo, New York, found that while patients with endometrial cancer and healthy controls had used similar amounts of menopausal estrogens, estrogen users had a significantly higher frequency of low-grade tumors and a correspondingly better survival rate (90). Menopausal estrogens became popular much later in Europe, and relatively little evidence has emerged to complement the US findings. In 1983, however, when Persson in Sweden completed a very large cohort study, he found that while among women treated with estrogens there was no significant increase in endometrial cancer compared with the control population, there was indeed a significantly increased incidence of premalignant lesions among women who had used estrogens alone for more than 3 years (91). A protracted case-control study in a Swiss population pointed in the same direction; the use of HRT for 5 years or more created a mean relative risk of 1.9, and use for 5 years or more a relative risk of 5.1 (CI 2.7, 9.8) (92). This, as well as evidence that progestogens have some protective effect on the endometrium (93), emphasizes the need for prospective studies in different subpopulations taking different types of replacement therapy.

Some helpful evidence comes from related fields. It should be borne in mind, for example, that the question of an increased risk of endometrial hyperplasia and endometrial cancer also arises in patients with estrogen-producing tumors of the ovaries, obesity, and polycystic ovarian syndrome (94) and in patients with breast cancer who are using tamoxifen (95).

During one 3-year study, under 1% of 596 women taking placebo or an estrogen + a progestogen had an abnormal endometrial biopsy. Of women taking an unopposed estrogen, 12% developed typical hyperplasia, 23% complex hyperplasia, and 28% simple hyperplasia. Use of HRT for 15 or more years resulted in a significantly higher relative risk of 1.3 for breast cancer, but was also associated with a significantly lower total mortality (96). The use of combined therapy was not associated with an increased risk of endometrial carcinoma, unless the progestogen was added for less than 10 days each month (97).

Detailed studies may also help to clarify further the risks and the possible interaction of estrogens with other susceptibility factors for endometrial tumors; there is, for example, an impression that the risk is greater in lean than in overweight women, although upper abdominal obesity is thought to reflect a higher risk. Patients who develop endometrial cancer often have an increase in estrogen production, reduced ovulation, and a lower sex hormone binding globulin concentration, resulting in high concentrations of free estrogen. As regards subjects of low susceptibility, the cancer threat may be less in women who have used oral contraceptives earlier.

One can also recognize some correlations between the subtype of tumor and the type of hormonal exposure. Unopposed hyperestrogenism is most likely to be associated with the endometrioid type of endometrial carcinoma, rather than with clear-cell, serous-papillary, and mucinous carcinomas.

Remarkably, the survival curves for women taking estrogens and developing adenocarcinomas are actually better than in women not taking estrogens and not developing adenocarcinomas. In 1822 women with angiographically documented severe coronary artery disease, the mortality among estrogen users was 4% compared with 35% among non-users, suggesting that the benefit of postmenopausal estrogen replacement therapy may be even greater in women with established coronary artery disease than it is in healthy women. A possible explanation is that estrogen replacement therapy in postmenopausal women reduces the risk of coronary heart disease by 5% or more.

Like a history of breast cancer, a history of cancer of the endometrium is commonly regarded as a reason to avoid HRT with estrogens. One study, though limited in duration, provided encouraging evidence that such treatment at least does not adversely affect the rate of recurrence or the survival time (98).

Of 249 women with surgical stage I, II, and III endometrial cancer treated between 1984 and 1998, 130 used estrogen replacement after their primary cancer treatments and half of these used progesterone in addition to estrogen. Among this cohort, 75 matched treatment-control pairs were identified. The hormone users were followed for a mean of 83 months and the non-hormone users for a mean of 69 months. There were two recurrences among the 75 HRT users compared with 11 recurrences in the 75 non-hormone users. Hormone users had a statistically significant longer disease-free interval than untreated women. Whether this is sufficient to conclude that the effect is actually positive is not clear, but no evidence of an increase in risk came to the fore.

In view of the possibility that HRT can trigger malignancy in the endometrium itself, it is not surprising to find that it has also been reported to do so in endometriosis deposits elsewhere. An adenocarcinoma arose after many years of HRT in abdominal areas of endometriosis in a woman who had undergone hysterectomy and salpingo-oophorectomy 17 years before (99). It is of course known that some 1–2% of endometriosis deposits undergo malignant degeneration, and the link with HRT could therefore have been fortuitous.

The minimum dose of continuously administered norethindrone acetate needed to reduce significantly the incidence of endometrial hyperplasia associated with the use of 17-β-estradiol 1 mg/day has been investigated in a large, controlled, comparative study in 1146 women over 12 months (100). The results suggested that continuous norethindrone acetate at doses as low as 0.1 mg/day is fully effective, at least during the first year of treatment.

The evidence that concurrent use of progestogens reduces the risk of cancer induction needs to be further supplemented; if this beneficial effect of progestogens truly exists, one must still determine how they can best be used. They are widely used, but not consistently, and increase the risk of endometrial cancer both during and after treatment. Some workers have recommended that for partial protection of the endometrium, dosages of medroxyprogesterone acetate of 2.5 mg/day continuously or 5.0 mg/day given for 14 days per cycle are the minimum required to counteract the endometrial effects of continuous therapy with estrogens (101). The added medroxyprogesterone is claimed to have no effect on the efficacy of the estrogen in treating vasomotor symptoms or in preventing osteoporosis. Others have concluded that administration of continuous rather than cyclical estrogen + progestogen therapy is more likely to maintain the beneficial effects of the estrogen and yet protect against the increase in endometrial carcinoma that occurs with estrogen therapy alone (102). However, progestogens have a negative impact on circulating lipids (55); it is possible that this adverse effect is less when using natural progesterone, but this is hardly practicable. The risk of endometrial hyperplasia and endometrial cancer with estrogens given alone must therefore be balanced against this negative impact.

Thus, although our knowledge is still incomplete and needs to be extended, it is highly likely that estrogen replacement therapy given without progestogens considerably increases the risk of endometrial carcinoma. It seems likely that the use of concurrent progestogen treatment reduces the risk, but it is still uncertain how this supplementary treatment can best be administered.

The possibility that the risk of endometrial complications might have been incorrectly estimated and commonly underestimated has been examined with the hypothesis that the method of endometrial examination or sampling is crucial (103). Hysteroscopy was performed in 98 menopausal women with endometrial thickening, and the findings were matched with those of histopathology based on various means of tissue collection, including suction curettage, oriented-streak curettage, hysteroscopically targeted biopsies, or polypectomy and hysterectomy. There was an abnormal endometrium in 35 patients (65% in symptomatic and 22% in asymptomatic women) and there were six carcinomas, 18 polyps, and 11 cases of hyperplasia. Hysteroscopy had a sensitivity of 89% and a specificity of 98%. With blind sampling, tissue collection was too scant to make diagnosis possible in 29% of patients, while in 81% of patients in whom hysteroscopy showed cystic atrophy the pathologist failed to confirm this condition. Moreover, eight endometrial polyps (36%) detected by hysteroscopy were missed when samples were studied in the laboratory. Hysteroscopy with targeted sampling thus appears to be the most effective method for assessing the endometrial lining and detecting unwanted changes.

The endometrial effects of transdermal sequential combination therapy with estradiol and levonorgestrel in various doses has been examined over 1 year in 468 postmenopausal women, who each month used patches that released estradiol for 1 week followed later in the month by combined patches that released both estradiol and levonorgestrel, again for 1 week (104). The dose of estradiol was 50–100 micrograms/day and that of levonorgestrel 15–20 micrograms/day. Endometrial biopsies, obtained from 399 subjects, generally showed good tolerance for all the various combinations tested. However, there were two cases of endometrial hyperplasia at the highest doses, while the lowest dose was associated with less bleeding than the two higher doses and a somewhat different histological pattern.

Oral contraceptives and endometrial cancer

Suggestive case histories raised at an early phase the notion of a possible correlation of oral contraceptives with endometrial cancer. Among cases of endometrial cancer there seemed to be an excess of users of oral contraceptives, particularly of the early high-dose estrogen type. With the virtual demise of these early products, the situation seems to have reversed: a 1983 study from the Centers for Disease Control (CDC) in Atlanta showed that women who had used fixed combinations for oral contraception at some time in their lives had a relative risk of endometrial cancer of only 0.5 compared with never-users (105). The protective effect occurred only in women who had used oral contraception for at least 12 months, and lasted for at least 10 years after withdrawal. The WHO adopted the same view in 1988 in the light of multinational data (106). As in the case of hormonal replacement therapy, the protective effect seems to be due to the progestogen component.

Many studies have also shown a duration-related protective effect of combined oral contraceptives on endometrial cancer, the risk before age 60 being reduced by 38% after 2 years of use and up to a 70% reduction after 12 years (107). This beneficial effect continued for at least 15 years after the end of use. As with ovarian cancer, the CASH study results suggest that the lower-dose combined oral contraceptives have a protective effect similar to that of the higher-dose tablets (108).

Oral contraceptives, cervical neoplasms, and adenosis

A 1988 statistical analysis of data from the Royal College of General Practitioners study in Britain pointed clearly to an association between oral contraceptive use and cervical neoplasms (109); of 47 000 women followed since 1965, those who had at some time used oral contraceptives had a significantly higher incidence of cervical cancer than never-users after standardization of other variables, including a history of sexually transmitted disease. The incidence increased with duration of use, attaining four-fold control values after 10 years of use. Other studies (110,111) similarly showed an increased risk with increased duration of use but also with the use of formulations that contained a higher proportion of estrogen or in users with a history of genital infections or abnormal Papanicolaou smears. Benign cervical adenosis and adenomatous polyps have been seen in oral contraceptive users and were prominent in some early reports (SED-11, 857). They often (but not always) disappear when medication is stopped.

By the mid-1980s it was fair to conclude that: (a) oral contraceptive use did not appear to increase the subsequent incidence of abnormal cytology among women who had normal smears at the time they began to use the products; (b) extended oral contraceptive use (over 6 years) appeared to increase by several times the rate of conversion of pre-existing cervical dysplasia to carcinoma in situ. Generally speaking, subsequent data have tended to be compatible with those conclusions, for example pointing to an increased incidence of micro-invasive cervical carcinoma and again stressing the changes in cytology and the extent to which the effect differs with the strength and composition of the product. The average risk figures that emerge are generally in line with those found in a Norwegian study, in which, after correcting for other risk factors, relative rates were found of 1.5 for current users and 1.4 for past users as compared with never-users (112). Clearly, confounding factors, such as differences in sexual activity, age at first coitus, and the number of sexual partners, can confuse the issue and make interpretation more complex (113). In addition, any discussion of the issue must today take into account the current view of the human papilloma virus (HPV) as a sexually transmitted agent that is the main cause of cervical cancer (114), and the possible influence of Herpes simplex virus type 2, smoking, and other known or emergent risk factors.

The most authoritative view on cervical cancer at present is that expressed by the WHO in 1992: "Recent studies suggest that use of oral contraceptives for more than 5 years is associated with a modest increase in relative risk (ranging from 1.3 to 1.8). The extent to which this reflects a biological relationship is uncertain, particularly given the absence of reliable information on the role of possible infectious agents, such as the human papilloma viruses …" (115). In the present state of knowledge, all women taking oral contraceptives over long periods should undergo regular routine screening by cervical cytology to ensure early detection of premalignant and malignant processes.

In 2002 the Chief Medical Officer of the UK Department of Health issued an urgent communication to all Health Professionals that oral contraceptives may contribute to the development of cervical cancer in women with high-risk type HPV, because of an association between an increased risk of cervical cancer and increasing duration of use of oral contraceptives (116). There was a three-fold increase in risk after 5–9 years of oral contraceptive use versus a four-fold increase after 10 or more years in women with HPV, which is sexually transmitted. There are more than 80 HPV, only a few of which are associated with an increased risk of cervical cancer. With the current evidence it is difficult to state what the main precipitating factors for cervical cancer are—the use of oral contraceptives, sexual activity, the type of HPV, or the duration of infection. While cervical screening is not perfect, 80–90% of cervical abnormalities can be detected and treated in women who attend regular screening programmes. The Chief Medical Officer therefore advised that all sexually active women, especially those taking long-term oral contraceptives, should be encouraged to have regular cervical smears.

Oral contraceptives and uterine fibroids

In a long-term, follow-up study in Scandinavia, the risk of fibroids fell consistently with increasing duration of oral contraceptive use (117). A decade earlier, the British Royal College of Physicians study had similarly suggested a protective effect, while an Oxford study had not, but once more the issue is confused by the change in composition of oral contraceptives over the years; more recent papers thus carry the most weight. On the other hand a causal relation between apoplectic leiomyomas and oral contraceptive usage was strongly suggested by Myles and Hart in the light of their study of five histologically distinctive uterine smooth muscle neoplasms with multifocal hemorrhages (118). They thought that effects of hormonal steroids on the blood vessels in pre-existing leiomyomas might be responsible for intimal hyperplasia with or without accompanying thrombi.

Ovarian tumors

Hormone replacement therapy

While the risk that hormone replacement therapy may cause endometrial tumors has been widely discussed, less attention has been given to the possibility that it could increase the risk of epithelial ovarian cancer. Since cancer of the ovary has some risk factors in common with endometrial cancer (notably low parity and obesity), this possible risk needs to be considered, especially in view of the fact that the endometrioid epithelial type of ovarian tumor is histologically so similar to adenocarcinoma of the endometrium.

The issue has been examined in a large Australian case-control study. A total of 793 eligible incident diagnoses of epithelial ovarian cancer in 1990–93 among women living in Queensland, New South Wales, and Victoria were identified. These were compared with 855 eligible female controls selected at random. Standard questionnaires were used to obtain histories. There were no clear associations between the use of hormone replacement therapy overall and the risk of ovarian cancer. However, unopposed estrogen replacement therapy was associated with a significant increase in the risk of endometrioid or clear-cell epithelial ovarian tumors. In addition, the risk associated with estrogen replacement therapy was much larger in women with an intact genital tract than in those with a history of either hysterectomy or tubal ligation. The authors therefore suggested that postmenopausal estrogen replacement may be a risk factor associated with endometrioid and clear-cell tumors in particular.

The risk of ovarian cancer with various hormonal replacement regimens has been examined in a nationwide study in Sweden in relation to plain estrogen regimens as well as estrogen + sequentially added progestogens or continuously added progestogens (119). Between 1993 and 1995, the investigators enrolled 655 women with histologically verified ovarian cancers and 3899 randomly selected population controls, all aged 50–74. Data on the use of estrogen replacement therapy were collected by postal questionnaires. The risk of ovarian cancer was higher among ever-users than never-users as regards both plain estrogen supplementation (OR = 1.43, 95% CI = 1.02, 2.00) and estrogens with sequentially added progestogens (OR = 1.54, 95% CI = 1.15, 2.05); the increase in risk applied to the serous, mucinous, and endometrioid subtypes. For all cancer types combined, the greatest increases in risk were seen when hormone use exceeded 10 years. The odds ratios after ever use of low-potency estrogens were 1.18 (95% CI = 0.89, 1.55) for oral and 1.33 (95% CI = 1.03, 1.72) for vaginal use. There was no increase in risk among users of continuously added progestogens. In other words, the continuous addition of progestogens appeared to reduce or eliminate the risk.

Oral contraceptives

The results of two major British prospective studies of 1974 and 1976 (120,121) suggested that oral contraceptive treatment was unrelated to the development of benign ovarian tumors; these and other studies also suggested that follicular and lutein cysts are suppressed in women using oral contraceptives. With regard to ovarian cancer, somewhat later data suggested a reduced risk in oral contraceptive users; impressive case-control work from the USA in 1981 seemed to show this protective effect when oral contraceptives had been taken for 4 years or more, the risk of ovarian cancer then being decreased by a mean of some 40%; the effect was even greater when the contraceptives had been used for a longer period (122). Very similarly, in 1988, the results of a multi-country study backed by the WHO suggested that sometime users of combined oral contraceptives had a risk rate that was only 71% of that in non-users, while women who had used oral contraceptives for 5 or more years had about a 50% reduction in risk (106). It should be added, however, that not all reviewers find these trends significant.

A meta-analysis of epidemiological studies of ovarian cancer showed a summary estimated relative risk of 0.64 for ever-use of combined oral contraceptives, implying a 36% reduction in ovarian cancer risk (123). This protective effect increased with increasing duration of oral contraceptive use and continued for at least 10 years after discontinuation. Although most of the oral contraceptives reported in these studies were older, higher-dose formulations, the Cancer and Steroid Hormone (CASH) study included users of tablets containing ethinylestradiol 35 μg or less, and this subgroup of women had a reduced risk of ovarian cancer (108).

With conjugated estrogens, the risk of ovarian cancer was stated in 1977 to increase two- to three-fold (SED-12, 1026), but this conclusion was based primarily on findings in women who had also taken diethylstilbestrol, and it was therefore not generally accepted. A 1982 study in which there was an apparent slight increase in ovarian epithelial carcinoma among American women taking estrogens was similarly open to challenge (SEDA-7, 385) and the link cannot be regarded as having been established (124).

Breast neoplasms

Oral contraceptives

Shortly after the first oral contraceptives were introduced around 1959, the fact that some women noticed acute effects on the breast led to fears that the ultimate consequence might be induction of mammary disorders, particularly tumors; the same concerns were raised about estrogen replacement therapy (125). The debate on this issue has now continued for more than 30 years and it is characterized by contradictions, discrepancies in scientific findings, qualified statements, and controversies and a massive output of data and opinions. The present review will necessarily be confined to some of the highlights of the discussion, presented in Table 1, leading up to a summary of the present situation and the questions that still remain open.

It is clear from the studies reported in Table 1 (126–142) that there is no simple relation between treatment with hormonal oral contraceptives and the incidence of breast cancer. As in the case of other neoplasms, studies are confounded by the influence of many factors, including age, parity, age at first delivery, family history, pre-existent fibrocystic disease, geographical or environmental influences, the ages at which the menarche and menopause have occurred, and progressive changes in the spectrum of contraceptives in use. Information bias can easily mislead. The possible influence of the long latency likely to be involved in any effect has been heavily debated; breast tumors may have been present for many years by the time they become clinically detectable; many tumors induced by oral contraceptives may therefore so far have been missed, but conversely, oral contraceptives must often have been prescribed to women who unknowingly were already suffering from breast cancer. One must also bear in mind the apparently spontaneous increase in the incidence of breast cancer over the last 40 years. Finally, when cancers are found, there is little or nothing to distinguish them histologically from tumors that arise spontaneously (143).

Four meta-analyses have shown no increased risk of breast cancer in women who have ever taken an estrogen, compared with non-users. However, most studies suggest an increased risk of breast cancer among women who take estrogen for 5–10 years or longer. The summary relative risk estimate based on the findings of these studies is 1.32 (95% Cl = 1.16, 1.51) for women who reported long-term use compared with never-users. The increased risk of breast cancer may not persist after estrogen therapy is withdrawn, suggesting that estrogen acts as a promoter rather than a cause of breast cancer (144). In one publication from the Nurse's Health Study, the estimated risk of breast cancer associated with estrogen alone was 1.36 compared with 1.50 for estrogen + progestogen therapy (145). A later analysis from the same cohort showed that women who took unopposed estrogen had a 5% per year increased risk of breast cancer compared with 9% per year in women taking an estrogen + a progestogen. The

Table 1 The possible association of oral contraceptives with breast neoplasms

Type of study	Findings	Source
Review of nine major studies of oral contraceptives	Reduced risk of breast cancer in eight studies; greater effect with higher doses; clinically significant with 2 years of use	(126)
Case-control study	Link between oral contraceptives and breast cancer, but only in those aged 30–34 years; coincidental?	(127)
Prospective epidemiological study	Link between oral contraceptives and breast cancer if used before first full-term pregnancy; high doses→higher risk	(128)
Case-control study	No link between oral contraceptives and breast cancer	(129)
Historical study of breast cancer cases	Four-fold increased risk with injectable estrogens	(130)
Case-control study	No link between oral contraceptives and breast cancer	(131)
Case-control study	Ever-users of oral contraceptives had 1.1 risk compared with never-users; higher doses produce a slightly higher risk; duration of use irrelevant; family history: higher risk; use after age 40: risk increased by 50%	(132)
Editorial	Greater risk if oral contraceptives used long-term in early life?	(133)
Case-control study	Ever-users of oral contraceptives had 0.9 (0.8, 1.2) risk compared with never-users; family history and use of oral contraceptives before first pregnancy irrelevant	(105)
Epidemiological study (extension of Pike, 1981)	Link between oral contraceptives and breast cancer if used before first full-term pregnancy: high doses→higher risk	(128)
Case-control study	Pike's results not confirmed; may be some protective effect of oral contraceptives?	(129)
Case-control study	No link with oral contraceptives	(134)
Case-control study	No link with oral contraceptives, except for a 30% increase if taken before first full pregnancy	(135)
Epidemiological study	No link with oral contraceptives, even in subpopulations	(136)
Epidemiological study	No link with oral contraceptives, even in subpopulations	(137)
Case-control study	Evidence of risk if duration and dosage considered	(138)
International case-control study	Risk doubled by use of oral contraceptives for 12 years; risk increased by duration of use; risk increased by use before first pregnancy; results may only be valid for Swedish women under 40; not seen in older or Norwegian women	(139)
Population-based case control study	No link with oral contraceptives	(137)
Narrative review	No risk	(140)
Systematic review	Greater risk with oral contraceptives in women with a history of fibroadenomas	(141)
Case-control study	Significantly more cases of breast cancer with depot medroxyprogesterone; no link with oral contraceptives	(142)
Population-based, case-control study	12-fold risk increase when young women use oral contraceptives for 12 years or more	(141)
Narrative review	Most studies have found no link with oral contraceptives; no reason for serious concern; possibly slightly higher frequency in industrialized countries	(106)
Narrative review	No increased risk from past use of oral contraceptives in women aged over 45 years; weak link in younger women with long-term use	(115)

most promising marker is the increase in breast density that occurs in 15–50% of women who take replacement estrogen (144).

There are some circumstances in which it is prudent to avoid using oral contraceptives, or in which frequent control of the state of the breasts is essential. These include (a) very long-term use before the first full pregnancy; (b) prolonged use of high-dose formulations; (c) uninterrupted use in women with a family history of breast cancer or with a personal history of fibroadenoma.

Finally, it is clear that the increase in the use of estrogen-containing contraceptives during the last 30 years cannot be held responsible for the current population-wide increase in breast cancer; as the International Committee for Research in Reproduction pointed out in 1989, the overwhelming proportion of the current rise in cases of breast cancer is among women who are too old to have taken oral contraceptives when they were younger. In addition, calculations suggest that even if an adverse effect among younger users of oral contraceptives were proved, it would still only account for a few percent of all breast cancers occurring in Western countries.

Patients with breast cancer who have discontinued estrogens less than 1 year before diagnosis have a significantly higher survival rate (146). Current users of estrogens at breast cancer diagnosis have a survival rate 5 years longer than non-users. However, they also have an increased incidence of breast cancer. This increased survival disappears when corrected for stage at diagnosis, when one can see that estrogen use relates most strongly to early-stage tumors. One might therefore expect that these tumors are less aggressive and that they result in an increased survival after diagnosis. The effect of hormone replacement therapy on breast cancer mortality may even be beneficial (147,148). Indicators of biological aggressiveness are the c-er 6 B2 oncoprotein, ploidy, tumor proliferation rate, and the presence of estrogen receptors (149).

Hormone replacement therapy

As far as hormone replacement therapy is concerned (Table 2) one must provisionally conclude, with the authors of a major Canadian study published in 1992, that long-term past use of estrogens is not related to risk, but that current estrogen use increases the risk of breast cancer to a modest degree, and that the addition of progestogens probably does not remove the increased risk resulting from the use of unopposed estrogen (150).

In the Iowa Women's Health Study of postmenopausal women for 11 years, during which 1520 specific breast cancers occurred in the at-risk cohort of 37 105 women, it was concluded that exposure to hormone replacement therapy was associated most strongly with an increased risk of invasive breast cancer with a favorable prognosis. There was a more modest increase in the risk of invasive ductal or lobular carcinoma of the breast (159).

Many clinicians continue to withhold estrogen-based replacement therapy from women who have a history of breast cancer because they fear impairing their prognosis; the evidence is not firm, but experts continue to urge caution in the absence of firm data either way (161). A well-designed study from Finland in 131 such women, two-thirds of whom used HRT, showed no increase in the breast cancer recurrence rate after an average of 2.5 years (162). However, the limited size of the study (and the fact that various different forms of HRT were used) make it difficult to exclude the risk on the basis of these data alone.

Because hyperplastic or fibrocystic changes in the breast may be pre-malignant, there has been a study of 42 women who at breast biopsy had atypical hyperplasia, 74 age-matched women with proliferative fibrocystic changes, and 74 with non-proliferative fibrocystic changes (163). The patients were aged 26–77 years, and had taken predominantly HRT (usually conjugated estrogen) but sometimes oral contraceptives. There was a strong association between exogenous hormone use and the presence of atypical hyperplasia. The authors considered that their results were in line with the theory that there is a continuum between hyperplasia and carcinoma and considered that exogenous hormone use may influence the transition from one to the other in a (still undefined) subset of women.

It is difficult to interpret a Japanese report of a woman aged 62 years who developed a benign fibrous tumor of the breast. The mass, which had been noted 1 year before, progressively enlarged. Bearing in mind that such fibrous tumors of the breast are almost always premenopausal, it may be significant that she had been taking estrogens irregularly for the previous 10 years but had taken them

Table 2 Some studies of the association between hormone replacement therapy and breast neoplasms

Type of study	Findings	Source
Prospective comparative study of users and non-users	Positive link between breast cancer and HRT, provided the menopause was natural	(88)
Cohort study following up long-term users of HRT	Slight increase in breast cancer, possibly accentuated by progestogens; possible methodological problems	(SED-12, 1027) (151)
	Risk increased with HRT by up to 30%	(152)
	Link between HRT and breast cancer uncertain, but Nurse's Health Study suggested a relative risk of 1.36; adding a progestogen reduces the risk	(153)
17 relevant studies of HRT reviewed	Risk increased by 20% with use for over 10 years and 50% with use for over 20 years	(154)
Review	At least 10 acceptable epidemiological papers point to a link between long-term HRT and breast cancer	(155)
Case-control study	No increase in risk among users of combined estrogen + progestogen HRT	(156)
Large case-control study	No increased risk of breast cancer with HRT	(157)
Case-control study	Increased risk among users of any type of HRT for more than 10 years; odds ratio 2.1	(158)
Iowa Women's Health Study	HRT associated most strongly with an increased risk of invasive breast cancer and modest increases in risk of invasive ductal or lobular carcinoma of the breast	(159)
Million Women Study	Current users of HRT more likely than never-users to develop breast cancer	(160)

intensively during the last year. In addition, there was positive immunohistochemical nuclear staining for estrogen receptor antibodies in stromal cells (164).

By far the largest piece of evidence to emerge on the risk of breast cancer is that from the Million Women Study (160). In all, more than a million women aged 50–64 were recruited into this study between 1996 and 2001 and are being followed up with respect to cancer incidence and deaths. There were 9364 incident invasive breast cancers and 637 breast cancer deaths after an average of 2.6 and 4.1 years of follow-up respectively. Current users of HRT at recruitment were more likely than never-users to develop breast cancer (adjusted RR = 1.66; 95% CI = 1.58, 1.75) and die from it (1.22; 1.00, 1.48). Past users of hormone replacement therapy were not at an increased risk. The risk was significantly increased among current users of formulations containing estrogen only, estrogen + progestogen, and tibolone, but the risk was substantially greater for estrogen + progestogen than for other types of hormone replacement therapy. The risks were significantly increased separately for oral, transdermal, and implanted estrogen-only formulations. In current users of each type of hormone replacement therapy the risk of breast cancer increased with increasing total duration of use. Although the conclusions of this major study are roughly similar to those of the Women's Health Initiative, it has already been challenged on methodological and statistical grounds as presenting an unjustified threat to the continued use of HRT in women who need it (165).

When breast cancers occur in women taking estrogen replacement therapy they are sometimes claimed to be less aggressive than in other women. The effect of the duration or type of replacement therapy on the aggressiveness of such tumors has been studied in 1105 consecutive postmenopausal patients treated for operable breast cancer at the European Institute of Oncology (166). Tumors in women who had been exposed to estrogen replacement therapy were characterized by better stage distribution, a smaller diameter, and less extensive involvement of the axillary lymph nodes; histological grade III tumors were less common. The prognosis was generally better in women who took estrogen replacement therapy for more than 5 years. Tumors with estrogen-positive receptors were more common in the controls, but this tendency was reversed when the comparison was limited to those who had had particularly long exposure. Overall, these findings seem to confirm that prolonged use of estrogen replacement therapy does reduce the degree of aggressiveness of breast cancer, but they still have to be set against the evidence that the incidence of such cancers is increased.

A new approach to the study of the effects of hormone replacement therapy on the breast is to examine breast density, using mammography and the Wolfe classification. In a randomized study of 166 menopausal women, using this technique, there was increased breast density after 6 months of treatment; eight times more commonly in those who took estradiol and norethisterone acetate than in those who took tibolone (167). The significance of this increased density is not clear, but it should for the present be regarded as undesirable, perhaps representing the prodromal phase of more serious complications.

Malignant melanoma

Mortality and incidence rates of malignant melanoma and skin cancer have increased in most Western countries during the last 20 years, clearly for reasons unconnected with oral contraception. However, endocrinological factors can affect the melanocytes and the spread of malignant melanoma. Estrogen receptors have been noted in malignant melanoma cells, and estrogens are known to stimulate melanogenesis, an effect that is enhanced by simultaneous administration of progestogens. Oral contraceptives might therefore have an effect; the fact that chloasma has long been known to occur in some oral contraceptive users is perhaps relevant (168).

One large epidemiological study from California showed that women taking oral contraceptives, particularly long-term users, had a relatively high incidence of malignant melanoma (169). In Australia, there was a significant association with melanoma in women who had used oral contraceptives for at least 10 years before diagnosis (170). In a Canadian study, on the other hand, there was no association between the risk of superficially spreading melanoma or nodular melanoma and the use of either oral contraceptives or menopausal estrogens (SED-12, 1029) (171); however, it was suggested that there might be a risk in some subpopulations. One must be alert for confounding factors: for example, among oral contraceptive users there could be a relatively higher proportion of physically active and sporting women who are more susceptible than the average to expose themselves to sunlight. The results of a case control study in Philadelphia specifically on intraocular malignant melanoma showed that hormonal factors played only a limited role in the causation of this condition (SED-12, 1029) (172).

Pituitary tumors

A 1978 WHO report quoted an unpublished study by March in which pituitary adenomas were found in 26% of women with secondary amenorrhea following the use of oral contraceptives, yet in only 13% of cases who had not used these products (111). The difference was significant, but selection bias might have explained the results.

Second-Generation Effects

Fertility

In 1993, Sharpe and Skakkebaek published a theory that environmental and other forms of exposure of males to estrogens, particularly during fetal life, might explain the increasing incidence of reduced sperm counts and developmental disorders of the male genital system (173). Such exposure could be in part due, for example, to dietary changes in mothers: a low-fiber diet results in a great reabsorption of endogenous estrogens, and there is an increasing use in the diet of soya, which is a rich source of phytoestrogens. The topic goes beyond the scope of this volume, but it is not impossible that baseline exposure to estrogens in the diet or environment could increase the sensitivity of individuals to estrogens that are administered therapeutically or for purposes of contraception.

Teratogenicity

The best-known second-generation effects of estrogens are the genital complications that result from the formerly widespread use in pregnancy of diethylstilbestrol (q.v.), mainly between 1940 and 1975. Although it is difficult to reconstruct medical histories dating back to this period, evidence continues to emerge. The evidence is covered in the monograph on Oral contraceptives.

Hormone replacement therapy is generally given at a time when pregnancy can be excluded, but in principle some of the risks discussed in connection with oral contraceptives would arise if a women taking hormone replacement therapy were to become pregnant. In 1980, an authoritative Scientific Group of the World Health Organization (WHO) surveyed the entire question of the effects of female sex hormones on fetal development and infant health (174), and after 25 years one can conclude that later reports in the literature have almost entirely supported its conclusions.

Congenital abnormalities

Records available in Finland have been used to seek correlations between hormonal treatment (with diethylstilbestrol, estrogens, or progestogens) and adverse effects, including cancers in the mother or infant. A retrospective cohort of 2052 hormone-drug exposed mothers, 2038 control mothers, and their 4130 infants was collected from maternity centers in Helsinki covering the period from 1954 to 1963 (175). Cancer cases were sought in national registers through record linkage. Exposures were examined by the type of the drug (estrogen + progestogen or progestogen only) and by timing (early in pregnancy or only late in pregnancy). There were no statistically significant differences between the groups with regard to maternal cancers, whether total or specified hormone-dependent cancers. However, the total number of malformations recorded, as well as genital malformations in male infants, was higher among exposed children. The number of cancers among the offspring was small, and none of the differences between groups was statistically significant. The authors suggested that their study supported the conclusion that estrogen or progestogen therapy during pregnancy causes malformations among children who were exposed in utero, but not the hypothesis that it causes cancer later in life in the mother; the power to study cancers in offspring was too low to draw firm conclusions. Non-existence of the risk, negative confounding, weak exposure, or a low study power may have explained the negative findings.

Susceptibility Factors

Age

Occasionally, children are exposed unknowingly to estrogens. Precocious puberty has been observed in young girls after contact with hair lotions and other products containing estrogenic compounds (SED-12, 1032) (176,177).

The short-term complications of estrogens are unpleasant rather than dangerous. A questionnaire survey among American pediatric endocrinologists has showed that these effects commonly included weight gain, nausea or vomiting, areolar or nipple pigmentation, headache, and irregular menses (178). However, there seems to have been no methodical follow-up to determine the long-term consequences.

The longer-term consequences have in recent years given rise to rather greater concern. The use of estrogens to arrest excessive growth in height in girls was first reported in 1956 (179). While the estrogen is given continuously, the addition of a progestogen given cyclically around the time of the menarche is customary in order to induce (or permit) menstrual periods and to prevent metropathia hemorrhagica. The estrogen produces a mean reduction in predicted height, provided the treatment is begun at a bone age of 12 years and before the menarche (180). The duration of treatment is from 8 months to 3 years.

There has been an anecdotal report of thrombosis in a girl taking estrogens in addition to older evidence that they can reduce antithrombin activity, which could indeed raise the risk of thrombotic complications (181).

It was long thought that there was no impairment of subsequent fertility or of the pituitary–ovarian axis in tall healthy girls treated with estrogens, but this is now uncertain. In a retrospective cohort study in Tasmania, using medical record reviews and interviews, women who had been treated with estrogen to suppress growth were significantly more likely to be infertile and were more than twice as likely to have ever taken fertility drugs than women who were not treated in this way (182).

Estrogen treatment of girls in whom growth in height tends to be excessive is progressively losing favor. In 2002, after reviewing the possible risks, which in its view could include miscarriage, endometriosis, and ovarian cysts as well as infertility, the USA Physicians' Committee for Responsible Medicine petitioned the FDA to issue appropriate warnings (178).

Sex

Following castration for cancer of the prostate, a high proportion of men have hot flushes, and estrogens can provide relief. In a study in 12 such men, estrogen in a low dose (0.05 mg) or high dose (0.10 mg) given as patches twice-weekly for 4 weeks provided considerable improvement (183). In this dosage, mild painless breast swelling or nipple tenderness was noted in two and five of the 12 men treated with the low- and high-dose patches respectively. Estradiol concentrations increased from 12 pg/ml to 16 and 27 pg/ml with the low-dose and high-dose patches respectively. There were no significant changes in serum testosterone or luteinizing hormone concentrations. This was a small study, and data on the tolerability of this topical treatment in a larger series would be welcome.

There is evidence for a role of estrogen in male bone metabolism, notably from studies in a man with a genetic defect in estrogen receptors and in men with aromatase deficiencies. Estrogen is likely to affect bone turnover in men throughout life, and it has been suggested that older men could have reduced bone resorption in response to estrogen therapy. In a study of this possibility, in 14 men with osteopenia of the femoral neck using micronized estradiol 1 mg/day for 9 weeks, that is a dose that is effective in postmenopausal women, estradiol and estrone concentrations increased significantly by more than 6-fold and 15-fold respectively (184). Concentrations of serum hormone binding globulin increased significantly by 17%, but concentrations of total and unbound testosterone fell significantly, by 27% and 34% respectively. Markers of bone resorption showed wide variations both at baseline and during treatment; they were too inconsistent to justify conclusions as to the potential usefulness of the treatment. However, the adverse effects of treatment were minimal, including (as might be expected) breast tenderness and reduced libido, which reversed after treatment.

Hepatic disease

Women with even mild liver disease can have an increased risk of the adverse effects of some estrogens on the liver (185,186). Furthermore, estrogens can potentiate and aggravate the organic complications of liver disease in other systems, for example increased cholesterol or lithogenesis (187,188).

Other features of the patient

Estrogens should be avoided in individuals with current thrombophlebitis or thromboembolism, estrogen-dependent tumors, abnormal genital bleeding without a diagnosis, and pregnancy. They are also contraindicated in apparently healthy women if they have an earlier history of jaundice in pregnancy, hepatic disease, thromboembolism, or porphyria.

Swedish workers have sought to develop a test system to define men who have a higher risk of cardiovascular complications when they take estrogens for cancer of the prostate (189). An investigational battery using exercise stress testing, evaluation of the peripheral circulation, blood volume estimation, chest X-ray, blood tests including hormonal status, lipoproteins, and antithrombin III, and history and physical examination taken by a cardiologist is claimed to make it possible to classify 84% of estrogen-treated patients as individuals with or without a particular risk of a cardiovascular complication and to identify an extremely high-risk subgroup.

Drug Administration

Drug administration route

Intranasal administration

Intranasal estradiol gives results comparable to transdermal estradiol, but substantially higher doses are needed. In 300 postmenopausal women, 17-β-estradiol 300 micrograms/day was as effective as two patches per week delivering 50 micrograms/day (190). Adverse events rates were similar but moderate, and severe mastalgia was significantly less frequent with intranasal estradiol (7.2%) than with the patch (15.5%); 66% of the patients chose to continue the intranasal therapy and 34% the transdermal therapy.

Subcutaneous implants

Implantable formulations of estrogens have been reviewed (191). Subcutaneous implants have as a rule durations of action of 4–12 months, depending on the dosage and formulation used; variations can be due to technical problems, such as disintegration or migration of an implant.

Transdermal patches

Typical patches of estradiol contain 50 micrograms, but there are important differences between the wanted and unwanted effects of the available products, because of the ways in which they are formulated. The wash-out period of estradiol after transdermal administration is about 6 weeks. Transdermal estrogens can also be supplemented periodically by an oral progestogen (192). New topical formulations of estrogens continue to be studied and marketed, although most studies have shown little difference between the various formulations available (193).

The reported incidence of adverse skin reactions to transdermal estradiol varies from 2% to over 25%, depending on the transdermal system, climatic conditions, and individual sensitivity. Of 78 women 29 reported one or more adverse events and eight discontinued prematurely (194). The main reasons for premature withdrawal included problems of adhesion, skin reactions, or undesirable systemic effects, such as headache, breast tenderness, weight gain, leg cramps, and unacceptable withdrawal bleeding.

Poor adhesion and skin irritation, with erythema and itching, are the principal drawbacks of transdermal therapy (195). Skin irritation can be overcome in some cases by changing the application site every day. In a direct comparison of transdermal patches, the duration, severity, and number of skin reactions depended on the individual formulation and excipients.

Allergic contact dermatitis from transdermal estrogen has been described in Korea, where the reaction was found to be due to 17-β-estradiol itself and not to an excipient (196). In some cases, allergic reactions and systemic contact dermatitis are clearly attributable to the patch material or to excipients. Even natural estradiol given in this way can occasionally cause hypersensitivity reactions, as determined by patch tests (197).

All the systemic effects of estrogens can occur with transdermal administration, subject to some modification as a result of the liver being bypassed (198).

Transdermal absorption of estrogen can lead to pseudoprecocious puberty in young girls, and to symptoms in young boys and adult men such as gynecomastia, loss of libido, impotence, and galactorrhea (199–201).

In a randomized, placebo-controlled, crossover study for 12 weeks, the estrogen matrix patch Estraderm MX, which unlike some other patches contains no alcohol, significantly relieved climacteric symptoms in both lower and higher strengths (50 and 100 micrograms of estradiol) (202). Local tolerability was good, but there was a slight increase in estrogen-related adverse effects (breast tenderness, leukorrhea) with the higher dose; there was a 4.8% overall incidence of endometrial hyperplasia in patients with an intact uterus. In women who have local reactions to alcohol, a patch of this type may be helpful.

Other work has confirmed the similar value of two patch formulations, Menorest and Climara; the latter has been reported to cause a much higher incidence of local reactions, but they are mild (203). The Fem 7 patch, which delivers estradiol 50 micrograms/day, was also well tolerated (204). Another effective and well-accepted variant on the patch theme is Demestril, which releases estradiol 25 or 37.5 micrograms/day depending on the formulation used (205). Differences in effect and tolerability between all these various estradiol patches are primarily a question of dosage and release rate, but it also seems that acceptance may be better when the drug is incorporated into the adhesive rather than being stored in a separate reservoir. The former type of patch shows better adhesion and is cosmetically more acceptable (206).

When low-dose patch therapy results in breakthrough bleeding it is supposedly more likely to occur in women with large, thin-walled, superficial endometrial vessels (82). If this finding is correct it might also apply to breakthrough bleeding with other forms of hormonal therapy.

Vaginal administration

Because weak estrogens, such as estriol and estrone (the main component of conjugated estrogens), are claimed to act primarily on the lower part of the genital tract, they have long been used topically for atrophic conditions of the vagina and vulva, and are reputed to have useful effects in doses that do not cause marked endometrial or systemic changes. However, everything may in fact be a question of dosage; it could well be that even a low dose of a potent estrogen would have a similarly selective effect. In 159 menopausal women with atrophic vaginitis who used either a conjugated equine estrogen vaginal cream (2 g/day containing conjugated estrogens 1.25 mg) or 17-β-estradiol pessaries 25 μg (one daily for 2 weeks), the two treatments provided equivalent relief of the symptoms of atrophic vaginitis, but at weeks 2, 12, and 24 there were increases in serum estradiol concentrations and suppression of follicle-stimulating hormone in significantly more patients who used the conjugated estrogen cream than in those who used the estradiol pessaries; the patients themselves rated the estradiol treatment more highly (207).

Another effective alternative to the use of weak estrogens is the administration of estradiol from an estradiol-releasing vaginal ring, which offers efficacy, safety, and tolerability with improved comfort and acceptability. The most frequent adverse events were vaginitis, breast tenderness, abdominal pain, pruritus, and vaginal discomfort (208). However, the incidence of these adverse events was similar to those of other estrogen vaginal delivery systems. In women with lower urinary tract symptoms after the menopause an estradiol-releasing vaginal ring was well tolerated and enjoyed better patient acceptance than local estriol (209).

With vaginal creams, used primarily in order to secure a marked local effect in arresting atrophy of the vulva and vagina, the degree of systemic effect can be variable, because of variations from day to day in vaginal vascularization and secretions (198).

References

1. Studd J, Pornel B, Marton I, Bringer J, Varin C, Tsouderos Y, Christiansen C. Efficacy and acceptability of intranasal 17 beta-oestradiol for menopausal symptoms: randomised dose–response study. Aerodiol Study Group. Lancet 1999;353(9164):1574–8.
2. Schmidt-Elmendorff H, Kammerling R. Vergleichende klinische Untersuchungen von Clomiphen. Cyclofenil und Epimestrol. [Comparative clinical studies on clomiphen, cyclofenil and epimestrol.] Geburtshilfe Frauenheilkd 1977;37(6):531–41.
3. Iida H, Miyamoto I, Noda Y, Sawaki M, Nagai Y. Adrenocortical insufficiency associated with long-term high-dose fosfestrol therapy for prostatic carcinoma. Intern Med 1999;38(10):804–7.
4. Ockene JK, Barad DH, Cochrane BB, Larson JC, Gass M, Wassertheil-Smoller S, Manson JE, Barnabei VM, Lane DS, Brzyski RG, Rosal MC, Wylie-Rosett J, Hays J. Symptom experience after discounting use of estrogen plus progestin. JAMA 2005;294(2):183–93.
5. Liu YK, Kosfeld RE, Marcum SG. Treatment of uraemic bleeding with conjugated oestrogen. Lancet 1984; 2(8408):887–90.
6. Livio M, Mannucci PM, Vigano G, Mingardi G, Lombardi R, Mecca G, Remuzzi G. Conjugated estrogens for the management of bleeding associated with renal failure. N Engl J Med 1986;315(12):731–5.
7. Koch HJ Jr, Escher GC, Lewis JS. Hormonal management of hereditary hemorrhagic talangiectasia. JAMA 1952;149(15):1376–80.
8. Vase P. Estrogen treatment of hereditary hemorrhagic telangiectasia. A double-blind controlled clinical trial. Acta Med Scand 1981;209(5):393–6.
9. Iversen P. Orchidectomy and oestrogen therapy revisited. Eur Urol 1998;34(Suppl 3):7–11.
10. Sonnenschein C, Soto AM. An updated review of environmental estrogen and androgen mimics and antagonists. J Steroid Biochem Mol Biol 1998;65(1–6):143–50.
11. Perez Gutthann S, Garcia Rodriguez LA, Castellsague J, Duque Oliart A. Hormone replacement therapy and risk of venous thromboembolism: population based case-control study. BMJ 1997;314(7083):796–800.
12. The Coronary Drug Project Research Group. The Coronary Drug Project. Findings leading to discontinuation of the 2.5-mg day estrogen group. JAMA 1973; 226(6):652–7.
13. Aitken DA, Daw EG. Allergic reaction to quinestrol. Br Med J 1970;2(702):177.
14. Lake SR, Vernon SA. Emergency contraception and retinal vein thrombosis. Br J Ophthalmol 1999;83(5):630–1.
15. Murray DC, Christopoulou D, Hero M. Combined central retinal vein occlusion and cilioretinal artery occlusion in a patient on hormone replacement therapy. Br J Ophthalmol 2000;84(5):549–50.
16. Cahill M, O'Toole L, Acheson RW. Hormone replacement therapy and retinal vein occlusion. Eye 1999;13(Pt 6): 798–800.
17. Kirwan JF, Tsaloumas MD, Vinall H, Prior P, Kritzinger EE, Dodson PM. Sex hormone preparations and retinal vein occlusion. Eye 1997;11(Pt 1):53–6.
18. Vastag O, Tornoczky J. Oralis anticoncipiens szedese soran kialakult szemfeneki arterias occlusio. [Arterial occlusion in the ocular fundus induced by oral contraceptives.] Orv Hetil 1984;125(51):3121–5.
19. Zeydler-Grzedzielewska L, Baszczynska-Zielinska B. Powiklania oczne po doustnym stosowaniu srodkow antykoncepcyjnych. [Ophthalmological complications after oral contraceptives.] Klin Oczna 1978;48(5):239–42.
20. Huismans H. Monolaterale rezidivierende Neuritis N. optici unter Langzeittherapie mit dem hormonalen Kontrazeptivum Anacyclin 28. [Recurring inflammation of optic nerve after long-time therapy with hormonal contraceptive anacyclin 28.] Klin Monatsbl Augenheilkd 1982;180(2):173–5.
21. Gierkowa A, Szaflik J, Samochowiec E, Halatek R. Estrogeny a cisnienie Wewntrz-gallkowc. [Oestrogens and intraocular pressure.] Klin Oczna 1977;47(3):113–15.
22. Kimura D. Estrogen replacement therapy may protect against intellectual decline in postmenopausal women. Horm Behav 1995;29(3):312–21.
23. Saletu B, Brandstatter N, Metka M, Stamenkovic M, Anderer P, Semlitsch HV, Heytmanek G, Huber J,

Grunberger J, Linzmayer L, Kurz CH, Decker K, Binder G, Knogler W, Koll B. Double-blind, placebo-controlled, hormonal, syndromal and EEG mapping studies with transdermal oestradiol therapy in menopausal depression. Psychopharmacology (Berl) 1995;122(4):321–9.
24. Kay PAJ, Yurkow J, Forman LJ, Chopra A, Cavalieri T. Transdermal estradiol in the management of aggressive behavior in male patients with dementia. Clin Gerontol 1995;15:54–8.
25. Abdalla HI, Hart DM, Beastall GH. Reduced serum free thyroxine concentration in postmenopausal women receiving oestrogen treatment. BMJ (Clin Res Ed) 1984;288(6419):754–5.
26. Sturdee DW, Gustafson RC, Moore B. Glucose tolerance and hormone replacement therapy. A preliminary study. Postgrad Med J 1976;52(Suppl 6):52–4.
27. Weimann E, Brack C. Severe thrombosis during treatment with ethinylestradiol for tall stature. Horm Res 1996;45(6):261–3.
28. Malina L, Chlumsky J. Oestrogen-induced familial porphyria cutanea tarda. Br J Dermatol 1975;92(6):707–9.
29. Heinemann G. [Plasma iron, serum copper, and serum zinc during therapy with ovulation inhibitors.] Med Klin 1974;69(20):892–6.
30. Henriksson P, Blomback M, Bratt G, Edhag O, Eriksson A, Vesterqvist O. Effects of oestrogen therapy and orchidectomy on coagulation and prostanoid synthesis in patients with prostatic cancer. Med Oncol Tumor Pharmacother 1989;6(3):219–25.
31. Rosendaal FR, Helmerhorst FM, Vandenbroucke JP. Oral contraceptives, hormone replacement therapy and thrombosis. Thromb Haemost 2001;86(1):112–23.
32. Scarabin PY, Oger E, Plu-Bureau G.EStrogen and THromboEmbolism Risk Study Group. Differential association of oral and transdermal oestrogen-replacement therapy with venous thromboembolism risk. Lancet 2003; 362(9382):428–32.
33. Douketis JD, Julian JA, Kearon C, Anderson DR, Crowther MA, Bates SM, Barone M, Piovella F, Turpie AG, Middeldorp S, van Nguyen P, Prandoni P, Wells PS, Kovacs MJ, Macgillavry MR, Costantini L, Ginsberg JS. Does the type of hormone replacement therapy influence the risk of deep vein thrombosis? A prospective case-control study. J Thromb Haemost 2005;3(5):943–8.
34. Astedt B. Low fibrinolytic activity of veins during treatment with ethinyloestradiol. Acta Obstet Gynecol Scand 1971;50(3):279–83.
35. Beller FK, Nachtigall L, Rosenberg M. Coagulation studies of menopausal women taking estrogen replacement. Obstet Gynecol 1972;39(5):775–8.
36. Kroon UB, Silfverstolpe G, Tengborn L. The effects of transdermal estradiol and oral conjugated estrogens on haemostasis variables. Thromb Haemost 1994; 71(4):420–3.
37. Casson PR, Carson SA. Androgen replacement therapy in women: myths and realities. Int J Fertil Menopausal Stud 1996;41(4):412–22.
38. Barlow DH. HRT and the risk of deep vein thrombosis. Int J Gynaecol Obstet 1997;59(Suppl 1):S29–33.
39. Barrett-Connor E, Timmons C, Young R, Wiita B; Estra Test Working Group. Interim safety analysis of a two year study comparing oral estrogen–androgen and conjugated estrogens in surgically menopausal women. J Women's Health 1996;5:593–602.
40. Sahdev P, Wolff M, Widmann WD. Mesenteric venous thrombosis associated with estrogen therapy for treatment of prostatic carcinoma. J Urol 1985;134(3):563–4.
41. McClennan BL. Ischemic colitis secondary to Premarin: report of a case. Dis Colon Rectum 1976;19(7):618–20.
42. Parker WA, Morris ME, Shearer CA. Oral contraceptive-induced ischemic bowel disease. Am J Hosp Pharm 1979; 36(8):1103–7.
43. Grimaud JC, Bourliere M. Contraception et hépato-gastro-entérologie. [Contraception and hepatogastroenterology.] Fertil Contracept Sex 1989;17(5):407–13.
44. Eisalo A, Heino A, Rasanen V. Oestrogen, proestogen and liver function tests. Acta Obstet Gynecol Scand 1968;47(1):58–65.
45. Ottosson UB, Carlstrom K, Johansson BG, von Schoultz B. Estrogen induction of liver proteins and high-density lipoprotein cholesterol: comparison between estradiol valerate and ethinyl estradiol. Gynecol Obstet Invest 1986;22(4):198–205.
46. Underwood TW, Frye CB. Drug-induced pancreatitis. Clin Pharm 1993;12(6):440–8.
47. Orlander JD, Jick SS, Dean AD, Jick H. Urinary tract infections and estrogen use in older women. J Am Geriatr Soc 1992;40(8):817–20.
48. Kok AL, Burger CW, van de Weijer PH, Voetberg GA, Peters-Muller ER, Kenemans P. Micturition complaints in postmenopausal women treated with continuously combined hormone replacement therapy: a prospective study. Maturitas 1999;31(2):143–9.
49. Cooper SM, George S. Photosensitivity reaction associated with use of the combined oral contraceptive. Br J Dermatol 2001;144(3):641–2.
50. Horkay I, Tamasi P, Prekopa A, Dalmy L. Photodermatoses induced by oral contraceptives. Arch Dermatol Res 1975;253(1):53–61.
51. Corazza M, Mantovani L, Montanari A, Virgili A. Allergic contact dermatitis from transdermal estradiol and systemic contact dermatitis from oral estradiol. A case report. J Reprod Med 2002;47(6):507–9.
52. Smith AG, Shuster S, Thody AJ, Peberdy M. Chloasma, oral contraceptives, and plasma immunoreactive beta-melanocyte-stimulating hormone. J Invest Dermatol 1977;68(4):169–70.
53. Morgan MB, Raley BA, Vannarath RL, Lightfoot SL, Everett MA. Papillomatous melanocytic nevi: an estrogen related phenomenon. J Cutan Pathol 1995;22(5):446–9.
54. Ellis DL, Wheeland RG, Solomon H. Estrogen and progesterone receptors in melanocytic lesions. Occurrence in patients with dysplastic nevus syndrome. Arch Dermatol 1985;121(10):1282–5.
55. Baker VL. Alternatives to oral estrogen replacement. Transdermal patches, percutaneous gels, vaginal creams and rings, implants, other methods of delivery. Obstet Gynecol Clin North Am 1994;21(2):271–97.
56. Yang SG, Han KH, Cho KH, Lee AY. Development of erythema nodosum in the course of oestrogen replacement therapy. Br J Dermatol 1997;137(2):319–20.
57. Schmidt JB, Binder M, Demschik G, Bieglmayer C, Reiner A. Treatment of skin aging with topical estrogens. Int J Dermatol 1996;35(9):669–74.
58. Dei M, Verni A, Bigozzi L, Bruni V. Sex steroids and libido. Eur J Contracept Reprod Health Care 1997; 2(4):253–8.
59. Graziottin A. Libido: the biologic scenario. Maturitas 2000;34(Suppl 1):S9–16.
60. Lethaby A, Suckling J, Barlow D, Farquhar CM, Jepson RG, Roberts H. Hormone replacement therapy in postmenopausal women: endometrial hyperplasia and irregular bleeding. Cochrane Database Syst Rev 2004;(3):CD000402.
61. Bazex A, Salvador R, Dupré A, et al. Gynécomastie et hyperpigmentation aréolaire après locale anti-séborrhéique. Bull Soc Fr Dermatol Syphiligr 1967; 74:466.

62. Styrt B, Sugarman B. Estrogens and infection. Rev Infect Dis 1991;13(6):1139–50.
63. Klinger G, Graser T, Mellinger U, Moore C, Vogelsang H, Groh A, Latterman C, Klinger G. A comparative study of the effects of two oral contraceptives containing dienogest or desogestrel on the human immune system. Gynecol Endocrinol 2000;14(1):15–24.
64. Searcy CJ, Kushner M, Nell P, Beckmann CR. Anaphylactic reaction to intravenous conjugated estrogens. Clin Pharm 1987;6(1):74–6.
65. Ford LG, Brawley OW, Perlman JA, Nayfield SG, Johnson KA, Kramer BS. The potential for hormonal prevention trials. Cancer 1994;74(Suppl 9):2726–33.
66. Coker AL, Harlap S, Fortney JA. Oral contraceptives and reproductive cancers: weighing the risks and benefits. Fam Plann Perspect 1993;25(1):17–21, 36.
67. Oda K, Oguma N, Kawano M, Kimura A, Kuramoto A, Tokumo K. Hepatocellular carcinoma associated with long-term anabolic steroid therapy in two patients with aplastic anemia. Nippon Ketsueki Gakkai Zasshi 1987;50(1):29–36.
68. Greer T. Hepatic adenoma and oral contraceptive use. J Fam Pract 1989;28(3):322–6.
69. Brooks JJ. Hepatoma associated with diethylstilbestrol therapy for prostatic carcinoma. J Urol 1982;128(5): 1044–5.
70. Heresbach D, Deugnier Y, Brissot P, Bourel M. Dilatations sinusoidales et prise de contraceptifs oraux. A propos d'un casavec revue de la litterature. [Sinusoid dilatation and the use of oral contraceptives. Apropos of a case with a review of the literature.] Ann Gastroenterol Hepatol (Paris) 1988;24(4):189–91.
71. Christopherson WM. Liver tumours and the pill. BMJ 1975;4(5999):756.
72. Buhler H, Pirovino M, Akobiantz A, Altorfer J, Weitzel M, Maranta E, Schmid M. Regression of liver cell adenoma. A follow-up study of three consecutive patients after discontinuation of oral contraceptive use. Gastroenterology 1982;82(4):775–82.
73. Marks WH, Thompson N, Appleman H. Failure of hepatic adenomas (HCA) to regress after discontinuance of oral contraceptives. An association with focal nodular hyperplasia (FNH) and uterine leiomyoma. Ann Surg 1988;208(2):190–5.
74. Ross RK, Bernstein L, Garabrant D, Henderson BE. Avoidable nondietary risk factors for cancer. Am Fam Physician 1988;38(2):153–60.
75. La Vecchia C, Negri E, Parazzini F. Oral contraceptives and primary liver cancer. Br J Cancer 1989;59(3):460–1.
76. Neuberger J, Forman D, Doll R, Williams R. Oral contraceptives and hepatocellular carcinoma. BMJ (Clin Res Ed) 1986;292(6532):1355–7.
77. World Health Organization. Combined oral contraceptives and liver cancer. The WHO Collaborative Study of Neoplasia and Steroid Contraceptives. Int J Cancer 1989;43(2):254–9.
78. Hsing AW, Hoover RN, McLaughlin JK, Co-Chien HT, Wacholder S, Blot WJ, Fraumeni JF Jr. Oral contraceptives and primary liver cancer among young women. Cancer Causes Control 1992;3(1):43–8.
79. Prentice RL, Thomas DB. On the epidemiology of oral contraceptives and disease. Adv Cancer Res 1987;49: 285–401.
80. Stanford JL, Thomas DB. Reproductive factors in the etiology of hepatocellular carcinoma. The WHO Collaborative Study of Neoplasia and Steroid Contraceptives. Cancer Causes Control 1992;3(1):37–42.
81. Parazzini F, Negri E, La Vecchia C, Bruzzi P, Decarli A. Population attributable risk for endometrial cancer in northern Italy. Eur J Cancer Clin Oncol 1989;25(10): 1451–6.
82. McGavigan CJ, Metaxa-Mariatou V, Dockery P, Rodger MW, Cameron IT, Campbell S. Large, thin walled, superficial endometrial vessels: the cause of breakthrough bleeding in women with Mirena? Br J Fam Plann 2000;26:235–6.
83. Horwitz RI, Feinstein AR. Estrogens and endometrial cancer. Responses to arguments and current status of an epidemiologic controversy. Am J Med 1986;81(3):503–7.
84. Rubin GL, Peterson HB, Lee NC, Maes EF, Wingo PA, Becker S. Estrogen replacement therapy and the risk of endometrial cancer: remaining controversies. Am J Obstet Gynecol 1990;162(1):148–54.
85. Horwitz RI, Feinstein AR. Alternative analytic methods for case-control studies of estrogens and endometrial cancer. N Engl J Med 1978;299(20):1089–94.
86. Antunes CM, Strolley PD, Rosenshein NB, Davies JL, Tonascia JA, Brown C, Burnett L, Rutledge A, Pokempner M, Garcia R. Endometrial cancer and estrogen use. Report of a large case-control study. N Engl J Med 1979;300(1):9–13.
87. Buring JE, Bain CJ, Ehrmann RL. Conjugated estrogen use and risk of endometrial cancer. Am J Epidemiol 1986;124(3):434–41.
88. Jick H, Watkins RN, Hunter JR, Dinan BJ, Madsen S, Rothman KJ, Walker AM. Replacement estrogens and endometrial cancer. N Engl J Med 1979;300(5):218–22.
89. Ziel HK, Finkle WD. Association of estrone with the development of endometrial carcinoma. Am J Obstet Gynecol 1976;124(7):735–40.
90. Spengler RF, Clarke EA, Woolever CA, Newman AM, Osborn RW. Exogenous estrogens and endometrial cancer: a case-control study and assessment of potential biases. Am J Epidemiol 1981;114(4):497–506.
91. Persson I. Climacteric Treatment with Estrogens and Estrogen–Progestogen Combinations: the Risk of Endometrial Neoplasia. Results of a Cohort Study. Thesis, University of Uppsala. Stockholm: Almqvist and Wiksell, 1983.
92. Levi F, La Vecchia C, Gulie C, Franceschi S, Negri E. Oestrogen replacement treatment and the risk of endometrial cancer: an assessment of the role of covariates. Eur J Cancer 1993;29A(10):1445–9.
93. Jacobs HS, Loeffler FE. Postmenopausal hormone replacement therapy. BMJ 1992;305(6866):1403–8.
94. Woodruff JD, Pickar JH. Incidence of endometrial hyperplasia in postmenopausal women taking conjugated estrogens (Premarin) with medroxyprogesterone acetate or conjugated estrogens alone. The Menopause Study Group. Am J Obstet Gynecol 1994;170(5 Pt 1): 1213–23.
95. Sulak PJ. Endometrial cancer and hormone replacement therapy. Appropriate use of progestins to oppose endogenous and exogenous estrogen. Endocrinol Metab Clin North Am 1997;26(2):399–412.
96. Battistini M. Estrogen and the prevention and treatment of osteoporosis. J Clin Rheumatol 1997;3:S28–33.
97. Beresford SA, Weiss NS, Voigt LF, McKnight B. Risk of endometrial cancer in relation to use of oestrogen combined with cyclic progestagen therapy in postmenopausal women. Lancet 1997;349(9050):458–61.
98. Suriano KA, McHale M, McLaren CE, Li KT, Re A, DiSaia PJ. Estrogen replacement therapy in endometrial cancer patients: a matched control study. Obstet Gynecol 2001;97(4):555–60.
99. Debus G, Schuhmacher I. Endometrial adenocarcinoma arising during estrogenic treatment 17 years after total abdominal hysterectomy and bilateral salpingo-oophorectomy: a case report. Acta Obstet Gynecol Scand 2001; 80(6):589–90.

100. Kurman RJ, Felix JC, Archer DF, Nanavati N, Arce J, Moyer DL. Norethindrone acetate and estradiol-induced endometrial hyperplasia. Obstet Gynecol 2000;96(3): 373–9.
101. Turner RT, Riggs BL, Spelsberg TC. Skeletal effects of estrogen. Endocr Rev 1994;15(3):275–300.
102. Kafonek SD. Postmenopausal hormone replacement therapy and cardiovascular risk reduction. A review. Drugs 1994;47(Suppl 2):16–24.
103. Garuti G, Grossi F, Cellani F, Centinaio G, Colonnelli M, Luerti M. Hysteroscopic assessment of menopausal breast-cancer patients taking tamoxifen; there is a bias from the mode of endometrial sampling in estimating endometrial morbidity? Breast Cancer Res Treat 2002;72(3):245–53.
104. Sturdee DW, van de Weijer P, von Holst T. Endometrial safety of a transdermal sequential estradiol–levonorgestrel combination. Climacteric 2002;5(2):170–7.
105. The Centers for Disease Control Cancer and Steroid Hormone Study. Oral contraceptive use and the risk of endometrial cancer. JAMA 1983;249(12):1600–4.
106. The WHO Collaborative Study of Neoplasia and Steroid Contraceptives. Epithelial ovarian cancer and combined oral contraceptives. The WHO Collaborative Study of Neoplasia and Steroid Contraceptives. Int J Epidemiol 1989;18(3):538–45.
107. Schlesselman JJ. Oral contraceptives and neoplasia of the uterine corpus. Contraception 1991;43(6):557–79.
108. The Cancer and Steroid Hormone Study of the Centers for Disease Control and the National Institute of Child Health and Human Development. The reduction in risk of ovarian cancer associated with oral-contraceptive use. N Engl J Med 1987;316(11):650–5.
109. Beral V, Hannaford P, Kay C. Oral contraceptive use and malignancies of the genital tract. Results from the Royal College of General Practitioners' Oral Contraception Study. Lancet 1988;2(8624):1331–5.
110. Brinton LA, Huggins GR, Lehman HF, Mallin K, Savitz DA, Trapido E, Rosenthal J, Hoover R. Long-term use of oral contraceptives and risk of invasive cervical cancer. Int J Cancer 1986;38(3):339–44.
111. Slattery ML, Overall JC Jr, Abbott TM, French TK, Robison LM, Gardner J. Sexual activity, contraception, genital infections, and cervical cancer: support for a sexually transmitted disease hypothesis. Am J Epidemiol 1989;130(2):248–58.
112. Gram IT, Macaluso M, Stalsberg H. Oral contraceptive use and the incidence of cervical intraepithelial neoplasia. Am J Obstet Gynecol 1992;167(1):40–4.
113. Bosch FX, Munoz N, de Sanjose S, Izarzugaza I, Gili M, Viladiu P, Tormo MJ, Moreo P, Ascunce N, Gonzalez LC, et al. Risk factors for cervical cancer in Colombia and Spain. Int J Cancer 1992;52(5):750–8.
114. Macnab JC, Walkinshaw SA, Cordiner JW, Clements JB. Human papillomavirus in clinically and histologically normal tissue of patients with genital cancer. N Engl J Med 1986;315(17):1052–8.
115. World Health Organization. Oral contraceptives and neoplasia: report of a WHO Scientific Group. WHO Tech Rep Ser 1992:817.
116. Anonymous. Oral contraceptives. Risk of cervical cancer with long-term use in woman with high risk type of HPV. WHO Pharmaceuticals Newslett 2002;2:3–4.
117. Kjaeldgaard A, Larsson B. Long-term treatment with combined oral contraceptives and cigarette smoking associated with impaired activity of tissue plasminogen activator. Acta Obstet Gynecol Scand 1986;65(3):219–22.
118. Myles JL, Hart WR. Apoplectic leiomyomas of the uterus. A clinicopathologic study of five distinctive hemorrhagic leiomyomas associated with oral contraceptive usage. Am J Surg Pathol 1985;9(11):798–805.
119. Riman T, Dickman PW, Nilsson S, Correia N, Nordlinder H, Magnusson CM, Weiderpass E, Persson IR. Hormone replacement therapy and the risk of invasive epithelial ovarian cancer in Swedish women. J Natl Cancer Inst 2002;94(7):497–504.
120. Royal College of General Practitioners. Oral Contraceptives and Health. London: RCGP, 1974.
121. Vessey M, Doll R, Peto R, Johnson B, Wiggins P. A long-term follow-up study of women using different methods of contraception—an interim report. J Biosoc Sci 1976;8(4): 373–427.
122. Weiss NS, Lyon JL, Liff JM, Vollmer WM, Daling JR. Incidence of ovarian cancer in relation to the use of oral contraceptives. Int J Cancer 1981;28(6):669–71.
123. Hankinson SE, Colditz GA, Hunter DJ, Spencer TL, Rosner B, Stampfer MJ. A quantitative assessment of oral contraceptive use and risk of ovarian cancer. Obstet Gynecol 1992;80(4):708–14.
124. Mack TM. Hormone replacement therapy and cancer. Baillières Clin Endocrinol Metab 1993;7(1):113–49.
125. Nisker JA, Siiteri PK. Estrogens and breast cancer. Clin Obstet Gynecol 1981;24(1):301–22.
126. WHO Scientific Group. Steroid contraception and the risk of neoplasia. World Health Organ Tech Rep Ser 1978;619:1–54.
127. Royal College of General Practitioners. Oral Contraceptive Study. London: RCGP, 1981.
128. Pike MC, Henderson BE, Casagrande JT, Rosario I, Gray GE. Oral contraceptive use and early abortion as risk factors for breast cancer in young women. Br J Cancer 1981;43(1):72–6.
129. Vessey MP, McPherson K, Doll R. Breast cancer and oral contraceptives: findings in Oxford–Family Planning Association contraceptive study. BMJ (Clin Res Ed) 1981;282(6282):2093–4.
130. Hulka BS, Chambless LE, Deubner DC, Wilkinson WE. Breast cancer and estrogen replacement therapy. Am J Obstet Gynecol 1982;143(6):638–44.
131. Ory GW, Layde OM, et al. Long term oral contraceptive use and the risk of breast cancer. Paper presented at 31st Annual Epidemic Service Conference. Atlanta, Georgia, 1982.
132. Brinton LA, Hoover R, Szklo M, Fraumeni JF Jr. Oral contraceptives and breast cancer. Int J Epidemiol 1982;11(4):316–22.
133. Drife J. Which pill? BMJ (Clin Res Ed) 1983;287(6403): 1397–9.
134. Janerich DT, Polednak AP, Glebatis DM, Lawrence CE. Breast cancer and oral contraceptive use: a case-control study. J Chronic Dis 1983;36(9):639–46.
135. Rosenberg L, Miller DR, Kaufman DW, Helmrich SP, Stolley PD, Schottenfeld D, Shapiro S. Breast cancer and oral contraceptive use. Am J Epidemiol 1984;119(2):167–76.
136. Stadel BV, Rubin GL, Webster LA, Schlesselman JJ, Wingo PA. Oral contraceptives and breast cancer in young women. Lancet 1985;2(8462):970–3.
137. The Cancer and Steroid Hormone Study of the Centers for Disease Control and the National Institute of Child Health and Human Development. Oral-contraceptive use and the risk of breast cancer. N Engl J Med 1986;315(7):405–11.
138. Ellery C, MacLennan R, Berry G, Shearman RP. A case-control study of breast cancer in relation to the use of steroid contraceptive agents. Med J Aust 1986;144(4):173–6.
139. Meirik O, Lund E, Adami HO, Bergstrom R, Christoffersen T, Bergsjo P. Oral contraceptive use and breast cancer in young women. A joint national

case-control study in Sweden and Norway. Lancet 1986;2(8508):650–4.
140. Shapiro S. Oral contraceptives—time to take stock. N Engl J Med 1986;315(7):450–1.
141. Stadel BV, Lai SH, Schlesselman JJ, Murray P. Oral contraceptives and premenopausal breast cancer in nulliparous women. Contraception 1988;38(3):287–99.
142. Lee NC, Rosero-Bixby L, Oberle MW, Grimaldo C, Whatley AS, Rovira EZ. A case-control study of breast cancer and hormonal contraception in Costa Rica. J Natl Cancer Inst 1987;79(6):1247–54.
143. Hulman G, Trowbridge P, Taylor CN, Chilvers CE, Sloane JP. Oral contraceptive use and histopathology of cancerous breasts in young women. Members of the U.K. National Case-Control Study Group. J Pathol 1992;167(4):407–11.
144. Barrett-Connor E, Grady D. Hormone replacement therapy, heart disease, and other considerations. Annu Rev Public Health 1998;19:55–72.
145. Colditz GA, Hankinson SE, Hunter DJ, Willett WC, Manson JE, Stampfer MJ, Hennekens C, Rosner B, Speizer FE. The use of estrogens and progestins and the risk of breast cancer in postmenopausal women. N Engl J Med 1995;332(24):1589–93.
146. Brinton LA. Hormone replacement therapy and risk for breast cancer. Endocrinol Metab Clin North Am 1997;26(2):361–78.
147. Willis DB, Calle EE, Miracle-McMahill HL, Heath CW Jr. Estrogen replacement therapy and risk of fatal breast cancer in a prospective cohort of postmenopausal women in the United States. Cancer Causes Control 1996;7(4):449–57.
148. Grodstein F, Stampfer MJ, Colditz GA, Willett WC, Manson JE, Joffe M, Rosner B, Fuchs C, Hankinson SE, Hunter DJ, Hennekens CH, Speizer FE. Postmenopausal hormone therapy and mortality. N Engl J Med 1997;336(25):1769–75.
149. Holli K, Isola J, Cuzick J. Hormone replacement therapy and biological aggressiveness of breast cancer. Lancet 1997;350(9092):1704–5.
150. Colditz GA, Stampfer MJ, Willett WC, Hunter DJ, Manson JE, Hennekens CK, Rosner BA, Speizer FE. Type of postmenopausal hormone use and risk of breast cancer. 12-year follow-up from the Nurses' Health Study. Cancer Causes Control 1992;3:433–9.
151. Bergkvist L, Adami HO, Persson I, Hoover R, Schairer C. The risk of breast cancer after estrogen and estrogen-progestin replacement. N Engl J Med 1989;321(5):293–7.
152. MacLennan AH. Hormone replacement therapy and the menopause. Australian Menopause Society. Med J Aust 1991;155(1):43–4.
153. Gambrell RD. Estrogen replacement therapy and breast cancer risk. A new look at the data. Female Patient 1993;18:55.
154. Colditz GA, Egan KM, Stampfer MJ. Hormone replacement therapy and risk of breast cancer: results from epidemiologic studies Am J Obstet Gynecol 1993;168(5): 1473–80.
155. Stewart GR. Hormone replacement therapy and breast cancer. Med J Aust 1993;158:146.
156. Stanford JL, Weiss NS, Voigt LF, Daling JR, Habel LA, Rossing MA. Combined estrogen and progestin hormone replacement therapy in relation to risk of breast cancer in middle-aged women. JAMA 1995;274(2):137–42.
157. Newcomb PA, Longnecker MP, Storer BE, Mittendorf R, Baron J, Clapp RW, Bogdan G, Willett WC. Long-term hormone replacement therapy and risk of breast cancer in postmenopausal women. Am J Epidemiol 1995; 142(8):788–95.
158. Persson I, Thurfjell E, Bergstrom R, Holmberg L. Hormone replacement therapy and the risk of breast cancer. Nested case-control study in a cohort of Swedish women attending mammography screening. Int J Cancer 1997;72(5):758–61.
159. Gapstur SM, Morrow M, Sellers TA. Hormone replacement therapy and risk of breast cancer with a favorable histology: results of the Iowa Women's Health Study. JAMA 1999;281(22):2091–7.
160. Beral V; Million Women Study Collaborators. Breast cancer and hormone-replacement therapy in the Million Women Study. Lancet 2003;362(9382):419–27.
161. Pritchard KI. Hormone replacement in women with a history of breast cancer. Oncologist 2001;6(4):353–62.
162. Marttunen MB, Hietanen P, Pyrhonen S, Tiitinen A, Ylikorkala O. A prospective study on women with a history of breast cancer and with or without estrogen replacement therapy. Maturitas 2001;39(3):217–25.
163. Zera RT, Danielson D, Van Camp JM, Schmidt-Steinbrunn B, Hong J, McCoy M, Anderson WR, Linzie BM, Rodriguez JL. Atypical hyperplasia, proliferative fibrocystic change, and exogenous hormone use. Surgery 2001;130(4):732–7.
164. Miyagawa A, Yuba Y, Haga H, Nishimura S, Kobashi Y. Fibrous tumor of the breast in a postmenopausal woman receiving estrogen. Pathol Int 2001;51(2):123–6.
165. Garton M. Breast cancer and hormone-replacement therapy: the Million Women Study. Lancet 2003; 362(9392):1328.
166. Sacchini V, Zurrida S, Andreoni G, Luini A, Galimberti V, Veronesi P, Intra M, Viale G, Veronesi U. Pathologic and biological prognostic factors of breast cancers in short- and long-term hormone replacement therapy users. Ann Surg Oncol 2002;9(3):266–71.
167. Lundstrom E, Christow A, Kersemaekers W, Svane G, Azavedo E, Soderqvist G, Mol-Arts M, Barkfeldt J, von Schoultz B. Effects of tibolone and continuous combined hormone replacement therapy on mammographic breast density. Am J Obstet Gynecol 2002;186(4):717–22.
168. Carruthers R. Chloasma and oral contraceptives. Med J Aust 1966;2(1):17–20.
169. Beral V, Ramcharan S, Faris R. Malignant melanoma and oral contraceptive use among women in California. Br J Cancer 1977;36(6):804–9.
170. Beral V, Evans S, Shaw H, Milton G. Oral contraceptive use and malignant melanoma in Australia. Br J Cancer 1984;50(5):681–5.
171. Gallagher RP, Elwood JM, Hill GB, Coldman AJ, Threlfall WJ, Spinelli JJ. Reproductive factors, oral contraceptives and risk of malignant melanoma: Western Canada Melanoma Study. Br J Cancer 1985;52(6):901–7.
172. Hartge P, Tucker MA, Shields JA, Augsburger J, Hoover RN, Fraumeni JF Jr. Case-control study of female hormones and eye melanoma. Cancer Res 1989;49(16): 4622–5.
173. Sharpe RM, Skakkebaek NE. Are oestrogens involved in falling sperm counts and disorders of the male reproductive tract? Lancet 1993;341(8857):1392–5.
174. World Health Organization Scientific Group. The effect of female sex hormones on fetal development and infant health. World Health Organ Tech Rep Ser 1981;657:1–76.
175. Hemminki E, Gissler M, Toukomaa H. Exposure to female hormone drugs during pregnancy: effect on malformations and cancer. Br J Cancer 1999;80(7):1092–7.
176. Ramos AS, Bower BF. Pseudoisosexual precocity due to cosmetic ingestion. JAMA 1969;207(2):368–9.
177. Landolt R, Murset G. Vorzeitige Pubertatsmerkmale als Folge unbeabsichitiger Ostrogenverabreichung. [Premature puberty signs as result of unintensional estrogen administration.] Schweiz Med Wochenschr 1968;98(17):638–41.

178. Barnard ND, Scialli AR, Bobela S. The current use of estrogens for growth-suppressant therapy in adolescent girls. J Pediatr Adolesc Gynecol 2002;15(1):23–6.
179. Denke MA. Hormone replacement therapy: benefit and safety issues. Curr Opin Lipidol 1996;7(6):369–73.
180 Sotos JF. Overgrowth disorders. Clin Pediatr (Phila) 1996; 35(10):517–29.
181. Blomback M, Hall K, Ritzen EM. Estrogen treatment of tall girls: risk of thrombosis? Pediatrics 1983;72(3):416–19.
182. Venn A, Bruinsma F, Werther G, Pyett P, Baird D, Jones P, Rayner J, Lumley J. Oestrogen treatment to reduce the adult height of tall girls: long-term effects on fertility. Lancet 2004;364(9444):1513–18.
183. Gerber GS, Zagaja GP, Ray PS, Rukstalis DB. Transdermal estrogen in the treatment of hot flushes in men with prostate cancer. Urology 2000;55(1):97–101.
184. Taxel P, Kennedy D, Fall P, Willard A, Shoukri K, Clive J, Raisz LG. The effect of short-term treatment with micronized estradiol on bone turnover and gonadotrophins in older men. Endocr Res 2000;26(3):381–98.
185. O'Donohue J, Williams R. Hormone replacement therapy in women with liver disease. Br J Obstet Gynaecol 1997;104(1):1–3.
186. Hannaford PC, Kay CR, Vessey MP, Painter R, Mant J. Combined oral contraceptives and liver disease. Contraception 1997;55(3):145–51.
187. Lindberg MC. Hepatobiliary complications of oral contraceptives. J Gen Intern Med 1992;7(2):199–209.
188. Knopp RH. Cardiovascular effects of endogenous and exogenous sex hormones over a woman's lifetime. Am J Obstet Gynecol 1988;158(6 Pt 2):1630–43.
189. Henriksson P, Johansson SE. Prediction of cardiovascular complications in patients with prostatic cancer treated with estrogen. Am J Epidemiol 1987;125(6):970–8.
190. Lopes P, Merkus HM, Nauman J, Bruschi F, Foidart JM, Calaf J. Randomized comparison of intranasal and transdermal estradiol. Obstet Gynecol 2000;96(6):906–12.
191. French RS, Cowan FM, Mansour DJ, Morris S, Procter T, Hughes D, Robinson A, Guillebaud J. Implantable contraceptives (subdermal implants and hormonally impregnated intrauterine systems) versus other forms of reversible contraceptives: two systematic reviews to assess relative effectiveness, acceptability, tolerability and cost-effectiveness. Health Technol Assess 2000;4(7):1–107.
192. Cerin A, Heldaas K, Moeller B. Adverse endometrial effects of long-cycle estrogen and progestogen replacement therapy. The Scandinavian LongCycle Study Group. N Engl J Med 1996;334(10):668–9.
193. Rovati LC, Setnikar I, Genazzani AR. Dose–response efficacy of a new estradiol transdermal matrix patch for 7-day application: a randomized, double-blind, placebo-controlled study. Italian Menopause Research Group. Gynecol Endocrinol 2000;14(4):282–91.
194. Young P, Purdie D, Jackman L, Molloy D, Green A. A study of infertility treatment and melanoma. Melanoma Res 2001;11(5):535–41.
195. Selby PL, Peacock M. The effect of transdermal oestrogen on bone, calcium-regulating hormones and liver in postmenopausal women. Clin Endocrinol (Oxf) 1986;25(5): 543–7.
196. Shin Taek Oh, Dong Won Lee, Jun Young Lee, Baik Kee Cho. A case of allergic contact dermatitis to transdermal estradiol system. Korean J Dermatol 2001;39:111–13.
197. Goncalo M, Oliveira HS, Monteiro C, Clerins I, Figueiredo A. Allergic and systemic contact dermatitis from estradiol. Contact Dermatitis 1999;40(1):58–9.
198. Jewelewicz R. New developments in topical estrogen therapy. Fertil Steril 1997;67(1):1–12.
199. Schmidt KU, Wagner G, Mensing H. Ostrogen-induzierte Gynakomastie nach Anwendung ostrogenhaltiger Lokaltherapeutika. [Estrogen-induced gynecomastia following use of estrogen-containing local agents.] Dtsch Med Wochenschr 1987;112(23):926–8.
200. Gottswinto JM, Korth-Schutz S, Tummers B, Ziegler R. Gynäkomastie durch östrogen-haltiges Haarwasser. Med Klin 1984;79:181–3.
201. Langer J. Gynäkomastie durch Pharmaka. [Gynecomastia caused by drugs.] Derm Beruf Umwelt 1989;37(4):121–47.
202. de Vrijer B, Snijders MP, Troostwijk AL, The S, Iding RJ, Friese S, Smit DA, Schierbeek JM, Brandts H, van Kempen PJ, van Buuren I, Monza G. Efficacy and tolerability of a new estradiol delivering matrix patch (Estraderm MX) in postmenopausal women. Maturitas 2000;34(1):47–55.
203. Andersson TL, Stehle B, Davidsson B, Hoglund P. Bioavailability of estradiol from two matrix transdermal delivery systems: Menorest and Climara. Maturitas 2000;34(1):57–64.
204. von Holst T, Salbach B. Efficacy and tolerability of a new 7-day transdermal estradiol patch versus placebo in hysterectomized women with postmenopausal complaints. Maturitas 2000;34(2):143–53.
205. De Aloysio D, Rovati LC, Giacovelli G, Setnikar I, Bottiglioni F. Efficacy on climacteric symptoms and safety of low dose estradiol transdermal matrix patches. A randomized, double-blind placebo-controlled study. Arzneimittelforschung 2000;50(3):293–300.
206. Lake Y, Pinnock S. Improved patient acceptability with a transdermal drug-in-adhesive oestradiol patch. Aust NZ J Obstet Gynaecol 2000;40(3):313–16.
207. Rioux JE, Devlin C, Gelfand MM, Steinberg WM, Hepburn DS. 17 beta-estradiol vaginal tablet versus conjugated equine estrogen vaginal cream to relieve menopausal atrophic vaginitis. Menopause 2000;7(3):156–61.
208. Bachmann G. Estradiol-releasing vaginal ring delivery system for urogenital atrophy. Experience over the past decade. J Reprod Med 1998;43(11):991–8.
209. Lose G, Englev E. Oestradiol-releasing vaginal ring versus oestriol vaginal pessaries in the treatment of bothersome lower urinary tract symptoms. BJOG 2000; 107(8):1029–34.

Etacrynic acid

See also Diuretics

General Information

Etacrynic acid (ethacrynic acid) is a loop diuretic with similar actions to furosemide and bumetanide. However, it has more adverse effects than the other loop diuretics and offers no clear advantages.

Organs and Systems

Sensory systems

Etacrynic acid is ototoxic after intravenous administration (1–3), an effect that is dose-related. It can sometimes be permanent (3,4). An association with nystagmus has also been reported (3,5). The risk has been estimated to be about seven per 1000 injections (6). The risk is increased in renal insufficiency and in patients who are also being given aminoglycoside antibiotics. Animal data suggest that etacrynic acid is more ototoxic than furosemide (7).

Metabolism

Like other diuretics etacrynic acid can impair glucose tolerance in patients with type 2 diabetes mellitus (8). Non-ketotic hyperglycemia has also been reported (9). However, hypoglycemia has also been reported in two patients with uremia (10).

There has been an anecdotal report of hyperuricemia and acute gout in a patient taking etacrynic acid (11).

Electrolyte balance

Etacrynic acid can cause excessive diuresis, natriuresis, and kaliuresis, leading respectively to dehydration and sodium and potassium depletion (12–17).

Mineral balance

Etacrynic acid can cause hypocalcemia and hypomagnesemia (18).

Hematologic

There have been anecdotal reports of agranulocytosis (12,19), hemolytic anemia (20), and thrombocytopenia (16,21).

Gastrointestinal

Nausea, abdominal pain (22), and diarrhea are relatively common with etacrynic acid (23,24), more so than with other loop diuretics. Data from the Boston Drug Surveillance Program showed that intravenous etacrynic acid was associated with an increased incidence of gastrointestinal bleeding (25,26). Overall 20% of the patients treated with etacrynic acid bled, compared with 5% of those who received furosemide. With intravenous etacrynic acid the risk of gastrointestinal hemorrhage was 26%, compared with 10% after oral administration. However, 12 of 28 patients who bled did so before etacrynic acid had been given (27), and it is not clear whether there is a true difference in risk with the different routes of administration.

Liver

Like other diuretics etacrynic acid can precipitate hepatic encephalopathy in the treatment of ascites in patients with hepatic cirrhosis (28). There has been an anecdotal report of focal hepatic necrosis in a patient taking etacrynic acid (29).

Pancreas

There has been an anecdotal report of necrotizing pancreatitis in a patient taking etacrynic acid (30).

Immunologic

Two patients developed a Henoch-Schönlein type of necrotic hemorrhagic rash of the legs and lower part of the body accompanied by histological evidence of vasculitis (31). In both cases the lesions appeared about 2–3 weeks after the start of treatment; in another case a hemorrhagic rash was accompanied by acute gastric and duodenal ulceration (32).

Drug Administration

Drug administration route

Intravenous administration of etacrynic acid causes burning at the site of injection (18).

Drug–Drug Interactions

Aminoglycoside antibiotics

Etacrynic acid potentiates aminoglycoside ototoxicity by facilitating the entry of the antibiotics from the systemic circulation into the endolymph (33). Animal evidence suggests that this effect may be potentiated by glutathione depletion (34). Conversely, neomycin can enhance the penetration of etacrynic acid into the inner ear (35).

Cardiac glycosides

Etacrynic acid potentiates the actions of cardiac glycosides if it causes potassium depletion.

- A patient developed digitalis intoxication and quinidine-induced cardiac dysrhythmias when hypokalemia occurred during etacrynic acid therapy (36).

In rats etacrynic acid inhibited the absorption of digitoxin from the small intestine (37), but an interaction of this sort has not been described in man.

Cefaloridine

Etacrynic potentiated the nephrotoxic effects of cefaloridine in mice, causing renal tubular necrosis (38).

Glucocorticoids

In a survey of the effects of etacrynic acid in 16 646 patients with gastrointestinal bleeding, the risk of major bleeding was increased in patients taking etacrynic acid (4.5% of 111 patients versus 0.2% of 10 637 patients taking no drugs). The risk was further increased in patients taking etacrynic acid plus glucocorticoids (9.1% of 22 patients) (25).

Glyceryl trinitrate

Etacrynic acid inhibited relaxation of large coronary microvessels in response to glyceryl trinitrate in pigs (39). The relevance of this to the clinical use of these drugs is not known.

Lithium

The loop diuretics increase the renal excretion of lithium after single-dose intravenous administration in both animals (40) and man (41). Furosemide has been used to treat lithium intoxication (42). The effect of etacrynic acid is larger than those of furosemide and bumetanide (41). However, long-term treatment with furosemide and bumetanide can cause lithium intoxication in some patients (43,44), perhaps by causing sodium depletion and a secondary increase in lithium reabsorption. An adverse interaction of lithium during long-term therapy with etacrynic acid is therefore theoretically likely.

Methotrexate

Etacrynic acid interacts with human serum albumin and modifies its binding properties (45). Since it binds to two binding sites on albumin, the benzodiazepine binding site and the warfarin binding site, it can displace drugs that bind at those sites (46). It competitively displaced 7-hydroxymethotrexate from its binding proteins in vitro (47). The clinical significance of this effect is not known.

Warfarin

Etacrynic acid interacts with human serum albumin and modifies its binding properties (45). Since it binds to two binding sites on albumin, the benzodiazepine binding site and the warfarin binding site, it can displace drugs that bind at those sites (46,48). This has been described for warfarin, whose anticoagulant effect it potentiated (49).

References

1. Beauchamp GD, Crouch TC. Deafness. Review of intravenous ethacrynic acid. J Kans Med Soc 1975;76(7):166–8, 180.
2. Schneider WJ, Becker EL. Acute transient hearing loss after ethacrynic acid therapy. Arch Intern Med 1966;117(5):715–17.
3. Schwartz FD, Pillay VK, Kark RM. Ethacrynic acid: its usefulness and untoward effects. Am Heart J 1970;79(3):427–8.
4. Meriwether WD, Mangi RJ, Serpick AA. Deafness following standard intravenous dose of ethacrynic acid. JAMA 1971;216(5):795–8.
5. Gomolin IH, Garschick E. Ethacrynic acid-induced deafness accompanied by nystagmus. N Engl J Med 1980;303(12):702.
6. Boston Collaborative Drug Surveillance Program. A cooperative study. Drug-induced deafness. JAMA 1973;224(4):515–16.
7. Brown RD. Comparison of the cochlear toxicity of sodium ethacrynate, furosemide, and the cysteine adduct of sodium ethacrynate in cats. Toxicol Appl Pharmacol 1975;31(2):270–82.
8. Russell RP, Lindeman RD, Prescott LF. Metabolic and hypotensive effects of ethacrynic acid. Comparative study with hydrochlorothiazide. JAMA 1968;205(1):81–5.
9. Cowley AJ, Elkeles RS. Diabetes and therapy with potent diuretics. Lancet 1978;1(8056):154.
10. Maher JF, Schreiner GE. Studies on ethacrynic acid in patients with refractory edema. Ann Intern Med 1965;62:15–29.
11. Melvin KE, Farrelly RO, North JD. Ethacrynic acid: a new oral diuretic. BMJ 1963;5344:1521–4.
12. Ledingham JG, Bayliss RI. Ethacrynic acid: two years' experience with a new diuretic. BMJ 1965;5464:732–5.
13. Daley D, Evans B. Diuretic action of ethacrynic acid in congestive heart failure. BMJ 1963;5366:1169–71.
14. DeRubertis FR, Michelis MF, Beck N, Davis BB. Complications of diuretic therapy: severe alkalosis and syndrome resembling inappropriate secretion of antidiuretic hormone. Metabolism 1970;19(9):709–19.
15. Fort AT, Morrison JC, Fish SA. Iatrogenic hypokalemia of pregnancy by furosemide and ethacrynic acid. J Reprod Med 1971;6(5):207–8.
16. Schroeder G, Sannerstedt R, Werkoe L. Clinical experiences with ethacrynic acid, a new non-thiazide saluretic agent (MK-595). Acta Med Scand 1964;175:781–6.
17. Sullivan RC, Freemon FR, Caranasos GJ. Complications from diuretic therapy with ethacrynic acid and furosemide. South Med J 1971;64(7):869–72.
18. Lacreta FP, Brennan JM, Nash SL, Comis RL, Tew KD, O'Dwyer PJ. Pharmacokinetics and bioavailability study of ethacrynic acid as a modulator of drug resistance in patients with cancer. J Pharmacol Exp Ther 1994;270(3): 1186–91.
19. Walker JG. Fatal agranulocytosis complicating treatment with ethacrynic acid. Report of a case. Ann Intern Med 1966;64(6):1303–5.
20. Hanna M. Ethacrynic acid (MK595) as a diuretic—some early observations. Med J Aust 1966;1(13):534–7.
21. O'Dwyer PJ, LaCreta F, Nash S, Tinsley PW, Schilder R, Clapper ML, Tew KD, Panting L, Litwin S, Comis RL, et al. Phase I study of thiotepa in combination with the glutathione transferase inhibitor ethacrynic acid. Cancer Res 1991;51(22):6059–65.
22. Hagedorn CW, Kaplan AA, Hulet WH. Prolonged administration of ethacrynic acid in patients with chronic renal disease. N Engl J Med 1965;272:1152–5.
23. Dollery CT, Parry EH, Young DS. Diuretic and hypotensive properties of ethacrynic acid: a comparison with hydrochlorothiazide. Lancet 1964;41:947–52.
24. Lauwers L. Clinical experience with a new diuretic: ethacrinic acid. Acta Cardiol 1966;21(1):79–89.
25. Jick H, Porter J. Drug-induced gastrointestinal bleeding. Report from the Boston Collaborative Drug Surveillance Program, Boston University Medical Center. Lancet 1978;2(8080):87–9.
26. Slone D, Jick H, Lewis GP, Shapiro S, Miettinen OS. Intravenously given ethacrynic acid and gastrointestinal bleeding. A finding resulting from comprehensive drug surveillance. JAMA 1969;209(11):1668–71.
27. Wilkinson WH, Ciminera JL, Simpkins GT. Intravenously given ethacrynic acid and gastrointestinal bleeding. JAMA 1969;210:347.
28. Sherlock S, Senewiratne B, Scott A, Walker JG. Complications of diuretic therapy in hepatic cirrhosis. Lancet 1966;1(7446):1049–52.
29. Datey KK, Deshmukh SN, Dalvi CP, Purandare NM. Hepatocellular damage with ethacrynic acid. BMJ 1967;3(558):152–3.
30. Schmidt P, Friedman IS. Adverse effects of ethacrynic acid. NY State J Med 1967;67(11):1438–42.
31. Bar-On H, Eisenberg S, Eliakim M. Clinical experience with ethacrynic acid with reference to a possible complication of the Schoenlein–Henoch type. Isr J Med Sci 1967;3(1):113–18.
32. Pain AK. Acute gastric ulceration associated with drug therapy. BMJ 1967;1(540):634.
33. Conlon BJ, McSwain SD, Smith DW. Topical gentamicin and ethacrynic acid: effects on cochlear function. Laryngoscope 1998;108(7):1087–9.
34. Hoffman DW, Whitworth CA, Jones-King KL, Rybak LP. Potentiation of ototoxicity by glutathione depletion. Ann Otol Rhinol Laryngol 1988;97(1):36–41.
35. Orsulakova A, Schacht J. A biochemical mechanism of the ototoxic interaction between neomycin and ethacrynic acid. Acta Otolaryngol 1982;93(1–2):43–8.

36. Oravetz J, Slodki SJ. Recurrent ventricular fibrillation precipitated by quinidine. Report of a patient with recovery after 28 paroxysms. Arch Intern Med 1968;122(1):63–5.
37. Braun W, Damm KH. Drug interactions in intestinal absorption of ^{3}H-digitoxin in rats. Experientia 1976;32(5):613–14.
38. Dodds MG, Foord RD. Enhancement by potent diuretics of renal tubular necrosis induced by cephaloridine. Br J Pharmacol 1970;40(2):227–36.
39. Sellke FW, Tomanek RJ, Harrison DG. L-cysteine selectively potentiates nitroglycerin-induced dilation of small coronary microvessels. J Pharmacol Exp Ther 1991;258(1): 365–9.
40. Stokke ES, Ostensen J, Hartmann A, Kiil F. Loop diuretics reduce lithium reabsorption without affecting bicarbonate and phosphate reabsorption. Acta Physiol Scand 1990;140(1):111–18.
41. Beutler JJ, Boer WH, Koomans HA, Dorhout Mees EJ. Comparative study of the effects of furosemide, ethacrynic acid and bumetanide on the lithium clearance and diluting segment reabsorption in humans. J Pharmacol Exp Ther 1992;260(2):768–72.
42. Hansen HE, Amdisen A. Lithium intoxication. (Report of 23 cases and review of 100 cases from the literature). Q J Med 1978;47(186):123–44.
43. Jefferson JW, Kalin NH. Serum lithium levels and long-term diuretic use. JAMA 1979;241(11):1134–6.
44. Huang LG. Lithium intoxication with coadministration of a loop-diuretic. J Clin Psychopharmacol 1990;10(3):228.
45. Bertucci C, Wainer IW. Improved chromatographic performance of a modified human albumin based stationary phase. Chirality 1997;9(4):335–40.
46. Fehske KJ, Muller WE. High-affinity binding of ethacrynic acid is mediated by the two most important drug binding sites of human serum albumin. Pharmacology 1986;32(4): 208–13.
47. Slordal L, Sager G, Jaeger R, Aarbakke J. Interactions with the protein binding of 7-hydroxy-methotrexate in human serum in vitro. Biochem Pharmacol 1988;37(4): 607–11.
48. Sellers EM, Koch-Weser J. Displacement of warfarin from human albumin by diazoxide and ethacrynic, mefenamic, and nalidixic acids. Clin Pharmacol Ther 1970;11(4):524–9.
49. Petrick RJ, Kronacher N, Alcena V. Interaction between warfarin and ethacrynic acid. JAMA 1975;231(8):843–4.

Etamivan

General Information

Etamivan has actions similar to doxapram hydrochloride and has been used as a respiratory stimulant. However, it has a low therapeutic index and the incidence of adverse effects from intravenous etamivan is high. Laryngospasm, sneezing, and substernal chest pain have been among the reactions recorded after intravenous infusion.

Drug Administration

Drug overdose

If it is given too rapidly or in too high a dose; generalized convulsions sometimes occur (1). Epilepsy is a contraindication to etamivan.

Drug–Drug Interactions

Monoamine oxidase inhibitors

Concurrent use of monoamine oxidase inhibitors, which lower the seizure threshold, is a contraindication to etamivan.

Reference

1. Couch RB, Cate TR, Chanock RM. Evaluation of a new analeptic: etamivan (emivan). JAMA 1964;187:448–9.

Etamsylate

General Information

Etamsylate (formerly also known as cyclonamine) is a synthetic water-soluble non-steroidal drug (diethylamine 2,5-dihydroxybenzenesulphonate), which was shown many years ago to increase platelet adhesion to glass beads. Subsequent clinical studies in animals reported dose-related reduced blood loss after experimental injury associated with etamsylate (1). In a small, randomized, double-blind trial, etamsylate reduced the prolongation of bleeding time and associated blood loss caused by aspirin (2). Treatment with etamsylate does not boost the platelet count or concentrations of coagulation factors (3). Etamsylate improves hemostasis by improving platelet adhesiveness and restoring capillary resistance through enhancement of the expression of P-selectin (4). It has also been suggested that it increases capillary vascular wall resistance (5).

Uses

Etamsylate is licensed for the prophylaxis and treatment of periventricular hemorrhage in neonates, in whom it is apparently effective (6,7). In a multicenter, double-blind, placebo-controlled trial in 330 infants, intraventricular and parenchymal hemorrhages developed in 30/162 infants in the treated group (etamsylate 12.5 mg/kg 6-hourly from within 1 hour of delivery for 4 days), compared with 50/168 in the control group (8). The incidence of intraventricular and parenchymal hemorrhage in survivors was 20/137 after etamsylate and 37/146 in the controls. No adverse effects were attributed to etamsylate. In a double-blind, prospective follow-up of this study, 268 of 276 survivors of the original study were seen at 3.5–4.2 years of age (9). There was no difference between the groups in neuromotor outcome (cerebral palsy) or in the general cognitive index of the McCarthy scales; fewer of the children who were given etamsylate had squints or required surgery for patent ductus arteriosus.

Etamsylate is more widely used to treat menorrhagia, including that associated with use of intrauterine contraceptive devices (10–12), although its efficacy has been challenged. A meta-analysis of drugs available in primary care showed that tranexamic acid was the most effective agent available for treatment of menorrhagia, while etamsylate was not associated with significant benefit (13). Guidelines published by the Royal College of Obstetricians and Gynaecologists in the UK stated that "at currently recommended doses, etamsylate is not an effective treatment for menorrhagia" (14). A significant proportion of women with primary menorrhagia turn out to have congenital disorders of coagulation, such as von Willebrand disease, and these cases do not respond to etamsylate (3).

No clinical benefit for patients without bleeding disorders undergoing surgical procedures has been established (15–17), although results in tonsillectomy have yielded conflicting results (18,19).

General adverse effects

Whatever the merits of etamsylate in reducing blood loss in various clinical conditions, it is at least clear that no serious adverse reactions have been attributed to it. A few patients experience nausea, but this is usually avoided by taking the drug after food. Minor adverse effects that have been reported include indigestion, headache, and vertigo (20). Toxicity studies in mice have also shown no adverse effects.

Organs and Systems

Cardiovascular

Modest but transient hypotension has occasionally been observed after intravenous injection, and elderly subjects appear to be more susceptible (21).

Hematologic

Marked leukopenia was reported in one retrospective study in children receiving etamsylate, but a causal link was not firmly established (1,22).

Skin

Skin rashes have occasionally been observed in patients taking etamsylate (23).

References

1. Deacock AR, Birley DM. The anti-haemorrhagic activity of ethamsylate (Dicynene). An experimental study. Br J Anaesth 1969;41(1):18–24.
2. Hutton RA, Wickham EA, Reed JV, Tuddenham EG. Studies on the action of ethamsylate (Dicynene) on haemostasis. Thromb Haemost 1986;56(1):6–8.
3. Hutton RA, Hales M, Kernoff PB. A study of the effect of ethamsylate (Dicynene) on the bleeding time, von Willebrand factor level and fibrinolysis in patients with von Willebrand's disease. Thromb Haemost 1988;60(3):506–7.
4. Alvarez-Guerra M, Hernandez MR, Escolar G, Chiavaroli C, Garay RP, Hannaert P. The hemostatic agent ethamsylate enhances P-selectin membrane expression in human platelets and cultured endothelial cells. Thromb Res 2002;107(6):329–35.
5. Vinazzer H. Clinical and experimental studies on the action of ethamsylate on haemostasis and on platelet functions. Thromb Res 1980;19(6):783–91.
6. Morgan ME, Benson JW, Cooke RW. Ethamsylate reduces the incidence of periventricular haemorrhage in very low birth-weight babies. Lancet 1981;2(8251):830–1.
7. Harrison RF, Matthews T. Intrapartum ethamsylate. Lancet 1984;2(8397):296.
8. Benson JW, Drayton MR, Hayward C, Murphy JF, Osborne JP, Rennie JM, Schulte JF, Speidel BD, Cooke RW. Multicentre trial of ethamsylate for prevention of periventricular haemorrhage in very low birthweight infants. Lancet 1986;2(8519):1297–300.
9. Schulte J, Osborne J, Benson JW, Cooke R, Drayton M, Murphy J, Rennie J, Speidel B. Developmental outcome of the use of etamsylate for prevention of periventricular haemorrhage in a randomised controlled trial. Arch Dis Child Fetal Neonatal Ed 2005;90(1):F31–5.
10. Jaffe G, Wickham A. A double-blind pilot study of Dicynene in the control of menorrhagia. J Intern Med Res 1973;1:127.
11. Harrison RF, Cambell S. A double-blind trial of ethamsylate in the treatment of primary and intrauterine-device menorrhagia. Lancet 1976;2(7980):283–5.
12. Kovacs L, Annus J. Effectiveness of etamsylate in intrauterine-device menorrhagia. Gynecol Invest 1978; 9(4):161–5.
13. Coulter A, Kelland J, Peto V, Rees MC. Treating menorrhagia in primary care. An overview of drug trials and a survey of prescribing practice. Int J Technol Assess Health Care 1995;11(3):456–71.
14. Royal College of Obstetricians and Gynaecologists (UK) Menorrhagia Guideline Group. The initial management of menorrhagia, 1998.
15. Keith I. Ethamsylate and blood loss in total hip replacement. Anaesthesia 1979;34(7):666–70.
16. Martin JP. Effect of ethamsylate on blood loss during cataract surgery. Trans Ophthalmol Soc U K 1974; 94(2):610–13.
17. Lyth DR, Booth CM. Does ethamsylate reduce haemorrhage in transurethral prostatectomy? Br J Urol 1990; 66(6):631–4.
18. Verstraete M, Tyberghein J, De Greef Y, Daems L, Van Hoof A. Double-blind trials with ethamsylate, batroxobin or tranexamic acid on blood loss after adenotonsillectomy. Acta Clin Belg 1977;32(2):136–41.
19. Arora YR, Manford ML. Operative blood loss and the frequency of haemorrhage associated with adenotonsillectomy in children: a double-blind trial of ethamsylate. Br J Anaesth 1979;51(6):557–61.
20. Sevin R, Cuendet JF. Résistance capillaire et rétinopathie diabetique. Effect de l'etamsylate (Cyclonamine ou Dicynone). [Capillary resistance and diabetic retinopathy. Effect of etamsylate (Cyclonamine or Dicynone).] Ophthalmologica 1968; 155(3):186–93.
21. Watson B. Transient hypotension following intravenous ethamsylate (Dicynene) BMJ 1977;1(6077):1664.
22. Ritter L, Schlosser H, Boos J, Heyen P. Einfluss von Etamsylat auf die Blutungsneigung von Kindern mit onkologischen Erkrankungen—Retrospektive Matched-pair-Analyse von 64 Patienten bei Untersuchung von 100 Patienten der Universitätskinderklinik Münster. [Effect of etamsylate on hemorrhagic diathesis of children with oncologic diseases. Retrospective matched-pair analysis of 64 patients in a study of 100 patients of the Munster University Pediatric Clinic.] Klin Padiatr 1991; 203(4):296–301.
23. Roy SN, Bhattacharya S. Benefits and risks of pharmacological agents used for the treatment of menorrhagia. Drug Saf 2004;27(2):75–90.

Etanercept

General Information

Etanercept is a dimeric fusion protein consisting of two recombinant p75 tumor necrosis factor receptors fused with the Fc portion of human IgG1. It inhibits the binding of tumor necrosis factor alfa to its receptor and thereby neutralizes its biological activity. It has been used in the treatment of moderate to severe active rheumatoid arthritis, ankylosing spondylitis, psoriatic arthropathy, and juvenile rheumatoid arthritis in patients who have failed to respond to previous disease-modifying antirheumatic drugs. The clinical pharmacology and adverse effects of etanercept in patients with rheumatoid disorders have been reviewed (1).

Comparative studies

In a study of weekly oral methotrexate in two different doses (10 or 25 mg) or twice-weekly etanercept in 632 patients, etanercept produced fewer systemic adverse effects than methotrexate, but a higher incidence of injection site reactions (2). Despite theoretical concerns about the development of autoimmune reactions in patients taking etanercept, no evidence of clinical autoimmune disease emerged from this large trial.

General adverse effects

The therapeutic use and safety of etanercept have been reviewed (3). Mild-to-moderate injection site reactions were the most common adverse effects (42–49%), with a frequency 3.8 to 6 times greater than with placebo. Non-neutralizing antibodies to etanercept were rarely detected. Etanercept-treated patients more often developed new antinuclear antibodies or anti-double-stranded DNA antibodies, but no patient developed symptoms suggestive of an autoimmune disease during clinical trials.

Organs and Systems

Respiratory

The typical histological morphology of pulmonary rheumatoid nodules that developed during etanercept treatment has been reported (4,5). Pulmonary granulomas during etanercept treatment can be coincidental and difficult to distinguish from other pulmonary complications, such as relapse of tuberculosis. In two patients with rheumatoid arthritis who underwent lung biopsy for etanercept-associated pulmonary granulomas, there were non-caseating granulomas containing birefringent particulate in one (6) and caseating necrosis in the other (7). Infectious causes were ruled out. After etanercept withdrawal, the lesions resolved completely with steroid treatment in the first patient but persisted over 1 year despite antituberculosis treatment in the other.

Nervous system

Postmarketing warnings about etanercept that have been issued by regulatory agencies and the manufacturers relate to a possible increased risk of demyelinating disorders, such as multiple sclerosis, myelitis, and optic neuritis, in patients with pre-existing or a recent history of demyelinating disorders (SEDA-26, 399). This was in keeping with the results obtained in a placebo-controlled trial of lenercept, another recombinant tumor necrosis factor alfa receptor immunoglobulin fusion protein, in 168 patients with multiple sclerosis; compared with placebo, significantly more patients randomized to lenercept had exacerbation of multiple sclerosis, and exacerbation also occurred earlier (8).

Transverse myelitis of abrupt onset has also been reported (9).

- A 45-year-old woman with resistant rheumatoid arthritis was given etanercept 25 mg twice weekly. Nine days later she developed total acute sensory loss, with flaccid paraplegia, fecal incontinence, and urinary retention. MRI imaging and cerebrospinal fluid analysis were consistent with a diagnosis of transverse myelitis. She also had positive antinuclear and anticardiolipin antibodies. After etanercept withdrawal and treatment with dexamethasone and cyclophosphamide, her motor function improved with no change in sensory function.

Neurological events suggestive of demyelinating disorders in patients treated with tumor necrosis factor alfa antagonists and reported to the FDA's Adverse Events Reporting System have been reviewed (10). These included 17 cases temporarily associated with etanercept and two with infliximab, but complete information was lacking in a number of cases. One additional case with etanercept was more extensively detailed. The first symptoms occurred after a large range of delay after first drug administration (1 week to 15 months; mean 5 months) and mostly included paresthesia, optic neuritis, and confusion. MRI scans in 19 patients showed demyelination in various brain areas in 16. Although a causal relation was not proven, it is noteworthy that most patients improved after withdrawal and one patient had recurrent neurological symptoms after etanercept readministration. The various hypothetical mechanisms by which tumor necrosis factor alfa antagonists might produce demyelinating events have been discussed elsewhere (11). Briefly, they cause increased peripheral T cell autoreactivity, and their inability to cross the blood–brain barrier may account for exacerbation of central demyelinating disorders.

Endocrine

- Transient hyperthyroidism occurred after 6 months of etanercept treatment in a 37-year-old woman with rheumatoid arthritis (12).

However, a direct causal relation with etanercept was debatable, because there was complete resolution with propranolol and despite continuation of etanercept.

Metabolism

Type 1 diabetes mellitus occurred after 5 months treatment with etanercept for juvenile rheumatoid arthritis in a 7-year-old girl (13). Antiglutamic acid decarboxylase antibodies were positive both before and during treatment, suggesting that etanercept may have prematurely triggered an underlying disease.

Hematologic

Postmarketing warnings about etanercept that have been issued by regulatory agencies and the manufacturers relate to a possible risk of aplastic anemia and pancytopenia (10 reported cases, of which 5 ended in fatal sepsis) (8).

Etanercept has reportedly caused abrupt exacerbation of the macrophage activation syndrome (14).

- A 22-year-old woman with adult-onset Still's disease developed symptoms suggestive of the macrophage activation syndrome. After initial glucocorticoid treatment, she received two doses of etanercept, and within 6 days her white blood cell count fell from $6.4 \times 10^9/l$ to $2.5 \times 10^9/l$ and the neutrophil count from $0.8 \times 10^9/l$ to $0.2 \times 10^9/l$. There was also thrombocytopenia and impaired coagulation and her liver enzymes were raised. A bone marrow aspirate showed delayed myelopoiesis. She received multiple transfusions, intravenous immunoglobulin, and granulocyte-macrophage colony-stimulating factor. The macrophage activation syndrome was diagnosed at that time and she was successfully treated with pulse methylprednisolone and ciclosporin. Epstein–Barr virus infection was subsequently confirmed.

Because soluble tumor necrosis factor alfa receptors are supposedly involved in the macrophage activation syndrome, the authors speculated that the administration of additional soluble receptors may have been the cause of a prolonged and exacerbated syndrome.

Urinary tract

Glomerulonephritis has been discussed as a possible consequence of etanercept treatment in two patients, with biopsy-proven mesangial deposits of IgA in one (15).

Skin

Injection site reactions are very common during the first month of treatment with etanercept. Histological findings in one patient showed a mild transient inflammatory response that did not suggest sensitization (16). The clinical and histological characteristics of these lesions have been analysed in a retrospective review of 103 etanercept-treated patients and in three other patients assessed prospectively (17). Of 103 patients, 21 had injection site reactions (erythema, pain, pruritus, or edema) within the first 2 months of treatment, and typically within 1–2 days after the last injection. In addition, eight patients developed recall reactions while continuing to take etanercept. Skin biopsies and immunohistological analysis of reaction sites in three patients showed an inflammatory infiltrate consistent with a T cell-mediated delayed hypersensitivity reaction.

There have been several descriptions of new cutaneous or pulmonary nodulosis in patients with rheumatoid arthritis treated with etanercept (4,18); concomitant cutaneous vasculitis was also reported in two patients (18). Although this may have been due to the natural history of rheumatoid arthritis or a lack of response to treatment, the short time to the occurrence of cutaneous nodulosis after the start of therapy in some patients implicated the etanercept.

Cutaneous vasculitis can also be the sole cutaneous manifestation of etanercept treatment (19). Purpuric lesions with histological features of leukocytoclastic vasculitis have been reported in a 58-year-old man (20) and a necrotizing vasculitis with eosinophils in a skin biopsy in a woman with rheumatoid arthritis (21). However, it is not known whether this resulted from the deposition of specific immune complexes.

- A 13-year-old girl developed a slowly reversible purpuric rash after 6 weeks of etanercept treatment, and the lesions recurred on re-administration (22). However, further administration of a gradually increasing dose of etanercept, with concomitant high-dose glucocorticoids, and antihistamines, was well tolerated, suggesting that tolerance can be obtained.

One patient who had separate episodes of vascular purpura during each of three sequences of treatment with etanercept, with leukocytoclastic vasculitis during the third episode, later developed similar cutaneous lesions after a third injection of infliximab (19).

Other types of skin reactions that have been described in isolated reports include urticaria-like eruptions with prurigo in two patients with juvenile arthritis (23) and discoid lupus erythematosus in a woman with rheumatoid arthritis (21). Erythema multiforme in three patients and a lichenoid eruption in one were attributed to infliximab; however, one patient had similar lesions after etanercept (24).

Musculoskeletal

Painless orbital myositis has been reported in a 42-year-old woman taking etanercept, but a causal relation was not established (25).

Immunologic

Although patients treated with etanercept commonly develop new antinuclear antibodies or anti-double-stranded DNA antibodies, there were no reports of cutaneous or systemic lupus erythematosus in early clinical trials. However, since then, at least eight cases have been reported, including five patients with a lupus-like syndrome, two with acute discoid lupus, and one with subacute cutaneous lupus erythematosus (26–29). All were women and they developed their first symptoms 6 weeks to 14 months after the first injection of etanercept. Antinuclear and/or anti-DNA antibodies were positive in most of them. Etanercept was withdrawn in all patients with features of systemic lupus erythematosus, and the symptoms resolved within 2–8 weeks. The skin lesions also improved with local glucocorticoids, despite continued etanercept treatment in two patients with discoid lupus or subacute cutaneous lupus erythematosus. This suggests that etanercept-induced autoantibodies are sometimes associated with clinical autoimmune disease.

Infection risk

In contrast to infliximab, etanercept is rarely associated with severe infectious complications. This has been attributed to different mechanisms of tumor necrosis factor alfa neutralization by the two drugs. Indeed, only nine cases of tuberculosis have previously been reported to the FDA from more than 100 000 patients treated worldwide (30). However, severe or uncommon infectious complications (severe viral pneumonia, fatal pneumococcal sepsis due to necrotizing fasciitis, osteoarticular tuberculosis) have been described in patients taking etanercept and long-term glucocorticoids (31–33).

Long-Term Effects

Tumorigenicity

There is great concern about the potential development of malignancy after blockade of tumor necrosis factor alfa, and it is biologically plausible. The FDA received reports of 26 cases of lymphoproliferative disorders in patients treated with etanercept ($n = 18$) or infliximab ($n = 8$) over 20 months (34). Although this reporting rate does not exceed the age-adjusted incidence of lymphomas in the USA, spontaneous reporting underestimates the true incidence. In addition, several findings were similar to those reported in patients taking immunosuppressive drugs after transplantation. For example, 81% of the reported cases were non-Hodgkin's lymphomas. Also, the median time to occurrence after the start of anti-TNF-alfa treatment was only 8 weeks. Finally, lymphoma regressed in two patients after withdrawal and without specific cytotoxic therapy. Although the actual incidence of neoplasia was low, additional long-term data that take into account concomitant or previous immunosuppressive treatment are needed before firm conclusions can be reached.

Susceptibility Factors

Age

In eight children with juvenile rheumatoid arthritis, who had failed to respond to disease-modifying anti-rheumatic drugs, high-dose etanercept was well tolerated (35). None withdrew because of etanercept-related adverse events. One child reported transient erythema at the injection site after the first injection. Three had mild transient upper respiratory tract infections. There were no laboratory abnormalities.

Interference with Diagnostic Tests

Troponin concentration

Non-neutralizing antibodies to etanercept have been identified in clinical trials. Although there was no correlation between these antibodies and the development of adverse effects (2), their presence was suggested as a likely explanation of false-positive rises in troponin concentrations in an assay that used mouse antihuman troponin (36).

References

1. Culy CR, Keating GM. Etanercept: an updated review of its use in rheumatoid arthritis, psoriatic arthritis and juvenile rheumatoid arthritis. Drugs 2002;62(17):2493–537.
2. Bathon JM, Martin RW, Fleischmann RM, Tesser JR, Schiff MH, Keystone EC, Genovese MC, Wasko MC, Moreland LW, Weaver AL, Markenson J, Finck BK. A comparison of etanercept and methotrexate in patients with early rheumatoid arthritis. N Engl J Med 2000;343(22):1586–93.
3. Jarvis B, Faulds D. Etanercept: a review of its use in rheumatoid arthritis. Drugs 1999;57(6):945–66.
4. Kekow J, Welte T, Kellner U, Pap T. Development of rheumatoid nodules during anti-tumor necrosis factor alpha therapy with etanercept. Arthritis Rheum 2002;46(3):843–4.
5. Hubscher O, Re R, Iotti R. Pulmonary rheumatoid nodules in an etanercept-treated patient. Arthritis Rheum 2003;48(7):2077–8.
6. Peno-Green L, Lluberas G, Kingsley T, Brantley S. Lung injury linked to etanercept therapy. Chest 2002;122(5):1858–60.
7. Vavricka SR, Wettstein T, Speich R, Gaspert A, Bachli EB. Pulmonary granulomas after tumour necrosis factor alpha antagonist therapy. Thorax 2003;58(3):278–9.
8. Arnason BGW; The Lenercept Multiple Sclerosis Study Group and The University of British Columbia MS/MRI Analysis Group. TNF neutralization in MS: results of a randomized, placebo-controlled multicenter study. Neurology 1999;53(3):457–65.
9. van der Laken CJ, Lems WF, van Soesbergen RM, van der Sande JJ, Dijkmans BA. Paraplegia in a patient receiving anti-tumor necrosis factor therapy for rheumatoid arthritis: comment on the article by Mohan et al. Arthritis Rheum 2003;48(1):269–70.
10. Mohan N, Edwards ET, Cupps TR, Oliverio PJ, Sandberg G, Crayton H, Richert JR, Siegel JN. Demyelination occurring during anti-tumor necrosis factor alpha therapy for inflammatory arthritides. Arthritis Rheum 2001;44(12):2862–9.
11. Robinson WH, Genovese MC, Moreland LW. Demyelinating and neurologic events reported in association with tumor necrosis factor alpha antagonism: by what mechanisms could tumor necrosis factor alpha antagonists improve rheumatoid arthritis but exacerbate multiple sclerosis? Arthritis Rheum 2001;44(9):1977–83.
12. Allanore Y, Bremont C, Kahan A, Menkes CJ. Transient hyperthyroidism in a patient with rheumatoid arthritis treated by etanercept. Clin Exp Rheumatol 2001;19(3):356–7.
13. Bloom BJ. Development of diabetes mellitus during etanercept therapy in a child with systemic-onset juvenile rheumatoid arthritis. Arthritis Rheum 2000;43(11):2606–8.
14. Stern A, Buckley L. Worsening of macrophage activation syndrome in a patient with adult onset Still's disease after initiation of etanercept therapy. J Clin Rheumatol 2001;7:252–6.
15. Kemp E, Nielsen H, Petersen LJ, Gam AN, Dahlager J, Horn T, Larsen S, Olsen S. Newer immunomodulating drugs in rheumatoid arthritis may precipitate glomerulonephritis. Clin Nephrol 2001;55(1):87–8.
16. Murphy FT, Enzenauer RJ, Battafarano DF, David-Bajar K. Etanercept-associated injection-site reactions. Arch Dermatol 2000;136(4):556–7.
17. Zeltser R, Valle L, Tanck C, Holyst MM, Ritchlin C, Gaspari AA. Clinical, histological, and immunophenotypic characteristics of injection site reactions associated with etanercept: a recombinant tumor necrosis factor alpha receptor: Fc fusion protein. Arch Dermatol 2001;137(7):893–9.
18. Cunnane G, Warnock M, Fye KH, Daikh DI. Accelerated nodulosis and vasculitis following etanercept therapy for rheumatoid arthritis. Arthritis Rheum 2002;47(4):445–9.
19. McCain ME, Quinet RJ, Davis WE. Etanercept and infliximab associated with cutaneous vasculitis. Rheumatology (Oxford) 2002;41(1):116–17.
20. Galaria NA, Werth VP, Schumacher HR. Leukocytoclastic vasculitis due to etanercept. J Rheumatol 2000;27(8):2041–4.
21. Brion PH, Mittal-Henkle A, Kalunian KC. Autoimmune skin rashes associated with etanercept for rheumatoid arthritis. Ann Intern Med 1999;131(8):634.
22. Livermore PA, Murray KJ. Anti-tumour necrosis factor therapy associated with cutaneous vasculitis. Rheumatology (Oxford) 2002;41(12):1450–2.
23. Skytta E, Pohjankoski H, Savolainen A. Etanercept and urticaria in patients with juvenile idiopathic arthritis. Clin Exp Rheumatol 2000;18(4):533–4.

24. Vergara G, Silvestre JF, Betlloch I, Vela P, Albares MP, Pascual JC. Cutaneous drug eruption to infliximab: report of 4 cases with an interface dermatitis pattern. Arch Dermatol 2002;138(9):1258–9.
25. Caramaschi P, Biasi D, Carletto A, Bambara LM. Orbital myositis in a rheumatoid arthritis patient during etanercept treatment. Clin Exp Rheumatol 2003;21(1):136–7.
26. Bleumink GS, ter Borg EJ, Ramselaar CG, Ch Stricker BH. Etanercept-induced subacute cutaneous lupus erythematosus. Rheumatology (Oxford) 2001;40(11):1317–19.
27. De Bandt MJ, Descamps V, Meyer O. Two cases of etanercept-induced systemic lupus erythematosus in patients with rheumatoid arthritis. Ann Rheum Dis 2001;60:175.
28. Misery L, Perrot JL, Gentil-Perret A, Pallot-Prades B, Cambazard F, Alexandre C. Dermatological complications of etanercept therapy for rheumatoid arthritis. Br J Dermatol 2002;146(2):334–5.
29. Shakoor N, Michalska M, Harris CA, Block JA. Drug-induced systemic lupus erythematosus associated with etanercept therapy. Lancet 2002;359(9306):579–80.
30. Keane J, Gershon S, Wise RP, Mirabile-Levens E, Kasznica J, Schwieterman WD, Siegel JN, Braun MM. Tuberculosis associated with infliximab, a tumor necrosis factor alpha-neutralizing agent. N Engl J Med 2001;345(15):1098–104.
31. Baghai M, Osmon DR, Wolk DM, Wold LE, Haidukewych GJ, Matteson EL. Fatal sepsis in a patient with rheumatoid arthritis treated with etanercept. Mayo Clin Proc 2001;76(6):653–6.
32. Myers A, Clark J, Foster H. Tuberculosis and treatment with infliximab. N Engl J Med 2002;346(8):623–6.
33. Smith D, Letendre S. Viral pneumonia as a serious complication of etanercept therapy. Ann Intern Med 2002;136(2):174.
34. Brown SL, Greene MH, Gershon SK, Edwards ET, Braun MM. Tumor necrosis factor antagonist therapy and lymphoma development: twenty-six cases reported to the Food and Drug Administration. Arthritis Rheum 2002;46(12):3151–8.
35. Takei S, Groh D, Bernstein B, Shaham B, Gallagher K, Reiff A. Safety and efficacy of high dose etanercept in treatment of juvenile rheumatoid arthritis. J Rheumatol 2001;28(7):1677–80.
36. Russell E, Zeihen M, Wergin S, Litton T. Patients receiving etanercept may develop antibodies that interfere with monoclonal antibody laboratory assays. Arthritis Rheum 2000;43(4):944.

Ethacridine

See also Disinfectants and antiseptics

General Information

Ethacridine (6,9-diamino-2-ethoxyacridine) is widely used in the local treatment of inflammatory or ulcerative conditions of the skin, particularly crural eczema due to venous stasis. Many publications point to the high frequency of exacerbation involving local allergic reactions and also generalized eczematous reactions (SEDA-11, 474).

Ethacridine has also been given by slow extra-amniotic instillation of 150 ml of a 0.1% solution to induce abortion or delivery in patients with missed abortion or fetal death, and during the second and third trimester without or in combination with drip infusion of oxytocin or dinoprost (prostaglandin $F_{2\alpha}$) (SEDA-11, 474).

In 56 women (18–20 weeks gestation), treated at the Marie Stopes Clinic in Jodhpur, India, who underwent termination of pregnancy with 0.1% ethacridine lactate 150 ml injected into the intrauterine extra-amniotic space and in whom intravenous oxytocin was used to expedite the delivery of the abortus, ethacridine lactate induced successful abortion in 52 cases (1). Abortion failure occurred in the other four cases because of transverse lie of fetus ($n = 2$), cervical dystocia ($n = 1$), and uterine inertia ($n = 1$). In 41 women the abortion occurred at 12–24 hours after induction (mean 20 hours) which was shorter than that of previous reports (29.5–38 hours). There were complications in six cases: three women had cervical tears and three had incomplete expulsion. There was one case each of severe bleeding and vaginal laceration. There were no cases of sepsis. The authors concluded that ethacridine lactate performed better than other instillation abortion methods.

In a prospective, placebo-controlled study, tannin albuminate 500 mg plus ethacridine lactate 50 mg was given to 30 patients with Crohn's disease and chronic diarrhea for 5 days, followed by a 5-day break, and then a further 5 days treatment (2). Stool frequency was significantly reduced, albeit by only a small amount, with an improvement in the consistency of the stools.

References

1. Gupta S, Sachdeva L, Gupta R. Ethacridine lactate—a safe and effective drug for termination of pregnancy. Indian J Matern Child Health 1993;4(2):59–61.
2. Plein K, Burkard G, Hotz J. Behandlung der chronischen Diarrhoe beim Morbus Crohn. Eine Pilotstudie zur klinischen Wirkung von Tanninalbuminat und Ethacridinlactat. [Treatment of chronic diarrhea in Crohn disease. A pilot study of the clinical effect of tannin albuminate and ethacridine lactate.] Fortschr Med 1993;111(7):114–18.

Ethambutol

See also Antituberculosis drugs

General Information

Ethambutol is tuberculostatic and acts against *Mycobacterium tuberculosis* and *Mycobacterium kansasii* as well as some strains of *Mycobacterium avium* complex. It has no effect on other bacteria. The sensitivities of non-tuberculous mycobacteria are variable. Ethambutol suppresses the growth of most isoniazid-resistant and streptomycin-resistant tubercle bacilli (1).

The adverse effects of ethambutol are mainly seen in patients taking very high doses, that is over 25 mg/kg/day. Dosages over 25 mg/kg/day should be administered for only about 2 weeks at the beginning of therapy. Treatment can then be continued with 15 mg/kg/day. If initial problems arise and ethambutol is essential, the daily dose should not exceed 10 mg/kg.

About 80% of an oral dose of ethambutol is absorbed from the gastrointestinal tract. Peak plasma concentrations are reached in 2–4 hours and the half-life is 3–4 hours. Within 24 hours, about 60% is excreted unchanged in the urine. In patients with renal insufficiency, the dose has to be altered (2). There is no indication for ethambutol monotherapy.

General adverse effects

Visual disturbances are the most common adverse effects and also the most important. These include diminished visual acuity, retrobulbar neuritis, retinal pigment displacement, and (rarely) hemorrhages. Gastrointestinal symptoms (abdominal pain or vomiting), and headache, dizziness, mental confusion, and hallucinations are all rarely seen. Adverse effects are more frequent in elderly patients and patients with alcoholism, diabetes, or renal insufficiency. Stevens–Johnson syndrome, toxic epidermal necrolysis (3), purpura-like vasculitis, acute thrombogenic purpura, joint pain, drug fever, tachycardia, and leukopenia have been attributed to allergy. As these reactions often arise during combined treatment with other tuberculostatic drugs, it is difficult or impossible to determine which drug is responsible. Tumor-inducing and teratogenic effects have not been described.

Organs and Systems

Nervous system

Peripheral neuropathy can precede or accompany ocular damage from ethambutol. These symptoms can serve as warning of impending eye damage (4). Loss of sensitivity, with numbness and tingling of the fingers, are relatively rare adverse effects (5). Electroneuromyography in ethambutol-induced neuropathy has confirmed that elderly patients are at increased risk (6). Sensory changes are more severe than motor dysfunction (5).

Sensory systems

Ocular disturbances due to ethambutol are dose-related. Dosages not over 25 mg/kg/day during the first 2 months of treatment and 15 mg/kg/day thereafter are generally accepted as adequate (7). At a dosage of 15 mg/kg/day, which should be regarded as a maximum for maintenance therapy, ocular toxicity developed in only 1.6% of patients (8). Advanced age (9), renal insufficiency, and diabetes can enhance ocular damage.

- The earliest onset of visual disturbance occurred in a 26-year-old man 3 days after beginning combined treatment including 15 mg/kg/day ethambutol, suggesting an idiosyncratic reaction (10).

Biochemical research has shown the importance of zinc metabolism in the retina (9). Zinc is found in high concentrations in the choroid, the retina, and especially the ganglion cells. Retinol dehydrogenase, a zinc-containing enzyme, interferes with the transformation of retinol (vitamin A_1), which is essential for color sensation and conal vision. Furthermore, zinc is involved in the biosynthesis of the specific transport of retinol from the liver to the effector cells. Ethambutol is a chelating agent and makes zinc unavailable for axoplasmic transport, provoking optic or retrobulbar neuritis (11). Patients with zinc blood concentrations below 0.7 μg/ml (reference range 0.9–1.0 μg/ml) before the use of ethambutol are at high risk of ocular disturbances (12).

The onset of visual loss can be sudden and dramatic, with color vision defects in the red–green or blue–yellow spectra, as well as variable field defects. In acute cases, disc edema is accompanied by splinter hemorrhages. Retrobulbar neuritis with ethambutol can be predominantly axial, presenting with reduced visual acuity and central scotoma, or periaxial, with peripheral field defects. In non-acute types the fundi and discs appear normal (13). Visual defects can be unilateral or bilateral.

Visual-evoked potential tests, such as flash electroretinography, flash and pattern visual-evoked responses, flicker fusion thresholds, and visual field perimetry, are reported to be the most reliable methods for early detection of ocular abnormalities (8,11,14). The routine use of visual-evoked potentials in the systematic follow-up of ethambutol-treated patients has been recommended (15).

Color vision and visual acuity should be examined before beginning ethambutol and every 2–4 weeks during treatment, using color tables and reading tests (SED-9, 525). Some recommend computerized perimetry of the central visual fields (SED-10, 581) (16,17). In patients with diabetes with retinopathy monthly monitoring of the fundi and visual acuity are mandatory. Early childhood, when visual examination is difficult or impossible, is a major indication for electroretinography. As a rule, ethambutol is not recommended for children under 5 years of age, because of the difficulty in reliably testing their visual acuity, unless the severity of tuberculosis makes the use of ethambutol necessary (15).

If ethambutol is not withdrawn when visual symptoms occur, optic atrophy or permanent blindness can occur. Patients therefore have to be instructed to interrupt treatment if they experience any visual abnormality. Hydroxocobalamin can accelerate recovery (18).

Metabolism

Blood urate concentrations can be increased because of reduced excretion of uric acid in patients taking ethambutol (19). This is probably enhanced by combined treatment with isoniazid and pyridoxine. Special attention should be paid when tuberculostatic drug combinations include pyrazinamide. However, severe untoward clinical effects are rare, except in patients with gout or renal insufficiency (2,20).

Hematologic

Acute thrombocytopenia, probably due to an immunological mechanism, has been described in a single patient (21).

Liver

Jaundice and non-icteric liver disturbances probably occur in under 0.1% of patients, as long as isoniazid and rifampicin are not given simultaneously (22).

Second-Generation Effects

Pregnancy

Ethambutol in combination with isoniazid in pregnancy has been suspected of causing one case of gastrointestinal malformation, but other factors may have been implicated (SEDA-12, 256).

Teratogenicity

Fetal damage has not been attributed to ethambutol (23).

Fetotoxicity

Toxic effects in the newborn have not been attributed to ethambutol (24).

Lactation

No adverse effects during lactation have been attributed to ethambutol (24).

Susceptibility Factors

Renal disease

In patients with impaired glomerular filtration or any other renal dysfunction, ethambutol dosages have to be altered (25).

Drug–Drug Interactions

Antacids

In 13 patients with tuberculosis, aluminium hydroxide significantly lowered serum ethambutol concentrations during the first 4 hours after a dose; in healthy volunteers, both aluminium hydroxide and glycopyrrhonium, alone or in combination, reduced ethambutol absorption (26).

Isoniazid

The risk of optic neuropathy due to ethambutol may be increased when it is combined with isoniazid.

- A 40-year-old patient underwent unsuccessful cadaver kidney transplantation and was treated with ethambutol and isoniazid (27). Bilateral retrobulbar neuropathy with an unusual central bitemporal hemianopic scotoma developed and ethambutol was withdrawn, but there was only a small improvement. When isoniazid was also withdrawn, there was dramatic improvement in visual acuity.

In another patient taking isoniazid and ethambutol, optic neuropathy improved only when both drugs were withdrawn (28).

Isoniazid 300 mg/day orally for 7 days increased serum ethambutol concentrations at 4, 6, and 8 hours after a daily dose of 20 mg/kg; the cumulative percentage dose excreted was significantly reduced at 4, 6, and 24 hours (29). In another study from the same center, ethambutol 20 mg/kg did not alter the pharmacokinetics of a single dose of isoniazid 300 mg in 10 patients with tuberculosis (30).

References

1. Dickinson JM, Aber VR, Mitchison DA. Bactericidal activity of streptomycin, isoniazid, rifampin, ethambutol, and pyrazinamide alone and in combination against *Mycobacterium tuberculosis*. Am Rev Respir Dis 1977;116(4):627–35.
2. Mandell GL, Sande MA. Antimicrobial agents: drugs used in the chemotherapy of tuberculosis and leprosy. In: Goodman Gilman A, Rall TW, Nies AS, Taylor P, editors. Goodman and Gilman's The Pharmacological Basis of Therapeutics. 8th ed. Chapter 49. New York: Pergamon Press, 1990:1146 .
3. Pegram PS Jr, Mountz JD, O'Bar PR. Ethambutol-induced toxic epidermal necrolysis. Arch Intern Med 1981;141(12):1677–8.
4. Nair VS, LeBrun M, Kass I. Peripheral neuropathy associated with ethambutol. Chest 1980;77(1):98–100.
5. Takeuchi H, Takahashi M, Tarui S, Sanagi S, Takenaka H. Peripheral nerve conduction function in patients treated with antituberculotic agents, with special reference to ethambutol and isoniazid. Folia Psychiatr Neurol Jpn 1980;34(1):57–64.
6. Takeuchi H, Takahashi M, Kang J, Ueno S, Tarui S, Nakao Y, Otori T. Ethambutol neurophathy: clinical and electroneuromyographic studies. Folia Psychiatr Neurol Jpn 1980;34(1):45–55.
7. Otori T. Drug-induced ocular side effects. Asian Med J 1981;24:141.
8. Garrett CR. Optic neuritis in a patient on ethambutol and isoniazid evaluated by visual evoked potentials: case report. Mil Med 1985;150(1):43–6.
9. Cole A, May PM, Williams DR. Metal binding by pharmaceuticals. Part 1. Copper(II) and zinc(II) interactions following ethambutol administration. Agents Actions 1981;11(3):296–305.
10. Karnik AM, Al-Shamali MA, Fenech FF. A case of ocular toxicity to ethambutol—an idiosyncratic reaction? Postgrad Med J 1985;61(719):811–13.
11. Yolton DP. Nutritional effects of zinc on ocular and systemic physiology. J Am Optom Assoc 1981;52(5):409–14.
12. Delacoux E, Moreau Y, Godefroy A, Evstigneeff T. Prévention de la toxicité oculaire de l'éthambutol: intérêt de la zincémie et de l'analyse du sens chromatique. [Prevention of ocular toxicity of ethambutol: study of zincaemia and chromatic analysis.] J Fr Ophtalmol 1978;1(3): 191–6.
13. Baciewicz AM, Self TH, Bekemeyer WB. Update on rifampin drug interactions. Arch Intern Med 1987;147(3):565–8.
14. Williams DE. Visual electrophysiology and psychophysics in chronic alcoholics and in patients on tuberculostatic chemotherapy. Am J Optom Physiol Opt 1984;61(9):576–85.
15. Trebucq A. Should ethambutol be recommended for routine treatment of tuberculosis in children? A review of the literature. Int J Tuberc Lung Dis 1997;1(1):12–15.
16. Trau R, Salu P, Jonckheere P, Leysen R. Early diagnosis of Myambutol (ethambutol) ocular toxicity by electrophysiological examination. Bull Soc Belge Ophtalmol 1981;193: 201–12.
17. Gramer E, Jeschke R, Krieglstein GK. Zur computergesteuerten Gesichtsfeldkontrolle bei Kindern mit Ethambutol-Medikation. [Computerized perimetry in infants treated with ethambutol.] Klin Padiatr 1982;194(1):52–5.
18. Guerra R, Casu L. Hydroxycobalamin for ethambutol-induced optic neuropathy. Lancet 1981;2(8256):1176.
19. Khanna BK, Gupta VP, Singh MP. Ethambutol-induced hyperuricaemia. Tubercle 1984;65(3):195–9.
20. Khanna BK. Acute gouty arthritis following ethambutol therapy. Br J Dis Chest 1980;74(4):409–10.

21. Rabinovitz M, Pitlik SD, Halevy J, Rosenfeld JB. Ethambutol-induced thrombocytopenia. Chest 1982;81(6):765–6.
22. Ansari MM, Beg MH, Haleem S. Hepatitis in patients with surgical complications of pulmonary tuberculosis. Indian J Chest Dis Allied Sci 1991;33(3):133–8.
23. Lewit T, Nebel L, Terracina S, Karman S. Ethambutol in pregnancy: observations on embryogenesis. Chest 1974;66(1):25–6.
24. Kunz J, Schreiner WE. Pharmakotherapie während Schwangerschaft und Stillperiode. Stuttgart-New York: G Thieme, 1982.
25. Strauss I, Erhardt F. Ethambutol absorption, excretion and dosage in patients with renal tuberculosis. Chemotherapy 1970;15(3):148–57.
26. Mattila MJ, Linnoila M, Seppala T, Koskinen R. Effect of aluminium hydroxide and glycopyrrhonium on the absorption of ethambutol and alcohol in man. Br J Clin Pharmacol 1978;5(2):161–6.
27. Karmon G, Savir H, Zevin D, Levi J. Bilateral optic neuropathy due to combined ethambutol and isoniazid treatment. Ann Ophthalmol 1979;11(7):1013–17.
28. Jimenez-Lucho VE, del Busto R, Odel J. Isoniazid and ethambutol as a cause of optic neuropathy. Eur J Respir Dis 1987;71(1):42–5.
29. Singhal KC, Rathi R, Varshney DP, Kishore K. Serum concentration and urinary excretion of ethambutol administered alone and in combination with isoniazid in patients of pulmonary tuberculosis. Indian J Physiol Pharmacol 1985;29(4):223–6.
30. Singhal KC, Varshney DP, Rathi R, Kishore K, Varshney SC. Serum concentration of isoniazid administered with & without ethambutol in pulmonary tuberculosis patients. Indian J Med Res 1986;83:360–2.

Ethanol

General Information

Ethanol (alcohol) is a drug of frequent abuse, and has long-term adverse effects that will not be discussed here. It is sometimes used therapeutically in the following ways:

- topically as an astringent.
- by direct instillation to embolize arteries.
- by direct injection into nerve ganglia or around nerve trunks to destroy them and relieve severe or chronic pain (for example trigeminal neuralgia); however, the results are generally only short-lasting.
- to swab the skin before venepuncture and other surgical procedures.
- as a rubefacient in some liniments.
- to harden the skin to prevent bedsores, and to harden the nipples before breastfeeding.
- to reduce sweating.
- in the treatment of acute methanol poisoning, since ethyl alcohol competes with methyl alcohol (methanol) for hepatic metabolism.

Alcohol is also widely used as a solvent in pharmaceutical preparations.

In 28 children from Argentina there was alcohol intoxication when ethyl alcohol was applied to the abdomen in alcohol-soaked cloths, as a home-remedy for disturbance of the gastrointestinal tract (1). The symptoms and signs included nervous system depression (100%), abdominal erythema (89%), alcoholic breath (86%), miosis (86%), hypoglycemia (54%), convulsions (18%), respiratory depression (18%), mydriasis (14%), acidosis (11%), and death (7%).

A danger of embolization of arteries is reflux of the instilled ethanol and the possibility of embolization of arteries other than the targeted ones. Infarction of the left testis secondary to transcatheter embolization of a malignant left renal tumor with ethanol has been reported (2). Colonic infarction following ethanol embolization of a renal tumor has been attributed to a reflux of ethanol from the renal artery into the aorta (3).

In combination therapy of unresectable hepatocellular carcinoma with transcatheter embolization and percutaneous injection of alcohol in 24 patients, 18 developed transient local pain and a burning sensation after the injection of alcohol, 16 had mild fever, and two had transient hypotension (4).

Organs and Systems

Cardiovascular

Alcohol is one of many drugs that cause or aggravate systemic hypertension. Acute alcohol exposure has an inconsistent effect on blood pressure, but cross-sectional population studies have shown a relation between chronic alcohol consumption and blood pressure, and the prevalence of hypertension up to three times higher in heavy drinkers (5). Although the mechanism of hypertension caused by chronic alcohol consumption is not known, it is suspected that it is partly related to repeated episodes of acute withdrawal, causing increased sympathoadrenomedullary activity, an increase in plasma renin activity, and increased ACTH secretion, which may be sufficient to have a mineralocorticoid effect (6).

Respiratory

In 36 patients with inoperable cancers of the esophagus who were treated by endoscopic injection of alcohol, complications included mediastinitis in one patient and tracheoesophageal fistulas in two (7).

Nervous system

Peripheral nerve block is created by injecting ethanol around the selected nerve. The effect of alcohol on nerve tissue has been examined in animal models and in postmortem specimens from patients who received neurolytic blocks (8,9). In general, alcohol causes destruction of nerve fibers, with subsequent Wallerian degeneration. The basal lamina around the Schwann cell usually remains intact. This leaves a tract available for axon regeneration without the formation of a neuroma. If the cell bodies are completely destroyed, regeneration will not occur. Contact of alcohol with unintended nerve roots underlies many of the more serious complications. Involvement of anterior rootlets sufficient to interrupt motor nerve function will result in muscle weakness or paralysis. Interruption of parasympathetic fibers in the anterior roots of the three middle sacral segments can result in bowel and bladder dysfunction and can cause urinary retention and anal sphincter paralysis.

In one study of 82 patients over a 20-year period who received repeated peripheral alcohol nerve blocks for trigeminal neuralgia, although moderate swelling and discomfort were invariable, significant complications occurred in only three of 413 nerve blocks (10):

- avascular necrosis, leading to a sequestrum, possibly due to repeated injections;
- necrosis of the lateral aspect of the nose, attributed to intravascular injection of alcohol;
- pallor and faintness after the injection followed by diplopia, which took 5 months to resolve.

Alcohol relatively commonly causes less serious complications, such as vomiting, headache, and paresthesia, which are but fortunately of limited duration, while loss of proprioception and profound numbness are disconcerting but almost always preferable to the pain that the alcohol injection has relieved (11).

Liver

Injection of ethanol into the liver to treat hepatocellular carcinoma commonly causes severe pain, fever, and hepatic dysfunction; there can also be pleural effusion, pneumothorax, ascites, vasovagal reaction, transient hypotension, myoglobinuria, and portal thrombosis. Fatal massive hepatic necrosis distant from the injection site has also been attributed to this treatment (SEDA-18, 377).

There have been three studies of the effects of percutaneous ethanol injections in the treatment of hepatocellular carcinoma, either alone (12,13) or in combination with transcatheter arterial embolization (14). The procedure was effective and safe and improved long-term survival. Adverse effects were generally mild and of short duration, and commonly included abdominal pain, fever, intoxication (especially among non-drinkers), transient rises in serum transaminases, and chemical thrombosis of the tributary branch of the portal vein. Hepatic infarction has been reported in two patients with hepatocellular carcinoma after percutaneous ethanol injection of the tumors (15). Both patients had previously been treated with transcatheter arterial infusion using a suspension of styrene maleic acid neocarzinostatin, and the liver damage may have occurred through a combination of arterial damage due to the neocarzinostatin and vasculitis caused by flow of the injected ethanol into a portal vein branch.

In an open trial, percutaneous ethanol injections into the liver improved prognosis compared with conservative treatment in 63 patients with cirrhosis and hepatocellular carcinoma who were not suitable for surgery or transcatheter arterial chemoembolization (16). Most of the patients had mild to moderate local pain during or immediately after injection and 29% developed fever.

Urinary tract

When 99% ethanol was instilled into renal cysts under ultrasound guidance in 25 cases, there were 12 complications after puncture, either related to the puncture itself or caused by the ethanol (17). They included flank pain, nausea, causalgia, and a feeling of drunkenness, which occurred immediately after instillation.

References

1. Gimenez ER, Vallejo NE, Roy E, et al. Percutaneous alcohol intoxication. Clin Toxicol 1968;1:39.
2. Siniluoto TM, Hellstrom PA, Paivansalo MJ, Leinonen AS. Testicular infarction following ethanol embolization of a renal neoplasm. Cardiovasc Intervent Radiol 1988;11(3): 162–4.
3. Cox GG, Lee KR, Price HI, Gunter K, Noble MJ, Mebust WK. Colonic infarction following ethanol embolization of renal-cell carcinoma. Radiology 1982;145(2):343–5.
4. Kato T, Saito Y, Niwa M, Ishiguro J, Ogoshi K. Combination therapy of transcatheter chemoembolization and percutaneous ethanol injection therapy for unresectable hepatocellular carcinoma. Cancer Chemother Pharmacol 1994;33(Suppl):S115–18.
5. Kaysen G, Noth RH. The effects of alcohol on blood pressure and electrolytes. Med Clin North Am 1984;68(1): 221–46.
6. Thomas SHL. Drug induced systemic hypertension. Adv Drug React Bull 1993;150:559–62.
7. Chung SC, Leong HT, Choi CY, Leung JW, Li AK. Palliation of malignant oesophageal obstruction by endoscopic alcohol injection. Endoscopy 1994;26(3):275–7.
8. Merrick RL. Degeneration and recovery of autonomic neurons following alcoholic block. Ann Surg 1941;113:298–305.
9. Woolsey RM, Taylor JJ, Nagel JH. Acute effects of topical ethyl alcohol on the sciatic nerve of the mouse. Arch Phys Med Rehabil 1972;53(9):410–14.
10. Fardy MJ, Patton DW. Complications associated with peripheral alcohol injections in the management of trigeminal neuralgia. Br J Oral Maxillofac Surg 1994;32(6):387–91.
11. Kemp JR, Kilbride MJ, Winnie AP. Intrathecal alcohol neurolysis for the treatment of injectable pain. Pain Digest 1995;5:186–91.
12. Livraghi T. Percutaneous ethanol injection in the treatment of hepatocellular carcinoma in cirrhosis. Minimally Invasive Ther Allied Technol 1998;7:553–8.
13. Livraghi T, Benedini V, Lazzaroni S, Meloni F, Torzilli G, Vettori C. Long term results of single session percutaneous ethanol injection in patients with large hepatocellular carcinoma. Cancer 1998;83(1):48–57.
14. Tanaka K, Nakamura S, Numata K, Kondo M, Morita K, Kitamura T, Saito S, Kiba T, Okazaki H, Sekihara H. The long term efficacy of combined transcatheter arterial embolization and percutaneous ethanol injection in the treatment of patients with large hepatocellular carcinoma and cirrhosis. Cancer 1998;82(1):78–85.
15. Seki T, Wakabayashi M, Nakagawa T, Imamura M, Tamai T, Nishimura A, Yamashiki N, Okamura A, Inoue K. Hepatic infarction following percutaneous ethanol injection therapy for hepatocellular carcinoma. Eur J Gastroenterol Hepatol 1998;10(11):915–18.
16. Huo TI, Huang YH, Wu JC, Lee PC, Chang FY, Lee SD. Survival benefit of cirrhotic patients with hepatocellular carcinoma treated by percutaneous ethanol injection as a salvage therapy. Scand J Gastroenterol 2002;37(3):350–5.
17. Furuta H, Nakada T, Akiya T, Ishikawa N, Satomi S, Sakamoto M, Kohno T, Kazama T, Umeda K, Sasagawa I, et al. [Renal cyst puncture under ultrasound guidance: complications of ethanol injection.] Hinyokika Kiyo 1988;34(9):1575–8.

Etherified starches

General Information

Etherified starches are synthetic colloids containing over 90% amylopectin, a waxy starch derived from maize, that has been variably etherified. There are two major forms, hetastarch and pentastarch (both BAN and USAN). They are produced synthetically by introducing hydroxyethyl groups into glucose units of starch molecules, followed by acid hydrolysis, which results in a product with a molecular weight of several thousands of daltons. In hetastarch 7 or 8 and in pentastarch 4 or 5 of the hydroxyl groups in each glucose molecule are etherified.

The etherified starches are used in solution as plasma substitutes. They are good alternatives to albumin, because they have an extended shelf-life, carry no risk of transmitting blood-borne diseases, and can be infused into patients who refuse blood products on religious grounds.

The elimination of etherified starches is complex and related to the size of the particles. The smaller molecules, with a molecular weight of less than 50 000 daltons, are excreted unchanged by glomerular filtration. The larger molecules are metabolized to smaller molecules and distributed to various body tissues, where they may undergo hydrolysis in the reticuloendothelial system or enzymatic degradation by amylases.

A detailed histological and immunohistochemical study of deposits of hetastarch in rat tissues has thrown some light on the relation between its adverse effects and its fate in the body (1). Thirteen days after a single intravenous injection the rats were sacrificed and their liver, spleen, lymph node, lung, kidney, and skin were studied. In all these organs anti-etherified starch antibody stained cells that were mainly regarded as mononuclear phagocytes (confirmed by the use of antimacrophage monoclonal antibody ED1). These findings suggested a degree of prolonged tissue storage of either etherified starch or of a degradation product that stains with the antibody, and this may account for persistent complications such as pruritus. However, in this histochemical study there was no mast cell degranulation or accumulation of inflammatory cells.

Nomenclature

Different types of etherified starch are designated by a number that indicates the molecular weight in kilodaltons followed by a number that indicates the degree of substitution of glucose units with hydroxyethyl groups. Thus, etherified starch with a molecular weight of 200 kDa and 62% substitution is designated 200/0.62.

Comparative studies

The efficacy and safety of hetastarch and albumin have been compared in 85 patients with postaneurysmal subarachnoid hemorrhage (2). Of 26 patients who developed clinical symptoms of vasospasm, 14 were treated with hetastarch, while the other 12 received albumin. In all patients who received hetastarch there was significant prolongation of the partial thromboplastin time after transfusion (pretransfusion mean 24 seconds, post-transfusion 33 seconds), while in patients treated with albumin the partial thromboplastin time was not significantly altered. The prolongation of the partial thromboplastin time resulted in increased occult blood loss in the hetastarch-treated patients, requiring blood transfusion in four patients. On the basis of hetastarch-associated coagulopathy and data that show that albumin may be the most effective agent for increasing cerebral blood flow and preventing infarction, the authors stopped using hetastarch in these patients and decided to recommend albumin exclusively.

Some authors have concluded that etherified starches and albumin do not differ with respect to efficacy and adverse effects on coagulation and renal function (3), but etherified starches clearly do have a distinct adverse reactions profile. Some of the problems that they cause, such as anaphylaxis, volume overload, cerebral hemorrhage, and acute renal insufficiency, are sufficient reason to avoid hetastarch when benefit is doubtful, such as ischemic brain infarction (4).

Placebo-controlled studies

Hypervolemic hemodilution with agents such as etherified starches or dextran increases cerebral blood flow and can therefore reduce ischemic tissue damage in the penumbra zones when given within the therapeutic time window. However, the clinical benefit of such therapy has yet to be proven. Since etherified starch is considered to be the safer choice, in particular the recently developed lower molecular weight form (etherified starch 130/0.4), an explorative, randomized, placebo-controlled, safety trial of etherified starch for hypervolemic hemodilution in patients with acute ischemic stroke has been undertaken (5). This was a double-blind, randomized, placebo-controlled, parallel-group, multicenter study in 106 patients with acute ischemic stroke, who were recruited over 3 years. Treatment comprised high-dose hypervolemic hemodilution with either etherified starch 130/0.4 or placebo within 6 hours of the start of symptoms, with a randomization ratio of 2:1 in favor of etherified starch. There were no significant differences between the groups with regard to the incidence of specific adverse events (cardiovascular, bleeding complications, allergic reactions), assessed over days 1–30, or of deaths over days 1–8. The author, on behalf of the Hydroxyethyl Starch in Acute Stroke Study Group in Germany, noted that while the study was not designed to prove efficacy, the global tests of efficacy suggested a slight but insignificant trend toward better functional outcome with etherified starch.

General adverse effects

Transitory hyperamylasemia, chills, and mild increases in body temperature, pruritus, enlargement of the submandibular and parotid glands, and erythema multiforme can occur (6). The risk of anaphylactic reactions to hetastarch is very small (about 5 per million) (7).

Organs and Systems

Cardiovascular

In a comprehensive comparison of the pharmacokinetics and pharmacodynamics of dextran and etherified starch (8), the effects of etherified starch on the cardiovascular system have been delineated. The mean arterial pressure, central venous pressure, wedge pressure, cardiac index, left ventricular stroke work index, and stroke output all rise, whereas the pulmonary vascular resistance falls. Oxygen availability to the tissues is improved. The effects of etherified starch on blood viscosity and erythrocyte aggregation, in particular, are more pronounced than with dextran.

Nervous system

The effect of hemodilution with colloids on somatosensory-evoked potentials in non-premedicated volunteers has been reported (9). In seven subjects, blood (20 ml/kg within 30 minutes) was removed and simultaneously replaced by gelatine 3% or etherified starches 6%. After 30 minutes, blood was retransfused. Median and posterior tibial nerve somatosensory-evoked potentials were recorded from the cortex, second cervical vertebra, Erb's point, and first lumbar vertebra. Hemodilution with gelatine or etherified starches or retransfusion did not affect somatosensory-evoked potentials, provided normovolemic conditions were maintained.

Acid–base balance

Two prospective, randomized studies of acid-base changes induced by etherified starches have been reported. In the first study (10), healthy volunteers were given 15 ml/kg of hetastarch 6% or albumin 5% intravenously over 30 minutes. Four weeks later they were given the other colloid. Arterial blood gases and electrolyte parameters were measured at baseline and at 30-minute intervals for 5 hours. There were statistically significant changes in bicarbonate, chloride ion, and albumin concentrations, base excess, and arterial carbon dioxide tension 30 minutes after infusion of hetastarch, but only the albumin concentration changed significantly in the albumin-treated group.

In the second study (11) there were acid–base changes caused by the same two colloids in patients undergoing acute normovolemic hemodilution during gynecological surgery. Two groups of 10 patients were randomly assigned to receive either albumin 5% or etherified starch 6%, containing chloride ion concentrations of 150 and 154 mmol/l respectively. The blood volume was well maintained in both groups. Acute normovolemic hemodilution caused slight metabolic acidosis with hyperchloremia. Plasma albumin concentrations fell after hemofiltration with etherified starches but increased after albumin. The authors concluded that acute normovolemic hemodilution with albumin or etherified starches led to some degree of metabolic acidosis, but not of clinical relevance.

Hematologic

After intravenous administration, hetastarch alters the rheological properties (12) of blood and increases the erythrocyte sedimentation rate (13).

Coagulation

Etherified starch can cause coagulation disorders. Administration of 10% hydroxyethyl starch 200/0.62 to 10 patients with cerebrovascular diseases over 10 days (a loading dose of 500 ml administered once over 45–60 minutes followed by 500 ml/day) had a markedly unfavorable effect on blood coagulation (14). There was a significant 43% increase in activated partial thromboplastin time. Factor VIII:C, von Willebrand ristocetin co-factor, and von Willebrand factor antigen fell during therapy below the limit required for hemostasis (30%), and in some patients below 10%. This was thought to be due to accumulation of large molecules that are difficult to break down and which unfavorably affect rheological and coagulation function.

The pathogenic mechanism that affects factor VIII/vWF complex has not been elucidated. There may be accelerated elimination after attachment of factor VIII/vWF complex to starch molecules. The significant fall in factor XI and factor XII shows that impairment of the intrinsic system of coagulation is not limited to factor VII/vWF complex (14). Even a small volume of 6% etherified starches (average molecular weight 450 kDa; 2.5 litres in 3 days) can cause a significant coagulation disorder (15).

In another study, administration for 24 hours of hetastarch (6%) or human serum albumin to 12 patients with septic shock caused moderate effects on hemostasis (prothrombin time, partial thromboplastin time, and quantitative platelet count). There was no increase in bleeding, and there were no statistically significant differences between these effects and those produced by human serum albumin (16); however, it should be noted that the number of subjects was so small as effectively to preclude a finding of significant difference between the groups studied. The authors' conclusion that hetastarch is a safe and effective volume expander in patients with sepsis and shock needs to be considered cautiously, particularly as the authors pointed out that there is an immediate fall in factor VIII coagulant to about half normal in patients receiving hetastarch. Furthermore, a patient with von Willebrand's disease had a markedly prolonged bleeding time and reduced platelet adhesiveness, although there was no overt bleeding.

- A man of 33 developed von Willebrand's disease shortly after he had been given 3 liters of hetastarch over 3 days after acute sensorineural hearing loss. He had a history of a prolonged activated partial thromboplastin time (APTT), although he had previously undergone bilateral hip arthroplasties with no evidence of abnormal bleeding. He had an episode of epistaxis and experienced weakness and pain in his leg. When hetastarch was withdrawn, it was noted that he had a raised APTT concentration, and reduced concentrations of factors XII and VIII:C. Over the next few months, the von Willebrand's syndrome was reversed, although his factor XII concentration remained reduced (17).

This case is typical of many others. In six patients with cerebral circulatory disturbances who received hemodilution therapy for 9–10 days with etherified starches (molecular weight 200 kDa and a high degree of substitution, 0.62), all the multimers of von Willebrand factor fell to the same extent. This corresponds to type 1 von

Willebrand's syndrome (18). This potential hemorrhagic complication is treatable, since type 1 von Willebrand's syndrome can be controlled with the vasopressin derivative desmopressin.

A survey of formulations containing etherified starch, and particularly Elohes 6% (molecular weight about 200 kDa), carried out by the French Agency for Health Products identified eight cases of acquired von Willebrand disease (19). Three cases were fatal and in two cases there were hematomas with prolongation of the activated cephalin clotting time. All these effects were observed during the administration of Elohes for vasospasm secondary to meningeal hemorrhage due to rupture of a cerebral aneurysm in patients with no relevant previous history. Duration of treatment of more than 4 days appears to be a risk factor. Nine cases of hepatic overload were also reported, and could cause or aggravate portal hypertension. The Agency announced that the product information for products containing hetastarch would be revised, with a contraindication to the use of Elohes in patients with severe hepatic insufficiency, the stipulation of a maximum dose, a restriction on the duration of treatment, and instructions on the monitoring of hemostasis.

Of nine patients with hemostatic disorders, all treated with medium molecular weight etherified starch (Elohes), six developed type I von Willebrand's disease (20). Before the abnormalities in coagulation were discovered, the patients had received a mean dose of pentastarch of 121 ml/kg. The abnormalities resolved each time pentastarch was withdrawn. The authors hypothesized that accumulation of starch probably led to quantitative defects of complex factor VIII and von Willebrand factor by accelerated elimination from the circulation of complexes attached to starch molecules. Because Elohes is highly substituted, it is difficult to break down and is therefore eliminated more slowly. Accumulation of Elohes after repeated administration may explain why its adverse effects on coagulation resemble those of high molecular weight starch, while other medium molecular weight starches affect coagulation much less. The authors recommended that the dose of Elohes should be limited to 33 ml/kg/day and the cumulative dose to 80 ml/kg. Treatment should be given over no more than 3 days and Elohes is contraindicated in patients with coagulation disorders.

Etherified starch shortens the thrombin time by a fibrinoplastic effect. This accelerates the conversion of fibrinogen to fibrin, resulting in a less stable thrombus, which is more susceptible to lysis. The macromolecules in etherified starch induce an acquired von Willebrand's syndrome with reduced concentrations of all three main forms of factor VIII: factor VIII:C, von Willebrand factor, and von Willebrand factor antigen (vWFag).

Platelets

Plasma substitutes in general reduce the platelet count partly by a dilutional effect, even after a single dose. However, there are other mechanisms. In a study of the effects on platelet number and function of etherified starches, given for 10 days to 20 patients with cerebrovascular diseases, both medium- and low-molecular weight etherified starches caused a significant reduction in the number of platelets on the first day, in excess of a dilutional effect. During the course of treatment the platelet number increased, recovering its initial value. The number of large platelets fell disproportionately and significantly. Etherified starch did not affect spontaneous platelet aggregation. The fall in platelets was probably caused by colloid-osmotic shrinkage and increased degradation. There were no signs of impaired platelet function, as determined by spontaneous platelet aggregation (21). Patients suffering from thrombocytopenia or impaired platelet function should be carefully monitored when they are receiving large doses of etherified starches.

Macromolecules may coat the outer membrane of circulating platelets and cause a qualitative functional defect, thus prolonging bleeding time. Minor abnormalities of platelet aggregation have been observed after infusion of low volumes of etherified starches, and platelet defects probably contribute to the hemorrhagic state.

Etherified starch altered hemostasis in vitro in blood taken from patients undergoing abdominal surgery; the effect was more pronounced in patients with blood group O (22). The authors recommended that the intraoperative administration of etherified starches should be restricted in patients with blood group O undergoing surgical procedures with a high risk of bleeding.

Urinary tract

In a patient with normal renal function it is possible that the kidneys present a selective barrier to all but the smallest of starch molecules. The breakdown products are then eliminated by urinary excretion. Etherified starch can be associated with increasing serum creatinine concentrations (23). Associated clinical symptoms and signs include pain in the renal region and swelling of kidney parenchyma. In a study of 25 patients randomly allocated to control and treatment groups (the latter received 10% etherified starch 12 ml/kg) there were differences in renal tubular function in the latter. Those who received etherified starch had increased excretion of alpha$_1$-microglobulin, Tamm-Horsfall protein, and brush border enzyme acetyl-beta-glucosaminidase. There were no significant differences in glomerular function. The findings suggest a primary renal tubular lesion caused by etherified starch (23).

The risk of acute renal insufficiency associated with the use of etherified starch in volume replacement therapy has been critically reviewed (24). The author made the important point that not all etherified starch formulations are the same—they differ widely in physicochemical characteristics. Such differences have consequences for adverse events, including impaired renal function. Furthermore, all volume replacement therapies have potential hazards. The author therefore concluded that etherified starch, in particular products containing etherified starch with a low or medium molecular weight (for example 70, 130, or 200 kDa) and a low degree of substitution (0.4 or 0.5), can be considered for use in patients without pre-existing kidney dysfunction. It is recommended that all formulations of etherified starch, including the latest (molecular weight 130, degree of substitution 0.4), should be used only very cautiously in patients with some degree of renal impairment (plasma creatinine concentration greater than 365 μmol/l, 3 mg/l) and are probably best avoided for alternative regimens.

Osmotic nephrosis-like lesions have been reported in kidney transplant recipients, attributed to etherified starches that had been used in brainstem-dead patients before organ procurement (25). The incidence of these lesions was not influenced by cold ischemia time, the presence and length of delayed graft function, or the immunosuppressive regimen (including the use of ciclosporin). The lesions had no significant deleterious influence on the occurrence of delayed graft function or on serum creatinine at 3 and 6 months after transplantation. Osmotic nephrosis-like lesions can be long-lasting, since in three patients they were still present at 3 months after transplantation on routine renal biopsy. In patients without osmotic nephrosis-like lesions no kidney was lost, whereas among those with such lesions, seven of 31 were lost. Although there was no obvious short-term detrimental influence on renal function, these lesions might cloud the already difficult interpretation of renal transplant biopsies, especially for ciclosporin-induced nephrotoxicity. The authors recommended avoiding etherified starches in potential organ donors.

Two cases of osmotic nephrosis-like lesions have been reported in which similar changes have been noted, accompanied by evidence of renal insufficiency. The first case occurred after the administration of etherified starch during surgery (26).

- A 67-year-old woman with no history of nephritis was given etherified starch (500 ml) and Ringer's lactate (2.5 litres) for hypotension during surgery. Postoperatively she developed acute renal insufficiency (urine output below 600 ml/day) and her serum creatinine rose to 443 μmol/l, despite fluid challenge. Ultrasound showed no urinary obstruction, no thrombosis in the renal vessels, and normal kidneys. A renal biopsy showed major osmotic nephrosis-like lesions in the proximal tubules, but no lesions suggestive of acute tubular necrosis. Renal function returned to normal within 14 days after surgery.

The authors suggested that the renal insufficiency was due to the perioperative infusion of etherified starch, even though she received a much smaller dose (less than 10 ml/kg) than kidney donors usually receive. They further suggested that nephrotoxicity can occur within a few hours after even low-dose infusion of etherified starches.

- A 20-year-old man from Mali with polymyositis that had not responded to prednisolone, monthly infusions of immunoglobulin, and plasma exchanges with albumin and modified gelatin, was given ciclosporin, which led to marked improvement (27). When he developed hepatic cirrhosis the ciclosporin was withdrawn and glucocorticoids were reintroduced in association with plasma exchanges three times a week with 6% etherified starches and 4% albumin. After seven plasma exchanges (cumulative dose 320 g) his serum creatinine rose to 216 μmol/l without proteinuria or hematuria. Renal biopsy showed diffuse microvacuolization of the tubular epithelial cells (osmotic nephrosis-like lesions). Plasma exchange was restarted with 4% albumin alone, after which his renal function improved and the polymyositis stabilized.

The authors concluded that the most likely cause of renal insufficiency was etherified starch-induced tubulopathy and hypothesized that even low amounts of etherified starch as replacement fluid in plasma exchange can cause renal tubular lesions in patients predisposed for other reasons (such as drugs or renal hypoperfusion) to renal insufficiency. In this context, albumin should be combined with replacement fluids other than etherified starch.

The lesions of osmotic nephrosis involve the proximal and distal tubules. Severe changes in proximal tubules have been described in dogs after complete blood exchange with etherified starches. It is believed that smaller molecules (molecular weight under 50 kDa) are excreted unchanged by glomerular filtration, leading to a large amount of osmotically active small molecules in the ultrafiltrate. As a result of reduced glomerular filtration in these patients, a highly viscous ultrafiltrate, complicated by tubular stasis and osmotic nephrosis of tubular cells, may have been caused by reabsorption of etherified starches, resulting in acute renal insufficiency. In the two cases described in this report, and in the absence of either significant hypotension or oliguria, acute renal insufficiency due to purely prerenal (hypovolemic) causes was improbable (28).

Hetastarch can cause a discrepancy between urinary specific gravity and osmolality (29). High-molecular weight molecules present in the hetastarch solution produced a disproportionate rise in urine specific gravity compared with osmolality. In two patients, the combined effects of acute tubular necrosis secondary to hypotension and abnormal glomerular permeability were thought to have allowed high-molecular weight particles of hetastarch to be excreted in the urine. The hetastarch particles increased the urine specific gravity, but had a correspondingly smaller effect on osmolality. It was not thought that hetastarch itself was nephrotoxic. The authors concluded that in the setting of pre-existing renal disease, hetastarch may increase the urinary specific gravity without unduly affecting the ability of the kidney to concentrate urine. They recommended that urinary osmolality, rather than specific gravity, should be regarded as the preferred method of evaluating the urine after the administration of high-molecular weight colloid solutions.

Hemodilution therapy with etherified starch caused acute deterioration of an already existing nephropathy in two cases (29). The authors suggested, on theoretical grounds, that the deterioration in renal function was likely to have been the result of increased permeability caused by damage to the glomerular basement membrane. Etherified starch molecules are filtered above the physiological renal threshold, and this increases the viscosity of the urine. This can be counteracted by promoting diuresis. The authors managed to avoid precipitating renal insufficiency by ensuring a fluid intake of about 3 l/day. Without an adequate diuresis etherified starches accumulate in patients with renal dysfunction, with consequences that include further damage to the diseased kidneys.

Conclusions have differed as to whether use of etherified starch in brain-dead organ donors influences kidney graft function at 1, 3, and 6 months after transplantation (30–32). In one report (33), during the first 10 days after transplantation there was reduced kidney graft function with higher creatininemia or increased requirements for hemodialysis in recipients in those given etherified starch plus gelatin. Some other workers have not confirmed this finding (30,31), but it is not unique. In 69 other brain-dead patients followed up prospectively over a period of 18 months 33% of those who received etherified starch up to 33 ml/kg during the first 8 days after transplantation for colloid plasma volume expansion required extrarenal hemodialysis or hemodiafiltration, compared with 5% in a control gelatin-only group (33). Serum creatinine concentrations were significantly lower in the controls. The results suggested that etherified starch used as a plasma volume expander in brain-dead donors impairs renal function.

Skin

Severe pruritus after infusion of etherified starch is common and troublesome. In skin biopsies taken from 93 patients who had received etherified starches, half of whom had pruritus, immunoelectron microscopy was conducted using an antibody highly specific for etherified starches. After infusion of etherified starches, formation of intracytoplasmic storage vacuoles in the skin was demonstrated in all cases. Dose-related uptake of etherified starches was first detectable in macrophages and afterwards in endothelial and epithelial cells. There were vacuoles that reacted to etherified starches in the Schwann cells of unmyelinated as well as small myelinated nerve fibers, and in endoneural and perineural cells. Neural devacuolization paralleled the clinical improvement in itch (34). The authors of this study suggest that deposits of etherified starches in cutaneous nerves, as a consequence of a high cumulative dose, may account for the itching seen after infusion of etherified starch.

In 481 patients with diseases of the microcirculation of the cochleovestibular system, 149 of whom were treated with etherified starch, 43 (29%) complained of pruritus, compared with only 5.7% of another group of patients who were treated with dextran 40 (35). In more than 40% of the patients pruritus started in normal skin 1–3 weeks after therapy and lasted between 6 weeks and 6 months; the itching was resistant to therapy with antihistamines. Pruritus can be socially embarrassing, particularly when etherified starch has been given in high doses. The resistance of etherified starch-induced pruritus to standard therapy, including antihistamines, glucocorticoids, ultraviolet light, and other measures, has been described in a single case (36). This resistance to treatment is not unusual. Four patients with nausea or tinnitus who received intravenous etherified starch developed severe pruritus, especially on the trunk, without skin eruptions, 1–3 weeks after the start of treatment. The pruritus was refractory to treatment, and neither oral nor topical antihistamines were effective; only ultraviolet phototherapy or topical glucocorticoids gradually alleviated the pruritus after periods ranging from several weeks to 1 year (37).

In a retrospective study of 491 patients treated for various cochleovestibular disorders, 25 of 59 patients (42%) treated with etherified starch complained of pruritus, compared with four of 35 (11%) treated with dextran-40 (38).

Generalized itching occurred in 43 of 149 patients treated with etherified starch for acute or chronic microcirculatory disease causing neuro-otological disturbances (39).

In another retrospective study of 266 patients receiving etherified starch for otological indications 32% developed pruritus, which characteristically appeared as a pruritic crisis. In 55% of the patients the onset of symptoms was after the etherified starch had been withdrawn. The symptoms persisted on average for 8.8 weeks. Pruritus was generalized, but with a predilection for the trunk and genitalia. Coincidental atopic disease or higher age were not predisposing factors. The incidence of pruritus correlated well with the cumulative dosage and also depended on the type and molecular weight of the etherified starch given (6 or 10%, molecular weight 40 or 200 kDa). Light and electron microscopy showed deposits of etherified starch, especially within dermal macrophages and endothelial cells adjacent to nerve fibers (40). The authors suggested that a histamine-independent pathway is probably responsible for pruritus due to etherified starch. Antihistamines had no therapeutic effect on the patients reported.

After etherified starches treatment, vacuoles in the cells of various organs in humans occur, predominantly affecting the mononuclear phagocyte system (41). These vacuoles are indirect evidence for phagocytosis of etherified starch particles. In skin biopsies of patients who had received etherified starch and later suffered from itching, light and electron microscopy, immunohistochemistry, and immunoelectron microscopy using a polyclonal anti-hetastarch antiserum showed that storage of etherified starch was present in the skin of all patients. This was mainly in dermal macrophages, endothelial cells of blood and lymph vessels, some perineural cells and endoneural macrophages of larger nerve fascicles, some keratinocytes, and Langerhans cells. There were no morphological signs of histamine release from mast cells. The authors concluded that mediators other than histamine, released from hetastarch-affected cells, must be responsible for the itching.

In three patients with persistent pruritus after the administration of etherified starches during and after heart surgery, there was histopathological evidence of storage vacuoles containing etherified starch in the dermis (42). Etherified starch solutions are heterogeneous, containing molecules with a wide range of molecular weights. The smaller molecules (<50 kDa) are rapidly excreted by the kidneys, whereas larger molecules persist intravascularly until they are slowly hydrolysed or taken up by the mononuclear phagocyte system and other cells in various tissues. The mechanism by which storage of etherified starch causes pruritus is not adequately understood. It does not seem to be an allergic reaction mediated by the immune system, as there is usually little or no inflammatory cell infiltration, and the incidence of pruritus is dose-related. Whether macrophages, endothelial cells, keratinocytes, Langerhans cells, or other cells in which the starch molecules are deposited release mediators that induce itching, or whether there is a more direct effect on sensory nerve fibers, is uncertain. In this small series the number of mast cells was increased and mast cells were degranulated on electron microscopy. These features have not been seen in other studies. The resistance of the pruritus to treatment suggests that it is not simply mediated by histamine and indeed etherified starch does not release histamine (42).

- A 68-year-old woman developed marked and persistent periocular swelling after infusion of etherified starch for sudden hearing loss. In both the affected periocular skin and healthy skin there was lysosomal storage of etherified starches with a specific antibody in histiocytes, endothelial cells, basal keratinocytes, and small nerves. In the periocular skin there was more deposition of etherified starches, in addition to distinct xanthomatous changes and features of lymphedema. In addition, there was a 50% reduction in the pH-dependent activity of the lysosomal alpha-glucosidase in cultured fibroblasts.

This finding is consistent with a heterozygous glycogenosis type II (Pompe's disease) and is of potential pathogenic relevance for the intralysosomal accumulation of etherified starch. It is possible that alpha-glucosidase has a role in the elimination of tissue-stored etherified starch. Patients with reduced alpha-glucosidase activity may be at risk of unusual adverse effects after extraordinary and prolonged tissue storage of etherified starches, especially if it is infused in large quantities. There may be unusual lysosomal accumulation of etherified starches in endothelial cells and macrophages, which may in turn account for the higher risk of pruritus and other unusual adverse effects (43).

In a prospective, randomized, controlled, epidemiological comparison of 6% etherified starch solution (200/0.5) and lactated Ringer's solution, there were no more serious complications with the former than the latter. There was a greater than 10% incidence of pruritus in both groups (44).

In 26 patients who had received etherified starch (varying widely in both dose and duration), storage of etherified starch was dose-related, and fell in all organs over time; tissues deposits were greater in patients with pruritus (45). The authors concluded that tissue deposition is transitory and dose-related, but varies widely between subjects in both severity and duration. In a retrospective postal questionnaire in 100 consecutive intensive care patients who had previously received etherified starch, of 73 patients who replied, 34% had pruritus after discharge, of whom 44% had persistent pruritus that did not resolve with conventional treatments (46). There was a significant relation between the volume of etherified starch infused and the occurrence of pruritus.

In 120 patients who had received plasma substitutes (including 93 who had received etherified starch) skin biopsies showed lysosomal deposits in the histiocytes, some of them also in the cutaneous epithelium and endothelium (47). The extent of lysosomal storage correlated with the amount of etherified starch infused. Consecutive biopsies in some cases showed a slow reduction (over years) of etherified starch deposits in vacuoles. The authors suggested that pruritus after high cumulative doses of etherified starches was closely related to deposition of etherified starch in cutaneous nerves.

In a retrospective study of the dose-relatedness of pruritus caused by etherified starch, 50 consecutive patients were evaluated by questionnaire about 6 months after treatment; 37 returned the questionnaires, of whom 20 reported pruritus, lasting an average of 15 weeks (48). There was significantly more pruritus in patients who had received more than 5 liters of etherified starch compared with those who had received less than 5 liters. The pruritus had a delayed onset and occurred in acute bouts lasting 2–30 minutes. The authors concluded that hetastarch-induced pruritus is dose-related, and that in some cases it can be prolonged and severe.

Reproductive system

Ovarian hyperstimulation syndrome has been attributed to etherified starch (49).

- A 32-year-old Caucasian woman underwent IVF for primary tubal sterility and hyperandrogenemia as reflected by polycystic disease. Follicle formation was stimulated with FSH. The first stimulation cycle had to be discontinued because of threatened ovarian hyperstimulation syndrome. During the second attempt the dose of FSH was reduced to 100 IU/day for 10 days then 150 IU/day for 7 days, when follicles were observed. Ovulation was induced with a reduced dose of HCG (5000 IU). She was given crystalloids, 50 ml of serum albumin 20%, and 500 ml of medium molecular weight etherified starch 10% (HEAS, Fresenius). This was repeated on days 5–8 and 11–15, this time with high molecular weight etherified starch 6% (Plasmasteril, Fresenius), together with other fluids. After 4 days she developed massive ascites, abdominal pain, dyspnea, hemoconcentration, and a leukocytosis of $27 \times 10^9/l$. Her girth increased between days 7 and 12, and continuous abdominal paracentesis over 6 days was necessary. Her renal function was supported using diuretics and by a continuous infusion of dopamine. On day 17 she developed increased dyspnea and headache and a pleural effusion. Her anemia was severe (hemoglobin 7.8 g/dl) and nearly all the factors in the intrinsic coagulation cascade were greatly reduced. Disseminated intravascular coagulopathy and primary liver disease were excluded. The pleural effusion contained a high concentration of etherified starch (74% of the plasma concentration). She gradually improved and was discharged on day 36.

The authors concluded that the most likely cause of severe ovarian hyperstimulation syndrome was overinfusion of etherified starch.

Immunologic

Starch derivatives are relatively safer in terms of adverse reactions than other colloid plasma substitutes, but there is an incidence of anaphylactic reactions of 4–6 per million.

- An anaphylactic reaction has been attributed to etherified starches during re-infusion of autologous bone marrow in a man treated for malignant lymphoma (6). The re-infused material had been processed using etherified starches. The patient reported pruritus and carpal spasm. Edema and erythema of the hands were present, together with hypotension and tachycardia. A very small amount of etherified starches was present in the processed bone autograft.

However, in this case other causes such as dimethylsulfoxide (DMSO) or plasma used while processing the autologous bone marrow for freezing could not be excluded.

- A 43-year-old male non-smoker, with a history of asthma, hypertension, and angina pectoris, was admitted to an intensive care unit for mechanical ventilation for acute severe asthma (50). He was given an inhaled bronchodilator, aminophylline, and prednisolone. His condition improved slowly but he became hypovolemic. Within 60 seconds of a fluid challenge with pentastarch 200 ml he had a severe anaphylactoid reaction.

Patients with allergy and atopy have an exaggerated response to chemical mediators released during adverse reactions. The incidence of allergy, atopy, and asthma in patients who have anaphylactic reactions is substantially greater than in non-reacting controls, which may have explained this incident. This sudden unanticipated severe reaction demanded immediate intervention, and its occurrence in a patient with pre-existing bronchospasm posed problems in maintaining ventilation and oxygenation.

Volume therapy with etherified starches in trauma patients results in a reduction in circulating adhesion molecules, an effect that is not observed with albumin infusion (51). Continuous infusion of pentoxifylline did not have a beneficial modulating action on circulating adhesion molecules. Adhesion molecules appear to play an important role in tissue damage secondary to the inflammatory process. Besides neutrophil- and endothelium-bound adhesion molecules, soluble forms have been detected in the circulating blood in trauma patients. They seem to be markers of endothelial damage, but they may also have other biological functions.

Of 1004 patients assessed at least 14 days after starch administration, using a highly sensitive enzyme-linked immunoadsorbent assay technique, one had a low titer (1:10) of etherified starch-reactive antibodies of the immunoglobulin M (IgM) class. Despite repeated infusions, no clinical reaction could be detected in this patient. The authors concluded that antibodies to etherified starches are extremely rare and that they do not necessarily cause anaphylaxis. This low antigenicity of etherified starches might explain their excellent tolerance, compared with other plasma expanders (52).

The reason for the considerable tolerability of etherified starch may be the raw material: etherified starch is synthesized from amylopectin by attaching hydroxyethyl groups. Amylopectin is very similar to glycogen, but whereas glycogen occurs in the cells of warm-blooded organisms, amylopectin is the lower-branched analogue in cells of plant origin. The human immune system is replete with this molecular structure. This may explain why the etherified starch-induced antibody was directed against the hydroxyethyl group and not against the starch molecule itself.

Second-Generation Effects

Pregnancy

Two healthy, full-term primigravidae with uneventful pregnancies and without a previous history of renal disease developed acute transient non-oliguric renal insufficiency after cesarean section under epidural anesthesia. During the procedure etherified starch 6% (70/0.5) was administered, 500 ml to one patient and 1000 ml to the other, for volume substitution after moderate blood loss (less than 800 ml). Acute non-oliguric renal insufficiency occurred on day 3 after cesarean section in the first patient and on day 2 in the second. Renal function recovered spontaneously.

Drug–Drug Interactions

Metamizole

- After plastic reconstruction with a neurovascular pedicular cutaneous sliding flap a healthy 46-year-old man developed acute renal insufficiency (53). He had received two 500 mg doses of the pyrazolone metamizole and two 500 ml infusions of 6% etherified starches.

A causative link between acute renal insufficiency and etherified starch in this case was tenuous, as it was with the metamizole. Simultaneous administration of the two is not advised.

References

1. Parth E, Jurecka W, Szepfalusi Z, Schimetta W, Gebhart W, Scheiner O, Kraft D. Histological and immunohistochemical investigations of hydroxyethyl-starch deposits in rat tissues. Eur Surg Res 1992;24(1):13–21.
2. Ljungstrom KG, Willman B, Hedin H. Hapten inhibition of dextran anaphylaxis. Nine years of post-marketing surveillance of dextran 1. Ann Fr Anesth Reanim 1993;12(2):219–22.
3. Vogt NH, Bothner U, Lerch G, Lindner KH, Georgieff M. Large-dose administration of 6% hydroxyethyl starch 200/0.5 total hip arthroplasty: plasma homeostasis, hemostasis, and renal function compared to use of 5% human albumin. Anesth Analg 1996;83(2):262–8.
4. Lang C. Risiken und Nebenwirkungen der Hämodilutionstherapie. Nervenheilkunde 1992;11:44.
5. Rudolf J; HES in Acute Stroke Study Group. Hydroxyethyl starch for hypervolemic hemodilution in patients with acute ischemic stroke: a randomized, placebo-controlled phase II safety study. Cerebrovasc Dis 2002;14(1):33–41.
6. Putarek K, Minigo H, Planinc-Peraica A, Jaksic B. Allergic reaction during reinfusion of autologous bone marrow related to treatment of Hodgkin's lymphoma; possible role of hydroxyethyl starch—a case report. Libri Oncol 1996;25:53–5.
7. Trumble ER, Muizelaar JP, Myseros JS, Choi SC, Warren BB. Coagulopathy with the use of hetastarch in the treatment of vasospasm. J Neurosurg 1995;82(1):44–7.
8. Schulze VH, Berlin-Buch VH. Plasmaersatzstoffe: Dextran und Hydroxyethylstärke im Vergleich. Krankenhauspharmazie 1991;12:551.
9. Detsch O, Muhling J, Bachmann-Mennenga B, Thiel A, Heesen M, Hempelmann G. Volume replacement with gelatin or hydroxyethylstarch solutions does not impair somatosensory evoked potential monitoring: a haemodilution study in conscious volunteers. Eur J Anaesthesiol 1996;13(6):599–605.
10. Waters JH, Bernstein CA. Dilutional acidosis following hetastarch or albumin in healthy volunteers. Anesthesiology 2000;93(5):1184–7.

11. Rehm M, Orth V, Scheingraber S, Kreimeier U, Brechtelsbauer H, Finsterer U. Acid–base changes caused by 5% albumin versus 6% hydroxyethyl starch solution in patients undergoing acute normovolemic hemodilution: a randomized prospective study. Anesthesiology 2000;93(5): 1174–83.
12. Corry WD, Jackson LJ, Seaman GV. Action of hydroxyethyl starch on the flow properties of human erythrocyte suspensions. Biorheology 1983;20(5):705–17.
13. Sumpelmann R, Gunther A, Zander R. Haemoconcentration by gelatin-induced acceleration of erythrocyte sedimentation rate. Anaesthesia 2000;55(3):217–20.
14. Treib J, Haass A, Pindur G, Grauer MT, Jung F, Wenzel E, Schimrigk K. Increased haemorrhagic risk after repeated infusion of highly substituted medium molecular weight hydroxyethyl starch. Arzneimittelforschung 1997;47(1):18–22.
15. Baldassarre S, Vincent JL. Coagulopathy induced by hydroxyethyl starch. Anesth Analg 1997;84(2):451–3.
16. Falk JL, Rackow EC, Astiz ME, Weil MH. Effects of hetastarch and albumin on coagulation in patients with septic shock. J Clin Pharmacol 1988;28(5):412–15.
17. Dalrymple-Hay M, Aitchison R, Collins P, Sekhar M, Colvin B. Hydroxyethyl starch induced acquired von Willebrand's disease. Clin Lab Haematol 1992;14(3):209–11.
18. Treib J, Haass A, Pindur G, Miyachita C, Grauer MT, Jung F, Wenzel E, Schimrigk K. Highly substituted hydroxyethyl starch (HES200/0.62) leads to Type-I von Willebrand syndrome after repeated administration. Haemostasis 1996;26(4):210–13.
19. Anonymous. Hetastarch (hydroxyethyl-starch)—fatal haemorrhages. WHO Pharm Newslett 1999;7/8:2.
20. Jonville-Bera AP, Autret-Leca E, Gruel Y. Acquired type I von Willebrand's disease associated with highly substituted hydroxyethyl starch. N Engl J Med 2001;345(8):622–3.
21. Treib J, Haass A, Pindur G, Grauer MT, Treib W, Wenzel E, Schimrigk K. Influence of low and medium molecular weight hydroxyethyl starch on platelets during a long-term hemodilution in patients with cerebrovascular diseases. Arzneimittelforschung 1996;46(11):1064–6.
22. Huraux C, Ankri AA, Eyraud D, Sevin O, Menegaux F, Coriat P, Samama CM. Hemostatic changes in patients receiving hydroxyethyl starch: the influence of ABO blood group. Anesth Analg 2001;92(6):1396–401.
23. Dehne MG, Muhling J, Sablotzki A, Papke G, Kuntzsch U, Hempelmann G. Einfluss von Hydroxyethylstärke - Losung auf die Nieseufunktion bei operativen Intensivpatienten. [Effect of hydroxyethyl starch solution on kidney function in surgical intensive care patients.] Anasthesiol Intensivmed Notfallmed Schmerzther 1997;32(6):348–54.
24. Boldt J. Hydroxyethylstarch as a risk factor for acute renal failure: is a change of clinical practice indicated? Drug Saf 2002;25(12):837–46.
25. Legendre C, Thervet E, Page B, Percheron A, Noel LH, Kreis H. Hydroxyethylstarch and osmotic-nephrosis-like lesions in kidney transplantation. Lancet 1993;342(8865): 248–9.
26. De Labarthe A, Jacobs F, Blot F, Glotz D. Acute renal failure secondary to hydroxyethylstarch administration in a surgical patient. Am J Med 2001;111(5):417–8.
27. Peron S, Mouthon L, Guettier C, Brechignac S, Cohen P, Guillevin L. Hydroxyethyl starch-induced renal insufficiency after plasma exchange in a patient with polymyositis and liver cirrhosis. Clin Nephrol 2001;55(5):408–11.
28. Inoko M, Konishi T, Matsusue S, Kobashi Y. Midmural fibrosis of left ventricle due to selenium deficiency. Circulation 1998;98(23):2638–9.
29. Haskell LP, Tannenberg AM. Elevated urinary specific gravity in acute oliguric renal failure due to hetastarch administration. NY State J Med 1988;88(7):387–8.
30. Holzheimer R. Hydroxyethylstarch and renal function in kidney transplant recipients. Lancet 1997;349(9055): 883–4.
31. Coronel B, Mercatello A, Martin X, Lefrancois N. Hydroxyethylstarch and renal function in kidney transplant recipients. Lancet 1997;349(9055):884.
32. Cittanova ML, Legendre C. Hydroxyethylstarch and renal function in kidney transplant recipients. Lancet 1997;349(9055):884.
33. Cittanova ML, Leblanc I, Legendre C, Mouquet C, Riou B, Coriat P. Effect of hydroxyethylstarch in brain-dead kidney donors on renal function in kidney-transplant recipients. Lancet 1996;348(9042):1620–2.
34. Metze D, Reimann S, Szepfalusi Z, Bohle B, Kraft D, Luger TA. Persistent pruritus after hydroxyethyl starch infusion therapy: a result of long-term storage in cutaneous nerves. Br J Dermatol 1997;136(4):553–9.
35. Albegger K, Schneeberger R, Franke V, Oberascher G, Miller K. Juckreiz nach Therapie mit Hydroxyäthylstärke (HES) bei otoneurologischen Erkrankungen. [Itching following therapy with hydroxyethyl starch (HES) in otoneurological diseases.] Wien Med Wochenschr 1992;142(1):1–7.
36. Vente C, Schulze HJ. Persistierender Pruritus nach niedrigmolekulärer Hydroxyethylstärke (HES)-Infusionen. Kolner Dermatol 1991;53:733.
37. Lentner A, Warmke S, Genzel I, Jansen W. Persistierender Pruritus nach Hydroxyethylstärke-Infusionen? Z Hautkr 1991;66:214–21.
38. Schneeberger R, Albegger K, Oberascher G, Miller K. Juckreiz-Eine Nebenwirkung von Hydroxyäthylstärke (HES)? [Pruritus—a side effect of hydroxyethyl starch? First report.] HNO 1990;38(8):298–303.
39. Schneeberger R. Auftreten von Juckreiz als Nebenwirkung einer hochdosierten Hämodilutionstherapie mit Hydroxyäthylstarke. Akt Ernahr-Med 1993;18:263–5.
40. Gall H, Kaufmann R, von Ehr M, Schumann K, Sterry W. Persistierender Pruritus nach Hydroxyäthylstärke-Infusionen. [Persistent pruritus after hydroxyethyl starch infusions. Retrospective long-term study of 266 cases.] Hautarzt 1993;44(11):713–16.
41. Jurecka W, Szepfalusi Z, Parth E, Schimetta W, Gebhart W, Scheiner O, Kraft D. Hydroxyethylstarch deposits in human skin—a model for pruritus? Arch Dermatol Res 1993;285(1–2):13–19.
42. Speight EL, MacSween RM, Stevens A. Persistent itching due to etherified starch plasma expander. BMJ 1997;314(7092):1466–7.
43. Kiehl P, Metze D, Kresse H, Reimann S, Kraft D, Kapp A. Decreased activity of acid alpha-glucosidase in a patient with persistent periocular swelling after infusions of hydroxyethyl starch. Br J Dermatol 1998;138(4):672–7.
44. Bothner U, Georgieff M, Vogt NH. Assessment of the safety and tolerance of 6% hydroxyethyl starch (200/0.5) solution: a randomized, controlled epidemiology study. Anesth Analg 1998;86(4):850–5.
45. Sirtl C, Laubenthal H, Zumtobel V, Kraft D, Jurecka W. Tissue deposits of hydroxyethyl starch (HES): dose-dependent and time-related. Br J Anaesth 1999;82(4): 510–15.
46. Sharland C, Huggett A, Nielson MS, Friedmann PS. Persistent pruritis after pentastarch infusions in intensive care patients. Anaesthesia 1999;54(5):500–1.
47. Reimann S, Szepfalusi Z, Kraft D, Luger T, Metze D. Hydroxyethylstärke-speicherung in der haut unter besonder Berucksichtigung des Hydroxyethylstarke-assoziierten Juckreizes. [Hydroxyethyl starch accumulation in the skin with special reference to hydroxyethyl starch-associated pruritus.] Dtsch Med Wochenschr 2000;125(10):280–5.

48. Kimme P, Jannsen B, Ledin T, Gupta A, Vegfors M. High incidence of pruritus after large doses of hydroxyethyl starch (HES) infusions. Acta Anaesthesiol Scand 2001;45(6):686–9.
49. Kissler S, Neidhardt B, Siebzehnrubl E, Schmitt H, Tschaikowsky K, Wildt L. The detrimental role of colloidal volume substitutes in severe ovarian hyperstimulation syndrome: a case report. Eur J Obstet Gynecol Reprod Biol 2001;99(1):131–4.
50. Kannan S, Milligan KR. Moderately severe anaphylactoid reaction to pentastarch (200/0.5) in a patient with acute severe asthma. Intensive Care Med 1999;25(2):220–2.
51. Boldt J, Heesen M, Padberg W, Martin K, Hempelmann G. The influence of volume therapy and pentoxifylline infusion on circulating adhesion molecules in trauma patients. Anaesthesia 1996;51(6):529–35.
52. Dieterich HJ, Kraft D, Sirtl C, Laubenthal H, Schimetta W, Polz W, Gerlach E, Peter K. Hydroxyethyl starch antibodies in humans: incidence and clinical relevance. Anesth Analg 1998;86(5):1123–6.
53. Schumacher S, Ruland WO. Acute renal failure following haemodilution with HES in combination with metamizole? Aktuel Chir 1996;31:244–6.

Ethionamide and protionamide

See also Antituberculosis drugs

General Information

Ethionamide is a synthetic derivative of thio-isonicotinamide. The initial oral dosage for adults is 250 mg/day, slowly increasing up to 15–20 mg/kg/day (maximum 1 g/day).

Protionamide is a pyridine derivative of ethionamide. The dosage is 250–300 mg/day.

Ethionamide and protionamide have often proved to be effective in non-tuberculous mycobacterial infections. Acute rheumatic symptoms and difficulty in the management of diabetes have been reported (1).

Organs and Systems

Nervous system

Mental depression, weakness, drowsiness, and hypotension are not rare in patients taking ethionamide or protionamide (1,2). Other neurological reactions include diplopia, olfactory disturbances, metallic taste, dizziness, paresthesia, headache, and tremor (3).

Psychological, psychiatric

Psychotic reactions have been described in patients taking ethionamide (4,5) and may be exacerbated by alcohol (6).

Endocrine

Goitrous hypothyroidism has rarely been described in patients taking ethionamide (7), with recovery after withdrawal (8). Ethionamide inhibits both the uptake of iodine and its incorporation into trichloroacetic acid-precipitable protein (9).

Metabolism

Thionamides lower the blood glucose concentration and also suppress appetite, which influences carbohydrate intake (10).

Gastrointestinal

Nausea, vomiting, and anorexia reflect gastric intolerance, and ethionamide is best taken with meals (1,2). Protionamide has better gastric tolerance, but patients with a history of stomach ulcer are susceptible to gastric problems (11).

Skin

Severe allergic skin reactions, alopecia, acne, and purpura can occur in patients taking ethionamide (1,12). Other adverse effects include acneiform eruptions, photodermatitis, and hair loss (13).

Sexual function

Gynecomastia, impotence, and menorrhagia have been observed in patients taking ethionamide (7,14).

Second-Generation Effects

Teratogenicity

Ethionamide is teratogenic (15,16), and neither ethionamide nor protionamide should be administered during the first trimester of pregnancy.

Susceptibility Factors

Hepatic disease

Since hepatitis occurs in about 5% of patients treated with ethionamide or protionamide, frequent monitoring of liver function is compulsory (17).

Drug–Drug Interactions

Rifamycins

When thionamides are used in combination with rifampicin, hepatotoxicity is more common and severe (18,19). There was a 13% incidence of hepatotoxicity in patients with multibacillary leprosy treated with dapsone, rifampicin, and protionamide 10 mg/kg/day, and a 17% incidence in 110 patients treated with dapsone, rifampicin, and protionamide 5 mg/kg/day; however, although the lower dose of protionamide did not reduce the incidence of hepatotoxicity, it did reduce its severity (20). Protionamide does not affect the pharmacokinetics of rifampicin (21).

References

1. Council on Drugs. Ethionamide. A tuberculostatic agent (Trecator). JAMA 1964;187(7):527.
2. Schwartz WS. Comparison of ethionamide with isoniazid in original treatment cases of pulmonary tuberculosis. XIV. A report of the Veterans Administration—Armed Forces cooperative study. Am Rev Respir Dis 1966;93(5): 685–92.
3. Verbist L, Prignot J, Cosemans J, Gyselen A. Tolerance to ethionamid and PAS in original treatment of tuberculous patients. Scand J Respir Dis 1966;47(4):225–35.
4. Narang RK. Acute psychotic reaction probably caused by ethionamide. Tubercle 1972;53(2):137–8.
5. Sharma GS, Gupta PK, Jain NK, Shanker A, Nanawati V. Toxic psychosis to isoniazid and ethionamide in a patient with pulmonary tuberculosis. Tubercle 1979;60(3):171–2.
6. Lansdown FS, Beran M, Litwak T. Psychotoxic reaction during ethionamide therapy. Am Rev Respir Dis 1967;95(6):1053–5.
7. Moulding T, Fraser R. Hypothyroidism related to ethionamide. Am Rev Respir Dis 1970;101(1):90–4.
8. Drucker D, Eggo MC, Salit IE, Burrow GN. Ethionamide-induced goitrous hypothyroidism. Ann Intern Med 1984;100(6):837–9.
9. Danan G, Pessayre D, Larrey D, Benhamou JP. Pyrazinamide fulminant hepatitis: an old hepatotoxin strikes again. Lancet 1981;2(8254):1056–7.
10. Filla E, Comenale D. La terapia con PAS, rifamicina ed etionamide per via endovenosa e sue ripercussioni sul ricambio glucidico in diabetici affetti da tubercolosi polmonare. [Therapy with PAS, rifamycin and ethionamide administered intravenously and its effects on glucide metabolism in diabetics affected by pulmonary tuberculosis.] Minerva Med 1965;56(103):4570–3.
11. Samtsov VS. [Treatment of patients with pulmonary tuberculosis, complicated by peptic ulcer, with ethionamide and prothionamide.] Probl Tuberk 1973;51(7):67–70.
12. Desmons MT. Aspect pseudolupique provoqué par l'éthionamide (Trecator). Bull Soc Franc Derm Syph 1973;80:168.
13. Holdiness MR. Adverse cutaneous reactions to antituberculosis drugs. Int J Dermatol 1985;24(5):280–5.
14. Hussey HH. Editorial: Gynecomastia. JAMA 1974;228(11):1423.
15. Potworowska M. Leczenie etionamidem a ciaza. Gruzlica Chor Pluc 1966;34(4):345.
16. Jentgens H. Ethionamid und teratogene Wirkung. [Ethionamide and teratogenic effect.] Prax Pneumol 1968;22(11):699–704.
17. Mitchell I, Wendon J, Fitt S, Williams R. Anti-tuberculous therapy and acute liver failure. Lancet 1995;345(8949):555–6.
18. Braude AL, Davis Ch E, Fierer J. Infectious Diseases and Medical Microbiology. 2nd ed. Philadelphia: WB Saunders, 1966:1171.
19. Pattyn SR, Janssens L, Bourland J, Saylan T, Davies EM, Grillone S, Feracci C. Hepatotoxicity of the combination of rifampin–ethionamide in the treatment of multibacillary leprosy. Int J Lepr Other Mycobact Dis 1984;52(1):1–6.
20. Cartel JL, Naudillon Y, Artus JC, Grosset JH. Hepatotoxicity of the daily combination of 5 mg/kg prothionamide + 10 mg/kg rifampin Int J Lepr Other Mycobact Dis 1985;53(1):15–18.
21. Mathur A, Venkatesan K, Girdhar BK, Bharadwaj VP, Girdhar A, Bagga AK. A study of drug interactions in leprosy—1. Effect of simultaneous administration of prothionamide on metabolic disposition of rifampicin and dapsone. Lepr Rev 1986;57(1):33–7.

Ethosuximide

See also Antiepileptic drugs

General Information

The main adverse effects of ethosuximide include gastrointestinal disturbances, anorexia, dizziness, fatigue, drowsiness, headache, mood and behavioral disturbances, dyskinesias, and hiccups (1). Skin rashes (including Stevens–Johnson syndrome), systemic lupus erythematosus, scleroderma, nephrotic syndrome, blood dyscrasias, liver dysfunction, and autoimmune thyroiditis are rare.

Organs and Systems

Immunologic

Patients who develop antinuclear antibodies should be watched for the subsequent development of systemic lupus erythematosus (SEDA-19, 67) (SEDA-22, 83).

Reference

1. Perucca E. Succinimides. In: Dam M, Gram L, editors. Comprehensive Epileptology. New York: Raven Press, 1990::603–11

Ethylene oxide

See also Disinfectants and antiseptics

General Information

Ethylene oxide is a gas that is used in the sterilization of equipment too large for other techniques, and for sterilizing rubber, plastic goods, and other materials that are damaged by heat and not adequately disinfected by other cold methods.

Ethylene oxide is highly toxic. If it is not eliminated after sterilization it can produce severe irritation and burns. In addition, it forms ethylene glycol with moisture and ethylene chlorhydrine with free chlorine atoms. Both products, also irritants, are absorbed by the sterilized object, from which they elute very slowly. The rate of elimination of ethylene oxide and its irritant reaction products depends on a variety of factors, such as the nature and thickness of the material, the duration and temperature of aeration, and the material used for wrapping the sterilized item. Ethylene oxide is also an alkylating agent, a directly acting mutagen and carcinogen.

Exposure

Exposure to ethylene oxide has been reported predominantly in workers in sterilization units, and should be kept as low as feasible. Health personnel working in close proximity to ethylene oxide should be given information about its dangers, and should be informed of the known and uncertain risks of exposure. Sterilizing equipment should be regularly checked, proper ventilation established, and alarm systems installed. These procedures must guarantee that the content of ethylene oxide is lower than 1 ppm, and that the content of halogenated ethylene hydrines is lower than 150 ppm on materials that have been sterilized by ethylene oxide at the time of use. The manufacturer of each device or instrument that should be sterilized by ethylene oxide must declare the conditions necessary for sterilization and decontamination (SEDA-11, 479).

Occupational exposure of sterilizing staff to ethylene oxide in hospitals, tissue banks, and research facilities can result during any of the following operations and conditions (1):

- changing pressurized ethylene oxide gas cylinders
- leaking valves, firings, and piping
- leaking sterilizer-door gaskets
- opening sterilizer doors at the end of a cycle
- improper ventilation at the sterilizer door
- improperly ventilated or unventilated air gap between the discharge line and the sewer drain
- removal of items from sterilizers and transfer of sterilized loads to aerators
- improper ventilation of aerators and aeration areas
- incomplete aeration items
- inadequate general room ventilation
- passing near sterilizers and aerators during operation.

In most studies, exposure appears to result mostly from peak emissions during such operations as opening the door of a sterilizer and unloading and transferring sterilized material. Although much smaller amounts are used in sterilizing medicinal instruments and supplies in hospitals and industrially, it is during these uses that the highest occupational exposures have been measured. On the other hand, proper engineering controls and work practices are reported to result in full-shift exposure of less than 0.1 ppm (0.18 mg/m^3) and short-term exposure of less than 2 ppm (3.6 mg/m^3) (1). Regular medical follow-up is advisable for sterilizing staff.

Monitoring exposure

Measurement of the concentration of ethylene oxide in workplace air is commonly used for exposure control. A standard of 1 ppm for workplace air is currently accepted as a threshold limit (SEDA-21, 254).

In 12 workers who were occupationally exposed to ethylene oxide during the sterilization of medical equipment, concentrations of 0.2–8.5 ppm were detected (2). This study also confirmed the relation between the ethylene oxide concentration in ambient air and the amount of *N*-2-hydroxyethylvaline in human globin, which has been used as a biological marker of carcinogenicity.

Disposition

Ethylene oxide is readily taken up by the lung. At steady state, 20–25% of inhaled ethylene oxide reaching the alveolar space is exhaled as unchanged compound and 75–80% is taken up by the body and metabolized. Aqueous ethylene oxide solutions can penetrate human skin.

Ethylene oxide is rapidly and uniformly distributed throughout the body. It is eliminated metabolically by hydrolysis and by conjugation with glutathione and glycol. The half-life has been estimated at 14 minutes to 3.3 hours (3–6). It is excreted mainly in the urine as thioethers; at higher doses, the proportion of thioethers is reduced, while the proportion of ethylene glycol increases.

Ethylene oxide alkylates nucleophilic groups in biological macromolecules. Hemoglobin adducts have been used to monitor tissue doses of ethylene oxide (7).

Local irritant effects

Some communications report irritating effects caused by liberation of residue of ethylene oxide and its reaction products in industrial materials, for example (SEDA-11, 479):

- tracheal stenosis by tracheotomy cannulae
- severe bronchospasm and asthmatic attacks after endotracheal anesthesia by endotracheal tubes
- anaphylaxis in a hemodialysis patient from plastic and rubber connecting tubes in an arteriovenous shunt
- postoperative inflammatory reactions to intraocular lenses
- allergic contact dermatitis
- hemolysis after exposure to plastic tubing sterilized with ethylene oxide.

Organs and Systems

Nervous system

In 12 men who were exposed to ethylene oxide after a sterilizer developed a leak, although the concentrations of ethylene oxide were not monitored, all four operators intermittently smelled the ethylene oxide gas, roughly indicating a concentration of more than 700 ppm (8). All four operators developed neurological disorders. One operator who had been working for only 3 weeks developed headache, nausea, vomiting, and lethargy, followed by major motor seizures. The other three had all been working for more than 2 years and had headache, limb numbness and weakness, increased fatigue, trouble with memory, and slurred speech. Three of them developed cataracts and one required bilateral cataract extractions. Four men, two of whom had not worked directly with the leaking sterilizer, had increased central corneal thickness with normal endothelial cell counts (SEDA-11, 479).

Other reports of neurological dysfunction related to acute and chronic exposure to ethylene oxide have appeared (9–15).

Sensory systems

Of 16 hospital sterilization operators who had been exposed to ethylene oxide and underwent medical and ocular examinations, 14 had lens opacities and 12 had abnormal contrast vision (an abnormality that is nonspecific to cataracts but which often supports the diagnosis) (16).

Hematologic

Epidemiological studies have associated ethylene oxide with hematological diseases (mainly anemia, leukopenia, and leukemia) (SEDA-24, 271). To determine whether occupational exposure to low concentrations of ethylene oxide can cause hematological abnormalities and whether blood monitoring could be used as health surveillance, a cross-sectional study was undertaken (17). Blood samples were collected from 47 hospital workers who were exposed to ethylene oxide during a mean period of 6.6 years. Ethylene oxide concentrations were in the range <0.01–0.06 ppm. The control group, individually matched by age, sex, and smoking habits, consisted of 88 workers from the administrative sector who had never been occupationally exposed to ethylene oxide. There were significant differences between the exposed and the control groups in the frequency of workers with low leukocyte counts. There was no significant difference in the absolute mean number of total leukocytes, but there was an increase in the mean number of monocytes and eosinophils and a reduction in the absolute mean number of lymphocytes in the exposed group compared with the controls. There was an increase in the percentage hematocrit and the mean absolute number of erythrocytes and a fall in the mean absolute number of platelets in the exposed group compared with the controls. The mean absolute numbers of eosinophils and erythrocytes were significantly higher, as was the hematocrit, and the mean absolute numbers of lymphocytes and platelets were significantly lower in the subgroups with a higher cumulative dose of exposure. There was a dose relation between cumulative exposure and the absolute mean number of eosinophils. The results of this study suggest that the total leukocyte count and the eosinophil count could be used to monitor for early detection of health problems in ethylene oxide workers.

Immunologic

Dialyser hypersensitivity syndrome (SEDA-11, 219) (SEDA-11, 479) presents as an acute anaphylactic reaction, the symptoms of which range from mild to life-threatening. The cause of the syndrome is unknown, but affected patients appear to have a high incidence of positive radioabsorbent tests to a conjugate of human serum albumin and ethylene oxide used to sterilize artificial kidneys. This conjugate may be the allergen responsible.

Immediate hypersensitivity reactions occurred in six of 600 donors who underwent automated platelet pheresis; skin-prick testing in four of them (but in none of 40 controls) was positive when an ethylene oxide human serum albumin reagent was used (18). Radioallergosorbent testing showed that serum from four of the six donors, but only one of 145 controls, contained IgE antibodies to ethylene oxide-albumin.

Long-Term Effects

Mutagenicity

There is overwhelming evidence that ethylene oxide produces genetic damage in a wide range of organisms and cells, including somatic cells of exposed humans (7,19). Ethylene oxide is a germ-cell mutagen in rodents. In male mice it induces chromosome breakage, leading to dominant lethal mutations and heritable translocations. Sensitive stages appear to be restricted to late spermatocytes and early spermatozoa.

In females, ethylene oxide also induces presumed, dominant, lethal mutations. When females are exposed shortly after mating or during the early pronuclear stage of the zygote, high frequencies of fetal anomalies are induced.

Ethylene oxide was ineffective in inducing morphological-specific locus mutations in spermatogonial stem cells; however, it produced dominant visible and electrophoresis-specific locus mutants in male mice, assumed to be derived from poststem cells.

The effectiveness of ethylene oxide in inducing chromosome breakage in germ cells of male mice is strongly influenced by varying degrees or rates of exposure. Since there was a dose-rate effect for ethylene oxide-induced, dominant, lethal mutations at high concentrations and over long exposure periods, considering the short burst exposure and low TWA exposure in humans, the question of whether significant dose-rate effects also exist at low exposures is unanswered.

Cytogenetic studies have been performed in the peripheral lymphocytes of humans exposed to ethylene oxide (SEDA-12, 574). Several studies in workers in hospital ethylene oxide sterilization units or plants have suggested that these workers have increased frequencies of chromosomal aberrations, including micronuclei and sister chromatid exchanges in peripheral lymphocytes.

The International Agency for Research on Cancer (IARC) Working Group reviewed the published studies of workers exposed to ethylene oxide in hospital and factory sterilization units and in ethylene manufacturing and processing plants (9). The studies consistently showed chromosomal damage in peripheral blood lymphocytes, including chromosomal aberrations in 11 of 14 studies, sister chromatid exchange in 20 of 23 studies, micronuclei in three of eight studies, and gene mutation in one study. In general, the degree of damage is correlated with the degree and duration of exposure. The induction of sister chromatid exchange appears to be more sensitive to exposure to ethylene oxide than is induction of either chromosomal aberrations or micronuclei. In one study, chromosomal aberrations were observed in the peripheral lymphocytes of workers 2 years after cessation of exposure to ethylene oxide, and sister chromatid exchanges 6 months after cessation of exposure. However, in one study, incidental exposure to high concentrations of ethylene oxide did not cause any measurable permanent mutational/cytogenetic damage in lymphocytes of exposed persons (20).

The effects of glutathione-*S*-transferase T1 and M1 genotypes on hemoglobin adducts in erythrocytes and sister chromatid exchange in lymphocytes have been examined in 58 hospital operators of sterilizers that used ethylene oxide and non-exposed workers (21). The results suggested that the glutathione-*S*-transferase T1 null genotype was associated with increased formation of ethylene oxide-hemoglobin adducts in relation to occupational exposure. This suggests that individuals with the glutathione-*S*-transferase T1 null genotype may be more susceptible to the genotoxic effects of ethylene oxide.

Tumorigenicity

Ethylene oxide is carcinogenic, assigned to Group 1 of the IARC (7). There is limited evidence of carcinogenicity in humans, but much evidence in experimental animals, and the IARC has classified ethylene oxide in category 1 ("carcinogenic in humans"), based primarily on evidence in animals and genotoxic considerations. The overall evaluation of the Working group of the IARC, updated in 1995, is based on the following supporting evidence.

Ethylene oxide is a directly acting alkylating agent that:

- induces a sensitive, persistent, dose-related increase in the frequency of chromosomal aberrations and sister chromatid exchange in peripheral lymphocytes and micronuclei in bone marrow cells of exposed workers;
- has been associated with malignancies of the lymphatic and hemopoietic systems in both humans and experimental animals;
- induces a dose-related increase in the frequency of hemoglobin adducts in exposed humans and a dose-related increase in the numbers of adducts in both DNA and hemoglobin in exposed rodents;
- induces gene mutations and heritable translocations in germ cells of exposed rodents;
- is a powerful mutagen and clastogen at all phylogenetic levels.

In 1979, three cases of hemopoietic cancer that had occurred between 1972 and 1977 were reported in workers at a Swedish factory where 50% ethylene oxide and 50% methyl formate had been used since 1968 to sterilize hospital equipment (22).

In epidemiological studies of exposure to ethylene oxide, the most frequently reported association has been with lymphatic and hemopoietic cancer. Two populations were studied: people using ethylene oxide as a sterilizing agent and chemical workers manufacturing or using ethylene oxide. Of studies of sterilization personnel, the largest and most informative is that conducted in the USA (23,24). Overall, mortality from lymphatic and hemopoietic cancers was only marginally raised, but there was a significant trend, especially for lymphatic leukemia and non-Hodgkin's lymphoma, in relation to estimated cumulative exposure. For exposure to 1 ppm (1.8 mg/m^3) over a working lifetime of 45 years, a ratio of 1.2 was estimated for lymphatic and hemopoietic cancers. The other studies of workers involved in sterilization in Sweden (25–27) and in the UK (28) each showed non-significant excesses of lymphatic and hemopoietic cancers. An assessment based on epidemiological data showed no increase in leukemia in those who had been exposed to ethylene oxide (29).

Because of the possibility of confounding occupational exposure in the studies of chemical workers exposed to ethylene oxide (20,25,26,28,30–38), less weight can be given to the positive findings. Nevertheless, they are compatible with a small but consistent excess of lymphatic and hemopoietic cancers found in studies of sterilization personnel. Some of the epidemiological studies have shown an additional risk of cancer of the stomach, which was significant only in one study from Sweden (25,26,30).

Second-Generation Effects

Teratogenicity

In animals, ethylene oxide has toxic effects on reproduction and is teratogenic, but the relevance of animal and epidemiological studies to occupational exposure of humans in the environment of sterilization units is unclear (SEDA-12, 576) (39).

References

1. Mortimer VD Jr, Kercher SL. Control Technology for 668 Ethylene Oxide Sterilization in hospitals. Cincinnati, OH: National Institute for Occupational Safety and Health, 1989.
2. Leonardos G, Kendak D, Barnard N. Odor threshold déterminations of 53 odorant chemicals. J Air Pollut Control Assoc 1969;19:51.
3. Brugnone F, Perbellini L, Faccini G, Pasini F. Concentration of ethylene oxide in the alveolar air of occupationally exposed workers. Am J Ind Med 1985;8(1):67–72.
4. Osterman-Golkar S, Bergmark E. Occupational exposure to ethylene oxide. Relation between in vivo dose and exposure dose. Scand J Work Environ Health 1988;14(6):372–7.
5. Osterman-Golkar S. Dosimetry of ethylene oxide. In: Bartsch H, Hemminki K, O'Neill IK, editors. Methods for detecting DNA Damaging Agents in Humans: Applications in Cancer Epidemiology and Prevention. Lyon: IARC, 1988;89:249–57.
6. Filser JG, Denk B, Tornqvist M, Kessler W, Ehrenberg L. Pharmacokinetics of ethylene in man; body burden with ethylene oxide and hydroxyethylation of hemoglobin due to endogenous and environmental ethylene. Arch Toxicol 1992;66(3):157–63.
7. WHO International Agency for Research of Cancer. Ethylene oxide. IARC Monogr Eval Carcinog Risks Hum 1994;60:73–159.
8. Jay WM, Swift TR, Hull DS. Possible relationship of ethylene oxide exposure to cataract formation. Am J Ophthalmol 1982;93(6):727–32.
9. Schroder JM, Hoheneck M, Weis J, Deist H. Ethylene oxide polyneuropathy: clinical follow-up study with morphometric and electron microscopic findings in a sural nerve biopsy. J Neurol 1985;232(2):83–90.
10. Fukushima T, Abe K, Nakagawa A, Osaki Y, Yoshida N, Yamane Y. Chronic ethylene oxide poisoning in a factory manufacturing medical appliances. J Soc Occup Med 1986;36(4):118–23.
11. Estrin WJ, Cavalieri SA, Wald P, Becker CE, Jones JR, Cone JE. Evidence of neurologic dysfunction related to long-term ethylene oxide exposure. Arch Neurol 1987;44(12):1283–6.
12. Estrin WJ, Bowler RM, Lash A, Becker CE. Neurotoxicological evaluation of hospital sterilizer workers exposed to ethylene oxide. J Toxicol Clin Toxicol 1990;28(1):1–20.
13. Crystal HA, Schaumburg HH, Grober E, Fuld PA, Lipton RB. Cognitive impairment and sensory loss associated with chronic low-level ethylene oxide exposure. Neurology 1988;38(4):567–9.
14. Klees JE, Lash A, Bowler RM, Shore M, Becker CE. Neuropsychologic "impairment" in a cohort of hospital workers chronically exposed to ethylene oxide. J Toxicol Clin Toxicol 1990;28(1):21–8.
15. Grober E, Crystal H, Lipton RB, Schaumburg H. Authors' commentary. EtO is associated with cognitive dysfunction. J Occup Med 1992;34(11):1114–16.
16. Sobaszek A, Hache JC, Frimat P, Akakpo V, Victoire G, Furon D. Working conditions and health effects of ethylene oxide exposure at hospital sterilization sites. J Occup Environ Med 1999;41(6):492–9.
17. Shaham J, Levi Z, Gurvich R, Shain R, Ribak J. Hematological changes in hospital workers due to chronic exposure to low levels of ethylene oxide. J Occup Environ Med 2000;42(8):843–50.

18. Leitman SF, Boltansky H, Alter HJ, Pearson FC, Kaliner MA. Allergic reactions in healthy plateletpheresis donors caused by sensitization to ethylene oxide gas. N Engl J Med 1986;315(19):1192–6.
19. Dellarco VL, Generoso WM, Sega GA, Fowle JR 3rd, Jacobson-Kram D. Review of the mutagenicity of ethylene oxide. Environ Mol Mutagen 1990;16(2):85–103.
20. Tates AD, Boogaard PJ, Darroudi F, Natarajan AT, Caubo ME, van Sittert NJ. Biological effect monitoring in industrial workers following incidental exposure to high concentrations of ethylene oxide. Mutat Res 1995;329(1):63–77.
21. Yong LC, Schulte PA, Wiencke JK, Boeniger MF, Connally LB, Walker JT, Whelan EA, Ward EM. Hemoglobin adducts and sister chromatid exchanges in hospital workers exposed to ethylene oxide: effects of glutathione S-transferase T1 and M1 genotypes. Cancer Epidemiol Biomarkers Prev 2001;10(5):539–50.
22. Hogstedt C, Malmqvist N, Wadman B. Leukemia in workers exposed to ethylene oxide. JAMA 1979;241(11): 1132–3.
23. Stayner L, Steenland K, Greife A, Hornung R, Hayes RB, Nowlin S, Morawetz J, Ringenburg V, Elliot L, Halperin W. Exposure-response analysis of cancer mortality in a cohort of workers exposed to ethylene oxide. Am J Epidemiol 1993;138(10):787–98.
24. Steenland K, Stayner L, Greife A, Halperin W, Hayes R, Hornung R, Nowlin S. Mortality among workers exposed to ethylene oxide. N Engl J Med 1991;324(20):1402–7.
25. Hogstedt C, Aringer L, Gustavsson A. Epidemiologic support for ethylene oxide as a cancer-causing agent. JAMA 1986;255(12):1575–8.
26. Hogstedt C. Epidemiological studies on ethylene oxide and cancer: an updating. In: Bartsch H, Hemminki K, O'Neill, editors. Methods for Detecting DNA Damaging Agents in Humans: Applications in Cancer Epidemiology and Prevention. Lyon: IARC, 1988;89:265–70.
27. Hagmar L, Welinder H, Linden K, Attewell R, Osterman-Golkar S, Tornqvist M. An epidemiological study of cancer risk among workers exposed to ethylene oxide using hemoglobin adducts to validate environmental exposure assessments. Int Arch Occup Environ Health 1991;63(4):271–7.
28. Gardner MJ, Coggon D, Pannett B, Harris EC. Workers exposed to ethylene oxide: a follow up study. Br J Ind Med 1989;46(12):860–5.
29. Baca D, Drexler C, Cullen E. Obstructive laryngotracheitis secondary to gentian violet exposure. Clin Pediatr (Phila) 2001;40(4):233–5.
30. Hogstedt C, Rohlen O, Berndtsson BS, Axelson O, Ehrenberg L. A cohort study of mortality and cancer incidence in ethylene oxide production workers. Br J Ind Med 1979;36(4):276–80.
31. Morgan RW, Claxton KW, Divine BJ, Kaplan SD, Harris VB. Mortality among ethylene oxide workers. J Occup Med 1981;23(11):767–70.
32. Shore RE, Gardner MJ, Pannett B. Ethylene oxide: an assessment of the epidemiological evidence on carcinogenicity. Br J Ind Med 1993;50(11):971–97.
33. Kiesselbach N, Ulm K, Lange HJ, Korallus U. A multicentre mortality study of workers exposed to ethylene oxide. Br J Ind Med 1990;47(3):182–8.
34. Benson LO, Teta MJ. Mortality due to pancreatic and lymphopoietic cancers in chlorohydrin production workers. Br J Ind Med 1993;50(8):710–16.
35. Teta MJ, Benson LO, Vitale JN. Mortality study of ethylene oxide workers in chemical manufacturing: a 10 year update. Br J Ind Med 1993;50(8):704–9.
36. Bisanti L, Maggini M, Raschetti R, Alegiani SS, Ippolito FM, Caffari B, Segnan N, Ponti A. Cancer mortality in ethylene oxide workers. Br J Ind Med 1993;50(4):317–24.
37. Thiess AM, Schwegler H, Fleig I, Stocker WG. Mutagenicity study of workers exposed to alkylene oxides (ethylene oxide/propylene oxide) and derivatives. J Occup Med 1981;23(5):343–7.
38. Greenberg HL, Ott MG, Shore RE. Men assigned to ethylene oxide production or other ethylene oxide related chemical manufacturing: a mortality study. Br J Ind Med 1990;47(4):221–30.
39. Florack EI, Zielhuis GA. Occupational ethylene oxide exposure and reproduction. Int Arch Occup Environ Health 1990;62(4):273–7.

Ethylenediamine

General Information

Ethylenediamine is used to improve the solubility of theophylline in the formulation known as aminophylline (theophylline ethylenediamine). Aminophylline is converted to theophylline after oral and intravenous administration.

Ethylenediamine is also used as a stabilizer in creams and ointments.

Ethylenediamine tetra-acetic acid is a chelating agent that is used as an anticoagulant for collecting blood samples and for removing calcium from experimental fluids in laboratories.

Organs and Systems

Respiratory

Asthma has been reported after occupational exposure to ethylenediamine (1).

Skin

Cutaneous reactions have been reported with ethylenediamine (2).

Immunologic

Systemic contact dermatitis is a delayed hypersensitivity skin reaction that results from systemic exposure. Exanthematous systemic contact dermatitis from ethylenediamine has been reported with aminophylline. Disodium edetate (ethylenediamine tetra-acetic acid) has caused contact dermatitis after local application (SEDA-23, 242), and ethylenediamine cross-reacted in a patch test in a patient who had had contact dermatitis with hydroxyzine, an ethylenediamine derivative (SEDA-22, 178). Prior sensitization can occur to ethylenediamine in creams and ointments (SED-14, 485).

Originally described in 1984, baboon syndrome is a form of systemic contact dermatitis involving the buttocks and adjacent skin in a distribution reminiscent of the erythematous buttocks seen in baboons (3). Areas under the underwear, the inner thighs, and the axillae can also be affected. Most cases are caused by oral agents, suggesting that excretion of the antigen may be a factor. In one case systemic administration caused a reaction at a site that may have been previously exposed to topical ethylenediamine (2).

- A 64-year-old man developed a pruritic erythematous eruption in the perineal area a few hours after a stress test, during which he received dipyridamole and intravenous aminophylline. He had a morbilliform erythema of the perineal area under his underclothing anteriorly, with still more prominent erythema posteriorly. The measles-like rash lacked epidermal changes of exudation of scaling. A series of 20 standard patch tests were negative, except for a +++ response to ethylenediamine. On being questioned, he remembered using a topical medicament prescribed for his wife on this area in the distant past. He improved uneventfully with time and avoidance.

The authors proposed that the topical medicament had contained ethylenediamine.

- A 30-year-old woman developed a generalized urticarial reaction immediately after the intravenous administration of aminophylline (4). Skin intradermal testing was positive to ethylenediamine. Rechallenge was positive with intravenous aminophylline but negative with diprophylline, which does not contain ethylenediamine.

Most reports of aminophylline hypersensitivity reactions in the English language literature were delayed reactions. However, most of the Japanese cases were immediate reactions. Acetylation is the main metabolic pathway of ethylenediamine. Most Japanese are rapid or intermediate acetylators, while 50% of Caucasians are slow acetylators. This difference suggests an explanation for the different incidences of immediate and delayed reactions to ethylenediamine in Japanese and Caucasians.

References

1. Asakawa H, Araki T, Yamamoto N, Imai I, Yamane M, Tsutsumi Y, Kawakami F. Allergy to ethylenediamine and steroid. J Investig Allergol Clin Immunol 2000;10(6):372–4.
2. Guin JD, Fields P, Thomas KL. Baboon syndrome from i.v. aminophylline in a patient allergic to ethylenediamine. Contact Dermatitis 1999;40(3):170–1.
3. Andersen KE, Hjorth N, Menne T. The baboon syndrome: systemically-induced allergic contact dermatitis. Contact Dermatitis 1984;10(2):97–100.
4. Yoshizawa A, Araki Y, Kobayashi N, Kudo K. [A case of aminophylline hypersensitivity reaction due to ethylenediamine.] Arerugi 1999;48(11):1206–11.

Etidocaine

See also Local anesthetics

General Information

Etidocaine is a highly lipid-soluble, long-acting aminoamide. It has a similar toxicity profile to that of bupivacaine and there is an increased risk of life-threatening cardiac events compared with lidocaine (1).

Reference

1. Bacsik CJ, Swift JQ, Havgreaves KM. Toxic systemic reactions of bupivacaine and etidocaine. Oral Surg Oral Med Oral Pathol Oral Radiol Endod 1995;79(1):18–23.

Etifoxine

General Information

Etifoxine is a non-benzodiazepine drug, licensed in France for psychosomatic manifestations of anxiety.

Organs and Systems

Psychological, psychiatric

The psychomotor and amnesic effects of single oral doses of etifoxine (50 mg and 100 mg) and lorazepam (2 mg) were studied in 48 healthy subjects in a double-blind, placebo-controlled, randomized, parallel-group study (1). Its effects were assessed by a battery of subjective and objective tests that explored mood and vigilance, attention, psychomotor performance, and memory. Whereas vigilance, psychomotor performance, and free recall were significantly impaired by lorazepam, neither dose of etifoxine (50 mg and 100 mg) produced such effects. The results suggested that 50 mg and 100 mg single doses of etifoxine do not induce amnesia and sedation compared with lorazepam.

Reference

1. Micallef J, Soubrouillard C, Guet F, Le Guern ME, Alquier C, Bruguerolle B, Blin O. A double blind parallel group placebo controlled comparison of sedative and amnesic effects of etifoxine and lorazepam in healthy subjects. Fundam Clin Pharmacol 2001;15(3):209–16.

Etodolac

See also Non-steroidal anti-inflammatory drugs

General Information

Etodolac, a pyranocarboxylic acid, was first marketed in the UK in 1986. By 1988, etodolac had been reported 27 times to the UK Committee on Safety of Medicines as being suspected of causing serious adverse reactions (1). In a French postmarketing safety study in 51 355 patients taking 200–600 mg/day, 10% of patients reported a total of 6236 adverse reactions and 9% dropped out because of adverse reactions, 21 of which were judged severe (2). In another four postmarketing surveillance studies in 8334 patients with rheumatic conditions who took 200–600 mg/day of etodolac for periods ranging from 4 weeks to 1 year, 23% reported adverse events and 9%

stopped taking the drug because of adverse reactions; gastrointestinal events were the most commonly reported (3).

Organs and Systems

Nervous system

Nervous system effects of etodolac include dizziness (4.4%), headache (6.0%), and tinnitus (2.6%).

Hematologic

One case of agranulocytosis, probably induced by etodolac, with the pattern common to the other NSAIDs, has been reported (4).

Gastrointestinal

Animal experiments, as well as endoscopic and ^{51}Cr blood loss studies in man, suggest that the gastric irritancy of etodolac is low (5,6), but such claims have to be regarded with the reservations expressed about all NSAIDs. Etodolac in short-term dosages of 200, 400, and 600 mg bd caused significantly less damage to both the gastric and the duodenal mucosa than aspirin 3.9 g/day (SEDA-12, 85). It had a less damaging effect on the stomach than naproxen in a short-term endoscopic study in rheumatoid arthritis (7). The most frequent adverse effects in 1379 patients in trials were gastrointestinal symptoms: 8.9% of patients had nausea, 5.8% epigastric pain, 5.7% heartburn, and 5.2% indigestion; 1.9% of patients had to be withdrawn because of these adverse effects.

Acute colitis demonstrated by endoscopy and rechallenge was reported in two patients taking etodolac for arthritis (8). Colonic strictures have been described in another report (SEDA-22, 115).

Skin

Skin rashes occur in 3% of patients who take etodolac (SEDA-12, 85).

Susceptibility Factors

Age

The safety profiles of etodolac in elderly and younger patients are similar (SEDA-19, 98).

Drug Administration

Drug formulations

The long-term treatment safety profile of a modified-release formulation of etodolac was similar to that of the standard formulation (SEDA-18, 104).

Drug dosage regimens

In 1986, the UK Drug Safety Research Unit at Southampton published a report on its prescription event monitoring study of etodolac (SEDA-13, 80). Etodolac was rated effective in only 56% of 9109 patients, and the Unit concluded that the average dosage used (400 mg/day) was too low to be effective. Consequently, the adverse reaction figures should be viewed with great caution. Indeed, at an adequate dosage they might actually be unfavorable, since in this study the rate of dyspepsia during the first month was 16 per 1000 compared with 3 per 1000 for piroxicam. After the first month, the rates were similar for etodolac and piroxicam. Few serious events were recorded: exfoliative dermatitis in one patient with psoriatic arthritis and 20 cases of hematemesis or melena.

References

1. Bem JL, Breckenridge AM, Mann RD, Rawlins MD. Review of yellow cards (1986): report to the Committee on the Safety of Medicines. Br J Clin Pharmacol 1988;26(6):679–89.
2. Benhamou CL. Large-scale open trials with etodolac (Lodine) in France: an assessment of safety. Rheumatol Int 1990;10(Suppl):29–34.
3. Serni U. Global safety of etodolac: reports from worldwide postmarketing surveillance studies. Rheumatol Int 1990;10(Suppl):23–7.
4. Cramer RL, Aboko-Cole VC, Gualtieri RJ. Agranulocytosis associated with etodolac. Ann Pharmacother 1994;28(4):458–60.
5. Jacob G, Messina M, Kennedy J, Epstein C, Sanda M, Mullane J. Minimum effective dose of etodolac for the treatment of rheumatoid arthritis. J Clin Pharmacol 1986;26(3):195–202.
6. Lanza FL, Arnold JD. Etodolac, a new nonsteroidal anti-inflammatory drug: gastrointestinal microbleeding and endoscopic studies. Clin Rheumatol 1989;8(Suppl 1):5–15.
7. Taha AS, McLaughlin S, Sturrock RD, Russell RI. Evaluation of the efficacy and comparative effects on gastric and duodenal mucosa of etodolac and naproxen in patients with rheumatoid arthritis using endoscopy. Br J Rheumatol 1989;28(4):329–32.
8. Wilcox GM, Porensky RS. Acute colitis associated with etodolac. J Clin Gastroenterol 1997;25(1):367–8.

Etomidate

See also General anesthetics

General Information

Etomidate, a non-barbiturate anesthetic, is considered to be safe, especially in patients with hemodynamic instability. The most common complications of using etomidate are venous sequelae, pain on injection (1), and involuntary muscle movements (SED-11, 211) (2).

Organs and Systems

Cardiovascular

The cardiorespiratory tolerance of etomidate is usually excellent (3), but cardiovascular instability has been described after a bolus dose (4).

Nervous system

In 104 patients, the frequency of pain on injection of etomidate was 32–53% and was severe in 5–20% of patients (5). The frequency of involuntary movements was 15–35%. The frequency of both pain and involuntary muscle movements was least when fentanyl 2.5 μg/kg was given before etomidate. There was no significant relation between pain and muscle movement. A medium-chain triglyceride and soya bean emulsion formulation has been used for anesthetic induction, in an attempt to reduce the unwanted adverse effects of pain on injection and thrombophlebitis (6).

Myoclonus has been noted, and can be dangerous in open eye surgery (7).

Etomidate produced activation of epileptiform activity, and electrographic seizures during craniotomy in epileptic patients (8). Generalized seizures were noted after etomidate induction in 20% of 30 patients without a history of epilepsy (9). Cerebral excitation can also occur after recovery from etomidate anesthesia, with potential respiratory disturbance (10,11). Caution should be exercised when giving etomidate to patients with a history of seizures (SEDA-18, 113).

When etomidate was given to 12 patients who had seizures of short duration during electroconvulsive therapy conducted previously under propofol anesthesia, mean seizure duration was significantly increased with etomidate anesthesia (12). However, there is no evidence that this observation is associated with an improved psychiatric outcome.

Endocrine

Adrenocortical function has been assessed in a randomized trial after intravenous etomidate in 30 patients who required rapid-sequence induction and tracheal intubation (13). The controls received midazolam. Etomidate caused adrenocortical dysfunction, which resolved after 12 hours.

Cortisol and aldosterone concentrations were reduced by etomidate in adults (14,15), but the clinical relevance was minimal after a single bolus (16). A reduction in cortisol was reported 2 hours after delivery in 40 infants whose mothers received etomidate for cesarean section. There were also nine cases of severe to moderate hypoglycemia in this study, but the changes in blood glucose concentration were not significantly different from those in controls (17).

Hematologic

Hemolysis has been reported after the administration of etomidate (18). It may be related to the use of propylene glycol as a solvent (19,20).

Platelet hyperaggregability after general anesthesia has been reported in patients undergoing vascular surgery. The effect of etomidate and thiopental on platelet function has now been examined in 46 patients undergoing infrainguinal vascular surgery (21). Etomidate caused significant platelet inhibitory effects, whereas the effects of thiopental were minor. This may affect the choice of anesthetic in patients with compromised hemostasis.

Immunologic

Transient erythema has been described, but histamine release does not occur (22).

Etomidate is the induction agent of choice in atopic patients, in whom etomidate, fentanyl, and vecuronium comprise the safest combination of drugs for general anesthesia. However, non-allergic anaphylactic (anaphylactoid) reactions have been observed, even with this combination (23,24), and it can even be life-threatening; one patient also had a myocardial infarction (24).

Drug Administration

Drug formulations

An oral transmucosal formulation of etomidate, which is absorbed over 15 minutes, has been studied in 10 healthy adults at four doses: 12.5, 25, 50, and 100 mg (25). Dose-related drowsiness and light sleep occurred 10–20 minutes after administration. Peak serum concentrations and clinical effects were noted at about 20 minutes, with no clinical effect noticeable by 60 minutes. There was no vomiting and only four patients had transient nausea. Two patients had brief episodes of involuntary tremor with the 100 mg dose. Of note was the increasingly unpleasant taste with increasing dose and the apparent reduction in absorption with higher doses.

References

1. Kawar P, Dundee JW. Frequency of pain on injection and venous sequelae following the I.V. administration of certain anaesthetics and sedatives. Br J Anaesth 1982;54(9):935–9.
2. Holdcroft A, Morgan M, Whitwam JG, Lumley J. Effect of dose and premedication on induction complications with etomidate. Br J Anaesth 1976;48(3):199–205.
3. Colvin MP, Savege TM, Newland PE, Weaver EJ, Waters AF, Brookes JM, Inniss R. Cardiorespiratory changes following induction of anaesthesia with etomidate in patients with cardiac disease. Br J Anaesth 1979;51(6):551–6.
4. Price ML, Millar B, Grounds M, Cashman J. Changes in cardiac index and estimated systemic vascular resistance during induction of anaesthesia with thiopentone, methohexitone, propofol and etomidate. Br J Anaesth 1992;69(2):172–6.
5. Korttila K, Tammisto T, Aromaa U. Comparison of etomidate in combination with fentanyl or diazepam, with thiopentone as an induction agent for general anaesthesia. Br J Anaesth 1979;51(12):1151–7.
6. Mayer M, Doenicke A, Nebauer AE, Hepting L. Propofol und Etomidat-Lipuro zur Einleitung einer Allgemeinanästhesie. Hämodynamik, Venenverträglichkeit, subjektives Empfinden und postoperative Übelkeit. [Propofol and etomidate-Lipuro for induction of general anesthesia. Hemodynamics, vascular compatibility,

subjective findings and postoperative nausea.] Anaesthesist 1996;45(11):1082–4.
7. Berry JM, Merin RG. Etomidate myoclonus and the open globe. Anesth Analg 1989;69(2):256–9.
8. Krieger W, Koerner M. Generalized grand mal seizure after recovery from uncomplicated fentanyl–etomidate anesthesia. Anesth Analg 1987;66(3):284–5.
9. Nickel B, Schmickaly R. Gesteigerte Anfallsbereitschaft unter Etomidatlangzeitinfusion beim Delirium tremens. [Increased tendency to seizures as affected by long-term infusions of etomidate in delirium tremens.] Anaesthesist 1985;34(9):462–9.
10. Parker CJ. Respiratory disturbance during recovery from etomidate anaesthesia. Anaesthesia 1988;43(1):16–17.
11. Hansen HC, Drenck NE. Generalised seizures after etomidate anaesthesia. Anaesthesia 1988;43(9):805–6.
12. Stadtland C, Erfurth A, Ruta U, Michael N. A switch from propofol to etomidate during an ECT course increases EEG and motor seizure duration. J ECT 2002;18(1):22–5.
13. Schenarts CL, Burton JH, Riker RR. Adrenocortical dysfunction following etomidate induction in emergency department patients. Acad Emerg Med 2001;8(1):1–7.
14. Weber MM, Lang J, Abedinpour F, Zeilberger K, Adelmann B, Engelhardt D. Different inhibitory effect of etomidate and ketoconazole on the human adrenal steroid biosynthesis. Clin Investig 1993;71(11):933–8.
15. Varga I, Racz K, Kiss R, Futo L, Toth M, Sergev O, Glaz E. Direct inhibitory effect of etomidate on corticosteroid secretion in human pathologic adrenocortical cells. Steroids 1993;58(2):64–8.
16. Vanacker B, Wiebalck A, Van Aken H, Sermeus L, Bouillon R, Amery A. Induktionsqualität und Nebennierenrindenfunktion. Ein klinischer Vergleich von Etomidat-Lipuro und Hypnomidate. [Quality of induction and adrenocortical function. A clinical comparison of Etomidate-Lipuro and Hypnomidate.] Anaesthesist 1993;42(2):81–9.
17. Crozier TA, Flamm C, Speer CP, Rath W, Wuttke W, Kuhn W, Kettler D. Effects of etomidate on the adrenocortical and metabolic adaptation of the neonate. Br J Anaesth 1993;70(1):47–53.
18. Nebauer AE, Doenicke A, Hoernecke R, Angster R, Mayer M. Does etomidate cause haemolysis? Br J Anaesth 1992;69(1):58–60.
19. Wertz E. Does etomidate cause haemolysis? Br J Anaesth 1993;70(4):490–1.
20. Doenicke A, Nebauer AE, Hoernecke R, Angster R, Mayer M. Does etomidate cause haemolysis? In response. Br J Anaesth 1993;70:491.
21. Gries A, Weis S, Herr A, Graf BM, Seelos R, Martin E, Bohrer H. Etomidate and thiopental inhibit platelet function in patients undergoing infrainguinal vascular surgery. Acta Anaesthesiol Scand 2001;45(4):449–57.
22. Doenicke A, Hartel U, Buttner T, Kropp W. Anaesthesien für endoskopischdiagnostische Eingriffe unter besonderer Berücksichtigung von Etomidate. In: Proceedings, 8th International Anaesthesia Postgraduate Course. Vienna: p.l. Egermann.
23. Fazackerley EJ, Martin AJ, Tolhurst-Cleaver CL, Watkins J. Anaphylactoid reaction following the use of etomidate. Anaesthesia 1988;43(11):953–4.
24. Moorthy SS, Laurent B, Pandya P, Fry V. Anaphylactoid reaction to etomidate: report of a case. J Clin Anesth 2001;13(8):582–4.
25. Streisand JB, Jaarsma RL, Gay MA, Badger MJ, Maland L, Nordbrock E, Stanley TH. Oral transmucosal etomidate in volunteers. Anesthesiology 1998;88(1):89–95.

Euphorbiaceae

See also Herbal medicines

General Information

The genera in the family of Euphorbiaceae (Table 1) include various spurges, such as poinsettia and croton.

Breynia officinalis

Breynia officinalis (Chi R Yun) contains the saponin breynin, and terpenic and phenolic glycosides (1). Its Chinese name, Chi R Yun, means dizziness or vertigo for 7 days. It has been used to treat venereal diseases, contusions, heart failure, growth retardation, and

Table 1 The genera of Euphorbiaceae

Acalypha (copperleaf)
Adelia (wild lime)
Alchornea (alchornea)
Alchorneopsis (alchorneopsis)
Aleurites (aleurites)
Antidesma (china laurel)
Argythamnia (silverbush)
Bernardia (myrtle croton)
Bischofia (bishopwood)
Breynia (breynia)
Caperonia (false croton)
Chamaesyce (sandmat)
Chrozophora (chrozophora)
Claoxylon (claoxylon)
Cnidoscolusohl (cnidoscolus)
Codiaeum (codiaeum)
Croton (croton)
Dalechampia (dalechampia)
Ditta (ditta)
Drypetes (drypetes)
Euphorbia (spurge)
Flueggea (bushweed)
Gymnanthes (gymnanthes)
Hippomane (hippomane)
Hura (sandbox tree)
Hyeronima (hyeronima)
Jatropha (nettle spurge)
Leptopus (maidenbush)
Macaranga (macaranga)
Mallotus (mallotus)
Manihot (manihot)
Margaritaria (margaritaria)
Mercurialis (mercurialis)
Pedilanthus (pedilanthus)
Pera (pera)
Phyllanthus (leaf flower)
Reverchonia (reverchonia)
Ricinus (castor)
Sapium (milk tree)
Savia (savia)
Sebastiania (Sebastian bush)
Stillingia (toothleaf)
Tetracoccus (shrubby spurge)
Tragia (noseburn)
Triadica (tallow tree)
Vernicia (vernicia)

conjunctivitis in combination with other traditional Chinese medicines.

Adverse effects

Taiwanese doctors have reported two cases of hepatocellular injury after oral administration of infusions of *B. officinalis* (2).

- One of the two patients had taken 1500 mg of the lower stem and root of *B. officinalis* boiled in water in a suicide attempt. She was admitted with vomiting and headache and later developed gastritis, hematuria, and liver damage. Symptomatic treatment resulted in full recovery.
- A 51-year-old woman consumed 20 pieces of the lower stem and root of *B. officinalis* to treat dermatitis. She developed nausea, vomiting, and dizziness, and had raised liver enzymes. Her liver function recovered 1 month after withdrawal of *B. officinalis*.

When *B. officinalis* was mistaken for a similar plant, *Securinega suffruticosa*, and was cooked in a soup used for muscle aches, lumbago, or as a tonic by 19 patients, 14 developed diarrhea, 10 had nausea and felt cold, nine had sensations of abdominal fullness, and seven vomited (3). Liver enzymes rose and the median times to median peak activities were 3 days for alanine transaminase, 2 days for aspartate transaminase, 5 days for alkaline phosphatase, and 12 days for gamma glutamyltranspeptidase. The liver damage was hepatocellular liver injury rather than cholestatic and marked jaundice did not develop.

Croton tiglium

The oil of *Croton tiglium* (croton) has a violent purgative action and contains tumor-promoting phorbol diesters and triesters.

Adverse effects

Croton oil has been used as a peeling agent in phenol as a carrier; its use in concentrations of 2% and over is almost always associated with depigmentation of the skin and delays in healing in areas other than the thick skin of the lower nose and around the mouth (4).

Croton is also the name given to *Codiaeum variegatum*, a highly decorative potted plant. Handling this plant over a period of 6 months produced contact eczema of the hands in a nursery gardener. Patch tests with croton leaves were positive (5).

Ricinus communis

Castor oil is the fixed oil obtained from the seeds of *Ricinus communis* (castor) by cold expression. The whole beans contain a variety of substances that are not expressed with the oil, including the toxin ricin (6,7).

Adverse effects

When taken by mouth, especially in large doses, castor oil can cause violent purgation with nausea, vomiting, colic, and a risk of miscarriage.

Transdermal exposure to ricin is not serious, since it is not well absorbed through the skin. Oral exposure, for example by ingestion of castor beans, can cause severe gastroenteritis, gastrointestinal hemorrhage, and death due to circulatory collapse. Parenteral injection of ricin is rapidly fatal, as is aerosol exposure; the lethal dose by these routes is 5–10 micrograms/kg (8).

Immunologic

Anaphylaxis has been attributed to consumption of whole castor beans (9).

- A 44-year-old woman chewed a castor bean seed and within minutes developed urticaria, drowsiness, Quincke's edema, and extreme hypotension. Her anaphylactic shock was treated with adrenaline, intravenous glucocorticoids, antihistamines, and intravenous fluids. She quickly recovered and a subsequent blood test demonstrated CAP-RAST to castor beans.

Fetotoxicity

In 498 women who had recently taken castor oil and possibly herbal substances called "sihlambezo" before artificial rupture of membranes, fetal passage of meconium was more common (10). However, in a study of 100 women castor oil had no effect on the rate of meconium-stained liquor (11).

References

1. Morikawa H, Kasai R, Otsuka H, Hirata E, Shinzato T, Aramoto M, Takeda Y. Terpenic and phenolic glycosides from leaves of *Breynia officinalis* HEMSL. Chem Pharm Bull (Tokyo) 2004;52(9):1086–90.
2. Lin TJ, Tsai MS, Chiou NM, Deng JF, Chiu NY. Hepatotoxicity caused by *Breynia officinalis*. Vet Hum Toxicol 2002;44(2):87–8.
3. Lin TJ, Su CC, Lan CK, Jiang DD, Tsai JL, Tsai MS. Acute poisonings with *Breynia officinalis*—an outbreak of hepatotoxicity. J Toxicol Clin Toxicol 2003;41(5):591–4.
4. Hetter GP. An examination of the phenol-croton oil peel: part IV. Face peel results with different concentrations of phenol and croton oil. Plast Reconstr Surg 2000; 105(3):1061–83.
5. Hausen BM, Schulz KH. Occupational contact dermatitis due to croton (*Codiaeum variegatum* (L.) *A. Juss* var. *pictum* (Lodd.) Muell. Arg.). Sensitization by plants of the Euphorbiaceae. Contact Dermatitis 1977;3(6):289–92.
6. Marks JD. Medical aspects of biologic toxins. Anesthesiol Clin North America 2004;22(3):509–32.
7. Doan LG. Ricin: mechanism of toxicity, clinical manifestations, and vaccine development. A review. J Toxicol Clin Toxicol 2004;42(2):201–8.
8. Bradberry SM, Dickers KJ, Rice P, Griffiths GD, Vale JA. Ricin poisoning. Toxicol Rev 2003;22(1):65–70.
9. Navarro-Rouimi R, Charpin D. Anaphylactic reaction to castor bean seeds. Allergy 1999;54(10):1117.
10. Mitri F, Hofmeyr GJ, van Gelderen CJ. Meconium during labour—self-medication and other associations. S Afr Med J 1987;71(7):431–3.
11. Kelly AJ, Kavanagh J, Thomas J. Castor oil, bath and/or enema for cervical priming and induction of labour. Cochrane Database Syst Rev 2001;(2):CD003099.

Everolimus

General Information

Everolimus is an immunosuppressive macrolide that also has synergistic actions with ciclosporin and interrupts the proliferative responses of vascular and bronchial smooth muscle cells. In a phase I trial, its safety profile and pharmacokinetics were assessed during a 4-week course of once-daily sequential ascending doses (0.75, 2.5, or 7.5 mg/day) in renal transplant recipients on a stable regimen of ciclosporin and prednisone (1). Pharmacokinetic data showed dose proportionality, a good correlation between trough and AUC concentrations, and moderate accumulation (2.5-fold). Absorption was within 2 hours, and the half-life was 16–19 hours. There was no evidence of a pharmacokinetic interaction of ciclosporin with everolimus. Virtually every patient in this study had at least one adverse event and 43% of patients treated with everolimus 7.5 mg/day had serious adverse events. In all everolimus groups there was an increased incidence of infectious episodes (*Herpes simplex*, upper respiratory infections, pharyngitis, pneumonia, and sinusitis). Similarly, adverse events involving the gastrointestinal system (diarrhea, nausea, and vomiting) were more common. Serum concentrations of triglycerides and total cholesterol increased significantly over time. Individuals treated with everolimus 7.5 mg/day had significant falls in white cell count (–2.6%) and platelet count (–51%); the nadir occurred on day 19 and the cell counts recovered spontaneously without withdrawal of the drug. Serum creatinine concentrations and blood pressure did not change.

Drug–Drug Interactions

Ciclosporin

Both everolimus and ciclosporin are extensively biotransformed by CYP3A and are substrates for P-glycoprotein. However, in a multicenter randomized double-blind study in 101 patients, 1 year after kidney transplantation, who were randomly assigned to receive everolimus 0.5, 1, and 2 mg bd plus ciclosporin and prednisone, the pharmacokinetics of ciclosporin were similar to published values in patients not taking everolimus (2).

References

1. Kahan BD, Wong RL, Carter C, Katz SH, Von Fellenberg J, Van Buren CT, Appel-Dingemanse S. A phase I study of a 4-week course of SDZ-RAD (RAD) quiescent cyclosporine–prednisone-treated renal transplant recipients. Transplantation 1999;68(8):1100–6.
2. Kovarik JM, Kahan BD, Kaplan B, Lorber M, Winkler M, Rouilly M, Gerbeau C, Cambon N, Boger R, Rordorf C; Everolimus Phase 2 Study Group. Longitudinal assessment of everolimus in de novo renal transplant recipients over the first post-transplant year: pharmacokinetics, exposure-response relationships, and influence on cyclosporine. Clin Pharmacol Ther 2001;69(1):48–56.

Eye-drops and ointments

General Information

Eye-drops and ointments are specialized pharmaceutical formulations intended to produce therapeutic concentrations of the active drug in ocular structures; a lower dose can be used than would be necessary to obtain the same effect by systemic administration. They can cause local adverse effects in the eye due either to the active ingredient or to excipients in the liquid or solid vehicle. The excipients included in modern ophthalmic medicines increase the viscosity of the drug, help to maintain it in solution or suspension, and are thought to stay longer on the exterior of the eye, leading to a longer contact time and possibly greater absorption of the drug than is the case with a simple aqueous solution (1).

Excipients

Methylcellulose is a vehicle used in eye-drops and contact lens solutions (SEDA-1, 369). It is non-irritant and has a good refractive index. A 1% solution is well retained in the conjunctival sac. Corneal cultures have been stimulated by methylcellulose, resulting in increased growth of cells (2); tear-film break-up time was increased four-fold with 2% methylcellulose. Hydroxypropyl methylcellulose is also used as artificial tears for people with dry eyes (3).

Petrolatum-mineral oil ointment is retained longer on the eye than other vehicles. The large molecules of the petrolatum-mineral oil-base ointment are not easily removed by blinking, and a component of the corneal tear film is a non-polar oil. Ointments are oil bases and non-polar, which is why they are readily absorbed by the pre-corneal and conjunctival tear films. To maintain drug contact with the eye, patching is recommended (1).

Polyvinyl alcohol, a synthetic long-chain alcohol, has been used as a component of various ophthalmic drug vehicles. For retaining clear vision and longer drug contact with the eye, polyvinyl alcohol is superior to saline. Polyvinyl alcohol has good drug compatibility and it acts as a wetting agent, lowering surface tension; at a concentration of 1.4% it does not interfere with corneal wound healing (1).

Systemic effects of ophthalmic medications

Of the drug that is administered in eye-drops, 80% diffuses into the general circulation and can have systemic effects, even when low concentrations are used (1). The lacrimal pump is the essential route of diffusion from eye-drops into the systemic circulation, through active cellular absorption in the lacrimal secretory pathways. The active ingredient avoids first-pass metabolism and reaches its site of action directly, resulting in increased systemic availability. All the same, this form of treatment is generally very well tolerated, when one bears in mind the immense volume of eye-drops prescribed by ophthalmologists each day.

The systemic effects exerted by eye-drops are most pronounced in the case of agonists and antagonists in the autonomic nervous system. For example, beta-blockers in eye-drops can cause bronchospasm, heart failure, syncope, and psychiatric disorders (4–6), especially at high doses and with non-selective beta-blockers, although these adverse reactions are usually related to failure to observe prescribing precautions (1).

Alpha$_2$-adrenoceptor agonist eye-drops can cause hypotension (7).

Except in patients at special risk (children under the age of 30 months and the elderly) parasympathomimetic eye-drops cause few systemic adverse effects (SEDA-16, 543).

Cholinesterase inhibitors, which have curare-like properties, are contraindicated for 6 weeks before general anesthesia.

In the very young and the very old patients atropine eye-drops carry a risk of cardiovascular collapse and neuropsychiatric disturbances (SEDA-16, 543).

Systemic problems can also develop with antimicrobial eye-drops (8) and contact lens products (9,10).

Local adverse effects

Ophthalmic drugs can cause problems of local tolerance, but with variable frequency. They can cause pain on instillation, allergic reactions, delayed healing, punctate keratitis, and disturbances of lacrimal secretion and accommodation. These local problems may be responsible for poor patient adherence to therapy.

Contact dermatitis

Allergic contact dermatitis is the most common dermatological condition that affects the eyelids. Allergic contact dermatitis was found in a retrospective study in 151 (74%) of 203 patients with persistent or recurrent eyelid dermatitis with or without dermatitis elsewhere (11): 46 had protein-contact dermatitis, but only 14 had protein-contact dermatitis without concurrent allergic contact dermatitis; 23 patients had atopic eczema, of whom 16 also had allergic contact dermatitis, protein-contact dermatitis, or both. Other conditions included seborrheic dermatitis, psoriasis, dry eyes, and dermatomyositis or overlapping connective tissue disease. Important sources of contact sensitivity were topical ocular medications, including glucocorticoids, cosmetics, metals, dust mites, animal dander, and artificial nails; only five cases were caused by nail lacquer.

Susceptibility factors

Elderly people are particularly likely to make errors in the administration of ophthalmic medications, resulting in overdosage and adverse toxic effects or underdosage with inadequately controlled glaucoma (12). This may reflect impaired memory, mental confusion, impaired vision, hearing, and mobility, or a combination of these factors. It is wise to assess both adherence to therapy and administration technique to ensure the safe and effective use of ophthalmic formulations in these patients (SEDA-21, 487) (13).

Use of eye-drops

A few simple rules can reduce the incidence of adverse effects of eye-drops and improve adherence to therapy:

- respect the contraindications and precautions applicable to the drug (1);
- start with the lowest possible dose, especially in children and elderly people (12);
- never administer more than 30 μl of an eye-drop at any time, and give it only into the superolateral corner of the eye (13);
- close the medial canthus with the finger after instillation of the eye-drop to minimize systemic absorption (14).

References

1. Hugues FC, Le Jeunne C. Systemic and local tolerability of ophthalmic drug formulations. An update. Drug Saf 1993;8(5):365–80.
2. Burstein NL. Corneal cytotoxicity of topically applied drugs, vehicles and preservatives. Surv Ophthalmol 1980; 25(1):15–30.
3. Toda I, Shinozaki N, Tsubota K. Hydroxypropyl methylcellulose for the treatment of severe dry eye associated with Sjogren's syndrome. Cornea 1996;15(2):120–8.
4. Fraunfelder FT, Meyer SM. Systemic adverse reactions to glaucoma medications. Int Ophthalmol Clin 1989; 29(3):143–6.
5. Masche UP. Systemische Nebenwirkungen von Augentropfen. Pharma-Kritik 1989;11:17.
6. Shore JH, Fraunfelder FT, Meyer SM. Psychiatric side effects from topical ocular timolol, a beta-adrenergic blocker. J Clin Psychopharmacol 1987;7(4):264–7.
7. Yuksel N, Karabas L, Altintas O, Yildirim Y, Caglar Y. A comparison of the short-term hypotensive effects and side effects of unilateral brimonidine and apraclonidine in patients with elevated intraocular pressure. Ophthalmologica 2002;216(1):45–9.
8. Flach AJ. Systemic toxicity. Associated with topical ophthalmic medications. J Fla Med Assoc 1994;81(4):256–260.
9. Morgan JF. Complications associated with contact lens solutions. Ophthalmology 1979;86(6):1107–19.
10. Mondino BJ, Salamon SM, Zaidman GW. Allergic and toxic reactions of soft contact lens wearers. Surv Ophthalmol 1982;26(6):337–44.
11. Guin JD. Eyelid dermatitis: experience in 203 cases. J Am Acad Dermatol 2002;47(5):755–65.
12. Anand KB, Beizer JL. Extraocular effects of ophthalmic drugs in the geriatric patient. Geriatr Med Today 1990;9:15–23.
13. Diamond JP. Systemic adverse effects of topical ophthalmic agents. Implications for older patients. Drugs Aging 1997;11(5):352–60.
14. Bailey CS, Buckley RJ. Nedocromil sodium in contact-lens-associated papillary conjunctivitis. Eye 1993;7(Pt 3 Suppl): 29–33.

Ezetimibe

General Information

Ezetimibe is a selective potent inhibitor of the intestinal absorption of dietary and biliary cholesterol. A total of 432 patients were included in a pooled analysis of two phase-II studies, both lasting for 12 weeks; ezetimibe was well tolerated, with an adverse events profile similar to that of placebo (1). In 668 patients who took ezetimibe with simvastatin, the adverse effects were similar to those with simvastatin alone (2).

References

1. Bays HE, Moore PB, Drehobl MA, Rosenblatt S, Toth PD, Dujovne CA, Knopp RH, Lipka LJ, Lebeaut AP, Yang B, Mellars LE, Cuffie-Jackson C, Veltri EP. Ezetimibe Study Group. Effectiveness and tolerability of ezetimibe in patients with primary hypercholesterolemia: pooled analysis of two phase II studies. Clin Ther 2001;23(8):1209–30.
2. Davidson MH, McGarry T, Bettis R, Melani L, Lipka LJ, LeBeaut AP, Suresh R, Sun S, Veltri EP. Ezetimibe coadministered with simvastatin in patients with primary hypercholesterolemia. J Am Coll Cardiol 2002;40(12): 2125–34.

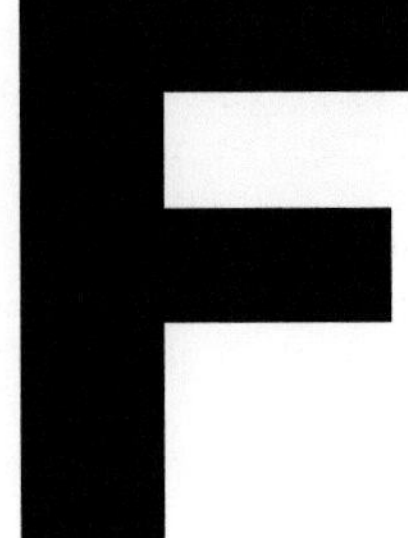

Fabaceae

See also Herbal medicines

General Information

The genera in the family of Fabaceae (Table 1) (formerly Leguminosae) include broom, liquorice, senna, tamarind, and a variety of pulses, such as fava beans, lentil, peas, and vetches.

Cassia species

The leaves and fruits of *Cassia angustifolia* and *Cassia senna* (senna) contain laxative anthranoid derivatives. Mutagenicity testing of sennosides has produced negative results in several bacterial and mammalian systems, except for a weak effect in *Salmonella typhimurium* strain TA102 (1,2). No evidence of reproductive toxicity of sennosides has been found in rats and rabbits (3).

Senna is widely used in fairly low doses without serious problems; it has also been used in a very high dosage form to clear the colon before radiological examination. In this form it is generally well tolerated, but it should not be used if there is any predisposition to colonic rupture.

Adverse effects

The safety and efficacy of senna have been reviewed (4). Its rhein-anthrone-induced laxative effects occur through two distinct mechanisms, an increase in intestinal fluid transport, which causes accumulation of fluid intraluminally, and an increase in intestinal motility. Senna can cause mild abdominal complaints, such as cramps or pain. Other adverse effects are discoloration of the urine and hemorrhoidal congestion. Prolonged use and overdose can result in diarrhea, extreme loss of electrolytes, especially potassium, damage to the surface epithelium, and impairment of bowel function by damage to autonomic nerves. Abuse of senna has also been associated with melanosis coli, but resolution occurs 8–11 months after withdrawal. Tolerance and genotoxicity do not seem to be problems associated with senna, especially when used periodically in therapeutic doses.

Liver

Abuse of senna can cause hepatitis (5,6).

Skin

Occupational allergic contact dermatitis has been attributed to a species of *Cassia* (7,8), as has contact urticaria (9).

Musculoskeletal

Finger clubbing (hypertrophic osteoarthropathy) has been reported in patients who have abused senna (10–15).

Lactation

When a standardized preparation containing senna pods (providing 15 mg of sennosides per day) was given to breastfeeding mothers, the suckling infants were only exposed to a non-laxative amount of rhein, which

Table 1 The genera of Fabaceae

Abrus (abrus)
Acacia (acacia)
Adenanthera (bead tree)
Aeschynomene (joint vetch)
Afzelia (mahogany)
Albizia (albizia)
Alhagi (alhagi)
Alysicarpus (moneywort)
Amorpha (false indigo)
Amphicarpaea (hog peanut)
Anadenanthera (anadenanthera)
Andira (andira)
Anthyllis (kidney vetch)
Apios (groundnut)
Arachis (peanut)
Aspalathus (aspalathus)
Astragalus (milk vetch)
Baphia (baphia)
Baptisia (wild indigo)
Barbieria (barbieria)
Bauhinia (bauhinia)
Bituminaria (bituminaria)
Brongniartia (green twig)
Brya (coccuswood)
Butea (butea)
Caesalpinia (nicker)
Cajanus (cajanus)
Calliandra (stick pea)
Calopogonium (calopogonium)
Canavalia (jackbean)
Caragana (peashrub)
Carmichaelia (carmichaelia)
Cassia (cassia)
Centrosema (butterfly pea)
Ceratonia (ceratonia)
Cercis (redbud)
Chamaecystis (chamaecystis)
Chamaecrista (sensitive pea)
Chapmannia (chapmannia)
Christia (island pea)
Cicer (cicer)
Cladrastis (yellowwood)
Clianthus (glory pea)
Clitoria (pigeon wings)
Codariocalyx. (tick trefoil)
Cojoba (cojoba)
Cologania (cologania)
Colutea (colutea)
Copaifera (copaifera)
Coronilla (crown vetch)
Coursetia (baby bonnets)
Crotalaria (rattlebox)
Crudia (bedstraw)
Cullen (scurf pea)
Cyamopsis (cyamopsis)
Cynometra (cynometra)
Cytisus (broom)
Dalbergia (Indian rosewood)
Dalea (prairie clover)
Daniellia (daniellia)
Delonix (delonix)
Derris (derris)
Desmanthus (bundle flower)
Desmodium (tick trefoil)
Dialium (dialium)

Continued

Table 1 Continued

Dichrostachys (dichrostachys)
Dioclea (dioclea)
Diphysa (diphysa)
Dipogon (dipogon)
Dipteryx (dipteryx)

Ebenopsis (Texas ebony)
Entada (callingcard vine)
Enterolobium (enterolobium)
Eriosema (sand pea)
Errazurizia (dunebroom)
Erythrina (erythrina)
Erythrophleum (sasswood)
Eysenhardtia (kidneywood)

Faidherbia (acacia)
Falcataria (peacock's plume)
Flemingia (flemingia)

Galactia (milk pea)
Galega (professor weed)
Genista (broom)
Genistidium (brush pea)
Gleditsia (locust)
Gliricidia (quickstick)
Glottidium (glottidium)
Glycine (soybean)
Glycyrrhiza (licorice)
Gymnocladus (coffee tree)

Haematoxylum (haematoxylum)
Halimodendron (halimodendron)
Havardia (havardia)
Hedysarum (sweet vetch)
Hippocrepis (hippocrepis)
Hoffmannseggia (rush pea)
Hoita (leather root)
Hymenaea (hymenaea)

Indigofera (indigo)
Inga (inga)
Inocarpus (chestnut)

Kanaloa (kanaloa)
Kummerowia (kummerowia)

Lablab (lablab)
Laburnum (golden chain tree)
Lathyrus (pea)
Lens (lentil)
Lespedeza (lespedeza)
Leucaena (lead tree)
Lonchocarpus (lance pod)
Lotononis (lotononis)
Lotus (trefoil)
Lupinus (lupin)
Lysiloma (falsetamarind)
Maackia (maackia)
Machaerium (machaerium)
Macroptilium (bush bean)
Macrotyloma (macrotyloma)
Marina (false prairie clover)
Medicago (alfalfa)
Melilotus (sweet clover)
Mimosa (sensitive plant)
Mucuna (mucuna)
Myrospermum (myrospermum)
Myroxylon (myroxylon)

Neonotonia (neonotonia)
Neorudolphia (neorudolphia)
Neptunia (puff)
Nissolia (yellowhood)

Olneya (olneya)
Onobrychis (sainfoin)
Ononis (restharrow)
Orbexilum (leather root)
Ormosia (ormosia)
Ornithopus (bird's foot)
Oxyrhynchus (oxyrhynchus)
Oxytropis (locoweed)

Pachyrhizus (pachyrhizus)
Paraserianthes (paraserianthes)
Parkinsonia (paloverde)
Parkia (parkia)
Parryella (parryella)
Pediomelum (Indian breadroot)
Peltophorum (peltophorum)
Pentaclethra (pentaclethra)
Pericopsis (peperomia)
Peteria (peteria)
Phaseolus (bean)
Physostigma (physostigma)
Pickeringia (chaparral pea)
Pictetia (pictetia)
Piscidia (piscidia)
Pisum (pea)
Pithecellobium (blackbead)
Poitea (wattapama)
Prosopis (mesquite)
Psophocarpus (psophocarpus)
Psoralidium (scurf pea)
Psorothamnus (dalea)
Pterocarpus (pterocarpus)
Pueraria (kudzu)

Retama (bridal broom)
Rhynchosia (snoutbean)
Robinia (locust)
Rupertia (rupertia)

Samanea (raintree)
Schizolobium (Brazilian firetree)
Schleinitzia (strand tangantangan)
Scorpiurus (scorpion's tail)
Senna (senna)
Serianthes (vaivai)
Sesbania (riverhemp)
Sophora (necklace pod)
Spartium (broom)
Sphaerophysa (sphaerophysa)
Sphenostylis (sphenostylis)
Sphinctospermum (sphinctospermum)
Stahlia (stahlia)
Strongylodon (strongylodon)
Strophostyles (fuzzy bean)
Stryphnodendron (stryphnodendron)
Stylosanthes (pencil flower)
Sutherlandia (sutherlandia)

Tamarindus (tamarind)
Taralea (taralea)
Tephrosia (hoarypea)
Teramnus (teramnus)
Tetragonolobus (tetragonolobus)
Thermopsis (golden banner)
Ticanto (gray nicker)
Trifolium (clover)
Trigonella (fenugreek)

Ulex (gorse)

Vicia (vetch)
Vigna (cowpea)
Virgilia (virgilia)
Wisteria (wisteria)
Zapoteca (white stick pea)
Zornia (zornia)

remained a factor of 10^{-3} below the maternal intake of this active metabolite (16).

Tumorigenicity
A well-defined purified senna extract was not carcinogenic, when administered orally to rats in daily doses up to 25 mg/kg for 2 years (17).

Drug interactions
An unusual Antabuse-type reaction reported on one occasion seems to have been due to an interaction of metronidazole with the alcohol present in the high-dosage form X-Prep (SEDA-15, 398).

Crotalaria species

Most of the members of the *Crotalaria* (rattlebox) species contain pyrrolizidine alkaloids, such as crotaline and monocrotaline, and therefore have hepatotoxic potential (18). These alkaloids are covered in a separate monograph.

Adverse effects
Pyrrolizidine alkaloids cause obstruction of the hepatic venous system and can lead to hepatic necrosis. Clinical manifestations include abdominal pain, ascites, hepatomegaly, and raised serum transaminases. The prognosis is often poor, death rates of 20–30% being reported. In an outbreak of veno-occlusive disease in the Sarguja district of India, probably caused by consumption of cereals mixed with *Crotalaria* seeds, 28 of 67 patients died (19).

It is prudent to avoid exposing unborn or suckling children to herbal remedies containing pyrrolizidine alkaloids. Animal studies have shown that transplacental passage and transfer to breast milk are possible, and there is a human case on record of fatal neonatal liver injury, in which the mother had used a herbal cough tea containing pyrrolizidine alkaloids throughout her pregnancy.

Cyamopsis tetragonoloba

Guar gum, which is covered in a separate monograph, comes from the endosperm of the seeds of *Cyamopsis tetragonoloba* (cluster bean). It has a small hypolipidemic effect (20) and a small blood glucose-lowering effect (21).

Adverse effects
Guar gum causes abdominal pain, flatulence, diarrhea, and cramps (22). It has been repeatedly associated with esophageal obstruction (23).

Guar gum can cause occupational rhinitis and asthma. Of 162 employees at a carpet-manufacturing plant, in which guar gum is used to adhere the dye to the fiber, 37 (23%) had a history suggestive of occupational asthma and 59 (36%) of occupational rhinitis (24). Eight (5%) had immediate skin reactivity to guar gum. Eleven (8.3%) had serum IgE antibodies to guar gum.

Guar gum reduces the speed but not the extent of absorption of digoxin (25), nitrofurantoin (26), and paracetamol (27). It reduces both the speed and extent of absorption of phenoxymethylpenicillin (25).

Cytisus scoparius

Cytisus scoparius (Scotch broom) contains the toxic alkaloid sparteine and related quinolizidine alkaloids, such as isosparteine and cytisine. Sparteine has been used as a marker of drug metabolism by CYP2D6 (28) and is covered in a separate monograph.

Adverse effects
Inexpert self-medication with a broom tea has resulted in fatal poisoning with clinical symptoms of ileus, heart failure, and circulatory weakness.

It is prudent to avoid broom formulations during pregnancy, not only because sparteine has abortifacient potential but also because of evidence that the plant produced malformed lambs in feeding trials.

Dipteryx species

The seeds of *Dipteryx odorata* (Dutch tonka bean) and *Dipteryx oppositofolia* (English tonka bean) are said to yield 1–3% of the non-anticoagulant coumarin, which is covered in a separate monograph.

Genista tinctoria

Genista tinctoria (dyer's broom) contains 0.3–0.8% of toxic quinolizidine alkaloids, such as anagyrin, cytisine, and *N*-methylcytisine. The last two constituents have peripheral effects similar to those of nicotine, whereas their central activity may be different. Anagyrine is a suspected animal teratogen and cytisine has teratogenic activity in rabbits.

Glycyrrhiza glabra

Glycyrrhiza glabra (licorice) (29) contains a wide variety of chalcones, coumarins, flavonoids, and triterpenoids, some of which mimic the mineralocorticoid actions of aldosterone. The saponin glycoside glycyrrhizinic acid (glycyrrhetinic acid, carbenoxolone) (30) and deglycyrrhizinized licorice (Caved-S) (31) have both been used to treat gastric ulceration, but have been displaced by better drugs.

Licorice is used widely and is found in a variety of sources (32):

Licorice sticks, bricks, cakes, toffee, pipes, bars, balls, tubes, Catherine wheels, pastilles, and Licorice Allsorts
Torpedos
Blackcurrant
Pomfret (Pontefract) cakes
Servez vous

Sorbits chewing gum
Stimorol chewing gum
Health products
Liquirizia naturale
Licorice-flavoured diet gum
Throat pearls
Licorice-flavored cough mixtures
Herbal cough mixtures
Antibron tablets
Licorice tea
All types of licorice root
Afghan, Chinese, Iranian, Russian, Turkish, and of unknown origin
Chewing tobacco
Alcoholic drinks
Belgian beers
Pastis brands
Anisettes (raki, ouzo, Pernod).

Adverse effects

Most individuals can consume 400 mg of glycyrrhizin daily without adverse effects, but some individuals develop adverse effects following regular daily intake of as little as 100 mg of glycyrrhizin (33).

Cardiovascular

In healthy volunteers who took licorice corresponding to glycyrrhizinic acid 75–540 mg/day for periods of 2–4 weeks, there was an average increase in systolic blood pressure of 3.1–14.4 mmHg (34). The increase in blood pressure was dose-related and the authors concluded that as little as 50 g/day of licorice for 2 weeks would have caused a significant rise in blood pressure.

Sensory systems

Five patients who had consumed large amounts (0.1–1 kg) of licorice subsequently had transient visual loss/aberrations (35). Glycyrrhizinic acid in licorice causes vasoconstriction in vascular smooth muscle and the authors therefore speculated that vasospasm of the retinal or occipital artery had caused the problems.

Electrolyte balance

The active ingredients of licorice inhibit the breakdown of mineralocorticoids by inhibiting 11-beta-hydroxysteroid dehydrogenase type 2, and its adverse effects relate mainly to mineralocorticoid excess, with sodium retention, potassium loss, and inhibition of the renin–angiotensin–aldosterone system (36).

In two cases prolonged intake of relatively small amounts of licorice resulted in hypertension, encephalopathy, and pseudohyperaldosteronism (37). Both patients were highly susceptible to the adverse effects of glycyrrhizinic acid because of 11-beta-hydroxysteroid dehydrogenase deficiency.

- A 44-year-old woman developed an irregular heart rhythm and repeated episodes of life-threatening torsade de pointes (38). Her serum potassium was 2.3 mmol/l. Treatment with an infusion of potassium and magnesium promptly restored normal rhythm. The cause of the problem was identified as the patient's habit of consuming large (but not more closely defined) quantities of licorice daily. One year after this episode she was still abstaining from licorice and showed no signs of cardiac disease.
- A 39-year-old woman had a potassium concentration of 2.9 mmol/l at a routine checkup (39). She denied taking any medications except a "cleansing tea" purchased from a health food company. The tea was analysed and found to contain significant amounts of licorice. Her potassium concentration normalized after withdrawal of the product and potassium supplementation.
- A 67-year-old Chinese man developed progressive muscular weakness (40). His medical history was unremarkable, but his urinary potassium excretion was high and he had hypokalemia and low plasma renin activity. He admitted taking a powdered Chinese herbal formulation for about 4 months, which was shown to contain large amounts of glycyrrhizinic acid (336 mg/day). He was treated with spironolactone, and 2 weeks later his potassium values had normalized.

Two patients who used licorice-flavored chewing gum developed severe hypokalemia (32).

- A 21-year-old woman who took licorice about 100 g/day developed a headache, hypertension (190/120 mmHg), and hypokalemia (2.6 mmol/l). She stopped eating licorice and instead used a chewing gum that also contained licorice (daily intake of glycyrrhizinic acid about 120 mg). Three weeks after she stopped using the gum her blood pressure was 110/80 mmHg and plasma potassium concentration 5.3 mmol/l.
- A 35-year-old woman developed pretibial edema and hypokalemia (2.2 mmol/1) after using a licorice-flavored chewing gum (about 50 mg of glycyrrhizinic acid per day). She stopped using the gum and improved within 2 weeks.

In six male volunteers who took glycyrrhizinic acid for 7 days, serum, urinary, and sweat electrolytes values were consistent with a mineralocorticoid-like effect (41). Plasma renin activity was suppressed, and plasma cortisol and aldosterone progressively fell during treatment. The authors proposed that glycyrrhizinic acid initially acts by increasing the effect of endogenous mineralocorticoids, and then when it or its metabolites accumulate it may also have a direct mineralocorticoid-like effect itself.

***Lupinus* species**

Lupinus (lupin) seeds are commonly taken as an appetizer in Southern Europe and the Middle East. Lupin flour has been used as a source of energy and protein (42,43). An extract of *Lupus termis* has been used to treat chronic eczema (44).

Adverse effects

Anticholinergic effects of lupin poisoning have been reported (45).

- A 72-year-old Portuguese woman presented to an emergency department with classic anticholinergic signs: sudden onset of nausea and vomiting, blurred vision, generalized weakness, and tachycardia (46). She had taken a herbal product containing lupin seeds in the belief that it would cure her recently diagnosed diabetes mellitus.

Analysis of the product identified the preponderant compound as oxosparteine, which has powerful anticholinergic effects.

Medicago species

Medicago sativa (alfalfa) sprouts are commonly used as a source of protein.

Adverse effects

Skin

Dermatitis has been recorded after the ingestion of infusions made from alfalfa seeds. Dermatitis has also been reported in horse handlers exposed to the straw itch mite, *Pyemotes tritici*, contaminating alfalfa seeds (47).

Immunologic

Prolonged ingestion of alfalfa seeds or alfalfa tablets has been associated with the induction or exacerbation of a lupus-like syndrome in humans, perhaps because of the canavanine alfalfa contains (48,49).

Infection risk

Alfalfa seeds are readily infected and there have been numerous reports of infections arising from the consumption of alfalfa sprouts grown from contaminated seeds. The most common infections are with *Salmonella* species, including *Salmonella enterica* (50), *Salmonella havana* (51), *Salmonella kottbus* (52,53), *Salmonella mbandaka* (54), *Salmonella muenchen* (55), *Salmonella paratyphi* (56), *Salmonella stanley* (57), and other serotypes (58,59). Occasionally, other organisms occur, such as *Listeria* (60) and *Escherichia coli* (61,62).

Melilotus officinalis

Melilotus officinalis (sweet clover) contains coumarin, 3,4-dihydrocoumarin (melilotine), ortho-coumaric acid, ortho-hydroxycoumaric acid, and the ortho-glucoside of ortho-coumaric acid (melilotoside). Withering of the plant leads to enzymatic glycoside hydrolysis and the resulting ortho-coumaric acid is spontaneously transformed to coumarin; the dried herb therefore smells strongly of coumarin (see separate monograph). *M. officinalis* has been used to treat lymphedema and the edema of chronic venous insufficiency.

Myroxylon species

Balsam of Peru is derived from species of *Myroxylon* such as *Myroxylon balsamum* and *Myroxylon pereirae* and has been used in medicinal and cosmetic ointments for centuries. It contains about 25 different substances, including triterpenoids, and can cause allergic reactions. Its sensitizing constituents have been determined (63).

Adverse effects

Balsam of Peru is a topical photosensitizer (SEDA-19, 162) and can cause contact urticaria (64,65). A systemic contact dermatitis has been reported after oral administration (66). In one case an allergic contact dermatitis in a patient sensitive to balsam of Peru caused a primary eruption on the face with secondary purpuric vasculitis-like eruptions on both legs (67).

In 60 patients with positive patch-test reactions to a fragrance mix or *M. pereirae* resin (balsam of Peru) there were positive immediate contact reactions to *M. pereirae* resin in 57% and to the fragrance mix in 12% (68). In a control group ($n = 50$) of eczematous, patch test-negative patients there were positive immediate reactions to *M. pereirae* resin in 58% and to the fragrance mix in 12%. The authors commented that the absence of a significant difference between the fragrance-allergic group and the control group was in keeping with a non-immunological basis for the immediate contact reactions.

Pithecollobium jiringa

Pithecollobium jiringa (jering fruit) is valued in Malaysia and Indonesia as a delicacy and for its antidiabetic properties.

Adverse effects

Acute renal insufficiency is a rare complication of the use of jering. In one case there was dysuria, hematuria, vomiting, abdominal pain, and blue urine (69). In two other cases there was bilateral loin pain, fever, nausea, vomiting, oliguria, hematuria, and passage of sandy particles in the urine (70). Blood urea and serum creatinine were markedly raised. With conservative therapy, which included rehydration with isotonic saline and alkalinization of the urine with sodium bicarbonate, the acute renal insufficiency resolved.

Sophora falvescens

Sophora falvescens (Ku shen) contains a variety of matrine alkaloids, such as aloperine, cytosine, lehmannine, matrine, oxymartine, oxysophocarpine, sophocarpine, sophoramine, and sophoridine, the flavonoid kushenol, and the saponin sophoraflavoside. Ku shen is a Chinese herbal remedy made from the root of *S. falvescens*. And Qing luo yin, a Chinese herbal remedy for rheumatoid arthritis, is a combination of extracts of *Dioscorea hypoglauca*, *Phellodendron amurense*, *Sinomenium acutum*, and *S. flavescens*.

Adverse effects

A herbal record lists the following adverse effects of Ku shen: salivation, abnormal gait, dyspnea, tachycardia (71). In larger doses, nervous system stimulation with muscle spasm and seizures can occur. There have been three reports of adverse reactions such as nausea, vomiting, dizziness, bradycardia, palpitation, ataxia, pallor, sweating, seizures, and dysphasia.

Trifolium pratense

Trifolium pratense (red clover) contains flavones (isorhamnetin, pratensein), phenolic coumarins, phytoestrogens, and demethylpterocarpin. It has been used to treat menopausal symptoms, without good evidence of efficacy (72).

Adverse effects

The coumarins in red clover may potentiate the effects of oral anticoagulants (73).

References

1. Mengs U. Toxic effects of sennosides in laboratory animals and in vitro. Pharmacology 1988;36(Suppl 1):180–7.
2. Sandnes D, Johansen T, Teien G, Ulsaker G. Mutagenicity of crude senna and senna glycosides in *Salmonella typhimurium*. Pharmacol Toxicol 1992;71(3 Pt 1):165–72.
3. Mengs U. Reproductive toxicological investigations with sennosides. Arzneimittelforschung 1986;36(9):1355–8.
4. Mascolo N, Capasso R, Capasso F. Senna. A safe and effective drug. Phytother Res 1998;12(Suppl 1):S143–5.
5. Beuers U, Spengler U, Pape GR. Hepatitis after chronic abuse of senna. Lancet 1991;337(8737):372–3.
6. Seybold U, Landauer N, Hillebrand S, Goebel FD. Senna-induced hepatitis in a poor metabolizer. Ann Intern Med 2004;141(8):650–1.
7. De Benito V, Alzaga R. Occupational allergic contact dermatitis from *Cassia* (Chinese cinnamon) as a flavouring agent in coffee. Contact Dermatitis 1999;40(3):165.
8. Rudzki E, Grzywa Z. Immediate reactions to balsam of Peru, cassia oil and ethyl vanillin. Contact Dermatitis 1976;2(6):360–1.
9. Rietschel RL. Contact urticaria from synthetic cassia oil and sorbic acid limited to the face. Contact Dermatitis 1978;4(6):347–9.
10. Silk DB, Gibson JA, Murray CR. Reversible finger clubbing in a case of purgative abuse. Gastroenterology 1975;68 (4 Pt 1):790–4.
11. Prior J, White I. Tetany and clubbing in patient who ingested large quantities of senna. Lancet 1978;2(8096):947.
12. Malmquist J, Ericsson B, Hulten-Nosslin MB, Jeppsson JO, Ljungberg O. Finger clubbing and aspartylglucosamine excretion in a laxative-abusing patient. Postgrad Med J 1980;56(662):862–4.
13. Levine D, Goode AW, Wingate DL. Purgative abuse associated with reversible cachexia, hypogammaglobulinaemia, and finger clubbing. Lancet 1981;1(8226):919–20.
14. Armstrong RD, Crisp AJ, Grahame R, Woolf DL. Hypertrophic osteoarthropathy and purgative abuse. BMJ (Clin Res Ed) 1981;282(6279):1836.
15. Fichter M, Chlond C. Hypertrophe Osteoarthropathie bei *Bulimia nervosa* mit chronischer Intoxikation mit Laxantien. [Hypertrophic osteoarthropathy in *Bulimia nervosa* with chronic poisoning by laxatives.] Nervenarzt 1988;59(4):244–7.
16. Faber P, Strenge-Hesse A. Relevance of rhein excretion into breast milk. Pharmacology 1988;36(Suppl 1):212–20.
17. Lyden-Sokolowski A, Nilsson A, Sjoberg P. Two-year carcinogenicity study with sennosides in the rat: emphasis on gastro-intestinal alterations. Pharmacology 1993; 47(Suppl 1):209–15.
18. Larrey D. Accidents hépatiques de la phytothérapie. [Liver involvement in the course of phytotherapy.] Presse Méd 1994;23(15):691–3.
19. Tandon BN, Tandon HD, Tandon RK, Narndranathan M, Joshi YK. An epidemic of veno-occlusive disease of liver in central India. Lancet 1976;2(7980):271–2.
20. Brown L, Rosner B, Willett WW, Sacks FM. Cholesterol-lowering effects of dietary fiber: a meta-analysis. Am J Clin Nutr 1999;69(1):30–42.
21. Fuessl HS, Williams G, Adrian TE, Bloom SR. Guar sprinkled on food: effect on glycaemic control, plasma lipids and gut hormones in non-insulin dependent diabetic patients. Diabet Med 1987;4(5):463–8.
22. Pittler MH, Ernst E. Guar gum for body weight reduction: meta-analysis of randomized trials. Am J Med 2001;110(9):724–30.
23. Lewis JH. Esophageal and small bowel obstruction from guar gum-containing "diet pills": analysis of 26 cases reported to the Food and Drug Administration. Am J Gastroenterol 1992;87(10):1424–8.
24. Malo JL, Cartier A, L'Archeveque J, Ghezzo H, Soucy F, Somers J, Dolovich J. Prevalence of occupational asthma and immunologic sensitization to guar gum among employees at a carpet-manufacturing plant. J Allergy Clin Immunol 1990;86(4 Pt 1):562–9.
25. Huupponen R, Seppala P, Iisalo E. Effect of guar gum, a fibre preparation, on digoxin and penicillin absorption in man. Eur J Clin Pharmacol 1984;26(2):279–81.
26. Soci MM, Parrott EL. Influence of viscosity on absorption from nitrofurantoin suspensions. J Pharm Sci 1980;69(4):403–6.
27. Holt S, Heading RC, Carter DC, Prescott LF, Tothill P. Effect of gel fibre on gastric emptying and absorption of glucose and paracetamol. Lancet 1979;1(8117):636–9.
28. Meyer UA, Skoda RC, Zanger UM. The genetic polymorphism of debrisoquine/sparteine metabolism—molecular mechanisms. Pharmacol Ther 1990;46(2):297–308.
29. Shibata S. A drug over the millennia: pharmacognosy, chemistry, and pharmacology of licorice. Yakugaku Zasshi 2000;120(10):849–62.
30. Bianchi Porro G, Petrillo M, Lazzaroni M, Mazzacca G, Sabbatini F, Piai G, Dobrilla G, De Pretis G, Daniotti S. Comparison of pirenzepine and carbenoxolone in the treatment of chronic gastric ulcer. A double-blind endoscopic trial. Hepatogastroenterology 1985;32(6):293–5.
31. Morgan AG, McAdam WA, Pacsoo C, Darnborough A. Comparison between cimetidine and Caved-S in the treatment of gastric ulceration, and subsequent maintenance therapy. Gut 1982;23(6):545–51.
32. de Klerk GJ, Nieuwenhuis MG, Beutler JJ. Hypokalaemia and hypertension associated with use of liquorice flavoured chewing gum. BMJ 1997;314(7082):731–2.
33. Stormer FC, Reistad R, Alexander J. Glycyrrhizic acid in liquorice—evaluation of health hazard. Food Chem Toxicol 1993;31(4):303–12.
34. Sigurjonsdottir HA, Franzson L, Manhem K, Ragnarsson J, Sigurdsson G, Wallerstedt S. Liquorice-induced rise in blood pressure: a linear dose-response relationship. J Hum Hypertens 2001;15(8):549–52.
35. Dobbins KR, Saul RF. Transient visual loss after licorice ingestion. J Neuroophthalmol 2000;20(1):38–41.
36. Olukoga A, Donaldson D. Liquorice and its health implications. J R Soc Health 2000;120(2):83–9.
37. Russo S, Mastropasqua M, Mosetti MA, Persegani C, Paggi A. Low doses of liquorice can induce hypertension encephalopathy. Am J Nephrol 2000;20(2):145–8.
38. Eriksson JW, Carlberg B, Hillorn V. Life-threatening ventricular tachycardia due to liquorice-induced hypokalaemia. J Intern Med 1999;245(3):307–10.
39. Feingold RM. Should we fear "health foods"? Arch Intern Med 1999;159(13):1502.
40. Lin SH, Chau T. A puzzling cause of hypokalaemia. Lancet 2002;360(9328):224.
41. Armanini D, Scali M, Zennaro MC, Karbowiak I, Wallace C, Lewicka S, Vecsei P, Mantero F. The pathogenesis of pseudohyperaldosteronism from carbenoxolone. J Endocrinol Invest 1989;12(5):337–41.
42. Gattas Zaror V, Barrera Acevedo G, Yanez Soto E, Uauy-Dagach Imbarack R. Evaluacion de la tolerancia y

aceptabilidad cronica de la harina de lupino (*Lupinus albus* var. multolupa) en la alimentacion de adultos jovenes. [Tolerance and chronic acceptability of lupine (*Lupinus albus* var. *multolupa*) flour for feeding of young adults.] Arch Latinoam Nutr 1990;40(4):490–502.

43. Gross R, Morales E, Gross U, von Baer E. Die Lupine, ein Beitrag zur Nahrungsversorgung in den Anden 3. Ernahrungsphysiologische Untersuchung mit dem Mehl der Susslupine (*Lupinus albus*). [Lupine, a contribution to the human food supply. 3. Nutritional physiological study with lupine (*Lupinus albus*) flour.] Z Ernahrungswiss 1976;15(4):391–5.
44. Antoun MD, Taha OM. Studies on Sudanese medicinal plants. II. Evaluation of an extract of *Lupinus termis* seeds in chronic eczema. J Nat Prod 1981;44(2):179–83.
45. Luque Marquez R, Gutierrez-Rave M, Infante Miranda F. Acute poisoning by lupine seed debittering water. Vet Hum Toxicol 1991;33(3):265–7.
46. Tsiodras S, Shin RK, Christian M, Shaw LM, Sass DA. Anticholinergic toxicity associated with lupine seeds as a home remedy for diabetes mellitus. Ann Emerg Med 1999;33(6):715–17.
47. Kunkle GA, Greiner EC. Dermatitis in horses and man caused by the straw itch mite. J Am Vet Med Assoc 1982;181(5):467–9.
48. Roberts JL, Hayashi JA. Exacerbation of SLE associated with alfalfa ingestion. N Engl J Med 1983;308(22):1361.
49. Alcocer-Varela J, Iglesias A, Llorente L, Alarcon-Segovia D. Effects of L-canavanine on T cells may explain the induction of systemic lupus erythematosus by alfalfa. Arthritis Rheum 1985;28(1):52–7.
50. Van Beneden CA, Keene WE, Strang RA, Werker DH, King AS, Mahon B, Hedberg K, Bell A, Kelly MT, Balan VK, Mac Kenzie WR, Fleming D. Multinational outbreak of *Salmonella enterica* serotype Newport infections due to contaminated alfalfa sprouts. JAMA 1999;281(2):158–62.
51. Backer HD, Mohle-Boetani JC, Werner SB, Abbott SL, Farrar J, Vugia DJ. High incidence of extra-intestinal infections in a *Salmonella havana* outbreak associated with alfalfa sprouts. Public Health Rep 2000;115(4):339–45.
52. Centers for Disease Control and Prevention (CDC). Outbreak of *Salmonella* serotype kottbus infections associated with eating alfalfa sprouts—Arizona, California, Colorado, and New Mexico, February–April 2001. MMWR Morb Mortal Wkly Rep 2002;51(1):7–9.
53. Winthrop KL, Palumbo MS, Farrar JA, Mohle-Boetani JC, Abbott S, Beatty ME, Inami G, Werner SB. Alfalfa sprouts and *Salmonella kottbus* infection: a multistate outbreak following inadequate seed disinfection with heat and chlorine. J Food Prot 2003;66(1):13–17.
54. Suslow TV, Wu J, Fett WF, Harris LJ. Detection and elimination of *Salmonella mbandaka* from naturally contaminated alfalfa seed by treatment with heat or calcium hypochlorite. J Food Prot 2002;65(3):452–8.
55. Proctor ME, Hamacher M, Tortorello ML, Archer JR, Davis JP. Multistate outbreak of *Salmonella* serovar muenchen infections associated with alfalfa sprouts grown from seeds pretreated with calcium hypochlorite. J Clin Microbiol 2001;39(10):3461–5.
56. Stratton J, Stefaniw L, Grimsrud K, Werker DH, Ellis A, Ashton E, Chui L, Blewett E, Ahmed R, Clark C, Rodgers F, Trottier L, Jensen B. Outbreak of *Salmonella paratyphi* B var *java* due to contaminated alfalfa sprouts in Alberta, British Columbia and Saskatchewan. Can Commun Dis Rep 2001;27(16):133–7.
57. Mahon BE, Ponka A, Hall WN, Komatsu K, Dietrich SE, Siitonen A, Cage G, Hayes PS, Lambert-Fair MA, Bean NH, Griffin PM, Slutsker L. An international outbreak of *Salmonella* infections caused by alfalfa sprouts grown from contaminated seeds. J Infect Dis 1997; 175(4):876–82.
58. Inami GB, Moler SE. Detection and isolation of *Salmonella* from naturally contaminated alfalfa seeds following an outbreak investigation. J Food Prot 1999;62(6):662–4.
59. Stewart DS, Reineke KF, Ulaszek JM, Tortorello ML. Growth of *Salmonella* during sprouting of alfalfa seeds associated with salmonellosis outbreaks. J Food Prot 2001;64(5):618–22.
60. Czajka J, Batt CA. Verification of causal relationships between *Listeria monocytogenes* isolates implicated in food-borne outbreaks of listeriosis by randomly amplified polymorphic DNA patterns. J Clin Microbiol 1994;32(5):1280–7.
61. Breuer T, Benkel DH, Shapiro RL, Hall WN, Winnett MM, Linn MJ, Neimann J, Barrett TJ, Dietrich S, Downes FP, Toney DM, Pearson JL, Rolka H, Slutsker L, Griffin PM; Investigation Team. A multistate outbreak of *Escherichia coli* O157:H7 infections linked to alfalfa sprouts grown from contaminated seeds. Emerg Infect Dis 2001;7(6):977–82.
62. Anonymous. From the Centers for Disease Control and Prevention. Outbreaks of *Escherichia coli* O157:H7 infection associated with eating alfalfa sprouts—Michigan and Virginia, June–July 1997. JAMA 1997;278(10):809–10.
63. Hausen BM, Simatupang T, Bruhn G, Evers P, Koenig WA. Identification of new allergenic constituents and proof of evidence for coniferyl benzoate in balsam of Peru. Am J Contact Dermatitis 1995;6:199–208.
64. Temesvari E, Soos G, Podanyi B, Kovacs I, Nemeth I. Contact urticaria provoked by balsam of Peru. Contact Dermatitis 1978;4(2):65–8.
65. Cancian M, Fortina AB, Peserico A. Contact urticaria syndrome from constituents of balsam of Peru and fragrance mix in a patient with chronic urticaria. Contact Dermatitis 1999;41(5):300.
66. Pfutzner W, Thomas P, Niedermeier A, Pfeiffer C, Sander C, Przybilla B. Systemic contact dermatitis elicited by oral intake of Balsam of Peru. Acta Derm Venereol 2003;83(4):294–5.
67. Bruynzeel DP, van den Hoogenband HM, Koedijk F. Purpuric vasculitis-like eruption in a patient sensitive to balsam of Peru. Contact Dermatitis 1984;11(4):207–9.
68. Tanaka S, Matsumoto Y, Dlova N, Ostlere LS, Goldsmith PC, Rycroft RJ, Basketter DA, White IR, Banerjee P, McFadden JP. Immediate contact reactions to fragrance mix constituents and *Myroxylon pereirae* resin. Contact Dermatitis 2004;51(1):20–1.
69. Yong M, Cheong I. Jering-induced acute renal failure with blue urine. Trop Doct 1995;25(1):31.
70. H'ng PK, Nayar SK, Lau WM, Segasothy M. Acute renal failure following jering ingestion. Singapore Med J 1991;32(2):148–9.
71. Drew AK, Bensoussan A, Whyte IM, Dawson AH, Zhu X, Myers SP. Chinese herbal medicine toxicology database: monograph on Radix Sophorae Flavescentis, "ku shen". J Toxicol Clin Toxicol 2002;40(2):173–6.
72. Baber RJ, Templeman C, Morton T, Kelly GE, West L. Randomized placebo-controlled trial of an isoflavone supplement and menopausal symptoms in women. Climacteric 1999;2(2):85–92.
73. Heck AM, DeWitt BA, Lukes AL. Potential interactions between alternative therapies and warfarin. Am J Health Syst Pharm 2000;57(13):1221–7.

Factor VII

See also Coagulation proteins

General Information

Factor VII is the most sensitive of the vitamin K-dependent clotting factors. The mode of action is tissue factor-dependent activation of factors Xa and IXa on the surfaces of activated platelets (1). Factor Xa leads to thrombin generation and hemostasis, by converting fibrinogen to fibrin. This process is limited to the site of injury, since exposure of tissue factor from the subendothelial matrix has a role in the action of recombinant factor VIIa, thereby reducing the risk of thromboembolic events (2).

Recombinant activated factor VII (factor VIIa) is indicated for patients with inhibitors of clotting factors VIII and IX (3–5). It has also been used to good effect preoperatively, in patients with severe thrombocytopenia, and in the treatment of life-threatening bleeding, including bleeding related to anticoagulant therapy or liver failure (3). The usefulness of recombinant factor VIIa for correcting the prothrombin time has been demonstrated in three neonates with liver failure undergoing liver biopsy and central venous catheter placement (6).

A disadvantage of recombinant factor VIIa is the need for frequent administration, because of its short half-life, about 2.7 hours with a clearance of 0.5 ml/kg/minute. The clearance is even faster in patients aged under 15 years. In one child the half-life was no more than 1 hour (7).

In general factor VII is well tolerated, with an incidence of non-serious adverse events of 3.6% (3). The most frequently reported adverse events are hypertension, skin reactions, fever, headache, epistaxis, reduced plasma fibrinogen, and prolonged prothrombin time (3,4).

Animal studies and case reports have suggested that recombinant factor VIIa should reduce the INR in patients taking oral anticoagulants and also has a hemostatic effect (8).

Organs and Systems

Cardiovascular

Thrombophlebitis at the infusion site is a common complication of continuous infusion of various clotting factor concentrates and has been noted after infusion of factor VIIa (9,10). Thrombophlebitis occurred in one of eight hemophiliacs with inhibitors who received continuous infusion of recombinant factor VIIa to allow elective surgery (11). In 25 hemophilia patients with inhibitors, who received recombinant factor VIIa for surgical procedures or spontaneous bleeding, there was one case of thrombophlebitis in 35 continuous infusion courses (12). In most instances, thrombophlebitis can be prevented by parallel infusion of saline or heparin.

- A 38-year-old patient with hemophilia A with factor VIII inhibitors was treated with recombinant factor VIIa for about 1 month and 18 days after the last infusion developed a distal deep venous thrombosis. An effect of the factor VIIa could not be ruled out, but long-term immobilization and severe infection could have contributed (13).

Angina pectoris and tachycardia have been reported after the use of recombinant factor VIIa (3). Among patients who had more than 2400 treatment episodes with recombinant factor VIIa, there were two cases of acute myocardial infarction (14). One of these patients had a history of cardiovascular disease and the other was very overweight and received massive transfusions, human factor VIII, activated prothrombin complex, and finally recombinant factor VIIa to treat severe intra-abdominal bleeding and shock.

Hematologic

Bleeding at sites other than the primary site (oozing at a central line insertion site, hemarthrosis, and epistaxis) has been reported during treatment with recombinant factor VIIa in four patients (7). The authors suggested that local fibrinolysis may have contributed to or actually caused bleeding from central line insertion sites. In three cases they found raised fibrin degradation products and in two cases a 15–35% fall in plasminogen activity.

No causality has been demonstrated between administration of recombinant factor VIIa and arterial thrombotic complications (15,16). However, venous thrombosis has been reported (17).

The risk of disseminated intravascular coagulation and other thrombotic events appears to be less with factor VII than with activated prothrombin complex products (1,18). However, disseminated intravascular coagulation after infusion of recombinant factor VIIa has been reported (19,20).

Urinary tract

In two patients with hemophilia with antibodies to both human and porcine factor VIII, continuous recombinant factor VIIa resulted in hematuria (21). In neither case was a cause of the hematuria found. The author suggested that mucosal bleeds, such as hematuria, are characterized by high fibrinolytic activity locally and may require higher peak concentrations of factor VII to generate sufficient thrombin to achieve and sustain hemostasis. The need for a full thrombin burst could relate to the role of thrombin in the activation of thrombin-activatable fibrinolysis inhibitor.

Immunologic

The development of antibodies against recombinant factor VIIa or hypersensitivity reactions to normal doses of recombinant factor VIIa have not so far been reported (7). No antibodies against recombinant factor VIIa were observed in a group of 222 hemophilia A and 16 hemophilia B patients with inhibitors treated with high doses of factor VIIa (14). However, antibodies to factor VII have been observed in a patient with factor VII deficiency who received 40 times the recommended dose of recombinant activated factor VIIa (3). Another case of low-titer and transient factor VII antibody formation has been reported in a patient with factor VII deficiency (10).

Drug Administration

Drug administration route

Continuous infusion of recombinant factor VII appears to offer advantages over bolus dosing, with a reduction in the total dose of recombinant factor VIIa by 50–75% (7,22).

Drug–Drug Interactions

Heparin

Small doses of heparin are used for the prophylaxis of infusion-related thrombophlebitis (23). Low molecular weight heparin is added to recombinant factor VIIa to prevent a 50% loss of activity of factor VII within 4 hours of storage (9). In one case, however, there was co-precipitation of reconstituted factor VIIa and low molecular weight heparin in syringes (24). The authors therefore suggested that a parallel saline infusion be used instead of heparin to prevent thrombophlebitis.

References

1. Shapiro AD. Recombinant factor VIIa: A viewpoint. BioDrugs 1999;12:78.
2. Veldman A, Fischer D, Voigt B, Beyer PA, Schlosser R, Allendorf A, Kreuz W. Life-threatening hemorrhage in neonates: management with recombinant activated factor VII. Intensive Care Med 2002;28(11):1635–7.
3. Roberts HR. Clinical experience with activated factor VII: focus on safety aspects. Blood Coagul Fibrinolysis 1998;9(Suppl 1):S115–18.
4. Key NS, Aledort LM, Beardsley D, Cooper HA, Davignon G, Ewenstein BM, Gilchrist GS, Gill JC, Glader B, Hoots WK, Kisker CT, Lusher JM, Rosenfield CG, Shapiro AD, Smith H, Taft E. Home treatment of mild to moderate bleeding episodes using recombinant factor VIIa (Novoseven) in haemophiliacs with inhibitors. Thromb Haemost 1998;80(6):912–18.
5. Hedner U, Kisiel W. Use of human factor VIIa in the treatment of two hemophilia A patients with high-titer inhibitors. J Clin Invest 1983;71(6):1836–41.
6. Young G, Nugent DJ. Prevention of bleeding complications in neonates with liver failure undergoing surgery using recombinant factor VIIa. Hematology 2001;6:341–6.
7. Shapiro AD. Recombinant factor VIIa in the treatment of bleeding in hemophilic children with inhibitors. Semin Thromb Hemost 2000;26(4):413–19.
8. Berntorp E. Recombinant FVIIa in the treatment of warfarin bleeding. Semin Thromb Hemost 2000;26(4):433–5.
9. Scharrer I. Recombinant factor VIIa for patients with inhibitors to factor VIII or IX or factor VII deficiency. Haemophilia 1999;5(4):253–9.
10. Barthels M. Clinical efficacy of prothrombin complex concentrates and recombinant factor VIIa in the treatment of bleeding episodes in patients with factor VII and IX inhibitors. Thromb Res 1999;95(4 Suppl 1):S31–8.
11. Smith MP, Ludlam CA, Collins PW, Hay CR, Wilde JT, Grigeri A, Melsen T, Savidge GF. Elective surgery on factor VIII inhibitor patients using continuous infusion of recombinant activated factor VII: plasma factor VII activity of 10 IU/ml is associated with an increased incidence of bleeding. Thromb Haemost 2001;86(4):949–53.
12. Santagostino E, Morfini M, Rocino A, Baudo F, Scaraggi FA, Gringeri A. Relationship between factor VII activity and clinical efficacy of recombinant factor VIIa given by continuous infusion to patients with factor VIII inhibitors. Thromb Haemost 2001;86(4):954–8.
13. Van der Planken MG, Schroyens W, Vertessen F, Michiels JJ, Berneman ZN. Distal deep venous thrombosis in a hemophilia A patient with inhibitor and severe infectious disease, 18 days after recombinant activated factor VII transfusion. Blood Coagul Fibrinolysis 2002;13(4):367–70.
14. Hedner U. Use of high dose factor VIIa in hemophilia patients. Adv Exp Med Biol 2001;489:75–88.
15. Ehrenforth S. Therapeutic potential of recombinant activated factor VII in intensive care medicine. J Anasth Intensivbehandl 2001;3:S110–12.
16. Kenet G. Recombinant FVIIa for profuse bleeding in trauma and surgery. J Anasth Intensivbehandl 2001;3:S112–13.
17. Ingerslev J. Efficacy and safety of recombinant factor VIIa in the prophylaxis of bleeding in various surgical procedures in hemophilic patients with factor VIII and factor IX inhibitors. Semin Thromb Hemost 2000; 26(4):425–32.
18. Santagostino E, Gringeri A, Mannucci PM. Home treatment with recombinant activated factor VII in patients with factor VIII inhibitors: the advantages of early intervention. Br J Haematol 1999;104(1):22–6.
19. Stein SF, Duncan A, Cutler D, et al. Disseminated intravascular coagulation (DIC) in a haemophiliac treated with recombinant Factor VIIa. Blood 1990;76:438a.
20. Penner JA. Management of haemophilia in patients with high-titre inhibitors: focus on the evolution of activated prothrombin complex concentrate AUTOPLEX T. Haemophilia 1999;5(Suppl 3):1–9.
21. Al-Trabolsi HA. Hematuria associated with continuous infusion of recombinant factor VIIa. Ann Saudi Med 2000;20:147–9.
22. Chuansumrit A, Isarangkura P, Angchaisuksiri P, Sriudomporn N, Tanpowpong K, Hathirat P, Jorgensen LN. Controlling acute bleeding episodes with recombinant factor VIIa in haemophiliacs with inhibitor: continuous infusion and bolus injection. Haemophilia 2000;6(2):61–5.
23. Rochat C, McFadyen ML, Schwyzer R, Gillham A, Cruickshank A. Continuous infusion of intermediate-purity factor VIII in haemophilia A patients undergoing elective surgery. Haemophilia 1999;5(3):181–6.
24. Lorenzo JI, Montoro JM, Aznar JA. Postoperative use of rFVIIa by continuous infusion in a haemophilic boy. Haemophilia 1999;5(2):135–8.

Factor VIII

See also Coagulation proteins

General Information

Lyophilized factor VIII has been used as substitution therapy in patients with hemophilia A. Most, but not all, recombinant factor VIII (recFVIII) is structurally and immunologically similar to plasma-derived factor VIII, and it has been well tolerated by patients in clinical trials. A major concern about recombinant factor VIII has been the occurrence inhibitors (1). However, there is evidence that there is no difference in the occurrence of inhibitors between recombinant factor VIII and plasma-derived factor VIII (2).

Highly purified animal coagulation factors, such as porcine factor VIII, continue to be used to good effect in patients with hemophilia with high-titer inhibitors. Adverse effects are relatively mild, consisting of fever and rare anaphylactoid reactions (3); platelet aggregation and progressive thrombocytopenia have also been observed (4).

Gene therapy

Trials of gene therapy in hemophilia A and B, to determine safety and efficacy, are under way (5). The hazards of current vectors include the development of inhibitors, as observed in substitution therapy, insertion mutagenesis (for example through disruption of a regulatory gene such as a tumor suppressor gene), and transmission of genes to germ cells (6). In the various phase I trials performed in patients with hemophilia such adverse events have not been observed (6). Other theoretical hazards are immunogenesis, hepatotoxicity, and carcinogenic effects. In particular, retroviral vectors have a considerable carcinogenic potential. Adenoviruses, which do not integrate into the genome and consequently have only a transient effect, are considered to be safer. Also adeno-associated viruses have a low pathogenic potential in humans, as do lentiviruses.

The death of a young patient who took part in a clinical gene therapy study, probably caused by an adverse reaction to the viral vector (7,8), has led to increased interest in the application of non-viral techniques for gene therapy. When factor VIII genes were introduced into autologous skin cells in culture by electroporation, and thereafter implanted in the omentum in six patients with hemophilia A, no adverse events were reported (9).

Organs and Systems

Cardiovascular

Thromboembolic complications developed in two of 81 patients with Von Willebrand disease treated with a high-purity factor VIII/Von Willebrand factor (VWF) concentrate (10). Four cases of venous thrombosis were reported in patients with Von Willebrand disease treated with an intermediate-purity factor VIII/VWF concentrate. Use of pure VWF concentrate without increased factor VIII:C is preferable (11).

Respiratory

In a retrospective study of 29 treatments with porcine factor VIII:C in 18 patients with hemophilia A with inhibitors, the initial bolus administration of porcine factor VIII:C before continuous infusion caused bronchospasm in one patient (12).

Nervous system

- A 71-year-old man with acquired hemophilia and high titers of antibodies to factor VIII developed a fatal thrombotic stroke while receiving porcine factor VIII (13).

Hematologic

Porcine factor VIII, used for the treatment of patients with inhibitors of factor VIII, can cause thrombocytopenia, which is dose-related and occurs during intensive treatment for severe bleeding or surgery (14,15).

During continuous infusion of porcine factor VIII:C in patients with hemophilia A with inhibitors there is a smaller fall in platelet count and fewer other adverse effects than during the period after the initial bolus administration, as was shown in a retrospective study of 29 treatments with porcine factor VIII:C of 18 patients with hemophilia A with inhibitors (13). The authors attributed these differences to the dose of factor VIII:C and the rate of administration.

Skin

Urticaria and periorbital edema after initial bolus administration of porcine factor VIII:C before continuous infusion have been observed in one of 18 patients with hemophilia with inhibitors receiving a total of 29 treatments with porcine factor VIII:C (13).

Immunologic

There has been some concern about the possible effects of factor VIII formulations on the immune system. In vitro experiments with coagulation factor concentrates have shown immunosuppressive effects (16,17), such as the impairment of Fc receptor-mediated phagocytosis and intracellular bacterial killing (18). Inhibition of IL-2 production, an impaired MLR, and impairment of PHA transformation have been demonstrated (19). A fall in the number of T4 lymphocytes has also been found. Whether these findings reflect functional impairment of the immune system is still unclear.

If the modulation of certain immune functions is in fact due to contaminating components in the preparations, one would expect the new generation of factor VIII preparations of very high purity to behave differently. Highly purified factor VIII with a specific activity of 100–150 U/mg protein is now available, as is factor VIII purified by immunoaffinity chromatography using mouse monoclonal antibodies.

In 58 previously treated patients with hemophilia treated with a recombinant factor VIII product for more than 5 years, there were neither allergic reactions to murine or hamster proteins nor any de novo formation of inhibitors of factor VIII (20).

Antibodies to factor VIII (factor VIII inhibitors)

Patients with bleeding disorders are at risk of developing antibodies against the coagulation protein that is absent, present in reduced amounts, or present in an inactive form in their blood. Such coagulation inhibitors make treatment very difficult. Gene deletions, truncations, and inversions of the factor VIII gene give rise to abnormal forms of the factor VIII protein, resulting in failure to induce tolerance against the normal form of factor VIII (21). Starting with factor VIII treatment at an early age is associated with an increased risk of developing inhibitors (22).

Frequency

Inhibitors of factor VIII are the most common and develop in 5–36% of patients with hemophilia A (23,24). Inhibitors of factor IX develop in 1–8% of patients with hemophilia B (24–26). Frequency varies with age (24). Patients with factor VIII inhibitors present clinically either as "high responders" who show a strong anamnestic response and a sharp rise in inhibitor concentrations after exposure to factor VIII, or "low responders", who show little or no anamnestic response (27).

Following the introduction of recombinant factor products, the incidence of antibody formation seemed to be higher than in patients using plasma products (28). However, after considering factors such as the number of exposure days, the severity of the disease, and the frequency of prospective monitoring, the prevalence and the incidence of antibody formation for both products were similar.

In two studies of previously untreated patients with severe hemophilia, who were given two different recombinant factor VIII products, the incidence of development of an inhibitor was comparable (about 30%) (29).

In 31 previously untreated and minimally treated children with severe hemophilia A, who received full-length recombinant factor VIII (formulated with sucrose) for home therapy and surgery, there was no difference in the incidence of inhibitor formation compared with other recombinant products or plasma-derived products (2).

Mechanism

Antibody formation in patients with mild and moderate hemophilia most likely results from the presence of structurally abnormal circulating factor VIII, so that administration of exogenous factor VIII leads to the development of antibodies by exposing the immune system to epitopes on factor VIII molecules not previously encountered (30). Data from the UK Haemophilia Centre Directors Organization have shown that 25% of patients who developed antibodies had mild or moderate hemophilia (30). It has been suggested that this high figure can be explained by improved data collection and by changes in clinical practice, namely the switch from lower purity to higher purity or recombinant products and the use of continuous infusion instead of repeated injections (30).

Novel molecular defects, Arg2163His and Phe2101Cys, were held responsible for inhibitor formation in two patients (31).

- Two patients (aged 60 and 73 years) with mild and moderate hemophilia respectively, without a family history of inhibitor formation, were exposed to factor VIII for more than 50 days. An inhibitor developed in both patients after an intermediate factor VIII product was replaced by a high-purity factor VIII product, which was given by continuous infusion during a surgical procedure.

Susceptibility factors

Six cases of factor VIII inhibitor development within the postoperative period have been described (32). Some patients have a greater tendency to develop inhibitors, such as patients with severe hemophilia who were sparingly treated, patients with moderate hemophilia and a family history of inhibitor development, patients who had transient inhibitors in the past, and patients with high-risk mutations in their factor VIII gene (32). It has been suggested that alteration of the immune system, by operative stress or the use of antibiotics, increases the risk of inhibitor development (32). Of 81 patients with Von Willebrand disease, who were treated with high-purity factor VIII/Von Willebrand factor concentrate, two had reduced in vivo recovery, suggesting antibody formation (10).

The formation of inhibitors of factor VIII is not restricted to patients with severe hemophilia. There have been two cases of high-titer factor VIII inhibitors in two children with mild hemophilia A; one occurred after only minimal exposure to factor VIII:C (33).

In 20 previously treated patients with severe or moderate hemophilia A treated with recombinant factor VIII formulated with sucrose, no inhibitors were found (34). The risk of forming inhibitors after treatment with B domain-deleted recombinant factor VIII was comparable to that seen with full-length recombinant products (35,36).

Management

Treatment options for patients with inhibitors are high dosages of clotting factor or recombinant factor VIIa for both hemophilia A and B or, in the case of hemophilia A, porcine factor VIII:C or activated prothrombin complex (37). Regular administration of intermediate or low-dose factor VIII concentrates leads to the rapid disappearance of factor VIII inhibitors in some high responders (27); this is thought to be due to the development of immune tolerance.

This may explain the effectiveness of treating patients with hemophilia who have inhibitors with high doses of factor VIII. Another approach involves the use of prothrombin complex concentrate to treat bleeding episodes in patients with factor VIII inhibitors (38); however, thromboembolic complications related to higher doses of prothrombin complex concentrate have been described, although these are relatively rare (39,40). Thrombotic events are extremely rare when highly purified factor IX is used. Activated prothrombin complex concentrate is also effective in patients with factor VIII inhibitors (41). Serious complications are rare, but disseminated intravascular coagulation has been reported (42).

If the inhibitor activity is under 10 Bethesda units/ml, patients can be treated with increased doses of factor VIII or IX concentrates (43). In addition, patients with hemophilia A with low or intermediate antibody titers can also be treated with porcine factor VIII (43). However, hemorrhagic episodes in patients with antibody activity over 10 Bethesda units/ml may result in life-threatening hemorrhage that cannot be treated by conventional therapy (26,43). Prevention or treatment of clinically significant bleeding episodes in these patients can be achieved by using so-called bypassing therapies, such as recombinant factor VIIa and activated prothrombin complex (23,26,43). Recombinant factor VIIa is both effective and safe in the treatment of inhibitors directed to either factor VIII or IX (44,45).

A less effective method of treating patients with inhibitors is to give them deamino-d-arginine vasopressin (DDAVP), which increases production of intrinsic factor VIII. This has a number of drawbacks, such as tachyphylaxis, flushing, headaches, myocardial ischemia, and fluid retention (46).

It has been recommended that non-hemophiliacs with autoantibodies be treated with porcine factor VIII products (14).

Inhibitor bypassing agents include prothrombin complex concentrates, activated prothrombin complex concentrates (such as FEIBA), porcine factor VIII, and recombinant factor VIIa. During 10 years usage of FEIBA (3.95×10^5 FEIBA units infused) a total of 16 thrombotic events were reported, corresponding to an incidence of 4.05 per 10^5

infusions. In 13 of these 16 events, known risk factors, such as FEIBA overdose, obesity, and serum lipid abnormalities, were present (47). Antibody reactivity against factor VIIa, which was detected in patients with hemophilia with high-titer antibodies, was a response to treatment with blood products or bypassing agents or due to cross-reactivity. This reactivity might hamper the hemostatic effect (48).

The production process of porcine factor VIII does not incorporate virus-eliminating steps. However, each batch is extensively screened to confirm the absence of viruses. In a pharmacovigilance study of 81 hemophiliacs treated with porcine factor VIII, there were no cases of transmission of porcine viruses (porcine parvovirus, encephalomyocarditis virus, porcine respiratory, and reproductive syndrome virus) (49).

Body temperature

Febrile reactions occurred in two patients after the initial bolus administration of porcine factor VIII:C in a retrospective study of 29 treatments with porcine factor VIII:C in 18 patients with hemophilia A with inhibitors (13).

Drug Administration

Drug formulations

Recombinant factor VIII is stabilized with human serum albumin during purification and in the final product. Although albumin has an excellent safety record and no recombinant antihemophilic factors have been associated with virus transmission, there is still concern about the safety of products that contain human- or animal-derived components (50). A second-generation recombinant factor VIII product has been developed with a modified manufacturing process and a formulation in which the recombinant factor VIII is stabilized by sucrose instead of albumin (50).

Drug contamination

Plasma-derived factor VIII concentrates have been implicated in the transmission of the non-enveloped hepatitis A and parvovirus B19 (28). The virus-inactivating procedures now in use (chemical inactivation, wet-heat treatment, and nanofiltration) should provide coagulation factors without risk of transmitting HIV and with a very high safety for hepatitis virus. Nevertheless, recombinant factor VIII is considered a safer alternative.

Patients with hemophilia have various disturbances of immune function, resulting not only from infections with HIV and hepatitis, but also from chronic exposure to extraneous proteins in clotting factor concentrates (51). Protein contaminants, such as immunoglobulins, fibrinogen, and fibronectin, can depress immune function. It has been postulated that high-purity concentrates in HIV-positive hemophiliacs are associated with better maintenance of $CD4^+$ cells and other indicators of immune function compared with products of intermediate purity (51).

One of 81 patients with Von Willebrand disease treated with a high-purity factor VIII/Von Willebrand factor concentrate was infected with parvovirus B19 after infusion of a solvent/detergent-treated formulation. Parvovirus B19 is not lipid-enveloped and is resistant to treatment by solvent detergent (10).

Parvovirus B19 transmission occurred in a child who had received vapor heat-treated prothrombin complex concentrate (60°C for 10 hours and 80°C for 1 hour) and in another child who received dry-heated factor VIII concentrate (80°C for 72 hours). Both children had severe hemophilia A and were treated for factor VIII inhibitors (52).

Second-generation recombinant factor VIII products, which contain lower amounts of human albumin, and third-generation products, which are free of human proteins and thereby carry a lower risk of pathogen transmission, are on the market.

Drug administration route

Hemophiliacs are traditionally treated with bolus injections of factor VIII. This kind of administration is associated with peak and trough concentrations of these factors, with a risk of bleeding when the concentration of factor VIII falls below a critical concentration (53).

Several studies of continuous infusions of factor VIIa, factor VIII, and factor IX in hemophiliacs undergoing surgery have shown that this mode of administration is safe and effective when steady plasma concentrations of the clotting factors can be achieved (53–56). The total dosage of clotting factor concentrates is reduced, and so continuous infusions are cost-effective (53,56).

References

1. Pipe SW. The promise and challenges of bioengineered recombinant clotting factors. J Thromb Haemost 2005; 3(8):1692–701.
2. Giangrande PL; KOGENATE Bayer Study Group. Safety and efficacy of KOGENATE Bayer in previously untreated patients (PUPs) and minimally treated patients (MTPs). Haemophilia 2002;8(Suppl 2):19–22.
3. Brettler DB, Forsberg AD, Levine PH, Aledort LM, Hilgartner MW, Kasper CK, Lusher JM, McMillan C, Roberts H. The use of porcine factor VIII concentrate (Hyate:C) in the treatment of patients with inhibitor antibodies to factor VIII. A multicenter US experience. Arch Intern Med 1989;149(6):1381–5.
4. Green D, Tuite GF Jr. Declining platelet counts platelet aggregation during porcine VIII:C infusions. Am J Med 1989;86(2):222–4.
5. Liras A. Gene therapy for haemophilia: the end of a "royal pathology" in the third millennium? Haemophilia 2001;7(5):441–5.
6. Manno CS. Gene therapy for bleeding disorders. Curr Opin Hematol 2002;9(6):511–15.
7. Dettweiler U, Simon P. Points to consider for ethics committees in human gene therapy trials. Bioethics 2001;15(5–6):491–500.
8. Rubanyi GM. The future of human gene therapy. Mol Aspects Med 2001;22(3):113–42.
9. Stephenson J. New therapies show promise for patients with leukemia, hemophilia, and heart disease. JAMA 2001;285(2):153–5.
10. Mannucci PM, Chediak J, Hanna W, Byrnes J, Ledford M, Ewenstein BM; Retzios AD, Kapelan BA, Schwartz RS, Kessler C; Alphanate Study Group. Treatment of von Willebrand disease with a high-purity factor VIII/von Willebrand factor concentrate: a prospective, multicenter study. Blood 2002;99(2):450–6.
11. Makris M, Colvin B, Gupta V, Shields ML, Smith MP. Venous thrombosis following the use of intermediate purity

FVIII concentrate to treat patients with von Willebrand's disease. Thromb Haemost 2002;88(3):387–8.
12. O'Gorman P, Dimichele DM, Kasper CK, Mannucci PM, Santagostini E, Hay CR. Continuous infusion of porcine factor VIII in patients with haemophilia A and high-responding inhibitors: stability and clinical experience. Haemophilia 2001;7(6):537–43.
13. Ashrani AA, Reding MT, Greeno EW, Shet A, Key NS. Thrombotic stroke associated with the use of porcine factor VIII in a patient with acquired haemophilia. Haemophilia 2002;8(1):56–8.
14. Penner JA. Management of haemophilia in patients with high-titre inhibitors: focus on the evolution of activated prothrombin complex concentrate AUTOPLEX T. Haemophilia 1999;5(Suppl 3):1–9.
15. Santagostino E, Gringeri A, Mannucci PM. Home treatment with recombinant activated factor VII in patients with factor VIII inhibitors: the advantages of early intervention. Br J Haematol 1999;104(1):22–6.
16. Aledort LM. Blood products and immune changes: impacts without HIV infection. Semin Hematol 1988;25(2 Suppl 1):14–19.
17. Carr R, Veitch SE, Edmond E, Peutherer JF, Prescott RJ, Steel CM, Ludlam CA. Abnormalities of circulating lymphocyte subsets in haemophiliacs in an AIDS-free population. Lancet 1984;1(8392):1431–4.
18. Mannhalter JW, Ahmad R, Leibl H, Gottlicher J, Wolf HM, Eibl MM. Comparable modulation of human monocyte functions by commercial factor VIII concentrates of varying purity. Blood 1988;71(6):1662–8.
19. Thorpe R, Dilger P, Dawson NJ, Barrowcliffe TW. Inhibition of interleukin-2 secretion by factor VIII concentrates: a possible cause of immunosuppression in haemophiliacs. Br J Haematol 1989;71(3):387–91.
20. Seremetis S, Lusher JM, Abildgaard CF, Kasper CK, Allred R, Hurst D. Human recombinant DNA-derived antihaemophilic factor (factor VIII) in the treatment of haemophilia A: conclusions of a 5-year study of home therapy. The KOGENATE Study Group. Haemophilia 1999;5(1):9–16.
21. Spiegel PC Jr, Stoddard BL. Optimization of factor VIII replacement therapy: can structural studies help in evading antibody inhibitors? Br J Haematol 2002;119(2):310–22.
22. van der Bom JG, Mauser-Bunschoten EP, Fischer K, van den Berg HM. Age at first treatment and immune tolerance to factor VIII in severe hemophilia. Thromb Haemost 2003;89(3):475–9.
23. DellaCroce FJ, Kountakis S, Aguilar EF 3rd. Manifestations of factor VIII inhibitor in the head and neck. Arch Otolaryngol Head Neck Surg 1999;125(11):1258–61.
24. Darby SC, Kerling DM, Spooner RJ, Wan Kan S, Giangrande PL, Collins PW, Hill FG, Hay CR. The incidence of factor VIII and factor IX inhibitors in the hemophilia population of the UK and their effect on subsequent mortality, 1977–99. J Thromb Haemost 2004;2(7):1047–54.
25. Hasegawa DK, Edson JR. Detection of factor VIII and IX inhibitors after first exposure to heat-treated concentrates. Lancet 1987;1(8530):449.
26. Pasi KJ, Hamon MD, Perry DJ, Hill FG. Factor VIII and IX inhibitors after exposure to heat-treated concentrates. Lancet 1987;1(8534):689.
27. Van Leeuwen EF, Mauser-Bunschoten EP, Van Dijken PJ, Kok AJ, Sjamsoedin-Visser EJ, Sixma JJ. Disappearance of factor VIII:C antibodies in patients with haemophilia A upon frequent administration of factor VIII in intermediate or low dose. Br J Haematol 1986;64(2):291–7.
28. Abshire TC, Brackmann HH, Scharrer I, Hoots K, Gazengel C, Powell JS, Gorina E, Kellermann E, Vosburgh E. Sucrose formulated recombinant human antihemophilic factor VIII is safe and efficacious for treatment of hemophilia A in home therapy—International Kogenate-FS Study Group. Thromb Haemost 2000;83(6):811–16.
29. Berntorp E. Other ongoing rFVIII PUP studies. Vox Sang 1999;77(Suppl 1):10–12.
30. White B, Cotter M, Byrne M, O'Shea E, Smith OP. High responding factor VIII inhibitors in mild haemophilia—is there a link with recent changes in clinical practice? Haemophilia 2000;6(2):113–15.
31. Yee TT, Lee CA. Is a change of factor VIII product a risk factor for the development of a factor VIII inhibitor? Thromb Haemost 1999;81(5):852.
32. Ghosh K, Jijina F, Shetty S, Madkaikar M, Mohanty D. First-time development of FVIII inhibitor in haemophilia patients during the postoperative period. Haemophilia 2002;8(6):776–80.
33. Puetz JJ, Bouhasin JD. High-titre factor VIII inhibitor in two children with mild haemophilia A. Haemophilia 2001;7(2):215–19.
34. Yoshioka A, Shima M, Fukutake K, Takamatsu J, Shirahata A; Coganate FS Study Group. Safety and efficacy of a new recombinant FVIII formulated with sucrose (rFVIII-FS) in patients with haemophilia A: a long-term, multicentre clinical study in Japan. Haemophilia 2001;7(3):242–9.
35. Courter SG, Bedrosian CL. Clinical evaluation of B-domain deleted recombinant factor VIII in previously treated patients. Semin Hematol 2001;38(2 Suppl 4):44–51.
36. Courter SG, Bedrosian CL. Clinical evaluation of B-domain deleted recombinant factor VIII in previously untreated patients. Semin Hematol 2001;38(2 Suppl 4):52–9.
37. Penner JA. Haemophilic patients with inhibitors to factor VIII or IX: variables affecting treatment response. Haemophilia 2001;7(1):103–8.
38. Chandra S, Brummelhuis HG. Prothrombin complex concentrates for clinical use. Vox Sang 1981;41(5–6):257–73.
39. Fuerth JH, Mahrer P. Myocardial infarction after factor IX therapy. JAMA 1981;245(14):1455–6.
40. Small M, Lowe GD, Douglas JT, Forbes CD, Prentice CR, Factor IX thrombogenicity: in vivo effects on coagulation activation and a case report of disseminated intravascular coagulation. Thromb Haemost 1982;48(1):76–7.
41. Abildgaard CF, Penner JA, Watson-Williams EJ. Anti-inhibitor Coagulant Complex (Autoplex) for treatment of factor VIII inhibitors in hemophilia. Blood 1980;56(6):978–84.
42. Rodeghiero F, Castronovo S, Dini E. Disseminated intravascular coagulation after infusion of FEIBA (factor VIII inhibitor bypassing activity) in a patient with acquired haemophilia. Thromb Haemost 1982;48(3):339–40.
43. Ingerslev J. Efficacy and safety of recombinant factor VIIa in the prophylaxis of bleeding in various surgical procedures in hemophilic patients with factor VIII and factor IX inhibitors. Semin Thromb Hemost 2000;26(4):425–32.
44. Roberts HR. The use of agents that by-pass factor VIII inhibitors in patients with haemophilia. Vox Sang 1999;77(Suppl 1):38–41.
45. Shapiro AD. Recombinant factor VIIa: a viewpoint. BioDrugs 1999;12:78.
46. Mannucci PM, Lusher JM. Desmopressin and thrombosis. Lancet 1989;2(8664):675–6.
47. Ehrlich HJ, Henzl MJ, Gomperts ED. Safety of factor VIII inhibitor bypass activity (FEIBA): 10-year compilation of thrombotic adverse events. Haemophilia 2002;8(2):83–90.
48. Astermark J, Ekman M, Berntorp E. Antibodies to factor VIIa in patients with haemophilia and high-responding inhibitors. Br J Haematol 2002;119(2):342–7.
49. Giangrande PL, Kessler CM, Jenkins CE, Weatherill PJ, Webb PD. Viral pharmacovigilance study of haemophiliacs receiving porcine factor VIII. Haemophilia 2002;8(6):798–801.

50. Scharrer I, Brackmann HH, Sultan Y, Abshire T, Gazengel C, Ragni M, Gorina E, Vosburgh E, Kellermann E. Efficacy of a sucrose-formulated recombinant factor VIII used for 22 surgical procedures in patients with severe haemophilia A. Haemophilia 2000;6(6):614–18.
51. Hoots K, Canty D. Clotting factor concentrates and immune function in haemophilic patients. Haemophilia 1998; 4(5):704–13.
52. Blumel J, Schmidt I, Effenberger W, Seitz H, Willkommen H, Brackmann HH, Lower J, Eis-Hubinger AM. Parvovirus B19 transmission by heat-treated clotting factor concentrates. Transfusion 2002;42(11):1473–81.
53. Tagariello G, Davoli PG, Gajo GB, De Biasi E, Risato R, Baggio R, Traldi A. Safety and efficacy of high-purity concentrates in haemophiliac patients undergoing surgery by continuous infusion. Haemophilia 1999;5(6):426–30.
54. Lorenzo JI, Montoro JM, Aznar JA. Postoperative use of rFVIIa by continuous infusion in a haemophilic boy. Haemophilia 1999;5(2):135–8.
55. Rochat C, McFadyen ML, Schwyzer R, Gillham A, Cruickshank A. Continuous infusion of intermediate-purity factor VIII in haemophilia A patients undergoing elective surgery. Haemophilia 1999;5(3):181–6.
56. Schulman S, Wallensten R, White B, Smith OP. Efficacy of a high purity, chemically treated and nanofiltered factor IX concentrate for continuous infusion in haemophilia patients undergoing surgery. Haemophilia 1999; 5(2):96–100.

Factor IX

See also Coagulation proteins

General Information

Factor IX is used as substitution therapy in patients with hemophilia B. Although the half-lives of recombinant and plasma factor IX products are comparable, the in vivo recovery of recombinant factor IX is 28% lower than a highly purified plasma-derived product. To treat hemorrhage the dosage of recombinant factor IX needs to be 20% higher than plasma-derived products to increase the circulating factor IX activity to 1% per IU of recombinant factor IX given (1).

General adverse effects

Mild adverse effects of factor IX include discomfort at the infusion site, fever, dizziness, allergic rhinitis, and lightheadedness (1).

Gene therapy

Trials of gene therapy in hemophilia A and B, to determine safety and efficacy, are under way (2). Three patients with hemophilia B were treated in a phase I trial with a recombinant adenovirus-associated vector expressing human blood-coagulation factor IX (3). There was no evidence of formation of inhibitory antibodies against factor IX. In a phase I trial with a recombinant adenovirus-associated vector expressing human blood-coagulation factor IX, there was no evidence of germ-line transmission of vector sequences (3).

The hazards of current vectors include insertion mutagenesis, immunogenesis, hepatotoxicity, and carcinogenic effects. In particular, retroviral vectors have a considerable carcinogenic potential. Adenoviruses, which do not integrate into the genome and consequently have only a transient effect, are considered to be safer. Also adeno-associated viruses have a low pathogenic potential in humans, as do lentiviruses.

Organs and Systems

Cardiovascular

Thrombophlebitis at the infusion site is a common complication of continuous infusion of various clotting factor concentrates. Continuous infusion of recombinant factor IX in six patients with hemophilia B undergoing surgery or suffering bleeding was complicated in two cases by thrombophlebitis (4). In most instances, thrombophlebitis can be prevented by parallel infusion of saline or heparin.

Respiratory

Shortness of breath was observed in a young patient with hemophilia B with inhibitors after a number of attempts to induce immune tolerance with a high dose of factor IX:C (5).

Urinary tract

During treatment with extremely high doses of factor IX concentrate, to induce immune tolerance, nephrotic syndrome has been described (6,7). Withdrawal or dosage reduction is of crucial importance for the resolution of nephrosis (6). Renal biopsy in one of these patients showed peripheral capillary wall thickening and deposits throughout the basement membrane (7). In addition minimal interstitial fibrosis and tubular atrophy were present. There were no deposits of factor IX in the glomeruli, which the authors attributed to absence of free factor IX epitope in the tissue (7).

In patients with hemophilia B with antibodies who undergo immune tolerance induction there is a risk of nephrotic syndrome (8).

Skin

A young patient with hemophilia B with inhibitors developed an urticarial rash after several attempts to induce immune tolerance with a high dose of factor IX:C (5). Recombinant factor IX gave rise to urticaria in patients with hemophilia B undergoing surgery (9).

Immunologic

Allergic and anaphylactic reactions due to factor IX inhibitor have been described (SEDA-21, 343) (6). Anaphylactic reactions occur particularly in patients with undetectable concentrations of factor IX, because of major disruptions in the factor IX gene (10). In patients with factor IX inhibitor, IgG1 subclass antibodies have been found, which may activate complement, resulting in allergic reactions (SEDA-21, 343) (10). However, it has also been suggested that allergic reactions to factor IX products are IgE-mediated.

- In two patients with severe factor IX deficiency and high concentrations of factor IX inhibitors who developed anaphylaxis to factor IX, RAST and skin test reactions to factor IX were positive (10). After desensitization, the circulating IgE antibodies to factor IX fell.

Treatment with high dosages of clotting factors to induce immune tolerance brings a risk of allergic reactions, as has been observed in a 4-year-old child with hemophilia B (5).

Antibodies to factor IX (factor IX inhibitors)
Patients with bleeding disorders are at risk of developing antibodies against the coagulation protein that is absent, present in reduced amounts, or present in an inactive form in their blood. Such coagulation inhibitors make treatment very difficult.

Inhibitors of factor VIII are the most common and develop in 5–15% of patients with hemophilia A. Inhibitors of factor IX develop in 1–4% of patients with hemophilia B (11,12). Patients with hemophilia B with complete gene deletions or derangement of the factor IX gene are particularly at risk of developing antibodies after the administration of factor IX concentrate (8). In patients with hemophilia B with antibodies, treatment with factor IX concentrate can result in an anaphylactic response.

Anaphylaxis in conjunction with inhibitor development has been described. Patients with hemophilia B with complete gene deletions have the greatest risk of anaphylaxis, with a minimum risk of 26%, whereas the risk in patients with null mutations was 2.4% and nearly zero for mis-sense mutations (13). Predisposing factors for the development of anaphylaxis, besides mutation type, are genetic predisposition and environmental experience, such as the type and frequency of factor IX product (13).

Drug Administration

Drug administration route

Hemophiliacs are traditionally treated with bolus injections of factor IX, which is associated with peak and trough concentrations of these factors, with a risk of bleeding when the concentration of factor IX falls below a critical concentration (14).

Several studies of continuous infusions of factor VIIa, factor VIII, and factor IX in hemophiliacs undergoing surgery have shown that this mode of administration is safe and effective when steady plasma concentrations of the clotting factors can be achieved (14–17). The total dosage of clotting factor concentrates is reduced, and so continuous infusions are cost effective (14,17).

References

1. White G, Shapiro A, Ragni M, Garzone P, Goodfellow J, Tubridy K, Courter S. Clinical evaluation of recombinant factor IX. Semin Hematol 1998;35(2 Suppl 2):33–8.
2. Liras A. Gene therapy for haemophilia: the end of a 'royal pathology' in the third millennium? Haemophilia 2001;7(5):441–5.
3. Fabb SA, Dickson JG. Technology evaluation: AAV factor IX gene therapy, Avigen Inc. Curr Opin Mol Ther 2000;2(5):601–6.
4. Chowdary P, Dasani H, Jones JA, Loran CM, Eldridge A, Hughes S, Collins PW. Recombinant factor IX (BeneFix) by adjusted continuous infusion: a study of stability, sterility and clinical experience. Haemophilia 2001;7(2):140–5.
5. Barnes C, Brewin T, Ekert H. Induction of immune tolerance and suppression of anaphylaxis in a child with haemophilia B by simple plasmapheresis and antigen exposure: progress report. Haemophilia 2001;7(4):439–40.
6. Tengborn L, Hansson S, Fasth A, Lubeck PO, Berg A, Ljung R. Anaphylactoid reactions and nephrotic syndrome—a considerable risk during factor IX treatment in patients with haemophilia B and inhibitors: a report on the outcome in two brothers. Haemophilia 1998;4(6):854–9.
7. Dharnidharka VR, Takemoto C, Ewenstein BM, Rosen S, Harris HW. Membranous glomerulonephritis and nephrosis post factor IX infusions in hemophilia B. Pediatr Nephrol 1998;12(8):654–7.
8. Shapiro AD. Recombinant factor VIIa in the treatment of bleeding in hemophilic children with inhibitors. Semin Thromb Hemost 2000;26(4):413–19.
9. Ragni MV, Pasi KJ, White GC, Giangrande PL, Courter SG, Tubridy KL; Recombinant FIX Surgical Study Group. Use of recombinant factor IX in subjects with haemophilia B undergoing surgery. Haemophilia 2002;8(2):91–7.
10. Dioun AF, Ewenstein BM, Geha RS, Schneider LC. IgE-mediated allergy and desensitization to factor IX in hemophilia B. J Allergy Clin Immunol 1998;102(1):113–17.
11. Hasegawa DK, Edson JR. Detection of factor VIII and IX inhibitors after first exposure to heat-treated concentrates. Lancet 1987;1(8530):449.
12. Pasi KJ, Hamon MD, Perry DJ, Hill FG. Factor VIII and IX inhibitors after exposure to heat-treated concentrates. Lancet 1987;1(8534):689.
13. Thorland EC, Drost JB, Lusher JM, Warrier I, Shapiro A, Koerper MA, Dimichele D, Westman J, Key NS, Sommer SS. Anaphylactic response to factor IX replacement therapy in haemophilia B patients: complete gene deletions confer the highest risk. Haemophilia 1999;5(2):101–5.
14. Tagariello G, Davoli PG, Gajo GB, De Biasi E, Risato R, Baggio R, Traldi A. Safety and efficacy of high-purity concentrates in haemophiliac patients undergoing surgery by continuous infusion. Haemophilia 1999;5(6):426–30.
15. Lorenzo JI, Montoro JM, Aznar JA. Postoperative use of rFVIIa by continuous infusion in a haemophilic boy. Haemophilia 1999;5(2):135–8.
16. Rochat C, McFadyen ML, Schwyzer R, Gillham A, Cruickshank A. Continuous infusion of intermediate-purity factor VIII in haemophilia A patients undergoing elective surgery. Haemophilia 1999;5(3):181–6.
17. Schulman S, Wallensten R, White B, Smith OP. Efficacy of a high purity, chemically treated and nanofiltered factor IX concentrate for continuous infusion in haemophilia patients undergoing surgery. Haemophilia 1999; 5(2):96–100.

Famciclovir

General Information

Famciclovir is an oral prodrug of penciclovir, a selective antiviral drug with activity against *Varicella zoster* virus, *Herpes simplex* virus types 1 and 2, and Epstein–Barr virus, as well as human hepatitis B virus.

After oral administration, famciclovir is well absorbed (systemic availability 77%), with little intersubject variability, and is rapidly converted to penciclovir. This compares favorably with aciclovir, the absorption of which is slow and incomplete, with a highly variable systemic availability of only 10–20%.

Comparative studies

In a study of oral famciclovir versus oral aciclovir, designed to demonstrate equivalence of efficacy of the two drugs in the treatment of mucocutaneous *Herpes simplex* infection in HIV-infected individuals, there was no difference in the incidence or nature of adverse effects in the two groups (1). None of the withdrawals from the trial was considered by the investigator to be related to the study medication.

Placebo-controlled studies

In an integrated safety analysis of 1607 patients who had taken famciclovir for the treatment of *Herpes zoster* or genital herpes, famciclovir was extremely well tolerated with an adverse effect profile similar to placebo (2). Headache, nausea, and diarrhea were the most frequently reported adverse events in those taking both famciclovir and placebo.

In an experimental study of *Herpes simplex* labialis, adverse events (diarrhea and nausea) occurred with similar frequency with famciclovir and placebo (3). No laboratory abnormalities were consistently associated with famciclovir.

In a randomized, placebo-controlled study in 455 patients oral famciclovir (125 or 250 mg tds or 250 mg bd) used to suppress recurrent genital *Herpes simplex* infections, the toxicity profile of famciclovir was comparable to placebo (4). The only serious adverse effects reported as being possibly related to famciclovir were raised bilirubin concentration and lipase activity in one patient after 10 months of treatment with famciclovir 125 mg tds. However, these laboratory abnormalities resolved on therapy after 7 days and did not recur during the rest of the study.

Organs and Systems

Gastrointestinal

Adverse effects associated with famciclovir have been collected in over 6000 patients in two postmarketing surveillance studies (5). Only headache, abdominal symptoms, dizziness, vomiting, and diarrhea were associated with the drug. Two prospective trials have confirmed the low frequency of adverse effects, the more common ones being nausea, headache, vomiting, and diarrhea (6,7).

Sexual function

Prolonged administration of high dosages of famciclovir has been associated with reversible dose-dependent adverse effects on testicular function in rats and dogs. However, in a double-blind, placebo-controlled trial in which 34 men with recurrent genital herpes took famciclovir 250 mg bd for 18 weeks, there were no significant effects on sperm production or function (8).

References

1. Romanowski B, Aoki FY, Martel AY, Lavender EA, Parsons JE, Saltzman RL. Efficacy and safety of famciclovir for treating mucocutaneous *Herpes simplex* infection in HIV-infected individuals. Collaborative Famciclovir HIV Study Group. AIDS 2000;14(9):1211–17.
2. Saltzman R, Jurewicz R, Boon R. Safety of famciclovir in patients with *Herpes zoster* and genital herpes. Antimicrob Agents Chemother 1994;38(10):2454–7.
3. Spruance SL, Rowe NH, Raborn GW, Thibodeau EA, D'Ambrosio JA, Bernstein DI. Peroral famciclovir in the treatment of experimental ultraviolet radiation-induced *Herpes simplex* labialis: a double-blind, dose-ranging, placebo-controlled, multicenter trial. J Infect Dis 1999;179(2):303–10.
4. Diaz-Mitoma F, Sibbald RG, Shafran SD, Boon R, Saltzman RL. Oral famciclovir for the suppression of recurrent genital herpes: a randomized controlled trial. Collaborative Famciclovir Genital Herpes Research Group. JAMA 1998;280(10):887–92.
5. Engst R, Schiewe U, Hobel W, Machka K, Meister W. Famciclovir in treatment of acute *Herpes zoster*: results of two post-marketing surveillance studies in Germany. Acta Derm Venereol 2001;81(1):59–60.
6. Tyring S, Engst R, Corriveau C, Robillard N, Trottier S, Van Slycken S, Crann RA, Locke LA, Saltzman R, Palestine AG; Collaborative Famciclovir Ophthalmic Zoster Research Group. Famciclovir for ophthalmic zoster: a randomised aciclovir controlled study. Br J Ophthalmol 2001;85(5):576–81.
7. Manns MP, Neuhaus P, Atkinson GF, Griffin KE, Barnass S, Vollmar J, Yeang Y, Young CL; Famciclovir Liver Transplant Study Group. Famciclovir treatment of hepatitis B infection following liver transplantation: a long-term, multi-centre study. Transpl Infect Dis 2001;3(1):16–23.
8. Perry CM, Wagstaff AJ. Famciclovir. A review of its pharmacological properties and therapeutic efficacy in herpesvirus infections. Drugs 1995;50(2):396–415.

Famotidine

See also Histamine H_2 receptor antagonists

General Information

Famotidine is a histamine H_2 receptor antagonist. It does not affect drug metabolism and it has been claimed to be free of the antiandrogenic effect of cimetidine; however in one woman who accidentally took double doses of the drug for some months it did cause hyperprolactinemia and breast engorgement (SEDA-18, 372). In other ways it bears a very close resemblance to cimetidine; for example, headache and confusion with intravenous use are reported, as are thrombocytopenia and pancytopenia (SEDA-15, 395).

The effects of famotidine 20 mg bd and omeprazole 20 mg/day for 8 weeks have been compared in the treatment of reflux esophagitis in a randomized trial in 56 patients (1). Omeprazole was more effective in healing esophagitis and providing symptom relief. Adverse events, which were rare, were similar in the two groups, and consisted of nausea, palpitation, abdominal pain, and mild abnormalities of liver function tests.

Organs and Systems

Nervous system

Histamine receptor antagonists can cause a variety of reactions involving the central nervous system. These are rare with famotidine.

- Five elderly patients (61–85-years-old) developed acute central nervous system reactions, consisting of confusion, agitation, hallucinations, and disorientation, 24 hours to a few days after starting to take famotidine 40 mg/day (2). These features resolved completely 24–48 hours after withdrawal. Rechallenge was not attempted.

Hematologic

Although it is hard to make a direct comparison between famotidine and cimetidine, since the former has been less extensively used, it is possible that the hematological problems occur more often with famotidine; there have been frequent well-documented reports of both thrombocytopenia and neutropenia, sometimes severe (SEDA-17, 417).

Liver

- Famotidine-induced cholestatic hepatitis has been reported in a previously healthy 13-year-old boy who had taken famotidine 40 mg/day for 30 days for epigastric pain (3). Other possible causes were excluded. He had a gradual and complete recovery 2 months after drug withdrawal.

Musculoskeletal

Rhabdomyolysis has been attributed to famotidine and might reflect its immunomodulating action (SEDA-17, 418).

Immunologic

Vasculitis occurred in a patient taking famotidine who had tolerated cimetidine well (4).

Body temperature

Hyperpyrexia has been attributed to famotidine, but the patient had pre-existing cerebral trauma as a facilitating factor (SEDA-16, 422).

Drug Administration

Drug overdose

After overdosage famotidine has a wide margin of safety; deliberate ingestion of very high doses did not appear to be associated with adverse sequelae (SEDA-21, 363) (5).

Drug–Drug Interactions

Omeprazole

Intragastric acid control by omeprazole 20 mg taken in the morning after variable dosing of over-the-counter famotidine 10 mg has been assessed in 12 healthy volunteers negative for *Helicobacter pylori* (6). Famotidine did not reduce the daytime efficacy of the next-morning dose of omeprazole.

References

1. Kawano S, Murata H, Tsuji S, Kubo M, Tatsuta M, Iishi H, Kanda T, Sato T, Yoshihara H, Masuda E, Noguchi M, Kashio S, Ikeda M, Kaneko A. Randomized comparative study of omeprazole and famotidine in reflux esophagitis. J Gastroenterol Hepatol 2002;17(9):955–9.
2. Odeh M, Oliven A. Central nervous system reactions associated with famotidine: report of five cases. J Clin Gastroenterol 1998;27(3):253–4.
3. Jimenez-Saenz M, Arguelles-Arias F, Herrerias-Gutierrez JM, Duran-Quintana JA. Acute cholestatic hepatitis in a child treated with famotidine. Am J Gastroenterol 2000;95(12):3665–6.
4. Andreo JA, Vivancos F, Lopez VM, Soriano J. Vasculitis leucocitoclastica y famotidina. [Leukocytoclastic vasculitis and famotidine.] Med Clin (Barc) 1990;95(6):234–5.
5. Howden CW, Tytgat GN. The tolerability and safety profile of famotidine. Clin Ther 1996;18(1):36–54.
6. Tutuian R, Katz PO, Ahmed F, Korn S, Castell DO. Over-the-counter H(2)-receptor antagonists do not compromise intragastric pH control with proton pump inhibitors. Aliment Pharmacol Ther 2002;16(3):473–7.

Fazadinium

See also Neuromuscular blocking drugs

General Information

Originally claimed, from animal experiments, to be of rapid onset, short duration, and free from important adverse effects, this non-depolarizing relaxant has been found to be less satisfactory in man. The usual doses are 0.5–0.75 mg/kg, although 1 mg/kg is sometimes advocated for fast intubation (within 1–2 minutes). The duration of action is similar in man to that of D-tubocurarine and pancuronium. Excretion is primarily in the urine (50–80%, mostly in the first 6 hours), although a biliary route has also been suggested. Metabolism occurs, probably to a minor extent, 1–3% being detected in the urine as inactive metabolites.

Organs and Systems

Cardiovascular

Cardiovascular effects account for the relative unpopularity of fazadinium. It has some ganglion-blocking activity (1) and blocks cardiac muscarinic receptors in the therapeutic dose range (2). Its vagolytic potency is about the same as that of gallamine. Fazadinium, like pancuronium, also blocks the reuptake of noradrenaline into sympathetic nerve endings. These actions explain its major cardiac adverse effect, namely significant tachycardia (3), which occurs even with small doses and is persistent.

It is dose-related (4), the increase in heart rate varying between 30 and 100%, and is associated with a rise in cardiac output and falls in stroke volume and peripheral resistance. Hypertension or hypotension can occur (5,6). If fazadinium is used injudiciously, extreme and dangerous cardiovascular changes can ensue (7).

Immunologic

Histamine release from fazadinium is very uncommon, but hypotension associated with an urticarial rash and two cases of severe bronchospasm and cardiac arrest (in patients who had also received thiopental) have been reported (8) as probably being due to fazadinium.

Immunological investigations combined with positive intradermal tests have been used to confirm fazadinium as the causative agent in a severe reaction (9).

Second-Generation Effects

Fetotoxicity

Placental transfer occurs and, though there may be some fetal uptake, Apgar scores did not appear to be affected (10,11).

References

1. Hughes R, Chapple DJ. Effects on non-depolarizing neuromuscular blocking agents on peripheral autonomic mechanisms in cats. Br J Anaesth 1976;48(2):59–68.
2. Marshall IG. The ganglion blocking and vagolytic actions of three short-acting neuromuscular blocking drugs in the cat. J Pharm Pharmacol 1973;25(7):530–6.
3. Hughes R, Payne JP, Sugai N. Studies on fazadinium bromide (AH 8165): a new non-depolarizing neuromuscular blocking agent. Can Anaesth Soc J 1976;23(1):36–47.
4. Schuh FT. Clinical neuromuscular pharmacology of AH 8165 D, an azobis-arylimidazo-pyridinium-compound. Anaesthesist 1975;24(4):151–6.
5. Lyons SM, Clarke RS, Young HS. A clinical comparison of AH8165 and pancuronium as muscle relaxants in patients undergoing cardiac surgery. Br J Anaesth 1975;47(6):725–9.
6. Lienhart A, Tauvent A, Guggiari M. Effets hemodynamiques des curares. [Hemodynamic effects of curares.] In: Curares et Curarisation. Paris: Librairie Arnette, 1979;1:384.
7. Pinaud M, Arnould F, Souron R, Nicolas F. Influence of cardiac rhythm on the haemodynamic effects of fazadinium in patients with heart failure. Br J Anaesth 1983;55(6):507–12.
8. Alexander JP. Adverse reactions following fazadinium–thiopentone induction. Anaesthesia 1979;34(7):661–5.
9. Baldassare M, Mastroianni A. Su un grave caso di shock da bromuro di fazadinio. [On a severe case of shock caused by fazadinium bromide.] Acta Anaesthesiol Ital 1983;34:91.
10. Bertrand JC, Duvaldestin P, Henzel D, Desmonts JM. Quantitative assessment of placental transfer of fazadinium in obstetric anaesthesia. Acta Anaesthesiol Scand 1980;24(2):135–7.
11. Rainaldi MP, Busi T, Melloni C, Boschi S. Pharmacokinetics and placental transmission of fazadinium in elective caesarean sections. Acta Anaesthesiol Scand 1984;28(2):222–5.

Felbamate

See also Antiepileptic drugs

General Information

Felbamate is a broad-spectrum antiepileptic drug, whose use has been drastically curtailed owing to the risks of aplastic anemia and hepatotoxicity.

Benefit to harm balance

The Quality Standards Subcommittee of the American Academy of Neurology and the American Epilepsy Society (1) has reviewed efficacy and safety data to establish recommendations for felbamate use in the light of the risk of aplastic anemia and liver toxicity (SEDA-22, 86). Felbamate was considered to have a favorable benefit to harm balance in patients with Lennox–Gastaut syndrome aged over 4 years who were unresponsive to primary anticonvulsants, in patients over 18 years of age with intractable partial seizures that have not responded to standard antiepileptic drugs in therapeutic concentrations, and in patients who are already taking felbamate and benefit from it for more than 18 months. There are conditions in which the benefit:harm balance is unclear, but for which use may be appropriate under certain circumstances, depending on the nature and severity of the seizure disorder; these include children with intractable partial epilepsy, patients with other generalized epilepsies unresponsive to primary agents, patients who have unacceptable sedative or cognitive effects with traditional antiepileptic drugs, and patients under 4 years with Lennox–Gastaut syndrome unresponsive to other antiepileptic drugs.

Assessment of its benefit to harm balance does not support the use of felbamate in new-onset epilepsy in children and adults, in patients who have significant prior hematological adverse events, in patients in whom follow-up and compliance will not allow careful monitoring, and in patients who are unable to discuss risk/benefits and for whom no parent or legal guardian is available to provide consent.

In patients taking felbamate, the benefit to harm balance should be constantly assessed. Patients should be educated about early signs of liver and bone-marrow toxicity, and about the manufacturers' recommendations. Laboratory monitoring has not been proven efficacious, but the manufacturer and the FDA suggest liver function and hematology testing at baseline and every 1–2 weeks for the first year. After that, the risk of aplastic anemia falls and the need for regular testing is less clear. A registry has been set up by the manufacturers to collect further safety data in patients started on the drug.

An open trial with 3-year follow up has been conducted in 36 patients with catastrophic childhood onset epilepsy (2). The overall responder rate (more than a 50% reduction in seizure frequency) fell with time: 69% at 3 months, 66% at 6 months, 47% at 1 year, and 41% at the end of the study. The most frequent adverse effects were anorexia, weight loss, urinary retention, somnolence, nervousness, and insomnia. Other reported adverse effects include skin reactions (including Stevens–Johnson syndrome), various blood dyscrasias, hepatotoxicity, and systemic lupus erythematosus (3).

Organs and Systems

Nervous system

Central nervous system adverse effects are common with felbamate, and consist mainly of insomnia, headache, impaired concentration, ataxia, dizziness, somnolence, behavioral disturbances, and mood changes. Movement disorders, psychosis, increased seizures, status epilepticus, and withdrawal seizures are less common (SEDA-19, 67) (SEDA-20, 61). The incidence of these effects is increased in the elderly, possibly owing to reduced drug clearance (4), whereas patients with mental retardation may be more prone to behavioral disorders (SEDA-19, 68).

Hematologic

Aplastic anemia affects 1 in 5000, or even 1 in 2000 patients (5), although a more recent estimate is 27–209 per million, compared with 2–2.5 per million in the general population (6). The underlying mechanism is unknown, although a deficiency in free radical scavenging activity may play a role (SEDA-22, 86).

Of 34 cases of aplastic anemia (mean age 41 years, mean time of felbamate exposure 154 days), 20 occurred in combination with other compounds implicated as a possible cause of aplastic anemia and 5 occurred concurrently with viral infections (7). Although 5 patients were taking felbamate monotherapy, 13 of the 34 suffered from autoimmune disease, and 1 was receiving cytostatic therapy. Past allergic or toxic reactions to other anticonvulsants were reported by 65% of the patients and blood dyscrasias by 45%, while 32% had serological evidence of a previous immune disorder. Eight of nine patients tested had experienced at least one episode of aplastic anemia associated with HLA antigens.

Felbamate is currently reserved for patients who are refractory to other drugs after careful consideration of the benefit:harm balance. In some countries the indication has been restricted to refractory Lennox–Gastaut syndrome. It is wise to avoid felbamate in patients with previous blood dyscrasias or autoimmune disorders, especially lupus erythematosus. Before they start to take it, patients should be informed about the potential risks and early symptoms of bone-marrow toxicity, such as bruisability, petechiae, fever of unknown origin, weakness, and fatigue. Hematology tests should be performed at baseline and during treatment, and dose escalation should be slow.

Because felbamate-induced aplastic anemia might be linked to the formation of atropaldehyde, a urine screening test has been developed that indirectly assesses the formation of this toxic metabolite (8). The risk of serious toxicity may also be related to HLA status, and HLA typing is being performed in patients entered in the manufacturer's felbamate registry. The potential value of these tests in reducing the risk of toxicity remains to be established.

Gastrointestinal

Felbamate is commonly associated with anorexia, nausea, and vomiting (9,10). Constipation and abdominal pain also occur. In 36 patients (12 men) aged 11–68 (mean 30) years in whom felbamate dosage was titrated gradually from 300 mg/day to a mean total daily maintenance dose of 1936 mg, the most frequent adverse events were: nausea, vomiting, anorexia, and weight loss (11).

Weight loss can occur. Of 65 patients with intractable seizures who received felbamate for a mean treatment time of 23 (range 6–116) weeks 49 lost weight (12). Among those over 15 years, there was a mean weight loss of 3.2 kg or 4.1% of body weight; 22 lost more than 4 kg, and 7 lost more than 8 kg. Among those aged 15 years or younger there was a non-significant mean weight loss of 0.20 kg or 1.8% of body weight.

However, in another study of 30 children aged 2–17 years with refractory partial seizures, felbamate up to a maximum of 45 mg/kg caused transient weight loss in 57%, maximal after 12 weeks and abating after 20 weeks (13). Anorexia and insomnia occurred in 20% and 16% of the patients respectively.

Liver

Of 23 reported cases of hepatic failure, only 10 (including 5 who died) were considered to be probably related to the drug (7,14). There have also been 20 cases of hepatitis in which no deaths occurred; in five of these a relation to felbamate was unlikely. Overall the incidence of fatal liver toxicity is estimated at 1 per 26 000–34 000. A careful history of past hepatic toxicity with other drugs should be taken and liver function tests are recommended before starting felbamate. Patients should have hepatic function monitored regularly and should be alerted to the signs and symptoms of hepatotoxicity.

Urinary tract

Urolithiasis has been associated with felbamate (15).

- A 15-year-old boy with Lennox–Gastaut syndrome taking felbamate(3000 mg/day), topiramate(200 mg/day), and lorazepam developed painful hematuria, bilateral urethral obstruction, and urinary retention. Kidney, bladder, and urethral stones were found. The stone material was identified as felbamate by chemical analysis. However, as the patient was also taking topiramate the association with felbamate was uncertain.

Susceptibility Factors

It is wise to avoid felbamate in patients with previous blood dyscrasias or autoimmune disorders, especially lupus erythematosus.

Drug–Drug Interactions

Carbamazepine-10,11-epoxide

Felbamate is a metabolic inhibitor and significantly increases blood concentrations of carbamazepine-10,11-epoxide (SEDA-19, 69) (SEDA-20, 61).

Clonazepam

Although felbamate increases the plasma concentrations of clonazepam only slightly, patients taking this combination are more vulnerable to central nervous system adverse effects (16).

Gestodene

Felbamate reduces the plasma concentrations of gestodene and may reduce its contraceptive efficacy (SEDA-20, 61).

Phenobarbital

Felbamate is a metabolic inhibitor and significantly increases blood concentrations of phenobarbital (SEDA-19, 69) (SEDA-20, 61).

Phenytoin

Felbamate is a metabolic inhibitor and significantly increases blood concentrations of phenytoin (SEDA-19, 69) (SEDA-20, 61).

The dose dependency and clinical relevance of the inhibition of phenytoin metabolism by felbamate has been examined in 10 patients (17). Phenytoin concentrations increased from 64 μmol/l at baseline to 84 and 107 μmol/l after felbamate 1200 and 1800 mg/day respectively. Owing to adverse effects, a reduction in phenytoin dosage was required in four patients after felbamate 1800 mg/day and in six patients after felbamate 2400 mg/day. Felbamate titration to doses of 3600 mg/day required overall phenytoin dosage reductions of 40% on average (range 20–72%), based on tolerability. Based on these findings, phenytoin dosage should be reduced by 20% when felbamate is added, and further dosage reductions are likely to be required when felbamate dosage is increased. Requirements for dosage reductions may be predicted by clinical signs of phenytoin intolerance, such as mental slowing, nausea, fatigue, and somnolence. The same study showed that in patients taking phenytoin co-medication serum felbamate concentrations are reduced by about 60% compared with those achieved in monotherapy.

Valproate

Felbamate is a metabolic inhibitor and significantly increases blood concentrations of valproic acid (SEDA-19, 69) (SEDA-20, 61).

References

1. French J, Smith M, Faught E, Brown L. Practice advisory: the use of felbamate in the treatment of patients with intractable epilepsy. Epilepsia 1999;40:803–8.
2. Cilio MR, Kartashov AI, Vigevano F. The long-term use of felbamate in children with severe refractory epilepsy. Epilepsy Res 2001;47(1–2):1–7.
3. Brodie MJ. Felbamate: a new antiepileptic drug. Lancet 1993;341(8858):1445–6.
4. Richens A, Banfield CR, Salfi M, Nomeir A, Lin CC, Jensen P, Affrime MB, Glue P. Single and multiple dose pharmacokinetics of felbamate in the elderly. Br J Clin Pharmacol 1997;44(2):129–34.
5. Pennell PB, Ogaily MS, Macdonald RL. Aplastic anemia in a patient receiving felbamate for complex partial seizures. Neurology 1995;45(3 Pt 1):456–60.
6. Kaufman DW, Kelly JP, Anderson T, Harmon DC, Shapiro S. Evaluation of case reports of aplastic anemia among patients treated with felbamate. Epilepsia 1997;38(12):1265–9.
7. Pellock JM, Brodie MJ. Felbamate: 1997 update. Epilepsia 1997;38(12):1261–4.
8. Pellock J. Progress in felbamate research: toxic metabolite test and HLA typing. Epilepsia 1999;40(Suppl 2):251.
9. Wagner ML. Felbamate: a new antiepileptic drug. Am J Hosp Pharm 1994;51(13):1657–66.
10. Palmer KJ, McTavish D. Felbamate. A review of its pharmacodynamic and pharmacokinetic properties, and therapeutic efficacy in epilepsy. Drugs 1993;45(6):1041–65.
11. Canger R, Vignoli A, Bonardi R, Guidolin L. Felbamate in refractory partial epilepsy. Epilepsy Res 1999;34(1):43–8.
12. Bergen DC, Ristanovic RK, Waicosky K, Kanner A, Hoeppner TJ. Weight loss in patients taking felbamate. Clin Neuropharmacol 1995;18(1):23–7.
13. Carmant L, Holmes GL, Sawyer S, Rifai N, Anderson J, Mikati MA. Efficacy of felbamate in therapy for partial epilepsy in children. J Pediatr 1994;125(3):481–6.
14. O'Neil MG, Perdun CS, Wilson MB, McGown ST, Patel S. Felbamate-associated fatal acute hepatic necrosis. Neurology 1996;46(5):1457–9.
15. Sparagana SP, Strand WR, Adams RC. Felbamate urolithiasis. Epilepsia 2001;42(5):682–5.
16. Colucci R, Glue P, Banfield C, Reidenberg P, Meehan J, Radwanski E, Korduba C, Lin C, Dogterom P, Ebels T, Hendriks G, Jonkman J, Affrime M. Effect of felbamate on the pharmacokinetics of clonazepam. Am J Ther 1996; 3(4):294–7.
17. Sachdeo R, Wagner ML, Sachdeo S, Shumaker RC, Lyness WH, Rosenberg A, Ward D, Perhach JL. Coadministration of phenytoin and felbamate: evidence of additional phenytoin dose-reduction requirements based on pharmacokinetics and tolerability with increasing doses of felbamate. Epilepsia 1999;40(8):1122–8.

Felbinac

See also Non-steroidal anti-inflammatory drugs

General Information

Felbinac, an active metabolite of fenbufen, is used as a gel for topical treatment (1).

Organs and Systems

Skin

Felbinac can cause itching, rash, and eosinophilia (SEDA-16, 110).

Reference

1. Hosie G, Bird H. The topical NSAID felbinac versus oral NSAIDS: a critical review. Eur J Rheumatol Inflamm 1994;14(4):21–8.

Felodipine

See also Calcium channel blockers

General Information

Felodipine is a dihydropyridine derivative with diuretic properties (1). Its diuretic properties are not unique but are shared by other dihydropyridines. Its vasodilator-related adverse effects include flushing, headache, and tachycardia (2,3). Reduced arterial oxygen saturation has been seen in patients given intravenous felodipine for pulmonary hypertension (4,5). Along with amlodipine, but unlike other calcium channel blockers, felodipine may be safer in severe chronic heart failure accompanied by angina or hypertension.

Organs and Systems

Skin

Different skin reactions have been reported with calcium antagonists, and in particular telangiectases in light-exposed areas of the skin with nifedipine and amlodipine (6).

- A 70-year-old woman took felodipine 10 mg/day and enalapril for about 1 year for hypertension. She developed telangiectatic lesions of both sides of the trunk. After excluding other causes, felodipine was withdrawn. After 2 months the lesions slightly abated, but never completely disappeared. The diagnosis was confirmed by histological evidence of enlarged capillaries parallel to the skin surface, in the absence of mast cells.
- Photodistributed telangiectases, made worse by solar radiation have been reported in a 67-year-old man taking felodipine 5 mg/day (7). Rosacea was also present. Felodipine was withdrawn and the telangiectases improved. Rechallenge was not performed.
- A 67-year-old man who had taken felodipine 5 mg/day for 4 years developed facial telangiectatic lesions that worsened with solar exposure for 9 months before felodipine was withdrawn; 2 months later the lesions had markedly diminished (7).

Drug–Drug Interactions

Erythromycin

The metabolism of felodipine is inhibited by erythromycin (SEDA-17, 239).

Grapefruit juice

In 12 elderly people (aged 70 years and over), grapefruit juice increased the AUC of felodipine three-fold and its peak concentration four-fold (8). Blood pressure was lower with grapefruit juice after a single dose of felodipine, but not at steady state. Heart rate was higher with grapefruit juice after both single and multiple doses. Elderly patients should avoid taking grapefruit juice during treatment with felodipine because of this marked and unpredictable interaction.

References

1. Edgar B, Bengtsson B, Elmfeldt D, Lundborg P, Nyberg G, Raner S, Ronn O. Acute diuretic/natriuretic properties of felodipine in man. Drugs 1985;29(Suppl 2):176–84.
2. Sluiter HE, Huysmans FT, Thien TA, Koene RA. Haemodynamic effects of intravenous felodipine in normotensive and hypertensive subjects. Drugs 1985;29 (Suppl 2):144–53.
3. Agner E, Rehling M, Trap-Jensen J. Haemodynamic effects of single-dose felodipine in normal man. Drugs 1985; 29(Suppl 2):36–40.
4. Bratel T, Hedenstierna G, Nyquist O, Ripe E. The effect of a new calcium antagonist, felodipine, on pulmonary hypertension and gas exchange in chronic obstructive lung disease. Eur J Respir Dis 1985;67(4):244–53.
5. Cohn JN, Ziesche S, Smith R, Anand I, Dunkman WB, Loeb H, Cintron G, Boden W, Baruch L, Rochin P, Loss L. Effect of the calcium antagonist felodipine as supplementary vasodilator therapy in patients with chronic heart failure treated with enalapril: V-HeFT III. Vasodilator-Heart Failure Trial (V-HeFT) Study Group. Circulation 1997;96(3):856–63.
6. Karonen T, Stubb S, Keski-Oja J. Truncal telangiectases coinciding with felodipine. Dermatology 1998;196(2):272–3.
7. Silvestre JF, Albares MP, Carnero L, Botella R. Photodistributed felodipine-induced facial telangiectasia. J Am Acad Dermatol 2001;45(2):323–4.
8. Love JN. Acebutolol overdose resulting in fatalities. J Emerg Med 2000;18(3):341–4.

Fenbendazole

General Information

The antiprotozoal activity of fenbendazole, a benzimidazole derivative, is similar to that of mebendazole; the target seems to be the microtubule protein beta-tubulin. Its adverse effects are comparable to those of mebendazole (1).

Reference

1. Katiyar SK, Gordon VR, McLaughlin GL, Edlind TD. Antiprotozoal activities of benzimidazoles and correlations with beta-tubulin sequence. Antimicrob Agents Chemother 1994;38(9):2086–90.

Fenbufen

See also Non-steroidal anti-inflammatory drugs

General Information

The profile of fenbufen is similar to the profiles of other NSAIDs (1). The dropout rate due to adverse reactions was 12–22% in different studies.

Organs and Systems

Respiratory

Fenbufen can cause a pulmonary alveolitis with rash, dry cough, breathlessness, fever, hypoxia, sometimes eosinophilia, and bilateral alveolar shadowing or infiltrates, which regress after withdrawal (SEDA-12, 85) (SEDA-13, 80) (SEDA-15, 100).

Nervous system

Headache has been reported with fenbufen (2).

Severe encephalitis, with generalized erythema and maculopapular rash on the trunk, has been reported (SEDA-19, 98).

Hematologic

Hemolytic anemia, in some cases with signs of hypersensitivity, has been reported (SEDA-14, 94). Aplastic anemia has been described in two patients (SEDA-18, 104), but both recovered fully after withdrawal.

Liver

The incidence of hepatotoxicity with fenbufen varies greatly. Changes in liver function tests were recorded in 25% patients in an early study (SEDA-4, 68), but were not confirmed later (SEDA-5, 194) (SEDA-6, 96). Abnormalities in the liver function of patients with rheumatoid arthritis may be a non-specific reaction to inflammation; however, hepatotoxicity should be watched for in patients taking fenbufen.

Skin

About 5% of patients have itching, rashes, or erythema multiforme (3). Circulating immune complexes have been found (4). The UK's Committee on Safety of Medicines issued a warning about the high rate of cutaneous adverse reactions with fenbufen and noted that some are followed by severe illnesses (SEDA-13, 72) (SEDA-14, 94) (SEDA-15, 100). Toxic epidermal necrolysis, a life-threatening reaction, has also been reported (SEDA-6, 96) (SEDA-8, 106) and a 1981–85 review on its incidence in France identified fenbufen as the third most common NSAID, after isoxicam and oxyphenbutazone, as a causal factor (5). Another severe skin reaction with laboratory evidence of hepatotoxicity has been described (SEDA-22, 115).

Drug–Drug Interactions

Enoxacin

Many cases of epileptic seizures have been reported in Japan in patients taking a combination of fenbufen and enoxacin (SEDA-12, 85) (SEDA-15, 100).

Quinolones

Fenbufen can cause convulsions, which has mainly been described in patients taking quinolone antibiotics (SEDA-18, 104).

References

1. Brogden RN, Heel RC, Speight TM, Avery GS. Fenbufen: a review of its pharmacological properties and therapeutic use in rheumatic diseases and acute pain. Drugs 1981;21(1):22.
2. Deodhar SD, Sethi R. A comparative study of fenbufen and indomethacin in patients with rheumatoid arthritis. Curr Med Res Opin 1979;6(4):263–6.
3. Peacock A, Ledingham J. Fenbufen-induced erythema multiforme. BMJ (Clin Res Ed) 1981;283(6291):582.
4. Nicolas C, Chouvet B, Cambazard F, Bernollin C, Thivolet J. Accidents cutanés lies à un nouvel anti-inflammatoire: fenbufenc. [Skin lesions related to a new anti-inflammatory agent: fenbufen. Apropos of 3 clinical cases.] Ann Dermatol Venereol 1983;110(5):419–23.
5. Roujeau JC, Guillaume JC, Fabre JP, Penso D, Flechet ML, Girre JP. Toxic epidermal necrolysis (Lyell syndrome). Incidence and drug etiology in France, 1981–1985. Arch Dermatol 1990;126(1):37–42.

Fenclofenac

See also Non-steroidal anti-inflammatory drugs

General Information

Fenclofenac was withdrawn in the UK after its license was not renewed because of its adverse drug reaction profile (1). Data from the UK's Committee on Safety of Medicines included records of seven deaths and 895 adverse effects in patients taking fenclofenac. Shortly afterwards it was withdrawn in all other countries in which it had been marketed.

Organs and Systems

Skin

Fenclofenac has the second highest incidence of complications and ranks first in the number and severity of skin reactions (2).

References

1. Anonymous. Fenclofenac withdrawn. Lancet 1984;2:56.
2. Weber JCP. Epidemiology of adverse reactions to non-steroidal anti-inflammatory drugs. Adv Inflam Res 1984;6:1.

Fenfluramines

See also Anorectic drugs

General Information

Although it resembles amfetamine structurally, the appetite suppressant fenfluramine does not produce central nervous system stimulation in therapeutic doses.

Dexfenfluramine, the dextrorotatory isomer, was previously widely marketed as an appetite suppressant in the management of obesity. It appears to be a pure serotonin receptor agonist without the dopaminergic and sympathetic activity of the racemic mixture.

Fenfluramine, dexfenfluramine, and phentermine have been used alone or in combination as an alternative to diet and surgery in the management of obesity. This therapy was halted in 1997 after reports of valvular lesions affecting almost one-third of patients treated with these drugs. The combination of fenfluramine and phentermine is called fen–phen.

General Adverse Effects

Dexfenfluramine

During both short-term and long-term therapy the adverse effects of dexfenfluramine seen with greater frequency than with placebo were tiredness, nausea, diarrhea, and dry mouth (1,2). Mydriasis, depression, withdrawal depression, insomnia, nervousness, headache, and increased urinary frequency have also been reported. So far, published clinical experience suggests that the greater selectivity of the dextrorotatory isomer leads to better tolerability. There has been only one long-term, that is longer than 6 months, trial on which to base this opinion (2). Since weight increase is common after withdrawal of treatment, long-term treatment is likely to be sought and given. Because studies on laboratory animals, including squirrel monkeys, suggest that there is a dose-dependent depletion of serotonin and metabolites along with a persistently reduced number of uptake sites, there has always been concern about a neurotoxic response with both isomers. However, it has also been pointed out that dexfenfluramine was used by more than 5 million patients for 6 years, and the parent compound by more than 20 million patients for 26 years, and yet it has not been associated with any serotonergic-mediated functional nervous system pathology in humans (SEDA-17, 1).

Fenfluramine

The main adverse effects of fenfluramine in two double-blind studies were sedation and drowsiness in addition to abdominal discomfort and dry mouth (3). Very rarely were these severe enough to justify withdrawal. At fairly high doses, the above-mentioned adverse effects became more severe and frequent. Drowsiness and gastrointestinal disturbances, consisting of colicky abdominal pain, were among the outstanding adverse effects in several other studies, most of them double blind; dizziness, light-headedness, and headaches were less frequent but occasionally quite marked (4). Shivering, teeth grinding, and alopecia have occasionally been reported as adverse effects of fenfluramine (4).

Phentermine

Phentermine is a central nervous system stimulant that can increase brain dopamine concentrations and has a structure similar to amfetamine.

Phentermine is indicated only for short-term treatment, and tolerance often develops. Its common adverse effects are dry mouth, insomnia, increased blood pressure, and constipation (5). It is the subject of a separate monograph (p. 2804).

Organs and Systems

Cardiovascular

Spontaneous rupture of a retroperitoneal aneurysm occurred in a 70-year-old woman who had been taking phentermine hydrochloride, 30 mg/day, for about 1 month (6). Other long-term medications included fluoxetine and amitriptyline, and she had no history of coronary artery disease, hypertension, diabetes, or complications of pregnancy. Although it is plausible that phentermine could have contributed to the ruptured aneurysm, other possibilities should be considered, particularly rupture of an anomalous retroperitoneal blood vessel.

Cardiomyopathy

Restrictive cardiomyopathy due to endocardial fibrosis occurred in a 35-year-old woman 5 months after she had started to take fenfluramine 10 mg tds and phentermine 15 mg/day (7). The endocardial findings strongly resembled the valvular lesions associated with the use of fenfluramine–phentermine. Endocardial and valvular fibrosis associated with anorectic drugs is strikingly similar to the plaque material found in patients with carcinoid syndrome and those exposed to methysergide, and all possibly arise from a common mechanism.

Valvulopathy

The fenfluramines and phentermine can cause valvular heart disease (8–10), and this has been reviewed (11). Fenfluramine was voluntarily withdrawn by the manufacturers on 15 September 1997, and the US Department of Health and Human Services issued interim recommendations for people previously exposed to fenfluramine or dexfenfluramine with cardiac valvulopathies (SEDA-22, 3).

The use of fenfluramine or dexfenfluramine alone or in combination with phentermine, in 2524 adult participants in the population-based Hypertension Genetic Epidemiology Network Study, was associated with aortic regurgitation independent of aortic dilatation or fibrocalcification (12). The association between the use of fenfluramine or dexfenfluramine (alone or with phentermine) and aortic regurgitation adjusted for potential confounders was analysed. Nineteen participants, all of whom had hypertension, were being treated with fenfluramine or dexfenfluramine (5 on these agents alone, 14 also with phentermine). Aortic regurgitation was present in 32% ($n = 6$) of those taking fenfluramine/dexfenfluramine versus 6% (162/2505) of the remaining subjects. In multivariate analyses, after adjusting for important confounders, in particular aortic root structure, treatment with fenfluramine or dexfenfluramine was associated with aortic regurgitation (OR, 5.2; 95% CI, 1.7–14) and fibrocalcification (OR, 5.2; 95% CI, 1.9–15).

The autopsy findings in the heart and lungs of a patient with pulmonary hypertension associated with fenfluramine and phentermine have been described (13).

- A 36-year-old woman with a body mass index of 47.5 kg/m^2, took fen–phen for 7 months and developed pulmonary hypertension. Her pulmonary arterial pressure was 56 mmHg and echocardiography showed right ventricular dilatation and hypokinesia. She had a cardiopulmonary arrest during right-heart catheterization and died 3 days later. At autopsy, there was right ventricular dilatation with a fibroproliferative tricuspid valve. The pulmonary arteries had fibroproliferative plaques which were more severe and prominent in the upper lobes than in the lower lobes.

More autopsy cases of patients with a history of fen–phen use are warranted to document the frequency of combined cardiac valvular disease and pulmonary hypertension.

Progressive pulmonary hypertension occurred in two patients who took fenfluramine for only 8 months (SEDA-6, 9). The symptoms abated on withdrawal but returned in one patient when rechallenged.

In 1996, in a case-control study, 95 patients from 35 centers in France, Belgium, the UK, and the Netherlands were compared with 355 age- and sex-matched controls (14). The use of anorexic drugs (mainly derivatives of fenfluramine) was associated with an increased risk of primary pulmonary hypertension. Association with recognized risk factors such as a family history of primary pulmonary hypertension, infection with HIV, or the use of intravenous drugs was also confirmed. The absolute risk for obese patients who took anorexic agents for more than 3 months was 30 times higher than in non-users.

Echocardiography with color Doppler in 22 patients aged 25–69 years (19 women and three men) who had taken fen–phen for more than 3 months showed that one patient with newly discovered aortic insufficiency was asymptomatic. Some were taking several other drugs, none of which is known to precipitate valvular heart disease. Echocardiography was normal in 12 cases and abnormal in 10 including significant aortic insufficiency and significant mitral regurgitation. Ten of the patients had significant aortic insufficiency and nine had at least mild mitral insufficiency. The author inferred that fenfluramine was the likely offending agent, because (a) while it is known to cause release of serotonin, phentermine does not; (b) carcinoid tumors, which secrete serotonin and ergotamine, a serotonergic drug, are known to cause valvular heart disease; *and* (c) none of the obese patients who took phentermine and fluoxetine for more than 2 years developed pulmonary hypertension (15) and the author found no valvular heart disease in this cohort either (16). The recommendation that phentermine should be combined with fluoxetine, sertraline, or fluvoxamine as safer alternatives (16) requires prospective studies.

It was suggested that in patients who met the FDA criteria for cardiac valvular abnormalities on echocardiography performed soon after the withdrawal of appetite suppressants, there was a possibility (ranging from as low as 5% to as high as 67%) that the abnormality was a naturally occurring phenomenon and not a consequence of drug use (17). However, various studies have supported earlier reports of an association between fenfluramine or its d-isomer and cardiac valvular regurgitation, although they have differed with regard to the strength and clinical significance of the association (17). Differences in design, including a lack of baseline cardiac evaluation in echocardiographic assessment (9,10,18), have precluded comparisons. Additional evidence linking the use of fenfluramine or dexfenfluramine to cardiac valvular regurgitation has reaffirmed the wisdom of the FDA's decision to withdraw them from the market.

Why was this type of valvulopathy not recognized sooner? Changes in medical practice seem to have played a role as long-term and widespread use of these drugs evolved in the 1990s. Furthermore, cardiac murmurs can be more difficult to detect in obese patients (19).

Prevalence

Although initially a prevalence of up to 30% was estimated, subsequent reports have suggested much lower rates. There are several reasons for this disparity including uncontrolled data and the limitations of echocardiography (20–22). The FDA surveys and the University of Minnesota study reported point prevalences and inherently overestimated the association of appetite suppressants with valvulopathy because a certain percentage of patients have pre-existing valvular lesions. The method of detection also plays a crucial role. Echocardiography is far more sensitive than clinical examination in detecting valvular regurgitation. The issue may also be confounded by lesion regression after withdrawal of therapy (23). Moreover, case-control studies are no substitute for objective evidence of the status of cardiac valves before drug exposure (8). Also the duration of exposure has varied widely in different reports.

Pulmonary hypertension and valvular heart disease associated with anorexigens have been described predominantly in women, which raises important questions about biological and psychological risk factors and ethical practice. Do women respond differently to these drugs because of genetic or physiological factors or are these drugs being prescribed almost exclusively for women? Was it realistic for the regulatory authorities to believe that these drugs would be used only to treat morbid obesity? Most important, what view of the benefit to harm balance of using anorexigenic drugs has allowed women and their physicians to justify the use of potentially lethal drugs to deal with concerns about body image and weight? These questions (24) are pertinent to the current scenario of appetite-suppressant drug-related concerns.

Studies in which baseline echocardiography was carried out before the drug was used showed that the risk of new or prospective valvular heart disease was much lower than implied by previous prevalence studies (8). In 46 patients who used fenfluramine or dexfenfluramine for 14 days or more, the primary outcome was new or worsening valvulopathy, defined as progression of either aortic regurgitation or mitral regurgitation by at least one degree of severity and disease that met FDA criteria. Two patients taking fen–phen developed valvular heart disease. One had mild aortic regurgitation that progressed to moderate regurgitation and the second developed new moderate aortic insufficiency. The authors argued that the referral bias in their study, which required an echocardiogram for inclusion, would have tended to result in a higher incidence of valvular disease.

In an amended randomized double-blind placebo-controlled comparison of dexfenfluramine with an investigational modified-release formulation of dexfenfluramine, the study medication was discontinued and echocardiographic examinations were performed on 1072 overweight patients within a median of 1 month after withdrawal of treatment (18). These patients, 80% of whom were women, had been randomly assigned to receive dexfenfluramine (366 patients), modified-release dexfenfluramine (352 patients), or placebo (354 patients). The average duration of treatment was 71–72 days in each group. Echocardiograms were assessed blind. Pooling the fenfluramine groups, there was a higher prevalence of any degree of aortic regurgitation (17 versus 12%) and mitral regurgitation (61 versus 54%) with fenfluramine. Analyses carried out using the criteria set by the FDA showed that aortic regurgitation of mild or greater severity occurred in 5% of the patients taking dexfenfluramine, 5.4% of those in the two fenfluramine groups combined, and 3.6% of those in the placebo group. Moderate or severe mitral regurgitation occurred in 1.7 and 1.8% of those taking fenfluramine and 1.2% of those taking placebo. Aortic regurgitation of mild or greater severity, mitral regurgitation of moderate or greater severity, or both occurred in 6.5, 6.9, and 4.5% respectively.

This was an unusual study because patients enrolled for a different purpose were analysed mid-way through the study in response to withdrawal of fenfluramine. Exposure to fenfluramine in this study was relatively short (2–3 months) and the prevalences of mitral regurgitation and aortic regurgitation in this study were much lower than previously described (25).

Although the findings of this study may be reassuring for patients who have taken dexfenfluramine for 2–3 months, they should not preclude the appropriate investigation of a new murmur or new symptoms in any patient with a history of exposure to dexfenfluramine as specified in the American College of Cardiology Guidelines (26).

In 24 women who were evaluated an average of 12 months after starting to take fen–phen, echocardiography showed that all had unusual valvular morphology and regurgitation affecting valves on the right and left sides (27). Eight women also had newly documented pulmonary hypertension. Histopathological findings included plaque-like encasement of the leaflets and chordal structures with intact valve architecture. The histopathological features were like those seen in carcinoid or ergotamine-induced valve disease. As of the end of September 1997, the FDA had received 144 individual spontaneous reports (including the 24 cases reported earlier) involving fenfluramine or dexfenfluramine with or without phentermine in association with valvulopathy, 113 with complete information (28). Of these, 98% occurred in women of whom 2% used fenfluramine alone, 14% used dexfenfluramine alone, 79% used fenfluramine with phentermine, and 5% used a combination of all three; none had used phentermine alone. The median duration of drug use was 9 months (range 1–39 months). Cardiac valve replacement surgery was required in 24% and there was an 11% mortality.

Based on a prospective study carried out in 226 obese subjects (183 women and 43 men) with a mean body mass index of 40 kg/m^2, therapy with fen–phen was associated with low prevalence of significant valvular regurgitation (29). The authors suggested that valvular regurgitation in these subjects may have reflected age-related degenerative changes. However, several limitations of this study have been pointed out: (a) there was no control group and not all the subjects had echocardiography; (b) multiple readers interpreted the echocardiograms, rendering the comparison less accurate; (c) there was inherent inaccuracy in differentiating mild degrees of valvular regurgitation especially using qualitative scoring systems; (d) there was selection bias; and (e) neither direct inspection nor histopathological confirmation of valvular lesions was performed on any patient.

The risk of a subsequent clinical diagnosis of a valvular disorder of uncertain origin has been assessed in a population-based follow-up study using nested case-control analysis of 6532 subjects who took dexfenfluramine, 2371 who took fenfluramine, and 862 who took phentermine (10). The control group comprised 9281 obese subjects who did not take appetite suppressants matched with the treated subjects for age, sex, and weight. No subject had cardiovascular disease at the start of the follow-up for an average duration of 5 years. There were 11 cases of newly diagnosed idiopathic valvular disorders, five with dexfenfluramine and six with fenfluramine. There were six cases of aortic regurgitation, two of mitral regurgitation, and three of combined aortic and mitral regurgitation. There were no cases of idiopathic cardiac valve abnormalities among the controls or those who took phentermine. The 5-year cumulative incidence of idiopathic cardiac valve disorders was 0 per 10 000 among both those who had not taken appetite suppressants (95 CI = 0, 15) and those who took phentermine alone (CI = 0, 77), 7.1 per 10 000 among those who took either fenfluramine or dexfenfluramine for less than 4 months (CI = 3.6, 18), and 35 per 10 000 among those who took either of these medications for 4 months or more (CI = 16, 76). The authors concluded that the use of fenfluramine or dexfenfluramine, particularly when used for 4 months or longer, is associated with an increased risk of newly diagnosed cardiac valve disorders, particularly aortic regurgitation.

The above study was based on information derived from the General Practice Research Database in the UK. Subjects who had been given at least one prescription for dexfenfluramine, fenfluramine, or phentermine after 1 January 1988, and who were 70 years or younger at the time of their first prescription were included. Subjects were considered to have a new cardiac abnormality if they had no history, on the basis of clinical records, of cardiac valvular abnormalities and if there was evidence of a new valvular disorder on the basis of echocardiography or clinical examination after exposure to appetite suppressants. All the data had been recorded before the publication of recent reports of an association between appetite suppressants and cardiac valve disorders (25,27,30–32) or primary pulmonary hypertension (14). Hence, it was possible to exclude the possibility that enhanced awareness of possible serious adverse effects of appetite suppressants had led to closer surveillance of patients who were taking these drugs. Nevertheless, the study did not provide information on the frequency of idiopathic cardiac valve disorders that are asymptomatic or otherwise not clinically diagnosed.

Using the FDA case definition of appetite-suppressant related valvulopathy, the prevalence was 31% (60/191) in a selected group of Mayo Clinic patients at Rochester (33). The most common finding was mild aortic regurgitation. Of asymptomatic patients 28% had abnormal echocardiographic findings. This study emphasized the spectrum of diet- or drug-related cardiac disease and the potential for valvulopathy in asymptomatic patients.

In patients who had taken dexfenfluramine ($n = 479$) or fen–phen ($n = 455$) continuously for 30 days or more in the previous 14 months, there was an increase in the prevalence of aortic regurgitation compared with 539 control subjects (34). There was no increase in the prevalence of moderate or severe aortic regurgitation in treated patients, and no difference in the prevalence of mitral regurgitation between the untreated and treated groups, irrespective of duration of therapy. All evaluations were carried out using the FDA criteria. The authors were careful to point out that their study was not specifically designed or adequately powered to evaluate specific categories of anorexigen therapy duration.

Further evidence that the prevalence of significant valvular regurgitation is low in patients who take fen–phen has been reported (35). Transthoracic echocardiography was performed in 343 obese patients in a 3-year prospective study that began within 4 months from the withdrawal of fenfluramine and dexfenfluramine from the market. There were 281 women and 62 men, mean age 47 years, and mean body mass index 40 kg/m^2. Using the FDA's criteria, only 21 subjects (6.1%) had significant valvular lesions. Aortic regurgitation was detected in 18 subjects, mitral regurgitation in 3, and both aortic and mitral regurgitation in 1. Significant valvular disease did not correlate with age, sex, initial or final body mass index, drug dose, or the duration of therapy.

Mechanisms and risk factors

The determinants of valvulopathy in patients treated with dexfenfluramine have been investigated: age and blood pressure can also affect the prevalence of regurgitation (36,37), as can duration of exposure (36). Others have found no correlation between valvular disease associated with appetite suppressants and either dose or duration of drug exposure (29).

Cases of severe diffuse multivalvular disease associated with fen–phen have been described (38,39).

- A 52-year-old woman had a transesophageal echocardiogram 1 year before starting to take fen–phen, and had no significant valvular disease. She presented a year later with a new heart murmur and eventually required isolated aortic valve replacement. Pathological evaluation of the excised aortic valve was consistent with that described with fen–phen use.
- A 44-year-old woman who had previously taken appetite suppressants, developed valvular disease consistent with the effects of fen–phen. She had an identical twin who, despite having been treated with the same medication, remained symptom-free and without abnormal echocardiography. Both the patient and her sister took fen–phen for 2 years. However, the patient took a daily dose of fenfluramine of 60–120 mg (and often as much as 240 mg) and phentermine 90 mg (at times 180 mg), whereas her twin sister adhered to the daily amount prescribed (fenfluramine 60 mg and phentermine 24 mg).

The latter case suggests that dosage is important in the production of the valvular pathology. Mitral and tricuspid insufficiency developed in a 36-year-old woman who had taken fen–phen for 24 months (40). Transmission electron microscopy of the mitral and tricuspid valves showed many areas that appeared to contain intracellular, virus-like particles clustered in the cytoplasm, with a mean diameter of 32 nm. Whether this finding was incidental or related to the underlying pathology was uncertain.

There is further evidence, from an uncontrolled observational study in 85 patients, that the dose and duration of administration of fen–phen affects the risk of significant valvular disease (41). The authors suggested that it would be prudent to consider diagnostic echocardiography in patients who have used fen–phen either in a dosage of at least 60 mg/day or for at least 9 months. They also raised concerns that for patients with mild obesity, the prolonged use of larger cumulative amounts may lead to a higher risk of valve regurgitation.

There is further evidence of the relation between the duration of treatment with fen–phen and the prevalence of valvular abnormalities (42). In 1163 patients who had taken anorexigens within the previous 5 years and 672 control patients who had not, valvular abnormalities primarily involved those who had taken anorexigens for more than 6 months, and predominantly resulted in mild aortic regurgitation. The study had some noteworthy limitations: since fenfluramine has been withdrawn from use, a randomized trial was impossible; also the lack of baseline echocardiograms before treatment implies that one cannot be certain that the valvular regurgitation developed subsequent to drug treatment.

Diagnosis

It has been proposed that valvular disease can be attributable to appetite suppressants only if the following criteria are satisfied:

- the macroscopic and microscopic features are consistent with fenfluramine-related valvulopathy;
- clinical, echocardiographic, and intraoperative findings support the diagnosis;
- the history of drug exposure predates the development or exacerbation of valvular dysfunction (43).

It is obvious that these criteria can be applicable only in cases in which cardiac valves are explanted and are available for histopathological studies.

The prevalence and diagnostic value of cardiac murmurs for valvular regurgitation has been determined in 223 patients taking dexfenfluramine for 6.9 months and 189 matched controls. Experienced physicians, non-cardiologists, who were unaware of the echocardiographic findings, took a history and performed cardiac auscultation. Based on their findings the authors recommended that cardiac auscultation should be the screening method of choice for detecting valvular regurgitation in users of anorexigens (44). In this study, the absence of cardiac murmurs predicted the absence of clinically important valvular regurgitation in 93% of dexfenfluramine users. These results support the recommendation by the American Heart Association and American College of Cardiology (45) that asymptomatic users of anorexigens without a cardiac murmur do not warrant echocardiography. The data also suggest that in users of anorexigens with a 10% prevalence of valvular regurgitation and a 10–15% prevalence of cardiac murmurs, cardiac auscultation will prevent 85–90% of patients from undergoing unnecessary echocardiography. These implications may apply to all users of anorexigens because the prevalence of valvular regurgitation in recent large series is similar to that in this study (SEDA-24, 4). There are therefore large potential cost savings of cardiac auscultation, by preventing a large proportion of the more than 6 million Americans who are exposed to anorexigens from undergoing initial and follow-up echocardiography or from receiving empiric antibiotic prophylaxis for emergency procedures that preclude further cardiac evaluation.

Effects of withdrawal of therapy on valvulopathy

In a patient who was followed-up for 2 years after withdrawal, multivalvular regurgitation associated with fenfluramine and phentermine may have regressed (23).

- A 44-year-old woman with morbid obesity but no history of cardiac disease developed atypical chest pain. Myocardial infarction was ruled out, and an echocardiogram showed normal chamber sizes and mildly reduced global systolic function. However, moderate to moderately severe aortic regurgitation, mild mitral regurgitation, and moderate tricuspid regurgitation were present. The estimated pulmonary artery pressure was slightly raised. Her only medications were fenfluramine 60 mg/day and phentermine 30 mg/day, which she had taken for the previous 50 weeks, during which time she had lost 40 kg. These drugs were withdrawn and 6 months later an echocardiogram showed improved left ventricular function and a reduction in the severity of all her valvular lesions with no clinically significant change in the estimated pulmonary artery pressure. An echocardiogram obtained 2 years after the initial study showed only trace aortic and tricuspid regurgitation without mitral regurgitation.

In this case, serial echocardiography over 2 years documented regression of multivalvular regurgitation, first discovered while the patient was taking fenfluramine and phentermine. The authors argued that although she was also given lisinopril, the marked degree of improvement in all the valvular lesions after withdrawal of the appetite suppressants was unlikely to be attributable to this alone (46).

The small increase in prevalence of minor degrees of aortic regurgitation and mitral regurgitation in 941 patients treated with dexfenfluramine for 2–3 months was no longer present 3–5 months (median 137 days) after withdrawal (47). Echocardiograms were acquired using a standardized protocol and were assessed blindly.

In 50 patients with fenfluramine-associated valvular heart disease followed by serial echocardiography for 6–24 months after withdrawal of therapy (48), in most cases valvular heart disease either did not change or improved at least by one grade. Mitral and aortic regurgitation improved in some patients, and tricuspid and pulmonic regurgitation improved in most patients after withdrawal. When improvement did occur, regression of regurgitation often involved multiple valves on both the left and right sides of the heart, rather than affecting one valve in isolation. Although most of the patients stabilized or improved, a few had worsening of valvular regurgitation despite withdrawal.

Comparable results were also reported in a larger series in another study (49). Sequential echocardiographic evaluation 1 year after withdrawal of dexfenfluramine showed a significant reduction in aortic regurgitation. There were no significant changes in mitral regurgitation or any other valvular variables. Although these results can be applied only to the population studied (predominantly middle-aged, obese, white women who took dexfenfluramine for 2–3 months), the implications are considerable. Because valvular regurgitation remained stable or improved in most of the patients, surgical referral for patients with severe regurgitation may be delayed. Improvement in valvular regurgitation often occurred within months after drug withdrawal. Watchful waiting with serial echocardiography, prophylaxis against endocarditis, and medical therapy may be a reasonable management strategy in patients with severe regurgitation, minimal symptoms, and no evidence of left ventricular dysfunction (48).

However, reversibility may not occur in all cases (50).

- Cardiac allograft transplantation was carried out from a 35-year-old hypertensive donor with prolonged exposure to fenfluramine and phentermine. There was non-specific mitral valve thickening, with trivial mitral regurgitation and poor approximation of the mitral valve leaflets, due to reduced posterior leaflet mobility. There was no evidence of any other valvular lesion. Examination of the donor heart during cardiac implantation showed three discontinuous lesions along the left atrial surface of the mitral valve annulus and another firm nodular lesion of the annular endocardium. Transplantation of the heart was uneventful and intraoperative transesophageal echocardiography, performed after weaning from cardiopulmonary bypass, showed trivial mitral regurgitation with excellent allograft contractility. The postoperative course was uneventful and the patient was discharged on the eighth postoperative day. Histological examination of the specimen showed a glistening appearance with proliferating myofibroblasts and associated fibrinous vegetations. There was no evidence of acute or chronic inflammation, and Gram staining did not show bacterial or fungal elements. A transthoracic echocardiogram 6 weeks after transplantation showed only trivial mitral regurgitation with improved mobility of the posterior leaflet. Hemodynamic data showed normal allograft function. However, after 6 months of follow-up, Doppler echocardiography showed worsening of mitral regurgitation to moderate severity, but no adverse effects of this hemodynamic load were noted and the patient remained stable.

Although conclusions based on single cases have limitations, they can often provide useful insights and act as catalysts for further studies. This report illustrates a few important features of cardiac valvulopathy associated with anorexigen use. There was no involvement of chordal apparatus and so the pathological changes within the valve leaflets and annulus represented the earliest site of an anorexigen-induced valvulopathy. This opportunity to observe a case of "early" valvulopathy visually and histopathologically offered insight into pathogenesis, and may have been helpful in staging the lesions temporally.

Of 120 patients who had follow-up echocardiography at least twice after stopping fen–phen, 99 met FDA criteria for valvulopathy (51). On second echocardiography, 57 of these 99 had no change in valvulopathy, 33 had improved, and 9 had deteriorated; nine patients no longer met FDA criteria for valvulopathy. The authors suggested that physicians must continue to be vigilant with patients who develop valvulopathy after taking fen–phen.

Obesity as a confounding factor in cardiac valvulopathy
It is not clear whether valvular insufficiency is related to the use of appetite suppressants or is simply a consequence of obesity. Obese patients who took dexfenfluramine alone, dexfenfluramine in combination with phentermine, or fenfluramine in combination with phentermine have been compared with a matched group of obese-control subjects who had not taken these medications (9). A total of 1.3% of the controls (3 of 233) and 23% of the patients (53 of 233) met the case definition for cardiac valve abnormalities (OR=23). The odds ratios for such cardiac valve abnormalities were 13 with dexfenfluramine alone, 25 with dexfenfluramine and phentermine, and 26 with fenfluramine and phentermine. This study showed that the prevalence of valvular insufficiency is significantly higher among obese patients who have taken appetite suppressants than among subjects matched for age, sex, and body mass index who did not take such drugs. Since a higher percentage of patients than controls had trace aortic valve insufficiency, the authors questioned whether the case definition threshold for cardiac valve abnormalities in association with appetite suppressants set by the FDA and Centers for Disease Control and Prevention is perhaps too high. In this study the factors that predisposed patients to valvular insufficiency were (a) age at the start of therapy, (b) use of dexfenfluramine, (c) combination of dexfenfluramine with phentermine, and (d) combination of fenfluramine with phentermine. Hence, neither the clinical significance nor the natural history of this type of valvular disease has been defined.

Other epidemiological studies have ruled out the possibility that obesity itself causes a high prevalence of cardiac valvular regurgitation (52–54).

Pulmonary hypertension
Pulmonary hypertension associated with fenfluramine was first reported in the early 1980s. A retrospective study further established the link (55). Subsequently a multicenter case-control study in 95 patients showed a high incidence of pulmonary hypertension in patients who had used fenfluramine or dexfenfluramine (14). Moreover, there was a strong suggestion of a dose–response effect, longer periods of use being associated with a progressive increase in the relative risk of pulmonary hypertension. In 1997, the first case of pulmonary hypertension in association with fen–phen was reported (56). Eight of the 24 patients with valvular disease had newly diagnosed pulmonary hypertension, although in most cases it was attributable to valvular abnormalities (57). It is not clear whether a combination of these agents poses a higher risk in predisposed individuals.

The results of a Belgian study in 35 patients with pulmonary hypertension and 85 matched controls have been published (58). The data were collected when there was no restriction on prescribing of appetite suppressants. Of the patients, 23 had previously taken appetite suppressants, mainly fenfluramines, compared with 5 controls. Moreover, the patients who had been exposed to appetite suppressants tended to be on an average more severely ill and to have a shorter median delay between the onset of symptoms and diagnosis.

Pulmonary artery pressure and cardiac valvular status were determined in a series of 156 mostly asymptomatic patients taking fenfluramine and phentermine (59). The anorexigen was withdrawn when abnormalities were noted. Pulmonary artery pressure was estimated and valvular examination was performed using Doppler echocardiography. There was borderline or mildly elevated pulmonary artery pressure in 21 patients and 31 patients had notable valvular abnormalities. It has therefore been established that asymptomatic patients may have significant echocardiographic abnormalities, representing early lesions.

- A 30-year-old woman who had taken dexfenfluramine for 7 months developed pulmonary hypertension and right heart failure during late pregnancy. She died of septicemia with multiorgan failure 4 days after a cesarean section (60).
- Pulmonary hypertension and multivalvular damage after prolonged use of fenfluramine with phentermine have been reported in a 70-year-old Israeli woman (61).
- Fatal pulmonary hypertension occurred in a 32-year-old man who had been taking phentermine in unknown doses for 4 months (62).

Incidence
The epidemiological association of pulmonary hypertension with aminorex and dexfenfluramine, both with respect to the strength of the association (estimate of relative risk) and its impact on public health, has been investigated (63). Control rates of exposure were used to estimate population exposure prevalences. The estimated odds ratio for the association between pulmonary hypertension and any exposure to aminorex was 98 and for dexfenfluramine 3.7. The strong association between aminorex and pulmonary hypertension projected a fivefold increase in the incidence of pulmonary hypertension, and thus a very noticeable epidemic. In contrast, the association with dexfenfluramine is expected to result in an incidence of only 20% and thus a repeat epidemic seems unlikely.

In a prospective surveillance study of 579 patients with pulmonary hypertension at 12 large referral centers in North America, 205 had primary pulmonary hypertension and 374 had secondary pulmonary hypertension (64). Among the drugs surveyed, only fenfluramine had a significant association with primary pulmonary hypertension compared with secondary pulmonary hypertension (adjusted odds ratio for use for more than 6 months = 7.5; 95% CI = 1.7, 32). The association was stronger with longer duration of use compared with shorter duration of use and was more pronounced in recent users than in remote users. An unexpectedly high (11%) number of patients with secondary pulmonary hypertension had used anorexigens. The high prevalence of anorexigen use in patients with secondary pulmonary hypertension also raised the possibility that these drugs precipitate pulmonary hypertension in patients with underlying conditions associated with secondary pulmonary hypertension.

The age-adjusted mortality rates from primary pulmonary hypertension in the years immediately preceding the use of fen–phen were not different from those reported during the years of widespread use among patients aged 20–54 years. This analysis failed to support the hypothesis that the widespread use of fen–phen in the years 1992–1997 increased the incidence of primary pulmonary hypertension. "If the use [of fen–phen] during these years created an epidemic of primary pulmonary hypertension, as some have declared, such an epidemic is not reflected in the mortality database maintained by CDC" (65).

Prognosis

Of 62 patients (61 women) exposed to fenfluramine compared with 125 sex-matched patients with primary pulmonary hypertension, 33 had used dexfenfluramine alone, 7 had used fenfluramine alone, and 5 had used both (66). In 17 cases fenfluramines were taken with amphetamines. Most of the patients (81%) had taken fenfluramines for at least 3 months. The interval between the start of therapy and the onset of dyspnea was 49 months (range 27 days to 23 years). The two groups differed significantly in terms of age and body mass index. Both groups had similar severe baseline hemodynamics, but the percentage of responders to an acute vasodilator was higher in patients with primary pulmonary hypertension. Hence, more patients with primary pulmonary hypertension were treated with oral vasodilators, and long-term epoprostenol infusion was more often used in fenfluramine users. Overall survival was similar in the two groups, with a 3-year survival rate of 50%.

Mechanism and pathophysiology

The mechanism of fenfluramine-associated pulmonary hypertension has been reviewed (SEDA-21, 3). Since only a minority of patients exposed to fenfluramines develop pulmonary hypertension, it has been postulated that a subset may be genetically susceptible. Whether there is a related genetic abnormality in the familial PPH gene located on chromosome 2q (67) or an abnormality of the angiotensin-converting enzyme gene (68) has yet to be explored.

Anorexigenic drugs accumulate in the lung and other tissues, especially in cellular organelles with an internal acid pH, such as lysosomes, where they bind to acidic enzymes. Lipid enzyme inhibition, lysosomal lipidosis, and associated myeloidosis are key events in the pathological cascade (69). Since several stimulants and other psychotropic drugs are cationic amphiphilic compounds that accumulate in the lung, brain, and other tissues, the variety of pathological mechanisms involved in the effects of this group of drugs should be kept in mind during long-term use (70,71).

The hypothesis that nitric oxide deficiency predisposes affected individuals to anorexigen-associated pulmonary hypertension has been tested in a prospective case-control comparison with two sex-matched sets of controls: patients with primary pulmonary hypertension ($n = 8$) and healthy volunteers ($n = 12$) (72). Lung production of nitric oxide and systemic plasma oxidation products of nitric oxide were measured at rest and during exercise, and were lower in patients with anorexigen-associated pulmonary hypertension than in patients with primary pulmonary hypertension. This deficiency may have resulted from increased oxidative inactivation of nitric oxide, as the concentrations of their oxidative products were raised in inverse proportion to nitric oxide. These findings, and earlier evidence from animal studies (73), have given support to the hypothesis incriminating nitric oxide as a determinant of individual susceptibility to anorexigen-associated pulmonary hypertension.

The pressure response to endothelin-1 in the canine circulation has been investigated in isolated perfused dog lung (74). Acute treatment of the isolated lobes with fenfluramine increased pulmonary arterial pressure. Chronic treatment with fenfluramine potentiated the pulmonary vasoconstrictor response to endothelin-1. Based on these findings, the authors proposed that the pulmonary vasculature becomes hyper-reactive to vasoactive substances, such as serotonin and endothelin-1, possibly leading to pulmonary hypertension.

Anorexigen-associated severe pulmonary hypertension is clinically and histopathologically indistinguishable from idiopathic or primary pulmonary hypertension. Analysis of clonality in microdissected endothelial cells of plexiform lesions in two patients with anorexigen-associated pulmonary hypertension showed a monoclonal expansion of pulmonary endothelial cells. Accelerated growth of pulmonary endothelial cells in response to anorexigens in patients with predisposition to primary pulmonary hypertension has been speculated (75).

Hypertension

In a few patients, hypertension was induced or aggravated by fenfluramine. The hypertension disappeared on withdrawal, but could not in all instances be reinduced by rechallenge (76).

Nervous system

The frequent occurrence of sedation, drowsiness, lightheadedness, and headaches has been referred to in the general section above.

Impaired powers of concentration during the first week, insomnia, apathy, tiredness, reduction in general memory, and a feeling of derealization, but not mood elevation, were noted in healthy people who took fenfluramine (SEDA-13, 3) (77).

Of special interest are studies on the effects of fenfluramine on sleep. After administration of 40 or 80 mg of fenfluramine, patients with chronic psychiatric disorders fell asleep normally, but a few hours later were troubled with a peculiar feeling of uneasiness that kept them awake for the rest of the night. The following night, however, they fell asleep more quickly, regardless of the medication. Moreover, one patient had nightmares after taking two tablets a day; when the dosage was reduced to a single tablet in the morning, the nightmares ceased (78). About half of a group of 50 obese women treated for 20 weeks with various doses, increasing gradually up to the maximum tolerated dose of

160 mg/day and then reduced again, reported of increased dreaming (79). In other studies vivid and disturbing dreams were reported by patients who tools fenfluramine 20–60 mg/day (80,81).

A 43-year-old woman had tightening movements of the head and neck with tongue and throat muscle spasm after a single fenfluramine tablet (82).

With phentermine, adverse effects due to stimulation of the central nervous system are less than with dexamphetamine, although in one study withdrawal because of adverse effects was as high as 16 of 177 patients (9%); 2 of 13 healthy young volunteers withdrew because of unacceptable stimulation (83).

Insomnia is one of the most common adverse effects of phentermine. In a survey in Edinburgh, 20% of the subjects taking phentermine reported insomnia compared with 6% of those taking placebo (4).

Psychological, psychiatric

The effect of fenfluramine is usually not one of stimulation but of calmness or drowsiness. However, in predisposed subjects, it can precipitate psychotic illness. Several published cases illustrate this (84). It is wise to avoid fenfluramine in patients prone to endogenous depression or psychosis.

A schizophreniform-like psychotic disorder was attributed to phentermine in a young woman without a personal or family history of psychiatric disorders (85).

Metabolism

Fenfluramine tends to improve glucose tolerance and to cause small but significant reductions in fasting blood cholesterol and beta-lipoprotein concentrations. Although it has been suggested that metabolic effects may play a role in weight reduction, and that fenfluramine might even be used to reduce blood lipids, the metabolic effects observed are slight and of dubious clinical importance.

Hematologic

Hemolytic anemia has been attributed to fenfluramine (86).

- A 46-year-old woman took fenfluramine for 5 months without incident. Some time later she restarted therapy and after 2 months developed a hemoglobin concentration of 5.1 g/dl, a reticulocyte count of 8.6%, a white cell count of 17.1×10^9/l, and a positive direct Coombs' test, with IgG rhesus antibodies (anti-e and anti-nl). Fenfluramine was withdrawn and the Coombs' test became negative and the patient recovered after prednisolone infusion.

Two other cases are known of anemia in patients who received fenfluramine and propranolol (SED-9, 13).

A clotting disorder has been attributed to fen–phen (87).

- A 35-year-old woman developed calf-pain while taking fen–phen. It resolved when the medications were withdrawn, but her pain returned when fenfluramine was restarted. She had slight rises in aspartate transaminase and lactate dehydrogenase activities and a remarkably shortened prothrombin time. The clot was composed of very thin fibrin fibers. All laboratory abnormalities, including the abnormal fibrin structure, completely resolved when fen–phen was withdrawn.

Thin fibrin fibers are more resistant to lysis and can result from a variety of factors and increase the risk of thrombosis. Whether abnormal fibrin structure and an increased thrombotic tendency play a role in patients who develop fenfluramine-associated pulmonary hypertension and valvular heart disease is a question that deserves further investigation.

Gastrointestinal

Diarrhea, dry mouth, and nausea have been reported (88).

Urinary tract

Phentermine can cause allergic interstitial nephritis (89).

- A 47-year-old mildly obese woman began a weight-reduction program that included anorectic therapy with phentermine and phendimetrazine. She had normal renal function at the start of therapy. After 3 weeks of treatment she fell ill and discontinued treatment. She was subsequently found to have leukocyturia, a rash on her face and chest, and a rise in serum creatinine from 67 to 175 μmol/l (0.8–2.1 mg/dl). Renal biopsy confirmed the diagnosis of acute interstitial nephritis. She was treated with corticosteroids and her renal function returned to normal.

Sexual function

There have been occasional reports of erectile impotence that disappeared on withdrawal. Very high dose regimens of 240 mg/day seem to produce a fairly high incidence of loss of libido, especially in women (90).

Immunologic

Shortly after starting dexfenfluramine 30 mg/day, an 18-year-old woman died of sclerodermal renal crisis (91). Although there have been reports linking long-term fenfluramine use and the development of scleroderma (92,93), this is perhaps the first report implicating dexfenfluramine.

Long-Term Effects

Drug abuse

Fenfluramine has the potential to become a drug of abuse when used in high dosages. Of 438 drug-dependent subjects, 60 gave a history of fenfluramine abuse and experienced euphoria, depersonalization, and perceptual changes after taking up to 400 mg (SED-9, 13). In another report, three of the eight subjects taking fenfluramine 240 mg/day experienced psychedelic states (SED-9, 13). A 28-year-old woman became dependent on fenfluramine at an average dose of 240 mg/day (SEDA-1, 5).

Some cases of toxic psychosis have been reported with abuse doses of phentermine (94).

Drug tolerance

While tolerance to the anorectic effects of fenfluramine appears to set in after 6–12 months, tolerance to its adverse effects is much more rapid in onset (90).

Drug withdrawal

Depression can occur but is more common during the first few days following sudden withdrawal (SED-9, 12). An explanation for the depression and irritability encountered after sudden withdrawal may be a rapid reduction in 5-hydroxytryptamine through which the central effect of fenfluramine is mediated.

Second-Generation Effects

Pregnancy

In a prospective cohort study of 98 women who had taken fen–phen at the recommended daily dose during the first trimester of pregnancy and 233 women who had not taken it, there was no evidence of an increased risk of spontaneous abortion or of major or minor anomalies in the offspring of women who took fen–phen (95). These findings are similar to those of a previous French Collaborative Study (96). However, the risk to the offspring of women who take fen–phen for more prolonged periods and at higher dosages during pregnancy is unknown.

Drug Administration

Drug contamination

There have been reports of herbal remedies adulterated with fenfluramine. There was public health concern in the UK after the referral of a 44-year-old woman with new-onset hypertension, palpitation, anxiety, and a body mass index of 19 kg/m^2. It became apparent that an alarming number of the local population had been attending a particular Chinese herbalist for weight loss remedies. Most had been taking multiple formulations and described "spectacular" results. Several reported considerable cardiovascular symptoms, but they were reassured that Chinese medicines are natural and can cause no harm. Analysis by gas chromatography showed a high concentration of fenfluramine in two of the products (sold as Qian Er and Ma Zin Dol, presumably mimicking the brand name Mazindol). Fenfluramine was also found in the patients' urine. Subsequently, a student nurse was admitted with severe fenfluramine toxicity which developed 2 hours after her first dose of a herbal slimming remedy (97). Following an investigation of this case the Medicines Control Agency published a report on traditional ethnic medicines and the current law (98). Stringent regulation of traditional medicines, at least to the standards of conventional practice, is urgently needed. The hazards associated with the use of dietary supplements containing ma huang, a herbal source of ephedrine, have also been reported (99).

Drug overdose

A systematic study of fenfluramine poisoning in 96 human subjects (38 in detail) has been reported (100). Convulsions and coma occurred in 75% of those who took more than 15 mg/kg. Increased muscle tone, hyper-reflexia, or clonus were common; one-third had hyperthermia, but less than 10% died of it; symptoms could last for days. Blood concentrations of 240–850 ng/ml were associated with tachycardia, mydriasis, and confusion. Deaths occurred beginning at 650 ng/ml. Early gastric lavage, activated charcoal, diazepam for seizures, chlorpromazine and cooling for malignant hyperthermia, and lidocaine and constant electrocardiographic monitoring for extra beats were recommended.

Drug–Drug Interactions

Fluoxetine

Following the withdrawal of the fenfluramines, alternative combinations have been explored as appetite suppressants. In an open study of a combination of phentermine + fluoxetine in 16 obese patients with binge-eating disorder, in the setting of cognitive behavioral therapy, there were significant reductions in weight, binge frequency, and psychological distress by the end of treatment; however, the patients regained most of the weight within 1 year (101). At follow-up at 18 months there was still a reduction in binge eating in patients who continued maintenance treatment. The results did not support the long-term value of adding phentermine/fluoxetine to cognitive behavioral therapy for binge-eating disorder. It is worth emphasizing that it is not known whether phentermine/fluoxetine is also associated with cardiac valvulopathy. Moreover, the recognition that phentermine is a monoamine oxidase inhibitor (102) raises further concerns about its safety.

Halothane

Following a report of death after an anesthetic in a 23-year-old woman who had been taking fenfluramine, a study was undertaken in rabbits to investigate the possibility of an interaction of fenfluramine with halothane. Electrocardiographic and phonocardiographic changes were recorded in rabbits given the combined treatment, and could not readily be reversed with beta-blockers and resuscitative drugs. It was recommended that fenfluramine be discontinued a week before anesthesia (SED-9, 13).

Monoamine oxidase inhibitors

Fenfluramine can cause acute confusion if it is given together with monoamine oxidase inhibitors (SED-9, 9).

References

1. Guy-Grand B. Therapeutic use of dexfenfluramine in obesity. In: Bender, et al., editors. Body Weight Control. The Physiology, Clinical Treatment and Prevention of Obesity. London: Churchill Livingstone, 1987:384.

2. Guy-Grand B, Apfelbaum M, Crepaldi G, Gries A, Lefebvre P, Turner P. International trial of long-term dexfenfluramine in obesity. Lancet 1989;2(8672):1142–5.
3. Owen JH. Acceptability of prolonged release fenfluramine capsules in obese patients in general practice. Postgrad Med J 1975;51(Suppl. 1):176–7.
4. Steel JM, Munro JF, Duncan LJ. A comparative trial of different regimens of fenfluramine and phentermine in obesity. Practitioner 1973;211(262):232–6.
5. Campbell ML, Mathys ML. Pharmacologic options for the treatment of obesity. Am J Health Syst Pharm 2001;58(14):1301–8.
6. Sobel RM. Ruptured retroperitoneal aneurysm in a patient taking phentermine hydrochloride. Am J Emerg Med 1999;17(1):102–3.
7. Fowles RE, Cloward TV, Yowell RL. Endocardial fibrosis associated with fenfluramine–phentermine. N Engl J Med 1998;338(18):1316.
8. Wee CC, Phillips RS, Aurigemma G, Erban S, Kriegel G, Riley M, Douglas PS. Risk for valvular heart disease among users of fenfluramine and dexfenfluramine who underwent echocardiography before use of medication. Ann Intern Med 1998;129(11):870–4.
9. Khan MA, Herzog CA, St Peter JV, Hartley GG, Madlon-Kay R, Dick CD, Asinger RW, Vessey JT. The prevalence of cardiac valvular insufficiency assessed by transthoracic echocardiography in obese patients treated with appetite-suppressant drugs. N Engl J Med 1998;339(11):713–18.
10. Jick H, Vasilakis C, Weinrauch LA, Meier CR, Jick SS, Derby LE. A population-based study of appetite-suppressant drugs and the risk of cardiac-valve regurgitation. N Engl J Med 1998;339(11):719–24.
11. Murthy TH, Weissman NJ. Diet-drug valvulopathy. ACC Curr J Rev 2002;11:17–20.
12. Palmieri V, Arnett DK, Roman MJ, Liu JE, Bella JN, Oberman A, Kitzman DW, Hopkins PN, Morgan D, de Simone G, Devereux RB. Appetite suppressants and valvular heart disease in a population-based sample: the HyperGEN study. Am J Med 2002;112(9):710–15.
13. Tomita T, Zhao Q. Autopsy findings of heart and lungs in a patient with primary pulmonary hypertension associated with use of fenfluramine and phentermine. Chest 2002;121(2):649–52.
14. Abenhaim L, Moride Y, Brenot F, Rich S, Benichou J, Kurz X, Higenbottam T, Oakley C, Wouters E, Aubier M, Simonneau G, Begaud B. Appetite-suppressant drugs and the risk of primary pulmonary hypertension. International Primary Pulmonary Hypertension Study Group. N Engl J Med 1996;335(9):609–16.
15. Anchors M. Fluoxetine is a safer alternative to fenfluramine in the medical treatment of obesity. Arch Intern Med 1997;157(11):1270.
16. Griffen L, Anchors M. Asymptomatic mitral and aortic valve disease is seen in half of the patients taking "phen-fen". Arch Intern Med 1998;158(1):102.
17. Devereux RB. Appetite suppressants and valvular heart disease. N Engl J Med 1998;339(11):765–6.
18. Weissman NJ, Tighe JF Jr, Gottdiener JS, Gwynne JT. An assessment of heart-valve abnormalities in obese patients taking dexfenfluramine, sustained-release dexfenfluramine, or placebo. Sustained-Release Dexfenfluramine Study Group. N Engl J Med 1998;339(11):725–32.
19. Parisi AF. Diet-drug debacle. Ann Intern Med 1998;129(11):903–5.
20. Weissman NJ. Appetite suppressant valvulopathy: a review of current data. Cardiovasc Rev Rep 1999;20:146–55.
21. Adams C, Cohen A. Appetite suppressants and heart valve disorders. Arch Mal Coeur Vaiss 1999;92(9):1213–19.
22. Ewalenko M, Richard C, Vandenbossche JL. Fenfluramines and cardiac valvular lesions. Rev Med Brux 1999;20(5):419–26.
23. Cannistra LB, Cannistra AJ. Regression of multivalvular regurgitation after the cessation of fenfluramine and phentermine treatment. N Engl J Med 1998;339(11):771.
24. Day A. Lessons in women's health: body image and pulmonary disease. CMAJ 1998;159(4):346–9.
25. Anonymous. Cardiac valvulopathy associated with exposure to fenfluramine or dexfenfluramine: U.S. Department of Health and Human Services interim public health recommendations. MMWR Morb Mortal Wkly Rep November 1997;46(45):1061–6.
26. Anonymous. Statement of the American College of Cardiology on recommendations for patients who have used anorectic drugs. Bethesda MD: American College of Cardiology, October 18, 1997.
27. Connolly HM, Crary JL, McGoon MD, Hensrud DD, Edwards BS, Edwards WD, Schaff HV. Valvular heart disease associated with fenfluramine–phentermine. N Engl J Med 1997;337(9):581–8.
28. Redmon B, Raatz S, Bantle JP. Valvular heart disease associated with fenfluramine–phentermine. N Engl J Med 1997;337(24):1773–4.
29. Burger AJ, Sherman HB, Charlamb MJ, Kim J, Asinas LA, Flickner SR, Blackburn GL. Low prevalence of valvular heart disease in 226 phentermine–fenfluramine protocol subjects prospectively followed for up to 30 months J Am Coll Cardiol 1999;34(4):1153–830.
30. Graham DJ, Green L. Further cases of valvular heart disease associated with fenfluramine–phentermine. N Engl J Med 1997;337(9):635.
31. Kurz X, Van Ermen A. Valvular heart disease associated with fenfluramine–phentermine. N Engl J Med 1997;337(24):1772–3.
32. Rasmussen S, Corya BC, Glassman RD. Valvular heart disease associated with fenfluramine–phentermine. N Engl J Med 1997;337(24):1773.
33. Teramae CY, Connolly HM, Grogan M, Miller FA Jr. Diet drug-related cardiac valve disease: the Mayo Clinic echocardiographic laboratory experience. Mayo Clin Proc 2000;75(5):456–61.
34. Gardin JM, Schumacher D, Constantine G, Davis KD, Leung C, Reid CL. Valvular abnormalities and cardiovascular status following exposure to dexfenfluramine or phentermine/fenfluramine. JAMA 2000;283(13):1703–9.
35. Burger AJ, Charlamb MJ, Singh S, Notarianni M, Blackburn GL, Sherman HB. Low risk of significant echocardiographic valvulopathy in patients treated with anorectic drugs. Int J Cardiol 2001;79(2–3):159–65.
36. Shively BK, Roldan CA, Gill EA, Najarian T, Loar SB. Prevalence and determinants of valvulopathy in patients treated with dexfenfluramine. Circulation 1999;100(21):2161–7.
37. Weissman NJ, Tighe. JF Jr, Gottdiener JS, Gwynne JT. Prevalence of valvular-regurgitation associated with dexfenfluramine three to five months after discontinuation of treatment. J Am Coll Cardiol 1999;34(7):2088–95.
38. Mangion JR, Habboub AA, Kamat BR, Tam SK. Transesophageal echocardiography with pathological correlation in severe valvular disease associated with fenfluramine–phentermine. Echocardiography 1999;16(1): 27–30.
39. Tovar EA, Landa DW, Borsari BE. Dose effect of fenfluramine–phentermine in the production of valvular heart disease. Ann Thorac Surg 1999;67(4):1213–14.
40. Garon CF, Oury JH, Duran CM. Virus-like particles in the mitral and tricuspid valves explanted from a patient treated with fenfluramine–phentermine. J Heart Valve Dis 1999;8(2):232.

41. Lepor NE, Gross SB, Daley WL, Samuels BA, Rizzo MJ, Luko SP, Hickey A, Buchbinder NA, Naqvi TZ. Dose and duration of fenfluramine–phentermine therapy impacts the risk of significant valvular heart disease. Am J Cardiol 2000;86(1):107–10.
42. Jollis JG, Landolfo CK, Kisslo J, Constantine GD, Davis KD, Ryan T. Fenfluramine and phentermine and cardiovascular findings: effect of treatment duration on prevalence of valve abnormalities. Circulation 2000;101(17): 2071–77.
43. Steffee CH, Singh HK, Chitwood WR. Histologic changes in three explanted native cardiac valves following use of fenfluramines. Cardiovasc Pathol 1999;8(5):245–53.
44. Roldan CA, Gill EA, Shively BK. Prevalence and diagnostic value of precordial murmurs for valvular regurgitation in obese patients treated with dexfenfluramine. Am J Cardiol 2000;86(5):535–9.
45. Bonow RO, Carabello B, de Leon AC Jr, Edmunds LH Jr, Fedderly BJ, Freed MD, Gaasch WH, McKay CR, Nishimura RA, O'Gara PT, O'Rourke RA, Rahimtoola SH, Ritchie JL, Cheitlin MD, Eagle KA, Gardner TJ, Garson A Jr, Gibbons RJ, Russell RO, Ryan TJ, Smith SC Jr. Guidelines for the management of patients with valvular heart disease: executive summary. A report of the American College of Cardiology/American Heart Association Task Force on Practice Guidelines (Committee on Management of Patients with Valvular Heart Disease). Circulation 1998;98(18):1949–84.
46. Levine HJ, Gaasch WH. Vasoactive drugs in chronic regurgitant lesions of the mitral and aortic valves. J Am Coll Cardiol 1996;28(5):1083–91.
47. Kancherla MK, Salti HI, Mulderink TA, Parker M, Bonow RO, Mehlman DJ. Echocardiographic prevalence of mitral and/or aortic regurgitation in patients exposed to either fenfluramine–phentermine combination or to dexfenfluramine. Am J Cardiol 1999;84(11):1335–8.
48. Mast ST, Jollis JG, Ryan T, Anstrom KJ, Crary JL. The progression of fenfluramine-associated valvular heart disease assessed by echocardiography. Ann Intern Med 2001;134(4):261–6.
49. Weissman NJ, Panza JA, Tighe JF, Gwynne JT. Natural history of valvular regurgitation 1 year after discontinuation of dexfenfluramine therapy. A randomized, double-blind, placebo-controlled trial. Ann Intern Med 2001;134(4):267–73.
50. Prasad A, Mehra M, Park M, Scott R, Uber PA, McFadden PM. Cardiac allograft valvulopathy: a case of donor-anorexigen-induced valvular disease. Ann Thorac Surg 1999;68(5):1840–1.
51. Dahl CF, Allen MR. Regression and progression of valvulopathy associated with fenfluramine and phentermine. Ann Intern Med 2002;136(6):489.
52. Singh JP, Evans JC, Levy D, Larson MG, Freed LA, Fuller DL, Lehman B, Benjamin EJ. Prevalence and clinical determinants of mitral, tricuspid, and aortic regurgitation (the Framingham Heart Study). Am J Cardiol 1999;83(6):897–902.
53. Klein AL, Burstow DJ, Tajik AJ, Zachariah PK, Taliercio CP, Taylor CL, Bailey KR, Seward JB. Age-related prevalence of valvular regurgitation in normal subjects: a comprehensive color flow examination of 118 volunteers. J Am Soc Echocardiogr 1990;3(1):54–63.
54. Bella JN, Devereux RB, Roman MJ, O'Grady MJ, Welty TK, Lee ET, Fabsitz RR, Howard BV. Relations of left ventricular mass to fat-free and adipose body mass: the strong heart study. The Strong Heart Study Investigators Circulation 1998;98(23):2538–44.
55. Brenot F, Herve P, Petitpretz P, Parent F, Duroux P, Simonneau G. Primary pulmonary hypertension and fenfluramine use. Br Heart J 1993;70(6):537–41.
56. Mark EJ, Patalas ED, Chang HT, Evans RJ, Kessler SC. Fatal pulmonary hypertension associated with short-term use of fenfluramine and phentermine. N Engl J Med 1997;337(9):602–6.
57. Bruce CJ, Connolly HM. Valvular heart disease, pulmonary hypertension and fenfluramine–phentermine use. Cardiol Rev 1998;15:17–19.
58. Delcroix M, Kurz X, Walckiers D, Demedts M, Naeije R. High incidence of primary pulmonary hypertension associated with appetite suppressants in Belgium. Eur Respir J 1998;12(2):271–6.
59. Fisher EA, Ruden R. Pulmonary artery pressures and valvular lesions in patients taking diet suppressants. Cardiovasc Rev Rep 1998;19:13–16.
60. Hellermann J, Salomon F. Appetite depressants and pulmonary hypertension. Ther Umsch 1998;55(9):548–50.
61. Goldstein SE, Levy Y, Shoenfeld Y. Development of pulmonary hypertension and multi-valvular damage caused by appetite depressants. Harefuah 1998;135(11):489–92, 568.
62. Heuer L, Benoit W, Heydrich D, Kummer D, Schick J. Pulmonale Hypertonie durch Appetitzügler (Mirapront). [Pulmonary hypertension caused by appetite suppressants (Mirapront).] Chir Praxis 1978;23:497.
63. Kramer MS, Lane DA. Aminorex, dexfenfluramine, and primary pulmonary hypertension. J Clin Epidemiol 1998;51(4):361–4.
64. Rich S, Rubin L, Walker AM, Schneeweiss S, Abenhaim L. Anorexigens and pulmonary hypertension in the United States results from the surveillance of North American pulmonary hypertension. Chest 2000;117(3):870–4.
65. Rothman RB. The age-adjusted mortality rate from primary pulmonary hypertension, in age range 20–54 years, did not increase during the years of peak "phen/fen" use. Chest 2000;118(5):1516–17.
66. Simonneau G, Fartoukh M, Sitbon O, Humbert M, Jagot JL, Herve P. Primary pulmonary hypertension associated with the use of fenfluramine derivatives. Chest 1998;114(Suppl. 3):195S–9S.
67. Nichols WC, Koller DL, Slovis B, Foroud T, Terry VH, Arnold ND, Siemieniak DR, Wheeler L, Phillips JA 3rd, Newman JH, Conneally PM, Ginsburg D, Loyd JE. Localization of the gene for familial primary pulmonary hypertension to chromosome 2q31–32. Nat Genet 1997;15(3):277–80.
68. Morrell NW, Sarybaev AS, Alikhan A, Mirrakhimov MM, Aldashev AA. ACE genotype and risk of high altitude pulmonary hypertension in Kyrghyz highlanders. Lancet 1999;353(9155):814.
69. Lullmann H, Lullmann-Rauch R, Wassermann O. Drug-induced phospholipidoses. II. Tissue distribution of the amphiphilic drug chlorphentermine. CRC Crit Rev Toxicol 1975;4(2):185–218.
70. Hruban Z. Pulmonary and generalized lysosomal storage induced by amphiphilic drugs. Environ Health Perspect 1984;55:53–76.
71. Halliwell WH. Cationic amphiphilic drug-induced phospholipidosis. Toxicol Pathol 1997;25(1):53–60.
72. Archer SL, Djaballah K, Humbert M, Weir KE, Fartoukh M, Dall'ava-Santucci J, Mercier JC, Simonneau G, Dinh-Xuan AT. Nitric oxide deficiency in fenfluramine- and dexfenfluramine-induced pulmonary hypertension. Am J Respir Crit Care Med 1998;158(4):1061–7.
73. Weir EK, Reeve HL, Huang JM, Michelakis E, Nelson DP, Hampl V, Archer SL. Anorexic agents aminorex, fenfluramine, and dexfenfluramine inhibit potassium current in rat pulmonary vascular smooth muscle and cause pulmonary vasoconstriction. Circulation 1996; 94(9):2216–20.

74. Barman SA, Isales CM. Fenfluramine potentiates canine pulmonary vasoreactivity to endothelin-1. Pulm Pharmacol Ther 1998;11(2–3):183–7.
75. Tuder RM, Radisavljevic Z, Shroyer KR, Polak JM, Voelkel NF. Monoclonal endothelial cells in appetite suppressant-associated pulmonary hypertension. Am J Respir Crit Care Med 1998;158(6):1999–2001.
76. Mabadeje AF. Fenfluramine-associated hypertension. West Afr J Pharmacol Drug Res 1975;2(2):145–52.
77. Holmstrand J, Jonsson J. Subjective effects of two anorexigenic agents – fenfluramine and AN 448 in normal subjects. Postgrad Med J 1975;51(Suppl. 1):183–6.
78. Alvi MY. Unusual effect of fenfluramine. BMJ 1969;4(677):237.
79. Innes JA, Watson ML, Ford MJ, Munro JF, Stoddart ME, Campbell DB. Plasma fenfluramine levels, weight loss, and side effects. BMJ 1977;2(6098):1322–5.
80. Hooper AC. Fenfluramine and dreaming. BMJ 1971;3:305.
81. Mullen A, Wilson CWM. Fenfluramine and dreaming. Lancet 1974;2:594.
82. Sananman ML. Letter: dyskinesia after fenfluramine. N Engl J Med 1974;291(8):422.
83. Malcolm AD, Mace PM, Outar KP, Pawan GL. Experimental evaluation of anorexigenic agents in man: a pilot study. Proc Nutr Soc 1972;31(1):12A–14A.
84. Shannon PJ, Leonard D, Kidson MA. Letter: fenfluramine and psychosis. BMJ 1974;3(5930):576.
85. Lee SH, Liu CY, Yang YY. Schizophreniform-like psychotic disorder induced by phentermine: a case report Zhonghua Yi Xue Za Zhi . (Taipei) 1998;61(1):44–7.
86. Nussey AM. Fenfluramine and haemolytic anaemia. BMJ 1973;1(5846):177–8.
87. Carr ME Jr, Carr SL, Martin EJ, Johnson BA. Rapid clot formation and abnormal fibrin structure in a symptomatic patient taking fenfluramine – a case report. Angiology 2001;52(5):361–6.
88. Weintraub M, Sriwatanakul K, Sundaresan PR, Weis OF, Dorn M. Extended-release fenfluramine: patient acceptance and efficacy of evening dosing. Clin Pharmacol Ther 1983;33(5):621–7.
89. Markowitz GS, Tartini A, D'Agati VD. Acute interstitial nephritis following treatment with anorectic agents phentermine and phendimetrazine. Clin Nephrol 1998;50(4):252–4.
90. Pinder RM, Brogden RN, Sawyer PR, Speight TM, Avery GS. Fenfluramine: a review of its pharmacological properties and therapeutic efficacy in obesity. Drugs 1975;10(4):241–323.
91. Jefferson HJ, Jayne DR. Peripheral vasculopathy and nephropathy in association with phentermine. Nephrol Dial Transplant 1999;14(7):1761–3.
92. Korkmaz C, Fresko I, Yazici H. A case of systemic sclerosis that developed under dexfenfluramine use. Rheumatology (Oxford) 1999;38(4):379–80.
93. Aeschlimann A, de Truchis P, Kahn MF. Scleroderma after therapy with appetite suppressants. Report on four cases. Scand J Rheumatol 1990;19(1):87–90.
94. Munro JF. Clinical aspects of the treatment of obesity by drugs: a review. Int J Obes 1979;3(2):171–80.
95. Jones KL, Johnson KA, Dick LM, Felix RJ, Kao KK, Chambers CD. Pregnancy outcomes after first trimester exposure to phentermine/fenfluramine. Teratology 2002;65(3):125–30.
96. Vial T, Robert E, Cartier P, Bertolotti E, Burn A. First-trimester in utero exposure to anorectics: a French collaborative study with special reference to dexfenfluramine. Int J Risk Saf Medical 1992;3:207–14.
97. Metcalfe K, Corns C, Fahie-Wilson M, Mackenzie P. Chinese medicines for slimming still cause health problems. BMJ 2002;324(7338):679.
98. Medicines Control Agency. Traditional ethnic medicines: Public health and compliance with medicines law. London: MCA, 2001.
99. Samenuk D, Link MS, Homoud MK, Contreras R, Theoharides TC, Wang PJ, Estes. NA 3rd. Adverse cardiovascular events temporally associated with ma huang, an herbal source of ephedrine. Mayo Clin Proc 2002;77(1):12–16.
100. Von Muhlendahl KE, Krienke EG. Fenfluramine poisoning. Clin Toxicol 1979;14(1):97–106.
101. Devlin MJ, Goldfein JA, Carino JS, Wolk SL. Open treatment of overweight binge eaters with phentermine and fluoxetine as an adjunct to cognitive-behavioral therapy. Int J Eat Disord 2000;28(3):325–32.
102. Maher TJ, Ulus IH, Wurtman RJ. Phentermine and other monoamine-oxidase inhibitors may increase plasma serotonin when given with fenfluramines. Lancet 1999;353(9146):38.

Fenoterol

See also Beta$_2$-adrenoceptor agonists

General Information

Fenoterol is a beta$_2$-adrenoceptor agonist with higher intrinsic activity than salbutamol; it produces a greater maximal effect and has greater systemic effects at higher than conventional doses. It is available as a multidose pressurized aerosol 100 and 200 micrograms/puff and as a nebulizer solution, respules, 4 ml containing 1.25 mg. A formulation for injection is available in some countries.

Like other beta$_2$-agonists fenoterol has been used in premature labor as well as in asthma.

The safety of fenoterol in severe asthma

Debate continues about the safety of fenoterol in the treatment of severe asthma. A sharp rise in asthma mortality in 1977 in New Zealand provoked debate about the safety of beta$_2$-adrenoceptor agonists, especially the short-acting compound fenoterol. This led to the withdrawal of fenoterol in New Zealand and amendment of the American Asthma Guidelines, suggesting caution in the regular use of beta$_2$-adrenoceptor agonists (1). Although there is evidence linking fenoterol to increased morbidity and mortality in asthma (2), the underlying mechanisms were not known. It was suggested that the increase in mortality might be linked to fatal cardiac dysrhythmias, developing under conditions of asthma-induced hypoxia and high doses of beta$_2$-adrenoceptor agonists (3).

In a report the manufacturers have discussed the epidemiological data linking the use of fenoterol to asthma mortality in New Zealand. They pointed out that asthma mortality started to fall in 1979 while fenoterol sales were still increasing. Sales of fenoterol in Austria, Belgium, and Germany were similar to those in New Zealand at the peak of the New Zealand asthma death epidemic, but asthma mortality in the other countries did not rise. The confounding problem that fenoterol was preferentially prescribed for the more severe cases of asthma was again mentioned. Researchers who adjust their data appropriately for asthma severity have concluded that the increased risk of death from asthma reported in patients using fenoterol is due to underlying severe disease in the patients using fenoterol. The proponents of the hypothesis have responded by pointing out that four case-control studies all showed a significantly higher death rate in patients taking fenoterol than in patients taking other $beta_2$ agonists. They have acknowledged that there is some evidence of selective prescribing of fenoterol in populations studied in New Zealand and Canada. However, they do not agree that the association between fenoterol and asthma deaths is due to confounding by asthma severity. A third group has concluded that the association between fenoterol and severe life-threatening asthma is explained by the preferential prescribing of fenoterol for patients with more severe disease. They have pointed out that doses of fenoterol (up to 3200 micrograms) or salbutamol (up to 1600 micrograms) failed to produce clinically relevant cardiac dysrhythmias in patients with acute severe asthma. This was despite the fact that the two-fold higher dose of fenoterol caused greater systemic $beta_2$ effects. They have concluded that although epidemiological evidence may implicate fenoterol as a cause of asthma deaths it can only generate a hypothesis. The hypothesis is not substantiated by data from carefully controlled pharmacodynamic and pharmacoepidemiological studies. They have supported the view that excessive use of $beta_2$ agonists, including fenoterol, in severe asthma is a marker of inadequate suppression of the underlying inflammatory process, indicating the need to introduce or optimize the dose of glucocorticoids.

It is interesting to reflect that a similar debate followed the rise in asthma deaths in the UK in the 1960s. Most physicians now accept that excessive use of beta-adrenoceptor agonists in worsening asthma indicates inadequate treatment rather than a toxic effect of the drugs.

Organs and Systems

Cardiovascular

The cardiovascular safety of high doses of inhaled fenoterol and salbutamol has been compared in acute severe asthma (SEDA-21, 183). It was concluded that in adequately oxygenated patients a total dose of 3.2 mg of fenoterol or 1.6 mg of salbutamol given over 60 minutes was safe in terms of cardiovascular effects in acute severe asthma.

Electrolyte balance

In one study, an intravenous infusion of fenoterol 0.5–2.0 micrograms/minute was given to 83 patients (aged 28–34 years) in premature labor (SEDA-22, 189). Pretreatment plasma potassium concentrations were normal (median 4.10 mmol/l; 25–75 percentiles 4.10–4.40 mmol/l). During the first 2 hours the serum potassium fell significantly to 2.88 mmol/l (2.80–3.00 mmol/l), but returned to normal during the first day and then remained in the reference range, despite continuous fenoterol administration. No potassium supplements were given. No clinical abnormalities, including cardiac dysrhythmias, due to hypokalemia were seen.

Liver

Liver damage has been attributed to fenoterol (SEDA-21, 183).

- A 27-year-old woman at 31 weeks of a second pregnancy was admitted in premature labor and treated with intravenous fenoterol 7.5 mg/day. Within 48 hours her liver enzymes were raised. Because the liver function tests became progressively worse and she had epigastric pain and severe nausea, the fenoterol was withdrawn after 9 days. The liver function tests quickly normalized and there appeared to be a clear relation between the administration of fenoterol and the occurrence of liver damage.

References

1. Bremner P, Burgess CD, Crane J, McHaffie D, Galletly D, Pearce N, Woodman K, Beasley R. Cardiovascular effects of fenoterol under conditions of hypoxaemia. Thorax 1992;47(10):814–17.
2. Burggraaf J, Westendorp RG, in't Veen JC, Schoemaker RC, Sterk PJ, Cohen AF, Blauw GJ. Cardiovascular side effects of inhaled salbutamol in hypoxic asthmatic patients. Thorax 2001;56(7):567–9.
3. Lowe MD, Rowland E, Brown MJ, Grace AA. Beta(2) adrenergic receptors mediate important electrophysiological effects in human ventricular myocardium. Heart 2001;86(1):45–51.

Fenproporex hydrochloride

See also Anorectic drugs

General Information

Fenproporex, one of the lesser known anorectic drugs, is structurally related to amfetamine, to which it is rapidly metabolized after oral ingestion. Stimulatory effects, somnolence, and electroencephalographic abnormalities are reported to be the major undesired reactions (1).

Reference

1. Choteau P. Deux cas d'iatrogénie paradoxales par médications encéphalotropes. [Two cases of paradoxical iatrogenic effects induced by encephalotropic drugs.] J Sci Méd Lille 1977;95:287.

Fenspiride

General Information

Fenspiride is a bronchodilator and anti-inflammatory drug. Two in vitro studies have suggested possible mechanisms for these effects.

Functional studies in human isolated bronchi showed that fenspiride causes a shift to the left of concentration effect curves for relaxation induced by isoprenaline and sodium nitroprusside. Biochemical studies confirmed that phosphodiesterase type IV (cyclic AMP-specific) and phosphodiesterase type V (cyclic GMP-specific) are the main phosphodiesterase isoforms present in human bronchi. Fenspiride inhibited both isoforms. Fenspiride facilitates relaxation of human bronchial smooth muscle in vitro, and this effect may be due to inhibition of phosphodiesterases IV and V.

In a human lung epithelial cell line, in which histamine increased the intracellular calcium concentration and the formation of eicosanoids, this response was antagonized by the histamine H_1 receptor antagonist diphenhydramine but unaffected by the H_2 receptor antagonist cimetidine. Fenspiride inhibited H_1 receptor-induced calcium increase. Histamine also caused a biphasic increase in arachidonic acid release, which was inhibited by fenspiride. This study suggests a further mechanism that would promote anti-inflammatory and bronchodilator properties.

The findings in several thousand patients treated by 800 general practitioners have been reported (1). There were mild adverse effects in 10% of the patients, but they were not thought to be specific to the drug (gastrointestinal, neurovegetative).

Fenspiride has been used to treat 392 adults with acute respiratory tract infections, most of whom were considered to have a moderate symptom score that improved with 7 days of treatment with fenspiride. Adverse reactions were classified as mild and tolerance was excellent; only 20 of 392 patients discontinued the drug.

Reference

1. Brems H, Pauly N, Thomas J. Fenspiride (Pneumorel 80) dans le traitement des affections aiguës des voies respiratoires. Ars Med 1984;39:55–8.

Fentanyl

General Information

Fentanyl citrate is a synthetic opioid 1000 times more potent than pethidine. It has a relatively short duration of action, and its effects are rapidly reversed by opioid antagonists (1). It is useful (2) but has typical opioid adverse effects.

The analgesic effect of fentanyl 1.5 μg/kg has been compared with that of tramadol 1.5 mg/kg in 61 patients receiving standardized anesthetics for day-case arthroscopic knee surgery (3). Opioid adverse effects and analgesia were similar in the two groups.

The analgesic effects and adverse effects profiles of subcutaneous fentanyl and subcutaneous morphine have been compared in a double-blind, crossover, 6-day study in 23 patients with cancer pain (4). There were no significant differences in pain scores between the two drugs and no changes in the level of acute confusion (using the Saskatoon Delirium Checklist) or cognitive impairment (in tests of semantic fluency and trail-making tests). Fentanyl caused significantly less constipation. The patients in this study were highly stable and compliant, and the results cannot be generalized.

Organs and Systems

Cardiovascular

A hypertensive crisis occurred in a patient with a previously unknown pheochromocytoma (5).

Respiratory

Even small doses of fentanyl can cause respiratory depression. Delayed respiratory depression can be a particular problem in the elderly, in whom the half-life is approximately three times longer than in younger patients (6). Respiratory depression has been reversed with nalbuphine; doxapram could only antagonize this effect for 2–5 minutes (7). However, the need for prolonged treatment of respiratory depression with naloxone, because of pharmacokinetic variability and/or transdermal drug reservoir, has been emphasized by several authors (SEDA-16, 80) (SEDA-17, 80).

Fentanyl can evoke the pulmonary chemoreflex, as evidenced by 50% of patients in one study and 28% in another, who coughed after the administration of fentanyl through a central line (SEDA-16, 79) (8). The coughing caused by fentanyl is inhibited by terbutaline (SEDA-21, 88).

Cough has been attributed to fentanyl (9).

- A 7-year-old boy with trisomy 21 (Down syndrome) had explosive coughing, 30 seconds after fentanyl 50 μg (2 μg/kg) had been injected and flushed through an intravenous cannula. The cough was unproductive and persisted in spasmodic bursts for a further 2–3 minutes until anesthesia was induced with propofol 60 mg and atracurium 15 mg intravenously. The coughing immediately ceased. A petechial rash in the conjunctivae and periorbital regions was subsequently noted and disappeared by the end of the first postoperative day.

Nervous system

Movement disorders after withdrawal of continuous infusion, without the characteristic autonomic signs of opioid withdrawal, have been reported in children (SEDA-17, 80).

Fentanyl-induced seizures have been reported (10).

Life-threatening complications have included raised intracranial pressure and critically reducing cerebral perfusion (11).

- A 55-year-old man was given fentanyl 0.05 mg for treatment of left chest pain and immediately developed an acute confusional state and fluctuating tetraparesis (12). The symptoms abated 12 hours after withdrawal. A provocation test confirmed that fentanyl 0.1 mg was enough to cause myoclonic and dystonic reactions with increased agitation. Administration of intravenous naloxone 0.8 mg improved the condition.
- A 14-year-old girl developed a dystonic reaction to fentanyl 50 μg given as a general anesthesia for dental extraction; her abnormal movements stopped completely after 3 days (13).

Fentanyl can displace bilirubin from albumin in neonates, with a risk of kernicterus; other drugs should be used (SEDA-17, 81).

Psychological, psychiatric

Mood alteration during patient-controlled epidural anesthesia with either morphine or fentanyl was compared in a randomized, double-blind study of 52 patients undergoing elective hip or knee joint arthroplasty under general anesthesia (14). Mood was assessed preoperatively and at 24, 48, and 72 hours, using the bipolar version of the Profile of Mood States. Pain intensity postoperatively did not vary with morphine or fentanyl and, as expected, both fentanyl and morphine users had significant somnolence, pruritus, and nausea compared with baseline. With morphine, the mean score for measures of composure/anxiety, elation/depression and clear-headedness/confusion increased, indicating a change toward the more positive pole, but there were negative changes for the fentanyl users' scores for five of the six components of the Profile of Mood States. The difference in test scores between morphine and fentanyl was significant at 48 hours of patient-controlled anesthesia and 24 hours after withdrawal. There was no correlation between mood scores and pain scores, and mood scores with fentanyl fell with increasing plasma concentrations. Previous investigations have shown transient positive feelings with intravenous fentanyl, followed by more negative feelings in the longer term. The authors suggested that the differences in mood between the two groups may have been explained by differences in the lipid solubility and pharmacokinetics of epidural morphine and fentanyl.

Urinary tract

There have been two cases of urinary retention leading to renal pelvocalyceal dilatation as a result of continuous infusion of fentanyl (3 μg/kg/hour) in premature neonates (15). In both cases the problem was resolved by inserting an indwelling catheter.

Skin

A rash has been attributed to fentanyl (16).

- A 70-year-old man with metastatic cancer of the colon was given transdermal fentanyl 50 mg for analgesia. After 10 days he developed an itchy pustular eruption on the trunk and limbs. The lesions subsided on withdrawal of fentanyl. When he restarted transdermal fentanyl 2 months later, the skin lesions reappeared and became more generalized. The pustules were scattered, sparse, and superficial, and included the tongue and buccal mucosa, but not the conjunctivae or genitalia. A history of eosinophilia suggested an immunoallergic origin.

Like other opioids, fentanyl can cause pruritus. Prophylactic intravenous ondansetron 8 mg with hyperbaric bupivacaine 7–10 mg and fentanyl 25 μg significantly reduced the incidence of intrathecal fentanyl-induced pruritus in 125 patients undergoing knee arthroscopy or urological surgery in a randomized, double-blind, placebo-controlled trial (17). The incidence of pruritus was 39% with ondansetron and 68% with placebo.

Musculoskeletal

There have been three reports and a prospective study of muscle rigidity after fentanyl administration in neonates (18,19).

- Two neonates had transient (0.5–2 minutes) chest wall rigidity after intravenous boluses of fentanyl 2 and 4 μg/kg. They were already compromised, one with a respiratory distress syndrome and one with a diaphragmatic hernia.
- A premature male infant of 28 weeks gestation was given an intravenous bolus of fentanyl 3 μg/kg before intubation and this was followed by isolated rigidity of the tongue lasting 20 seconds (18).

In a prospective case series study of 89 preterm and term infants who received fentanyl out of a total of 404 neonatal intensive care patients in one year, eight neonates (9%) had chest wall rigidity (19). The spectrum of neuromuscular activity extends from mild muscle rigidity through abnormal muscle movements (chewing) to tonic-clonic movements. In two cases there was laryngospasm with chest wall rigidity. In all cases low-dose fentanyl (3–6 μg/kg) had been given for analgesia or sedation.

Chest wall rigidity, sometimes lasting for more than 24 hours and causing hypoxia, can occur postoperatively; it can be attenuated with naloxone or neuromuscular blockers (SEDA-22, 98) (20).

Second-Generation Effects

Pregnancy

The efficacy of intrathecal fentanyl and sufentanil for labor analgesia has been studied in 75 nulliparous women in a two-part comparison (21). In the first phase, 20 subjects received varying doses of fentanyl; the ED_{50} of intrathecal fentanyl for 60 minutes of labor analgesia was 18 μg, with a potency ratio of intrathecal sufentanil to intrathecal fentanyl of 4.4. In the second phase, 55 subjects participated in a double-blind, randomized comparison of the efficacy and safety of either intrathecal fentanyl 36 μg or sufentanil 8 μg. Sufentanil gave 25 minutes longer analgesia than fentanyl. There were no significant differences in adverse effects between the two groups: 83% had pruritus and 27% of those given sufentanil and 10% of those given fentanyl had nausea.

In a randomized, double-blind, placebo-controlled study of whether patient-controlled epidural fentanyl could produce effective and safe postoperative analgesia following 25 μg of spinal fentanyl at cesarean section in 36 patients, the fentanyl group used a mean of 23 μg/hour of fentanyl compared with 27 μg/hour in the control group (22). There was pruritus in 15 patients given fentanyl compared with one control; 9 given fentanyl had mild or moderate drowsiness during the operation compared with 8 controls. Postoperative nausea, pruritus, and drowsiness did not differ between the two groups.

In a randomized, controlled trial, 52 patients in labor were randomly given either intrathecal fentanyl 25 μg with saline or fentanyl 25 μg with magnesium sulfate 50 mg as part of a combined spinal-epidural technique

(21). The incidence of pruritus with fentanyl alone was 65%, significantly lower than with fentanyl plus magnesium sulfate (77%). However, fentanyl plus magnesium sulfate produced significantly better and longer-lasting pain control, potentially reducing postoperative opioid requirements.

Susceptibility Factors

Other features of the patient

When the concentration of α_1-acid glycoprotein is reduced, with reduced binding, highly protein-bound basic drugs, such as fentanyl, should be given with caution in order to avoid high unbound concentrations and unwanted effects (SEDA-17, 81).

Drug Administration

Drug formulations

- A woman suffered sedation, localized erythematous lesions on the hands, and reduced appetite with weight loss after removing transdermal fentanyl patches from her daughter's skin and replacing them without wearing protective gloves (23). She had severe headaches, night sweats, irritability, nausea, and insomnia. When she used gloves, her weight gradually increased and the sedation abated.
- A 57-year-old woman using transdermal fentanyl (75 μg/hour) developed a reduced respiratory rate and bilateral pinpoint pupils when an upper body warming blanket was used as a normal postoperative procedure (24). The resultant increase in skin temperature significantly enhanced skin perfusion, and increased the systemic absorption of fentanyl from the intracutaneous fentanyl depot, leading to symptoms of opioid overdose. She recovered after removal of the fentanyl patch and the intravenous administration of naloxone 60 μg.

Oral transmucosal fentanyl administration, avoiding first-pass metabolism, produces analgesia and sedation in both adults and children undergoing short painful outpatient procedures. The quality of analgesia is good, and the adverse effects are those typical of the opioids. However, an unusual reaction, with agitation and hyperactivity, progressing over a week to delirium, has been reported. Mild impairment of hepatic and renal function, with accumulation of norfentanyl, has been postulated as a possible mechanism (SEDA-20, 77).

Drug additives

Bupivacaine and/or adrenaline

The addition of bupivacaine and/or adrenaline to epidural fentanyl analgesia has also been studied in 100 women after elective cesarean section. All received fentanyl (3 μg/ml) by patient-controlled analgesia (PCA) for 48 hours and were randomly assigned double-blind to receive either bupivacaine 0.01%, ephedrine 0.5 μg/ml, both, or neither (25). Patients who received fentanyl alone made more attempts at PCA than the other groups, suggesting that this regimen was less effective and the higher dose of fentanyl used perhaps contributed to a higher incidence of nausea and urinary retention and to a higher frequency of severe pruritus. The authors suggested that with lower doses of fentanyl there was less rostral spread of the drug and lower concentrations at the brain stem, thus reducing adverse effects. Breast-fed neonates were neurologically assessed at 2 and 48 hours by a pediatrician and, despite the different fentanyl requirements of mothers, neurobehavioral scores were equally high in the different groups.

Bupivacaine

Effective postoperative pain relief can be obtained with a mixture of fentanyl and bupivacaine, which not only provides better analgesia than either drug alone, but also fewer adverse effects. There have been several studies of the efficacy of this mixture, using different doses and routes of administration, the addition of clonidine, and in comparison with morphine.

In a randomized, double-blind study in 56 patients, continuous infusion of fentanyl (1 μg/kg/hour or 0.5 μg/kg/hour) and bupivacaine 0.1 mg/kg/hour, with intravenous morphine PCA as rescue analgesia, produced better pain relief after knee ligament operations than epidural saline combined with intravenous morphine PCA (26). There was a non-significant increase in nausea in the fentanyl group.

In another randomized, double-blind study, 84 parturients requesting epidural analgesia were given either bupivacaine 20 ml only, followed by intravenous fentanyl 60 μg or bupivacaine 20 ml with fentanyl 60 μg followed by intravenous saline (27). The minimum local analgesia concentration (MLAC) of bupivacaine + intravenous fentanyl was 0.064% w/v and the MLAC of bupivacaine + epidural fentanyl was 0.034% w/v. The epidural fentanyl solution significantly increased the analgesic potency of bupivacaine by a factor of 1.88 compared with intravenous fentanyl. This was associated with increased pruritus with epidural fentanyl.

Women scheduled for cesarean section (n = 32) were given spinal bupivacaine 10 mg (0.5%) or spinal bupivacaine 5 mg (0.5%) plus fentanyl 25 μg (28). Those given fentanyl had adequate spinal anesthesia for cesarean section with fewer adverse effects (nausea and hypotension). This observation was reproduced by spinal anesthesia with bupivacaine 4 mg plus fentanyl 20 μg, which provided adequate spinal anesthesia for surgical repair of hip fracture in elderly patients, with fewer adverse effects than bupivacaine 10 mg (29).

Bupivacaine, clonidine

Different combinations of fentanyl, bupivacaine, and clonidine were investigated in a multicenter (6 sites) trial of 78 women undergoing elective cesarean section under "spinal block" (30). In some cases, this appeared to imply intrathecal administration, and in others combined intrathecal and epidural administration. Patients received hyperbaric bupivacaine alone, or with 75 μg of clonidine, or with 75 μg of clonidine and 12.5 μg of fentanyl. There were no reported hemodynamic differences between the groups, but sedation and pruritus were significantly more common in those who received fentanyl, occurring in 65% and 25% of subjects respectively. Apgar scores and umbilical artery blood pH were unaffected by the drug regimens.

Bupivacaine or ropivacaine

The addition of fentanyl 1 μg/ml to ropivacaine 7.5 mg/ml did not improve nerve blockade by axillary brachial plexus anesthesia in a double-blind, randomized study in 30 patients undergoing orthopedic procedures (31). In another double-blind, randomized study, 60 patients receiving axillary brachial plexus blockade were given 0.25% bupivacaine 40 mg, 0.25% bupivacaine 40 mg plus fentanyl 2.5 μg/ml, or 0.125% bupivacaine 40 mg plus fentanyl 2.5 μg/ml (32). The addition of fentanyl 2.5 μg/ml prolonged sensory and motor blockade without any improvement in the onset of anesthesia and no significant increase in adverse effects. These two studies have reaffirmed the current position of conflicting results in studies of the benefits of adding fentanyl to local anesthetics for peripheral nerve blockade.

Ropivacaine

In a randomized, placebo-controlled study, a mixture of ropivacaine 0.2% and fentanyl 2 μg/ml plus a background infusion of 5 ml/hour was given to 20 patients for postoperative patient-controlled epidural analgesia after gynecological surgery. Another 21 patients were given the same mixture without the background infusion. Both groups were monitored hourly for arterial blood pressure, heart rate, and respiratory rate, and pain, sedation, motor blockade, and sensory levels were monitored every 6 hours (33). There was no difference in pain scores or patient satisfaction scores between the two groups, but the patients who received the background infusion had a higher incidence of adverse effects (71 versus 30%). The authors suggested that there was no additional benefit in using a background infusion.

Fentanyl 2 μg/ml has been used in combination with ropivacaine 2 mg/ml to determine its impact on the quality of postoperative analgesia and the incidence of adverse effects after colonic surgery in 155 patients scheduled for elective colonic surgery in a multicenter, double-blind, randomized study (34). The incidences of hypotension and pruritus in those given fentanyl were significantly increased, although they had better analgesic control. They also had an increased incidence of serious adverse effects affecting the respiratory, cardiovascular, and genitourinary systems.

The ideal combination strength of ropivacaine with fentanyl for postoperative epidural analgesia has been investigated in two studies. In a double-blind, randomized study, 30 patients undergoing lower abdominal surgery received one of three solutions for PCA after a standardized combined epidural and general anesthetic: ropivacaine 0.2% plus fentanyl 4 μg, ropivacaine 0.1% plus fentanyl 2 μg, or ropivacaine 0.05% plus fentanyl 1 μg (35). All three solutions produced equivalent analgesia. Motor block secondary to the ropivacaine was significantly more frequent and intense with ropivacaine 0.2% plus fentanyl 4 μg. Pruritus, nausea, sedation, and hypotension occurred equally often in the three groups and were mild. It was therefore inferred that ropivacaine 0.2% plus fentanyl 4 μg is preferable for analgesia after lower abdominal surgery.

Sufentanil

There was no difference in analgesic efficacy or the incidence of adverse effects when fentanyl 100 μg was compared with sufentanil 20 μg in women in labor who requested epidural analgesia (36).

Bupivacaine or lidocaine

The addition of clonidine or fentanyl to local anesthetics for single shot caudal blocks has been studied in 64 children undergoing bilateral correction of vesicoureteral reflux randomized into four groups (37). The control group received a mixture of 0.25% bupivacaine with adrenaline plus 1% lidocaine; other groups received the same combination plus 1.5 μg/kg of clonidine, or the control combination plus 1 μg/kg of fentanyl, or the control combination plus 0.5 μg/kg of fentanyl plus 0.75 μg/kg of clonidine. The addition of either clonidine or fentanyl significantly prolonged anesthesia, and during recovery the groups receiving local anesthetics alone or with the addition of fentanyl alone had significantly increased heart rates. Two of the children who received extradural fentanyl had a transient reduction in oxygen of saturation to 92% in the first hour of recovery. One of these was from those who received fentanyl alone, while one had received fentanyl plus clonidine. Vomiting occurred only in children exposed to fentanyl (nine of 29 subjects). This is the first report of respiratory depression in children after the caudal administration of fentanyl or clonidine, this adverse effect having been previously described with extradural opioids and clonidine in adults.

Lidocaine

In 100 patients undergoing arthroscopic outpatient surgery minidose spinal lidocaine plus fentanyl (0.5% lidocaine 20 mg plus fentanyl 20 μg) has been compared with traditional spinal anesthesia (1% lidocaine 30 ml with titrated intravenous propofol infusion) (38). The study was randomized and prospective but unblinded. Whereas those given local anesthesia were more likely to have pain requiring analgesic medication before discharge (44 versus 20%), those given spinal anesthesia group were more likely to have nausea (8 versus 22%) or pruritus (8 versus 68%). Both techniques provided a high degree of patient satisfaction, with comparable efficacy both intraoperatively and postoperatively.

Drug dosage regimens

Fentanyl is widely used for obstetric analgesia and the dose–response relation for intrathecal fentanyl has been examined in a randomized study of 84 nulliparous full-term parturients in labor (39). They received intrathecal doses of fentanyl of 5–45 μg and visual analogue scales were used to measure analgesia and adverse effects. The mean duration of anesthesia increased in the dose range 5–25 μg of fentanyl and then reached a plateau. Adequate analgesia was obtained with all doses of fentanyl above 10 μg. Maternal systolic blood pressure was not significantly affected at any dose, although diastolic blood pressure fell significantly at 10–30 minutes after fentanyl. Nausea and vomiting were uncommon, but pruritus was common in all groups and was more severe with higher doses of fentanyl. Fetal heart rate did not change significantly with fentanyl at any dose, although the authors acknowledged that they did not undertake continuous fetal heart tracing. They concluded that there is no benefit in using doses of intrathecal fentanyl above 25 μg when fentanyl is used as the sole analgesic agent in labor.

Drug administration route

Opioids have traditionally been given intramuscularly and intravenously. Other methods of administration are oral, subcutaneous, rectal, intrathecal, and extradural. Novel routes include intranasal, inhalational, intra-articular, and transdermal.

Buccal

Oral transmucosal fentanyl citrate has two advantages: it is more acceptable as a flavored lozenge than an oral elixir or tablet would be, especially in children, and 25% goes directly into the systemic circulation without first-pass metabolism (SEDA-20, 77). Its main adverse effect is dose-dependent nausea and/or vomiting, which occurs in 25–50% of patients. In a double-blind, placebo-controlled comparison of oral transmucosal fentanyl citrate (10 μg/kg) and oral oxycodone (0.2 mg/kg) in outpatient wound care procedures in 22 children, there were similar outcomes and no adverse effects in either group (40).

Transdermal

Fentanyl can be used transdermally because of its high solubility in both fat and water, low molecular weight, high analgesic potency, and fewer adverse effects, especially gastrointestinal symptoms (41). It is easy to administer and can be given at 3-day intervals. Transdermal fentanyl has been extensively reviewed in patients with chronic cancer pain (22) and in a review in which the possibilities and techniques available for acute and/or chronic pain relief were considered (42).

Transdermal fentanyl has an adverse effects profile similar to that associated with parenteral administration (SEDA-20, 77). Local erythema and rash have been reported (43), as well as the usual opioid adverse effects. However, an unusual reaction, with progressive agitation to acute delirium, has occurred (SEDA-20, 79).

Local heating and cutaneous hyperthermia of the patch area can cause lethal problems of overdose, owing to increased release and absorption (SEDA-18, 80) (SEDA-19, 83).

Transdermal administration of fentanyl has been extensively reviewed (44). In systemic availability studies, 92% of the fentanyl dose delivered from the transdermal therapeutic system into the skin reached the systemic circulation as unchanged unmetabolized fentanyl (41). Morphine, codeine, and hydromorphone are not good candidates for transdermal administration. Pethidine has a high transdermal permeability but poor analgesic potency. Besides fentanyl, only sufentanil and buprenorphine would be suitable opioids for transdermal administration (45).

There are three techniques used for the transdermal administration of fentanyl. The transdermal therapeutic system (TTS) is a membrane-controlled system designed to release fentanyl at a constant rate for up to 3 days, and is useful in patients with chronic cancer pain (46). There are still limited and predominantly uncontrolled studies that show that TTS fentanyl is useful in chronic pain of neuropathic or somatic origin. An open randomized, crossover trial in 18 patients with painful chronic pancreatitis concluded that TTS fentanyl should not be the first-choice analgesic, because of a high incidence of skin adverse effects and low analgesic effects compared with morphine (47).

TTS fentanyl is not useful in acute or postoperative pain, because of the risk of respiratory depression due to the long delay and decay time, which do not allow adequate dose finding (44). Some patients have acute symptoms of morphine withdrawal, in spite of adequate pain control, when they are converted from morphine to transdermal fentanyl. The mechanism has not yet been determined (48,49).

Transdermal fentanyl was the cause of an opioid overdose when a 77-year-old man with a history of severe arthritis developed respiratory failure after starting epidural diamorphine–bupivacaine mixture for postoperative pain (50). The fentanyl patch was removed, the epidural infusion was stopped, and naloxone was given to counteract the excessive opioid effects.

Fentanyl transdermal delivery systems (FTDS) use an unsealed multilaminate system containing a solid matrix, in which fentanyl is embedded instead of the reservoir designed in the TTS. FTDS is not to be recommended for routine postoperative pain treatment, even though it has a faster onset of action (4–6 hours) after cases of fentanyl toxicity, especially respiratory depression. FTDS has not been investigated adequately in chronic pain and is not expected to be superior to the TTS technique.

Iontophoretic transdermal application of opioids is another technique that is currently being tested. The factors that affect the delivery of opioids like fentanyl and sufentanil by this technique include the physicochemical nature of the drug solution, the voltage used, and the duration and nature of the current used (51,52).

An electrotransport therapeutic system (ETS) for fentanyl has been developed. Preliminary studies show that ETS of fentanyl may be useful for the treatment of acute pain (53).

Transdermal fentanyl has been compared with modified-release oral formulations of morphine among 504 patients with advanced cancer in a multicenter, cross-sectional quality-of-life study using four widely validated scales plus original scales, generated and validated for this study (54). The authors used conversion rates "often reported in the literature" to calculate that the fentanyl group used significantly more opiate (200–300 mg of morphine-equivalent units/day) than the oral morphine users (195 mg/day). Despite this, transdermal fentanyl patients reported fewer and less bothersome adverse effects, although these were not separately identified; 50% reported never having any adverse effects compared with 36% of morphine users without adverse effects, although measures of pain intensity showed no significant difference between the two groups. Subgroup analysis by sex showed that the difference in adverse effects between the two modes of administration was significant only in men. However, it should be noted that the mean ages of the two treatment groups were significantly different, a fact that may qualify the reported results.

Transdermal fentanyl avoids the discomfort of injections and reduces fluctuations in drug concentrations. In an open study of transdermal fentanyl patches 50 μg for postoperative pain management in 15 thoracotomy patients, two patients had nausea and one had erythema over the site of application of the patch (55).

Transdermal fentanyl in chronic cancer pain control has been extensively reviewed (22). Data from non-blinded, randomized trials suggest that it is as effective as modified-release oral morphine and that the most common adverse effects include nausea, vomiting, and constipation. The most serious adverse effect reported was hypoventilation, which occurred in about 2% of patients. Skin reactions occurred in 1–3%. A number of non-comparative trials have described the use of transdermal fentanyl for periods of at least a year without serious adverse effects.

In a follow-up study of 78 patients with cancer who participated in a crossover, randomized study of transdermal fentanyl (mean final dose 100 μg/hour) and oral morphine for 4 weeks, the incidences of skin reactions and gastrointestinal symptoms were low (56). Other adverse effects reported were breakthrough pain, light-headedness, and diarrhea. In the original randomized study, which lasted 15 days, there was significantly less constipation with fentanyl than with morphine (57). These results suggest that many patients have stable analgesic requirements with transdermal fentanyl up to the time of death, with no need for additional medication.

In a questionnaire survey of 1005 patients, only 11 had chronic pain from non-malignant disease while taking transdermal fentanyl (58). Their physicians were asked to provide information about their reasons for switching to transdermal fentanyl and were then surveyed until withdrawal of fentanyl because of death, change in analgesic regimen, or serious adverse effects. Modified-release morphine (median dose 90 mg/day) was used in 72% of patients before switching to fentanyl. More than 20% of the cohort had received no continuous opioid medication before the start of transdermal therapy. Most of the patients were switched to fentanyl because of inadequate analgesia or opioid-induced gastrointestinal symptoms. The simplicity of administration and patients' wishes were also contributory factors. Transdermal fentanyl was discontinued primarily because patients died (46%); other reasons included inadequate pain relief (10%), pain relief with another analgesic regimen (10%), adverse effects (5%), rejection of transdermal therapy by the patient (6%), and other unspecified causes, such as pathological fractures and anemia (16%). There were opioid-related adverse effects in 26% of the patients. Serious neurotoxic effects, such as hallucinations (0.2%), withdrawal symptoms (0.1%), or convulsions (0.1%), were rare.

Under controlled conditions, transdermal fentanyl is a useful option for direct conversion from mild to strong opioids in cancer patients. In addition, 25 μg/hour daily incremental steps of transdermal fentanyl can be made by palliative care specialists, if it is required for cancer pain management (59).

Transdermal fentanyl for chronic non-cancer pain control has been studied in two open trials (60,61). In a multicenter, open, randomized study of 256 patients with a history of chronic non-cancer pain, 65% preferred transdermal fentanyl, whereas 28% preferred modified-release oral morphine. Subjective pain control and quality of life were significantly better in the patients who used transdermal fentanyl. Despite a preference for transdermal fentanyl, more patients withdrew because of adverse effects in the first fentanyl period (16%) than in the first morphine period (9%). The difference could have been related to patients' previous experience of morphine, with enhanced tolerance of its adverse effects.

In the second study, 35 patients with severe AIDS-related chronic pain were recruited in a prospective, open, before/after comparison of the analgesic efficacy and adverse effects profile of a stable dose of transdermal fentanyl (25–300 μg/hour) or oral morphine (less than 45 mg/day) for 15 consecutive days (61). Transdermal fentanyl alleviated chronic pain and those who were already dependent on an opioid needed less fentanyl for the same analgesic result.

The long-term use of transdermal fentanyl in patients with chronic non-cancer pain (back pain, leg pain, arthritic pain, trigeminal neuralgia, and intestinal cystitis), which is controversial, has been discussed (62). Transdermal fentanyl was effective and safe and improved quality of life and independent living. However, these case reports were collected by authors closely associated with the company that manufactures transdermal fentanyl patches; a degree of case selectivity and bias might have occurred.

In a prospective study, 64 patients with a recent history of at least one vertebral fracture caused by primary and secondary osteoporosis were recruited from six osteoporosis centers in Germany between December 1999 and April 2001 (63). Transdermal fentanyl 25 μg/hour was the recommended starting dose, with incremental steps of 25 μg/hour if there was insufficient analgesia. Treatment was stopped after less than 28 days in 15 patients (23%). In 10 of these, fentanyl was stopped because of nausea and/or vomiting and/or dizziness. In 49 patients, pain at rest (55% reduction) and on motion (47% reduction) abated significantly from baseline. The starting dose of 25 μg/hour of fentanyl was sufficient in most patients (70%).

The use of transdermal fentanyl in 113 patients with undertreated chronic cancer pain was studied in a non-randomized, uncontrolled, open study for 42 days (64). The mean dose of fentanyl increased from 25 μg/hour to 117 μg/hour between the start and end of the study. By day 3, six patients reported sleepiness and two reported dizziness; five reported nausea and two had vomiting, and by days 21–42 four of the 100 patients who completed the study had severe nausea and vomiting. Non-compliance was not related to the adverse effects of fentanyl, but to insufficient pain control (nine patients) and/or death (three patients).

Epidural

In view of the popularity of fentanyl as an epidural analgesic in labor, its site of action is of some interest, and this has been examined in a randomized study in 55 parturients who received 0.125% bupivacaine plus one of three treatments: epidural saline plus intravenous saline; epidural fentanyl (20 μg/hour) plus intravenous saline; epidural saline plus intravenous fentanyl (20 μg/hour) (65). Study treatments were continuously infused, while epidural bupivacaine was patient-controlled. There was a significant reduction (28%) in bupivacaine use with epidural but not intravenous fentanyl, but there was no significant difference in the incidence of adverse effects. This result suggested that the analgesic effects of epidural fentanyl in labor are due to a spinal mechanism, rather than to systemic absorption and a supraspinal effect. However, the authors acknowledged various limitations of their study and commented that they were able to use low doses of fentanyl because of the concomitant use of bupivacaine, which acts synergistically. It is possible that this synergy allows effective analgesia of the visceral afferents at a spinal level without the need for the higher doses that are required for analgesia with fentanyl alone. Higher doses of fentanyl may mask this spinal effect.

In a prospective study of 1030 mixed surgical patients receiving patient-controlled epidural analgesia with 0.05% bupivacaine and fentanyl 4 μg/ml, the incidence of adverse effects was broadly as expected (66): 17% had pruritus, 15% nausea, 13% sedation, 6.8% hypotension, 2% motor block, and 0.3% respiratory depression. Two patients required naloxone for respiratory depression and sedation. Analgesia was terminated electively in 82%, 12% of cases were terminated owing to a displaced catheter, and 3% of cases required anticoagulation, while infection, adverse effects, and inadequate analgesia each accounted for termination of epidural analgesia in 1% of cases. Risk factors for adverse effects were identified as: patient age under 58 years, weight under 73 kg, being female, high fentanyl consumption (over 9 ml/hour), and lumbar placement of the epidural catheter. There was a significant association between patient age and pruritus, and between female sex and nausea, hypotension, and sedation.

The relations between fentanyl and local anesthetics and their adverse effects profiles in epidural analgesia (67) further demonstrate the need for well-controlled, double-blind studies (68,69).

The use of a continuous epidural infusion of lidocaine 0.4% plus fentanyl 1 μg/ml in combination with intravenous metamizol 40 mg/kg provided significantly better analgesia than epidural morphine 20 μg/kg plus intravenous metamizol 40 mg/kg during the first 3 postoperative days in 30 children undergoing orthopedic surgery, without increasing the incidence of adverse effects; however, the difference in beneficial effect was small (70).

Prophylactic nalbuphine 4 mg and droperidol 0.625 mg with minidose lidocaine + fentanyl spinal anesthesia in a randomized, double-blinded, controlled study in 62 patients having outpatient knee arthroscopy provided significantly better analgesia and reduced nausea and pruritus than in another 62 patients who received only nalbuphine 4 mg with minidose lidocaine + fentanyl spinal anesthesia (71).

Intravenous patient-controlled analgesia

In a randomized, double-blind, multicenter trial, 150 postoperative patients who had undergone major surgery received demand doses of fentanyl 20, 40, or 60 μg delivered intravenously by PCA (72); higher doses of fentanyl were associated with improved analgesic effect. Adverse effects were reported in 70 patients; the most commonly reported were nausea and vomiting and most adverse effects were described as mild to moderate. Bradypnea occurred in 6% of patients who received fentanyl 60 μg, in one case sufficiently severe to warrant temporary withdrawal of treatment; respiratory depression and moderate hypoxia occurred in one patient on 40 μg and in one on 60 μg, again requiring withdrawal. Overall, mean respiratory rates in the 60 μg group were significantly lower than in the 20 μg group throughout the study, and at 6 hours after initiation compared with the 40 μg group. One patient developed acute confusion and aggression while receiving fentanyl 40 μg. The authors concluded that 40 μg of fentanyl is an appropriate dose for PCA, as this balances analgesic efficacy against the incidence of adverse effects.

Drug overdose

Accidental overdose can be caused by fentanyl patches.

- A 71-year-old woman was found unconscious, with reduced respiration and miotic pupils, having previously had nausea, dizziness, and drowsiness (73). She had inappropriately applied a fentanyl patch 100 μg/hour a day before the symptoms occurred. She recovered fully after treatment with intravenous naloxone 0.4 mg.
- A 24-year-old woman, with a history of polysubstance abuse and extensive psychiatric history, presented with acute opioid overdose caused by the intentional oral ingestion of a fentanyl patch (Duragesic) (74).

Drug–Drug Interactions

Bupivacaine

Bupivacaine is increasingly being used in combination with fentanyl for obstetric analgesia and has been reported to reduce the incidence of pruritus. In a prospective study, 65 parturients in labor were randomly assigned to receive intrathecal fentanyl (25 μg), intrathecal bupivacaine (2.5 mg), or both as part of epidural anesthesia (75). The group that received both drugs had more prolonged analgesia and significantly less pruritus than those who received fentanyl alone (36 versus 95%). However, the incidence of facial pruritus was not significantly different. The type of analgesia did not affect the outcome of labor, although one patient in the combined treatment group required ephedrine for reduced blood pressure. It was proposed that pruritus is the result of stimulation of mu receptors supraspinally and in the dorsal horn of the spinal cord, and that facial itching is associated with mu receptor activation in the medullary dorsal horn, affecting the trigeminal nerve. Local anesthetics may alter this adverse effect by local neuronal blockade or by direct modulation of mu-opioid receptors. Bupivacaine also promotes opioid binding to kappa-opioid receptors, which reduce pruritus. The failure to relieve facial pruritus suggests a direct effect of fentanyl in the brain stem.

Cimetidine

The hepatic metabolism of fentanyl can be inhibited by cimetidine, leading to respiratory depression and sedation (76,77).

Droperidol

The addition of droperidol 2.5 mg to fentanyl 0.4 mg in 40 ml of 0.125% bupivacaine lowered the incidence of postoperative nausea and vomiting compared with a solution without droperidol or with butorphanol added instead in patients undergoing anorectal surgery in a prospective randomized, single-blind study (78).

Fentanyl plus droperidol (neuroleptanalgesia) was more effective than morphine in relieving anginal pain during unstable angina. However, the patients who received the neuroleptanalgesia also had longer hospital stays, because of significantly more cardiac instability and anginal episodes, and a higher total mortality (79).

Etodimate

Used as a pretreatment for anesthetic induction with etomidate, fentanyl 500 μg produced apnea in all patients, with a 67% incidence of nausea and a 47% incidence of postoperative vomiting (80).

Itraconazole

Oral itraconazole 200 mg did not alter the pharmacokinetics of intravenous fentanyl 3 μg/kg, despite being a strong inhibitor of CYP3A4 in vitro (81). In vitro research suggests that itraconazole should inhibit the elimination of fentanyl, as it has been shown to do to alfentanil. This difference can be accounted for by the higher hepatic extraction ratio of fentanyl (0.8–1.0) compared with alfentanil (0.3–0.5), so that even large changes in the activity of enzymes that metabolize fentanyl significantly affect its pharmacokinetics.

Midazolam

Several adverse effects have been reported with the combined use of fentanyl and midazolam, including chest wall rigidity, making ventilation with a bag and mask impossible (SEDA-16, 79).

In neonates, hypotension can occur (SEDA-16, 80), and respiratory arrest in a child and sudden cardiac arrest have been reported (SEDA-16, 80). However, in one study there were no cardiac electrophysiological effects of midazolam combined with fentanyl in subjects undergoing cardiac electrophysiological studies (SEDA-18, 80).

Monoamine oxidase inhibitors

There is a risk of hypertension, tachycardia, hyperpyrexia, and coma with the concurrent administration of opioids and monoamine oxidase inhibitors (SEDA-19, 83).

Prilocaine

The addition of fentanyl to the local anesthetic prilocaine does not seem to cause major analgesic benefits, but increases the incidence of adverse effects, particularly affecting the nervous system (82).

Propofol

The interaction between propofol and fentanyl has been studied in relation to suppressing the somatic or hemodynamic responses to three types of surgical event—skin incision, peritoneum incision, and abdominal retraction (83). Three of ninety-nine subjects were withdrawn from the study after bradycardia of under 50/minute occurred when intravenous fentanyl (dose not stated) was given to those already anesthetized with propofol. Propofol and fentanyl (concentration range 0.5–9 ng/ml maintained by computer-assisted continuous infusion for at least 30 minutes) had a predictable synergistic effect and caused a fall in systolic blood pressure. After stimulation, the different concentrations of fentanyl required to block somatic responses to surgery in 50% of subjects were 9.7 ng/ml, 15 ng/ml, and 28 ng/ml respectively for skin incision, peritoneum incision, and abdominal retraction. Concentrations required to give a 15% or less increase in post-incision systolic blood pressure were 5.3 ng/ml, 9.7 ng/ml, and 12 ng/ml respectively. At doses of less than 3 ng/ml of fentanyl the hemodynamic response to peritoneal incision or abdominal retraction was inadequate, even when sufficient propofol was present to suppress somatic responses. Somatic response suppression correlated with fentanyl for skin incision, fentanyl and propofol for peritoneal incision, and propofol for abdominal retraction. Prestimulation propofol reduced systolic blood pressure in a concentration-dependent fashion, while post-stimulation fentanyl significantly suppressed increases in systolic blood pressure. This difference in effect was attributed to propofol's mainly sedative and hypnotic effects, while fentanyl is primarily analgesic.

Ritonavir

Ritonavir is an inhibitor of HIV protease and a potent inhibitor of CYP3A4 and CYP2D6. The interaction between ritonavir and intravenous fentanyl has been investigated in 12 healthy volunteers in a double-blind, placebo-controlled, crossover study (84). The volunteers took ritonavir 600 mg on day 1, ritonavir 900 mg and intravenous fentanyl 5 μg/kg on day 2, and ritonavir 300 mg or placebo on day 3. Ritonavir reduced the clearance of fentanyl by 67% by inhibiting its metabolism. This could result in prolongation of fentanyl-induced respiratory depression in a patient with an already compromised cardiorespiratory system.

Ropivacaine

In a prospective, randomized, double-blind study, the analgesic effect and adverse effects profile of epidural ropivacaine (2 mg/ml) alone was compared with three different fentanyl/ropivacaine combinations (fentanyl 1, 2, and 4 μg/ml) for up to 72 hours of postoperative analgesia in 244 patients after major abdominal surgery, most commonly colorectal surgery (85). Hypotension was significantly more common with fentanyl 4 μg (52%) compared with the other three groups (31–34%) in the first 24 hours, but not later. Nausea was not significantly different among the groups, although there was more antiemetic drug use in patients given fentanyl 2 and 4 μg by day 3. Pruritus was significantly more common in patients who received fentanyl 4 μg throughout the whole 72 hours.

Ropivacaine 2 μg/ml plus fentanyl 4 μg/ml provided the most effective pain relief over the 3 days.

References

1. Anonymous. High-dose fentanyl. Lancet 1979;1(8107):81–2.
2. Chudnofsky CR, Wright SW, Dronen SC, Borron SW, Wright MB. The safety of fentanyl use in the emergency department. Ann Emerg Med 1989;18(6):635–9.
3. Cagney B, Williams O, Jennings L, Buggy D. Tramadol or fentanyl analgesia for ambulatory knee arthroscopy. Eur J Anaesthesiol 1999;16(3):182–5.
4. Hunt R, Fazekas B, Thorne D, Brooksbank M. A comparison of subcutaneous morphine and fentanyl in hospice cancer patients. J Pain Symptom Manage 1999;18(2):111–19.
5. Barancik M. Inadvertent diagnosis of pheochromocytoma after endoscopic premedication. Dig Dis Sci 1989;34(1):136–8.
6. Chung F, Evans D. Low-dose fentanyl: haemodynamic response during induction and intubation in geriatric patients. Can Anaesth Soc J 1985;32(6):622–8.
7. Grote B, Kugler J, Gutzeit M, Doenicke A. Einfluss von Doxapram auf eine fentanylinduzierte Atemdepression bein Menshen. [The influence of doxapram in human on the respiratory depression by fentanyl.] Anaesthesist 1978;27(6):287–90.
8. Bohrer H, Fleischer F, Werning P. Tussive effect of a fentanyl bolus administered through a central venous catheter. Anaesthesia 1990;45(1):18–21.
9. Tweed WA, Dakin D. Explosive coughing after bolus fentanyl injection. Anesth Analg 2001;92(6):1442–3.
10. Scott JC, Sarnquist FH. Seizure-like movements during a fentanyl infusion with absence of seizure activity in a simultaneous EEG recording. Anesthesiology 1985;62(6):812–14.
11. Knuttgen D, Doehn M, Eymer D, Muller MR. Hirudrucksteigerung nach Fentanyl. [An increase in intracranial pressure following fentanyl.] Anaesthesist 1989;38(2):73–5.
12. Stuerenburg HJ, Claassen J, Eggers C, Hansen HC. Acute adverse reaction to fentanyl in a 55 year old man. J Neurol Neurosurg Psychiatry 2000;69(2):281–2.
13. Bragonier R, Bartle D, Langton-Hewer S. Acute dystonia in a 14-yr-old following propofol and fentanyl anaesthesia. Br J Anaesth 2000;84(6):828–9.
14. Tsueda K, Mosca PJ, Heine MF, Loyd GE, Durkis DA, Malkani AL, Hurst HE. Mood during epidural patient-controlled analgesia with morphine or fentanyl. Anesthesiology 1998;88(4):885–91.
15. Das UG, Sasidharan P. Bladder retention of urine as a result of continuous intravenous infusion of fentanyl: 2 case reports. Pediatrics 2001;108(4):1012–15.
16. Mancuso G, Berdondini RM, Passarini B. Eosinophilic pustular eruption associated with transdermal fentanyl. J Eur Acad Dermatol Venereol 2001;15(1):70–2.
17. Gurkan Y, Toker K. Prophylactic ondansetron reduces the incidence of intrathecal fentanyl-induced pruritus. Anesth Analg 2002;95(6):1763–6.
18. Muller P, Vogtmann C. Three cases with different presentation of fentanyl-induced muscle rigidity—a rare problem in intensive care of neonates. Am J Perinatol 2000;17(1):23–6.
19. Fahnenstich H, Steffan J, Kau N, Bartmann P. Fentanyl-induced chest wall rigidity and laryngospasm in preterm and term infants. Crit Care Med 2000;28(3):836–9.
20. Christian CM 2nd, Waller JL, Moldenhauer CC. Postoperative rigidity following fentanyl anesthesia. Anesthesiology 1983;58(3):275–7.
21. Buvanendran A, McCarthy RJ, Kroin JS, Leong W, Perry P, Tuman KJ. Intrathecal magnesium prolongs fentanyl analgesia: a prospective, randomized, controlled trial. Anesth Analg 2002;95(3):661–6.
22. Muijsers RB, Wagstaff AJ. Transdermal fentanyl: an updated review of its pharmacological properties and therapeutic efficacy in chronic cancer pain control. Drugs 2001;61(15):2289–307.
23. Gardner-Nix J. Caregiver toxicity from transdermal fentanyl. J Pain Symptom Manage 2001;21(6):447–8.
24. Frolich MA, Giannotti A, Modell JH, Frolich M. Opioid overdose in a patient using a fentanyl patch during treatment with a warming blanket. Anesth Analg 2001;93(3):647–8.
25. Cohen S, Lowenwirt I, Pantuck CB, Amar D, Pantuck EJ. Bupivacaine 0.01% and/or epinephrine 0.5 microg/ml improve epidural fentanyl analgesia after cesarean section. Anesthesiology 1998;89(6):1354–61.
26. Silvasti M, Pitkanen M. Continuous epidural analgesia with bupivacaine–fentanyl versus patient-controlled analgesia with i.v. morphine for postoperative pain relief after knee ligament surgery. Acta Anaesthesiol Scand 2000;44(1):37–42.
27. Polley LS, Columb MO, Naughton NN, Wagner DS, Dorantes DM, van de Ven CJ. Effect of intravenous versus epidural fentanyl on the minimum local analgesic concentration of epidural bupivacaine in labor. Anesthesiology 2000;93(1):122–8.
28. Ben-David B, Miller G, Gavriel R, Gurevitch A. Low-dose bupivacaine-fentanyl spinal anesthesia for cesarean delivery. Reg Anesth Pain Med 2000;25(3):235–9.
29. Ben-David B, Frankel R, Arzumonov T, Marchevsky Y, Volpin G. Minidose bupivacaine–fentanyl spinal anesthesia for surgical repair of hip fracture in the aged. Anesthesiology 2000;92(1):6–10.
30. Benhamou D, Thorin D, Brichant JF, Dailland P, Milon D, Schneider M. Intrathecal clonidine and fentanyl with hyperbaric bupivacaine improves analgesia during cesarean section. Anesth Analg 1998;87(3):609–13.
31. Fanelli G, Casati A, Magistris L, Berti M, Albertin A, Scarioni M, Torri G. Fentanyl does not improve the nerve block characteristics of axillary brachial plexus anaesthesia performed with ropivacaine. Acta Anaesthesiol Scand 2001;45(5):590–4.
32. Karakaya D, Buyukgoz F, Baris S, Guldogus F, Tur A. Addition of fentanyl to bupivacaine prolongs anesthesia and analgesia in axillary brachial plexus block. Reg Anesth Pain Med 2001;26(5):434–8.
33. Wong K, Chong JL, Lo WK, Sia AT. A comparison of patient-controlled epidural analgesia following gynaecological surgery with and without a background infusion. Anaesthesia 2000;55(3):212–16.
34. Finucane BT, Ganapathy S, Carli F, Pridham JN, Ong BY, Shukla RC, Kristoffersson AH, Huizar KM, Nevin K, Ahlen KG; Canadian Ropivacaine Research Group. Prolonged epidural infusions of ropivacaine (2 mg/ml) after colonic surgery: the impact of adding fentanyl. Anesth Analg 2001;92(5):1276–85.
35. Liu SS, Moore JM, Luo AM, Trautman WJ, Carpenter RL. Comparison of three solutions of ropivacaine/fentanyl for postoperative patient-controlled epidural analgesia. Anesthesiology 1999;90(3):727–33.
36. Connelly NR, Parker RK, Vallurupalli V, Bhopatkar S, Dunn S. Comparison of epidural fentanyl versus epidural sufentanil for analgesia in ambulatory patients in early labor. Anesth Analg 2000;91(2):374–8.
37. Constant I, Gall O, Gouyet L, Chauvin M, Murat I. Addition of clonidine or fentanyl to local anaesthetics prolongs the duration of surgical analgesia after single shot caudal block in children. Br J Anaesth 1998;80(3):294–8.
38. Ben-David B, DeMeo PJ, Lucyk C, Solosko D. A comparison of minidose lidocaine–fentanyl spinal anesthesia and

local anesthesia/propofol infusion for outpatient knee arthroscopy. Anesth Analg 2001;93(2):319–25.
39. Palmer CM, Cork RC, Hays R, Van Maren G, Alves D. The dose–response relation of intrathecal fentanyl for labor analgesia. Anesthesiology 1998;88(2):355–61.
40. Sharar SR, Carrougher GJ, Selzer K, O'Donnell F, Vavilala MS, Lee LA. A comparison of oral transmucosal fentanyl citrate and oral oxycodone for pediatric outpatient wound care. J Burn Care Rehabil 2002;23(1):27–31.
41. Varvel JR, Shafer SL, Hwang SS, Coen PA, Stanski DR. Absorption characteristics of transdermally administered fentanyl. Anesthesiology 1989;70(6):928–34.
42. Alexander-Williams JM, Rowbotham DJ. Novel routes of opioid administration. Br J Anaesth 1998;81(1):3–7.
43. Caplan RA, Ready LB, Oden RV, Matsen FA 3rd, Nessly ML, Olsson GL. Transdermal fentanyl for post-operative pain management. A double-blind placebo study. JAMA 1989;261(7):1036–9.
44. Grond S, Radbruch L, Lehmann KA. Clinical pharmacokinetics of transdermal opioids: focus on transdermal fentanyl. Clin Pharmacokinet 2000;38(1):59–89.
45. Roy SD, Flynn GL. Transdermal delivery of narcotic analgesics: comparative permeabilities of narcotic analgesics through human cadaver skin. Pharm Res 1989;6(10):825–32.
46. Vielvoye-Kerkmeer AP, Mattern C, Uitendaal MP. Transdermal fentanyl in opioid-naive cancer pain patients: an open trial using transdermal fentanyl for the treatment of chronic cancer pain in opioid-naive patients and a group using codeine. J Pain Symptom Manage 2000;19(3):185–92.
47. Niemann T, Madsen LG, Larsen S, Thorsgaard N. Opioid treatment of painful chronic pancreatitis. Int J Pancreatol 2000;27(3):235–40.
48. Davies AN, Bond C. Transdermal fentanyl and the opioid withdrawal syndrome. Palliat Med 1996;10(4):348.
49. Zenz M, Donner B, Strumpf M. Withdrawal symptoms during therapy with transdermal fentanyl (fentanyl TTS)? J Pain Symptom Manage 1994;9(1):54–5.
50. Alsahaf MH, Stockwell M. Respiratory failure due to the combined effects of transdermal fentanyl and epidural bupivacaine/diamorphine following radical nephrectomy. J Pain Symptom Manage 2000;20(3):210–13.
51. Vanbever R, LeBoulenge E, Preat V. Transdermal delivery of fentanyl by electroporation. I. Influence of electrical factors. Pharm Res 1996;13(4):559–65.
52. Vanbever R, Morre ND, Preat V. Transdermal delivery of fentanyl by electroporation. II. Mechanisms involved in drug transport. Pharm Res 1996;13(9):1360–6.
53. Dunn C. "Touch of a button" delivers transdermal fentanyl. In Pharm 1997;1087:19–20.
54. Payne R, Mathias SD, Pasta DJ, Wanke LA, Williams R, Mahmoud R. Quality of life and cancer pain: satisfaction and side effects with transdermal fentanyl versus oral morphine. J Clin Oncol 1998;16(4):1588–93.
55. Pereira B, Jain PN, Kakhandki V, Dasgupta D. Transdermal fentanyl in post-thoracotomy pain. J Anaesthesiol Clin Pharmacol 1999;115:169–72.
56. Nugent M, Davis C, Brooks D, Ahmedzai SH. Long-term observations of patients receiving transdermal fentanyl after a randomized trial. J Pain Symptom Manage 2001;21(5):385–91.
57. Ahmedzai S, Brooks D. Transdermal fentanyl versus sustained-release oral morphine in cancer pain: preference, efficacy, and quality of life. The TTS–Fentanyl Comparative Trial Group. J Pain Symptom Manage 1997;13(5):254–61.
58. Radbruch L, Sabatowski R, Petzke F, Brunsch-Radbruch A, Grond S, Lehmann KA. Transdermal fentanyl for the management of cancer pain: a survey of 1005 patients. Palliat Med 2001;15(4):309–21.
59. Mystakidou K, Befon S, Kouskouni E, Gerolymatos K, Georgaki S, Tsilika E, Vlahos L. From codeine to transdermal fentanyl for cancer pain control: a safety and efficacy clinical trial. Anticancer Res 2001;21(3C):2225–30.
60. Allan L, Hays H, Jensen NH, de Waroux BL, Bolt M, Donald R, Kalso E. Randomised crossover trial of transdermal fentanyl and sustained release oral morphine for treating chronic non-cancer pain. BMJ 2001;322(7295):1154–8.
61. Newshan G, Lefkowitz M. Transdermal fentanyl for chronic pain in AIDS: a pilot study. J Pain Symptom Manage 2001;21(1):69–77.
62. Libretto SE. Use of transdermal fentanyl in patients with continuous non-malignant pain: a case report series. Clin Drug Invest 2002;22:473–83.
63. Ringe JD, Faber H, Bock O, Valentine S, Felsenberg D, Pfeifer M, Minne HW, Schwalen S. Transdermal fentanyl for the treatment of back pain caused by vertebral osteoporosis. Rheumatol Int 2002;22(5):199–203.
64. Mystakidou K, Befon S, Tsilika E, Dardoufas K, Georgaki S, Vlahos L. Use of TTS fentanyl as a single opioid for cancer pain relief: a safety and efficacy clinical trial in patients naive to mild or strong opioids. Oncology 2002;62(1):9–16.
65. D'Angelo R, Gerancher JC, Eisenach JC, Raphael BL. Epidural fentanyl produces labor analgesia by a spinal mechanism. Anesthesiology 1998;88(6):1519–23.
66. Liu SS, Allen HW, Olsson GL. Patient-controlled epidural analgesia with bupivacaine and fentanyl on hospital wards: prospective experience with 1030 surgical patients. Anesthesiology 1998;88(3):688–95.
67. Niemi G, Breivik H. Epidural fentanyl markedly improves thoracic epidural analgesia in a low-dose infusion of bupivacaine, adrenaline and fentanyl. A randomized, double-blind crossover study with and without fentanyl. Acta Anaesthesiol Scand 2001;45(2):221–32.
68. Wigfull J, Welchew E. Survey of 1057 patients receiving postoperative patient-controlled epidural analgesia. Anaesthesia 2001;56(1):70–5.
69. Lovstad RZ, Stoen R. Postoperative epidural analgesia in children after major orthopaedic surgery. A randomised study of the effect on PONV of two anaesthetic techniques: low and high dose i.v. fentanyl and epidural infusions with and without fentanyl. Acta Anaesthesiol Scand 2001;45(4):482–8.
70. Reinoso-Barbero F, Saavedra B, Hervilla S, de Vicente J, Tabares B, Gomez-Criado MS. Lidocaine with fentanyl, compared to morphine, marginally improves postoperative epidural analgesia in children. Can J Anaesth 2002;49(1):67–71.
71. Mendelson JH, Mello NK. Plasma testosterone levels during chronic heroin use and protracted abstinence. A study of Hong Kong addicts. Clin Pharmacol Ther 1975;17(5):529–33.
72. Camu F, Van Aken H, Bovill JG. Postoperative analgesic effects of three demand-dose sizes of fentanyl administered by patient-controlled analgesia. Anesth Analg 1998;87(4):890–5.
73. Klockgether-Radke AP, Gaus P, Neumann P. Opioidintoxikation durch transdermales Fentanyl. [Opioid intoxication following transdermal administration of fentanyl.] Anaesthesist 2002;51(4):269–71.
74. Purucker M, Swann W. Potential for Duragesic patch abuse. Ann Emerg Med 2000;35(3):314.
75. Asokumar B, Newman LM, McCarthy RJ, Ivankovich AD, Tuman KJ. Intrathecal bupivacaine reduces pruritus and prolongs duration of fentanyl analgesia during labor: a prospective, randomized controlled trial. Anesth Analg 1998;87(6):1309–15.
76. Knodell RG, Holtzman JL, Crankshaw DL, Steele NM, Stanley LN. Drug metabolism by rat and human hepatic microsomes in response to interaction with H_2-receptor antagonists. Gastroenterology 1982;82(1):84–8.

77. Lee HR, et al. Effect of histamine H_2-receptors on fentanyl metabolism. Pharmacology 1982;24:145.
78. Kotake Y, Matsumoto M, Ai K, Morisaki H, Takeda J. Additional droperidol, not butorphanol, augments epidural fentanyl analgesia following anorectal surgery. J Clin Anesth 2000;12(1):9–13.
79. Burduk P, Guzik P, Piechocka M, Bronisz M, Rozek A, Jazdon M, Jordan MR. Comparison of fentanyl and droperidol mixture (neuroleptanalgesia II) with morphine on clinical outcomes in unstable angina patients. Cardiovasc Drugs Ther 2000;14(3):259–69.
80. Stockham RJ, Stanley TH, Pace NL, Gillmor S, Groen F, Hilkens P. Fentanyl pretreatment modifies anaesthetic induction with etomidate. Anaesth Intensive Care 1988;16(2):171–6.
81. Palkama VJ, Neuvonen PJ, Olkkola KT. The CYP 3A4 inhibitor itraconazole has no effect on the pharmacokinetics of i.v. fentanyl. Br J Anaesth 1998;81(4):598–600.
82. Pitkanen MT, Rosenberg PH, Pere PJ, Tuominen MK, Seppala TA. Fentanyl–prilocaine mixture for intravenous regional anaesthesia in patients undergoing surgery. Anaesthesia 1992;47(5):395–8.
83. Kazama T, Ikeda K, Morita K. The pharmacodynamic interaction between propofol and fentanyl with respect to the suppression of somatic or hemodynamic responses to skin incision, peritoneum incision, and abdominal wall retraction. Anesthesiology 1998;89(4):894–906.
84. Olkkola KT, Palkama VJ, Neuvonen PJ. Ritonavir's role in reducing fentanyl clearance and prolonging its half-life. Anesthesiology 1999;91(3):681–5.
85. Scott DA, Blake D, Buckland M, Etches R, Halliwell R, Marsland C, Merridew G, Murphy D, Paech M, Schug SA, Turner G, Walker S, Huizar K, Gustafsson U, Deam RK, Blyth C, Wallace M, Buckland M, Downey G, Etches R, Bignell S, Pavy T, Orlikowski C, Ryan C, Eugster D, Lim W, Dillenbeck C, Sidebotham D. A comparison of epidural ropivacaine infusion alone and in combination with 1, 2, and 4 microgram/ml fentanyl for seventy-two hours of postoperative analgesia after major abdominal surgery. Anesth Analg 1999;88(4):857–64.

Fentiazac

See also Non-steroidal anti-inflammatory drugs

General Information

Fentiazac, a thiazoleacetic acid derivative, has the same adverse reactions profile as other NSAIDs. Adverse effects in as many as 56% of patients (5-56%), are even more frequent than with phenylbutazone (1).

In 40 patients with rheumatoid arthritis enrolled in a double-blind trial of fentiazac 400 mg/day or sulindac 200 mg/day for 3 months, adverse effects were reported in three patients taking fentiazac (rash, headache, epigastric pain) (2).

Organs and Systems

Nervous system

Adverse effects involving the central nervous system include headache, dizziness, mental confusion, sedation, giddiness, and blurred vision; dysesthesia and oral paresthesia have also been reported (3).

Gastrointestinal

Pyrosis, epigastric pain, nausea, constipation/diarrhea, and occult bleeding are the most frequent gastrointestinal effects of fentiazac (3). Rectal administration can cause both local and systemic adverse effects.

Liver

In one study, seven of 20 patients with rheumatoid arthritis had significant rises in aspartate transaminase and alkaline phosphatase activities (4). Reversible hepatotoxicity occurred in three of 33 patients who took fentiazac during long-term therapy (2).

References

1. Buerklin EM, Ballard IM. A double blind comparison of fentiazac and phenylbutazone in the treatment of acute tendinitis and bursitis. Curr Med Res Opin 1979;6(Suppl 2):90.
2. Bunde B, Deckers Y, Dequeker J. Fentiazac in rheumatoid arthritis: comparison with sulindac and long-term tolerance. Curr Med Res Opin 1983;8(5):310–14.
3. Teixeira MA, Da Silva AP, Lourenco I, Teixeira ML. Fentiazac in the treatment of some rheumatic disorders. Curr Med Res Opin 1979;(Suppl 2):97–106.
4. Katona G, Boudani A. Efficacy and tolerability of fentiazac in rheumatoid arthritis: double blind study versus indometacine. Curr Med Res Opin 1979;6(Suppl 2):71.

Feprazone

See also Non-steroidal anti-inflammatory drugs

General Information

Feprazone is an NSAID that is related to phenylbutazone. Feprazone was withdrawn in the UK because of its adverse effects, which resemble those of phenylbutazone. It was designated as a last-resort drug by the Japanese Committee on Safety of Drugs (SEDA-12, 83).

In an 8-week trial in 2693 patients with rheumatoid arthritis and osteoarthritis, 30% reported adverse effects and 11% failed to complete the study. However, two large short-term multicenter studies in general practices in 11 000 patients in Italy reported a very low percentage (1.2–9.8%) of adverse effects (1,2).

Gastrotoxicity, nephrotoxicity, edema, headache, tinnitus, and depression have been attributed to feprazone (3).

Organs and Systems

Hematologic

Thrombocytopenia and immune complex-mediated hemolytic anemia have been reported with feprazone (SEDA-7, 108).

Skin

Skin reactions (including severe bullous dermatosis) have been attributed to feprazone (SEDA-9, 87). Contact dermatitis has been described with feprazone cream (SEDA-18, 101).

References

1. Montanari C. Large cooperative multicentric trial with feprazone in the inflammatory process of dental tissues. Curr Ther Res Clin Exp 1975;17(2):166–74.
2. Chierichetti S. Esempio di monitoraggio attivo su un farmaco: il feprazone. Emerg Med 1976;500.
3. Sturrock R, Isaacs A, Hart FD. Feprazone compared with indomethacin in the management of rheumatoid arthritis. Practitioner 1975;215(1285):94–7.

Fexofenadine

See also Antihistamines

General Information

Fexofenadine is the active metabolite of terfenadine. It has antihistaminic but not dysrhythmogenic properties. It is not metabolized by the liver, but eliminated unchanged in the urine. It is efficacious and well tolerated in seasonal allergic rhinitis (1), with positive effects on nasal blockade (2), and in chronic idiopathic urticaria (1,3).

Organs and Systems

Cardiovascular

Fexofenadine is said to have little cardiotoxicity (4). In one study fexofenadine was well tolerated, and there were no statistically significant changes in PR interval, QT interval, QRS complex, or heart rate (5).

There has been a report of ventricular fibrillation during fexofenadine administration in a man with a pre-existing long QT interval (6). However, causality between fexofenadine and the cardiac effects was unclear.

The safety of fexofenadine in children aged 6–11 years with seasonal allergic rhinitis has been assessed in a large double-blind, randomized, placebo-controlled, parallel study (7). There were no statistically significant electrocardiographic effects, suggesting that fexofenadine is both efficacious and well tolerated in children with allergic disease.

Nervous system

The effects of fexofenadine (120, 180, and 240 mg) on performance and sleepiness have been studied in healthy volunteers. There were no changes at any time compared with placebo, and the authors suggested that fexofenadine may prove to be suitable for use by air personnel (8).

Psychological, psychiatric

Even in a high dose (360 mg bd versus the recommended dose of 60 mg bd) fexofenadine had no disruptive effects on psychomotor performance and cognitive function in healthy volunteers (9).

In one study fexofenadine did not alter driving and psychomotor performance when taken in the recommended dosage of 60 mg bd (10).

Skin

Eight episodes of a fixed drug eruption occurred in a 45-year-old man who was taking fexofenadine for seasonal allergies; after withdrawal of fexofenadine the rash did not recur (11).

Drug–Drug Interactions

Azithromycin

The effect of co-administration of azithromycin on plasma concentrations of fexofenadine 60 mg bd has been examined in a randomized third-party-blind, placebo-controlled, parallel-group study in 98 healthy volunteers (5). An initial loading dose of azithromycin (500 mg) was given on day 3, followed by 250 mg od for 4 days. Concomitant azithromycin caused increases in the C_{max} and AUC of fexofenadine (69 and 67% respectively). However, there were no statistically significant increases in the PR, QT, QT_c interval, QRS complex duration, or ventricular rate after administration of fexofenadine with or without azithromycin.

Grapefruit juice

In a non-blinded, randomized, single-dose, crossover study in 24 healthy adults, grapefruit juice reduced the rate of absorption and the systemic availability of oral fexofenadine by 30% (12). However, there were no clinically significant electrocardiographic changes after co-administration of grapefruit juice with fexofenadine compared with fexofenadine alone. The authors concluded that the systemic availability of drugs that do not undergo significant intestinal or hepatic metabolism, such as fexofenadine, may nevertheless be altered when they are given with agents that affect drug transport mechanisms.

St John's wort

St John's wort (*Hypericum perforatum*) is a popular and widely available herbal extract used as a remedy for anxiety, depression, and sleep disorders. Fexofenadine is transported by P glycoprotein in vitro (13) and there is evidence that St John's wort can alter P glycoprotein activity (14). The effects of St John's wort on the pharmacokinetics of fexofenadine have therefore been studied (15). Fexofenadine 60 mg was given orally twice—before a single dose of St John's wort 900 mg and again after 3 weeks treatment with 300 mg tds. A single dose of St John's wort significantly inhibited intestinal P glycoprotein activity and increased the maximum plasma concentration of fexofenadine by 45%. In contrast, long-term St John's wort caused a 35% reduction in the C_{max} of fexofenadine and increased its oral clearance. However, the authors concluded that these pharmacokinetic changes alone are unlikely to be clinically significant.

In addition to their effects on P glycoprotein, fruit juices and St John's wort can also inhibit organic anion transporting polypeptides (16). These findings suggest new models of intestinal drug absorption and mechanisms of drug interactions.

References

1. Simpson K, Jarvis B. Fexofenadine: a review of its use in the management of seasonal allergic rhinitis and chronic idiopathic urticaria. Drugs 2000;59(2):301–21.
2. Wilson AM, Orr LC, Coutie WJ, Sims EJ, Lipworth BJ. A comparison of once daily fexofenadine versus the combination of montelukast plus loratadine on domiciliary nasal peak flow and symptoms in seasonal allergic rhinitis. Clin Exp Allergy 2002;32(1):126–32.
3. Kawashima M, Harada S, Tango T. Review of fexofenadine in the treatment of chronic idiopathic urticaria. Int J Dermatol 2002;41(10):701–6.
4. Eseverri J. Proyeccion de los nuevos antihistaminicos. [Projection of new antihistamines.] Allergol Immunopathol (Madr) 2000;28(3):143–52.
5. Gupta S, Banfield C, Kantesaria B, Marino M, Clement R, Affrime M, Batra V. Pharmacokinetic and safety profile of desloratadine and fexofenadine when coadministered with azithromycin: a randomized, placebo-controlled, parallel-group study. Clin Ther 2001;23(3):451–66.
6. Anonymous. Severe cardiac arrhythmia on fexofenadine? Prescrire Int 2000;9(45):212.
7. Graft DF, Bernstein DI, Goldsobel A, Meltzer EO, Portnoy J, Long J. Safety of fexofenadine in children treated for seasonal allergic rhinitis. Ann Allergy Asthma Immunol 2001;87(1):22–6.
8. Nicholson AN, Stone BM, Turner C, Mills SL. Antihistamines and aircrew: usefulness of fexofenadine. Aviat Space Environ Med 2000;71(1):2–6.
9. Hindmarch I, Shamsi Z, Kimber S. An evaluation of the effects of high-dose fexofenadine on the central nervous system: a double-blind, placebo-controlled study in healthy volunteers. Clin Exp Allergy 2002;32(1):133–9.
10. Vermeeren A, O'Hanlon JF. Fexofenadine's effects, alone and with alcohol, on actual driving and psychomotor performance. J Allergy Clin Immunol 1998;101(3):306.
11. Anonymous. Reaction to fexofenadine. Consultant 2001;41:154.
12. Banfield C, Gupta S, Marino M, Lim J, Affrime M. Grapefruit juice reduces the oral bioavailability of fexofenadine but not desloratadine. Clin Pharmacokinet 2002;41(4):311–18.
13. Cvetkovic M, Leake B, Fromm MF, Wilkinson GR, Kim RB. OATP and P-glycoprotein transporters mediate the cellular uptake and excretion of fexofenadine. Drug Metab Dispos 1999;27(8):866–71.
14. Johne A, Brockmoller J, Bauer S, Maurer A, Langheinrich M, Roots I. Pharmacokinetic interaction of digoxin with an herbal extract from St John's wort (*Hypericum perforatum*). Clin Pharmacol Ther 1999;66(4):338–45.
15. Wang Z, Hamman MA, Huang SM, Lesko LJ, Hall SD. Effect of St John's wort on the pharmacokinetics of fexofenadine. Clin Pharmacol Ther 2002;71(6):414–20.
16. Dresser GK, Bailey DG, Leake BF, Schwarz UI, Dawson PA, Freeman DJ, Kim RB. Fruit juices inhibit organic anion transporting polypeptide-mediated drug uptake to decrease the oral availability of fexofenadine. Clin Pharmacol Ther 2002;71(1):11–20.

Fibrates

General Information

Fibrates reduce plasma triglycerides by inhibiting their hepatic synthesis and increasing their catabolism. They reduce the synthesis of triglyceride–very low density lipoprotein (VLDL) by increasing the beta-oxidation of fatty acids in the liver. They increase triglyceride catabolism by inducing lipoprotein lipase gene transcription and reducing apoC-III gene transcription. Fibrates increase high-density lipoprotein (HDL) cholesterol by increasing apoA-I and apoA-II gene transcription. These effects are due to activation of peroxisome proliferator-activated receptors (PPAR) alpha and induction of the over-expression of genes containing a peroxisome proliferator response element (PPRE) in their promoter (1).

The fibrates include beclobrate, bezafibrate, biclofibrate, binifibrate, ciprofibrate, clinofibrate, clofibrate, dulofibrate, etofibrate, fenirofibrate, fenofibrate, gemfibrozil, lifibrate, nicofibrate, picafibrate, pirifibrate, ponfibrate, ronifibrate, salafibrate, serfibrate, simfibrate, sitofibrate, tiafibrate, timofibrate, tocofibrate, urefibrate, and xantifibrate (all rINNs).

The adverse events of the fibrates are essentially the same with all members of the class and are generally mild or absent during short-term treatment. The observed frequency of adverse effects with a micronized formulation of fenofibrate is comparable to that associated with the usual formulation (SEDA-22, 490).

Organs and Systems

Nervous system

Nervous system adverse effects are rare, constituting 0.5% of all adverse effects (2). Gemfibrozil-induced headache has been reported (3) and occurred in one patient who had taken bezafibrate for 24 hours (4). Peripheral neuropathy has been observed with bezafibrate (SEDA-13, 1324) (5).

Metabolism

Of 70 patients with cutaneous T cell lymphomas, three who were taking gemfibrozil had to have it withdrawn because of increases in serum triglycerides (6).

- A 76-year-old woman with type 2 diabetes taking gemfibrozil for pronounced hypertriglyceridemia had recurrent episodes of hypoglycemia; her insulin requirements fell by 65% and her HbA_{1c} concentration fell from 9 to 6.5% over 5 months (7).

In patients taking fenofibrate and atorvastatin, increased concentrations of plasma homocysteine were attributed to an action of the fibrates themselves and not indirectly via their lipid-lowering effect (8). Concomitant administration of folic acid, at least in part, offset this adverse effect

(9). The degree of rise in homocysteine differs among the various fibrates. It has been reported with fenofibrate and bezafibrate, and a study of fenofibrate and gemfibrozil substantiated a difference between the drugs (10). Because the concentration of plasma homocysteine depends on renal function, increased plasma homocysteine concentrations could result from renal function impairment caused by fenofibrate. In contrast, gemfibrozil does not affect renal function. This was tested in a crossover study in 22 patients who had hypertriglyceridemia, by giving them gemfibrozil 900 mg/day or fenofibrate 200 mg/day for 6 weeks (11). Lipids were altered similarly, but homocysteine, creatinine, and cystatin C were raised by fenofibrate but not by gemfibrozil. In another report, there was a 57% increase in homocysteine in 26 individuals who took ciprofibrate and a 17% reduction in homocysteine in 12 patients who took bezafibrate.

Fluid balance

Clofibrate has a mild antidiuretic effect (12), and animal studies suggest that this is due to release of antidiuretic hormone (ADH) (13). This effect has been used in the treatment of cranial diabetes insipidus (14).

Hematologic

Leukopenia has been reported with bezafibrate (15), clofibrate (16), and fenofibrate (17).

Gastrointestinal

Abdominal discomfort occurs in 5–10% of all patients taking fibrates. Epigastric fullness, nausea, meteorism, and mild diarrhea have been repeatedly described, and stomatitis has been incidentally mentioned. There are wide discrepancies in the figures given for such complications, ranging as they do from 2 (2) to 20%; the truth appears to be that during the first few days and weeks of treatment, mild discomfort of one sort or another is quite common, although some of it is due to a placebo effect; serious symptoms are most unusual. Bezafibrate is better tolerated than gemfibrozil (18). In a double-blind trial with fenofibrate, the incidence of gastrointestinal adverse effects was not different from that seen with placebo (19). Five of 1213 individuals taking beclobrate complained of diarrhea (20).

Liver

Assurance of good renal and hepatic function is mandatory before beginning treatment with the fibrates (21). Serum transaminase changes are regularly seen and hepatitis occurs (22). Several cases of hepatitis due to fenofibrate have been reviewed (23) and it has also been observed with etofibrate (24). One case of liver failure, probably due to beclobrate, has been reported (SEDA-13, 1324) (25). Liver biopsies showed a lymphoplasmocytic infiltrate in all of five cases of chronic hepatitis associated with fibrates (26).

Biliary tract

Fibrates produce bile that is supersaturated with cholesterol. Although gallstones are common with clofibrate, no excess frequency has been observed with fenofibrate (22). In the WHO study, 59 patients taking clofibrate had to be operated on for gallstones, compared with 24 and 25 respectively in the two placebo groups (27).

Pancreas

Pancreatitis has been attributed to bezafibrate.

- A 75-year-old white woman had fever and raised amylase on three consecutive occasions after taking a tablet of bezafibrate (28). After stopping taking the drug, she remained free of symptoms.

Urinary tract

Unexpected acute renal insufficiency occurred in four patients after uncomplicated cardiac surgery; each was taking a fibrate (29). Renal insufficiency occurred rapidly within 3 days of surgery and was associated with increased concentrations of skeletal muscle-derived creatine kinase. One patient developed myoglobinuria. Presumably, patients taking lipid-lowering drugs are at higher risk of acute renal insufficiency after cardiac surgery, because of rhabdomyolysis. This suggests that patients taking either statins or fibrates should discontinue them before cardiac surgery.

Fenofibrate was the probable cause of rises in serum creatinine concentrations in six patients in one clinic (30). The authors therefore recommended routine serum creatinine monitoring at baseline and at 1 month after starting fenofibrate.

Severe reversible renal insufficiency has been reported with fibrates (31).

Skin

Non-specific rashes have been reported in patients taking fibrates. With fenofibrate, rashes are reported significantly more often than with placebo (32), and occur in some 0.6% of patients (22). In a double-blind trial, the incidence of cutaneous adverse effects was 11% with fenofibrate and less than 1% with placebo; they included hives and urticaria (19). In another study, the difference was 6% (33).

- Chronic radiodermatitis after cardiac catheterization has been observed in a 62-year-old woman taking ciprofibrate. A second catheterization performed when she had stopped taking it did not provoke new lesions (34).

Photosensitivity due to fenofibrate (35) was confirmed by systemic photochallenge (36). Photodermatitis has been associated with cross-reactivity between ketoprofen and fenofibrate; this was thought to be due to chemical similarities between these two drugs (37).

Psoriasis was exacerbated by gemfibrozil in one case (38).

Stevens–Johnson syndrome has been associated with bezafibrate (39) and clofibrate (40).

Musculoskeletal

Rhabdomyolysis is a problem with several lipid-lowering drugs (SEDA-13, 1325) (SEDA-13, 1328) (SEDA-13, 1330) (SEDA-19, 409) (41–43), especially when they are used in combination (44). In individuals with pre-existing renal insufficiency, this can lead to an earlier need for chronic dialysis (45). Also, interactions between various hypolipidemic drugs and other drugs sometimes cause rhabdomyolysis (SEDA-18, 426).

Creatine kinase activity increased in five out of 1213 patients taking beclobrate (20). Myopathy during treatment has been reported with gemfibrozil (46) and ciprofibrate (47,48).

Hypothyroidism predisposes to rhabdomyolysis (49,50) and screening of thyroid function has been advocated before starting hypolipidemic drugs (SEDA-21, 458). This notion has been supported by observations in a 69-year-old man taking fenofibrate 200 mg daily (51). The muscular syndrome appears to be a special risk in patients with nephrotic syndrome (SEDA-13, 1325) (52).

- Two women, 55 and 57 years old, with renal insufficiency, had rhabdomyolysis after taking micronized fenofibrate in dosages a little higher than recommended (53). Both had mild hypothyroidism.

Reduced renal function in the elderly appears to be a risk factor for myopathy (SEDA-23, 472).

- A 73-year-old woman had an increase in serum creatinine concentration while she was taking long-acting bezafibrate and again when she was re-challenged by self-medication (54).
- Low-dose bezafibrate was associated with myositis in a patient with mild chronic renal insufficiency (serum creatinine 210 μmol/l) (55). She was a 58-year-old obese diabetic with isolated hypertriglyceridemia.

Sexual function

Erectile dysfunction has been reported in 12% of 339 men treated with fibrate derivatives or statins, compared with 5.6% of similar patients not taking these drugs (57). The mechanism is unknown and should be confirmed in randomized studies.

Gemfibrozil was suspected to have reduced libido in two cases (58,59), an effect that is well-known with clofibrate, and four cases of loss of libido and impotence involving gemfibrozil have previously been reported (SEDA-13, 1325) (60,61).

Immunologic

Vasculitis, Raynaud's phenomenon, and polyarthritis have been reported with gemfibrozil (62).

Allergic reactions have been reported with some fibrates.

- A 61-year-old woman with penicillin allergy suffered generalized urticaria, chest tightness, wheezing, nausea, vomiting, hypotension, and loss of consciousness (63). Two hours earlier, she had taken Eulitop Retard after lunch. She had intense positive responses to intradermal Eulitop Retard and its active component, bezafibrate; skin tests in control subjects were negative. Specific IgE tests (RAST) to Eulitop Retard were negative. The positive skin tests suggested that an IgE mechanism was responsible for this adverse reaction.
- A 69-year-old woman developed a major allergic reaction after taking fenofibrate 300 mg/day for 10 days (64). The clinical features included weakness, hyperthermia, and slight muscular pain. Biological abnormalities were mildly raised muscle enzymes and pancytopenia, which developed rapidly.

Long-Term Effects

Tumorigenicity

It has been suspected that low concentrations of serum cholesterol might be associated with an increased risk of cancer or overall mortality. All fibrates and statins cause cancer in rodents, but the relevance of this finding to man has been questioned (65). In an epidemiological study these risks were almost non-existent after adjusting for confounding factors.

Second-Generation Effects

Fetotoxicity

In pregnant mice given etofylline clofibrate and fenofibrate in doses of 12, 117, and 586 mg/kg orally from day 7 to day 16 of gestation, terminal maternal body weight was significantly reduced by all doses of etofylline clofibrate (66). The low and middle doses of etofylline clofibrate and fenofibrate had no adverse effects on embryofetal development, but the highest dose of etofylline clofibrate significantly reduced fetal weight at term. Postimplantation loss was significantly higher after the highest dose of fenofibrate. There were no teratogenic effects. The significance of these results to human pregnancy is unknown.

Drug–Drug Interactions

Bexarotene

Of 70 patients with cutaneous T cell lymphomas, three who were taking gemfibrozil had to have it withdrawn because of increases in serum concentrations of triglycerides and bexarotene, an RXR-selective retinoid "rexinoid", which is used for all stages of cutaneous T cell lymphoma (6).

Colchicine

Rhabdomyolysis due to the combination of colchicine with gemfibrozil has been reported in a 40-year-old man with amyloidosis and chronic liver disease (67).

Ibuprofen

Acute renal insufficiency occurred in one patient taking ciprofibrate 100 mg/day and ibuprofen 400 mg/day (68). Both drugs are highly protein-bound and contain propionic acid groups. Thus, ibuprofen may displace ciprofibrate.

Statins

The increased risk of myopathy observed during concomitant treatment with statins and fibrates may be partly pharmacokinetic in origin. In interactions between fibrates and statins there may be differences between the various fibrates (69). Eleven healthy volunteers took bezafibrate 400 mg/day, gemfibrozil 1200 mg/day, or placebo for 3 days. On day 3, each took a single dose of lovastatin 40 mg. Plasma concentrations of lovastatin, lovastatin acid, gemfibrozil, and bezafibrate were measured for up to 24 hours. Gemfibrozil markedly increased plasma concentrations of lovastatin acid, but bezafibrate did not. The risk of myopathy during concomitant therapy with lovastatin and a fibrate may be smaller with bezafibrate than with gemfibrozil.

In 80 patients with primary mixed hyperlipidemia, gemfibrozil used together with lovastatin resulted in 3% discontinuation because of myositis, but none attributable to rhabdomyolysis or myoglobinuria (70).

Sulfonylureas

Fibrates are highly bound to albumin and displace other similarly bound drugs. This can affect treatment with sulfonylureas. Hypoglycemia occurred in a diabetic patient taking glibenclamide plus gemfibrozil (71).

In 10 healthy volunteers, gemfibrozil 600 mg bd increased the mean total AUC of a single dose of glimepiride 0.5 mg by 23% (range 6–56%) (72). The mean half-life of glimepiride was prolonged from 2.1 to 2.3 hours. This effect may have been caused by inhibition of CYP2C9. However, there were no statistically significant effects on serum insulin or blood glucose variables.

Warfarin

Several interactions between warfarin and hypolipidemic drugs have been described (SEDA-21, 459), including clinically important potentiation of warfarin by bezafibrate (73) and gemfibrozil (74). Two patients developed a significantly increased anticoagulant effect of warfarin while taking fenofibrate (75).

References

1. Duriez P. Mécanismes d'action des statines et des fibrates. [Mechanisms of actions of statins and fibrates.] Therapie 2003;58(1):5–14.
2. Adkins JC, Faulds D. Micronised fenofibrate: a review of its pharmacodynamic properties and clinical efficacy in the management of dyslipidaemia. Drugs 1997;54(4):615–33.
3. Alvarez-Sabin J, Codina A, Rodriguez C, Laporte JR. Gemfibrozil-induced headache. Lancet 1988;2(8622):1246.
4. Hodgetts TJ, Tunnicliffe C. Bezafibrate-induced headache. Lancet 1989;1(8630):163.
5. Ellis CJ, Wallis WE, Caruana M. Peripheral neuropathy with bezafibrate. BMJ 1994;309(6959):929.
6. Talpur R, Ward S, Apisarnthanarax N, Breuer-Mcham J, Duvic M. Optimizing bexarotene therapy for cutaneous T cell lymphoma. J Am Acad Dermatol 2002;47(5):672–84.
7. Klein J, Ott V, Schutt M, Klein HH. Recurrent hypoglycaemic episodes in a patient with Type 2 diabetes under fibrate therapy. J Diabetes Complications 2002;16(3):246–8.
8. Giral P, Bruckert E, Jacob N, Chapman MJ, Foglietti MJ, Turpin G. Homocysteine and lipid lowering agents. A comparison between atorvastatin and fenofibrate in patients with mixed hyperlipidemia. Atherosclerosis 2001;154(2):421–7.
9. Stulc T, Melenovsky V, Grauova B, Kozich V, Ceska R. Folate supplementation prevents plasma homocysteine increase after fenofibrate therapy. Nutrition 2001;17(9): 721–3.
10. Westphal S, Dierkes J, Luley C. Effects of fenofibrate and gemfibrozil on plasma homocysteine. Lancet 2001;358(9275):39–40.
11. Harats D, Yodfat O, Doolman R, Gavendo S, Marko D, Shaish A, Sela BA. Homocysteine elevation with fibrates: is it a class effect? Isr Med Assoc J 2001;3(4):243–6.
12. Rado JP. Evidence for permanent enhancement of residual ADH induced by antidiuretic agents (chlorpropamide, carbamazepine, clofibrate) in patients with pituitary diabetes insipidus. Endokrinologie 1975;64(2):217–22.
13. Czako L, Nagy E, Szilagyi I, Laszlo FA. Study of the antidiuretic effect of clofibrate in rat. Endokrinologie 1976;68(2):235–8.
14. Perlemuter L, Hazard J, Kazatchkine M, Guilhaume B, Bernheim R. Action comparée de la carbamazepine et du clofibrate dans le diabète insipide. Etude de 7 cas. [Comparative action of carbamazepine and clofibrate in diabetes insipidus. Study of 7 cases.] Nouv Presse Méd 1975;4(32):2307–10.
15. Ariad S, Hechtlinger V. Bezafibrate-induced neutropenia. Eur J Haematol 1993;50(3):179.
16. Janke EM. Reaction to clofibrate. Can Med Assoc J 1974;111(8):752.
17. Roberts WC. Safety of fenofibrate–US and worldwide experience. Cardiology 1989;76(3):169–79.
18. Kremer P, Marowski C, Jones C, Acacia E. Therapeutic effects of bezafibrate and gemfibrozil in hyperlipoproteinaemia type IIa and IIb. Curr Med Res Opin 1989;11(5):293–303.
19. Brown WV. Treatment of hypercholesterolaemia with fenofibrate: a review. Curr Med Res Opin 1989;11(5):321–30.
20. Capurso A. Drugs affecting triglycerides. Cardiology 1991;78(3):218–25.
21. Brown WV. Fibric acid derivatives. J Drug Dev 1990;3:211–16.
22. Roberts WC. Safety of fenofibrate—US and worldwide experience. Cardiology 1989;76(3):169–79.
23. Rigal J, Furet Y, Autret E, Breteau M. Hépatite mixte sévère au fénofibrate? Revue de la littérature à propos d'un cas. [Severe mixed hepatitis caused by fenofibrate? A review of the literature apropos of a case.] Rev Med Interne 1989;10(1):65–7.
24. Macedo G, Ribeiro T. Etofibrate induced acute hepatitis mimicking biliary tract disease. Arch Med 1996;10:185–6.
25. Vartiainen E, Puska P, Pekkanen J, Tuomilehto J, Lonnqvist J, Ehnholm C. Serum cholesterol concentration and mortality from accidents, suicide, and other violent causes. BMJ 1994;309(6952):445–7.
26. Ganne-Carrie N, de Leusse A, Guettier C, Castera L, Levecq H, Bertrand HJ, Plumet Y, Trinchet JC, Beaugrand M. Hépatites d'allure auto-immune induites par les fibrates. [Autoimmune hepatitis induced by fibrates.] Gastroenterol Clin Biol 1998;22(5):525–9.
27. Anonymous. Trial of clofibrate in the treatment of ischaemic heart disease. Five-year study by a group of physicians of the Newcastle upon Tyne region. BMJ 1971;4(5790):767–75.
28. Gang N, Langevitz P, Livneh A. Relapsing acute pancreatitis induced by re-exposure to the cholestrol lowering agent bezafibrate. Am J Gastroenterol 1999;94(12):3626–8.
29. Sharobeem KM, Madden BP, Millner R, Rolfe LM, Seymour CA, Parker J. Acute renal failure after cardiopulmonary bypass: a possible association with drugs of the fibrate group. J Cardiovasc Pharmacol Ther 2000;5(1):33–9.
30. Ritter JL, Nabulsi S. Fenofibrate-induced elevation in serum creatinine. Pharmacotherapy 2001;21(9):1145–9.
31. Lipkin GW, Tomson CR. Severe reversible renal failure with bezafibrate. Lancet 1993;341(8841):371.

32. Zimetbaum P, Frishman WH, Kahn S. Effects of gemfibrozil and other fibric acid derivatives on blood lipids and lipoproteins. J Clin Pharmacol 1991;31(1):25–37.
33. Knopp RH. Review of the effects of fenofibrate on lipoproteins, apoproteins, and bile saturation: US studies. Cardiology 1989;76(Suppl 1):14–22.
34. Gironet N, Jan V, Machet MC, Machet L, Lorette G, Vaillant L. Radiodermite chronique post cathétérisme cardiaque: role favorisant du ciprofibrate (Lipanor)? [Chronic radiodermatitis after heart catheterization: the contributing role of ciprofibrate (Lipanor)?] Ann Dermatol Venereol 1998;125(9):598–600.
35. Leroy D, Dompmartin A, Lorier E, Leport Y, Audebert C. Photosensitivity induced by fenofibrate. Photodermatol Photoimmunol Photomed 1990;7(3):136–7.
36. Leenutaphong V, Manuskiatti W. Fenofibrate-induced photosensitivity. J Am Acad Dermatol 1996;35(5 Pt 1):775–7.
37. Leroy D, Dompmartin A, Szczurko C, Michel M, Louvet S. Photodermatitis from ketoprofen with cross-reactivity to fenofibrate and benzophenones. Photodermatol Photoimmunol Photomed 1997;13(3):93–7.
38. Fisher DA, Elias PM, LeBoit PL. Exacerbation of psoriasis by the hypolipidemic agent, gemfibrozil. Arch Dermatol 1988;124(6):854–5.
39. Sawamura D, Umeki K. Stevens–Johnson syndrome associated with bezafibrate. Acta Dermatol Venereol 2000;80(6):457.
40. Wong SS. Stevens–Johnson syndrome induced by clofibrate. Acta Dermatol Venereol 1994;74(6):475.
41. Ory JP, Cleau D, Jobard JM, Bourscheid D. Interaction miconazole–cipofibrate responsable d'une rhabdomyolyse. A propos d'un cas. Ann Med Nancy Est 1993;32:305.
42. Mantell G, Burke MT, Staggers J. Extended clinical safety profile of lovastatin. Am J Cardiol 1990;66(8):B11–15.
43. Reaven P, Witztum JL. Lovastatin, nicotinic acid, and rhabdomyolysis. Ann Intern Med 1988;109(7):597–8.
44. van Puijenbroek EP, Du Buf-Vereijken PW, Spooren PF, van Doormaal JJ. Possible increased risk of rhabdomyolysis during concomitant use of simvastatin and gemfibrozil. J Intern Med 1996;240(6):403–4.
45. Biesenbach G, Janko O, Stuby U, Zazgornik J. Terminales myoglobinurisches Nierenversagen unter Lovastatintherapie bei präexistenter chronischer Nierenfunktionsstorung. [Terminal myoglobinuric renal failure in lovastatin therapy with pre-existing chronic renal insufficiency.] Wien Klin Wochenschr 1996;108(11):334–7.
46. Magarian GJ, Lucas LM, Colley C. Gemfibrozil-induced myopathy. Arch Intern Med 1991;151(9):1873–4.
47. Harvengt C. Drugs recently released in Belgium. Mefloquine—ciprofibrate. Acta Clin Belg 1991;46(2):117–19.
48. Buck N, Devlin HB, Lunn JN. The Report of A Confidental Enquiry into Perioperative Deaths. London: Buttfield Provincial Hospitals Trust and King's Fund, 1987.
49. Tregouet B. L'hypothyroïdie favorise-t-elle la toxicité musculaire des fibrates? [Does hypothyroidism predispose muscular toxicity of fibrates?] Rev Med Interne 1991;12(2):159.
50. Hattori N, Shimatsu A, Murabe H, Nishimura M, Nakamura H, Imura H. Clofibrate-induced myopathy in a patient with primary hypothyroidism. Jpn J Med 1990;29(5):545–7.
51. Neuvonen PJ, Jalava KM. Itraconazole drastically increases plasma concentrations of lovastatin and lovastatin acid. Clin Pharmacol Ther 1996;60(1):54–61.
52. Bridgman JF, Rosen SM, Thorp JM. Complications during clofibrate treatment of nephrotic-syndrome hyperlipoproteinaemia. Lancet 1972;2(7776):506–9.
53. Clouatre Y, Leblanc M, Ouimet D, Pichette V. Fenofibrate-induced rhabdomyolysis in two dialysis patients with hypothyroidism. Nephrol Dial Transplant 1999;14(4):1047–8.
54. Terrovitou CT, Milionis HJ, Elisaf MS. Acute rhabdomyolysis after bezafibrate re-exposure. Nephron 1998;78(3):336–7.
55. Gotsman I, Haviv YS, Nir-Paz R. Low-dose bezafibrate-associated myositis in a patient with chronic renal failure. Clin Drug Invest 1999;18:481–3.
56. Chow LT, Chow WH. Acute compartment syndrome: an unusual presentation of gemfibrozil induced myositis. Med J Aust 1993;158(1):48–9.
57. Bruckert E, Giral P, Heshmati HM, Turpin G. Men treated with hypolipidaemic drugs complain more frequently of erectile dysfunction. J Clin Pharm Ther 1996;21(2):89–94.
58. Bain SC, Lemon M, Jones AF. Gemfibrozil-induced impotence. Lancet 1990;336(8727):1389.
59. Pizarro S, Bargay J, D'Agosto P. Gemfibrozil-induced impotence. Lancet 1990;336(8723):1135.
60. Figueras A, Castel JM, LaPorte JR, Capella D. Gemfibrozil-induced impotence. Ann Pharmacother 1993;27(7–8):982.
61. Alcala Pedrajas JN, Prada Pardal JL. Impotencia por gemfibrozil. [Gemfibrozil induced impotence.] An Med Interna 1998;15(3):175–6.
62. Smith GW, Hurst NP. Vasculitis, Raynaud's phenomenon and polyarthritis associated with gemfibrozil therapy. Br J Rheumatol 1993;32(1):84–5.
63. de Barrio M, Matheu V, Baeza ML, Tornero P, Rubio M, Zubeldia JM. Bezafibrate-induced anaphylactic shock: unusual clinical presentation. J Investig Allergol Clin Immunol 2001;11(1):53–5.
64. Rabasa-Lhoret R, Rasamisoa M, Avignon A, Monnier L. Rare side-effects of fenofibrate. Diabetes Metab 2001;27(1):66–8.
65. Cattley RC. Carcinogenicity of lipid-lowering drugs. JAMA 1996;275(19):1479.
66. Ujhazy E, Onderova E, Horakova M, Bencova E, Durisova M, Nosal R, Balonova T, Zeljenkova D. Teratological study of the hypolipidaemic drugs etofylline clofibrate (VULM) and fenofibrate in Swiss mice. Pharmacol Toxicol 1989;64(3):286–90.
67. Atmaca H, Sayarlioglu H, Kulah E, Demircan N, Akpolat T. Rhabdomyolysis associated with gemfibrozil–colchicine therapy. Ann Pharmacother 2002;36(11):1719–21.
68. Ramachandran S, Giles PD, Hartland A. Acute renal failure due to rhabdomyolysis in presence of concurrent ciprofibrate and ibuprofen treatment. BMJ 1997; 314(7094):1593.
69. Kyrklund C, Backman JT, Kivisto KT, Neuvonen M, Laitila J, Neuvonen PJ. Plasma concentrations of active lovastatin acid are markedly increased by gemfibrozil but not by bezafibrate. Clin Pharmacol Ther 2001;69(5):340–5.
70. Jacobson RH, Wang P, Glueck CJ. Myositis and rhabdomyolysis associated with concurrent use of simvastatin and nefazodone. JAMA 1997;277(4):296–7.
71. Ahmad S. Gemfibrozil: interaction with glyburide. South Med J 1991;84(1):102.
72. Niemi M, Neuvonen PJ, Kivisto KT. Effect of gemfibrozil on the pharmacokinetics and pharmacodynamics of glimepiride. Clin Pharmacol Ther 2001;70(5):439–45.
73. Beringer TR. Warfarin potentiation with bezafibrate. Postgrad Med J 1997;73(864):657–8.
74. Rindone JP, Keng HC. Gemfibrozil–warfarin drug interaction resulting in profound hypoprothrombinemia. Chest 1998;114(2):641–2.
75. Ascah KJ, Rock GA, Wells PS. Interaction between fenofibrate and warfarin. Ann Pharmacother 1998;32(7–8):765–8.

Fibrin glue

General Information

Fibrin glue is a topical tissue adhesive, a two-component system. One component contains highly concentrated fibrinogen, factor VIII, fibronectin, and traces of other plasma proteins. The other component contains thrombin, calcium chloride, and antifibrinolytic agents such as aprotinin. Mixing the two components promotes clotting. Fibrinogen is activated by thrombin in the presence of calcium, and the resultant clot aids hemostasis and tissue sealing and is completely absorbed during wound healing without foreign body reaction or extensive fibrosis. Fibrin glue thus imitates the final stages of coagulation (1) and is used for tissue sealing, hemostasis, and wound healing.

Because of its adverse effects, the original topical fibrin glue, which contained thrombin of bovine origin, has been withdrawn and replaced by a product (Quixil) whose components are all human in origin and not bovine or recombinant. Tranexamic acid is added in order to increase stabilization of the clot. The fibrinogen component is made from pooled plasma and is not highly purified; it therefore contains factor XIII, which also stabilizes the clot. Methods involving precipitation of fibrinogen by cryoprecipitation, polyethylene glycol, or ammonium sulfate have been described and evaluated.

All the components of fibrin glue are subjected to virucidal treatment (solvent/detergent treatment for fibrinogen and nanofiltration for thrombin).

Uses

The primary purpose of using fibrin glue is to reduce blood loss and hence the need for transfusion. It is sprayed on to a surgical field in aerosolized form with a double-barrelled syringe, using either compressed air or nitrogen. Its hemostatic and adhesive properties can be used in any surgical specialty, for example to control bleeding after organ injury (2). Its usefulness is particularly well documented in the fields of cardiovascular surgery (3,4), ENT surgery (5), neurosurgery (6), and thoracic surgery (7).

Fibrin glue has been widely used to treat anal fistulae. In a systematic review of 19 studies the reported success rates ranged from 0 to 100%, which may have been due to differences in patient selection (including fistula aetiology and type), treatment protocols, and follow-up duration (8).

The hemostatic efficacy of fibrin glue in a nasal spray has been studied in 24 patients with hereditary hemorrhagic telangiectasia and epistaxis (9). Fibrin glue produced immediate hemostasis and good healing of bleeding sites, no secondary bleeding, and no inflammation. Adverse events, including local swelling, pain, and slow healing of the bleeding site with atrophy of the nasal mucosa, were more frequent in those who were given foam nasal packing rather than fibrin glue spray.

Fibrin glue has also been used experimentally to deliver a high concentration of drug to a local site, as in the example of the use of losartan to prevent neointimal hyperplasia in pig saphenous artery (10).

Organs and Systems

Nervous system

The use of bovine fibrin glue in neurosurgery was associated with fatal neurotoxicity if the glue came into contact with the cerebrospinal fluid or dura (11,12); this has not been reported with fibrin glue of human origin.

Hematologic

In three patients who underwent cardiovascular surgery subsequent abnormalities in hemostasis, characterized by increased activated partial thromboplastin time, prothrombin time, and bovine thrombin time, and by a markedly reduced concentration of factor V, developed between the seventh and eighth postoperative days after exposure to fibrin glue containing bovine thrombin (13). It was suggested that the glue also contains small amounts of factor V and that this may have caused the abnormalities.

Immunologic

An anaphylactic reaction occurred after the use of bovine fibrin glue as a sealant after mastectomy, probably due to the presence of bovine aprotinin (14).

The use of preparations of fibrin glue containing bovine thrombin resulted in the development of antibovine thrombin antibodies. In a prospective study, 13 of 34 patients developed a thrombin inhibitor and reduced factor V activity (15,16). In another study a factor V inhibitor developed after cardiac surgery (17).

Severe hypotension has been reported after the use of bovine fibrin glue for hemostasis in hepatic injury (18). In one there was cardiac arrest and death. These effects may have been the result of an anaphylactic reaction to one or more components of the glue. Of the three ingredients used to prepare fibrin glue, cryoprecipitate and bovine thrombin are antigenic and potentially the most likely causes of anaphylaxis.

References

1. Canonico S. The use of human fibrin glue in the surgical operations. Acta Biomed Ateneo Parmense 2003;74(Suppl 2):21–5.
2. Kram HB, Reuben BI, Fleming AW, Shoemaker WC. Use of fibrin glue in hepatic trauma. J Trauma 1988;28(8):1195–201.
3. Solov'ev GM, Suprunov MV, Khorobrykh TV. Fibrinovyi klei v serdechno-sosudistoi khirurgii. [Fibrin glue in cardiovascular surgery.] Kardiologiia 2003;43(4):4–5.
4. Spotnitz WD, Dalton MS, Baker JW, Nolan SP. Reduction of perioperative hemorrhage by anterior mediastinal spray application of fibrin glue during cardiac operations. Ann Thorac Surg 1987;44(5):529–31.
5. Vaiman M, Eviatar E, Shlamkovich N, Segal S. Effect of modern fibrin glue on bleeding after tonsillectomy and adenoidectomy. Ann Otol Rhinol Laryngol 2003;112(5):410–14.
6. Brennan M. Fibrin glue. Blood Rev 1991;5(4):240–4.
7. Jessen C, Sharma P. Use of fibrin glue in thoracic surgery. Ann Thorac Surg 1985;39(6):521–4.
8. Hammond TM, Grahn MF, Lunniss PJ. Fibrin glue in the management of anal fistulae. Colorectal Dis 2004;6(5):308–19.
9. Vaiman M, Martinovich U, Eviatar E, Kessler A, Segal S. Fibrin glue in initial treatment of epistaxis in hereditary

haemorrhagic telangiectasia (Rendu-Osler-Weber disease). Blood Coagul Fibrinolysis 2004;15(4):359–63.
10. Moon MC, Molnar K, Yau L, Zahradka P. Perivascular delivery of losartan with surgical fibrin glue prevents neointimal hyperplasia after arterial injury. J Vasc Surg 2004;40(1):130–7.
11. Committee on Safety of Medicines/Medicines Control Agency. Quixil human surgical sealant: reports of fatal reactions. Current Problems 1999;25:19.
12. Committee on Safety of Medicines/Medicines Control Agency. Quixil human surgical sealant: update on fatal neurotoxic reactions. Current Problems 2000;26:10.
13. Berruyer M, Amiral J, Ffrench P, Belleville J, Bastien O, Clerc J, Kassir A, Estanove S, Dechavanne M. Immunization by bovine thrombin used with fibrin glue during cardiovascular operations. Development of thrombin and factor V inhibitors. J Thorac Cardiovasc Surg 1993;105(5):892–7.
14. Kon NF, Masumo H, Nakajima S, Tozawa R, Kimura M, Maeda S. [Anaphylactic reaction to aprotinin following topical use of biological tissue sealant.] Masui 1994;43(10):1606–10.
15. Banninger H, Hardegger T, Tobler A, Barth A, Schupbach P, Reinhart W, Lammle B, Furlan M. Fibrin glue in surgery: frequent development of inhibitors of bovine thrombin and human factor V. Br J Haematol 1993;85(3):528–32.
16. Ortel TL, Charles LA, Keller FG, Marcom PK, Oldham HN Jr, Kane WH, Macik BG. Topical thrombin and acquired coagulation factor inhibitors: clinical spectrum and laboratory diagnosis. Am J Hematol 1994;45(2):128–35.
17. Muntean W, Zenz W, Finding K, Zobel G, Beitzke A. Inhibitor to factor V after exposure to fibrin sealant during cardiac surgery in a two-year-old child. Acta Paediatr 1994;83(1):84–7.
18. Berguer R, Staerkel RL, Moore EE, Moore FA, Galloway WB, Mockus MB. Warning: fatal reaction to the use of fibrin glue in deep hepatic wounds. Case reports. J Trauma 1991;31(3):408–11.

Fish oils

General Information

Omega-3 fatty acids are long-chain polyunsaturated fatty acids. The parent fatty acid of this group is alpha-linolenic acid, an essential fatty acid that the body is unable to synthesize; alpha-linolenic acid can be converted in the body to eicosapentaenoic acid (EPA) and docosahexaenoic acid (DHA). In animals and man, these acids reduce the production of several compounds that are involved in inflammation and thrombosis, such as eicosanoids (prostaglandins, thromboxanes, prostacyclin, and leukotrienes) and cytokines (interleukin II-1) (1). The extent of the conversion of alpha-linolenic acid to EPA and DHA is unclear. The conversion process appears to be inhibited by a high intake of linoleic acid, another essential fatty acid (2). In addition, alpha-linolenic acid is found in dark green vegetables and the oils of certain nuts and seeds, especially rape seeds and soya beans.

Oily fish and extracted fish oils contain high concentrations of EPA and DHA. Fish oils also contain vitamins A and D. Oil derived from cod, halibut, or shark liver, or from fish body, typically contains about 200 mg/ml of long-chain omega-3 fatty acids. In addition, cod liver oil provides 50 μg/ml of vitamin A and 2 μg/ml of vitamin D. Many fish oil supplements are artificially enriched with omega-3 fatty acids.

The safety of drugs containing EPA and DHA has been reviewed; the reported adverse effects were similar to those in control groups (3). Even 3–7 g/day for several months did not change liver enzyme activities, and there were no bleeding problems. Consumption of fish oils reduces the resistance of LDL to oxidative modification, and this is partly opposed by the addition of vitamin E (4). Belching or eructation with a fishy taste or smell, vomiting, flatulence, diarrhea, and constipation are relatively common.

Organs and Systems

Respiratory

Fish oils can cause exacerbation of asthma in aspirin-sensitive patients (5).

Cod liver oil supplements can cause lipoid pneumonia (6).

Metabolism

In high doses, fish oils can cause a rise in blood glucose concentration in patients with non-insulin-dependent diabetes mellitus (7).

Hematologic

Bleeding times can increase in patients taking fish oils (8), leading to more prolonged and frequent nose-bleeds (9). Fish oil supplements should be used with care in patients with hemophilia and anyone taking high doses of anticoagulants or aspirin.

Gastrointestinal

Of 39 patients with Crohn's disease, treated with an enteric-coated fish oil formulation, 4 were withdrawn because of diarrhea, the only reported adverse effect in this investigation (10).

In 814 patients randomly allocated to fish oils for 18 weeks for the reduction of re-stenosis after percutaneous transluminal coronary angioplasty, gastrointestinal adverse effects, most commonly bloating and burping, were reported in 37% of patients taking fish oils, versus 31% of those taking placebo (11).

Second-Generation Effects

Pregnancy

During early pregnancy, high doses of vitamin A (as found in halibut and shark liver oils) can lead to birth defects (12). Fish oil supplements rich in vitamin A should therefore be avoided by women in the first trimester and those who might become pregnant.

Drug–Drug Interactions

Acetylsalicylic acid

In eight healthy men who took a total of 485 mg of aspirin over 3 days before beginning 2 weeks of fish oil supplementation (4.5 g of n-3 fatty acids/day), aspirin alone prolonged the bleeding time by 34% and fish oil alone prolonged it by only 9%; however, aspirin + fish oil prolonged the bleeding time by 78% (13). Although fish oil alone did not significantly raise aggregation thresholds for collagen, arachidonic acid, or platelet activating factor, it did reduce the extent of aggregation with collagen. When challenged by single or dual agonists, the combination of fish oil and aspirin did not make platelets less sensitive than aspirin alone.

However, in 18 healthy men randomly allocated to N-3 polyunsaturated fatty acids 10 g/day or placebo for 14 days, the addition of a single intravenous dose of acetylsalicylic acid 100 mg did not alter the small effect of polyunsaturated fatty acids on platelet aggregation (14).

In four subjects given a single oral dose of aspirin 37.5 mg before and after a natural stable fish oil daily for 1 week, serum thromboxane A_2 fell by 40% after aspirin alone, but by 62% after fish oil + aspirin, and leukotriene B_4 rose by 19% after aspirin and fell by 69% after fish oil + aspirin; serum prostacyclin fell equally in both cases (15).

In healthy subjects who took either fish oil or olive oil (control) daily for 3 weeks before exposure to aspirin or no aspirin, fish oil had no significant effect on mucosal prostaglandin E_2 or $F_{2\alpha}$ content or on the damaging effect of aspirin on the stomach, despite the fact that fish oil reduced serum triglyceride concentrations significantly (16).

Warfarin

In a placebo-controlled, randomized, double-blind study of the effect of fish oil supplements 3–6 g/day for 4 weeks on the International Normalized Ratio (INR) in 16 patients taking chronic warfarin therapy there was no statistically significant effect on anticoagulation (17).

However, fish oils can affect hemostasis, and there has been an anecdotal report of a possible interaction.

- A 67-year-old white woman who had been taking warfarin for 18 months doubled her dose of fish oil from 1000 to 2000 mg/day. The INR increased from 2.8 to 4.3 within 1 month and fell to 1.6 within 1 week of reduction of the dose of fish oil (18).

References

1. Sanders TA. Marine oils: metabolic effects and role in human nutrition. Proc Nutr Soc 1993;52(3):457–72.
2. Sanders TA, Roshanai F. The influence of different types of omega 3 polyunsaturated fatty acids on blood lipids and platelet function in healthy volunteers. Clin Sci (Lond) 1983;64(1):91–9.
3. Harris WS. Dietary fish oil and blood lipids. Curr Opin Lipidol 1996;7(1):3–7.
4. Wander RC, Du SH, Ketchum SO, Rowe KE. Effects of interaction of RRR-alpha-tocopheryl acetate and fish oil on low-density-lipoprotein oxidation in postmenopausal women with and without hormone-replacement therapy. Am J Clin Nutr 1996;63(2):184–93.
5. Ritter JM, Taylor GW. Fish oil in asthma. Thorax 1988;43(2):81–3.
6. Dawson JK, Abernethy VE, Graham DR, Lynch MP. A woman who took cod-liver oil and smoked. Lancet 1996;347(9018):1804.
7. Vessby B, Boberg M. Dietary supplementation with n-3 fatty acids may impair glucose homeostasis in patients with non-insulin-dependent diabetes mellitus. J Intern Med 1990;228(2):165–71.
8. Tracy RP. Diet and hemostatic factors. Curr Atheroscler Rep 1999;1(3):243–8.
9. Clarke JT, Cullen-Dean G, Regelink E, Chan L, Rose V. Increased incidence of epistaxis in adolescents with familial hypercholesterolemia treated with fish oil. J Pediatr 1990;116(1):139–41.
10. Belluzzi A, Brignola C, Campieri M, Pera A, Boschi S, Miglioli M. Effect of an enteric-coated fish-oil preparation on relapses in Crohn's disease. N Engl J Med 1996;334(24):1557–60.
11. Cairns JA, Gill J, Morton B, Roberts R, Gent M, Hirsh J, Holder D, Finnie K, Marquis JF, Naqvi S, Cohen E. Fish oils and low-molecular-weight heparin for the reduction of restenosis after percutaneous transluminal coronary angioplasty. The EMPAR Study. Circulation 1996;94(7):1553–60.
12. Rothman KJ, Moore LL, Singer MR, Nguyen US, Mannino S, Milunsky A. Teratogenicity of high vitamin A intake. N Engl J Med 1995;333(21):1369–73.
13. Harris WS, Silveira S, Dujovne CA. The combined effects of N-3 fatty acids and aspirin on hemostatic parameters in man. Thromb Res 1990;57(4):517–26.
14. Svaneborg N, Kristensen SD, Hansen LM, Bullow I, Husted SE, Schmidt EB. The acute and short-time effect of supplementation with the combination of N-3 fatty acids and acetylsalicylic acid on platelet function and plasma lipids. Thromb Res 2002;105(4):311–16.
15. Engstrom K, Wallin R, Saldeen T. Effect of low-dose aspirin in combination with stable fish oil on whole blood production of eicosanoids. Prostaglandins Leukot Essent Fatty Acids 2001;64(6):291–7.
16. Faust TW, Redfern JS, Podolsky I, Lee E, Grundy SM, Feldman M. Effects of aspirin on gastric mucosal prostaglandin E2 and F2 alpha content and on gastric mucosal injury in humans receiving fish oil or olive oil. Gastroenterology 1990;98(3):586–91.
17. Bender NK, Kraynak MA, Chiquette E, Linn WD, Clark GM, Bussey HI. Effects of marine fish oils on the anticoagulation status of patients receiving chronic warfarin therapy. J Thromb Thrombolysis 1998;5(3):257–61.
18. Buckley MS, Goff AD, Knapp WE. Fish oil interaction with warfarin. Ann Pharmacother 2004;38(1):50–2.

5-HT_3 receptor antagonists

General Information

The 5-HT_3 antagonists, alosetron, granisetron, ondansetron, and tropisetron (all rINNs), are effective antiemetics used in treating cytotoxic-induced and postoperative vomiting.

There have been several reviews of the pharmacology and use of alosetron (1–5). In patients with irritable bowel syndrome, alosetron increases colonic transit time and colonic compliance. It produces significant improvement in abdominal pain, stool consistency, and frequency and urgency of defecation in non-constipated women with irritable bowel syndrome, but not in men. Constipation is the most common adverse effect. It occurs more commonly at higher doses and is more common in women, which is consistent with reported bowel function data.

Granisetron and tropisetron appear to have the same safety profile as ondansetron (6). Their adverse reactions include mild rises in transaminases (up to 17%), slight headache (8–42%), transient diarrhea (2–5%), which may be followed during longer-term therapy by constipation, dizziness (5%), and dry mouth (5–17%); the incidence of xerostomia is higher than with metoclopramide. Other reported adverse effects include anorexia, paresthesia, constipation or abdominal discomfort, changes in blood pressure, fever, facial edema, leg cramps, hot flushes, and enlargement of the spleen (7).

Observational studies

Granisetron

In 59 patients who were given intravenous granisetron 1 mg 30 minutes before treatment on days of chemotherapy, the most common adverse effects were headache, somnolence, and weakness (8).

In another open trial the combination of intravenous granisetron (1 mg) plus dexamethasone (10 mg) was effective and well tolerated for antiemetic control in 100 bone-marrow transplant patients receiving highly emetogenic chemotherapy with or without irradiation (9). Adverse effects were mild; headache, diarrhea, and constipation were the most frequent.

Tropisetron

The safety and efficacy of tropisetron in the prevention of chemotherapy-induced nausea and vomiting has been reviewed (10). Tropisetron monotherapy is effective for the control of acute, and to some extent delayed, nausea and vomiting in patients receiving emetogenic chemotherapy. Combining it with dexamethasone increases its efficacy.

The antiemetic efficacy of tropisetron has been confirmed in 22 children (median age 14 years) who received a total of 125 courses of highly emetogenic chemotherapy (11). The only reported adverse effects attributable to tropisetron were mild diarrhea during two treatment courses and dry mouth during three courses.

Comparative studies

Granisetron versus ondansetron

The efficacy and safety of oral granisetron (2 mg od) and oral ondansetron (8 mg tds for 3 days and bd on day 4) in the prophylaxis of nausea and vomiting have been studied in 34 patients receiving hyperfractionated total body irradiation in a randomized, double-blind trial (12). A historical group of 90 patients who received a similar irradiation regimen but no 5HT$_3$ receptor antagonists acted as a control group. Both drugs were safe and effective in preventing nausea and vomiting resulting from irradiation. The most frequent adverse effects were headache and diarrhea.

Oral granisetron (1 mg bd) plus intravenous dexamethasone (10 mg) have been compared with intravenous ondansetron (8 mg tds) plus dexamethasone (10 mg) for the control of nausea and vomiting in a randomized, open trial in 51 patients receiving emetogenic chemotherapy (13). The two combinations were equally effective, and the frequencies of adverse events (none serious) in the two groups were comparable. The most frequent were diarrhea with granisetron and constipation with ondansetron.

The efficacy of converting from intravenous ondansetron to oral granisetron in preventing chemotherapy-induced nausea and vomiting has been assessed in 608 patient interviews (14). There was no difference in the control of nausea and vomiting between the two treatments. Patient adherence to treatment increased from 48 to 78% after the use of oral granisetron. The costs of preventing acute chemotherapy-induced nausea and vomiting also fell, from US$107 to US$65 per treatment.

In a large double-blind study comparison of single-dose oral granisetron versus intravenous ondansetron in the prevention of nausea and vomiting induced by chemotherapy in 1085 patients, the drugs were equally effective and gave rise to a similar frequency of adverse effects, commonly headache, weakness, and constipation (15). Dizziness and blurred vision were reported by significantly more of the patients who received ondansetron.

Granisetron and ondansetron were also effective in controlling nausea and vomiting related to emetogenic chemotherapy in a crossover study in 40 oriental patients (16). Adverse effects were similar to those reported in Western studies, constipation and headache being the commonest. In another placebo-controlled study of the efficacy and safety of granisetron (3 mg), droperidol (1.25 mg), and metoclopramide (10 mg) intravenously for the prevention of nausea and vomiting in 120 parturients undergoing cesarean section under spinal anesthesia, granisetron was the most effective antiemetic (17). The adverse events profiles of all three drugs were similar to that of placebo.

Granisetron versus ramosetron

Oral ramosetron 0.1 mg without water has been compared with oral granisetron 2 mg with water given 1 hour before infusion of chemotherapy in a multicenter, randomized, single-blind, crossover study in 73 patients with cancer (18). The two regimens had similar efficacy in the prevention of chemotherapy-induced anorexia, nausea, and vomiting. The incidence of adverse effects was similar in the two treatment groups. More patients given ramosetron (10%) complained of headache than those given granisetron (1.3%). The other important adverse effects were dry mouth, insomnia, heavy-headedness, and dizziness. In another multicenter, randomized, single-blind study in 194 patients receiving cisplatin chemotherapy for cancer, intravenous ramosetron 3 mg was as effective as intravenous granisetron 3 mg in preventing nausea and vomiting (19). Although the incidence of adverse effects was similar in the two groups, significantly more patients who received granisetron than ramosetron complained of dull headache.

Granisetron versus droperidol

In a randomized trial in 60 patients who underwent elective laparoscopic cholecystectomy the combination of intravenous granisetron 3 mg plus droperidol 1.25 mg was more effective in preventing postoperative nausea and vomiting than granisetron 3 mg alone (20). No significant adverse effects were reported in either group.

Granisetron versus droperidol and metoclopramide

The efficacy of intravenous granisetron 40 micrograms/kg, droperidol 20 micrograms/kg, and metoclopramide 0.2 mg/kg have been compared in the treatment of nausea and vomiting after laparoscopic cholecystectomy in a double-blind trial in 120 patients (21). The patients were observed for 24 hours after administration. Granisetron was significantly more effective than the other two drugs. All three drugs were equally well tolerated. The common adverse effects were headache and dizziness.

Ondansetron versus droperidol

Intravenous ondansetron (4 mg at induction of anesthesia and 0.13 mg with each 1 mg bolus of morphine) has been compared with intravenous droperidol (0.5 mg at induction and 0.05 mg with each bolus of morphine) in a double-blind trial in 142 patients (22). The two regimens had similar efficacy in the prevention of postoperative nausea and vomiting. The most important adverse effect was sedation; significantly more patients given droperidol (15%) had excessive sedation than patients given ondansetron (5%).

Ondansetron versus metoclopramide

The antiemetic effect of combined intravenous ondansetron 8 mg, oral dexamethasone 20 mg, and oral lorazepam 0.5 mg was significantly better than that of intravenous metoclopramide 10 mg, dexamethasone 20 mg, and oral lorazepam 0.5 mg in 30 patients receiving chemotherapy for ovarian cancer in a randomized trial (23). All the antiemetics were given 30 minutes before and 6 hours after chemotherapy. Significantly more patients given metoclopramide (40% versus 13%) complained of adverse effects. The most frequent adverse effects with both regimens were sedation and headache.

The antiemetic effects of intravenous metoclopramide 1 mg/kg tds and ondansetron 8 mg/kg tds, alone or in combination with dexamethasone or methylprednisolone, have been compared in an open study in 101 patients receiving several cycles of moderately emetogenic chemotherapy (24). The regimens had similar efficacy in controlling emesis during the first course of chemotherapy. However, ondansetron alone, ondansetron plus glucocorticoids, and metoclopramide plus glucocorticoids were more effective than metoclopramide alone during the next two cycles. All the antiemetic regimens were well tolerated and caused similar frequencies of adverse effects. The most common were headache, constipation, and diarrhea.

Ondansetron or tropisetron versus metoclopramide

In a randomized, double-blind trial in 179 patients undergoing thyroid or parathyroid surgery, premedication with oral tropisetron 5 mg was more effective in preventing postoperative nausea and vomiting in the initial postoperative period (0–2 hours) than either oral ondansetron 16 mg or oral metoclopramide 10 mg when given 1 hour before the operation (25). When the entire 24-hour postoperative period was considered, the incidence of vomiting was lower with ondansetron and tropisetron than with metoclopramide. The adverse effects profiles were similar in the three groups. Common adverse effects were headache, dizziness, pruritus, and visual disturbances.

Placebo-controlled studies

Alosetron

Alosetron (1 mg bd) was well tolerated and effective in alleviating abdominal pain, urgency, and stool frequency in a randomized, double-blind, placebo-controlled trial in 647 women with irritable bowel syndrome (26). Constipation occurred in 30% of patients taking alosetron and 3% of those taking placebo. Laboratory values, including liver function tests, were unchanged by alosetron.

The efficacy of alosetron in the treatment of irritable bowel syndrome has been evaluated in a double-blind, placebo controlled, dose-ranging study in 462 patients (27). In women, but not in men, alosetron 2 mg bd significantly increased the proportion of pain-free days and reduced the visual analogue scale score for diarrhea. Alosetron 0.5–2 mg bd led to significant hardening of stools and reduced stool frequency in the total population. The overall incidence of adverse effects was similar with alosetron and placebo. However, the incidence of constipation was significantly higher during treatment with alosetron 0.5 mg bd and 2 mg bd. There were no changes in laboratory values associated with alosetron.

In a randomized, double-blind, placebo-controlled, crossover trial, alosetron (2 mg bd) delayed left colonic transit in both patients with irritable bowel syndrome ($n = 13$) and healthy volunteers ($n = 12$) (28). In another double-blind, placebo-controlled trial in 25 non-constipated patients with irritable bowel syndrome, alosetron (1 and 4 mg bd) had no significant effect on gastrointestinal transit or rectal sensory and motor mechanisms (29).

Granisetron

Oral granisetron 2 mg has been studied in the prophylaxis of nausea and vomiting following fractionated upper abdominal radiotherapy in a double-blind, placebo-controlled trial in 160 patients (30). Granisetron was significantly more effective than placebo. The common adverse effects attributed to granisetron were diarrhea, weakness, and constipation.

In a crossover study in 90 patients receiving cisplatin-based chemotherapy, prednisolone 50 mg significantly improved the antiemetic effects of granisetron (3 mg intravenously) compared with placebo (31).

Tropisetron

In a randomized, double-blind, placebo-controlled study, intravenous tropisetron 2 mg and 5 mg was effective in preventing emesis in 60 patients who underwent general anesthesia (32). Both doses of tropisetron were equally effective. Adverse effects were not mentioned.

Organs and Systems

Cardiovascular

Hypertension or disturbances of cardiac rhythm can occur with 5HT$_3$ receptor antagonistsT3 antagnists HT, especially in elderly patients (SEDA-20, 316).

Some patients have electrocardiographic changes, such as prolongation of the QT interval. In a double-blind, placebo-controlled, randomized study of the effects of dolasetron mesylate 0.6–5.0 mg/kg in 80 subjects, there were transient and asymptomatic electrocardiographic changes (small mean increases in PR interval and QRS complex duration versus baseline) in several subjects at 1–2 hours after infusion at doses of 3.0 mg/kg and over (33).

In one trial a patient who took ondansetron had syncope, presumably because of a change in blood pressure (SEDA-18, 370).

Nervous system

Ondansetron can cause extrapyramidal reactions (34). In two cases the reaction did not recur after a reduction in dosage or a change in the infusion time.

Hematologic

Thrombocytopenia has been observed in patients who were given 5 HT3 receptor antagonists, but was probably coincidental, since they were also given cytostatic drugs (35,36).

Gastrointestinal

Constipation is the commonest adverse effect of alosetron. In women with irritable bowel syndrome, alosetron 1 mg bd was more effective than placebo and mebeverine in relieving abdominal pain, discomfort, and diarrhea. The most frequent adverse effect was constipation (1–4). In 30 patients (15 men, 15 women) using scintigraphy to measure bowel transit, alosetron 1 mg bd for 6 weeks caused significantly delayed small bowel and colonic transit times (37). This effect was significantly greater in women. Alosetron 1 mg bd was significantly more effective than placebo in the treatment of diarrhea-predominant irritable bowel syndrome in a multicenter, double-blind, placebo-controlled study in 801 women (38). Constipation was the most frequently reported adverse effect. The tolerability and safety of alosetron 1 mg bd during long-term administration (48 weeks) has been studied in a multicenter, double-blind, placebo-controlled trial in 859 subjects (39). Alosetron was generally well tolerated. The frequencies of adverse events were similar in the two groups, with the exception of constipation, which occurred significantly more often in the treatment group (32% compared with 5%). In most cases (72%) constipation was mild to moderate. There were two deaths in subjects with pre-existing cardiovascular risk factors in the treatment group, but neither was attributed to alosetron. In a dose-ranging, randomized, placebo-controlled, multicenter trial in 320 patients with functional dyspepsia, alosetron 0.5 mg bd and 1 mg bd was better than placebo in symptom control (40). Women had significantly greater responses than men. Constipation was the most commonly reported adverse effect of alosetron (49% compared with 13% in the placebo group). In a randomized, double-blind, placebo-controlled trial in 626 women with diarrhea-predominant irritable bowel syndrome, alosetron 1 mg bd was significantly more effective than placebo in controlling symptoms (41). Constipation was the most common adverse effect of alosetron (25% compared with 5% in the placebo group).

Ischemic colitis has been attributed to alosetron (42).

- A 55-year-old man with irritable bowel syndrome who took alosetron 1 mg bd for 4 days developed symptoms of ischemic colitis, including rectal bleeding, and the diagnosis was confirmed macroscopically and histologically at colonoscopy. The symptoms suggestive of colitis abated on withdrawal of alosetron, but the symptoms of irritable bowel syndrome returned. Colonoscopy 2 weeks later showed a normal colon and biopsies showed normal colonic histology.

The combination of intravenous granisetron (40 micrograms/kg) and dexamethasone (8 mg) was more effective than granisetron alone for prophylaxis of postoperative nausea and vomiting after laparoscopic cholecystectomy in a randomized, double-blind trial in 120 patients (43). There was no difference in the incidence of adverse effects between the two groups. The most frequent were nausea, retching, and vomiting.

Drug Administration

Drug administration route

In a randomized, double-blind study, oral granisetron (1 mg) was more effective than intravenous granisetron (1 mg) in preventing emesis caused by high-dose chemotherapy in 51 patients who underwent peripheral blood progenitor cell or bone-marrow transplantation (44). There was no significant difference in adverse events. The more frequent were headache, diarrhea, extrapyramidal symptoms, and sedation.

Drug–Drug Interactions

Fluoxetine

In an open, non-randomized, crossover study in 12 healthy female and male volunteers alosetron 1 mg bd had no effect on the pharmacokinetics of fluoxetine 20 mg/day (45). Co-administration of the two drugs was well tolerated by all the subjects.

Zenoplatin

Data from a single trial suggest that ondansetron can enhance the nephrotoxicity of the cytostatic drug zenoplatin (SEDA-17, 415).

References

1. Balfour JA, Goa KL, Perry CM. Alosetron. Drugs 2000;59(3):511–18.
2. Mucke H, Cole P, Rabasseda X. Alosetron. Drugs Today (Barc) 2000;36(9):595–607.
3. Reddy P. Alosetron: A 5-HT3 receptor antagonist for treatment of irritable bowel syndrome. Formulary 2000;35: 404–11.
4. Camilleri M. Pharmacology and clinical experience with alosetron. Expert Opin Investig Drugs 2000;9(1):147–59.
5. Mangel AW, Northcutt AR. Review article: the safety and efficacy of alosetron, a 5-HT3 receptor antagonist, in female irritable bowel syndrome patients. Aliment Pharmacol Ther 1999;13(Suppl 2):77–82.

6. Del Favero A, Roila F, Tonato M. Reducing chemotherapy-induced nausea and vomiting. Current perspectives and future possibilities. Drug Saf 1993;9(6):410–28.
7. Finn AL. Toxicity and side effects of ondansetron. Semin Oncol 1992;19(4 Suppl 10):53–60.
8. Trovato JA, Stull DM, Finley RS. Outcomes of antiemetic therapy after the administration of high-dose antineoplastic agents. Am J Health Syst Pharm 1998;55(12):1269–74.
9. Abbott B, Ippoliti C, Hecth D, Bruton J, Whaley B, Champlin R. Granisetron (Kytril) plus dexamethasone for antiemetic control in bone marrow transplant patients receiving highly emetogenic chemotherapy with or without total body irradiation. Bone Marrow Transplant 2000;25(12):1279–83.
10. Simpson K, Spencer CM, McClellan KJ. Tropisetron: an update of its use in the prevention of chemotherapy-induced nausea and vomiting. Drugs 2000;59(6):1297–315.
11. Uysal KM, Olgun N, Sarialioglu F. Tropisetron in the prevention of chemotherapy-induced acute emesis in pediatric patients. Turk J Pediatr 1999;41(2):207–18.
12. Spitzer TR, Friedman CJ, Bushnell W, Frankel SR, Raschko J. Double-blind, randomized, parallel-group study on the efficacy and safety of oral granisetron and oral ondansetron in the prophylaxis of nausea and vomiting in patients receiving hyperfractionated total body irradiation. Bone Marrow Transplant 2000;26(2):203–10.
13. Chiou TJ, Tzeng WF, Wang WS, Yen CC, Fan FS, Liu JH, Chen PM. Comparison of the efficacy and safety of oral granisetron plus dexamethasone with intravenous ondansetron plus dexamethasone to control nausea and vomiting induced by moderate/severe emetogenic chemotherapy Zhonghua Yi Xue Za Zhi (Taipei) 2000;63(10):729–36.
14. McCune JS, Oertel MD, Pfeifer D, Houston SA, Bingham A, Sawyer WT, Lindley CM. Evaluation of outcomes in converting from intravenous ondansetron to oral granisetron: an observational study. Ann Pharmacother 2001;35(1):14–20.
15. Perez EA, Hesketh P, Sandbach J, Reeves J, Chawla S, Markman M, Hainsworth J, Bushnell W, Friedman C. Comparison of single-dose oral granisetron versus intravenous ondansetron in the prevention of nausea and vomiting induced by moderately emetogenic chemotherapy: a multicenter, double-blind, randomized parallel study. J Clin Oncol 1998;16(2):754–60.
16. Poon RT, Chow LW. Comparison of antiemetic efficacy of granisetron and ondansetron in Oriental patients: a randomized crossover study. Br J Cancer 1998;77(10):1683–5.
17. Fujii Y, Tanaka H, Toyooka H. Prevention of nausea and vomiting with granisetron, droperidol and metoclopramide during and after spinal anaesthesia for caesarean section: a randomized, double-blind, placebo-controlled trial. Acta Anaesthesiol Scand 1998;42(8):921–5.
18. Feng FY, Zhang P, He YJ, Li YH, Zhou MZ, Cheng G, Chen Y, Kikkawa T, Yamamoto M. Oral formulations of the selective serotonin 3 antagonists ramosetron (intraoral disintegrator formulation) and granisetron hydrochloride (standard tablet) in treating acute chemotherapy-induced emesis, nausea and anorexia: a multicenter, randomized, single-blind, crossover, comparison study. Curr Ther Res Clin Exp 2002;63:725–35.
19. Kang YK, Park YH, Ryoo BY, Bang YJ, Cho KS, Shin DB, Kim HC, Lee KH, Park YS, Lee KS, Heo DS, Kim SY, Cho EK, Lim HY, Kim WK, Lee JA, Kim TY, Lee JC, Yoon HJ, Kim NK. Ramosetron for the prevention of cisplatin-induced acute emesis: a prospective randomized comparison with granisetron. J Int Med Res 2002;30(3):220–9.
20. Ozmen S, Yavuz L, Ceylan BG, Tarhan O, Aydin C. Comparison of granisetron with granisetron plus droperidol combination prophylaxis in post-operative nausea and vomiting after laparoscopic cholecystectomy. J Int Med Res 2002;30(5):520–4.
21. Fujii Y, Tanaka H, Kawasaki T. Randomized clinical trial of granisetron, droperidol and metoclopramide for the treatment of nausea and vomiting after laparoscopic cholecystectomy. Br J Surg 2000;87(3):285–8.
22. Millo J, Siddons M, Innes R, Laurie PS. Randomised double-blind comparison of ondansetron and droperidol to prevent postoperative nausea and vomiting associated with patient-controlled analgesia. Anaesthesia 2001;56(1):60–5.
23. Manusirivithaya S, Chareoniam V, Isariyodom P, Sungsab D. Comparison of ondansetron–dexamethasone–lorazepam versus metoclopramide–dexamethasone–lorazepam in the control of cisplatin induced emesis. J Med Assoc Thai 2001;84(7):966–72.
24. Raynov J, Danon S, Valerianova Z. Control of acute emesis in repeated courses of moderately emetogenic chemotherapy. J BUON 2002;7:57–60.
25. Jokela R, Koivuranta M, Kangas-Saarela T, Purhonen S, Alahuhta S. Oral ondansetron, tropisetron or metoclopramide to prevent postoperative nausea and vomiting: a comparison in high-risk patients undergoing thyroid or parathyroid surgery. Acta Anaesthesiol Scand 2002;46(5):519–24.
26. Camilleri M, Northcutt AR, Kong S, Dukes GE, McSorley D, Mangel AW. Efficacy and safety of alosetron in women with irritable bowel syndrome: a randomised, placebo-controlled trial. Lancet 2000;355(9209):1035–40.
27. Bardhan KD, Bodemar G, Geldof H, Schutz E, Heath A, Mills JG, Jacques LA. A double-blind, randomized, placebo-controlled dose-ranging study to evaluate the efficacy of alosetron in the treatment of irritable bowel syndrome. Aliment Pharmacol Ther 2000;14(1):23–34.
28. Houghton LA, Foster JM, Whorwell PJ. Alosetron, a 5-HT3 receptor antagonist, delays colonic transit in patients with irritable bowel syndrome and healthy volunteers. Aliment Pharmacol Ther 2000;14(6):775–82.
29. Thumshirn M, Coulie B, Camilleri M, Zinsmeister AR, Burton DD, Van Dyke C. Effects of alosetron on gastrointestinal transit time and rectal sensation in patients with irritable bowel syndrome. Aliment Pharmacol Ther 2000;14(7):869–78.
30. Lanciano R, Sherman DM, Michalski J, Preston AJ, Yocom K, Friedman C. The efficacy and safety of once-daily Kytril (granisetron hydrochloride) tablets in the prophylaxis of nausea and emesis following fractionated upper abdominal radiotherapy. Cancer Invest 2001;19(8):763–72.
31. Handberg J, Wessel V, Larsen L, Herrstedt J, Hansen HH. Randomized, double-blind comparison of granisetron versus granisetron plus prednisolone as antiemetic prophylaxis during multiple-day cisplatin-based chemotherapy. Support Care Cancer 1998;6(1):63–7.
32. Yilmazlar A, Tokat O, Kutlay O, Yilmazlar T, Turker G. Comparison of the efficacy of 2 mg versus 5 mg tropisetron in the management of post-operative nausea and vomiting. J Int Med Res 2001;29(5):385–8.
33. Hunt TL, Cramer M, Shah A, Stewart W, Benedict CR, Hahne WF. A double-blind, placebo-controlled, dose-ranging safety evaluation of single-dose intravenous dolasetron in healthy male volunteers. J Clin Pharmacol 1995;35(7):705–12.
34. Skoglund RR, Ware LL Jr, Schanberger JE. Prolonged seizures due to contact and inhalation exposure to camphor. A case report. Clin Pediatr (Phila) 1977;16(10):901–2.
35. Sorensen JB, Wedervang K, Dombernowsky P. Preliminary results of a phase II study of paclitaxel and cisplatin in patients with non-small cell lung cancer. Semin Oncol 1997;24(4 Suppl 12):S12–18, S12–20.
36. Abratt RP, Bezwoda WR, Falkson G, Goedhals L, Hacking D, Rugg TA. Efficacy and safety profile of

gemcitabine in non-small-cell lung cancer: a phase II study. J Clin Oncol 1994;12(8):1535–40.
37. Viramontes BE, Camilleri M, McKinzie S, Pardi DS, Burton D, Thomforde GM. Gender-related differences in slowing colonic transit by a 5-HT3 antagonist in subjects with diarrhea-predominant irritable bowel syndrome. Am J Gastroenterol 2001;96(9):2671–6.
38. Lembo T, Wright RA, Bagby B, Decker C, Gordon S, Jhingran P, Carter E; Lotronex Investigator Team. Alosetron controls bowel urgency and provides global symptom improvement in women with diarrhea-predominant irritable bowel syndrome Am J Gastroenterol 2001;96(9):2662–70.
39. Wolfe SG, Chey WY, Washington MK, Harding J, Heath AT, McSorley DJ, Dukes GE, Hunt CM. Tolerability and safety of alosetron during long-term administration in female and male irritable bowel syndrome patients. Am J Gastroenterol 2001;96(3):803–11.
40. Talley NJ, Van Zanten SV, Saez LR, Dukes G, Perschy T, Heath M, Kleoudis C, Mangel AW. A dose-ranging, placebo-controlled, randomized trial of alosetron in patients with functional dyspepsia. Aliment Pharmacol Ther 2001;15(4):525–37.
41. Camilleri M, Chey WY, Mayer EA, Northcutt AR, Heath A, Dukes GE, McSorley D, Mangel AM. A randomized controlled clinical trial of the serotonin type 3 receptor antagonist alosetron in women with diarrhea-predominant irritable bowel syndrome. Arch Intern Med 2001;161(14):1733–40.
42. Friedel D, Thomas R, Fisher RS. Ischemic colitis during treatment with alosetron. Gastroenterology 2001;120(2): 557–60.
43. Fujii Y, Saitoh Y, Tanaka H, Toyooka H. Granisetron/dexamethasone combination for the prevention of postoperative nausea and vomiting after laparoscopic cholecystectomy. Eur J Anaesthesiol 2000;17(1):64–8.
44. Abang AM, Takemoto MH, Pham T, Mandanas RA, Roy V, Selby GB, Carter TH. Efficacy and safety of oral granisetron versus i.v. granisetron in patients undergoing peripheral blood progenitor cell and bone marrow transplantation Anticancer Drugs 2000;11(2):137–42.
45. D'Souza DL, Dimmitt DC, Robbins DK, Nezamis J, Simms L, Koch KM. Effect of alosetron on the pharmacokinetics of fluoxetine. J Clin Pharmacol 2001;41(4):455–8.

Flavoxate

See also Anticholinergic drugs

General Information

Flavoxate is an anticholinergic drug that is used to treat bladder detrusor instability. It can cause all the adverse effects that would be expected from its anticholinergic action.

Organs and Systems

Skin

- An 83-year-old man developed a generalized pruritic erythematous reaction with a fever after taking flavoxate 200 mg tds for 6 months in combination with tamsulosin hydrochloride and allylestrenol for prostatic hyperplasia (1). Patch tests with these drugs showed a positive reaction on flavoxate 10% on day 3. Rechallenge with flavoxate caused generalized pruritic erythema with fever.

Reference

1. Enomoto U, Ohnishi Y, Kimura M, Kawada A, Ishibashi A. Drug eruption due to flavoxate hydrochloride. Contact Dermatitis 1999;40(6):337–8.

Flecainide

See also Antidysrhythmic drugs

General Information

Flecainide is a class Ic antidysrhythmic drug. Its clinical pharmacology, clinical use, and adverse effects have been reviewed (1–3).

Comparative studies

In some patients treatment with a class I antidysrhythmic drug converts atrial fibrillation to atrial flutter. Of 187 patients with paroxysmal atrial fibrillation who were treated with flecainide or propafenone, 24 developed atrial flutter, which was typical in 20 cases (4). These patients underwent radiofrequency ablation, which failed in only one case. All the patients continued to take their preexisting drugs, and during a mean follow-up period of 11 months the incidence of atrial fibrillation was higher in patients who were taking combined therapy than in those taking monotherapy. The authors suggested that in patients with atrial fibrillation who developed typical atrial flutter due to class Ic antidysrhythmic drugs, combined catheter ablation and continued drug treatment is highly effective in reducing the occurrence and duration of atrial tachydysrhythmias. They did not report adverse effects.

In 33 patients with symptomatic and inducible supraventricular tachycardias single doses of placebo, flecainide 3 mg/kg, or diltiazem 120 mg plus propranolol 80 mg were used to terminate the dysrhythmia (5). Conversion to sinus rhythm was achieved within 2 hours in 17 patients with placebo, in 20 with flecainide, and in 31 with diltiazem plus propranolol. Time to conversion was shorter with diltiazem plus propranolol (32 minutes) than with flecainide (74 minutes) or placebo (77 minutes). Of those who were given flecainide, two had hypotension and one had sinus bradycardia.

Systematic reviews

A systematic review of 22 studies of the effects of flecainide used for at least 3 months in the treatment of supraventricular dysrhythmias suggested that flecainide is associated with a variety of adverse reactions, many of which are well tolerated, but carries a small risk of serious cardiac events (2%), which can lead to death (0.13%) (SEDA-21, 200).

In a meta-analysis of 122 prospective studies of the use of flecainide in 4811 patients with supraventricular

Table 1 Numbers (%) of cardiac and non-cardiac adverse effects of flecainide in a meta-analysis of 4375 treatment courses compared with 1818 treatment courses in controls

System	Adverse effect	Flecainide	Controls
Cardiovascular	Angina pectoris	43 (1.0)	25 (1.3)
	Palpitation	17 (0.4)	6 (0.3)
	Hypotension	33 (0.8)	24 (1.3)*
	Syncope	5 (0.1)	3 (0.2)
	Heart failure/ dyspnea	40 (0.9)	13 (0.7)
	Sinus node dysfunction	52 (1.2)	22 (1.2)
	Bundle branch block	29 (0.7)	7 (0.4)
	Atrioventricular block	24 (0.5)	7 (0.4)
Nervous system	Total	412 (9.4)	65 (3.4)*
	Headache	88 (2.0)	53 (2.9)*
	Dizziness	148 (3.4)	45 (2.5)
	Vertigo	137 (3.1)	42 (2.3)
Sensory systems	Visual disturbances	175 (4.0)	16 (0.9)*
Gastrointestinal	Total	144 (3.3)	121 (6.7)*
	Diarrhea	29 (0.7)	50 (2.8)*
	Nausea	71 (1.6)	33 (1.8)

*Significantly different.

dysrhythmias, 21 were placebo-controlled and 37 were comparative studies with other antidysrhythmic drugs (6). The total exposure time was 2015 patient-years, with a mean oral flecainide dose of 216 mg/day. There were eight deaths (total mortality 0.17%, fatality rate per 100 patient-years 0.40; 95% CI = 0.17, 0.78), confirming the earlier finding. Three deaths were non-cardiac (cancer, suicide, urinary sepsis). Of the cardiac deaths, all but two occurred in patients with coronary heart disease. In controls, there was one death. There were prodysrhythmic events in 120 patients taking flecainide (2.7%) and 88 controls (4.8%), 58 (7.4%) of which occurred in patients taking placebo. Non-cardiac adverse effects are listed in Table 1. Thus, flecainide is safe in patients with supraventricular dysrhythmias with no cardiac damage, in contrast to patients with ventricular dysrhythmias after myocardial infarction.

Organs and Systems

Cardiovascular

In a review of 60 original articles detailing 1835 courses of intravenous and/or oral flecainide in both placebo-controlled and comparative studies as well as a large number of uncontrolled studies, unwanted cardiac events occurred in 8% of patients (7). The cardiac events were hypotension (1.3%), heart failure (0.4%), sinus node dysfunction (1.6%), bundle branch block (1.0%), atrial dysrhythmias (1.6%), and ventricular dysrhythmias (1.3%). However, in 8505 patients, 5507 of whom were administered flecainide for more than 4 weeks and most of whom took dosages of 100–300 mg/day, cardiac adverse effects occurred in only about 2% and non-cardiac effects in about 10% (8). The most common cardiac adverse effects were angina pectoris, dysrhythmias, worsening of heart failure, and hemodynamic changes. Of the long-term non-cardiac adverse effects the most common were nausea, vomiting, dizziness, bowel disturbances, headache, and visual disturbances.

Cardiac dysrhythmias

In the wake of the preliminary and final reports of the Cardiac Arrhythmia Suppression Trial (CAST) (9,10), which showed that there was an increased risk of death among patients who took encainide and flecainide after myocardial infarction, there have been many publications in which the implications of these findings have been thoroughly discussed (11–15). The relative risk of death or cardiac arrest due to dysrhythmias in the treated patients was 2.6 and the relative risk due to all causes was 2.4. The risk of non-fatal cardiac adverse effects was no different in treated patients from that in those taking placebo and there was no difference between the groups in the use of other drugs.

Although there is a consensus that encainide and flecainide were associated with an increase in the rate of mortality in CAST, there are still some open questions. First, all the patients recruited to CAST had asymptomatic ventricular dysrhythmias after myocardial infarction, and it is not clear whether the results can be extrapolated to other patients. Secondly, the reasons for the increased mortality in the treated patients are not clear: ventricular dysrhythmias and worsening of left ventricular function are both possible. Thirdly, it is not clear whether the results of CAST in patients with asymptomatic ventricular dysrhythmias after myocardial infarction can also be applied to other Class I antidysrhythmic drugs.

The prodysrhythmic effects of flecainide, by prolongation of the QT_c interval, have been widely discussed (SEDA-15, 175) (16–20). However, overall, cardiac dysrhythmias are less common with flecainide than with other antidysrhythmic drugs of Class I, and the dysrhythmogenic effects of flecainide in patients with supraventricular dysrhythmias may not be great (SEDA-22, 207). When dysrhythmias occur, prolongation of the QT interval is an important mechanism, but in a recent case it was suggested that tachycardia was due to re-entry within the His-Purkinje system (21). In another case flecainide reportedly caused a wide-complex tachycardia due to atypical atrial flutter with 1:1 conduction and aberrant QRS complexes (22). Although drugs of Class Ic, such as flecainide, can slow atrial and atrioventricular nodal conduction in patients with atrial fibrillation or atrial flutter, they do not alter the refractoriness of the atrioventricular node, and this allows 1:1 atrioventricular conduction as the atrial rate slows. This happens despite prolongation of the PR interval.

- Syncope occurred in a patient whose QRS complex duration was prolonged (23).
- In a 67-year-old woman taking flecainide 150 mg bd, widening of the QRS complex occurred during exercise; the effect did not occur at rest or with a dose of 50 mg bd (24).

Hypokalemia can increase the risk of torsade de pointes with flecainide, as with other antidysrhythmic drugs.

- Torsade pointes has been attributed to mosapride (which is related to cisapride) and flecainide in a 68-year-old man with a plasma potassium concentration of 3.2 mmol/l and prolongation of the QT_c interval from 0.48 to 0.56 seconds (25). His plasma flecainide concentration was just above the target range at 1013 ng/ml, but the mosapride concentration was not reported.

The authors speculated that mosapride may have inhibited the metabolism of flecainide by CYP2D6.

In a retrospective analysis of 24 patients who developed atrial flutter while taking flecainide ($n = 12$) or propafenone ($n = 12$), the electrocardiogram was classified as typical atrial flutter in 13 cases, atypical atrial flutter in eight, or coarse atrial fibrillation in three (26). Counterclockwise atrial flutter was the predominant dysrhythmia. The acute results of ablation suggested that the flutter circuit was located in the right atrium and that the isthmus was involved in the re-entry mechanism. There was better long-term control of recurrent atrial fibrillation in patients with typical atrial flutter (85%) compared with atypical atrial flutter (50%). The authors suggested that patients who develop coarse drug-induced atrial fibrillation may not be candidates for ablation.

Cardioversion

In 24 patients with atrial fibrillation who underwent elective transvenous cardioversion for atrial fibrillation, flecainide reduced the energy requirements for further defibrillation after induction of atrial fibrillation by atrial pacing (27). There were no ventricular dysrhythmias, but transient bradycardia requiring ventricular pacing occurred in two patients. Two patients had transient asymptomatic hypotension after flecainide and one reported transient dizziness and some light-headedness.

Antidysrhythmic drugs increase the pacing threshold, but failure to capture is a rare consequence. It has, however, been reported twice with flecainide (28,29).

Electrocardiographic changes

ST segment elevation in leads II, III, and aVf, resembling an acute inferior myocardial infarction, have been reported with oral flecainide (30). Brugada syndrome is partial right bundle branch block with ST segment elevation in the right precordial leads of the electrocardiogram; it is due to an abnormality of sodium channels and occurs in 0.05–0.1% of the population; some cases are inherited (31). Flecainide can bring out Brugada-type changes on the electrocardiogram (32–34).

Hypotension

Flecainide has been reported to cause acute hypotension after intravenous administration (35).

Respiratory

Interstitial pneumonitis has only rarely been attributed to flecainide (SEDA-16, 181).

- Interstitial pneumonitis with acute respiratory failure was attributed to flecainide in a 59-year-old man with congenital heart disease related to the LEOPARD syndrome, in which there are multiple freckles (Lentigines), Electrocardiographic abnormalities, Ocular hypertelorism, Pulmonic stenosis, Abnormalities of the genitalia, Retarded growth, and sensorineural Deafness (36). A CT scan showed diffuse interstitial injury characterized by thickening of the intralobular septa, with areas of ground-glass pattern. Flecainide was withdrawn and within 2 weeks the changes on CT scan had almost completely disappeared.
- A 75-year-old man, who had taken flecainide 100 mg/day for 22 months, developed fever, headache, and a dry cough (37). A CT scan of the lungs was normal and he responded to prednisone. His symptoms disappeared, but when prednisone was withdrawn they returned, with breathlessness, a dry cough, and weight loss. A chest X-ray showed bilateral patchy opacities and a CT scan subpleural ground-glass opacities and septal thickening. He had impaired lung function, including a reduced diffusion capacity. Biopsy showed diffuse interstitial thickening with lymphocytic and eosinophilic infiltrates. Flecainide was withdrawn and prednisone given, and he made a full recovery within 1 month.
- A 73-year-old man, who had taken flecainide 100 mg/day for 4 months, developed fever, weight loss, breathlessness, and a dry cough (37). A chest X-ray showed patchy infiltrates and a CT scan ground-glass opacities and subpleural septal thickening. He had normal lung function, apart from a reduced diffusion capacity. Flecainide was withdrawn and prednisone given, and he made a full recovery within a few months.

Nervous system

The most common non-cardiac adverse effects of flecainide are on the central nervous system and include dizziness, drowsiness, visual disturbances, headache, nausea, paresthesia, nervousness, and tremor. The incidence of these adverse effects has varied widely (38,39).

Other reported effects of flecainide include dysarthria and visual hallucinations (40), abnormal taste sensations, flushing, a glove-and-stocking type of peripheral neuropathy, and dystonia (SEDA-17, 223).

Sensory systems

Ocular adverse effects of flecainide have included corneal deposits in two patients, due to deposition of flecainide (41). In 38 patients taking flecainide 100–300 mg/day there were brown corneal epithelial deposits in 11 eyes, dryness in eight eyes, and slight blurring of vision on lateral gaze in four patients (42). Four patients had local symptoms, including tearing, itching, and burning. Color vision, contrast sensitivity, and visual fields were all unaffected.

Hematologic

Flecainide can cause neutropenia (43).

Liver

Flecainide can cause increases in the serum activities of transaminases (44). In one case cholestasis and jaundice occurred (45).

Urinary tract

Flecainide can cause acute urinary retention, perhaps due to a local anesthetic effect on the bladder mucosa (46).

Skin

Flecainide reportedly caused a psoriasiform eruption (47).

Sexual function

Flecainide inhibits sperm motility in vitro (48), but this has not been reported to be of clinical relevance.

Flecainide can cause erectile impotence (49).

Second-Generation Effects

Pregnancy

Flecainide is occasionally used to treat fetal cardiac dysrhythmias by administration to the mother (50,51), although occasionally it can cause adverse effects in the child (SEDA-25, 184) and in the mother (52).

- At 30 weeks of gestation in a 41-year-old woman the fetus had hydrops, ascites, a pericardial effusion, and bilateral hydroceles. A supraventricular tachycardia with 1:1 conduction was treated by giving the mother oral flecainide 150 mg bd. However, during the next few weeks the mother developed evidence of hepatic cholestasis. The dosage of flecainide was reduced to 50 mg bd and the liver damage resolved. The child was born healthy but later required sotalol for a re-entry tachycardia.

Fetotoxicity

- A pregnant woman was given digoxin and flecainide at 29 weeks of gestation for fetal tachycardia and hydrops fetalis (53). The child was delivered spontaneously at 33 weeks and had mild respiratory distress. His electrocardiogram showed bifid P waves, a prolonged PR interval, deep wide Q waves, and raised ST segments. The QT interval was not prolonged. The serum digoxin concentration in the neonate was 1.2 mg/ml. The abnormalities resolved within 3 weeks of birth, despite continued digoxin therapy.

The authors attributed the electrocardiographic abnormalities to maternal use of flecainide.

Susceptibility Factors

Age

Reports of the use of flecainide in children suggest that the risk of adverse effects is low, although these studies have been very small (54–56).

Renal disease

Flecainide is cleared partly by dose-dependent hydroxylation and partly unchanged via the kidneys. Therefore, severe renal impairment and hepatic impairment both cause a reduction in its rate of clearance (57,58). Dosages should be reduced in these circumstances.

Hepatic disease

Flecainide is cleared partly by dose-dependent hydroxylation and partly unchanged via the kidneys. Therefore, severe renal impairment and hepatic impairment both cause a reduction in its rate of clearance (57,58). Dosages should be reduced in these circumstances.

Other features of the patient

Flecainide half-life is prolonged in poor hydroxylators (59) and poor metabolizers may be at an increased risk of adverse effects.

Drug Administration

Drug overdose

There have been a few reports of the effects of overdosage of flecainide (60–65). Various treatments have been used in these circumstances; none is specific.

- A 20-year-old woman took 3–4 g of flecainide and developed circulatory failure unresponsive to pacing, inotropic drugs, and sodium bicarbonate (66). She was then successfully treated with cardiopulmonary bypass for 30 hours. At peak, the plasma flecainide concentration was in excess of 4000 μg/ml, and although this fell during bypass to below 3.5 μg/ml, clinical recovery preceded this fall. Other complications included a coagulopathy with intravascular hemolysis, requiring the use of blood products, and renal insufficiency requiring hemodiafiltration.

The authors proposed that extracorporeal circulatory support had allowed increased perfusion of the liver and therefore more effective metabolism of the flecainide.

- Death has been reported in two patients who took flecainide (67). The postmortem femoral blood flecainide concentrations were 5.4 and 1.2 μg/ml (target range 0.2–1.0).
- Fatal flecainide overdose has been reported in a 65-year-old man who probably took 20 tablets of 100 mg each (68). However, no clinical details were available, because he was found dead. Flecainide was detected in his blood, gastric contents, and liver. *O*-dealkylated flecainide was found in his urine.

Of other fatal cases reviewed in the paper, in only one was there a slightly lower blood concentration of flecainide (7.3 compared with 7.7 mg/kg). The authors proposed that pre-existing cardiac damage could have predisposed this man to a dysrhythmic death.

Drug–Drug Interactions

Amiodarone

The combination of flecainide with amiodarone can result in reduced conduction, predisposing to bundle branch block and dysrhythmias (69,70).

Beta-adrenoceptor antagonists

The combination of flecainide with propranolol results in additive hypotensive and negative inotropic effects (71).

Lipophilic beta-adrenoceptor antagonists are metabolized to varying degrees by oxidation by liver microsomal cytochrome P450 (for example propranolol by CYP1A2 and CYP2D6 and metoprolol by CYP2D6). They can therefore reduce the clearance and increase the steady-state plasma concentrations of other drugs that undergo similar metabolism, potentiating their effects. Drugs that interact in this way include flecainide (72).

Digoxin

Despite an early report that flecainide might alter the pharmacokinetics of digoxin, this action is minimal and probably of no clinical significance (72). The combination causes a significant increase in the PR interval; but the clinical significance of this is unclear, it may be important for patients with impaired sinus node function (73).

Quinidine

Flecainide is metabolized by CYP2D6, and is subject to polymorphic metabolism. In extensive metabolizers its clearance is reduced by quinine (74). Quinidine reduces the clearance of *R*-flecainide but not that of *S*-flecainide (75).

Verapamil

Although verapamil reduces the clearance of flecainide, this is probably not clinically important (76). However, there is also a pharmacodynamic interaction, since both drugs increase the PR interval and have additive effects on myocardial contractility and atrioventricular conduction (77).

References

1. International Symposium on Supraventricular Arrhythmias: Focus on Flecainide. October 23–26, 1987, Paradise Island, Nassau, Bahamas. Proceedings. Am J Cardiol 1988;62(6):D1–D67.
2. Schneeweiss A. New antiarrhythmic drugs. II Flecainide. Pediatr Cardiol 1990;11(3):143–6.
3. Falk RH, Fogel RI. Flecainide. J Cardiovasc Electrophysiol 1994;5(11):964–81.
4. Schumacher B, Jung W, Lewalter T, Vahlhaus C, Wolpert C, Luderitz B. Radiofrequency ablation of atrial flutter due to administration of class IC antiarrhythmic drugs for atrial fibrillation. Am J Cardiol 1999;83(5):710–13.
5. Alboni P, Menozzi C. Episodic drug therapy for paroxysmal supraventricular tachycardia. Cardiol Rev 2002;19:44–6.
6. Wehling M. Meta-analysis of flecainide safety in patients with supraventricular arrhythmias. Arzneimittelforschung 2002;52(7):507–14.
7. Hohnloser SH, Zabel M. Short- and long-term efficacy and safety of flecainide acetate for supraventricular arrhythmias. Am J Cardiol 1992;70(5):A3–10.
8. Schulze JJ, Inhester B. Arrhythmiebehandlung unter Praxisbedingungen. Therapiewoche 1985;35:5898.
9. The Cardiac Arrhythmia Suppression Trial (CAST) Investigators. Preliminary report: effect of encainide and flecainide on mortality in a randomized trial of arrhythmia suppression after myocardial infarction. N Engl J Med 1989;321(6):406–12.
10. Echt DS, Liebson PR, Mitchell LB, Peters RW, Obias-Manno D, Barker AH, Arensberg D, Baker A, Friedman L, Greene HL, Huther ML, Richardson DW. Mortality and morbidity in patients receiving encainide, flecainide, or placebo. The Cardiac Arrhythmia Suppression Trial. N Engl J Med 1991;324(12):781–8.
11. Gottlieb SS. The use of antiarrhythmic agents in heart failure: implications of CAST. Am Heart J 1989;118(5 Pt 1):1074–7.
12. Podrid PJ, Marcus FI. Lessons to be learned from the Cardiac Arrhythmia Suppression Trial. Am J Cardiol 1989;64(18):1189–91.
13. Bigger JT Jr. The events surrounding the removal of encainide and flecainide from the Cardiac Arrhythmia Suppression Trial (CAST) and why CAST is continuing with moricizine. J Am Coll Cardiol 1990;15(1):243–5.
14. Akhtar M, Breithardt G, Camm AJ, Coumel P, Janse MJ, Lazzara R, Myerburg RJ, Schwartz PJ, Waldo AL, Wellens HJ, et al. CAST and beyond. Implications of the Cardiac Arrhythmia Suppression Trial. Task Force of the Working Group on Arrhythmias of the European Society of Cardiology. Circulation 1990;81(3):1123–7.
15. Thomis JA. Encainide—an updated safety profile. Cardiovasc Drugs Ther 1990;4(Suppl 3):585–94.
16. Anderson JL, Jolivette DM, Fredell PA. Summary of efficacy and safety of flecainide for supraventricular arrhythmias. Am J Cardiol 1988;62(6):D62–6.
17. Morganroth J, Horowitz LN. Flecainide: its proarrhythmic effect and expected changes on the surface electrocardiogram. Am J Cardiol 1984;53(5):B89–94.
18. Nathan AW, Hellestrand KJ, Bexton RS, Spurrell RA, Camm AJ. The proarrhythmic effects of flecainide. Drugs 1985;29(Suppl 4):45–53.
19. Podrid PJ, Morganroth J. Aggravation of arrhythmia during drug therapy: experience with flecainide acetate. Pract Cardiol 1985;11:55–70.
20. Wehr M, Noll B, Krappe J. Flecainide-induced aggravation of ventricular arrhythmias. Am J Cardiol 1985;55(13 Pt 1):1643–4.
21. Chalvidan T, Cellarier G, Deharo JC, Colin R, Savon N, Barra N, Peyre JP, Djiane P. His–Purkinje system reentry as a proarrhythmic effect of flecainide. Pacing Clin Electrophysiol 2000;23(4 Pt 1):530–3.
22. Mackstaller LL, Marcus FI. Rapid ventricular response due to treatment of atrial flutter or fibrillation with Class I antiarrhythmic drugs. Ann Noninvasive Electrocardiol 2000;5:101–4.
23. Kawabata M, Hirao K, Horikawa T, Suzuki K, Motokawa K, Suzuki F, Azegami K, Hiejima K. Syncope in patients with atrial flutter during treatment with class Ic antiarrhythmic drugs. J Electrocardiol 2001;34(1):65–72.
24. Turner N, Thwaites BC. Exercise induced widening of the QRS complex in a patient on flecainide. Heart 2001;85(4):423.
25. Ohki R, Takahashi M, Mizuno O, Fujikawa H, Mitsuhashi T, Katsuki T, Ikeda U, Shimada K. Torsades de pointes ventricular tachycardia induced by mosapride and flecainide in the presence of hypokalemia. Pacing Clin Electrophysiol 2001;24(1):119–21.
26. Nabar A, Rodriguez LM, Timmermans C, van Mechelen R, Wellens HJ. Class IC antiarrhythmic drug induced atrial flutter: electrocardiographic and electrophysiological findings and their importance for long term outcome after right atrial isthmus ablation. Heart 2001;85(4):424–9.
27. Boriani G, Biffi M, Capucci A, Bronzetti G, Ayers GM, Zannoli R, Branzi A, Magnani B. Favorable effects of flecainide in transvenous internal cardioversion of atrial fibrillation. J Am Coll Cardiol 1999;33(2):333–41.
28. Walker PR, Papouchado M, James MA, Clarke LM. Pacing failure due to flecainide acetate. Pacing Clin Electrophysiol 1985;8(6):900–2.
29. Antonelli D, Freedberg NA, Rosenfeld T. Acute loss of capture due to flecainide acetate. Pacing Clin Electrophysiol 2001;24(7):1170.
30. Nakamura W, Segawa K, Ito H, Tanaka S, Yoshimoto N. Class IC antiarrhythmic drugs, flecainide and pilsicainide, produce ST segment elevation simulating inferior myocardial ischemia. J Cardiovasc Electrophysiol 1998;9(8):855–8.
31. Chandrasekaran B, Kurbaan AS. Brugada syndrome: a review. Br J Cardiol 2002;9:406–10.
32. Priori SG, Napolitano C, Terrence L, et al. Incomplete penetrance and variable response to sodium channel blockade in Brugada's syndrome. Eur Heart J 1999; 20(Suppl):465A.
33. Brugada R, Brugada J, Antzelevitch C, Kirsch GE, Potenza D, Towbin JA, Brugada P. Sodium channel blockers identify risk for sudden death in patients with ST-segment elevation and right bundle branch block but structurally normal hearts. Circulation 2000;101(5):510–15.

34. Priori SG, Napolitano C, Schwartz PJ, Bloise R, Crotti L, Ronchetti E. The elusive link between LQT3 and Brugada syndrome: the role of flecainide challenge. Circulation 2000;102(9):945–7.
35. Saishu T, Iwatsuki N, Tajima T, Hashimoto Y. Flecainide is effective against premature supraventricular and ventricular contractions during general anesthesia. J Anesth 1994;8:284–7.
36. Robain A, Perchet H, Fuhrman C. Flecainide-associated pneumonitis with acute respiratory failure in a patient with the LEOPARD syndrome. Acta Cardiol 2000;55(1):45–7.
37. Pesenti S, Lauque D, Daste G, Boulay V, Pujazon MC, Carles P. Diffuse infiltrative lung disease associated with flecainide. Report of two cases. Respiration 2002;69(2):182–5.
38. Gentzkow GD, Sullivan JY. Extracardiac adverse effects of flecainide. Am J Cardiol 1984;53(5):B101–5.
39. Epstein M, Jardine RM, Obel IW. Flecainide acetate in the treatment of resistant supraventricular arrhythmias. S Afr Med J 1988;74(11):559–62.
40. Ramhamadany E, Mackenzie S, Ramsdale DR. Dysarthria and visual hallucinations due to flecainide toxicity. Postgrad Med J 1986;62(723):61–2.
41. Moller HU, Thygesen K, Kruit PJ. Corneal deposits associated with flecainide. BMJ 1991;302(6775):506–7.
42. Ikaheimo K, Kettunen R, Mantyjarvi M. Adverse ocular effects of flecainide. Acta Ophthalmol Scand 2001;79(2):175–6.
43. Samlowski WE, Frame RN, Logue GL. Flecanide-induced immune neutropenia. Documentation of a hapten-mediated mechanism of cell destruction. Arch Intern Med 1987;147(2):383–4.
44. Kuhlkamp V, Haasis R, Seipel L. Flecainidinduzierte Hepatitis. [Flecainide-induced hepatitis.] Z Kardiol 1988;77(10):678–80.
45. Mikloweit P, Bienmuller H. Medikamentös induzierte intrahepatische Cholestase durch Flecainidacetat und Enalapril. [Drug-induced intrahepatic cholestasis caused by flecainide acetate and enalapril.] Internist (Berl) 1987;28(3):193–5.
46. Ziegelbaum M, Lever H. Acute urinary retention associated with flecainide. Cleve Clin J Med 1990;57(1):86–7.
47. Mancuso G, Tampieri E, Berdondini RM. Eruzione psoriasiforme da flecainide. [Psoriasis-like eruption caused by flecainide.] G Ital Dermatol Venereol 1988;123(4):171–2.
48. Penhall RK, Hong CY, Muhiddin KA. The effect of flecainide on human sperm motility. Br J Clin Pharmacol 1982;14:147P.
49. Zehender M, Treese N, Kasper W, Pop T, Meinertz T. Effectiveness and tolerance in long-term treatment with flecainide. Circulation 1982;66(Suppl II):144.
50. Allan LD, Chita SK, Sharland GK, Maxwell D, Priestley K. Flecainide in the treatment of fetal tachycardias. Br Heart J 1991;65(1):46–8.
51. Edwards A, Peek MJ, Curren J. Transplacental flecainide therapy for fetal supraventricular tachycardia in a twin pregnancy. Aust NZ J Obstet Gynaecol 1999;39(1):110–12.
52. D'Souza D, MacKenzie WE, Martin WL. Transplacental flecainide therapy in the treatment of fetal supraventricular tachycardia. J Obstet Gynaecol 2002;22(3):320–2.
53. Trotter A, Kaestner M, Pohlandt F, Lang D. Unusual electrocardiogram findings in a preterm infant after fetal tachycardia with hydrops fetalis treated with flecainide. Pediatr Cardiol 2000;21(3):259–62.
54. Musto B, D'Onofrio A, Cavallaro C, Musto A, Greco R. Electrophysiologic effects and clinical efficacy of flecainide in children with recurrent paroxysmal supraventricular tachycardia. Am J Cardiol 1988;62(4):229–33.
55. Priestley KA, Ladusans EJ, Rosenthal E, Holt DW, Tynan MJ, Jones OD, Curry PV. Experience with flecainide for the treatment of cardiac arrhythmias in children. Eur Heart J 1988;9(12):1284–90.
56. Perry JC, McQuinn RL, Smith RT Jr, Gothing C, Fredell P, Garson A Jr. Flecainide acetate for resistant arrhythmias in the young: efficacy and pharmacokinetics. J Am Coll Cardiol 1989;14(1):185–91.
57. Williams AJ, McQuinn RL, Walls J. Pharmacokinetics of flecainide acetate in patients with severe renal impairment. Clin Pharmacol Ther 1988;43(4):449–55.
58. McQuinn RL, Pentikainen PJ, Chang SF, Conard GJ. Pharmacokinetics of flecainide in patients with cirrhosis of the liver. Clin Pharmacol Ther 1988;44(5):566–72.
59. Beckmann J, Hertrampf R, Gundert-Remy U, Mikus G, Gross AS, Eichelbaum M. Is there a genetic factor in flecainide toxicity? BMJ 1988;297(6659):1316.
60. Rodin SM, Johnson BF, Wilson J, Ritchie P, Johnson J. Comparative effects of verapamil and isradipine on steady-state digoxin kinetics. Clin Pharmacol Ther 1988;43(6):668–72.
61. Kirch W, Logemann C, Heidemann H, Santos SR, Ohnhaus EE. Nitrendipine/digoxin interaction. J Cardiovasc Pharmacol 1987;10(Suppl 10):S74–5.
62. Dunselman PH, Scaf AH, Kuntze CE, Lie KI, Wesseling H. Digoxin–felodipine interaction in patients with congestive heart failure. Eur J Clin Pharmacol 1988;35(5):461–5.
63. Bruserud O, Skadberg BT, Ohm OJ. Combined intoxication with digitoxin and verapamil. The possible inhibition of sensitisation to digitalis-specific antiserum by toxic drug concentrations. J Clin Lab Immunol 1988;25(4):167–71.
64. Ferrari E, Fournier JP, Gibelin P, Drici MD, Morand P. Le traitement par le lactate molaire de l'intoxication par le flécainide est-il sans danger? [Is treatment with molar lactate in flecainide poisoning safe?] Presse Méd 1989;18(28):1395.
65. Yang XS, Sun JP, Zhi GN. Acute flecainide toxicity. Chin Med J (Engl) 1990;103(7):606–7.
66. Corkeron MA, van Heerden PV, Newman SM, Dusci L. Extracorporeal circulatory support in near-fatal flecainide overdose. Anaesth Intensive Care 1999;27(4):405–8.
67. Lynch MJ, Gerostamoulos J. Flecainide toxicity: cause and contribution to death. Leg Med (Tokyo) 2001;3(4):233–6.
68. Romain N, Giroud C, Michaud K, Augsburger M, Mangin P. Fatal flecainide intoxication. Forensic Sci Int 1999;106(2):115–23.
69. Chouty F, Coumel P. Oral flecainide for prophylaxis of paroxysmal atrial fibrillation. Am J Cardiol 1988; 62(6):D35–7.
70. Saoudi N, Galtier M, Hidden F, Gerber L, Letac B. Bundle-branch reentrant ventricular tachycardia: a possible mechanism of flecainide proarrhythmic effect. J Electrophysiol 1988;2:365–71.
71. Almeyda J, Levantine A. Cutaneous reactions to cardiovascular drugs. Br J Dermatol 1973;88(3):313–19.
72. Lewis GP, Holtzman JL. Interaction of flecainide with digoxin and propranolol. Am J Cardiol 1984;53(5):B52–7.
73. Hellestrand KJ, Nathan AW, Bexton RS, Camm AJ. Response of an abnormal sinus node to intravenous flecainide acetate. Pacing Clin Electrophysiol 1984;7(3 Pt 1):436–9.
74. Munafo A, Reymond-Michel G, Biollaz J. Altered flecainide disposition in healthy volunteers taking quinine. Eur J Clin Pharmacol 1990;38(3):269–73.
75. Birgersdotter UM, Wong W, Turgeon J, Roden DM. Stereoselective genetically-determined interaction between chronic flecainide and quinidine in patients with arrhythmias. Br J Clin Pharmacol 1992;33(3):275–80.
76. Holtzman JL, Finley D, Mottonen L, Berry DA, Ekholm BP, Kvam DC, McQuinn RL, Miller AM. The pharmacodynamic and pharmacokinetic interaction between single doses of flecainide acetate and verapamil: effects on cardiac function and drug clearance. Clin Pharmacol Ther 1989;46(1):26–32.
77. Buss J, Lasserre JJ, Heene DL. Asystole and cardiogenic shock due to combined treatment with verapamil and flecainide. Lancet 1992;340(8818):546.

Floctafenine

See also Non-steroidal anti-inflammatory drugs

General Information

Floctafenine is a 4-aminoquinoline NSAID, closely related to antrafenine and glafenine, and its adverse effects profile is similar (1).

Organs and Systems

Urinary tract

Floctafenine has been detected in a urinary calculus (2).

Immunologic

Floctafenine has frequently been associated with anaphylactic reactions (3).

Drug Interactions

Cimetidine

Coma has been reported in a patient taking diuretics and cimetidine, who was given floctafenine (4).

Coumarin anticoagulants

Floctafenine may increase the action of coumarin anticoagulants (5).

References

1. Cheymol G, Biour M, Bruneel M, Albengres E, Hamel JD. Bilan d'une enquête nationale prospective sur les effets indesirables de la glafénine, de l'antrafênine et de la floctafénine. [Evaluation of a national prospective survey on the undesirable effects of glafenine, antrafenine and floctafenine.] Therapie 1985;40(1):45–50.
2. Moesch C, Rince M, Raby C, Leroux-Robert C. Identification d'un metabolite de la floctafénine dans un calcul urinaire. [Identification of metabolite of floctafenine in urinary calculi.] Ann Biol Clin (Paris) 1987;45(5):546–50.
3. van der Klauw MM, Wilson JH, Stricker BH. Drug-associated anaphylaxis: 20 years of reporting in The Netherlands (1974–1994) and review of the literature. Clin Exp Allergy 1996;26(12):1355–63.
4. Pasqua P, Craxi A, Pagliara L. Floctafenine and coma in cirrhosis. Ann Intern Med 1982;96(2):253.
5. Boeijinga JK, van de Broeke RN, Jochemsen R, Breimer DD, Hoogslag MA, Jeletich-Bastiaanse A. De involved van floctafenine (Idalon) op antistollingsbehandeling met coumarinederivaten. [The effect of floctafenine (Idalon) on anticoagulant treatment with coumarin derivatives.] Ned Tijdschr Geneeskd 1981;125(47):1931–5.

Flosulide

General Information

Flosulide is a COX-2 inhibitor.

Organs and Systems

Gastrointestinal

Flosulide caused less damage to the mucosa and was better tolerated than naproxen in a 2-week endoscopic study, but the clinical relevance of endoscopic studies of this sort is debatable (SEDA-14, 79).

Urinary tract

Clinical development of flosulide, a COX-2 selective inhibitor, has been discontinued because of nephrotoxicity (1). Measurement of renal prostaglandin synthesis did not predict the nephrotoxicity of flosulide in single-dose and short-term studies (2).

References

1. Kaplan-Machlis B, Klostermeyer BS. The cyclooxygenase-2 inhibitors: safety and effectiveness. Ann Pharmacother 1999;33(9):979–88.
2. Brunel P, Hornych A, Guyene TT, Sioufi A, Turri M, Menard J. Renal and endocrine effects of flosulide, after single and repeated administration to healthy volunteers. Eur J Clin Pharmacol 1995;49(3):193–201.

Floxuridine

See also Cytostatic and immunosuppressant drugs

General Information

Floxuridine is a pyrimidine analogue that is used in regional arterial chemotherapy for primary and metastatic malignancies, delivered using an implantable pump.

Organs and Systems

Gastrointestinal

Nine patients who received hepatic arterial infusion chemotherapy developed gastritis heralded by epigastric pain and tenderness, nausea, vomiting, weakness, and anorexia (1). In 7 patients, 18 gastric ulcers were detected endoscopically. Mucosal damage developed despite prophylactic antiulcer therapy and healed only on withdrawal. In 17 biopsy specimens there were variously inflammatory changes, reactive glandular changes, and cell necrosis, even in patients without ulcers. In addition, there was floxuridine-induced glandular atypia in eight biopsy samples from six patients; the crowded glands were distorted and lined by large cells that included bizarre forms with pleomorphic nuclei.

- A patient who received regional intrahepatic chemotherapy from a continuous infusion pump for 31 months developed a gastroduodenal artery–duodenal fistula, and presented with signs and symptoms of upper gastrointestinal bleeding.

Six patients who had received an infusion of floxuridine, either via the hepatic artery or intravenously, developed severe diarrhea (2). In four, the entire ileum or its more distal part was markedly narrowed and in the other two there was thickening or effacement of the mucosal folds in the distal ileum. The symptoms resolved and the radiographic appearances improved after withdrawal.

Biliary tract

The principle of hepatic arterial infusion is based on the fact that hepatic tumors derive much of their blood supply from the hepatic artery, whereas the liver parenchyma receives its supply from the portal venous circulation.

- Acute and chronic cholecystitis has been reported after floxuridine hepatic artery infusion (3). Chemotherapy in this patient was associated with persistent epigastric pain with radiation to the back which was not accompanied by any fever or white blood cell elevation. Cholecystectomy showed a shrunken, thickened fibrotic gallbladder that was filled with thick, pasty, hemorrhagic material. There were no gallstones.

In 27 patients who received intrahepatic floxuridine, total dose 20–41 mg/kg extrahepatic biliary sclerosis was discovered by CT scan and ultrasound, followed by endoscopic retrograde cholangiopancreatography and/or percutaneous cholangiography in three cases (4). Radiological findings included complete obstruction of the common hepatic duct in one case, common hepatic duct stenosis in two cases, common bile duct obstruction in one case, and intrahepatic bile duct dilatation without identifiable obstruction in one case

References

1. Doria MI Jr, Doria LK, Faintuch J, Levin B. Gastric mucosal injury after hepatic arterial infusion chemotherapy with floxuridine. A clinical and pathologic study. Cancer 1994;73(8):2042–7.
2. Kelvin FM, Gramm HF, Gluck WL, Lokich JJ. Radiologic manifestations of small-bowel toxicity due to floxuridine therapy. Am J Roentgenol 1986;146(1):39–43.
3. Pietrafitta JJ, Anderson BG, O'Brien MJ, Deckers PJ. Cholecystitis secondary to infusion chemotherapy. J Surg Oncol 1986;31(4):287–93.
4. Aldrighetti L, Arru M, Ronzoni M, Salvioni M, Villa E, Ferla G. Extrahepatic biliary stenoses after hepatic arterial infusion (HAI) of floxuridine (FUdR) for liver metastases from colorectal cancer. Hepatogastroenterology 2001;48(41):1302–7.

Fluconazole

See also Antifungal azoles

General Information

Fluconazole is an antifungal triazole that was derived from the older imidazoles. It has a lower molecular weight and is soluble in water. It can be administered orally and parenterally.

Pharmacokinetics

After oral administration, its systemic availability is about 90%; maximum plasma concentrations are seen in 1–2 hours, its half-life is about 30 hours and steady state is reached within 5–7 days. Fluconazole has low protein binding (about 12%), is hardly metabolized, and about 80% of it is excreted in the urine. Hemodialysis reduces plasma concentrations by about half in 3 hours (1–3). Tissue and body fluid penetration is good (2,4–9). The CSF concentration ratio is 0.5–0.9, the resultant concentrations being adequate for the treatment of cryptococcal meningitis (10–12). Penetration into the eye is good (13), and fluconazole has been used successfully in fungal endophthalmitis (14–17). In a patient in whom the concentrations of fluconazole in bile were studied, the concentrations after the first dose were about the same as in serum, but 10–12 hours after the dose, bile concentrations were higher than serum concentrations (18). Sputum concentrations are similar to plasma concentrations. Concentrations in vaginal secretions are slightly lower than in plasma, but persist for longer (19,20).

Like ketoconazole, fluconazole is a potent inhibitor of cytochrome P450, but with much higher specificity for fungal enzymes compared with human enzymes (21,22). Clinical interaction studies and some in vitro studies have suggested that azole antifungal drugs inhibit P glycoprotein. In a cell line in which human P glycoprotein was overexpressed, itraconazole and ketoconazole inhibited P glycoprotein function, with 50% inhibitory concentrations of about 2 and 6 μmol/l respectively; however, fluconazole had no effect (23).

Observational studies

The prophylactic use of oral fluconazole to prevent invasive *Candida* infections in 260 critically ill surgical patients has been investigated in a prospective, randomized, placebo-controlled trial in a single-center, tertiary-care surgical intensive care unit (24). The patients were randomly assigned to receive either oral fluconazole 400 mg/day or placebo. The risk of presumed and proven *Candida* infections in the patients who received fluconazole was significantly less than the risk in those who received placebo. After adjusting for several potentially confounding effects, fluconazole reduced the risk of presumed and proven fungal infection by 55%. There was no difference in death rate between fluconazole and placebo. The authors concluded that enteral fluconazole safely reduced the incidence of fungal infections in this high-risk population.

Comparative studies

Amphotericin

Fluconazole and amphotericin as empirical antifungal drugs in febrile neutropenic patients have been investigated in a prospective, randomized, multicenter study in 317 patients randomized to either fluconazole (400 mg qds) or amphotericin deoxycholate (0.5 mg/kg qds) (25). Adverse events (fever, chills, renal insufficiency, electrolyte disturbances, and respiratory distress) occurred significantly more often in patients who were given amphotericin (128/151 patients, 81%) than in those given fluconazole (20/158 patients, 13%). Eleven patients treated with amphotericin, but only one treated with fluconazole, were withdrawn because of an adverse event. Overall mortality and mortality from fungal infections were similar in both groups. There was a satisfactory response in 68% of the patients treated with fluconazole and 67% of those treated with amphotericin. Thus, fluconazole may be a safe and effective alternative to amphotericin for empirical therapy of febrile neutropenic patients; however, since fluconazole is ineffective against opportunistic molds, the possibility of an invasive infection by a filamentous fungus should be excluded before starting empirical therapy. Similarly, patients who take azoles for prophylaxis are not candidates for empirical therapy with fluconazole.

Conventional amphotericin deoxycholate (0.2 mg/kg qds) and fluconazole (400 mg qds) have been compared in a prospective, randomized study in 355 patients with allogeneic and autologous bone marrow transplantation (26). The drugs were given prophylactically from day –1 until engraftment. There was no difference in the occurrence of invasive fungal infections, but amphotericin was significantly more toxic than fluconazole, especially in related allogeneic transplantation, after which 19% of patients developed toxicity compared with none of those who received fluconazole.

Echinocandins

Caspofungin and fluconazole have been compared in adults with *Candida* esophagitis in a double-blind, randomized trial (27). Eligible patients had symptoms compatible with esophagitis, endoscopic mucosal plaques, and microscopic *Candida*. They were randomized to receive caspofungin (50 mg) or fluconazole (200 mg) intravenously once a day for 7–21 days. Most of them (154/177) had HIV infection, with a median CD4 count of 30×10^6/l. Favorable response rates were achieved in 66 of the 81 patients in the caspofungin arm and in 80 of the 94 patients in the fluconazole arm; symptoms had resolved in over 50% of the patients in both groups by the fifth day of treatment. Drug-related adverse effects were reported in 41% of patients given caspofungin and 32% of those given fluconazole; the most common events in both groups were phlebitis, headache, fever, nausea, diarrhea, abdominal pain, and rashes. Drug-related laboratory abnormalities developed in 29% of patients given caspofungin and in 34% of those given fluconazole. The most frequent laboratory abnormalities included reduced white blood cell count, hemoglobin concentration, and serum albumin concentration, and increased alkaline phosphatase and transaminases. No patient given caspofungin developed a serious drug-related adverse effect; therapy was withdrawn in only one patient (who was receiving fluconazole), because of an unspecified adverse effect.

Placebo-controlled studies

In a randomized, double-blind, placebo-controlled study in Saudi Arabia of oral fluconazole (200 mg/day for 6 weeks) in the treatment of cutaneous leishmaniasis, 106 patients were assigned to fluconazole and 103 to placebo (28). Follow-up data were available for 80 and 65 patients respectively. At the 3-month follow-up, healing of lesions was complete in 63 of the 80 patients who took fluconazole and 22 of the 65 patients who took placebo (relative risk of complete healing, 2.33; 95% CI = 1.63, 3.33). Adverse effects were mild and similar in the two groups.

General adverse effects

Fluconazole is generally well tolerated. The most common adverse effects are nausea and vomiting. Abnormal liver function tests and slight increases in hepatic enzymes have been reported, and there have been anecdotal reports of hepatitis and hepatic failure. Early studies have shown no changes in testosterone concentrations or in the adrenal response to ACTH. Rashes and a few cases of exfoliative skin disorder have been reported (SED-12, 681) and have been seen more frequently in patients with AIDS (29). Alopecia has been reported in a few cases with the use of high doses for prolonged periods of time (SEDA-18, 281). Rare instances of anaphylactoid reactions have been reported (SED-12, 681) (30). Rare instances of hypersensitivity reactions have occurred in other individuals (SEDA-16, 293) (SEDA-17, 320). Tumor-inducing effects have not been reported.

In a study using the UK General Practice Research Database to determine rates of drug-induced, rare, serious adverse effects on the liver, kidneys, skin, or blood, occurring within 45 days of completing a prescription or refill in 54 803 users of either fluconazole or itraconazole, three had illnesses for which a fluconazole-induced cause could not be ruled out; one with thrombocytopenia, one with neutropenia, and one with an abnormal liver function test just after receiving fluconazole (31). The rates were 2.8/100 000 prescriptions (95% CI = 0.8, 10) for serious, adverse blood events and 1.4/100 000 prescriptions (95% CI = 0.25, 8.2) for serious, adverse liver events. These results suggest that fluconazole does not commonly have serious adverse effects on the liver, kidneys, skin, or blood.

Organs and Systems

Cardiovascular

Prolongation of the QT interval is a class effect of the antifungal azoles and has occasionally been reported with fluconazole, with a risk of torsade de pointes.

- A 68-year-old woman with *Candida glabrata* isolated from a presacral abscess developed torsade de pointes after 8 days treatment with oral fluconazole 150 mg/day (32). She had no other risk factors for torsade de pointes, including coronary artery disease, cardiomyopathy, congestive heart failure, or electrolyte abnormalities. The dysrhythmia resolved when fluconazole was withdrawn, but she continued to have ventricular extra beats and non-sustained ventricular tachycardia for 6 days.

- A 59-year-old woman with liver cirrhosis and *Candida* peritonitis developed long QT syndrome and torsade de pointes after intravenous therapy with 400–800 mg/day of fluconazole for 65 weeks, followed by intraperitoneal administration (150 mg/day) (33). One day after the second intraperitoneal administration, she developed palpitation, multifocal ventricular extra beats, and syncope. In contrast to a normal electrocardiogram on admission, electrocardiography showed polymorphic ventricular extra beats, T wave inversion, alternating T wave amplitude, and a prolonged QT_c interval of 606 ms. Torsade de pointes required cardiopulmonary resuscitation. The fluconazole plasma concentration was 216 μg/ml (usual target range at 400–800 mg/day: 18–28 μg/ml). Fluconazole was withdrawn and all conduction abnormalities reversed fully within 3 weeks.

These patients were not taking any concomitant drugs that prolong the QT interval, suggesting that fluconazole was to blame.

- A 25-year-old woman with worsening endocarditis had a prolonged QT interval at baseline and developed monomorphic ventricular dysrhythmias, which were managed successfully with pacing and antidysrhythmic therapy, including amiodarone (34). Several days later, she was given high-dose fluconazole (800 mg/day) for fungemia and after 3 days had episodes of torsade de pointes.

In this case torsade de pointes developed in the presence of known risk factors—hypokalemia, hypomagnesemia, female sex, baseline QT interval prolongation, and ventricular dysrhythmias.

Nervous system

Central nervous system abnormalities constitute the major dose-limiting adverse effects of fluconazole and are observed at dosages over 1200 mg/day (35).

Dizziness, headache, and seizures were seen in 2–5% of 232 patients with severe systemic fungal infections taking fluconazole (36). In the same group there were three cases each of delirium and dysesthesia (1.3%). A possible effect of the underlying illness has to be considered. In 14 patients treated with fluconazole for cryptococcal meningitis, dizziness was reported in 14% (SED-12, 681).

Two Japanese patients developed clonic convulsions while taking fluconazole 800 mg/day (37).

- A 66-year-old woman with complicated invasive *Candida tropicalis* infection but no renal impairment took fluconazole 800 mg/day. On the 21st day she developed clonic convulsions. The fluconazole trough concentration at the time of the event was 82 μg/ml.
- A 62-year-old man with deteriorating renal and hepatic function after coronary artery bypass surgery was given fluconazole 400 mg bd for a fungal sternal wound infection. On the 15th day he developed seizures. His trough plasma fluconazole concentration was 88 μg/ml. Nineteen days after dosage adjustment to 400 mg qds, he had another seizure. The trough fluconazole concentration was 103 μg/ml, probably because of deteriorating renal function.

In both cases, the seizures abated after dosage reduction. These case reports suggest an association between trough plasma fluconazole concentrations of 80 μg/ml and central nervous system toxicity; they re-emphasize the need for careful monitoring and dosage adjustment of fluconazole in patients with reduced renal function.

Endocrine

Preliminary studies concerning a possible effect on testosterone concentrations and the adrenal response to adrenocorticotropic hormone did not show any changes. However, determinations were performed after only 14 days of fluconazole administration.

- Two critically ill patients, a 77-year-old man with esophageal cancer and a 66-year-old woman with multiple organ failure, developed reversible adrenal insufficiency temporally related to the use of high-dose fluconazole (800 mg loading dose followed by 400 mg/day), as assessed by short stimulation tests with cosyntropin (ACTH) (38). Although anecdotal, these data suggest that the possibility that high-dose fluconazole can cause adrenal insufficiency in already compromised critically ill patients needs to be investigated further.
- A 63-year-old man received high-dose cyclophosphamide for peripheral blood stem-cell harvesting, having been taking fluconazole 200 mg/day (39). On day 3 he developed atrial fibrillation and his blood pressure fell to 78 mmHg. A rapid ACTH stimulation test showed a blunted adrenal response. He was suspected of having adrenal failure, and fluconazole was withdrawn. A rapid ACTH test was normal on day 14. To clarify the association between adrenal failure and fluconazole, he was rechallenged with fluconazole 400 mg/day from day 16 and a rapid ACTH test was performed on day 21; it showed a blunted adrenal response.

Mineral balance

Hypokalemia was observed in only a few patients taking fluconazole, which contrasts with experience with itraconazole (36,40). However, hyperkalemia was reported in one paper (SED-12, 681) (40).

Hematologic

Cytopenias occur but seem to be mild. Occasionally, more marked changes have been described, but these could have been connected with the underlying disease (SED-12, 681) (40,41). In a single placebo-controlled study of fluconazole prophylaxis using a relatively high dose of 400 mg/day, a post-hoc analysis suggested prolongation of granulocytopenia after intensive chemotherapy for hematological neoplasms in the fluconazole group. This may have been due to an interaction with the antineoplastic drug (42).

Leukopenia with eosinophilia has been attributed to fluconazole (43).

- A 75-year-old man with non-Hodgkin's lymphoma and cryptococcal meningoencephalitis developed neutropenia with eosinophilia associated with fluconazole. After 1 week of fluconazole 400 mg/day his total leukocyte count began to fall and his eosinophil count increased. Concurrent medications included levothyroxine, famotidine, and co-trimoxazole. The last two drugs were withdrawn and he was given G-CSF.

However, his leukocyte count continued to fall and 4 days later reached a nadir of 700×10^6/l; the platelet count remained normal. The leukopenia and eosinophilia resolved promptly after withdrawal of fluconazole.

Since the leukopenia and eosinophilia did not resolve until fluconazole was withdrawn, an effect of the compound was plausible. This case and two other reported cases (44,45) emphasize the importance of recognizing fluconazole as a rare but potential cause of bone marrow suppression in patients in whom drug-induced agranulocytosis is suspected.

In one study in patients with AIDS taking prophylactic maintenance fluconazole for cryptococcal meningitis, there was a higher rate of hematological toxicity with fluconazole than with placebo, but this probably reflected the greater proportional and absolute amounts of zidovudine used in the fluconazole group; there was no serious hematotoxicity (SED-12, 682).

Gastrointestinal

Nausea and vomiting are mentioned in most reports of patients taking fluconazole, with an incidence of 10–15% (SED-12, 682) (36,40,41,46,47). Anorexia, mild abdominal pain, and diarrhea have been reported, but none was severe.

Liver

Raised liver enzyme activities have been reported in most studies. In some articles this effect was described as transient, in others as disappearing after withdrawal. The incidence varies from a few percent of cases to 35–45%, but occasionally the effect has been recorded in all cases treated. A temporal relation between these liver function changes and fluconazole treatment has been shown in many cases. Severe liver toxicity has not been reported (SED-12, 681) (21). While asymptomatic rises in transaminases were noted in some children with neoplastic disease who were treated concomitantly with fluconazole in a small study (48), there were no significant changes in a larger study in cancer patients treated with placebo or fluconazole 400 mg (42).

- A 45-year-old woman with protracted cryptococcal meningoencephalitis developed fulminant hepatic failure secondary to high fluconazole serum concentrations, possibly precipitated by renal dysfunction induced by concomitant amphotericin therapy or concomitant therapy with lisinopril, atenolol, or amlodipine (49). Four days after the withdrawal of fluconazole 400 mg/day the serum concentration of fluconazole was 40 μg/ml.

This case points to the potential risks of fluconazole therapy in the setting of renal insufficiency, in particular with higher dosages (400 mg/day and more).

Skin

Rashes of several types occur with fluconazole and are more frequent in immunocompromised patients.

The risk of serious skin disorders has been estimated in 61 858 users of oral antifungal drugs, aged 20–79 years, identified in the UK General Practice Research Database (50). They had received at least one prescription for oral fluconazole, griseofulvin, itraconazole, ketoconazole, or terbinafine. The background rate of serious cutaneous adverse reactions (corresponding to non-use of oral antifungal drugs) was 3.9 per 10 000 person-years (95% CI = 2.9, 5.2). Incidence rates for current use were 15 per 10 000 person-years (1.9, 56) for itraconazole, 11.1 (3.0, 29) for terbinafine, 10 (1.3, 38) for fluconazole, and 4.6 (0.1, 26) for griseofulvin. Cutaneous disorders associated with the use of oral antifungal drugs in this study were all mild.

Pruritus has also been reported (51). A few cases of Stevens–Johnson disease have been reported worldwide (SED-12, 682) (22,46,52), as well as a few instances of fixed-drug eruption (53). In cases of hypersensitivity, desensitization has reportedly been used with success (54).

Fixed drug eruption caused by systemic fluconazole has been reported (55).

- A 36-year-old woman with a history of atopy and recurrent *Candida* vaginitis developed a fixed drug eruption while taking fluconazole 150 mg/day. Local provocation with 10% fluconazole in petrolatum applied at the site of a previous site of fixed drug eruption reproduced the eruption clinically and histopathologically.

Nails

A patient developed a longitudinal band of pigmentation in the diseased nail after fluconazole therapy for onychomycosis at a dosage of 150 mg once a week for 4 weeks (56).

Second-Generation Effects

Teratogenicity

The teratogenic activity of triazole and two triazole derivatives, flusilazole (an agricultural triazole monoderivative fungicide) and fluconazole, has been studied in vitro (57). Rat embryos 9.5 days old (1–3 somites) were exposed in vitro to triazole 500–5000 μmol/l, flusilazole 3.125–250 μmol/l, or fluconazole 62.5–500 μmol/l and examined after 48 hours in culture. There were similar teratogenic effects (abnormalities at the branchial apparatus level and cell death at the level of the branchial mesenchyme) at 6.25 μmol/l and higher for flusilazole and 125 μmol/l and higher for fluconazole. In contrast, there was little effect at the highest concentrations of triazole, suggesting no teratogenic activity. These investigations have confirmed the embryotoxic potential of antifungal triazole derivatives, specifically on the branchial apparatus.

However, teratogenic effects have not been found in humans. The risk of malformations and other outcomes in children exposed to fluconazole in utero has been examined in 165 women who had taken fluconazole just before or during pregnancy, mostly in the form of a single dose of 150 mg to treat vaginal candidiasis (58). Birth outcomes (malformations, low birth weight, and preterm delivery) were compared with the outcomes among 13 327 women who did not receive any prescriptions during their pregnancies. The prevalence of malformation was 3.3% (four cases) among the 121 women who had used fluconazole in the first trimester, and 5.2% (697 cases) in offspring to controls (OR = 0.65; CI = 0.24, 1.77). The risks of preterm delivery (OR = 1.17; CI = 0.63, 2.17) and low birth weight (OR = 1.19; CI = 0.37, 3.79) were not significantly increased in association with fluconazole. Thus, the study showed no increased risk of congenital malformations, low birth weight, or preterm birth in offspring to women who had used single doses of fluconazole before conception or during pregnancy.

The potential ability of fluconazole to modulate phenytoin teratogenesis has been studied in Swiss mice (59). Pretreatment with a non-embryotoxic dosage of fluconazole (10 mg) potentiated phenytoin teratogenesis; combined treatment of fluconazole 50 mg with phenytoin resulted in a significant increase in embryo deaths. The mechanism of this teratological interaction remains to be established.

Lactation

Fluconazole is found in breast milk at concentrations comparable with those found in the blood after single or multiple doses (2); this may be of clinical relevance (60).

Susceptibility Factors

Age

In a group of children with fever, neutropenia, and neoplastic disease, there was an increase in renal fluconazole clearance (45). In infants and children, the volume of distribution of fluconazole is significantly higher and falls with age. With the exception of infants, who have a slower clearance rate, children clear the compound more rapidly (61). However, a second larger study reported slower elimination in children under 1 year of age, requiring dosage adjustments (62). Low birth-weight neonates have a particularly low clearance rate, which increases within weeks (63).

The use of fluconazole in 726 children under 1 year of age, reported in 78 publications, has been reviewed (64). They received a wide range of dosages for up to 162 days. Fluconazole was well tolerated and efficacious in the therapy of systemic candidiasis and candidemia in children under 1 year of age, including neonates and very low birth-weight infants. The daily dosage recommended by the manufacturers is 6 mg/kg, to be reduced in patients with impaired renal function in accordance with the guidelines given for adults.

The efficacy and safety of fluconazole in neonates with *Candida* fungemia has been evaluated in a multicenter prospective study (65). Fluconazole was safe and effective even in complicated cases, including infants of very low birth weights. Two of 50 neonates developed raised liver enzymes during fluconazole therapy and two others had raised serum creatinine concentrations. In none of them did these abnormalities necessitate discontinuation of antifungal therapy.

The safety profile of fluconazole has been assessed in 562 children (aged 0–17 years; 323 boys and 239 girls), enrolled into 12 clinical studies of prophylactic or therapeutic fluconazole in predominantly immunocompromised patients (66). Most of the children received multiple doses of fluconazole 1–12 mg/kg, given as oral suspension or intravenously. Overall, 58 children reported 80 treatment-related adverse effects. The most common adverse effects were associated with the gastrointestinal tract (7.7%), the skin (1.2%), or the liver and biliary system (0.5% or three patients). Overall, 18 patients discontinued treatment owing to adverse effects, mainly gastrointestinal. Dosage and age did not affect the incidence and pattern of adverse effects. Treatment-related laboratory abnormalities included transiently raised alanine transaminase (4.9%), aspartate transaminase (2.7%), and alkaline phosphatase (2.3%). Although 99% of patients were taking concomitant drugs, there were no clinical or laboratory interactions. The safety profile of fluconazole was compared with those of other antifungal agents, mostly oral polyenes, by using a subset of data from five controlled studies. Adverse effects were reported by more patients treated with fluconazole (45 of 382; 12%) than by patients treated with comparator agents (25 of 381; 6.6%); vomiting and diarrhea were the most common events in both groups. The incidence and type of treatment-related laboratory abnormalities were similar in the two groups. Fluconazole was well tolerated, mirroring the favorable safety profile seen in adults.

In 34 otherwise healthy infants with oral candidiasis randomized to either nystatin oral suspension qds for 10 days or fluconazole suspension 3 mg/kg in a single daily dose for 7 days, 6 of 19 were cured by nystatin and all of 15 by fluconazole (67). Fluconazole was tolerated without apparent adverse events.

Renal disease

If the creatinine clearance is below 40 ml/minute fluconazole doses should be adjusted (SED-12, 682) (7).

Drug–Drug Interactions

Alfentanil

In a randomized, double-blind, placebo-controlled, cross-over study in nine subjects, fluconazole 400 mg reduced the clearance of alfentanil 20 micrograms/kg by 55% and increased alfentanil-induced subjective effects (68).

Amitriptyline

An interaction of fluconazole with amitriptyline has been reported (69).

- A 12-year-old boy with prostatic rhabdomyosarcoma had episodes of syncope periodically over 7 months while taking fluconazole for chemotherapy-induced mucositis. He had taken fluconazole in the past without problems but had also taken a stable dose of amitriptyline for neuropathic pain. On withdrawal of amitriptyline he had no further episodes. The effect was confirmed by readministration.

Concurrent administration of fluconazole probably causes increased exposure to amitriptyline. Three reports of adults have shown increased amitriptyline plasma concentrations with concurrent administration of fluconazole; in one patient, a 57-year-old woman, the QT interval was prolonged and torsade de pointes occurred (70).

Amphotericin

In vitro studies and experiments in animals have given conflicting results relating to potential antagonism between the effects of fluconazole and amphotericin on *Candida* species (71). However, large, randomized, double-blind comparisons of fluconazole with and without amphotericin for 5 days in non-neutropenic patients with candidemia showed no evidence of antagonism, but faster clearance of the organism from the blood and a trend toward an improved outcome in those who received the combination (72).

Antacids

Fluconazole absorption after oral administration is not influenced by gastric pH; thus there is no effect of antacids such as co-magaldrox (SED-12, 682) (73).

Antihistamines

The concurrent use of terfenadine with fluconazole can lead to dangerously high terfenadine concentrations, with resulting cardiotoxicity (74). It is suspected that the same may happen with astemizole (75).

Benzodiazepines

The interaction of fluconazole with bromazepam has been studied in 12 healthy men in a randomized, double-blind, four-way, crossover study (76). They received single oral or rectal doses of bromazepam (3 mg) after 4-day pretreatment with oral fluconazole (100 mg/day) or placebo. Fluconazole caused no significant changes in the pharmacokinetics and pharmacodynamics of oral or rectal bromazepam.

Fluconazole increased blood concentrations of midazolam (77) and triazolam (78).

The effects of fluconazole (400 mg loading dose followed by 200 mg/day) on the kinetics of midazolam have been studied in 10 mechanically ventilated adults receiving a stable infusion of midazolam (79). Concentrations of midazolam were increased up to four-fold after the start of fluconazole therapy; these changes were most marked in patients with renal insufficiency. During the study, the ratio of α-hydroxymidazolam to midazolam progressively fell. The authors concluded that in ICU patients receiving fluconazole, reduction of the dose of midazolam should be considered if the degree of sedation is increasing.

In a study of the pharmacokinetics and pharmacodynamics of oral midazolam 7.5–15 mg, switching from inhibition of metabolism by itraconazole 200 mg/day to induction of metabolism by rifampicin 600 mg/day caused an up to 400-fold change in the AUC of oral midazolam (80).

Calcium channel blockers

- Fluconazole enhanced the blood pressure-lowering effects of nifedipine by increasing its plasma concentrations in a 16-year-old patient with malignant pheochromocytoma taking chronic nifedipine for arterial hypertension who was given fluconazole for *Candida* septicemia (81).

Carbamazepime

Fluconazole can cause carbamazepine toxicity, presumably by inhibition of CYP3A4 (82).

- A 33-year-old man on stable therapy with carbamazepine (400 mg tds) for a seizure disorder became stuporose due to carbamazepine toxicity after taking fluconazole 150 mg/day for 3 days. Withdrawal of both drugs resulted in a fall in carbamazepine concentrations (maximum concentration 25 μg/ml) and return of the patient's baseline mental status. Carbamazepine was restarted and the patient had no further adverse events.
- Carbamazepine serum concentrations increased during concomitant fluconazole administration (400 mg/day) in a 38-year-old man (83).

Ciclosporin

Fluconazole can increase concentrations of ciclosporin by inhibiting CYP3A4. In some studies, minimal or no effects were recorded, but in others ciclosporin concentrations were increased by fluconazole. Differences in the dosage and duration of fluconazole treatment could have explained these discrepancies (SED-12, 682) (21,84–87). For example, there was no interaction at a fluconazole dosage of 100 mg/day, but high dosages of fluconazole (400 mg/day or more) increase blood ciclosporin and tacrolimus concentrations (88,89).

The interaction of ciclosporin with fluconazole has been retrospectively evaluated in 19 kidney and pancreas/kidney transplant recipients (90). Both intravenous and oral fluconazole altered the blood concentration of ciclosporin. Five subjects did not have a significant interaction and 15 did. No patient had nephrotoxicity or transplant rejection related to antifungal therapy.

The effects of higher dosages of fluconazole on ciclosporin immunosuppression have been investigated in six renal transplant patients in a prospective, unblinded, crossover study (91). Baseline renal function, ciclosporin AUC, C_{max}, C_{min}, t_{max}, and clearance were compared with those 2, 4, and 7 days after starting fluconazole orally in a dosage of 200 mg/day. From day 8 onwards the ciclosporin dose was reduced by 50% and the above parameters were repeated on day 14. The results are shown in Table 1. On repeated-measures ANOVA only the AUC and C_{max} on day 4 of fluconazole were significantly higher than on day 0. There were no significant changes in ciclosporin clearance and t_{max}. The authors concluded that changes in C_{min} may not be sensitive enough to detect the described interaction and suggested monitoring the AUC near day 4 of treatment to guide ciclosporin dosage adjustments in all patients taking concomitant fluconazole.

Table 1 Changes in ciclosporin kinetics during co-administration of fluconazole

Parameter	Day 0	Day 4	Day 7	Day 14
AUC (hours.ng/ml)	2887	4750	4052	2330
C_{max} (ng/ml)	701	941	768	498
C_{min} (ng/ml)	207	274	293	174
Clearance (ml/minute/kg)	17	13	12	30
t_{max} (hours)	3.0	2.0	2.5	3.0

Cimetidine

Fluconazole absorption after oral administration is not influenced by gastric pH; thus there is no effect of cimetidine.

Clarithromycin

The effects of fluconazole and clarithromycin on the pharmacokinetics of rifabutin and 25-*O*-desacetylrifabutin have been studied in 10 HIV-infected patients who were given rifabutin 300 mg qds in addition to fluconazole 200 mg qds and clarithromycin 500 mg qds (92). There was a 76% increase in the plasma AUC of rifabutin when either fluconazole or clarithromycin was given alone and a 152% increase when both drugs were given together. The authors concluded that patients should be monitored for adverse effects of rifabutin when it is co-administered with fluconazole or clarithromycin.

Cyclophosphamide

Cyclophosphamide is a prodrug that is metabolized by CYP450 enzymes to produce alkylating species, which are cytotoxic, and the extent of cyclophosphamide metabolism correlates with both treatment efficacy and toxicity. In vitro studies in six human liver microsomes showed that the IC_{50} of fluconazole for reduction of 4-hydroxycyclophosphamide production was 9–80 μmol/l (93).

A retrospective study in 22 children with cancers addressed the potential interaction between fluconazole and cyclophosphamide. Children with an established profile of cyclophosphamide metabolism who were not receiving other drugs known to affect drug metabolism were selected; 9 were taking fluconazole and 13 were controls. The plasma clearance was significantly lower in patients taking concomitant fluconazole (2.4 versus 4.2 l/hour/m^2). It is unclear whether this interaction is associated with a reduction in the therapeutic efficacy of cyclophosphamide.

Doxorubicin

The effect of fluconazole on the plasma pharmacokinetics of doxorubicin has been investigated in a randomized, crossover study in non-human primates (94). Fluconazole (10 mg/kg/day) was given intravenously for 4 days before doxorubicin (2.0 mg/kg intravenously). Pretreatment with fluconazole had no effect on the pharmacokinetics of doxorubicin, and the incidence of severe neutropenia (absolute neutrophil count below 0.5×10^9/l) was higher with doxorubicin alone than with the combination of doxorubicin and fluconazole. Thus, fluconazole does not appear to contribute to the marrow-suppressive effects of doxorubicin.

Flucytosine

The concurrent use of fluconazole with flucytosine may have an additive effect (95). This combination could be useful in the treatment of cryptococcal meningitis (21).

HIV protease inhibitors

The pharmacokinetic interaction of fluconazole 400 mg od and indinavir 1000 mg tds has been evaluated in a placebo-controlled, crossover study for 8 days; there was no significant interaction (96).

The effect of fluconazole on the steady-state pharmacokinetics of ritonavir and saquinavir has been studied in patients infected with HIV-1 (97). They received the protease inhibitor (saquinavir 1200 mg tds, $n = 5$, or ritonavir 600 mg bd, $n = 3$) alone on day 1 and then with fluconazole 400 mg on day 2 and 200 mg on days 3–8. The median increase in saquinavir AUC was 50%, and the median increase in C_{max} was 56%. In contrast, fluconazole had no effect on the disposition of ritonavir.

Methadone

An interaction between fluconazole and methadone (a substrate of CYP3A4, CYP2C9, and CYP2C19) has been reported.

- While taking a stable dose of methadone, a 60-year-old man with advanced cancer developed respiratory depression 2 days after receiving intravenous fluconazole for refractory oral candidiasis (98). Intravenous naloxone reversed the respiratory depression.

In a randomized, double-blind, placebo-controlled study in 25 patients, fluconazole 200 mg/day increased methadone concentrations, but patients treated with fluconazole did not have signs or symptoms of significant narcotic overdose (99).

Omeprazole

Fluconazole absorption after oral administration is not influenced by gastric pH; thus there is no effect of omeprazole (100). Omeprazole is extensively metabolized in the liver by 5-hydroxylation and sulfoxidation reactions, catalysed predominantly by CYP2C19 and CYP3A4 respectively. Fluconazole is a potent competitive inhibitor of CYP2C19 and a weak inhibitor of CYP3A4. The effect of fluconazole on the pharmacokinetics of a single oral dose of omeprazole 20 mg has been evaluated after a single oral dose of fluconazole 100 mg and after 4 days of oral administration of 100 mg/day in 18 healthy male volunteers (101). Fluconazole increased the C_{max} and the mean AUC of omeprazole and prolonged its half-life (2.59 versus 0.85 hours).

Oral contraceptives

Fluconazole did not significantly alter the pharmacokinetics of ethinylestradiol or norgestrel, and this finding was interpreted by the investigators as suggesting that treatment with fluconazole in a user of oral contraceptives would not increase the risk of pregnancy (102). However, the study was carried out using a 50 mg dose of fluconazole, and experience with higher dosages has shown different results (SED-12, 682).

In another study, fluconazole reduced the systemic availability of ethinylestradiol in an oral contraceptive, but there was no information about the doses used (75).

In an open, crossover study in 10 young healthy subjects, fluconazole 150 mg increased the serum concentrations of ethinylestradiol 30–35 μg/day (103).

The potential pharmacokinetic interaction between fluconazole 300 mg once weekly and an oral contraceptive containing ethinylestradiol and norethindrone (Ortho Novum 7/7/7; Ortho-McNeil Pharmaceutical Inc, Raritan, NJ) has been studied in a placebo-controlled, double-blind, randomized, two-way, crossover study in 26 healthy women aged 18–36 years (104). During the first cycle they took the oral contraceptive only. During the second cycle they were assigned randomly to oral contraceptive + fluconazole or oral contraceptive + placebo. In the third cycle they were given the other treatment. Fluconazole caused small but statistically significant increases in the AUC_{0-24} of both ethinylestradiol and norethindrone. There were no adverse events related to treatment in those given fluconazole.

It therefore appears that there is no threat of contraceptive failure because of concomitant fluconazole administration.

Phenytoin

Co-administration of fluconazole and phenytoin resulted in markedly higher phenytoin concentrations (SED-12, 682) (21,84,87,105).

Rifamycins

The combination of rifampicin with fluconazole has insignificant effects (SED-12, 682) (21,87,106).

Statins

The effects of fluconazole on plasma fluvastatin and pravastatin concentrations have been studied in two separate, randomized, double-blind, two-phase, crossover studies (107). Healthy volunteers were given oral fluconazole (400 mg on day 1 and 200 mg on days 2–4) or placebo. On day 4, they took a single oral dose of fluvastatin 40 mg or pravastatin 40 mg. Fluconazole increased the plasma AUC and the half-life of fluvastatin by 80% but had no significant effects on the pharmacokinetics of pravastatin. The mechanism of the prolonged elimination of fluvastatin was probably inhibition of CYP2C9. Pravastatin, in contrast, appears not to be susceptible to interactions with fluconazole and other CYP2C9 inhibitors.

The effect of fluconazole on the pharmacokinetics of rosuvastatin has been investigated in a randomized, double-blind, two-way, crossover, placebo-controlled study (108). Healthy male volunteers ($n = 14$) were given fluconazole 200 mg/day or matching placebo for 11 days; rosuvastatin 80 mg was co-administered on day 8. Plasma concentrations of rosuvastatin, *N*-desmethylrosuvastatin, and active and total HMG-CoA reductase inhibitors were measured up to 96 hours after the dose. Fluconazole increased the AUC and C_{max} of rosuvastatin by 14% and 9% respectively. Limited data available for the *N*-desmethylated metabolite showed that the C_{max} fell by about 25%. Fluconazole did not affect the proportion of circulating active or total HMG-CoA reductase inhibitors accounted for by circulating rosuvastatin. Thus, fluconazole produced only small changes in rosuvastatin kinetics, which were not considered to be of clinical relevance.

Sulfonylureas

The concurrent administration of fluconazole with tolbutamide resulted in increased tolbutamide concentrations (SED-12, 682) (71).

- A 56-year-old HIV-positive patient with diabetes mellitus taking gliclazide 160 mg/day developed severe hypoglycemia when treated with co-trimoxazole 480 mg/day and fluconazole 200 mg/day (109). The authors speculated that fluconazole might have inhibited gliclazide metabolism by inhibiting CYP2C9.

The effects of fluconazole and fluvoxamine on the pharmacokinetics and pharmacodynamics of glimepiride have been studied in a randomized, double-blind, crossover study in 12 healthy volunteers who took fluconazole 200 mg/day (400 mg on day 1), fluvoxamine 100 mg/day, or placebo once daily for 4 days (110). On day 4 they took a single oral dose of glimepiride 0.5 mg. Fluconazole increased the mean total AUC of glimepiride to 238% and the peak plasma concentration to 151% of control values, and the half-life of glimepiride was prolonged from 2.0 to 3.3 hours. This was probably due to inhibition of CYP2C9-mediated biotransformation of glimepiride by fluconazole. However, fluconazole did not cause statistically significant changes in the effects of glimepiride on blood glucose concentrations.

Tacrolimus

Since tacrolimus (FK506) is metabolized by intestinal and hepatic CYP3A4, drugs that inhibit CYP3A4 can reduce the metabolism of tacrolimus and increase tacrolimus blood concentrations (111). The effect of fluconazole on the blood concentrations of tacrolimus have been investigated in eight liver transplant patients in whom prophylactic fluconazole (200 mg/day) was withdrawn because of rises in hepatic transaminases ($n = 6$), renal dysfunction, or eosinophilia ($n = 1$ each) (112). Calculated tacrolimus concentrations fell by 13–81% (median 41%) between the fourth and ninth days after withdrawal of fluconazole. Tacrolimus blood concentrations should be carefully monitored and dosages increased as necessary after withdrawal of fluconazole.

The interaction of tacrolimus with fluconazole has been retrospectively evaluated in 19 kidney and pancreas/kidney transplant recipients (90). Both intravenous and oral fluconazole altered the blood concentration of tacrolimus. Five subjects did not have a significant interaction and 15 did. No patient had nephrotoxicity or transplant rejection related to antifungal therapy.

- A 17-year-old man with cystic fibrosis who took itraconazole after a lung-liver transplant had high trough concentrations of tacrolimus, despite the relatively low dosage (0.1–0.3 mg/kg/day) (113).
- A patient taking tacrolimus 0.085 mg/kg bd with itraconazole 200–400 mg/day developed ketoacidosis, neutropenia, and thrombocytopenia, requiring the withdrawal of both drugs (114).
- A 34-year-old renal transplant recipient taking a stable regimen of tacrolimus and methylprednisolone was given itraconazole 100 mg bd for a yeast infection of the urinary tract (115). Concomitant therapy with itraconazole led to a marked increase in tacrolimus trough concentrations on the second day of therapy (from 13 to 21 ng/ml) and an increase in serum creatinine concentrations, necessitating dosage reduction of tacrolimus by 50%.

When itraconazole was withdrawn the effect of itraconazole on the kinetics of tacrolimus took 12 days to reverse.

The inhibitory effect of itraconazole occurred quickly, while the time of disappearance was much longer, which is important for clinical management. Thus, during co-administration of itraconazole with tacrolimus, close monitoring of tacrolimus blood concentrations and careful dosage adjustments are essential to avoid toxicity.

Warfarin

Co-administration of fluconazole and warfarin has led in some cases to prolongation of the prothrombin time (21,87,106,116).

Zidovudine

Zidovudine glucuronidation in human hepatic microsomes in vitro was inhibited more by the combination of fluconazole with valproic acid than with other drugs, such as atovaquone and methadone (117).

References

1. Berl T, Wilner KD, Gardner M, Hansen RA, Farmer B, Baris BA, Henrich WL. Pharmacokinetics of fluconazole in renal failure. J Am Soc Nephrol 1995;6(2):242–7.
2. Debruyne D. Clinical pharmacokinetics of fluconazole in superficial and systemic mycoses. Clin Pharmacokinet 1997;33(1):52–77.
3. Pittrow L, Penk A. Dosage adjustment of fluconazole during continuous renal replacement therapy (CAVH, CVVH, CAVHD, CVVHD). Mycoses 1999;42(1–2):17–19.
4. Schafer-Korting M. Pharmacokinetic optimisation of oral antifungal therapy. Clin Pharmacokinet 1993;25(4):329–41.
5. Grant SM, Clissold SP. Fluconazole. A review of its pharmacodynamic and pharmacokinetic properties, and therapeutic potential in superficial and systemic mycoses. Drugs 1990;39(6):877–916. Erratum in: Drugs 1990;40(6):862.
6. Lazar JD, Hilligoss DM. The clinical pharmacology of fluconazole. Semin Oncol 1990;17(3 Suppl 6):14–18.
7. Brammer KW, Farrow PR, Faulkner JK. Pharmacokinetics and tissue penetration of fluconazole in humans. Rev Infect Dis 1990;12(Suppl 3):S318–26.
8. Goa KL, Barradell LB. Fluconazole. An update of its pharmacodynamic and pharmacokinetic properties and therapeutic use in major superficial and systemic mycoses in immunocompromised patients. Drugs 1995;50(4):658–90. Erratum in: Drugs 1996;51(3):505.
9. Debruyne D, Ryckelynck JP. Clinical pharmacokinetics of fluconazole. Clin Pharmacokinet 1993;24(1):10–27.
10. Tucker RM, Williams PL, Arathoon EG, Levine BE, Hartstein AI, Hanson LH, Stevens DA. Pharmacokinetics of fluconazole in cerebrospinal fluid and serum in human coccidioidal meningitis. Antimicrob Agents Chemother 1988;32(3):369–73.
11. Arndt CA, Walsh TJ, McCully CL, Balis FM, Pizzo PA, Poplack DG. Fluconazole penetration into cerebrospinal fluid: implications for treating fungal infections of the central nervous system. J Infect Dis 1988;157(1):178–80.
12. Menichetti F, Fiorio M, Tosti A, Gatti G, Bruna Pasticci M, Miletich F, Marroni M, Bassetti D, Pauluzzi S. High-dose fluconazole therapy for cryptococcal meningitis in patients with AIDS. Clin Infect Dis 1996;22(5):838–40.
13. Mian UK, Mayers M, Garg Y, Liu QF, Newcomer G, Madu C, Liu W, Louie A, Miller MH. Comparison of fluconazole pharmacokinetics in serum, aqueous humor, vitreous humor, and cerebrospinal fluid following a single dose and at steady state. J Ocul Pharmacol Ther 1998;14(5):459–71.
14. Christmas NJ, Smiddy WE. Vitrectomy and systemic fluconazole for treatment of endogenous fungal endophthalmitis. Ophthalmic Surg Lasers 1996;27(12):1012–18.
15. Zarbin MA, Becker E, Witcher J, Yamani A, Irvine AR. Treatment of presumed fungal endophthalmitis with oral fluconazole. Ophthalmic Surg Lasers 1996;27(7):628–31.
16. Luttrull JK, Wan WL, Kubak BM, Smith MD, Oster HA. Treatment of ocular fungal infections with oral fluconazole. Am J Ophthalmol 1995;119(4):477–81.
17. Akler ME, Vellend H, McNeely DM, Walmsley SL, Gold WL. Use of fluconazole in the treatment of candidal endophthalmitis. Clin Infect Dis 1995;20(3):657–64.
18. Bozzette SA, Gordon RL, Yen A, Rinaldi M, Ito MK, Fierer J. Biliary concentrations of fluconazole in a patient with candidal cholecystitis: case report. Clin Infect Dis 1992;15(4):701–3.
19. Edelman DA, Grant S. One-day therapy for vaginal candidiasis. A review. J Reprod Med 1999;44(6):543–7.
20. Houang ET, Chappatte O, Byrne D, Macrae PV, Thorpe JE. Fluconazole levels in plasma and vaginal secretions of patients after a 150-milligram single oral dose and rate of eradication of infection in vaginal candidiasis. Antimicrob Agents Chemother 1990;34(5):909–10.
21. Francis P, Walsh TJ. Evolving role of flucytosine in immunocompromised patients: new insights into safety, pharmacokinetics, and antifungal therapy. Clin Infect Dis 1992;15(6):1003–18.
22. Azon-Masoliver A, Vilaplana J. Fluconazole-induced toxic epidermal necrolysis in a patient with human immunodeficiency virus infection. Dermatology 1993;187(4):268–9.
23. Wang EJ, Lew K, Casciano CN, Clement RP, Johnson WW. Interaction of common azole antifungals with P glycoprotein. Antimicrob Agents Chemother 2002;46(1):160–5.
24. Pelz RK, Hendrix CW, Swoboda SM, Diener-West M, Merz WG, Hammond J, Lipsett PA. Double-blind placebo-controlled trial of fluconazole to prevent candidal infections in critically ill surgical patients. Ann Surg 2001;233(4):542–8.
25. Winston DJ, Hathorn JW, Schuster MG, Schiller GJ, Territo MC. A multicenter, randomized trial of fluconazole versus amphotericin B for empiric antifungal therapy of febrile neutropenic patients with cancer. Am J Med 2000;108(4):282–9.
26. Wolff SN, Fay J, Stevens D, Herzig RH, Pohlman B, Bolwell B, Lynch J, Ericson S, Freytes CO, LeMaistre F, Collins R, Pineiro L, Greer J, Stein R, Goodman SA, Dummer S. Fluconazole vs low-dose amphotericin B for the prevention of fungal infections in patients undergoing bone marrow transplantation: a study of the North American Marrow Transplant Group. Bone Marrow Transplant 2000;25(8):853–9.
27. Villanueva A, Gotuzzo E, Arathoon EG, Noriega LM, Kartsonis NA, Lupinacci RJ, Smietana JM, DiNubile MJ, Sable CA. A randomized double-blind study of caspofungin versus fluconazole for the treatment of esophageal candidiasis. Am J Med 2002;113(4):294–9.
28. Alrajhi AA, Ibrahim EA, De Vol EB, Khairat M, Faris RM, Maguire JH. Fluconazole for the treatment of cutaneous leishmaniasis caused by Leishmania major. N Engl J Med 2002;346(12):891–5.
29. Gupta AK, Katz HI, Shear NH. Drug interactions with itraconazole, fluconazole, and terbinafine and their management. J Am Acad Dermatol 1999;41(2 Pt 1):237–49.
30. Neuhaus G, Pavic N, Pletscher M. Anaphylactic reaction after oral fluconazole. BMJ 1991;302(6788):1341.
31. Bradbury BD, Jick SS. Itraconazole and fluconazole and certain rare, serious adverse events. Pharmacotherapy 2002;22(6):697–700.
32. Tholakanahalli VN, Potti A, Hanley JF, Merliss AD. Fluconazole-induced torsade de pointes. Ann Pharmacother 2001;35(4):432–4.

33. Wassmann S, Nickenig G, Bohm M. Long QT syndrome and torsade de pointes in a patient receiving fluconazole. Ann Intern Med 1999;131(10):797.
34. Khazan M, Mathis AS. Probable case of torsades de pointes induced by fluconazole. Pharmacotherapy 2002;22(12):1632–7.
35. Anaissie EJ, Kontoyiannis DP, Huls C, Vartivarian SE, Karl C, Prince RA, Bosso J, Bodey GP. Safety, plasma concentrations, and efficacy of high-dose fluconazole in invasive mold infections. J Infect Dis 1995;172(2):599–602.
36. Robinson PA, Knirsch AK, Joseph JA. Fluconazole for life-threatening fungal infections in patients who cannot be treated with conventional antifungal agents. Rev Infect Dis 1990;12(Suppl 3):S349–63.
37. Matsumoto K, Ueno K, Yoshimura H, Morii M, Takada M, Sawai T, Mitsutake K, Shibakawa M. Fluconazole-induced convulsions at serum trough concentrations of approximately 80 microg/mL. Ther Drug Monit 2000;22(5):635–6.
38. Albert SG, DeLeon MJ, Silverberg AB. Possible association between high-dose fluconazole and adrenal insufficiency in critically ill patients. Crit Care Med 2001;29(3):668–70.
39. Shibata S, Kami M, Kanda Y, Machida U, Iwata H, Kishi Y, Takeshita A, Miyakoshi S, Ueyama J, Morinaga S, Mutou Y. Acute adrenal failure associated with fluconazole after administration of high-dose cyclophosphamide. Am J Hematol 2001;66(4):303–5.
40. Larsen RA, Leal MA, Chan LS. Fluconazole compared with amphotericin B plus flucytosine for cryptococcal meningitis in AIDS. A randomized trial. Ann Intern Med 1990;113(3):183–7.
41. Bozzette SA, Larsen RA, Chiu J, Leal MA, Jacobsen J, Rothman P, Robinson P, Gilbert G, McCutchan JA, Tilles J, et al. A placebo-controlled trial of maintenance therapy with fluconazole after treatment of cryptococcal meningitis in the acquired immunodeficiency syndrome. California Collaborative Treatment Group. N Engl J Med 1991;324(9):580–4.
42. Schaffner A, Schaffner M. Effect of prophylactic fluconazole on the frequency of fungal infections, amphotericin B use, and health care costs in patients undergoing intensive chemotherapy for hematologic neoplasias. J Infect Dis 1995;172(4):1035–41.
43. Wong-Beringer A, Shriner K. Fluconazole-induced agranulocytosis with eosinophilia. Pharmacotherapy 2000;20(4):484–6.
44. Chuncharunee S, Sathapatayavongs B, Singhasivanon P, Singhasivanon V. Fluconazole-induced agranulocytosis. Therapie 1994;49(6):517–18.
45. Murakami H, Katahira H, Matsushima T, Sakura T, Tamura J, Sawamura M, Tsuchiya J. Agranulocytosis during treatment with fluconazole. J Int Med Res 1992;20(6):492–4.
46. Sugar AM, Stern JJ, Dupont B. Overview: treatment of cryptococcal meningitis. Rev Infect Dis 1990;12(Suppl 3):S338–48.
47. Chabot GG, Pazdur R, Valeriote FA, Baker LH. Pharmacokinetics and toxicity of continuous infusion amphotericin B in cancer patients. J Pharm Sci 1989; 78(4):307–10.
48. Lee JW, Seibel NL, Amantea M, Whitcomb P, Pizzo PA, Walsh TJ. Safety and pharmacokinetics of fluconazole in children with neoplastic diseases. J Pediatr 1992; 120(6):987–93.
49. Crerar-Gilbert A, Boots R, Fraenkel D, MacDonald GA. Survival following fulminant hepatic failure from fluconazole induced hepatitis. Anaesth Intensive Care 1999;27(6):650–2.
50. Castellsague J, Garcia-Rodriguez LA, Duque A, Perez S. Risk of serious skin disorders among users of oral antifungals: a population-based study. BMC Dermatol 2002;2(1):14.
51. Haria M, Bryson HM, Goa KL. Itraconazole. A reappraisal of its pharmacological properties and therapeutic use in the management of superficial fungal infections. Drugs 1996;51(4):585–620. Erratum in: Drugs. 1996;52(2):253.
52. Gussenhoven MJ, Haak A, Peereboom-Wynia JD, van 't Wout JW. Stevens–Johnson syndrome after fluconazole. Lancet 1991;338(8759):120.
53. Morgan JM, Carmichael AJ. Fixed drug eruption with fluconazole. BMJ 1994;308(6926):454.
54. Craig TJ, Peralta F, Boggavarapu J. Desensitization for fluconazole hypersensitivity. J Allergy Clin Immunol 1996;98(4):845–6.
55. Heikkila H, Timonen K, Stubb S. Fixed drug eruption due to fluconazole. J Am Acad Dermatol 2000;42(5 Pt 2):883–4.
56. Kar HK. Longitudinal melanonychia associated with fluconazole therapy. Int J Dermatol 1998;37(9):719–20.
57. Menegola E, Broccia ML, Di Renzo F, Giavini E. Antifungal triazoles induce malformations in vitro. Reprod Toxicol 2001;15(4):421–7.
58. Sorensen HT, Nielsen GL, Olesen C, Larsen H, Steffensen FH, Schonheyder HC, Olsen J, Czeizel AE. Risk of malformations and other outcomes in children exposed to fluconazole in utero. Br J Clin Pharmacol 1999;48(2):234–8.
59. Tiboni GM, Iammarrone E, Giampietro F, Lamonaca D, Bellati U, Di Ilio C. Teratological interaction between the bis-triazole antifungal agent fluconazole and the anticonvulsant drug phenytoin. Teratology 1999;59(2):81–7.
60. Force RW. Fluconazole concentrations in breast milk. Pediatr Infect Dis J 1995;14(3):235–6.
61. Brammer KW, Coates PE. Pharmacokinetics of fluconazole in pediatric patients. Eur J Clin Microbiol Infect Dis 1994;13(4):325–9.
62. Schwarze R, Penk A, Pittrow L. Administration of fluconazole in children below 1 year of age. Mycoses 1999;42 (1–2):3–16.
63. Saxen H, Hoppu K, Pohjavuori M. Pharmacokinetics of fluconazole in very low birth weight infants during the first two weeks of life. Clin Pharmacol Ther 1993;54(3):269–77.
64. Schwarze R, Penk A, Pittrow L. Anwendung von Fluconazol bei Kinden <1 Jahr: Ubersicht. [Use of fluconazole in children less than 1 year old: review.] Mycoses 1998;41(Suppl 1):61–70.
65. Huttova M, Hartmanova I, Kralinsky K, Filka J, Uher J, Kurak J, Krizan S, Krcmery V Jr. Candida fungemia in neonates treated with fluconazole: report of forty cases, including eight with meningitis. Pediatr Infect Dis J 1998;17(11):1012–15.
66. Novelli V, Holzel H. Safety and tolerability of fluconazole in children. Antimicrob Agents Chemother 1999;43(8):1955–60.
67. Goins RA, Ascher D, Waecker N, Arnold J, Moorefield E. Comparison of fluconazole and nystatin oral suspensions for treatment of oral candidiasis in infants. Pediatr Infect Dis J 2002;21(12):1165–7.
68. Palkama VJ, Isohanni MH, Neuvonen PJ, Olkkola KT. The effect of intravenous and oral fluconazole on the pharmacokinetics and pharmacodynamics of intravenous alfentanil. Anesth Analg 1998;87(1):190–4.
69. Robinson RF, Nahata MC, Olshefski RS. Syncope associated with concurrent amitriptyline and fluconazole therapy. Ann Pharmacother 2000;34(12):1406–9.
70. Dorsey ST, Biblo LA. Prolonged QT interval and torsades de pointes caused by the combination of fluconazole and amitriptyline. Am J Emerg Med 2000;18(2):227–9.
71. Pahls S, Schaffner A. Aspergillus fumigatus pneumonia in neutropenic patients receiving fluconazole for infection

due to *Candida* species: is amphotericin B combined with fluconazole the appropriate answer? Clin Infect Dis 1994;18(3):484–6.

72. Rex JH, Pappas PG, Karchmer AW, Sobel J, Edwards JE, Hadley S, Brass C, Vazquez JA, Chapman SW, Horowitz HW, Zervos M, McKinsey D, Lee J, Babinchak T, Bradsher RW, Cleary JD, Cohen DM, Danziger L, Goldman M, Goodman J, Hilton E, Hyslop NE, Kett DH, Lutz J, Rubin RH, Scheld WM, Schuster M, Simmons B, Stein DK, Washburn RG, Mautner L, Chu TC, Panzer H, Rosenstein RB, Booth J; National Institute of Allergy and Infectious Diseases Mycoses Study Group. A randomized and blinded multicenter trial of high-dose fluconazole plus placebo versus fluconazole plus amphotericin B as therapy for candidemia and its consequences in nonneutropenic subjects. Clin Infect Dis 2003;36(10):1221–8.
73. Thorpe JE, Baker N, Bromet-Petit M. Effect of oral antacid administration on the pharmacokinetics of oral fluconazole. Antimicrob Agents Chemother 1990;34(10):2032–3.
74. Venkatakrishnan K, von Moltke LL, Greenblatt DJ. Effects of the antifungal agents on oxidative drug metabolism: clinical relevance. Clin Pharmacokinet 2000;38(2):111–80.
75. Bickers DR. Antifungal therapy: potential interactions with other classes of drugs. J Am Acad Dermatol 1994;31(3 Pt 2):S87–90.
76. Ohtani Y, Kotegawa T, Tsutsumi K, Morimoto T, Hirose Y, Nakano S. Effect of fluconazole on the pharmacokinetics and pharmacodynamics of oral and rectal bromazepam: an application of electroencephalography as the pharmacodynamic method. J Clin Pharmacol 2002;42(2):183–91.
77. Olkkola KT, Ahonen J, Neuvonen PJ. The effects of the systemic antimycotics, itraconazole and fluconazole, on the pharmacokinetics and pharmacodynamics of intravenous and oral midazolam. Anesth Analg 1996;82(3):511–16.
78. Varhe A, Olkkola KT, Neuvonen PJ. Effect of fluconazole dose on the extent of fluconazole–triazolam interaction. Br J Clin Pharmacol 1996;42(4):465–70.
79. Ahonen J, Olkkola KT, Takala A, Neuvonen PJ. Interaction between fluconazole and midazolam in intensive care patients. Acta Anaesthesiol Scand 1999;43(5):509–14.
80. Backman JT, Kivisto KT, Olkkola KT, Neuvonen PJ. The area under the plasma concentration-time curve for oral midazolam is 400-fold larger during treatment with itraconazole than with rifampicin. Eur J Clin Pharmacol 1998;54(1):53–8.
81. Kremens B, Brendel E, Bald M, Czyborra P, Michel MC. Loss of blood pressure control on withdrawal of fluconazole during nifedipine therapy. Br J Clin Pharmacol 1999;47(6):707–8.
82. Nair DR, Morris HH. Potential fluconazole-induced carbamazepine toxicity. Ann Pharmacother 1999;33(7–8):790–2.
83. Finch CK, Green CA, Self TH. Fluconazole–carbamazepine interaction. South Med J 2002;95(9):1099–100.
84. Lazar JD, Wilner KD. Drug interactions with fluconazole. Rev Infect Dis 1990;12(Suppl 3):S327–33.
85. Milliken ST, Powles RL. Antifungal prophylaxis in bone marrow transplantation. Rev Infect Dis 1990;12(Suppl 3):S374–9.
86. Sugar AM, Saunders C, Idelson BA, Bernard DB. Interaction of fluconazole and cyclosporine. Ann Intern Med 1989;110(10):844.
87. Lyman CA, Walsh TJ. Systemically administered antifungal agents. A review of their clinical pharmacology and therapeutic applications. Drugs 1992;44(1):9–35.
88. Osowski CL, Dix SP, Lin LS, Mullins RE, Geller RB, Wingard JR. Evaluation of the drug interaction between intravenous high-dose fluconazole and cyclosporine or tacrolimus in bone marrow transplant patients. Transplantation 1996;61(8):1268–72.
89. Lopez-Gil JA. Fluconazole–cyclosporine interaction: a dose-dependent effect? Ann Pharmacother 1993;27(4):427–30.
90. Mathis AS, DiRenzo T, Friedman GS, Kaplan B, Adamson R. Sex and ethnicity may chiefly influence the interaction of fluconazole with calcineurin inhibitors. Transplantation 2001;71(8):1069–75.
91. Sud K, Singh B, Krishna VS, Thennarasu K, Kohli HS, Jha V, Gupta KL, Sakhuja V. Unpredictable cyclosporin–fluconazole interaction in renal transplant recipients. Nephrol Dial Transplant 1999;14(7):1698–703.
92. Jordan MK, Polis MA, Kelly G, Narang PK, Masur H, Piscitelli SC. Effects of fluconazole and clarithromycin on rifabutin and 25-O-desacetylrifabutin pharmacokinetics. Antimicrob Agents Chemother 2000;44(8):2170–2.
93. Yule SM, Walker D, Cole M, McSorley L, Cholerton S, Daly AK, Pearson AD, Boddy AV. The effect of fluconazole on cyclophosphamide metabolism in children. Drug Metab Dispos 1999;27(3):417–21.
94. Warren KE, McCully CM, Walsh TJ, Balis FM. Effect of fluconazole on the pharmacokinetics of doxorubicin in nonhuman primates. Antimicrob Agents Chemother 2000;44(4):1100–1.
95. Mikami Y, Scalarone GM, Kurita N, Yazawa K, Uno J, Miyaji M. Synergistic postantifungal effect of flucytosine and fluconazole on *Candida albicans*. J Med Vet Mycol 1992;30(3):197–206.
96. De Wit S, Debier M, De Smet M, McCrea J, Stone J, Carides A, Matthews C, Deutsch P, Clumeck N. Effect of fluconazole on indinavir pharmacokinetics in human immunodeficiency virus-infected patients. Antimicrob Agents Chemother 1998;42(2):223–7.
97. Koks CH, Crommentuyn KM, Hoetelmans RM, Burger DM, Koopmans PP, Mathot RA, Mulder JW, Meenhorst PL, Beijnen JH. The effect of fluconazole on ritonavir and saquinavir pharmacokinetics in HIV-1-infected individuals. Br J Clin Pharmacol 2001;51(6):631–5.
98. Tarumi Y, Pereira J, Watanabe S. Methadone and fluconazole: respiratory depression by drug interaction. J Pain Symptom Manage 2002;23(2):148–53.
99. Cobb MN, Desai J, Brown LS Jr, Zannikos PN, Rainey PM. The effect of fluconazole on the clinical pharmacokinetics of methadone. Clin Pharmacol Ther 1998;63(6):655–62.
100. Zimmermann T, Yeates RA, Riedel KD, Lach P, Laufen H. The influence of gastric pH on the pharmacokinetics of fluconazole: the effect of omeprazole. Int J Clin Pharmacol Ther 1994;32(9):491–6.
101. Kang BC, Yang CQ, Cho HK, Suh OK, Shin WG. Influence of fluconazole on the pharmacokinetics of omeprazole in healthy volunteers. Biopharm Drug Dispos 2002;23(2):77–81.
102. Devenport MH, Crook D, Wynn V, Lees LJ. Metabolic effects of low-dose fluconazole in healthy female users and non-users of oral contraceptives. Br J Clin Pharmacol 1989;27(6):851–9.
103. Sinofsky FE, Pasquale SA. The effect of fluconazole on circulating ethinyl estradiol levels in women taking oral contraceptives. Am J Obstet Gynecol 1998;178(2):300–4.
104. Hilbert J, Messig M, Kuye O, Friedman H. Evaluation of interaction between fluconazole and an oral contraceptive in healthy women. Obstet Gynecol 2001;98(2):218–23.
105. Mitchell AS, Holland JT. Fluconazole and phenytoin: a predictable interaction. BMJ 1989;298(6683):1315.
106. Gericke KR. Possible interaction between warfarin and fluconazole. Pharmacotherapy 1993;13(5):508–9.

107. Kantola T, Backman JT, Niemi M, Kivisto KT, Neuvonen PJ. Effect of fluconazole on plasma fluvastatin and pravastatin concentrations. Eur J Clin Pharmacol 2000;56(3):225–9.
108. Cooper KJ, Martin PD, Dane AL, Warwick MJ, Schneck DW, Cantarini MV. The effect of fluconazole on the pharmacokinetics of rosuvastatin. Eur J Clin Pharmacol 2002;58(8):527–31.
109. Abad S, Moachon L, Blanche P, Bavoux F, Sicard D, Salmon-Ceron D. Possible interaction between gliclazide, fluconazole and sulfamethoxazole resulting in severe hypoglycaemia. Br J Clin Pharmacol 2001;52(4):456–7.
110. Niemi M, Backman JT, Neuvonen M, Laitila J, Neuvonen PJ, Kivisto KT. Effects of fluconazole and fluvoxamine on the pharmacokinetics and pharmacodynamics of glimepiride. Clin Pharmacol Ther 2001;69(4):194–200.
111. Moreno M, Latorre A, Manzanares C, Morales E, Herrero JC, Dominguez-Gil B, Carreno A, Cubas A, Delgado M, Andres A, Morales JM. Clinical management of tacrolimus drug interactions in renal transplant patients. Transplant Proc 1999;31(6):2252–3.
112. Hairhara Y, Makuuchi M, Kawarasaki H, Takayama T, Kubota K, Ito M, Tanaka H, Yoshino H, Hirata M, Kita Y, Kusaka K, Sano K, Saiura A, Ijichi M, Matsukura A, Watanabe M, Hashizume K, Nakatsuka T. Effect of fluconazole on blood levels of tacrolimus. Transplant Proc 1999;31(7):2767.
113. Billaud EM, Guillemain R, Tacco F, Chevalier P. Evidence for a pharmacokinetic interaction between itraconazole and tacrolimus in organ transplant patients. Br J Clin Pharmacol 1998;46(3):271–2.
114. Furlan V, Parquin F, Penaud JF, Cerrina J, Ladurie FL, Dartevelle P, Taburet AM. Interaction between tacrolimus and itraconazole in a heart–lung transplant recipient. Transplant Proc 1998;30(1):187–8.
115. Capone D, Gentile A, Imperatore P, Palmiero G, Basile V. Effects of itraconazole on tacrolimus blood concentrations in a renal transplant recipient. Ann Pharmacother 1999;33(10):1124–5.
116. Black DJ, Kunze KL, Wienkers LC, Gidal BE, Seaton TL, McDonnell ND, Evans JS, Bauwens JE, Trager WF. Warfarin–fluconazole. II. A metabolically based drug interaction: in vivo studies. Drug Metab Dispos 1996;24(4):422–8.
117. Trapnell CB, Klecker RW, Jamis-Dow C, Collins JM. Glucuronidation of 3'-azido-3'-deoxythymidine (zidovudine) by human liver microsomes: relevance to clinical pharmacokinetic interactions with atovaquone, fluconazole, methadone, and valproic acid. Antimicrob Agents Chemother 1998;42(7):1592–6.

Flucytosine

General Information

Flucytosine is an antimetabolite of the fluoropyrimidine type. The principle of selectivity of flucytosine for the fungal cell is dual: it depends on an enzyme in order to penetrate the cell (fungal cytosine permease) and a fungal enzyme that deaminates flucytosine to the active antimetabolite 5-fluorouracil, which is metabolized to 5-fluoruridine. Replacement of 5-fluorouracil in RNA results in the disruption of protein synthesis in the fungus. Flucytosine has selective activity against pathogenic yeasts such as Candida, but only moderate activity against Aspergillus and chromoblastomycosis. There is synergy between flucytosine and amphotericin, and the combination is effective against meningeal cryptococcosis and pheohyphomycosis of the central nervous system, specifically disease caused by *Xylohypha bantiana* (1–3). Flucytosine can be given orally as well as parenterally. For most fungal infections it should not be given as a single agent, because of the development of secondary drug resistance (4), with the possible exception of urinary tract infection (5), in which secondary resistance does however also occur.

The mechanism of toxicity of flucytosine is not fully understood. Conversion of flucytosine to certain metabolites, in particular 5-fluorouracil, in the liver or by the intestinal microflora after oral administration has been proposed. Toxicity may also occur through impurities in the raw material and the formation of fluorouracil from flucytosine after sterilization and storage.

Pharmacokinetics

Flucytosine can be given orally, and peak serum concentrations occur within 1–2 hours in patients with normal renal function. The absorption of flucytosine can be delayed by food or antacids. Flucytosine is minimally bound to plasma proteins. It penetrates into the CSF, vitreous humor, peritoneal fluid, inflamed joints, and other fluid compartments. There are several methods for determining serum concentrations, particularly the creatinine iminohydrolase assay, which makes use of the spurious creatinine increase in serum, as measured by the Kodak Ektachem analyser, an apparatus widely available and providing a low cost method compared with HPLC (6). Flucytosine accumulates in patients with renal insufficiency, resulting in potentially toxic serum concentrations. About 90% of the dose is excreted unchanged in the urine. Dose adjustments in renal insufficiency can be made in proportion to the reduction in creatinine clearance (7). Metabolism occurs to a limited extent (8). There is evidence that some flucytosine (5-fluorocytosine) is converted into 5-fluorouracil by the intestinal flora (9,10); 5-fluorouracil may also be present as an impurity in the original formulation or after prolonged storage (11).

Observational studies

Experience with flucytosine monotherapy of cryptococcosis has been reviewed in 27 patients treated between 1968 and 1973 who were selected for this form of therapy on the basis of criteria associated with good prognosis (4). Flucytosine was given as primary therapy to 18 patients and as secondary therapy (following failure of amphotericin deoxycholate) to nine patients in dosages of 4–10 g/day in four divided doses for 8 weeks. Toxicity associated with flucytosine was uncommon and mild. Mild leukopenia (nadir 3–4 $\times$ 10^9/l) developed in three patients, and mild thrombocytopenia (101 $\times$ 10^9/l) and worsening anemia occurred in one patient each. Therapy was stopped early or changed in two patients. In the first, therapy was stopped after 31 days because of a white cell count of 4.1 $\times$ 10^9/l; despite the shortened course of therapy, the patient achieved a long-term cure, and the leukopenia was ultimately believed to be secondary to sarcoidosis.

There was bone marrow suppression in the second patient shortly after the withdrawal of flucytosine (because of failure to respond); later resumption of flucytosine during amphotericin therapy for this critically ill patient was associated with severe bone marrow suppression and death.

Comparative studies

Combination therapy with fluconazole (200 mg/day for 2 months) and flucytosine (150 mg/kg/day for the first 2 weeks; $n = 30$) has been compared with fluconazole monotherapy (200 mg/day for 2 months; $n = 28$) in a randomized open trial in Ugandan patients with AIDS-associated cryptococcal meningitis (12). Patients in both groups who survived for 2 months received maintenance therapy with fluconazole (200 mg three times per week for 4 months). There were no serious adverse events in any of the patients. The combination therapy prevented death within 2 weeks and significantly increased the survival rate at 6 months (32 versus 12%). However, the rate of positive cryptococcal antigen titers remained high at 2 months after treatment in both groups.

General adverse effects

The toxicity and drug interactions of flucytosine have been reviewed (13). Nausea, vomiting, and diarrhea are common. Enterocolitis is infrequent. Hepatic dysfunction, hepatitis, and even hepatic necrosis and blood disorders, including fatal aplastic anemia, can occur (14). Severe reactions mainly occurred at a time when the importance of high serum concentrations (in excess of 100 μg/ml) of flucytosine in causing these adverse effects was not recognized. The importance of parenteral versus intravenous administration in the development of enterocolitis is unclear. Patients have been described who suffered adverse effects, such as hepatotoxicity or eosinophilia, that were idiosyncratic and not related to flucytosine concentrations. Hypersensitivity reactions can occur. Neither teratogenic nor tumor-inducing effects have been recorded.

Organs and Systems

Cardiovascular

Life-threatening fluorouracil-like cardiotoxicity has been attributed to flucytosine (15).

- A 34-year-old woman took flucytosine, 500 mg 12 times a day for 2 days, for vaginal candidiasis. After the last dose she complained of chest pain, which persisted for a week and was associated with ST segment elevation during exercise. Coronary angiography showed normal coronary arteries. One month later she was rechallenged with 500 mg 12 times a day for 2 days. The day after completion of this regimen, she developed severe chest pain. Electrocardiography showed widespread ST segment elevation and echocardiography showed apicolateral septal hypokinesia with a left ventricular ejection fraction of less than 15%. Her flucytosine plasma concentration 48 hours after the last dose was not high, but the fluorouracil concentration was similar to that found during a 5-day continuous infusion of 5-fluorouracil. Her lymphocytes showed no abnormalities of intracellular flucytosine clearance, and cytosine deaminase, the enzyme that converts flucytosine to fluorouracil, was not detectable.

Similar cardiotoxicity has been reported with 5-fluorouracil. The reported events were generally consistent with a drug- or metabolite-induced increase in coronary vasomotor tone and spasm, leading to myocardial ischemia. The authors concluded that more attention should be given to the conversion of flucytosine to fluorouracil; however, it is not clear whether flucytosine should be contraindicated in patients with vasospastic or exertional angina.

Nervous system

Headaches, confusion, hallucinations, somnolence, and vertigo can occur. There have also been a few reports of peripheral neuropathy. However, it is difficult to establish the role of flucytosine in these adverse reactions (SED-12, 674). An acute cerebellopathy has been attributed to flucytosine (16).

Hematologic

Bone marrow suppression is a recognized toxic effect of flucytosine; anemia, leukopenia, and thrombocytopenia occur in about 5% of cases. The hematological effects are dose-related and occur after prolonged high blood concentrations of flucytosine (over 100 μg/ml). Hematotoxicity is seen more often in the presence of renal insufficiency and hence during the use of flucytosine in combination with amphotericin. If bone marrow reserve has already been depleted by underlying disease or by medications, the risk of hematotoxicity increases.

The relation between the toxicity and pharmacokinetics of flucytosine has been investigated in a retrospective study in 53 patients in an intensive care unit (17). Thrombocytopenia, as a marker of bone marrow depression, was associated with a reduced clearance of flucytosine; the lowest thrombocyte count was linearly related to the clearance of flucytosine. Patients with flucytosine concentrations over 100 μg/ml were at higher risk of thrombocytopenia and raised hepatic transaminases than those who did not exceed this threshold. In a second study, the authors corroborated their earlier findings and showed a significant relation between the lowest thrombocyte counts and thrombocyte counts predicted on the basis of the creatinine clearance in a new set of patients admitted to the intensive care unit (18).

In a pilot study in six patients receiving intravenous flucytosine, hematotoxicity was monitored by measuring platelet and leukocyte counts; flucytosine and 5-fluorouracil serum concentrations were measured using HPLC (19). The concentrations of 5-fluorouracil in the 34 available serum samples were below the limit of quantification (0.05 μg/ml), but flucytosine was detectable in all samples and the 5-fluorouracil metabolite, α-fluoro-β-alanine (FBAL), was detected at low concentrations in several samples. One patient developed thrombocytopenia (50×10^9/l) during therapy, and one developed leukopenia (2.6×10^9/l). The fact that 5-fluorouracil was not detected in the serum made it unlikely that the toxic effects of intravenous flucytosine resulted from exposure to 5-fluorouracil.

Patients with AIDS, treated for antifungal disease with flucytosine and amphotericin, are particularly susceptible to develop bone marrow depression (1,3). On the other hand, flucytosine can be safely administered to patients with cancer (6) or AIDS (12,20), if toxic concentrations are avoided and blood counts monitored.

Gastrointestinal

Nausea, vomiting, and diarrhea are the most common adverse effects of flucytosine.

Enterocolitis, usually sparing the rectosigmoid, has been described in some cases (21). This type of flucytosine toxicity may be associated with deamination of flucytosine to 5-fluorouracil in the gut (1). Potentially fatal ulcerative colitis has been suspected in a few patients; however, in most cases there were no diagnostic data to back up the diagnosis.

Liver

Abnormal liver function tests (above normal serum alkaline phosphatase and transaminases and, less often, raised serum bilirubin concentrations) have all been reported. Hepatic involvement is rarely serious (SED-12, 675) (22).

Liver cell necrosis, detected by means of liver biopsy, has been rarely described (SED-9, 477) (23).

The reason for antifungal treatment and the concurrent use of other medication may contribute to hepatotoxicity (SED-12, 675) (1,6).

Urinary tract

Crystalluria has been reported, with urinary gravel, consisting of a co-precipitate of flucytosine and uric acid (24).

Skin

Maculopapular and urticarial rashes severe enough to require drug withdrawal have been reported (SEDA-2, 242). The incidence is low.

Acquired photosensitivity has been described in two cases (25).

Immunologic

Anaphylaxis has been reported in a patient with AIDS (26).

Second-Generation Effects

Teratogenicity

Flucytosine is teratogenic in rats, and its close chemical relation to antimetabolites plus the fact that 5-fluorouracil is a metabolite make it inadvisable to administer flucytosine during pregnancy or to fertile women taking no contraceptive precautions.

Drug–Drug Interactions

Amphotericin

Amphotericin in combination with flucytosine results in an increased risk of hematological complications, because amphotericin often impairs renal function, causing retention of flucytosine (7). This combination also delays hematopoietic recovery after cytotoxic chemotherapy; it should not be used as empirical antifungal therapy in febrile patients with neutropenia (27).

Antifungal azoles

Flucytosine has been successfully used in combination with ketoconazole, fluconazole, and itraconazole. Flucytosine and ketoconazole were synergistic in about 40% of yeast isolates resistant to flucytosine alone. The synergistic action of flucytosine with the triazoles against *Candida* species was seen both in vitro and in vivo (3–6).

Cytarabine

The suggested interaction of cytarabine with flucytosine, in which there is competitive inhibition of antifungal activity, has not been confirmed (28).

Monitoring Therapy

Monitoring blood concentrations of flucytosine is essential, so that the dosage can be altered according to changing renal function and to avoid toxicity. Peak plasma concentrations should be 40–60 μg/ml after an oral dose, and under 100 μg/ml after intravenous infusion. To avoid fungal resistance, trough concentrations below 20 μg/ml are recommended (7).

References

1. Lyman CA, Walsh TJ. Systemically administered antifungal agents. A review of their clinical pharmacology and therapeutic applications. Drugs 1992;44(1):9–35.
2. Vanden Bossche H, Dromer F, Improvisi I, Lozano-Chiu M, Rex JH, Sanglard D. Antifungal drug resistance in pathogenic fungi. Med Mycol 1998;36(Suppl 1):119–28.
3. Viviani MA. Flucytosine—what is its future? J Antimicrob Chemother 1995;35(2):241–4.
4. Hospenthal DR, Bennett JE. Flucytosine monotherapy for cryptococcosis. Clin Infect Dis 1998;27(2):260–4.
5. Wise GJ, Kozinn PJ, Goldberg P. Flucytosine in the management of genitourinary candidiasis: 5 years of experience. J Urol 1980;124(1):70–2.
6. Francis P, Walsh TJ. Evolving role of flucytosine in immunocompromised patients: new insights into safety, pharmacokinetics, and antifungal therapy. Clin Infect Dis 1992;15(6):1003–18.
7. Polak A. Pharmacokinetics of amphotericin B and flucytosine. Postgrad Med J 1979;55(647):667–70.
8. Chouini-Lalanne N, Malet-Martino MC, Gilard V, Ader JC, Martino R. Structural determination of a glucuronide conjugate of flucytosine in humans. Drug Metab Dispos 1995;23(8):813–7.
9. Malet-Martino MC, Martino R, de Forni M, Andremont A, Hartmann O, Armand JP. Flucytosine conversion to fluorouracil in humans: does a correlation with gut flora status

exist? A report of two cases using fluorine-19 magnetic resonance spectroscopy. Infection 1991;19(3):178–80.
10. Harris BE, Manning BW, Federle TW, Diasio RB. Conversion of 5-fluorocytosine to 5-fluorouracil by human intestinal microflora. Antimicrob Agents Chemother 1986;29(1):44–8.
11. Vermes A, van der Sijs H, Guchelaar HJ. An accelerated stability study of 5-flucytosine in intravenous solution. Pharm World Sci 1999;21(1):35–9.
12. Mayanja-Kizza H, Oishi K, Mitarai S, Yamashita H, Nalongo K, Watanabe K, Izumi T, Ococi-Jungala K, Augustine K, Mugerwa R, Nagatake T, Matsumoto K. Combination therapy with fluconazole and flucytosine for cryptococcal meningitis in Ugandan patients with AIDS. Clin Infect Dis 1998;26(6):1362–6.
13. Vermes A, Guchelaar HJ, Dankert J. Flucytosine: a review of its pharmacology, clinical indications, pharmacokinetics, toxicity and drug interactions. J Antimicrob Chemother 2000;46(2):171–9.
14. Groll AH, Gea-Banacloche JC, Glasmacher A, Just-Nuebling G, Maschmeyer G, Walsh TJ. Clinical pharmacology of antifungal compounds. Infect Dis Clin North Am 2003;17(1):159–91.
15. Isetta C, Garaffo R, Bastian G, Jourdan J, Baudouy M, Milano G. Life-threatening 5-fluorouracil-like cardiac toxicity after treatment with 5-fluorocytosine. Clin Pharmacol Ther 2000;67(3):323–5.
16. Cubo Delgado E, Sanz Boza R, Garcia Urra D, Barquero Jimenez S, Vargas Castrillon E. Acute cerebellopathy as a probable toxic effect of flucytosine. Eur J Clin Pharmacol 1997;51(6):505–6.
17. Vermes A, van Der Sijs H, Guchelaar HJ. Flucytosine: correlation between toxicity and pharmacokinetic parameters. Chemotherapy 2000;46(2):86–94.
18. Vermes A, Guchelaar HJ, Dankert J. Prediction of flucytosine-induced thrombocytopenia using creatinine clearance. Chemotherapy 2000;46(5):335–41.
19. Vermes A, Guchelaar HJ, van Kuilenburg AB, Dankert J. 5-fluorocytosine-related bone-marrow depression and conversion to fluorouracil: a pilot study. Fundam Clin Pharmacol 2002;16(1):39–47.
20. van der Horst CM, Saag MS, Cloud GA, Hamill RJ, Graybill JR, Sobel JD, Johnson PC, Tuazon CU, Kerkering T, Moskovitz BL, Powderly WG, Dismukes WE. Treatment of cryptococcal meningitis associated with the acquired immunodeficiency syndrome. National Institute of Allergy and Infectious Diseases Mycoses Study Group and AIDS Clinical Trials Group. N Engl J Med 1997;337(1):15–21.
21. Cappell MS, Simon T. Colonic toxicity of administered medications and chemicals. Am J Gastroenterol 1993;88(10):1684–99.
22. Larsen RA, Leal MA, Chan LS. Fluconazole compared with amphotericin B plus flucytosine for cryptococcal meningitis in AIDS. A randomized trial. Ann Intern Med 1990;113(3):183–7.
23. Bennet JE. Flucytosine. Ann Intern Med 1977;86(3):319–21.
24. Williams KM, Chinwah PM, Cobcroft R. Crystalluria during flucytosine therapy. Med J Aust 1979;2(11):617.
25. Shelley WB, Sica PA Jr. Disseminate sporotrichosis of skin and bone cured with 5-fluorocytosine: Photosensitivity as a complication. J Am Acad Dermatol 1983;8(2):229–35.
26. Kotani S, Hirose S, Niiya K, Kubonishi I, Miyoshi I. Anaphylaxis to flucytosine in a patient with AIDS. JAMA 1988;260(22):3275–6.
27. Hiddemann W, Essink ME, Fegeler W, Zuhlsdorf M, Sauerland C, Buchner T. Antifungal treatment by amphotericin B and 5-fluorocytosine delays the recovery of normal hematopoietic cells after intensive cytostatic therapy for acute myeloid leukemia. Cancer 1991;68(1):9–14.
28. Wingfield HJ. Absence of fungistatic antagonism between flucytosine and cytarabine in vitro and in vivo. J Antimicrob Chemother 1987;20(4):523–7.

Fludarabine

See also Cytostatic and immunosuppressant drugs

General Information

Fludarabine phosphate is a purine nucleoside antitumor agent, which inhibits adenosine deaminase. It is mainly used to treat chronic lymphocytic leukemia. Dose-limiting myelotoxicity, nausea and vomiting, and raised liver enzymes were observed during early clinical studies. The most common adverse effect is myelosuppression (WHO grade 3 or 4), and other common adverse effects include infections and gastrointestinal disturbances, although these are usually of mild to moderate intensity (WHO grade 1 or 2) (1).

Organs and Systems

Respiratory

Fludarabine can cause interstitial pneumonitis (2,3).

- A 73-year-old woman developed fever and cough 2 weeks after completing a third cycle of fludarabine for chronic lymphocytic leukemia. A chest X-ray showed multiple pulmonary nodules and a biopsy showed a mononuclear interstitial infiltrate without evidence of malignant, infectious, granulomatous, or vascular causes. Her symptoms and pulmonary nodules resolved after treatment with glucocorticoids (4).

There has also been a report of an acute eosinophilic pneumonia associated with peripheral blood eosinophilia in a patient with follicular lymphoma (5).

Nervous system

Dose-intensified fludarabine causes severe central nervous system toxicity. In 70 patients with acute leukemia who received 95 courses of fludarabine 20–220 mg/m^2 for 5–7 days there was neurotoxicity in 36% of those who received doses over 96 mg/m^2/day, but in only 0.2% of those who received lower doses (6). The onset of neurological symptoms was at 21–60 days after the last course of fludarabine. Visual symptoms were the most common. There was progressive deterioration of mental state or encephalopathy leading to a vegetative state in 11 patients. Progressive demyelination in the central nervous system was the main factor causing the neurotoxic symptoms; this can occur as a result of viral complications during drug-related immunosuppression.

Hematologic

Fludarabine can cause or exacerbate autoimmune thrombocytopenia in chronic lymphocytic leukemia. Two patients with chronic lymphatic leukemia who developed thrombocytopenia while taking fludarabine were treated with high-dose glucocorticoids and initially responded with recovery of platelet counts (7). One developed recurrent thrombocytopenia on two occasions after re-exposure to fludarabine when his disease had become refractory to all other treatments. Of 45 patients with lymphoproliferative disorders treated with fludarabine over the previous 6 years, retrospectively reviewed, 2 had developed autoimmune thrombocytopenia and 3 had developed autoimmune hemolytic anemia.

In three patients with chronic lymphatic leukemia, fludarabine-associated thrombocytopenia responded to rituximab 375 mg/m^2/week for 4 weeks (8). Other similar cases have been reported (9). However, when rituximab was added to a regimen of fludarabine plus cyclophosphamide in patients with relapsed follicular lymphoma, there was unexpected severe hematological toxicity, with significant, prolonged thrombocytopenia WHO grade 3/4 in six of 17 patients (10). Older patients (mean age 65 versus 57 years) were significantly more likely to have this adverse effect, and no other clinical or hematological parameters differed between the patients with thrombocytopenia and those without.

Peripheral blood eosinophilia, in one case up to 7.9×10^9/l, has been attributed to fludarabine (11).

- A 58-year-old man who took fludarabine for 5 months developed a peripheral eosinophilia with a peak value of 1.7×10^9/l; thorough investigation for other causes of eosinophilia was negative (12).

A patient with a high-grade B cell non-Hodgkin's lymphoma treated with fludarabine developed a high-titer antibody to factor VIII while the lymphoma was in remission; the authors speculated that the occurrence of the inhibitor was an autoimmune adverse effect of fludarabine (13).

Gastrointestinal

Intestinal pseudo-obstruction has been attributed to fludarabine in a 66-year-old man with non-Hodgkin's lymphoma; it was successfully managed with a combination of parasympathomimetic drugs and mechanical decompression (14).

Immunologic

Treatment with fludarabine results in prolonged immunosuppression lasting over 6 months (15). Patients who are immunocompromised are at risk of infection with chemotherapy. Infection with JC virus, a human polyoma virus, occurred in two patients after fludarabine treatment of a low-grade lymphoma, which led to a progressive multifocal leukoencephalopathy (16). In one series of 27 patients who received fludarabine, serious infections developed in 24 (17).

Drug–Drug Interactions

Melphalan

Cardiotoxicity has rarely been reported with melphalan or fludarabine alone, but severe left ventricular failure developed in three of 21 patients treated with a combination of these two drugs (18).

References

1. Plosker GL, Figgitt DP. Oral fludarabine. Drugs 2003;63(21):2317–23.
2. Hurst PG, Habib MP, Garewal H, Bluestein M, Paquin M, Greenberg BR. Pulmonary toxicity associated with fludarabine monophosphate. Invest New Drugs 1987;5(2):207–10.
3. Levin M, Aziz M, Opitz L. Steroid-responsive interstitial pneumonitis after fludarabine therapy. Chest 1997;111(5):1472–3.
4. Garg S, Garg MS, Basmaji N. Multiple pulmonary nodules: an unusual presentation of fludarabine pulmonary toxicity: case report and review of literature. Am J Hematol 2002;70(3):241–5.
5. Trojan A, Meier R, Licht A, Taverna C. Eosinophilic pneumonia after administration of fludarabine for the treatment of non-Hodgkin's lymphoma. Ann Hematol 2002;81(9):535–7.
6. 2. Chun HG, Leyland-Jones BR, Caryk SM, Hoth DF. Central nervous system toxicity of fludarabine phosphate. Cancer Treat Rep 1986;70(10):1225–8.
7. Leach M, Parsons RM, Reilly JT, Winfield DA. Autoimmune thrombocytopenia: a complication of fludarabine therapy in lymphoproliferative disorders. Clin Lab Haematol 2000;22(3):175–8.
8. Hegde UP, Wilson WH, White T, Cheson BD. Rituximab treatment of refractory fludarabine-associated immune thrombocytopenia in chronic lymphocytic leukemia. Blood 2002;100(6):2260–2.
9. Fernandez MJ, Llopis I, Pastor E, Real E, Grau E. Immune thrombocytopenia induced by fludarabine successfully treated with rituximab. Haematologica 2003;88(2):ELT02.
10. Leo E, Scheuer L, Schmidt-Wolf IG, Kerowgan M, Schmitt C, Leo A, Baumbach T, Kraemer A, Mey U, Benner A, Parwaresch R, Ho AD. Significant thrombocytopenia associated with the addition of rituximab to a combination of fludarabine and cyclophosphamide in the treatment of relapsed follicular lymphoma. Eur J Haematol 2004;73(4):251–7.
11. Sezer O, Schmid P, Hallek M, Schweigert M, Beinert T, Langelotz C, Mergenthaler HG, Possinger K. Eosinophilia during fludarabine treatment of chronic lymphocytic leukemia. Ann Hematol 1999;78(10):475–7.
12. Voutsadakis IA. Fludarabine-induced eosinophilia: case report. Ann Hematol 2002;81(5):292–3.
13. Tiplady CW, Hamilton PJ, Galloway MJ. Acquired haemophilia complicating the remission of a patient with high grade non-Hodgkin's lymphoma treated by fludarabine. Clin Lab Haematol 2000;22(3):163–5.
14. Campbell S, Thomas R, Parker A, Ghosh S. Fludarabine induced intestinal pseudo-obstruction: case report and literature review. Eur J Gastroenterol Hepatol 2000;12(6):711–13.
15. Samonis G, Kontoyiannis DP. Infectious complications of purine analogue therapy. Curr Opin Infect Dis 2001;14(4):409–13.
16. Vidarsson B, Mosher DF, Salamat MS, Isaksson HJ, Onundarson PT. Progressive multifocal leukoencephalopathy after fludarabine therapy for low-grade lymphoproliferative disease. Am J Hematol 2002;70(1):51–4.
17. Perkins JG, Flynn JM, Howard RS, Byrd JC. Frequency and type of serious infections in fludarabine-refractory B-cell chronic lymphocytic leukemia and small lymphocytic lymphoma: implications for clinical trials in this patient population. Cancer 2002;94(7):2033–9.
18. Ritchie DS, Seymour JF, Roberts AW, Szer J, Grigg AP. Acute left ventricular failure following melphalan and fludarabine conditioning. Bone Marrow Transplant 2001;28(1):101–3.

Flufenamic acid and meclofenamic acid

See also Non-steroidal anti-inflammatory drugs

General Information

Flufenamic acid and meclofenamic acid are anthranilic acid derivatives similar to mefenamic acid. The withdrawal rate because of adverse effects is 7–31% and is higher in long-term studies. Flufenamic acid and meclofenamic acid are not widely prescribed and so there is little evidence to show whether they have any advantages over other NSAIDs. Both have a high incidence of gastrointestinal adverse effects (30–60% of patients at recommended doses). Diarrhea affects 11–46% of patients (SEDA-4, 68) (SEDA-6, 99) (SEDA-7, 116) (SEDA-14, 95). Thrombocytopenia with positive rechallenge has been described (1). Rashes occur in under 10% of patients. Meclofenamic acid exacerbates psoriasis in psoriatic arthropathy (2).

References

1. Rodriguez J. Thrombocytopenia associated with meclofenamate. Drug Intell Clin Pharm 1981;5(12):999.
2. Meyerhoff JO. Exacerbation of psoriasis with meclofenamate. N Engl J Med 1983;309(8):496.

Flumazenil

General Information

Flumazenil is used as a benzodiazepine antagonist in the treatment of poisoning or the reversal of benzodiazepine effects in anesthesia (1,2) or in neonates (3). Guidelines for its use have been summarized (4). The problems in its use are those of dose adjustment, the risks of panic anxiety, seizures, or other signs of excessively rapid benzodiazepine withdrawal, and pharmacokinetic problems due to the short half-life of flumazenil (about 1 hour) compared with the longer half-lives of most benzodiazepines (5). Its use is also commonly associated with vomiting and headache, and rarely with psychosis or sudden cardiac death (SEDA-17, 46), especially in mixed overdoses. Flumazenil was not effective in reversing the amnesic effects of midazolam (6), but it may be useful in hepatic coma, regardless of cause (7). In patients with a history of seizures or chronic benzodiazepine dependence, or after mixed drug overdose, flumazenil can trigger convulsions, which are occasionally fatal. It is not generally helpful to measure benzodiazepine plasma concentrations, but they can assist in the diagnosis of overdose and thus guide the use of antagonists (8).

Midazolam can cause paradoxical reactions, including increased agitation and poor cooperation (9,10). Often other drugs are required to continue the procedure successfully. Reversal of these reactions by flumazenil has been reported. In 58 patients undergoing surgery under spinal or epidural anesthesia, flumazenil 0.1 mg over 10 seconds abolished the agitation without reversing sedation (total dose range 0.1–0.5 mg) (11). In 30 patients who had been given midazolam, flumazenil 0.15–0.5 mg resulted in cessation of the agitation without reversal of sedation (9). Adverse effects of flumazenil were not reported in these studies.

The usefulness and relative safety of midazolam in children have been reviewed (12). Myoclonic-like movements associated with midazolam in three full-term newborns were reversed by flumazenil (13). However, care must be taken when considering the use of flumazenil for reversal of midazolam-induced agitation, as no controlled trials have been published.

Organs and Systems

Nervous system

A case of opisthotonos after flumazenil has been reported (14).

- A healthy 17-year-old man received an interscalene brachial plexus block using mepivacaine 600 mg and bupivacaine 150 mg. He became disorientated and showed signs of local anesthetic toxicity, for which he was given midazolam 5 mg. Flumazenil 0.5 mg was given 23 minutes after the end of the procedure, causing opisthotonos.

Similar reports have appeared in the past in patients with seizure disorders. It is recommended that flumazenil not be used in patients predisposed to seizures.

Endocrine

The effects of flumazenil and midazolam on adrenocorticotrophic hormone and cortisol responses to a corticotrophin-releasing hormone challenge have been assessed in eight healthy men (15). Flumazenil significantly reduced adrenocorticotrophic responses compared with midazolam or placebo, but had no effects on cortisol secretion. The authors suggested that this agonist effect of flumazenil on the pituitary–adrenal axis might account for the anxiolytic activity of flumazenil, which has been observed during simulated stress.

Long-Term Effects

Drug withdrawal

Flumazenil can provoke acute withdrawal reactions and extreme anxiety (16). Its duration of action (less than 1 hour) is generally shorter than that of the original benzodiazepine, whose effects can therefore return while the patient is unobserved.

References

1. Gaudreault P, Guay J, Thivierge RL, Verdy I. Benzodiazepine poisoning. Clinical and pharmacological considerations and treatment. Drug Saf 1991;6(4):247–65.
2. Brogden RN, Goa KL. Flumazenil. A reappraisal of its pharmacological properties and therapeutic efficacy as a benzodiazepine antagonist. Drugs 1991;42(6):1061–89.
3. Richard P, Autret E, Bardol J, Soyez C, Barbier P, Jonville AP, Ramponi N. The use of flumazenil in a neonate. J Toxicol Clin Toxicol 1991;29(1):137–40.

4. Cone AM, Stott SA. Flumazenil. Br J Hosp Med 1994;51(7):346–8.
5. Geller E, Halpern P. Benzodiazepine antagonists and inverse agonists. Curr Opin Anaesthesiol 1990;3:568.
6. Curran HV, Birch B. Differentiating the sedative, psychomotor and amnesic effects of benzodiazepines: a study with midazolam and the benzodiazepine antagonist, flumazenil. Psychopharmacology (Berl) 1991;103(4):519–23.
7. Ananth J, Swartz R, Burgoyne K, Gadasally R. Hepatic disease and psychiatric illness. relationships and treatment. Psychother Psychosom 1994;62(3–4):146–59.
8. Nishikawa T, Suzuki S, Ohtani H, Eizawa NW, Sugiyama T, Kawaguchi T, Miura S. Benzodiazepine concentrations in sera determined by radioreceptor assay for therapeutic-dose recipients. Am J Clin Pathol 1994;102(5):605–10.
9. Fulton SA, Mullen KD. Completion of upper endoscopic procedures despite paradoxical reaction to midazolam: a role for flumazenil? Am J Gastroenterol 2000;95(3): 809–11.
10. Saltik IN, Ozen H. Role of flumazenil for paradoxical reaction to midazolam during endoscopic procedures in children. Am J Gastroenterol 2000;95(10):3011–12.
11. Weinbroum AA, Szold O, Ogorek D, Flaishon R. The midazolam-induced paradox phenomenon is reversible by flumazenil. Epidemiology, patient characteristics and review of the literature. Eur J Anaesthesiol 2001;18(12):789–97.
12. Aviram EE, Ben-Abraham R, Weinbroum AA. Flumazenil use in children. Paediatr Perinatal Drug Ther 2003;5(4):202–9.
13. Zaw W, Knoppert DC, da Silva O. Flumazenil's reversal of myoclonic-like movements associated with midazolam in term newborns. Pharmacotherapy 2001;21(5):642–6.
14. Watanabe S, Satumae T, Takeshima R, Taguchi N. Opisthotonos after flumazenil administered to antagonize midazolam previously administered to treat developing local anesthetic toxicity. Anesth Analg 1998;86(3):677–8.
15. Strohle A, Wiedemann K. Flumazenil attenuates the pituitary response to CRH in healthy males. Eur Neuropsychopharmacol 1996;6(4):323–5.
16. Lopez A, Rebollo J. Benzodiazepine withdrawal syndrome after a benzodiazepine antagonist. Crit Care Med 1990;18(12):1480–1.

Flunitrazepam

See also Benzodiazepines

General Information

Flunitrazepam has acquired a reputation for toxicity, abuse potential (1) and associated forensic problems (2), including being implicated in sexual assault ("date rape") (3). It has been withdrawn from general availability in various countries, including the USA, Australia, and New Zealand, and it is considered to be a narcotic in various European countries. It has a rapid onset of action but a long half-life. The earlier recommended hypnotic dose (1–2 mg) is excessive, and like some other benzodiazepines, such as triazolam, flunitrazepam is safer in a smaller dose (4). Like triazolam, it has been associated with nocturnal binge eating (5). Although its outpatient use in individuals who are susceptible to abuse is hazardous, intravenous flunitrazepam is useful for alcohol withdrawal delirium, but assisted ventilation should be available.

Long-Term Effects

Drug withdrawal

Withdrawal syndrome and delirium has been attributed to flunitrazepam (6).

- A 69-year-old man developed acute benzodiazepine withdrawal delirium following a short course of flunitrazepam after an acute exacerbation of chronic obstructive pulmonary disease. He was not an alcohol- or drug-abuser and he had not previously taken benzodiazepines. Six days after withdrawal of flunitrazepam he became agitated and confused, and had visual hallucinations, disorganized thinking, insomnia, increased psychomotor activity, disorientation in time and place, and memory impairment. Tachycardia and significant anxiety were also noted. He fulfilled the DSM IV criteria for withdrawal syndrome and delirium, and had spontaneous remission of symptoms within 48 hours.

The authors commented that physicians should be more aware of drug withdrawal syndromes, even after limited periods of administration of sedative drugs.

References

1. Bond A, Seijas D, Dawling S, Lader M. Systemic absorption and abuse liability of snorted flunitrazepam. Addiction 1994;89(7):821–30.
2. Michel L, Lang JP. Benzodiazepines et passage à l'acte criminel. [Benzodiazepines and forensic aspects.] Encephale 2003;29(6):479–85.
3. Smith KM, Larive LL, Romanelli F. Club drugs: methylenedioxymethamphetamine, flunitrazepam, ketamine hydrochloride, and gamma-hydroxybutyrate. Am J Health Syst Pharm 2002;59(11):1067–76.
4. Grahnen A, Wennerlund P, Dahlstrom B, Eckernas SA. Inter- and intraindividual variability in the concentration-effect (sedation) relationship of flunitrazepam. Br J Clin Pharmacol 1991;31(1):89–92.
5. Lowenstein W, LeJeunne C, Fadlallah JP, Hughes FC, Haas C, Durand H. Binge eating and flunitrazepam. Eur J Intern Med 1994;5:57.
6. Diehl JL, Guillibert E, Guerot E, Kimounn E, Labrousse J. Acute benzodiazepine withdrawal delirium after a short course of flunitrazepam in an intensive care patient. Ann Med Interne (Paris) 2000;151(Suppl. A):A44–46.

Flunoxaprofen

See also Non-steroidal anti-inflammatory drugs

General Information

Flunoxaprofen is an NSAID, an arylalkanoic acid derivative. Its adverse effects profile is similar to the profiles of other NSAIDs, including gastrointestinal disturbances (1).

Reference

1. Forgione A, Zanoboni A, Zanoboni-Muciaccia W, et al. Long-term tolerability of flunoxaprofen in elderly subjects with normal or impaired renal function. Curr Ther Res 1985;37:77.

Fluoride salts and derivatives

General Information

Fluoride is the single most potent bone-forming agent currently available for therapeutic use (1). The active moiety is the fluoride ion itself, and its main pharmacological effect is on dental enamel and bone. Fluoride ions bind to calcium ions, stimulating trabecular bone formation. Different fluoride products have been used for the therapy of osteoporosis. The first was sodium fluoride (NaF), but that had several adverse effects, such as epigastric pain, gastric hemorrhage, leg pain, and so-called stress fractures (2).

In a study of the adverse effects of fluorinated drinking water (3), a few patients had non-specific ailments of varying duration, involving different systems. Severe headache, loss of strength, and abdominal cramps were noted, sometimes with polydipsia and polyuria. The symptoms disappeared promptly when fluorinated water was withdrawn, and reappeared immediately after rechallenge.

Therapeutic studies

There are currently no trial-based recommendations for the treatment of idiopathic osteoporosis in men. The effects of intermittent low-dose fluoride combined with continuous calcium supplementation on bone mass and future fracture events have been evaluated in 64 men with idiopathic osteoporosis (4). They were randomized to intermittent treatment with monofluorophosphate plus calcium or calcium supplementation alone for 3 years. Seven of the patients given fluoride had leg pain. In most cases the pain, which was generally confined to the ankle, disappeared during the fluoride-free month. In a few cases, the fluoride-free month had to be prolonged to 7 or 8 weeks before the symptoms subsided. During fluoride therapy, two patients had mild epigastric symptoms and one had diarrhea, but these appeared to be related to calcium; seven of the patients who were given calcium alone complained of epigastric discomfort and two had diarrhea. All the adverse events were mild to moderate and transient, and none led to discontinuation of treatment.

A 3-year, open study (5) has been performed with monofluorophosphate in 60 patients under 75 years old (average age 62 years, body weight 42–84 kg, height 148–174 cm) with established postmenopausal vertebral osteoporosis and a lumbar t-score lower than –2.5 BDM (measured by dual-energy X-ray absorptiometry) and at least one vertebral fracture diagnosed according to WHO criteria (6). The patients had taken hormone replacement therapy for an average of 2 years. Patients with inflammatory rheumatic diseases and those who were taking other medications that can modify bone metabolism, such as calcitonins, bisphosphonates, vitamin D, or anabolic agents, were excluded. There were adverse events in 19 patients, 10 of which were probably due to the monofluorophosphate or calcium components, three with gastrointestinal symptoms and seven with leg pain. The other nine adverse events were probably due to the hormone replacement therapy component: three with vaginal bleeding, four with breast tenderness, one with "heavy legs," and one with increased body weight. All the adverse events were of mild or moderate intensity and resolved spontaneously; none required withdrawal of treatment.

Organs and Systems

Nervous system

In a child, there were tetanic spasms and a convulsion more than 12 hours after fluoride ingestion, with a normal serum calcium. It is advisable that patients with intoxication should remain under surveillance for at least 24 hours, after the usual acute symptoms such as vomiting and diarrhea have settled (SEDA-10, 439).

Mouth and teeth

Fluoride poisoning can occur: after chronic ingestion of excessive amounts of fluoride, causing osteosclerosis and dental fluorosis (mottled enamel), due to accidental ingestion of fluoride mixtures during dental treatment (7,8), or after ingestion of insecticides or rodenticides containing fluoride salts.

Gastrointestinal

Fluoride can cause gastrointestinal damage (9). In 10 subjects, 3 g of a 0.42% fluoride gel caused mucosal petechiae and erosions in 7 cases; there were histopathological changes in nine cases, mostly affecting the surface epithelium (8). The authors advocated the use of a low concentration of fluoride gel instead of a 1.23% gel in small children, in order to avoid adverse gastric effects.

Skin

Fluoride in therapeutic doses can cause atopic dermatitis (9). Two patients who used fluoride gel preparations applied to the teeth developed papulonodular eruptions similar to halogenodermas (10).

Musculoskeletal

Although sodium fluoride can be used to treat osteoporosis, there is a risk of stress fractures (11–14). Fluoride has a dual effect on osteoblasts: it increases the rate of production of osteoblasts by a mitogenic effect on their precursors but also has a toxic effect on individual cells, causing impairment of mineralization and a reduced rate of apposition resembling osteomalacia (15). Fluoride increases axial bone density, but without matching changes in cortical bone. The effect on fracture rates of adding fluoride to the drinking water is not clear, but it probably only has a small impact. In two controlled studies the incidence of vertebral fractures fell, while in two other studies it increased.

Chronic ingestion of excessive amounts of fluoride can cause osteosclerosis (15). Severe dental fluorosis, hypersensitivity of teeth, and skeletal fluorosis have been reported in rural communities exposed over a long period of time to high concentrations of fluoride in the water (10 ppm) (16). There were deformities of the arms and legs with resultant genu valgum. There was osteosclerosis of the axial bones and osteoporosis in the appendicular bones. Serum calcium and inorganic phosphate were normal, but serum alkaline phosphatase was increased.

Perimalleolar pain with swelling (SED-12, 1243) and extremity pain after fluoride treatment in postmenopausal osteoporosis (17) have been reported.

Second-Generation Effects

Fertility

In a US study designed to determine whether fluoride affects human birth rate (18) the annual total fertility rate in women aged 10–49 years was calculated for 1970–88 in counties with water fluoride concentrations of at least 3 parts per million (ppm). For each region separately, the annual total fertility rate was tested by regression against the water fluoride content and sociodemographic co-variables. In most regions there was an association between increasing fluoride concentrations in drinking water and a falling total fertility rate. The study was based on population means rather than individual data, but there was no indication that the result was influenced by selection bias, inaccurate data, or inappropriate analytical methods. It does not necessarily follow that the effect of fluoride on fertility rate also applies to individual women, and that is a matter for further research.

Drug Administration

Drug overdose

Although 5–10 g of fluoride is considered to be the acute lethal dose, a fatality has been reported in a patient who took less than 50 mg, suggesting a wide variation in the lethal dose.

References

1. Baylink DJ, Duane PB, Farley SM, Farley JR. Monofluorophosphate physiology: the effects of fluoride on bone. Caries Res 1983;17(Suppl 1):56–76.
2. Riggs BL, Hodgson SF, O'Fallon WM, Chao EY, Wahner HW, Muhs JM, Cedel SL, Melton LJ 3rd. Effect of fluoride treatment on the fracture rate in postmenopausal women with osteoporosis. N Engl J Med 1990;322(12):802–9.
3. Waldbott GL. Fluoridation: a clinician's experience. South Med J 1980;73(3):301–6.
4. Ringe JD, Dorst A, Kipshoven C, Rovati LC, Setnikar I. Avoidance of vertebral fractures in men with idiopathic osteoporosis by a three year therapy with calcium and low-dose intermittent monofluorophosphate. Osteoporos Int 1998;8(1):47–52.
5. Ringe JD, Setnikar I. Monofluorophosphate combined with hormone replacement therapy in postmenopausal osteoporosis. An open-label pilot efficacy and safety study. Rheumatol Int 2002;22(1):27–32.
6. WHO Study Group. Assessment of fracture risk and its application to screening for postmenopausal osteoporosis. World Health Organ Tech Rep Ser 1994;843:66–73.
7. Stadtler P. Fluorides. Int J Clin Pharmacol Ther Toxicol 1990;28(1):20–6.
8. Spak CJ, Sjostedt S, Eleborg L, Veress B, Perbeck L, Ekstrand J. Studies of human gastric mucosa after application of 0.42% fluoride gel. J Dent Res 1990;69(2):426–9.
9. Editorial. Another fluoride fatality: a physician's dilemma. Fluoride 1979;12:55.
10. Blasik LG, Spencer SK. Fluoroderma. Arch Dermatol 1979;115(11):1334–5.
11. Harrison JE. Fluoride treatment for osteoporosis. Calcif Tissue Int 1990;46(5):287–8.
12. Schnitzler CM, Wing JR, Mesquita JM, Gear AK, Robson HJ, Smyth AE. Risk factors for the development of stress fractures during fluoride therapy for osteoporosis. J Bone Miner Res 1990;5(Suppl 1):S195–200.
13. Bayley TA, Harrison JE, Murray TM, Josse RG, Sturtridge W, Pritzker KP, Strauss A, Vieth R, Goodwin S. Fluoride-induced fractures: relation to osteogenic effect. J Bone Miner Res 1990;5(Suppl 1):S217–22.
14. Orcel P, de Vernejoul MC, Prier A, Miravet L, Kuntz D, Kaplan G. Stress fractures of the lower limbs in osteoporotic patients treated with fluoride. J Bone Miner Res 1990;5(Suppl 1):S191–94.
15. Dequeker J, Declerck K. Fluor in the treatment of osteoporosis. An overview of thirty years clinical research. Schweiz Med Wochenschr 1993;123(47):2228–34.
16. Opinya GN, Imalingat B. Skeletal and dental fluorosis: two case reports. East Afr Med J 1991;68(4):304–11.
17. Weingrad TR, Eymontt MJ, Martin JH, Steltz MD. Periostitis due to low-dose fluoride intoxication demonstrated by bone scanning. Clin Nucl Med 1991;16(1):59–61.
18. Freni SC. Exposure to high fluoride concentrations in drinking water is associated with decreased birth rates. J Toxicol Environ Health 1994;42(1):109–21.

Fluoroquinolones

See also Individual agents

General Information

Following the introduction of the first quinolone antibiotic (nalidixic acid, see separate monograph), structural modifications to the basic quinolone and naphthyridone nucleus and to the side-chains produced fluoroquinolones with improved coverage of bacterial pathogens, with high activity against Gram-negative species and a number of atypical pathogens, and good-to-moderate activity against Gram-positive species. However, despite their broad spectrum and clinical success, defects became evident, and compounds developed in recent years have targeted improvements in pharmacokinetic properties (improved systemic availability, once-daily dosing), greater activity against Gram-positive cocci and anerobes, activity against fluoroquinolone-resistant strains, and better coverage of non-fermenting Gram-negative species (1–4).

The following fluoroquinolones are covered in separate monographs: alatrofloxacin and trovafloxacin, ciprofloxacin, garenoxacin, gatifloxacin, gemifloxacin, grepafloxacin, levofloxacin, lomefloxacin, moxifloxacin, norfloxacin, ofloxacin, pazufloxacin, pefloxacin, sitafloxacin, sparfloxacin, and tosufloxacin (all rINNs).

Fluoroquinolones are administered by several routes (5). The duration of therapy can vary from a single dose to several weeks or months. Owing to their adverse effects (including severe anaphylaxis, QT interval prolongation, and potential cardiotoxicity), several fluoroquinolones have had to be withdrawn (for example temafloxacin and grepafloxacin) or strictly limited in their use (for example trovafloxacin) after marketing (6). A serious idiosyncratic reaction profile may be related to the immunologically reactive 1-difluorophenyl substituent that characterizes temafloxacin, trovafloxacin, and tosufloxacin (1).

Withdrawal of fluoroquinolones

Owing to adverse effects (including severe anaphylaxis, QT interval prolongation, and potential cardiotoxicity), several fluoroquinolones have had to be withdrawn (for example temafloxacin and grepafloxacin) or strictly limited in their uses (for example trovafloxacin) after marketing. A serious idiosyncratic reaction profile is possibly related to the immunologically reactive 1-difluorophenyl substituent that characterizes temafloxacin, tosufloxacin, and trovafloxacin (7).

The withdrawal of temafloxacin in 1992, only 6 months after its introduction, followed the observation of serious adverse events that were labeled the "temafloxacin syndrome" (8). Adverse effects, including hemolysis, renal dysfunction, coagulopathy, and hepatic dysfunction, were estimated to occur in one in 3500 patients. For comparison, incidence rates for these adverse events were about one in 17 000 patients treated with ciprofloxacin and one in 33 000 patients treated with ofloxacin.

In 1999 trovafloxacin was withdrawn after reports of lethal hepatic damage. Before this development, several studies had been published describing impressive clinical efficacy coupled with an almost flawless safety profile (9,10).

Grepafloxacin was withdrawn from the market in 1999 because of its adverse cardiovascular events, which included dysrhythmias (11).

Clinafloxacin has been withdrawn because of phototoxicity and hypoglycemia and sparfloxacin because of phototoxicity (12).

These experiences demonstrate the need to be vigilant about any untoward events associated with large-scale use of new fluoroquinolones.

Comparative studies

In a crossover, randomized study, 16 fasted volunteers (8 men, 8 women) took single oral doses of gemifloxacin 320 mg and ofloxacin 400 mg on two separate occasions, in order to assess urinary excretion (13). Urine concentrations of ofloxacin were higher than those of gemifloxacin. There were no adverse effects.

General adverse effects

In spite of widely publicized negative experiences, most fluoroquinolones are safe, and adverse events are, compared with other groups of antimicrobial agents, relatively rare (14). The rates of overall adverse events were similar in several comparisons of individual quinolones among themselves or with other antimicrobial agents. In one multicenter, double-blind, randomized study drug-related adverse events were reported by 8.9% of those taking levofloxacin and 8.2% of those taking ciprofloxacin for 7–10 days (15). A meta-analysis of data from 20 phase II and III studies in 4926 patients treated with moxifloxacin showed that adverse events led to withdrawal of treatment in 3.8% of patients (16). In a comparison of grepafloxacin and ciprofloxacin for exacerbations of chronic bronchitis withdrawal was precipitated by adverse events in 3% of 624 patients; there was no difference between ciprofloxacin and grepafloxacin (17). The most frequent causes of withdrawal were nausea, vomiting, dysgeusia, dizziness, and diarrhea. In smaller studies, adverse events are occasionally observed more often. In a prospective, double-blind comparison of ciprofloxacin, ofloxacin, and co-trimoxazole for short-course treatment of acute urinary tract infections, there were drug-related adverse events in 26% of patients treated with ciprofloxacin and 34% of patients treated with ofloxacin (18).

If analysis of the frequency of adverse events is based on prescription event monitoring (PEM), the rates of adverse events are usually substantially lower. In one study, over 11 000 patients taking each antibiotic were monitored (19). Among the fluoroquinolones, ciprofloxacin, norfloxacin, and ofloxacin were used. Adverse events resulted in withdrawal of norfloxacin or ofloxacin in under 1% of patients (19).

The main systems affected by adverse effects of the quinolones are the skin, liver, and nervous system. The best-known adverse effect is phototoxicity, the risk of which varies markedly among the quinolones; lomefloxacin and sparfloxacin carry a particularly high risk. The development of phototoxicity is based on an interaction between light and the drug. Neurotoxicity also occurs, with marked variation of incidence between the various compounds. Hypersensitivity reactions to quinolones are rare, and include anaphylactic shock and anaphylactoid reactions. Organ-specific reactions attributed to hypersensitivity involve the liver and kidneys. If hypersensitivity reactions occur, switching from one quinolone compound to another is probably not advisable, since there is cross-reactivity.

The risk of neoplastic disease is minimal, even during long-term use, but may be increased by exposure to UVA light.

Using electron spin resonance spectroscopy and spin trapping, ciprofloxacin has been shown to cause free radical production in a dose- and time-dependent manner; the authors suggested that this effect may contribute to drug-related adverse effects, including phototoxicity and cartilage defects (20).

The most common drug interactions include malabsorption interactions associated with multivalent cations and CYP450 interactions (21).

Pharmacoeconomics

The pharmacoeconomic impact of adverse effects of antimicrobial drugs is enormous. Antibacterial drug reactions account for about 25% of adverse drug reactions. The adverse effects profile of an antimicrobial agent can contribute significantly to its overall direct costs (monitoring costs, prolonged hospitalization due to complications or treatment failures) and indirect costs (quality of life, loss of productivity, time spent by families and patients receiving medical care). In one study an adverse event in a hospitalized patient was associated on average with an excess of 1.9 days in the length of stay, extra costs of $US2262 (1990–93 values), and an almost two-fold increase in the risk of death. In the outpatient setting, adverse drug reactions result in 2–6% of hospitalizations, and most of them were thought to be avoidable if appropriate interventions had been taken. In a review, economic aspects of antibacterial therapy with fluoroquinolones have been summarized and critically evaluated (22).

Organs and Systems

Cardiovascular

Some quinolones can prolong the QT interval, with a risk of cardiac dysrhythmias. In an in vitro study in isolated canine cardiac Purkinje fibers the rank order of potency in prolonging action potential duration was sparfloxacin > grepafloxacin = moxifloxacin > ciprofloxacin (23). In guinea-pig ventricular myocardium sparfloxacin prolonged the action potential duration by about 8% at 10 μmol/l and 41% at 100 μmol/l (24). Gatifloxacin, grepafloxacin, and moxifloxacin were less potent, but prolonged the action potential duration at 100 μmol/l by about 13%, 24%, and 25% respectively. In contrast, ciprofloxacin, gemifloxacin, levofloxacin, sitafloxacin, tosufloxacin, and trovafloxacin had little or no effect on the action potential at concentrations as high as 100 μmol/l.

Preclinical and clinical trial data and data from phase IV studies have shown that levofloxacin, moxifloxacin, and gatifloxacin cause prolongation of the QT interval, but that the potential for torsade de pointes is rare and is influenced by several independent variables (for example concurrent administration of class Ia and III antidysrhythmic agents) (25). There is a moderate increase in the QT interval associated with sparfloxacin, averaging 3%, and the few serious adverse cardiovascular events that have been reported during postmarketing surveillance all occurred in patients with underlying heart disease (26).

In patients taking quinolones (ciprofloxacin 11 477, enoxacin 2790, ofloxacin 11 033, and norfloxacin 11 110; mean ages 49–57 years) there was no evidence of drug-induced dysrhythmias associated with enoxacin within 42 days of drug administration (27). Of the other quinolones, atrial fibrillation was reported most often within 42 days of ciprofloxacin administration, with no change in event rate over that time. The crude rate of palpitation did not change significantly with ciprofloxacin, norfloxacin, or ofloxacin. Syncope and tachycardia were also reported with ciprofloxacin and ofloxacin. There was no evidence of drug-induced hepatic dysfunction within 42 days of drug administration with any of the quinolones used.

In a retrospective database analysis 25 cases of torsade de pointes associated with ciprofloxacin ($n = 2$), ofloxacin ($n = 2$), levofloxacin ($n = 13$), and gatifloxacin ($n = 8$) were identified in the USA (28). Ciprofloxacin was associated with a significantly lower rate of torsade de pointes (0.3 cases/10 million prescriptions) than levofloxacin (5.4/10 million) or gatifloxacin (27/10 million). When the analysis was limited to the first 16 months after initial approval of the drug, the rates for levofloxacin (16/10 million) and gatifloxacin (27/10 million) were similar.

Nervous system

The main central nervous system adverse effects of the fluoroquinolones include dizziness, convulsions, psychosis, and insomnia; levofloxacin, moxifloxacin, and ofloxacin are reportedly least likely to cause these effects, based on a study of European and international data from about 130 million prescriptions (29).

A review has suggested that fluoroquinolone-associated peripheral nervous system events are mild and short-term (30). Among 60 courses of quinolones in 45 patients (levofloxacin 33 courses, ciprofloxacin 11 courses, ofloxacin 6 courses, lomefloxacin 1 course, trovafloxacin 1 course; in eight cases the same antibiotic was prescribed twice) there were 36 severe events that typically involved multiple organ systems. The symptoms lasted more than 3 months in 71% of cases and more than 1 year in 58%. The onset of the adverse events in the 45 patients was usually rapid: 15 events began within 24 hours of the start of treatment, 26 within 72 hours, and 38 within 1 week.

Dizziness is not rare in patients taking fluoroquinolones, and was observed in 2.8% of patients taking moxifloxacin (16), in 8 and 9% of patients taking grepafloxacin 400 mg/day and 600 mg/day, and in 6% of patients taking ciprofloxacin (17). Prescription event monitoring found markedly lower rates of this adverse event during treatment with ciprofloxacin, norfloxacin, or ofloxacin (19).

Headache was recorded in 8% of patients taking ciprofloxacin and 9% taking ofloxacin during short-course treatment of urinary tract infections (18). Similar rates are reported for grepafloxacin (17).

In two patients with myasthenia gravis, ciprofloxacin and norfloxacin exacerbated the symptoms (31).

Encephalopathy with unconsciousness has been reported in a 48-year-old woman with Machado–Joseph disease after the administration of fleroxacin (200 mg/day) for 3 days (32). She recovered after withdrawal. The serum and cerebrospinal fluid concentrations of fleroxacin were within normal limits.

Seizures

Quinolone antibiotics vary in their ability to cause seizures. Trovafloxacin has the greatest potential and levofloxacin possibly the least. Ciprofloxacin can cause confusion and general seizures (33,34). Seizures also occurred in patients taking ofloxacin (35) and levofloxacin (34). However, this must be rare, since there have only been isolated case reports.

Among over 30 000 patients treated with ciprofloxacin, norfloxacin, or ofloxacin, no seizures were detected during prescription event monitoring (19). The risk of seizures during treatment with individual quinolones is currently unknown. Electrophysiological field potentials in animals are affected to varying degrees by different quinolones; the smallest effect was observed with ofloxacin, followed by ciprofloxacin and nalidixic acid, whereas there was an increasing excitatory effect with clinafloxacin, enoxacin, fleroxacin, lomefloxacin, moxifloxacin, and trovafloxacin (36). The pathophysiological basis for the triggering of seizures probably lies in the binding of fluoroquinolones to $GABA_A$ receptors in the brain, blocking the natural ligand GABA; this results in nervous system stimulation (37). Binding to this receptor is strongly influenced by the side chain in the 7-position; quinolones with bulky moieties, such as temafloxacin and sparfloxacin, bind less efficiently to GABA receptors.

Sensory systems

Taste

Dysgeusia is reported with many quinolones. This was observed more often with higher doses of grepafloxacin (600 mg/day; 17%) than with lower doses (400 mg/day; 9%) (38). In another study there was a similar dose–response relation: 13% of patients taking 400 mg/day and 27% of those taking 600 mg/day (17).

In 135 unmedicated young volunteers, 13 elderly volunteers and 14 unmedicated HIV-infected patients, enoxacin applied to the tongue was described as metallic by young subjects, but bitter by elderly subjects; lefloxacin and ofloxacin were described as bitter (39).

Psychological, psychiatric

Isolated cases of depression (18) and psychosis have been described in temporal association with fluoroquinolones (40).

Hematologic

In over 33 000 patients treated with ciprofloxacin, norfloxacin, or ofloxacin, no case of hemolytic anemia was discovered by prescription event monitoring (19). However, ciprofloxacin has been associated with hemolysis in combination with a severe skin reaction in a young adult (41).

Leukopenia has been observed in 0.1–0.7% of patients given fluoroquinolones in Japan and eosinophilia was observed in 0.5–2.2% of these patients (42). Leukopenia was generally mild and reversible after dosage reduction or withdrawal (43,44).

Anemia, thrombocytopenia, and thrombocytosis have only rarely been reported (45–48).

Gastrointestinal

Adverse gastrointestinal events are not uncommon during treatment with fluoroquinolones. There may be some dose-dependency, since with grepafloxacin 600 mg/day the rates of the following adverse events were noticeably higher than with 400 mg/day: nausea (15 versus 11%), vomiting (6 versus 1%), and diarrhea (4 versus 3%) (38). In a randomized, double-blind comparison of prulifloxacin 600 mg/day and ciprofloxacin 500 mg bd in 235 patients with acute exacerbations of chronic bronchitis, the most common treatment-related adverse event was gastric pain of mild or moderate intensity, reported in 8.5% of the patients taking prulifloxacin and 6.8% of those taking ciprofloxacin (49).

Liver

Transient rises in serum transaminase and serum alkaline phosphatase activities have been observed with all fluoroquinolones. This occurred in 0.9–4.3% of patients in Japan. In the vast majority of the cases this alteration was self-limited and reversible without withdrawal of the drug (42).

Urinary tract

In a Medline search to investigate the incidence and features of fluoroquinolone nephrotoxicity only primarily case reports and temporally related events could be identified (50). Ciprofloxacin was associated with an increased risk of renal insufficiency, probably because it has been in use longer and more widely than the newer agents. Raised serum creatinine or blood urea nitrogen concentrations have been observed in 0.1–0.7% of patients (42).

Single cases of reversible, acute non-oliguric or oliguric renal insufficiency, probably due to tubulointerstitial nephritis, have been reported (51,52), as well as isolated cases of hematuria (53). The newer fluoroquinolones have only rarely been associated with nephrotoxicity, with an estimated incidence of 0.4–0.8%.

Rare cases of possibly drug-related crystalluria have been described in patients taking fluoroquinolones (54–56).

Skin

Skin rashes are relatively common with fluoroquinolones. A retrospective cohort study in patients in general practice in the Netherlands focused on the use of antibacterial agents and the occurrence of adverse cutaneous events covered 469 505 consultations with 87 475 patients, of whom 13 679 received prescriptions for antibiotics (57). After adjustment for age, sex, and co-medications, the incidence density ratio (incidence density per 1000 exposed days) for various groups of antibacterial agents was as follows: tetracyclines 1.0, macrolides 1.1, fluoroquinolones 2.8, penicillins 2.9, and co-trimoxazole 4.4 (57). No details of the types of skin reactions were given, and it is therefore possible that phototoxic events were included. Compared with other studies, the reported rate of antibiotic-associated adverse cutaneous events in this outpatient population was rather low.

Exposure to light causes photosensitivity reactions in patients taking quinolones and fluoroquinolones. In guinea-pigs the phototoxic potencies were: enoxacin, lomefloxacin > ofloxacin > nalidixic acid, tosufloxacin > norfloxacin, ciprofloxacin (58). Photosensitivity reactions to ofloxacin may be initiated by oxygen radicals and/or by ofloxacin radicals acting as haptens (59). In a mouse model pefloxacin and ciprofloxacin augmented the effect of ultraviolet A by increasing sunburn and apoptosis, depleting Langerhans cells, and suppressing local immune responses (60).

A combination of primary ear swelling analysis and cell counting of ear-draining lymph nodes after UV irradiation in mice was fast and highly predictive of the risks of photosensitization and photoirritancy of fluoroquinolones, depending on the route of exposure (oral or dermal) and may therefore be good tools for preclinical risk assessment in terms of discriminating photoreactions (61).

Tosufloxacin has been associated with a fixed drug eruption (62).

In a phase III, randomized, investigator-blinded comparison of the safety and efficacy of clinafloxacin with those of piperacillin/tazobactam in the treatment of adults with severe skin and soft-tissue infections, four of 84 patients randomized to clinafloxacin developed phototoxicity (63).

Photosensitivity

Photosensitivity is a common adverse effect of the fluoroquinolones. It results from an abnormal reaction of the skin to natural or artificial light sources, usually associated with the UVA part of the electromagnetic spectrum (315–400 nm), mediated by the absorption of light energy into fluoroquinolones, followed by degradation of the molecule and formation of cytotoxic photoproducts (64).

The chemical structure at position 8 in the quinolone ring probably determines the phototoxic potential, since the introduction of a methoxy group at this position markedly reduces the phototoxicity of individual drugs (65).

The early fluoroquinolones, that is ciprofloxacin, norfloxacin, and ofloxacin, are mild photosensitizers (66–70). Clinically relevant photosensitivity was generally only observed when high dosages were used and the patient was exposed to large amounts of sunlight. The phototoxic potential of lomefloxacin, sparfloxacin, and fleroxacin is far greater than that of earlier compounds (71–76). However, even with fluoroquinolones that are reported to have a relatively high rate of phototoxicity, the incidence is low. In a Japanese study of 4276 patients, photosensitivity was found in 44 (1.03%) and was typically not severe (77). Patients with co-morbidity or those over 60 years were at higher risk. The risk may be further increased by a long duration of treatment.

The photosensitizing effect of grepafloxacin is relatively weak and similar to that of ciprofloxacin (38). In one study, one of 207 patients taking grepafloxacin 400 mg/day and six of 204 taking 600 mg/day developed phototoxicity (17). Moxifloxacin is not phototoxic (78). Data obtained in albino mice have suggested that the phototoxic potential of sitafloxacin is milder than that of lomefloxacin or sparfloxacin (79).

Musculoskeletal

Tendinopathy

Tendinopathy and partial or complete tendon rupture as adverse events of fluoroquinolones have been reported during or shortly after the use of fluoroquinolones (80–84). Pefloxacin and ofloxacin have been implicated, as has ciprofloxacin (85,86). In six patients taking fluoroquinolones risk factors included renal insufficiency, glucocorticoid therapy, secondary hyperparathyroidism, advanced age, and diabetes mellitus (87). Cases have also been reported among immunocompromised renal transplant recipients (88).

In 42 spontaneous reports of fluoroquinolone-associated tendon disorders, 32 patients had tendinitis, 24 bilaterally, and 10 had a tendon rupture; most affected the Achilles tendon (89). The median age was 68 years and there was a male predominance. In 16 cases ofloxacin was implicated, in 13 ciprofloxacin, in eight norfloxacin, and in five pefloxacin. The delay between the start of treatment and the appearance of the first symptoms was 1–510 (median 6) days. Most patients recovered within 2 months after withdrawal, but 26% had not yet recovered at follow-up.

In a retrospective analysis, quinolone arthropathy developed during the first 3 weeks, and depended on the patient's age and history (90). It resolved fully within 7 days to 3 months after drug withdrawal.

In a study of fibroblast metabolism in vitro, ciprofloxacin stimulated matrix-degrading protease activity and inhibited fibroblast metabolism; these effects may both contribute to the tendinopathy that is associated with fluoroquinolones (91).

Animal studies show that the propensity to induce tendon lesions varies among fluoroquinolones. Fleroxacin, pefloxacin, levofloxacin, and ofloxacin were the most toxic, while enoxacin, norfloxacin, and ciprofloxacin had little or no effect (92). The structure of the substituent at position 7 seems to be a determining factor. Quinolones with toxic effects in animals share a methylpiperadinyl substituent at the position 7 of the fluoroquinolone core structure, while this position is occupied by a piperadinyl substituent in ciprofloxacin, norfloxacin, and enoxacin (92). It is recommended that quinolones be discontinued at the first sign of tendon pain or inflammation and that the patient should not exercise until the diagnosis of tendonitis can be confidently excluded.

In rodents, pefloxacin (400 mg/kg for several days) caused oxidative damage to the type I collagen in the Achilles tendon; these alterations were identical to those observed in experimental tendinous ischemia and a reperfusion model (93). Oxidative damage was prevented by the co-administration of *N*-acetylcysteine (150 mg/kg).

Arthropathy

Arthropathy has been reported with various fluoroquinolones, particularly in children. In a Russian study in children with cystic fibrosis five were withdrawn (four taking ciprofloxacin and one taking pefloxacin) (94). Two had an arthropathy that was drug- and age-dependent. Quinolone-induced arthropathy was more common with pefloxacin and occurred only in children over 10 years old with a history of joint problems. The arthropathy fully recovered within 7 days to 3 months and there was no cartilage damage.

In Wistar rats treated with ciprofloxacin, there was poor healing of experimental fractures during the early stages of repair, suggesting that fluoroquinolones may compromise the clinical course of fracture healing (95).

Sexual function

In a large study vaginitis and vulvitis were detected by prescription event monitoring in a significantly higher proportion of women taking fluoroquinolones than women taking azithromycin or cefixime (19).

Immunologic

Fluoroquinolones have immunomodulatory effects, at least partly at the gene transcription level, demonstrated by inhibition of cytokine (IL-1α, TNF-α, IL-6, and IL-8) mRNA and cytokine (IL-1α and IL-1β) concentrations by grepafloxacin (1–30 mg/l) in vitro (96).

Anaphylactic shock associated with cinoxacin was reported in three patients by the Netherlands Center for Monitoring of Adverse Reactions to Drugs (97). Another 17 cases were reported to the WHO Collaborating Center for International Drug Monitoring. In some cases the reaction was observed immediately after the first dose of a repeat cycle of treatment. Anaphylactoid reactions to ciprofloxacin have been reported in patients with cystic fibrosis (98–100).

Organ-specific reactions attributed to hypersensitivity involve the liver and kidneys. In one instance centrilobular hepatic necrosis developed during treatment of a urinary tract infection with ciprofloxacin (101). Among 14 cases of drug-induced allergic nephritis, two were associated with quinolones (102). Isolated case reports of allergic nephropathy associated with norfloxacin and ciprofloxacin therapy suggest that this type of reaction is probably very rare (103), since the authors were able to find only 28 other reported cases. If hypersensitivity reactions occur, switching from one quinolone compound to another is probably not advisable, since oral provocation using different agents reproduced the initially observed hypersensitivity reaction (104). This clinical observation is supported by the results of in vitro lymphocyte transformation tests, which were positive with ofloxacin in two patients with allergy to ciprofloxacin (105).

Infection risk

Ciprofloxacin, norfloxacin, and ofloxacin increased gastrointestinal colonization by *Candida albicans* in 17 patients (106). Ciprofloxacin caused the largest increase, but the difference was not statistically significant.

In a retrospective cohort study of patients hospitalized in a Canadian teaching hospital during January 2003 to June 2004 there were 7421 episodes of care in 5619 patients, who were observed until they developed *Clostridium difficile*-associated diarrhea, or died, or for 60 days after discharge (107). Fluoroquinolones were the antibiotics that were most strongly associated with *Clostridium difficile*-associated diarrhea (adjusted hazard ratio = 3.44; 95% CI = 2.65, 4.47). Almost one-quarter of all in-patients received quinolones, for which the population-attributable fraction of *Clostridium difficile*-associated diarrhea was 36%. All three generations of cephalosporins, macrolides, clindamycin, and intravenous beta-lactam/beta-lactamase inhibitors were intermediate-risk antibiotics, with similar hazard ratios (1.56–1.89).

Long-Term Effects

Drug tolerance

To study the impact on the normal intestinal microflora, gatifloxacin was given to 18 healthy volunteers (400 mg/day orally). In the aerobic intestinal microflora *E. coli* strains were eliminated or strongly suppressed and the number of enterococci fell significantly, while the number of staphylococci increased. In the anerobic microflora the numbers of *Clostridia* and fusobacteria fell significantly. The microflora normalized 40 days after the gatifloxacin withdrawal. No selection or overgrowth of resistant bacterial strains or yeasts occurred (108).

Salmonella typhimurium DT104 is usually resistant to ampicillin, chloramphenicol, streptomycin, sulfonamides, and tetracycline. An outbreak of 25 culture-confirmed cases of multidrug-resistant *Salmonella typhimurium* DT104 has been identified in Denmark. The strain was resistant to the abovementioned antibiotics and nalidixic acid and had reduced susceptibility to fluoroquinolones. A swineherd was identified as the primary source (109). The DT104 strain was also found in cases of salmonellosis in Washington State, and soft cheese made with unpasteurized milk was identified as an important vehicle of its transmission (110).

From 8419 worldwide clinical isolates of *Streptococcus pneumoniae* associated with lower respiratory tract or blood infections obtained from 519 geographically distinct hospital laboratories during 1997–98, 69 had reduced susceptibility or resistance to fluoroquinolones. Only mutations in parC and gyrA (especially in combination), but not in gyrB or parE, contributed significantly to resistance. Efflux is probably crucial in reduced susceptibility for new hydrophilic fluoroquinolones (111).

In an in vitro study, ciprofloxacin, grepafloxacin, levofloxacin, moxifloxacin, ofloxacin, and sparfloxacin had similar good activity against *Haemophilus influenzae* and *Moraxella catarrhalis* (112). Against *S. pneumoniae* (irrespective of the strain's susceptibility to penicillin), grepafloxacin, levofloxacin, moxifloxacin, and sparfloxacin had better activity than ciprofloxacin and ofloxacin.

Clinafloxacin, moxifloxacin, sparfloxacin, and trovafloxacin were significantly more active in vitro than ciprofloxacin and levofloxacin against *Stenotrophomonas maltophilia*, a microorganism with inherent resistance to many antibiotics; new-generation quinolones may become very useful in the treatment of certain severe or life-threatening infectious conditions due to this bacterium (113).

In over 90 000 routine samples of *Escherichia coli* in five Dutch laboratories during 1989–98 resistance to norfloxacin increased from 1.3% to 5.8% (114). In addition, multiresistance, defined as resistance to norfloxacin and at least two other antibiotics (from a group consisting of amoxicillin, trimethoprim, and nitrofurantoin), increased from 0.5% to 4.0%.

Mutagenicity

In vitro lomefloxacin photochemically produced oxidative DNA damage, an effect known to be of mutagenic potential (115). This may be the basis of the photochemical mutagenicity and photochemical carcinogenicity of quinolones.

Tumorigenicity

Results of carcinogenicity studies have suggested that the risk of neoplastic disease is minimal, even during long-term use (116). However, the risk may be increased by exposure to UVA light. Skin tumors, only a minority of them malignant, developed in mice after treatment with various quinolones for up to 78 weeks and exposure to UV light. It therefore appears that fluoroquinolones have the potential to enhance the UVA-induced phototumorigenic effect (117).

Second-Generation Effects

Teratogenicity

Possible adverse outcomes were investigated in the newborns of 38 mothers who had received quinolones during pregnancy between 1989 and 1992. The majority (35 women) took norfloxacin or ciprofloxacin for urinary tract infections during the first trimester of pregnancy. There were no malformations in the quinolone group, whereas one child in the control group had a ventricular septal defect. There were no differences between the groups in the achievement of developmental milestones or in the musculoskeletal system (118). However, the authors of the study pointed out that the duration of follow-up may have been too short to draw firm conclusions regarding the safety of quinolones during pregnancy. In addition, the size of the study population was probably inadequate for statistically meaningful comparisons.

Treatment with fluoroquinolones during embryogenesis was not associated with an increased risk of major malformations in a multicenter, prospective, controlled trial in 400 women (119). There was a higher rate of therapeutic abortions in quinolone-exposed women. This may have been explained by the misperception of a major risk related to quinolones during pregnancy.

In pregnant rats fed with norfloxacin, there was DNA fragmentation in fetal tissues (14). Even though this effect was attributed to general toxicity rather than genotoxicity, quinolones should be avoided during pregnancy (120).

Lactation

Given the potential for untoward effects on the cartilage of breast-feeding infants, fluoroquinolones should be avoided by nursing mothers.

Susceptibility Factors

Genetic factors

The pharmacokinetics of fleroxacin (200 mg intravenously or 200 mg orally) have been studied in 19 Nigerian men. C_{max} and AUC were 3–4 fold lower than previously reported after identical doses, but systemic availability profile was as previously reported (121).

Age

Children

The use of fluoroquinolones in children is controversial. Fluoroquinolones have greatly facilitated the management of exacerbations of pulmonary infections in cystic fibrosis. Apart from this indication, they have rarely been used in children for other indications, such as urinary tract infection, prophylaxis in neutropenia, gastrointestinal infections, and nervous system infections (122). Thorough reviews of published experience suggest that fluoroquinolones can be used without increased risks of short-term or long-term adverse events. A study of adverse events within 45 days of receiving a prescription for ciprofloxacin was remarkable for the fact that among over 1700 children, no cases of newly diagnosed acute arthritis or other serious disturbances of liver or kidney function were recorded (123). One patient with hemolytic–uremic syndrome had an exacerbation that was possibly caused by ciprofloxacin.

Renal disease

Based on their predominant renal elimination, dosage adjustment is necessary in the presence of renal disease for ciprofloxacin, gatifloxacin, levofloxacin, and sitafloxacin (124).

Hepatic disease

The penetration of routinely used fluoroquinolones into ascitic fluid after intravenous administration has been studied in patients with uncompensated hepatic cirrhosis (125). Three patients received three doses of ciprofloxacin 200 mg, six received three doses of ciprofloxacin 300 mg, seven received three doses of pefloxacin 400 mg, and six received three doses of ofloxacin 400 mg. Pefloxacin and ofloxacin produced serum and ascitic fluid concentrations above the MICs of the common pathogens that cause spontaneous bacterial peritonitis, and the authors concluded that they could be given to cirrhotic patients in dosage regimens similar to those in patients with normal hepatic function.

Other features of the patient

Given the well-described risk of phototoxicity associated with fluoroquinolones, sunlight and direct exposure to the sun are risk factors. Patients therefore need to be instructed about protective measures.

In patients with leg ischemia fleroxacin diffused into both ischemic and non-ischemic tissues (bone, subcutaneous fat, muscle, and tendons) after a 400 mg intravenous dose (126). Since the maximum antibiotic concentrations were lower than the MICs of various relevant pathogens, the dose used for perioperative prophylaxis in these patients should be increased to 800 mg.

Drug–Drug Interactions

Antacids

Concurrent treatment with antacids reduces the oral absorption of many quinolones, such as ciprofloxacin and enoxacin (127), moxifloxacin (16), norfloxacin (128), ofloxacin (129), and sparfloxacin (130).

Caffeine

CYP1A2 participates in the metabolism of both enoxacin and caffeine, and inhibition of caffeine metabolism by enoxacin can cause adverse effects (131).

In 24 healthy volunteers, 12 men and 12 women, the women had significantly different caffeine pharmacokinetics in the presence of ciprofloxacin and fleroxacin compared with the men (132). There were also significant differences between the sexes in the pharmacokinetics of ciprofloxacin and fleroxacin in the presence of caffeine. The differences were in part due to different body weights.

Clinafloxacin 200 or 400 mg reduced the mean clearance of caffeine by 84% (133).

Cimetidine

Cimetidine reduces the metabolic clearance of both enoxacin and pefloxacin by about 20% (134,135).

Digoxin

The pharmacokinetics of digoxin were not altered by sparfloxacin (136).

Drugs that prolong the QT interval

In order to prevent any untoward effect on cardiac repolarization, agents that prolong the QT interval, such as terfenadine, astemizole, erythromycin, and agents with Class Ia and Class III antidysrhythmic activity, should not be used together with sparfloxacin (137).

Furosemide

The renal excretion of lomefloxacin and ofloxacin was reduced and plasma concentrations increased by furosemide, resulting in higher concentrations (138).

Iron

All of the fluoroquinolones interact with polyvalent cations, and their systematic availability is reduced by 50% when they are co-administered with iron compounds; ciprofloxacin and moxifloxacin (16) are more affected than gemifloxacin or levofloxacin (139).

Ferrous salts reduce the systemic availability of fluoroquinolones (127), including sparfloxacin (140).

NSAIDs

Co-administration of fenbufen and fluoroquinolones has been associated with seizures (141). The structure at the 7-position greatly affects the risk of NSAID-potentiated nervous system effects. Fluoroquinolones with unsubstituted piperazinyl rings (ciprofloxacin, enoxacin, and norfloxacin) have a strong interaction with NSAIDs (142). The increased risk of seizures is not caused by increased serum concentrations of fluoroquinolones, since their pharmacokinetics are not altered by NSAIDs (143). The mechanism has been suggested to be facilitation by fenbufen of the fluoroquinolone-induced inhibition of $GABA_A$ receptor function in the hippocampus and frontal cortex (144).

Probenecid

Probenecid increases the serum concentrations of cinoxacin (145), enoxacin (146), and nalidixic acid (147) probably by inhibiting their renal tubular secretion.

Sucralfate

Sucralfate markedly reduces the systemic availability of fluoroquinolones (127,148,149).

Theophylline

Fluoroquinolones are potent inhibitors of hepatic cytochrome P450 isozymes (150). They inhibit theophylline metabolism, and accumulation of theophylline has led to seizures (151). Theophylline clearance is reduced by about 10% by norfloxacin, 30% by ciprofloxacin, and 70% by enoxacin (152–162). In a comparison of grepafloxacin (400 and 600 mg/day) and ciprofloxacin, increased theophylline concentrations associated with clinical symptoms were found with both doses of grepafloxacin but not in patients taking ciprofloxacin (17). The dosage of theophylline should be reduced when a quinolone is given.

No interaction has been reported with levofloxacin (139) or sparfloxacin (137,161).

Warfarin

The anticoagulant effect of warfarin was altered by ciprofloxacin (162) but not by sparfloxacin (149) or moxifloxacin (16).

Interference with Diagnostic Tests

Opioid immunoassays

The reactivity of 13 quinolones and fluoroquinolones (ciprofloxacin, clinafloxacin, enoxacin, gatifloxacin, levofloxacin, lomefloxacin, moxifloxacin, nalidixic acid, norfloxacin, ofloxacin, pefloxacin, sparfloxacin, and trovafloxacin) with five commercial opiate immunoassays has been tested in vitro and in three healthy volunteers (163). In vitro, levofloxacin and ofloxacin (using Abbott AxSYM, CEDIA, EMIT II, and Roche OnLine assays), pefloxacin (using CEDIA, EMIT II, and Roche OnLine assays), enoxacin (using CEDIA and EMIT II assays), gatifloxacin (using EMIT II assay), and ciprofloxacin, lomefloxacin, moxifloxacin, and norfloxacin (using Roche OnLine assay) cross-reacted and cause a positive test result for opiates. Clinafloxacin, nalidixic acid, sparfloxacin, and trovafloxacin did not cross-react in any of the assays. A single dose of levofloxacin 500 mg caused a false-positive test result using the EMIT II assay within 2 hours for as long as 22 hours in all three volunteers. Ofloxacin (a single dose of 400 mg) produced a similar pattern. Detectable opiate activity in the urine was seen for more than 30 hours with both levofloxacin and ofloxacin.

References

1. Ball P. New antibiotics for community-acquired lower respiratory tract infections: improved activity at a cost? Int J Antimicrob Agents 2000;16(3):263–72 .
2. Hooper DC. The fluoroquinolones after ciprofloxacin and ofloxacin. Curr Clin Top Infect Dis 2000;20:63–91.
3. O'Donnell JA, Gelone SP. Fluoroquinolones. Infect Dis Clin North Am 2000;14(2):489–513.
4. King DE, Malone R, Lilley SH. New classification and update on the quinolone antibiotics. Am Fam Physician 2000;61(9):2741–8.
5. Hooper DC. Expanding uses of fluoroquinolones: opportunities and challenges. Ann Intern Med 1998;129(11):908–10.
6. Bertino J Jr, Fish D. The safety profile of the fluoroquinolones. Clin Ther 2000;22(7):798–817.
7. Rubinstein E. History of quinolones and their side effects. Chemotherapy 2001;47(Suppl 3):3–8; discussion 44–8.
8. Lietman PS. Fluoroquinolone toxicities. An update. Drugs 1995;49(Suppl 2):159–63.
9. Williams DJ, Hopkins S. Safety and tolerability of intravenous-to-oral treatment and single-dose intravenous or oral prophylaxis with trovafloxacin. Am J Surg 1998;176(Suppl 6A):S74–9.
10. Donahue PE, Smith DL, Yellin AE, Mintz SJ, Bur F, Luke DR. Trovafloxacin in the treatment of intra-abdominal infections: results of a double-blind, multicenter comparison with imipenem/cilastatin. Trovafloxacin Surgical Group Am J Surg 1998;176(Suppl 6A):S53–61.
11. Gibaldi M. Grepafloxacin withdrawn from market. Drug Ther Topics Suppl 2000;29:6.
12. Zhanel GG, Ennis K, Vercaigne L, Walkty A, Gin AS, Embil J, Smith H, Hoban DJ. A critical review of the fluoroquinolones: focus on respiratory infections. Drugs 2002;62(1):13–59.
13. Barker PJ, Sheehan R, Teillol-Foo M, Palmgren AC, Nord CE. Impact of gemifloxacin on the normal human intestinal microflora. J Chemother 2001;13(1):47–51.
14. Norrby SR, Lietman PS. Safety and tolerability of fluoroquinolones. Drugs 1993;45(Suppl 3):59–64.
15. Nicodemo AC, Robledo JA, Jasovich A, Neto W. A multicentre, double-blind, randomised study comparing the efficacy and safety of oral levofloxacin versus ciprofloxacin in the treatment of uncomplicated skin and skin structure infections. Int J Clin Pract 1998;52(2):69–74.

16. Balfour JA, Wiseman LR. Moxifloxacin. Drugs 1999;57(3):363–73.
17. Chodosh S, Lakshminarayan S, Swarz H, Breisch S. Efficacy and safety of a 10-day course of 400 or 600 milligrams of grepafloxacin once daily for treatment of acute bacterial exacerbations of chronic bronchitis: comparison with a 10-day course of 500 milligrams of ciprofloxacin twice daily. Antimicrob Agents Chemother 1998;42(1):114–20.
18. McCarty JM, Richard G, Huck W, Tucker RM, Tosiello RL, Shan M, Heyd A, Echols RM. A randomized trial of short-course ciprofloxacin, ofloxacin, or trimethoprim/sulfamethoxazole for the treatment of acute urinary tract infection in women. Ciprofloxacin Urinary Tract Infection Group. Am J Med 1999;106(3):292–9.
19. Wilton LV, Pearce GL, Mann RD. A comparison of ciprofloxacin, norfloxacin, ofloxacin, azithromycin and cefixime examined by observational cohort studies. Br J Clin Pharmacol 1996;41(4):277–84.
20. Gurbay A, Gonthier B, Daveloose D, Favier A, Hincal F. Microsomal metabolism of ciprofloxacin generates free radicals. Free Radic Biol Med 2001;30(10):1118–21.
21. Berning SE. The role of fluoroquinolones in tuberculosis today. Drugs 2001;61(1):9–18.
22. Beringer PM, Wong-Beringer A, Rho JP. Economic aspects of antibacterial adverse effects. Pharmacoeconomics 1998;13(1 Pt 1):35–49.
23. Patmore L, Fraser S, Mair D, Templeton A. Effects of sparfloxacin, grepafloxacin, moxifloxacin, and ciprofloxacin on cardiac action potential duration. Eur J Pharmacol 2000;406(3):449–52.
24. Hagiwara T, Satoh S, Kasai Y, Takasuna K. A comparative study of the fluoroquinolone antibacterial agents on the action potential duration in guinea pig ventricular myocardia. Jpn J Pharmacol 2001;87(3):231–4.
25. Owens RC Jr, Ambrose PG. Torsades de pointes associated with fluoroquinolones. Pharmacotherapy 2002;22(5):663–8; discussion 668–72.
26. Jaillon P, Morganroth J, Brumpt I, Talbot G. Overview of electrocardiographic and cardiovascular safety data for sparfloxacin. Sparfloxacin Safety Group. J Antimicrob Chemother 1996;37(Suppl A):161–7.
27. Clark DW, Layton D, Wilton LV, Pearce GL, Shakir SA. Profiles of hepatic and dysrhythmic cardiovascular events following use of fluoroquinolone antibacterials: experience from large cohorts from the Drug Safety Research Unit Prescription-Event Monitoring database. Drug Saf 2001;24(15):1143–54.
28. Frothingham R. Rates of torsades de pointes associated with ciprofloxacin, ofloxacin, levofloxacin, gatifloxacin, and moxifloxacin. Pharmacotherapy 2001;21(12):1468–72.
29. Carbon C. Comparison of side effects of levofloxacin versus other fluoroquinolones. Chemotherapy 2001;47(Suppl 3):9–14;discussion 44–8.
30. Cohen JS. Peripheral neuropathy associated with fluoroquinolones. Ann Pharmacother 2001;35(12):1540–7.
31. Moore B, Safani M, Keesey J. Possible exacerbation of myasthenia gravis by ciprofloxacin. Lancet 1988;1(8590):882.
32. Kimura M, Fujiyama J, Nagai A, Hirayama M, Kuriyama M. [Encephalopathy induced by fleroxacin in a patient with Machado–Joseph disease.] Rinsho Shinkeigaku 1998;38(9):846–8.
33. Tattevin P, Messiaen T, Pras V, Ronco P, Biour M. Confusion and general seizures following ciprofloxacin administration. Nephrol Dial Transplant 1998;13(10):2712–13.
34. Kushner JM, Peckman HJ, Snyder CR. Seizures associated with fluoroquinolones. Ann Pharmacother 2001;35(10): 1194–8.
35. Walton GD, Hon JK, Mulpur TG. Ofloxacin-induced seizure. Ann Pharmacother 1997;31(12):1475–7.
36. Schmuck G, Schurmann A, Schluter G. Determination of the excitatory potencies of fluoroquinolones in the central nervous system by an in vitro model. Antimicrob Agents Chemother 1998;42(7):1831–6.
37. Bryskier A, Chantot JF. Classification and structure–activity relationships of fluoroquinolones. Drugs 1995;49(Suppl 2):16–28.
38. Stahlmann R, Schwabe R. Safety profile of grepafloxacin compared with other fluoroquinolones. J Antimicrob Chemother 1997;40(Suppl A):83–92.
39. Schiffman SS, Zervakis J, Westall HL, Graham BG, Metz A, Bennett JL, Heald AE. Effect of antimicrobial and anti-inflammatory medications on the sense of taste. Physiol Behav 2000;69(4–5):413–24.
40. Reeves RR. Ciprofloxacin-induced psychosis. Ann Pharmacother 1992;26(7–8):930–1.
41. Kundu AK. Ciprofloxacin-induced severe cutaneous reaction and haemolysis in a young adult. J Assoc Physicians India 2000;48(6):649–50.
42. Shimada J, Hori S. Adverse effects of fluoroquinolones. Prog Drug Res 1992;38:133–43.
43. Eron LJ, Harvey L, Hixon DL, Poretz DM. Ciprofloxacin therapy of infections caused by *Pseudomonas aeruginosa* and other resistant bacteria. Antimicrob Agents Chemother 1985;28(2):308–10.
44. Patoia L, Guerciolini R, Menichetti F, Bucaneve G, Del Favero A. Norfloxacin and neutropenia. Ann Intern Med 1987;107(5):788–9.
45. Wang C, Sabbaj J, Corrado M, Hoagland V. World-wide clinical experience with norfloxacin: efficacy and safety. Scand J Infect Dis Suppl 1986;48:81–9.
46. Ball P. Ciprofloxacin: an overview of adverse experiences. J Antimicrob Chemother 1986;18(Suppl D):187–93.
47. Sawada M, Nakamura S, Yamada A, Kobayashi T, Okada S. Phase IV study and post-marketing surveillance of ofloxacin in Japan. Chemotherapy 1991;37(2):134–42.
48. Simon J, Guyot A. Pefloxacin: safety in man. J Antimicrob Chemother 1990;26(Suppl B):215–18.
49. Grassi C, Salvatori E, Rosignoli MT, Dionisio P; Prulifloxacin Study Group. Randomized, double-blind study of prulifloxacin versus ciprofloxacin in patients with acute exacerbations of chronic bronchitis. Respiration 2002;69(3):217–22.
50. Lomaestro BM. Fluoroquinolone-induced renal failure. Drug Saf 2000;22(6):479–85.
51. Hootkins R, Fenves AZ, Stephens MK. Acute renal failure secondary to oral ciprofloxacin therapy: a presentation of three cases and a review of the literature. Clin Nephrol 1989;32(2):75–8.
52. Hatton J, Haagensen D. Renal dysfunction associated with ciprofloxacin. Pharmacotherapy 1990;10(5):337–40.
53. Rastogi S, Atkinson JL, McCarthy JT. Allergic nephropathy associated with ciprofloxacin. Mayo Clin Proc 1990;65(7):987–9.
54. Swanson BN, Boppana VK, Vlasses PH, Rotmensch HH, Ferguson RK. Norfloxacin disposition after sequentially increasing oral doses. Antimicrob Agents Chemother 1983;23(2):284–8.
55. Schaeffer AJ. Multiclinic study of norfloxacin for treatment of urinary tract infections. Am J Med 1987;82(6B):53–8.
56. Campoli-Richards DM, Monk JP, Price A, Benfield P, Todd PA, Ward A. Ciprofloxacin. A review of its antibacterial activity, pharmacokinetic properties and therapeutic use. Drugs 1988;35(4):373–447.
57. van der Linden PD, van der Lei J, Vlug AE, Stricker BH. Skin reactions to antibacterial agents in general practice. J Clin Epidemiol 1998;51(8):703–8.
58. Horio T, Miyauchi H, Asada Y, Aoki Y, Harada M. Phototoxicity and photoallergenicity of quinolones in guinea pigs. J Dermatol Sci 1994;7(2):130–5.

59. Navaratnam S, Claridge J. Primary photophysical properties of ofloxacin. Photochem Photobiol 2000;72(3):283–90.
60. Sun YW, Heo EP, Cho YH, Bark KM, Yoon TJ, Kim TH. Pefloxacin and ciprofloxacin increase UVA-induced edema and immune suppression. Photodermatol Photoimmunol Photomed 2001;17(4):172–7.
61. Blotz A, Michel L, Moysan A, Blumel J, Dubertret L, Ahr HJ, Vohr HW. Analyses of cutaneous fluoroquinolones photoreactivity using the integrated model for the differentiation of skin reactions. J Photochem Photobiol B 2000;58(1):46–53.
62. Sangen Y, Kawada A, Asai M, Aragane Y, Yudate T, Tezuka T. Fixed drug eruption induced by tosufloxacin tosilate. Contact Dermatitis 2000;42(5):285.
63. Siami FS, LaFleur BJ, Siami GA. Clinafloxacin versus piperacillin/tazobactam in the treatment of severe skin and soft-tissue infections in adults at a Veterans Affairs medical center. Clin Ther 2002;24(1):59–72.
64. Matsumoto M, Kojima K, Nagano H, Matsubara S, Yokota T. Photostability and biological activity of fluoroquinolones substituted at the 8 position after UV irradiation. Antimicrob Agents Chemother 1992;36(8):1715–19.
65. Marutani K, Matsumoto M, Otabe Y, Nagamuta M, Tanaka K, Miyoshi A, Hasegawa T, Nagano H, Matsubara S, Kamide R, et al. Reduced phototoxicity of a fluoroquinolone antibacterial agent with a methoxy group at the 8 position in mice irradiated with long-wavelength UV light. Antimicrob Agents Chemother 1993;37(10):2217–23.
66. Wainwright NJ, Collins P, Ferguson J. Photosensitivity associated with antibacterial agents. Drug Saf 1993;9(6):437–40.
67. Ferguson J, Johnson BE. Clinical and laboratory studies of the photosensitizing potential of norfloxacin, a 4-quinolone broad-spectrum antibiotic. Br J Dermatol 1993;128(3):285–95.
68. Jensen T, Pedersen SS, Nielsen CH, Hoiby N, Koch C. The efficacy and safety of ciprofloxacin and ofloxacin in chronic *Pseudomonas aeruginosa* infection in cystic fibrosis. J Antimicrob Chemother 1987;20(4):585–94.
69. Jungst G, Mohr R. Side effects of ofloxacin in clinical trials and in postmarketing surveillance. Drugs 1987;34(Suppl 1):144–9.
70. Scheife RT, Cramer WR, Decker EL. Photosensitizing potential of ofloxacin. Int J Dermatol 1993;32(6):413–16.
71. Lopitaux R, Hermet R, Sirot J, Filiu P, Terver S. Tolérance de la péfloxacine au cours du traitement d'une série d'infections ostéo-articulaires. [Tolerance to pefloxacine during treatment of a series of osteoarticular infections. 36 cases.] Therapie 1985;40(5):349–52.
72. Stahlmann R. Safety profile of the quinolones. J Antimicrob Chemother 1990;26(Suppl D):31–44.
73. Bowie WR, Willetts V, Jewesson PJ. Adverse reactions in a dose-ranging study with a new long-acting fluoroquinolone, fleroxacin. Antimicrob Agents Chemother 1989;33(10):1778–82.
74. Cohen JB, Bergstresser PR. Inadvertent phototoxicity from home tanning equipment. Arch Dermatol 1994;130(6):804–6.
75. Correia O, Delgado L, Barros MA. Bullous photodermatosis after lomefloxacin. Arch Dermatol 1994;130(6):808–9.
76. Kurumaji Y, Shono M. Scarified photopatch testing in lomefloxacin photosensitivity. Contact Dermatitis 1992;26(1):5–10.
77. Arata J, Horio T, Soejima R, Ohara K. Photosensitivity reactions caused by lomefloxacin hydrochloride: a multicenter survey. Antimicrob Agents Chemother 1998;42(12):3141–5.
78. Man I, Murphy J, Ferguson J. Fluoroquinolone phototoxicity: a comparison of moxifloxacin and lomefloxacin in normal volunteers. J Antimicrob Chemother 1999;43(Suppl B):77–82.
79. Shimoda K, Ikeda T, Okawara S, Kato M. Possible relationship between phototoxicity and photodegradation of sitafloxacin, a quinolone antibacterial agent, in the auricular skin of albino mice. Toxicol Sci 2000;56(2):290–6.
80. Ribard P, Audisio F, Kahn MF, De Bandt M, Jorgensen C, Hayem G, Meyer O, Palazzo E. Seven Achilles tendinitis including 3 complicated by rupture during fluoroquinolone therapy. J Rheumatol 1992;19(9):1479–81.
81. Blanco Andres C, Bravo Toledo R. Tendinitis bilateral secundaria a ciprofloxacino. [Bilateral tendinitis caused by ciprofloxacin.] Aten Primaria 1998;21(3):184–5.
82. West MB, Gow P. Ciprofloxacin, bilateral Achilles tendonitis and unilateral tendon rupture—a case report. NZ Med J 1998;111(1058):18–19.
83. Stahlmann R. Clinical toxicological aspects of fluoroquinolones. Toxicol Lett 2002;127(1–3):269–77.
84. Burstein GR, Berman SM, Blumer JL, Moran JS. Ciprofloxacin for the treatment of uncomplicated gonorrhea infection in adolescents: does the benefit outweigh the risk? Clin Infect Dis 2002;35(Suppl 2):S191–9.
85. Casparian JM, Luchi M, Moffat RE, Hinthorn D. Quinolones and tendon ruptures. South Med J 2000;93(5):488–91.
86. Saint F, Gueguen G, Biserte J, Fontaine C, Mazeman E. Rupture du ligament patellaire un mois après traitement par fluoroquinolone. [Rupture of the patellar ligament one month after treatment with fluoroquinolone.] Rev Chir Orthop Reparatrice Appar Mot 2000;86(5):495–7.
87. Gabutti L, Stoller R, Marti HP. Fluoroquinolone als Ursache von Tendinopathien. [Fluoroquinolones as etiology of tendinopathy.] Ther Umsch 1998;55(9):558–61.
88. Donck JB, Segaert MF, Vanrenterghem YF. Fluoroquinolones and Achilles tendinopathy in renal transplant recipients. Transplantation 1994;58(6):736–7.
89. van der Linden PD, van Puijenbroek EP, Feenstra J, Veld BA, Sturkenboom MC, Herings RM, Leufkens HG, Stricker BH. Tendon disorders attributed to fluoroquinolones: a study on 42 spontaneous reports in the period 1988 to 1998. Arthritis Rheum 2001;45(3):235–9.
90. Postnikov SS, Semykin SIu, Nazhimov VP, Novichkova GA. Mesto pefloksatsina v lechenii bol'nykh mukovistsidozom. [On fluoroquinolones treatment safety in children (clinical, morphological and catamnesis data).] Antibiot Khimioter 2002;47(9):14–17.
91. Williams RJ 3rd, Attia E, Wickiewicz TL, Hannafin JA. The effect of ciprofloxacin on tendon, paratenon, and capsular fibroblast metabolism. Am J Sports Med 2000;28(3):364–9.
92. Kashida Y, Kato M. Characterization of fluoroquinolone-induced Achilles tendon toxicity in rats: comparison of toxicities of 10 fluoroquinolones and effects of anti-inflammatory compounds. Antimicrob Agents Chemother 1997;41(11):2389–93.
93. Simonin MA, Gegout-Pottie P, Minn A, Gillet P, Netter P, Terlain B. Pefloxacin-induced achilles tendon toxicity in rodents: biochemical changes in proteoglycan synthesis and oxidative damage to collagen. Antimicrob Agents Chemother 2000;44(4):867–72.
94. Postnikov SS. Sravnitel'naia effektivnost' i bezopasnost' tsiprofloksatsina, ofloksatsina i pefloksatsina pri lechenii infektsii dykhatel'nykh putei u detei s mukovitsidozom. [Comparative efficacy and safety of ciprofloxacin, ofloxacin, and pefloxacin in treatment of respiratory infections in children with cystic fibrosis.] Antibiot Khimioter 2001;46(3):16–20.
95. Huddleston PM, Steckelberg JM, Hanssen AD, Rouse MS, Bolander ME, Patel R. Ciprofloxacin inhibition of experimental fracture healing. J Bone Joint Surg Am 2000;82(2):161–73.
96. Ono Y, Ohmoto Y, Ono K, Sakata Y, Murata K. Effect of grepafloxacin on cytokine production in vitro. J Antimicrob Chemother 2000;46(1):91–4.

97. Stricker BH, Slagboom G, Demaeseneer R, Slootmaekers V, Thijs I, Olsson S. Anaphylactic reactions to cinoxacin. BMJ 1988;297(6661):1434–5.
98. Davis H, McGoodwin E, Reed TG. Anaphylactoid reactions reported after treatment with ciprofloxacin. Ann Intern Med 1989;111(12):1041–3.
99. Kennedy CA, Goetz MB, Mathisen GE. Ciprofloxacin-induced anaphylactoid reactions in patients infected with the human immunodeficiency virus. West J Med 1990;153(5):563–4.
100. Miller MS, Gaido F, Rourk MH Jr, Spock A. Anaphylactoid reactions to ciprofloxacin in cystic fibrosis patients. Pediatr Infect Dis J 1991;10(2):164–5.
101. Grassmick BK, Lehr VT, Sundareson AS. Fulminant hepatic failure possibly related to ciprofloxacin. Ann Pharmacother 1992;26(5):636–9.
102. Shibasaki T, Ishimoto F, Sakai O, Joh K, Aizawa S. Clinical characterization of drug-induced allergic nephritis. Am J Nephrol 1991;11(3):174–80.
103. Hadimeri H, Almroth G, Cederbrant K, Enestrom S, Hultman P, Lindell A. Allergic nephropathy associated with norfloxacin and ciprofloxacin therapy. Report of two cases and review of the literature. Scand J Urol Nephrol 1997;31(5):481–5.
104. Davila I, Diez ML, Quirce S, Fraj J, De La Hoz B, Lazaro M. Cross-reactivity between quinolones. Report of three cases. Allergy 1993;48(5):388–90.
105. Ronnau AC, Sachs B, von Schmiedeberg S, Hunzelmann N, Ruzicka T, Gleichmann E, Schuppe HC. Cutaneous adverse reaction to ciprofloxacin: demonstration of specific lymphocyte proliferation and cross-reactivity to ofloxacin in vitro. Acta Derm Venereol 1997;77(4):285–8.
106. Mavromanolakis E, Maraki S, Cranidis A, Tselentis Y, Kontoyiannis DP, Samonis G. The impact of norfloxacin, ciprofloxacin and ofloxacin on human gut colonization by *Candida albicans*. Scand J Infect Dis 2001;33(6):477–8.
107. Pepin J, Saheb N, Coulombe MA, Alary ME, Corriveau MP, Authier S, Leblanc M, Rivard G, Bettez M, Primeau V, Nguyen M, Jocob CE, Lanthier L. Emergence of fluoroquinolones as the prodominant risk factor for *Clostridium difficile*-associated diarrhea: a cohort study during an epidemic in Quebec. Clin Infect Dis 2005;41(9):1254–60.
108. Edlund C, Nord CE. Ecological effect of gatifloxacin on the normal human intestinal microflora. J Chemother 1999;11(1):50–3.
109. Molbak K, Baggesen DL, Aarestrup FM, Ebbesen JM, Engberg J, Frydendahl K, Gerner-smidt P, Petersen AM, Wegener HC. An outbreak of multidrug-resistant, quinolone-resistant *Salmonella enterica* serotype typhimurium DT104 N Engl J Med 1999;341(19):1420–5.
110. Villar RG, Macek MD, Simons S, Hayes PS, Goldoft MJ, Lewis JH, Rowan LL, Hursh D, Patnode M, Mead PS. Investigation of multidurg-resistant *Salmonella* serotype typhimurium DT104 infections linked to raw-milk cheese in Washington State JAMA 1999;281(19):1811–6.
111. Jones ME, Sahm DF, Martin N, Scheuring S, Heisig P, Thornsberry C, Kohrer K, Schmitz FJ. Prevalence of gyrA, gyrB, parC, and parE mutations in clinical isolates of *Streptococcus pneumoniae* with decreased susceptibilities to different fluoroquinolones and originating from worldwide surveillance studies during the 1997–1998 respiratory season. Antimicrob Agents Chemother 2000;44(2):462–6.
112. Esposito S, Noviello S, Ianniello F. Comparative in vitro activity of older and newer fluoroquinolones against respiratory tract pathogens. Chemotherapy 2000;46(5):309–14.
113. Weiss K, Restieri C, De Carolis E, Laverdiere M, Guay H. Comparative activity of new quinolones against 326 clinical isolates of *Stenotrophomonas maltophilia*. J Antimicrob Chemother 2000;45(3):363–5.
114. Goettsch W, van Pelt W, Nagelkerke N, Hendrix MG, Buiting AG, Petit PL, Sabbe LJ, van Griethuysen AJ, de Neeling AJ. Increasing resistance to fluoroquinolones in *Escherichia coli* from urinary tract infections in the netherlands. J Antimicrob Chemother 2000;46(2):223–8.
115. Jeffrey AM, Shao L, Brendler-Schwaab SY, Schluter G, Williams GM. Photochemical mutagenicity of phototoxic and photochemically carcinogenic fluoroquinolones in comparison with the photostable moxifloxacin. Arch Toxicol 2000;74(9):555–9.
116. Fort FL. Mutagenicity of quinolone antibacterials. Drug Saf 1992;7(3):214–22.
117. Klecak G, Urbach F, Urwyler H. Fluoroquinolone antibacterials enhance UVA-induced skin tumors. J Photochem Photobiol B 1997;37(3):174–81.
118. Berkovitch M, Pastuszak A, Gazarian M, Lewis M, Koren G. Safety of the new quinolones in pregnancy. Obstet Gynecol 1994;84(4):535–8.
119. Loebstein R, Addis A, Ho E, Andreou R, Sage S, Donnenfeld AE, Schick B, Bonati M, Moretti M, Lalkin A, Pastuszak A, Koren G. Pregnancy outcome following gestational exposure to fluoroquinolones: a multicenter prospective controlled study. Antimicrob Agents Chemother 1998;42(6):1336–9.
120. Cukierski MA, Prahalada S, Zacchei AG, Peter CP, Rodgers JD, Hess DL, Cukierski MJ, Tarantal AF, Nyland T, Robertson RT, et al. Embryotoxicity studies of norfloxacin in cynomolgus monkeys: I. Teratology studies and norfloxacin plasma concentration in pregnant and nonpregnant monkeys. Teratology 1989;39(1):39–52.
121. Chukwuani CM, Coker HA, Oduola AM, Sowunmi A, Ifudu ND. Bioavailability of ciprofloxacin and fleroxacin: results of a preliminary investigation in healthy adult Nigerian male volunteers. Biol Pharm Bull 2000;23(8):968–72.
122. Dagan R. Fluoroquinolones in paediatrics—1995. Drugs 1995;49(Suppl 2):92–9.
123. Jick S. Ciprofloxacin safety in a pediatric population. Pediatr Infect Dis J 1997;16(1):130–3.
124. Aminimanizani A, Beringer P, Jelliffe R. Comparative pharmacokinetics and pharmacodynamics of the newer fluoroquinolone antibacterials. Clin Pharmacokinet 2001;40(3):169–87.
125. Sambatakou H, Giamarellos-Bourboulis EJ, Galanakis N, Giamarellou H. Pharmacokinetics of fluoroquinolones in uncompensated cirrhosis: the significance of penetration in the ascitic fluid. Int J Antimicrob Agents 2001;18(5):441–4.
126. Miglioli PA, Kafka R, Bonatti H, Fraedrich G, Allerberger F, Schoeffel U. Fleroxacin uptake in ischaemic limb tissue. Acta Microbiol Immunol Hung 2001;48(1):11–15.
127. Deppermann KM, Lode H. Fluoroquinolones: interaction profile during enteral absorption. Drugs 1993;45(Suppl 3):65–72.
128. Cordoba-Diaz M, Cordoba-Borrego M, Cordoba-Diaz D. Influence of pharmacotechnical design on the interaction and availability of norfloxacin in directly compressed tablets with certain antacids. Drug Dev Ind Pharm 2000;26(2):159–66.
129. Flor S, Guay DR, Opsahl JA, Tack K, Matzke GR. Effects of magnesium–aluminum hydroxide and calcium carbonate antacids on bioavailability of ofloxacin. Antimicrob Agents Chemother 1990;34(12):2436–8.
130. Johnson RD, Dorr MB, Talbot GH, Caille G. Effect of Maalox on the oral absorption of sparfloxacin. Clin Ther 1998;20(6):1149–58.
131. Carrillo JA, Benitez J. Clinically significant pharmacokinetic interactions between dietary caffeine and medications. Clin Pharmacokinet 2000;39(2):127–53.
132. Kim MK, Nightingale C, Nicolau D. Influence of sex on the pharmacokinetic interaction of fleroxacin and ciprofloxacin with caffeine. Clin Pharmacokinet 2003;42(11):985–96.

133. Randinitis EJ, Alvey CW, Koup JR, Rausch G, Abel R, Bron NJ, Hounslow NJ, Vassos AB, Sedman AJ. Drug interactions with clinafloxacin. Antimicrob Agents Chemother 2001;45(9):2543–52.
134. Misiak PM, Eldon MA, Toothaker RD, Sedman AJ. Effects of oral cimetidine or ranitidine on the pharmacokinetics of intravenous enoxacin. J Clin Pharmacol 1993;33(1):53–6.
135. Bressolle F, Goncalves F, Gouby A, Galtier M. Pefloxacin clinical pharmacokinetics. Clin Pharmacokinet 1994;27(6):418–46.
136. Johnson R, Wilson J, Talbot G. The effect of sparfloxacin on the steady-state pharmacokinetics of digoxin in healthy male volunteers. Pharm Res 1994;11(Suppl):429.
137. Goa KL, Bryson HM, Markham A. Sparfloxacin. A review of its antibacterial activity, pharmacokinetic properties, clinical efficacy and tolerability in lower respiratory tract infections. Drugs 1997;53(4):700–25.
138. Sudoh T, Fujimura A, Shiga T, Sasaki M, Harada K, Tateishi T, Ohashi K, Ebihara A. Renal clearance of lomefloxacin is decreased by furosemide. Eur J Clin Pharmacol 1994;46(3):267–9.
139. Lode H. Evidence of different profiles of side effects and drug–drug interactions among the quinolones—the pharmacokinetic standpoint. Chemotherapy 2001;47(Suppl 3):24–31; discussion 44–8.
140. Kanemitsu K, Hori S, Yanagawa A, Shimada J. Effect of ferrous sulfate on the absorption of sparfloxacin in healthy volunteers and rats. Drugs 1995;49(Suppl 2):352–6.
141. Morita H, Maemura K, Sakai Y, Kaneda Y. [A case of convulsion, loss of consciousness and subsequent acute renal failure caused by enoxacin and fenbufen.] Nippon Naika Gakkai Zasshi 1988;77(5):744–5.
142. Furuhama K, Akahane K, Iawara K, Takayama S. Interaction of the new quinolone antibacterial agent levofloxacin with fenbufen in mice. Arzneimittelforschung 1992;43(3A):406–8.
143. Fillastre JP, Leroy A, Borsa-Lebas F, Etienne I, Gy C, Humbert G. Effects of ketoprofen (NSAID) on the pharmacokinetics of pefloxacin and ofloxacin in healthy volunteers. Drugs Exp Clin Res 1992;18(11–12):487–92.
144. Motomura M, Kataoka Y, Takeo G, Shibayama K, Ohishi K, Nakamura T, Niwa M, Tsujihata M, Nagataki S. Hippocampus and frontal cortex are the potential mediatory sites for convulsions induced by new quinolones and non-steroidal anti-inflammatory drugs. Int J Clin Pharmacol Ther Toxicol 1991;29(6):223–7.
145. Rodriguez N, Madsen PO, Welling PG. Influence of probenecid on serum levels and urinary excertion of cinoxacin. Antimicrob Agents Chemother 1979;15(3):465–9.
146. Wijnands WJ, Vree TB, Baars AM, van Herwaarden CL. Pharmacokinetics of enoxacin and its penetration into bronchial secretions and lung tissue. J Antimicrob Chemother 1988;21(Suppl B):67–77.
147. Vree TB, Van den Biggelaar-Martea M, Van Ewijk-Beneken Kolmer EW, Hekster YA. Probenecid inhibits the renal clearance and renal glucuronidation of nalidixic acid. A pilot experiment. Pharm World Sci 1993;15(4):165–70.
148. Zix JA, Geerdes-Fenge HF, Rau M, Vockler J, Borner K, Koeppe P, Lode H. Pharmacokinetics of sparfloxacin and interaction with cisapride and sucralfate. Antimicrob Agents Chemother 1997;41(8):1668–72.
149. Lee LJ, Hafkin B, Lee ID, Hoh J, Dix R. Effects of food and sucralfate on a single oral dose of 500 milligrams of levofloxacin in healthy subjects. Antimicrob Agents Chemother 1997;41(10):2196–200.
150. Polk RE. Drug–drug interactions with ciprofloxacin and other fluoroquinolones. Am J Med 1989;87(5A):S76–81.
151. Grasela TH Jr, Dreis MW. An evaluation of the quinolone–theophylline interaction using the Food and Drug Administration spontaneous reporting system. Arch Intern Med 1992;152(3):617–21.
152. Takagi K, Hasegawa T, Yamaki K, Suzuki R, Watanabe T, Satake T. Interaction between theophylline and enoxacin. Int J Clin Pharmacol Ther Toxicol 1988;26(6):288–92.
153. Beckmann J, Elsasser W, Gundert-Remy U, Hertrampf R. Enoxacin—a potent inhibitor of theophylline metabolism. Eur J Clin Pharmacol 1987;33(3):227–30.
154. Wijnands WJ, Vree TB, van Herwaarden CL. The influence of quinolone derivatives on theophylline clearance. Br J Clin Pharmacol 1986;22(6):677–83.
155. Nix DE, DeVito JM, Whitbread MA, Schentag JJ. Effect of multiple dose oral ciprofloxacin on the pharmacokinetics of theophylline and indocyanine green. J Antimicrob Chemother 1987;19(2):263–9.
156. Schwartz J, Jauregui L, Lettieri J, Bachmann K. Impact of ciprofloxacin on theophylline clearance and steady-state concentrations in serum. Antimicrob Agents Chemother 1988;32(1):75–7.
157. Bowles SK, Popovski Z, Rybak MJ, Beckman HB, Edwards DJ. Effect of norfloxacin on theophylline pharmacokinetics at steady state. Antimicrob Agents Chemother 1988;32(4):510–12.
158. Ho G, Tierney MG, Dales RE. Evaluation of the effect of norfloxacin on the pharmacokinetics of theophylline. Clin Pharmacol Ther 1988;44(1):35–8.
159. Davis RL, Kelly HW, Quenzer RW, Standefer J, Steinberg B, Gallegos J. Effect of norfloxacin on theophylline metabolism. Antimicrob Agents Chemother 1989;33(2):212–14.
160. Prince RA, Casabar E, Adair CG, Wexler DB, Lettieri J, Kasik JE. Effect of quinolone antimicrobials on theophylline pharmacokinetics. J Clin Pharmacol 1989;29(7):650–4.
161. Takagi K, Yamaki K, Nadai M, Kuzuya T, Hasegawa T. Effect of a new quinolone, sparfloxacin, on the pharmacokinetics of theophylline in asthmatic patients. Antimicrob Agents Chemother 1991;35(6):1137–41.
162. Ellis RJ, Mayo MS, Bodensteiner DM. Ciprofloxacin–warfarin coagulopathy: a case series. Am J Hematol 2000;63(1):28–31.
163. Baden LR, Horowitz G, Jacoby H, Eliopoulos GM. Quinolones and false-positive urine screening for opiates by immunoassay technology. JAMA 2001;286(24):3115–19.

Fluorouracil

See also Cytostatic and immunosuppressant drugs

General Information

Fluorouracil is a fluorinated pyrimidine, which is converted intracellularly to the active form, fluorodeoxyuridine monophosphate, which inhibits thymidylate synthetase and hence reduces the production of thymidylic acid, the deoxyribonucleotide of thymine (5-methyluracil), a DNA pyrimidine base, blocking DNA synthesis. In addition, intracellular conversion to 5-fluorouridine monophosphate results in incorporation of the activated antimetabolite into RNA and consequent RNA dysfunction.

Fluorouracil is specific to the S phase of the cell cycle. It is primarily used intravenously to treat carcinoma of the breast and adenocarcinomas of the gastrointestinal tract (1). In addition, topical fluorouracil is used to treat actinic keratoses.

General adverse effects

The dose-limiting toxic effects of fluorouracil vary with the dose and mode of administration.

- With five consecutive daily bolus injections of 450–600 mg/m^2, the dose-limiting effects are myelosuppression, mucositis, and diarrhea.
- With weekly injections of 450–600 mg/m^2, myelosuppression is dose-limiting.
- With continuous five-day infusion of 1000 mg/m^2/day, mucositis and diarrhea are dose-limiting.
- With protracted continuous infusion of 200–400 mg/m^2/day, mucositis and palmar–plantar erythrodysesthesia syndrome are the most common dose-limiting adverse effects (2).

Some very high-dose, short-exposure studies have been reported, including 14 g over 24 hours (3) and 2.6 g/m^2 weekly (4); in the latter study, neurotoxicity was dose-limiting; with 24-hour infusion of 2.6 g/m^2 weekly, palmar–plantar erythrodysesthesia syndrome is a major adverse effect.

Relation of toxicity to pharmacokinetics

The pharmacokinetics of fluorouracil have been determined in 19 patients receiving fluorouracil by protracted intravenous infusion of 190–600 mg/m^2/day (5). The steady-state fluorouracil plasma concentration and AUC were significantly lower in the nine patients who had WHO grade 2 toxicity or less compared with the nine patients who had greater than grade 2 toxicity. In contrast, there was no difference in fluorouracil plasma concentrations between the 10 responders and the nine patients who had no evidence of a clinical response. These investigations confirm previous observations that correlations can be drawn between fluorouracil pharmacokinetics and clinical toxicity (6). Furthermore, the data suggest that pharmacokinetic monitoring might permit identification of patients at increased risk of toxicity.

Organs and Systems

Cardiovascular

Fluorouracil can cause anginal chest pain, with non-specific ST–T electrocardiographic changes, during infusion (7). The outcome is favourable if the drug is withdrawn. Re-introduction of the drug has been associated with occasional fatal outcomes and is not recommended (8). The cardiotoxicity of 5-fluorouracil in 135 reported cases has been reviewed (9).

Presentation

More frequent use of fluorouracil by continuous infusion, increased awareness of the problems, and more sophisticated monitoring have increased the reported incidence. By 1990, more than 67 clinical cases had been described (10) and an incidence ranging up to 68% of silent ischemic electrocardiographic changes was identified in patients monitored by continuous 24-hour ambulatory electrocardiography during fluorouracil infusion (11). The clinical features include the following:

- Precordial pain (both non-specific and anginal) (10).
- Electrocardiographic ST–T wave changes (non-specific and ischemic) (10,11).
- Acute myocardial infarction (rare) (12,13).
- Atrial dysrhythmias (including atrial fibrillation) and less often, ventricular extra beats (including refractory ventricular tachycardia and fibrillation) (11–13).
- Ventricular dysfunction (usually global, less frequently segmental).
- Cardiac failure, pulmonary edema, and cardiogenic shock (with and without ischemic symptoms) (13–16).
- Sudden death, presumed to be caused by ventricular fibrillation (13,17,18).

In most patients with chest pain, with or without electrocardiographic changes, the creatinine kinase MB fraction remained normal (10,13,15).

Acute dilated cardiomyopathy with left ventricular dysfunction related temporally to fluorouracil and cisplatin infusion, with subsequent complete recovery, has been tentatively linked to fluorouracil (19). Other similar events have been reported (20,21). The association is more striking in patients who receive a continuous infusion of fluorouracil and in patients who receive concomitant cisplatin (22,23). For example, myocardial ischemia and infarction occur in about 10% of patients who receive fluorouracil by infusion and sudden death has occurred (24).

Five cases of paroxysmal atrial fibrillation and sinus bradycardia attributed to fluorouracil have been reported (25).

Acute pulmonary edema leading to lethal cardiogenic shock has been reported with fluorouracil. This occurred despite the fact that the patient had received eight infusions of leucovorin 100 mg/m^2 at weekly intervals (26).

Most often, cardiotoxicity develops during the second or later course of treatment, but some patients have problems during the first course (10). Those who develop cardiac toxicity and recover usually have symptoms again when re-challenged with another infusion (10,13).

Fluorouracil has also been associated with a number of vascular effects, particularly thromboembolic or circulatory in nature (27). Although Raynaud's phenomenon has been reported after cisplatin-based chemotherapy, the first case of digital ischemia and Raynaud's phenomenon has been reported with fluorouracil given in a De Gramond type schedule (28).

Mechanisms and pathophysiology

The mechanisms of fluorouracil cardiotoxicity are not known. Those that have been suggested include:

- direct uncoupling of electromechanical myocardial function at the level of ATP generation (20);
- an immunoallergic reaction following sensitization by a complex of fluorouracil and cardiac cells;
- vasospasm secondary either to fluorouracil or to released products;
- a direct toxic effect of the drug on the myocardium.

Most reports have attributed chest pain to vasospasm (29). Certainly, the ischemic-like pains and electrocardiographic findings, lack of changes in creatine kinase, and frequent responses to nitrates and at times to calcium antagonists in the setting of anatomically normal coronary angiography, plus reversible contractility defects suggest coronary vasospasm as a mechanism of fluorouracil cardiotoxicity. However, global dysfunction possibly due to stunned myocardium and the lack of universal response to coronary vasodilators leaves some questions about this hypothesis. Some investigators have postulated myocarditis or myocardiopathy (30–32). In 43 patients it did not interfere with the electrical properties of myocardial fibers (33).

Findings on autopsy and endomyocardial biopsy have shown diffuse, interstitial edema, intracytoplasmic vacuolization of myocytes, and no inflammatory infiltrate (34). Acute myocardial infarction has been demonstrated pathologically in some, but not all, patients with clinical infarction (10).

In patients with fluorouracil cardiotoxicity endothelin plasma concentrations were raised (35).

Susceptibility factors

With regard to susceptibility factors for cardiotoxicity with fluorouracil, there was no effect of age or sex on incidence (10). Symptoms have been reported in a 38-year-old man (16) and in several women in their forties (10,14) with no prior cardiac history. Cardiac findings have occurred when fluorouracil was given by infusion or bolus as a single agent or with cisplatin and other drugs (10,21). Although some felt that cardiac irradiation and pre-existing heart disease were susceptibility factors (11,36), others did not (10,37). Several investigators have documented normal coronary arteries in patients with severe symptoms (13,14).

Frequency

The cardiotoxicity of fluorouracil was first identified in 1975 (38). Of 140 patients treated with intravenous 5-fluorouracil, 4 developed ischemic chest pain within 18 hours of either the second or third dose. In three of these patients the pain recurred after subsequent doses. Predose electrocardiograms in two cases were normal. None of the four patients had a history of ischemic heart disease, although all had received left ventricular irradiation (39).

A 5% incidence of cardiotoxicity-complicating high-dose infusion of fluorouracil 1000 mg/m^2/day for 4 days has been reported and correlated with plasma fluorouracil concentrations in excess of 450 mg/ml (40).

In 910 patients toxicity was life-threatening in 0.55% (41). A combination of cisplatin, fluorouracil, and etoposide given for advanced non-small cell cancer of the lung caused only the expected amount of hematological toxicity, but was associated with a higher than expected incidence of cardiac, pulmonary, and cerebrovascular toxicity, including two myocardial infarctions, two cases of congestive heart failure, one pulmonary embolus, and one cerebrovascular accident in a study of 35 patients (42).

In 1083 patients there was cardiotoxicity in 1.1% of all patients and in 4.6% of patients with prior evidence of heart disease (36).

Management

Some investigators have reported success in preventing cardiotoxicity with calcium antagonists, such as nifedipine and diltiazem (29), while others had less success (15,43). Two patients with proven fluorouracil cardiotoxicity did not have cardiotoxicity when treated with the specific thymidylate synthase inhibitor raltitrexed 3 mg/m^2 every 3 weeks (44). The authors commented that fluorouracil cardiotoxicity is therefore not mediated via thymidylate synthase.

In most cases, fluorouracil-induced dysrhythmias were treatable and the ischemic-like symptoms and electrocardiographic changes disappeared if the infusion was discontinued or responded to nitrates, allowing the infusion to continue. The abnormalities of segmental and global ventricular function reverted to normal within days to weeks of withdrawal. In some patients intravenous inotropic and vasodilator support was needed during the initial period (14–16,19).

However, in one case, both oral nitrates and calcium antagonists failed to prevent chest pain associated with 5-fluorouracil (45).

- About 48 hours after starting her first course of 5-fluorouracil (1000 mg/m^2/day) a woman developed anginal chest pain and electrocardiographic changes that eventually normalized. She was readmitted for her second cycle whilst taking amlodipine 10 mg/day and isosorbide dinitrate 40 mg/day, and after 42 hours into the second cycle had the same chest pain and electrocardiographic changes. These were only controlled by withdrawal of the 5-fluorouracil and the intravenous administration of glyceryl trinitrate.

Respiratory

Pulmonary toxicity in the form of fibrosing alveolitis has been attributed to fluorouracil.

- A 55-year-old man with gastric adenocarcinoma received fluorouracil 1 g intravenously each week for 9 weeks and mitomycin 10 mg intravenously every 3 weeks (46). After 12 treatments he developed severe dyspnea.

Although mitomycin C was most likely the agent responsible for pulmonary toxicity in this patient, combined use with fluorouracil as a contributing factor cannot be ruled out. Necropsy confirmed that the patient had interstitial fibrosis (47).

Nervous system

Fluorouracil can cause neurotoxicity (48), with an incidence of 5–15% and with all schedules of administration in common use (49,50). The toxicity is acute in onset and cumulative dose-dependency has not been observed.

Acute cerebellar dysfunction, with gait ataxia, nystagmus, dysmetria, and dysarthria, is the most common form of neurotoxicity (48,49). A rare problem is optic neuropathy and impaired vision (51).

The acute cerebellar syndrome is considered to be associated with peak concentrations of fluorouracil (48,52). Continuous 5-day infusions appear not to cause neurological toxicity, even when the total dose is higher, although high-dose infusions can cause encephalopathy, with symptoms varying from lethargy to coma (53).

Cerebral demyelination has been reported in a patient receiving fluorouracil and levamisole (54).

Two patients with some of the classic neurological complications of fluorouracil have been reported. One had a cerebellar syndrome in association with global motor weakness and bulbar palsy and the other a bilateral third cranial nerve palsy (55).

Peripheral neuropathy, possibly caused by fluorouracil, has been reported (56).

Five patients developed ischemic stroke within 2–5 days of finishing a 4-day course of fluorouracil plus low-dose cisplatin by continuous infusion (57). Whilst cisplatin has been implicated as having produced central ischemic events, most commonly in combination with vindesine and bleomycin, there has only been one other report involving fluorouracil. Although the causal link was not conclusive, the circumstantial evidence was strong.

The cause of neurotoxicity is not well understood. Acute neurological symptoms, including somnolence, cerebellar ataxia, and upper motor neuron signs, are primarily seen in patients receiving intracarotid infusions for head and neck tumors and also in patients receiving fluorouracil monotherapy in high doses. This syndrome has been reproduced in animals by a neurotoxic metabolite of fluorouracil, fluorocitrate, which has been believed to cause neurotoxicity (52,58). However, several patients have developed severe toxic symptoms due to deficiency of dihydropyrimidine dehydrogenase, the enzyme that is mainly responsible for metabolizing fluorouracil (59). This toxicity appears to be due to the parent compound and not metabolites. Patients with complete or partial deficiency of the enzyme are particularly subject to fluorouracil neurotoxicity.

The neurotoxicity is usually reversible by withdrawing fluorouracil. Since there is no cumulative effect, therapy can be resumed later if desired, usually with either a lower dose or a less frequent dosing schedule to prevent recurrence.

Sensory systems

Fluorouracil-containing regimens have been linked with several ocular adverse effects, including marked lacrimation, ocular pruritus, and a burning sensation in the eyes (60).

Striate melanokeratosis of the retina has been associated with 5-fluorouracil in reports from a number of centers; there has been no consistent explanation of the pathogenesis of this adverse effect (61–63).

Excessive lacrimation and other ocular disturbances have been reported secondary to intravenous fluorouracil (64–66). In a review of this subject, blurred vision, excessive lacrimation, excessive nasal discharge, and conjunctivitis were the most commonly reported ocular effects of fluorouracil (67). The symptoms, eye irritation and excessive tear production, can be aggravated by cold weather. The onset of symptoms varies from 15 minutes to 14 months after the start of treatment (64). The symptoms usually resolve 2–3 weeks after withdrawal of therapy, with or without the use of topical antibiotic-glucocorticoid combinations (64,67).

More severe toxic effects, including tear duct fibrosis and eversion of the lower eye lid, have been reported (64). Tear duct fibrosis develops in one of six patients with excessive lacrimation from fluorouracil (66). The eversion of the lower eyelid is reversible with conservative management (68) while the tear duct fibrosis may not be (69). Persistent lacrimation has been described in six patients receiving intravenous fluorouracil weekly for 6–10 months (69). Lacrimation persisted in five patients after the withdrawal of fluorouracil, suggesting an irreversible dacryostenosis. Lacrimal duct stenosis has also been reported (70). Bilateral cicatricial ectropion was also reported in a patient after topical administration of fluorouracil for the treatment of multiple facial actinic keratoses (71). If ectropion and tear duct stenosis progress, surgical correction may be required.

Three women developed lacrimal outflow obstruction while receiving fluorouracil, cyclophosphamide, and methotrexate for breast cancer (72). The authors commented on both the high incidence of excessive tearing in patients given fluorouracil, a probable precondition, and the rarity of permanent damage (12 patients reported worldwide), but counselled on the need for vigilance and early referral to an ophthalmologist. Others have suggested that the prevalence of tearing and canalicular fibrosis in patients receiving fluorouracil is related to total dose and duration of treatment, and that the risks become significant at 20–60 weeks of therapy and a total fluorouracil dose of 20–50 g (73).

- Ankyloblepharon (adherence of the eyelids resulting in narrowing of palpebral apertures) was reported in a 59-year-old man during fluorouracil therapy for metastatic adenocarcinoma of the stomach (74). It appeared that bilateral conjunctival ulcers, secondary to fluorouracil and ulcerative blepharitis, resulted in ankyloblepharon. Withdrawal of chemotherapy resulted in improvement and re-initiation of therapy resulted in recurrence of ocular lesions.

Transient, non-infectious, crystalline, intrastromal corneal deposits have been reported after subconjunctival administration of 5-fluorouracil (75). The deposits were treated with glucocorticoids and completely resolved in 4 days.

Psychological, psychiatric

Confusion and cerebral cognitive defects have been attributed to fluorouracil (49,76).

Metabolism

Patients with poorly controlled diabetes are at risk of greater or more severe fluorouracil toxicity, causing hyperglycemia, which has been fatal. This effect seems to be independent of previous diabetic control and or fluorouracil dosage schedules (77)

There have been attempts to unravel the mechanism of fluorouracil-induced hyperammonemia, lactic acidosis, and encephalopathy, a rare adverse effect associated with high-dose therapy. The cause is not known, although Krebs cycle metabolism is almost certainly involved (78,79).

Hematologic

The hematological toxicity of fluorouracil is dose- and schedule-related (80). Leukocytes and platelets are affected, although the latter less so. Myelosuppression begins 4–7 days after the first dose, with recovery usually 14 days after the last dose (2). With continued treatment, anemia can develop in 3–4 months (81). Severe bone marrow depression causing death has been reported (82).

Leukopenia is the most common blood dyscrasia secondary to fluorouracil and usually occurs after every course. The lowest white cell counts are usually seen at 9–14 days after the first course of treatment, but can be delayed for up to 20 days (83,84). Leukopenia usually resolves after drug withdrawal. Leukopenia is often followed by megaloblastic anemia (85). Agranulocytosis has been reported during fluorouracil therapy (84).

Thrombocytopenia has occurred during fluorouracil therapy but is much less frequent than leukopenia (59).

The following summarizes the dose-relatedness of the hematological effects of fluorouracil (86,87):

- With a daily bolus of 12 mg/kg for 5 days, leukopenia (under 4×10^9/l) occurred in all of 70 patients; 31% had marked leukopenia (under 2×10^9/l).
- With a continuous infusion of 30 mg/kg/day for 5 days, the leukopenia was mild and occurred in only 12% of patients.
- A protracted continuous infusion of 300 mg/m^2/day caused one case of moderate leukopenia and four cases of mild/moderate thrombocytopenia.
- With a daily bolus of 500 mg/m^2 for 5 days there was a 38% incidence of leukopenia (with 20% below 2×10^9/l and an 8% incidence of thrombocytopenia (1% severe).

Gastrointestinal

The gastrointestinal toxicity of 5-fluorouracil is well documented and often dose-limiting. However, in a retrospective 10-year survey of gastrointestinal function in 19 patients who also had inflammatory bowel disease, although it did appear to increase the risk of exacerbation of diarrhea, it was not totally conclusive, as it was difficult to evaluate the contribution of other potentially causative factors, such as radiation (88).

Any site along the gastrointestinal tract can be affected, resulting in symptoms such as nausea and vomiting, stomatitis, dysphagia, retrosternal burning, abdominal pain, diarrhea, and proctitis.

Stomatitis is common and can be severe and life-threatening (84). Stomatitis may be preceded by a dry mouth and erythema of the mucosa followed by a white patchy membrane. In severe cases this is followed by ulceration and necrosis. Breakdown of the mucosa is very painful and can act as a focus for infection (2). Xerostomia at the start of therapy and a baseline neutrophil count of under 4×10^9/l are significantly associated with dose-limiting oral mucositis later in chemotherapy, according to the results of a logistic regression analysis of 63 patients (89). Mouth-cooling with oral ice chips for 30 minutes starting immediately before fluorouracil substantially reduced the severity of mucositis.

Nausea and vomiting are common but generally mild (84).

Gastric ulceration has been reported in patients receiving fluorouracil by intrahepatic infusion via percutaneous catheterization in doses of 20–30 mg/kg for 4 days followed by 15 mg/kg over 17 days. Symptoms were observed from 4 to 20 days after starting therapy (90). Gastrointestinal bleeding in three patients and death in one patient were also reported following intra-arterial fluorouracil (91).

Diarrhea is common, particularly in patients who receive a 5-day regimen. The diarrhea can be watery or bloody and life-threatening in severe cases. Repeated episodes of watery diarrhea (more than three movements per day) for several days should alert the oncologist to the potential dangers of dehydration and sepsis, which are potentially fatal adverse effects. Life-threatening diarrhea, with hematemesis, high intestinal obstruction, melena, septicemia, and shock, have been reported after total doses of 4–4.5 g of fluorouracil (92). Similarly, diarrhea followed by neutropenia and life-threatening or fatal sepsis occurred in two of 55 patients with advanced colorectal carcinoma in a pilot study of continuous infusion of fluorouracil (750 mg/m^2/day for 5 days) plus subcutaneous recombinant interferon alfa-2a (6–18 million units/day) (93). Severe diarrhea and mucosal ulceration of the colon with necrosis has also been reported (94).

- A 53-year-old man had a side-to-side ileo-descending colostomy for disseminated carcinoma. Fluorouracil was given in doses of 15 mg/kg for 4 days, then 7.5 mg/kg intravenously on days 6 and 8. He developed severe diarrhea and severe ulceration of the bypassed portion of the colon, resulting in necrosis, and death occurred as the result of bronchopneumonia. Autopsy showed ulcers from the ileocecal valve to the ileo-colostomy site. The mucosa of the stomach, small intestine, and colon distal to the colostomy were not involved.

In two cases the diarrhea and colitis associated with fluorouracil therapy were caused by toxigenic *Clostridium difficile*. Both patients responded to oral vancomycin (95).

Colitis has been reported as a rare complication of fluorouracil treatment. Two cases have been reported after intra-arterial chemotherapy (96). A further case has been reported, described by the authors as neutropenic enterocolitis, presenting as abdominal pain, diarrhea, and neutropenia (97). Proven pseudomembranous colitis followed 36 weekly doses of fluorouracil (700 mg) and folinic acid (150 mg); the authors believed that this was only the second reported case (98).

Liver

It has been suggested that handling cytostatic agents can insidiously cause hepatic damage and possibly irreversible fibrosis. Three case reports of hepatic injury in nurses after years of handling cytotoxic drugs (bleomycin, vincristine, cyclophosphamide, doxorubicin, dacarbazine, fluorouracil, and methotrexate) have been described (99). All had neurological symptoms associated with raised serum alanine transaminase and alkaline phosphatase activities. Liver biopsy showed portal hepatitis, with piecemeal necrosis in one and hepatic fibrosis and fat accumulation in the others.

- Diffuse hepatic necrosis has been described in a 29-year-old man receiving 500 mg/day fluorouracil for 4 days (route of administration unspecified) for adenocarcinoma (100). He developed nausea, vomiting, diarrhea, and massive and diffuse hepatic necrosis. The drug was withdrawn and he died 2 days later (6 days after starting medication).

However, the role of fluorouracil in inducing hepatic disease in this patient is unclear.

In a retrospective analysis of a study of *N*-phosphonoacetyl-L-aspartate (250 mg/m^2) followed by weekly boluses of fluorouracil (600–800 mg/m^2) in 44 patients with metastatic colorectal cancer, five of 17 patients with complete or partial responses to therapy developed transient ascites (with or without associated hypoalbuminemia) compared with one of 27 without such a response (101). Other significant findings in some of the responders included raised bilirubin concentrations and transaminase activities from metastasis. The authors cautioned that the adverse effects observed do not necessarily represent disease progression.

Biliary tract

Intrahepatic infusion of fluorouracil can cause biliary sclerosis (102), believed to result from perfusion of the blood supply to the gall bladder and upper bile duct with high local concentrations of the drug. The median time to onset of biliary sclerosis is three treatment cycles, and although fluorouracil may be restarted at a lower dose after normalization of serum hepatic enzyme activities, most patients become progressively less tolerant.

Of 57 consecutive patients treated with implanted hepatic arterial infusion pumps with a regimen of alternating floxuridine (0.1 mg/kg/day for 7 days) followed by a weekly pump bolus of 5-fluorouracil (15 mg/kg for 3 weeks), two developed biliary sclerosis and 12 had mild transient liver function abnormalities (103). The liver alone or in combination with another area was the site of first progression of disease in 40 patients.

Skin

Two types of skin rashes occur with fluorouracil. The more common form involves erythema of exposed skin areas. With continued fluorouracil therapy the skin becomes hyperpigmented, thin, and atrophic (82). Patients treated with fluorouracil also have an increased susceptibility to sunburn (104). Less commonly (about 1.5%), a severe seborrheic pruritic dermatitis occurs (82). These rashes are usually reversible on withdrawal of fluorouracil. Acute, painful, swollen, and self-limiting erythema of the hands and soles has been reported in association with protracted infusion of fluorouracil (105).

Fluorouracil commonly causes hyperpigmentation and multiple pigmented macules (106). Serpentine supravenous hyperpigmentation is a peculiar dermatological effect seen with continuous infusions of fluorouracil (82,107). Residual macular pigmentation can persist for 3 months after withdrawal. Hyperpigmentation occurs only in the tissues overlying the veins proximal to the infusion site in the limb used. The veins are not sclerosed and usually remain patent (108). This has also been reported in a 56-year-old black man after intravenous fluorouracil 750 mg/m^2/week over 24 weeks for stage-D prostatic carcinoma (109). The patient developed nasal mucosal friability, diffuse pigmentation of the face and hands, and markedly increased pigmentation of the skin immediately overlying the veins that had been used for multiple fluorouracil infusions. Many irregular dark streaks were noted, extending from the hand to the shoulder. These streaks were 1–1.5 cm wide and serpiginous in their course.

Fluorouracil, alone or in combination regimens, via continuous or intermittent infusions or bolus doses, has been associated with hand–foot syndrome or palmar–plantar erythrodysesthesia, a rare syndrome of unknown cause, characterized by varying degrees of painful, erythematous, swollen palms of the hand and soles of the feet (110). Tingling, tenderness, and desquamation can also occur. The pain can be so severe as to inhibit walking and hand grasping (110). The onset of the reaction has ranged from 3 days to 10 months (110,111). Severity appeared to be dose-related in one case (112). The condition gradually subsides over 5–7 days when the drug is withdrawn (112). However, it may recur on rechallenge (111). Pyridoxine 100–150 mg/day has been used to manage this syndrome, allowing continued treatment in a small number of patients (113,114). Topical 5-fluorouracil often causes skin irritation. However, allergic contact dermatitis is only infrequently reported, although it may be underdiagnosed.

- A 64-year-old man was treated with Efudix ointment (containing 5% fluorouracil) for actinic keratosis (115). Patch-testing with the constituents of the cream showed a doubtful reaction to fluorouracil 5% in petroleum jelly; however, intradermal injection of fluorouracil 10 mg/ml gave a positive reaction.

Topical fluorouracil has been associated with allergic contact dermatitis in patients with actinic keratosis and basal cell epitheliomas (116). Topical fluorouracil ointment (5%) was reported to exacerbate dermatitis when it was mistakenly given instead of fluocinonide ointment (117).

Telangiectasia and herpes labialis have been reported in four patients receiving topical 1% fluorouracil in propylene glycol applied three times a day for 7–28 days. Two patients developed herpes labialis 7–10 days after the start of therapy and two developed persistent telangiectasia at the application site (118).

- Bullous pemphigoid has been reported in an 84-year-old man after topical therapy with fluorouracil 1% solution daily over several days for actinic keratosis. All treated lesions became bullous, with the development of a few bullae on untreated areas of normal skin. Bullous lesions were pruritic and sore and some contained hemorrhagic fluid. There was a leukocytosis (11.7×10^9/l). The blister fluid contained predominantly eosinophils, and immunofluorescent studies of the serum and blister fluid showed anti-basement membrane antibody titers of 1:640 and 1:160 respectively. Fluorouracil was discontinued and the patient was treated with steroids and saline compresses, with abatement of symptoms (119).

Fluorouracil not only augments the therapeutic effect of ionizing radiation on tumors, but also increases its mucocutaneous toxicity. The likelihood of severe toxicity within the radiation field is increased significantly and relates to the area irradiated (for example oral stomatitis, esophagitis, enteritis, and skin desquamation). The onset of these effects is within 7 days of the start of radiation.

Hair

Partial reversible alopecia is common after systemic fluorouracil therapy (84).

Nails

Diffuse blue superficial pigmentation, onycholysis, dystrophy, pain and thickening of the nail bed, transverse striations, paronychial inflammation, hyperpigmentation, and nail loss have all been reported with fluorouracil therapy (120–122). It has further been reported that the blue pigment may be scraped off (120).

Sexual function

Vaginitis (shedding of the vaginal epithelium) may be nearly as common as mucositis in women receiving systemic fluorouracil-based chemotherapy regimens (123).

Immunologic

- An anaphylactic reaction with shock after a 10th dose of fluorouracil 900 mg intravenously was reported in a 60-year-old man with colorectal adenocarcinoma (124). Two minutes after his 10th dose of fluorouracil, he became cyanotic and collapsed, with a rapid thready pulse of 120. His blood pressure was 30/0 mmHg. Adrenaline 1:1000, 1 ml, was given, with immediate and prompt signs of recovery. Within 25 minutes, his blood pressure, pulse, and skin color had returned to normal.

Second-Generation Effects

Pregnancy

Fluorouracil is contraindicated throughout pregnancy. The literature on pregnancy and cytotoxic drugs is necessarily limited, but it appears in general that risk of teratogenesis diminishes with the advancement of pregnancy. Therefore, most cytotoxic drugs are absolutely contraindicated in the first trimester, and when fluorouracil has been used in the first trimester it has been reported to cause multiple congenital abnormalities (125).

Administration of fluorouracil to pregnant rats on day 14 of gestation resulted in dose-dependent growth retardation and numerous malformations in near-term fetuses, including hind limb defects and cleft palate (126). After treatment, a number of rapid biochemical and cellular alterations were detectable in embryonic hind limbs and in craniofacial and other tissues, including inhibition of thymidylate synthetase and altered cell cycle progression. In order to assess the importance of these early events in fluorouracil-induced dysmorphogenesis, embryonic mid-facial tissues and hind limbs were dissected 3 or 6 hours after administration of fluorouracil to the dam and placed in explant culture. After 5 days in culture, craniofacial explants were evaluated morphologically for palatal closure, and growth was assessed by measuring total protein and DNA contents. Hind-limb explants were stained for cartilage using Alcian blue to evaluate development of digits. Craniofacial explants cultured at either 3 or 6 hours after exposure showed dose-dependent growth retardation and defects of palatal fusion at the end of the culture period. Deficits in protein and DNA content were similar to those in craniofacial tissues that continued to develop in utero after treatment, although morphological defects in cultured explants did not correlate well with the incidence of cleft palate in vivo. Dose-dependent deficits in metatarsal and phalanx development were observed in hind-limb explants dissected either 3 or 6 hours after maternal treatment.

Susceptibility Factors

Genetic factors

Anabolism of fluorouracil to pyrimidine nucleotide analogues is required for its cytotoxic effects and pyrimidine catabolism is important in the regulation of fluorouracil availability and its subsequent anabolism. Dihydropyrimidine dehydrogenase is the initial enzyme of pyrimidine catabolism, accounting for degradation of greater than 80% of a dose of fluorouracil. The importance of catabolism and particularly dihydropyrimidine dehydrogenase in fluorouracil chemotherapy has previously been demonstrated in studies with competitive inhibitors of dihydropyrimidine dehydrogenase and in patients with suspected or proven dihydropyrimidine dehydrogenase deficiency. Before 1991, only two cases of dihydropyrimidine dehydrogenase deficiency associated with fluorouracil toxicity in adults were reported, and in both cases it was the fluorouracil toxicity that focused attention on pyrimidine catabolism. In 1991 a third case of dihydropyrimidine dehydrogenase deficiency was reported (127), suggesting that it may be more frequent than initially thought. There was complete deficiency of dihydropyrimidine dehydrogenase in the affected patient, with evidence of partial deficiency in the patient's parents, daughter, brother, and the brother's children. This pattern of dihydropyrimidine dehydrogenase activity was consistent with the previous two reports, suggesting an autosomal recessive pattern of inheritance.

- A 35-year-old woman with breast carcinoma treated with doses of fluorouracil that were not unusually high. Chemotherapy with cyclophosphamide, fluorouracil, and methotrexate started 3 weeks after surgery. Following day 8 of the protocol, the patient had severe gastrointestinal adverse effects (nausea, prolonged vomiting, diarrhea, stomatitis), hematological toxicity (neutropenia), and fever. She also had mild neurological toxicity causing unsteadiness and difficulty in spelling simple words, which persisted for about 2 weeks.

The neurotoxicity of fluorouracil seems to be more prolonged and severe in patients with dihydropyrimidine dehydrogenase deficiency (128).

Only a few cases of dihydropyrimidine dehydrogenase deficiency have been identified: however, all cases exhibited remarkable toxicity. Enhanced toxicity occurring at normal doses is what usually sets these patients apart. The authors suggested that monitoring dihydropyrimidine dehydrogenase activity may be appropriate in the management of those who have severe toxicity from fluorouracil (127).

Additional studies are needed to characterize this genetic defect, in order to answer the following questions:

- What is the frequency of this gene defect in the general population?
- Does dihydropyrimidine dehydrogenase deficiency correlate with the occurrence of severe fluorouracil toxicity?
- Do individuals with partial dihydropyrimidine dehydrogenase deficiency (that is heterozygotes) have altered metabolism of fluorouracil?
- Is monitoring dihydropyrimidine dehydrogenase activity helpful in the management of patients experiencing severe toxicity to fluorouracil chemotherapy?

Age

Cancer is most common in older people, but little information is available with regard to the impact of age on the toxicity of chemotherapy. A study has been undertaken to determine if age is an independent risk factor for fluorouracil toxicity (129). Toxicity data from a prospective, randomized, multi-institution trial of fluorouracil-based treatment for advanced colorectal carcinoma were analysed. Toxicity for each organ system was graded. The results showed that advanced age was significantly associated with the occurrence of any severe toxicity (58 versus 36%), leukopenia (24 versus 10%), diarrhea (24 versus 14%), vomiting (15 versus 5%), severe toxicity in more than two organ systems (10 versus 3%), and treatment mortality (9 versus 2%). Age and sex were independent predictors of severe toxicity. Advanced age does not contraindicate the use of this type of chemotherapy, but monitoring for multiple organ toxicity and vigorous supportive care of those with toxicity are required.

Dosing decisions in older patients are difficult and must integrate assessments of organ function, co-morbidity, overall physical status, and goals of treatment, in an effort to ensure the best possible outcome for these patients.

Other features of the patient

Circadian variation in toxicity

If the rhythm in fluorouracil toxicity is linked to the asleep–awake circadian cycle across species, the least toxic time in man would correspond to 0400 hours. This hypothesis has been tested using a single-reservoir, programmable-in-time, external ambulatory pump (Chronopump, Autosyringe, Hooksett, USA) in 35 patients with metastatic colorectal cancer (130). Fluorouracil was infused for 5 days via an implanted venous access port, with peak drug delivery at 0400 hours and no infusion from 1800 to 2200 hours. Each course was repeated after a drug-free interval of 16 days. Intrapatient dose escalation was planned from 4 to 9 g/m^2/course (800–1800 mg/m^2/day for 5 days) if toxicity was less than grade 2 according to the World Health Organization (WHO). There was grade 2 or greater toxicity in under 5% of the courses, indicating adequate control of toxicity via dose escalation, and their incidence was dose-dependent. The median maximal tolerated dose was 7.5 mg/m^2/course in 30 patients assessed for this end point.

Cellular glutathione concentrations and fluorouracil toxicity

Little is known about whether components of the diet can modulate the efficacy of fluorouracil in patients with colon carcinoma. Glutathione, an important antioxidant and anticarcinogen, is present in many foods in varying amounts.

The effect of cellular glutathione concentration on the growth of human colon adenocarcinoma cells HT-29 and on the cytotoxic activity of fluorouracil in these cells has been studied (131). Glutathione and buthionine sulfoximine were used respectively to enhance or reduce the glutathione concentration in these cells. A 34% increase in cellular glutathione concentration had no effect on the growth of HT-29 cells, nor on the cytotoxic activity of fluorouracil. A 50% reduction in the cellular glutathione concentration enhanced fluorouracil cytotoxicity by 20–31%, depending on the fluorouracil concentration.

Drug Administration

Drug dosage regimens

Stomatitis and diarrhea are particularly frequent in patients who received a 5-day regimen. An alternative regimen using continuous intravenous infusion of fluorouracil at doses of 30 mg/kg/day for 5 days gives equivalent therapeutic results but a different pattern of toxicity (132). Gastrointestinal symptoms, such as stomatitis and diarrhea, are the principal dose-limiting toxic effects, but myelosuppression is less intense. When fluorouracil is given in combination with leucovorin in patients with metastatic colon cancer, there is enhanced gastrointestinal toxicity, irrespective of the fluorouracil schedule.

Drug administration route

Intravenous administration of fluorouracil 1 g has been compared with hepatic arterial infusion (133). When fluorouracil was administered over 2 hours, systemic drug exposure was 0.7 times lower and clearance 1.5 times higher with hepatic arterial infusion. When the duration of infusion was extended to 24 hours, systemic drug exposure was 0.4 times lower and the clearance was two- to three-fold higher with hepatic arterial infusion. For the 24-hour infusion, co-treatment with angiotensin II (given temporarily to increase tumor blood flow) and albumin microspheres, given to increase drug uptake by the liver via the hepatic artery produced an additional two-fold reduction in systemic fluorouracil exposure. Further evaluation is planned to determine if this will improve the therapeutic index of regionally administered fluorouracil.

Intraperitoneal administration of fluorouracil has been reported to produce a desirable regional advantage (134). The results of a phase I trial of intraperitoneal fluorouracil in escalating concentrations for 4 hours, along with a fixed dose of cisplatin 90 mg/m^2 every 28 days, has been used (135). There was dose-limiting neutropenia at a fluorouracil concentration of 20 mmol/l, although individual patients tolerated concentrations as high as 30 mmol/l.

Other toxic effects included mild-to-moderate nausea and vomiting; diarrhea occurred less often. Peak plasma concentrations occurred 1 hour after instillation and there was a significant linear relation between the intraperitoneal fluorouracil dose and the peak plasma fluorouracil concentration. At every dose, the mean peak intraperitoneal fluorouracil concentration exceeded that in the plasma by two to three log units.

Drug overdose

Cases of deliberate overdosage are unknown, but excessive duration or dosage of therapy will produce life-threatening toxicity because of the hematological effects and other symptoms and signs that are qualitatively similar to the adverse effects. There is no specific antidote to fluorouracil toxicity; treatment consists of supportive care, including G-CSF and antidiarrheal agents.

Drug–Drug Interactions

Allopurinol

Concurrent administration of allopurinol with fluorouracil inhibits the intracellular formation of fluorouridine monophosphate from fluorouracil in normal tissues. In tumor cells that activate fluorouracil by alternative pathways, antitumor responses are still seen (2). Allopurinol increased the half-life of high-dose fluorouracil when it was given by intravenous bolus but not when it was given by 5-day continuous infusion (2).

Allopurinol ameliorates fluorouracil-induced granulocytopenia and possibly lessens the severity of mucositis (136). Allopurinol mouthwash (450 mg total in methylcellulose) given immediately and 1, 2, and 3 hours after fluorouracil reduced the incidence and severity of mucositis in six patients (137) and in another study of 42 patients there was significant reduction of oral toxicity and prolonged pain relief (138). In a randomized, double-blind, placebo-controlled trial, in 44 patients, allopurinol mouthwashes resolved stomatitis in nine of 22 treated patients, and diminished its intensity in 10 (139). However, in another randomized, double-blind, crossover study of allopurinol, mouthwash in 77 patients did not ameliorate fluorouracil-induced mucositis (140), nor did allopurinol reduce the toxicity of intravenously administered fluorouracil (141). Allopurinol is not currently recommended in the prophylaxis of fluorouracil-induced mucositis.

Cimetidine

Pre-treatment for 4 weeks with cimetidine 1 g/day increased the oral systemic availability of fluorouracil by 74%; the AUC was increased by 27% and total body clearance was reduced by 28% (142).

Dipyridamole

The pharmacokinetics of fluorouracil have been studied with escalating doses as a 72-hour intravenous infusion alone or in combination with a fixed dose of dipyridamole, a nucleoside transport inhibitor, and an enhancer of fluorouracil cytotoxicity (143). Stomatitis was dose-limiting at a fluorouracil dose of 2300 mg/m^2/day. For courses given with fluorouracil alone, the pharmacokinetics were linear for doses of 185–2300 mg/m^2/day; however, above this dose total body clearance fell significantly. Dipyridamole increased the total body clearance of fluorouracil, resulting in significantly lower mean steady-state fluorouracil plasma concentrations over the dose range studied. The clinical observation that dipyridamole did not appear to modulate fluorouracil-induced mucositis or leukopenia can be explained by lower exposure to fluorouracil. The basis for this pharmacokinetic interaction is not understood but it serves to underscore the importance of incorporating pharmacokinetic analysis in clinical trials involving new drug combinations.

Interferons

Initial studies have suggested that interferons may have synergistic activity with fluorouracil (144,145). Interferon alfa-2b has also been associated with an 80% increase in fluorouracil AUC (146).

Leucovorin

When combined with fluorouracil, leucovorin enhances the binding of the fluorouracil metabolite fluorouridine monophosphate to thymidylate synthetase. DNA-directed toxicity is increased, whilst RNA-directed toxicity is not affected (146). A qualitative alteration in toxicity is reported with increased gastrointestinal toxicity (2).

Methotrexate

There is sequence-dependent synergy between fluorouracil and methotrexate. Pretreatment with methotrexate enhances the formation of fluorouridine monophosphate and hence fluorouridine triphosphate and RNA-directed toxicity. In studies in which methotrexate has been given 1 hour before fluorouracil, response rates did not differ significantly. However, when it was given 4 hours or more before, there were significantly better response rates (147).

Metronidazole

Pretreatment with metronidazole increased the toxicity of fluorouracil given by daily bolus dose (148). The clinical significance of this is yet to be determined.

Pyridoxine

The dose and duration of protracted infusional fluorouracil is limited by mucositis, diarrhea, and/or palmar–plantar erythrodysesthesia. Typically, palmar–plantar dysesthesia begins several weeks to months after starting treatment. Although the dysesthesia abates within several weeks of discontinuing the infusion, it rapidly recurs when the infusion is resumed. Five patients who developed palmar–plantar dysesthesia during infusion of fluorouracil were treated with oral pyridoxine, 50 or 150 mg/day, once it reached moderate severity (149). The severity of the skin toxicity improved, with resolution of pain in four of the five patients, despite continued administration of fluorouracil. The ability of pyridoxine to modulate fluorouracil-induced cutaneous toxicity is currently undergoing evaluation in the randomized trial (150).

Other Environmental Interactions

Ionizing radiation

Fluorouracil increases the activity and toxicity of ionizing radiation (2).

References

1. Leichman CG, Fleming TR, Muggia FM, Tangen CM, Ardalan B, Doroshow JH, Meyers FJ, Holcombe RF, Weiss GR, Mangalik A, et al. Phase II study of fluorouracil and its modulation in advanced colorectal cancer: a Southwest Oncology Group study. J Clin Oncol 1995;13(6):1303–11.
2. Chabner BA, Myers CE. Clinical pharmacology of cancer chemotherapy. In: Devita VT, Hellman S, Rosenberg SA, editors. Cancer: Principles and Practice of Oncology. 3rd ed. Philadelphia: Lippincoft, 1990:349–95.
3. Sullivan RD, Young CW, Miller E, Glatstein N, Clarkson B, Burchenal JH. The clinical effects of the continuous administration of fluorinated pyrimidines (5-fluorouracil and 5-fluoro-2′-deoxyuridine). Cancer Chemother Rep 1960; 8:77–83.
4. Ardalan B, Singh G, Silberman H. A randomized phase I and II study of short-term infusion of high-dose fluorouracil with or without N-(phosphonacetyl)-L-aspartic acid in patients with advanced pancreatic and colorectal cancers. J Clin Oncol 1988;6(6):1053–8.
5. Yoshida T, Araki E, Iigo M, Fujii T, Yoshino M, Shimada Y, Saito D, Tajiri H, Yamaguchi H, Yoshida S, Ohkura H, Yoshimori M, Okazaki N. Clinical significance of monitoring serum levels of 5-fluorouracil by continuous infusion in patients with advanced colonic cancer. Cancer Chemother Pharmacol 1990;26(5):352–4.
6. Thyss A, Milano G, Renee N, Vallicioni J, Schneider M, Demard F. Clinical pharmacokinetic study of 5-FU in continuous 5-day infusions for head and neck cancer. Cancer Chemother Pharmacol 1986;16(1):64–6.
7. Farooqi IS, Aronson JK. Iatrogenic chest pain: a case of 5-fluorouracil cardiotoxicity. QJM 1996;89(12):953–5.
8. Clavel M, Simeone P, Grivet B. Toxicité cardiaqué du 5-fluorouracile. Revue de la litterature, cinq nouveaux cas. [Cardiac toxicity of 5-fluorouracil. Review of the literature, 5 new cases.] Presse Méd 1988;17(33):1675–8.
9. Robben NC, Pippas AW, Moore JO. The syndrome of 5-fluorouracil cardiotoxicity. An elusive cardiopathy. Cancer 1993;71(2):493–509.
10. Lomeo AM, Avolio C, Iacobellis G, Manzione L. 5-Fluorouracil cardiotoxicity. Eur J Gynaecol Oncol 1990;11(3):237–41.
11. Rezkalla S, Kloner RA, Ensley J, al-Sarraf M, Revels S, Olivenstein A, Bhasin S, Kerpel-Fronious S, Turi ZG. Continuous ambulatory ECG monitoring during fluorouracil therapy: a prospective study. J Clin Oncol 1989;7(4):509–14.
12. Collins C, Weiden PL. Cardiotoxicity of 5-fluorouracil. Cancer Treat Rep 1987;71(7–8):733–6.
13. Freeman NJ, Costanza ME. 5-Fluorouracil-associated cardiotoxicity. Cancer 1988;61(1):36–45.
14. McKendall GR, Shurman A, Anamur M, Most AS. Toxic cardiogenic shock associated with infusion of 5-fluorouracil Am Heart J 1989;118(1):184–6.
15. Patel B, Kloner RA, Ensley J, Al-Sarraf M, Kish J, Wynne J. 5-Fluorouracil cardiotoxicity: left ventricular dysfunction and effect of coronary vasodilators. Am J Med Sci 1987;294(4):238–43.
16. Misset B, Escudier B, Leclercq B, Rivara D, Rougier P, Nitenberg G. Acute myocardiotoxicity during 5-fluorouracil therapy. Intensive Care Med 1990;16(3):210–11.
17. Eskilsson J, Albertsson M, Mercke C. Adverse cardiac effects during induction chemotherapy treatment with cisplatin and 5-fluorouracil. Radiother Oncol 1988;13(1):41–6.
18. Mortimer JE, Higano C. Continuous infusion 5-fluorouracil and folinic acid in disseminated colorectal cancer. Cancer Invest 1988;6(2):129–32.
19. Coronel B, Madonna O, Mercatello A, Caillette A, Moskovtchenko JF. Myocardiotoxicity of 5 fluorouracil. Intensive Care Med 1988;14(4):429–30.
20. Chaudary S, Song SY, Jaski BE. Profound, yet reversible, heart failure secondary to 5-fluorouracil. Am J Med 1988;85(3):454–6.
21. Jakubowski AA, Kemeny N. Hypotension as a manifestation of cardiotoxicity in three patients receiving cisplatin and 5-fluorouracil. Cancer 1988;62(2):266–9.
22. de Forni M, Malet-Martino MC, Jaillais P, Shubinski RE, Bachaud JM, Lemaire L, Canal P, Chevreau C, Carrie D, Soulie P, Roche H, Boudjema B, Mihura J, Martino R, Bernadet P, Bugat R. Cardiotoxicity of high-dose continuous infusion fluorouracil: a prospective clinical study. J Clin Oncol 1992;10(11):1795–801.
23. Ensley J, Kish J, Tapazoglou E, et al. 5-FU infusions associated with an ischaemic cardiotoxicity syndrome. Proc Am Soc Clin Oncol 1986;5:142.
24. Gradishar WJ, Vokes EE. 5-Fluorouracil cardiotoxicity: a critical review. Ann Oncol 1990;1(6):409–14.
25. Aziz SA, Tramboo NA, Mohi-ud-Din K, Iqbal K, Jalal S, Ahmad M. Supraventricular arrhythmia: a complication of 5-fluorouracil therapy. Clin Oncol (R Coll Radiol) 1998;10(6):377–8.
26. Wang WS, Hsieh RK, Chiou TJ, Liu JH, Fan FS, Yen CC, Tung SL, Chen PM. Toxic cardiogenic shock in a patient receiving weekly 24-h infusion of high-dose 5-fluorouracil and leucovorin. Jpn J Clin Oncol 1998;28(9):551–4.
27. Doll DC, Yarbro JW. Vascular toxicity associated with chemotherapy and hormonotherapy. Curr Opin Oncol 1994;6(4):345–50.
28. Papamichael D, Amft N, Slevin ML, D'Cruz D. 5-Fluorouracil-induced Raynaud's phenomenon. Eur J Cancer 1998;34(12):1983.
29. Kleiman NS, Lehane DE, Geyer CE Jr, Pratt CM, Young JB. Prinzmetal's angina during 5-fluorouracil chemotherapy. Am J Med 1987;82(3):566–8.
30. Liss RH, Chadwick M. Correlation of 5-fluorouracil (NSC-19893) distribution in rodents with toxicity and chemotherapy in man. Cancer Chemother Rep 1974;58(6):777–86.
31. Suzuki T, Nakanishi H, Hayashi A, et al. Cardiac toxicity of 5-FU in rabbits. Jpn J Pharmacol 1972;27(Suppl):137.
32. Matsubara I, Kamiya J, Imai S. Cardiotoxic effects of 5-fluorouracil in the guinea pig. Jpn J Pharmacol 1980;30(6):871–9.
33. Orditura M, De Vita F, Sarubbi B, Ducceschi V, Auriemma A, Infusino S, Iacono A, Catalano G. Analysis of recovery time indexes in 5-fluorouracil-treated cancer patients. Oncol Rep 1998;5(3):645–7.
34. Martin M, Diaz-Rubio E, Furio V, Blazquez J, Almenarez J, Farina J. Lethal cardiac toxicity after cisplatin and 5-fluorouracil chemotherapy. Report of a case with necropsy study. Am J Clin Oncol 1989;12(3):229–34.
35. Thyss A, Gaspard MH, Marsault R, Milano G, Frelin C, Schneider M. Very high endothelin plasma levels in patients with 5-FU cardiotoxicity. Ann Oncol 1992;3(1):88.
36. Labianca R, Beretta G, Clerici M, Fraschini P, Luporini G. Cardiac toxicity of 5-fluorouracil: a study on 1083 patients. Tumori 1982;68(6):505–10.

37. Jeremic B, Jevremovic S, Djuric L, Mijatovic L. Cardiotoxicity during chemotherapy treatment with 5-fluorouracil and cisplatin. J Chemother 1990;2(4):264–7.
38. Dent RG, McColl I. Letter: 5-Fluorouracil and angina. Lancet 1975;1(7902):347–8.
39. Pottage A, Holt S, Ludgate S, Langlands AO. Fluorouracil cardiotoxicity. BMJ 1978;1(6112):547.
40. Gamelin E, Gamelin L, Larra F, Turcant A, Alain P, Maillart P, Allain YM, Minier JF, Dubin J. Toxicité cardiaque aiguë du 5-fluorouracile: correlation pharmacocinétique. [Acute cardiac toxicity of 5-fluorouracil: pharmacokinetic correlation.] Bull Cancer 1991;78(12):1147–53.
41. Keefe DL, Roistacher N, Pierri MK. Clinical cardiotoxicity of 5-fluorouracil. J Clin Pharmacol 1993;33(11):1060–70.
42. Lynch TJ Jr, Kass F, Kalish LA, Elias AD, Strauss G, Shulman LN, Sugarbaker DJ, Skarin A, Frei E 3rd. Cisplatin, 5-fluorouracil, and etoposide for advanced non-small cell lung cancer. Cancer 1993;71(10):2953–7.
43. Burger AJ, Mannino S. 5-Fluorouracil-induced coronary vasospasm. Am Heart J 1987;114(2):433–6.
44. Kohne CH, Thuss-Patience P, Friedrich M, Daniel PT, Kretzschmar A, Benter T, Bauer B, Dietz R, Dorken B. Raltitrexed (Tomudex): an alternative drug for patients with colorectal cancer and 5-fluorouracil associated cardiotoxicity. Br J Cancer 1998;77(6):973–7.
45. Akpek G, Hartshorn KL. Failure of oral nitrate and calcium channel blocker therapy to prevent 5-fluorouracil-related myocardial ischemia: a case report. Cancer Chemother Pharmacol 1999;43(2):157–61.
46. Fielding JW, Stockley RA, Brookes VS. Interstitial lung disease in a patient treated with 5-fluorouracil and mitomycin C. BMJ 1978;2(6137):602.
47. Fielding JW, Crocker J, Stockley RA, Brookes VS. Interstitial fibrosis in a patient treated with 5-fluorouracil and mitomycin C. BMJ 1979;2(6189):551–2.
48. Moertel CG, Reitemeier RJ, Bolton CF, Shorter RG. Cerebellar ataxia associated with fluorinated pyrimidine therapy. Cancer Chemother Rep 1964;41:15–18.
49. Tuxen MK, Hansen SW. Neurotoxicity secondary to antineoplastic drugs. Cancer Treat Rev 1994;20(2): 191–214.
50. Ranuzzi M, Taddei A. Neurotoxicity of antineoplastic agents in chemotherapy. Nuova Riv Neurol 1996;6: 55–63.
51. Adams JW, Bofenkamp TM, Kobrin J, Wirtschafter JD, Zeese JA. Recurrent acute toxic optic neuropathy secondary to 5-FU. Cancer Treat Rep 1984;68(3):565–6.
52. Weiss HD, Walker MD, Wiernik PH. Neurotoxicity of commonly used antineoplastic agents. N Engl J Med 1974;291(2):75–81;1974;291(3):127–33.
53. Shapiro WR, Young DF. Neurological complications of antineoplastic therapy. Acta Neurol Scand Suppl 1984;100:125–32.
54. Fassas AB, Gattani AM, Morgello S. Cerebral demyelination with 5-fluorouracil and levamisole. Cancer Invest 1994;12(4):379–83.
55. Bygrave HA, Geh JI, Jani Y, Glynne-Jones R. Neurological complications of 5-fluorouracil chemotherapy: case report and review of the literature. Clin Oncol (R Coll Radiol) 1998;10(5):334–6.
56. Stein ME, Drumea K, Yarnitsky D, Benny A, Tzuk-Shina T. A rare event of 5-fluorouracil-associated peripheral neuropathy: a report of two patients. Am J Clin Oncol 1998;21(3):248–9.
57. El Amrani M, Heinzlef O, Debroucker T, Roullet E, Bousser MG, Amarenco P. Brain infarction following 5-fluorouracil and cisplatin therapy. Neurology 1998;51(3):899–901.
58. Koenig H, Patel A. Biochemical basis for fluorouracil neurotoxicity. The role of Krebs cycle inhibition by fluoroacetate. Arch Neurol 1970;23(2):155–60.
59. Diasio RB, Beavers TL, Carpenter JT. Familial deficiency of dihydropyrimidine dehydrogenase. Biochemical basis for familial pyrimidinemia and severe 5-fluorouracil-induced toxicity. J Clin Invest 1988;81(1):47–51.
60. Loprinzi CL, Love RR, Garrity JA, Ames MM. Cyclophosphamide, methotrexate, and 5-fluorouracil (CMF)-induced ocular toxicity. Cancer Invest 1990;8(5):459–65.
61. Peterson MR, Skuta GL, Phelan MJ, Stanley SA. Striate melanokeratosis following trabeculectomy with 5-fluorouracil. Arch Ophthalmol 1990;108(9):1216–17.
62. Stank TM, Krupin T, Feitl ME. Subconjunctival 5-fluorouracil-induced transient striate melanokeratosis. Arch Ophthalmol 1990;108(9):1210.
63. Lemp MA. Striate melanokeratosis. Arch Ophthalmol 1991;109(7):917.
64. Christophidis N, Vajda FJ, Lucas I, Louis WJ. Ocular side effects with 5-fluorouracil. Aust NZ J Med 1979;9(2):143–4.
65. Hamersley J, Luce JK, Florentz TR, Burkholder MM, Pepper JJ. Excessive lacrimation from fluorouracil treatment. JAMA 1973;225(7):747–8.
66. Griffin JD, Garnick MB. Eye toxicity of cancer chemotherapy: a review of the literature. Cancer 1981;48(7):1539–49.
67. Imperia PS, Lazarus HM, Lass JH. Ocular complications of systemic cancer chemotherapy. Surv Ophthalmol 1989;34(3):209–30.
68. Straus DJ, Mausolf FA, Ellerby RA, McCracken JD. Cicatricial ectropion secondary to 5-fluorouracil therapy. Med Pediatr Oncol 1977;3(1):15–19.
69. Haidak DJ, Hurwitz BS, Yeung KY. Tear-duct fibrosis (dacryostenosis) due to 5-fluorouracil. Ann Intern Med 1978;88(5):657.
70. Prasad S, Kamath GG, Phillips RP. Lacrimal canalicular stenosis associated with systemic 5-fluorouacil therapy. Acta Ophthalmol Scand 2000;78(1):110–3.
71. Galentine P, Sloas H, Hargett N, Cupples HP. Bilateral cicatricial ectropion following topical administration of 5-fluorouracil. Ann Ophthalmol 1981;13(5):575–7.
72. Lee V, Bentley CR, Olver JM. Sclerosing canaliculitis after 5-fluorouracil breast cancer chemotherapy. Eye 1998;12 (Pt 3a):343–9.
73. Hassan A, Hurwitz JJ, Burkes RL. Epiphora in patients receiving systemic 5-fluorouracil therapy. Can J Ophthalmol 1998;33(1):14–19.
74. Insler MS, Helm CJ. Ankyloblepharon associated with systemic 5-fluorouracil treatment. Ann Ophthalmol 1987;19(10):374–5.
75. Rothman RF, Liebmann JM, Ritch R. Noninfectious crystalline keratopathy after postoperative subconjunctival 5-fluorouracil. Am J Ophthalmol 1999;128(2):236–7.
76. Lynch HT, Droszcz CP, Albano WA, Lynch JF. "Organic brain syndrome" secondary to 5-fluorouracil toxicity. Dis Colon Rectum 1981;24(2):130–1.
77. Sadoff L. Overwhelming 5-fluorouracil toxicity in patients whose diabetes is poorly controlled. Am J Clin Oncol 1998;21(6):605–7.
78. Yeh KH, Cheng AL. High-dose 5-fluorouracil infusional therapy is associated with hyperammonaemia, lactic acidosis and encephalopathy. Br J Cancer 1997;75(3):464–5.
79. Valik D, Yeh KH, Cheng AL. Encephalopathy, lactic acidosis, hyperammonaemia and 5-fluorouracil toxicity. Br J Cancer 1998;77(10):1710–12.
80. Grem JL. Fluorinated pyrimidines. In: Chabner BA, Collins JM, editors. Cancer Chemotherapy: Principles and Practice. Philadelphia: Lippincoft, 1990:180–225.
81. Vaitkevicius VK, Brennan MJ, Beckett VL, Kelly JE, Talley RW. Clinical evaluation of cancer chemotherapy with 5-fluorouracil. Cancer 1961;14:131–52.

82. Reitemeier RJ, Moertel CG, Hahn RG. Comparison of 5-fluorouracil (NSC-19893) and 2′-deoxy-5-fluorouridine (NSC-27640) in treatment of patients with advanced adenocarcinoma of colon or rectum. Cancer Chemother Rep 1965;44:39–43.
83. Piro AJ, Wilson RE, Hall TC, Aliapoulios MA, Nevinny HB, Moore FD. Toxicity studies of fluorouracil used with adrenalectomy in breast cancer. Arch Surg 1972;105(1):95–9.
84. Cohn I Jr. Complications and toxic manifestations of surgical adjuvant chemotherapy for breast cancer. Surg Gynecol Obstet 1968;127(6):1201–9.
85. Scott JM, Weir DG. Drug-induced megaloblastic change. Clin Haematol 1980;9(3):587–606.
86. Seifert P, Baker LH, Reed ML, Vaitkevicius VK. Comparison of continuously infused 5-fluorouracil with bolus injection in treatment of patients with colorectal adenocarcinoma. Cancer 1975;36(1):123–8.
87. Lokich JJ, Ahlgren JD, Gullo JJ, Philips JA, Fryer JG. A prospective randomized comparison of continuous infusion fluorouracil with a conventional bolus schedule in metastatic colorectal carcinoma: a Mid-Atlantic Oncology Program Study. J Clin Oncol 1989;7(4):425–32.
88. Tiersten A, Saltz LB. Influence of inflammatory bowel disease on the ability of patients to tolerate systemic fluorouracil-based chemotherapy. J Clin Oncol 1996;14(7):2043–6.
89. McCarthy GM, Awde JD, Ghandi H, Vincent M, Kocha WI. Risk factors associated with mucositis in cancer patients receiving 5-fluorouracil. Oral Oncol 1998;34(6):484–90.
90. Narsete T, Ansfield F, Wirtanen G, Ramirez G, Wolberg W, Jarrett F. Gastric ulceration in patients receiving intrahepatic infusion of 5-fluorouracil. Ann Surg 1977;186(6):734–6.
91. Rousselot LM, Cole DR, Grossi CE. Gastrointestinal bleeding as a sequel to cancer chemotherapy. Am J Gastroenterol 1965;43:311–16.
92. Biran S, krasnokuki D, Brufman G. [Life-threatening gastrointestinal toxicity during 5-fluorouracil therapy.] Harefuah 1977;93(3–4):77.
93. Wadler S, Lyver A, Wiernik PH. Clinical toxicities of the combination of 5-fluorouracil and recombinant interferon alfa-2a: an unusual toxicity profile. Oncol Nurs Forum 1989;16(Suppl 6):12–15.
94. Barrett O Jr, Bourgeois C, Plecha FR. Fluorouracil toxicity following gastrointestinal surgery. Arch Surg 1965;91(6):1002–4.
95. Cudmore MA, Silva J Jr, Fekety R, Liepman MK, Kim KH. Clostridium difficile colitis associated with cancer chemotherapy. Arch Intern Med 1982;142(2):333–5.
96. Abe H, Tsunaga N, Yamashita S, Ishiguro K, Mitani I. [Anticancer drug-induced colitis—case report and review of the literature.] Gan To Kagaku Ryoho 1997;24(5): 619–24.
97. Kronawitter U, Kemeny NE, Blumgart L. Neutropenic enterocolitis in a patient with colorectal carcinoma: unusual course after treatment with 5-fluorouracil and leucovorin—a case report. Cancer 1997;80(4):656–60.
98. Trevisani F, Simoncini M, Alampi G, Bernardi M. Colitis associated to chemotherapy with 5-fluorouracil. Hepatogastroenterology 1997;44(15):710–12.
99. Sotaniemi EA, Sutinen S, Arranto AJ, Sutinen S, Sotaniemi KA, Lehtola J, Pelkonen RO. Liver damage in nurses handling cytostatic agents. Acta Med Scand 1983;214(3):181–9.
100. Vestfrid MA, Castelleto L, Gimenez PO. Necrosis hepatica diffusa en el tratamiento con 5-fluorouracilo. [Diffuse liver necrosis in treatment with 5-fluorouracil.] Rev Clin Esp 1972;125(6):549–50.
101. Kemeny N, Seiter K, Martin D, Urmacher C, Niedzwiecki D, Kurtz RC, Costa P, Murray M. A new syndrome: ascites, hyperbilirubinemia, and hypoalbuminemia after biochemical modulation of fluorouracil with N-phosphonacetyl-L-aspartate (PALA) Ann Intern Med 1991;115(12):946–51.
102. Lorenz M, Hottenrott C, Reimann-Kirkowa M, Encke A. Regionale Therapie von isolierten Mamma-karzinom-Lebermetastasen. [Regional therapy of isolated liver metastases from breast cancer.] Geburtshilfe Frauenheilkd 1988;48(6):425–9.
103. Davidson BS, Izzo F, Chase JL, DuBrow RA, Patt Y, Hohn DC, Curley SA. Alternating floxuridine and 5-fluorouracil hepatic arterial chemotherapy for colorectal liver metastases minimizes biliary toxicity. Am J Surg 1996;172(3):244–7.
104. Falkson G, Schulz EJ. Skin changes in patients treated with 5-fluorouracil. Br J Dermatol 1962;74:229–36.
105. Bellmunt J, Navarro M, Hidalgo R, Sole LA. Palmar-plantar erythrodysesthesia syndrome associated with short-term continuous infusion (5 days) of 5-fluorouracil. Tumori 1988;74(3):329–31.
106. Cho KH, Chung JH, Lee AY, Lee YS, Kim NK, Kim CW. Pigmented macules in patients treated with systemic 5-fluorouracil. J Dermatol 1988;15(4):342–6.
107. Pujol RM, Rocamora V, Lopez-Pousa A, Taberner R, Alomar A. Persistent supravenous erythematous eruption: a rare local complication of intravenous 5-fluorouracil therapy. J Am Acad Dermatol 1998;39(5 Pt 2):839–42.
108. Dunagin WO. Dermatologic toxicity. In: Perry MC, Yarbro JW, editors. Toxicity of Chemotherapy. Orlando: Grune and Stratton, 1984:125–54.
109. Hrushesky WJ. Unusual pigmentary changes associated with 5-fluorouracil therapy. Cutis 1980;26(2):181–2.
110. Curran CF, Luce JK. Fluorouracil and palmar-plantar erythrodysesthesia. Ann Intern Med 1989;111(10):858.
111. Jorda E, Galan A, Betlloch I, Ramon D, Revert A, Torres V. Painful, red hands. A side effect of 5-fluorouracil by continuous perfusion. Int J Dermatol 1991;30(9):653.
112. Feldman LD, Ajani JA. Fluorouracil-associated dermatitis of the hands and feet. JAMA 1985;254(24):3479.
113. Vukelja SJ, Lombardo FA, James WD, Weiss RB. Pyridoxine for the palmar-plantar erythrodysesthesia syndrome. Ann Intern Med 1989;111(8):688–9.
114. Molina R, Fabian C, Slavik M, et al. Reversal of palmar-plantar erythrodysesthesia SPPE by B6 without loss of response in colon cancer patients receiving 200 mg/m^2/day continuous 5-FU. Proc Am Soc Clin Oncol 1987;6:90.
115. Sanchez-Perez J, Bartolome B, del Rio MJ, Garcia-Diez A. Allergic contact dermatitis from 5-fluorouracil with positive intradermal test and doubtful patch test reactions. Contact Dermatitis 1999;41(2):106–7.
116. Sams WM. Untoward response with topical fluorouracil. Arch Dermatol 1968;97(1):14–22.
117. Clemons DE, Aeling JL, Nuss DD. Dermatitis medicamentosa: a pitfall for the unwary. Arch Dermatol 1976;112(8):1179.
118. Burnett JW. Letter: Two unusual complications of topical fluorouracil therapy. Arch Dermatol 1975;111(3):398.
119. Bart BJ, Bean SF. Bullous pemphigoid following the topical use of fluorouracil. Arch Dermatol 1970;102(4):457–60.
120. Nixon DW, Pirozzi D, York RM, Black M, Lawson DH. Dermatologic changes after systemic cancer therapy. Cutis 1981;27(2):181–94.
121. Norton LA. Nail disorders. A review. J Am Acad Dermatol 1980;2(6):451–67.
122. Katz ME, Hansen TW. Nail plate-nail bed separation. An unusual side effect of systemic fluorouracil administration. Arch Dermatol 1979;115(7):860–1.
123. Moroni M, Porta C. Possible efficacy of allopurinol vaginal washings in the treatment of chemotherapy-induced vaginitis. Cancer Chemother Pharmacol 1998;41(2):171–2.

124. DeBeer R, Kabakow B. Anaphylactoid reaction. Associated with intravenous administration of 5-fluorouracil. NY State J Med 1979;79(11):1750–1.
125. Stephens JD, Golbus MS, Miller TR, Wilber RR, Epstein CJ. Multiple congenital anomalies in a fetus exposed to 5-fluorouracil during the first trimester. Am J Obstet Gynecol 1980;137(6):747–9.
126. Shuey DL, Buckalew AR, Wilke TS, Rogers JM, Abbott BD. Early events following maternal exposure to 5-fluorouracil lead to dysmorphology in cultured embryonic tissues. Teratology 1994;50(6):379–86.
127. Harris BE, Carpenter JT, Diasio RB. Severe 5-fluorouracil toxicity secondary to dihydropyrimidine dehydrogenase deficiency. A potentially more common pharmacogenetic syndrome. Cancer 1991;68(3):499–501.
128. Shehata N, Pater A, Tang SC. Prolonged severe 5-fluorouracil-associated neurotoxicity in a patient with dihydropyrimidine dehydrogenase deficiency. Cancer Invest 1999;17(3):201–5.
129. Stein BN, Petrelli NJ, Douglass HO, Driscoll DL, Arcangeli G, Meropol NJ. Age and sex are independent predictors of 5-fluorouracil toxicity. Analysis of a large scale phase III trial. Cancer 1995;75(1):11–17.
130. Levi F, Soussan A, Adam R, Caussanel JP, Metzger G, Jasmin C, Bismuth H, Smolensky M, Misset JL. A phase I-II trial of five-day continuous intravenous infusion of 5-fluorouracil delivered at circadian rhythm modulated rate in patients with metastatic colorectal cancer. J Infus Chemother 1995;5(3 Suppl 1):153–8.
131. Chen MF, Chen LT, Boyce HW Jr. 5-Fluorouracil cytotoxicity in human colon HT-29 cells with moderately increased or decreased cellular glutathione level. Anticancer Res 1995;15(1):163–7.
132. Lokich J, Bothe A, Fine N, Perri J. Phase I study of protracted venous infusion of 5-fluorouracil. Cancer 1981;48(12):2565–8.
133. Goldberg JA, Kerr DJ, Watson DG, Willmott N, Bates CD, McKillop JH, McArdle CS. The pharmacokinetics of 5-fluorouracil administered by arterial infusion in advanced colorectal hepatic metastases. Br J Cancer 1990;61(6):913–15.
134. Speyer JL, Collins JM, Dedrick RL, Brennan MF, Buckpitt AR, Londer H, DeVita VT Jr, Myers CE. Phase I and pharmacological studies of 5-fluorouracil administered intraperitoneally. Cancer Res 1980;40(3):567–72.
135. Schilsky RL, Choi KE, Grayhack J, Grimmer D, Guarnieri C, Fullem L. Phase I clinical and pharmacologic study of intraperitoneal cisplatin and fluorouracil in patients with advanced intraabdominal cancer. J Clin Oncol 1990;8(12):2054–61.
136. Woolley PV, Ayoob MJ, Smith FP, Lokey JL, DeGreen P, Marantz A, Schein PS. A controlled trial of the effect of 4-hydroxypyrazolopyrimidine (allopurinol) on the toxicity of a single bolus dose of 5-fluorouracil. J Clin Oncol 1985;3(1):103–9.
137. Clark PI, Slevin ML. Allopurinol mouthwashes and 5-fluorouracil induced oral toxicity. Eur J Surg Oncol 1985;11(3):267–8.
138. Tsavaris NB, Komitsopoulou P, Tzannou I, Loucatou P, Tsaroucha-Noutsou A, Kilafis G, Kosmidis P. Decreased oral toxicity with the local use of allopurinol in patients who received high dose 5-fluorouracil. Sel Cancer Ther 1991;7(3):113–17.
139. Porta C, Moroni M, Nastasi G. Allopurinol mouthwashes in the treatment of 5-fluorouracil-induced stomatitis. Am J Clin Oncol 1994;17(3):246–7.
140. Loprinzi CL, Cianflone SG, Dose AM, Etzell PS, Burnham NL, Therneau TM, Hagen L, Gainey DK, Cross M, Athmann LM, et al. A controlled evaluation of an allopurinol mouthwash as prophylaxis against 5-fluorouracil-induced stomatitis. Cancer 1990;65(8):1879–82.
141. Howell SB, Pfeifle CE, Wung WE. Effect of allopurinol on the toxicity of high-dose 5-fluorouracil administered by intermittent bolus injection. Cancer 1983;51(2):220–5.
142. Harvey VJ, Slevin ML, Dilloway MR, Clark PI, Johnston A, Lant AF. The influence of cimetidine on the pharmacokinetics of 5-fluorouracil. Br J Clin Pharmacol 1984;18(3):421–30.
143. Remick SC, Grem JL, Fischer PH, Tutsch KD, Alberti DB, Nieting LM, Tombes MB, Bruggink J, Willson JK, Trump DL. Phase I trial of 5-fluorouracil and dipyridamole administered by seventy-two-hour concurrent continuous infusion. Cancer Res 1990;50(9):2667–72.
144. Elias L, Crissman HA. Interferon effects upon the adenocarcinoma 38 and HL-60 cell lines: antiproliferative responses and synergistic interactions with halogenated pyrimidine antimetabolites. Cancer Res 1988;48(17):4868–73.
145. Wadler S, Wiernik PH. Clinical update on the role of fluorouracil and recombinant interferon alfa-2a in the treatment of colorectal carcinoma. Semin Oncol 1990;17(1 Suppl 1):16–21.
146. Schuller J, Czejka M, Miksche M, et al. Influence of interferon alpha-2b leucovorin on pharmacokinetics of 5-fluorouracil. Proc Am Soc Clin Oncol 1991;10:98.
147. Damon LE, Cadman E, Benz C. Enhancement of 5-fluorouracil antitumor effects by the prior administration of methotrexate. Pharmacol Ther 1989;43(2):155–85.
148. Bardakji Z, Jolivet J, Langelier Y, Besner JG, Ayoub J. 5-Fluorouracil–metronidazole combination therapy in metastatic colorectal cancer. Clinical, pharmacokinetic and in vitro cytotoxicity studies. Cancer Chemother Pharmacol 1986;18(2):140–4.
149. Fabian CJ, Molina R, Slavik M, Dahlberg S, Giri S, Stephens R. Pyridoxine therapy for palmar-plantar erythrodysesthesia associated with continuous 5-fluorouracil infusion. Invest New Drugs 1990;8(1):57–63.
150. Beveridge RA, Kales AN, Binder RA, Miller JA, Virts SG. Pyridoxine (B6) and amelioration of hand/foot syndrome. Proc Am Soc Clin Oncol 1990;9:102.

Fluoxetine

See also Selective serotonin re-uptake inhibitors (SSRIs)

General Information

Fluoxetine is a selective serotonin re-uptake inhibitor (SSRI). The manufacturers of fluoxetine have published a review of the adverse effects that were noted in 1378 patients who took it for up to 2 years (1).

In a meta-analysis based on 9087 patients in 87 different randomized clinical trials fluoxetine was more effective than placebo from the first week of therapy (2). In bulimia nervosa, fluoxetine was as effective as other agents. It was as effective as clomipramine in the treatment of obsessive-compulsive disorder.

The major adverse effects of fluoxetine confirm its stimulant profile and its relative lack of anticholinergic actions. The most frequent adverse effects, which occurred in 10–25% of patients, were nausea (25%), nervousness, insomnia, headache, tremor, anxiety, drowsiness, dry mouth, sweating, and diarrhea (10%). Most of these adverse effects occurred early in treatment and seldom led to drug withdrawal.

Organs and Systems

Cardiovascular

Fluoxetine appears not to have the cardiovascular effects associated with tricyclic compounds, but 10 patients did discontinue treatment because of tachycardia, palpitation, and dyspnea (3). Two older women each had a myocardial infarction and subsequently died, although these events may not have been drug-related.

In general, SSRIs are assumed to be safe in patients with cardiovascular disease, although there have been few systematic investigations in these patients. In a prospective study of 27 depressed patients with established cardiac disease, fluoxetine (up to 60 mg/day for 7 weeks) produced a statistically significant reduction in heart rate (6%) and an increase in supine systolic blood pressure (2%) (4). One patient had worsening of a pre-existing dysrhythmia and this persisted after fluoxetine withdrawal. These findings suggest that, relative to tricyclic antidepressants, fluoxetine may have a relatively benign profile in patients with cardiovascular disease. However, the authors cautioned that in view of the small number of patients studied, these findings cannot be widely generalized.

The effects of fluoxetine (20 mg/day for 12 weeks) on sitting and standing blood pressures have been reported (5). Fluoxetine modestly but significantly lowered sitting and standing systolic and diastolic blood pressures by about 2 mmHg. Patients with pre-existing cardiovascular disease showed no change. This study confirms that fluoxetine has little effect on blood pressure in physically healthy depressed patients and in those with moderate cardiovascular disease.

Fluoxetine-induced remission of Raynaud's phenomenon has been reported (SEDA-18, 20) (6).

Cardiac dysrhythmias

Fluoxetine has reportedly caused prolongation of the QT_c interval (7).

- A 52-year-old man had an abnormally prolonged QT_c interval of 560 ms, with broad-based T-waves. He had taken fluoxetine 40 mg/day over the previous 3 months, before which an electrocardiogram had shown a normal QT_c interval (380 ms). The fluoxetine was withdrawn, and 10 days later the QT_c interval was 380 ms. His only other medication was verapamil which he had taken for 3 years for hypertension.

Systematic studies of fluoxetine as monotherapy have not shown evidence of QT_c prolongation. It is possible in this case that fluoxetine interacted with verapamil to produce a conduction disorder.

An elderly man developed atrial fibrillation and bradycardia shortly after starting fluoxetine, and again on rechallenge (SEDA-16, 9). Dose-dependent bradycardia with dizziness and syncope has also been reported in a few patients taking fluoxetine (SEDA-16, 9) and in a presenile patient (8).

Nervous system

Several cases in which fluoxetine worsened parkinsonian disability have been described, and the problem of exacerbation of Parkinson's disease by fluoxetine has been reviewed (SEDA-18, 19).

Five patients taking fluoxetine developed akathisia, perhaps due to enhanced serotonergic inhibition of dopamine neurons (9). A causal link between fluoxetine-induced akathisia and suicidal behavior has been suggested (SEDA-17, 19) (SEDA-18, 19), and akathisia has also been associated with "indifference" (SEDA-18, 19).

One case of neuroleptic malignant syndrome has been described with fluoxetine (10).

One case of tics after long-term fluoxetine therapy has been described; the symptoms subsided several months after withdrawal (SEDA-18, 19).

One case of migraine associated with fluoxetine has been reported, with no further attacks when the drug was withdrawn (SEDA-18, 20).

Stuttering has been reported with fluoxetine (11).

Two patients who had been maintained successfully on fluoxetine (20 mg/day) for 6 and 10 years respectively began to have agitation, tension, and sleep disturbance (12). There had been no recent changes in medications or life events to explain these symptoms, which closely resembled the kind of adverse effects that can occur shortly after the start of SSRI treatment. Both patients improved after downward titration of the dose of fluoxetine. Blood concentrations of fluoxetine were not reported, so it is possible that for some reason (for example a change in diet or activity) plasma fluoxetine concentrations had recently increased in these subjects. However, the development of characteristic adverse effects after such a long trouble-free period suggests that patients taking maintenance medication need long-term follow-up, or at least ready access to specialist advice.

Seizures

Fluoxetine has been associated with seizures, both in therapeutic doses (3,13) and in overdose (3,14). It has also been shown to lengthen seizure duration during electroconvulsive therapy (SEDA-17, 20). Four patients had suspected seizures during studies (3) and one who took a 3000 mg overdose (3) had unequivocal convulsions but recovered.

Sensory systems

Tricyclic antidepressants can precipitate acute glaucoma through their anticholinergic effects. There are also reports that SSRIs can cause acute glaucoma, presumably by pupillary dilatation (see the monograph on Paroxetine).

In a placebo-controlled study in depressed patients a single dose of fluoxetine (20 mg) increased intraocular pressure by 4 mmHg (15). This increase is within the normal diurnal range, but could be of clinical consequence in individuals predisposed to glaucoma. However, post-marketing surveillance has not suggested an association between the use of fluoxetine and glaucoma (16).

Blurred vision has occasionally required withdrawal of fluoxetine (3).

Psychological, psychiatric

An analysis of severe adverse effects that caused drug withdrawal showed that psychotic reactions occurred in nine of 1378 patients; in four cases this appeared to be a stimulant psychosis and in three a conversion to mania (3).

Cognitive function can be impaired by fluoxetine; a negative effect on learning and memory has been described (SEDA-17, 20).

Reports of acute mania and manic-like behavior after treatment with fluoxetine or fluvoxamine have appeared (SEDA-13, 12) (SEDA-17, 20) (SEDA-18, 20), but there are not enough data to estimate the incidence.

Suicidal ideation has been described after 2–7 weeks of fluoxetine (17) and other case reports (SEDA-16, 9) (SEDA-17, 19). A causal link was initially questioned (SED-12, 57) (SEDA-15, 15) (SEDA-17, 19), and in one controlled trial there was no increase (SEDA-16, 9). Furthermore, a meta-analysis of controlled trials did not point to a greater risk of suicide attempts or suicidal ideation with fluoxetine than with tricyclic antidepressants (1).

In a meta-analysis based on 9087 patients in 87 different randomized clinical trials with fluoxetine there was no increased risk of suicide (2).

In an analysis of data from the National Institute of Mental Health Collaborative Depression Study in 643 patients with affective disorders who were followed up after fluoxetine was approved by the FDA in December 1987 for the treatment of depression, nearly 30% (n = 185) took fluoxetine at some point (18). There was an increased rate of suicide attempts before fluoxetine treatment in those who subsequently took fluoxetine. Relative to no treatment, fluoxetine and other antidepressants were associated with non-significant reductions in the likelihood of suicide attempts or completions. Severity of psychopathology was strongly associated with increased risk, and each suicide attempt after admission to the study was associated with a marginally significant increase in the risk of suicidal behavior. The authors concluded that the results did not support the speculation that fluoxetine increases the risk of suicide.

Endocrine

Fluoxetine causes weight loss, in contrast to tricyclic antidepressants (19). In one study there was a mean fall in weight of 3.88 pounds over 6 weeks compared with a gain of 4.6 pounds with amitriptyline (20).

Serotonin pathways are involved in the regulation of prolactin secretion. Amenorrhea, galactorrhea, and hyperprolactinemia have been reported in a patient taking SSRIs.

- A 71-year-old woman who had taken fluoxetine (dose unspecified) for a number of weeks noted unilateral galactorrhea and had a raised prolactin of 37 ng/ml (reference range 1.2–24 ng/ml) (21). She was also taking estrogen hormonal replacement therapy, benazapril, and occasional alprazolam. Withdrawal of the fluoxetine led to normalization of the prolactin concentration and resolution of the galactorrhea.

Estrogens also facilitate prolactin release, and so hormone replacement therapy may have played a part in this case.

Hematologic

Petechiae and prolongation of bleeding time have been reported in association with fluoxetine (SEDA-16, 10). In one case a 31-year-old woman taking fluoxetine developed bruising (22).

Aplastic anemia with fever, pleuritic chest pain, and pancytopenia developed in a 28-year-old woman (23) after 6 weeks of fluoxetine therapy. Bone-marrow examination confirmed acute marrow aplasia. She recovered 19 days after withdrawal. Neutropenia occurred rapidly after rechallenge. Another report described severe neutropenia during fluoxetine treatment (24).

Gastrointestinal

Gastrointestinal adverse effects are one of the major disadvantages of SSRIs (see General section). Two women developed stomatitis while taking fluoxetine; in one it recurred on rechallenge (25).

Liver

Chronic hepatitis associated with fluoxetine has been reported in a 35-year-old man (26).

In a post-marketing surveillance study there were some cases in which fluoxetine alone appeared to have precipitated hepatitis, which remitted when treatment was withdrawn (27). Fluoxetine can cause mild increases in liver enzymes, with a rate in clinical trials of about 0.5%. Rarely this can progress to hepatitis.

Skin

Rashes due to fluoxetine occur in a few percent of patients (28). Fluoxetine has been implicated in two cases of psoriasis (SEDA-17, 20). A woman taking fluoxetine monotherapy had painful burning, persistent erythema, and blisters on sun-exposed areas (SEDA-20, 8).

Hair

Reversible hair loss has been reported in patients taking fluoxetine (SEDA-16, 10) (SEDA-17, 20).

Sexual function

Fluoxetine can impair sexual function in both sexes, and particularly causes delayed orgasm or anorgasmia (SEDA-14, 14) (SEDA-17, 21) (SEDA-18, 21), in 5–10% of patients (29,30).

Fluoxetine has been implicated in one case of prolonged erection (SEDA-18, 21).

Yawning, clitoral engorgement, and spontaneous orgasm have been associated with fluoxetine (31).

Penile anesthesia has been reported in association with fluoxetine and sertraline (SEDA-17, 20).

Immunologic

Vasculitis has been attributed to fluoxetine (32,33).

- A patient who took fluoxetine for a manic-depressive disorder developed pulmonary inflammatory nodules with non-caseating giant cell granulomas, interstitial pneumonia, and non-necrotizing vasculitis, but remained asymptomatic (34). The diagnosis was made by open lung biopsy. The pulmonary nodules progressively resolved after withdrawal and the chest X-ray returned to normal in 9 months.

Second-Generation Effects

Fetotoxicity

Fluoxetine can occasionally cause cardiac dysrhythmias in adults, and may have done so in a fetus, whose mother took fluoxetine during pregnancy.

A woman took fluoxetine (20–30 mg/day) from the 28th week of pregnancy (35). The fluoxetine was withdrawn during the 37th week, and at 38 weeks a male infant (2700 g) was born by spontaneous vaginal delivery. Both before and after delivery the baby was noted to have multiple atrial and ventricular extra beats. Echocardiography showed a normal heart and the baby was otherwise well. By discharge on day 5 the frequency of extra beats had fallen, and on follow-up 1 month later they were no longer present.

The long half-life of fluoxetine and its active metabolite, norfluoxetine, means that the active drug would have been present in the mother and baby for some weeks after withdrawal. However, as the authors pointed out, the baseline incidence of atrial extra beats in a fetus in utero is about 1–2%. It is therefore possible that treatment with fluoxetine in this case was coincidental.

Fluoxetine-related withdrawal effects have been reported in a neonate whose mother had taken fluoxetine during pregnancy (SEDA-18, 21).

Drug Administration

Drug overdose

Nine patients took overdoses of fluoxetine in amounts up to 3000 mg (37 times the recommended dose) (3). One, who also took several other drugs, including amitriptyline, died, but the other eight all recovered with relatively minor symptoms in most cases. Four patients had suspected seizures during studies (3) and one who took a 3000 mg overdose had unequivocal convulsions but recovered.

Overdosage of fluoxetine has been implicated in the development of seizures, but usually only when taken with other substances.

- A 15-year-old girl had a tonic-clonic seizure after overdosage of fluoxetine alone; she recovered uneventfully (36).

Drug–Drug Interactions

Beta-blockers

An interaction between metoprolol and fluoxetine with severe bradycardia has been described (SEDA-18, 23).

Carbamazepine

Fluoxetine can increase plasma concentrations of carbamazepine (SEDA-17, 21) (SEDA-18, 23).

Digoxin

Fluoxetine has been reported to increase serum digoxin concentrations (37).

- A 93-year-old woman with congestive cardiac failure, paroxysmal atrial fibrillation, and hypertension developed depression after the death of her daughter. For several months she had been taking captopril 25 mg bd, furosemide 40 mg/day, digoxin 0.125 mg/day, and ranitidine 150 mg bd. She was in sinus rhythm and her serum digoxin concentration was 1.0–1.4 nmol/l. She was treated with fluoxetine (10 mg/day), but a week later she developed anorexia. At that time the serum digoxin concentration was 4.2 nmol/l. Both digoxin and fluoxetine were withdrawn and the digoxin concentration returned to the target range within 5 days, with resolution of the anorexia. Digoxin was restarted and concentrations in the usual target range were achieved during the next 3 weeks (0.9–1.4 nmol/l). Because of persisting depressive symptoms, fluoxetine (10 mg/day) was given again, but the digoxin concentrations rose and after 4 days were 2.8 nmol/l. Both digoxin and fluoxetine were then withdrawn.

Because digoxin has a narrow therapeutic range, this interaction, if confirmed, may be of clinical significance. The mechanism is not clear, because digoxin is not a substrate for the cytochrome P450 enzymes that are inhibited by fluoxetine. The authors speculated that fluoxetine may reduce the renal clearance of digoxin; if so, it might do that by inhibiting the P-glycoprotein that is responsible for the active tubular secretion of digoxin.

Lithium

A report has been published of lithium toxicity induced by combined treatment with fluoxetine (38).

Monoamine oxidase inhibitors

The problem of the long half-life of fluoxetine, leading to interactions with monoamine oxidase inhibitors, even after withdrawal, has been discussed previously (SEDA-13, 12), and caused the manufacturer to circulate a warning to that effect.

Pseudopheochromocytoma, with hypertension, palpitation, and headache, has been reported in a patient taking fluoxetine and selegiline (SEDA-18, 23).

Phenytoin

Several case reports and one in vitro study have suggested that combined administration of fluoxetine with phenytoin can significantly increase phenytoin serum concentrations, leading to toxicity (19,39,40).

Risperidone

Combined treatment with atypical neuroleptic drugs and SSRIs is common and case reports have suggested that SSRIs can increase risperidone concentrations and increase the risk of extrapyramidal disorders (SEDA-23, 18).

- Severe parkinsonism with urinary retention occurred when fluoxetine 20 mg/day was added to risperidone 2 mg/day in a 46-year-old man with schizophrenia. Risperidone had been prescribed at this dose for 1 month without any adverse effects, and the authors considered that a pharmacokinetic interaction between fluoxetine and risperidone was the most likely mechanism (41).

In a systematic open study in 11 hospitalized patients taking a steady dose of risperidone (4–6 mg/day), fluoxetine (20 mg/day) increased plasma concentrations of active antipsychotic medication (combined concentrations of risperidone and 9-hydroxyrisperidone) by 50% after treatment for 25 days (42). Despite this, the treatment was well tolerated and there were improvements in rating scales of psychosis and depressed mood. Whether this was due to the introduction of fluoxetine or the higher plasma concentrations of risperidone is not clear. Fluoxetine and norfluoxetine would require at least a further 2 weeks to reach steady state, so additional increases in risperidone concentrations might be anticipated over this time.

Triptans

Caution has been advocated when SSRIs such as fluoxetine are combined with the triptans that are used to treat acute episodes of migraine (SEDA-24, 16). There are case reports of symptoms suggestive of serotonin toxicity when fluoxetine has been combined with sumatriptan, perhaps because the SSRI can potentiate the $5\text{-HT}_{1B/1D}$ agonist effects of the triptan (SEDA-22, 14).

The effect of fluoxetine 60 mg/day for 8 days on the pharmacokinetics of almotriptan has been studied in 14 healthy volunteers (43). Fluoxetine produced a significant increase in the peak concentration of almotriptan, but the AUC was not altered. These results suggest that CYP2D6 plays a minor role in the metabolism of almotriptan. The combined treatment was reported to be well tolerated, but this does not exclude the possibility of occasional cases of serotonin toxicity in some individuals.

References

1. Beasley CM, Jr. Dornseif BE, Bosomworth JC, Sayler ME, Rampey AH, Jr. Heiligenstein JH, Thompson VL, Murphy DJ, Masica DN. Fluoxetine and suicide: a meta-analysis of controlled trials of treatment for depression. BMJ 1991;303(6804):685–92.
2. Rossi A, Barraco A, Donda P. Fluoxetine: a review on evidence based medicine. Ann Gen Hosp Psychiatry 2004;3(1):2.
3. Wernicke JF. The side effect profile and safety of fluoxetine. J Clin Psychiatry 1985;46(3 Part 2):59–67.
4. Roose SP, Glassman AH, Attia E, Woodring S, Giardina EG, Bigger JT, Jr. Cardiovascular effects of fluoxetine in depressed patients with heart disease. Am J Psychiatry 1998;155(5):660–5.
5. Amsterdam JD, Garcia-Espana F, Fawcett J, Quitkin FM, Reimherr FW, Rosenbaum JF, Beasley C. Blood pressure changes during short-term fluoxetine treatment. J Clin Psychopharmacol 1999;19(1):9–14.
6. Rudnick A, Modai I, Zelikovski A. Fluoxetine-induced Raynaud's phenomenon. Biol Psychiatry 1997;41(12):1218–21.
7. Varriale P. Fluoxetine (Prozac) as a cause of QT prolongation. Arch Intern Med 2001;161(4):12.
8. Anderson J, Compton SA. Fluoxetine induced bradycardia in presenile dementia. Ulster Med J 1997;66(2):144–5.
9. Lipinski JF, Jr. Mallya G, Zimmerman P, Pope HG Jr. Fluoxetine-induced akathisia: clinical and theoretical implications. J Clin Psychiatry 1989;50(9):339–42.
10. Halman M, Goldbloom DS. Fluoxetine and neuroleptic malignant syndrome. Biol Psychiatry 1990;28(6):518–21.
11. Guthrie S, Grunhaus L. Fluoxetine-induced stuttering. J Clin Psychiatry 1990;51(2):85.
12. Buchman N, Strous RD, Baruch Y. Side effects of long-term treatment with fluoxetine. Clin Neuropharmacol 2002;25(1):55–7.
13. Weber JJ. Seizure activity associated with fluoxetine therapy. Clin Pharm 1989;8(4):296–8.
14. Riddle MA, Brown N, Dzubinski D, Jetmalani AN, Law Y, Woolston JL. Fluoxetine overdose in an adolescent. J Am Acad Child Adolesc Psychiatry 1989;28(4):587–8.
15. Costagliola C, Mastropasqua L, Steardo L, Testa N. Fluoxetine oral administration increases intraocular pressure. Br J Ophthalmol 1996;80(7):678.
16. Eke T, Carr S, Costagliola C, Mastropasqua L, Steardo L. Acute glaucoma, chronic glaucoma, and serotoninergic drugs. Br J Ophthalmol 1998;82(8):976–8.
17. Teicher MH, Glod C, Cole JO. Emergence of intense suicidal preoccupation during fluoxetine treatment. Am J Psychiatry 1990;147(2):207–10.
18. Leon AC, Keller MB, Warshaw MG, Mueller TI. Solomon DA, Coryell W, Endicott J. Prospective study of fluoxetine treatment and suicidal behavior in affectively ill subjects. Am J Psychiatry 1999;156(2):195–201.
19. Jalil P. Toxic reaction following the combined administration of fluoxetine and phenytoin: two case reports. J Neurol Neurosurg Psychiatry 1992;55(5):412–13.
20. Fawcett J, Zajecka JM, Kravitz HM, et al. Fluoxetine versus amitriptyline in adult outpatients with major depression. Psychiatry Res 1989;45:821.
21. Peterson MC. Reversible galactorrhea and prolactin elevation related to fluoxetine use. Mayo Clin Proc 2001;76(2):215–16.
22. Bottlender R, Dobmeier P, Moller HJ. Der Einfluss von selektiven Serotonin-Wiederaufnahmeinhibitoren auf die Blutgerinnung. [The effect of selective serotonin-reuptake inhibitors in blood coagulation.] Fortschr Neurol Psychiatr 1998;66(1):32–5.
23. Calhoun JW, Calhoun DD. Prolonged bleeding time in a patient treated with setraline. Am J Psychiatry 1996;153:443.
24. Vilinsky FD, Lubin A. Severe neutropenia associated with fluoxetine hydrochloride. Ann Intern Med 1997;127(7):573–4.
25. Palop V, Sancho A, Morales-Olivas FJ, Martinez-Mir I. Fluoxetine-associated stomatitis. Ann Pharmacother 1997;31(12):1478–80.
26. Johnston DE, Wheeler DE. Chronic hepatitis related to use of fluoxetine. Am J Gastroenterol 1997;92(7):1225–6.
27. Capella D, Bruguera M, Figueras A, Laporte J. Fluoxetine-induced hepatitis: why is postmarketing surveillance needed? Eur J Clin Pharmacol 1999;55(7):545–6.
28. Cooper GL. The safety of fluoxetine – an update. Br J Psychiatry Suppl. 1988;3:77–86.
29. Stark P, Hardison CD. A review of multicenter controlled studies of fluoxetine vs. imipramine and placebo in outpatients with major depressive disorder. J Clin Psychiatry 1985;46(3 Part 2):53–8.
30. Herman JB, Brotman AW, Pollack MH, Falk WE, Biederman J, Rosenbaum JF. Fluoxetine-induced sexual dysfunction. J Clin Psychiatry 1990;51(1):25–7.
31. Modell JG. Repeated observations of yawning, clitoral engorgement, and orgasm associated with fluoxetine administration. J Clin Psychopharmacol 1989;9(1):63–5.
32. Roger D, Rolle F, Mausset J, Lavignac C, Bonnetblanc JM. Urticarial vasculitis induced by fluoxetine. Dermatology 1995;191(2):164.
33. Fisher A, McLean AJ, Purcell P, Herdson PB, Dahlstrom JE, Le Couteur DG. Focal necrotising vasculitis with secondary myositis following fluoxetine administration. Aust NZ J Med 1999;29(3):375–6.

34. de Kerviler E, Tredaniel J, Revlon G, Groussard O, Zalcman G, Ortoli JM, Espie M, Hirsch A, Frija J. Fluoxetin-induced pulmonary granulomatosis. Eur Respir J 1996;9(3):615–17.
35. Abebe-Campino G, Offer D, Stahl B, Merlob P. Cardiac arrhythmia in a newborn infant associated with fluoxetine use during pregnancy. Ann Pharmacother 2002;36(3):533–4.
36. Brosen K. The pharmacogenetics of the selective serotonin reuptake inhibitors. Clin Investig 1993;71(12):1002–9.
37. Leibovitz A, Bilchinsky T, Gil I, Habot B. Elevated serum digoxin level associated with coadministered fluoxetine. Arch Intern Med 1998;158(10):1152–3.
38. Salama AA, Shafey M. A case of severe lithium toxicity induced by combined fluoxetine and lithium carbonate. Am J Psychiatry 1989;146(2):278.
39. Woods DJ, Coulter DM, Pillans P. Interaction of phenytoin and fluoxetine. NZ Med J 1994;107(970):19.
40. Schmider J, Greenblatt DJ, von Moltke LL, Karsov D, Shader RI. Inhibition of CYP2C9 by selective serotonin reuptake inhibitors in vitro: studies of phenytoin *p*-hydroxylation. Br J Clin Pharmacol 1997;44(5):495–8.
41. Bozikas V, Petrikis P, Karavatos A. Urinary retention caused after fluoxetine–risperidone combination. J Psychopharmacol 2001;15(2):142–3.
42. Bondolfi G, Eap CB, Bertschy G, Zullino D, Vermeulen A, Baumann P. The effect of fluoxetine on the pharmacokinetics and safety of risperidone in psychiatric patients. Pharmacopsychiatry 2002;35(2):50–6.
43. Fleishaker JC, Ryan KK, Carel BJ, Azie NE. Evaluation of the potential pharmacokinetic interaction between almotriptan and fluoxetine in healthy volunteers. J Clin Pharmacol 2001;41(2):217–23.

Flupentixol

See also Neuroleptic drugs

General Information

Flupentixol is a thioxanthene neuroleptic drug.

Organs and Systems

Nervous system

Autoamputation of the tongue in a patient who was taking flupentixol has been explained as being secondary to an acute, atypical, neuroleptic drug-induced orolingual dyskinesia (1).

- A 21-year-old man, who had been mentally retarded from birth, was given intramuscular flupentixol 50 mg/day and oral diazepam 7.5 mg/day for disruptive and inappropriate behavior, and 84 hours later began chewing his tongue repetitively, with resultant edema and bleeding from multiple lacerations. The biting abated within 2 hours after intravenous biperiden 5 mg and diazepam 5 mg; ampicillin, cloxacillin, and metronidazole were also given. One week after admission to hospital, he had an autoamputation of the distal one-third of his tongue.

Reference

1. Pantanowitz L, Berk M. Auto-amputation of the tongue associated with flupenthixol induced extrapyramidal symptoms. Int Clin Psychopharmacol 1999;14(2):129–31.

Fluphenazine

See also Neuroleptic drugs

General Information

Fluphenazine is a phenothiazine neuroleptic drug.

In a double-blind comparison of a group of stabilized outpatients taking a low dosage of fluphenazine enanthate (1.25–5 mg every 2 weeks) with a group taking a standard dosage (12.5–50 mg every 2 weeks), relapse rates were higher in the low-dose group (56%) than in the standard-dose group (7%) (1). However, patients in the low-dose group had a better outcome in terms of some measures of psychosocial adjustment and family satisfaction. Patients in the low-dose group had fewer signs of tardive dyskinesia, and relapses led less often to re-admission to hospital; they also responded more readily to treatment with temporary increases in medication than patients treated with standard doses.

In a comparison of a low dose of fluphenazine decanoate (5 mg) with a standard dose (25 mg) every 2 weeks, there was no significant difference in relapse at 1 year (2), nor was there a difference in survival at 1 year, but at 2 years, survival was significantly better with the 25 mg dose (64%) than with the 5 mg dose (31%) (3).

Organs and Systems

Gastrointestinal

Neuroleptic drugs, particularly phenothiazine derivatives, have been reported to cause colitis (SED-14, 150) (4) (SEDA-20, 43). The mechanism was thought to be an anticholinergic effect. Two other cases have been reported (5,6), one with positive rechallenge.

- A 41-year-old man developed acute abdominal pain with profuse diarrhea and fever (39°C) while receiving intramuscular fluphenazine decanoate 125 mg once every 3 weeks. During the previous 3 months he had also taken oral alimemazine 50 mg/day, levomepromazine 50 mg/day, and amitriptyline 100 mg/day. Colonoscopy showed necrotic ulcers in the mucosa of the sigmoid and descending colon. After three weeks of parenteral nutrition, there was a marked reduction in the colonic lesions and he recovered. Levomepromazine 50 mg/day and fluphenazine decanoate 100 mg/day were reintroduced. Two days later he complained again of abdominal pain, and tomodensitometry confirmed distension.

Second-Generation Effects

Fetotoxicity

Severe rhinorrhea and respiratory distress occurred in a neonate exposed to fluphenazine hydrochloride prenatally (7).

Drug–Drug Interactions

Vitamin C

In one patient, ascorbic acid reduced serum fluphenazine concentrations, perhaps by liver enzyme induction or by reduced absorption (8).

References

1. Kane JM, Rifkin A, Woerner M, Reardon G, Sarantakos S, Schiebel D, Ramos-Lorenzi J. Low-dose neuroleptic treatment of outpatient schizophrenics. I. Preliminary results for relapse rates. Arch Gen Psychiatry 1983;40(8):893–6.
2. Marder SR, Van Putten T, Mintz J, McKenzie J, Lebell M, Faltico G, May PR. Costs and benefits of two doses of fluphenazine. Arch Gen Psychiatry 1984;41(11):1025–9.
3. Marder SR, Van Putten T, Mintz J, Lebell M, McKenzie J, May PR. Low- and conventional-dose maintenance therapy with fluphenazine decanoate. Two-year outcome. Arch Gen Psychiatry 1987;44(6):518–21.
4. Larrey D, Lainey E, Blanc P, Diaz D, David R, Biaggi A, Barneon G, Bottai T, Potet F, Michel H. Acute colitis associated with prolonged administration of neuroleptics. J Clin Gastroenterol 1992;14(1):64–7.
5. Capron M, Lafitte B, Benedit M, Camard CN, Nicolas F, Beligon C, Baillet C. Colite nécrosante chez un homme de 29 ans sous forte dose de neuroleptiques. [Necrotizing colitis in a 29-year-old man following high doses of neuroleptics.] Reanim Urgences 1999;8:701–4.
6. Filloux MC, Marechal K, Bagheri H, Morales J, Nouvel A, Laurencin G, Montastruc JL. Phenothiazine-induced acute colitis: a positive rechallenge case report. Clin Neuropharmacol 1999;22(4):244–5.
7. Nath SP, Miller DA, Muraskas JK. Severe rhinorrhea and respiratory distress in a neonate exposed to fluphenazine hydrochloride prenatally. Ann Pharmacother 1996;30(1): 35–7.
8. Dysken MW, Cumming RJ, Channon RA, Davis JM. Drug interaction between ascorbic acid and fluphenazine. JAMA 1979;241(19):2008.

Flupirtine

General Information

Flupirtine is a non-opiate, centrally acting analgesic, with muscle relaxant properties. It causes predominantly nervous system adverse effects (visual, disorientation, confusion, tremor). About 26% of patients develop minor adverse reactions (1).

Reference

1. Galasko CS, Courtenay PM, Jane M, Stamp TC. Trial of oral flupirtine maleate in the treatment of pain after orthopaedic surgery. Curr Med Res Opin 1985;9(9):594–601.

Fluproquazone and proquazone

See also Non-steroidal anti-inflammatory drugs

General Information

Fluproquazone and proquazone, quinazoline derivatives, are analgesics of minor importance. Gastrointestinal adverse effects are the most frequent (SEDA-4, 69) (SEDA-5, 197) (SEDA-10, 88). Because fluproquazone caused hepatic injury in 14% of patients in clinical trials, evaluation was halted (1).

Reference

1. Lewis JH. Hepatic toxicity of nonsteroidal anti-inflammatory drugs. Clin Pharm 1984;3(2):128–38.

Flurbiprofen

See also Non-steroidal anti-inflammatory drugs

General Information

In a short-term multicenter study of flurbiprofen only 6% of patients were withdrawn because of adverse effects (1). However, in a prolonged open study in 1200 patients, more than 50% reported adverse reactions and therapy had to be withdrawn in 19% (2).

Organs and Systems

Nervous system

Nervous system effects with flurbiprofen are less common than with indometacin (3). Flurbiprofen precipitates extrapyramidal reactions, albeit rarely (SEDA-15, 101), and a parkinsonian syndrome has been reported in a predisposed patient (SEDA-15, 101).

Gastrointestinal

Flurbiprofen causes more gastrointestinal adverse effects than naproxen or ibuprofen. In a series of controlled double-blind studies, adverse reactions occurred in 27–42% of patients and were most commonly gastrointestinal in origin (18–28%) (SEDA-12, 85).

Local tolerance of flurbiprofen suppositories is often satisfactory, but discomfort, irritation, tenesmus, and diarrhea have been observed (4).

Urinary tract

Interstitial nephritis with the nephrotic syndrome and one case of renal papillary necrosis have been recorded (SEDA-12, 86) (SEDA-17, 110). Flurbiprofen can cause a membranous nephropathy (SEDA-21, 105).

Skin

There have been two reports of a dermatitis herpetiformis-like eruption in patients taking flurbiprofen (SEDA-18, 104).

Immunologic

Leukocytoclastic vasculitis caused by flurbiprofen has been observed in a patient with rheumatoid arthritis (SEDA-15, 101).

Susceptibility Factors

Age

Elderly patients seem to be particularly sensitive to and intolerant of flurbiprofen; one study reported adverse effects in 80% (SED-11, 183) (5).

Drug Administration

Drug administration route

Intramuscular flurbiprofen was effective and well tolerated in ureteric colic; local adverse effects were slight (SEDA-20, 93).

Drug–Drug Interactions

Acenocoumarol

Flurbiprofen potentiates the anticoagulant effect of acenocoumarol (SEDA-7, 112).

Furosemide

Flurbiprofen reduces the diuretic action of furosemide (6).

Quinolone antibiotics

The Japanese regulatory authority has suggested that the data sheet for flurbiprofen should include a warning that it can cause convulsions, which has mainly been described in patients taking quinolone antibiotics (SEDA-18, 104); quinolones should not be used concomitantly (SEDA-18, 104).

References

1. Benvenuti C, Longoni L. Multicentre study on effectiveness and safety of flurbiprofen versus alternative therapy in 738 rheumatic patients. Curr Ther Res 1983;34:30.
2. Sheldrake FE, Webber JM, Marsh BD. A long-term assessment of flurbiprofen. Curr Med Res Opin 1977;5(1):106–16.
3. De Moor M, Ooghe R. A double-blind comparison of flurbiprofen and indomethacin suppositories in the treatment of osteoarthrosis and rheumatoid disease. J Int Med Res 1981;9(6):495–500.
4. Huskisson EC, Woolf DL, Boyle DV, Scott J. A trial of naproxen, flurbiprofen, indometacin and placebo in the treatment of osteoarthritis. Eur J Rheumatol Inflamm 1980;2:69.
5. Innes EH. Efficacy and tolerance of flurbiprofen in the elderly using liquid and tablet formulations. Curr Med Res Opin 1977;5(1):122–6.
6. Rawles JM. Antagonism between non-steroidal anti-inflammatory drugs and diuretics. Scott Med J 1982;27(1):37–40.

Flurotyl

General Information

Flurotyl, a hexafluorinated ether, has been used as a therapeutic inhalational convulsant in psychiatry (SED-13, 11). Its intravenous use in a polyethylene glycol solution has been discontinued because of possible renal damage. In most Western and North American countries, flurotyl is not recommended because of variations in response and dosing difficulties.

Organs and Systems

Respiratory

Flurotyl is excreted via the lungs and there has been concern about the possibility of apnea, cardiac arrest, or vascular collapse; it has therefore been recommended that resuscitation facilities be available when it is used (1).

Nervous system

The main adverse effects of flurotyl are restlessness, confusion, dysphasia, headache, and dysmelia (SED-8, 5). Prolonged muscle twitching can occur, as can intermittent jerky movements of the limbs (SED-9, 2).

Psychological, psychiatric

Flurotyl caused toxic delirium in two of 135 patients with schizophrenia (SED-13, 12).

Drug–Drug Interactions

General

Flurotyl should not be used in combination with drugs that lower the seizure threshold, such as monoamine oxidase inhibitors and phenothiazines.

Reference

1. Council on Drugs. A convulsant agent for psychiatric use. Flurotyl (Indoklon) JAMA 1966;196(1):29–30.

Flutamide

See also Cytostatic and immunosuppressant drugs

General Information

Flutamide is a non-steroidal antiandrogen that is used to treat prostatic cancer. Its most common adverse effects are liver damage and photosensitivity.

Organs and Systems

Respiratory

Flutamide has been associated with interstitial pneumonitis.

- An 88-year-old man with prostate cancer took flutamide 375 mg/day for 3 weeks and developed dyspnea and bilateral pulmonary interstitial infiltrates; glucocorticoid therapy and withdrawal of flutamide resulted in clinical improvement (1).

Metabolism

Flutamide has been implicated in cases of pseudoporphyria (2,3).

- A 75-year-old man with prostatic carcinoma took flutamide for 18 months and developed blisters on the back of the hands and fingers after exposure to the sun (4). The bullae were associated with skin fragility and atrophic scarring. Histopathology and direct immunofluorescence showed ultrastructural features similar to those described in porphyria cutanea tarda. However, porphyrin concentrations in the urine and blood were normal. Flutamide was withdrawn and the lesions healed, without relapse after 11 months.

Hematologic

Although it is the commonest of all antineoplastic adverse effects, there are sometimes peculiarities of hematological toxicity that make it worthy of comment (5).

Flutamide can cause methemoglobinemia (6–8) or sulfhemoglobinemia (5). The latter occurred in a 70-year-old man who had taken flutamide 150 mg tds for 1 month and developed cyanosis and anemia that was not responsive to methylthioninium chloride (methylene blue).

In 45 patients with prostatic cancer taking flutamide 250 mg tds, there was no evidence of methemoglobinemia (9). It is possible that anecdotal reports of this adverse effect are in patients with a particular susceptibility that was not represented in this study.

Gastrointestinal

Among 440 patients taking flutamide, gastrointestinal adverse effects (abdominal pain/distension, diarrhea, constipation, nausea/vomiting, and anorexia) occurred in about 22% (10).

Ischemic colitis has been attributed to flutamide (11).

Liver

Flutamide can cause liver damage, which can occasionally be fatal (12).

- A 74-year-old man developed life-threatening acute liver failure while taking flutamide (13). Other causes of acute liver failure were ruled out and there was no evidence of active prostate cancer or liver metastases.

The authors suggested that mitochondrial dysfunction is implicated in flutamide-associated liver damage.

Three patients with advanced prostate carcinoma who took flutamide 250 mg tds for 20–22 weeks developed signs of liver damage (jaundice, anorexia, nausea, dark urine) and changes in liver function tests (high transaminases and bilirubin), indicative of acute hepatitis; flutamide was withdrawn and there was spontaneous remission over the next 8 weeks (14).

In a retrospective study of 185 patients who had taken flutamide for 151 (range 4–443) days, 9 had liver damage (15). The most common features were weakness, anorexia, weight loss, nausea, vomiting, and jaundice. No patient had evidence of hypersensitivity. In two patients there was fulminant liver failure; one had a liver transplant and the other died. The authors suggested that liver function tests should be monitored during the first months of flutamide therapy and that the drug should be withdrawn if transaminases begin to rise.

Of 123 patients who had taken flutamide, 33 had liver disorders, mostly within 9 months (16). Three variables, body mass index, a past history of liver disorders, and raised transaminases were significantly related to the incidence of liver disorders. Smoking was related to a lower incidence.

Urinary tract

Flutamide rarely causes renal damage.

- A 54-year-old man with metastatic prostate cancer developed non-oliguric acute renal insufficiency while taking flutamide; after withdrawal his renal function returned to normal within 4 weeks (17). After rechallenge his blood urea nitrogen and serum creatinine rose again and recovered completely after withdrawal.

Skin

Flutamide can cause photosensitivity reactions (18–20) and can cause residual vitiligo (21,22). The spectrum of the effect is in the UVA range (23).

- A 68-year-old man had a photosensitive drug eruption while taking flutamide (24). The minimal erythema dose with ultraviolet A light was reduced to 2 J/cm^2 and recovered to over 16 J/cm^2 after withdrawal, without changing reactivity to ultraviolet B. The absorption spectrum of flutamide was not altered after ultraviolet A irradiation.

The authors thought that flutamide has low potency to act as a photohapten, and that a non-photohaptenic mechanism is responsible for this photosensitivity or that its active metabolite may act as a photosensitizer.

Musculoskeletal

In 26 men who took androgen deprivation therapy for prostate cancer for 10 years there was reduced bone mineral density with increasing duration of androgen deprivation therapy across the whole 10-year period (25). The authors also noted that patients taking intermittent therapy had similar loss of bone mineral density at years 2 and 4, but less bone loss from year 6 onwards.

Susceptibility Factors

Renal disease

The pharmacokinetics of flutamide and its pharmacologically active metabolite, hydroxyflutamide, have been studied in 26 men with normal or reduced renal function, some of whom were undergoing hemodialysis; the pharmacokinetics were not altered by renal impairment or hemodialysis (26).

References

1. Nomura M, Sato H, Fujimoto N, Matsumoto T. Interstitial pneumonitis related to flutamide monotherapy for prostate cancer. Int J Urol 2004;11(9):798–800.
2. Schmutz JL, Barbaud A, Trechot P. Flutamide et pseudoporphyrie. [Flutamide and pseudoporphyria.] Ann Dermatol Venereol 1999;126(4):374.
3. Borroni G, Brazzelli V, Baldini F, Borghini F, Gaviglio MR, Beltrami B, Nolli G. Flutamide-induced pseudoporphyria. Br J Dermatol 1998;138(4):711–12.
4. Mantoux F, Bahadoran P, Perrin C, Bermon C, Lacour JP, Ortonne JP. Pseudo-porphyrie cutanée tardive induite par le flutamide. [Flutamide-induced late cutaneous pseudoporphyria.] Ann Dermatol Venereol 1999;126(2):150–2.
5. Kouides PA, Abboud CN, Fairbanks VF. Flutamide-induced cyanosis refractory to methylene blue therapy. Br J Haematol 1996;94(1):73–5.
6. Schott AM, Vial T, Gozzo I, Chareyre S, Delmas PD. Flutamide-induced methemoglobinemia. DICP 1991;25(6):600–1.
7. Jackson SH, Barker SJ. Methemoglobinemia in a patient receiving flutamide. Anesthesiology 1995;82(4):1065–7.
8. Khan AM, Singh NT, Bilgrami S. Flutamide induced methemoglobinemia. J Urol 1997;157(4):1363.
9. Schulz M, Schmoldt A, Donn F, Becker H. Lack of methemoglobinemia with flutamide. Ann Pharmacother 2001;35(1):21–5.
10. Langenstroer P, Porter HJ 2nd, McLeod DG, Thrasher JB. Direct gastrointestinal toxicity of flutamide: comparison of irradiated and nonirradiated cases. J Urol 2004;171(2 Pt 1):684–6.
11. Barouk J, Doubremelle M, Faroux R, Schnee M, Lafargue JP. Colite ischémique après prise de flutamide. [Ischemic colitis after taking flutamide.] Gastroenterol Clin Biol 1998;22(10):841.
12. Lubbert C, Wiese M, Haupt R, Ruf BR. Ikterus und schwere Leberfunktionsstorung bei der hormonablativen Behandlung des Prostatakarzinoms. [Toxic hepatitis and liver failure under therapy with flutamide.] Internist (Berl) 2004;45(3):333–40.
13. Famularo G, De Simone C, Minisola G, Nicotra GC. Flutamide-associated acute liver failure. Ann Ital Med Int 2003;18(4):250–3.
14. Kraus I, Vitezic D, Oguic R. Flutamide-induced acute hepatitis in advanced prostate cancer patients. Int J Clin Pharmacol Ther 2001;39(9):395–9.
15. Garcia Cortes M, Andrade RJ, Lucena MI, Sanchez Martinez H, Fernandez MC, Ferrer T, Martin-Vivaldi R, Pelaez G, Suarez F, Romero-Gomez M, Montero JL, Fraga E, Camargo R, Alcantara R, Pizarro MA, Garcia-Ruiz E, Rosemary-Gomez M. Flutamide-induced hepatotoxicity: report of a case series. Rev Esp Enferm Dig 2001;93(7):423–32.
16. Wada T, Ueda M, Abe K, Kobari T, Yamazaki H, Nakata J, Ikemoto I, Ohishi Y, Aizawa Y. [Risk factor of liver disorders caused by flutamide—statistical analysis using multivariate logistic regression analysis.] Hinyokika Kiyo 1999;45(8):521–6.
17. Altiparmak MR, Bilici A, Kisacik B, Ozguroglu M. Flutamide-induced acute renal failure in a patient with metastatic prostate cancer. Med Oncol 2002;19(2):117–19.
18. Tsien C, Souhami L. Flutamide photosensitivity. J Urol 1999;162(2):494.
19. Kaur C, Thami GP. Flutamide-induced photosensitivity: is it a forme fruste of lupus? Br J Dermatol 2003;148(3):603–4.
20. Martin-Lazaro J, Bujan JG, Arrondo AP, Lozano JR, Galindo EC, Capdevila EF. Is photopatch testing useful in the investigation of photosensitivity due to flutamide? Contact Dermatitis 2004;50(5):325–6.
21. Vilaplana J, Romaguera C, Azon A, Lecha M. Flutamide photosensitivity—residual vitiliginous lesions. Contact Dermatitis 1998;38(2):68–70.
22. Rafael JP, Manuel GG, Antonio V, Carlos MJ. Widespread vitiligo after erythroderma caused by photosensitivity to flutamide. Contact Dermatitis 2004;50(2):98–100.
23. Leroy D, Dompmartin A, Szczurko C. Flutamide photosensitivity. Photodermatol Photoimmunol Photomed 1996;12(5):216–18.
24. Yokote R, Tokura Y, Igarashi N, Ishikawa O, Miyachi Y. Photosensitive drug eruption induced by flutamide. Eur J Dermatol 1998;8(6):427–9.
25. Kiratli BJ, Srinivas S, Perkash I, Terris MK. Progressive decrease in bone density over 10 years of androgen deprivation therapy in patients with prostate cancer. Urology 2001;57(1):127–32.
26. Anjum S, Swan SK, Lambrecht LJ, Radwanski E, Cutler DL, Affrime MB, Halstenson CE. Pharmacokinetics of flutamide in patients with renal insufficiency. Br J Clin Pharmacol 1999;47(1):43–7.

Fluvastatin

See also HMG Co-A reductase inhibitors

General Information

It has been suggested that the pharmacokinetics of fluvastatin, including extensive biliary excretion and absence of circulating active metabolites, might be associated with a low incidence of systemic adverse effects compared with other statins. In over 1800 patients treated for an average of 61 weeks, fluvastatin was safe and tolerable (SEDA-19, 408). Pooled data from clinical trials have shown that gastrointestinal symptoms occurred in 14% of fluvastatin recipients compared with 9% taking placebo; other complaints occurred

0.5–5% more often with fluvastatin, including insomnia, sinusitis, hypesthesia, tooth disorders, and urinary tract infections. Fluvastatin was withdrawn because of adverse events in 3.5% of 2585 patients taking monotherapy and in 3.2% of 842 patients taking placebo (1).

Organs and Systems

Liver

Hepatotoxicity has been reported with fluvastatin.

- Cholestatic hepatitis developed in a 71-year-old man with nephrotic syndrome (2). Hepatic function was normal after several months of fluvastatin 20 mg/day. Some weeks after the dose was increased to 40 mg/day, his gamma-glutamyl transpeptidase activity rose from normal to 1818 IU/l, with negative serology for viruses. After normalization, re-introduction of fluvastatin 20 mg/day was not tolerated, but he did tolerate simvastatin 20 mg/day.
- A 61-year-old woman developed symptoms of acute hepatitis 6 weeks after she began to take fluvastatin sodium 20 mg/day for hypercholesterolemia (3). Ultrasonography and liver biopsy confirmed the diagnosis of non-obstructive intrahepatic jaundice. Studies of viral markers and autoimmune factors excluded viral hepatitis and autoimmune hepatitis. There was a high serum concentration of a metabolite of fluvastatin, suggesting a possible anomaly of drug metabolism. All liver function tests normalized 8 weeks after the withdrawal of fluvastatin.

Pancreas

Acute pancreatitis has been attributed to fluvastatin (4).

- A 36-year-old man took fluvastatin 40 mg/day for 3 months and developed mild acute pancreatitis, which settled with medical treatment. Other causes were ruled out. Some months later, he started taking fluvastatin again and had a recurrence of pancreatitis within a few days.

According to the authors, statin-induced acute pancreatitis can occur on the first day of therapy or after several months. It is generally mild and runs a benign course; no deaths have been reported. Its frequency is unknown but it is probably rare.

Musculoskeletal

In a pooled analysis of a large population of patients with hypercholesterolemia taking fluvastatin 20 mg/day, 40 mg/day, and fluvastatin modified-release 80 mg/day, the frequency of significant rises in creatine kinase activity was low and not different from placebo (5). This applied to men and women both above and below the age of 65 years. There were no increases in the frequency of rises in creatine kinase activity with higher doses of fluvastatin.

Immunologic

- A 67-year-old woman had a fatal reaction 1 week after she started to take fluvastatin 20 mg/day. When the drug was withdrawn 10 weeks later, she had arthralgia, myalgia, an erythematous maculopapular rash, and breathlessness due to a widespread alveolitis (6).

Drug Administration

Drug formulations

Once-daily administration of modified-release formulation of fluvastatin 80–320 mg/day was generally safe and well tolerated in 40 patients with primary hypercholesterolemia over 13 days (7). However, fluvastatin 640 mg in this formulation was not well tolerated: six of seven patients had adverse events, including diarrhea, headache, and rises in serum transaminases. In addition, the pharmacokinetics of fluvastatin were non-linear at this dose, possibly because of saturation of first-pass metabolism, causing higher than expected serum drug concentrations.

Drug–Drug Interactions

Bezafibrate

Concomitant administration of fluvastatin and bezafibrate resulted in a 50% increase in the AUC of fluvastatin (SEDA-21, 460).

Ion-exchange resins

The systemic availability of fluvastatin is reduced by bile acid sequestrants (1).

Rifampicin

The systemic availability of fluvastatin is reduced by the hepatic enzyme inducer rifampicin (1).

References

1. Plosker GL, Wagstaff AJ. Fluvastatin: a review of its pharmacology and use in the management of hypercholesterolaemia. Drugs 1996;51(3):433–59.
2. Gascon A, Zabala S, Iglesias E. Acute cholestasis during long-term treatment with fluvastatin in a nephrotic patient. Nephrol Dial Transplant 1999;14(4):1038.
3. Wachi K, Ishii K, Ikehara T, Shinohara M, Kawafune T, Sumino Y, Nonaka H. A case of acute cholestatic hepatitis associated with fluvastatin sodium. J Med Soc Toho 2001;48:153–8.
4. Tysk C, Al-Eryani AY, Shawabkeh AA. Acute pancreatitis induced by fluvastatin therapy. J Clin Gastroenterol 2002;35(5):406–8.
5. Benghozi R, Bortolini M, Jia Y, Isaacsohn JL, Troendle AJ, Gonasun L. Frequency of creatine kinase elevation during treatment with fluvastatin. Am J Cardiol 2002;89(2):231–3.
6. Sridhar MK, Abdulla A. Fatal lupus-like syndrome and ARDS induced by fluvastatin. Lancet 1998;352(9122):114.
7. Sabia H, Prasad P, Smith HT, Stoltz RR, Rothenberg P. Safety, tolerability, and pharmacokinetics of an extended-release formulation of fluvastatin administered once daily to patients with primary hypercholesterolemia. J Cardiovasc Pharmacol 2001;37(5):502–11.

Fluvoxamine

See also Selective serotonin re-uptake inhibitors (SSRIs)

General Information

Fluvoxamine is a non-sedating antidepressant with fewer anticholinergic adverse effects than clomipramine or imipramine (1–3). Its major adverse effects, like those of other SSRIs, include nausea and vomiting. It has a half-life of 15 hours, and peak plasma concentrations occur at 1–8 hours after oral administration (4). It is metabolized (by oxidation, oxidative deamination, and hydrolysis) to nine metabolites, none of which is pharmacologically active (5). Studies of single versus multiple dosing have shown no significant differences (6,7). Usual doses are in the range of 150–300 mg/day, and once-a-day dosing is possible.

Fluvoxamine appears to have no specific effects on laboratory tests (4,8,9); although some have reported a significant fall in platelet count and an increase in serum creatinine, most of the values remained well within the reference ranges (10).

Organs and Systems

Cardiovascular

A slight, clinically unimportant reduction in heart rate has been reported with fluvoxamine (11,12). There has been one report of supraventricular tachycardia in a woman with no previous cardiovascular disease, but the association with fluvoxamine was unclear since there was no rechallenge (SEDA-16, 9).

Nervous system

In a yearlong study of 31 patients there was agitation, which required withdrawal in two patients early in treatment, dry mouth, tremor, and insomnia (13). Increased agitation and insomnia may require the addition of a sedative or hypnotic.

Acute dystonia has been described in association with fluvoxamine (SEDA-18, 20).

Seizures have been reported in a predisposed subject given fluvoxamine (SEDA-17, 20).

Treatment with serotonin-potentiating drugs in usual therapeutic doses can sometimes produce the serotonin syndrome. There are also case reports of this reaction with single doses of SSRIs (see also the monograph on Sertraline) (14).

- An 11-year-old boy was brought to the emergency room about 2 hours after taking a single tablet of fluvoxamine (50 mg) prescribed for treatment of attention-deficit disorder. He was also taking benzatropine and perphenazine (dosages not stated). On arrival, he was agitated and unresponsive, with bilateral ankle clonus, muscle rigidity, fasciculations, and profuse sweating. His temperature rose to 39.7°C. He was paralysed, intubated, and ventilated, after which his condition improved. Two days after admission, he had fully recovered.

The dopamine receptor antagonist properties of perphenazine may have played a part in producing the syndrome in this case.

SSRIs can cause insomnia and daytime somnolence; however, the symptoms seem to reflect a sleep–wake cycle disorder. It is conceivable that disruptions in the normal pattern of melatonin secretion, particularly a delay in the normal early morning fall in plasma concentrations, could be involved in the pathophysiology of these symptoms. The fact that these sleep disorders were seen only with fluvoxamine would also support a role of melatonin (see the section on Endocrine in this monograph).

Psychological, psychiatric

Reports of acute mania and manic-like behavior after treatment with fluoxetine or fluvoxamine have appeared (SEDA-13, 12) (SEDA-17, 20) (SEDA-18, 20), but there are not enough data to estimate the incidence.

Endocrine

Fluvoxamine causes increased plasma melatonin concentrations. In an in vitro preparation, melatonin was metabolized to 6-hydroxymelatonin by CYP1A2, which was inhibited by fluvoxamine at concentrations similar to those found in the plasma during therapy (15). This effect was not shared by other SSRIs or by tricyclic antidepressants, which do not have prominent effects on melatonin secretion. Whether increased concentrations of melatonin and loss of its normal circadian rhythm might cause symptoms is unclear. However, melatonin is believed to play a role in the regulation of circadian rhythms, including entrainment of the sleep–wake cycle. There have been 10 cases of circadian rhythm sleep disorder associated with fluvoxamine (16). All the patients had delayed sleep-phase syndrome, which is characterized by delayed-sleep onset and late awakening. The delay in falling asleep and waking up in the morning was 2.5–4 hours. In nine of the cases withdrawal of fluvoxamine or a reduced dosage led to resolution of the sleep disorder. When the patients were given alternative serotonin potentiating agents, such as clomipramine or fluoxetine, the sleep disorder did not recur.

Serotonin pathways are involved in the regulation of prolactin secretion. Amenorrhea, galactorrhea, and hyperprolactinemia have been reported in a patient who was already taking an antipsychotic drug after starting treatment with fluvoxamine (SEDA-17, 20).

Three cases of fluvoxamine-induced polydipsia, attributed to the syndrome of inappropriate ADH secretion (SIADH), have been reported (SEDA-18, 20).

Hematologic

Fluvoxamine-associated bleeding has been described (17–19).

Skin

A case of toxic epidermal necrolysis after fluvoxamine has been described; although the patient was taking other drugs, the authors concluded that the skin reaction was probably due to fluvoxamine (SEDA-18, 20).

Hair

Hair loss has been associated with fluvoxamine (20).

Long-Term Effects

Drug withdrawal

Withdrawal symptoms have been reported with fluvoxamine (SEDA-17, 20) (SEDA-18, 21).

Second-Generation Effects

Lactation

In two cases, treatment of breast-feeding mothers with fluvoxamine (300 mg/day) was associated with undetectable concentrations of fluvoxamine (below 2.5 ng/ml) in the plasma of both infants (21). These results are encouraging, but further data will be needed before it can be concluded that fluvoxamine has an advantage over other SSRIs in this respect.

Drug Administrations

Drug overdose

There have been four cases of overdosage with fluvoxamine in amounts ranging from 600 to 2500 mg (22).

Drug–Drug Interactions

Buspirone

In 10 healthy volunteers, fluvoxamine (100 mg/day for 5 days) significantly increased the peak concentrations of the anxiolytic drug buspirone. Concentrations of the active metabolite, 1-(2-pyrimidinyl)-piperazine, were reduced (23). These effects were probably mediated through inhibition of CYP3A4 by fluvoxamine.

Clozapine

In a prospective study fluvoxamine, in a low dosage of 50 mg/day, produced a threefold increase in plasma clozapine concentrations ($n = 16$) (24).

Other reports have confirmed that fluvoxamine increases plasma concentrations of clozapine and its metabolites (25,26) (SEDA-21, 12). The mechanism is probably inhibition of CYP1A2.

Methadone

Fluvoxamine increases methadone concentrations in patients taking methadone maintenance treatment for the management of opioid dependence (SEDA-19, 11). The addition of sertraline (200 mg/day) produced a modest (16%) increase in methadone concentrations in 31 depressed opioid-dependent subjects after 6 but not 12 weeks of combined treatment (27). The increase in methadone concentrations was more modest than that reported with fluvoxamine, presumably because sertraline is a less potent inhibitor of CYP1A2 and CYP3A4, both of which are involved in methadone metabolism.

Olanzapine

The atypical antipsychotic drug olanzapine is also metabolized by CYP1A2.

- A 21-year-old woman with schizophrenia and depression, who had been taking fluvoxamine (150 mg/day) and olanzapine (15 mg/day) for several months, developed an extrapyramidal movement disorder, including rigidity and tremor (28). The plasma fluvoxamine concentration was 70 ng/ml (usual target range is 20–500 ng/ml), while that of olanzapine was 120 ng/ml (usual target range is 9–25 ng/ml). The dosage of olanzapine was reduced to 5 mg/day and the plasma olanzapine concentration fell to 38 ng/ml, with resolution of the tremor and rigidity. When fluvoxamine was replaced with paroxetine (20 mg/day) the olanzapine concentration fell further to 22 ng/ml.

Of the SSRIs, fluvoxamine is the most potent inhibitor of CYP1A2 and is therefore likely to increase plasma olanzapine concentrations. The extrapyramidal effects in this case were presumably due to excessive blockade of dopamine D_2 receptors by raised olanzapine concentrations.

Phenytoin

Fluvoxamine inhibits CYP2C9 and CYP2C19, the enzymes responsible for the metabolism of phenytoin.

- A 45-year-old woman taking phenytoin 300 mg/day had a plasma phenytoin concentration of 66 μmol/l (29). When she became depressed fluvoxamine 50 mg/day was added. A month later her depressive symptoms had improved, but she was ataxic and the plasma phenytoin concentration was 196 μmol/l. The fluvoxamine was withdrawn and the phenytoin dose reduced to 150 mg/day. Her plasma phenytoin concentration fell to 99 μmol/l, with resolution of the ataxia.

In vitro studies suggest that fluvoxamine is the most potent SSRI in terms of its ability to inhibit phenytoin metabolism. Inhibition of CYP2C19 or CYP2C9 could be responsible, although fluvoxamine is a relatively weak in vitro inhibitor of CYP2C9. However, in 14 healthy volunteers fluvoxamine (150–300 mg/day for 5 days) significantly reduced the clearance of tolbutamide (30). This suggests that fluvoxamine should be used with caution when it is co-administered with drugs such as tolbutamide, phenytoin, and warfarin, which are substrates for CYP2C9.

Thioridazine

Fluvoxamine inhibits CYP1A2, and a low dosage (50 mg/day) produced a 225% increase in plasma thioridazine concentrations in 10 patients with schizophrenia (31). This was not reflected in an increased incidence of clinical adverse events; however, thioridazine prolongs the QT_c interval, which was not measured.

Tolbutamide

In 14 healthy volunteers fluvoxamine (150–300 mg/day for 5 days) significantly reduced the clearance of tolbutamide (30). This suggests that fluvoxamine should be used with caution when it is co-administered with drugs that are substrates for CYP2C9, such as tolbutamide, phenytoin, and warfarin.

Tricyclic antidepressants

Fluvoxamine is a potent inhibitor of cytochrome CYP1A2, which may lead to interactions with several tricyclic antidepressants and theophylline (32).

References

1. De Wilde JE, Mertens C, Wakelin JS. Clinical trials of fluvoxamine vs chlorimipramine with single and three times daily dosing. Br J Clin Pharmacol 1983;15(Suppl. 3):427S–31S.
2. Itil TM, Shrivastava RK, Mukherjee S, Coleman BS, Michael ST. A double-blind placebo-controlled study of fluvoxamine and imipramine in out-patients with primary depression. Br J Clin Pharmacol 1983;15(Suppl. 3):433S–8S.
3. Klok CJ, Brouwer GJ, van Praag HM, Doogan D. Fluvoxamine and clomipramine in depressed patients. A double-blind clinical study. Acta Psychiatr Scand 1981;64(1):1–11.
4. Claassen V. Review of the animal pharmacology and pharmacokinetics of fluvoxamine. Br J Clin Pharmacol 1983;15(Suppl. 3):349S–55S.
5. Kinney-Parker JL, Smith D, Ingle SF. Fluoxetine and weight: something lost and something gained? Clin Pharm 1989;8(10):727–33.
6. Doogan DP. Fluvoxamine as an antidepressant drug. Neuropharmacology 1980;19(12):1215–16.
7. Siddiqui UA, Chakravarti SK, Jesinger DK. The tolerance and antidepressive activity of fluvoxamine as a single dose compared to a twice daily dose. Curr Med Res Opin 1985;9(10):681–90.
8. Coleman BS, Block BA. Fluvoxamine maleate, a serotonergic antidepressant; a comparison with chlorimipramine. Prog Neuropsychopharmacol Biol Psychiatry 1982;6(4–6):475–8.
9. De Wilde JE, Doogan DP. Fluvoxamine and chlorimipramine in endogenous depression. J Affect Disord 1982;4(3):249–59.
10. Guelfi JD, Dreyfus JF, Pichot P. A double-blind controlled clinical trial comparing fluvoxamine with imipramine. Br J Clin Pharmacol 1983;15(Suppl. 3):411S–17S.
11. Roos JC. Cardiac effects of antidepressant drugs. A comparison of the tricyclic antidepressants and fluvoxamine. Br J Clin Pharmacol 1983;15(Suppl. 3):439S–45S.
12. Robinson JF, Doogan DP. A placebo controlled study of the cardiovascular effects of fluvoxamine and clovoxamine in human volunteers. Br J Clin Pharmacol 1982;4(6):805–8.
13. Feldmann HS, Denber HC. Long-term study of fluvoxamine: a new rapid-acting antidepressant. Int Pharmacopsychiatry 1982;17(2):114–22.
14. Gill M, LoVecchio F, Selden B. Serotonin syndrome in a child after a single dose of fluvoxamine. Ann Emerg Med 1999;33(4):457–9.
15. Peterson MC. Reversible galactorrhea and prolactin elevation related to fluoxetine use. Mayo Clin Proc 2001;76(2):215–16.
16. Morrison J, Remick RA, Leung M, Wrixon KJ, Bebb RA. Galactorrhea induced by paroxetine. Can J Psychiatry 2001;46(1):88–9.
17. Calhoun JW, Calhoun DD. Two other published reports describing fluvoxamine-associated bleeding.
18. Leung M, Shore R. Fluvoxamine-associated bleeding. Can J Psychiatry 1996;41(9):604–5.
19. Wilmshurst PT, Kumar AV. Subhyaloid haemorrhage with fluoxetine. Eye 1996;10(Pt 1):141.
20. Parameshwar E. Hair loss associated with fluvoxamine use. Am J Psychiatry 1996;153(4):581–2.
21. Piontek CM, Wisner KL, Perel JM, Peindl KS. Serum fluvoxamine levels in breastfed infants. J Clin Psychiatry 2001;62(2):111–13.
22. Bradford LD, Coleman BS, Hoeve L. Summary of the properties of fluvoxamine maleate. Duphar Report no. H114.058. 1984.
23. Lamberg TS, Kivisto KT, Laitila J, Martensson K, Neuvonen PJ. The effect of fluvoxamine on the pharmacokinetics and pharmacodynamics of buspirone. Eur J Clin Pharmacol 1998;54(9–10):761–6.
24. Wetzel H, Anghelescu I, Szegedi A, Wiesner J, Weigmann H, Harter S, Hiemke C. Pharmacokinetic interactions of clozapine with selective serotonin reuptake inhibitors: differential effects of fluvoxamine and paroxetine in a prospective study. J Clin Psychopharmacol 1998;18(1):2–9.
25. Fabrazzo M, La Pia S, Monteleone P, Mennella R, Esposito G, Pinto A, Maj M. Fluvoxamine increases plasma and urinary levels of clozapine and its major metabolites in a time- and dose-dependent manner. J Clin Psychopharmacol 2000;20(6):708–10.
26. Lu ML, Lane HY, Chen KP, Jann MW, Su MH, Chang WH. Fluvoxamine reduces the clozapine dosage needed in refractory schizophrenic patients. J Clin Psychiatry 2000;61(8):594–9.
27. Hamilton SP, Nunes EV, Janal M, Weber L. The effect of sertraline on methadone plasma levels in methadone-maintenance patients. Am J Addict 2000;9(1):63–9.
28. de Jong J, Hoogenboom B, van Troostwijk LD, de Haan L. Interaction of olanzapine with fluvoxamine. Psychopharmacology (Berl) 2001;155(2):219–20.
29. Mamiya K, Kojima K, Yukawa E, Higuchi S, Ieiri I, Ninomiya H, Tashiro N. Phenytoin intoxication induced by fluvoxamine. Ther Drug Monit 2001;23(1):75–7.
30. Madsen H, Enggaard TP, Hansen LL, Klitgaard NA, Brosen K. Fluvoxamine inhibits the CYP2C9 catalysed biotransformation of tolbutamide. Clin Pharmacol Ther 2001;69(1):41–7.
31. Carrillo JA, Ramos SI, Herraiz AG, Llerena A, Agundez JA, Berecz R, Duran M, Benitez J. Pharmacokinetic interaction of fluvoxamine and thioridazine in schizophrenic patients. J Clin Psychopharmacol 1999;19(6):494–9.
32. Barnes TR, Kidger T, Greenwood DT. Viloxazine and migraine. Lancet 1979;2(8156–8157):1368.

Folic acid, folinic acid, and calcium folinate

See also Vitamins

General Information

Folic acid (pteroylglutamic acid) is a vitamin of the B group, whose Average Dietary Requirement in adults has been set at 140 micrograms/day, with a Population Reference Intake of 200 micrograms/day. Red cell folate concentrations above 150 ng/ml indicate sufficiency (1). However, higher doses are used for specific purposes, including in pregnancy, apparently without ill effects. Neural tube defects can be prevented in offspring by periconceptual ingestion of

400 micrograms/day (2). One aspect of folate metabolism concerns the recycling of the putatively atherogenic amino acid, homocysteine (3). For reasons that are not clear, homocysteine accumulates in the blood of dialysis patients, and this accumulation is inversely related to folate status. Because of the association of folate with a risk factor for atherosclerosis—it is the major cause of morbidity and mortality in dialysis patients—folate supplementation has been widely recommended as a strategy to reduce homocysteine concentrations, and a daily dose of 800 micrograms has been proposed as part of a mass strategy to reduce the risk of heart attacks and strokes by over 80% (4).

Folinic acid is a reduced form of folic acid. The adverse effects of antifolate drugs that are tetrahydrofolate reductase inhibitors, such as methotrexate, cannot be prevented by giving folic acid, since antifolate drugs inhibit the conversion of folic acid to folinic acid. Folinic acid is therefore given instead, as calcium folinate (leucovorin). However, in patients who take antifolate drugs intermittently (for example methotrexate once a week in psoriasis or rheumatoid arthritis) folic acid taken on another day is adequate.

Recommendations that women who plan to become or have just become pregnant should take daily oral folic acid supplements in order to prevent neural tube defects were issued by health authorities in several European countries from 1991 onwards (5). The recommendations generally follow the lead of the US Public Health authorities which recommended a supplementation dose of 400 micrograms/day (6). This is what a woman would consume if she followed the US Dietary Guidelines and Dietary Pyramid (7). The etiology of neural tube defects is not entirely clear; the condition may have several different causes, only some of which may be responsive to folate (8,9). Rates of neural tube defects vary considerably between countries; in the USA rates of neural tube defects isolated from other birth anomalies fell over the period 1968–89 (10). The justification for a recommendation for general high-dose supplementation or food fortification is still under discussion (11). The debate elicited by this recommendation has spurred interest in possible adverse effects, and a thorough review published in 1998 (12) identified the following potential safety issues of folic acid supplementation in addition to those mentioned above: folate neurotoxicity, reduced zinc absorption, association with malignant neoplasms, hypersensitivity reactions, and increased susceptibility to malaria. However, the data are weak and consist predominantly of case series and individual reports. Furthermore, it is likely that even if such adverse effects did occur, the benefit to harm balance would still be highly favorable.

The main argument against an increase in folic acid supply to the population as a whole is the possible masking of vitamin B_{12} deficiency by normalization of the blood count (see the section *Does folic acid mask vitamin B_{12} deficiency?* in this monograph). However, while certain animal findings and some case reports have actually suggested worsening of the neurological effects of vitamin B_{12} deficiency when patients are treated with folic acid, these do not prove a causal relation (see the section *Does folic acid enhance the neurological symptoms of vitamin B_{12} deficiency?* in this monograph). Nevertheless, because the available data do not exclude such an effect, in the US-Canadian "Dietary Reference Intakes" in adults the upper limit has been set at 1000 micrograms/day folic acid in supplements or enriched food preparations and in children (1–18 years of age) the upper limit has been set at 300–800 micrograms. At doses of 5 mg/day in more than 100 patients there was progression of neurological complications, but there have only been eight case reports of the effect of lower doses of folic acid. Because there is no NOAEL (no observed adverse effect level), a LOAEL (lowest observed adverse effect level) of 5 mg/day had to be used for the upper limit. In contrast, in 1996 the FDA fixed an upper limit of 1000 micrograms/day folic acid (natural and synthetic preparations) (6,13). It was also argued that in children of vegetarians natural folate had masked vitamin B_{12} deficiency. These previous values have now been re-evaluated by the FDA. Dietary supplementation with both folic acid and vitamin B_{12} offers a solution to this problem. No risks of increasing the supply of vitamin B_{12} are expected, but the dosage that would correct vitamin B_{12} deficiency remains to be defined (6,12).

General adverse effects

Negative effects resulting from dietary intake of high concentrations of folic acid have only rarely been documented in some older case reports and uncontrolled intervention studies. Some of these negative effects were not confirmed in subsequent randomized, controlled intervention studies (14).

In humans the toxicity of folic acid is low, even after long-term use (12,15,16). Only in one trial in 14 volunteers (six women, eight men, aged 22–57 years) were there adverse effects, such as gastrointestinal disturbances, insomnia, irritability, or depressive states (17). As a possible cause the authors suggested a high folic acid concentration in the cerebrospinal fluid (5–10 times higher than that in serum). However, these findings were not confirmed in subsequent trials with high-dose folic acid supplementation.

Does folic acid mask vitamin B_{12} deficiency?

Vitamin B_{12} deficiency most frequently is seen in people over 60 years of age (11). Deficiency of vitamin B_{12} in younger adults is rare, but can occur as a result of reduced absorption of vitamin B_{12}, for example in pernicious anemia, atrophic gastritis type B, long-term use of blockers of acid secretion, or short bowel syndrome after resection of the terminal ileum (18,19). Vitamin B_{12} deficiency in children usually depends on inborn defects of vitamin B_{12} metabolism or on insufficient support during pregnancy and breastfeeding.

Vitamin B_{12} deficiency can present as hematological, gastrointestinal, and neurological disturbances. The anemia of B_{12} deficiency is actually due to functional deficiency of folic acid, and results from accumulation of folic acid derivatives in the form of 5-methyltetrahydrofolate, which prevents regeneration of tetrahydrofolic acid and consequently, by interfering with the synthesis of purines and DNA, reduces cell proliferation. Therefore, giving folic acid to patients with vitamin B_{12} deficiency can abolish the hematological effects but will not affect the neurological symptoms. Normalization of the blood count requires high doses of folic acid in the absence of B_{12} replacement therapy. Treatment with folic acid 0.3–1 mg/day normalizes the blood count in 50% of patients with B_{12} deficiency, while at doses over 5 mg/day the hematological changes are normalized in most patients (20). However, the hematological effects can recur, even after treatment with high doses of folic acid (5–500 mg/day), if the vitamin B_{12} deficiency is not treated.

Concerning possible masking of vitamin B_{12} deficiency by folic acid, blood counts in 11–33% of the patients with neurological symptoms of vitamin B_{12} deficiency are in the reference range. That means that in patients with severe funicular myelosis, a vitamin B_{12} deficiency psychosis, changes in the blood count may not occur, while on the other hand in patients with severe pernicious anemia neurological symptoms are not inevitably present.

Organs and Systems

Nervous system

Does folic acid enhance the neurological symptoms of vitamin B_{12} deficiency?

The results of some animal experiments and case reports have suggested that high doses of folic acid can enhance or worsen the neurological effects of vitamin B_{12} deficiency. Thus, in animals with vitamin B_{12} deficiency being treated with folic acid, neurotoxicity developed more rapidly than in the untreated controls (21–23). Some unproven hypotheses about how folic acid could enhance the neurological symptoms of vitamin B_{12} deficiency have been discussed, for example redistribution of B_{12} from the nervous system into the bone marrow, accompanied by a fall in serum concentration and reticulocytosis (20). There have also been some reports that in patients with vitamin B_{12} deficiency neurological complications occurred for the first time or increased in severity when folic acid was given, the severity and onset of the complications correlating with the dose of folic acid.

Whether folic acid is responsible for these observations or whether the neuropathy depends on progressive vitamin B_{12} deficiency and simply coincides with the administration of high doses of folic acid cannot be determined from these reports. In patients who were treated beforehand with liver extracts the neurological changes were weaker and occurred later than in patients who were treated with folic acid exclusively. This suggests that progressive reduction in cobalamin pools is as important for the development of the neurological complications as the supply of folic acid. Furthermore, rapid worsening of neurological changes in patients with cobalamin deficiency has also been seen in patients who have not received folic acid.

Because there have been no double-blind, placebo-controlled intervention studies of the effect of folic acid, the question of whether folic acid in patients with vitamin B_{12} deficiency aggravates the neurological complications cannot be answered definitively. From the data at hand we cannot exclude the possibility that folic acid may exacerbate the effects of vitamin B_{12} deficiency. For that reason an upper limit of 1 mg/day folic acid (in supplements or a vitamin-enriched diet) has been set in the "Dietary Reference Intakes" (15).

Folic acid and seizures

In patients with a history of seizures, worsening of the seizures and an increase in their frequency have been reported in relation to folic acid (24).

- A 26-year-old woman with a family history of spinal amyotrophy and multiple sclerosis sought prepregnancy counselling and was given folic acid 800 micrograms/day to prevent neural tube defects. At 2 years of age, 6 months after a chickenpox infection, she had had recurrent fits and language regression, successfully treated with ethosuximide. At 12 years of age she developed seizures nearly every month, characterized by sensations of fear, loss of contact, fixed eyes, motor automatism, and post-ictal aphasia. This had responded to carbamazepine. After starting to take folic acid she had a generalized tonic-clonic seizure for the first time and a significant increase in seizure frequency.

There has been some discussion as to whether an adverse effect of folic acid on seizures represents a direct epileptogenic effect or results from interference with the effects of anticonvulsants. Initially, it was supposed that folic acid provokes seizures, and the first report of an epileptic patient with megaloblastic anemia in whom folate therapy resulted in an exacerbation of seizures was published in 1960. Although several subsequent controlled studies failed to show any adverse effect on seizure frequency linked to folic acid supplementation, case reports and uncontrolled studies have documented worsening seizure frequency in some patients given folic acid, but the susceptibility factors at play have not been identified.

Antiepileptic drugs reduce serum folate concentrations. Conversely, the use of folic acid can reduce the effects of antiepileptic drugs such as phenytoin and can reduce their serum concentrations (25,26).

Besides its effect on antiepileptic drugs, folic acid in animal experiments was neurotoxic and epileptogenic (27). However, when the neurotoxicity of folic acid was investigated in two groups of patients—the newborns of mothers who had taken folic acid during pregnancy and patients with parkinsonian syndromes—neurotoxicity was not found in either group (12).

Metal metabolism

The authors of the "Dietary Reference Intakes" (15) have concluded that reports of the effect of folic acid supplementation on the intestinal absorption of zinc are controversial, but that the recent literature shows that folic acid supplementation has either no effect or an extremely weak effect on zinc supply.

Hematologic

High doses of folic acid and vitamin B_{12} increase the reticulocyte count. Use of either of these vitamins can therefore mask a deficiency of the other (SEDA 17, 440). If anemia due to deficiency of either of these nutrients is suspected, serum concentrations of both vitamin B_{12} and folic acid should be assessed (28).

Immunologic

There have been some reports of hypersensitivity after oral, parenteral, and intradermal administration of folic acid, and a case has recently been reported with folinic acid (29).

- An 80-year-old woman had a colonic resection for Duke's C stage adenocarcinoma and was then given fluorouracil 400 mg/m^2/day and folinic acid 200 mg/m^2/day for 5 days every 4 weeks. She later developed metastases and a second course of chemotherapy included irinotecan (180 mg/m^2), fluorouracil 400 mg/m^2, followed by a continuous infusion of 2400 mg/m^2 over 2 days, folinic acid 200 mg/m^2, ondansetron, and atropine. During the first course of chemotherapy she developed urticaria following the administration of ondansetron and folinic acid. The ondansetron was withdrawn and replaced by metoclopramide and prednisone. During the next course, just after the administration of folinic acid, metoclopramide, and prednisone, she had more urticaria and profound hypotension and required intravenous adrenaline. Folinic acid was withdrawn and subsequent courses were uneventful.

Using a published method (30) the reaction in this case was considered to be very probably due to folinic acid.

IgE-antibodies to folic acid have been demonstrated in a woman with anaphylactic reactions to two multivitamin formulations containing folic acid (31).

Long-Term Effects

Tumorigenicity

In a large US cohort study folic acid was associated with an increased risk of cancer in general and of cancers of the oropharynx and hypopharynx (32). However, the authors pointed to the possibility that the observed association could have depended on confounding by alcohol and smoking.

Second-Generation Effects

Pregnancy

High doses of folic acid (commonly 4–5 mg) have been used in pregnancy to prevent neural tube defects, without apparent ill effects (33). In a non-randomized, Swedish study in 2569 women the number of twin births in those who took folic acid supplements during early pregnancy was increased (34). In those who took folic acid the rate of twin births was 2.8% compared with 1.5% overall. However, in the large, randomized, multicenter MRC study with high doses of folic acid (4 mg/day) there was no increase in the frequency of twin births (33). Because of the higher rate of complications in twin pregnancies and twin births, the authors suggested that folic acid prophylaxis in countries with low frequencies of spina bifida might be harmful rather than useful. Similar results have also been seen in other studies (35,36).

Drug–Drug Interactions

Anticonvulsant drugs

An interaction of anticonvulsant drugs with the metabolism of folate has been described (SEDA-13, 348) (see also the section on *Nervous system* in this monograph).

Folic acid can alter the metabolism of phenytoin. In one case folic acid 5 mg/day reduced the serum phenytoin concentration to below the target range, and a breakthrough seizure occurred (25). The Km of phenytoin metabolism was significantly reduced, suggesting competitive inhibition of metabolism. In another series folic acid reduced the serum concentrations of phenytoin (37). Furthermore, the administration of folic acid to treat folate deficiency can reduce the beneficial effects of anticonvulsants (38). Rare but serious cases in which this epileptogenic effect of folic acid has been very pronounced have been reported (39). However, folic acid is well tolerated by many other patients with epilepsy who require folic acid.

Fluorouracil

Reduced folates are co-factors for the 5-fluorodeoxyuridine monophosphate-thymidilate synthetase reaction. Leucovorin (calcium folinate) therefore potentiates the toxicity of 5-fluorouracil, and fatal adverse effects have been reported in patients over 65 years of age receiving high-dose treatment with leucovorin simultaneously with fluorouracil. This has led some groups to recommend that initial dose levels of fluorouracil should be lowered by 20% and that therapy be stopped temporarily at the first sign of distal gastrointestinal adverse effects (SEDA-15, 414).

Methotrexate

Methotrexate is an antagonist of folic acid and is used for treating neoplastic diseases and non-neoplastic diseases such as rheumatoid arthritis and psoriasis. As methotrexate reduces the activity of dihydrofolate reductase, supplementation with folic acid and especially with folinic acid could reduce the beneficial effects of methotrexate. This assumption has been supported by the results of an intervention study (40). Patients with rheumatoid arthritis treated with methotrexate (15 g/week) had an increase in symptoms. An open intervention trial of folinic acid 45 mg/week also showed an increase in arthritis symptoms (41). However, other trials showed no effects of this sort, and administration of folic acid or folinic acid is important in preventing methotrexate-induced blood dyscrasias.

References

1. Chanarin I. The Megaloblastic Anaemias. 2nd ed. Oxford: Blackwell Scientific Publications, 1979.
2. Oakley GP Jr, Johnston RB Jr. Balancing benefits and harms in public health prevention programmes mandated by governments. BMJ 2004;329(7456):41–3.
3. Westhuyzen J. Folate supplementation in the dialysis patient—fragmentary evidence and tentative recommendations. Nephrol Dial Transplant 1998;13(11):2748–50.
4. Wald NJ, Law MR. A strategy to reduce cardiovascular disease by more than 80%. BMJ 2003;326(7404):1419.

5. Acheson D, Poole AAB. Folic acid in the prevention of neural tube defect. Circular letter to all doctors in England. Issued by the Department of Health. London, 1991.
6. United States Public Heath Service. US Public Health Says B Vitamin Can Cut Birth Defects Risk (Press release). 14/09/1992.
7. Scott JM, Kirke P, O'Broin S, Weir DG, et al. Folic acid to prevent neural tube defects. Lancet 1991;338(8765):505–6.
8. Holmes LB. Prevention of neural tube defects. J Pediatr 1992;120(6):918–19.
9. Gaull GE, Testa CA, Thomas PR, Weinreich DA. Fortification of the food supply with folic acid to prevent neural tube defects is not yet warranted. J Nutr 1996;126(3):S773–80.
10. Yen IH, Khoury MJ, Erickson JD, James LM, Waters GD, Berry RJ. The changing epidemiology of neural tube defects. United States, 1968–1989. Am J Dis Child 1992;146(7):857–61.
11. Rothenberg SP. Increasing the dietary intake of folate: pros and cons. Semin Hematol 1999;36(1):65–74.
12. Campbell NR. How safe are folic acid supplements? Arch Intern Med 1996;156(15):1638–44.
13. FDA (Food and Drug Administration). Food additives permitted for direct addition to food for human consumption; folic acid (folacin). Federal Register, Rules and Regulations 1996;61:8797–807. Internet release: http://vm.cfsan.fda.gov/~lrd/fr96305c.html.
14. Eichholzer M, Luthy J, Moser U, Stahelin HB, Gutzwiller F. Sicherheitsaspekte der Folsäure fur die Gesamtbevolkerung. [Safety aspects of folic acid for the general population.] Schweiz Rundsch Med Prax 2002;91(1–2):7–16.
15. Standing Committee on the Scientific Evaluation of Dietary Reference Intakes and its Panel on Folate, other B vitamins, and Choline and Subcommittee on Upper Reference Levels of Nutrients. Dietary reference intakes for thiamin, riboflavin, niacin, vitamin B6, folate, vitamin B12, pantothenic acid, biotin, and choline. Washington DC: National Academy Press, 1998.
16. Bässler KH, Golly I, Loew D, Pietrzik K. Vitamin-Lexikon. Stuttgart, Jena, Lubeck, Ulm: Fischer Verlag, 1999.
17. Hunter R, Barnes J, Oakeley HF, Matthews DM. Toxicity of folic acid given in pharmacological doses to healthy volunteers. Lancet 1970;1(7637):61–3.
18. Bayer W, Schmidt K. Vitamine in Prävention und Therapie. Stuttgart: Hippokrates, 1991.
19. Bachli E, Fehr J. Diagnose eines Vitamin-B12—Mangels nur scheinbar ein Kinderspiel. [Diagnosis of vitamin B12 deficiency: only apparently child's play.] Schweiz Med Wochenschr 1999;129(23):861–72.
20. Savage DG, Lindenbaum J. Folate–cobalamin interactions. In: Bailey LB, editor. Folate in Health and Disease. New York: Marcel Dekker Inc, 1994:237–85.
21. Agamanolis DP, Chester EM, Victor M, Kark JA, Hines JD, Harris JW. Neuropathology of experimental vitamin B12 deficiency in monkeys. Neurology 1976;26(10):905–14.
22. van der Westhuyzen J, Metz J. Tissue S-adenosylmethionine levels in fruit bats (*Rousettus aegyptiacus*) with nitrous oxide-induced neuropathy. Br J Nutr 1983;50(2):325–30.
23. van der Westhuyzen J, Fernandes-Costa F, Metz J. Cobalamin inactivation by nitrous oxide produces severe neurological impairment in fruit bats : protection by methionine and aggravation by folates. Life Sci 1982;31(18):2001–10.
24. Guidolin L, Vignoli A, Canger R. Worsening in seizure frequency and severity in relation to folic acid administration. Eur J Neurol 1998;5(3):301–3.
25. Seligmann H, Potasman I, Weller B, Schwartz M, Prokocimer M. Phenytoin–folic acid interaction: a lesson to be learned. Clin Neuropharmacol 1999;22(5):268–72.
26. Furlanut M, Benetello P, Avogaro A, Dainese R. Effects of folic acid on phenytoin kinetics in healthy subjects. Clin Pharmacol Ther 1978;24(3):294–7.
27. Weller M, Marini AM, Martin B, Paul SM. The reduced unsubstituted pteroate moiety is required for folate toxicity of cultured cerebellar granule neurons. J Pharmacol Exp Ther 1994;269(1):393–401.
28. Wald NJ, Bower C. Folic acid and the prevention of neural tube defects. BMJ 1995;310(6986):1019–20.
29. Benchalal M, Yahchouchy-Chouillard E, Fouere S, Fingerhut A. Anaphylactic shock secondary to intravenous administration of folinic acid: a first report. Ann Oncol 2002;13(3):480–1.
30. Moore N, Biour M, Paux G, Loupi E, Begaud B, Boismare F, Royer RJ. Adverse drug reaction monitoring: doing it the French way. Lancet 1985;2(8463):1056–8.
31. Dykewicz MS, Orfan NA, Sun W. In vitro demonstration of IgE antibody to folate–albumin in anaphylaxis from folic acid. J Allergy Clin Immunol 2000;106(2):386–9.
32. Selby JV, Friedman GD, Fireman BH. Screening prescription drugs for possible carcinogenicity: eleven to fifteen years of follow-up. Cancer Res 1989;49(20):5736–47.
33. Mathews F, Murphy M, Wald NJ, Hackshaw A. Twinning and folic acid use. Lancet 1999;353(9149):291–2.
34. Ericson A, Kallen B, Aberg A. Use of multivitamins and folic acid in early pregnancy and multiple births in Sweden. Twin Res 2001;4(2):63–6.
35. Czeizel AE, Metneki J, Dudas I. Higher rate of multiple births after periconceptional vitamin supplementation. N Engl J Med 1994;330(23):1687–8.
36. Werler MM, Cragan JD, Wasserman CR, Shaw GM, Erickson JD, Mitchell AA. Multivitamin supplementation and multiple births. Am J Med Genet 1997;71(1):93–6.
37. Baylis EM, Crowley JM, Preece JM, Sylvester PE, Marks V. Influence of folic acid on blood-phenytoin levels. Lancet 1971;1(7689):62–4.
38. Reynolds EH. Effects of folic acid on the mental state and fit-frequency of drug-treated epileptic patients. Lancet 1967;1(7499):1086–8.
39. Bramanti P, Ricci RM, Bagala S, Candela L, De Luca GP, Di Bella P, Di Perri R. Does folic acid exert a provocative action on the EEG of epileptic patients? A preliminary report. Acta Neurol (Napoli) 1987;9(4):250–5.
40. Joyce DA, Will RK, Hoffman DM, Laing B, Blackbourn SJ. Exacerbation of rheumatoid arthritis in patients treated with methotrexate after administration of folinic acid. Ann Rheum Dis 1991;50(12):913–14.
41. Tishler M, Caspi D, Fishel B, Yaron M. The effects of leucovorin (folinic acid) on methotrexate therapy in rheumatoid arthritis patients. Arthritis Rheum 1988;31(7):906–8.

Follitropin

General Information

The first gonadotropins available for clinical use were extracted from the urine of postmenopausal women. Human menopausal gonadotropin (hMG) is in limited supply and contains other proteins, which may be allergenic, as well as luteinizing hormone. Purified preparations of follicle-stimulating hormone (FSH; urofollitropin and highly purified urofollitropin) are also extracted from human urine. Recombinant FSH (follitropin-alfa) prepared from a Chinese hamster ovarian cell line is likely to replace other gonadotropins because of its purity and ease of patient self-administration.

Follitropin treatment for infertility has been reviewed in detail (1,2). Multiple pregnancy occurs in 20% of patients, 80% being twin pregnancies. There is no documented increase in congenital abnormalities in children conceived after ovulation induction with follitropin.

Organs and Systems

Nervous system

- A 32-year-old woman who was not obese developed benign intracranial hypertension in association with ovarian hyperstimulation syndrome after ovulation induction using goserelin, follitropin, and human chorionic gonadotropin (hCG) (3). The syndrome did not recur during a second pregnancy in which follitropin and hCG were not used

Reproductive system

Ovarian hyperstimulation syndrome (OHSS) is characterized by massive ovarian enlargement and fluid shift from the intravascular space to the peritoneal, pleural, and pericardial cavities. Rates of up to 20% for all grades and 1–2% for severe OHSS have been documented and do not differ between preparations of follitropin. Women with polycystic ovarian syndrome are at higher risk of this complication. In rare cases women have died of pulmonary embolism, disseminated intravascular coagulation, or adult respiratory distress syndrome. If the patient is pregnant, OHSS is more severe and prolonged (1). Generally, it resolves within 7 days if the patient is not pregnant or in 10–20 days if she is. The underlying cause of this adverse effect is not known.

References

1. Vollenhoven BJ, Healy DL. Short- and long-term effects of ovulation induction. Endocrinol Metab Clin North Am 1998;27(4):903–14.
2. Goa KL, Wagstaff AJ. Follitropin alpha in infertility. Biodrugs 1998;9:235–60.
3. Lesny P, Maguiness SD, Hay DM, Robinson J, Clarke CE, Killick SR. Ovarian hyperstimulation syndrome and benign intracranial hypertension in pregnancy after in-vitro fertilization and embryo transfer: case report. Hum Reprod 1999;14(8):1953–5.

Fomivirsen

General Information

Fomivirsen (ISIS 2922) is an antisense oligonucleotide that specifically inhibits replication of human cytomegalovirus. It has been developed for intravitreal administration to treat cytomegalovirus retinitis in patients with AIDS.

Organs and Systems

Sensory systems

The most common adverse effects of fomivirsen reported in clinical trials have been increased intraocular pressure and mild to moderate uveitis (1,2). These events were generally transient or reversible with topical glucocorticoids.

In 150 patients who were given intravitreous fomivirsen 165 micrograms/injection (35 eyes, 30 patients) or two different regimens of 330 micrograms/injection (142 eyes, 110 patients), anterior chamber inflammation and increased intraocular pressure were dose-related and schedule-dependent: 165 micrograms/injection, 4.1 events/patient-year; 330 micrograms/injection, 6.6 events/patient-year (less intense regimen) and 8.4 events/patient-year (more intense regimen) (3). A large number of other ocular adverse events may not have been related to the drug.

In 309 eyes of 238 patients there were two cases of bull's-eye maculopathy, which resolved after withdrawal (4).

Retinal pigment epithelial changes have been noted at doses of fomivirsen that overlap with those used to treat CMV retinitis (2). In one case there was nyctalopia and reduced visual acuity (20/50 OD) in conjunction with mid-peripheral epithelial pigmentation and cotton-wool spots around the perifoveal capillary network (5).

References

1. Perry CM, Balfour JA, Johnson DW, De Clercq E. Fomivirsen. Drugs 1999;57(3):375–81.
2. Freeman WR. Retinal toxic effects associated with intravitreal fomivirsen. Arch Ophthalmol 2001;119(3):458.
3. Boyer DS, Cowen SJ, Danis RP, Diamond JG, Fish RH, Goldstein DA, Jaffe GJ, Lelezari JP, Lieberman RM, Belfort R Jr, Muccioli C, Palestine AG, Perez JE, Territo C, Johnson DW, Mansour SE, Sheppard JD, Mora-Durate J, Chan CK, Andreu-Andreu D, Deschenes JG, deSmet MD, Fisher M, Gastaut J-A, Gazzard BG, Lightman B, Johnson MA, Klauss V, Gumbel H, et al. Vitravene Study Group. Safety of intravitreous fomivirsen for treatment of cytomegalovirus retinitis in patients with AIDS. Am J Ophthalmol 2002;133(4):484–98.
4. Stone TW, Jaffe GJ. Reversible bull's-eye maculopathy associated with intravitreal fomivirsen therapy for cytomegalovirus retinitis. Am J Ophthalmol 2000;130(2):242–3.
5. Amin HI, Ai E, McDonald HR, Johnson RN. Retinal toxic effects associated with intravitreal fomivirsen. Arch Ophthalmol 2000;118(3):426–7.

Fondaparinux

General Information

Fondaparinux is a synthetic pentasaccharide that mimics the site of heparin that binds to antithrombin III and inhibits factor Xa activity, which in turn inhibits thrombin generation. It does not release tissue factor pathway inhibitor. It is nearly completely absorbed after subcutaneous administration, has a rapid onset of action and a long half-life (14–20 hours), and is excreted by the kidneys. Its pharmacology, clinical pharmacology, and uses have been reviewed (1–16).

Fondaparinux has been approved in some countries for the prophylaxis of venous thrombosis after orthopedic surgery in a fixed dose of 2.5 mg/day without monitoring. A structural analogue, idraparinux sodium, has additional methyl groups, a long half-life, and once-weekly administration. Both drugs are being developed as antithrombotic drugs for venous and arterial thrombosis, acute coronary syndrome, and stroke, and as adjuncts to thrombolytic therapy.

There is currently no specific antidote for fondaparinux: it is not neutralized by protamine sulfate. Fondaparinux shows no cross-reactivity with antibodies associated with heparin-induced thrombocytopenia.

Comparative studies

There have been two double-blind, randomized comparisons of fondaparinux 2.5 mg/day or enoxaparin 40 mg/day after hip fracture surgery (17), or elective major knee surgery (18). Fondaparinux reduced the risk of thromboembolism by 56% in the first study ($n = 1250$) and by 55% in the second ($n = 724$). There were no significant differences between the two groups in the first study in the incidence of death or clinically important bleeding. In the second study, major bleeding occurred more often with fondaparinux, but there were no significant differences between the two groups in the incidence of bleeding leading to death or reoperation, or occurring in a critical organ.

In a double-blind, randomized study of 2309 consecutive patients undergoing elective hip replacement, postoperative subcutaneous fondaparinux 2.5 mg/day was compared with preoperative enoxaparin 40 mg/day (19). By day 11, venous thromboembolism had occurred in 85 (9%) of 919 patients assigned to enoxaparin and in 37 (4%) of 908 patients assigned to fondaparinux, a relative risk reduction of 56% (95% CI = 33, 73). In a similar comparison of postoperative fondaparinux 2.5 mg/day and enoxaparin 30 mg bd in 2275 consecutive patients undergoing elective hip replacement, by day 11 venous thromboembolism had occurred in 48 (6%) of 787 patients assigned to fondaparinux and in 66 (8%) of 797 patients assigned to enoxaparin, a relative risk reduction of 26% (95% CI = 11, 53) (20).

In a meta-analysis of these studies, bleeding was slightly, but not significantly, more frequent with fondaparinux than with enoxaparin (21,22).

Drug–Drug Interactions

Aspirin

In healthy volunteers, steady-state fondaparinux did not alter the pharmacodynamic effects of a single dose of aspirin 975 mg (23). Aspirin did not alter the pharmacokinetics of fondaparinux.

Digoxin

In a randomized, crossover study in 24 healthy volunteers, the pharmacokinetics of fondaparinux sodium 10 mg/day subcutaneously for 7 days were unaffected by digoxin 0.25 mg/day orally for 7 days (24).

Piroxicam

In healthy volunteers, steady-state fondaparinux did not alter the pharmacodynamic effects of a single dose of piroxicam 20 mg (23). Piroxicam did not alter the pharmacokinetics of fondaparinux.

Warfarin

There was no pharmacodynamic interaction of subcutaneous fondaparinux 4 mg with warfarin in 12 healthy men (25).

References

1. Keam SJ, Goa KL. Fondaparinux sodium. Drugs 2002;62(11):1673–85.
2. Walenga JM, Jeske WP, Samama MM, Frapaise FX, Bick RL, Fareed J. Fondaparinux: a synthetic heparin pentasaccharide as a new antithrombotic agent. Expert Opin Investig Drugs 2002;11(3):397–407.
3. Regazzoni S, de Moerloose P. Deux nouveaux agents antithrombotiques très prometteurs: le pentasaccharide et le ximelagatran. [Two new very promising antithrombotic agents: pentasaccharide and ximelagatran.] Rev Med Suisse Romande 2002;122(1):29–33.
4. Bounameaux H, Perneger T. Fondaparinux: a new synthetic pentasaccharide for thrombosis prevention. Lancet 2002;359(9319):1710–11.
5. Bauer KA, Hawkins DW, Peters PC, Petitou M, Herbert JM, van Boeckel CA, Meuleman DG. Fondaparinux, a synthetic pentasaccharide: the first in a new class of antithrombotic agents—the selective factor Xa inhibitors. Cardiovasc Drug Rev 2002;20(1):37–52.
6. Bauer KA. Selective inhibition of coagulation factors: advances in antithrombotic therapy. Semin Thromb Hemost 2002;28(Suppl 2):15–24.
7. Turpie AG. Optimizing prophylaxis of venous thromboembolism. Semin Thromb Hemost 2002;28(Suppl 2):25–32.
8. Buller HR. Treatment of symptomatic venous thromboembolism: improving outcomes. Semin Thromb Hemost 2002;28(Suppl 2):41–8.
9. Turpie AG. Pentasaccharides. Semin Hematol 2002;39(3):158–71.
10. Gallus AS, Coghlan DW. Heparin pentasaccharide. Curr Opin Hematol 2002;9(5):422–9.
11. Bauer KA, Eriksson BI, Lassen MR, Turpie AG. Factor Xa inhibition in the prevention of venous thromboembolism and treatment of patients with venous thromboembolism. Curr Opin Pulm Med 2002;8(5):398–404.
12. Garces K. Fondaparinux for post-operative venous thrombosis prophylaxis. Issues Emerg Health Technol 2002;(37):1–4.
13. Petitou M, Duchaussoy P, Herbert JM, Duc G, El Hajji M, Branellec JF, Donat F, Necciari J, Cariou R, Bouthier J, Garrigou E. The synthetic pentasaccharide fondaparinux: first in the class of antithrombotic agents that selectively inhibit coagulation factor Xa. Semin Thromb Hemost 2002;28(4):393–402.
14. Cheng JW. Fondaparinux: a new antithrombotic agent. Clin Ther 2002;24(11):1757–69.

15. Reverter JC. Fondaparinux sodium. Drugs Today (Barc) 2002;38(3):185–94.
16. Samama MM, Gerotziafas GT, Elalamy I, Horellou MH, Conard J. Biochemistry and clinical pharmacology of new anticoagulant agents. Pathophysiol Haemost Thromb 2002;32(5–6):218–24.
17. Eriksson BI, Bauer KA, Lassen MR, Turpie AG; Steering Committee of the Pentasaccharide in Hip-Fracture Surgery Study. Fondaparinux compared with enoxaparin for the prevention of venous thromboembolism after hip-fracture surgery. N Engl J Med 2001;345(18):1298–304.
18. Bauer KA, Eriksson BI, Lassen MR, Turpie AG; Steering Committee of the Pentasaccharide in Major Knee Surgery Study. Fondaparinux compared with enoxaparin for the prevention of venous thromboembolism after elective major knee surgery. N Engl J Med 2001;345(18):1305–10.
19. Lassen MR, Bauer KA, Eriksson BI, Turpie AG; European Pentasaccharide Elective Surgery Study (EPHESUS) Steering Committee. Postoperative fondaparinux versus preoperative enoxaparin for prevention of venous thromboembolism in elective hip-replacement surgery: a randomised double-blind comparison. Lancet 2002;359(9319):1715–20.
20. Turpie AG, Bauer KA, Eriksson BI, Lassen MR; PENTATHALON 2000 Study Steering Committee. Postoperative fondaparinux versus postoperative enoxaparin for prevention of venous thromboembolism after elective hip-replacement surgery: a randomised double-blind trial. Lancet 2002;359(9319):1721–6.
21. Turpie AG, Bauer KA, Eriksson BI, Lassen MR. Fondaparinux vs enoxaparin for the prevention of venous thromboembolism in major orthopedic surgery: a meta-analysis of 4 randomized double-blind studies. Arch Intern Med 2002;162(16):1833–40.
22. Turpie AG, Eriksson BI, Lassen MR, Bauer KA. A meta-analysis of fondaparinux versus enoxaparin in the prevention of venous thromboembolism after major orthopaedic surgery. J South Orthop Assoc 2002;11(4):182–8.
23. Ollier C, Faaij RA, Santoni A, Duvauchelle T, van Haard PM, Schoemaker RC, Cohen AF, de Greef R, Burggraaf J. Absence of interaction of fondaparinux sodium with aspirin and piroxicam in healthy male volunteers. Clin Pharmacokinet 2002;41(Suppl 2):31–7.
24. Mant T, Fournie P, Ollier C, Donat F, Necciari J. Absence of interaction of fondaparinux sodium with digoxin in healthy volunteers. Clin Pharmacokinet 2002;41(Suppl 2):39–45.
25. Faaij RA, Burggraaf J, Schoemaker RC, Van Amsterdam RG, Cohen AF. Absence of an interaction between the synthetic pentasaccharide fondaparinux and oral warfarin. Br J Clin Pharmacol 2002;54(3):304–8.

Formaldehyde

See also Disinfectants and antiseptics

General Information

Aldehydes such as formaldehyde, glyoxal, and glutaral (glutaraldehyde) are used as solutions and vapours for disinfection and sterilization. They are irritating and sensitizing and cause contact dermatitis in health-care workers (SEDA-21, 254).

Formulations

Formaldehyde is released by numerous agents, such as paraformaldehyde, dichlorophene, Dowicil 75 and Dowicil 200 (*cis*-1-(3-chloroalkyl)-3,5,7-triaza-l-azonia-adamantane chloride), bronopol, Biocide DS 52–49 (1,2-benzoisothiazoline-3-one plus a formaldehyde releaser), and Bakzid (cyclic aminoacetal). Formalin is an alternative name for an aqueous solution of formaldehyde, but the latter name is preferred, since formalin is also used as a brand name in some countries.

Free formaldehyde is used in cosmetics, especially in hair shampoos, and in many disinfectants and antiseptics. The solid paraformaldehyde is used as a source of formaldehyde vapor for the disinfection of rooms. Noxythiolin, polynoxylin, hexamidine, and taurolidine act by slow release of formaldehyde. Formaldehyde solution contains 34–38% of formaldehyde methanol as a stabilizing agent to delay polymerization of the formaldehyde. Formaldehyde gel contains 0.75% of formaldehyde and is used to treat warts.

Formaldehyde cannot be applied safely to the skin or the mucous membranes in the concentration necessary to rapidly kill microbes, and formaldehyde solutions have to be diluted before use to a 2–8% solution to disinfect inanimate objects and to a 1–2% solution for disinfection by scrubbing. For fumigation of air a concentration of 1–2% is used.

General adverse effects

Discussion about the toxicity, mutagenicity, and potential carcinogenicity of formaldehyde relates more to occupational and environmental exposure, caused by its release from urea formaldehyde resins used for wood products and from foams for cavity-wall insulation, than its use in disinfection and sterilization (SEDA-11, 476) (SEDA-12, 569). However, the concentrations of formaldehyde that are found in the air after scrubbing with formaldehyde-containing disinfectants can be several hundred percentage higher than the maximum safe workplace concentration, even when scrubbing is carried out properly (1). Very high concentrations have also been found in pathologists' workrooms. In the pathology departments of two Italian hospitals the highest values of 2.6 and 6.0 ppm were measured in the dissection laboratories; in the histology and cytology laboratories, concentrations were less than 1 ppm, except when technicians handled formaldehyde solutions (2).

Primary irritant effects of formaldehyde

The minimum amount of formaldehyde that can be detected by odor varies considerably between individuals and ranges from 0.1 to 1.0 ppm (0.12–1.2 mg/m^3), close to the concentration at which minimal irritant effects are felt in the eyes and in the pulmonary airways (3). Thus, the fundamental toxicity of formaldehyde lies in primary irritation to the eyes, nose, and throat when the subject is exposed to concentrations in the range of 1–5 ppm. Concentrations above 2–5 ppm cause irritation of the pharynx, lungs, and eyes, and some erythema of vaporized areas of the skin, such as the face and neck. Acute exposure to concentrations of formaldehyde of the order of three times the maximum threshold of detection of the odor will most likely produce severe acute pulmonary edema after only a few minutes.

Acute toxicity after local administration of formaldehyde-containing solutions

Dilute solutions of 1–10% formalin have been instilled into the bladder to treat inoperable profusely bleeding tumors or intractable hemorrhagic cystitis. Anuria was a severe complication. This was due either to edematous obstruction of the ureter or to tubular or papillary necrosis, probably caused by systemic absorption. Bladder perforation with intraperitoneal spillage, peritonitis, and finally death was described in an elderly patient with a carcinoma of the uterine cervix (SEDA-11, 476).

In 1983, Godec and Gleich reviewed all published results of treatment of intractable hematuria with formalin. Dilutions of 1–10% formalin (containing 0.37–3.7% formaldehyde) were used; the most commonly used concentration of formalin was 10%. The authors concluded that formalin was probably the most effective tool for controlling massive hematuria, but also probably the most dangerous. The review covered 23 articles and 118 patients; in 104 cases, treatment was successful. However, in only 10 reports had the treatment been used without serious adverse effects; the other 13 articles listed four deaths and many serious local and systemic complications. The complication rate increased when the formalin concentration was higher, but the contact time and the volume instilled did not influence the occurrence of adverse effects. The most frequent local complications were reflux and hydronephrosis. Fibrosis of the bladder with reduced capacity was the usual clinical outcome. A systemic effect was tubular necrosis with anuria, with two deaths. Another complication was ureteric obstruction, which was not related to ureteric fibrosis or bladder wall fibrosis obstructing the intramural ureter; in two cases the obstruction appeared to be due to retroperitoneal fibrosis (SEDA-11, 476) (4).

In 1989, Donahue and Frank (SEDA-12, 569) (SEDA-14, 205) (5) published a systematic review of 235 cases of intravesical hemorrhagic cystitis treated with intravesical instillations of diluted formalin in concentrations of 1, 5, or 10%. Complete response rates were 71, 78, and 83% respectively. The average duration of a complete response was 3–4 months; the recurrence rate fell gradually with the use of higher concentrations. Complications were divided into two groups: "minor complications" included all mild or transient problems not requiring surgical intervention (fever, tachycardia, transient or minor rises in blood urea nitrogen or creatinine, mild hydronephrosis, grades I and II uricourethral reflux, increased urinary frequency, urgency, incontinence, suprapubic pain, or a reduction in bladder capacity not requiring urinary diversion); "major complications" were those that required surgical intervention, resulting in loss of renal function or causing damage to the supravesical urinary tracts (stricture formation), including anuria, acute tubular necrosis, papillary necrosis, ureteric or retroperitoneal fibrosis, uterovesical or uteropelvic junction obstruction, severe hydronephrosis, grades III or IV vesicoureteric reflux, any vesical fistula, or a reduction in bladder capacity requiring urinary diversion. Major complications occurred in all treatment groups, including those treated with 1% formalin. The higher rate observed with 10% formalin was not significantly different from the rates associated with the use of 1 or 5% formalin. The mortality rates were 2.2% in all the formalin groups, but the rates were not significantly different. Formalin 10% resulted in a higher and favorable response rate, a lower recurrence rate, equal numbers of major complications and mortality rate, and a three-fold higher rate of minor complications than 5% formalin in patients with hemorrhagic cystitis due to radiotherapy for bladder tumors. In contrast, formalin 5% was more effective than formalin 10% in treating patients with intractable hematuria due to unresectable bladder tumors or cyclophosphamide-induced cystitis.

The use of 2 or 4% formaldehyde as a scolecidal agent for injection into hydatid cysts and for peritoneal lavage was followed by shock in seven cases and resulted in death in three. All three patients who died had undergone a peritoneal lavage with 2–8 liters of 2 or 4% formaldehyde (SEDA-11, 476).

Immunogenicity

Formaldehyde is one of the most frequent contact allergens. If the responses in some individuals to acute exposure to formaldehyde are immunogenically mediated, they are of serious clinical significance. These individuals should not be exposed to any concentration of the agent. However, the intensity and nature of the immunogenic response can so resemble a primary irritant effect that a different diagnosis is not possible.

Mutagenicity and carcinogenicity

Formaldehyde is mutagenic in vitro and although there is conflicting evidence about its carcinogenicity, this should be taken seriously.

Organs and Systems

Respiratory

Formaldehyde-induced bronchial asthma occurred in a laboratory technician and in a neurologist preparing brain specimens for a student demonstration (6).

In a renal dialysis unit, five of 28 members of the staff had respiratory symptoms associated with formaldehyde, and in two cases, attacks of wheezing could be provoked by exposure to formaldehyde. One nurse was particularly affected, the asthmatic wheeze persisting for 8 days after exposure (7).

Of 230 people who had been exposed to formaldehyde and had asthma-like respiratory symptoms with a bronchial provocation test, 12 were considered to be caused by specific sensitization to formaldehyde, 11 were triggered by a concentration of 2.5 mg/m^3, and one by 1.2 mg/m^3 (SEDA-11, 477) (8). The authors concluded that formaldehyde-induced asthma, although apparently rare, is under-reported.

Biliary tract

Three cases of secondary sclerosing cholangitis developed during the early postoperative phase of surgical treatment of hydatid liver cysts in which formaldehyde was used; one patient died within 3 months and the remaining two underwent liver transplantation following biliary sclerosis. Another group also reported three cases of sclerosing cholangitis. Both groups of authors concluded that because of the risk of complication and the unproven efficacy of intracystic injection of a scolecidal solution in preventing dissemination of the parasite, this technique should be abandoned in the surgical treatment of hydatid disease of the liver. However, in 560 patients, there were no cases of sclerosing cholangitis when the concentration was not more than 2% and the solution was injected only into cysts that contained clear fluid content (SEDA-11, 476) (9).

Skin

Formaldehyde-releasing preservatives, such as quaternium-15, diazolidinyl urea, and imidazolidinyl urea, are widely used in cosmetics and topical medications and are well-known contact sensitizers. In spite of positive patch test reactions to these preservatives in a number of patients, only some of these patients will react when they use the corresponding commercial formulations. This is because the concentrations of preservatives in the commercial products are often below the threshold necessary to produce a clinical reaction. This finding confirms the importance of using commercial formulations of topical agents in estimating the clinical relevance of patch test results (10).

The formaldehyde concentration in patch-testing, which has been lowered to 1% in the standard series in recent years, has been studied in a comparison of concentrations of 1% and 2% in 3734 consecutively patch-tested patients (11). Since there was no significant difference between 1 and 2% formaldehyde with respect to the frequency of positive patch test reactions, while there were more irritant reactions with 2%, a 1% patch test concentration can still be recommended.

Allergic dermatitis has been demonstrated from direct skin contact and from exposure to gaseous formaldehyde in the air. Various forms of reaction occur, from simple erythema to maculopapular lesions, hyperesthesia, and angioedema. Five patients developed an allergic contact dermatitis to plaster casts, caused by free formaldehyde released by a melamine–formaldehyde resin incorporated in the plaster.

Urticaria with acute Quincke's edema was reported following the use of a formaldehyde-containing dental paste (SEDA-11, 477) (12).

The first published case of photosensitivity to formaldehyde was reported in 1982 in a man who developed pruritus, burning, and redness of the skin within minutes of exposure to sunlight; photopatch tests showed specific photosensitivity to formaldehyde (13).

Immunologic

Aldehydes are irritating and sensitizing and cause contact dermatitis in health-care workers (SEDA-21, 254). The incidence of allergy to aldehydes has been examined in 280 health-care workers with skin lesions (14). Allergy was diagnosed in 64 (23%). Most (86%) were sensitive to only one aldehyde. Formaldehyde caused allergy slightly more often (14%) than glutaraldehyde (12%). Only five (1.9%) were sensitive to glyoxal. This hierarchy of sensitivity was also confirmed in animal testing.

Immediate-type allergy to formaldehyde mediated by ice occurred during the use of a formaldehyde reconditioned dialyser in a 20-year-old woman without a personal or familiar history of atopy.

A specific cold agglutinin cross-reacting with anti-N was detected in the sera of 68 (21%) of 325 hemodialysis patients; each had used a dialyser that had been sterilized with formaldehyde. The results of transfusion experiments suggested in vivo hemolytic activity of this antibody. The authors postulated that such in vivo exposure to formaldehyde might make the MN-receptor on erythrocytes immunogenic, thus inducing the formation of the anti-N-like antibody.

The commonly used Clinitest reaction for residual formaldehyde in reused dialysers fails to detect concentrations below 50 ppm (15). The use of Schiff reagent in ratios of 1:1 to 3:1, which can detect formaldehyde at concentrations of 3.6–5.0 ppm, has therefore been recommended (SEDA-12, 571) (16). It can also be used in combination with a glucose-containing dialysate.

Long-Term Effects

Mutagenicity

Formaldehyde is mutagenic in many laboratory test systems, for example fruit flies (Drosophila), grasshoppers, flowering plants, fungi, bacteria, and cultured human bronchial fibroblasts.

Formaldehyde may be genotoxic by a dual mechanism: direct damage to DNA and inhibition of repair of mutagenic and carcinogenic DNA lesions by other chemical and physical carcinogens.

Marked chromosomal abnormalities and chromosomal breaks were found in metaphases in direct bone marrow preparations from 40 patients undergoing maintenance hemodialysis (SEDA-11, 477) (17). During the period of these cytogenetic studies, the dialysers were reused after sterilization with formaldehyde, and each patient may have received residual amounts of as much as 127 (sd 51) mg of formaldehyde during each dialysis.

Tumorigenicity

There is evidence of possible carcinogenicity of formaldehyde from two inhalation studies on rats and mice (SEDA-10, 423) (SEDA-11, 477) (SEDA-12, 571) (13).

In man, a number of epidemiological studies using different designs have been conducted (17) on the health risks of non-medical exposure to formaldehyde and also in health-care professionals (18–23), with contradictory results. Cancers in excess in more than one study were: Hodgkin's disease (24,25), leukemia (18,19,22,23,26), cancers of the buccal cavity and pharynx (particular the nasopharynx) (18,19,25,27,28), lung (18,24,27,29–31), nose (32–36), prostate (19,24,26), bladder (19,23,26), brain (20), colon (18–20,25,27), skin (18,25), and kidney (27).

There was no association between formaldehyde exposure and lung cancer in a case-referral study among Danish physicians working in departments of pathology, forensic medicine, and anatomy (21).

Mortality from prostatic cancer was increased among embalmers (19) and industrial workers (24,26), but the excess was statistically significant only among embalmers (19). A slight excess of mortality from bladder cancer (19,22,26), a significant excess of colon cancers (18,19,27), and a significant excess mortality from skin cancer (18,25) were noted among British pathologists (22), embalmers (18,19), and industrial workers (25–27).

Excess mortality from leukemia and cancer of the brain was generally not seen among industrial workers, which suggests that the increased rates of these cancers among professionals (anatomists (20), pathologists (22), embalmers (18,19), and undertakers (23)) is due to factors other than just formaldehyde.

It is of course possible that the studies that have provided positive evidence of a link between formaldehyde and cancer related to more intensive exposure; for example, reports on the risk associated with chronic exposure to low concentrations of formaldehyde suggest that formaldehyde cannot be a potent carcinogen; if it were, the high degree of environmental exposure would result in much clearer evidence of risk. However, any compound that produces cancer in experimental animals or mutagenicity in several test systems should be considered as a potential cancer risk to human subjects, even though humans and animals may differ in their susceptibility to formaldehyde. The contradictory evidence from human studies should therefore be taken seriously and efforts should be made to reduce exposure.

The need to re-evaluate the rationale underlying the use of formaldehyde, formocresol, and paraformaldehyde in dentistry has been stressed, since the clinical use and delivery of these products are considered to be arbitrary and unscientific (37).

References

1. Ponsold B, Schulze B, Kirsch H. Hygienische Probleme bei des Anwendung formaldehydheltiger Desinfektionsmitted. [Hygienic problems in the use of formaldehyde containing disinfectants.] Z Gesamte Hyg 1977;23(6):408–11.
2. De Zotti R, Petronio L, Negro C, Gabelli A. Inquinamento da formaldeide in anatomia patologica: esperienze in due ospedali regionali. [Formaldehyde pollution in pathologic anatomy: experiences at 2 regional hospitals.] Med Lav 1986;77(5):523–8.
3. Leonardos G, Kendak D, Barnard N. Odor threshold déterminations of 53 odorant chemicals. J Air Pollut Control Assoc 1969;19:51.
4. Ferrie BG, Smith PJ, Kirk D. Retroperitoneal fibrosis complicating intravesical formalin therapy. J R Soc Med 1983;76(10):831–2.
5. Donahue LA, Frank IN. Intravesical formalin for hemorrhagic cystitis: analysis of therapy. J Urol 1989;141(4):809–12.
6. Sakula A. Formalin asthma in hospital laboratory staff. Lancet 1975;2(7939):816.
7. Hendrick DJ, Lane DJ. Formalin asthma in hospital staff. BMJ 1975;1(5958):607–8.
8. Nordman H, Keskinen H, Tuppurainen M. Formaldehyde asthma—rare or overlooked? J Allergy Clin Immunol 1985;75(1 Pt 1):91–9.
9. Bourgeon R. Cholangite sclérosante due au formol dans le traitement du kyste hydatique du foie. [Sclerosing cholangitis caused by formol in the treatment of hydatid cyst of the liver.] Gastroenterol Clin Biol 1985;9(8–9):644–5.
10. Skinner SL, Marks JG. Allergic contact dermatitis to preservatives in topical medicaments. Am J Contact Dermat 1998;9(4):199–201.
11. Trattner A, Johansen JD, Menne T. Formaldehyde concentration in diagnostic patch testing: comparison of 1% with 2%. Contact Dermatitis 1998;38(1):9–13.
12. Burri C, Wüthrich B. Quincke-Ödem mit Urtikaria nach Zahnwurzelbehandlung mit einem Paraformaldehyd-haltigen Dentalantiseptikum bei Spättyp-Sensibilisierung auf Paraformaldehyd. Allergologie 1985;8:264.
13. Shelley WB. Immediate sunburn-like reaction in a patient with formaldehyde photosensitivity. Arch Dermatol 1982;118(2):117–18.
14. Kiec-Swierczynska M, Krecisz B, Krysiak B, Kuchowicz E, Rydzynski K. Occupational allergy to aldehydes in health care workers. Clinical observations. Experiments. Int J Occup Med Environ Health 1998;11(4):349–58.
15. Friedman EA, Lundin AP 3rd. Environmental and iatrogenic obstacles to long life on hemodialysis. N Engl J Med 1982;306(3):167–9.
16. Zasuwa G, Levin NW. Problems in hemodialysis. N Engl J Med 1982;306(25):1550.
17. IARC Monographs updating of Vol. 1 to 42, Supplement, 1987:211–16.
18. Walrath J, Fraumeni JF Jr. Mortality patterns among embalmers. Int J Cancer 1983;31(4):407–11.
19. Walrath J, Fraumeni JF Jr. Cancer and other causes of death among embalmers. Cancer Res 1984;44(10):4638–41.
20. Stroup NE, Blair A, Erikson GE. Brain cancer and other causes of death in anatomists. J Natl Cancer Inst 1986;77(6):1217–24.
21. Jensen OM, Andersen SK. Lung cancer risk from formaldehyde. Lancet 1982;1(8277):913.
22. Harrington JM, Oakes D. Mortality study of British pathologists 1974–80. Br J Ind Med 1984;41(2):188–91.
23. Levine RJ, Andjelkovich DA, Shaw LK. The mortality of Ontario undertakers and a review of formaldehyde-related mortality studies. J Occup Med 1984;26(10):740–6.
24. Blair A, Stewart P, O'Berg M, Gaffey W, Walrath J, Ward J, Bales R, Kaplan S, Cubit D. Mortality among industrial workers exposed to formaldehyde. J Natl Cancer Inst 1986;76(6):1071–84.
25. Stayner L, Smith AB, Reeve G, Blade L, Elliott L, Keenlyside R, Halperin W. Proportionate mortality study of workers in the garment industry exposed to formaldehyde. Am J Ind Med 1985;7(3):229–40.
26. Fayerweather WE, Pell S, Bender JB. Case-control study of cancer deaths in DuPont workers with potential exposure to formaldehyde. In: Clary JJ, Gibson JE, Waritz RS, editors. Formaldehyde: Toxicology, Epidemiology, Mechanisms. New York: Marcel Dekker, 1983:47–125.
27. Liebling T, Rosenman KD, Pastides H, Griffith RG, Lemeshow S. Cancer mortality among workers exposed to formaldehyde. Am J Ind Med 1984;5(6):423–8.
28. Vaughan TL, Strader C, Davis S, Daling JR. Formaldehyde and cancers of the pharynx, sinus and nasal cavity: I. Occupational exposures. Int J Cancer 1986;38(5):677–83.
29. Partanen T, Kauppinen T, Nurminen M, Nickels J, Hernberg S, Hakulinen T, Pukkala E, Savonen E. Formaldehyde exposure and respiratory and related cancers. A case-referent study among Finnish woodworkers. Scand J Work Environ Health 1985;11(6):409–15.
30. Coggon D, Pannett B, Acheson ED. Use of job-exposure matrix in an occupational analysis of lung and bladder cancers on the basis of death certificates. J Natl Cancer Inst 1984;72(1):61–5.

31. Bertazzi PA, Pesatori AC, Radice L, Zocchetti C, Vai T. Exposure to formaldehyde and cancer mortality in a cohort of workers producing resins. Scand J Work Environ Health 1986;12(5):461–8.
32. Hayes RB, Raatgever JW, de Bruyn A, Gerin M. Cancer of the nasal cavity and paranasal sinuses, and formaldehyde exposure. Int J Cancer 1986;37(4):487–92.
33. Olsen JH, Jensen SP, Hink M, Faurbo K, Breum NO, Jensen OM. Occupational formaldehyde exposure and increased nasal cancer risk in man. Int J Cancer 1984;34(5):639–44.
34. Olsen JH, Asnaes S. Formaldehyde and the risk of squamous cell carcinoma of the sinonasal cavities. Br J Ind Med 1986;43(11):769–74.
35. Acheson ED, Barnes HR, Gardner MJ, Osmond C, Pannett B, Taylor CP. Formaldehyde in the British chemical industry. An occupational cohort study. Lancet 1984;1(8377):611–16.
36. Vaughan TL, Strader C, Davis S, Daling JR. Formaldehyde and cancers of the pharynx, sinus and nasal cavity: II. Residential exposures. Int J Cancer 1986;38(5):685–8.
37. Lewis BB, Chestner SB. Formaldehyde in dentistry: a review of mutagenic and carcinogenic potential. J Am Dent Assoc 1981;103(3):429–34.

Formoterol

See also Beta$_2$-adrenoceptor agonists

General Information

Formoterol is a long-acting selective beta$_2$-adrenoceptor agonist that is more potent than salmeterol (1) and has a similar duration of action (12 hours) but a rapid onset of effect similar to that of salbutamol. It is available as a multidose, pressurized aerosol and as a dry powder inhaler, delivering 0.006 or 0.012 mg per dose. The usual dose is 0.012 mg bd.

The pharmacokinetics and pharmacodynamics of a single oral dose of formoterol 168 μg have been studied in eight healthy men. Plasma concentrations reached a maximum of 94 pg/ml 70 minutes after administration. The biological effects peaked later, at 4 hours. Plasma potassium fell from 3.98 mmol/l to 2.33 mmol/l. There was a fall in blood eosinophil count from 277×10^6/l to 47×10^6/l (2).

In a postmarketing surveillance study of the long-acting beta$_2$-adrenoceptor agonist formoterol in the UK using the technique of prescription event monitoring, exposure and outcome data in 5777 patients aged 3–96 years were collected (3). The most commonly reported events, excluding those related to respiratory disease, were headache, tremor, palpitation, cramp, and nausea and vomiting, events known to be associated with beta$_2$-adrenoceptor agonists (4). However, the frequencies of nausea and vomiting (1.3%) and pruritus (0.5%) differed from the frequencies reported in the premarketing trials.

Therapeutic studies

Observational studies

The cardiovascular and metabolic responses to increasing doses of formoterol 12, 24, 48, and 96 μg administered from a dry powder inhaler have been assessed in a randomized, double-blind, crossover study in 20 patients with mild to moderate asthma. There was no difference in the maximum effects of formoterol 12 micrograms and placebo. The 24 micrograms dose significantly reduced plasma potassium (average fall 0.2 mmol/l) and increased blood glucose (average rise 1.8 mmol/l). After formoterol 96 micrograms the rise in heart rate was 9/minute greater than after placebo, systolic blood pressure rose by an average of 4 mmHg, and diastolic pressure fell by an average of 3 mmHg. Plasma potassium fell by an average of 0.5 mmol/l and blood glucose rose by an average of 2.6 mmol/l. The effects on extrapulmonary parameters would only be of clinical significance at the highest dose of formoterol studied (5).

A 3-month, open, uncontrolled, multicenter trial has been carried out in 1380 patients with moderate to severe persistent asthma taking inhaled corticosteroids (6). Formoterol was given via a single-dose, breath-activated device (Foradil). There were significant increases in peak flow and a three-fold reduction in the need for rescue treatment with short acting beta$_2$-adrenoceptor agonists. By the end of the study, 72% of the patients were taking formoterol 12 micrograms bd and 29% were taking 24 micrograms bd. Physician evaluation indicated that tolerability was very good or good in 93% of the patients. There were only minor drug-related adverse events similar to those produced by other beta$_2$-agonists.

Placebo-controlled studies

In a double-blind, crossover study 12 healthy subjects were randomized to receive either inhaled placebo or inhaled budesonide 1.2 mg bd for 7 days, with a minimum 7-day washout period between the two treatments (7). They used formoterol 24 micrograms bd during both treatment periods. A dose-response curve for systemic beta$_2$-adrenoceptor responses to inhaled salbutamol (0.8–3.2 mg) was carried out before and after 7 days of each treatment. The pretreatment value of plasma cortisol averaged 407 nmol/l and fell to 22 nmol/l after 7 days of budesonide; placebo had no effect. There was a significant reduction in the peak heart rate response to salbutamol when formoterol was given with placebo. This was partially reversed when formoterol was combined with budesonide. The peak rise in heart rate with salbutamol after formoterol and placebo was 24/minute and increased to 35/minute when formoterol was given with budesonide. The peak fall in potassium with salbutamol after formoterol and placebo was 0.48 mmol/l and did not change significantly when formoterol was combined with budesonide (0.36 mmol/l).

In multiple dose studies with formoterol (Oxis, Turbuhaler, Astra) 6, 12, and 24 micrograms bd, terbutaline 0.5 mg qds, or placebo in a total of 1199 patients, at least one adverse event was reported by 65% of the patients in each treatment group (8). Adverse events related to the respiratory system were reported by 37% of the patients and were attributed to underlying disease. Tremor was reported by 2% of patients taking formoterol 6 micrograms bd, by 4% with 12 micrograms bd, and by 12% with 24 micrograms bd. Tremor was reported by 5% of patients taking terbutaline 0.5 mg qds. No patient reported tremor with placebo.

In 397 adults with mild to moderate asthma randomly allocated to one of three treatments for 12 weeks (formoterol 6 micrograms bd, terbutaline 0.5 mg qds, and placebo), formoterol was significantly more effective than either terbutaline or placebo in reducing asthma symptoms (9). It also resulted in significantly higher evening peak flow readings and less use of rescue medication. The bronchodilator response to the study drugs and an additional 1.25 mg of terbutaline was similar before and at the end of the 12 weeks. This suggested that there was no loss of beta-adrenoceptor mediated bronchodilatation in any of the treatment groups. No patient in any group reported a clinically relevant adverse effect.

Of 31 patients with asthma and a mean FEV_1 of 1.97 litres in a double-blind, randomized, placebo-controlled, crossover study of single inhaled doses of placebo or formoterol, 6, 12, 24, or 48 micrograms on five separate days, most had at least a 50% increase in specific airway conductance within 1–4 minutes (10). The maximum increase in FEV_1 was dose-dependent, rising by 12% (6 micrograms), 18% (12 micrograms), 19% (24 micrograms), and 26% (48 micrograms). At 12 hours after the administration of 6, 12, 24, and 48 micrograms of formoterol, the mean increases in FEV_1 were still 7, 15, 18, and 27%, respectively, above the value seen with placebo. The most frequently reported adverse effect was headache, which occurred with all treatments, including placebo. After inhalation of formoterol 48 micrograms, three patients had mild tremor lasting for less than 1 hour. One patient had the same effect for 3 hours after placebo.

Comparative studies

Formoterol has been compared with various other beta$_2$-adrenoceptor agonists.

Fenoterol and salbutamol

Formoterol 24 micrograms, fenoterol 0.4 mg, and salbutamol 0.4 mg all caused an increase in heart rate and plasma glucose, and a fall in diastolic blood pressure and plasma potassium (1). Fenoterol had a greater maximum effect on heart rate than either salbutamol or formoterol. Formoterol and fenoterol caused a similar maximum reduction in plasma potassium greater than that seen with salbutamol.

Salmeterol

The relative efficacy of the long-acting beta$_2$-adrenoceptor agonists formoterol and salmeterol has been studied in a randomized, double-blind, crossover trial in 15 patients with asthma taking regular corticosteroids and salbutamol (11). The patients had methacholine challenges performed after varying single doses of formoterol (12, 60, and 120 micrograms) and salmeterol (50, 250, and 500 micrograms). The maximal protective effect of salmeterol against methacholine challenge was reached at 250 micrograms, whereas formoterol showed a dose-response relation, with maximum protection at the highest dose. This confirmed the authors' hypothesis that salmeterol is a partial agonist at beta-adrenoceptors compared with formoterol. The higher affinity of formoterol for beta-adrenoceptors also produced more adverse effects. There was a significant fall in serum potassium concentration after 60 micrograms of formoterol but not after 250 micrograms of salmeterol. The serum potassium concentration was also significantly lower with the highest dose of formoterol compared with the highest dose of salmeterol (minimum concentration 3.1 mmol/l). The highest dose of formoterol also resulted in more tremor than the highest dose of salmeterol. The increases in heart rate and QT interval were similar with the two drugs. It should be noted that the doses used in this study were higher than recommended. It is unclear whether the partial agonist activity of salmeterol is clinically important, but this seems unlikely.

Terbutaline

In 12 stable asthmatic patients who took high doses of formoterol or terbutaline, terbutaline had significantly greater systemic effects than formoterol, as indicated by pulse, blood pressure, and heart rate. Baseline serum potassium concentrations were all within the reference range (3.7–5.3 mmol/l). There was no significant difference between the mean potassium-lowering effects of formoterol 72 micrograms and terbutaline 6 mg. Mean maximal systolic blood pressure rose from 150 to 155 mmHg with formoterol 72 micrograms and from 139 to 153 mmHg with terbutaline 6 mg. The difference between treatment groups, 5 mmHg, was statistically significant. Diastolic blood pressure fell significantly with both formoterol (from 86 to 70 mmHg) and terbutaline (from 85 to 66 mmHg). Heart rate rose from 61/minute to 79/minute on day 3 in patients taking formoterol 72 micrograms/day compared with a rise from 63/minute to 86/minute with terbutaline 6 mg; this difference was statistically significant.

Formoterol 120 micrograms had significantly smaller effects than terbutaline 10 mg/day on serum potassium concentrations, pulse, and heart rate. During treatment with formoterol 120 micrograms/day, potassium concentrations were under 3.7 mmol/l in 10 patients on day 1, six patients on day 2, and five patients on day 3. With terbutaline 10 mg the corresponding numbers were 12, 10, and 9. However, the effect of terbutaline 10 mg was significantly greater than formoterol 120 micrograms over the three treatment days. Formoterol 120 micrograms/day caused a rise in baseline systolic blood pressure from 134 to 145 mmHg; terbutaline 10 mg produced a rise from 131 to 141 mmHg. The difference between the groups, 0.6 mmHg, was not statistically significant. With formoterol 120 micrograms/day the heart rate rose from 65/minute to 78/minute, and with terbutaline 10 mg/day it rose from 63/minute to 86/minute. The difference in mean heart rate rise of 8/minute was statistically significant. A patient taking formoterol 72 micrograms/day developed atrial fibrillation on day 1. Minor adverse events occurred in seven patients taking formoterol 72 micrograms/day and six patients taking terbutaline 6 mg/day. Eight patients reported adverse events when taking formoterol 120 micrograms/day, as did 10 patients taking terbutaline 10 mg/day. Minor adverse effects included headache, muscle cramps, fatigue, and tremor with all four treatments. Tremor was reported in two of 12 patients taking terbutaline 6 mg and in five of 15 patients taking terbutaline 10 mg. The corresponding numbers for formoterol were none with formoterol 72 micrograms and one of 15 with formoterol 120 micrograms (12).

High-dose formoterol (Oxis Turbuhaler) and terbutaline (Bricanyl Turbuhaler) have been compared in a randomized, double-blind trial in 48 patients with obstructive airways disease (mean FEV_1 0.98 liter or 33% predicted) (13). Patients with acute bronchoconstriction received either a cumulative dose of 90 micrograms inhaled formoterol or 10 mg inhaled terbutaline (corresponding to 20 puffs each) within the first 3 hours of admission. Treatment included intravenous prednisolone 40 mg after 1.5 hours and oxygen during the first 3 hours. FEV_1 improved similarly in both treatment groups, serum potassium concentration fell in both groups but to the same extent, and the mean 12-hour pulse rate was significantly higher with terbutaline. The authors concluded that formoterol is at least as safe and equally well tolerated as terbutaline.

Organs and Systems

Cardiovascular

The cardiac effects of formoterol and salmeterol have been studied in 12 patients with COPD, hypoxemia (PaO_2 below 60 mmHg), and cardiac disease. Holter monitoring showed that the heart rate was higher after formoterol 24 micrograms than after either formoterol 12 micrograms or salmeterol 50 micrograms. Supraventricular or ventricular extra beats occurred more often after formoterol 24 micrograms. Formoterol 24 micrograms caused a significant reduction in the plasma potassium concentration for 9 hours after administration. The authors suggested that in patients with COPD, hypoxemia, and pre-existing cardiac dysrhythmias, long-acting $beta_2$-adrenoceptor agonists can cause adverse cardiac effects. However, the recommended single dose of salmeterol or formoterol allows a higher safety margin than inhaled formoterol 24 micrograms (14).

The non-pulmonary effects of formoterol have been carefully studied in an uncontrolled observational trial in 10 patients with asthma who were already taking regular inhaled budesonide (400 micrograms bd) (15). A 24-hour Holter recording was taken at baseline, and after a 2-week treatment period with formoterol 12 micrograms bd, there were no significant changes in blood pressure, heart rate, cardiac morphology, or the circadian rhythm of autonomic regulation as assessed by measurements taken from the Holter monitor after the treatment period.

Respiratory

The effect of formoterol 18 micrograms on histamine-induced plasma exudation into sputum has been investigated in 16 healthy subjects in a double-blind, placebo-controlled, crossover study. Plasma exudation into the airways was produced by inhalation of histamine. Sputum was induced by inhalation of hypertonic (4.5%) saline. Induced sputum was obtained at baseline and then at 30 minutes and 8 hours after histamine inhalation. Sputum concentrations of $alpha_2$-macroglobulin were measured as a marker of microvascular-epithelial exudation of bulk plasma. Histamine-induced plasma exudation 30 minutes after placebo was considerably greater than at baseline. The median difference was 11 μg/ml (95% CI = 0.9, 90) expressed as $alpha_2$-macroglobulin. The effect of histamine was reduced by 5.1 μg/ml (CI = 0.9, 62) 30 minutes after formoterol compared with placebo. At 8 hours, histamine exudation was much less and was no longer inhibited by formoterol (16).

Nervous system

The non-pulmonary effects of formoterol have been carefully studied in an uncontrolled observational trial in 10 patients with asthma who were already taking regular inhaled budesonide (400 micrograms bd) (15) There was a significant increase in upper limb tremor with formoterol and this was assessed as discomfort by one patient. This was considered due to stimulation of $beta_2$-adrenoceptors in skeletal muscle.

Long-Term Effects

Drug tolerance

Several studies have shown that regular use of formoterol results in the development of tolerance to its bronchoprotective effects, even with treatment periods as short as 1 week. The significance of this tolerance is unclear, but it is potentially important clinically.

A randomized, double-blind, placebo-controlled, crossover trial was designed to see whether formoterol given once daily was associated with less subsensitivity. Ten asthmatics using inhaled steroids were given inhaled formoterol dry powder 24 micrograms od or bd or identical placebo for 1 week. Bronchoprotection was estimated by measuring the PC_{20} for adenosine monophosphate (AMP) 12 hours after the first and last doses of each treatment. The PC_{20} is the concentration of AMP that causes a 20% fall in the FEV_1 and is directly proportional to the degree of bronchoprotection. With placebo, the PC_{20} values for AMP at the start and end of one week were 71 μg/ml and 75 μg/ml. There was a significant loss of bronchoprotection after 1 week of treatment with twice-daily formoterol. The PC_{20} for AMP at the start was 475 μg/ml, indicating significant bronchoprotection by formoterol compared with placebo. After 1 week the PC_{20} had fallen to 127 μg/ml, a near four-fold loss of the bronchoprotective effect of formoterol. When formoterol was given daily for a week the PC_{20} values were 367 μg/ml and 127 μg/ml, a three-fold loss of bronchoprotection. There was no significant difference in the effects of formoterol given once or twice a day (17).

A randomized, parallel-group, double-blind study in 67 patients with stable asthma requiring inhaled glucocorticoids used the PC_{20} for inhaled methacholine as a measure of bronchoprotection. The patients were treated for 2 weeks with formoterol 12 micrograms od, 6 micrograms bd, or 24 micrograms bd, terbutaline 500 micrograms qds, or placebo. Each of the four active treatments caused a significant fall in the PC_{20} for metacholine, and there was no significant difference between them. In contrast to the reduced bronchoprotective effect the bronchodilator effect of formoterol was maintained over the 2-week treatment period (18).

The effect of a bolus of inhaled budesonide on formoterol-induced subsensitivity in airway beta-adrenoceptors has been studied in a randomized, double-blind, crossover study in 10 asthmatic patients taking regular inhaled glucocorticoids (19). Challenge testing with AMP was performed at baseline and after one week of regular formoterol (24 micrograms bd). Before the second challenge the patients were given either a dose of inhaled budesonide (1600 micrograms) or placebo via a dry powder inhaler. After one week of formoterol, the PC_{20} for the second challenge fell significantly (by a factor of 3.9). However, when the second challenge was performed after a bolus of budesonide, there was no fall in the PC_{20}, suggesting protection against formoterol-induced tolerance. Lymphocyte beta-adrenoceptor density fell with regular formoterol, but not after a bolus of budesonide. These results have implications for the treatment of acute severe asthma in patients taking regular long-acting $beta_2$-adrenoceptor agonists. It may be appropriate to give a bolus dose of inhaled glucocorticoids to these patients early in an acute asthma attack, particularly if they are poorly responsive to initial therapy with short-acting bronchodilators.

Susceptibility Factors

Age

The use of long-acting beta-adrenoceptor agonists in the management of asthma in children has been comprehensively reviewed (20). In children, as in adults, regular long-acting beta-adrenoceptor agonists can produce bronchodilator subsensitivity to short-acting beta-agonists and tolerance to the bronchoprotective effects of long-acting beta-agonists against challenges with exercise and methacholine. The clinical significance of these findings is unclear. Formoterol and salmeterol have similar adverse effects profiles, similar to that of salbutamol. The most common medication-related adverse effects are cardiovascular, such as increased heart rate and palpitation, or tremor and headache. Small changes in serum potassium and glucose can also be seen, but all changes are minor. The exact role of long-acting beta-adrenoceptor agonists in childhood asthma remains to be defined.

Drug Administration

Drug formulations

Formoterol 12 and 24 micrograms, delivered from either a multidose pressurized aerosol or a dry powder inhaler, did not affect heart rate. However, at doses of 48 and 96 micrograms the heart rate rose significantly after the dry powder formulation. Tremor was significantly higher after the 48 micrograms dose of dry powder compared with the multidose pressurized aerosol. The two formulations were equipotent in producing bronchodilatation (SEDA-21, 184).

Drug–Drug Interactions

Salbutamol

The interaction of formoterol and salmeterol with salbutamol has been studied in a randomized, double-blind, crossover study in 16 asthmatic patients (21). The patients were taking regular inhaled corticosteroids and were responsive to methacholine challenge, with a PD_{20} (that is the dose of methacholine that produced a fall in FEV_1 of 20%) of less than 500 μg. The patients had methacholine challenges performed 12 hours after a single dose of formoterol 12 micrograms, salmeterol 50 micrograms, placebo, and either a low dose (400 micrograms) or a high dose (1600 micrograms) of salbutamol. With placebo, challenge after high-dose salbutamol resulted in a higher PD_{20} than after low-dose salbutamol (as expected). However, after both formoterol and salmeterol, the higher dose of salbutamol did not give as great an increase in PD_{20} over the lower dose of salbutamol. This suggests that prior treatment with formoterol and salmeterol can antagonize the protective effect of salbutamol against bronchoconstriction. This effect may be important in patients with acute asthma.

References

1. Bremner P, Woodman K, Burgess C, Crane J, Purdie G, Pearce N, Beasley R. A comparison of the cardiovascular and metabolic effects of formoterol, salbutamol and fenoterol. Eur Respir J 1993;6(2):204–10.
2. van den Berg BT, Braat MC, van Boxtel CJ. Pharmacokinetics and effects of formoterol fumarate in healthy human subjects after oral dosing. Eur J Clin Pharmacol 1998;54(6):463–8.
3. Wilton LV, Shakir SA. A post-marketing surveillance study of formoterol (Foradil): its use in general practice in England. Drug Saf 2002;25(3):213–23.
4. Sears MR. Adverse effects of beta-agonists. J Allergy Clin Immunol 2002;110(Suppl 6):S322–8.
5. Burgess C, Ayson M, Rajasingham S, Crane J, Della Cioppa G, Till MD. The extrapulmonary effects of increasing doses of formoterol in patients with asthma. Eur J Clin Pharmacol 1998;54(2):141–7.
6. Clauzel AM, Molimard M, Le Gros V, Lepere E, Febvre N, Michel FB. Use of formoterol dry powder administered for three months via a single-dose inhaler in 1,380 asthmatic patients. J Investig Allergol Clin Immunol 1998;8(5):265–70.
7. Aziz I, McFarlane LC, Lipworth BJ. Concomitant inhaled corticosteroid resensitises cardiac beta2-adrenoceptors in the presence of long-acting beta2-agonist therapy. Eur J Clin Pharmacol 1998;54(5):377–81.
8. Selroos O. The pharmacologic and clinical properties of Oxis (formoterol) Turbuhaler. Allergy 1998;53(Suppl 42):14–19.
9. Ekstrom T, Ringdal N, Sobradillo V, Runnerstrom E, Soliman S. Low-dose formoterol Turbuhaler (Oxis) b.i.d., a 3-month placebo-controlled comparison with terbutaline (q.i.d.). Respir Med 1998;92(8):1040–5.
10. Ringdal N, Derom E, Wahlin-Boll E, Pauwels R. Onset and duration of action of single doses of formoterol inhaled via Turbuhaler. Respir Med 1998;92(8):1017–21.
11. Palmqvist M, Ibsen T, Mellen A, Lotvall J. Comparison of the relative efficacy of formoterol and salmeterol in asthmatic patients. Am J Respir Crit Care Med 1999;160(1):244–9.
12. Totterman KJ, Huhti L, Sutinen E, Backman R, Pietinalho A, Falck M, Larsson P, Selroos O. Tolerability to high doses of formoterol and terbutaline via Turbuhaler for 3 days in stable asthmatic patients. Eur Respir J 1998;12(3):573–9.
13. Handley DA. Single-isomer beta-agonists. Pharmacotherapy 2001;21(3 Pt 2):S21–7.
14. Cazzola M, Imperatore F, Salzillo A, Di Perna F, Calderaro F, Imperatore A, Matera MG. Cardiac effects of formoterol and salmeterol in patients suffering from

COPD with pre-existing cardiac arrhythmias and hypoxemia. Chest 1998;114(2):411–15.
15. Centanni S, Carlucci P, Santus P, Boveri B, Tarricone D, Fiorentini C, Lombardi F, Cazzola M. Non-pulmonary effects induced by the addition of formoterol to budesonide therapy in patients with mild or moderate persistent asthma. Respiration 2000;67(1):60–4.
16. Greiff L, Wollmer P, Andersson M, Svensson C, Persson CG. Effects of formoterol on histamine induced plasma exudation in induced sputum from normal subjects. Thorax 1998;53(12):1010–13.
17. Aziz I, Tan KS, Hall IP, Devlin MM, Lipworth BJ. Subsensitivity to bronchoprotection against adenosine monophosphate challenge following regular once-daily formoterol. Eur Respir J 1998;12(3):580–4.
18. Lipworth B, Tan S, Devlin M, Aiken T, Baker R, Hendrick D. Effects of treatment with formoterol on bronchoprotection against methacholine. Am J Med 1998;104(5):431–8.
19. Aziz I, Lipworth BJ. A bolus of inhaled budesonide rapidly reverses airway subsensitivity and beta2-adrenoceptor down-regulation after regular inhaled formoterol. Chest 1999;115(3):623–8.
20. Bisgaard H. Long-acting beta(2)-agonists in management of childhood asthma: a critical review of the literature. Pediatr Pulmonol 2000;29(3):221–34.
21. Aziz I, Lipworth BJ. In vivo effect of albuterol on methacholine-contracted bronchi in conjunction with salmeterol and formoterol. J Allergy Clin Immunol 1999;103(5 Pt 1):816–22.

Foscarnet

General Information

Foscarnet (trisodium phosphonoformate hexahydrate) is a pyrophosphate analogue that interacts with the enzymatic action of polymerases and inhibits the cleavage of pyrophosphate from the nucleoside triphosphate. Because of this mechanism, the antiviral activity of the drug is broad. Foscarnet is a non-competitive inhibitor of herpesvirus DNA polymerase, hepatitis B virus DNA polymerase, and reverse transcriptases (1). Intravenous foscarnet has been used for the treatment of mucocutaneous disease due to acyclovir-resistant *Herpes simplex* (2) and for the treatment of severe CMV infection (3,4). Foscarnet has been shown to be as effective as ganciclovir in the treatment of gastrointestinal CMV and CMV retinitis in patients with AIDS (5). The two drugs differ, however, in their respective toxicity profile, and in a comparison in CMV retinitis, ganciclovir was better tolerated (6). Treatment-limiting adverse effects are renal toxicity, hypocalcemia, and mucosal ulceration.

Organs and Systems

Electrolyte balance

Significant electrolyte abnormalities have been attributed to foscarnet in a bone marrow transplant recipient on parenteral nutrition (7).

- A 39-year-old man with acute myelogenous leukemia developed a fever after allogeneic bone marrow transplantation and was given prophylactic ganciclovir and antibiotics. Parenteral nutrition was started when severe mucositis and diarrhea limited oral nutrition. On the 18th day after transplantation CMV DNA was detected in his blood and he was given foscarnet. His requirements for potassium, calcium, magnesium, and phosphorus increased dramatically, while his sodium requirements fell. Electrolyte depletion occurred within 24 hours and was accompanied by deteriorating renal function (serum creatinine 106–220, reference range 60–125 μmol/l). On withdrawal of foscarnet, the serum creatinine fell within 24 hours and the electrolyte concentrations returned to normal.

Mineral balance

The second most common adverse effect of foscarnet is symptomatic hypocalcemia, which may be responsible for the cardiac dysrhythmias and seizures that occur after acute overdose or excessively rapid infusion of foscarnet. Foscarnet stimulates the release of parathyroid hormone, which raised concerns about long-term administration (8). However, in a study of seven patients receiving a 14-day foscarnet induction regimen, there were no changes in calcium or phosphate metabolism (9).

Recognizing that foscarnet is a potent chelator of divalent cations, and that acute ionized hypocalcemia and hypomagnesemia are common adverse effects, a trial of intravenous magnesium sulfate has been conducted for foscarnet-induced hypocalcemia and hypomagnesemia in 12 AIDS patients with CMV infection (10). Increasing doses of magnesium sulfate reduced or eliminated foscarnet-induced ionized hypomagnesemia but had no discernible effect on ionized hypocalcemia, despite significant increases in serum parathyroid hormone concentrations. On this basis, intravenous supplementation for patients with normal serum magnesium concentrations was not recommended during treatment with foscarnet.

Urinary tract

Alterations in creatinine clearance or acute renal insufficiency occur in 10–20% of patients with AIDS receiving intravenous foscarnet (11), due to acute tubular damage. Severe renal insufficiency can be prevented in most cases by careful hydration before and during therapy (12). To minimize the residual incidence of nephrotoxicity, the dose of foscarnet should be frequently recalculated, based on the estimated creatinine clearance.

Patients who have undergone renal transplantation and then require treatment for cytomegalovirus infection are at special risk of renal damage due to foscarnet.

- One renal transplant recipient developed the nephrotic syndrome, with microscopic hematuria and non-oliguric acute renal insufficiency within 15 days after starting foscarnet therapy for cytomegalovirus infection (13). A kidney biopsy showed crystals in all glomeruli and in the proximal tubules. The crystals consisted of several forms of foscarnet salts. Renal function and proteinuria nevertheless improved progressively, and a second transplant biopsy 8 months after the first one showed fibrotic organization of half of the glomeruli and of the interstitial tissues, and a reduction in the amount of crystals.

The renal damage caused by foscarnet can itself alter the drug's kinetics; the dosage needs to be substantially reduced when renal complications occur, and appropriate guidelines have been developed (14).

Skin

Painful oral, penile, and vulvar ulceration can occur during foscarnet therapy (15), most probably due to local accumulation of the drug (SEDA-17, 338). Penile ulcers have been reported to be the reason for discontinuation of foscarnet therapy in up to 10% of patients (16).

Eosinophilic folliculitis is a common skin manifestation associated with HIV infection, but not commonly associated with medications.

- A 38-year-old patient with AIDS was given intravenous foscarnet 400 mg tds and no other medications (17). On the second day, a pruritic, erythematous, maculopapular, urticarial rash was noted on the limbs and trunk. The infusion was stopped and the reaction disappeared. On restarting the infusion, the reaction recurred but did not clear after withdrawal. Histology showed a pattern consistent with eosinophilic folliculitis. After UVB phototherapy for 2 months the folliculitis resolved.

References

1. Oberg B. Molecular basis of foscarnet action in human herpesvirus infections. In: Lopez C, Roizman B, editors. Human Herpesvirus Infections. New York: Raven Press 1986:141.
2. Chatis PA, Miller CH, Schrager LE, Crumpacker CS. Successful treatment with foscarnet of an acyclovir-resistant mucocutaneous infection with *Herpes simplex* virus in a patient with acquired immunodeficiency syndrome. N Engl J Med 1989;320(5):297–300.
3. Klintmalm G, Lonnqvist B, Oberg B, Gahrton G, Lernestedt JO, Lundgren G, Ringden O, Robert KH, Wahren B, Groth CG. Intravenous foscarnet for the treatment of severe cytomegalovirus infection in allograft recipients. Scand J Infect Dis 1985;17(2):157–63.
4. Jacobson MA, Drew WL, Feinberg J, O'Donnell JJ, Whitmore PV, Miner RD, Parenti D. Foscarnet therapy for ganciclovir-resistant cytomegalovirus retinitis in patients with AIDS. J Infect Dis 1991;163(6):1348–51.
5. Blanshard C, Benhamou Y, Dohin E, Lernestedt JO, Gazzard BG, Katlama C. Treatment of AIDS-associated gastrointestinal cytomegalovirus infection with foscarnet and ganciclovir: a randomized comparison. J Infect Dis 1995;172(3):622–8.
6. Lewis RA, Clogston P, Fainstein V, et al. Morbidity and toxic effects associated with ganciclovir or foscarnet therapy in a randomized cytomegalovirus retinitis trial. Studies of ocular complications of AIDS Research Group, in collaboration with the AIDS Clinical Trials Group. Arch Intern Med 1995;155(1):65–74.
7. Matarese LE, Speerhas R, Seidner DL, Steiger E. Foscarnet-induced electrolyte abnormalities in a bone marrow transplant patient receiving parenteral nutrition. JPEN J Parenter Enteral Nutr 2000;24(3):170–3.
8. Richman DD. HIV and other human retroviruses. In: Galasso GJ, Whitley RJ, Merigan TC, editors. Antiviral Agents and Viral Diseases of Man. New York: Raven Press 1990;581.
9. Jacobson MA. Maintenance therapy for cytomegalovirus retinitis in patients with acquired immunodeficiency syndrome: foscarnet. Am J Med 1992;92(2A):S26–9.
10. Huycke MM, Naguib MT, Stroemmel MM, Blick K, Monti K, Martin-Munley S, Kaufman C. A double-blind placebo-controlled crossover trial of intravenous magnesium sulfate for foscarnet-induced ionized hypocalcemia and hypomagnesemia in patients with AIDS and cytomegalovirus infection. Antimicrob Agents Chemother 2000;44(8):2143–8.
11. Katlama C, Dohin E, Caumes E, Cochereau-Massin I, Brancon C, Robinet M, Rogeaux O, Dahan R, Gentilini M. Foscarnet induction therapy for cytomegalovirus retinitis in AIDS: comparison of twice-daily and three-times-daily regimens. J Acquir Immune Defic Syndr 1992;5(Suppl 1):S18–24.
12. Deray G, Martinez F, Katlama C, Levaltier B, Beaufils H, Danis M, Rozenheim M, Baumelou A, Dohin E, Gentilini M, et al. Foscarnet nephrotoxicity: mechanism, incidence and prevention. Am J Nephrol 1989;9(4):316–21.
13. Zanetta G, Maurice-Estepa L, Mousson C, Justrabo E, Daudon M, Rifle G, Tanter Y. Foscarnet-induced crystalline glomerulonephritis with nephrotic syndrome and acute renal failure after kidney transplantation. Transplantation 1999;67(10):1376–8.
14. Aweeka FT, Jacobson MA, Martin-Munley S, Hedman A, Schoenfeld P, Omachi R, Tsunoda S, Gambertoglio JG. Effect of renal disease and hemodialysis on foscarnet pharmacokinetics and dosing recommendations. J Acquir Immune Defic Syndr Hum Retrovirol 1999;20(4):350–7.
15. Lacey HB, Ness A, Mandal BK. Vulval ulceration associated with foscarnet. Genitourin Med 1992;68(3):182.
16. Moyle G, Barton S, Gazzard BG. Penile ulceration with foscarnet therapy. AIDS 1993;7(1):140–1.
17. Roos TC, Albrecht H. Foscarnet-associated eosinophilic folliculitis in a patient with AIDS. J Am Acad Dermatol 2001;44(3):546–7.

Fosfomycin

General Information

Fosfomycin is a broad-spectrum antibiotic used to treat uncomplicated lower urinary tract infections. It penetrates interstitial space fluids of soft tissues well and reaches concentrations sufficient to substantially inhibit the growth of relevant bacteria at the target site (1).

Fosfomycin has relatively low toxicity. Its penetration into tissues, including bones and joints, and into the cerebrospinal fluid is good. When given orally (2–3 g/day), it can produce gastrointestinal distress; when injected intramuscularly, it can cause local pain. Fosfomycin is recommended in daily doses of 4–16 g intravenously for the treatment of severe infections resistant to other commonly used antibiotics. Fosfomycin diffuses moderately well into bone tissue (2).

During systemic administration, rises in the activities of serum transaminases and lactate dehydrogenase, skin reactions, eosinophilia, and altered vision have been noted (3).

Comparative studies

In a multicenter trial in 749 ambulatory women aged at least 12 years with an acute uncomplicated urinary tract infection, a single dose of fosfomycin tromethamine 3 g had an equivalent bacteriological and clinical cure rate as a 7-day course of nitrofurantoin (4). Adverse events were reported by 5.3% of fosfomycin-treated patients (versus 5.6%). The most common adverse effects were diarrhea (2.4%), vaginitis (1.8%), and nausea (0.8%), and 1.9% of fosfomycin-treated patients were withdrawn owing to adverse events (versus 4.3%).

Organs and Systems

Nervous system

Fosfomycin concentrations in brain interstitium were measured in two patients after the intravenous administration of 4 g (5). Brain C_{max} values were above MIC for relevant pathogens, such as *Streptococcus pneumoniae* and *Neisseria meningitidis*. Variability in brain penetration might be explained by the degree to which the integrity of the blood–brain barrier is disrupted by the underlying disease.

Hematologic

The effects of fosfomycin on several indices of neutrophil function have been studied in vitro (6). Phagocytosis was unaffected but there was enhanced bactericidal ability, increased intracellular calcium concentrations, raised extracellular reactive oxygen intermediate production, and reduced chemotaxis; fosfomycin did not affect intracellular oxygen intermediate production or chemokinesis.

Liver

Fosfomycin-induced recurrent liver toxicity occurred in a patient with cystic fibrosis (7).

Urinary tract

In Japanese children the use of fosfomycin within the first two days for treatment of illness caused by *Escherichia coli* O157 reduced the risk of subsequent hemolytic–uremic syndrome (8). However, treatment with oral fluoroquinolones may be preferable (9).

In rats, co-administration of fosfomycin significantly reduced the nephrotoxicity of vancomycin (10).

Immunologic

The immunomodulatory effect of fosfomycin may in part be explained by an effect on cytokine production, as shown in mice in vivo (11).

Infection risk

Bacterial biofilms develop on a number of living and inert surfaces within the urinary tract, producing chronic intractable urinary tract infections. Combination therapy with fosfomycin and a fluoroquinolone (or a fluoroquinolone and a macrolide) may be the most effective regimen available at present. Nevertheless, management of the local urinary condition and removal of the local underlying disease are the most effective approaches for treating urinary biofilm infection (12).

Long-Term Effects

Drug tolerance

There is a serious reduction in the susceptibility of strains of *E. coli* to amoxicillin (due to R-TEM enzymes), to co-trimoxazole, and to trimethoprim. However, fosfomycin trometamol remains highly active against urinary *Enterobacteriaceae*, and over 90% of *E. coli* are susceptible (13). Fosfomycin is as active as fluoroquinolones or better for treating intestinal infections caused by *Salmonella* species, pathogenic *E. coli*, *Campylobacter* species, and *Shigella* species (14).

Drug–Drug Interactions

Cisplatin

Fosfomycin is both otoprotective and nephroprotective against cisplatin-induced toxicity, without inhibiting the tumoricidal activity of cisplatin (15). Mice treated with cisplatin and fosfomycin also survived longer than animals treated with cisplatin alone, probably owing to lessening of immediate cisplatin systemic toxicity (16).

References

1. Frossard M, Joukhadar C, Erovic BM, Dittrich P, Mrass PE, Van Houte M, Burgmann H, Georgopoulos A, Muller M. Distribution and antimicrobial activity of fosfomycin in the interstitial fluid of human soft tissues. Antimicrob Agents Chemother 2000;44(10):2728–32.
2. Boselli E, Allaouchiche B. Diffusion osseuse des antibiotiques. [Diffusion in bone tissue of antibiotics.] Presse Méd 1999;28(40):2265–76.
3. Reports of fosfomycin (76 laboratory and clinical studies in Japanese, with summaries in English). Chemotherapy (Tokyo) 1975;23:1649.
4. Stein GE. Comparison of single-dose fosfomycin and a 7-day course of nitrofurantoin in female patients with uncomplicated urinary tract infection. Clin Ther 1999;21(11):1864–72.
5. Brunner M, Reinprecht A, Illievich U, Spiss CK, Dittrich P, van Houte M, Muller M. Penetration of fosfomycin into the parenchyma of human brain: a case study in three patients. Br J Clin Pharmacol 2002;54(5):548–50.
6. Krause R, Patruta S, Daxbock F, Fladerer P, Wenisch C. The effect of fosfomycin on neutrophil function. J Antimicrob Chemother 2001;47(2):141–6.
7. Durupt S, Josserand RN, Sibille M, Durieu I. Acute, recurrent fosfomycin-induced liver toxicity in an adult patient with cystic fibrosis. Scand J Infect Dis 2001;33(5):391–2.
8. Ikeda K, Ida O, Kimoto K, Takatorige T, Nakanishi N, Tatara K. Effect of early fosfomycin treatment on prevention of hemolytic uremic syndrome accompanying Escherichia coli O157:H7 infection. Clin Nephrol 1999;52(6):357–62.
9. Shiomi M, Togawa M, Fujita K, Murata R. Effect of early oral fluoroquinolones in hemorrhagic colitis due to *Escherichia coli* O157:H7. Pediatr Int 1999;41(2):228–32.
10. Nakamura T, Kokuryo T, Hashimoto Y, Inui KI. Effects of fosfomycin and imipenem–cilastatin on the nephrotoxicity

of vancomycin and cisplatin in rats. J Pharm Pharmacol 1999;51(2):227–32.
11. Matsumoto T, Tateda K, Miyazaki S, Furuya N, Ohno A, Ishii Y, Hirakata Y, Yamaguchi K. Fosfomycin alters lipopolysaccharide-induced inflammatory cytokine production in mice. Antimicrob Agents Chemother 1999;43(3):697–8.
12. Kumon H. Management of biofilm infections in the urinary tract. World J Surg 2000;24(10):1193–6.
13. Chomarat M. Resistance of bacteria in urinary tract infections. Int J Antimicrob Agents 2000;16(4):483–7.
14. Fukuyama M, Furuhata K, Oonaka K, Hara T, Sunakawa K. [Antibacterial activity of fosfomycin against the causative bacteria isolated from bacterial enteritis.] Jpn J Antibiot 2000;53(7):522–31.
15. Sakamoto M, Kaga K, Kamio T. Extended high-frequency ototoxicity induced by the first administration of cisplatin. Otolaryngol Head Neck Surg 2000;122(6):828–33.
16. Tandy JR, Tandy RD, Farris P, Truelson JM. In vivo interaction of cis-platinum and fosfomycin on squamous cell carcinoma. Laryngoscope 2000;110(7):1222–4.

Fosinopril

See also Angiotensin converting enzyme inhibitors

General Information

Fosinopril is a phosphorus-containing ester prodrug of the ACE inhibitor fosinoprilat. Its clinical pharmacology, clinical use, and safety profile have been reviewed (1).

Organs and Systems

Respiratory

Claims that cough is less often observed with fosinopril than with other ACE inhibitors are primarily based on a single open unconvincing study (2).

Liver

Hepatic injury has been described from time to time with ACE inhibitors. Severe, prolonged cholestatic jaundice has been reported with fosinopril (3). The evidence of a link to fosinopril was convincing.

- A 61-year-old man developed weakness, severe jaundice, pruritus, and weight loss over 2 weeks. He had started to take metoprolol, fosinopril, and diazepam for hypertension 5 weeks before. He had raised hepatic transaminases and bilirubin. A liver biopsy showed cholestasis in a normal cellular architecture. A lymphocyte transformation assay showed reactivity to fosinopril but not diazepam or metoprolol. Bilirubin concentrations took 4 months to normalize and pruritus persisted for 6 months.

Skin

There is a recognized association between the use of ACE inhibitors and the development of pemphigus vulgaris, for example with enalapril (SEDA-26, 235). A case of worsening of pemphigus vulgaris with fosinopril, and a subsequent in vitro mechanistic study, has been published (4).

- A 64-year-old woman with insulin-dependent diabetes mellitus and pemphigus vulgaris controlled by deflazacort 12 mg/day was given fosinopril 10 mg/day for hypertension. Within 1 month her skin lesions worsened and an indirect immunofluorescence test became positive. Fosinopril was withdrawn and her skin lesions improved without modification of her steroid regimen; 10 months later the immunofluorescence test was negative.

Following this, normal human skin slices (obtained after informed consent from mammoplasty patients) were incubated with increasing concentrations of either fosinopril or captopril for 2–24 hours. Sera from patients with pemphigus vulgaris, containing antidesmoglein-3 antibodies (anti-Dsg3) were tested on the skin samples incubated with fosinopril and captopril, as well as control skin samples incubated with 0.9% saline. Indirect immunofluorescence testing showed that captopril at a concentration of 1.7×10^{-9} mmol/l blocked the binding of anti-Dsg3 to the keratinocyte surface, probably because captopril blocked adhesion molecules. In contrast, fosinopril only had this effect at a concentration of 1.7×10^{-2} mmol/l, a concentration much higher than would occur in vivo. The authors proposed that captopril produces acantholysis by blocking adhesion molecules, but that fosinopril does not have this effect, and that another mechanism must have been involved in the case that they reported.

References

1. Shionoiri H, Naruse M, Minamisawa K, Ueda S, Himeno H, Hiroto S, Takasaki I. Fosinopril. Clinical pharmacokinetics and clinical potential. Clin Pharmacokinet 1997;32(6):460–80.
2. Punzi HA. Safety update: focus on cough. Am J Cardiol 1993;72(20):H45–8.
3. Nunes AC, Amaro P, Mac as F, Cipriano A, Martins I, Rosa A, Pimenta I, Donato A, Freitas D. Fosinopril-induced prolonged cholestatic jaundice and pruritus: first case report. Eur J Gastroenterol Hepatol 2001;13(3):279–82.
4. Parodi A, Cozzani E, Milesi G, Drosera M, Rebora A. Fosinopril as a possible pemphigus-inducing drug. Dermatology 2002;204(2):139–41.

Fosmidomycin

General Information

Fosmidomycin is an antimicrobial drug that acts by inhibiting 1-deoxy-D-xylulose 5-phosphate reductoisomerase, a key enzyme of the non-mevalonate pathway of isoprenoid biosynthesis. It inhibits the synthesis of isoprenoids by *Plasmodium falciparum* and suppresses the growth of multidrug-resistant strains in vitro.

In an open, uncontrolled study, fosmidomycin was administered for 3–5 days (1.2 g every 8 hours) to 27 adults with malaria, of whom 16 reported possibly drug-related adverse events (1). The most frequent adverse events were headache, weakness, myalgia, abdominal pain, and loose stools. There were two cases of raised alanine transaminase activity.

Reference

1. Missinou MA, Borrmann S, Schindler A, Issifou S, Adegnika AA, Matsiegui PB, Binder R, Lell B, Wiesner J, Baranek T, Jomaa H, Kremsner PG. Fosmidomycin for malaria. Lancet 2002;360(9349):1941–2.

Fragrances

General Information

The fragrance mix, introduced in 1977 by Larsen (1), is used to detect sensitivity to fragrances in, for example, cosmetics and household products (SEDA-20, 149) (2). The mix contains eight widely used fragrance compounds. Additional indicators of fragrance allergy are balsam of Peru and colophony.

Organs and Systems

Immunologic

Contact sensitivity to fragrance mix is not infrequent and reflects the ubiquitous presence of these substances (3). The frequency of positive patch tests to the fragrance mix has increased over recent years. However, the mix has been estimated to miss 15% of relevant contact allergies (4). In a study of 1855 consecutive patients, patch tests with additional fragrance allergens has shown that lyral (2.7% positive reactions), citral (1.1%), and farnesol P (0.5%) are valuable additions when patch-testing to detect a fragrance allergy. Several other compounds that were tested at the same time were positive less often (5). A similar study in 1606 consecutively tested patients showed that ylang-ylang oil I (2.6% positive patch tests), ylang-ylang oil II (2.5%), lemongrass oil (1.6%), narcissus absolute (1.3%), jasmine absolute (1.2%), and sandalwood oil (0.9%) are the most important ingredients (6). In this series, limonene was positive in 0.6% of cases, but in another series of 2273 consecutive patients it was positive in 2.8%, of whom 57% did not react to the fragrance mix (7).

These and other compounds were patch-tested in another series of fragrance-sensitive patients (8). Of the 218 subjects tested, 76% were positive to the fragrance mix. Ten fragrances were not detected by the fragrance mix: benzenepropanol; beta, beta, 3-methylhexylsalicylate; dl-citronellol; synthetic ylang-ylang oil; benzyl mixture (containing benzyl alcohol, benzyl salicylate, and benzyl acetate); cyclohexylacetate; eugenyl methyl ether; isoeugenyl methyl ether; 3-phenyl-1-propanol; and 3,7-dimethyl-7-methoxyoctan-2-ol. In earlier studies by this group, significant additional reactions were found to sandela, geranium oil bourbon, spearmint oil, galaxolide (1,3,4,6,7,8-hexahydro-4,6,6,7,8,8-hexamethylcyclopenta-gamma-2-benzopyran), omega-6-hexadecenlactone, and tripal (dimethyltetrahydrobenzaldehyde) (9,10).

Patients with chronic venous insufficiency and venous leg ulcers are at risk of sensitization to topical medications. The frequency of sensitization in these patients is up to 67% (11). In a study using an expanded European standard series and 20 different wound dressings for patch-testing in 36 patients with chronic venous insufficiency, sensitization to fragrance mix was found in three cases (12).

References

1. Pasche-Koo F, Piletta PA, Hunziker N, Hauser C. High sensitization rate to emulsifiers in patients with chronic leg ulcers. Contact Dermatitis 1994;31(4):226–8.
2. de Groot AC, Frosch PJ. Adverse reactions to fragrances. A clinical review. Contact Dermatitis 1997;36(2):57–86.
3. Marren P, Wojnarowska F, Powell S. Allergic contact dermatitis and vulvar dermatoses. Br J Dermatol 1992;126(1):52–6.
4. De Groot AC, Weyland JW, Nater JP. Unwanted Effects of Cosmetics and Drugs Used in Dermatology. 3rd ed. Amsterdam: Elsevier, 1994.
5. Frosch PJ, Johansen JD, Menne T, Pirker C, Rastogi SC, Andersen KE, Bruze M, Goossens A, Lepoittevin JP, White IR. Further important sensitizers in patients sensitive to fragrances. I. Reactivity to 14 frequently used chemicals. Contact Dermatitis 2002;47(2):78–85.
6. Frosch PJ, Johansen JD, Menne T, Pirker C, Rastogi SC, Andersen KE, Bruze M, Goossens A, Lepoittevin JP, White IR. Further important sensitizers in patients sensitive to fragrances. II. Reactivity to essential oils. Contact Dermatitis 2002;47(5):279–87.
7. Matura M, Goossens A, Bordalo O, Garcia-Bravo B, Magnusson K, Wrangsjo K, Karlberg AT. Oxidized citrus oil (R-limonene): a frequent skin sensitizer in Europe. J Am Acad Dermatol 2002;47(5):709–14.
8. Larsen W, Nakayama H, Fischer T, Elsner P, Frosch P, Burrows D, Jordan W, Shaw S, Wilkinson J, Marks J, Sugawara M, Nethercott M, Nethercott J. Fragrance contact dermatitis—a worldwide multicenter investigation (Part III). Contact Dermatitis 2002;46(3):141–4.
9. Larsen W, Nakayama H, Lindberg M, Fischer T, Elsner P, Burrows D, Jordan W, Shaw S, Wilkinson J, Marks J Jr, Sugawara M, Nethercott J. Fragrance contact dermatitis: a worldwide multicenter investigation (Part I). Am J Contact Dermat 1996;7(2):77–83.
10. Larsen W, Nakayama H, Fischer T, Elsner P, Frosch P, Burrows D, Jordan W, Shaw S, Wilkinson J, Marks J Jr, Sugawara M, Nethercott M, Nethercott J. Fragrance contact dermatitis: a worldwide multicenter investigation (Part II). Contact Dermatitis 2001;44(6):344–6.
11. Wilson CL, Cameron J, Powell SM, Cherry G, Ryan TJ. High incidence of contact dermatitis in leg-ulcer patients—implications for management. Clin Exp Dermatol 1991;16(4):250–3.
12. Gallenkemper G, Rabe E, Bauer R. Contact sensitization in chronic venous insufficiency: modern wound dressings. Contact Dermatitis 1998;38(5):274–8.

Fructose and sorbitol

General Information

Attention has been drawn to the use of fructose-based and sorbitol-based solutions for parenteral administration in Germany and German-speaking countries, where they are available for routine fluid replacement and intravenous feeding, and are widely prescribed, even after minor surgical procedures (1). Their main advantage is claimed to be the avoidance of a blood glucose raising effect, particularly in severely ill patients with glucose intolerance. In such cases it may be possible to avoid insulin therapy, since the first steps in the metabolism of these carbohydrates are insulin-dependent.

Organs and Systems

Metabolism

Infusions of fructose or sorbitol can cause lactic acidosis (2,3), particularly in combination with ethanol.

- In one patient, blood lactate concentration was monitored frequently over 5 days during intravenous feeding with a sorbitol-ethanol-amino acid mixture. During the first five infusions, blood lactate rose only moderately, but with the final infusion, lactate rose to 11 mmol/l and the patient had a severe metabolic acidosis. In retrospect the patient had had worsening renal and hepatic function tests during the preceding 24 hours. On ending the infusions, the blood lactate concentration fell rapidly.

The problems that can result from the administration in total parenteral fluid infusions of D-fructose or sorbitol have been reviewed (4). Either of these can cause life-threatening hypoglycemia, unless glucose is administered concurrently, in patients who have underlying hereditary fructose intolerance. Unless there is a clear clinical history of the condition, it may not be readily identified. In some countries, fructose and D-glucitol (sorbitol) have been eliminated from the pharmacopoeia for this reason.

Acid–base balance

The combination of fructose with sorbitol (which is converted to fructose by sorbitol dehydrogenase) causes lactic acidosis and hyperuricemia (reflecting purine nucleotide breakdown in the liver). The assimilation of fructose (as the free monosaccharide or derived from the oxidation of sorbitol or hydrolysis of sucrose) differs from that of sucrose. Fructose is phosphorylated rapidly in the intestine and liver by the catalytic action of ketohexose kinase (fructokinase) at the 1-carbon position. Cleavage of fructose-1-phosphate by aldolase B ensures its metabolic incorporation into the pathways of glycolysis and gluconeogenesis. Inherited deficiency of aldolase B occurs in hereditary fructose intolerance, an autosomal recessive condition (5). After ingestion of fructose and related sugars in this disorder, high concentrations of fructose-1-phosphate accumulate in the liver, intestine, and proximal renal tubules, and a profound metabolic disturbance occurs. Metabolic acidosis, hypophosphatemia, hypoglycemia, and hyperuricemia result, and functional impairment and pathological injury occur in these tissues with continued administration (6).

Severe lactic acidosis, with serum lactate concentrations of 8.7, 8.6, and 7.9 ml developed in three patients with hyperosmolar syndromes (7). Each had received rehydration treatment with 5% fructose in water (fructose dosage was 0.5 g/kg/hour). After correction of the electrolyte disturbances, continued infusion of fructose in the same dosage increased the plasma lactate concentration in two of the patients to 4.9 and 4.0 mmol/l, indicating near normalization of hepatic lactate utilization. In addition to peripheral insulin resistance and reduced muscular glucose utilization, the hyperosmolar state was also associated with reduced tolerance to fructose. It follows that in rehydration therapy for hyperosmolar syndromes infusion solutions containing fructose should not be used. This "functional fructose intolerance" is thought to be due to impaired gluconeogenesis. In order to administer 50 g of fructose, infusion rates up to 1000 ml/hour are necessary to achieve a positive fluid balance and to match the osmotic diuresis that is produced. Failure to maintain proper balance can cause serious metabolic complications, such as hyperlactemia, lactic acidosis, and circulatory shock.

Hereditary fructose intolerance affects one in 21 000 persons, and there have been more than 12 severe complications caused by these solutions, several lethal. Since a prior history of fructose intolerance is often not obtained, it has been argued that the use of fructose- and sorbitol-containing infusion fluids must be regarded as offering doubtful advantage but carrying definite lethal risk, and that their use should be discontinued. A modified intravenous fructose tolerance test should at least be carried out before infusions of fructose or sorbitol are given (8).

Liver

Four children aged 2.5–14 years were given infusions of fructose, sorbitol, and xylitol after sustaining head trauma ($n = 3$) or after attempting suicide with carbromal ($n = 1$). After transitory polyuria, renal insufficiency of varying severity set in 3–6 days after the start of treatment. Serum osmolality fell to 265–274 mosmol/kg, the hematocrit to 0.25–0.31, and hyponatremia developed. Serum creatinine rose to a maximum of 256–930 μmol/l. Liver damage developed in parallel with renal insufficiency. Two of the children died of acute liver atrophy. The other patients were given symptomatic treatment with balanced equalization of the hyponatremia, administration of furosemide, and carbohydrate substitution. They were discharged after 4 and 8 weeks respectively, with normal renal and hepatic function. Dialysis was not required. The hepatic and renal abnormalities were attributed to the large amounts of fructose, sorbitol, and xylitol that had been administered, to totals of 7.1–23.0 g/kg on the first day (9).

Susceptibility Factors

Genetic factors

Hereditary fructose intolerance is an autosomal recessive disorder with reduced activity of aldolase B in the liver, kidney, and small intestine. Ingestion of only a few grams of fructose, sorbitol, or sucrose causes abdominal pain and vomiting (SEDA-13, 479). Affected individuals develop an aversion to sugary foods and drinks, and in severe cases exposure during infancy may result in progressive liver damage and death. Exclusion of fructose from the diet allows them to develop and grow normally.

- A 16-year-old girl died after an uncomplicated appendicectomy (10). She had undiagnosed hereditary fructose intolerance and had been given sorbitol and fructose postoperatively.

References

1. Cox TM. Therapeutic use of fructose: professional freedom, "pharmacovigilance" and Europe. QJM 1995;88(4):225–7.
2. Batstone GF, Alberti KG, Dewar AK. Reversible lactic acidosis associated with repeated intravenous infusions of sorbitol and ethanol. Postgrad Med J 1977;53(623):567–9.
3. Coarse JF, Cardoni AA. Use of fructose in the treatment of acute alcoholic intoxication. Am J Hosp Pharm 1975;32(5):518–19.
4. Palyza V, Bockova M. Poruchy metabolismu fruktozy a infuze. [Fructose metabolism disorders and infusions.] Vnitr Lek 1992;38(8):814–21.
5. Keller U. Zuckerersatzstoffe Fructose und Sorbit: ein unnötiges Risiko in der parenteralen Ernöhrung. [The sugar substitutes fructose and sorbite: an unnecessary risk in parenteral nutrition.] Schweiz Med Wochenschr 1989;119(4):101–6.
6. Sachs M, Asskali F, Forster H, Encke A. Wiederholte perioperative Application von Fructose und sorbit bei einer Patientin mit hereditarer fructoseintoleranz (HFI). [Repeated perioperative administration of fructose and sorbitol in a female patient with hereditary fructose intolerance (HFI).] Z Ernahrungswiss 1993;32(1):56–66.
7. Druml W, Kleinberger G, Lenz K, Laggner A, Schneeweiss B. Fructose-induced hyperlactemia in hyperosmolar syndromes. Klin Wochenschr 1986;64(13):615–18.
8. Panning B, Piepenbrock S. Kritische Bemerkungen zu Berichten über Todesfölle durch hereditäre Fructose intoleranz im Erwachsenenalter aus der Sicht der Neuroanästhesie. [Critical comments on reports of fatalities in hereditary fructose intolerance in adulthood from the viewpoint of neuroanesthesia.] Anasth Intensivther Notfallmed 1988;23(4):217–19.
9. Galaske RG, Burdelski M, Brodehl J. Primär polyurisches Nierenversagen und akute gelbe Leberdystrophie nach Infusion von Zuckeraustauschstoffen im Kindesalter. [Primary polyuric kidney failure and acute yellow liver dystrophy following infusion of glucose substitutes in children.] Dtsch Med Wochenschr 1986;111(25):978–83.
10. Collins J. Metabolic disease. Time for fructose solutions to go. Lancet 1993;341(8845):600.

Fumaric acid esters

General Information

Fumaric acid esters are used to treat a variety of skin disorders, including psoriasis (1), cutaneous sarcoidosis (2), necrobiosis lipoidica diabeticorum (3), and disseminated granuloma annulare (4).

In 39 patients with psoriasis (12 women, 27 men) in a randomized, double-blind, placebo-controlled study, three different treatments were used: (a) tablets containing a combination of topical dimethylfumarate plus different salts of monoethylfumarate, (b) octylhydrogen fumarate tablets, and (c) placebo (5). Five patients dropped out because of adverse effects or aggravation of the skin lesions. The patients who used the combination of monoethylfumarate plus dimethylfumarate had a significantly better therapeutic response than those who took placebo or octylhydrogen fumarate. Adverse effects of the fumarate-containing tablets were flushing, diarrhea, a reversible rise in transaminases, lymphocytopenia, and eosinophilia. One patient developed impaired renal function, which normalized after withdrawal.

In 83 patients with severe psoriasis vulgaris, the fumaric acid ester formulations Fumaderm initial and Fumaderm caused adverse effects in 62%, mainly flushing and gastrointestinal complaints, which decreased in frequency during the course of the study (6).

Of 101 patients with severe psoriasis vulgaris, 70 completed the treatment period of 4 months (7). Discontinuation was due to adverse events in 7, lack of efficacy in 2, and other reasons, such as non-attendance, in 22. There was a slight overall reduction in lymphocyte count, which was more than 50% below baseline in 10 patients. During weeks 4 and 8, mean eosinophil counts were above the reference range, but by the end of the therapy the eosinophil counts had returned to normal. None of the patients had changes in renal function. Adverse events were reported in 69%, consisting mainly of gastrointestinal complaints (56%) and flushing (31%). In five patients gastrointestinal complaints and in two patients flushing led to withdrawal from the study.

In 66 patients with severe psoriasis who took fumaric acid esters for up to 14 years, there were adverse events in 73%, usually mild and mainly consisting of flushing (55%), diarrhea (42%), nausea (14%), tiredness (14%), and stomach complaints (12%) (8). There was a relative lymphocytopenia in 76%, resulting in permanent withdrawal in four patients. There were transient eosinophilia in 14%, and moderate liver enzyme rises were observed in 25%.

The effect of systemically and/or topically administered ethyl fumarate on psoriasis was studied in six patients. Two patients who had been treated with locally applied ointments, consisting of 3 or 5% ethyl fumarate in petrolatum, developed symptoms of renal toxicity (9).

Organs and Systems

Skin

Topical monoethyl fumarate caused contact dermatitis in a patient with atopic eczema and a generalized, partly pustulous, exanthema in a patient with psoriasis (10). The authors suggested that the mechanism was nonimmunological contact urticaria.

In 12 healthy volunteers, topical monoethyl fumarate caused spontaneous persistent erythema and systemic administration caused flushing (11). In patients with urticaria pigmentosa the effect was significantly greater in the diseased skin than in the healthy skin, suggesting that monoethyl fumarate causes mast cell degranulation.

References

1. Werdenberg D, Joshi R, Wolffram S, Merkle HP, Langguth P. Presystemic metabolism and intestinal absorption of antipsoriatic fumaric acid esters. Biopharm Drug Dispos 2003;24(6):259–73.
2. Nowack U, Gambichler T, Hanefeld C, Kastner U, Altmeyer P. Successful treatment of recalcitrant cutaneous sarcoidosis with fumaric acid esters. BMC Dermatol 2002;2(1):15.
3. Gambichler T, Kreuter A, Freitag M, Pawlak FM, Brockmeyer NH, Altmeyer P. Clearance of necrobiosis lipoidica with fumaric acid esters. Dermatology 2003;207(4):422–4.
4. Kreuter A, Gambichler T, Altmeyer P, Brockmeyer NH. Treatment of disseminated granuloma annulare with fumaric acid esters. BMC Dermatol 2002;2(1):5.
5. Nugteren-Huying WM, van der Schroeff JG, Hermans J, Suurmond D. Fumaarzuurtherapie tegen psoriasis; een dubbelblind, placebo-gecontroleerd onderzoek. [Fumaric acid therapy in psoriasis; a double-blind, placebo-controlled study.] Ned Tijdschr Geneeskd 1990;134(49):2387–91.
6. Altmeyer P, Hartwig R, Matthes U. Das Wirkuns- und Sicherheitsprofil von Fumarsaureestern in der oralen Langzeittherapie bei schwerer therapieresistenter Psoriasis vulgaris. [Efficacy and safety profile of fumaric acid esters in oral long-term therapy with severe treatment refractory psoriasis vulgaris. A study of 83 patients.] Hautarzt 1996;47(3):190–6.
7. Mrowietz U, Christophers E, Altmeyer P. Treatment of psoriasis with fumaric acid esters: results of a prospective multicentre study. German Multicentre Study. Br J Dermatol 1998;138(3):456–60.
8. Hoefnagel JJ, Thio HB, Willemze R, Bouwes Bavinck JN. Long-term safety aspects of systemic therapy with fumaric acid esters in severe psoriasis. Br J Dermatol 2003;149(2):363–9.
9. Dubiel W, Happle R. Behandlungsversuch mit Fumarsäure monoäthylester bei Psoriasis vulgaris. [Experimental treatment with fumaric acid monoethylester in psoriasis vulgaris.] Z Haut Geschlechtskr 1972;47(13):545–50.
10. Ducker P, Pfeiff B. Zwei Falle von Nebenwirkungen einer Fumarsaureester—Lokaltherapie. [Two cases of side effects of a fumaric acid ester—local therapy.] Z Hautkr 1990;65(8):734–6.
11. Gehring W, Gloor M. Persistierende Spontanerytheme durch topische Anwendung von Fumarsauremonoethylester—eine obligate Mastzelldegranulation? [Persistent spontaneous erythema caused by topical use of fumaric acid monoethyl ester—an obligate mast cell degranulation?] Dermatol Monatsschr 1990;176(2–3):123–8.

Furaltadone

General Information

Furaltadone, 5-morpholinomethyl-3-(5-nitrofurfurylidenamino)oxazolidin-2-one), is a crystalline antibiotic powder, which is added to animal feeds.

Organs and Systems

Immunologic

Furaltadone can provoke contact allergic reactions (1). A case of contact allergy to the antibiotic in eardrops, with positive patch tests, has been reported (2).

References

1. Neldner KH. Contact dermatitis from animal feed additives. Arch Dermatol 1972;106(5):722–3.
2. Sanchez-Perez J, Cordoba S, del Rio MJ, Garcia-Dies A. Allergic contact dermatitis from furaltadone in eardrops. Contact Dermatitis 1999;40(4):222.

Furazolidone

General Information

Furazolidone is used in the treatment of giardiasis. Its adverse effects are usually mild and transient: abdominal discomfort, nausea, and vomiting. The urine may be dark-colored (SEDA-11, 597). Metabolites of furazolidone inhibit monoamine oxidase (1) and there is therefore the potential for interactions with foods containing tyramine (2) and with opioid analgesics; hyperpyrexia has been reported in rabbits that were given furazolidone and pethidine (3).

References

1. Timperio AM, Kuiper HA, Zolla L. Identification of a furazolidone metabolite responsible for the inhibition of amino oxidases. Xenobiotica 2003;33(2):153–67.
2. Pettinger WA, Oates JA. Supersensitivity to tyramine during monoamine oxidase inhibition in man. Mechanism at the level of the adrenergic neuron. Clin Pharmacol Ther 1968;9(3):341–4.
3. Eltayeb IB, Osman OH. Furazolidone–pethidine interaction in rabbits. Br J Pharmacol 1975;55(4):497–501.

Furosemide

See also Diuretics

General Information

Furosemide is the classic member of the group of so-called high-ceiling or loop diuretics, which can achieve a much greater peak diuresis than the thiazides. It is widely and frequently used both orally and parenterally over a wider dosage range than the thiazide diuretics, because its concentration-effect curve is steeper and because it is effective in patients with moderate renal insufficiency (creatinine clearance 5–25 ml/minute), in whom the thiazide diuretics and most related compounds are ineffective.

Furosemide is quickly and almost completely excreted by kidney unmetabolized. The usual oral dose is 20–120 mg, but much larger doses (for example 1000 mg) have been used in renal insufficiency. It is very effective after intravenous injection, and doses of 500 mg and more can be used in emergencies (renal insufficiency, pulmonary edema). The majority of adverse effects occur with the use of high doses, 95% of the reactions being dose dependent (1).

General adverse effects

Disturbances of fluid and electrolyte balance, such as hyponatremia, hypokalemia, and dehydration with circulatory disturbances (such as dizziness, postural hypotension, and syncope), have been reported. Rarely gastrointestinal symptoms are problems with high dosages and in the elderly. Pancreatitis and jaundice seem to occur more often than with the thiazide diuretics, but deterioration of glucose tolerance seems to be less common. At serum concentrations over 50 μg/ml, tinnitus, vertigo, and deafness, sometimes permanent, have been reported. Hematological disorders, particularly thrombocytopenia, and serious skin disorders occur occasionally, as do hypersensitivity reactions. Neither tumor-inducing effects nor second-generation effects have been documented.

Organs and Systems

Cardiovascular

Because furosemide, apart from its diuretic effect, has transient but pronounced vasodilator properties (changes in both venous capacitance and peripheral arteriolar resistance have been described in anephric patients), it can cause postural hypotension and syncope, particularly if given together with other blood pressure-lowering drugs (SED-8, 458) (SED-9, 349) (SED-9, 350). Ischemic complications have been reported in elderly patients. Reactions due to extracellular volume depletion accounted for 9% of all adverse effects observed in 535 patients treated with furosemide (1). Neuroendocrine activation and resultant increased peripheral resistance (afterload) after furosemide reduce cardiac output and stroke volume and increase cardiac work, with the possibility of worsening myocardial and tissue ischemia. Since many patients with heart failure have underlying myocardial ischemia or infarction, initial symptomatic benefit from furosemide can be followed by detrimental effects on myocardial perfusion, with extension or completion of myocardial necrosis.

When it is used in cardiac failure, furosemide acts in two ways: besides its diuretic effect it produces an immediate fall in left ventricular filling pressure, which is independent of and precedes diuresis. If furosemide is given intravenously in stable chronic heart failure (which it normally is not), this can be an unwanted effect, causing deterioration (SEDA-11, 199), particularly in patients with pure right ventricular failure.

Nervous system

Visual disturbances and drowsiness have been described, but it is not clear whether these were caused by reduced cerebral perfusion or by a direct effect of the drug itself.

Sensory systems

At high doses, and especially if serum concentrations are over 50 μg/ml, furosemide can cause ototoxic reactions, such as tinnitus, vertigo, and even deafness, sometimes permanent (SED-9, 351). Subclinical, audiometrically determined, high-tone deafness has been reported to occur in 6.4% of furosemide-treated patients (2). It is generally considered advisable to use another diuretic in patients whose hearing is already impaired, and to avoid using furosemide along with other ototoxic drugs, such as the aminoglycosides.

Sensorineural hearing loss occurs in a small proportion of very premature babies who are given furosemide. Various causative mechanisms have been suggested, including bilirubin, drugs, infection, and/or hypoxic brainstem injury. In a case-control study of 15 children and 30 controls born before 33 weeks of gestation, renal insufficiency and/or aminoglycoside use in conjunction with furosemide was associated with sensorineural hearing loss (3).

Endocrine

Furosemide rarely causes the syndrome of inappropriate antidiuretic hormone secretion (SIADH) (although it has been found useful in treating some patients with SIADH who cannot tolerate water restriction (4)). In furosemide-induced cases (SEDA-7, 246), serum ADH concentrations were raised, total body sodium was normal, total body potassium greatly reduced, and intracellular water raised at the expense of extracellular fluid volume. However, such cases are rare, and no new cases have been published since this complication was reported in SEDA-7.

Nutrition

Patients with congestive heart failure taking high doses of furosemide can develop thiamine deficiency, which is improved by thiamine supplementation. There is whole-blood thiamine phosphate deficiency, but no reduction in the storage form of thiamine, thiamine diphosphate. These observations suggest that thiamine supplementation may not be necessary in elderly patients taking furosemide for congestive heart failure (5).

Hematologic

Agranulocytosis, thrombocytopenia, and hemolytic anemia have been reported occasionally (SED-8, 484) (SED-9, 350) (SEDA-1, 180). The commonest complication is thrombocytopenia (6), although it is often mild and asymptomatic (7).

Gastrointestinal

With normal doses, nausea, vomiting, and diarrhea are very uncommon, accounting for less than 1% of all adverse reactions (SED-9, 350). The incidence rises with higher doses and in the presence of uremia.

Liver

Although furosemide is very hepatotoxic in experimental animals, only a few cases of jaundice have been reported (SED-8, 484) (SED-8, 485), and no fully documented cases have so far been published. However, in patients with cirrhosis furosemide readily precipitates hepatic encephalopathy (SED-8, 485), even when low doses are used (1).

Biliary tract

Biliary colic has been attributed to furosemide (SED-11, 427).

Pancreas

Increases in serum isoamylase (SEDA-6, 213) and pancreatitis have been reported in patients taking furosemide.

Urinary tract

Excessive diuresis and dehydration often cause a transient reduction in glomerular filtration rate and a rise in serum urea (about 8% of all adverse reactions) (SED-8, 350). The sudden diuresis can cause loin pain, particularly in elderly patients, and acute urinary retention and overflow incontinence in elderly men with prostatic hyperplasia.

Although it is often described in children, medullary nephrocalcinosis with furosemide has been rarely described in adults.

- A 40-year-old woman who had taken furosemide (40–160 mg/day) for 15 years developed medullary nephrocalcinosis (8).

Chronic tubulointerstitial nephritis has been reported with furosemide.

- A 25-year-old woman developed biopsy-proven chronic tubulointerstitial nephritis with accompanying distal renal tubular acidosis in association with furosemide abuse (up to 1.2 g/day for several months) (9).

Four children with the nephrotic syndrome developed transient hypercalciuria and intraluminal calcification in renal histopathological specimens without radiological evidence of renal calcification. These children were resistant to corticosteroids and were receiving furosemide plus albumin for the management of edema (10). This result stresses the pervasive effect of furosemide, and probably all loop diuretics, in increasing urinary calcium excretion, with resultant nephrocalcinosis. Whenever possible, steps should be taken to limit the hypercalciuric effect of loop diuretics. Such maneuvers could include limiting the sodium content of the diet and/or combining the loop diuretic with a thiazide diuretic.

Skin

Rashes seem to be just as common with furosemide (SED-8, 484) as with other oral diuretics, but severe skin reactions (exfoliative dermatitis, erythema multiforme, acquired epidermolysis bullosa), which are rare with other diuretics, have been occasionally reported with high doses of furosemide in renal insufficiency (SED-12, 503) (SEDA-18, 234).

Cases of furosemide-induced lupus-like syndrome (11), bullous pemphigoid (12,13), and lichenoid drug eruptions (14) have been reported.

A review of furosemide-induced skin reactions included a description of a unique case of an 88-year-old man who developed an eruption that clinically and histologically simulated Sweet's syndrome (acute febrile neutrophilic vasculitis) after 6 weeks (15). Atypical features and rapid resolution suggested a drug eruption rather than true Sweet's syndrome. However, a similar mechanism may have been implicated a hypersensitivity reaction involving immune complexes.

Linear IgA bullous dermatosis associated with the administration of furosemide has been reported (16).

- An 86-year-old woman, with a history of stable schizophrenia, chronic obstructive pulmonary disease, ischemic cardiomyopathy, and type 2 diabetes, was admitted with cardiac insufficiency, which was treated by introduction of enalapril. A chest infection was treated with co-amoxiclav with gradual alleviation of symptoms over 10 days. At this point, furosemide was begun, because of persistent signs of heart failure. After 3 days, erythema and bullae were noted on her palms and soles, and later on the trunk, extremities, hard palate, and buccal mucosa. Biopsy showed the characteristic features of linear IgA bullous dermatosis, with linear deposition of IgA along the basement membrane. Co-amoxiclav and furosemide were withdrawn; no new lesions were noted thereafter.

Furosemide has previously been related to other bullous dermatoses, particularly bullous pemphigoid (SED-14, 671). In this case only a temporal relation was demonstrated, as rechallenge was judged to be unethical. The other putative offending drug, co-amoxiclav, was regarded as unlikely to be causative, because it had been given many times before without noticeable skin lesions.

Furosemide has been associated with disseminated superficial porokeratosis, a heritable disorder of cornification (17).

A man developed acute generalized exanthematous pustulosis while taking furosemide (18). A positive lymphocyte transformation test suggested an immunological mechanism.

Immunologic

It has long been thought that loop and thiazide diuretics pose a theoretical risk of cross-sensitivity in patients with sulfonamide allergy because of their common structures. However, the available literature does not provide sufficient numbers of well-documented cases to support this impression (19). It seems that careful administration of diuretics is permissible in patients with documented sulfonamide allergy, but as always such a drug challenge should not be attempted without careful follow-up. A furosemide rechallenge protocol, based on a method that has been used to rechallenge with a sulfa-containing antimicrobial agent, safely allowed the long-term reinstitution of loop diuretic therapy with furosemide (20).

Body temperature

Several cases of furosemide-associated fever have been reported (SEDA-20, 204) (SEDA-21, 229) (SEDA-22, 238). These had certain features in common: (1) the affected infants were in their first year of life; (2) there was congestive heart failure as a result of congenital abnormalities or cardiomyopathy; (3) the temperature was raised to 38.5–40°C and there was a resemblance to septic fever; (4) concomitant treatment with digoxin; (5) negative physical examination and investigations for a source of infection; (6) withdrawal of furosemide was followed by disappearance of fever within 1–2 days. In some cases, the use of furosemide in lower dosages or on alternate days avoided fever. The mechanism of this adverse effect is unclear, but it appears to be dose-related. Consideration of furosemide as a cause of fever in such patients may save unnecessary laboratory studies and lead to early resolution.

Long-Term Effects

Drug withdrawal

The more intensive diuretic treatment is the greater the risk from sudden withdrawal. In one series of 38 patients, taking 20–40 mg furosemide or equivalent, generally for heart failure, withdrawal was attempted when all had been free of heart failure or hypertension for at least 3 months; it was followed by clinical or radiological relapse in 29% and one of the patients died (21). In another five patients, withdrawal in three led to severe symptoms necessitating admission to hospital (SEDA-10, 192) (SEDA-10, 193). The best advice is to withdraw intensive diuretic treatment only with the utmost caution and not to attempt withdrawal at all if there is any radiological evidence of heart failure. In patients with congestive heart failure, independent predictors of the need for continued diuretic were furosemide dosage greater than 40 mg/day, a left ventricular ejection fraction less than 0.27, and hypertension (22).

The effects of furosemide withdrawal on postprandial blood pressure have been assessed in 20 elderly patients (mean age 73 years) with heart failure and preserved left ventricular systolic function (ejection fraction 61%) (23). In 13 who were able to discontinue furosemide (mean dose 32 mg/day), maximum systolic blood pressure fell significantly from 25 mmHg to 11 mmHg and diastolic blood pressure from 18 to 9 mmHg over 3 months. In the continuation group (mean furosemide dose 21 mg/day), there was no change in the postprandial fall.

However, there are sometimes opportunities for withdrawal of furosemide (SEDA-22, 237). If diuretics are withdrawn suddenly in patients with a normal sodium intake, there will be rebound retention of sodium and water, because compensatory mechanisms that maintain sodium balance in the face of diuretics continue to act for several days after the diuresis has worn off. There are two methods of mitigating rebound retention of sodium and water: gradual reduction of the dosage or institution of a low sodium diet so that only a small amount of sodium can be retained when the diuretic is withdrawn. Rebound retention of sodium and water, with consequent edema, may convince the doctor that continued diuretic therapy is necessary, and the patient is then committed to life-time exposure. Even in patients with heart failure, reduced intake of salt may remove the need for diuretics or allow the use of lower dosages.

Second-Generation Effects

Pregnancy

Although furosemide has embryotoxic properties in some animal species, it has been widely used in pregnant women without any adverse effects. Nevertheless, it should be used with great caution, since hypovolemia can lead to reduced uterine and placental blood flow. Careful monitoring of fetal heart action is necessary. Furosemide passes the placenta and increases fetal urine production. It can also increase acid concentrations in maternal serum, fetal serum, and amniotic fluid, thus masking a useful index for the development of pre-eclampsia (24). Its use in pregnant women should therefore be restricted to the treatment of cardiac failure.

Lactation

Furosemide passes into the breast milk in a concentration 80% of that in serum at pH 7.0, but the total amount of drug ingested is probably too low to affect the neonate (25).

Susceptibility Factors

Age

In premature infants furosemide can cause persistent patent ductus arteriosus (SEDA-9, 208). The use of furosemide in this age group needs to be re-evaluated (SEDA-14, 182) (SEDA-15, 217).

Renal disease

High doses of furosemide in uremia are potentially ototoxic (26).

Hepatic disease

Although high-dose furosemide can be very useful in incipient acute renal insufficiency, it should be used with extreme caution in patients with severe hepatic insufficiency (SEDA-14, 183) and not at all in hepatic coma.

Drug–Drug Interactions

ACE inhibitors

Acute renal insufficiency with severe hyponatremia has been attributed to vigorous diuretic treatment (metolazone, furosemide, spironolactone) with an ACE inhibitor (27). Because ACE inhibition impairs renal protection against reduced perfusion, the combination of an ACE inhibitor with high-dose furosemide causes a reduction in glomerular filtration rate linearly related to the change in blood pressure.

In congestive heart failure, single conventional doses of captopril (25–75 mg) attenuated the natriuretic response to furosemide, while a low dose (1 mg) significantly enhanced furosemide-induced natriuresis (SEDA-17, 268) (SEDA-18, 236). The mechanism of this interaction is uncertain, but captopril did not affect delivery of furosemide to its site of action (28). In the long-term, intensive treatment with captopril enhanced the natriuretic response to furosemide (SEDA-17, 268).

Allopurinol

Interstitial nephritis with granulomatous hepatitis has been attributed to an interaction of furosemide with allopurinol (29). As in previous reports (SEDA-11, 198) the evidence for this interaction is not convincing. The role of allopurinol in causing the illness is credible, but the role of furosemide is doubtful.

Aminoglycoside antibiotics

Furosemide increases the ototoxic risks of aminoglycoside antibiotics (30,31) by reducing their clearance by about 35% (32); permanent deafness has resulted from the use of this combination.

- A 60-year-old woman developed moderately severe sensorineural hearing loss bilaterally after receiving five doses of gentamicin and one of furosemide 20 mg (33).

The cumulative dose and duration of aminoglycoside therapy are more important than serum concentrations in the development of gentamicin ototoxicity, except when interacting medications such as furosemide are co-administered.

Aspirin

Furosemide inhibits the absorption of aspirin (34), and aspirin 75 mg/day and 300 mg/day inhibits the venodilator effect of furosemide (35). These data raise the issue of whether aspirin should be routinely used in patients with congestive heart failure using furosemide.

Cephaloridine

The nephrotoxic effects of cefaloridine are potentiated by concurrent administration of furosemide (36,37), perhaps by a direct interaction and probably also because furosemide lowers the clearance of the antibiotic (38). Such combinations are better avoided.

Digoxin

It is advisable to monitor serum potassium concentrations closely if furosemide is combined with any cardiac glycoside.

Lithium

Furosemide can cause lithium toxicity by inhibiting the renal tubular excretion of lithium ions (39).

Mannitol

The combination of furosemide with mannitol can rapidly cause acute renal insufficiency (40) and potentiate the effect of curare (41).

NSAIDs

Furosemide inhibits the absorption of indometacin (42), while the diuretic and hypotensive effects of most diuretics are blunted by indometacin and probably also other NSAIDs (43). Intravenous furosemide is commonly given to patients with acute heart failure to relieve pulmonary congestion. Symptomatic relief occurs before the onset of diuresis, and the beneficial effect is believed to result from a venodilator action of furosemide, which precedes its diuretic effect. This venodilator response is inhibited by indometacin, suggesting that it occurs through local prostaglandin release.

Furosemide inhibits the absorption of meloxicam (44), an NSAID that is relatively selective for COX-2, sparing the physiologically important isoform that mediates vasodilator prostaglandins, which maintain renal function.

Phenytoin

The diuretic response to furosemide is reduced by approximately 50% during concurrent administration of phenytoin (45), probably through reduction of furosemide absorption (46).

Potassium-wasting drugs

The hypokalemic effects of furosemide can be potentiated by drugs such as licorice (47) and carbenoxolone (48).

Theophylline

Furosemide increases steady-state theophylline concentrations (SED-11, 428) (SED-14, 673).

A randomized, controlled study has shown an enhanced diuretic response to furosemide in infants taking theophylline during extracorporeal membrane oxygenation (49). The underlying mechanism was uncertain, but may have been an increase in glomerular filtration rate.

Thiazide diuretics

The use of thiazide and loop diuretics in combination to treat resistant hypertension often causes severe deterioration in renal function (50,51). It is not clear whether this is the result of excess diuresis or excessive blood pressure reduction.

Vancomycin

Ten preterm infants receiving regular theophylline for apnea of prematurity, who subsequently received vancomycin and furosemide, have been studied (52). When vancomycin was introduced in the infants who were established on furosemide and theophylline, there was a consistent failure to achieve therapeutic concentrations. Starting furosemide in infants who were already receiving vancomycin resulted in falls in serum vancomycin to subtherapeutic concentrations in all but one case. Serum concentrations fell by a mean of 24% (range 12–43%), in the 24 hours after the start of furosemide treatment. Two of the 10 infants had persistence of coagulase-negative staphylococcal sepsis while vancomycin concentrations were suboptimal. While the mechanism of this interaction is uncertain, the changes in serum vancomycin concentration may indicate acute changes in glomerular filtration rate. Preterm infants receiving theophylline and furosemide need shorter vancomycin dosage intervals to avoid therapeutic failure.

Warfarin

In patients taking warfarin, furosemide, like other diuretics, reduces the prothrombin time without changing the plasma warfarin concentration (SEDA-22, 238). The reduced anticoagulant effect is probably secondary to diuretic-induced volume depletion, mediating increases in clotting factors. Any effect is likely to be short-lived.

References

1. Naranjo CA, Busto U, Cassis L. Furosemide-induced adverse reactions during hospitalization. Am J Hosp Pharm 1978;35(7):794–8.
2. Tuzel IH. Comparison of adverse reactions to bumetanide and furosemide. J Clin Pharmacol 1981;21(11–12 Pt 2): 615–19.
3. Marlow ES, Hunt LP, Marlow N. Sensorineural hearing loss and prematurity. Arch Dis Child Fetal Neonatal Ed 2000;82(2):F141–4.
4. Decaux G, Waterlot Y, Genette F, Hallemans R, Demanet JC. Inappropriate secretion of antidiuretic hormone treated with frusemide. BMJ (Clin Res Ed) 1982;285(6335):89–90.
5. Hardig L, Daae C, Dellborg M, Kontny F, Bohmer T. Reduced thiamine phosphate, but not thiamine diphosphate, in erythrocytes in elderly patients with congestive heart failure treated with furosemide. J Intern Med 2000;247(5):597–600.
6. Bottiger LE, Westerholm B. Thrombocytopenia. II. Drug-induced thrombocytopenia. Acta Med Scand 1972;191(6):541–8.
7. De Gruchy GC. Thrombocytopenia. In: Drug-Induced Blood-Disorders. Oxford: Blackwell, 1975:118.
8. Simoes A, Domingos F, Prata MM. Nephrocalcinosis induced by furosemide in an adult patient with incomplete renal tubular acidosis. Nephrol Dial Transplant 2001;16(5):1073–4.
9. Park CW, You HY, Kim YK, Chang YS, Shin YS, Hong CK, Kim YC, Bang BK. Chronic tubulointerstitial nephritis and distal renal tubular acidosis in a patient with frusemide abuse. Nephrol Dial Transplant 2001;16(4):867–9.
10. Mocan H, Yildiran A, Camlibel T, Kuzey GM. Microscopic nephrocalcinosis and hypercalciuria in nephrotic syndrome. Hum Pathol 2000;31(11):1363–7.
11. Lin RY. Unusual autoimmune manifestations in furosemide-associated hypersensitivity angiitis. NY State J Med 1988;88(8):439–40.
12. Ihu H, Shimozuma H. Bullous pemphigoid induced by furosemide. Nishinihon J Dermatol 1993;55:890–3.
13. Guerrera V, Carbone RL. Bullous pemphigoid induced by furosemide. G Ital Dermatol Venereol 1994;129:239–41.
14. Eom SC, Chae YS, Suh KS, Kim ST. The clinical features of lichenoid drug eruption and the histopathological differentiation between lichenoid drug eruption and lichen planus. Korean J Dermatol 1994;32:1019–25.
15. Cobb MW. Furosemide-induced eruption simulating Sweet's syndrome. J Am Acad Dermatol 1989;21(2 Pt 2):339–43.
16. Cerottini JP, Ricci C, Guggisberg D, Panizzon RG. Drug-induced linear IgA bullous dermatosis probably induced by furosemide. J Am Acad Dermatol 1999;41(1):103–5.
17. Kroiss MM, Stolz W, Hohenleutner U, Landthaler M. Disseminated superficial porokeratosis induced by furosemide. Acta Derm Venereol 2000;80(1):52–3.
18. Noce R, Paredes BE, Pichler WJ, Krahenbuhl S. Acute generalized exanthematic pustulosis (AGEP) in a patient treated with furosemide. Am J Med Sci 2000;320(5):331–3.
19. Phipatanakul W, Adkinson NF Jr. Cross-reactivity between sulfonamides and loop or thiazide diuretics: a theoretical or actual risk? Allergy Clin Immunol Int 2000;12:26–8.
20. Earl G, Davenport J, Narula J. Furosemide challenge in patients with heart failure and adverse reactions to sulfa-containing diuretics. Ann Intern Med 2003;138(4):358–9.
21. Taggart AJ, McDevitt DG. Diuretic withdrawal—a need for caution. Curr Med Res Opin 1983;8(7):501–8.
22. Grinstead WC, Francis MJ, Marks GF, Tawa CB, Zoghbi WA, Young JB. Discontinuation of chronic diuretic therapy in stable congestive heart failure secondary to coronary artery disease or to idiopathic dilated cardiomyopathy. Am J Cardiol 1994;73(12):881–6.
23. van Kraaij DJ, Jansen RW, Bouwels LH, Hoefnagels WH. Furosemide withdrawal improves postprandial hypotension in elderly patients with heart failure and preserved left ventricular systolic function. Arch Intern Med 1999;159(14):1599–605.
24. Berkowitz RL, Coustan DR, Mochizuki TK. Furosemide (Lasix). In: Handbook for Prescribing Medications during Pregnancy. Boston, MA: Little, Brown and Co, 1981:95.
25. Dailey JW. Anticoagulant and cardiovascular drugs. In: Wilson JT, editor. Drugs in Breast Milk. Lancaster: MTP Press, 1981:61.
26. Wigand ME, Heidland A. Ototoxic side-effects of high doses of frusemide in patients with uraemia. Postgrad Med J 1971;47(Suppl):54–6.
27. Hogg KJ, Hillis WS. Captopril/metolazone induced renal failure. Lancet 1986;1(8479):501–2.
28. Reed S, Greene P, Ryan T, Cerimele B, Schwertschlag U, Weinberger M, Voelker J. The renin angiotensin aldosterone system and frusemide response in congestive heart failure. Br J Clin Pharmacol 1995;39(1):51–7.
29. Mousson C, Justrabo E, Tanter Y, Chalopin JM, Rifle G. Néphrite interstitielle et hépatite aiguës granulomateuses d'origine médicamenteuse: rôle possible de l'association allopurinol–furosémide. [Acute granulomatous interstitial nephritis and hepatitis caused by drugs. Possible role of an allopurinol–furosemide combination.] Nephrologie 1986;7(5):199–203.
30. Brown CB, Ogg CS, Cameron JS, Bewick M. High dose frusemide in acute reversible intrinsic renal failure. A preliminary communication. Scott Med J 1974;19(Suppl 1):35–9.
31. Thomsen J, Bech P, Szpirt W. Otologic symptoms in chronic renal failure. The possible role of aminoglycoside–furosemide interaction. Arch Otorhinolaryngol 1976;214(1):71–9.
32. Lawson DH, Tilstone WJ, Gray JM, Srivastava PK. Effect of furosemide on the pharmacokinetics of gentamicin in patients. J Clin Pharmacol 1982;22(5–6):254–8.
33. Bates DE, Beaumont SJ, Baylis BW. Ototoxicity induced by gentamicin and furosemide. Ann Pharmacother 2002;36(3):446–51.
34. Bartoli E, Arras S, Faedda R, Soggia G, Satta A, Olmeo NA. Blunting of furosemide diuresis by aspirin in man. J Clin Pharmacol 1980;20(7):452–8.
35. Jhund PS, Davie AP, McMurray JJ. Aspirin inhibits the acute venodilator response to furosemide in patients with chronic heart failure. J Am Coll Cardiol 2001;37(5): 1234–8.
36. Dodds MG, Foord RD. Enhancement by potent diuretics of renal tubular necrosis induced by cephaloridine. Br J Pharmacol 1970;40(2):227–36.

37. Simpson IJ. Nephrotoxicity and acute renal failure associated with cephalothin and cephaloridine. NZ Med J 1971;74(474):312–15.
38. Norrby R, Stenqvist K, Elgefors B. Interaction between cephaloridine and furosemide in man. Scand J Infect Dis 1976;8(3):209–12.
39. Hurtig HI, Dyson WL. Letter: Lithium toxicity enhanced by diuresis. N Engl J Med 1974;290(13):748–9.
40. Plouvier B, Baclet JL, de Coninck P. Une association néphrotoxique: mannitol et furosémide. [A nephrotoxic combination: mannitol and furosemide.] Nouv Presse Méd 1981;10(21):1744–5.
41. Miller RD, Sohn YJ, Matteo RS. Enhancement of d-tubocurarine neuromuscular blockade by diuretics in man. Anesthesiology 1976;45(4):442–5.
42. Brooks PM, Bell P, Lee P, et al. The effect of frusemide on indomethacin plasma levels. Br J Clin Pharmacol 1974;1:485.
43. Benet LZ. Pharmacokinetics/pharmacodynamics of furosemide in man: a review. J Pharmacokinet Biopharm 1979;7(1):1–27.
44. Muller FO, Middle MV, Schall R, Terblanche J, Hundt HK, Groenewoud G. An evaluation of the interaction of meloxicam with frusemide in patients with compensated chronic cardiac failure. Br J Clin Pharmacol 1997;44(4):393–8.
45. Ahmad S. Renal insensitivity to frusemide caused by chronic anticonvulsant therapy. BMJ 1974;3(5932):657–9.
46. Fine A, Henderson IS, Morgan DR, Tilstone WJ. Malabsorption of frusemide caused by phenytoin. BMJ 1977;2(6094):1061–2.
47. Famularo G, Corsi FM, Giacanelli M. Iatrogenic worsening of hypokalemia and neuromuscular paralysis associated with the use of glucose solutions for potassium replacement in a young woman with licorice intoxication and furosemide abuse. Acad Emerg Med 1999;6(9):960–4.
48. Sarkar SK. Stridor due to drug-induced hypokalaemic alkalosis. J Laryngol Otol 1987;101(2):197–8.
49. Lochan SR, Adeniyi-Jones S, Assadi FK, Frey BM, Marcus S, Baumgart S. Coadministration of theophylline enhances diuretic response to furosemide in infants during extracorporeal membrane oxygenation: a randomized controlled pilot study. J Pediatr 1998;133(1):86–9.
50. Freestone S, Ramsay LE. Frusemide and spironolactone in resistant hypertension: a controlled trial. J Hypertens 1983;1(Suppl 2):326.
51. Wollam GL, Tarazi RC, Bravo EL, Dustan HP. Diuretic potency of combined hydrochlorothiazide and furosemide therapy in patients with azotemia. Am J Med 1982;72(6):929–38.
52. Yeung MY, Smyth JP. Concurrent frusemide–theophylline dosing reduces serum vancomycin concentrations in preterm infants. Aust J Hosp Pharm 1999;29:269–72.

Fusidic acid

General Information

Fusidic acid is the best-known representative of a group of antibiotics with steroid structures, which are eliminated primarily by biliary excretion as microbiologically inactive metabolites. The antibacterial action of fusidic acid is bacteriostatic, although it can be bactericidal at higher concentrations. It exerts its antibacterial effect by inhibiting protein synthesis, but the exact mechanism by which this inhibition occurs has not yet been elucidated. It has a narrow antibiotic spectrum, with a bacteriostatic or slow bactericidal effect mainly directed at both coagulase-negative staphylococci and *Staphylococcus aureus* (1). Fusidic acid may also have a role as a clinically useful suppressor of immunoinflammatory processes (2).

Fusidic acid is adequately absorbed from the gastrointestinal tract, but has also been used topically. It has the important property of good tissue penetration, including entry into bones and joints, but does not reach the cerebrospinal fluid. Elimination of fusidic acid is primarily by non-renal mechanisms, and a proportion is metabolized to several breakdown products detectable in bile. Systemic clearance is increased by hypoalbuminemia, reduced by severe cholestasis, and is unchanged in renal insufficiency (3).

General adverse effects

The most common adverse effects of fusidic acid are minor and are related to the gastrointestinal tract (discomfort, diarrhea). Rare adverse events include granulocytopenia, thrombocytopenia, venous spasm, and skin reactions (4). Fusidic acid has detergent properties and can cause hemolysis when injected intravenously or can induce tissue damage when given intramuscularly. However, its systemic toxicity is relatively low.

Bacterial resistance has been an obstacle to the widespread use of fusidic acid; it develops in a single step in vitro and has also been observed in patients, particularly during prolonged administration (5).

Organs and Systems

Gastrointestinal

Oral fusidic acid can cause *Klebsiella oxytoca*-associated colitis (6).

Liver

Fusidic acid is chemically very similar to bile acids and hence competes with them for elimination and metabolism. A patient with a past history of alcohol-induced cirrhosis developed cholestatic jaundice after taking oral fusidic acid for 2 days (7).

Urinary tract

Severe hypocalcemia and acute renal insufficiency developed in two diabetic patients who took oral fusidic acid 500 mg tds (8).

Skin

Acanthosis nigricans has been associated with fusidic acid (9).

Sensitization to sodium fusidate is rare, and most often found in patients with stasis dermatitis or atopic dermatitis.

- Allergic contact dermatitis has been reported in a 26-year-old Korean woman after treatment of an abrasion on the left knee with fusidic acid ointment and povidone iodine (Betadine) (10). The diagnosis was confirmed by a strongly positive patch test for sodium fusidate.

Immunologic

Fusidic acid may have an immunomodulatory effect that seems to be partly mediated by suppression of cytokine production. The effect on several diseases has been investigated, but it remains to be characterized more in detail whether there is any therapeutic usefulness (4).

Positive patch tests occurred in three of 1119 patients who had used topical fusidic acid (11). In the second part of this study, all cases of positive patch tests to fusidic acid over the previous 20 years were reviewed; the average frequency was 1.62 patch-tested patients per year (1.45%) of those who were patch-tested.

Long-Term Effects

Drug tolerance

Mechanisms of resistance to fusidic acid include alterations in elongation factor G (whose inhibition at the ribosome level mediates the effect of fusidic acid), altered drug permeability, binding by chloramphenicol acetyltransferase type 1, and enhanced efflux (12).

Most studies show low levels of resistance in staphylococci, with a slightly higher rate in methicillin-resistant *S. aureus* (MRSA) (12). This has been confirmed in recent studies. Only 1 of 106 isolates of methicillin-resistant *S. aureus* was also resistant to fusidic acid (13). Only very little resistance to fusidic acid has been reported from Wales (14). However, clonal spread of fusidic acid-resistant methicillin-resistant *S. aureus* has been documented in Norway (15). A resistance rate of about 50% has been found in coagulase-negative staphylococci isolated in eight Swedish intensive care units between 1995 and 1997 (16). A high rate of resistance to fusidic acid was also found in bacteria that were cultured from blood after dental treatment (17).

Pathogenic nocardia may inactivate fusidic acid (18). In an in vitro study, salicylate and related compounds increased the MIC in strains of *S. aureus* both resistant and susceptible to fusidic acid (19).

In a prospective randomized trial, oral fusidic acid alone (500 mg tds for 7 days) failed to eradicate methicillin-resistant *S. aureus* colonization but resulted in the emergence of fusidic acid-resistant strains (20).

In an in vitro susceptibility study of 170 clinical isolates of *Mycobacterium tuberculosis* to fusidic acid, 19 isolates were resistant to at least one first-line antituberculosis drug (21). In all, 1.8% of the isolates were resistant to fusidic acid. Fusidic acid can be a potential supplementary drug for the treatment of infections due to multidrug-resistant strains of *M. tuberculosis*.

Susceptibility Factors

Other features of the patient

The half-life of fusidic acid was shortened in ten patients with severe burns treated with 500 mg tds intravenously (22). This effect may be explained by translesional extrahepatic clearance and an increase in hepatic clearance.

Drug–Drug Interactions

HIV protease inhibitors

In a 32-year-old man infected with HIV plasma concentrations of ritonavir, saquinavir, and fusidic acid were significantly raised when these drugs were administered in combination, possibly from mutual inhibition of metabolism (23).

Phenazone

Activation of the CYP450 enzyme system, demonstrated by an increase in the metabolism of phenazone (antipyrine), has been found in 30 HIV-positive drug abusers (24). This activating effect was demonstrated after 28 but not after 14 days of treatment with fusidic acid 500 mg/day, suggesting time dependency.

Statins

Acute rhabdomyolysis has been attributed to an interaction of fusidic acid with simvastatin (25).

- A 66-year-old kidney transplant recipient developed a gangrenous lesion on the left foot infected with *S. aureus* and *Escherichia coli*. He was given ciprofloxacin and clindamycin for 6 weeks and then fusidic acid 1500 mg/day for 2 weeks. He became ill, with myalgia and no active movement of his legs, and rhabdomyolysis was established by laboratory tests. He had also taken atorvastatin 10 mg/day and he slowly recovered after withdrawal of both atorvastatin and fusidic acid.

The authors identified only one previous report of a patient with rhabdomyolysis who had taken simvastatin and fusidic acid.

References

1. Collignon P, Turnidge J. Fusidic acid in vitro activity. Int J Antimicrob Agents 1999;12(Suppl 2):S45–58.
2. Bendtzen K, Diamant M, Faber V. Fusidic acid, an immunosuppressive drug with functions similar to cyclosporin A. Cytokine 1990;2(6):423–9.
3. Turnidge J. Fusidic acid pharmacology, pharmacokinetics and pharmacodynamics. Int J Antimicrob Agents 1999;12(Suppl 2):S23–34.
4. Christiansen K. Fusidic acid adverse drug reactions. Int J Antimicrob Agents 1999;12(Suppl 2):S3–9.
5. Shanson DC. Clinical relevance of resistance to fusidic acid in Staphylococcus aureus. J Antimicrob Chemother 1990;25(Suppl B):15–21.
6. Seksik P, Galula G, Maury E, Levy VG, Offenstadt G. [Klebsiella oxytoca-associated colitis after oral administration of fusidic acid.] Gastroenterol Clin Biol 2000;24(5):587–8.
7. Carbonell N, Thabut D, Podevin P, Biour M, Serfaty L, Poupon R. Ictère choléstatique induit par la prise d'acide fucidique chez un patient cirphotique. [Cholestatic icterus induced by the administration of fusidic acid in a cirrhotic patient.] Presse Méd 2002;31(23):1083–4.

8. Biswas M, Owen K, Jones MK. Hypocalcaemia during fusidic acid therapy. J R Soc Med 2002;95(2):91–3.
9. Cairo F, Rubino I, Rotundo R, Prato GP, Ficarra G. Oral acanthosis nigricans as a marker of internal malignancy. A case report. J Periodontol 2001;72(9):1271–5.
10. Lee AY, Joo HJ, Oh JG, Kim YG. Allergic contact dermatitis from sodium fusidate with no underlying dermatosis. Contact Dermatitis 2000;42(1):53.
11. Morris SD, Rycroft RJ, White IR, Wakelin SH, McFadden JP. Comparative frequency of patch test reactions to topical antibiotics. Br J Dermatol 2002;146(6):1047–51.
12. Turnidge J, Collignon P. Resistance to fusidic acid. Int J Antimicrob Agents 1999;12(Suppl 2):S35–44.
13. Liu CP, Lee CM, Su SC, Li YT. Susceptibility testing and clinical effect of fusidic acid in oxacillin-resistant Staphylococcus aureus infections. J Microbiol Immunol Infect 1999;32(3):194–8.
14. Morgan M, Salmon R, Keppie N, Evans-Williams D, Hosein I, Looker DN. All Wales surveillance of methicillin-resistant *Staphylococcus aureus* (MRSA): the first year's results. J Hosp Infect 1999;41(3):173–9.
15. Andersen BM, Bergh K, Steinbakk M, Syversen G, Magnaes B, Dalen H, Bruun JN. A Norwegian nosocomial outbreak of methicillin-resistant *Staphylococcus aureus* resistant to fusidic acid and susceptible to other antistaphylococcal agents. J Hosp Infect 1999;41(2):123–32.
16. Erlandsson CM, Hanberger H, Eliasson I, Hoffmann M, Isaksson B, Lindgren S, Nilsson LE, Soren L, Walther SM. Surveillance of antibiotic resistance in ICUs in southeastern Sweden. ICU Study Group of the South East of Sweden. Acta Anaesthesiol Scand 1999;43(8):815–20.
17. Messini M, Skourti I, Markopulos E, Koutsia-Carouzou C, Kyriakopoulou E, Kostaki S, Lambraki D, Georgopoulos A. Bacteremia after dental treatment in mentally handicapped people. J Clin Periodontol 1999;26(7):469–73.
18. Harada K, Tomita K, Fujii K, Sato N, Uchida H, Yazawa K, Mikami Y. Inactivation of fusidic acid by pathogenic Nocardia. J Antibiot (Tokyo) 1999;52(3):335–9.
19. Price CT, O'Brien FG, Shelton BP, Warmington JR, Grubb WB, Gustafson JE. Effects of salicylate and related compounds on fusidic acid MICs in *Staphylococcus aureus*. J Antimicrob Chemother 1999;44(1):57–64.
20. Chang SC, Hsieh SM, Chen ML, Sheng WH, Chen YC. Oral fusidic acid fails to eradicate methicillin-resistant *Staphylococcus aureus* colonization and results in emergence of fusidic acid-resistant strains. Diagn Microbiol Infect Dis 2000;36(2):131–6.
21. Cicek-Saydam C, Cavusoglu C, Burhanoglu D, Hilmioglu S, Ozkalay N, Bilgic A. In vitro susceptibility of *Mycobacterium tuberculosis* to fusidic acid. Clin Microbiol Infect 2001;7(12):700–2.
22. Lesne-Hulin A, Bourget P, Le Bever H, Carsin H. Pharmacocinetique de l'acide fusidique administre au sujet gravement brule infecte. [Pharmacokinetics of fusidic acid in patients with seriously infected burns.] Pathol Biol (Paris) 1999;47(5):486–90.
23. Reimann G, Barthel B, Rockstroh JK, Spatz D, Brockmeyer NH. Effect of fusidic acid on the hepatic cytochrome P450 enzyme system. Int J Clin Pharmacol Ther 1999;37(11):562–6.
24. Khaliq Y, Gallicano K, Leger R, Foster B, Badley A. A drug interaction between fusidic acid and a combination of ritonavir and saquinavir. Br J Clin Pharmacol 2000;50(1):82–3.
25. Wenisch C, Krause R, Fladerer P, El Menjawi I, Pohanka E. Acute rhabdomyolysis after atorvastatin and fusidic acid therapy. Am J Med 2000;109(1):78.

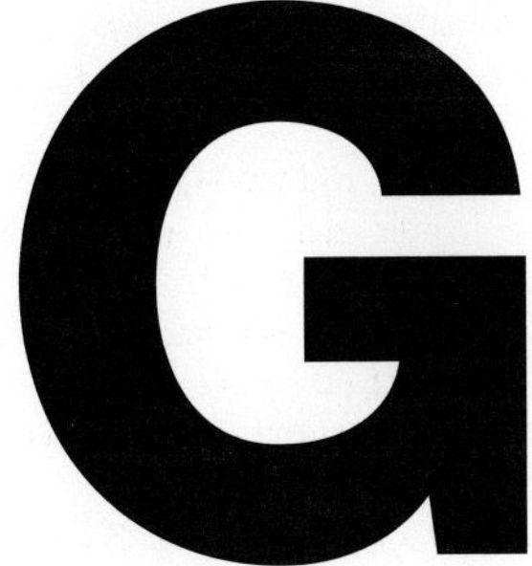

Gabapentin

See also Antiepileptic drugs

General Information

Gabapentin is used as adjunctive treatment for partial seizures and may be useful in some non-epileptic disorders, such as neuropathic pain. It has a favorable tolerability profile and is devoid of significant interactions with other anticonvulsants (1).

The use of gabapentin has been reviewed (2). Its adverse effects are limited to neuropsychological disorders, namely dizzy spells, drowsiness, fatigue, and headache. The risk of interactions is also limited.

The efficacy of gabapentin in dosages up to 3600 mg/day as adjunctive therapy has been studied in 2016 patients with partial seizures (3). The four most commonly reported adverse events were somnolence (15%), dizziness (10%), weakness (5.8%), and headache (4.5%).

In an uncontrolled trial using dosages up to 6000 mg/day in 50 patients with refractory partial epilepsy, tiredness, dizziness, headache, and diplopia were the most common adverse effects (4). At dosages above 3600 mg/day three patients developed flatulence and diarrhea and two had myoclonic jerks. At least in some patients, gabapentin gastrointestinal absorption did not become saturated within the explored dosage range.

The effectiveness of gabapentin has been studied in 22 patients with bipolar disorder who had an incomplete response to other mood stabilizers (5). Somnolence was common (six patients); adverse events that occurred in two patients each included irritability, memory impairment, headache, and tremor. One patient dropped out because of a mild rash.

In 237 children aged 3–12 years with refractory partial seizures gabapentin 24–70 mg/kg/day was used as add-on therapy over 6 months (6). There was a more than 50% reduction in partial seizures in 34% of the children. Somnolence was the most common adverse event related to gabapentin. Emotional lability and hostility were related to gabapentin in 3.4 and 3.0% of the patients respectively.

In a non-interventional observational cohort study, using the technique of prescription-event monitoring, patients taking gabapentin were identified from dispensed National Health Service prescriptions (7). Outcome data were obtained from questionnaires sent to the doctor 6 months after the initial gabapentin prescription. The cohort included 3100 patients, of whom 136 (4%) were children. The median duration of treatment was 8.1 months. The most frequently reported adverse events during the first month of treatment were neurological: drowsiness/sedation (6.7% of patients), headache/migraine (3.6%), malaise/lassitude (3.5%), dizziness (2.4%), and nausea/vomiting (2.6%). These events were also the commonest reasons for withdrawal of gabapentin and were reported as suspected adverse drug reactions. There were no congenital anomalies in the 11 babies born to women who used gabapentin during the first trimester of pregnancy. The crude mortality rate was five times that in the general population but similar to that in other published studies in patients with epilepsy. Thus, this report does not disclose new unrecognized adverse effects of gabapentin.

Comparative studies

Gabapentin and lamotrigine have been compared in an open, parallel-group, add-on, randomized study in 109 patients with uncontrolled partial epilepsy and learning disabilities (8). The two drugs were similarly efficacious, with similar incidences of adverse events and serious adverse events. Neither lamotrigine nor gabapentin exacerbated any of the challenging behaviors observed in these patients. The most common adverse effect of gabapentin was somnolence, which was mostly reported during the initial titration phase.

In a double-blind comparison of gabapentin and lamotrigine in 309 patients with new-onset partial or generalized seizures, the target doses were gabapentin 1800 mg/day and lamotrigine 150 mg/day (9). Severe adverse events were reported in 11% of patients taking gabapentin and 9.3% of patients taking lamotrigine. Two patients had serious adverse events thought to be related to the study drug; one took an overdose of gabapentin and the other had convulsions with lamotrigine. The most frequent treatment-related adverse events in both treatment groups were dizziness, weakness, and headache; 11% of patients taking gabapentin and 15% of those taking lamotrigine withdrew because of adverse events. There was an increase of over 7% in body weight from baseline in 14% of the patients taking gabapentin and 6.6% of those taking lamotrigine. There were benign skin rashes in 4.4% of those taking gabapentin and 11% of those taking lamotrigine.

Organs and Systems

Ear, nose, throat

Rhinitis is uncommon with gabapentin (10).

Nervous system

Drowsiness, dizziness, fatigue, or ataxia are seen in 10–20% of patients who use gabapentin (SEDA-19, 70) (SEDA-20, 62) (10). Of 240 adults followed for about 1 year, only 4% discontinued treatment because of adverse events (SEDA-19, 70). Adverse effects reported by more than 10% of patients were nystagmus, somnolence, diplopia, tremor, ataxia, and dizziness.

Gabapentin occasionally exacerbates absence and myoclonic seizures and causes de novo myoclonus (SEDA-21, 71). Myoclonus has been studied in 104 patients taking gabapentin for epilepsy (11). There were 13 cases of mild myoclonus, which did not significantly interfere with daily activities. All the patients had refractory epilepsy and were taking other antiepileptic drugs. Six had a severe chronic static encephalopathy; five had no medical diagnosis other than seizures. Ten developed multifocal myoclonus and three developed focal myoclonus, contralateral to their epileptic focus. Two had an exacerbation of pre-existing myoclonus. Withdrawal led to rapid resolution.

Choreoathetosis, dyskinesias, dystonic or myoclonic movement disorders (including oculogyric crises), and stuttering have been reported rarely (SEDA-21, 71) (SEDA-22, 87).

- Sensory neuropathy occurred in a 58-year-old man who had been given up to 2400 mg/day for over 5 months for the treatment of head pain (12). A mild pruritic rash had been present since starting treatment. Neuropathic symptoms included a burning sensation in the legs and hips. After withdrawal, reduced perception of tactile and noxious stimuli and neurogenic bladder dysfunction (with an associated syncopal episode) were recorded. The neuropathy improved over several months.

Gabapentin is used often to treat neuropathic pain, and its role in causing the sensory neuropathy in this patient was uncertain.

Gabapentin-induced myoclonus may be more common than initially thought. In a retrospective survey, 13 of 104 consecutive patients developed myoclonus at gabapentin dosages of 800–3200 mg/day (11). Six of the patients had severe chronic static encephalopathy. Three had focal myoclonus, contralateral to the epileptic focus, and two had exacerbation of pre-existent myoclonus. In all cases the myoclonus was mild and did not interfere with daily activities. The fact that in three patients the electroencephalogram did not show epileptiform discharges suggests that, at least in some cases, the myoclonus is non-epileptic in nature.

In a comparison of twice- and thrice-daily gabapentin, 29 stable responders were selected and followed for 3 months (13). The mean number of seizures per month was 4.2 at baseline, 1.0 during the thrice-daily and 0.9 during the twice-daily period. Adverse effects were reported by 11 patients during the thrice-daily period and by five patients during the twice-daily period; sedation and vertigo were the most frequent.

The efficacy and safety of gabapentin in relieving the symptoms of panic disorder have been studied in 103 patients in a randomized, placebo-controlled, double-blind study for 8 weeks (14). Adverse events included somnolence, headache, and dizziness. One patient had a serious adverse event, a car accident, while taking gabapentin.

Of 12 patients with moderate to severe dementia and severe behavioral disorders given gabapentin (200–1200 mg/day) for 8 weeks, 5 had adverse events such as gait instability, emotional instability, and sedation; two patients discontinued treatment prematurely because of severe adverse effects (15).

The role of gabapentin in patients with neuropathic pain has been evaluated in a systematic review (16). The most common adverse events were dizziness and somnolence, which occurred in about 25% of patients; ataxia occurred in about 8%. Adverse effects were dose-related.

- A 68-year-old man with essential tremor who was taking propranolol 80 mg/day had several daily episodes of paroxysmal dystonic movements in both hands 2 days after the addition of gabapentin 900 mg/day (17). The dose of propranolol was reduced to 40 mg/day and the dystonic movements resolved. The authors suggested that there had been a synergistic effect between propranolol and gabapentin.
- A 60-year-old woman with post-herpetic neuralgia developed asterixis after having taken gabapentin for 4 days (18). The authors proposed that the mechanism was GABAergic.

Two cases of gabapentin-related dyskinesia have been reported (19). The patients were 60 and 41 years old and took gabapentin 900–1200 mg/day for generalized anxiety. Generalized dyskinetic movements and facial tics appeared after 3 days and disappeared after 2 days of withdrawal.

Psychological, psychiatric

Gabapentin has rarely been implicated in psychiatric reactions. Two cases, one of mania (20) and one of catatonia (21), have been reported.

- A 35-year-old woman with epilepsy without a history of psychiatric disorders developed elevated mood after being stabilized on gabapentin monotherapy (3200 mg/day). After 5 months she developed a manic episode, which remitted when gabapentin was withdrawn.
- Catatonia was reported in a 48-year-old woman with bipolar disorder within 48 hours of withdrawal of gabapentin, 500 mg/day. The condition lasted for several days and disappeared after treatment with a benzodiazepine.

In the first case the presentation was strongly suggestive for a causative role of the drug. In the second it was speculated that the condition might have been provoked by altered GABAergic transmission after gabapentin withdrawal.

Two women, aged 37 and 38 years, took gabapentin and after a few days developed behavioral changes associated with euphoria (22). In one case the symptoms were transient and in the other they resolved after withdrawal. The behavioral changes were not related to seizure activity.

In a double-blind, crossover comparison of the cognitive effects of carbamazepine (mean dose 731 mg/day) and gabapentin (2400 mg/day), each given for 5 weeks, in 35 healthy volunteers performance on gabapentin was better than on carbamazepine for 8 of 31 variables (visual serial addition test, choice reaction times at initiation and total, memory paragraph I and delayed recall, Stroop Word and Interference, Vigor measure), whereas carbamazepine was better than gabapentin on none (23). Although these data suggest that gabapentin produces fewer cognitive effects than carbamazepine, the applicability of the findings to long-term therapy in epileptic patients is uncertain.

Behavioral disturbances, including aggressiveness, irritability, hyperactivity, and/or dysphoric changes, occur in up to 22% of patients. Children and patients with mental retardation or a history of similar disorders may be at special risk (SEDA-20, 61). In a recent study, hyperactivity, irritability, and agitation occurred in 15 of 32 mostly mentally retarded children, and required drug withdrawal in four (24).

The cognitive effects of carbamazepine and gabapentin have been compared in a double-blind, crossover, randomized study in 34 healthy elderly adults, of whom 19 subjects withdrew (15 while taking carbamazepine, probably due to excessively rapid dosage titration) (25). The primary outcome measures were standardized neuropsychological and mood state tests, yielding 17 variables. Each subject had cognitive testing at baseline (pre-drug), the end of the first drug phase, the end of the second drug phase, and 4 weeks after completion of the second drug phase. Adverse events were frequently reported with both antiepileptic drugs, although they were more common with carbamazepine. There were significant differences between carbamazepine and gabapentin for only 1 of 11 cognitive variables, with better attention/vigilance for gabapentin, although the effect was modest. Both carbamazepine and gabapentin can cause mild cognitive deficits in elderly subjects, and gabapentin has a slightly better profile.

Gabapentin has been associated with hostility, especially in children. Two cases of aggression in adults taking gabapentin for bipolar disorder have been reported (26). Neither patient had a history of aggression. In one the symptoms appeared after 3 days of treatment (1200 mg/day), and in the other after 48 hours (600 mg/day). In the second case, aggression was associated with auditory hallucinations. It is hard to associate new antiepileptic drugs with psychiatric adverse effects in patients with severe psychiatric disorders, and rechallenge with the offending drug should ideally have been tried before postulating a causal relation.

Endocrine

A 28-year-old woman with bipolar depression developed clinical and biochemical evidence of hyperthyroidism, ascribed to thyroiditis, while taking gabapentin (4800 mg/day) in a clinical trial (27). The condition cleared after withdrawal, and subsequent exposure to a lower dose of gabapentin (1500 mg/day) was uneventful.

Whether gabapentin was responsible for the thyroiditis is doubtful.

Metabolism

Weight gain occurs in up to about one-third of patients and may be more frequent at high dosages (SEDA-20, 61) (SEDA-22, 87). Of 44 patients given mean dosages of 3520 mg/day for at least 12 months, 10 gained more than 10% and 15 gained between 5 and 10% of their initial weight (28). The weight gain started after 2–3 months and tended to stabilize after 6–9 months.

Hematologic

In one case of reversible granulocytopenia attributed to gabapentin, cause and effect was dubious (SEDA-22, 88).

Gastrointestinal

Nausea and vomiting are uncommon with gabapentin (10).

Liver

Hepatotoxicity is exceedingly rare. The role of gabapentin in one patient with markedly raised liver enzymes after 12 weeks of treatment was unclear (SEDA-22, 88).

Gabapentin-induced cholestasis has been reported (29).

- A 50-year-old man was given gabapentin for diabetic neuropathic pain. He had also taken metformin, amitriptyline, dihydrocodeine (30 mg as required), and ramipril for over 12 months. After taking the gabapentin for 2 weeks, he developed clinical and biochemical evidence of cholestasis. Liver function tests were: bilirubin 199 μmol/l, aspartate transaminase 104 U/l, alkaline phosphatase 210 U/l, and gamma-glutamyltransferase 839 U/l. He had negative hepatitis A, B, and C serology and negative antinuclear antibody and anti-smooth muscle antibody. A blood count, renal profile, and liver ultrasound scan were also normal. A liver biopsy showed normal liver architecture with evidence of patchy steatosis, cholestasis, and some foci of chronic inflammation, thought to be consistent with a drug-induced etiology. Gabapentin was withdrawn and his symptoms and liver function tests improved gradually over 7–12 weeks.

The authors attributed the cholestasis to gabapentin because of the temporal relation. However, they failed to mention whether they withdrew other concomitant medications that could also have caused liver damage, a more likely explanation. Moreover, the number of dihydrocodeine tablets the patient took before admission was not stated.

Urinary tract

Urinary incontinence occurs rarely (SEDA-22, 88). Of 119 adults with partial seizures, 5 (4%) developed urinary incontinence which resolved after gabapentin withdrawal (30). Four of the five patients had signs of spasticity, suggesting that this may be a predisposing factor.

- A 27-year-old man with bipolar disorder had an increased serum creatinine concentration (up to 1.7 mg/dl, 150 μmol/l) after taking gabapentin 2000 mg/day for several weeks, the change being reversible after drug withdrawal (31).

The possibility of renal dysfunction as a rare adverse effect should be considered. The patient had a history of allergic reactions to lithium, carbamazepine, clozapine, haloperidol, and lamotrigine.

A renal transplant recipient with a long-term stable functioning allograft developed reversible acute renal dysfunction after beginning gabapentin therapy for chronic pain in diabetic neuropathy (32). The authors suggested that this was due to renal afferent vasoconstriction.

Patients on chronic hemodialysis are at risk of gabapentin toxicity. A patient undergoing hemodialysis and taking gabapentin 400 mg/day developed a very high serum concentration (56 μg/ml) and clinical toxicity manifested by stupor (33). A subsequent pharmacokinetic analysis suggested that in patients undergoing chronic hemodialysis, gabapentin should be started at 300 mg/day and post-hemodialysis dosing should be reduced to 100 mg/day, at least in some patients.

Skin

Skin rashes are rare with gabapentin.

There has been one case of diffuse alopecia reversible after drug withdrawal (SEDA-22, 88).

- A 32-year-old woman with HIV infection and cerebral toxoplasmosis developed histologically confirmed Stevens–Johnson syndrome after taking gabapentin (300–900 mg/day) for 3 days (34). Although other drugs were given, the condition resolved after withdrawal of gabapentin alone.

Whether the underlying condition played a role is open to speculation.

- In a 26-year-old woman who had severe Stevens–Johnson syndrome induced by phenytoin and later by carbamazepine, gabapentin resulted in an erythematous pruriginous skin eruption limited to the legs without mucosal involvement (35).

Although gabapentin has a lower allergenic potential than most other anticonvulsants, patients with a history of severe drug-induced idiosyncratic reactions may be at higher risk of gabapentin-induced skin reactions.

Sexual function

Anorgasmia has been quoted in the Physicians Desk Reference as an infrequent adverse effect.

- Anorgasmia was reported by a 52-year-old man while he was taking gabapentin, 900–1500 mg/day, for the treatment of neuropathic pain (36). The condition lasted for over 2 months and remitted when gabapentin was replaced with mexiletine.
- A 25-year-old man taking gabapentin 900 mg/day reported anorgasmia during sexual intercourse (37). He was given valproate instead and his symptom resolved within 12 days.
- Gabapentin-induced anorgasmia and reduced libido have been reported in two women (38). Both were taking relatively low doses of gabapentin (900–1800 mg). In one case the symptoms disappeared with dosage reduction but in the other gabapentin had to be withdrawn.

Immunologic

- A hypersensitivity syndrome secondary to gabapentin has been described in a 72-year-old patient after 9 days (39). The symptoms (altered mental status, fever, diffuse macular rash, and an enlarged spleen) resolved after withdrawal.

However, the concomitant use of levofloxacin made the association of gabapentin with the hypersensitivity syndrome unclear.

Body temperature

Gabapentin may be effective in the treatment of hot flushes (hot flashes), and by the same token has been reported to have increased the frequency of hypothermic episodes in a 38-year-old man with hypothalamic dysfunction (40).

Long-Term Effects

Drug withdrawal

Three cases of withdrawal symptoms after abrupt withdrawal of high-dose gabapentin have been reported in adults with psychiatric conditions (41). The patients were restless and anxious, with sweating and tachycardia. The symptoms improved after gabapentin was reintroduced.

Drug Administration

Drug dosage regimens

Two different regimens of add-on gabapentin have been compared in a double-blind, randomized trial (42). In 574 patients randomized to either slow initiation (300 mg on day 1, 600 mg on day 2, then 900 mg/day) or rapid initiation (900 mg/day immediately after the placebo lead-in), the four most common adverse events, which occurred equally in the two groups, were somnolence, dizziness, ataxia, and fatigue. The frequency of adverse events in a subgroup of elderly patients was similar to that in younger adults.

Drug overdose

- A 30-year-old woman with renal insufficiency on hemodialysis three times a week suffered no significant toxicity after ingesting 600 mg tds of gabapentin for 3 weeks, a large dose in view of her impaired kidney function (43). The blood gabapentin concentration was 496 μmol/l.

These data suggest that gabapentin poses no major risk in overdose, partly because large doses are poorly absorbed.

References

1. Andrews CO, Fischer JH. Gabapentin: a new agent for the management of epilepsy. Ann Pharmacother 1994;28(10):1188–96.
2. Anonymous. Gabapentin monotherapy: new indication. Sometimes helpful. Prescrire Int 2000;9(46):40–2.
3. Morrell MJ, McLean MJ, Willmore LJ, Privitera MD, Faught RE, Holmes GL, Magnus L, Bernstein P. Rose-Legatt. Efficacy of gabapentin as adjunctive therapy in a large, multicenter study. The Steps Study Group. Seizure 2000;9(4):241–8.
4. Wilson EA, Sills GJ, Forrest G, Brodie MJ. High dose gabapentin in refractory partial epilepsy: clinical observations in 50 patients. Epilepsy Res 1998;29(2):161–6.
5. Vieta E, Martinez-Aran A, Nieto E, Colom F, Reinares M, Benabarre A, Gasto C. Adjunctive gabapentin treatment of bipolar disorder. Eur Psychiatry 2000;15(7):433–7.

6. Appleton R, Fichtner K, LaMoreaux L, Alexander J, Maton S, Murray G, Garofalo E. Gabapentin as add-on therapy in children with refractory partial seizures: a 24-week, multicentre, open-label study. Dev Med Child Neurol 2001;43(4):269–73.
7. Wilton LV, Shakir S. A postmarketing surveillance study of gabapentin as add-on therapy for 3,100 patients in England. Epilepsia 2002;43(9):983–92.
8. Crawford P, Brown S, Kerr M; Parke Davis Clinical Trials Group. A randomized open-label study of gabapentin and lamotrigine in adults with learning disability and resistant epilepsy. Seizure 2001;10(2):107–15.
9. Brodie MJ, Chadwick DW, Anhut H, Otte A, Messmer SL, Maton S, Sauermann W, Murray G, Garofalo EA; Gabapentin Study Group 945-212. Gabapentin versus lamotrigine monotherapy: a double-blind comparison in newly diagnosed epilepsy. Epilepsia 2002;43(9):993–1000.
10. Goa KL, Sorkin EM. Gabapentin. A review of its pharmacological properties and clinical potential in epilepsy. Drugs 1993;46(3):409–27.
11. Asconape J, Diedrich A, DellaBadia J. Myoclonus associated with the use of gabapentin. Epilepsia 2000;41(4):479–81.
12. Gould HJ. Gabapentin induced polyneuropathy. Pain 1998;74(2–3):341–3.
13. Muscas GC, Chiroli S, Luceri F, Mastio MD, Balestrieri F, Arnetoli G. Conversion from thrice daily to twice daily administration of gabapentin (GBP) in partial epilepsy: analysis of clinical efficacy and plasma levels. Seizure 2000;9(1):47–50.
14. Pande AC, Pollack MH, Crockatt J, Greiner M, Chouinard G, Lydiard RB, Taylor CB, Dager SR, Shiovitz T. Placebo-controlled study of gabapentin treatment of panic disorder. J Clin Psychopharmacol 2000;20(4):467–71.
15. Herrmann N, Lanctot K, Myszak M. Effectiveness of gabapentin for the treatment of behavioral disorders in dementia. J Clin Psychopharmacol 2000;20(1):90–3.
16. Laird MA, Gidal BE. Use of gabapentin in the treatment of neuropathic pain. Ann Pharmacother 2000;34(6):802–7.
17. Palomeras E, Sanz P, Cano A, Fossas P. Dystonia in a patient treated with propranolol and gabapentin. Arch Neurol 2000;57(4):570–1.
18. Jacob PC, Chand RP, Omeima el-S. Asterixis induced by gabapentin. Clin Neuropharmacol 2000;23(1):53.
19. Norton JW, Quarles E. Gabapentin-related dyskinesia. J Clin Psychopharmacol 2001;21(6):623–4.
20. Leweke FM, Bauer J, Elger CE. Manic episode due to gabapentin treatment. Br J Psychiatry 1999;175:291.
21. Rosebush PI, MacQueen GM, Mazurek MF. Catatonia following gabapentin withdrawal. J Clin Psychopharmacol 1999;19(2):188–9.
22. Trinka E, Niedermuller U, Thaler C, Doering S, Moroder T, Ladurner G, Bauer G. Gabapentin-induced mood changes with hypomanic features in adults. Seizure 2000;9(7):505–8.
23. Meador KJ, Loring DW, Ray PG, Murro AM, King DW, Nichols ME, Deer EM, Goff WT. Differential cognitive effects of carbamazepine and gabapentin. Epilepsia 1999;40(9):1279–85.
24. Khurana DS, Riviello J, Helmers S, Holmes G, Anderson J, Mikati MA. Efficacy of gabapentin therapy in children with refractory partial seizures. J Pediatr 1996;128(6):829–33.
25. Mujica R, Weiden P. Neuroleptic malignant syndrome after addition of haloperidol to atypical antipsychotic. Am J Psychiatry 2001;158(4):650–1.
26. Pinninti NR, Mahajan DS. Gabapentin-associated aggression. J Neuropsychiatry Clin Neurosci 2001;13(3):424.
27. Frye MA, Luckenbaugh D, Kimbrell TA, Constantino C, Grothe D, Cora-Locatelli G, Ketter TA. Possible gabapentin-induced thyroiditis. J Clin Psychopharmacol 1999;19(1):94–5.
28. DeToledo JC, Toledo C, DeCerce J, Ramsay RE. Changes in body weight with chronic, high-dose gabapentin therapy. Ther Drug Monit 1997;19(4):394–6.
29. Richardson CE, Williams DW, Kingham JG. Gabapentin induced cholestasis. BMJ 2002;325(7365):635.
30. Doherty K, Gates JR, Penovich P, Moriarty M. Gabapentin in a medically refractory epilepsy population: seizure response and unusual side effects. Epilepsia 1995;36(Suppl 4):71.
31. Grunze H, Dittert S, Bungert M, Erfurth A. Renal impairment as a possible side effect of gabapentin. A single case report. Neuropsychobiology 1998;38(3):198–9.
32. Gallay BJ, de Mattos AM, Norman DJ. Reversible acute renal allograft dysfunction due to gabapentin. Transplantation 2000;70(1):208–9.
33. Bassilios N, Launay-Vacher V, Khoury N, Rondeau E, Deray G, Sraer JD. Gabapentin neurotoxicity in a chronic haemodialysis patient. Nephrol Dial Transplant 2001;16(10):2112–13.
34. Gonzalez-Sicilia L, Cano A, Serrano M, Hernandez J. Stevens–Johnson syndrome associated with gabapentin. Am J Med 1998;105(5):455.
35. DeToledo JC, Minagar A, Lowe MR, Ramsay RE. Skin eruption with gabapentin in a patient with repeated AED-induced Stevens–Johnson's syndrome. Ther Drug Monit 1999;21(1):137–8.
36. Clark JD, Elliott J. Gabapentin-induced anorgasmia. Neurology 1999;53(9):2209.
37. Brannon GE, Rolland PD. Anorgasmia in a patient with bipolar disorder type 1 treated with gabapentin. J Clin Psychopharmacol 2000;20(3):379–81.
38. Grant AC, Oh H. Gabapentin-induced anorgasmia in women. Am J Psychiatry 2002;159(7):1247.
39. Ragucci MV, Cohen JM. Gabapentin-induced hypersensitivity syndrome. Clin Neuropharmacol 2001;24(2):103–5.
40. Guttuso TJ Jr. Gabapentin's effects on hot flashes and hypothermia. Neurology 2000;54(11):2161–3.
41. Norton JW. Gabapentin withdrawal syndrome. Clin Neuropharmacol 2001;24(4):245–6.
42. Fisher RS, Sachdeo RC, Pellock J, Penovich PE, Magnus L, Bernstein P. Rapid initiation of gabapentin: a randomized, controlled trial. Neurology 2001;56(6):743–8.
43. Verma A, Miller P, Carwile ST, Husain AM, Radtke RA. Lamotrigine-induced blepharospasm. Pharmacotherapy 1999;19(7):877–80.

Gadolinium

General Information

Gadolinium chelates for MRI (SEDA 18, 446) (SEDA-20, 419) (SEDA-21, 475) (SEDA-22, 503) are inert, non-metabolized, small molecules, with essentially the same pharmacokinetic properties as the iodinated contrast agents. They are rapidly distributed in the extracellular fluid spaces, both intravascular and extravascular, although they do not cross the normal blood–brain barrier, and are almost entirely excreted by glomerular filtration, with no significant active tubular excretion or re-absorption. Hepatic excretion occurs in patients with severely impaired renal function, and trace amounts are normally excreted in the saliva, sweat, and tears (SEDA-21, 475).

Gadolinium-based contrast agents of intermediate size act like blood-pool contrast agents during the first pass (1). However, because they diffuse into the interstitium, they later act like extracellular agents. Examples are P760 (gadolinium tetra-azacyclododecanetetra-acetic acid, Gd-DOTA) and Gadomer-17 (gadolinium diethylenetriaminepenta-acetic acid, Gd-DTPA). Intermediate-sized agents are used for the following purposes:

- the detection of small, slow-flowing, tortuous vessels;
- the detection of increased capillary permeability in sufficiently injured tissues;
- improved and prolonged demonstration of zones of myocardial ischemia;
- estimating myocardial blood flow;
- tumor characterization.

The classical macromolecular blood-pool contrast agents are based on gadolinium DTPA or gadobenate dimeglumine, which are linked to albumin, dextran, or polylysine (1). Albumin-based agents are not considered optimal for clinical development, as it is difficult to obtain highly consistent synthetic products. There are also problems with cardiovascular toxicity and retention of gadolinium in bones and liver. Dextran-based agents appear to be safer, and an agent called CMD-A2-gadobenate dimeglumine (CMD = carboxymethyldextran) has a favorable toxicity profile.

Gadolinium chelates include ionic high-osmolar agents, such as gadolinium pentetate dimeglumine (Gd-DTPA) and low osmolar non-ionic agents, such as gadodiamide. They generally have similar MR relaxivities, pharmacokinetics, and biodistribution, behaving as non-specific extracellular fluid space agents analogues to iodinated contrast media. The similar safety and efficacy of ionic and non-ionic gadolinium-based extracellular contrast agents suggests that the choice of contrast medium will in future be determined by economic rather than clinical considerations (2).

The use of gadolinium-based contrast agents as an alternative to iodinated contrast agents has been reported in a patient with a history of allergy to the latter (3).

- A 77-year-old woman had a gadolinium-enhanced MRI scan followed by gadolinium-enhanced spiral CT pulmonary angiography for suspected pulmonary embolism. Gadodiamide 0.4 mmol/kg (60 ml) was injected intravenously at a rate of 2 ml/second. There were no adverse reactions.

Note on brand names

The various gadolinium salts are often known by their brand names, because their chemical names are complex. The following is a key to various brand names:

- AngioMARK: gadofosveset
- Dotarem, Guerbet SA: gadolinium tetra-azacyclododecanetetra-acetic acid (Gd-DOTA)
- Gadovist: gadobutrol (Gd-BT-DO3A)
- Magnevist: gadopentetate dimeglumine; the di-*N*-methylglucamine salt of gadopentetate (gadolinium diethylenetriamine penta-acetic acid, Gd-DTPA)
- MultiHance: gadobenate dimeglumine (Gd-BOPTA)
- Omniscan: gadodiamide
- OptiMARK: gadoversetamide (Gd-DTPA-BMEA).
- Primovist (Eovist): gadoxetic acid
- ProHance: gadoteridol.

Comparative studies

In a multicenter, randomized, double-blind comparison of the safety, tolerability, and efficacy of gadoversetamide (a non-ionic gadolinium chelate) and gadolinium DTPA in 99 patients during contrast-enhanced hepatic imaging, both agents were well tolerated and there were no serious or unexpected adverse events (2). A total of 154 adverse events were recorded in 82 patients, of which 33 (21%) were thought to be related to either agent. Headache and taste disturbances were the most common adverse effects; they occurred in about equal frequency in the two groups. There were no clinically relevant changes in electrocardiography or any laboratory parameter in either group.

The efficacy and the safety of gadoversetamide and gadopentetate dimeglumine have been compared in a multicenter, randomized, double-blind, parallel-group study in patients with suspected central nervous system pathology who required MRI examination (4). They were randomized to receive 0.1 mmol/kg of either gadoversetamide ($n = 262$, aged 1–80 years, mean volume of contrast medium injected 15 ml) or gadopentetate dimeglumine ($n = 133$, aged 20–73 years, mean volume of contrast medium injected 16 ml). There were no significant differences in adverse effects or diagnostic efficacy between the two groups. Of those given gadoversetamide, 71 patients (27%) had adverse events, severe in only 5 (1.9%). Of those given gadopentetate dimeglumine, 31 patients (23%) had adverse events, severe in only 5 (3.8%). The adverse effects included headache, chest pain, taste disturbance, and leg cramps.

In controlled studies, gadobenate dimeglumine has been compared with gadolinium chelates in 222 patients and with placebo in 189 patients (5). There were no serious events and no differences in the incidence of adverse effects between the groups. Adverse effects included vomiting, dizziness, and rashes. Similarly, there were no differences between children and adults or between subjects with renal or liver insufficiency. The authors concluded that gadobenate dimeglumine is safe, with a very low incidence of serious events, and that it compares favorably with other MR contrast agents, such as gadolinium DTPA.

Gadobenate dimeglumine, in cumulative doses of 0.15 and 0.2 mmol/kg, has been compared with gadodiamide 0.3 mmol/kg in 205 patients (aged 20–88 years) with suspected central nervous system lesions (6). Gadobenate dimeglumine was well tolerated and the safety profile was similar to that observed with gadodiamide. In the three groups, adverse effects occurred in 28, 23, and 32% respectively. The most common adverse events of gadobenate dimeglumine were headache (16%), dizziness (4.6%), and taste disturbances (4.6%); the most common adverse events of gadodiamide were headache (7.2%), nausea (5.8%), and taste disturbances (5.8%). All adverse events were classified as mild to moderate. There were no significant changes in vital signs, hematology, or serum chemistry in any group. There were no significant differences in the diagnostic quality of the examination.

General adverse effects

The reported rate of adverse reactions of gadolinium chelates at a dose of 0.1 mmol/kg is 2.4%. Most of these reactions tend to be mild and do not require treatment (SEDA-15, 505). Serious reactions are extremely rare. However, several severe anaphylactoid reactions and angioedema have been reported (SED-12, 1187) (SEDA-16, 537) (SEDA-17, 538) (SEDA-18, 446) (7). The incidence of adverse effects is slightly higher in patients with a history of asthma or allergy (3.7%). For patients with a history of a previous reaction to an MRI or iodinated X-ray contrast agent, the reported adverse reaction rates were 21 and 6% respectively (SEDA-20, 419). Adverse effects at a dose of 0.3 mmol/kg included urticaria, vomiting, diarrhea, flushing, paresthesia, and headache, which have previously been reported with standard doses. The most common adverse effects were nausea and a metallic taste. In a study of 79 patients given 0.3 mmol/kg no adverse effects were recorded (SEDA-22, 503).

There is no significant difference in the incidence of adverse effects between ionic and non-ionic gadolinium chelates (SEDA-21, 483).

Gadobenate dimeglumine (Gd-BOPTA)

Gadobenate dimeglumine is a novel paramagnetic contrast agent that combines the properties of a conventional extracellular contrast agent with those of a liver-specific contrast agent. It has potential for both hepatic and non-hepatic targeted imaging. Unlike standard gadolinium chelates, which are excreted by the kidneys, 3–5% of gadobenate dimeglumine is taken up by functioning hepatocytes and is excreted unchanged in the bile. It also has an inherently higher T1 relaxivity than conventional gadolinium chelates, and so causes very marked enhancement of the liver parenchyma on T1 images, which persists for up to 2 hours. Liver tumors generally do not contain functioning hepatocytes and therefore do not take up gadobenate dimeglumine; they therefore appear as unenhanced hypointense lesions.

In 74 patients over the age of 18 years with possible metastatic brain disease, a total cumulative dose of 0.2 mmol/kg of gadobenate dimeglumine injected intravenously over 20 minutes was safe and enhanced the assessment of brain secondaries (8).

The safety and efficacy of gadobenate dimeglumine in phase 1, 2, and 3 studies have been reviewed in 732 patients, of whom 168 received 0.05 mmol/kg and 564 received 0.1 mmol/kg (9). The overall incidence of adverse events was 14% with the lower dose and 9.9% with the higher dose. The vast majority of events were mild, transient, and self-limiting. There were no sex-, age-, or dose-related differences and no clinically important effects on vital signs or laboratory parameters. The most common adverse events were hypertension (1.37%), nausea (1.09%), tachycardia (0.96%), and albuminuria (0.75%). The authors concluded that gadobenate dimeglumine is safe and efficacious as a contrast agent for use in hepatic MRI.

The safety of gadobenate dimeglumine has been confirmed in phase 2 and phase 3 studies in Japan (10,11). The overall adverse reaction rate was 3.5–5% and all the reactions were mild or moderate. There were no differences in the rates of adverse reactions with different dosage regimens (0.05–2.0 mmol/kg).

A safety evaluation of gadobenate dimeglumine in patients with renal impairment has also been reported (12). In a placebo-controlled, double-blind study there were no changes in laboratory parameters or vital signs and no clinically important adverse events.

The safety of gadobenate dimeglumine has been evaluated in 2367 adults aged 18-88 years and 173 children. The overall incidence of adverse events was 20%. Events related to the contrast agent were reported in 15% of the adults. Most of the adverse events were mild and transient and resolved spontaneously. Headache, injection site reactions, nausea, taste disturbance, and vasodilatation were the most common, with frequencies of 1.0–2.6%. Serious adverse events potentially related to the contrast agent were reported in 0.2%. These events included laryngospasm, which developed 10 minutes after the contrast injection in a 51-year-old woman, severe vomiting in a 5-year-old child, and pulmonary edema in a 65-year-old patient.

Gadobenate dimeglumine (intravenous bolus injection of 0.05 mmol/kg) was well tolerated by 103 patients (mean age 56 years) with acute myocardial infarction (13). Minor adverse effects in 27 patients included injection site reactions (13%), paresthesia (6.8%), dry mouth (6.8%), taste disturbance (2.9%), and headache (1.9%). The authors concluded that the use of a bolus dose of gadobenate dimeglumine 0.05 mmol/kg up to 6 days after acute myocardial infarction is safe.

The safety of intravenous gadobenate dimeglumine 0.025, 0.05, 0.1, and 0.2 mmol/kg in MR angiography has been assessed in 94 patients (mean age 58 years). Diagnostic accuracy was optimal at a dose of 0.1 mmol/kg (14). All the doses were well tolerated and there were no significant changes in safety parameters. Six patients reported mild adverse effects related to the contrast agent, including urticaria ($n = 2$), nausea ($n = 2$), and mild increases in liver enzymes (gamma-glutamyl transpeptidase, alanine transaminase, and aspartate transaminase) ($n = 2$). All the adverse events resolved spontaneously.

Similar observations were made in another study using similar doses of gadobenate dimeglumine for MR angiography (15). There were no important adverse effects, and the authors concluded that gadobenate dimeglumine is safe for MR angiography and that the optimal diagnostic dose is 0.1 mmol/kg.

Gadobutrol

Gadobutrol 1.0 is an extracellular neutral gadolinium chelate belonging to the class of macrocyclic neutral gadolinium complexes. It has the lowest osmolality of gadolinium-based contrast agents (1.60 osmol/kg). In preclinical evaluation there was good tolerance up to a dose of 0.5 mmol/kg, and this has been confirmed in phase I clinical studies. In a phase II study, 89 patients with suspected cerebrovascular insufficiency received Gadovist 1.0 in doses of 0.1 ($n = 11$), 0.2 ($n = 21$), 0.3 ($n = 21$), 0.4 ($n = 21$), or 0.5 ($n = 15$) mmol/kg (16). There were no significant changes in vital signs or any serious adverse reactions. Two patients had nausea and dry mouth. A dose of 0.3 mmol/kg was diagnostically adequate.

Gadodiamide

Adverse events associated with the non-ionic, gadolinium-based contrast agent gadodiamide have been reported in 1–2% of patients. Most of the commonly reported adverse events have been headache, dizziness, or nausea and vomiting.

The safety and effectiveness of gadodiamide-enhanced magnetic resonance angiography (MRA) with single and triple doses in the assessment of abdominal arterial stenosis has been investigated in 105 patients, of whom 53 (aged 45–83 years) received 0.1 mmol/kg and 52 (aged 38–85 years) received 0.3 mmol/kg (17). There were no serious adverse events. Six patients in the single-dose group felt a sensation of heat or warmth in the abdomen, lumbar spine, upper legs, hips, or groin; five of these events were mild and one was moderate; one patient felt a mild cold sensation at the injection site. Six patients in the triple-dose group felt a warm discomfort in the abdomen, pelvis, or buttocks (two mild and four moderate); four other patients felt a cold sensation at the injection site or in the arm (three mild and one moderate). The authors concluded that gadodiamide-enhanced MRA performed with single and triple doses is safe and effective in assessing major abdominal arterial stenosis. Triple-dose MRA was better at evaluating image quality and the degree of arterial stenosis.

The safety of gadodiamide-enhanced MRI in staging suspected or recurrent soft tissue tumors of the head and neck has been investigated in 48 patients (aged 37–86) (18). There was only one adverse event, moderate thirst. The authors concluded that the use of gadodiamide for MRI contrast-enhanced examination of the head and neck is safe and provides more diagnostic information than unenhanced images.

Gadofosveset

Gadofosveset (MS-325) is a gadolinium-based small molecular weight chelate, which binds strongly and reversibly to human serum albumin after injection (19). Because of albumin binding it has a long half-life and increased relaxivity (RI = 48 $mM^{-1}sec^{-1}$ at 0.47 T and 37°C, which is 10 times higher than gadolinium DTPA). These properties are particularly useful for contrast-enhanced, three-dimensional MRA. Furthermore, MS-325 can be given as a bolus, allowing dynamic arterial imaging. Prolonged blood-pool retention also allows steady-state imaging. There are promising results from early studies of carotid and coronary arteries. No serious adverse effects have been reported after the injection of gadofosveset, although transient nausea and paresthesia were reported in two of seven volunteers (1).

The safety and diagnostic efficacy of gadofosveset in MRA of the carotid arteries has been investigated in 26 patients aged 42–81 years with suspected carotid artery stenosis. It was given intravenously to 4, 9, and 13 patients in single doses of 0.01, 0.03, or 0.05 mmol/kg respectively. There were no serious or severe adverse events. Two patients who received 0.05 mmol/kg had five adverse events within 3 hours after the injection (nausea, cramps, metallic taste, and pruritus), which were rated as mild. There were no significant changes in serum chemistry. High-quality MRA scans were obtained in all the patients.

Gadopentetate dimeglumine

Gadopentetate dimeglumine (1 ml mixed with 4 ml of 5% saline) has been used in myelocisternography in four patients (aged 28–62 years) to demonstrate the exact site of cerebrospinal fluid (CSF) leakage in patients with CSF rhinorrhea (20). All tolerated the examination without adverse effects or complications.

Gadoversetamide

The safety of intravenous gadoversetamide, 0.1, 0.3, and 0.5 mmol/kg, has been confirmed in a study of its pharmacokinetics, safety, and tolerability in 163 patients with nervous system or liver pathology and varying degrees of renal function (21). All the adverse events that were thought to be related to gadoversetamide were mild or moderate, and there was no difference between doses. There were no changes in laboratory parameters. Gadoversetamide was well tolerated, even in patients with prolonged elimination due to renal impairment.

The safety of gadoversetamide at doses of 0.1–0.7 mmol/kg has been evaluated in 18 clinical studies (22). Adverse events related to the contrast agent were reported in 31% of injections. There were no serious adverse events.

Gadoxetic acid

Gadoxetic acid (gadolinium ethoxybenzyl diethylenetriaminepenta-acetic acid) was developed as a tissue-specific contrast agent for the liver and biliary system to be used in MRI and is a derivative of gadolinium DTPA with higher lipophilicity. It is taken up into hepatocytes and undergoes biliary excretion. Intravenous gadoxetic acid disodium has been used to assess liver enhancement and detect lesions in CT scanning of 15 patients with known liver metastases. The contrast agent was administered as an intravenous infusion over 20 or 30 minutes in doses of 0.2, 0.35, and 0.5 mmol/kg. There were three mild adverse reactions and one moderate reaction. Two patients reported a burning sensation at the site of infusion or retrosternally, which resolved when the flow rate of the infusion was reduced. Two other patients reported right upper quadrant pain, which began 4 hours after the infusion; this resolved spontaneously after a few hours. There were also minor reversible alterations in liver enzymes in some patients. Overall patient tolerance was acceptable and the images showed good or excellent liver enhancement, liver to tumor attenuation difference, and tumor visualization in the majority of cases with doses of 0.35 and 0.5 mmol/kg (SEDA-22, 504).

Uses of gadolinium other than in MRI scanning

Gadolinium can sufficiently attenuate X-rays to be visualized with digital subtraction angiography, although the quality of image is consistently inferior to that produced by iodinated agents. Of 13 patients who underwent transplant angiography with 16–20 ml of either gadopentetate dimeglumine (0.5 mmol/ml) or gadolinium (0.5 mmol/ml), there was no significant deterioration in renal function in 11 patients (23). In the other two there were significant increases that were not considered to be due to either gadolinium or the administration of CO_2. These findings are consistent with previous studies (SEDA 22, 504) showing that gadolinium compounds are not nephrotoxic.

Organs and Systems

Pancreas

Acute pancreatitis has been attributed to gadodiamide.

- A 58-year-old man was given intravenous gadodiamide (non-ionic gadolinium chelate) 16 ml (0.2 mmol/kg) for hepatic MRI and immediately after the injection developed fatigue, nausea, vomiting, sweating, and later intense upper abdominal pain (24). His serum amylase was 4262 IU/l and abdominal MRI showed a diffusely enlarged pancreas, confirming the diagnosis of acute pancreatitis. A full history and biliary tract ultrasound excluded other causes. The attack was mild and the clinical course uneventful.
- A 68-year-old woman with long-standing peripheral vascular disease and chronic renal insufficiency (serum creatinine 334 μmol/l) underwent peripheral angiography with gadodiamide (dose not stated) and 6 hours later developed nausea, epigastric pain, and two episodes of vomiting, with further epigastric pain 5 hours later (25). Her serum amylase and lipase activities were 246 and 1314 U/l respectively (reference ranges 0–140 and 0–200 U/l). The next morning they were 684 and 1646 U/l respectively. Ultrasound scan of the liver and gallbladder was normal. She subsequently developed acute renal insufficiency, electrolyte imbalance, and pulmonary edema. Urine microscopy showed muddy brown casts consistent with acute tubular necrosis. Her pancreatitis resolved without any further complications.

The authors of the second case highlighted the fact that there is no recommended maximum safe dose of gadolinium, nor a minimum creatinine clearance below which gadolinium should not be used.

Urinary tract

Intravenous gadoterate meglumine 35 ml has been used as a contrast agent for arm venography using digital fluorography in 45 patients with end-stage renal insufficiency (age 26–88 years, serum creatinine 262–1360 μmol/l) before the creation of an arteriovenous fistula (26). The mean serum creatinine did not change significantly. There were no significant adverse effects. Only one patient developed vomiting. A good diagnostic examination was obtained in all cases.

The use of gadolinium-DTPA as a suitable contrast agent in patients with renal insufficiency undergoing vascular intervention with standard X-ray screening has been reported (SEDA-22, 504). During angiography two patients received gadolinium DTPA 50–60 ml without alterations in serum creatinine or any other adverse effect.

- A 55-year-old woman with polycystic kidney disease and chronic renal impairment (serum creatinine concentration 181 μmol/l) received gadodiamide (Omniscan) for cerebral angiography; there were no adverse effects and the serum creatinine was unchanged. (27)

The authors concluded that gadodiamide is a safe alternative to iodinated contrast media in patients with renal impairment.

However, the use of large volumes of gadolinium-based contrast agents can cause deterioration in renal function, and the safety of these agents in relation to the kidney when a large volume is used is not known (27).

The use of gadolinium-DTPA has been described in 28 patients (22 men, 6 women, mean age 51 years) for angiography (28). The mean dose of gadolinium was 35 (range 20–60) ml. All the patients had renal impairment (serum creatinine over 133 μmol/l). Gadolinium was well tolerated, but 17 patients noted a mild heat sensation and one complained of transient pain during the injection. Only one patient, who received 40 ml, developed worse renal function, with an increase in serum creatinine from 360 to 450 μmol/l. Although the gadolinium was well tolerated in this group of patients, gadolinium-based contrast agents should be used with extreme care, particularly in patients with renal impairment, as they can be nephrotoxic in large doses.

A prospective, randomized, double-blind, placebo-controlled trial has also confirmed the safety of gadolinium infusion in 32 patients with renal impairment in dosages typically used during MRI examination (29). Nine patients had moderate renal impairment (mean age 57 years, creatinine clearance 30–60 ml/minute) and 11 had severe renal impairment (mean age 63 years, creatinine clearance 10–29 ml/minute). They were given an intravenous bolus of gadobenate dimeglumine 0.2 mmol/kg. A comparable control group received an injection of isotonic saline. There was no significant deterioration in renal function in any group during the following 7 days.

- A 67-year-old woman with chronic renal insufficiency secondary to interstitial nephritis had rapid deterioration over several months, with a rise in serum creatinine from 150 to 290 μmol/l (30). Renal artery stenosis was suspected. She had anaphylaxis during spiral CT angiography with an iodinated contrast medium (details not given), which showed right renal artery stenosis. After further deterioration in renal function (serum creatinine 480 μmol/l) she underwent renal arteriography with 30 ml of a gadolinium-based contrast agent (0.3 mmol/kg) injected into the abdominal aorta just above the renal arteries. Her renal function was monitored for 15 days after the procedure, and there was no further rise in serum creatinine.
- A 64-year-old obese man with a history of radiocontrast-induced nephropathy had an MRI scan, which confirmed the presence of an aortic aneurysm from just below the renal arteries to the aortic bifurcation (31). Percutaneous stenting of the aortic aneurysm

Table 1 European Society of Urogenital Radiology (ESUR) position statement on the use of gadolinium-based contrast media for radiographic examinations (34)

Legal position	Gadolinium-based contrast media are not approved for X-ray examinations
Reported uses of gadolinium-based contrast media for X-ray examinations	Significant renal impairment Prior severe generalized adverse reaction to iodinated contrast media Imminent thyroid treatment with radioactive iodine
ESUR position	The use of gadolinium-based contrast media for radiographic examinations is not recommended to avoid nephrotoxicity in patients with renal impairment, since they are more nephrotoxic than iodinated contrast media in equivalent X-ray attenuating doses The use of gadolinium-based contrast media in approved intravenous doses of up to 0.3 mmol/kg will not give diagnostic radiographic information in most cases

was carried out with 0.5 mol/l gadoteridol solution 90 ml (0.375 mmol/kg) instead of an iodinated contrast agent. There was no further deterioration in renal function.

The authors of the second report erroneously concluded that gadolinium-containing contrast agents are not nephrotoxic, and they recommended their use in patients in whom conventional iodinated contrast agents are contraindicated. However, gadolinium-based contrast agents have more nephrotoxic potential than iodinated contrast agents in equimolar concentrations. Their use in patients with renal impairment should be carried out with care and the dosage should not exceed 0.3 mmol/kg.

This case underlines the fact that there is still misunderstanding about the nephrotoxic potential of gadolinium-based contrast agents. They should not replace iodinated contrast agents in patients with renal insufficiency. The recommended doses of up to 0.3 mmol/kg will not give satisfactory radiographic diagnostic information in most cases.

Susceptibility Factors

Renal disease

The use of gadolinium-based contrast media for radiographic examination as an alternative to iodinated contrast media in patients with impaired renal function has been erroneously endorsed by several authors. For example, in a German study gadopentetate dimeglumine (average dose 0.34 mmol/kg) was used in 29 patients (mean age 61 years) with renal impairment (mean baseline serum creatinine 318 μmol/l) as an alternative to an iodinated contrast agent for angiographic procedures (32). Only one patient developed contrast medium-induced renal damage, defined as an increase in serum creatinine by more than 88 μmol/l within 72 hours of injection of the contrast agent. The authors suggested that gadopentetate dimeglumine is a safe alternative to iodinated contrast agents for radiographic examinations in patients with renal impairment.

In another study, gadodiamide was used as an alternative for angiographic procedures in patients with contraindications to iodinated contrast media; 17 patients (mean age 74 years) received a mean volume of 136 ml of gadodiamide (range 60–200 ml) (33). The contraindications to iodinated contrast injection were renal impairment (12 patients, serum creatinine 200–500 μmol/l), a history of iodinated contrast reaction ($n = 3$), and hyperthyroidism ($n = 4$). Several of the patients had renal artery stenosis, and renal function improved after successful angioplasty. There were no cases of nephrotoxicity. The authors concluded that patients with contraindications to iodinated contrast injection can safely receive gadolinium-based contrast media for radiographic examinations.

The authors of these reports have erroneously suggested that gadolinium-based contrast media are less nephrotoxic than iodinated contrast media. However, at equimolar concentrations gadolinium-based contrast media are more nephrotoxic than iodinated contrast media, and at equivalent X-ray attenuation gadolinium-based contrast media are actually more nephrotoxic. The Contrast Media Safety Committee of the European Society of Urogenital Radiology has recently produced a report on the use of gadolinium-based contrast media for radiographic examinations, and its position is summarized in Table 1.

The safety and dialysability of gadobutrol 0.1 or 0.3 mmol/kg have been investigated in 11 patients (median age 42 years) with end-stage renal insufficiency who required hemodialysis (35). The patients were monitored for 120 hours. There were no important changes in hematology, clinical chemistry, or vital signs. Hemodialysis was effective in removing the gadolinium contrast agent from the body, and by the third session, 98% of the injected dose had been eliminated.

Hepatic disease

The safety of gadobenate dimeglumine has been evaluated in 16 subjects with liver impairment, 11 of whom (mean age 48 years) received gadobenate dimeglumine (0.1 mmol/kg) intravenously and five of whom (mean age 42 years) received placebo (36). There were no important adverse effects and no significant changes in laboratory parameters. The pharmacokinetics of the contrast agent were not different from those with normal liver function.

Drug Administration

Drug administration route

The safety of intrathecal gadopentetate dimeglumine has been investigated in 95 patients (aged 1 month to 78 years) (37). The contrast agent was injected into the subarachnoid space via a lumbar puncture needle; 3–5 ml of cerebral spinal fluid were withdrawn and mixed with 0.5, 0.7, 0.8, or 1 ml of gadopentetate dimeglumine. There were no significant behavioral changes, neurological changes, or seizure activity, but 19 patients had headache after lumbar puncture, 6 had nausea, and 2 had vomiting. All the adverse effects resolved within the first 24 hours with bed rest.

References

1. Kroft LJ, de Roos A. Blood pool contrast agents for cardiovascular MR imaging. J Magn Reson Imaging 1999; 10(3):395–403.
2. Rubin DL, Desser TS, Semelka R, Brown J, Nghiem HV, Stevens WR, Bluemke D, Nelson R, Fultz P, Reimer P, Ho V, Kristy RM, Pierro JA. A multicenter, randomized, double-blind study to evaluate the safety, tolerability, and efficacy of OptiMARK (gadoversetamide injection) compared with Magnevist (gadopentetate dimeglumine) in patients with liver pathology: results of a Phase III clinical trial. J Magn Reson Imaging 1999;9(2):240–50.
3. Coche EE, Hammer FD, Goffette PP. Demonstration of pulmonary embolism with gadolinium-enhanced spiral CT. Eur Radiol 2001;11(11):2306–9.
4. Grossman RI, Rubin DL, Hunter G, Haughton VM, Lee D, Sze G, Kuhn MJ, Maravilla K, Tu R, Heindel W, Wippold FJ 2nd, Leeds N, Zelch J, Jinkins JR, Grodd W, Truwit C, Kanal E, Provenzale JM, Ramsey R, Simon J, Brunberg JA, Stevens GR, Kristy RM. Magnetic resonance imaging in patients with central nervous system pathology: a comparison of OptiMARK (Gd-DTPA-BMEA) and Magnevist (Gd-DTPA). Invest Radiol 2000;35(7):412–19.
5. Kirchin MA, Pirovano G, Venetianer C, Spinazzi A. Safety assessment of gadobenate dimeglumine (MultiHance): extended clinical experience from phase I studies to post-marketing surveillance. J Magn Reson Imaging 2001;14(3):281–94.
6. Runge VM, Armstrong MR, Barr RG, Berger BL, Czervionke LF, Gonzalez CF, Halford HH, Kanal E, Kuhn MJ, Levin JM, Low RN, Tanenbaum LN, Wang AM, Wong W, Yuh WT, Zoarski GH. A clinical comparison of the safety and efficacy of MultiHance (gadobenate dimeglumine) and Omniscan (gadodiamide) in magnetic resonance imaging in patients with central nervous system pathology. Invest Radiol 2001;36(2):65–71.
7. Takebayashi S, Sugiyama M, Nagase M, et al. Severe adverse reaction to I.V. gadopentate dimeglumine. Radiology 1993;160:65.
8. Baleriaux D, Colosimo C, Ruscalleda J, Korves M, Schneider G, Bohndorf K, Bongartz G, van Buchem MA, Reiser M, Sartor K, Bourne MW, Parizel PM, Cherryman GR, Salerio I, La Noce A, Pirovano G, Kirchin MA, Spinazzi A. Magnetic resonance imaging of metastatic disease to the brain with gadobenate dimeglumine. Neuroradiology 2002;44(3):191–203.
9. Hamm B, Kirchin M, Pirovano G, Spinazzi A. Clinical utility and safety of MultiHance in magnetic resonance imaging of liver cancer: results of multicenter studies in Europe and the USA. J Comput Assist Tomogr 1999;23(Suppl 1):S53–60.
10. Tanimoto A, Kuwatsuru R, Kadoya M, Ohtomo K, Hirohashi S, Murakami T, Hiramatsu K, Yoshikawa K, Katayama H. Evaluation of gadobenate dimeglumine in hepatocellular carcinoma: results from phase II and phase III clinical trials in Japan. J Magn Reson Imaging 1999;10(3):450–60.
11. Kuwatsuru R, Kadoya M, Ohtomo K, Tanimoto A, Hirohashi S, Murakami T, Tanaka Y, Yoshikawa K, Katayama H. Clinical late phase II trials of MultiHance (Gd-BOPTA) for the magnetic resonance imaging of liver tumors in Japan. J Comput Assist Tomogr 1999;23(Suppl 1):S65–74.
12. Swan SK, Lambrecht LJ, Townsend R, Davies BE, McCloud S, Parker JR, Bensel K, LaFrance ND. Safety and pharmacokinetic profile of gadobenate dimeglumine in subjects with renal impairment. Invest Radiol 1999; 34(7):443–8.
13. Cherryman GR, Pirovano G, Kirchin MA. Gadobenate dimeglumine in MRI of acute myocardial infarction: results of a phase III study comparing dynamic and delayed contrast enhanced magnetic resonance imaging with EKG, (201)Tl SPECT, and echocardiography. Invest Radiol 2002;37(3):135–45.
14. Kroencke TJ, Wasser MN, Pattynama PM, Barentsz JO, Grabbe E, Marchal G, Knopp MV, Schneider G, Bonomo L, Pennell DJ, del Maschio A, Hentrich HR, Dapra M, Kirchin MA, Spinazzi A, Taupitz M, Hamm B. Gadobenate dimeglumine-enhanced MR angiography of the abdominal aorta and renal arteries. AJR Am J Roentgenol 2002;179(6):1573–82.
15. La Ferla R, Dapra M, Hentrich HR, Pirovano G, Kirchin MA. Gadobenate dimeglumine (Multihance) in contrast-enhanced magnetic resonance angiography. Acad Radiol 2002;9(Suppl 2):S409–11.
16. Benner T, Reimer P, Erb G, Schuierer G, Heiland S, Fischer C, Geens V, Sartor K, Forsting M. Cerebral MR perfusion imaging: first clinical application of a 1 M gadolinium chelate (Gadovist 1.0) in a double-blinded randomized dose-finding study. J Magn Reson Imaging 2000;12(3):371–80.
17. Thurnher SA, Capelastegui A, Del Olmo FH, Dondelinger RF, Gervas C, Jassoy AG, Keto P, Loewe C, Ludman CN, Marti-Bonmati L, Meusel M, da Cruz JP, Pruvo JP, Sanjuan VM, Vogl T. Safety and effectiveness of single- versus triple-dose gadodiamide injection- enhanced MR angiography of the abdomen: a phase III double-blind multicenter study. Radiology 2001;219(1):137–46.
18. Ekholm SE, Bjork-Eriksson T, Western A, Nellstrom H, Jonsson E, Johansson A, Lonn L, Mercke C, Tollesson PO. MRI staging using gadodiamide for soft-tissue tumors of the head and neck region. Results from a phase II trial and a 5-year clinical follow-up. Eur J Radiol 2001;39(3):168–75.
19. Bluemke DA, Stillman AE, Bis KG, Grist TM, Baum RA, D'Agostino R, Malden ES, Pierro JA, Yucel EK. Carotid MR angiography: phase II study of safety and efficacy for MS-325. Radiology 2001;219(1):114–22.
20. Wenzel R, Leppien A. Gadolinium-myelocisternography for cerebrospinal fluid rhinorrhoea. Neuroradiology 2000;42(12):874–80.
21. Swan SK, Baker JF, Free R, Tucker RM, Barron B, Barr R, Seltzer S, Gazelle GS, Maravilla KR, Barr W, Stevens GR, Lambrecht LJ, Pierro JA. Pharmacokinetics, safety, and tolerability of gadoversetamide injection (OptiMARK) in subjects with central nervous system or liver pathology and varying degrees of renal function. J Magn Reson Imaging 1999;9(2):317–21.
22. Brown JJ, Kristy RM, Stevens GR, Pierro JA. The OptiMARK clinical development program: summary of safety data. J Magn Reson Imaging 2002;15(4):446–55.
23. Spinosa DJ, Matsumoto AH, Angle JF, Hagspiel KD, Isaacs RB, McCullough CS, Lobo PI. Gadolinium-based contrast and carbon dioxide angiography to evaluate renal transplants for vascular causes of renal insufficiency and

accelerated hypertension. J Vasc Interv Radiol 1998;9(6): 909–16.
24. Terzi C, Sokmen S. Acute pancreatitis induced by magnetic-resonance-imaging contrast agent. Lancet 1999;354(9192): 1789–90.
25. Schenker MP, Solomon JA, Roberts DA. Gadolinium arteriography complicated by acute pancreatitis and acute renal failure. J Vasc Interv Radiol 2001;12(3):393.
26. Geoffroy O, Tassart M, Le Blanche AF, Khalil A, Duedal V, Rossert J, Bigot JM, Boudghene FP. Upper extremity digital subtraction venography with gadoterate meglumine before fistula creation for hemodialysis. Kidney Int 2001;59(4):1491–7.
27. Slaba SG, El-Hajj LF, Abboud GA, Gebara VA. Selective angiography of cerebral aneurysm using gadodiamide in polycystic kidney disease with renal insufficiency. AJR Am J Roentgenol 2000;175(5):1467–8.
28. Hammer FD, Malaise J, Goffette PP, Mathurin P. Gadolinium dimeglumine: an alternative contrast agent for digital subtraction angiography in patients with renal failure. Transplant Proc 2000;32(2):432–3.
29. Townsend RR, Cohen DL, Katholi R, Swan SK, Davies BE, Bensel K, Lambrecht L, Parker J. Safety of intravenous gadolinium (Gd-BOPTA) infusion in patients with renal insufficiency. Am J Kidney Dis 2000;36(6):1207–12.
30. Bassilios N, Vantelon C, Cluzel P, Baumelou A, Deray G. Use of gadolinium-based contrast agent for renal angiography: case report and review of the literature. Ren Fail 2001;23(6):857–61.
31. Wagner HJ, Storck M. Endovaskulare stentgraftgestutzte Exklusion eines infrarenalen Aortenaneurysmas mit Gadolinium als Kontrastmittel bei Niereninsuffizienz. [Endovascular stent graft support exclusion of an infrarenal aortic aneurysm using gadolinium as contrast medium in kidney insufficiency.] Dtsch Med Wochenschr 2001;126 (21):616–20.
32. Rieger J, Sitter T, Toepfer M, Linsenmaier U, Pfeifer KJ, Schiffl H. Gadolinium as an alternative contrast agent for diagnostic and interventional angiographic procedures in patients with impaired renal function. Nephrol Dial ransplant 2002;17(5):824–8.
33. Zeller T, Muller C, Frank U, Burgelin K, Sinn L, Horn B, Flugel PC, Roskamm H. Gadodiamide as an alternative contrast agent during angioplasty in patients with contra-indications to iodinated media. J Endovasc Ther 2002;9(5):625–32.
34. Thomsen HS, Almen T, Morcos SK; Contrast Media Safety Committee Of The European Society Of Urogenital Radiology (ESUR). Gadolinium-containing contrast media for radiographic examinations: a position paper. Eur Radiol 2002;12(10):2600–5.
35. Tombach B, Bremer C, Reimer P, Matzkies F, Schaefer RM, Ebert W, Geens V, Eisele J, Heindel W. Using highly concentrated gadobutrol as an MR contrast agent in patients also requiring hemodialysis: safety and dialysability. AJR Am J Roentgenol 2002; 178(1):105–9.
36. Davies BE, Kirchin MA, Bensel K, Lorusso V, Davies A, Parker JR, Lafrance ND. Pharmacokinetics and safety of gadobenate dimeglumine (multihance) in subjects with impaired liver function. Invest Radiol 2002; 37(5):299–308.
37. Tali ET, Ercan N, Krumina G, Rudwan M, Mironov A, Zeng QY, Jinkins JR. Intrathecal gadolinium (gadopentetate dimeglumine) enhanced magnetic resonance myelography and cisternography: results of a multicenter study. Invest Radiol 2002;37(3):152–9.

Gallamine triethiodide

See also Neuromuscular blocking drugs

General Information

Gallamine is a non-depolarizing muscle relaxant. For intubation about 2 mg/kg (some authors say 3–4 mg/kg) are necessary, and the duration of effect is then similar to the usual intubating doses of D-tubocurarine or pancuronium. A dose of 1–1.5 mg/kg is usually sufficient to produce apnea and adequate abdominal relaxation. Such doses are said to be short-acting (20 minutes) but can provide clinical relaxation (75% or more depression of twitch height) for some 30–40 minutes. Individual variation is considerable, and complete spontaneous reversal of blockade is relatively slow.

Organs and Systems

Cardiovascular

Tachycardia invariably accompanies the use of gallamine. It is seen after doses as low as 20 mg and reaches a maximum at around 100 mg in adults (1). It is often extreme, rates above 120 per minute being not uncommon. The increase in heart rate outlasts the neuromuscular blocking effect (1). Usual clinical doses also result in a slight increase in mean arterial pressure, a slight fall in systemic vascular resistance, and a marked rise in cardiac index (2,3). These cardiovascular effects are principally accounted for by the strong vagolytic action of gallamine, the cardiac muscarinic receptors being almost as sensitive to its blocking action as the acetylcholine receptors of the neuromuscular junction (4). Blockade of noradrenaline reuptake and an increased release of noradrenaline from cardiac adrenergic nerve endings (5,6) may contribute, although an inotropic effect in man is disputed (7). Ganglion-blocking activity is slight and is not seen in the usual dose range. The possible mechanisms have been reviewed (8–10). Gallamine should therefore not be used when tachycardia has to be avoided.

Immunologic

Histamine release may be associated with the use of gallamine more often than was previously believed, according to several studies involving large numbers of patients (11–14). There have been several reports of reactions involving skin flushing, bronchospasm, or cardiovascular collapse possibly due to gallamine, including anaphylactoid reactions to small precurarizing doses (15,16).

Second-Generation Effects

Fetotoxicity

Placental transfer has been variously reported, usually only small amounts being detected in the umbilical blood, with no clinically obvious effects on the newborn (17).

Susceptibility Factors

Renal disease

Gallamine does not undergo biotransformation and depends entirely on glomerular filtration for its excretion (17). In renal insufficiency the neuromuscular blockade that it causes is considerably prolonged and gallamine is contraindicated.

Drug–Drug Interactions

Azathioprine

Azathioprine reduces sensitivity to gallamine in experimental animals, possibly as a result of phosphodiesterase inhibition, increasing transmitter release (SEDA-4, 87) (18), (SEDA-13, 104).

References

1. Eisele JH, Marta JA, Davis HS. Quantitative aspects of the chronotropic and neuromuscular effects of gallamine in anesthetized man. Anesthesiology 1971;35(6):630–3.
2. Stoelting RK. Hemodynamic effects of gallamine during halothane–nitrous oxide anesthesia. Anesthesiology 1973;39(6):645–7.
3. Kennedy BR, Farman JV. Cardiovascular effects of gallamine triethiodide in man. Br J Anaesth 1968;40(10):773–80.
4. Riker WF Jr, Wescoe WC. The pharmacology of Flaxedil, with observations on certain analogues. Ann NY Acad Sci 1951;54(3):373–94.
5. Brown BR Jr, Crout JR. The sympathomimetic effect of gallamine on the heart. J Pharmacol Exp Ther 1970;172(2):266–73.
6. Vercruysse P, Bossuyt P, Hanegreefs G, Verbeuren TJ, Vanhoutte PM. Gallamine and pancuronium inhibit pre- and postjunctional muscarine receptors in canine saphenous veins. J Pharmacol Exp Ther 1979;209(2):225–30.
7. Reitan JA, Fraser AI, Eisele JH. Lack of cardiac inotropic effects of gallamine in anesthetized man. Anesth Analg 1973;52(6):974–9.
8. Marshall IG. Pharmacological effects of neuromuscular blocking agents: interaction with cholinoceptors other than nicotinic receptors of the neuromuscular junction. Anest Rianim 1986;27:19.
9. Bowman WC. Non-relaxant properties of neuromuscular blocking drugs. Br J Anaesth 1982;54(2):147–60.
10. Bowman WC. Pharmacology of Neuromuscular Function. 2nd ed. London/Boston/Singapore/Sydney/Toronto/Wellington: Wright, 1990.
11. Hatton F, Tiret L, Maujol L, N'Doye P, Vourc'h G, Desmonts JM, Otteni JC, Scherpereel P. Enquête épidémiologique sur les anesthésies. [INSERM. Epidemiological survey of anesthesia. Initial results.] Ann Fr Anesth Réanim 1983;2(5):331–86.
12. Fisher MM, Munro I. Life-threatening anaphylactoid reactions to muscle relaxants. Anesth Analg 1983;62(6):559–64.
13. Laxenaire MC, Moneret-Vautrin DA, Vervloet D. The French experience of anaphylactoid reactions. Int Anesthesiol Clin 1985;23(3):145–60.
14. Galletly DC, Treuren BC. Anaphylactoid reactions during anaesthesia. Seven years' experience of intradermal testing. Anaesthesia 1985;40(4):329–33.
15. Harrison GR, Thompson ID. Adverse reaction to methohexitone and gallamine. Anaesthesia 1981;36(1):40–4.
16. Harrison JF, Bird AG. Anaphylaxis to precurarising doses of gallamine triethiodide. Anaesthesia 1986;41(6):600–4.
17. Ramzan MI, Somogyi AA, Walker JS, Shanks CA, Triggs EJ. Clinical pharmacokinetics of the non-depolarising muscle relaxants. Clin Pharmacokinet 1981;6(1):25–60.
18. Dretchen KL, Morgenroth VH 3rd, Standaert FG, Walts LF. Azathioprine: effects on neuromuscular transmission. Anesthesiology 1976;45(6):604–9.

Gallium

General Information

Gallium is a metallic element (symbol Ga; atomic no. 31) that has been used in the form of a radiopharmaceutical (^{67}Ga as the citrate) in diagnostic imaging of cancers, inflammation, and infection (1–3). The mechanisms of the therapeutic activity of gallium have been reviewed (4).

Gallium nitrate is being increasingly used as a therapeutic agent in certain malignancies (5), since it has been shown to be concentrated in various neoplasms in both animals and man and to have antitumor activity (6), and the anticancer activity of new compounds, such as gallium maltolate, doxorubicin gallium transferrin conjugate, and trisquinolinolato gallium, is being explored (7).

Abnormal uptake of ^{67}Ga is reported as an adverse effect in diagnostic procedures, as in three cases:

- A 72-year-old man with acute lymphocytic leukemia who had normal ^{67}Ga uptake in all tissues except the liver (8).
- A 26-year-old pregnant woman with a mediastinal lymphoma that did not accumulate ^{67}Ga (9).
- A 49-year-old man with fever and increased ^{67}Ga uptake in the lungs but no other evidence of infection or cancer (10).

Gallium nitrate has been used as an alternative to bisphosphonates in hypercalcemia of malignancy (11), in which it is effective but associated with a higher frequency of renal toxicity (10%) and of nausea and vomiting (14%) than the bisphosphonates. The pathophysiology and treatment of hypercalcemia of malignancy has been reviewed and the role of gallium nitrate considered (12,13).

An early Phase I evaluation and subsequent reports presented similar pictures, with predominant renal and hematological adverse effects (14,15), but as a rule gallium has been used alongside other cytostatics and it is not possible to determine which of these has produced any particular effect. Other adverse effects observed have been nausea and/or vomiting, maculopapular skin rash, a metallic taste, and diarrhea (16).

Gallium alloys are still considered to be useful alternatives to amalgams in dental medicine, in spite of their tendency to corrosion, their controversial biocompatibility, and lack of knowledge about gallium's environmental impact (17).

Organs and Systems

Sensory systems

- A patient developed bilateral visual loss after systemic administration of gallium nitrate (SEDA-22, 244) (18). The condition worsened after oral corticosteroid therapy and partial recovery of optic nerve function in both eyes was present only after 12 months of oral ferrous sulfate administration.

Ototoxicity has been reported in a few patients taking gallium nitrate (19).

Hematologic

Hematological toxicity of gallium nitrate has been noted, for example granulocytopenia and anemia (19).

Mouth and teeth

Gallium is used in dental prostheses and is a source of increased sensitivity to postoperative dental pain (20). In a pilot study of a direct-placement gallium alloy (Galloy) in nine patients, 30 dental restorations were inserted and assessed over 3 years (21). The initial 18-month results were encouraging, but at 21 months there was one fractured tooth and within another year two molars had the cracked-tooth syndrome (incomplete tooth fracture). The fractured teeth were restored with amalgam. Tarnish and a rough surface were noted on many of the gallium restorations. These results suggest that Galloy, used with either of two sealing resins, is not a suitable dental restorative material.

Urinary tract

An early Phase I clinical evaluation indicated dose-related nephrotoxicity and this has led to much caution in dosage (19). At least one death from kidney failure has been reported. Maintaining adequate diuresis with 5% dextrose/saline may reduce the risk of nephrotoxicity.

In a comparative study of gallium nitrate and etidronate in acute control of cancer-related hypercalcemia, a significantly higher proportion of the patients treated with gallium nitrate developed asymptomatic hypophosphatemia (22).

Reproductive system

Gallium used in semiconductors has been found in animal studies to adversely affect male sperm count and to raise the proportion of abnormal sperm (SEDA-21, 235).

Immunologic

- A 40-year-old woman had multiple bone injuries, severe sepsis, and coma after a car accident; a retroperitoneal hematoma caused by lumbar fractures was drained, but she continued to be pyrexial (23). She had prominent accumulation of ^{67}Ga, which had been used for bone scanning, in her multiple recent fractures and an area of accumulation in the soft tissue related to a fractured vertebra. Post-traumatic paravertebral calcifications had accumulated ^{67}Ga and simulated the presence of an infected hematoma.

Susceptibility Factors

Renal disease

Because it is nephrotoxic, gallium nitrate should be avoided in renal dysfunction and in patients taking nephrotoxic drugs. Renal dysfunction also alters the kinetics of gallium (SED-12, 519).

Drug–Drug Interactions

Aminoglycosides

Concomitant treatment with aminoglycoside antibiotics in two cases resulted in acute renal insufficiency (24).

References

1. Gardin I, Faraggi M, Le Guludec D, Bok B. Cell irradiation caused by diagnostic nuclear medicine procedures: dose heterogeneity and biological consequences. Eur J Nucl Med 1999;26(12):1617–26.
2. Delcambre C, Reman O, Henry-Amar M, Peny AM, Macro M, Cheze S, Genot JY, Tanguy A, Switsers O, Van HL, Couette JE, Leporrier M, Bardet S. Clinical relevance of gallium-67 scintigraphy in lymphoma before and after therapy. Eur J Nucl Med 2000;27(2):176–84.
3. Boerman OC, Rennen H, Oyen WJ, Corstens FH. Radiopharmaceuticals to image infection and inflammation. Semin Nucl Med 2001;31(4):286–95.
4. Bernstein LR. Mechanisms of therapeutic activity for gallium. Pharmacol Rev 1998;50(4):665–82.
5. Apseloff G. Therapeutic uses of gallium nitrate: past, present, and future. Am J Ther 1999;6(6):327–39.
6. Malfetano JH, Blessing JA, Homesley HD. A phase II trial of gallium nitrate (NSC #15200) in nonsquamous cell carcinoma of the cervix. A Gynecologic Oncology Group Study. Am J Clin Oncol 1995;18(6):495–7.
7. Collery P, Keppler B, Madoulet C, Desoize B. Gallium in cancer treatment. Crit Rev Oncol Hematol 2002;42(3):283–96.
8. Nakahara T, Fujii H, Nakamura K, Hashimoto J, Kubo A. Inexplicable suppression of hepatic uptake of gallium-67, a case report. Ann Nucl Med 2001;15(4):377–9.
9. Kurosaki H, Saito Y, Kawashima M, Ebara T, Yamakawa M, Mitsuhashi N. Accumulation of 67Ga citrate in early pregnancy. Ann Nucl Med 2001;15(3):289–91.
10. Bernstine H, Bar-Sever Z, Cohen M, Hardoff R. Misleading thoracic Ga-67 uptake caused by splenic displacement. Clin Nucl Med 2001;26(2):147–8.
11. Zojer N, Keck AV, Pecherstorfer M. Comparative tolerability of drug therapies for hypercalcaemia of malignancy. Drug Saf 1999;21(5):389–406.
12. Schaiff RA, Hall TG, Bar RS. Medical treatment of hypercalcemia. Clin Pharm 1989;8(2):108–21.
13. Hall TG, Schaiff RA. Update on the medical treatment of hypercalcemia of malignancy. Clin Pharm 1993;12(2):117–25.
14. Chitambar CR, Zahir SA, Ritch PS, Anderson T. Evaluation of continuous-infusion gallium nitrate and hydroxyurea in combination for the treatment of refractory non-Hodgkin's lymphoma. Am J Clin Oncol 1997;20(2):173–8.
15. Dreicer R, Propert KJ, Roth BJ, Einhorn LH, Loehrer PJ. Vinblastine, ifosfamide, and gallium nitrate—an active new regimen in patients with advanced carcinoma of the urothelium. A phase II trial of the Eastern Cooperative Oncology Group (E5892). Cancer 1997;79(1):110–14.

16. Samson MK, Fraile RJ, Baker LH, O'Bryan R. Phase I-II clinical trial of gallium nitrate (NSC-15200). Cancer Clin Trials 1980;3(2):131–6.
17. Ruiz JI, Baciero GR, Gonzalvo EC, Gil BG. Gamalgamation: current situation. Refuat Hapeh Vehashinayim 2002;19(3):6–15, 88.
18. Csaky KG, Caruso RC. Gallium nitrate optic neuropathy. Am J Ophthalmol 1997;124(4):567–8.
19. Einhorn LH, Roth BJ, Ansari R, Dreicer R, Gonin R, Loehrer PJ. Phase II trial of vinblastine, ifosfamide, and gallium combination chemotherapy in metastatic urothelial carcinoma. J Clin Oncol 1994;12(11):2271–6.
20. Dunne SM, Abraham R. Dental post-operative sensitivity associated with a gallium-based restorative material. Br Dent J 2000;189(6):310–13.
21. Osborne JW, Summitt JB. Direct-placement gallium restorative alloy: a 3-year clinical evaluation. Quintessence Int 1999;30(1):49–53.
22. Warrell RP. Jr., Murphy WK, Schulman P, O'Dwyer PJ, Heller G. A randomized double-blind study of gallium nitrate compared with etidronate for acute control of cancer-related hypercalcemia. J Clin Oncol 1991;9(8):1467–75.
23. Lantsberg S, Rachinsky I, Boguslavsky L. False-positive Ga-67 uptake in a septic patient after severe automobile trauma. Clin Nucl Med 1999;24(11):890–1.
24. Warrell RP, Coonley CJ, Straus DJ, et al. Clinical evaluation of gallium nitrate (NSC-15200) by 7-day continuous infusion in advanced malignant lymphoma. Proc Am Assoc Cancer Res 1982;1:160.

Gammahydroxybutyrate

General Information

Sodium gammahydroxybutyrate (GHB or sodium oxybate) is an endogenous compound, a precursor of GABA, which increases the release of dopamine and acetylcholine in the brain. It was first synthesized in 1960 as a potential anesthetic, and was popular in the late 1980s and early 1990s as a dietary supplement (as a replacement for L-tryptophan after it had been recalled from the market), an aid to sleep, and a bodybuilding agent. It was subsequently used in the treatment of narcolepsy. However, it has also been used as a party drug, since it causes alcohol-like effects and aroused sexuality. In large doses it can cause disorientation, nausea and vomiting, and muscle spasms. It is also known as BDO, Blue Nitro, Enliven, GBH, Liquid ecstasy, Midnight Blue, RenewTrient, Reviarent, Serenity, and SomatoPro. An analogue, gammavalerolactone (GVL), is a precursor and has also been used recreationally, but it is very expensive.

In 1990 the FDA limited the availability of gammahydroxybutyrate, and in March 2000, the Drug Enforcement Agency made it a Schedule I drug. In 2001 the Expert Advisory Committee on Drugs (EACD) in New Zealand advised the New Zealand Medicines and Medical Devices Safety Authority to schedule gammahydroxybutyrate under the Misuse of Drugs Act 1975 (1). In June 2003 gammahydroxybutyrate was categorized as a Class C drug in the UK.

Ingestion of 0.5–3 teaspoons of sodium gammahydroxybutyrate can produce vomiting, drowsiness, hypotonia, and/or vertigo; loss of consciousness, irregular respiration, tremors, or myoclonus can follow. Seizure-like activity, bradycardia, hypotension, and/or respiratory arrest have also been reported. The severity and duration of symptoms depend on the dose and on the presence of other nervous system depressants, such as alcohol.

In a double-blind, randomized, placebo-controlled, crossover study in 24 patients with narcolepsy, gammahydroxybutyrate 60 mg/kg in a single night-dose for 4 weeks reduced the daily number of hypnagogic hallucinations, daytime sleep attacks, and the severity of subjective daytime sleepiness, and tended to reduce the number of daily attacks of cataplexy (2). It reduced the percentage of wakefulness during REM sleep and the number of awakenings out of REM sleep, and tended to increase slow wave sleep. Adverse events were few and mild.

Organs and Systems

Nervous system

In a double-blind, double-dummy comparison of clomethiazole and gammahydroxybutyrate in ameliorating the symptoms of alcohol withdrawal, alcohol-dependent patients were randomized to receive either clomethiazole 1000 mg or gammahydroxybutyrate 50 mg/kg (3). There was no difference between the treatments in ratings of alcohol withdrawal symptoms or requests for additional medications. After tapering the active medication, there was no increase in withdrawal symptoms, suggesting that physical tolerance did not develop to either clomethiazole or gammahydroxybutyrate during the 5-day treatment period. The most frequently reported adverse effect of gammahydroxybutyrate was transient vertigo, particularly after the evening double dose.

Drug Administration

Drug overdose

Some who have taken gammahydroxybutyrate without knowing what it was have subsequently awakened in hospital having been deeply comatose for a few hours, without after-effects (4).

References

1. Anonymous. Gamma hydroxybutyrate. Fantasy drugs to be classified. WHO Pharm Newslett 2001;2:5–6.
2. Lammers GJ, Arends J, Declerck AC, Ferrari MD, Schouwink G, Troost J. Gammahydroxybutyrate and narcolepsy: a double-blind placebo-controlled study. Sleep 1993;16(3):216–20.
3. Nimmerrichter AA, Walter H, Gutierrez-Lobos KE, Lesch OM. Double-blind controlled trial of gamma-hydroxybutyrate and clomethiazole in the treatment of alcohol withdrawal. Alcohol Alcohol 2002;37(1):67–73.
4. Strange DG, Jensen D. Gammahydroxybutyrat, et nyt rusmiddel. [Gamma-hydroxybutyrate, a new central nervous system stimulant.] Ugeskr Laeger 1999;161(50):6934–6.

Ganciclovir

General Information

Ganciclovir (dihydroxypropoxymethylguanine) is a nucleoside analogue with antiviral activity in vitro against herpesviruses. Intracellular phosphorylation of ganciclovir to its triphosphate derivative, which acts as a competitive inhibitor of deoxyguanosine triphosphate, leads to the inhibition of viral DNA synthesis. Because its toxicity profile is more favorable than those of foscarnet and cidofovir, it should be considered first-line treatment of life-threatening or sight-threatening cytomegalovirus (CMV) infections in immunocompromised patients. Ganciclovir is administered by infusion or by intravitreal injection (1). Oral ganciclovir as maintenance therapy for CMV retinitis in patients with AIDS has been reviewed (2). Oral ganciclovir has also been the subject of a pilot study in hepatitis B infection (3).

Observational studies

In 261 patients with CMV retinitis given oral ganciclovir 3–6 g/day or intravenous ganciclovir 5 mg/kg/day the most common adverse effects were on the gastrointestinal tract (nausea in 29–43%, vomiting in 17–23%, diarrhea in 33–52%, and flatulence in 2–18%) (4). There were rashes in 9–32%, a low neutrophil count (below 0.5×10^9/l) in 12–16%, a low hemoglobin concentration (below 8 g/dl) in 8–15%, a low platelet count (below 25×10^9/l) in 0–3%, and a raised serum creatinine in 17–27%.

General adverse effects

The proportion of patients in whom ganciclovir therapy is subsequently interrupted or withdrawn because of adverse effects is estimated at 32% (1).

Fever, rash, and abnormal liver function values are each reported to occur in about 2% of ganciclovir recipients (1). Other infrequently reported adverse effects, which may or may not be associated with ganciclovir, include chills, edema, malaise, vomiting, anorexia, diarrhea, dyspnea, reduced blood glucose, alopecia, impaired renal function, inflammation, pain, or phlebitis at the infusion site (1). These effects may also be due to the underlying illness in such patients.

Organs and Systems

Nervous system

Adverse effects of ganciclovir involving the central nervous system occur in about 5% of patients and include confusion, seizures, abnormal thinking, psychosis, hallucinations, nightmares, anxiety, tremor, dysesthesia, ataxia, coma, headache, and somnolence (1,5,6).

- A clear case of encephalopathy has been described in a patient who had received a bone marrow transplant; the problem resolved on withdrawal (7).

Sensory systems

Adverse effects reported in patients receiving intravitreal ganciclovir include foreign body sensation, conjunctival hemorrhage, mild conjunctival scarring, scleral induration, bacterial endophthalmitis, and retinal detachment (1).

For HIV-infected patients who have failed the intravenous CMV treatment options, intravitreal injections may be the last line. In one case only mild iris atrophy was noted, despite high-dose intravitreal ganciclovir (3 mg twice weekly) and high-dose intravitreal foscarnet (2.4 mg twice weekly) (8).

Endophthalmitis with scleral damage has been associated with a ganciclovir implant (9).

- A 39-year-old woman complained of increasing pain and complete loss of vision in the left eye 1 month after insertion of a ganciclovir implant. The eye was enucleated and pathological examination showed a vitreous abscess; the implant suture tab was intrasclerally located.

The authors concluded that intraocular infection had resulted from a foreign body (the surgical implant) in the scleral gap.

Metabolism

Six infants with cholestasis (aged 3–16 weeks) and signs of CMV infection were given intravenous ganciclovir for 3–7 weeks (10). One patient with septo-optic dysplasia and hypothyroidism had episodes of symptomatic hypoglycemia during treatment, which was withdrawn.

Hematologic

The adverse hematological effects of ganciclovir are generally rapidly reversible after withdrawal (1).

Pure red cell aplasia has been reported in one bone marrow transplant recipient (11) and hemolysis has been observed in two other patients (5).

Neutropenia is the most frequent adverse effect of ganciclovir. It usually occurs before a total dose of 200 mg/kg has been given. Other hematological adverse effects include thrombocytopenia, anemia, and lymphopenia. Since ganciclovir maintenance treatment is often necessary, concomitant use of G-CSF is often required in patients with AIDS with ganciclovir-associated neutropenia (12).

In a study of oral ganciclovir in 36 severely immunocompromised HIV-positive children with CMV disease, toxicity was minimal and manageable and similar to that in adults in controlled trials of the oral formulation (13). About 20% of the children withdrew, mainly as a result of intolerance of the large volume of oral suspension or numerous capsules. As in adults, neutropenia was the main toxic effect and it was successfully treated with G-CSF.

Of 40 patients who had achieved engraftment after allogeneic hemopoietic stem cell transplantation, 23 of whom had high-risk features, including transplant from an HLA-mismatched or unrelated donor, or associated acute graft-versus-host disease, 19 had pre-emptive therapy with ganciclovir in an initial dose of 5 mg/kg/day (4). There were no significant adverse effects attributed to ganciclovir, except low total leukocyte counts (below $0.5 \times 10^9/l$) in three patients, lasting 3, 4, and 14 days, while they were treated with granulocyte colony-stimulating factor.

Second-Generation Effects

Fertility

Animal data suggest that ganciclovir can inhibit spermatogenesis and fertility (14), but in one study there was no significant change in serum gonadotropin hormone concentrations in 32 men during ganciclovir therapy (15).

Drug Administration

Drug administration route

Treatment options for CMV retinitis include the intravitreal insertion of ganciclovir implants. This method of drug delivery has the attraction of avoiding systemic drug toxicity, but the inherent danger of introducing bacterial infection has been highlighted (16).

- A 42-year-old man with AIDS and a history of CMV retinitis developed pain in his right eye and reduced visual acuity 10 days after receiving a ganciclovir intraocular implant into that eye. A therapeutic vitrectomy was performed and a vitreal tap produced frank pus and white fluffy debris. Cultures grew oxacillin-resistant *Staphylococcus aureus* sensitive only to vancomycin, rifampicin, and co-trimoxazole. The ganciclovir implants were removed and he was given a 4-week course of vancomycin and rifampicin. The bacterial endophthalmitis left him blind in his right eye.

Drug–Drug Interactions

Trimethoprim

The interaction kinetics and safety profile of oral ganciclovir when co-administered with trimethoprim have been investigated in HIV- and CMV-seropositive patients (17). Trimethoprim significantly reduced the renal clearance of ganciclovir and prolonged its half-life, although the changes are unlikely to be clinically important. Ganciclovir did not alter trimethoprim pharmacokinetics, with the exception of a 13% increase in C_{min}. Ganciclovir was well tolerated when given alone or in this combination.

Zidovudine

Zidovudine and ganciclovir have overlapping toxicity profiles with respect to adverse hematological effects. Severe life-threatening hematological toxicity has been reported in 82% of patients treated with a combination of zidovudine and ganciclovir (18). The combination of ganciclovir with didanosine was much better tolerated (19).

Food–Drug Interactions

A well-controlled investigation using high doses of oral ganciclovir in HIV- and CMV-seropositive subjects has shown that food markedly increases the systemic availability of ganciclovir. For example, there is a doubling of blood concentrations and AUC if the drug is given within 30 minutes after a meal rather than on an empty stomach (20). Whatever dosage instructions are given, it seems clear that the relation to meal times should be explained, for example with a firm recommendation to take the drug consistently with food.

References

1. Faulds D, Heel RC. Ganciclovir. A review of its antiviral activity, pharmacokinetic properties and therapeutic efficacy in cytomegalovirus infections. Drugs 1990; 39(4):597–638.
2. Spector SA, McKinley GF, Lalezari JP, Samo T, Andruczk R, Follansbee S, Sparti PD, Havlir DV, Simpson G, Buhles W, Wong R, Stempien M. Oral ganciclovir for the prevention of cytomegalovirus disease in persons with AIDS. Roche Cooperative Oral Ganciclovir Study Group. N Engl J Med 1996;334(23):1491–7.
3. Hadziyannis SJ, Manesis EK, Papakonstantinou A. Oral ganciclovir treatment in chronic hepatitis B virus infection: a pilot study. J Hepatol 1999;31(2):210–14.
4. Kanda Y, Mineishi S, Saito T, Saito A, Ohnishi M, Niiya H, Chizuka A, Nakai K, Takeuchi T, Matsubara H, Makimoto A, Tanosaki R, Kunitoh H, Tobinai K, Takaue Y. Response-oriented preemptive therapy against cytomegalovirus disease with low-dose ganciclovir: a prospective evaluation. Transplantation 2002;73(4):568–72.
5. Thomson MH, Jeffries DJ. Ganciclovir therapy in iatrogenically immunosuppressed patients with cytomegalovirus disease. J Antimicrob Chemother 1989;23(Suppl E):61–70.
6. Collaborative DHPG Treatment Study Group. Treatment of serious cytomegalovirus infections with 9-(1,3-dihydroxy-2-propoxymethyl)guanine in patients with AIDS and other immunodeficiencies. N Engl J Med 1986;314(13):801–5.
7. Sharathkumar A, Shaw P. Ganciclovir-induced encephalopathy in a bone marrow transplant recipient. Bone Marrow Transplant 1999;24(4):421–3.
8. Velez G, Roy CE, Whitcup SM, Chan CC, Robinson MR. High-dose intravitreal ganciclovir and foscarnet for cytomegalovirus retinitis. Am J Ophthalmol 2001;131(3):396–7.
9. Charles NC, Freisberg L. Endophthalmitis associated with extrusion of a ganciclovir implant. Am J Ophthalmol 2002;133(2):273–5.
10. Fischler B, Casswall TH, Malmborg P, Nemeth A. Ganciclovir treatment in infants with cytomegalovirus infection and cholestasis. J Pediatr Gastroenterol Nutr 2002;34(2):154–7.
11. Emanuel D, Cunningham I, Jules-Elysee K, Brochstein JA, Kernan NA, Laver J, Stover D, White DA, Fels A, Polsky B, et al. Cytomegalovirus pneumonia after bone marrow transplantation successfully treated with the combination of ganciclovir and high-dose intravenous immune globulin. Ann Intern Med 1988;109(10):777–82.
12. Hermans P. Haematopoietic growth factors as supportive therapy in HIV-infected patients. AIDS 1995;9(Suppl 2):S9–14.
13. Frenkel LM, Capparelli EV, Dankner WM, Xu J, Smith IL, Ballow A, Culnane M, Read JS, Thompson M, Mohan KM, Shaver A, Robinson CA, Stempien MJ, Burchett SK,

Melvin AJ, Borkowsky W, Petru A, Kovacs A, Yogev R, Goldsmith J, McFarland EJ, Spector SA. Oral ganciclovir in children: pharmacokinetics, safety, tolerance, and antiviral effects. The Pediatric AIDS Clinical Trials Group. J Infect Dis 2000;182(6):1616–24.
14. Faqi AS, Klug A, Merker HJ, Chahoud I. Ganciclovir induces reproductive hazards in male rats after short-term exposure. Hum Exp Toxicol 1997;16(9):505–11.
15. Dieterich DT, Chachoua A, Lafleur F, Worrell C. Ganciclovir treatment of gastrointestinal infections caused by cytomegalovirus in patients with AIDS. Rev Infect Dis 1988;10(Suppl 3):S532–7.
16. Rombos Y, Tzanetea R, Konstantopoulos K, Simitzis S, Zervas C, Kyriaki P, Kavouklis M, Aessopos A, Sakellaropoulos N, Karagiorga M, Kalotychou V, Loukopoulos D. Chelation therapy in patients with thalassemia using the orally active iron chelator deferiprone (L1). Haematologica 2000;85(2):115–17.
17. Jung D, AbdelHameed MH, Hunter J, Teitelbaum P, Dorr A, Griffy K. The pharmacokinetics and safety profile of oral ganciclovir in combination with trimethoprim in HIV- and CMV-seropositive patients. Br J Clin Pharmacol 1999;47(3):255–9.
18. Hochster H, Dieterich D, Bozzette S, Reichman RC, Connor JD, Liebes L, Sonke RL, Spector SA, Valentine F, Pettinelli C, et al. Toxicity of combined ganciclovir and zidovudine for cytomegalovirus disease associated with AIDS. An AIDS Clinical Trials Group Study. Ann Intern Med 1990;113(2):111–17.
19. Jacobson MA, Owen W, Campbell J, Brosgart C, Abrams DI. Tolerability of combined ganciclovir and didanosine for the treatment of cytomegalovirus disease associated with AIDS. Clin Infect Dis 1993;16(Suppl 1):S69–73.
20. Jung D, Griffy K, Dorr A. Effect of food on high-dose oral ganciclovir disposition in HIV-positive subjects. J Clin Pharmacol 1999;39(2):161–5.

Garenoxacin

See also Fluoroquinolones

General Information

Garenoxacin is an orally and parenterally available 6-des-fluorinated quinolone, which has a high degree of in vitro activity against a broad range of bacterial pathogens (1).

Organs and Systems

Musculoskeletal

In dogs garenoxacin concentrations in plasma and joint tissue were higher than those of ciprofloxacin and norfloxacin (2). However, the articular toxicity of garenoxacin was much less than that of the other two quinolones.

References

1. Wise R, Gee T, Marshall G, Andrews JM. Single-dose pharmacokinetics and penetration of BMS 284756 into an inflammatory exudate. Antimicrob Agents Chemother 2002;46(1):242–4.
2. Nagai A, Miyazaki M, Morita T, Furubo S, Kizawa K, Fukumoto H, Sanzen T, Hayakawa H, Kawamura Y. Comparative articular toxicity of garenoxacin, a novel quinolone antimicrobial agent, in juvenile beagle dogs. J Toxicol Sci 2002;27(3):219–28.

Gatifloxacin

See also Fluoroquinolones

General Information

Gatifloxacin is an 8-methoxyfluoroquinolone with enhanced activity against Gram-positive, atypical agents, and some anerobes, and broad-spectrum activity against Gram-negative bacteria (1–4). It is bactericidal and produces a post-antibiotic effect in Gram-positive and Gram-negative bacteria. Gatifloxacin is well absorbed from the gastrointestinal tract (oral availability almost 100%), and concomitant administration of a continental breakfast, 1050 kcal, had no effect on its availability (5). The standard dose is 400 mg od and both oral and intravenous formulations are available (6,7).

Since gatifloxacin has a high oral systemic availability (96%), oral and intravenous formulations are bioequivalent and interchangeable (8). It has a large volume of distribution (about 1.8 l/kg), low protein binding (about 20%), broad tissue distribution, and is primarily excreted unchanged in the urine (over 80%) (7). After daily repeated administration, there was predictable modest accumulation; steady state concentrations were reached after the third dose (9).

The in vitro antibacterial spectrum of gatifloxacin has been tested against a variety of clinically important microorganisms (10). It is two to four times more potent than ciprofloxacin and ofloxacin against staphylococci, streptococci, pneumococci, and enterococci. However, it is two times less potent than ciprofloxacin, but the same as or two times more potent than ofloxacin against *Enterobacteriaceae*. Gatifloxacin and ofloxacin have similar antipseudomonal activity, while ciprofloxacin is two to eight times more potent. Gatifloxacin is highly potent against *Hemophilus influenzae*, *Legionella* species, and *Helicobacter pylori*, and also has activity against *Bacteroides fragilis* and *Clostridium difficile*. Like other quinolones, it has poor activity against *Mycobacterium avium* intracellulare, but is 8–16 times more potent against *Mycobacterium tuberculosis*.

Intravenous gatifloxacin can cause dose-related local reactions (8).

Gatifloxacin does not interact with drugs metabolized by the CYP450 enzyme family, as assessed in 14 healthy adult men using midazolam as a probe (11).

Organs and Systems

Cardiovascular

Although early studies suggested that gatifloxacin has little effect on the QT interval of the electrocardiogram (7,12), clinical trial data and data from phase IV studies have shown that it prolongs the QT interval (13). Four cases of gatifloxacin-associated cardiac toxicity have been reported in patients with known risk factors for this adverse event (14).

Nervous system

In patients taking gatifloxacin there have been reports of myoclonus and generalized seizures (15) and ataxia and generalized seizures (16).

Metabolism

Gatifloxacin was well tolerated in patients with non-insulin-dependent diabetes mellitus maintained with diet and exercise (17). It had no significant effect on glucose homeostasis, beta cell function, or long-term fasting serum glucose concentrations, but it caused a brief increase in serum insulin concentrations.

Gastrointestinal

Diarrhea and nausea were the most common adverse events in several clinical studies of gatifloxacin (4,18–20).

Liver

Gatifloxacin can cause hepatitis (21,22).

- A 44-year-old woman developed acute hepatitis while taking gatifloxacin for chronic sinusitis (23). After 5 days she developed nausea, lethargy, and abdominal pain, all of which progressed over the next few days. Liver function tests were abnormal, and the bilirubin peaked at 161 μmol/l. A percutaneous liver biopsy showed acute hepatitis with eosinophilic infiltrates, consistent with drug-induced hepatitis.

Susceptibility Factors

Age

Gatifloxacin can be administered without dose modification in the elderly (24).

Sex

Gatifloxacin can be administered without dose modification in women (24).

Hepatic disease

Gatifloxacin can be administered without dose modification in patients with hepatic impairment (25).

Drug–Drug Interactions

Oral hypoglycemic drugs

Four cases of severe persistent hypoglycemia due to gatifloxacin 400 mg/day have been reported in adults with diabetes mellitus who were taking oral hypoglycemic agents (repaglinide, glibenclamide, glimepiride) (26,27).

Oxycodone

Oral oxycodone and gatifloxacin can be co-administered without a significant reduction in systemic availability (28).

Warfarin

Enhanced hypoprothrombinemia has been reported when gatifloxacin was given with warfarin (29).

References

1. Fish DN, North DS. Gatifloxacin, an advanced 8-methoxy fluoroquinolone. Pharmacotherapy 2001;21(1):35–59.
2. Naber CK, Steghafner M, Kinzig-Schippers M, Sauber C, Sorgel F, Stahlberg HJ, Naber KG. Concentrations of gatifloxacin in plasma and urine and penetration into prostatic and seminal fluid, ejaculate, and sperm cells after single oral administrations of 400 milligrams to volunteers. Antimicrob Agents Chemother 2001;45(1):293–7.
3. Honeybourne D, Banerjee D, Andrews J, Wise R. Concentrations of gatifloxacin in plasma and pulmonary compartments following a single 400 mg oral dose in patients undergoing fibre-optic bronchoscopy. J Antimicrob Chemother 2001;48(1):63–6.
4. Perry CM, Ormrod D, Hurst M, Onrust SV. Gatifloxacin: a review of its use in the management of bacterial infections. Drugs 2002;62(1):169–207.
5. Mignot A, Guillaume M, Gohler K, Stahlberg HJ. Oral bioavailability of gatifloxacin in healthy volunteers under fasting and fed conditions. Chemotherapy 2002;48(3): 111–15.
6. Blondeau JM. Gatifloxacin: a new fluoroquinolone. Expert Opin Investig Drugs 2000;9(8):1877–95.
7. Grasela DM. Clinical pharmacology of gatifloxacin, a new fluoroquinolone. Clin Infect Dis 2000;31(Suppl 2):S51–8.
8. LaCreta FP, Kaul S, Kollia GD, Duncan G, Randall DM, Grasela DM. Interchangeability of 400-mg intravenous and oral gatifloxacin in healthy adults. Pharmacotherapy 2000;20(6 Pt 2):S59–66.
9. Gajjar DA, LaCreta FP, Uderman HD, Kollia GD, Duncan G, Birkhofer MJ, Grasela DM. A dose-escalation study of the safety, tolerability, and pharmacokinetics of intravenous gatifloxacin in healthy adult men. Pharmacotherapy 2000;20(6 Pt 2):S49–58.
10. Fung-Tomc J, Minassian B, Kolek B, Washo T, Huczko E, Bonner D. In vitro antibacterial spectrum of a new broad-spectrum 8-methoxy fluoroquinolone, gatifloxacin. J Antimicrob Chemother 2000;45(4):437–46.
11. Grasela DM, LaCreta FP, Kollia GD, Randall DM, Uderman HD. Open-label, nonrandomized study of the effects of gatifloxacin on the pharmacokinetics of midazolam in healthy male volunteers. Pharmacotherapy 2000;20(3):330–5.
12. Lannini PB, Circiumaru I. Gatifloxacin-induced QTc prolongation and ventricular tachycardia. Pharmacotherapy 2001;21(3):361–2.
13. Owens RC Jr, Ambrose PG. Torsades de pointes associated with fluoroquinolones. Pharmacotherapy 2002;22(5):663–8; discussion 668–72.
14. Bertino JS Jr, Owens RC. Jr., Carnes TD, Iannini PB. Gatifloxacin-associated corrected QT interval prolongation, torsades de pointes, and ventricular fibrillation in patients with known risk factors. Clin Infect Dis 2002;34(6):861–3.
15. Marinella MA. Myoclonus and generalized seizures associated with gatifloxacin treatment. Arch Intern Med 2001;161(18):2261–2.

16. Mohan N, Menon K, Rao PG. Oral gatifloxacin-induced ataxia. Am J Health Syst Pharm 2002;59(19):1894.
17. Gajjar DA, LaCreta FP, Kollia GD, Stolz RR, Berger S, Smith WB, Swingle M, Grasela DM. Effect of multiple-dose gatifloxacin or ciprofloxacin on glucose homeostasis and insulin production in patients with noninsulin-dependent diabetes mellitus maintained with diet and exercise. Pharmacotherapy 2000;20(6 Pt 2):S76–86.
18. Jones RN, Andes DR, Mandell LA, Gothelf S, Ehrhardt AF, Nicholson SC. Gatifloxacin used for therapy of outpatient community-acquired pneumonia caused by *Streptococcus pneumoniae*. Diagn Microbiol Infect Dis 2002;44(1):93–100.
19. Nicholson SC, Wilson WR, Naughton BJ, Gothelf S, Webb CD. Efficacy and safety of gatifloxacin in elderly outpatients with community-acquired pneumonia. Diagn Microbiol Infect Dis 2002;44(1):117–25.
20. Nicholson SC, High KP, Gothelf S, Webb CD. Gatifloxacin in community-based treatment of acute respiratory tract infections in the elderly. Diagn Microbiol Infect Dis 2002;44(1):109–16.
21. Gotfried M, Quinn TC, Gothelf S, Wikler MA, Webb CD, Nicholson SC. Oral gatifloxacin in outpatient community-acquired pneumonia: results from TeqCES, a community-based, open-label, multicenter study. Diagn Microbiol Infect Dis 2002;44(1):85–91.
22. Nicholson SC, Webb CD, Moellering RC Jr. Antimicrobial-associated acute hepatitis. Pharmacotherapy 2002;22(6):794–6; discussion 796–7.
23. Henann NE, Zambie MF. Gatifloxacin-associated acute hepatitis. Pharmacotherapy 2001;21(12):1579–82.
24. LaCreta FP, Kollia GD, Duncan G, Behr D, Grasela DM. Age and gender effects on the pharmacokinetics of gatifloxacin. Pharmacotherapy 2000;20(6 Pt 2):S67–75.
25. Grasela DM, Christofalo B, Kollia GD, Duncan G, Noveck R, Manning JA Jr, LaCreta FP. Safety and pharmacokinetics of a single oral dose of gatifloxacin in patients with moderate to severe hepatic impairment. Pharmacotherapy 2000;20(6 Pt 2):S87–94.
26. Baker SE, Hangii MC. Possible gatifloxacin-induced hypoglycemia. Ann Pharmacother 2002;36(11):1722–6.
27. Menzies DJ, Dorsainvil PA, Cunha BA, Johnson DH. Severe and persistent hypoglycemia due to gatifloxacin interaction with oral hypoglycemic agents. Am J Med 2002;113(3):232–4.
28. Grant EM, Nicolau DR, Nightingale C, Quintiliani R. Minimal interaction between gatifloxacin and oxycodone. J Clin Pharmacol 2002;42(8):928–32.
29. Artymowicz RJ, Cino BJ, Rossi JG, Walker JL, Moore S. Possible interaction between gatifloxacin and warfarin. Am J Health Syst Pharm 2002;59(12):1205–6.

Gemcitabine

See also Cytostatic and immunosuppressant drugs

General Information

Gemcitabine is an S-phase-specific pyrimidine nucleoside analogue of deoxycytidine (2′,2′-difluorodeoxycytidine) that is structurally similar to cytosine arabinoside. It has been used to treat metastatic urothelial carcinoma of the bladder, pancreatic cancer, and some other solid tumors.

General adverse effects

In a retrospective study of the adverse effects of gemcitabine 1000 mg/m^2 on days 1 and 8 in patients with non-small cell lung cancers, the adverse effects of gemcitabine involved the gastrointestinal system (nausea, vomiting, and diarrhea) and the hemopoietic system (leukopenia, neutropenia, thrombocytopenia, and anemia), but only in the last (8th–11th) cycles (1). There was grade 4 vomiting in three patients, grade 4 thrombocytopenia in two, and grade 3 leukopenia in three. Other adverse effects were mild. None of the patients died during chemotherapy.

Organs and Systems

Cardiovascular

In a retrospective chart review of patients with gemcitabine-associated thrombotic microangiopathy diagnosed between January 1997 and February 2002, the cumulative incidence was 0.31% (8 cases among 2586 patients), higher than previously reported (0.015%) (2). The median age was 53 years, the median time to development was 8 (range 3–18) months, and the cumulative dose was 9–56 g/m^2. New or exacerbated hypertension was a prominent feature in seven of nine patients and preceded the diagnosis by 0.5–10 weeks. Treatment included withdrawal of gemcitabine, antihypertensive therapy, plasma exchange, and dialysis. Six patients survived and three died of disease progression; none died as a direct result of thrombotic microangiopathy, but two developed renal insufficiency requiring dialysis, and one developed chronic renal insufficiency.

Gemcitabine can occasionally cause systemic capillary leak syndrome (3,4).

Respiratory

Gemcitabine can cause pulmonary toxicity. The clinical presentation is subacute and often non-specific. Chest X-ray usually shows reticulonodular interstitial infiltrates (5).

- A 75-year-old man with non-small cell lung cancer developed acute respiratory distress syndrome after intravenous gemcitabine monotherapy (6). The total dose of gemcitabine was 1500 mg, and the latent period was 3 days. Chest X-rays and a high resolution CT scan showed bilateral ground-glass opacity. He died on the fourteenth postchemotherapeutic day in respiratory failure. Postmortem examination of the lung showed mixed exudative and fibrotic stages of diffuse alveolar damage.

In one study, the incidence was as high as 15%, even with low-dose gemcitabine 600 mg/m^2 on days 1, 8, and 15 and docetaxel 60 mg/m^2 on day 1; all resolved after withdrawal of treatment and administration of glucocorticoids (7).

In a retrospective review pulmonary toxicity was defined as dyspnea, interstitial pneumonitis, lung disorder, lung edema, lung fibrosis, pneumonia, respiratory disorder, and respiratory distress syndrome (8). Based on 4448 patients, the incidences of dyspnea and other serious pulmonary toxicity were 0.45 and 0.27% respectively. Based on an estimated 217 400 patients treated with commercial gemcitabine worldwide, the crude incidences of dyspnea and other serious pulmonary toxicity were 0.02 and 0.06% respectively.

In a retrospective study of 312 patients treated with gemcitabine over 5 years, 18 developed episodes of acute dyspnea; 6 were attributed to the drug; 4 had a notifiable industrial disease secondary to asbestos exposure (OR = 85, 95% CI = 13, 546); and 5 were active smokers (5).

Liver

- Fatal cholestatic liver failure occurred in a 45-year-old woman with metastatic breast cancer who was given gemcitabine and carboplatin and pre-existing liver damage. After four courses of gemcitabine + carboplatin she developed severe decompensated cholestatic hepatitis (9). Liver biopsy showed marked cholestasis and hepatocellular injury consistent with drug-induced hepatotoxicity.

Urinary tract

Hemolytic–uremic syndrome has occasionally been attributed to gemcitabine (10–12). The manufacturers reviewed their database of 78 800 patient exposures, which confirmed that gemcitabine causes hemolytic–uremic syndrome with a crude overall incidence rate of 0.015% (13).

Skin

Erythema multiforme has been attributed to gemcitabine (14). Toxic epidermal necrolysis has been reported in an elderly man receiving gemcitabine for a transitional cell carcinoma of the bladder (15).

- Scleroderma-like changes of the legs occurred after treatment with gemcitabine in a patient with metastatic carcinoma of the bladder (16). There was initial inflammatory edema and subsequent scleroderma-like changes after 2 cycles of gemcitabine. Cutaneous biopsies showed diffuse sclerosis without involvement of the fascia or muscle. Withdrawal of gemcitabine resulted in resolution of the edema, softening of the skin, and partial reversibility of the fibrotic process.

Patients occasionally develop erysipeloid skin reactions, often, although not always, associated with previous radiotherapy or lymphedema (17).

A cutaneous reaction mimicking acute lipodermatosclerosis has been attributed to gemcitabine (18).

Immunologic

Two patients developed necrotizing enterocolitis after a first cycle of chemotherapy for epithelial ovarian/peritoneal cancer; both were due to vasculitis (19).

- In a 56-year-old man with a transitional cell carcinoma of the bladder gemcitabine plus cisplatin caused extensive necrotizing vasculitis with muscle damage after the second course of therapy (20). Chemotherapy was withdrawn immediately but the symptoms of severe myalgia and swelling persisted, and he needed additional treatment, consisting of cyclophosphamide and prednisolone.

Other cases of vasculitis have been reported (21).

- A 70-year-old woman with a bladder cancer was given gemcitabine 1700 mg on days 1 and 8 and 3–4 days later developed paresthesia of the fingers, Raynaud's phenomenon, an intermittent fever, digital necrosis, and fingertip gangrene (22). Angiography showed occlusion of the digital arteries of the second, third, and fourth fingers. Skin biopsy showed hyperkeratosis, acanthosis, and papillomatosis, with endothelioangiitis and non-specific arterial inflammation.

Radiation recall consists of inflammatory reactions triggered by cytotoxic drugs in previously irradiated areas; most are skin reactions. Gemcitabine has been implicated in several cases. The authors of a literature review discovered 12 cases of radiation recall caused by gemcitabine and reported a case of myositis in the rectus abdominis muscle of a patient with pancreatic adenocarcinoma as an effect of radiation recall (23). Most of the cases had inflammation of internal organs or tissues and 30% had dermatitis or mucositis. This is different from the effect of other agents that commonly cause radiation recall (anthracyclines and taxanes), with which 63% are skin reactions. Compared with anthracyclines and taxanes, the interval from the completion of radiation therapy to the start of chemotherapy is less with gemcitabine (median time 56 days, compared with 218 days for the taxanes and 646 days for doxorubicin).

References

1. Gallelli L, Nardi M, Prantera T, Barbera S, Raffaele M, Arminio D, Pirritano D, Colosimo M, Maselli R, Pelaia G, De Gregorio P, De Sarro GB. Retrospective analysis of adverse drug reactions induced by gemcitabine treatment in patients with non-small cell lung cancer. Pharmacol Res 2004;49(3):259–63.
2. Humphreys BD, Sharman JP, Henderson JM, Clark JW, Marks PW, Rennke HG, Zhu AX, Magee CC. Gemcitabine-associated thrombotic microangiopathy. Cancer 2004;100(12):2664–70.
3. De Pas T, Curigliano G, Franceschelli L, Catania C, Spaggiari L, de Braud F. Gemcitabine-induced systemic capillary leak syndrome. Ann Oncol 2001;12(11):1651–2.
4. Pulkkanen K, Kataja V, Johansson R. Systemic capillary leak syndrome resulting from gemcitabine treatment in renal cell carcinoma: a case report. J Chemother 2003; 15(3):287–9.
5. Barlesi F, Villani P, Doddoli C, Gimenez C, Kleisbauer JP. Gemcitabine-induced severe pulmonary toxicity. Fundam Clin Pharmacol 2004;18(1):85–91.
6. Maniwa K, Tanaka E, Inoue T, Kato T, Sakuramoto M, Minakuchi M, Maeda Y, Noma S, Kobashi Y, Taguchi Y. An autopsy case of acute pulmonary toxicity associated with gemcitabine. Intern Med 2003;42(10):1022–5.
7. Ryan DP, Kulke MH, Fuchs CS, Grossbard ML, Grossman SR, Morgan JA, Earle CC, Shivdasani R, Kim H, Mayer RJ, Clark JW. A Phase II study of gemcitabine and docetaxel in patients with metastatic pancreatic carcinoma. Cancer 2002;94(1):97–103.

8. Roychowdhury DF, Cassidy CA, Peterson P, Arning M. A report on serious pulmonary toxicity associated with gemcitabine-based therapy. Invest New Drugs 2002; 20(3):311–15.
9. Robinson K, Lambiase L, Li J, Monteiro C, Schiff M. Fatal cholestatic liver failure associated with gemcitabine therapy. Dig Dis Sci 2003;48(9):1804–8.
10. Dilhuydy MS, Delclaux C, Pariente A, De Precigout V, Aparicio M. Syndrome hémolytique et urémique compliquant un traitement au long cours par gemcitabine. A propos d'un cas, revue de la litterature. [Hemolytic–uremic syndrome complicating a long-term treatment with gemcitabine. Report of a case and review of the literature.] Rev Med Interne 2002;23(2):189–92.
11. Citarrella P, Gebbia V, Teresi M, Miceli S, Sciortino G, Vaglica M, Pizzardi N, Palmeri S. Hemolytic uremic syndrome after chemotherapy with gemcitabine and taxotere: a case report. Anticancer Res 2002;22(2B):1183–5.
12. Serke S, Riess H, Oettle H, Huhn D. Elevated reticulocyte count—a clue to the diagnosis of haemolytic–uraemic syndrome (HUS) associated with gemcitabine therapy for metastatic duodenal papillary carcinoma: a case report. Br J Cancer 1999;79(9–10):1519–21.
13. Fung MC, Storniolo AM, Nguyen B, Arning M, Brookfield W, Vigil J. A review of hemolytic uremic syndrome in patients treated with gemcitabine therapy. Cancer 1999;85(9):2023–32.
14. Sommers KR, Kong KM, Bui DT, Fruehauf JP, Holcombe RF. Stevens–Johnson syndrome/toxic epidermal necrolysis in a patient receiving concurrent radiation and gemcitabine. Anticancer Drugs 2003;14(8):659–62.
15. Mermershtain W, Cohen AD, Lazarev I, Grunwald M, Ariad S. Toxic epidermal necrolysis associated with gemcitabine therapy in a patient with metastatic transitional cell carcinoma of the bladder. J Chemother 2003; 15(5):510–11.
16. Bessis D, Guillot B, Legouffe E, Guilhou JJ. Gemcitabine-associated scleroderma-like changes of the lower extremities. J Am Acad Dermatol 2004;51(Suppl 2):S73–6.
17. Kuku I, Kaya E, Sevinc A, Aydogdu I. Gemcitabine-induced erysipeloid skin lesions in a patient with malignant mesothelioma. J Eur Acad Dermatol Venereol 2002;16(3):271–2.
18. Chu CY, Yang CH, Chiu HC. Gemcitabine-induced acute lipodermatosclerosis-like reaction. Acta Dermatol Venereol 2001;81(6):426–8.
19. Geisler JP, Schraith DF, Manahan KJ, Sorosky JI. Gemcitabine associated vasculitis leading to necrotizing enterocolitis and death in women undergoing primary treatment for epithelial ovarian/peritoneal cancer. Gynecol Oncol 2004;92(2):705–7.
20. Birlik M, Akar S, Tuzel E, Onen F, Ozer E, Manisali M, Kirkali Z, Akkoc N. Gemcitabine-induced vasculitis in advanced transitional cell carcinoma of the bladder. J Cancer Res Clin Oncol 2004;130(2):122–5.
21. Voorburg AM, van Beek FT, Slee PH, Seldenrijk CA, Schramel FM. Vasculitis due to gemcitabine. Lung Cancer 2002;36(2):203–5.
22. D'Alessandro V, Errico M, Varriale A, Greco A, De Cata A, Carnevale V, Grilli M, De Luca P, Brucoli I, Susi M, Camagna A. Acronecrosi degli arti superiori da gemcitabina: segnalazione di un caso clinico. [Case report: Acro-necrosis of the upper limbs caused by gemcitabine therapy.] Clin Ter 2003;154(3):207–10.
23. Friedlander PA, Bansal R, Schwartz L, Wagman R, Posner J, Kemeny N. Gemcitabine-related radiation recall preferentially involves internal tissue and organs. Cancer 2004;100(9):1793–9.

Gemeprost

See also Prostaglandins

General Information

Gemeprost is an analogue of PGE_2. Vaginal gemeprost is effective in inducing first and second trimester abortion and in cervical priming before vacuum aspiration. Pyrexia, vomiting, and diarrhea were experienced in 20% of patients (1).

In a double-blind, randomized, controlled trial, 896 healthy women requesting a medical abortion (57–63 days gestation, mean age 25 years) were randomized to a single oral dose of mifepristone 200 or 600 mg, both followed in 48 hours by gemeprost 1 mg vaginally (2). The complete abortion rates were similar with the lower and higher doses of mifepristone (92 versus 92%). The incidences of adverse effects were similar, with the exception of nausea at 1 week, which was less frequent in the low-dose group (3.6 versus 7.6%).

Organs and Systems

Cardiovascular

Two women developed myocardial ischemia during treatment with gemeprost for termination of pregnancy (3).

- A 29-year-old woman, a smoker with a history of renal insufficiency, obesity, hypertension, hypercholesterolemia, and cardiac dysrhythmias, underwent termination of pregnancy at 10 weeks with a pessary of gemeprost 1 mg and 5 hours later dilatation and evacuation, followed by tubal ligation. After surgery, her blood pressure became unmeasurable, her heart rate dropped to 40/minute, and she developed ventricular fibrillation. She was given streptokinase and intravenous heparin for suspected pulmonary embolism; her blood pressure rose and was maintained with adrenaline and noradrenaline. Angiography showed an 80% stenosis of her right coronary artery and complete occlusion of the anterior interventricular branch. Blood flow was re-established by coronary angioplasty.
- A 32-year-old woman, a smoker, had an evacuation after the death of her fetus at 18 weeks. Two pessaries of gemeprost 1 mg were inserted 7.25 hours apart, and about 90 minutes later she became unconscious, apneic, and cyanotic, and had dilated pupils and no detectable blood pressure or pulse. She was given 100% oxygen, intravenous adrenaline and dobutamine, and a crystalloid infusion. Her systolic pressure rose to 100 mmHg. Coronary angiography showed left and circumflex coronary artery spasm.

The author commented that the myocardial ischemia experienced by both of these patients was thought to be due to prostaglandin-induced coronary spasm. It would be prudent to monitor every woman treated with gemeprost during the course of an abortion.

Skin

Toxic epidermal necrolysis has been attributed to mifepristone/gemeprost (4).

References

1. Thong KJ, Robertson AJ, Baird DT. A retrospective study of 932 second trimester terminations using gemeprost (16,16 dimethyl-trans delta 2 PGE1 methyl ester). Prostaglandins 1992;44(1):65–74.
2. Weston BC. Migraine headache associated with latanoprost. Arch Ophthalmol 2001;119(2):300–1.
3. Schulte-Sasse U. Life threatening myocardial ischaemia associated with the use of prostaglandin E1 to induce abortion. BJOG 2000;107(5):700–2.
4. Lecorvaisier-Pieto C, Joly P, Thomine E, Tanasescu S, Noblet C, Lauret P. Toxic epidermal necrolysis after mifepristone/gemeprost-induced abortion. J Am Acad Dermatol 1996;35(1):112.

Gemifloxacin

See also Fluoroquinolones

General Information

Gemifloxacin is a fluoroquinolone that has enhanced affinity for topoisomerase. Compared with other fluoroquinolones, gemifloxacin was the most potent against penicillin-intermediate and penicillin-resistant pneumococci, methicillin-susceptible and methicillin-resistant *Staphylococcus epidermidis* isolates, and coagulase-negative staphylococci (1,2). It has excellent activity against *Haemophilus influenzae* and *Moraxella catarrhalis* and is unaffected by beta-lactamases. It is generally two-fold less active than ciprofloxacin against most *Enterobacteriaceae* (3). Atypical respiratory pathogens (*Legionella*, *Mycoplasma*, and *Chlamydia* species) and *Neisseria gonorrheae* are highly susceptible (4).

The pharmacokinetics of oral gemifloxacin have been characterized in healthy male volunteers (5). About 20–30% of the dose was excreted unchanged in the urine. The renal clearance was 160 ml/minute on average after single and multiple doses, which was slightly greater than the accepted glomerular filtration rate. There were no adverse effects.

Observational studies

In phase II trials oral gemifloxacin 320 mg/day produced bacteriological responses in 94% of patients with acute exacerbations of chronic bronchitis (6–8) and in 95% of patients with uncomplicated urinary tract infections. Adverse events included nausea, abdominal pain, headache, and a mild rash in both patients and healthy volunteers.

After a single dose of 20–800 mg of gemifloxacin, there were no significant changes in clinical chemistry, hematology, or urinalysis, vital signs, or 12-lead electrocardiograms in healthy men, irrespective of dose (9).

Gemifloxacin 320 mg od and trovafloxacin 200 mg od have been compared in 571 patients with community-acquired pneumonia in a multicenter, double-blind, parallel-group, randomized study (10). Gemifloxacin was slightly more effective (88%) than trovafloxacin (81%). Gemifloxacin was well tolerated and the incidence of transient liver function abnormalities was very low.

The effect of oral gemifloxacin 320 mg for 7 days on the human intestinal microflora has been investigated in 10 healthy subjects (11). The numbers of enterobacteria, enterococci, and streptococci were reduced. No other aerobic microorganisms were affected. The numbers of anerobic cocci and lactobacilli were reduced. The microflora normalized 49 days after withdrawal. There was no selection or overgrowth of resistant bacterial strains or yeasts.

Organs and Systems

Hematologic

Gemifloxacin reached intracellular concentrations in human polymorphonuclear leukocytes eight times higher than extracellular concentrations. Uptake was rapid, reversible, and non-saturable and was affected by environmental temperature, cell viability, and membrane stimuli (12).

Gastrointestinal

In a randomized, double-blind, multicenter comparison of a 5-day course of gemifloxacin 320 mg/day with a standard 7-day regimen of clarithromycin 500 mg bd in 712 patients with acute exacerbations of chronic bronchitis, the most frequently reported gemifloxacin-related adverse events were diarrhea (5.1%) and nausea (4.3%) (13).

Liver

Gemifloxacin was generally well tolerated in a pharmacokinetic study, although one subject was withdrawn after 6 days at 640 mg because of mild, transient rises in alanine transaminase and aspartate transaminase not associated with signs or symptoms (5).

Skin

Gemifloxacin has a low potential for mild phototoxicity (14).

Drug–Drug Interactions

Iron

In an open, randomized, single-dose, five-way crossover study of the effects of ferrous sulfate on the systemic availability of gemifloxacin, there were no changes when gemifloxacin was given at least 2 hours before or at least 3 hours after ferrous sulfate (9).

Sucralfate

In an open, randomized, single-dose, five-way crossover study of the effects of sucralfate on the systemic availability of gemifloxacin, there were no changes when gemifloxacin was given at least 2 hours before sucralfate (9).

Food–Drug Interactions

Food had a minor and clinically insignificant effect on the systemic availability of gemifloxacin (320 and 640 mg) (15).

References

1. Hardy D, Amsterdam D, Mandell LA, Rotstein C. Comparative in vitro activities of ciprofloxacin, gemifloxacin, grepafloxacin, moxifloxacin, ofloxacin, sparfloxacin, trovafloxacin, and other antimicrobial agents against bloodstream isolates of gram-positive cocci. Antimicrob Agents Chemother 2000;44(3):802–5.
2. Jones RN, Pfaller MA, Erwin ME. Evaluation of gemifloxacin (SB-265805, LB20304a): in vitro activity against over 6000 gram-positive pathogens from diverse geographic areas. Int J Antimicrob Agents 2000;15(3):227–30.
3. Marchese A, Debbia EA, Schito GC. Comparative in vitro potency of gemifloxacin against European respiratory tract pathogens isolated in the Alexander Project. J Antimicrob Chemother 2000;46(Suppl T1):11–15.
4. Berron S, Vazquez JA, Gimenez MJ, de la Fuente L, Aguilar L. In vitro susceptibilities of 400 Spanish isolates of *Neisseria gonorrhoeae* to gemifloxacin and 11 other antimicrobial agents. Antimicrob Agents Chemother 2000;44(9):2543–4.
5. Allen A, Bygate E, Vousden M, Oliver S, Johnson M, Ward C, Cheon A, Choo YS, Kim I. Multiple-dose pharmacokinetics and tolerability of gemifloxacin administered orally to healthy volunteers. Antimicrob Agents Chemother 2001;45(2):540–5.
6. File T, Schlemmer B, Garau J, Lode H, Lynch S, Young C. Gemifloxacin versus amoxicillin/clavulanate in the treatment of acute exacerbations of chronic bronchitis. The 070 Clinical Study group. J Chemother 2000;12(4):314–25.
7. Hong CY. Discovery of gemifloxacin (Factive, LB20304a): a quinolone of a new generation. Farmaco 2001;56(1–2):41–4.
8. Ball P, File TM, Twynholm M, Henkel T. Efficacy and safety of gemifloxacin 320 mg once-daily for 7 days in the treatment of adult lower respiratory tract infections. Int J Antimicrob Agents 2001;18(1):19–27.
9. Allen A, Bygate E, Oliver S, Johnson M, Ward C, Cheon AJ, Choo YS, Kim IC. Pharmacokinetics and tolerability of gemifloxacin (SB-265805) after administration of single oral doses to healthy volunteers. Antimicrob Agents Chemother 2000;44(6):1604–8.
10. Naber CK, Hammer M, Kinzig-Schippers M, Sauber C, Sorgel F, Bygate EA, Fairless AJ, Machka K, Naber KG. Urinary excretion and bactericidal activities of gemifloxacin and ofloxacin after a single oral dose in healthy volunteers. Antimicrob Agents Chemother 2001; 45(12):3524–30.
11. File TM Jr, Schlemmer B, Garau J, Cupo M, Young C; 049 Clinical Study Group. Efficacy and safety of gemifloxacin in the treatment of community-acquired pneumonia: a randomized, double-blind comparison with trovafloxacin. J Antimicrob Chemother 2001;48(1):67–74.
12. Garcia I, Pascual A, Ballesta S, Joyanes P, Perea EJ. Intracellular penetration and activity of gemifloxacin in human polymorphonuclear leukocytes. Antimicrob Agents Chemother 2000;44(11):3193–5.
13. Wilson R, Schentag JJ, Ball P, Mandell L; 068 Study Group. A comparison of gemifloxacin and clarithromycin in acute exacerbations of chronic bronchitis and long-term clinical outcomes. Clin Ther 2002;24(4):639–52.
14. Lowe MN, Lamb HM. Gemifloxacin. Drugs 2000; 59(5):1137–47.
15. Allen A, Bygate E, Clark D, Lewis A, Pay V. The effect of food on the bioavailability of oral gemifloxacin in healthy volunteers. Int J Antimicrob Agents 2000; 16(1):45–50.

Gemtuzumab ozogamicin

See also Monoclonal antibodies

General Information

Gemtuzumab ozogamicin (Mylotarg) consists of a humanized anti-CD33 monoclonal antibody conjugated to the cytotoxic enediyne antibiotic calicheamicin. It has been used to treat a subset of patients with acute myeloid leukemia in association with topotecan + cytarabine. Its most common adverse effects are myelosuppression, increased hepatic enzyme activity, infections, fever and chills, bleeding, nausea and vomiting, and dyspnea.

Infusion-related adverse effects of gemtuzumab ozogamicin can be treated with a brief course of an intravenous glucocorticoid. Of 143 patients with refractory myeloid leukemia treated with gemtuzumab ozogamicin, 110 received paracetamol 650 mg orally with diphenhydramine 50 mg intravenously and 33 received the same premeditations plus methylprednisolone sodium succinate 50 mg intravenously before the infusion and repeated 1 hour later (1). There were grade 2 or worse infusion-related adverse events in 32 (29%) of the former, but in only one of the latter (3%).

Organs and Systems

Liver

Hepatotoxicity, with raised bilirubin and liver enzymes, is common with gemtuzumab (30–50%) and is mostly reversible. A more severe complication, hepatic veno-occlusive disease, a syndrome consisting of hyperbilirubinemia, painful hepatomegaly, and fluid retention or ascites, is less common and is mostly seen in patients previously undergoing bone marrow transplantation (4–5%). It occurs most commonly after high-dose chemotherapy and hemopoietic stem cell transplantation. Patients with severe veno-occlusive disease die from progressive multiorgan failure. Close monitoring of patients receiving gemtuzumab is necessary, even if they have not had previous bone marrow transplantation (2).

In 119 patients (92 with acute myeloid leukemia, 25 with advanced myelodysplastic syndrome, and two with chronic myeloid leukemia), who did not receive concomitant stem cell transplantation, 14 developed veno-occlusive disease (3). Five of these 14 patients had not received prior antileukemic therapy, and in two cases gemtuzumab ozogamicin was used as single-agent chemotherapy.

Of eight patients who were given an infusion of gemtuzumab 9 months after hemopoietic stem cell transplantation, seven had normal serum bilirubin concentrations, and all eight had transaminase and alkaline phosphatase activities that were less than 1.5 times the upper limit of the reference range (4). Six had no evidence of hepatotoxicity. One developed abdominal pain, ascites, and mildly raised transaminases. A CT scan showed no evidence of hepatic disease. This patient did not meet the criteria of veno-occlusive disease. Patient 8 did meet the criteria of veno-occlusive disease 3 days after infusion with gemtuzumab. She developed multi-organ failure and died.

Of 17 patients who were given gemtuzumab, three developed grade 3 hyperbilirubinemia, and five developed grade 3–4 hepatic transaminitis after a median of 13 days, including one who developed veno-occlusive disease (4). This patient had abrupt onset of weight gain, associated with ascites, abdominal distension, acute hepatic failure, and right upper quadrant pain, and died. As a possible mechanism gemtuzumab may selectively target CD33-expressing cells in hepatic sinusoids, activate stellated cells, damage sinusoidal endothelial cells, and cause sinusoidal vasoconstriction or ischemic hepatocyte necrosis. Liver histology showed sinusoidal injury with extensive sinusoidal fibrosis, centrilobular congestion, and hepatocyte necrosis (5).

Immunologic

There has been one report of an anaphylactic reaction in a patient receiving gemtuzumab (6).

References

1. Giles FJ, Cortes JE, Halliburton TA, Mallard SJ, Estey EH, Waddelow TA, Lim JT. Intravenous corticosteroids to reduce gemtuzumab ozogamicin infusion reactions. Ann Pharmacother 2003;37(9):1182–5.
2. Voutsadakis IA. Gemtuzumab Ozogamicin (CMA-676, Mylotarg) for the treatment of CD33+ acute myeloid leukemia. Anticancer Drugs 2002;13(7):685–92.
3. Giles FJ, Kantarjian HM, Kornblau SM, Thomas DA, Garcia-Manero G, Waddelow TA, David CL, Phan AT, Colburn DE, Rashid A, Estey EH. Mylotarg (gemtuzumab ozogamicin) therapy is associated with hepatic venoocclusive disease in patients who have not received stem cell transplantation. Cancer 2001;92(2):406–13.
4. Cohen AD, Luger SM, Sickles C, Mangan PA, Porter DL, Schuster SJ, Tsai DE, Nasta S, Gewirtz AM, Stadtmauer EA. Gemtuzumab ozogamicin (Mylotarg) monotherapy for relapsed AML after hematopoietic stem cell transplant: efficacy and incidence of hepatic veno-occlusive disease. Bone Marrow Transplant 2002;30(1):23–8.
5. Rajvanshi P, Shulman HM, Sievers EL, McDonald GB. Hepatic sinusoidal obstruction after gemtuzumab ozogamicin (Mylotarg) therapy. Blood 2002;99(7):2310–14.
6. Reinhardt D, Diekamp S, Fleischhack G, Corbacioglu C, Jurgens H, Dworzak M, Kaspers G, Creutzig U, Zwaan CM. Gemtuzumab ozogamicin (Mylotarg) in children with refractory or relapsed acute myeloid leukemia. Onkologie 2004;27(3):269–72.

Genaconazole

See also Antifungal azoles

General Information

Genaconazole is an *N*-substituted triazole with a wide antifungal spectrum. Its absorption is slow, with peak concentrations 2–4 hours after a single dose and mean peak concentrations markedly higher after 16 days of administration. The mean elimination half-life is about 90–100 hours (1). It has high tissue penetration, including the CNS, and good broad-spectrum antifungal activity. However, it causes hepatocellular carcinoma in animals and the manufacturers stopped developing it because of concerns about toxicity.

Reference

1. Lin C, Kim H, Radwanski E, Affrime M, Brannan M, Cayen MN. Pharmacokinetics and metabolism of genaconazole, a potent antifungal drug, in men. Antimicrob Agents Chemother 1996;40(1):92–6.

General anesthetics

See also Individual agents

General Information

The inhalational and injectable agents that are covered in separate monographs are listed in the table below.

Inhalational	Injectable
Halogenated	*Barbiturates*
Chloroform	Methohexital
Desflurane	Thiamylal
Enflurane	Thiopental
Halothane	*Others*
Isoflurane	Alfadolone/alfaxolone
Methoxyflurane	Etomidate
Sevoflurane	Ketamine
Trichloroethylene	Propanidid
Others	Propofol
Anesthetic ether	
Cyclopropane	
Nitrous oxide	
Xenon	

The inhalational agents in common use share similar adverse effects, albeit with differing incidences. Initial hopes that new agents will be less problematic generally fade as their use increases and familiarity with their adverse effects grows. Although some untoward reactions related to inhalational anesthetics are unpredictable, it is important for the anesthetist/anesthesiologist to determine which patients are primarily at risk, so that safer use of anesthetic agents and better supervision of surgical patients can be achieved.

Anesthetic combinations

The importance of multiple anesthetics should not be overlooked. For example, patients in whom halothane anesthesia is given twice, at an interval of less than 6 weeks, are at major risk of developing jaundice. Some anesthetists avoid any second exposure to this agent. However, there are several reasons why single agents are often insufficient in anesthesia: different problems require separate treatments; the severity of the adverse effects of individual drugs can sometimes be reduced by the use of combinations; and repeated administration of a single agent can lead to cumulative effects. Drug interactions in anesthesia are therefore potentially common and have been reviewed, both systematically (1) and as uncritical listings (2,3). Many of the interactions are beneficial, the concurrent use of two or more different agents improving the quality of anesthesia. Several reviews of this have appeared (4–6). Disadvantages of combinations include unpredictability of synergistic actions or toxicity, mutual alterations in pharmacokinetics, increased likelihood of errors in drug administration, and difficulties in planning drug therapy when adverse effects occur and are not attributable to a particular drug.

Dental anesthesia

Adverse effects of dental anesthesia represent a special problem, about which reliable data are hard to obtain. Several studies of the safety of dental anesthesia have been performed in the USA (SEDA-18, 113); unfortunately, all have weaknesses. More informative is an American survey in which 47 oral and maxillofacial surgeons were approached directly, and all responded (7). Among the 74 871 patients to whom they had given general anesthesia, there were 250 cases of laryngospasm, 51 of phlebitis, 30 of dysrhythmias sufficiently severe to require therapy, 17 of hypotension requiring drug therapy, and 13 of bronchospasm. A few patients had allergic reactions requiring drug therapy ($n = 4$), convulsions ($n = 4$), hypertension ($n = 2$), myocardial infarction ($n = 2$), or vomiting with aspiration ($n = 2$); in one case an injection was inadvertently given into an artery.

Sedation for endoscopy

Gastrointestinal endoscopy is one of the most commonly performed invasive procedures in clinical practice (for example about 500 000 procedures per annum in Australasia). Propofol is a short-acting intravenous anesthetic with a rapid onset of action and a short half-life, making it eminently suitable for day procedures. However, the use of propofol by non-anesthetists has been controversial because of the perceived risks of its low therapeutic ratio.

The incidence of adverse events related to an endoscopy sedation regimen that included propofol (in addition to midazolam and fentanyl), delivered by specially trained general practitioners, has been examined in a prospective audit (8); 28 472 procedures were performed over 5 years. There were 185 sedation-related adverse events, 107 with airway or ventilation problems; 123 interventions were necessary to maintain ventilation. No patients required tracheal intubation and there were no deaths. The authors concluded that appropriately trained general practitioners encountered a low incidence of adverse events and could safely use propofol for sedation during endoscopy. It should be noted that all the general practitioners had some experience in anesthesia or intensive care and were individually trained by the Director of Anesthesia.

Sedation for surgery under regional anesthesia

Sedation during prolonged surgical procedures under regional anesthesia can be quite challenging. The $beta_2$ adrenoceptor agonist dexmedetomidine has potent sedative and analgesic-sparing properties. In therapeutic doses it does not cause respiratory depression, making it attractive for infusion sedation. However, it causes reduced sympathetic outflow, which might cause untoward hemodynamic upset during intraoperative sedation. Dexmedetomidine has been compared with propofol in a prospective randomized trial in 40 patients (9). Dexmedetomidine provided slightly slower onset and offset of sedation, higher intraoperative blood pressure, and better postoperative analgesia.

Remifentanil is a highly selective OP_3 (μ) opioid receptor agonist with an extremely short onset and offset of action, allowing rapid and accurate titration of infusion rate to drug effect with rapid down-titration in case of respiratory adverse effects. This makes it attractive for sedation. The efficacy and adverse effects profiles of remifentanil and propofol have been compared in a randomized, single-blind trial in 125 patients undergoing surgery with regional anesthesia (10). In those given remifentanil, nausea and vomiting were more frequent (27 versus 2%) and there was significantly more respiratory depression (46 versus 19%).

Sedation in intensive care

It has been proposed that a combination of propofol and midazolam may have advantages over either drug alone, reducing adverse effects while preserving the potential benefits ("co-sedation"). Propofol combined with a constant low dose of midazolam (1.0 mg/hour) has been compared with propofol alone for postoperative sedation in a randomized, placebo-controlled, double-blind trial in 60 patients undergoing coronary artery surgery under high-dose fentanyl anesthesia (11). Target sedation was achieved more readily with co-sedation (91 versus 79%) but at the expense of prolonged weaning from mechanical ventilation (432 versus 319 minutes). However, it is not clear whether this slightly prolonged time on the ventilator affected length of stay in the ICU.

It remains a source of much concern that those working in operating theaters spend their time in such a polluted environment, in spite of attempts to introduce scavenging of waste anesthetic gases (12). This is not without its effects. There is, for example, a relation between asthma and occupational exposure to various respiratory hazards, including anesthetic gases (13).

Comparative studies

Halothane versus propofol

A randomized prospective trial in 60 children undergoing outpatient anesthesia showed a 30% shorter time from discontinuation of anesthesia to eye opening and return to full wakefulness in patients receiving propofol alone compared with halothane + nitrous oxide anesthesia (14). Propofol was associated with a 17% incidence of emesis compared with 58 and 53% for halothane + nitrous oxide and propofol + nitrous oxide anesthesia respectively.

Isoflurane + nitrous oxide versus propofol

The risk of postoperative nausea and vomiting has been studied in a randomized, controlled trial of total intravenous anesthesia with propofol versus inhalational anesthesia with isoflurane and nitrous oxide in 2010 patients (15). It was accompanied by an economic analysis. Propofol total intravenous anesthesia reduced the absolute risk of postoperative nausea and vomiting up to 72 hours postoperatively from 61 to 46%, in inpatients (NNT = 6) and from 46 to 28% in outpatients (NNT = 5). Both anesthetic techniques were otherwise similar. Anesthesia drug costs were more than three times higher for propofol total intravenous anesthesia (as propofol is substantially more expensive than isoflurane + nitrous oxide). However, the patients preferred propofol.

Isoflurane versus sevoflurane

A study of single vital-capacity breath inhalational induction using either isoflurane or sevoflurane combined with 67% nitrous oxide in 67 adults showed that isoflurane was unsuitable for this technique (16). There was an 87% incidence of induction complications with isoflurane, including involuntary movements, cough, laryngospasm, and failure of induction.

In 75 patients of ASA grades 1 or 2, recovery from anesthesia after maintenance with isoflurane + nitrous oxide was significantly slower than with sevoflurane + nitrous oxide (17).

Isoflurane and sevoflurane have been compared in a randomized study in 180 patients undergoing knee arthroscopy (18). In those given sevoflurane there were significantly more respiratory and cardiovascular complications and increased nausea and vomiting.

In a comparison of sevoflurane and isoflurane anesthesia in 2008 patients there was a 3–4 minute reduction in time to recovery end-points with sevoflurane (19). These differences became larger in anesthetics lasting over 3 hours and were trivial in cases less than 1 hour. Patients aged over 65 years had a 5-minute increase in recovery times after receiving isoflurane. There was no significant difference in the incidence of nausea or vomiting between isoflurane, sevoflurane, and propofol.

Propofol versus sevoflurane

Sevoflurane is pleasant to breathe and has a rapid onset and offset of action. It is challenging the tradition of intravenous anesthetic induction in adult patients. In a meta-analysis of 12 studies in 1102 adult patients, intravenous bolus doses of sevoflurane 7–8% and propofol for anesthetic induction were compared (20). Anesthesia maintenance included nitrous oxide 50–70% and either propofol infusion or sevoflurane inhalation, and spontaneous ventilation via a laryngeal mask. Patients in the sevoflurane group were significantly more likely to have postoperative nausea and vomiting (odds ratios 4.2 and 3.2). There were non-significant trends toward greater patient dissatisfaction and a longer induction time in the sevoflurane group, and more frequent apnea in the propofol group. There were no significant complications in either group. Both agents are suitable for anesthetic induction, but propofol retains a small advantage in having better recovery characteristics.

Single-agent induction and maintenance of anesthesia has been compared in a randomized study of 44 patients undergoing elective spinal surgery (21). Patients received either propofol 4–6 μg/ml via a target-controlled infusion or sevoflurane 8% for induction, and sevoflurane 3.5% + 67% nitrous oxide for maintenance plus alfentanil as required. Patients in the propofol group required a significantly larger dose of opiate during the procedure (2.2 mg versus 0.3 mg). Two patients who received propofol complained of pain on injection. There was no significant breath-holding or laryngospasm in either group. Heart rate was significantly lower in the sevoflurane group compared with propofol both before and after incision. The numbers of adjustments to the patient's depth of anesthesia were similar in both groups. The authors concluded that either technique was suitable for spinal surgery. The inclusion of nitrous oxide in the sevoflurane group accounted for the differences in opioid requirements.

The effects of hypercapnia on cerebral autoregulation during sevoflurane or propofol anesthesia have been studied in a randomized, crossover study in eight healthy patients (22). Hypercapnia began to inhibit cerebral autoregulation, as measured by transcranial Doppler at a mean value of 56 mmHg P_aCO_2 with sevoflurane 1.0–1.1% and at 61 mmHg P_aCO_2 with propofol 140 μg/kg/minute. Patients also received remifentanil for analgesia, a drug with no known effects on cerebral autoregulation. The study is important, because one advantage of both propofol anesthesia and sevoflurane anesthesia is the lack of inhibition of cerebral autoregulation at standard doses. Clearly, careful control of ventilation is required for this to be true.

The effects of isoflurane, sevoflurane, and propofol on jugular venous oxygen saturation (S_jO_2) in patients undergoing coronary artery bypass surgery have been studied (23). S_jO_2 values were significantly lower in the propofol group 1 hour after bypass, suggesting an imbalance of oxygen supply and demand with propofol. Because anesthetic agents also reduce the cerebral metabolic rate, the implications of this finding are uncertain. However, low S_jO_2 values have previously been associated with postoperative neuropsychiatric dysfunction after cardiopulmonary bypass.

Vital capacity inhalational induction of anesthesia with sevoflurane has been compared with intravenous induction using propofol in 56 adults undergoing ambulatory anesthesia (24). The patients were randomized to either sevoflurane 8% + nitrous oxide 75% mixture at 8 l/minute ($n = 32$), or propofol 2 mg/kg bolus ($n = 24$), without any premedication. Induction time was significantly shorter with sevoflurane (average 51 seconds) than propofol (average 81 seconds). Adverse effects were different in the two groups: sevoflurane caused cough and hiccups, while propofol caused a fall in blood pressure and reduced movements. The overall incidence of adverse effects was similar. Postoperatively, there was mild nausea in 78% of the patients who received sevoflurane compared with 50% for propofol. However, no antiemetics were needed and discharge times were not delayed.

The characteristics of sevoflurane anesthesia have been compared with those of target-controlled infusion of propofol in 61 day-case adults undergoing surgery (25). All received nitrous oxide 50% and fentanyl 1 μg/kg. After insertion of a laryngeal mask airway the propofol target concentration was reduced from 8 to 4 μg/ml and the inspired concentration of sevoflurane was reduced from 8 to 3% and subsequently titrated to clinical effects. Mean times to loss of consciousness and laryngeal mask airway insertion were significantly longer after sevoflurane (73 and 146 seconds respectively) than with propofol (50 and 116 seconds respectively). Sevoflurane was associated with a lower incidence of intraoperative movements (10 versus 55%), necessitating less adjustment to the dose. The incidence of movement in the propofol group was comparable to other studies. Emergence was faster after sevoflurane (5.3 versus 7.1 minutes) but sevoflurane was associated with more postoperative nausea (30 versus 17%) and vomiting (3 versus 0%), resulting in delayed discharge times (258 versus 193 minutes) and a higher total cost. The finding of significantly earlier discharge times after propofol anesthesia was unusual.

Propofol + alfentanil + nitrous oxide anesthesia has been compared with sevoflurane + nitrous oxide anesthesia in 44 patients undergoing dilatation and evacuation of the uterus (26). There was significantly less intraoperative uterine bleeding, as estimated by the gynecologist, with propofol. Above-average bleeding occurred in 5% of the patients with propofol anesthesia and 27% of patients with sevoflurane. This result was not surprising, given that sevoflurane reduces uterine tone, while propofol has no effect.

In a prospective randomized study of 120 day-surgery patients, desflurane and sevoflurane were associated with shorter times to awakening, extubation, and orientation than propofol infusion (27). Average times to awakening at the end of anesthesia were 5, 5, and 8 minutes respectively. There were no significant differences in time-to-home readiness or actual discharge times. A review of 436 patients undergoing either sevoflurane or propofol-based anesthesia showed no difference in similar recovery end-points (19).

There has been a prospective randomized comparison of 185 patients who received propofol 6–8 mg/kg/hour and sevoflurane 1.5% for maintenance of anesthesia (28). The patients were ventilated via a laryngeal mask and no muscle relaxants were given. Both agents were suitable for this technique. Emergence was significantly faster after sevoflurane but associated with more excitatory phenomena and tachycardia.

Sevoflurane versus thiopental

Sevoflurane 8% plus nitrous oxide 66% has been compared with thiopental 4 mg/kg for induction of anesthesia in brief outpatient procedures (29). Sevoflurane was safer, more efficacious, and better accepted by 78 unpremedicated adults with laryngeal cancer undergoing direct laryngoscopy for staging and biopsy. All received suxamethonium 50 mg on loss of the eyelash reflex and the surgeon then performed the laryngoscopy. Hemodynamic stability was greater and immediate recovery was faster after sevoflurane (9.7 versus 11.4 minutes). The incidence of dysrhythmias was also higher with thiopental (19 versus 12 patients). The dysrhythmias were predominantly ventricular extra beats with sevoflurane and ventricular bigemini with thiopental. The high incidence of dysrhythmias was partly due to the lack of opioid medication as part of the anesthetic.

Organs and Systems

Cardiovascular

Volatile anesthetic agents depress cardiac output, especially in the elderly. A study of 80 patients aged over 60 years compared the effects of halothane and isoflurane with and without nitrous oxide 50% (104). Doses were carefully adjusted to be equipotent in all four groups. Isoflurane caused a 30% reduction in systolic and diastolic arterial pressures compared with a 17% reduction with halothane. The reductions in cardiac index were similar with the two agents, about 17%. The addition of nitrous oxide attenuated the reductions in arterial pressure. In the case of the combination of isoflurane with nitrous oxide, there was a small increase in cardiac index and a small reduction in the halothane/nitrous oxide group. Systemic vascular resistance was reduced by a greater extent with isoflurane compared with halothane and little altered by the addition of nitrous oxide. The result suggests that nitrous oxide supplementation may be advantageous in the elderly, but interpretation is limited by the fact that it does not include the effects of surgery on these important cardiac parameters.

The long QT syndrome is associated with potentially fatal ventricular dysrhythmias under anesthesia. The effect of halothane and isoflurane on the QT interval was studied in 51 healthy children (31). Isoflurane 2.3–3.0% increased the average QT interval from 425 to 475 milliseconds at the time of induction. Halothane reduced the average QT interval from 428 to 407 milliseconds. The result suggested that halothane may be the more desirable agent in children with a prolonged QT interval.

The frequencies of cardiac dysrhythmias during halothane and sevoflurane inhalation have been compared in 150 children aged 3–15 years undergoing outpatient general anesthesia for dental extraction (32). They were randomized into three groups and received either halothane or sevoflurane in 66% nitrous oxide whilst breathing spontaneously. One group received 0.75% increments of halothane every two to three breaths to a maximum of 3.0% for induction, and then 1.5% for maintenance of anesthesia. One group received sevoflurane in 2% increments to a maximum of 8% and then a maintenance dose of 4%. The final group received 8% sevoflurane for induction and then a maintenance dose of 4%. The children who received halothane had a 48% incidence of dysrhythmias, significantly higher than the 16% incidence in the sevoflurane group and 8% in the incremental sevoflurane group. The halothane-associated dysrhythmias mainly occurred during dental extraction or emergence from anesthesia, and were usually ventricular. Six children in the halothane group had ventricular tachycardia. The longest run of ventricular tachycardia lasted 5.5 seconds, and one child had 13 separate episodes. Sevoflurane-associated dysrhythmias were mainly single supraventricular extra beats, and did not differ between the two administration methods. Although there was insufficient evidence to suggest that transient dysrhythmias associated with halothane in dental anesthesia can lead to cardiac arrest, sustained ectopic ventricular activity, including ventricular tachycardia, even if self-limiting, results in reduced cardiac output and cannot be ignored. These results imply that sevoflurane may be the preferable agent in this setting.

The hemodynamic responses to induction and maintenance of anesthesia with halothane have been compared with those of sevoflurane in 68 unpremedicated children aged 1–3 years undergoing adenoidectomy (30). The children received either sevoflurane 8% or halothane 5% + nitrous oxide 66% for induction of anesthesia and tracheal intubation, without neuromuscular blocking drugs. Anesthesia was maintained by adjusting the inspired concentration of the volatile anesthetic to maintain arterial blood pressure within 20% of baseline values, and the electrocardiogram was continuously recorded. The incidence of cardiac dysrhythmias was 23% with halothane and 6% with sevoflurane. Most of the dysrhythmias were short-lasting/self-limiting supraventricular extra beats or ventricular extra beats. Although the overall incidence of dysrhythmias was low in both groups, the result again shows that sevoflurane causes fewer dysrhythmias in children and may be the preferable agent.

QT dispersion, defined as the difference between QT_{max} and QT_{min} in the 12-lead electrocardiogram, is a measure of regional variation in ventricular repolarization (33). It is greater in patients with dysrhythmias. The effects of halothane and isoflurane on QT dispersion have been studied in 46 adult patients undergoing general anesthesia. QT dispersion was increased in both groups both with and without correction for heart rate. The increase was significantly greater with halothane than with isoflurane. The clinical significance of this finding is not known. In isolation, QT dispersion reflects an abnormality in ventricular repolarization and correlates with dysrhythmic events. Although there were no overt dysrhythmias in this study, the effect suggests a reason for the variable results of past studies of the QT interval: most studies showed prolongation of the QT interval, but some showed no change, or shortening. Larger studies are needed to elaborate on the possible clinical importance of this phenomenon, but it may be a significant cause of dysrhythmias with volatile anesthetics.

Respiratory

The incidence of perioperative respiratory complications has been studied prospectively in 602 children aged 1 month to 12 years undergoing elective surgery using a halothane-based anesthetic (34). Exposure to environmental smoke was assessed using the history of exposure to cigarette smoke and measurement of urinary cotinine concentrations, and the respiratory complications of laryngospasm, bronchospasm, stridor, breath holding, coughing, and excessive mucus production were recorded. The incidence of respiratory concentrations in patients with a urinary cotinine concentration over 40 ng/ml was 42%, dropping to 24% in patients with a urinary cotinine concentration less than 10 ng/ml. Female sex and lower socioeconomic status of the mother increased the incidence of respiratory complications. The study showed the importance of factors other than the anesthetic drugs and techniques used in determining complications precipitated by anesthesia.

The respiratory effects of sevoflurane and halothane have been investigated in 30 infants aged 6–24 months (35). Respiratory depression was greater in the sevoflurane group, with a mean minute ventilation of 4.5 compared with 5.4 l/minute/m^2 and respiratory rate was lower at 38 compared with 47 breaths/minute. There was a lower incidence of thoracoabdominal asynchrony with sevoflurane, but no difference in respiratory drive, as evidenced by the flow pressure generated during 100 milliseconds of occlusion of the airway.

The effects of desflurane and sevoflurane on bronchial smooth muscle reactivity have been compared in a randomized study of 40 patients (36). Anesthesia was induced with thiopental, followed by muscle relaxation and ventilation. Airway pressures were recorded during administration of desflurane or sevoflurane at one minimal alveolar concentration (MAC). Airway resistance increased by 5% in the desflurane group and fell by 15% in the sevoflurane group. The increase in airways resistance was greater in smokers and with desflurane, but did not differ with sevoflurane. The result was a surprise, given that desflurane stimulates the sympathetic nervous system. Thiopental also increased airways resistance by 10%. The result is important, because induction of anesthesia can cause bronchospasm and desflurane can exacerbate this.

Nervous system

The effects of sevoflurane and isoflurane anesthesia on interictal spike activity have been studied in 12 patients with refractory epilepsy (37). The patients were undergoing insertion of subdural electrodes and were also given fentanyl during surgery. Electroencephalogram spike frequency increased significantly in all patients during 1.5 MAC sevoflurane anesthesia compared with awake recordings; hypocapnia did not change this increased spike activity. The electrocorticographic interictal spike frequency was also significantly higher in all patients during 1.5 MAC sevoflurane anesthesia and in eight of 10 patients during 1.5 MAC isoflurane anesthesia, compared with 0.3 MAC isoflurane anesthesia. In susceptible individuals, both sevoflurane and isoflurane can provoke interictal spike activity. This effect is only well described for enflurane, but it is a dose-dependent feature of most volatile agents.

Convulsions during anesthesia are of concern because with the use of muscle relaxants they may go unrecognized. The epileptogenic properties of isoflurane and sevoflurane have been compared under a range of different ventilatory conditions in 24 ASA I or II mentally handicapped patients undergoing dental operations (38). Half had a history of epilepsy and half did not. Each patient was ventilated with 100% oxygen (end-tidal carbon dioxide = 40 mmHg; A), then 50% oxygen 50% nitrous oxide (end-tidal carbon dioxide = 40 mmHg; B), and then 100% oxygen (end-tidal carbon dioxide = 20 mmHg; C). With each different mode of ventilation, isoflurane was given at 1 MAC then at 1.5 and 2.0 MAC. The process was repeated 3 months later with sevoflurane. The electroencephalogram was concurrently recorded. The spike and wave index increased significantly from 2.0% during 1.0 MAC sevoflurane to 6.1% during 2.0 MAC in group A in those with epilepsy, while no spike activity was seen in those without epilepsy. Only a few spikes were observed in the isoflurane group in A, with none in B or C. Supplementation with nitrous oxide or hyperventilation suppressed the occurrence of spikes. The authors concluded that sevoflurane has stronger epileptogenic properties than isoflurane, but that this can be counteracted by nitrous oxide or hyperventilation.

There has been an impressive French study of the risks of occupational exposure of hospital personnel to anesthetics among the staff of 18 Paris hospitals (excluding doctors) over 12 years (39). Among 557 staff who had been exposed to anesthetics and 566 workers who had been less exposed, neuropsychological and neurological symptoms (tiredness, nausea, headaches, memory impairment, reduced reaction time, tingling, numbness, cramps) were reported some three times more commonly by workers in theaters that had been less often scavenged than by controls; no difference was found between workers from well-scavenging theaters and controls. Neuropsychological symptoms were reported in several earlier papers (40).

Neuromuscular function

Both desflurane and sevoflurane significantly increase the neuromuscular blocking effects of rocuronium compared with isoflurane or propofol (41,42). The effective doses of rocuronium for 50% depression of single twitch height were 95, 120, 130, and 150 μg/kg for desflurane, sevoflurane, isoflurane, and propofol respectively. There were no differences in recovery profiles between the four drugs using equieffective doses. Desflurane, sevoflurane, and to a lesser extent isoflurane, also potentiated the neuromuscular blocking effect of cisatracurium by 30% compared with propofol (43,44).

Hematologic

Hemostasis can be impaired by both surgery and general anesthetics (45). Fentanyl, halothane, and enflurane enhance fibrinolytic activity significantly (46). In addition, there was a raised plasma beta-thromboglobulin concentration (a good indicator of platelet activation) in 61 patients after the use of nitrous oxide, oxygen, and halothane compared with controls (47).

In an in vitro study of the inhibitory effects of thiopental, midazolam, and ketamine on human neutrophil function, thiopental and midazolam inhibited chemotaxis, phagocytosis, and reactive oxygen species production at clinically relevant concentrations (48). Ketamine only impaired chemotaxis. These results may be relevant in guiding anesthetic drug therapy in septic patients.

Gastrointestinal

In a prospective study of 556 adults using isoflurane-, halothane-, or enflurane-based anesthesia for ear, nose, throat, and eye procedures, the incidences of emesis in the various groups over the ensuing 24 hours were 36, 41, and 46% respectively (49). Other drugs given during anesthesia included midazolam, thiopental, morphine, and nitrous oxide. Antiemetic requirements were also less with isoflurane: 12% of patients required an antiemetic compared with 23% with halothane and enflurane. There were no differences in the overall incidences of headache or analgesic requirements in the three groups.

In another prospective study of nausea and vomiting in 50 patients undergoing arthroscopy, sevoflurane was compared with desflurane (50). Other drugs given during anesthesia included propofol and alfentanil. There was no difference in the incidence of nausea, 8 and 16% respectively, and no vomiting in either group. The desflurane group had a significantly higher incidence of sore throat (32 versus 8%). These studies have confirmed that the newer volatile anesthetics isoflurane, sevoflurane, and desflurane cause less nausea and vomiting than halothane or enflurane.

Because population measures of anesthetic dosages do not consider the individual's anesthetic needs, anesthetists often err on the side of relative overdosage during balanced anesthesia, in order to prevent the devastating consequences of unintentional awareness during surgery. This excessive depth of anesthesia contributes to delayed recovery and more adverse effects, which is particularly important in ambulatory surgery. Monitoring of the bispectral index-processed electroencephalogram has enabled anesthetists to monitor the depth of anesthesia and has brought greater precision to the administration of intravenous and inhaled anesthetics and opioids. The hypothesis that titration of the maintenance dose of sevoflurane during outpatient gynecological surgery using bispectral index monitoring reduces postoperative vomiting and improves recovery has been tested in a randomized, controlled study in 22 patients (51). The monitored patients had significantly less vomiting than the controls (16 versus 40%).

Several small clinical trials have suggested that total intravenous anesthesia with propofol reduces the incidence of postoperative nausea and vomiting and results in shorter emergence times. However, a systematic review (52) and a meta-analysis (53) have shown that most studies were small, did not have follow-up for more than 6 hours postoperatively, and were sponsored by industry. The results were difficult to combine, owing to heterogeneous definitions of postoperative nausea and vomiting.

A simplified risk score for predicting postoperative nausea and vomiting in adult patients undergoing general anesthesia has been developed. In a study of 520 adults from Finland and 2202 patients from Germany who had received anesthesia that included benzodiazepine premedication, thiopental, fentanyl or alfentanil, isoflurane, enflurane or sevoflurane, and non-steroidal or opioid drugs for postoperative analgesia no antiemetic prophylaxis was given (54). The final derived score consisted of four predictors: female sex, a history of motion sickness or postoperative nausea and vomiting, non-smoking, and the use of postoperative opioids. The incidence of postoperative nausea and vomiting was 10% when there were no risk factors, 21% (one risk factor), 39% (two risk factors), 61% (three risk factors), and 79% (four risk factors). Only one of the four risk factors related to the drugs used.

Postoperative nausea and vomiting in children has been reviewed in detail, including multimodal strategies for management and prevention (55).

Urinary tract

Methoxyflurane, enflurane, isoflurane, and sevoflurane all release inorganic fluoride ions as a result of hepatic metabolism. Fluoride is nephrotoxic.

Renal function and fluoride ion release after anesthesia using not more than 2.4% sevoflurane or 1.9% isoflurane have been studied in 50 patients of ASA grades 1–3 undergoing operations lasting at least 1 hour (56). Serum fluoride ion concentrations were significantly increased in both groups, peaking at 28 μmol/l after sevoflurane and 5 μmol/l after isoflurane, both at 1 hour. Of more concern, three of the patients in the sevoflurane group had peak fluoride ion concentrations above 50 μmol/l; two of them had increases in serum blood urea nitrogen and creatinine at 24 hours after surgery. The half-life of fluoride ion was 22 hours.

Nephrotoxicity has been found with methoxyflurane when serum fluoride ion concentrations exceeded 50 μmol/l (SEDA-20, 106). Although this safety threshold has been applied to other volatile anesthetics as well, renal toxicity has not been reported for the other three anesthetics, even though the threshold can be exceeded during prolonged anesthesia.

Volatile agents do not cause nephrotoxicity in adults with normal renal function (57). However, using sensitive urinary markers, both sevoflurane and isoflurane caused mild transient glomerular and tubular functional impairment in 13 patients aged 70 years or over undergoing gastrectomy. The patients received epidural analgesia combined with inhalation anesthesia using 5 l/minute fresh gas flow. The mean dose of sevoflurane was 5.1 MAC-hours and of isoflurane 3.7 MAC-hours. The mean urinary albumin excretion increased from 65 to 148 mg/g creatinine in the sevoflurane group and from 44 to 197 mg/g creatinine in the isoflurane group, and returned to preoperative values on the first postoperative day. The mean urinary β_1 and β_2 microglobulin concentrations also increased markedly in both groups, from 9.3 and 0.8 mg/g to 31 and 6.2 mg/g with sevoflurane and from 7.4 and 0.7 mg/g to 44 and 11 mg/g with isoflurane. These values had returned to normal by day 7 postoperatively. The mean urinary *N*-acetyl-β-D-glucosaminidase concentration also increased significantly. These changes suggest transient renal tubular injury in both groups. There has not been any agreement on how these results should be interpreted, and larger studies are warranted.

Musculoskeletal

A spectrum of muscle reactions to all inhalational agents has been described. Masseteric muscle spasm can occur as an isolated phenomenon or can progress either to rhabdomyolysis with renal insufficiency or to malignant hyperpyrexia (58–61).

Generalized muscle rigidity and hypercapnia, followed by raised creatine kinase activity, have been reported in a child undergoing general anesthesia (62).

- A 2-year-old girl with a past history of asthma, developmental delay, short neck, and lumbar lordosis, but no known genetic defect or syndrome underwent anesthesia with midazolam and paracetamol premedication, halothane and nitrous oxide induction, and isoflurane plus nitrous oxide for maintenance of anesthesia. Difficulty with mouth opening was noted and endotracheal intubation was difficult. Limb rigidity developed rapidly. Thiopental and cisatracurium were given and the muscle rigidity abated over the next 10 minutes. The procedure was continued with a propofol infusion. No treatment for malignant hyperpyrexia was undertaken and no other markers for malignant hyperpyrexia were observed. She made a normal recovery from anesthesia. Creatine kinase activities were raised at 2370 U/l intraoperatively and 18 046 U/l at 20 hours postoperatively.

The case is interesting in that although episodes of masseter spasm, rigidity, rhabdomyolysis, and malignant hyperpyrexia are well known after the use of halothane and suxamethonium, they have only rarely been reported when suxamethonium was not used.

Immunologic

The issue of hypersensitivity reactions during general anesthesia is a matter of concern. However, despite considerable work on the subject, there is divergence in interpretation (63). In patients with no pre-anesthetic immunological anomaly, general anesthesia is unlikely to affect immune status significantly (64).

Widespread erythema and edema, the most dangerous form of which affects the glottis, occur in some cases of hypersensitivity. Hypotension is also seen, together with compensatory tachycardia. Bronchospasm is a common respiratory finding (65).

There were significant immunological changes in the peripheral blood film of personnel working in unscavenged operating theaters in Croatia (66). Some of the effects persisted beyond a 4-week period away from that environment.

In a review of 23 444 anesthetics given during 12 months, one patient in 630 had generalized erythema and edema and one in 1230 had erythema and hypotension (67). One patient died of shock. Female patients aged 15–25 with a history of allergy, subjects with excessive anxiety, and those who had previously undergone general anesthesia had a statistically significant higher risk of developing non-allergic anaphylactic reactions. The incidence of allergic anaphylactic reactions (with IgE antibodies) is said to be one in 4500–20 000 general anesthetics per year (68). However, the diagnosis is often missed (69).

The patient's history is hardly helpful; neither the presence nor the absence of a previous reaction gives guidance as to the likelihood of its occurring on future exposure. The mechanisms underlying such reactions may or may not involve histamine release, but the distinction between allergic anaphylactic and non-allergic anaphylactic (anaphylactoid) reactions is often unclear, for lack of definitive and easily available investigations. Furthermore, because anesthetic drugs are often given rapidly and in combination, it can be impossible to decide which was responsible for the reaction. Intradermal injection of a test dose is of limited predictive value (70); false-positive and false-negative results are often obtained, particularly with opiates, tubocurarine, and atracurium. What is more, the test is dose-dependent and can itself precipitate a hypersensitivity reaction (71). It has been suggested that leukocyte histamine release on exposure to drugs can be used in combination with paper radioallergosorbent testing for IgE antibodies, to detect the precise cause of any anaphylactic reaction: these techniques point to neuromuscular blocking drugs as being most commonly implicated in anaphylaxis (70).

In a French study, 1585 patients underwent diagnostic investigations after anaphylactic shock during anesthesia; 813 of them had a reaction of immunological origin. The drugs involved were muscle relaxants (70%), latex (13%), anesthetic drugs (5.6%), opioids (1.7%), colloids (4.7%), and antibiotics (2.6%) (72). Among the 45 patients in whom anesthetics were involved, the agents implicated were thiopental ($n = 18$), propofol ($n = 10$), ketamine ($n = 1$), midazolam ($n = 7$), diazepam ($n = 5$), and flunitrazepam ($n = 4$). These data did not differ from those reported in a UK study (73). In both studies there was a high proportion of cases in which muscular relaxants were used alongside anesthetics, resulting in a two-fold risk of hypersensitivity.

Body temperature

Malignant hyperthermia

Malignant hyperpyrexia is a life-threatening condition that involves sustained muscle contraction, muscle damage, and the production of vast quantities of metabolic heat, carbon dioxide, and potassium. Although it is a rare complication of general anesthesia, it remains a topic of considerable interest (74).

The incidence is difficult to determine, but it is currently estimated at one in every 10 000–20 000 anesthetics.

Diagnosis

Generalized muscle rigidity (found in 70% of the patients involved) and a progressive rise in body temperature (sometimes beyond 43°C) are the main clinical features, often associated with tachycardia, hypoxia, metabolic acidosis, cardiac dysrhythmias and, less often, disseminated intravascular coagulation, cerebral edema, and acute renal insufficiency. Diagnosis relies on the clinical signs, that is muscle rigidity and hyperpyrexia, and on raised serum activities of skeletal and cardiac muscle enzymes, for example aldolase and creatine kinase.

Genetic markers for malignant hyperpyrexia may soon make identification of risk groups simpler than the currently used muscle biopsy technique (75).

Susceptibility factors and prophylaxis

Although malignant hyperthermia is usually associated with the muscle relaxant suxamethonium, all inhalational anesthetics have been implicated and will be unsafe if risk factors for this condition are present, for example a family history or one of the congenital muscle disorders (76). This must be considered in patients at risk, as there are readily acceptable alternatives, such as propofol (77) and midazolam (78).

Malignant hyperthermia is probably due to the inability of certain individuals to control calcium concentrations in the muscle fiber and may involve a generalized alteration in cellular or subcellular membrane permeability, as suggested from research on pigs. This anomaly is genetically determined, but pre-anesthetic evaluation of susceptibility to malignant hyperthermia is a matter of controversy: measurement of blood creatine kinase, ATP muscle depletion, or myophosphorylase A, histological examination of muscle fibers, and in vitro exposure to caffeine or halothane have all been proposed. However, if susceptible patients require general anesthesia, despite the risk, prophylactic use of intravenous dantrolene 2.4 mg/kg during induction of anesthesia has been recommended (79).

Treatment and prognosis

Around 1970, mortality was as high as 70%, but it is now less than 10%. This reduction in mortality has been due to the use of dantrolene, the only specific treatment available, and also to an increased understanding of the condition (74).

Treatment is by withdrawal of the anesthetic, hyperventilation with 100% oxygen, cooling, and dantrolene. Doses of dantrolene of 2.5–5 mg/kg are usually recommended, given as early as possible to ensure rapid and complete resolution of the hyperthermic response (80).

Death

Correct estimates of the incidence of anesthetic deaths are difficult to obtain, since many deaths are multifactorial. Mortality due to anesthetic drugs is one in 10 000–20 000 (81). The adverse effects of anesthetics have been reviewed (82). Dose-related reactions are common and carry a low mortality, while non-dose-related reactions are less common and carry a high mortality.

A national prospective survey of complications related to anesthesia was carried out in France from 1978 to 1982 (83,84). In 198 103 anesthetic procedures, only 63 deaths were recorded, of which only 15 were definitely attributed to anesthesia (85). The Confidential Enquiry into Perioperative Deaths, conducted a decade ago in three British Health Regions (86) and covering a total of 555 248 patients, showed that the incidence of death within 30 days of surgery and anesthesia was 0.73% (4034 cases). Only about 14 of these deaths were considered to be partly or totally attributable to the anesthesia, and indeed in most cases other factors were also involved, including the surgery itself, the presurgical condition, and intercurrent illnesses. In a review of 25 deaths during anesthesia in 1982–86, only six were considered to be drug-related; of these, two were due to overdose and two more were the result of adverse effects of non-anesthetic agents (87).

Finally, except for certain specific effects that have a clear relation to a particular agent (for example liver damage after halothane), it is difficult to designate one anesthetic as being more risky than another. It has been authoritatively concluded that "the current level of research effort cannot distinguish mortality and serious morbidity between the most common anesthetic agents, and the clear differences in hemodynamic patterns among these anesthetic agents have an unknown, perhaps non-existent, relationship with mortality and serious morbidity" (88).

Long-Term Effects

Mutagenicity

Genetic damage was demonstrated in 10 non-smoking veterinary surgeons exposed to isoflurane and nitrous oxide compared with 10 non-smoking, non-exposed veterinary physicians acting as controls (89). The surgeons were monitored for 1 week in a working environment comparable to that of pediatric anesthesia, with the use of uncuffed endotracheal tubes and open-circuit breathing systems during operations on small animals. The overall calculated 8-hour time-weighted average exposure of cases was 5.3 ppm for isoflurane and 13 ppm for nitrous oxide. The European exposure limits are 10 ppm and 100 ppm respectively, and the corresponding values recommended by USA-NIOSH are 2 ppm and 25 ppm respectively. These values therefore violated the USA-NIOSH limit for isoflurane. The mean frequency of sister chromatid exchanges in peripheral blood lymphocytes was significantly higher in exposed workers than in controls (10 versus 7.4) and the proportion of micronuclei was also significantly higher in exposed workers (8.7 versus 6.8 per 500 binucleated cells). These measures reflect the mutagenicity of isoflurane and nitrous oxide. The findings are comparable to smoking 11–20 cigarettes a day. However, this study did not distinguish between the potential genotoxic effects of isoflurane and nitrous oxide; nor did it show a dose-dependency of genotoxicity, owing to the small sample size.

Second-Generation Effects

Fertility

Nitrous oxide may be the most serious of anesthetic pollutants; female dental assistants exposed to large amounts of nitrous oxide (5 hours or more of exposure per week) are significantly less fertile than women who are not exposed or who are exposed to lower amounts (90).

Pregnancy

The pharmacology and adverse effects of anesthetic drugs used for cesarean section have been reviewed (91).

Teratogenicity

In an epidemiological study, anesthetists had significantly greater exposure and perhaps more adverse effects than other operating-room personnel (92). Among women, exposure certainly causes an increased risk of spontaneous abortions in the first trimester, although teratogenicity is less clear-cut (93).

Susceptibility Factors

Underlying disease

Underlying disease is probably one of the most complex risk factors. Although general anesthesia is potentially more hazardous in patients with underlying disease in general (94) or specifically suffering from intracardiac conduction disturbances (95), severe hypertension (96), hypothyroidism (97), or cancer (98), it is extremely difficult to provide clear-cut recommendations, because the relative severity of disease in a given patient and the patient's response to the pathological process needs to be taken into account: while, for instance, thiopental may precipitate cardiovascular collapse, both pre-existing cardiac status and the dose of the drug are relevant.

Critically ill patients

Drug metabolism is reduced in critically ill patients. When the serum from five critically ill patients was incubated with microsomes prepared from three different human livers, the activity of CYP3A4, assessed by metabolism of midazolam to 1-hydroxymidazolam, was significantly inhibited compared with serum from healthy volunteers (99). The authors pointed out that many other drugs are also metabolized by this enzyme, including alfentanil, ciclosporin, cortisol, erythromycin, lidocaine, and nifedipine. This observation accounts for past reports of very slow metabolism of midazolam in seriously ill patients, resulting in high blood concentrations and delayed awakening.

Pre-anesthetic drug therapy

The consequences of pre-anesthetic drug therapy as a risk factor are obviously closely related to those of the underlying disease. The problem has attracted considerable attention in recent years and has been extensively reviewed (100). Interactions of drugs with anesthesia are dealt with here primarily in monographs on the drugs concerned. Although many pharmacological interactions with general anesthesia are firmly established, others remain ill-explained or unpredictable. Individual factors are likely to play a major role. Moreover, pre-anesthetic drug withdrawal in itself can be more dangerous than continuation of therapy, as exemplified by the case of the antihypertensive drug clonidine (101) or beta-blockers (102).

Driving

The hazard of driving shortly after general anesthesia is still difficult to evaluate. Although abstention from driving has been recommended for 48 hours after general anesthesia (103), it is still difficult to draw clear-cut conclusions from the available data. The matter is also referred to under individual anesthetic drugs.

References

1. Hindle AT, Columb MO, Shah MV. Drug interactions and anaesthesia. Curr Anaesth Crit Care 1995;6:103–12.
2. McAuliffe MS, Hartshorn EA. Anesthetic drug interactions. CRNA 1995;6(2):103–7.
3. McAuliffe MS, Hartshorn EA. Anesthetic drug interactions. CRNA 1995;6(3):139–42.
4. Stoltzfus DP. Advantages and disadvantages of combining sedative agents. Crit Care Clin 1995;11(4):903–12.
5. Whitwam JG. Co-induction of anaesthesia: day-case surgery. Eur J Anaesthesiol Suppl 1995;12:25–34.
6. Amrein R, Hetzel W, Allen SR. Co-induction of anaesthesia: the rationale. Eur J Anaesthesiol Suppl 1995;12:5–11.
7. D'Eramo EM. Morbidity and mortality with outpatient anesthesia: the Massachusetts experience. J Oral Maxillofac Surg 1992;50(7):700–4.
8. Clarke AC, Chiragakis L, Hillman LC, Kaye GL. Sedation for endoscopy: the safe use of propofol by general practitioner sedationists. Med J Aust 2002;176(4):158–61.
9. Arain SR, Ebert TJ. The efficacy, side effects, and recovery characteristics of dexmedetomidine versus propofol

when used for intraoperative sedation. Anesth Analg 2002;95(2):461–6.
10. Servin FS, Raeder JC, Merle JC, Wattwil M, Hanson AL, Lauwers MH, Aitkenhead A, Marty J, Reite K, Martisson S, Wostyn L. Remifentanil sedation compared with propofol during regional anaesthesia. Acta Anaesthesiol Scand 2002;46(3):309–15.
11. Walder B, Borgeat A, Suter PM, Romand JA. Propofol and midazolam versus propofol alone for sedation following coronary artery bypass grafting: a randomized, placebo-controlled trial. Anaesth Intensive Care 2002;30(2):171–8.
12. Gray WM. Occupational exposure to nitrous oxide in four hospitals. Anaesthesia 1989;44(6):511–14.
13. Gold DR. Indoor air pollution. Clin Chest Med 1992;13(2):215–29.
14. Crawford MW, Lerman J, Sloan MH, Sikich N, Halpern L, Bissonnette B. Recovery characteristics of propofol anaesthesia, with and without nitrous oxide: a comparison with halothane/nitrous oxide anaesthesia in children. Paediatr Anaesth 1998;8(1):49–54.
15. Visser K, Hassink EA, Bonsel GJ, Moen J, Kalkman CJ. Randomized controlled trial of total intravenous anesthesia with propofol versus inhalation anesthesia with isoflurane–nitrous oxide: postoperative nausea with vomiting and economic analysis. Anesthesiology 2001; 95(3):616–26.
16. Ti LK, Pua HL, Lee TL. Single vital capacity inhalational anaesthetic induction in adults—isoflurane vs sevoflurane. Can J Anaesth 1998;45(10):949–53.
17. Smith I, Ding Y, White PF. Comparison of induction, maintenance, and recovery characteristics of sevoflurane–N_2O and propofol–sevoflurane–N_2O with propofol–isoflurane–N_2O anesthesia. Anesth Analg 1992;74(2):253–9.
18. Elcock DH, Sweeney BP. Sevoflurane vs. isoflurane: a clinical comparison in day surgery. Anaesthesia 2002;57(1):52–6.
19. Ebert TJ, Robinson BJ, Uhrich TD, Mackenthun A, Pichotta PJ. Recovery from sevoflurane anesthesia: a comparison to isoflurane and propofol anesthesia. Anesthesiology 1998;89(6):1524–31.
20. Joo HS, Perks WJ. Sevoflurane versus propofol for anesthetic induction: a meta-analysis. Anesth Analg 2000; 91(1):213–19.
21. Watson KR, Shah MV. Clinical comparison of "single agent" anaesthesia with sevoflurane versus target controlled infusion of propofol. Br J Anaesth 2000;85(4):541–6.
22. McCulloch TJ, Visco E, Lam AM. Graded hypercapnia and cerebral autoregulation during sevoflurane or propofol anesthesia. Anesthesiology 2000;93(5):1205–9.
23. Nandate K, Vuylsteke A, Ratsep I, Messahel S, Oduro-Dominah A, Menon DK, Matta BF. Effects of isoflurane, sevoflurane and propofol anaesthesia on jugular venous oxygen saturation in patients undergoing coronary artery bypass surgery. Br J Anaesth 2000;84(5):631–3.
24. Philip BK, Lombard LL, Roaf ER, Drager LR, Calalang I, Philip JH. Comparison of vital capacity induction with sevoflurane to intravenous induction with propofol for adult ambulatory anesthesia. Anesth Analg 1999;89(3):623–7.
25. Smith I, Thwaites AJ. Target-controlled propofol vs. sevoflurane: a double-blind, randomised comparison in day-case anaesthesia. Anaesthesia 1999;54(8):745–52.
26. Nelskyla K, Korttila K, Yli-Hankala A. Comparison of sevoflurane–nitrous oxide and propofol–alfentanil–nitrous oxide anaesthesia for minor gynaecological surgery. Br J Anaesth 1999;83(4):576–9.
27. Song D, Joshi GP, White PF. Fast-track eligibility after ambulatory anesthesia: a comparison of desflurane, sevoflurane, and propofol. Anesth Analg 1998;86(2):267–73.
28. Keller C, Sparr HJ, Brimacombe JR. Positive pressure ventilation with the laryngeal mask airway in non-paralysed patients: comparison of sevoflurane and propofol maintenance techniques. Br J Anaesth 1998;80(3):332–6.
29. Nishiyama T, Nakayama H, Hanaoka K. Sevoflurane or thiopental–isoflurane for induction and laryngeal mask insertion? Comparison by side effects, hemodynamics, and spectral analysis of heart rate variability. Anesth Resusc 1999;35:99–103.
30. Viitanen H, Baer G, Koivu H, Annila P. The hemodynamic and Holter-electrocardiogram changes during halothane and sevoflurane anesthesia for adenoidectomy in children aged one to three years. Anesth Analg 1999; 89(6):1423–5.
31. Michaloudis D, Fraidakis O, Petrou A, Gigourtsi C, Parthenakis F. Anaesthesia and the QT interval. Effects of isoflurane and halothane in unpremedicated children. Anaesthesia 1998;53(5):435–9.
32. Blayney MR, Malins AF, Cooper GM. Cardiac arrhythmias in children during outpatient general anaesthesia for dentistry: a prospective randomised trial. Lancet 1999; 354(9193):1864–6.
33. Guler N, Bilge M, Eryonucu B, Kati I, Demirel CB. The effects of halothane and sevoflurane on QT dispersion. Acta Cardiol 1999;54(6):311–15.
34. Skolnick ET, Vomvolakis MA, Buck KA, Mannino SF, Sun LS. Exposure to environmental tobacco smoke and the risk of adverse respiratory events in children receiving general anesthesia. Anesthesiology 1998; 88(5):1144–53.
35. Brown K, Aun C, Stocks J, Jackson E, Mackersie A, Hatch D. A comparison of the respiratory effects of sevoflurane and halothane in infants and young children. Anesthesiology 1998;89(1):86–92.
36. Goff MJ, Arain SR, Ficke DJ, Uhrich TD, Ebert TJ. Absence of bronchodilation during desflurane anesthesia: a comparison to sevoflurane and thiopental. Anesthesiology 2000;93(2):404–8.
37. Watts AD, Herrick IA, McLachlan RS, Craen RA, Gelb AW. The effect of sevoflurane and isoflurane anesthesia on interictal spike activity among patients with refractory epilepsy. Anesth Analg 1999;89(5):1275–81.
38. Iijima T, Nakamura Z, Iwao Y, Sankawa H. The epileptogenic properties of the volatile anesthetics sevoflurane and isoflurane in patients with epilepsy. Anesth Analg 2000;91(4):989–95.
39. Saurel-Cubizolles MJ, Estryn-Behar M, Maillard MF, Mugnier N, Masson A, Monod G. Neuropsychological symptoms and occupational exposure to anaesthetics. Br J Ind Med 1992;49(4):276–81.
40. Vaisman AI. Usloviia truda v operatisionnykh i ikh vliianie na zdorov'e anesteziologov. [Working conditions in the operating room and their effect on the health of anesthetists.] Eksp Khir Anesteziol 1967;12(3):44–9.
41. Lowry DW, Mirakhur RK, Carrol MT. Time course of action of rocuronium during sevoflurane, isoflurane or i.v. anaesthesia. Br J Anaesth 1998;80:544.
42. Wulf H, Ledowski T, Linstedt U, Proppe D, Sitzlack D. Neuromuscular blocking effects of rocuronium during desflurane, isoflurane, and sevoflurane anaesthesia. Can J Anaesth 1998;45(6):526–32.
43. Wulf H, Kahl M, Ledowski T. Augmentation of the neuromuscular blocking effects of cisatracurium during desflurane, isoflurane, and sevoflurane anaesthesia. Can J Anaesth 1998;45:526–32.
44. Tran TV, Fiset P, Varin F. Pharmacokinetics and pharmacodynamics of cisatracurium after a short infusion in patients under propofol anesthesia. Anesth Analg 1998; 87(5):1158–63.

45. Sparacia A, Mangione S, Sansone A. Alterazioni dell'emostasi in relazione al farmaci anestetici ed all'emostasi ed all'intervento chirurgico. [Hemostatic changes related to anesthetic drugs and surgical intervention.] Minerva Anestesiol 1980;46(7):791–814.
46. Simpson PJ, Radford SG, Forster SJ, et al. The fibrinolytic effects of anesthesia. Anesth Analg 1982;60:319.
47. Zahavi J, Price AJ, Kakkar VV. Enhanced platelet release reaction associated with general anaesthesia. Lancet 1980;1(8178):1132–3.
48. Nishina K, Akamatsu H, Mikawa K, Shiga M, Maekawa N, Obara H, Niwa Y. The inhibitory effects of thiopental, midazolam, and ketamine on human neutrophil functions. Anesth Analg 1998;86(1):159–65.
49. van den Berg AA, Honjol NM, Mphanza T, Rozario CJ, Joseph D. Vomiting, retching, headache and restlessness after halothane-, isoflurane- and enflurane-based anaesthesia. An analysis of pooled data following ear, nose, throat and eye surgery. Acta Anaesthesiol Scand 1998;42(6):658–63.
50. Naidu-Sjosvard K, Sjoberg F, Gupta A. Anaesthesia for videoarthroscopy of the knee. A comparison between desflurane and sevoflurane. Acta Anaesthesiol Scand 1998;42(4):464–71.
51. Nelskyla KA, Yli-Hankala AM, Puro PH, Korttila KT. Sevoflurane titration using bispectral index decreases postoperative vomiting in phase II recovery after ambulatory surgery. Anesth Analg 2001;93(5):1165–9.
52. Tramèr M, Moore A, McQuay H. Propofol anaesthesia and postoperative nausea and vomiting: quantitative systematic review of randomized controlled studies. Br J Anaesth 1997;78(3):247–55.
53. Sneyd JR, Carr A, Byrom WD, Bilski AJ. A meta-analysis of nausea and vomiting following maintenance of anaesthesia with propofol or inhalational agents. Eur J Anaesthesiol 1998;15(4):433–45.
54. Apfel CC, Laara E, Koivuranta M, Greim CA, Roewer N. A simplified risk score for predicting postoperative nausea and vomiting: conclusions from cross-validations between two centers. Anesthesiology 1999;91(3):693–700.
55. Rose JB, Watcha MF. Postoperative nausea and vomiting in paediatric patients. Br J Anaesth 1999;83(1):104–17.
56. Goldberg ME, Cantillo J, Larijani GE, Torjman M, Vekeman D, Schieren H. Sevoflurane versus isoflurane for maintenance of anesthesia: are serum inorganic fluoride ion concentrations of concern? Anesth Analg 1996; 82(6):1268–72.
57. Hase K, Meguro K, Nakamura T. Assessment of renal effects of sevoflurane in elderly patients using urinary markers. Anesth Analg 1999;88(6):1426–7.
58. McGuire N, Easy WR. Malignant hyperthermia during isoflurane anaesthesia. Anaesthesia 1990;45(2):124–7.
59. Rubiano R, Chang JL, Carroll J, Sonbolian N, Larson CE. Acute rhabdomyolysis following halothane anesthesia without succinylcholine. Anesthesiology 1987;67(5):856–7.
60. Littleford JA, Patel LR, Bose D, Cameron CB, McKillop C. Masseter muscle spasm in children: implications of continuing the triggering anesthetic. Anesth Analg 1991;72(2):151–60.
61. Lee SC, Abe T, Sato T. Rhabdomyolysis and acute renal failure following use of succinylcholine and enflurane: report of a case. J Oral Maxillofac Surg 1987;45(9): 789–92.
62. Medina KA, Mayhew JF. Generalized muscle rigidity and hypercarbia with halothane and isoflurane. Anesth Analg 1998;86(2):297–8.
63. Walton B. Anaesthesia, surgery and immunology. Anaesthesia 1978;33(4):322–48.
64. Ryhanen P. Effects of anaesthesia and operative surgery on the immune response of patients of different ages. Ann Clin Res 1977;19(Suppl):9.
65. Clarke RS. The clinical presentation of anaphylactoid reactions in anesthesia. Int Anesthesiol Clin 1985;23(3):1–16.
66. Peric M, Vranes Z, Marusic M. Immunological disturbances in anaesthetic personnel chronically exposed to high occupational concentrations of nitrous oxide and halothane. Anaesthesia 1991;46(7):531–7.
67. Laxenaire MC, Manel J, Borgo J, Moneret-Vautrin DA. Facteurs de risque d'histamino-libération: étude prospective dans une population anestésie. [Risk factors in histamine liberation: a prospective study in an anesthetized population.] Ann Fr Anesth Reanim 1985; 4(2):158–66.
68. Watkins J. Investigation of allergic and hypersensitivity reactions to anaesthetic agents. Br J Anaesth 1987; 59(1):104–11.
69. Youngman PR, Taylor KM, Wilson JD. Anaphylactoid reactions to neuromuscular blocking agents: a commonly undiagnosed condition? Lancet 1983;2(8350):597–9.
70. Assem ES. Anaphylactic anaesthetic reactions. The value of paper radioallergosorbent tests for IgE antibodies to muscle relaxants and thiopentone. Anaesthesia 1990; 45(12):1032–8.
71. Assem ES, Symons IE. Anaphylaxis due to suxamethonium in a 7-year-old child: a 14-year follow-up with allergy testing. Anaesthesia 1989;44(2):121–4.
72. Laxenaire MC, Moneret-Vautrin DA, Guéant JL, et al. Drugs and other agents involved in anaphylactic shock occurring during anaesthesia. A French multicenter epidemiological inquiry. Ann Fr Anesth Reanim 1993; 12(2):91–6.
73. Clarke RS, Watkins J. Drugs responsible for anaphylactoid reactions in anaesthesia in the United Kingdom. Ann Fr Anesth Reanim 1993;12(2):105–8.
74. Halsall PJ, Ellis FR. Malignant hyperthermia. Bailliere's Clin Anaesthesiol 1993;7:343–56.
75. MacKenzie AE, Allen G, Lahey D, Crossan ML, Nolan K, Mettler G, Worton RG, MacLennan DH, Korneluk R. A comparison of the caffeine halothane muscle contracture test with the molecular genetic diagnosis of malignant hyperthermia. Anesthesiology 1991;75(1):4–8.
76. Chalkiadis GA, Branch KG. Cardiac arrest after isoflurane anaesthesia in a patient with Duchenne's muscular dystrophy. Anaesthesia 1990;45(1):22–5.
77. Gallen JS. Propofol does not trigger malignant hyperthermia. Anesth Analg 1991;72(3):413–14.
78. Brooks JH. Midazolam in a malignant hyperthermia-susceptible patient. Anesthesiology 1989;70(1):167–8.
79. Flewellen EH, Nelson TE, Jones WP, Arens JF, Wagner DL. Dantrolene dose response in awake man: implications for management of malignant hyperthermia. Anesthesiology 1983;59(4):275–80.
80. Harrison GG. Malignant hyperthermia. Dantrolene—dynamics and kinetics. Br J Anaesth 1988;60(3):279–86.
81. Derrington MC, Smith G. A review of studies of anaesthetic risk, morbidity and mortality. Br J Anaesth 1987;59(7):815–33.
82. Berthoud MC, Reilly CS. Adverse effects of general anaesthetics. Drug Saf 1992;7(6):434–59.
83. Harrison GG. Death attributable to anaesthesia. A 10-year survey (1967–1976). Br J Anaesth 1978; 50(10):1041–6.
84. Saarnivaara L. Comparison of halothane and enflurane anaesthesia for tonsillectomy in adults. Acta Anaesthesiol Scand 1984;28(3):319–24.
85. Vourc'h G, Hatton F, Tiret L, Desmonts JM. Étude épidemiologique sur les complications de l'anesthésie

en France. [Epidemiologic study of anesthesia complications in France.] Bull Acad Natl Med 1983; 167(8):939–45.
86. Buck N, Devlin HB, Lunn JN. The Report of A Confidental Enquiry into Perioperative Deaths. London: Nuffield Provincial Hospitals Trust and The King's Fund, 1987.
87. Gannon K. Mortality associated with anaesthesia. A case review study. Anaesthesia 1991;46(11):962–6.
88. Pace NL. Adverse outcomes and the multicenter study of general anesthesia: II. Anesthesiology 1992; 77(2):394–6.
89. Hoerauf K, Lierz M, Wiesner G, Schroegendorfer K, Lierz P, Spacek A, Brunnberg L, Nusse M. Genetic damage in operating room personnel exposed to isoflurane and nitrous oxide. Occup Environ Med 1999;56(7):433–7.
90. Rowland AS, Baird DD, Weinberg CR, Shore DL, Shy CM, Wilcox AJ. Reduced fertility among women employed as dental assistants exposed to high levels of nitrous oxide. N Engl J Med 1992;327(14):993–7.
91. D'Alessio JG, Ramanathan J. Effects of maternal anesthesia in the neonate. Semin Perinatol 1998; 22(5):350–62.
92. Sass-Kortsak AM, Purdham JT, Bozek PR, Murphy JH. Exposure of hospital operating room personnel to potentially harmful environmental agents. Am Ind Hyg Assoc J 1992;53(3):203–9.
93. Eger EI, editor. Nitrous Oxide. New York: Edward Arnold, 1985.
94. Train M, Lepage JY, Le Forestier K, Dixneuf B, Duveau D. Incidents et accidents observés lors de l'anesthésie-réanimation en chirurgie coronaire. [Accidents and complications seen during anesthesia and postoperative recovery in coronary surgery.] Ann Anesthesiol Fr 1979;20(5):431–4.
95. Tachoires D, Poisot D, Erny P, Mourot F, Bergeron JL. Les troubles de la conduction intra-cardiaque en anesthésie-réanimation. [Disorders of intracardiac conduction in anesthesia-resuscitation.] Ann Anesthesiol Fr 1979;20(4):357–69.
96. Rodriguez PR, Mangans DT. Anesthesia and hypertension. Semin Anaesthesiol 1982;1:226.
97. Murkin JM. Anesthesia and hypothyroidism: a review of thyroxine physiology, pharmacology, and anesthetic implications. Anesth Analg 1982;61(4):371–83.
98. Chung F. Cancer, chemotherapy and anaesthesia. Can Anaesth Soc J 1982;29(4):364–71.
99. Park GR, Miller E, Navapurkar V. What changes drug metabolism in critically ill patients?—II Serum inhibits the metabolism of midazolam in human microsomes. Anaesthesia 1996;51(1):11–15.
100. Craig DB, Bose D. Drug interactions in anaesthesia: chronic antihypertensive therapy. Can Anaesth Soc J 1984;31(5):580–9.
101. Stevens JE. Rebound hypertension during anaesthesia. Anaesthesia 1980;35(5):490–1.
102. Ponten J, Biber B, Bjuro T, Henriksson BA, Hjalmarson A. Beta-receptor blocker withdrawal. A preoperative problem in general surgery? Acta Anaesthesiol Scand Suppl 1982;76:32–7.
103. Havard J. Medical Aspects of Fitness to Drive. 3rd ed. London: A Rapple, 1976:43.
104. Mckinney MS, Fee JP. Cardiovascular effects of 50% nitrous oxide in older adult patients anaesthetized with isoflurane or halothane. Br J Anaesth 1998; 80(2):169–73.

Gentamicin

See also Aminoglycoside antibiotics

General Information

Gentamicin is well established for the treatment of several bacterial infections, especially those caused by Gram-negative bacteria, including *Pseudomonas aeruginosa*, *Klebsiella* species, and *Serratia marcescens*. In adults, it is usually given in daily doses of 240–360 mg.

Observational studies

In 17 patients with suspected postoperative endophthalmitis treated with 0.2 mg vancomycin and 0.05 mg gentamicin intravitreally, there were adequate intravitreal vancomycin and gentamicin concentrations for over a week; there were no adverse effects (1).

Intratympanic gentamicin therapy has gained some popularity in the treatment of vertigo associated with Menière's disease, as it offers some advantages over traditional surgical treatment. In a 2-year follow-up of 15 patients with Menière's disease, gentamicin solution 0.5 ml (20 mg/ml) injected intratympanically once a week minimized the risk of hearing loss in the treated ear, allowing complete control of vertigo in eight patients after two doses and in 14 patients after four doses (2).

In an open, randomized, controlled trial, once-daily and thrice-daily gentamicin were compared in 173 children aged 1 month to 12 years; there was no nephrotoxicity or ototoxicity (3). Daily doses of gentamicin in both groups were 7.5 mg/kg (under 5 years old), 6.0 mg/kg (5–10 years old), and 4.5 mg/kg (over 10 years old).

Organs and Systems

Respiratory

Acute respiratory failure with near-fatal bronchoconstriction has been reported in an adult with bronchiectasis and chronic *P. aeruginosa* airways colonization immediately after the first inhalation of a commercially available gentamicin solution (4).

Nervous system

Intraventricular gentamicin can cause aseptic meningitis (5).

Sensory systems

The frequency of aminoglycoside-associated hearing loss is 2–45%. Since gentamicin-induced ototoxicity in most cases only involves vestibular function, the symptoms are easily overlooked in severely ill patients who are unable to sit. If diagnosed early, the vestibular damage is usually reversible. In some cases, severe long-term disability has been described (6). Six patients presented with unilateral vestibulotoxicity after systemic gentamicin therapy (7). All had ataxia and oscillopsia, but none had a history of vertigo. The authors suggested that a subacute course of vestibulotoxicity with time for compensation or asymmetrical recovery of vestibular function after bilateral vestibular loss could have explained the lack of vertigo in these patients.

The risk of ototoxicity from gentamicin in children is probably less than in adults. In many studies of serious neonatal infections treated with gentamicin there have been very few cases that have provided unequivocal evidence of gentamicin-induced ototoxicity. Gentamicin can be an excellent drug in neonatal sepsis, and its potential toxicity should not preclude its use when it is needed.

Gentamicin ear-drops can cause serious adverse effects (for example vertigo, imbalance, ataxia, oscillating vision, hearing loss, and tinnitus) when they are used by patients with perforated tympanic membranes or tympanostomy tubes (8).

The symptom complex known as visual vestibular mismatch can be caused by peripheral vestibular disease. In a retrospective study of 28 patients with Menière's disease, 17 had visual vestibular mismatch; gentamicin therapy increased the number of positive answers (9).

In a retrospective analysis of 85 patients treated with intratympanic gentamicin, using a fixed-dose regimen of 26.7 mg/ml tds on 4 consecutive days, hearing loss occurred in 26% of individuals (10).

The characteristics of ototoxicity of topical gentamicin have been studied retrospectively in 16 patients (11). All used ear-drops for more than 7 days before the development of symptoms, and all had some degree of vestibulotoxicity, but only one had a worsening of cochlear reserve. Even if the tympanic membrane is intact, one should hesitate to use gentamicin in ear-drops or in other topical forms for the treatment of otitis media.

In patients with acute bacterial conjunctivitis there were adverse drug reactions in 4 of 103 treated with gentamicin (12). The adverse effects included redness, itching, and burning, and none was serious.

In two animal studies methylcobalamin or dimethylsulfoxide inhibited the ototoxic adverse effects of gentamicin (13,14).

Psychological, psychiatric

There are several case reports of acute toxic psychoses due to gentamicin (15).

Mineral balance

Gentamicin-induced magnesium depletion is most likely to occur in older patients when large doses are used over long periods of time (16). Under these circumstances, serum concentrations and urinary electrolyte losses should be monitored.

Liver

Increases in alkaline phosphatase after gentamicin have been described (17).

Urinary tract

A full course of gentamicin therapy causes nephrotoxicity in 1–55% of patients. Two types of gentamicin-induced nephrotoxicity are recognized: (1) a gradual reduction in creatinine clearance, occurring after about 2 weeks, in about 5–10% of patients receiving the drug in full doses, the reduction being rapidly reversible in most cases as soon as gentamicin is withdrawn; (2) acute renal insufficiency due to tubular necrosis, usually associated with oliguria lasting 10–12 days, followed by a diuretic phase; this type of nephrotoxicity occurs far less often than the first type.

The following order of relative nephrotoxicity has been found in many animal experiments: neomycin > gentamicin > tobramycin > amikacin > netilmicin (18,19). However, in humans, conclusive data regarding the relative toxicity of the various aminoglycosides are still lacking. An analysis of 24 controlled trials showed the following average rates for nephrotoxicity: gentamicin 11%; tobramycin 11.5%; amikacin 8.5%; and netilmicin 2.8% (20). In contrast to this survey, direct comparison in similar patient groups showed no significant differences between the various agents in most trials (21–27). In fact, the relative advantage of lower nephrotoxicity rates observed with netilmicin in some studies may be limited to administration of low doses. One prospective trial showed a significant advantage of tobramycin over gentamicin (28). However, these findings could subsequently not be confirmed (29). The risk of gentamicin nephrotoxicity is increased in biliary obstruction (SEDA-20, 235).

In a few cases, gentamicin nephrotoxicity was associated with a Fanconi syndrome, with raised serum enzymes activities in the urine. Among these, muramidase seemed to be especially useful in checking for proximal tubular dysfunction (30).

Gentamicin is of considerable value in the management of sepsis in immunosuppressed patients and renal transplant recipients. Although it has been suggested that gentamicin should be avoided in such patients because of potential renal toxicity in the allograft (31,32), experienced physicians have felt that gentamicin may be given, provided the dosage schedule is adapted to the degree of allograft function and that blood concentrations are monitored.

After a full course of gentamicin 1–55% of patients have nephrotoxicity. The increased serum creatinine concentration peaks on day 6 of therapy and is reversible in most cases within 30 days. Nephrotoxicity appears to be more common among patients with pre-existing renal impairment, longer treatment duration (over 7 days), repeated courses of aminoglycosides, and after the co-administration of other nephrotoxic drugs (for example amphotericin, cisplatin, daunorubicin, furosemide, and vancomycin). Animal studies have suggested that hydrocortisone, angiotensin converting enzyme inhibitors, and hypercalcemia can also increase aminoglycoside nephrotoxicity, whereas acetazolamide, bicarbonate, ceftriaxone, lithium, magnesium, melatonin, piperacillin, polyaspartic acid, pyridoxal-5′-phosphate, and a high protein diet may be protective (33,34).

In 87 patients with intertrochanteric hip fractures, preoperative antibiotic prophylaxis (gentamicin 240 mg and dicloxacillin 2 g) had no significant effect on wound infections; however, there were 16 reversible cases of nephrotoxicity and 1 irreversible case among patients who received antibiotic prophylaxis, compared with only 4 cases of reversible kidney damage among 76 patients who did not receive antibiotics (35).

- Acute renal insufficiency occurred in an 83-year-old woman after two-stage revision of an infected knee prosthesis with gentamicin-impregnated beads and block spacers (36). The combined use of beads and a cement block spacer, both gentamicin impregnated, may have caused this severe complication.
- A 43-year-old black woman with a 13-year history of lupus developed severe acute tubular necrosis secondary to gentamicin (37).

Since serum creatinine does not accurately reflect renal function in patients with spinal cord injury, dosage regimens of gentamicin should be individualized, based on age, sex, weight, height, the level of spinal cord injury, and renal function (38).

In animals melatonin (39,40) or l-carnitine (41) protected the kidneys against oxidative damage and the nephrotoxic effect of gentamicin.

Nephrocalcinosis occurred in 16 of 101 babies born at less than 32 weeks gestation (42). Multivariate analysis showed that the strongest predictors of nephrocalcinosis were duration of ventilation, toxic gentamicin/vancomycin concentrations, low fluid intake, and male sex.

Skin

Erythema multiforme developed in a 4-year-old girl after treatment with topical aural gentamicin sulfate (0.3%) plus hydrocortisone acetate (1%) prescribed for otorrhea (43).

Immunologic

Allergic contact dermatitis due to gentamicin is rare in patients with eyelid dermatitis, but it can occur.

- A 55-year-old housewife developed pruritic, erythematous, scaly plaques on the eyelids, spreading in a few days periorbitally after treatment with gentamicin eye-drops (Colircusi Gentamicina) (44). A positive patch test reaction to kanamycin, to which the patient had not been previously exposed, suggested cross-reactivity.

Second-Generation Effects

Teratogenicity

During pregnancy the aminoglycosides cross the placenta and they might theoretically be expected to cause otological and perhaps nephrological damage to the fetus. However, no proven cases of intrauterine damage by gentamicin have been recorded.

Susceptibility Factors

Age

In premature neonates, gentamicin clearance depends on gestational age, with a cut-off at 30 weeks: younger neonates have lower gentamicin clearance, a slightly higher volume of distribution, and a longer half-life compared with the older neonates (45). Loading doses of 3.7 and 3.5 mg/kg followed by maintenance doses of 2.8 mg/kg/day and 2.6 mg/kg/18 hours have been recommended for younger and older neonates respectively.

Drug Administration

Drug contamination

Several patients developed severe shaking chills, often accompanied by fever, tachycardia, and/or a significant reduction in systolic blood pressure within 3 hours of receiving intravenous once-daily dosing regimens of gentamicin produced by Fujisawa USA, Inc (Deerfield, Illinois). Investigations showed that gentamicin formulations that contain concentrations of endotoxin that are within the USP standards may deliver amounts of endotoxin that are above the threshold for pyrogenic reactions with once-daily dosing (46).

Of 155 patients (38% men, mean age 41 years) with pyrogenic reactions due to gentamicin, 81% received once-daily dosing (70% in a dose of 5–7 mg/kg) and 10% received a conventional dose (3 mg/kg in three divided doses (47)). Reactions typically occurred within 3 hours after infusion (98%) and lasted for less than 3 hours (96%). Patients reported chills, shaking, or shivering (75%), rigors (23%), fever (68%), tachycardia (17%), hypertension or hypotension (17%), and respiratory symptoms (47%). More serious reactions also occurred, including cyanosis (4%), oxygen saturation below 80% (7%), and pulmonary edema (one patient); 8% had severe reactions leading to hospitalization (with intubation, resuscitation, or admission to the intensive care unit in five cases), but none died. An FDA investigation showed that 10% of gentamicin lots tested had raised endotoxin concentrations, and an additional 4% of the lots would have exposed a patient to concentrations above the acceptable threshold with once-daily dosing. The two products implicated in these clusters involved the same supplier of bulk gentamicin; inadequacies in manufacturing practices had led to an increase in overall impurities (48,49).

Drug dosage regimens

Once-daily regimens are appealing for cost saving and may have a therapeutic advantage and reduced toxicity. A prolonged distribution time has been noted with high-dose gentamicin (7 mg/kg). Higher doses are used for extended-interval aminoglycoside therapy. In 12 healthy volunteers receiving extended-interval high-dose gentamicin, sampling within 90 minutes after the start of the infusion provided information that led to overestimation of peak serum concentration/minimum inhibitory concentration and inaccurate pharmacokinetic calculations (50).

Although once-daily dosing appears to be effective in limited studies in children, its role in Gram-positive coccal endocarditis, in individuals with neutropenia or cystic fibrosis, and in individuals with altered volumes of distribution remains uncertain (51).

In 18 patients receiving empirical therapy for CAPD-related peritonitis, once-daily intraperitoneal gentamicin (0.6 mg/kg) had less therapeutic benefit and peak serum gentamicin concentrations were lower than the suggested value of 4 μg/ml, whereas trough serum gentamicin concentrations were higher than the minimum toxic concentration; dialysate gentamicin concentrations were higher than therapeutic concentrations for only 4.75 hours of each day (52).

In 45 neonates (53) and 123 older children (54) gentamicin 4–5 mg/kg once a day produced peak concentrations associated with greater efficacy and trough concentrations associated with less toxicity than 2.0–2.5 mg/kg bd.

In febrile neutropenic episodes after intensive chemotherapy, once-daily gentamicin (7 mg/kg/day) in combination with azlocillin was more effective than a multiple-daily dosing regimen, but the incidence of toxicity was low overall and was slightly but not significantly higher in the once-daily group (55).

For external otitis, therapeutic local antibiotic concentrations can be achieved by giving gentamicin ear-drops twice daily; more frequent administration is not needed (56).

Drug administration route

Oral administration of gentamicin in low dosages to reduce the intestinal flora is rarely practiced, although it is probably as effective as neomycin. In the presence of intestinal mucosal inflammation more than 10% of the dose can be absorbed.

Endotracheal administration of gentamicin can be used in patients with a tracheotomy. This route of administration does not produce toxic plasma concentrations, but in patients with renal insufficiency the absorption of a certain amount via the respiratory tract should be taken into account.

Topical application of gentamicin to large areas of burns has caused ototoxic effects, ranging from mild to severe loss of hearing, with decrease of vestibular function (57). Positional vertigo occurred in one patient (58). In another case a woman complained of tinnitus each time she treated her paronychia with gentamicin cream (59).

Intrathecal gentamicin can cause neurotoxic lesions (60).

Increased penetration of gentamicin through a thin sclera can lead to toxic concentrations of the drug in a localized area adjacent to the site of injection, as has been shown in rabbits (61). These toxic effects are also influenced by the degree of pigmentation and acute inflammation. In a case of accidental injection of gentamicin 20 mg into the vitreous in a 70-year-old man during vitrectomy, no toxic signs occurred after the operation (62).

There is uncertainty about the risk of ototoxicity after the topical administration of aminoglycosides into the ear when the indication was appropriate (63,64). Nine cases of iatrogenic topical vestibulotoxicity have been reported (65). All had used ear-drops containing gentamicin sulfate and betamethasone sodium phosphate for prolonged periods. Toxicity was primarily vestibular rather than cochlear. Although compensation occurred in unilateral cases, the disability in bilateral cases was typically severe and often resulted in litigation.

Drug overdose

Although aminoglycoside antibiotics are dialysable, peritoneal dialysis may not remove them from the blood after overdosage. However, hemodialysis is effective (66).

Drug–Drug Interactions

Beta-lactam antibiotics

Gentamicin and other aminoglycosides have increased activity when they are combined with beta-lactams, resulting in increased bacterial aminoglycoside uptake (33). The proposed mechanism of synergism is damage to the cell membrane by the beta-lactam, followed by improved diffusion of gentamicin across the outer bacterial membrane. A second type of synergism, pharmacodynamic synergism, occurs when high serum concentrations of aminoglycosides cause efficient bacterial killing, resulting in reduced bacterial concentrations, which are more effectively eliminated by beta-lactams, as they work more efficiently against lower bacterial concentrations. The action of gentamicin is inhibited by some antimicrobials, which are bacteriostatic rather than bactericidal; for example antagonism occurs with macrolides, tetracycline and doxycycline, and chloramphenicol. The clinical significance of this antagonism is unknown.

There are many reports of acute renal insufficiency from combined treatment with gentamicin and one of the cephalosporins (67–69). The potential nephrotoxic effect of this combination seems to be related mainly to the nephrotoxic effect of gentamicin.

Methylthioninium chloride

Gentamicin is synergistic with methylthioninium chloride (methylene blue) in vitro against *P. aeruginosa* (70).

Metronidazole

In guinea-pigs, metronidazole augmented gentamicin-induced ototoxicity, determined by the measurement of compound action potentials (71).

NSAIDs

Aminoglycosides used in combination with non-steroidal anti-inflammatory drugs can be associated with renal insufficiency.

- An adolescent with cystic fibrosis developed renal insufficiency and severe vestibular toxicity after treatment with gentamicin and standard-dose ibuprofen (72). A low intravascular volume was a possible contributing factor.

Monitoring Therapy

During multiple-daily dosing regimens peak serum concentrations of gentamicin over 5–7 μg/ml are associated with improved survival in patients with septicemia and pneumonia caused by Gram-negative bacteria (73,74). On the other hand, excessive peak concentrations (over 10–12 μg/ml) and trough concentrations (over 2 μg/ml) of gentamicin increase the risk of ototoxicity and nephrotoxicity (75).

Salivary sampling is of potential interest in monitoring drug therapy, especially in children. Although there was no correlation between serum gentamicin concentrations and salivary concentrations when gentamicin was given two or three times daily in children with uncomplicated infections, there was a good correlation after once-daily dosing (76).

References

1. Gan IM, van Dissel JT, Beekhuis WH, Swart W, van Meurs JC. Intravitreal vancomycin and gentamicin concentrations in patients with postoperative endophthalmitis. Br J Ophthalmol 2001;85(11):1289–93.
2. Quaranta A, Scaringi A, Aloidi A, Quaranta N, Salonna I. Intratympanic therapy for Menière's disease: effect of administration of low concentration of gentamicin. Acta Otolaryngol 2001;121(3):387–92.
3. Carapetis JR, Jaquiery AL, Buttery JP, Starr M, Cranswick NE, Kohn S, Hogg GG, Woods S, Grimwood K. Randomized, controlled trial comparing once daily and three times daily gentamicin in children with urinary tract infections. Pediatr Infect Dis J 2001;20(3):240–6.
4. Melani AS, Di Gregorio A. Acute respiratory failure due to gentamicin aerosolization. Monaldi Arch Chest Dis 1998;53(3):274–6.
5. Haase KK, Lapointe M, Haines SJ. Aseptic meningitis after intraventricular administration of gentamicin. Pharmacotherapy 2001;21(1):103–7.
6. Dayal VS, Chait GE, Fenton SS. Gentamicin vestibulotoxicity. Long term disability. Ann Otol Rhinol Laryngol 1979;88(1 Pt 1):36–9.
7. Waterston JA, Halmagyi GM. Unilateral vestibulotoxicity due to systemic gentamicin therapy. Acta Otolaryngol 1998;118(4):474–8.
8. Wooltorton E. Ototoxic effects from gentamicin ear drops. CMAJ 2002;167(1):56.
9. Longridge NS, Mallinson AI, Denton A. Visual vestibular mismatch in patients treated with intratympanic gentamicin for Meniere's disease. J Otolaryngol 2002;31(1):5–8.
10. Kaplan DM, Nedzelski JM, Al-Abidi A, Chen JM, Shipp DB. Hearing loss following intratympanic instillation of gentamicin for the treatment of unilateral Menière's disease. J Otolaryngol 2002;31(2):106–11.
11. Bath AP, Walsh RM, Bance ML, Rutka JA. Ototoxicity of topical gentamicin preparations. Laryngoscope 1999;109(7 Pt 1):1088–93.
12. Papa V, Aragona P, Scuderi AC, Blanco AR, Zola P, Di BA, Santocono M, Milazzo G. Treatment of acute bacterial conjunctivitis with topical netilmicin. Cornea 2002;21(1):43–7.
13. Ali BH, Mousa HM. Effect of dimethyl sulfoxide on gentamicin-induced nephrotoxicity in rats. Hum Exp Toxicol 2001;20(4):199–203.
14. Jin X, Jin X, Sheng X. Methylcobalamin as antagonist to transient ototoxic action of gentamicin. Acta Otolaryngol 2001;121(3):351–4.
15. Kane FJ. Jr., Byrd G. Acute toxic psychosis associated with gentamicin therapy. South Med J 1975;68(10):1283–5.
16. Kes P, Reiner Z. Symptomatic hypomagnesemia associated with gentamicin therapy. Magnes Trace Elem 1990;9(1):54–60.
17. Mor F, Leibovici L, Cohen O, Wysenbeek AJ. Prospective evaluation of liver function tests in patients treated with aminoglycosides. DICP 1990;24(2):135–7.
18. Luft FC, Yum MN, Kleit SA. Comparative nephrotoxicities of netilmicin and gentamicin in rats. Antimicrob Agents Chemother 1976;10(5):845–9.
19. Hottendorf GH, Gordon LL. Comparative low-dose nephrotoxicities of gentamicin, tobramycin, and amikacin. Antimicrob Agents Chemother 1980;18(1):176–81.
20. Cone LA. A survey of prospective, controlled clinical trials of gentamicin, tobramycin, amikacin, and netilmicin. Clin Ther 1982;5(2):155–62.
21. Smith CR, Baughman KL, Edwards CQ, Rogers JF, Lietman PS. Controlled comparison of amikacin and gentamicin. N Engl J Med 1977;296(7):349–53.
22. Feld R, Valdivieso M, Bodey GP, Rodriguez V. Comparison of amikacin and tobramycin in the treatment of infection in patients with cancer. J Infect Dis 1977;135(1):61–6.
23. Love LJ, Schimpff SC, Hahn DM, Young VM, Standiford HC, Bender JF, Fortner CL, Wiernik PH. Randomized trial of empiric antibiotic therapy with ticarcillin in combination with gentamicin, amikacin or netilmicin in febrile patients with granulocytopenia and cancer. Am J Med 1979;66(4):603–10.
24. Lau WK, Young LS, Black RE, Winston DJ, Linne SR, Weinstein RJ, Hewitt WL. Comparative efficacy and toxicity of amikacin/carbenicillin versus gentamicin/carbenicillin in leukopenic patients: a randomized prospective trail. Am J Med 1977;62(6):959–66.
25. Fong IW, Fenton RS, Bird R. Comparative toxicity of gentamicin versus tobramycin: a randomized prospective study. J Antimicrob Chemother 1981;7(1):81–8.
26. Bock BV, Edelstein PH, Meyer RD. Prospective comparative study of efficacy and toxicity of netilmicin and amikacin. Antimicrob Agents Chemother 1980;17(2):217–25.
27. Barza M, Lauermann MW, Tally FP, Gorbach SL. Prospective, randomized trial of netilmicin and amikacin, with emphasis on eighth-nerve toxicity. Antimicrob Agents Chemother 1980;17(4):707–14.
28. Smith CR, Lipsky JJ, Laskin OL, Hellmann DB, Mellits ED, Longstreth J, Lietman PS. Double-blind comparison of the nephrotoxicity and auditory toxicity of gentamicin and tobramycin. N Engl J Med 1980;302(20):1106–9.
29. Matzke GR, Lucarotti RL, Shapiro HS. Controlled comparison of gentamicin and tobramycin nephrotoxicity. Am J Nephrol 1983;3(1):11–17.
30. Russo JC, Adelman RD. Gentamicin-induced Fanconi syndrome. J Pediatr 1980;96(1):151–3.
31. Wellwood JM, Tighe JR. Proceedings: Evidence of gentamicin nephrotoxicity in patients with renal allografts. Br J Surg 1975;62(2):156.
32. Termeer A, Hoitsma AJ, Koene RA. Severe nephrotoxicity caused by the combined use of gentamicin and cyclosporine in renal allograft recipients. Transplantation 1986;42(2):220–1.
33. Santucci RA, Krieger JN. Gentamicin for the practicing urologist: review of efficacy, single daily dosing and "switch" therapy. J Urol 2000;163(4):1076–84.
34. Ozbek E, Turkoz Y, Sahna E, Ozugurlu F, Mizrak B, Ozbek M. Melatonin administration prevents the nephrotoxicity induced by gentamicin. BJU Int 2000;85(6):742–6.
35. Solgaard L, Tuxoe JI, Mafi M, Due Olsen S, Toftgaard Jensen T. Nephrotoxicity by dicloxacillin and gentamicin in 163 patients with intertrochanteric hip fractures. Int Orthop 2000;24(3):155–7.
36. van Raaij TM, Visser LE, Vulto AG, Verhaar JA. Acute renal failure after local gentamicin treatment in an infected total knee arthroplasty. J Arthroplasty 2002;17(7):948–50.
37. Fogo AB. Quiz page. Mesangial lupus nephritis, WHO IIb, and severe acute tubular necrosis, secondary to gentamycin toxicity. Am J Kidney Dis 2002;40(5):xlix.
38. Vaidyanathan S, Watt JW, Singh G, Soni BM, Sett P. Dosage of once-daily gentamicin in spinal cord injury patients. Spinal Cord 2000;38(3):197–8.
39. Sener G, Sehirli AO, Altunbas HZ, Ersoy Y, Paskaloglu K, Arbak S, Ayanoglu-Dulger G. Melatonin protects against gentamicin-induced nephrotoxicity in rats. J Pineal Res 2002;32(4):231–6.

40. Reiter RJ, Tan DX, Sainz RM, Mayo JC, Lopez-Burillo S. Melatonin: reducing the toxicity and increasing the efficacy of drugs. J Pharm Pharmacol 2002;54(10):1299–321.
41. Kopple JD, Ding H, Letoha A, Ivanyi B, Qing DP, Dux L, Wang HY, Sonkodi S. L-carnitine ameliorates gentamicin-induced renal injury in rats. Nephrol Dial Transplant 2002;17(12):2122–31.
42. Narendra A, White MP, Rolton HA, Alloub ZI, Wilkinson G, McColl JH, Beattie J. Nephrocalcinosis in preterm babies. Arch Dis Child Fetal Neonatal Ed 2001;85(3):F207–13.
43. Siddiq MA. Erythema multiforme after application of aural Gentisone HC drops. J Laryngol Otol 1999;113(11):1002–3.
44. Sanchez-Perez J, Lopez MP, De Vega Haro JM, Garcia-Diez A. Allergic contact dermatitis from gentamicin in eye-drops, with cross-reactivity to kanamycin but not neomycin. Contact Dermatitis 2001;44(1):54.
45. Rocha MJ, Almeida AM, Afonso E, Martins V, Santos J, Leitao F, Falcao AC. The kinetic profile of gentamicin in premature neonates. J Pharm Pharmacol 2000;52(9):1091–7.
46. Centers for Disease Control and Prevention (CDC). Endotoxin-like reactions associated with intravenous gentamicin—California, 1998. MMWR Morb Mortal Wkly Rep 1998;47(41):877–80.
47. Fanning MM, Wassel R, Piazza-Hepp T. Pyrogenic reactions to gentamicin therapy. N Engl J Med 2000;343(22):1658–9.
48. Chuck SK, Raber SR, Rodvold KA, Areff D. National survey of extended-interval aminoglycoside dosing. Clin Infect Dis 2000;30(3):433–9.
49. Buchholz U, Richards C, Murthy R, Arduino M, Pon D, Schwartz W, Fontanilla E, Pegues C, Boghossian N, Peterson C, Kool J, Mascola L, Jarvis WR. Pyrogenic reactions associated with single daily dosing of intravenous gentamicin. Infect Control Hosp Epidemiol 2000;21(12):771–4.
50. McNamara DR, Nafziger AN, Menhinick AM, Bertino JS. Jr. A dose-ranging study of gentamicin pharmacokinetics: implications for extended interval aminoglycoside therapy. J Clin Pharmacol 2001;41(4):374–7.
51. The ARDS Network. Ketoconazole for early treatment of acute lung injury and acute respiratory distress syndrome: a randomized controlled trial. JAMA 2000;283(15):1995–2002.
52. Tosukhowong T, Eiam-Ong S, Thamutok K, Wittayalertpanya S, Na Ayudhya DP. Pharmacokinetics of intraperitoneal cefazolin and gentamicin in empiric therapy of peritonitis in continuous ambulatory peritoneal dialysis patients. Perit Dial Int 2001;21(6):587–94.
53. Chotigeat U, Narongsanti A, Ayudhya DP. Gentamicin in neonatal infection: once versus twice daily dosage. J Med Assoc Thai 2001;84(8):1109–15.
54. Robinson RF, Nahata MC. Safety of intravenous bolus administration of gentamicin in pediatric patients. Ann Pharmacother 2001;35(11):1327–31.
55. Bakri FE, Pallett A, Smith AG, Duncombe AS. Once-daily versus multiple-daily gentamicin in empirical antibiotic therapy of febrile neutropenia following intensive chemotherapy. J Antimicrob Chemother 2000;45(3):383–6.
56. Rakover Y, Smuskovitz A, Colodner R, Keness Y, Rosen G. Duration of antibacterial effectiveness of gentamicin ear drops in external otitis. J Laryngol Otol 2000;114(11):827–9.
57. Dayal VS, Smith EL, McCain WG. Cochlear and vestibular gentamicin toxicity. A clinical study of systemic and topical usage. Arch Otolaryngol 1974;100(5):338–40.
58. Leliever WC. Topical gentamicin-induced positional vertigo. Otolaryngol Head Neck Surg 1985;93(4):553–5.
59. Drake TE. Letter: Reaction to gentamicin sulfate cream. Arch Dermatol 1974;110(4):638.
60. Watanabe I, Hodges GR, Dworzack DL, Kepes JJ, Duensing GF. Neurotoxicity of intrathecal gentamicin: a case report and experimental study. Ann Neurol 1978;4(6):564–72.
61. Loewenstein A, Zemel E, Vered Y, Lazar M, Perlman I. Retinal toxicity of gentamicin after subconjunctival injection performed adjacent to thinned sclera. Ophthalmology 2001;108(4):759–64.
62. Burgansky Z, Rock T, Bartov E. Inadvertent intravitreal gentamicin injection. Eur J Ophthalmol 2002;12(2):138–40.
63. Indudharan R. Ototopic aminoglycosides and ototoxicity. J Otolaryngol 1998;27(3):182.
64. Walby P, Stewart R, Kerr AG. Aminoglycoside ear drop ototoxicity: a topical dilemma? Clin Otolaryngol Allied Sci 1998;23(4):289–90.
65. Marais J, Rutka JA. Ototoxicity and topical eardrops. Clin Otolaryngol Allied Sci 1998;23(4):360–7.
66. Lu CM, James SH, Lien YH. Acute massive gentamicin intoxication in a patient with end-stage renal disease. Am J Kidney Dis 1996;28(5):767–71.
67. Bailey RR. Renal failure in combined gentamicin and cephalothin therapy. BMJ 1973;2(5869):776–7.
68. Cabanillas F, Burgos RC, Rodriguez C, Baldizon C. Nephrotoxicity of combined cephalothin–gentamicin regimen. Arch Intern Med 1975;135(6):850–2.
69. Tobias JS, Whitehouse JM, Wrigley PF. Letter: Severe renal dysfunction after tobramycin/cephalothin therapy. Lancet 1976;1(7956):425.
70. Gunics G, Motohashi N, Amaral L, Farkas S, Molnar J. Interaction between antibiotics and non-conventional antibiotics on bacteria. Int J Antimicrob Agents 2000; 14(3):239–42.
71. Riggs LC, Shofner WP, Shah AR, Young MR, Hain TC, Matz GJ. Ototoxicity resulting from combined administration of metronidazole and gentamicin. Am J Otol 1999; 20(4):430–4.
72. Scott CS, Retsch-Bogart GZ, Henry MM. Renal failure and vestibular toxicity in an adolescent with cystic fibrosis receiving gentamicin and standard-dose ibuprofen. Pediatr Pulmonol 2001;31(4):314–16.
73. Moore RD, Smith CR, Lietman PS. The association of aminoglycoside plasma levels with mortality in patients with Gram-negative bacteremia. J Infect Dis 1984;149(3):443–8.
74. Moore RD, Smith CR, Lietman PS. Association of aminoglycoside plasma levels with therapeutic outcome in Gram-negative pneumonia. Am J Med 1984;77(4):657–62.
75. Wenk M, Vozeh S, Follath F. Serum level monitoring of antibacterial drugs. A review. Clin Pharmacokinet 1984; 9(6):475–92.
76. Berkovitch M, Goldman M, Silverman R, Chen-Levi Z, Greenberg R, Marcus O, Lahat E. Therapeutic drug monitoring of once daily gentamicin in serum and saliva of children. Eur J Pediatr 2000;159(9):697–8.

Gentianaceae

See also Herbal medicines

General Information

The genera in the family of Gentianaceae (Table 1) include centaury and various types of gentian.

Gentiana species

Gentiana (gentian) root is mutagenic in bacteria, which is due to the xanthone derivatives, gentisin and isogentisin. In experimental animals *Gentiana olivieri* is

Table 1 The genera of Gentianaceae

Bartonia (screwstem)
Centaurium (centaury)
Cicendia (cicendia)
Enicostema (whitehead)
Eustoma (prairie gentian)
Frasera (green gentian)
Gentiana (gentian)
Gentianella (dwarf gentian)
Gentianopsis (fringed gentian)
Halenia (spurred gentian)
Lisianthius (lisianthius)
Lomatogonium (lomatogonium)
Obolaria (obolaria)
Sabatia (rose gentian)
Schultesia (wingcup)
Swertia (felwort)
Voyria (ghostplant)

hypoglycemic, an effect that has been attributed to isoorientin, which is present in several species of *Gentiana* (1) and which also has antinociceptive and anti-inflammatory effects in animals (2). Some species of *Gentiana* inhibit monoamine oxidase (3) and acetylcholinesterase (4) in vitro.

Gentian violet is a purple dye that is obtained from coal tar; it is so called because its color resembles that of the flower and it has nothing to do with *Gentiana* species.

Swertia species

Swertia species (felwort) are mutagenic in bacteria, because of the several xanthone derivatives that it contains. The clinical relevance of this remains to be established. They also have hypoglycemic effects in animals (5).

References

1. Sezik E, Aslan M, Yesilada E, Ito S. Hypoglycaemic activity of *Gentiana olivieri* and isolation of the active constituent through bioassay-directed fractionation techniques. Life Sci 2005;76(11):1223–38.
2. Kupeli E, Aslan M, Gurbuz I, Yesilada E. Evaluation of in vivo biological activity profile of isoorientin. Z Naturforsch [C] 2004;59(11–12):787–90.
3. Haraguchi H, Tanaka Y, Kabbash A, Fujioka T, Ishizu T, Yagi A. Monoamine oxidase inhibitors from *Gentiana lutea*. Phytochemistry 2004;65(15):2255–60.
4. Urbain A, Marston A, Queiroz EF, Ndjoko K, Hostettmann K. Xanthones from *Gentiana campestris* as new acetylcholinesterase inhibitors. Planta Med 2004; 70(10):1011–14.
5. Grover JK, Yadav S, Vats V. Medicinal plants of India with anti-diabetic potential. J Ethnopharmacol 2002; 81(1):81–100.

Germanium

General Information

Germanium is a metallic element (symbol Ge; atomic no. 32) that is found as the sulfide in the mineral argyrodite.

In several countries, organic or inorganic germanium has acquired a remarkable reputation in self-medication as a widely useful prophylactic and therapeutic agent, but with little scientific evidence to support it. Some germanium compounds, particularly spirogermanium, do have certain immunoregulatory activities, but germanium itself does not seem to play a role in this. There has been some attempt to use germanium in cancer chemotherapy. The unsupervised use of germanium-containing "health products" is of particular concern. Finally, there may be non-medicinal exposure, for example from some semiconductors.

Renal and other organ failure has been caused by germanium intoxication.

Organs and Systems

Nervous system

Nephropathy and neuropathy have been attributed to germanium toxicity (1).

- A 53-year-old man developed severe general weakness, anorexia, and weight loss (16 kg in 3 months). Over the preceding 17 months he had taken a total of 400 g of lysine germanium oxide in powder form. After 15 months he developed a tingling sensation in the palms and soles and weakness of the limbs, especially the legs. Neurological examination showed grade IV motor strength and negative deep tendon reflexes in the legs. Laboratory tests showed impaired renal function and anemia. Urinary concentration of beta$_2$-microglobulin was raised. The blood germanium concentration was 63 ng/ml and the urine concentration 2190 ng/l (normal less than 5 ng/ml). Renal sonography showed no morphological abnormalities. Nerve conduction studies and needle electromyography suggested a sensorimotor polyneuropathy, predominantly involving sensory nerves. Renal biopsy showed tubulointerstitial nephritis. Abstinence from germanium and conservative management of the chronic renal insufficiency resulted in slight improvement of the weakness and renal function.

Urinary tract

Occupational exposure to inorganic germanium compounds can cause slightly impaired renal function (2). However, severe nephrotoxic reactions have been described, and it has become clear that these can occur both with inorganic and organic germanium compounds (SEDA-21, 235).

A 58-year-old man developed nausea, vomiting, anorexia, and weight loss (3). He had taken germanium lactate citrate, illegally purchased in a pharmacy, recommended as a natural antioxidant, anticancer, and immunostimulatory remedy. He took a total dose of 426 g orally over

6 months and developed renal insufficiency and proteinuria, implying tubular damage. His serum TSH, fasting glucose, glycosylated haemoglobin, and C-peptide were increased. Abdominal ultrasound showed normal kidneys. Cardiac ultrasound showed a pericardial effusion. An electrocardiogram showed a sinus tachycardia. Nerve conduction studies and electromyography showed pathological spontaneous muscular activity and myotonic discharge. The neural conduction velocity was normal in the median nerve and delayed in the peroneal nerve. He received intravenous nutrition, insulin, and electrolytes. The pericardial effusion regressed but the sinus tachycardia continued. The renal dysfunction and the polyneuropathy persisted.

- A middle-aged woman who had taken germanium lactate-citrate for at least a year (with an estimated cumulative dose of 32.1 g of germanium) developed renal insufficiency with a creatinine clearance of 10 ml/minute, raised creatine kinase activity, and moderately raised liver enzymes. Biopsy showed highly vacuolated cytoplasm in the epithelial cells of the distal renal tubules and microvesicular and macrovesicular steatosis of centrilobular hepatocytes. After withdrawal of the germanium the laboratory values normalized but moderately severe renal impairment persisted (SEDA-16, 231).
- A 63-year-old man developed membranous glomerulonephritis after having taken 10–12 tablets of a germanium-containing ginseng formulation about 10 days before (4). He responded to diuretic treatment and was discharged in improved condition. However, on the day after discharge he restarted his intake of the formulation; over the next 14 days, his weight increased by 12 kg and he developed worsening edema and hypertension, despite an increase in the dosage of furosemide to 240 mg bd. He was re-admitted and given intravenous furosemide (240 mg every 8 hours). The nutritional supplements were withheld and after 48 hours diuresis took effect.

While other causes may have contributed in part to this man's poor response to furosemide, the facts strongly suggest that germanium played an important role in producing a diuretic-refractory renal dysfunction in this case.

References

1. Kim KM, Lim CS, Kim S, Kim SH, Park JH, Ahn C, Han JS, Lee JS. Nephropathy and neuropathy induced by a germanium-containing compound. Nephrol Dial Transplant 1998;13(12):3218–19.
2. Swennen B, Mallants A, Roels HA, Buchet JP, Bernard A, Lauwerys RR, Lison D. Epidemiological survey of workers exposed to inorganic germanium compounds. Occup Environ Med 2000;57(4):242–8.
3. Luck BE, Mann H, Melzer H, Dunemann L, Begerow J. Renal and other organ failure caused by germanium intoxication. Nephrol Dial Transplant 1999;14(10):2464–8.
4. Becker BN, Greene J, Evanson J, Chidsey G, Stone WJ. Ginseng-induced diuretic resistance. JAMA 1996;276(8):606–7.

Ginkgoaceae

See also Herbal medicines

General Information

The family of Ginkgoaceae contains the single genus, *Ginkgo*, and a single species, *Ginkgo biloba.*

Ginkgo biloba

Ginkgo biloba (maidenhair tree, silver apricot) contains ginkgolides, which inhibit platelet-activating factor, reducing aggregability; this may contribute to bleeding disorders in patients taking *G. biloba*. *Ginkgo* has small beneficial effects in patients with intermittent claudication (1) and dementias (1,2).

Extracts from the leaves of *G. biloba* are marketed in some countries for the treatment of cerebral dysfunction and of intermittent claudication. In a review it was concluded that seven out of eight controlled trials of good quality showed positive effects of *G. biloba* compared with placebo on the following symptoms: memory difficulties, dizziness, tinnitus, headache, and emotional instability with anxiety (3). For intermittent claudication, the evidence for efficacy was judged unconvincing.

No serious adverse effects have been noted in any trial. However, *G. biloba* has been associated with gastrointestinal complaints, headache, and allergic skin reactions (SED-13, 538). Bleeding has been associated with chronic *G. biloba* ingestion because of its adverse effects on platelet aggregability, since the ginkgolide constituents of *G. biloba* inhibit platelet-activating factor.

Adverse effects

Ginkgo biloba has been associated with gastrointestinal complaints, headache, antiplatelet effects, and allergic skin reactions.

Nervous system

Ginkgo biloba can precipitate seizures in patients with well-controlled epilepsy (4).

- A 78-year-old man and an 84-year-old woman with previously well-controlled epilepsy presented with recurrent seizures (4). There were no obvious reasons for these events, and the investigator suspected self-medication with *G. biloba* extracts. Both patients had started taking *G. biloba* within 2 weeks of the start of the seizures. The herbal remedy was withdrawn and both patients remained seizure-free several months later. No other change of medication was made.

The author postulated that 4-0-methylpyridoxine, a constituent of *G. biloba* and a known neurotoxin, had caused the seizures.

Hematologic

Ginkgo biloba has well-documented antiplatelet effects, and bleeding complications can occur, including strokes.

- A 59-year-old man developed bleeding complications after liver transplantation while taking *G. biloba* supplements (5). Postoperatively, he developed large hematomas in the subphrenic space and near the porta hepatis. They were drained and his hematocrit fell to 21%. Three weeks later he complained of blurring in the right eye, and a vitreous hemorrhage was diagnosed. He then admitted to taking an unknown amount of *G. biloba*, which was withdrawn. Subsequently, no further bleeding episodes occurred.
- A 78-year-old man developed progressive right-sided muscular weakness after a fall (6). A CT scan showed a subdural hematoma. He had taken 150 mg of *G. biloba* extract.
- A 56-year-old man had a stroke without apparent risk factors (7). A CT scan confirmed a right parietal hematoma. He had not taken any medications, except for a *G. biloba* extract (3 × 40 mg/day) which he had started 18 months before.
- A 34-year-old woman had a laparoscopic cholecystectomy and started bleeding into the surgical wound postoperatively (8). This led to a fall in hemoglobin from 16.5 to 12.4 g/dl. She was given blood transfusions and recovered uneventfully.
- Hyphema led to temporarily impaired vision in a man who had taken *G. biloba* for 2 weeks; no other cause was found; the lesion regressed after withdrawal and did not recur (9).
- A spontaneous cerebellar bleed occurred in a man who had taken *G. biloba* (10).

In each case the authors believed that self-medication with *G. biloba* had caused the bleeding through its effect on platelets. In some cases another factor that implicated the extract was the absence of recurrence after withdrawal, although this is a weak argument.

Spontaneous bilateral subdural hematomas and increased bleeding time have been associated with chronic ingestion of *G. biloba* (120 mg/day for 2 years) (11).

Skin

- A 40-year-old Afro-American woman developed an exfoliative rash and blistering and swelling of the tongue (12). A diagnosis of Stevens–Johnson syndrome was made. She had not taken any medications other than two doses of a formulation that contained *G. biloba*. Her condition responded to treatment with prednisolone, clotrimazole, and famotidine. *G. biloba* was withdrawn and no further events occurred. However, 5 months later she still had tenderness in the soles of the feet, peeling of the nails, and discoloration of the skin.

Formulations

Subarachnoid hemorrhage associated with *G. biloba* (13) stimulated a vigorous discussion on the differences between the usual extract sold over the counter and a ginkgolide mixture, and their respective (absence of) effects on platelet-aggregating factor and bleeding time (14,15). The dispute points to confusion that can arise when formulations of similar origin but with variable composition are available.

Drug overdose

Acute poisoning with *G. biloba* seeds is occasionally seen in East Asian countries.

- A 36-year-old woman, without any past or family history of epilepsy, developed frequent vomiting and generalized convulsions about 4 hours after taking about 70–80 ginkgo nuts, seeds of *G. biloba*, in an attempt to improve her health (16).
- A 2-year-old girl was admitted with vomiting, diarrhea, and irritability a few hours after eating a large quantity of *G. biloba* seeds and then developed an afebrile generalized clonic seizure (17). Her serum concentration of 4-methoxypyridoxine, the putative toxic agent in the seed, was extremely high at 360 ng/ml.

Administration of pyridoxal phosphate, a competitive antagonist of 4-methoxypyridoxine, which inhibits the formation of gamma-aminobutyric acid (GABA), prevented further seizures in this case.

Drug interactions

Because of its antiplatelet activity *G. biloba* can interact with anticoagulants.

- A 78-year-old woman who had taken warfarin for 5 years, took *G. biloba* for 2 months, when she developed signs of a stroke, diagnosed as intracerebral hemorrhage (13).

Even though it is impossible to establish causality in this case, it is conceivable that the stroke was the result of over-anticoagulation induced by the herbal medication (11).

References

1. Pittler MH, Ernst E. *Ginkgo biloba* extract for the treatment of intermittent claudication: a meta-analysis of randomized trials. Am J Med 2000;108(4):276–81.
2. Oken BS, Storzbach DM, Kaye JA. The efficacy of *Ginkgo biloba* on cognitive function in Alzheimer disease. Arch Neurol 1998;55(11):1409–15.
3. Kleijnen J, Knipschild P. *Ginkgo biloba*. Lancet 1992;340(8828):1136–9.
4. Granger AS. *Ginkgo biloba* precipitating epileptic seizures. Age Ageing 2001;30(6):523–5.
5. Hauser D, Gayowski T, Singh N. Bleeding complications precipitated by unrecognized *Ginkgo biloba* use after liver transplantation. Transpl Int 2002;15(7):377–9.
6. Miller LG, Freeman B. Possible subdural hematoma associated with *Ginkgo biloba*. J Herb Pharmacother 2002;2(2):57–63.
7. Benjamin J, Muir T, Briggs K, Pentland B. A case of cerebral haemorrhage—can *Ginkgo biloba* be implicated? Postgrad Med J 2001;77(904):112–13.
8. Fessenden JM, Wittenborn W, Clarke L. *Ginkgo biloba*: a case report of herbal medicine and bleeding postoperatively from a laparoscopic cholecystectomy. Am Surg 2001;67(1): 33–5.
9. Schneider C, Bord C, Misse P, Arnaud B, Schmitt-Bernard CF. Hyphéma spontané provoqué par l'extrait de *Ginkgo biloba*. [Spontaneous hyphema caused by *Ginkgo biloba* extract.] J Fr Ophtalmol 2002;25(7): 731–2.
10. Purroy Garcia F, Molina C, Alvarez Sabin J. Hemorragia cerebelosa esponetanea asociada a la ingestion de *Ginkgo*

biloba. [Spontaneous cerebellar haemorrhage associated with *Ginkgo biloba* ingestion.] Med Clin (Barc) 2002;119(15):596–7.
11. Rowin J, Lewis SL. Spontaneous bilateral subdural hematomas associated with chronic *Ginkgo biloba* ingestion. Neurology 1996;46(6):1775–6.
12. Davydov L, Stirling AL. Stevens–Johnson syndrome with *Ginkgo biloba*. J Herb Pharmacother 2001;1:65–9.
13. Vale S. Subarachnoid haemorrhage associated with *Ginkgo biloba*. Lancet 1998;352(9121):36.
14. Skogh M. Extracts of *Ginkgo biloba* and bleeding or haemorrhage. Lancet 1998;352(9134):1145–6.
15. Vale S. Reply. Lancet 1998;352(9134):1146.
16. Miwa H, Iijima M, Tanaka S, Mizuno Y. Generalized convulsions after consuming a large amount of gingko nuts. Epilepsia 2001;42(2):280–1.
17. Kajiyama Y, Fujii K, Takeuchi H, Manabe Y. Ginkgo seed poisoning. Pediatrics 2002;109(2):325–7.

Glafenine

See also Non-steroidal anti-inflammatory drugs

General Information

Glafenine, an anthranilic acid derivative, has been withdrawn in much of the world (1). Until 1991 it was sold in about 70 countries (although never marketed or accepted in others), despite a long history of severe reactions (particularly anaphylaxis, fatal hepatotoxicity, and nephrotoxicity, even with normal doses). As late as 1989 the EC Committee on Proprietary Medicinal Products (CPMP) astonishingly recommended keeping glafenine on the market but controlling its distribution and monitoring adverse effects more closely (2). Firm restrictions or prohibitions nevertheless preceded or followed this recommendation in several European countries, and the CPMP finally condemned glafenine early in 1992. See also floctafenine.

Organs and Systems

Cardiovascular

A rise in blood pressure coupled with renal adverse effects has been reported. Coronary artery spasm leading to myocardial infarction was described as part of an allergic reaction with Quincke's edema (SED-11, 190) (3).

Hematologic

Acute hemolytic anemia, probably as part of an allergic reaction (SED-9, 154) (4,5), leukopenia through an unknown mechanism, and thrombocytopenic purpura with hemorrhage have been documented (6).

Liver

Liver injury has repeatedly been described in patients taking glafenine (SEDA-4, 69) (SEDA-5, 106), with fatal hepatotoxicity as part of a general toxic reaction in several cases (7). Glafenine-associated hepatic injury is characterized by a high prevalence of jaundice, a high death rate, and a predominantly hepatocellular histological pattern of liver lesions, varying from spotty panlobular, centrilobular, and submassive necrosis (acute pattern) to fibrosis and cirrhosis (chronic pattern) (8).

Biliary tract

Gallstones containing glafenic acid have been reported in a patient taking long-term therapy (SEDA-14, 95).

Urinary tract

Many nephrotoxic features have been observed in preclinical and clinical studies of glafenine in therapeutic doses and more especially in overdosage (SEDA-4, 69). Acute oliguria, anuria, increased blood urea and creatinine, proteinuria, and raised blood pressure have been repeatedly reported. Glafenine stones have been documented in five patients (9).

Musculoskeletal

Symptoms of rhabdomyolysis, associated with other disorders, occurred in two patients a few hours after glafenine (10).

Immunologic

Although rash has sometimes occurred (11), hypersensitivity reactions have been much more serious. Many acute anaphylactic reactions have been observed (SEDA-4, 69) (SEDA-6, 98) (12,13), with shock in more than 50% of cases; it was recorded in 24 of 1517 reports on the drug collected by the Pharmacovigilance Unit in Lyons, France (11). Occasional isolated fever, confirmed by rechallenge (14), is probably also of hypersensitive origin. Interstitial nephritis, hepatitis, and pulmonary hypersensitivity have been reported.

Drug–Drug Interactions

Methotrexate

An interaction of glafenine with methotrexate has been described in a patient with rheumatoid arthritis (SEDA-14, 95).

References

1. Anonymous. Withdrawal of glafenine. Lancet 1992;339:357.
2. Herxheimer A. Belgium: withdrawal of glafenine. Lancet 1991;337:102.
3. Weber S, Genevray B, Pasquier G, Chapsal J, Bonnin A, Degeorges M. Severe coronary spasm during drug-induced immediate hypersensitivity reaction. Lancet 1982;2(8302):821.
4. Mallein R, Boucherat M, Rondelet J, Fillastre JP, Mantel O. Pharmacocinétique de la glafénine chez des sujets ayant une fonction rénale normale et chez des malades atteints d'insuffisance rénale chronique. [Pharmacokinetics of glaphenine in subjects with normal renal function and in patients with chronic renal insufficiency.] Therapie 1976;31(6):739–45.
5. Grand A, Despret P. Choc anaphylactique inuit par la glafenine. [Anaphylactic shock induced by glafenine.] Nouv Presse Méd 1973;2(16):1075.

6. Bosset JF, Perriguey G, Rozenbaum A, Leconte Des Floris R. Thrombopénie aiguë récidivante après prise de glafénine: une observation. [Recurrent acute thrombopenia after glaphenine. 1 case.] Nouv Presse Méd 1979;8(19):1606.
7. Ypma RT, Festen JJ, De Bruin CD. Hepatotoxicity of glafenine. Lancet 1978;2(8087):480–1.
8. Stricker BH, Blok AP, Bronkhorst FB. Glafenine-associated hepatic injury. Analysis of 38 cases and review of the literature. Liver 1986;6(2):63–72.
9. Daudon M, Protat MF, Reveillaud RJ. Toxicité rénale de la glafénine chez l'homme: calculs rénaux et insuffisance rénale aiguë. [Renal toxicity of glafenine in man: renal stones and acute renal failure.] Ann Biol Clin (Paris) 1983;41(2):105–11.
10. Rouveix B, Benhamed S, Regnier B. Rhabdomyolyse et glafénine. [Rhabdomyolysis and glafenine.] Therapie 1984;39(1):53–4.
11. Descotes J, Lery N, Vigneau C, Loupi E, Evreux JC. Bilan des effets secondaires dus a la glafénine au Centre de Pharmacovigilance de Lyon. [Overview of glafenin side-effects from the experience of Lyon Pharmacovigilance Unit.] Therapie 1980;35(3):405–8.
12. Stricker BH, de Groot RR, Wilson JH. Anaphylaxis to glafenine. Lancet 1990;336(8720):943–4.
13. Stricker BH, de Groot RR, Wilson JH. Glafenine-associated anaphylaxis as a cause of hospital admission in The Netherlands. Eur J Clin Pharmacol 1991;40(4):367–71.
14. Garre M, Youinou P, Burtin C, Rolland J, Deraedt R. Fièvre isolée: effet secondaire singulier de la glafénine. [Isolated fever: an unusual side effect of glafenine.] Therapie 1980;35(6):752–3.

Glaucine

General Information

Glaucine is a non-narcotic antitussive agent. The D-isomer of glaucine is an alkaloid from *Glaucium flavum Crantz*, a species of Papaveraceae. It is better tolerated in doses claimed to be equieffective with codeine. Glaucine (30 mg capsules 3 times daily for 28 days) caused mild constipation in five patients (1).

Reference

1. Gastpar H, Criscuolo D, Dieterich HA. Efficacy and tolerability of glaucine as an antitussive agent. Curr Med Res Opin 1984;9(1):21–7.

Glucagon

General Information

Glucagon, which is produced in the alpha cells of the islets of Langerhans, is used in diabetes mellitus type 1 to stimulate glucose output from the liver during hypoglycemia (1 mg subcutaneously, repeated once or twice) when glucose cannot be given intravenously. In some countries it is often used by personnel, such as family members, who are not medically qualified, as the first action when the patient cannot take sugar orally. The antihypoglycemic effect of an intramuscular injection is longer lasting and more potent than that of intravenous glucagon (1). It is sometimes given by infusion to treat chronic hypoglycemia. However, when there is insulin reserve in the pancreas, glucagon induces hypoglycemia by stimulating insulin release (2).

Glucagon has also been used to stimulate insulin and C-peptide secretion, to see whether the islets still produce insulin, as a stimulatory test during pheochromocytoma, hyperinsulinism, and Zollinger–Ellison syndrome, or as an additive in upper gastrointestinal X-ray investigations (0.5–1 mg). It has been used in myocardial infarction, although its inotropic effects may present a risk. It has also been used to treat overdoses with beta-blockers (3) and calcium channel blockers (4), although its efficacy in such cases has only been demonstrated in animals (5) and to treat overdose with tricyclic antidepressants (6,7).

During long-term administration glucagon can cause the same effects as a glucagonoma: hyperglycemia, necrolytic migratory erythema, weight loss, anemia, angular cheilitis, and venous thrombosis (8).

Organs and Systems

Cardiovascular

Glucagon has been reported to have caused myocardial ischemia (9).

Metabolism

When there is insulin reserve in the pancreas, glucagon can cause hypoglycemia by stimulating insulin secretion.

Electrolyte balance

Hyponatremia can occur during long-term administration of glucagon (10).

Hematologic

Thrombocytopenia can occur during long-term administration of glucagon (10).

Gastrointestinal

Glucagon can cause nausea, vomiting, and diarrhea (11).

Skin

Chronic administration of glucagon can cause an eczema-like maculopapular scaly rash, which can progress to necrolytic migratory erythema, as in glucagonoma (8,12,13). Erythema multiforme has also been reported (14).

Glucagon, used to treat persistent hyperinsulinemic hypoglycemia of infancy, caused erythema necrolyticum migrans in two neonates (15).

- In the first child, a monozygotic twin girl, delivered at 30 weeks, diazoxide, chlorothiazide, and nifedipine did not alter glucose requirements, but octreotide halved the need, and intravenous glucagon lowered it further. However, the child then developed a maculopapular rash on the face and trunk. After 4 weeks the lesions worsened, increased in size, and became superficially necrosed with thick-caked scales. The rash also involved the limbs and mucous membranes, making feeding almost impossible. When glucagon was withdrawn the skin lesions resolved from the center within 2 days and disappeared without scarring in 10 days.
- The second child, who was delivered at term, had a blood glucose of 0.8 mmol/l 6 hours after birth and suffered a seizure that was treated with subcutaneous glucagon, octreotide, and other drugs. It was impossible to give sufficient feeding, and notwithstanding subcutaneous glucagon 11 micrograms/kg/hour and octreotide 4.3 micrograms/kg/hour, she had a generalized seizure when the blood glucose was 1.4 mmol/l. At 6 months, subtotal pancreatectomy was performed. During glucagon therapy she had seborrheic skin with silvery scales and on the thoracic skin an area of pale lichenification with mild hyperkeratosis. Within 2 weeks after surgery (and withdrawal of glucagon) the skin became totally normal.

Susceptibility Factors

Age

Hypoglycemia often occurs in premature children and can usually be treated by intravenous glucose. For intractable hypoglycemia an infusion of glucagon can be used. However, it can cause thrombocytopenia and hyponatremia with convulsions (10).

- A female triplet was born at 35 weeks by cesarean section after a normal pregnancy, during which her mother had had normal glucose tolerance. At 2 hours the baby's serum glucose was 1.0 mmol/l. Intravenous glucose was not effective. At 36 hours, dexamethasone was added, but 24 hours later her blood glucose was below 2.0 mmol/l. Dexamethasone was withdrawn and glucagon 1 mg/day was added to the infusion. After 4 hours the blood glucose became stable at 4.0 mmol/l. Her serum sodium fell from 138 to 116 mmol/l at about 120 hours, her potassium rose to 7.6 mmol/l, and her platelet count fell to 13×10^9/l. The glucagon infusion was stopped and within 24 hours her sodium and platelets normalized.

Glucagon infusion in premature babies is risky; more information is necessary.

References

1. Namba M, Hanafusa T, Kono N, Tarui S. Clinical evaluation of biosynthetic glucagon treatment for recovery from hypoglycemia developed in diabetic patients. The GL-G Hypoglycemia Study Group. Diabetes Res Clin Pract 1993;19(2):133–8.
2. Thoma ME, Glauser J, Genuth S. Persistent hypoglycemia and hyperinsulinemia: caution in using glucagon. Am J Emerg Med 1996;14(1):99–101.
3. Hazouard E, Ferrandiere M, Lesire V, Joye F, Perrotin D, de Toffol B. Peduncular hallucinosis related to propranolol self-poisoning: efficacy of intravenous glucagon. Intensive Care Med 1999;25(3):336–7.
4. Salhanick SD, Shannon MW. Management of calcium channel antagonist overdose. Drug Saf 2003;26(2):65–79.
5. Bailey B. Glucagon in beta-blocker and calcium channel blocker overdoses: a systematic review. J Toxicol Clin Toxicol 2003;41(5):595–602.
6. Sensky PR, Olczak SA. High-dose intravenous glucagon in severe tricyclic poisoning. Postgrad Med J 1999;75(888):611–12.
7. Teece S, Hogg K. Towards evidence based emergency medicine: best BETs from the Manchester Royal Infirmary. Glucagon in tricyclic overdose. Emerg Med J 2003; 20(3):264–5.
8. Wermers RA, Fatourechi V, Wynne AG, Kvols LK, Lloyd RV. The glucagonoma syndrome. Clinical and pathologic features in 21 patients. Medicine (Baltimore) 1996;75(2):53–63.
9. Chin DT. Myocardial ischemia induced by glucagon. Ann Pharmacother 1996;30(1):84–5.
10. Belik J, Musey J, Trussell RA. Continuous infusion of glucagon induces severe hyponatremia and thrombocytopenia in a premature neonate. Pediatrics 2001;107(3):595–7.
11. Ranganath L, Schaper F, Gama R, Morgan L. Mechanism of glucagon-induced nausea. Clin Endocrinol (Oxf) 1999;51(2):260–1.
12. Beltzer-Garelli E, Cesarini JP, Cywiner-Golenzer C, Eskenazi A, Grupper C. Lesions cutanées révélatrices d'un glucagonome. [Skin lesions revealing a glucagonoma.] Sem Hop 1980;56(11–12):579–82.
13. Dai W, Shi Y, Cai L. [Report of a case of glucagonoma misdiagnosed as "eczema" and "hepatic angioma" for three years and review of literature.] Zhonghua Nei Ke Za Zhi 1995;34(3):190–2.
14. Edell SL. Erythema multiforme secondary to intravenous glucagon. AJR Am J Roentgenol 1980;134(2):385–6.
15. Wald M, Lawrenz K, Luckner D, Seimann R, Mohnike K, Schober E. Glucagon therapy as a possible cause of erythema necrolyticum migrans in two neonates with persistent hyperinsulinaemic hypoglycaemia. Eur J Pediatr 2002;161(11):600–3.

Glucagon-like peptide-1

General Information

Glucagon-like peptide-1 is an intestinal hormone that increases insulin secretion and biosynthesis, has a trophic effect on beta cells, suppresses glucagon secretion, delays gastric emptying, increases satiety, and reduces food intake (1). Its effects are glucose-dependent and it should not cause hypoglycemia. However, in healthy subjects hypoglycemia can occur after high doses or after fasting.

Although it is a candidate for the treatment of type 2 diabetes, it has to be injected and is extremely rapidly degraded by dipeptidyl peptidase IV. Analogues that are resistant to degradation and inhibitors of the degrading enzyme are being investigated.

In a randomized, crossover study with glucagon-like peptide-1, metformin, or the combination, there were no differences between the monotherapies (2). The combination had additive effects in lowering blood glucose and tended to reduce appetite.

In a crossover study, 20 patients with type 2 diabetes were treated for 6 weeks with glucagon-like peptide-1 or saline added to continuous subcutaneous insulin infusion; glucagon-like peptide-1 reduced appetite and caused nausea and reduced well-being (3).

In healthy volunteers, a fatty acid derivative of glucagon-like peptide-1, NN2211, which binds to albumin and has a half-life of about 12 hours, caused more dizziness, headache, nausea, and vomiting than placebo (4,5).

Organs and Systems

Metabolism

In a double-blind, randomized, crossover study in 10 healthy subjects, subcutaneous glucagon-like peptide-1 after a 16-hour fast caused a near five-fold rise in plasma insulin concentration and circulating plasma glucose concentrations fell below the reference range in all subjects (6). One subject had symptoms of hypoglycemia. A rise in pulse rate correlated with the fall in plasma glucose concentration and there was an increase in blood pressure.

In eight patients with type 2 diabetes and seven matched non-diabetics, subcutaneous glucagon-like peptide-1 and intravenous glucose caused reactive hypoglycemia in five controls but not in the patients (7). Glucagon was suppressed.

References

1. Holst JJ. Therapy of type 2 diabetes mellitus based on the actions of glucagon-like peptide-1. Diabetes Metab Res Rev 2002;18(6):430–41.
2. Zander M, Taskiran M, Toft-Nielsen MB, Madsbad S, Holst JJ. Additive glucose-lowering effects of glucagon-like peptide-1 and metformin in type 2 diabetes. Diabetes Care 2001;24(4):720–5.
3. Zander M, Madsbad S, Madsen JL, Holst JJ. Effect of 6-week course of glucagon-like peptide 1 on glycaemic control, insulin sensitivity, and beta-cell function in type 2 diabetes: a parallel-group study. Lancet 2002;359(9309):824–30.
4. Elbrond B, Jakobsen G, Larsen S, Agerso H, Jensen LB, Rolan P, Sturis J, Hatorp V, Zdravkovic M. Pharmacokinetics, pharmacodynamics, safety, and tolerability of a single-dose of NN2211, a long-acting glucagon-like peptide 1 derivative, in healthy male subjects. Diabetes Care 2002;25(8):1398–404.
5. Agerso H, Jensen LB, Elbrond B, Rolan P, Zdravkovic M. The pharmacokinetics, pharmacodynamics, safety and tolerability of NN2211, a new long-acting GLP-1 derivative, in healthy men. Diabetologia 2002;45(2):195–202.
6. Edwards CM, Todd JF, Ghatei MA, Bloom SR. Subcutaneous glucagon-like peptide-1 (7-36) amide is insulinotropic and can cause hypoglycaemia in fasted healthy subjects. Clin Sci (Lond) 1998;95(6):719–24.
7. Vilsboll T, Krarup T, Madsbad S, Holst JJ. No reactive hypoglycaemia in Type 2 diabetic patients after subcutaneous administration of GLP-1 and intravenous glucose. Diabet Med 2001;18(2):144–9.

Glucametacin

General Information

Glucametacin is a glucosamide derivative of indometacin, with no advantages over indometacin and the same pattern of adverse effects, the most common of which are nausea and heartburn (1).

Reference

1. Colombo B, Carrabba M, Paresce E. Glucamethacin in the treatment of rheumatoid arthritis and arthrosis. Clin Trials J 1978;15:66.

Glues

General Information

Hair bonds and hair extensions are being increasingly used both as cosmetic hair alterations and in localized or diffuse alopecia. The commercial glues used to affix the exogenous hair are gelatinous liquids that contain pigments, antioxidants, and natural latex.

Organs and Systems

Immunologic

Two patients developed severe type I allergic reactions to a hair bond.

- A 37-year-old atopic patient had generalized pruritus, diffuse urticaria, angioedema, rhinoconjunctivitis, and tachycardia within minutes of having glued a hair bond to her scalp. Skin tests with the glue (diluted 1:10 000 in saline) were positive, as was an IgE RAST on latex proteins (1).
- A 40-year-old woman noted palmar irritation, followed by generalized pruritus, a feeling of faintness, facial edema, and difficulty in breathing. A latex skin prick test was positive (2).

References

1. Cogen FC, Beezhold DH. Hair glue anaphylaxis: a hidden latex allergy. Ann Allergy Asthma Immunol 2002; 88(1):61–3.
2. Wakelin SH. Contact anaphylaxis from natural rubber latex used as an adhesive for hair extensions. Br J Dermatol 2002;146(2):340–1.

Glutaral

See also Disinfectants and antiseptics

General Information

Aldehydes such as glutaral, formaldehyde, and glyoxal are used as solutions and vapors for disinfection and sterilization.

The safety and biocidal efficacy of glutaral has led to its endorsement by the CDC and WHO as a substitute for formaldehyde in high-level disinfection and cold sterilization (1,2). Glutaral is used in a 2% aqueous solution buffered to a pH of about 8 for sterilization of endoscopic and dental equipment and for other equipment that cannot be sterilized by heat.

Occupational safety considerations for glutaral largely relate to its volatility, and stringent precautions in handling are especially needed in tropical climates (3). The lack of precautionary details for glutaral fumes, especially in warm climates is inadequate. Manufacturers should provide details of possible adverse effects that could arise from glutaral vapor, and of the precautions that should be taken to keep the air concentration below the recommended limit. The odor threshold for glutaral vapor is about 0.04 ppm, the irritation threshold about 0.3 ppm, and the recommended Ceiling Threshold Limit Value 0.2 ppm. It should not be exceeded at any time during the working day (4–6). It is likely that glutaral vapor will be smelt before reaching overexposure concentration, but there is an urgent need to develop affordable and effective methods of containing glutaral fumes.

Of 169 nurses working in 17 hospitals, especially in endoscope units, 68% had symptoms, 38% two or more. The major complaints were eye irritation in 49%, skin discoloration or irritation in 41%, and cough or shortness of breath in 34% (7). Complaints were not related to habits, atopic status, or duration of exposure. In two hospitals, the time-weighted average concentrations were estimated. The 10-minute time-weighted average was below the UK occupational exposure standard of 0.2 ppm. In a similar survey of 150 staff in two Middlesex hospitals who were exposed to glutaral, the rate of complaints was in the same range (8).

Organs and Systems

Cardiovascular

Nine of 184 implantations of glutaral-preserved mitral valves became incompetent (9). This incidence of dehiscence substantially exceeded that previously noted with synthetic valves, and the authors suggested that incomplete removal of glutaral from the prosthesis might have contributed to failure of healing. Collagen ultrastructure investigations of glutaral-treated porcine aortic valve tissue showed that the long-term mechanical durability of treated aortic valves can be substantially increased if careful consideration is given to the pressure at which initial fixation of glutaral is carried out.

Respiratory

Nurses working in endoscopy units complained of respiratory symptoms on exposure to glutaral (10). The provocation test was positive in two of these patients.

Sensory systems

The eye is particularly sensitive to glutaral. The threshold for conjunctival irritation is 0.2–0.5% and for corneal injury 0.5–1.0%. At 2%, eye injury is moderate, whereas at 5% and above it is severe (6,11). In one case, acute eye injury was caused by a leakage of retained glutaral in an anesthesia mask (SEDA-13, 648).

Gastrointestinal

Residues of glutaral in endoscopes can cause significant mucosal injury resulting in acute colitis within 12–48 hours. Symptoms include hematochezia, fever, and tenesmus. Histological findings in biopsy specimens are similar to those of ischemic colitis, with crypt dilatation followed by epithelial cell dropout and subsequent acute inflammation. It cannot be diagnosed by histological analysis alone (12,13). Distinct from the type of colitis that is caused by hydrogen peroxide, the detrimental effects of glutaral are not immediately recognizable during the endoscopic examination. It does not cause raised white mucosal plaques ("pseudolipomatosis") (13).

Colitis was observed during endoscopy of the lower gastrointestinal tract in 21 patients (14). Some patients developed rectal bleeding, tenesmus, and increased frequency of stools, lasting 12 days.

The histological findings in 12 patients with suspected glutaral-induced hemorrhagic colitis were similar to those in rats after colonic instillation of the sterilizing solution (15).

Skin

Solutions of glutaral can cause skin irritation. With sustained contact under occlusion or on sensitive skin, the threshold for producing irritation is 0.2–0.5% (6). However, concentrations up to 5% may not be irritant if applied only briefly to non-occluded skin. The site of skin contact, the length of contact time, and whether the area is occluded are factors that determine the likelihood and severity of irritation.

A few people develop allergic contact dermatitis to glutaral (SEDA-11, 478) (SEDA-12, 572) (6,16).

Immunologic

Aldehydes are irritating and sensitizing and cause contact dermatitis in health-care workers (SEDA-21, 254). The incidence of allergy to aldehydes has been examined in 280 health-care workers with skin lesions (17). Allergy was diagnosed in 64 (23%). Most (86%) were sensitive to only one aldehyde. Formaldehyde caused allergy slightly more often (14%) than glutaral (12%). Only 5 (1.9%) were sensitive to glyoxal. This hierarchy of sensitivity was also confirmed in animal testing.

Anaphylaxis occurred in a woman after the fourth intramuscular injection of a glutaral-containing pollen formulation (SEDA-11, 478) (18).

Drug Administration

Drug overdose

The symptoms of overexposure to glutaral vapor include watery and/or burning eyes, nose and throat irritation, and some respiratory discomfort. Glutaral also causes asthma-like symptoms in a few hypersensitive individuals. However, in none of these cases was there evidence that an immune-mediated process was present; these cases probably represent bronchial hyper-reactivity rather than respiratory sensitization (6).

References

1. Guidelines on sterilization and desinfection effective against human immunodeficiency virus (HIV). WHO AIDS series Geneva: WHO 1989.
2. Centers for Disease Control (CDC). Recommendations for preventing transmission of infection with human T-lymphotropic virus type III/lymphadenopathy-associated virus in the workplace. MMWR Morb Mortal Wkly Rep 1985;34(45):681–6,691–5.
3. Mwaniki DL, Guthua SW. Occupational exposure to glutaraldehyde in tropical climates. Lancet 1992; 340(8833):1476–7.
4. American Conference of Governmental Industrial Hygienists (1991), 1991.
5. Ballantyne B. Toxicology of glutaraldehyde. Review of studies and human health effects. Danbury, CT: Union Carbide Corporation, 1995.
6. Jordan SL. The correct use of glutaraldehyde in the healthcare environment. Gastroenterol Nurs 1995; 18(4):143–5.
7. Calder IM, Wright LP, Grimstone D. Glutaraldehyde allergy in endoscopy units. Lancet 1992;339(8790):433.
8. Waldron HA. Glutaraldehyde allergy in hospital workers. Lancet 1992;339(8797):880.
9. Wright JS, Newman DC. Complications with glutaraldehyde-preserved bioprostheses. Med J Aust 1980;1(11):542–3.
10. Corrado OJ, Osman J, Davies RJ. Asthma and rhinitis after exposure to glutaraldehyde in endoscopy units. Hum Toxicol 1986;5(5):325–8.
11. Ballantyne B, Berman B. Dermal sensitization potential of glutaraldehyde: a review and recent observations. J Toxicol Cut Ocul Toxicol 1984;3:251–62.
12. West AB, Kuan SF, Bennick M, Lagarde S. Glutaraldehyde colitis following endoscopy: clinical and pathological features and investigation of an outbreak. Gastroenterology 1995;108(4):1250–5.
13. Ryan CK, Potter GD. Disinfectant colitis. Rinse as well as you wash. J Clin Gastroenterol 1995;21(1):6–9.
14. Jonas G, Mahoney A, Murray J, Gertler S. Chemical colitis due to endoscope cleaning solutions: a mimic of pseudomembranous colitis. Gastroenterology 1988; 95(5):1403–8.
15. Durante L, Zulty JC, Israel E, Powers PJ, Russell RG, Qizilbash AH, Morris JG. Jr. Investigation of an outbreak of bloody diarrhea: association with endoscopic cleaning solution and demonstration of lesions in an animal model. Am J Med 1992;92(5):476–80.
16. Rahi AH, Hungerford JL, Ahmed AI. Ocular toxicity of desferrioxamine: light microscopic histochemical and ultrastructural findings. Br J Ophthalmol 1986;70(5):373–81.
17. Kiec-Swierczynska M, Krecisz B, Krysiak B, Kuchowicz E, Rydzynski K. Occupational allergy to aldehydes in health care workers. Clinical observations. Experiments. Int J Occup Med Environ Health 1998;11(4):349–58.
18. Small P. Modified ragweed extract. J Allergy Clin Immunol 1982;69(6):547.

Glycerol

General Information

Glycerol is a colorless syrupy liquid that is used medically as a laxative given orally, as an enema, or in the form of suppositories. Oral hypertonic glycerol has been used as a test for reversibility of the symptoms of Menière's disease (1); however, it causes headache, nausea, and vomiting and is of poor sensitivity and specificity.

Intravenous glycerol has been given to reduce cerebral edema and hence reduce intracranial pressure.

Iodinated glycerol is used as a mucolytic agent in respiratory disorders. Organically bound iodine is changed to unbound iodide after absorption. Iodide inhibits the binding of iodine to the tyrosine residue of the thyroglobulin molecule, inhibiting the synthesis of thyroxine and triiodothyronine. In patients with iodide-induced goiter, there is increased iodine transport, further reducing thyroid hormone synthesis and causing thyroid hyperplasia (2).

Glycerol has been injected into nerve ganglia to destroy them. In 139 patients, 260 consecutive retrogasserian glycerol rhizotomies for trigeminal neuralgia were retrospectively analysed for technical surgical difficulties and immediate and early complications (3). There were technical obstacles in 47%. In 21 cases, the surgical procedure had to be interrupted because of vasovagal reactions, cardiac arrest, or difficulty in finding the trigeminal cistern. There were either transient or persistent complications in 67%, in most cases mild sensory defects. Other complications included labial herpes (3.8%), anesthesia dolorosa (0.8%), moderately or severely impaired sensation (19%), dysesthesia (23%), chemical meningitis (1.5%), and infectious meningitis (1.5%). In five patients hearing was affected, including deterioration of pre-existing tinnitus in one case. Although the frequency of surgical difficulties was high, success was hampered only in a few procedures.

Organs and Systems

Nervous system

In 122 patients with trigeminal neuralgia who underwent percutaneous retrogasserian glycerol injection (4), complications associated with the treatment were significant: 63% had marked hyperesthesia of the face and 29% unpleasant dysesthesias, including two cases of anesthesia dolorosa. Sensory disturbances were most frequent in patients who had previously undergone an alcohol block procedure. Because of the high rates of recurrence and sensory disturbances, the authors preferred microvascular decompression for the management of trigeminal neuralgia. In a study of glycerol injection in trigeminal neuralgia, paresthesia and dysesthesia were reported (5).

Rotatory vertigo with vertical nystagmus has been attributed to glycerol (6).

Sensory systems

Temporary loss of hearing has been reported after the oral administration of hypertonic glycerol in the diagnosis of Menière's disease (7).

Endocrine

Reversible hypothyroidism has been reported in nursing-home residents without a history of thyroid disease, who had been taking iodinated glycerol as an expectorant (8). Hypothyroidism has been reported after long-term treatment with iodinated glycerol (9).

Metabolism

Glycerol can increase plasma insulin concentrations and thereby worsen diabetes; it can particularly cause hyperosmolar non-ketotic hyperglycemia in patients with type 2 diabetes (10,11).

Fluid balance

Large oral doses of glycerol can cause severe derangements of water balance, which can be dangerous in patients in poor physical condition.

Hematologic

Intravascular hemolysis occurred during intravenous glycerol therapy in patients with acute stroke (12).

Gastrointestinal

Oral glycerol can cause nausea and vomiting (SEDA-20, 440) and less commonly diarrhea. Rectal administration can cause mucosal erosion.

Skin

Moisturizing creams have beneficial effects in the treatment of dry, scaly skin, but they can cause adverse skin reactions. In a double-blind, randomized study, 197 patients with atopic dermatitis, none of whom had known allergy to ingredients in the test creams, were randomized to one of three creams: 20% glycerol (55 women and 13 men, mean age 35 years), 4% urea plus 4% sodium chloride (47 women and 16 men, mean age 32 years), and vehicle (49 women and 17 men, mean age 34 years); they were asked to apply the cream at least once daily for 30 days (13). After 2 weeks the patients were asked to score the degree of smarting sensation (a sharp, local, superficial effect), stinging, itching, and dryness/irritation on a five-point scale (0–4). They were also asked to note skin dryness at the beginning of the study and after 1 month on a visual analogue scale. A dermatologist assessed dry skin at the start and after 30 days using the product of the sum of severity scores and area affected in four body regions (14). Adverse skin reactions such as smarting were significantly less common among patients who used the 20% glycerol cream (10%) compared with the urea + saline cream (24%). There were no differences in other skin reactions, such as stinging, itching, and dryness/irritation.

References

1. Skalabrin TA, Mangham CA. Analysis of the glycerin test for Menière's disease. Otolaryngol Head Neck Surg 1987;96(3):282–8.
2. Kalant H, Roschlau WHE. Organically bound iodine. In: Principles of Medical Pharmacology. 5th ed. Washington DC: Decker, 1989:484–5.
3. Blomstedt PC, Bergenheim AT. Technical difficulties and perioperative complications of retrogasserian glycerol rhizotomy for trigeminal neuralgia. Stereotact Funct Neurosurg 2002;79(3-4):168–81.
4. Fujimaki T, Fukushima T, Miyazaki S. Percutaneous retrogasserian glycerol injection in the management of trigeminal neuralgia: long-term follow-up results. J Neurosurg 1990;73(2):212–16.
5. Orlandini G, Pareti A. Trattamento della neuragia del trigemino con glicerolizzazione retrogasseriana. Acta Anaesthesiol Ital 1990;41:617–24.
6. Mizuta K, Furuta M, Ito Y, Sawai S, Fujigaki M, Horibe M, Miyata H. A case of Menière's disease with vertical nystagmus after administration of glycerol. Auris Nasus Larynx 2000;27(3):271–4.
7. Mattox DE, Goode RL. Temporary loss of hearing after a glycerin test. Arch Otolaryngol 1978;104(6):359–61.
8. Drinka PJ, Nolten WE. Effects of iodinated glycerol on thyroid function studies in elderly nursing home residents. J Am Geriatr Soc 1988;36(10):911–13.
9. Mather JL, Baycliff CD, Paterson NAM. Hypothyroidism secondary to iodinated glycerol. Can J Hosp Pharm 1993;46:177–8.
10. Oakley DE, Ellis PP. Glycerol and hyperosmolar nonketotic coma. Am J Ophthalmol 1976;81(4):469–72.
11. Sears ES. Nonketotic hyperosmolar hyperglycemia during glycerol therapy for cerebral edema. Neurology 1976; 26(1):89–94.
12. Kumana CR, Chan GT, Yu YL, Lauder IJ, Chan TK, Kou M. Investigation of intravascular haemolysis during treatment of acute stroke with intravenous glycerol. Br J Clin Pharmacol 1990;29(3):347–53.
13. Loden M, Andersson AC, Anderson C, Bergbrant IM, Frodin T, Ohman H, Sandstrom MH, Sarnhult T, Voog E, Stenberg B, Pawlik E, Preisler-Haggqvist A, Svensson A, Lindberg M. A double-blind study comparing the effect of glycerin and urea on dry, eczematous skin in atopic patients. Acta Derm Venereol 2002; 82(1):45–7.
14. Serup J. EEMCO guidance for the assessment of dry skin (xerosis) and ichthyosis: clinical scoring system. Skin Res Technol 1995;1:109–14.

Glycine

General Information

Glycine is an amino acid that is often used during transurethral prostatectomy for bladder irrigation, sometimes continuously for 24 hours after surgery.

Transurethral resection syndrome

Systemic absorption of the fluid used for bladder irrigation during transurethral resection of the prostate can cause a variety of disturbances of the circulatory and nervous systems, which are often referred to as the transurethral resection syndrome. The lack of a consistent definition and varying degrees of awareness of mild forms of this complication probably explain the different figures given for the incidence of the syndrome in prospective studies, varying from 2 to 10% of all transurethral resections performed. Many urologists claim they have not encountered the transurethral resection syndrome for many years (1–3). However, the incidence and severity of symptoms of the transurethral resection syndrome on absorption of increasing volumes of glycine solution have been described (4).

The signs and symptoms of the transurethral resection syndrome were evaluated and recorded during and after 273 transurethral prostatic resections performed at two hospitals between 1984 and 1993. Glycine solution was used as the irrigant and ethanol served as a tracer for fluid absorption. The incidence and severity of symptoms that could possibly be related to the syndrome increased progressively as more glycine solution was absorbed. Patients who absorbed up to 300 ml of glycine solution had an average of 1.3 such symptoms. This number increased to 2.3 when 1000–2000 ml were absorbed, 3.1 when 2000–3000 ml were absorbed, and 5.8 for volumes greater than 3000 ml. Nausea and vomiting occurred significantly more often when 1000–2000 ml were absorbed compared with no absorption. Confusion and arterial hypotension were other prominent signs of fluid absorption, whereas hypertension was not. The severity of symptoms was markedly aggravated when more than 3000 ml were absorbed. Extravasation resulted in higher risks of bradycardia, hypotension, and failed spontaneous diuresis postoperatively than absorption by the intravascular route.

Nausea after glycine irrigation can be partly explained by toxic effects of glycine and its secondary metabolites in addition to the effects of water intoxication and hyponatremia (5).

The fact that glycine can act as an inhibitory neurotransmitter may explain why absorption of glycine-containing irrigating fluid from the pelvic cavity or directly into the blood during transurethral prostate resection has been linked to loss of sight and vivid postoperative hallucinations (6). Ammonia production due to accumulation of glycine in tissues, and the mentioned neuroinhibitory effects of glycine should be considered risk factors when deciding on glycine as an irrigating fluid (7).

Rapid and massive fluid absorption due to leakage of fluid into the peritoneal cavity has also been reported during percutaneous nephrolithotomy (8).

It has been recommended that glycine irrigation should be confined to the time of operation, and an adequate diuresis should be ensured postoperatively (9).

References

1. Mebust WK, Holtgrewe HL, Cockett AT, Peters PC. Transurethral prostatectomy: immediate and postoperative complications. A cooperative study of 13 participating institutions evaluating 3,885 patients. J Urol 1989;141(2): 243–7.
2. Olsson J, Rentzhog L, Hjertberg H, Hahn RG. Reliability of clinical assessment of fluid absorption in transurethral prostatic resection. Eur Urol 1993;24(2):262–6.
3. Hahn RG, Stalberg HP, Gustafsson SA. Intravenous infusion of irrigating fluids containing glycine or mannitol with and without ethanol. J Urol 1989;142(4):1102–5.
4. Olsson J, Nilsson A, Hahn RG. Symptoms of the transurethral resection syndrome using glycine as the irrigant. J Urol 1995;154(1):123–8.
5. Istre O, Jellum E, Skajaa K, Forman A. Changes in amino acids, ammonium, and coagulation factors after transcervical resection of the endometrium with a glycine solution used for uterine irrigation. Am J Obstet Gynecol 1995;172(3):939–45.
6. Hahn RG. Hallucination and visual disturbances in transurethral prostatic resection. Intensive Care Med 1988; 14(6):668–71.
7. Norlen H, Dimberg M, Allgen LG, Vinnars E. Water and electrolytes in muscle tissue and free amino acids in muscle and plasma in connection with transurethral resection of the prostate. II. Isotonic 2.2% glycine solution as an irrigating fluid. Scand J Urol Nephrol 1990;24(2):95–101.
8. Rao PN. Absorption of irrigating fluid during transcervical resection of endometrium. BMJ 1990;300(6726):748–9.
9. Fitzpatrick JM, Kasidas GP, Rose GA. Hyperoxaluria following glycine irrigation for transurethral prostatectomy. Br J Urol 1981;53(3):250–2.

Glycols

General Information

Glycols are aliphatic dihydric alcohols. Primary and secondary glycols are thick liquids, and tertiary glycols (pinacones) are crystalline solids. The principal glycols to which people are or have been exposed, either occupationally or in medicinal products, are:

- Diethylene glycol — $HO.CH_2.CH_2.O.CH_2.CH_2.OH$
- Ethylene glycol — $HO.CH_2.CH_2.OH$
- Ethyl glycol (ethylene glycol monoethyl ether) — $C_2H_5.O.CH_2.CH_2.OH$
- Methyl glycol (ethylene glycol monomethyl ether) — $CH_3.O.CH_2.CH_2.OH$
- Polyethylene glycol — $HO.CH_2.(CH_2.O.CH_2)_nCH_2OH$
- Propylene glycol — $CH_3CH(OH)CH_2OH$.

Diethylene glycol

Diethylene glycol is important in the history of adverse drug reactions.

The first major drug catastrophe in the 20th-century history of the public control of drugs occurred in 1937 in the USA and involved diethylene glycol. A pharmacist introduced a drug, Elixir Sulfanilamide, that consisted of sulfanilamide dissolved in diethylene glycol. It had been tested for flavor, appearance, and fragrance, but not for safety. After taking the drug, over 100 patients died in severe pain; many were children, who were given Elixir Sulfanilamide for sore throats and coughs. Public outrage created support for proposed legislation to reinforce the public control of drugs that was pending in the US Congress (1). And so, the US 1938 Food, Drug, and Cosmetic Act came into being, and is still the country's legal foundation for the public control of drugs and devices intended for use in the diagnosis, cure, mitigation, treatment, or prevention of disease in humans or animals. It has been a model for similar legislation in many other countries.

The 1938 Food, Drug, and Cosmetic Act prohibited traffic in new drugs, unless they were safe for use under the conditions of use prescribed on their labels. The Act also explicitly required the labelling of drug products with adequate directions for use.

The burden of proof of harm of new drugs was laid on the Federal Food and Drug Agency (FDA). Companies that wanted to manufacture and sell new drugs in interstate commerce had to investigate their safety and report to the FDA. Unless the FDA, within a specified period of time, found that the safety of a drug had not been established, the company could proceed with its marketing. The FDA was also authorized to remove from the market any drug it could prove to be unsafe (2).

The US Supreme Court also established in 1941, in a legal case over drug adulteration, that responsible individuals in a company can be held personally accountable for the quality of the products manufactured by the company, and that distributors of pharmaceuticals are responsible for the quality of their products, even if they are manufactured elsewhere (3).

After the World War II, the pharmaceuticals market changed radically, as many companies started industrial production of drugs that had previously been manufactured in pharmacies. Announcements of new industrially produced drugs were hailed as part of technological advancement, as significant a sign of progress as the launching of satellites and putting a man on the moon. However, public safeguards against the risks of drugs remained unchanged in most countries. Thus, control of the effects of drugs largely lay in the hands of the manufacturers, even though the responsibility for taking precautions rested with pharmacists and doctors.

Diethylene glycol has been reported to cause acidosis and renal insufficiency (SEDA-19, 446).

Ethylene glycol, ethylene glycol monoethyl ether, and ethylene monomethyl ether

Ethylene glycol is a colorless, sweet-tasting liquid that is used as an anti-freeze, in the manufacture of polyester fibers and films, as a heat-transfer fluid, in aircraft and runway de-icing mixtures, to provide freeze-thaw stabilization to latex coatings, to improve the flexibility and drying time of paints, as a dehydrating agent in natural gas, in motor oil additives, as an additive in inks, pesticides, wood stains, and adhesives, and as a solvent and suspending medium for ammonium perborate, the conductor in most electrolytic capacitors. The monoethyl ether of ethylene glycol, 2-ethoxyethanol or ethyl glycol, has been used as an excipient in some drug formulations, in the semiconductor industry, in duplicating fluids, epoxy resins, lacquers, paints, printing inks, varnish removers, and wood stains. The monomethyl ether of ethylene glycol, 2-methoxyethanol or methyl glycol, is used as a jet fuel de-icer and as a solvent for cellulose acetate, dyes, enamels, nail polishes, resins, varnishes, and wood stains.

In one study, occupational exposure to ethylene glycol was not associated with adverse effects (4). However, other adverse effects of occupational exposure have been noted, including anemia, subfertility, and renal stones.

Ethylene glycol is sometimes used in suicide attempts. It is not itself toxic, but is converted to toxic metabolites. Conversion to glycoaldehyde by alcohol dehydrogenase is the rate-limiting step, and further metabolism yields glycolate, glyoxylate, and oxalate.

Polyethylene glycol

Polyethylene glycol is a high molecular weight inert molecule that is commonly combined with electrolytes (potassium chloride, sodium bicarbonate, sodium chloride, and sodium sulfate) in colonic lavage systems. Owing to the osmotic properties of these solutions, there is little absorption or secretion of electrolytes or water, although small amounts of polyethylene glycol and sulfates have been detected in the urine of healthy patients and higher concentrations in the urine of patients with inflammatory bowel disease (5). Common adverse effects of solutions containing polyethylene glycol and electrolytes include nausea, abdominal fullness, and bloating in up to 50% of patients. These solutions are contraindicated in patients with gastric outlet obstruction or gastroparesis, gastrointestinal obstruction or perforation, ileus, or toxic colitis (6).

Polyethylene glycol (PEG) is also used to convert certain compounds of relatively high molecular weights to more soluble products, known as pegylated derivatives. Such compounds include pegylated interferons and interleukins. The safety and activity of outpatient-based continuous intravenous interleukin-2 (IL-2) or a modified-release pegylated IL-2 have been studied in 115 HIV-positive patients with CD4 cell counts of 200–500 $\times$ 10^6/l randomized to antiretroviral therapy plus cyclical continuous intravenous IL-2 ($n = 27$), subcutaneous pegylated IL-2 ($n = 58$), or no IL-2 ($n = 30$) (7). The termination rates due to adverse events were 4% with continuous intravenous IL-2 and 7% with pegylated IL-2. The frequency and severity of grade 3 and 4 adverse events were similar in both IL-2 groups, with the exception of local erythema and induration associated with subcutaneous injections of pegylated IL-2. Fever, fatigue, stomatitis, erythema, gastrointestinal symptoms, and mood alterations constituted the majority of clinically significant toxic effects. Most of the adverse events resolved by 8–15 days of each cycle. There were several unusual adverse effects of IL-2 that were not dose-related. These included worsening of pre-existing diarrhea, cardiomyopathy in a patient with a history of heroin abuse, and attempted suicide in a patient with a psychiatric history.

In 68 patients randomly assigned to receive either sulfate-free polyethylene glycol electrolyte lavage or sodium picosulfate plus magnesium sulfate, the day before colonoscopy, bowel cleansing was significantly better with picosulfate plus magnesium sulfate (8). Adverse effects were more common with polyethylene glycol electrolyte lavage, especially nausea, vomiting, and palpitation, and four patients did not complete treatment owing to adverse effects.

Propylene glycol

Propylene glycol is widely used as a solvent in topical glucocorticoids, other medicines (including diazepam, etomidate, and lorazepam), foodstuffs, cosmetics, household detergents, paints, and brake fluids.

Organs and Systems

Respiratory

Polyethylene glycol has reportedly caused fulminant pulmonary edema (9).

Nervous system

Polyethylene glycol has reportedly caused seizures (SEDA-20, 440).

Metabolism

Lactic acidosis and convulsions have been associated with the use of propylene glycol (SEDA-15, 537) and polyethylene glycol, the latter after the administration of a high dose of lorazepam (10).

Hematologic

Propylene glycol causes acute hemolysis with raised lactate dehydrogenase activity, and raised bilirubin and plasma hemoglobin concentrations after use of a stock solution during intravenous administration of glyceryl trinitrate (11).

In 53 impregnation workers from two factories making copper-clad laminate with ethylene glycol monomethyl ether as a solvent and 121 lamination workers with indirect exposure, hemoglobin, packed cell volume, and erythrocyte count in the exposed workers were significantly lower than in the controls, and the frequency of anemia was significantly higher (26 versus 3.2%); there was no difference in spermatogenesis (12).

Pancreas

Severe acute pancreatitis has been reported in a 75-year-old woman who had been given polyethylene glycol 4 litre rectally (13).

Urinary tract

In silkscreen printers exposed to glycol ethers, the excretion of calcium increased according to the urinary alkoxyacetic acid load. The excretion of ammonia and chloride was higher among exposed workers than among controls. The tendency to form urinary stones was 2.4 times higher among silkscreen printers than among office workers (14).

However, in 33 aviation workers exposed to de-icing fluid containing ethylene glycol there was no evidence of acute or chronic kidney damage that could be attributed to working in the presence of ethylene glycol (15).

Polyethylene glycol has been associated with raised creatinine concentrations in eight patients who were given a continuous intravenous infusion of lorazepam (range 2–28 mg/hour) (16).

- A 57-year-old man with a history of alcohol abuse developed acute respiratory failure and was given lorazepam up to 18 mg/hour during alcohol withdrawal (17). On day 43 (cumulative intravenous lorazepam dose 4089 mg, containing about 220 ml of polyethylene glycol 400), he developed oliguric acute tubular necrosis with proteinuria and granular casts.

The authors attributed the renal damage to polyethylene glycol, perhaps enhanced by concurrent administration of vancomycin.

Skin

Contact dermatitis has been reported after exposure to glue containing 25% 2-hydroxyethyl methacrylate and 0.4% ethylene glycol dimethacrylate (18).

Propylene glycol has also been reported to cause contact dermatitis (19–24).

Reproductive system

In one study, occupational exposure to ethylene glycol was associated with delayed fertility in women (25).

In 1150 pregnancies, 561 in female employees of semiconductor manufacturers and 589 in the wives of male employees the former had increased risks of spontaneous abortion (RR = 2.8; 95%CI = 1.4, 5.6) and subfertility (OR = 4.6; 95%CI = 1.6, 13); both of these risks had a dose-response relation with potential exposure to ethylene glycol (26).

Immunologic

Polyethylene glycol has reportedly caused anaphylaxis (SEDA-20, 440).

Propylene glycol can be used in allergic individuals, although propylene glycol itself can cause allergic skin reactions. The incidence of propylene glycol allergy among patients with eczema is thought to be greater than 2% (27). Used in dermatological formulations, propylene glycol can occasionally perpetuate eczema in hypersensitive patients (28).

Drug Administration

Drug formulations

In 1995, a topical solution of erythromycin (Erythromycine Balleul) was withdrawn from the market because of its high content of ethylene glycol monoethyl ether, which is easily absorbed via the skin, is teratogenic in animals, and alters spermatogenesis.

Drug overdose

Ethylene glycol poisoning can cause acidosis, central nervous system depression, pulmonary edema, acute oliguric renal failure with crystalluria, liver damage due to calcium oxalate deposition, nausea, abdominal pain, and cramping, acute colonic ischemia (29), and papilledema and abducens nerve palsy (30).

- Hemorrhage in the globus pallidus occurred in a 50-year-old Afro-Caribbean alcoholic man after ethylene glycol poisoning; there was evidence of lactic acidosis and the ethylene glycol concentration was 6.06 mmol/l (31).
- A 36-year-old long-distance truck driver took 200 ml of ethylene glycol in a suicide attempt (32). He vomited, lost consciousness, and had miosis and external ophthalmoplegia. There was a severe metabolic acidosis with a wide anion gap and many crystals in the urinary sediment. Acute oliguric renal failure required continuous hemodialysis for 6 days. A CT scan of the brain showed low-density areas in the bilateral basal ganglia, midbrain, and pons. A renal biopsy showed tubular oxalate deposits. He gradually recovered within 36 days.

Treatment of ethylene glycol toxicity is with ethanol, which inhibits alcohol dehydrogenase, fomepizole, which also inhibits alcohol dehydrogenase, and bicarbonate to treat acidosis (33). In some cases hemodialysis has been used (34,35).

Propylene glycol has been reported to cause lactic acidosis after overdose (36).

References

1. US Congress. House Committee on Interstate and Foreign Commerce and Its Subcommittee on Public Health and Environment, 1974. A Brief Legislative History of the Food, Drug, and Cosmetic Act. Committee Print No. 14. Washington DC: US Government Printing Office, 1974;1–4.
2. USA. 52 Stat. 1040, 75th Congress, 3rd session, 25 June 1938.
3. USA vs Dotterweich, 1941.
4. Wang RS, Suda M, Gao X, Wang B, Nakajima T, Honma T. Health effects of exposure to ethylene glycol monoethyl ether in female workers. Ind Health 2004;42(4):447–51.
5. Brady CE 3rd, DiPalma JA, Morawski SG, Santa Ana CA, Fordtran JS. Urinary excretion of polyethylene glycol 3350 and sulfate after gut lavage with a polyethylene glycol electrolyte lavage solution. Gastroenterology 1986;90(6):1914–18.
6. Anonymous. PEG electrolyte lavage solutions: drug evaluation monograph. Englewood (CO): Micromedex Inc, 1999:1–21.
7. Carr A, Emery S, Lloyd A, Hoy J, Garsia R, French M, Stewart G, Fyfe G, Cooper DA. Outpatient continuous intravenous interleukin-2 or subcutaneous, polyethylene glycol-modified interleukin-2 in human immunodeficiency virus-infected patients: a randomized, controlled, multicenter study. Australian IL-2 Study Group. J Infect Dis 1998;178(4):992–9.
8. Regev A, Fraser G, Delpre G, Leiser A, Neeman A, Maoz E, Anikin V, Niv Y. Comparison of two bowel preparations for colonoscopy: sodium picosulphate with magnesium citrate versus sulphate-free polyethylene glycol lavage solution. Am J Gastroenterol 1998;93(9):1478–82.
9. Argent A, Hatherill M, Reynolds L, Purves L. Fulminant pulmonary oedema after administration of a balanced electrolyte polyethylene glycol solution. Arch Dis Child 2002;86(3):209.
10. Cawley MJ. Short-term lorazepam infusion and concern for propylene glycol toxicity: case report and review. Pharmacotherapy 2001;21(9):1140–4.
11. Demey HE, Daelemans RA, Verpooten GA, De Broe ME, Van Campenhout CM, Lakiere FV, Schepens PJ, Bossaert LL. Propylene glycol-induced side effects during intravenous nitroglycerin therapy. Intensive Care Med 1988;14(3):221–6.
12. Shih TS, Hsieh AT, Liao GD, Chen YH, Liou SH. Haematological and spermatotoxic effects of ethylene glycol monomethyl ether in copper clad laminate factories. Occup Environ Med 2000;57(5):348–52.
13. Franga DL, Harris JA. Polyethylene glycol-induced pancreatitis. Gastrointest Endosc 2000;52(6):789–91.
14. Laitinen J, Liesivuori J, Savolainen H. Urinary alkoxyacetic acids and renal effects of exposure to ethylene glycol ethers. Occup Environ Med 1996;53(9):595–600.
15. Gerin M, Patrice S, Begin D, Goldberg MS, Vyskocil A, Adib G, Drolet D, Viau C. A study of ethylene glycol exposure and kidney function of aircraft de-icing workers. Int Arch Occup Environ Health 1997;69(4):255–65.
16. Yaucher NE, Fish JT, Smith HW, Wells JA. Propylene glycol-associated renal toxicity from lorazepam infusion. Pharmacotherapy 2003;23(9):1094–9.
17. Laine GA, Hossain SM, Solis RT, Adams SC. Polyethylene glycol nephrotoxicity secondary to prolonged high-dose intravenous lorazepam. Ann Pharmacother 1995;29(11): 1110–14.
18. Kanerva L, Jolanki R, Leino T, Estlander T. Occupational allergic contact dermatitis from 2-hydroxyethyl methacrylate and ethylene glycol dimethacrylate in a modified acrylic structural adhesive. Contact Dermatitis 1995;33(2):84–9.
19. Lu R, Katta R. Iatrogenic contact dermatitis due to propylene glycol. J Drugs Dermatol 2005;4(1):98–101.
20. Connolly M, Buckley DA. Contact dermatitis from propylene glycol in ECG electrodes, complicated by medicament allergy. Contact Dermatitis 2004;50(1):42.
21. Farrar CW, Bell HK, King CM. Allergic contact dermatitis from propylene glycol in Efudix cream. Contact Dermatitis 2003;48(6):345.
22. Sowa J, Suzuki K, Tsuruta K, Akamatsu H, Matsunaga K. Allergic contact dermatitis from propylene glycol ricinoleate in a lipstick. Contact Dermatitis 2003;48(4):228–9.
23. Lamb SR, Ardley HC, Wilkinson SM. Contact allergy to propylene glycol in brassiere padding inserts. Contact Dermatitis 2003;48(4):224–5.
24. Guijarro SC, Sanchez-Perez J, Garcia-Diez A. Allergic contact dermatitis to polyethylene glycol and nitrofurazone. Am J Contact Dermat 1999;10(4):226–7.
25. Chen PC, Hsieh GY, Wang JD, Cheng TJ. Prolonged time to pregnancy in female workers exposed to ethylene glycol ethers in semiconductor manufacturing. Epidemiology 2002;13(2):191–6.
26. Correa A, Gray RH, Cohen R, Rothman N, Shah F, Seacat H, Corn M. Ethylene glycol ethers and risks of spontaneous abortion and subfertility. Am J Epidemiol 1996;143(7):707–17.
27. Catanzaro JM, Smith JG Jr. Propylene glycol dermatitis. J Am Acad Dermatol 1991;24(1):90–5.
28. Andersen KE. Hudreaktioner fremkaldt af propylenglykol. [Skin reactions caused by propylene glycol.] Ugeskr Laeger 1980;142(38):2478–80.
29. Gardner TB, Manning HL, Beelen AP, Cimis RJ, Cates JM, Lewis LD. Ethylene glycol toxicity associated with ischemia, perforation, and colonic oxalate crystal deposition. J Clin Gastroenterol 2004;38(5):435–9.

30. Delany C, Jay WM. Papilledema and abducens nerve palsy following ethylene glycol ingestion. Semin Ophthalmol 2004;19(3-4):72–4.
31. Caparros-Lefebvre D, Policard J, Sengler C, Benabdallah E, Colombani S, Rigal M. Bipallidal haemorrhage after ethylene glycol intoxication. Neuroradiology 2005;47(2):105–7.
32. Ohmori K, Kumada K, Kimura F, Ishihara S, Fukuda M, Suzuki K, Kohama A. [Ethylene glycol poisoning complicated by central nervous system abnormalities.] Chudoku Kenkyu 2004;17(4):365–70.
33. Caravati EM, Heileson HL, Jones M. Treatment of severe pediatric ethylene glycol intoxication without hemodialysis. J Toxicol Clin Toxicol 2004;42(3):255–9.
34. Wallman P, Hogg K. Towards evidence based emergency medicine: best BETs from the Manchester Royal Infirmary. Management of acute ethylene glycol poisoning. Emerg Med J 2002;19(5):431–2.
35. Rydel JJ, Carlson A, Sharma J, Leikin J. An approach to dialysis for ethylene glycol intoxication. Vet Hum Toxicol 2002;44(1):36–9.
36. Jorens PG, Demey HE, Schepens PJ, Coucke V, Verpooten GA, Couttenye MM, Van Hoof V. Unusual D-lactic acid acidosis from propylene glycol metabolism in overdose. J Toxicol Clin Toxicol 2004;42(2):163–9.

Glycopyrronium

General Information

Glycopyrronium is a quaternary ammonium compound with anticholinergic properties (1).

In 22 patients with Frey syndrome (localized facial gustatory sweating and flushing) treated with topical glycopyrrolate 0.5–2% in a solution, cream or roll-on lotion, 1012 applications were recorded (SEDA-8, 160). There were seven adverse events: blurred vision (one), minor eye infections (two), itchy or dry eyes (one), and dry mouth (three). In the control group blurred vision and dry mouth were also recorded as adverse events.

Reference

1. Mirakhur RK, Dundee JW, Jones CJ. Evaluation of the anticholinergic actions of glycopyrronium bromide. Br J Clin Pharmacol 1978;5(1):77–84.

Gold and gold salts

General Information

Gold is a heavy yellow-colored element (symbol Au; atomic no. 79). Its symbol derives from the Latin word aurum. It is usually found as the metallic element but can occur as salts such gold telluride (sylvanite).

Metallic gold is used in dentistry, and gold salts still form one of the mainstays of treatment for rheumatoid arthritis. The radioactive isotope ^{198}Au is used therapeutically in the treatment of certain malignancies. In Japan, chrysotherapy has a reputation for efficacy in bronchial asthma. The antitumor activity of novel gold compounds is being pursued (1). The molecular mechanisms of action of gold have been reviewed (2).

Gold salts

Sodium aurothiomalate is water-soluble and is given intramuscularly as an aqueous solution. Aurothioglucose is water-soluble and is given intramuscularly in either an aqueous solution or an oily suspension. Sodium aurothiopropanol sulfonate, aurotioprol, and aurothiosulfate have similar actions and uses to those of sodium aurothiomalate. They are given by intramuscular injection.

Auranofin

Auranofin is a triethylphosphine gold derivative for oral administration. It is in some respects strikingly different from the rest. Some 25% of an oral dose is absorbed through the intestinal wall and blood concentrations are some 15–25% of those reached with parenteral therapy. Auranofin is bound to cellular elements of the blood, is excreted mainly in the feces, and exhibits less tissue retention and total body gold accumulation than parenteral forms. It is more effective in acute inflammatory models and is a potent inhibitor of lysosomal enzyme release, antibody-dependent cellular toxicity, and superoxide production. Auranofin also affects humoral and cellular immune reactions. However, some have found auranofin to be rather less effective than parenteral gold. Auranofin is used in doses of 2–9 mg/day (generally 6 mg/day), which is less than the dose originally recommended.

In view of all this it is not surprising that auranofin has a distinct profile of therapeutic and adverse effects, the differences being so great that one actually suspects differences in the mechanism of action between oral and parenteral forms. Like the latter, however, auranofin shows no clear correlation between whole blood gold concentrations and either efficacy or adverse effects.

Use in rheumatoid arthritis

In rheumatoid arthritis the most commonly used gold salts are sodium aurothiomalate and aurothioglucose (3). There is some reason to believe that adverse effects are less frequent with the suspensions (of aurothioglucose or aurothiosulfate) than with the more rapidly absorbed solution (of sodium gold thiomalate) (SEDA-16, 233) (4).

Whereas gold was previously regarded as one of the most toxic drugs in the pharmacopeia, many authors now share the view that its adverse effects can to an important extent be contained by individually adapted dosage regimens and careful monitoring. However, it is not strictly possible to predict the nature or timing of the complications that an individual may experience, and it has to be borne in mind that some reactions are immunological (SEDA-21, 236). The prevalence of adverse gold reactions seems to be similar in patients given 25 or 50 mg of gold weekly (SED-12, 520) (5). Some studies have suggested that the frequency of mucocutaneous and renal adverse reactions may be higher in the initial months of treatment. In one series of patients receiving gold sodium thiomalate, a plateau in the cumulative incidence of withdrawals due to rash was reached only after 40 months (45% of all patients), while withdrawals due to proteinuria reached a plateau after 18 months (15%) (6). Hematological complications can occur at any stage.

It is widely considered that the patients who are most likely to develop adverse reactions to gold salts are those who react most favorably. In the past, many rheumatologists intensified treatment with high doses of gold salts until a skin eruption occurred, only then seeking to reduce to a maintenance dosage.

After withdrawal due to adverse reactions, treatment with gold compounds can be cautiously reintroduced without the previous adverse effects necessarily reappearing. However, clearly one will not take this course if life-threatening reactions have occurred. It should always be borne in mind that many adverse reactions allegedly due to chrysotherapy may have other causes, particularly in the case of skin reactions. Most patients have been or are using other drugs at the same time. The concomitant use of penicillamine can be particularly confusing, since its pattern of adverse effects closely resembles that produced by gold.

Use in dentistry

Dental gold alloys continue to be used and remain a source of contact hypersensitivity (7), including contact stomatitis and skin eruptions at sites not usually associated with dentistry. Contact dermatitis to metallic gold, for example in jewellery, has also repeatedly been observed (SED-8, 510) (SEDA-22, 245). A gold surgical clip has also caused an apparently allergic reaction, characterized by sterile abscess formation (8). However, such reactions are rare and may in part be due to other metals contained in the alloy.

General adverse effects

Intravenous gold salts

Adverse effects of gold salts occur in about one-third of systemically treated patients, the incidence varying from 25 to 40%. The dropout rate due to adverse reactions has been assessed as 22–26% (9). Children are considered to show the same pattern of adverse reactions as adults.

Cutaneous lesions are the most frequent adverse effects of gold salts, followed by involvement of the mucous membranes and kidneys. Pruritus and a wide range of skin reactions can occur. In the gastrointestinal system inflammation can occur at all levels, from the buccal cavity to the colon. Glossitis, cheilitis, and stomatitis are less common than dermatitis. Enterocolitis is a rare but very serious complication. Mild proteinuria is often seen in patients receiving chrysotherapy, while severe nephrotic syndrome is much less common. Blood dyscrasias of any type can occur either during therapy or after withdrawal. Leukopenia and thrombocytopenia are the most common hematological complications, although both are clearly less common than the mucocutaneous and renal adverse effects. Unusual reactions include pulmonary infiltration, intrahepatic cholestasis, and peripheral neuropathy. By and large, undesirable effects are transient and mild, but occasional deaths continue to be reported, usually because of hematological complications.

Apart from the "nitritoid" cardiovascular reaction, which is unique to sodium aurothiomalate, and possible differences between slowly and rapidly absorbed gold salts in the relative frequency of adverse effects, the general pattern of adverse reactions is similar for all parenteral gold salts.

Although most adverse effects of gold have traditionally been characterized as toxic, various factors show that some of the complications due to chrysotherapy are, at least in part, manifestations of hypersensitivity. Eosinophilia, raised IgE concentrations, immune complexes, and a positive reaction to gold in the lymphocyte transformation test have been observed in association with many adverse reactions to chrysotherapy and point to immunological mechanisms (10). With aurothiomalate both pemphigus and erythroderma have been described (SEDA-22, 246). It may be that gold facilitates the development of autoimmunity in patients with rheumatoid arthritis. Gold-induced membranous glomerulonephritis is believed to be an immune complex (type III) reaction, although the role of gold in the development of proteinuria has not yet been clarified. Gold-induced antibody deficiency may be more common than is usually recognized. In 22 patients with rheumatoid arthritis subnormal serum immunoglobulin concentrations developed as a consequence of gold treatment (11). There were mild deficiencies of single immunoglobulin isotypes or severe deficiencies affecting two or three isotypes. There may be transient exacerbation of rheumatoid symptoms before a therapeutic response to gold occurs. In one series of 43 patients with rheumatoid arthritis serious exacerbation of the disease occurred in 17% (12). Tumor-inducing effects have not been observed.

Auranofin

Auranofin is well tolerated by most patients; its adverse effects resemble those of parenteral gold salts, but the pattern differs, with gastrointestinal reactions predominating. Adverse reactions to auranofin are also generally less severe. Where serious adverse effects have been attributed to auranofin, cause and effect has usually remained in doubt. Adverse effects on the lower gastrointestinal tract are the most common; early studies showed a change in bowel habit in some 40% of cases, but this does not often amount to frank diarrhea (13). The same authors noted proteinuria (4%) and hematological reactions (2%). Mucocutaneous reactions (pruritus, conjunctivitis, stomatitis) often occur but are rarely severe and are less problematic than with sodium aurothiomalate. Most adverse effects occur during the first few months; age, sex, and duration of disease do not influence the risk of developing an adverse effect. The adverse effect-related withdrawal rates for injectable gold, auranofin, and placebo were 40, 14, and 6% respectively. Rashes occur in some 20% of cases but rarely require withdrawal. Tumor-inducing effects have not been observed.

Metallic gold

Dental gold alloys can cause contact hypersensitivity (7). Contact dermatitis to metallic gold, for example in jewellery, has also repeatedly been observed (SED-8, 510) (SEDA-22, 245). A gold surgical clip has also caused an apparently allergic reaction, characterized by sterile abscess formation (8). However, such reactions are rare and may in part be due to other metals contained in the alloy.

Organs and Systems

Cardiovascular

Acute vasodilatory (nitritoid) reactions occur in a minority of patients receiving parenteral gold, especially sodium aurothiomalate (SEDA-22, 245). A few minutes after injection the patient experiences weakness, flushing, hypotension, tachycardia, palpitation, sweating, and sometimes syncope (14). Very rarely myocardial infarction and stroke follow (14,15). The mechanism is unknown, but it has been suggested that the vehicle might be responsible, and that aurothioglucose might therefore be preferable to sodium aurothiomalate in elderly patients or in those with a history of cardiovascular disease.

Respiratory

Gold-induced lung toxicity is an infrequent adverse effect in patients with rheumatoid arthritis and psoriatic arthritis. There are three types: interstitial pneumonitis, bronchiolitis obliterans with organizing pneumonia, and bronchiolitis obliterans; the first is the most frequent. There have been two reports of gold-induced lung toxicity in psoriatic arthritis (16).

- A 54-year-old woman with psoriatic polyarthritis was treated with aurothiomalate 50 mg/week. When the cumulative dose reached 250 mg she developed weakness, dyspnea, fever, nausea, vomiting and erythematous skin lesions. Chest X-ray and CT scan showed diffuse interstitial pneumonitis. Gold was withdrawn and she was given prednisone 60 mg/day. She recovered in 6 months.
- A 62-year old woman with psoriatic arthritis was given aurothiomalate 50 mg/week. After a cumulative dose of 135 mg she developed an itchy rash, dyspnea, and fever. Chest X-ray and CT scan suggested pneumonitis and she was given prednisone 40 mg/day. She recovered in 6 months.

More than 60 cases of "gold lung" have been reported and there must be many more unpublished cases. Beginning as a rule some weeks or months after starting treatment, the patient develops dyspnea on exertion, weakness, a dry cough, and malaise. Chest X-rays show bilateral pulmonary infiltrates of varying extent, but cases have been described in which the radiography is entirely normal (17). If chrysotherapy is continued, pulmonary insufficiency can follow. In fact two types of process need to be distinguished; fibrosing alveolitis and obliterative bronchiolitis occur and can co-exist (18); some patients develop proliferative and immunoallergic changes, perhaps even mimicking malignant processes. In treating rheumatism, it can be difficult to distinguish "gold lung" from rheumatoid lung disease (SEDA-21, 236).

Bronchoalveolar lavage in "gold lung" tends to show an increase in the total cell count and predominance of the percentage of lymphocytes with an inverse helper/suppressor ratio. The prognosis is generally good; if gold is immediately withdrawn, the pulmonary lesions as a rule subside, although incomplete regression or even persistence of dyspnea and impaired lung function have been described, despite glucocorticoid therapy (19).

The pulmonary toxicity of gold salts uncommonly causes life-threatening respiratory failure. Patients who suffer from this do not usually need mechanical ventilation, and the toxicity can be difficult to diagnose when it occurs in patients with an illness with pulmonary involvement. However, severe respiratory failure requiring mechanical ventilation has been attributed to gold salt toxicity in a patient with rheumatoid arthritis (20). Glucocorticoid therapy was life-saving and induced complete resolution of the lung damage.

Pneumonitis associated with gold has been reported in a woman with rheumatoid arthritis.

- A 77-year-old woman with rheumatoid arthritis was given sodium aurothiomalate 50 mg intramuscularly weekly, following a test dose of 10 mg (21). Her rheumatoid arthritis responded well, but after a cumulative dose of 560 mg she became progressively short of breath on exertion and generally felt unwell. She had bilateral basal inspiratory crackles and widespread ill-defined shadowing on the chest X-ray, predominantly in the middle and lower zones of both lungs. A high-resolution CT scan showed ground glass opacities, particularly in the upper zones, and thickening of the peribronchovascular interstitium and interlobular septa in the middle and lower zones. Pulmonary function tests showed a restrictive lung defect. The gold injections were discontinued and she responded well to methylprednisolone. A CT scan 10 months later showed almost complete resolution, with some heterogeneity of lung density posteriorly in the lower lobes.

Interstitial pneumonia has been described in an adult who had taken auranofin for only 6 days; glucocorticoids were required (SEDA-17, 276).

Nervous system

Gold can damage nervous tissue. Peripheral neuropathy due to gold is possibly not as rare as was previously assumed and can co-exist with a neuroencephalopathy or other symptoms, such as dizziness and nausea (22). Nervous damage can take other forms: peripheral pain, general malaise, psychiatric disorders, and insomnia can be the first uncharacteristic symptoms and can easily be overlooked as adverse effects. Acute polyneuropathy of the Guillain-Barré type (SED-12, 521) (23), myokymia (Morvan-type fibrillating chorea) (SEDA-6, 216) (24), and gold encephalopathy (25) are rare neurological complications of chrysotherapy that have, however, all been well documented from different sources (24).

- A woman in whom gold had been withdrawn because of a rash developed a severe parkinsonian tremor of the hands a week later (22).

An axonal polyneuropathy has been attributed to gold (26).

- A 63-year-old man with a 4-month history of rheumatoid arthritis developed progressive malaise, anorexia, and weight loss, and had a 2-day history of diarrhea, fever, and chills. He had epigastric and periumbilical pain radiating to the back, associated with nausea, abdominal distension, and jaundice. He was taking prednisone 5 mg bd and diclofenac sodium 100 mg bd. He had recently started weekly gold injections (total dose of gold 150 mg). He received two test doses before starting induction therapy, with no adverse effects. Both gold and diclofenac sodium were withdrawn and 2 weeks later he complained of symmetrical distal paresthesia in a glove and stocking distribution. There was no weakness, parallel reflexes were diminished, and the ankle reflexes were both absent. Nerve conduction studies showed a reduction in sensory nerve action potential amplitude in the sural and median nerves, with normal motor conduction. There was a slightly increased threshold for warm and cold sensations in the foot, with normal results in the hand. A liver needle biopsy showed preserved liver architecture with marked cholestasis mainly in the central and mid zones. A positive lymphocyte transformation test to gold suggested a cell-mediated hypersensitivity reaction.

Intrathecal colloidal gold has been used as an adjunct in the treatment of childhood neoplasms, including medulloblastoma and leukemia. Long-term follow-up of patients treated with intrathecal colloidal gold has been described and the high incidence of delayed cerebrovascular complications and their management has been emphasized (27).

Between 1967 and 1970, 14 children with a posterior fossa medulloblastoma underwent treatment consisting of surgical resection, external beam radiotherapy, and intrathecal colloidal gold. All had persistent or recurrent disease and six died within 2 years of treatment. The eight surviving patients developed significant neurovascular complications 5–20 years after treatment. Three patients died as a result of aneurysmal subarachnoid hemorrhage and five developed cerebral ischemic symptoms from a severe vasculopathy that resembled moyamoya disease. Although therapy with colloidal gold results in long-term survival in a number of cases of childhood medulloblastoma, this study suggests that its severe cerebrovascular adverse effects fail to justify its use. The authors recommended routine screening of any long-term survivors after colloidal gold therapy, to exclude the presence of an intracranial aneurysm and to document the possibility of moyamoya disease.

Sensory systems

Chryseosis corneae (deposition of gold crystals in the cornea) occurs rarely in patients treated with a cumulative dose of up to 500 mg of gold, but they occur in nearly all patients who have received 1500 mg or more (28). Deposition of gold as such has no clinical consequences. Gold can occasionally cause a keratitis or keratoconjunctivitis, but these are usually associated with skin involvement and are not a consequence of gold deposits in the cornea.

Gold keratopathy has been reported in a woman with rheumatoid arthritis (29).

- A-60-year-old woman with rheumatoid arthritis who was taking prednisone, azathioprine, sulindac, plaquenil, and receiving intramuscular injections of gold sodium thiomalate (50 mg once weekly) developed intense, bilateral ocular irritation and photophobia. She had received a total of 7.4 g of gold over the past 3 years. Her conjunctivae were mildly injected, with bilateral perilimbal chemosis. The peripheral corneae showed 360° stromal edema. Mid-stromal vessels were seen entering the edematous stroma from the limbus. She was given topical prednisolone acetate hourly for rheumatoid marginal keratitis. Over the next 2 months her symptoms gradually resolved, but granular, golden-brown, pigmented deposits appeared in the corneal stroma in the same peripheral ring-like distribution as the resolved stromal keratitis. Gold was discontinued. Over the next 6 months, the stromal deposits partially cleared. She then had a milder episode of photophobia and irritation, with stromal edema in the same distribution. This was controlled by topical prednisolone. One year later, she continued to use topical prednisolone once a day and was asymptomatic, with no stromal inflammation, but persistent fine golden granules.

Conjunctivitis has occurred in some 10% of patients treated with auranofin, either early or late in treatment, and has led to withdrawal in about in 1% (30).

Metabolism

In one case, diabetes was destabilized after 3 weeks of auranofin treatment (31).

Hematologic

Because of the hematological effects of gold salts, full blood counts should be monitored regularly at least during the first 2 years of treatment (32).

Pure red cell aplasia occurred in a patient with cholestatic jaundice taking sodium aurothiomalate (SEDA-17, 275). Anemia has been reported occasionally with auranofin (0.1%) either as a direct effect or secondary to hematuria.

Eosinophilia in the peripheral blood is the most frequent hematological effect of parenteral gold salts, affecting up to 40% of patients. It is no longer believed that it is a reliable advance marker of more serious reactions of any type (33). Among the latter are severe blood dyscrasias, which sometimes appear unexpectedly, despite regular blood counts.

Auranofin has been associated with eosinophilia (range of incidence in various reports 0.1–13%). In a retrospective study of 82 patients with rheumatoid arthritis there was eosinophilia in 21% taking sodium aurothiomalate and 13% taking auranofin (33). However, early eosinophilia is not a reliable indicator of potential toxicity.

Leukopenia is rare, sometimes very mild, and not always related to gold (SED-12, 522). Granulocytopenia can evolve slowly or suddenly, and its course can be transient or prolonged. Some workers have found gold-associated granulocytopenias to be brief and self-limiting; indeed, if other marrow elements are unimpaired, full recovery can occur even from severe agranulocytosis. Full-fledged aplastic anemia and pancytopenia are the most serious and feared conditions, and although they are today uncommon, deaths continue to occur (SEDA-13, 192), particularly because of superimposed infections or hemorrhage. Auranofin has been associated with leukopenia (0.1%), lymphopenia, and neutropenia (SEDA-10, 207).

Leukopenia with liver damage has been reported (34).

- A 62-year-old woman with rheumatoid arthritis developed swelling and pain of both knees. Aurothiomalate was given in a test dose of 12.5 mg, followed the next day by a dose of 25 mg, and then 50 mg twice weekly (total cumulative dose 137.5 mg). She had a leukocyte count of 2.2×10^9/l, a normochromic anemia, and a normal platelet count. Her liver enzyme activities were raised. Aurothiomalate was withdrawn and about 6 weeks later her liver function tests returned to normal and her white cell count rose to 6.9×10^9/l.

Thrombocytopenia occurs in 0.7–3% of cases and can be severe (35). It presents with petechiae, hematuria, oral mucosal bleeding, and other hemorrhagic phenomena. Some cases are due to immune reactions, others to a direct toxic effect of gold on the megakaryocytes, and it is important to distinguish the two types. For an immunologically mediated thrombocytopenia, high-dose steroid therapy should be used if necessary, followed or accompanied by immunosuppressive drugs, infusions of fresh frozen plasma or high-dose immunoglobulin, and even splenectomy. Toxic thrombocytopenia probably demands gold chelator therapy. There is no correlation between the appearance of thrombocytopenia and effects on the skin or kidney (36). Thrombocytopenia is known with auranofin but rare (0.5%). Three patients developed serious thrombocytopenia after taking auranofin for 3 months (35). Auranofin was withdrawn and two of the patients were given oral glucocorticoids; platelet counts normalized within 8 weeks.

It has been postulated that early treatment with very high doses of intravenous *N*-acetylcysteine and the use of immunomodulatory drugs, such as antithymocyte globulin and ciclosporin, can improve the recovery of hematological parameters, even in the case of pancytopenia (37). One case of gold-induced aplastic anemia, unresponsive to various treatments, recovered after therapy with antithymocyte globulin (SED-12, 522).

Lymphadenopathy is a rare complication of gold injections (SEDA-12, 188). In one case lymphadenopathy in association with a patient with rheumatoid arthritis; biopsy of the lymph nodes showed crystalline material containing gold (SEDA-16, 234).

- A 34-year-old woman was given intramuscular sodium aurothiomalate for rheumatoid arthritis after little response to anti-inflammatory drugs (38). After the sixth injection she developed enlarged neck and axillary lymph nodes. Biopsy showed subtotal infarction of a reactive node, confirmed by histochemical, immunohistochemical, and molecular techniques. Gold was withdrawn and the lymphadenopathy gradually resolved over the next 2 months. She continued to suffer from rheumatoid arthritis with no evidence of malignant lymphoma after 3 years.

This case provides strong evidence that gold salts can cause malignant lymphoma.

Although there is no direct evidence of potentiation of hematological toxicity, the concomitant use of drugs that are known to carry a risk of blood dyscrasias is unwise. Simultaneous use of glucocorticoids in small doses is not thought to detract from the beneficial effects of gold and can delay the onset of adverse reactions (39)

Mouth and teeth

Stomatitis, sometimes preceded by a metallic taste, is a frequent complication of gold. It can take the form of superficial buccal erosions, which produce mild symptoms but tend to run a protracted course (40).

There has been one unusual report of obstructive sialadenitis caused by local compression of the excretory ducts of the parotid glands due to deposits of gold in the intraparotid lymphoid tissues; there was swelling of both parotid glands on eating (41).

Gastrointestinal

Fulminant enterocolitis or panenteritis are rare manifestations of gold intolerance; more than 30 cases have been published since 1945 (42) and one-third of them have been fatal. The presenting symptoms are diarrhea, rectal bleeding, and vomiting. Bowel dilatation can develop. The course of the disease is occasionally complicated by overwhelming infection. The X-ray picture sometimes simulates regional or ischemic enteritis. Pathological findings include intense mucosal edema, ulceration, hemorrhage, and infiltration of lymphocytes and plasma cells. No treatment is known. However, there is a milder eosinophilic type of enterocolitis due to gold, which, it has been suggested, responds to treatment with cromoglicate. Two cases of ischemic colitis have also been described, presenting as abdominal pain and rectal bleeding (SEDA-21, 236) (43).

The most common adverse effects of auranofin are gastrointestinal. About half of all users have loose stools at some time during treatment; this effect can be transient, can occur at any time, and is rarely severe. No infective cause or signs of malabsorption has been found in any case and neither was gold absorption adversely affected. In a long-term study, diarrhea was mainly observed in the first 6 months of therapy with auranofin 6 mg/day; in 8% of the cases this was a reason for withdrawal (44). There is experimental evidence in animals of a direct effect of auranofin on ion and water absorption from the intestine with inhibition of enterocyte Na^+/K^+-ATPase activity (SED-12, 525).

Stomatitis occurs in about 10% of patients taking auranofin, generally early in treatment, demanding withdrawal in up to 1% (45) (SEDA-9, 217).

Two patients developed fulminant colitis with toxic megacolon during treatment with auranofin (46,47). Both recovered completely within 4–6 weeks with supportive treatment, including high doses of prednisone.

Liver

Liver injury is an extremely rare complication of gold therapy (SEDA-14, 189) (48). The underlying mechanisms are probably complex and certainly variable. Overdosage can cause centrilobular necrosis and bile stasis. With normal doses intrahepatic cholestasis with an absence of necrosis is more likely, although there can be both bile duct damage and canalicular damage (49); an immunological mechanism for this disorder has been suggested. Several cases of a severe form of idiosyncratic hepatic necrosis soon after starting chrysotherapy have been described (11,50). However, most hepatic lesions as a rule resolve rapidly after withdrawal of chrysotherapy, and mild or moderate liver injury of any type is not necessarily a contraindication to gold treatment.

- A 62-year-old man with rheumatoid factor positive rheumatoid arthritis developed painless icterus, nausea and vomiting, and discolored stools (51). He had previously been given methotrexate without effect, and was instead given aurothioglucose 50 mg/week (cumulative dose 160 mg). He reported sweating, fatigue, and myalgia shortly after each gold injection. The liver was tender but not enlarged, and there were no signs of splenomegaly. Liver function tests showed a cholestatic pattern and predominantly conjugated hyperbilirubinemia. All potentially hepatotoxic drugs (aurothioglucose, naproxen, and aspirin) were withdrawn and his dose of prednisone was increased to 15 mg/day. His liver function tests normalized 4 weeks later.

Mild and transient abnormalities in serum transaminase and alkaline phosphatase activities have been reported during therapy with auranofin (0.4%). This is noteworthy, since almost all patients were taking acetylsalicylic acid or other non-steroidal anti-inflammatory drugs, which also can cause increases in transaminases. There has been a report of two cases of toxic hepatosis in patients taking auranofin (52).

Urinary tract

Mild proteinuria develops in 2–3% of patients receiving chrysotherapy; it is usually benign and reversible within a few weeks after discontinuation of therapy (53). No deterioration in creatinine clearance has been found at periodic follow-up. It is not always necessary to stop gold treatment if a patient develops proteinuria, provided there is no marked loss of renal function and proteinuria is not in the nephrotic range. Gold therapy can be continued under close monitoring for at least 10 months without causing permanent renal damage (54).

Proteinuria has been observed in many trials of auranofin, but in contrast to cases associated with parenteral gold it has only rarely progressed to nephrotic syndrome. Of 1283 auranofin-treated patients, 38 had a raised urinary protein concentration, but only in nine it was heavy, and in most patients who continued treatment the proteinuria did not persist beyond the first 12 months of treatment; seven of eight who were rechallenged, after auranofin had been withdrawn and the protein had cleared, were able to continue treatment without relapse. Biopsy showed membranous glomerulonephritis, suggesting an underlying immunopathological mechanism (55).

Microhematuria has long been considered a manifestation of nephrotoxicity from chrysotherapy, but one multicenter study showed no higher an incidence than in patients receiving placebo (SED-12, 522). Hematuria associated with auranofin has been reported in a few patients, generally after at least 2–3 months of treatment (56).

Serious nephrotoxicity is uncommon, but nephrotic syndrome can develop in about 0.3% of patients, generally among those who have experienced mild proteinuria earlier in treatment. Very exceptionally, acute renal insufficiency can occur; peritoneal dialysis has been reported to promote recovery.

The histological findings in cases of gold nephropathy range from essentially normal glomeruli to a focal increase in mesangium, glomerular basement membrane thickening or splitting, membranous glomerulonephritis (57,58), periglomerular fibrosis with proliferation of Bowman's capsule, and even hyalinization of glomeruli. Chronic interstitial nephritis can also occur (59). Fortunately, many cases of renal complications run a benign course if gold is withdrawn (58).

Gold nephropathy is often considered to be an immunological disorder, and IgG and C3 are usually present in fine granular immune complex deposits along the capillary walls of the glomeruli. Oddly, however, X-ray microanalysis fails to detect gold as a component of the deposited immune complexes, throwing doubt on the concept that gold itself acts as an antigen or a hapten. Gold might however alter the proximal tubular cells in such a way that tubular autoantigens are released, resulting in the development of antigen–antibody complexes; these would then become attached to the glomerular basement membrane, inducing membranous glomerulopathy and proteinuria. That gold does damage the tubular cells is well known, although there appears to be no correlation with dosage and duration of therapy. Gold-containing, electron-dense, filamentous, cytoplasmic inclusions have been found in proximal tubular cells. The urinary excretion of beta-glucosaminidase, leucine aminopeptidase, beta$_2$-microglobulin, and other tubular proteins has often been found to be increased in patients treated with gold compounds (SEDA-15, 229). Tubular dysfunction can persist for up to 2 years after the end of chrysotherapy.

Skin

Skin reactions are the most frequent of all adverse effects of gold; they develop in about 25% of patients, sometimes in association with other forms of gold intolerance. Up to 30% of patients taking auranofin develop mucocutaneous adverse effects and 18–24% develop a rash or pruritus, meriting withdrawal in some 4% of cases (SEDA-10, 208).

Skin reactions to gold salts can be toxic or immunological, and patch-testing is often positive (51). No increase in gold concentration in the skin has been found, nor is there any correlation with blood concentrations of gold. Skin biopsies show that both macrophages and Langerhans cells are actively involved in the pathogenesis of gold dermatitis (61).

Pruritus is the commonest and earliest manifestation of such reactions and can precede an eruption by some weeks. Lesions are of every conceivable type, ranging from transient, non-specific, localized, or generalized dermatitis (eczema) and erythematous, maculopapular rash to lichen planus-like eruptions, discoid eczema, pityriasis rosacea, erythema multiforme, erythema nodosum, scaling eruptions, urticaria, photosensitivity, hyperkeratosis, seborrheic dermatitis, toxic epidermal necrolysis, and granuloma annulare. Exacerbation of pre-existing psoriasis has been reported (62). Patients receiving aurothioglucose have sometimes developed a dermatitis closely resembling contact dermatitis (SED-12, 523). More than one of these effects can occur in the same patient.

Gold can also cause pemphigus (63).

- A 53-year-old woman with rheumatoid arthritis who had reacted to D-penicillamine treatment by developing myasthenia gravis was given gold instead and 12 months later developed pemphigus vulgaris (60).

Not every gold-induced skin disorder is necessarily wholly disfiguring; in one curious case, the patient was seen to "glitter" with tiny specks of a gold-coloured (and gold-containing) material covering the skin of the neck, upper arms, and back (64).

Chrysiasis, a gray, blue, or purple pigmentation on light-exposed skin areas, is a complication that tends to be permanent (SEDA-20, 210). In one series of 40 patients receiving sodium aurothiomalate it appeared in 31 (65).

Inadvertent gold administration has reportedly caused an allergic skin rash (66).

- A 31-year-old woman developed a rash, similar to the rash she had experienced after wearing gold jewellery. The evening before she had taken about 90–120 ml of Goldschlager liquor, a cinnamon schnapps that can contain as much as 8–17 mg of gold in 750 ml. The rash was isolated to her neck, upper chest, and hands and was erythematous and pruritic with no borders or margins. Her rash resolved over 2 weeks without desquamation.

In patients with a history of localized hypersensitivity to metallic gold, allergic skin reactions can develop in the sensitized region after gold injections (SEDA-13, 193).

Worldwide experience with auranofin points to a 2% incidence of alopecia, but this included older experience at high doses; at current doses, alopecia is rather less common (30).

If skin reactions are not serious, withdrawal of gold is not essential, and some physicians deliberately increase the dosage to the point where some skin reaction occurs, as a means of securing the best possible therapeutic effect. Once troublesome reactions have appeared they can often be relieved simply by reducing the dosage or the frequency of administration. More troublesome reactions will demand withdrawal of gold, and in that case most skin lesions will begin to subside within a few days or a week, and disappear within several weeks more; it may then be possible to resume gold at a reduced dosage (67). On the other hand, some gold-induced skin lesions can run a protracted course, in certain cases necessitating topical or systemic glucocorticoid treatment. A patchy brown discoloration can persist after the disorders have resolved. When gold has been withdrawn it can often be restarted later without recurrence of the lesion.

Nails

Gold rarely causes yellow thickening of the nails and onycholysis, followed by irreversible nail dystrophy (SED-9, 373).

- A 34-year-old woman with severe rheumatoid arthritis developed yellow thickening of all 20 nails 2 years after starting gold therapy (68). She had received 50 mg of gold salts intramuscularly at intervals of 2–4 weeks after an initial course of weekly injections (total cumulative dose 90 mg/kg) over 4 years. There was associated thickening of the nail plate, increased transverse curvature, and mild subungual hyperkeratosis. There was onycholysis of both thumbnails and the right little fingernail. There was no associated chrysiasis. Gold was withdrawn. The yellow discoloration began to grow out and fingernail growth increased in the next 3 months. Six months later there was further improvement, although light yellow discoloration of all nails persisted and there was markedly increased longitudinal growth. Both thumbnails showed transverse depressions of the nail plate (Beau's lines) where the change in growth rate had presumably occurred.

Immunologic

Several patients with selective IgA deficiency and even a panhypogammaglobulinemia during intramuscular gold treatment have been described (SEDA-14, 190) (SEDA-15, 230) (SEDA-21, 237).

Polyarteritis (69) and systemic lupus erythematosus (70) have been reported after the administration of gold compounds.

- After taking sodium aurothiomalate for 10 months (cumulative dose 550 mg) a 12-year-old girl with severe exudative polyarthritis developed pericarditis, high titers of antinuclear antibodies, and antibodies to native double-stranded DNA (70). After withdrawal her symptoms rapidly disappeared and did not recur after a follow-up period of 5 years. The titers of autoantibodies fell to normal within 1 year.

In one series of some 5500 patients with juvenile rheumatoid arthritis, 105 were found to have developed secondary amyloidosis; 37 of the latter had been receiving sodium aurothiomalate. In 12 of these children the time between withdrawal of gold (because of adverse effects) and the finding of amyloid A was less than six months (SEDA-21, 237).

- A 63-year-old woman with rheumatoid arthritis was given intramuscular gold sodium thiomalate and began to have nausea, vomiting, anorexia, and watery diarrhea (71). A year later the watery diarrhea became more frequent (more than 10 times within a day) and she developed proteinuria. Biopsies from the stomach, duodenum, and kidney showed systemic amyloidosis. This was a rare case of secondary systemic amyloidosis associated with rheumatoid arthritis. It is not clear from the report what the role of gold was in this case.

Infection risk

An increased incidence of *Herpes zoster* was found in a series of patients receiving sodium aurothiomalate; the mechanism is unknown, but herpesvirus infection can also occur in association with some other heavy metals, for example in environmental poisoning.

The incidence of *H. zoster* infection in auranofin-treated patients was slightly higher (0.9%) than in patients with rheumatoid arthritis not receiving gold therapy (0.4%), but less frequent than in patients given parenteral gold compounds (3.1%).

Body temperature

There may be transient exacerbation of rheumatoid symptoms before a therapeutic response to gold occurs. In one series of 43 patients with rheumatoid arthritis serious exacerbation of the disease occurred in 17% (12).

Second-Generation Effects

Teratogenicity

In 1980, alarm was caused by a report of a seriously malformed child born to a mother who had been treated with sodium aurothiomalate during pregnancy (72), particularly since a partially congruent pattern of neural abnormalities had earlier been described in rats and rabbits, and given the fact that gold crosses the placenta. On the other hand, a Danish team in 1983 studied eight children born after exposure to gold in utero from weeks 2–9 or longer; no abnormalities were found, and the children appeared to develop normally during a follow-up period averaging 8.6 years (73). In view of the lack of further incriminating evidence some physicians today adopt the view that chrysotherapy can be continued in selected pregnant women whose rheumatoid arthritis is of such severity as to warrant treatment.

Lactation

Breastfeeding is not recommended since gold salts are excreted in the milk (SEDA-12, 188) (SEDA-13, 193).

Susceptibility Factors

Genetic factors

There is good evidence that patients with rheumatoid arthritis who carry the DR3 antigen run a greater risk of proteinuria (74), mucocutaneous reactions (75), and hematological actions (76) to parenteral gold compounds as well as to penicillamine, although such patients also tend to react rather better than others to aurothioglucose (77). The same applies to the B8, DR3 haplotype (81). The prevalence of the HLA antigens DR2 and DR7 is lower among rheumatoid arthritis patients with toxic reactions than among patients without toxic reactions or among controls (79). Because of conflicting results and the low relative risk, HLA typing has not been of much practical help as a guide to forecasting the risk of therapy.

Patients with rheumatoid arthritis and poor sulfoxidation state are six times more susceptible than others to the adverse effects of sodium aurothiomalate (80). This parallels an earlier similar finding with penicillamine, which has the same sulfhydryl group in its structure.

Age

Several studies have shown that in juvenile chronic arthritis auranofin gives rise to fewer adverse reactions than in adults, but the therapeutic effect is dubious and variable (SEDA-17, 277).

Elderly patients were once thought to be more likely than younger individuals to develop severe reactions (81) but this seems not to be so (82).

Other features of the patient

There are various contraindications to gold therapy (83): active hepatic disease, impaired renal function, colitis, patients with a history of hematological disorders, and patients who have recently had radiotherapy (because of the depressant action of radiotherapy on hemopoietic tissue).

Drug Administration

Drug overdose

- Severe overdosage of sodium aurothiopropanol sulfonate (1.1 g daily for 13 days) caused jaundice and skin eruptions. Liver biopsies showed modest centrilobular necrosis and significant bile stasis. Serum hepatic enzyme activities were increased. The patient was treated with dimercaprol and recovered after 2 months, although alkaline phosphatase and gamma-glutamyltransferase activities remained high for 6 months.

It seems advisable in cases of acute gold intoxication to adopt a conservative strategy. Should severe complications occur, supportive therapy can be given in combination with such treatments as chelation, glucocorticoids, or gamma-globulin.

Drug–Drug Interactions

Glucocorticoids

In a placebo-controlled study auranofin reduced the doses of glucocorticoids needed in asthma (84). This is perhaps a parallel effect rather than an interaction since, as noted above, gold itself may have an effect in asthma.

References

1. Tiekink ER. Gold derivatives for the treatment of cancer. Crit Rev Oncol Hematol 2002;42(3):225–48.
2. Burmester GR. Molekulare Wirkungsmechanismen von Gold bei der Behandlung der Rheumatoiden Arthritis—ein Update. [Molecular mechanisms of action of gold in treatment of rheumatoid arthritis—an update.] Z Rheumatol 2001;60(3):167–73.
3. Gabriel SE, Coyle D, Moreland LW. A clinical and economic review of disease-modifying antirheumatic drugs. Pharmacoeconomics 2001;19(7):715–28.
4. Rothermich NO, Philips VK, Bergen W, Thomas MH. Chrysotherapy. A prospective study. Arthritis Rheum 1976;19(6):1321–7.
5. Griffin AJ, Gibson T, Huston G. A comparison of conventional and low dose sodium aurothiomalate treatment in rheumatoid arthritis. Br J Rheumatol 1983;22(2):82–8.
6. Sambrook PN, Browne CD, Champion GD, Day RO, Vallance JB, Warwick N. Terminations of treatment with

gold sodium thiomalate in rheumatoid arthritios. J Rheumatol 1982;9(6):932–4.

7. Vamnes JS, Morken T, Helland S, Gjerdet NR. Dental gold alloys and contact hypersensitivity. Contact Dermatitis 2000;42(3):128–33.
8. Trathen WT, Stanley RJ. Allergic reaction to Hulka clips. Obstet Gynecol 1985;66(5):743–4.
9. Arrigoni-Martelli E. Antirheumatic drugs. Med Actual 1982;18:461.
10. Rau R. Hepatotoxicity of gold compounds. In: Schattenkirchner M, Muller W, editors. Modern Aspects of Gold Therapy. Rheumatology, an Annual Review. Basel-New York: Karger, 1983;8:188.
11. Watkins PB, Schade R, Mills AS, Carithers RL Jr, Van Thiel DH. Fatal hepatic necrosis associated with parenteral gold therapy. Dig Dis Sci 1988;33(8):1025–9.
12. Vlak T, Jajic I. Nepozeljni ucinci lijecenja solima zlata u bolesnika s reumatoidnim artritisom. [Side effects of gold salt therapy in patients with rheumatoid arthritis.] Reumatizam 1992;39(2):25–8.
13. Heuer MA, Pietrusko RG, Morris RW, Scheffler BJ. An analysis of worldwide safety experience with auranofin. J Rheumatol 1985;12(4):695–9.
14. Hill C, Pile K, Henderson D, Kirkham B. Neurological side effects in two patients receiving gold injections for rheumatoid arthritis. Br J Rheumatol 1995;34(10):989–90.
15. Gottlieb NL, Gray RG. Diagnosis and management of adverse reactions from gold compounds. J Anal Toxicol 1978;2:173.
16. Manero Ruiz FJ, Larraga Palacio R, Herrero Labarga I, Ferrer Peralta M. Neumonitis por sales de oro en la artritis psoriasica: a proposito de dos casos. [Pneumonitis caused by gold salts in psoriatic arthritis: report of 2 cases.] An Med Interna 2002;19(5):237–40.
17. Blackwell TS, Gossage JR. Gold pulmonary toxicity in a patient with a normal chest radiograph. South Med J 1995;88(6):644–6.
18. Evans RB, Ettensohn DB, Fawaz-Estrup F, Lally EV, Kaplan SR. Gold lung: recent developments in pathogenesis, diagnosis, and therapy. Semin Arthritis Rheum 1987;16(3):196–205.
19. Liebetrau G. Alveolitis-eine seltene Nebenwirkung der Goldtherapie. [Alveolitis—a rare side effect of gold therapy.] Z Erkr Atmungsorgane 1984;163(2):200–4.
20. Blancas R, Moreno JL, Martin F, de la Casa R, Onoro JJ, Gomez V, Prados J. Alveolar-interstitial pneumopathy after gold-salts compounds administration, requiring mechanical ventilation. Intensive Care Med 1998; 24(10):1110–12.
21. Sinha A, Silverstone EJ, O'Sullivan MM. Gold-induced pneumonitis: computed tomography findings in a patient with rheumatoid arthritis. Rheumatology (Oxford) 2001;40(6):712–14.
22. Machtey I. Neurological signs in RA patients receiving gold. Br J Rheumatol 1996;35(8):804.
23. Dick DJ, Raman D. The Guillain–Barré syndrome following gold therapy. Scand J Rheumatol 1982;11(2):119–20.
24. Fam AG, Gordon DA, Sarkozi J, Blair GR, Cooper PW, Harth M, Lewis AJ. Neurologic complications associated with gold therapy for rheumatoid arthritis. J Rheumatol 1984;11(5):700–6.
25. Perry RP, Jacobsen ES. Gold induced encephalopathy: case report. J Rheumatol 1984;11(2):233–4.
26. Ben-Ami H, Pollack S, Nagachandran P, Lashevsky I, Yarnitsky D, Edoute Y. Reversible pancreatitis, hepatitis, and peripheral polyneuropathy associated with parenteral gold therapy. J Rheumatol 1999;26(9):2049–50.
27. Nussbaum ES, Sebring LA, Neglia JP, Chu R, Mattsen ND, Erickson DL. Delayed cerebrovascular complications of intrathecal colloidal gold. Neurosurgery 2001;49(6): 1308–12.
28. Rodenhauser JH, Behrend T. Art und Häufigkeit der Augenbeteiligung nach parenteraler Goldtherapie. [Nature and frequency of ocular involvement after parenteral gold therapy.] Dtsch Med Wochenschr 1969;94(46): 2389–92.
29. Zamir E, Read RW, Affeldt JC, Ramaswamy D, Rao NA. Gold induced interstitial keratitis. Br J Ophthalmol 2001;85(11):1386–7.
30. Rau R, Kaik B, Muller-Fassbender H, et al. Auranofin (SK&F 39 162) and sodium aurothiomalate in the treatment of rheumatoid arthritis. Rheumatology 1983;8:162.
31. Anonymous. Auranofin–Diabetes situation impaired/ hypoglycemia. Bull SADRAC, June/October (English version), 3.
32. Cervi PL, Wright P, Casey EB. Audit of full blood count monitoring in patients on longterm gold therapy for rheumatoid arthritis. Ir J Med Sci 1992;161(3):73–4.
33. Edelman J, Davis P, Owen ET. Prevalence of eosinophilia during gold therapy for rheumatoid arthritis. J Rheumatol 1983;10(1):121–3.
34. Uhm WS, Yoo DH, Lee JH, Kim TH, Jun JB, Lee IH, Bae SC, Kim SY. Injectable gold-induced hepatitis and neutropenia in rheumatoid arthritis. Korean J Intern Med 2000;15(2):156–9.
35. Bakke E, Myklebust G, Gran JT. Trombocytopeni utlost ved auranofinbehandling. [Thrombocytopenia induced by auranofin treatment.] Tidsskr Nor Laegeforen 1997;117(28):4081–2.
36. Davis P. Undesirable effects of gold salts. J Rheumatol Suppl 1979;5:18–24.
37. Yan A, Davis P. Gold induced marrow suppression: a review of 10 cases. J Rheumatol 1990;17(1):47–51.
38. Roberts C, Batstone PJ, Goodlad JR. Lymphadenopathy and lymph node infarction as a result of gold injections. J Clin Pathol 2001;54(7):562–4.
39. Corkill MM, Kirkham BW, Chikanza IC, Gibson T, Panayi GS. Intramuscular depot methylprednisolone induction of chrysotherapy in rheumatoid arthritis: a 24-week randomized controlled trial. Br J Rheumatol 1990;29(4):274–9.
40. Glenert U. Drug stomatitis due to gold therapy. Oral Surg Oral Med Oral Pathol 1984;58(1):52–6.
41. Zuazua JS, de la Fuente AM, Rodriguez JC, Garcia GB, Rodriguez AP. Obstructive sialadenitis caused by intraparotid deposits of gold salts: a case report. Oral Surg Oral Med Oral Pathol Oral Radiol Endod 1996; 81(6):649–51.
42. Jackson CW, Haboubi NY, Whorwell PJ, Schofield PF. Gold induced enterocolitis. Gut 1986;27(4):452–6.
43. Cobeta Garcia JC, Ruiz Jimeno MT. Ischemic colitis associated with gold salts treatment. Rev Esp Reumatol 1996;23:105–7.
44. Wallin BA, McCafferty JP, Fox MJ, Cooper DR, Goldschmidt MS. Incidence and management of diarrhea during longterm auranofin therapy. J Rheumatol 1988;15(12):1755–8.
45. Furst DE. Mechanism of action, pharmacology, clinical efficacy and side effects of auranofin. An orally administered organic gold compound for the treatment of rheumatoid arthritis. Pharmacotherapy 1983;3(5):284–98.
46. Horing E. Goldinduzierte kolitis. Med Welt 1989;40:876.
47. Jarner D, Nielsen AM. Auranofin (SK + F 39162) induced enterocolitis in rheumatoid arthritis. A case report. Scand J Rheumatol 1983;12(3):254–6.
48. Harats N, Ehrenfeld M, Shalit M, Lijovetzky G. Gold-induced granulomatous hepatitis. Isr J Med Sci 1985;21(9):753–6.

49. Murphy M, Hunt S, McDonald GSA, et al. Intrahepatic cholestasis secondary to gold therapy. Eur J Gastroenterol Hepatol 1991;3:855–9.
50. Van Linthoudt D, Buss W, Beyner F, Ott H. Nécrose hépatique fatale au cours d'un traitement aux sels d'or d'une polyarthrite rheumatoide. [Fatal hepatic necrosis due to a treatment course of rheumatoid arthritis with gold salts.] Schweiz Med Wochenschr 1991; 121(30):1099–102.
51. te Boekhorst PA, Barrera P, Laan RF, van de Putte LB. Hepatotoxicity of parenteral gold therapy in rheumatoid arthritis: a case report and review of the literature. Clin Exp Rheumatol 1999;17(3):359–62.
52. Goebel KM, Storck U, Kohl FV, et al. Klinischer Effekt und unerwünschte Arzneimittelwirkungen von Auranofin bei rheumatoider Arthritis. Inn Med 1985;12:39.
53. Hall CL, Fothergill NJ, Blackwell MM, Harrison PR, MacKenzie JC, MacIver AG. The natural course of gold nephropathy: long term study of 21 patients. BMJ (Clin Res Ed) 1987;295(6601):745–8.
54. Hall CL, Tighe R. The effect of continuing penicillamine and gold treatment on the course of penicillamine and gold nephropathy. Br J Rheumatol 1989;28(1):53–7.
55. Katz WA, Blodgett RC. Jr., Pietrusko RG. Proteinuria in gold-treated rheumatoid arthritis. Ann Intern Med 1984;101(2):176–9.
56. Smith PR, Brown GM, Meyers OL. An open comparative study of auranofin vs. gold sodium thiomalate. J Rheumatol Suppl 1982;8:190–6.
57. Davenport A, Maciver AG, Hall CL, MacKenzie JC. Do mesangial immune complex deposits affect the renal prognosis in membranous glomerulonephritis? Clin Nephrol 1994;41(5):271–6.
58. Pospishil' IuA. Patogistologicheskie i ul'trastrukturnye osobennosti medikamentoznogo membranoznogo glomerulonefrita. [Pathohistologic and ultrastructural features of drug-induced membranous glomerulonephritis.] Arkh Patol 1996;58(5):52–6.
59. Cramer CR, Hagler HK, Silva FG, Eigenbrodt EH, Meltzer JI, Pirani CL. Chronic interstitial nephritis associated with gold therapy. Arch Pathol Lab Med 1983;107(5):258–63.
60. Ciompi ML, Marchetti G, Bazzichi L, Puccetti L, Agelli M. D-penicillamine and gold salt treatments were complicated by myasthenia and pemphigus, respectively, in the same patient with rheumatoid arthritis. Rheumatol Int 1995;15(3):95–7.
61. Ranki A, Niemi KM, Kanerva L. Clinical, immunohistochemical, and electron-microscopic findings in gold dermatitis. Am J Dermatopathol 1989;11(1):22–8.
62. Smith DL, Wernick R. Exacerbation of psoriasis by chrysotherapy. Arch Dermatol 1991;127(2):268–70.
63. Papacharalambous VG, Pramatarov KD, Tsankov NK. Development of pemphigus in a patient with rheumatoid arthritis during a course of gold therapy. Eur J Dermatol 1997;7(1):65–66.
64. Michalski JP, Isphording W, Parker S, Hardin JG. All that glitters may be gold. Arthritis Rheum 1991;34(8): 1069.
65. Smith RW, Leppard B, Barnett NL, Millward-Sadler GH, McCrae F, Cawley MI. Chrysiasis revisited: a clinical and pathological study. Br J Dermatol 1995; 133(5):671–8.
66. Guenthner T, Stork CM, Cantor RM. Goldschlager allergy in a gold allergic patient. Vet Hum Toxicol 1999;41(4):246.
67. Klinkhoff AV, Teufel A. How low can you go? Use of very low dosage of gold in patients with mucocutaneous reactions. J Rheumatol 1995;22(9):1657–9.
68. Roest MA, Ratnavel R. Yellow nails associated with gold therapy for rheumatoid arthritis. Br J Dermatol 2001;145(5):855–6.
69. Oochi N, Kbayashi K, Nanishi F, Tsuruda H, Onoyama K, Fujishima M, Omae T. [A case of gold nephropathy associated with polyarteritis nodosa.] Nippon Jinzo Gakkai Shi 1986;28(1):87–94.
70. Korholz D, Nurnberger W, Göbel U, Wahn V. Gold-induzierter systemischer Lupus erythematodes. [Gold-induced systemic lupus erythematosus.] Monatsschr Kinderheilkd 1988;136(9):644–6.
71. Tahara K, Nishiya K, Yoshida T, Matsubara Y, Matsumori A, Ito H, Kumon Y, Hashimoto K, Moriki T, Ookubo S. [A case of secondary systemic amyloidosis associated with rheumatoid arthritis after 3-year disease duration.] Ryumachi 1999;39(1):27–32.
72. Rogers JG, Anderson RM, Chow CW, Gillam GL, Markman L. Possible teratogenic effects of gold. Aust Paediatr J 1980;16(3):194–5.
73. Tarp U, Graudal H, Muller-Madsen B, et al. A follow-up study of children exposed to gold salts in utero. In: Abstracts, X European Congress of Rheumatology, Abstract No. 646. Moscow, 1983.
74. Hakala M, van Assendelft AH, Ilonen J, Jalava S, Tiilikainen A. Association of different HLA antigens with various toxic effects of gold salts in rheumatoid arthritis. Ann Rheum Dis 1986;45(3):177–82.
75. Speerstra F, van Riel PL, Reekers P, van de Putte LB, Vandenbroucke JP. The influence of HLA phenotypes on the response to parenteral gold in rheumatoid arthritis. Tissue Antigens 1986;28(1):1–7.
76. Speerstra F, Reekers P, van de Putte LB, Vandenbroucke JP. HLA associations in aurothioglucose- and D-penicillamine-induced haematotoxic reactions in rheumatoid arthritis. Tissue Antigens 1985;26(1):35–40.
77. van Riel PL, Reekers P, van de Putte LB, Gribnau FW. Association of HLA antigens, toxic reactions and therapeutic response to auranofin and aurothioglucose in patients with rheumatoid arthritis. Tissue Antigens 1983;22(3):194–9.
78. Singal DP, Green D, Reid B, Gladman DD, Buchanan WW. HLA-D region genes and rheumatoid arthritis (RA): importance of DR and DQ genes in conferring susceptibility to RA. Ann Rheum Dis 1992;51(1):23–8.
79. Rodriguez Perez M, Gonzalez Dominguez J, Mataran Perez L, Salvatierra Rios D. HLA DR7 como factor de proteccion frente a la toxicidad por sales de oro en la artritis reumatoide. [HLA DR7 as a protective factor against gold salt toxicity in rheumatoid arthritis.] An Med Interna 1993;10(10):484–6.
80. Madhok R, Capell HA, Waring R. Does sulphoxidation state predict gold toxicity in rheumatoid arthritis? BMJ (Clin Res Ed) 1987;294(6570):483.
81. Prupas HM. Stroke-like syndrome after gold sodium thiomalate induced vasomotor reaction. J Rheumatol 1984;11(2):235–6.
82. Kean WF, Bellamy N, Brooks PM. Gold therapy in the elderly rheumatoid arthritis patient. Arthritis Rheum 1983;26(6):705–11.
83. Wijnands MJ, van Riel PL, Gribnau FW, van de Putte LB. Risk factors of second-line antirheumatic drugs in rheumatoid arthritis. Semin Arthritis Rheum 1990;19(6):337–52.
84. Nierop G, Gijzel WP, Bel EH, Zwinderman AH, Dijkman JH. Auranofin in the treatment of steroid dependent asthma: a double blind study. Thorax 1992; 47(5):349–54.

Gonadorelin

General Information

The effects of gonadorelin depend on the duration of use. Gonadotropin release is stimulated in the short term, but is later suppressed owing to down-regulation of hypophyseal receptors. Its therapeutic indications have been summarized (SEDA-13, 1311) (1). Long-acting and depot formulations have the same adverse effects as shorter-acting analogues. The available gonadorelin analogues include buserelin, goserelin, leprorelin, nafarelin, and triptorelin (all rINNs).

Gonadorelin and its analogues cause an initial surge in follicle-stimulating hormone (FSH), luteinizing hormone (LH), and gonadal steroids. Receptor down-regulation and gonadotropin suppression occur after prolonged administration. Thus, both the clinical and adverse effects depend on the duration of administration. Biological activity and adverse effects also vary between gonadorelin agonists.

Comparative studies

In 67 premenopausal Japanese women randomized to 4-weekly, low-dose buserelin 1.8 mg or leuprorelin 1.88 mg, women given leuprorelin had a more rapid clinical response and a higher rate of hot flushes (2).

Adverse effects and quality of life have been compared in 431 men with prostate cancer treated with a gonadorelin agonist or orchidectomy (3). Of the men who reported normal sexual function before treatment, 51% had reduced libido and 69% became impotent. Of those given gonadorelin, 57% had hot flushes. Breast swelling was more common in those given gonadorelin (25% compared with 10% after orchidectomy).

Of 547 men randomized to leuprorelin plus flutamide for 3 or 8 months, those treated for 8 months had a higher overall rate of adverse events, and 87% had hot flushes, compared with 72% of those who were treated for 3 months (4).

Organs and Systems

Cardiovascular

Gonadorelin inhibits nitric oxide-mediated arterial relaxation, which disappears within 3 months after stopping treatment. This effect was abolished with "add-back" hormone replacement in a prospective, randomized study of 50 women treated for 6 months (5).

Respiratory

- A 75-year-old man developed a high fever and cough immediately after an injection of leuprorelin acetate 3.75 mg and 8 days after starting flutamide 375 mg/day (6). He died of respiratory failure after a month, and interstitial pneumonitis was confirmed postmortem.

There have been two other reports of pneumonitis associated with gonadorelin agonists.

Ear, nose, throat

Local irritation or rhinitis occurs uncommonly when gonadorelin agonists are taken intranasally.

- A 34-year-old woman had to stop using nafarelin nasal spray after 14 days because of exacerbation of maxillary sinusitis (7).

Nervous system

Pituitary apoplexy (hemorrhagic infarction presenting with sudden severe headache, often followed by pituitary hormone deficiency) has been reported after intravenous gonadorelin testing to investigate a pituitary macroadenoma and in several patients with gonadotropin-secreting pituitary macroadenomas who were given gonadorelin to treat prostate cancer (8). It may be advisable to assess gonadotropin status prior to therapy in such patients.

- A 43-year-old woman with a pituitary macroadenoma, who took quinagolide 37.5 micrograms/day for 33 months, developed a severe headache, nausea and vomiting, and photophobia 30 minutes after diagnostic testing with gonadorelin 50 micrograms intravenously (9). Although a CT scan at the time showed no evidence of hemorrhage, an MRI scan 18 months later showed a partial empty sella.
- A 67-year-old man with prostate cancer and an unsuspected pituitary macroadenoma developed a severe frontal headache, nausea and vomiting, and blindness within 12 hours of insertion of a goserelin implant (10).

Two further cases have been reported, in which gonadorelin was administered either alone (11) or with insulin (12). The mechanism of pituitary apoplexy in these cases is unclear. Gonadorelin may have a direct effect on vascular tone or may increase tumor metabolic activity.

There has been one previous report of seizure exacerbation during leuprorelin treatment, in a girl with pre-existing brain damage (13), and a case of de novo seizures has also been reported (14).

- A 13-year-old girl, who had previously had surgery and radiotherapy for a medulloblastoma, developed atypical absence seizures for the first time after 3 months of therapy with leuprorelin. The seizures stopped 1 month after treatment was withdrawn and did not recur until 30 months later. The seizures were not related to estradiol concentrations or the menstrual cycle.

Neuromuscular function

Prolonged administration of gonadorelin is commonly associated with reduced muscle bulk and voluntary muscle function. In a prospective, uncontrolled study of 62 men with prostate cancer, treatment with cyproterone acetate and goserelin caused an increase in fatigue scores and increased muscle fatiguability on objective testing within 6 weeks, in 66% of subjects (15). Fatigue was unrelated to psychological complaints or to self-reported functional ability.

Sensory systems

Blurred vision, sometimes associated with headache and dizziness, is common soon after the commencement of treatment and usually resolves within 2–3 weeks. It has recurred in some patients after rechallenge (16).

Psychological, psychiatric

Depressed mood and emotional lability occur in up to 75% of gonadorelin recipients, and there are rare reports of more severe mood disturbances (17). Defects of verbal memory have been described and may be reversed by "add-back" estrogen treatment (17) and sertraline (18).

- A 32-year-old woman had psychotic symptoms of persecutory delusions, agitation, and auditory hallucinations a few days after her second injection of triptorelin (19). Her symptoms recurred after a pregnancy, suggesting that they were due to the rapid fall in estrogen in both instances.

During a 6-month, randomized trial, men randomized to gonadorelin agonists had reduced attention and memory test scores, compared with men who were not given gonadorelin agonists but were closely monitored, in whom there was no change (20).

Endocrine

Symptoms of hypoestrogenism, including hot flushes, vaginal dryness, reduced libido, and mood changes, occur in almost all women on long-term gonadorelin. Men also experience hypogonadal symptoms with prolonged gonadorelin administration, including hot flushes and reduced libido, although this is a therapeutic effect rather than an adverse effect. Gynecomastia occasionally occurs in men.

"Add-back" estrogen replacement reduces the frequency and severity of these symptoms without apparently compromising the effectiveness of gonadorelin in women with endometriosis (18,21). In a randomized, multicenter, double-blind comparison of intranasal nafarelin twice daily and depot leuprolide acetate monthly for 6 months in 192 young women with endometriosis, nafarelin caused fewer hypoestrogenic symptoms, although the difference between the two groups was statistically significant only after 3 months of therapy (22).

"Draw-back" therapy, in which the dosage of nafarelin was reduced after 4 weeks, had similar efficacy, but a smaller degree of bone loss and fewer vasomotor adverse effects compared with full-dose therapy, in a randomized study in 15 premenopausal women (23).

- A 47-year-old woman developed symptoms of thyrotoxicosis (palpitation, tremor, tachycardia, and goiter) due to Graves' disease, after using goserelin acetate for 13 months (24).
- A 45-year-old woman developed transient thyroiditis associated with antithyroid antibodies in taking leuprorelin (25).

The second patient had other risk factors for autoimmune thyroid disease, and the association was probably coincidental, but the episode may have been precipitated by low estrogen concentrations, as is hypothesized in postpartum thyroiditis.

Metabolism

In 20 premenopausal women treated with triptorelin for 8 weeks, the mean LDL concentration rose from 2.7 to 3.9 mmol/l and HDL fell from 1.6 to 1.5 mmol/l (26). Although the change in HDL was not clinically relevant in isolation, the increases in LDL and LDL:HDL ratio were significant, suggesting an increased risk of atherogenesis. "Add-back" conjugated equine estrogen did not reverse these changes over 24 weeks.

- A woman with type 2 diabetes had worse glycemic control while receiving buserelin (27). Her blood glucose returned to its previous concentration after withdrawal.

Hematologic

Leuprolide acetate has been reported to cause normochromic normocytic anemia in patients with benign prostatic hyperplasia (28). The anemia is usually transient, and the hemoglobin returns to baseline 6 months after stopping androgen suppression. There is a single case report of more serious red cell aplasia in a patient receiving gonadorelin, with resolution after treatment was withdrawn (29).

Skin

Injection site reactions are common with gonadorelin receptor agonists. In 119 women randomized to subcutaneous triptorelin a local reaction (redness, pain, or bruising) was present after 1 hour in 24% and persisted for 24 hours in 9.5% (30). In another study in 105 women randomized to leuprorelin acetate, moderate local reactions occurred in 24% and severe reactions in 1% (31).

- A 48-year-old woman developed an itchy skin eruption and spotted dark brown pigmentation 3 weeks after starting nasal buserelin 900 micrograms/day. The lesions resolved when buserelin was withdrawn, and recurred with rechallenge; some persisted for up to 2 years (32).
- A 78-year-old man treated with subcutaneous leuprorelin acetate had repeated local reactions, with erythema, induration, abscesses, and an ulcer on one hip (33).

Altered skin pigmentation has been previously reported in pregnancy and after sex hormone administration, so the initial surge in gonadotropins after gonadorelin treatment was a probable cause for the first patient's presentation. In the second case the lactic acid/glycolic acid vehicle may have caused the reaction rather than leuprorelin.

Musculoskeletal

Osteoporosis, trabecular bone being most affected, has been regularly observed in both sexes with chronic gonadorelin agonist treatment (34), and the duration of therapy for prostate cancer is inversely related to bone mineral density (35,36). Intravenous pamidronate may prevent bone loss in these patients (37,38).

- A 44-year-old woman with no previous history of widespread pain, depression, or anxiety developed a diffuse pain syndrome consistent with fibromyalgia after leuprorelin treatment. Her symptoms increased in severity with three successive monthly injections, and persisted for several months (39).

In 47 children treated with depot leuprolide acetate for precocious puberty for 2 years, bone mineral density decreased significantly and markers of bone turnover increased significantly during treatment but were normal for age 2 years after treatment was withdrawn (40).

Since women have a lower initial bone mass than men their fracture risk is higher. Osteoporosis is reversible in premenopausal patients after gonadorelin withdrawal (41). However, the treatment period should be limited to 6 months.

Cross-sectional (42) and longitudinal (43) studies of men with prostate cancer have shown a significant relation between the duration of gonadorelin treatment and bone loss.

Estrogens, etidronate, and parathyroid hormone have been used with partial success to prevent gonadorelin-induced bone loss. In a prospective study of 49 women treated with goserelin and randomized to estradiol plus norethisterone or placebo, bone loss persisted 6 years after stopping therapy, and the hormone replacement therapy had only a minor protective effect (44).

- An 87-year-old man developed progressive proximal limb weakness 1 year after starting leuprolide therapy for prostate cancer (45). Electromyography showed a moderately severe non-inflammatory myopathy without evidence of fiber necrosis or associated biochemical changes. Within 6 months after stopping leuprolide he was able to resume his usual activities.

Three men developed rheumatoid arthritis 1–9 months after starting antiandrogen therapy with either cyproterone acetate or leuprolide acetate (46).

Reproductive system

Ovarian hyperstimulation syndrome (OHSS) affects up to 33% of women undergoing ovulation induction with gonadorelin receptor agonists and gonadotropins given in combination (47), or with gonadotropins alone (48). Gonadotropins are usually withheld if the diagnosis is made before conception (47,49).

OHSS is characterized by cystic ovarian enlargement, increased capillary permeability, and third space fluid accumulation (that is in an extracellular compartment that is not in equilibrium with either the extracellular or intracellular fluid, for example the bowel lumen, subcutaneous tissues, retroperitoneal space, or peritoneal cavity). Risk factors include a previous history of OHSS, age under 30 years (probably because more follicles are available), and polycystic ovary syndrome. Non-pregnant patients usually recover within 14 days with supportive treatment. The severe form (with ascites or pleural effusion and hemoconcentration) occurs in 1–10% of patients (49,50). In critical cases, hypoxemia, renal insufficiency, thromboembolism, and rarely death can occur (51).

- A 29-year-old woman with polycystic ovary syndrome had her first in vitro fertilization cycle of leuprorelin acetate, FSH, and human chorionic gonadotropin (hCG) (52). Within 2 days she complained of abdominal distension, shortness of breath, and abdominal pain. Over the next few days she developed massive ovarian enlargement, ascites, hyponatremia, respiratory failure, and renal insufficiency. This was further complicated by duodenal perforation, probably due to severe physical stress.
- Ovarian hyperstimulation syndrome occurred in a woman with polycystic ovarian syndrome, 3 weeks after an intramuscular injection of leuprorelin acetate for endometriosis (53). She was later given further courses of the drug without this complication.
- A 35-year-old obese woman with a previously undiagnosed pituitary gonadotroph adenoma developed multiple ovarian cysts and abdominal distension after 1 month of leuprolide therapy (54).
- A 32-year-old woman who was not obese developed benign intracranial hypertension in association with ovarian hyperstimulation syndrome after ovulation induction using goserelin, FSH, and hCG (55). The syndrome did not recur during a second pregnancy in which FSH and hCG were not used.

It is unclear which of the hormonal agents used was responsible for this complication in the last case.

Gonadorelin receptor antagonists have been reported to lower the risk of OHSS significantly. A meta-analysis showed that cetrorelix but not ganirelix reduced the incidence of OHSS by 75%, both overall and the severe form (56).

Thromboembolism is a serious complication of OHSS (57–60).

- A previously healthy 34-year-old woman who underwent ovulation induction with leuprorelin acetate and FSH developed abdominal ascites due to OHSS, followed by acute aphasia and right hemiparesis (61). The stroke was caused by a large intracardiac thrombus.

A review identified 54 other reports of thromboembolic disease associated with ovulation induction; 60% were in upper limb veins and two-thirds of the patients had OHSS (62). The mechanism for the increased risk of thrombosis in these patients has not been determined, but hemoconcentration or a hypercoagulable state associated with high estrogen concentrations could be responsible.

Immunologic

Altered immune function has been reported in several cases associated with gonadorelin agonist therapy. This is possibly related to the initial surge in sex steroids that occurs with these agents, but there is no evidence that this is the mechanism. Cardiac allograft rejection occurred in three men within months of starting gonadorelin therapy for prostate cancer. One died of heart failure, but the other two recovered cardiac function after the gonadorelin agonist was withdrawn (63).

Systemic lupus erythematosus can be exacerbated in the initial gonadotropin-stimulating phase of gonadorelin therapy: in one case this was fatal (64).

Long-Term Effects

Tumorigenicity

Tumor flare occurs in up to 30% of treated patients after the first 4–7 days of gonadorelin therapy, due to an initial surge in gonadotropin concentrations (65). For this reason antiandrogen treatment is often given before gonadorelin in men with prostate cancer. However, despite tumor flare there was no difference in survival in a prospective, multicenter comparison of gonadorelin and surgical oophorectomy in 136 patients (66).

Second-Generation Effects

Teratogenicity

Pregnancies have occurred both after low-dose gonadorelin agonist therapy for ovulation induction and after higher-dose therapy for endometriosis or other indications: these have been reviewed in the context of a report of a 36-year-old woman who stopped monthly goserelin injections at 16 weeks of gestation and delivered a healthy girl. Congenital abnormalities have been reported in a few cases, including one child with trisomy 13, one with trisomy 18, and an intrauterine death due to thrombosis; however most pregnancies have had normal outcomes (67).

Drug Administration

Drug formulations

There is no difference in the adverse effects profiles of long-acting or depot formulations compared with shorter-acting analogues used continuously.

Drug-Drug Interactions

Oral contraceptives

There were mild increases in serum triglyceride and cholesterol concentrations in 13 hirsute women treated with triptorelin and a triphasic oral contraceptive, in a randomized comparison of triptorelin with flutamide + cyproterone acetate (68). Altered lipid profiles have not been described before in patients receiving gonadorelin agonists and oral contraceptives.

References

1. Filicori M. Gonadotrophin-releasing hormone agonists. A guide to use and selection. Drugs 1994;48(1):41–58.
2. Takeuchi H, Kobori H, Kikuchi I, Sato Y, Mitsuhashi N. A prospective randomized study comparing endocrinological and clinical effects of two types of GnRH agonists in cases of uterine leiomyomas or endometriosis. J Obstet Gynaecol Res 2000;26(5):325–31.
3. Potosky AL, Knopf K, Clegg LX, Albertsen PC, Stanford JL, Hamilton AS, Gilliland FD, Eley JW, Stephenson RA, Hoffman RM. Quality-of-life outcomes after primary androgen deprivation therapy: results from the Prostate Cancer Outcomes Study. J Clin Oncol 2001;19(17):3750–7.
4. Gleave ME, Goldenberg SL, Chin JL, Warner J, Saad F, Klotz LH, Jewett M, Kassabian V, Chetner M, Dupont C, Van Rensselaer S; Canadian Uro-Oncology Group. Randomized comparative study of 3 versus 8-month neoadjuvant hormonal therapy before radical prostatectomy: biochemical and pathological effects. J Urol 2001; 166(2):500–6.
5. Yim SF, Lau TK, Sahota DS, Chung TK, Chang AM, Haines CJ. Prospective randomized study of the effect of "add-back" hormone replacement on vascular function during treatment with gonadotropin-releasing hormone agonists. Circulation 1998;98(16):1631–5.
6. Azuma T, Kurimoto S, Mikami K, Oshi M. Interstitial pneumonitis related to leuprorelin acetate and flutamide. J Urol 1999;161(1):221.
7. Heinig J, Coenen-Worch V, Cirkel U. Acute exacerbation of chronic maxillary sinusitis during therapy with nafarelin nasal spray. Eur J Obstet Gynecol Reprod Biol 2001;99(2):266–7.
8. Morsi A, Jamal S, Silverberg JD. Pituitary apoplexy after leuprolide administration for carcinoma of the prostate. Clin Endocrinol (Oxf) 1996;44(1):121–4.
9. Foppiani L, Piredda S, Guido R, Spaziante R, Giusti M. Gonadotropin-releasing hormone-induced partial empty sella clinically mimicking pituitary apoplexy in a woman with a suspected non-secreting macroadenoma J Endocrinol Invest 2000;23(2):118–21.
10. Eaton HJ, Phillips PJ, Hanieh A, Cooper J, Bolt J, Torpy DJ. Rapid onset of pituitary apoplexy after goserelin implant for prostate cancer: need for heightened awareness. Intern Med J 2001;31(5):313–14.
11. Hiroi N, Ichijo T, Shimojo M, Ueshiba H, Tsuboi K, Miyachi Y. Pituitary apoplexy caused by luteinizing hormone-releasing hormone in prolactin-producing adenoma. Intern Med 2001;40(8):747–50.
12. Matsuura I, Saeki N, Kubota M, Murai H, Yamaura A. Infarction followed by hemorrhage in pituitary adenoma due to endocrine stimulation test. Endocr J 2001;48(4): 493–8.
13. Minagawa K, Sueoka H. [Seizure exacerbation by the use of leuprorelin acetate for treatment of central precocious puberty in a female patient with symptomatic localization-related epilepsy.] No To Hattatsu 1999;31(5):466–8.
14. Akaboshi S, Takeshita K. A case of atypical absence seizures induced by leuprolide acetate. Pediatr Neurol 2000;23(3):266–8.
15. Stone P, Hardy J, Huddart R, A'Hern R, Richards M. Fatigue in patients with prostate cancer receiving hormone therapy. Eur J Cancer 2000;36(9):1134–41.
16. Fraunfelder FT, Edwards R. Possible ocular adverse effects associated with leuprolide injections. JAMA 1995;273(10):773–4.
17. Warnock JK, Bundren JC, Morris DW. Depressive symptoms associated with gonadotropin-releasing hormone agonists. Depress Anxiety 1998;7(4):171–7.
18. Moghissi KS, Schlaff WD, Olive DL, Skinner MA, Yin H. Goserelin acetate (Zoladex) with or without hormone replacement therapy for the treatment of endometriosis. Fertil Steril 1998;69(6):1056–62.
19. Mahe V, Nartowski J, Montagnon F, Dumaine A, Gluck N. Psychosis associated with gonadorelin agonist administration. Br J Psychiatry 1999;175:290–1.
20. Green HJ, Pakenham KI, Headley BC, Yaxley J, Nicol DL, Mactaggart PN, Swanson C, Watson RB, Gardiner RA. Altered cognitive function in men treated for prostate cancer with luteinizing hormone-releasing hormone analogues and cyproterone acetate: a randomized controlled trial. BJU Int 2002;90(4):427–32.
21. Freundl G, Godtke K, Gnoth C, Godehardt E, Kienle E. Steroidal "add-back" therapy in patients treated with GnRH agonists. Gynecol Obstet Invest 1998;45 Suppl 1:22–30; discussion 35.
22. Zhao SZ, Kellerman LA, Francisco CA, Wong JM. Impact of nafarelin and leuprolide for endometriosis on quality of life and subjective clinical measures. J Reprod Med 1999;44(12):1000–6.

23. Tahara M, Matsuoka T, Yokoi T, Tasaka K, Kurachi H, Murata Y. Treatment of endometriosis with a decreasing dosage of a gonadotropin-releasing hormone agonist (nafarelin): a pilot study with low-dose agonist therapy ("draw-back" therapy). Fertil Steril 2000;73(4):799–804.
24. Morita S, Ueda Y. Graves' disease associated with goserelin acetate. Acta Med Nagasaki 2002;47:79–80.
25. Kasayama S, Miyake S, Samejima Y. Transient thyrotoxicosis and hypothyroidism following administration of the GnRH agonist leuprolide acetate. Endocr J 2000;47(6): 783–5.
26. Al-Omari WR, Nassir UN, Izzat B. Estrogen "add-back" and lipid profile during GnRH agonist (triptorelin) therapy. Int J Gynaecol Obstet 2001;74(1):61–2.
27. Imai A, Takagi A, Horibe S, Fuseya T, Takagi H, Tamaya T. A gonadotropin-releasing hormone analogue impairs glucose tolerance in a diabetic patient. Eur J Obstet Gynecol Reprod Biol 1998;76(1):121–2.
28. Strum SB, McDermed JE, Scholz MC, Johnson H, Tisman G. Anaemia associated with androgen deprivation in patients with prostate cancer receiving combined hormone blockade. Br J Urol 1997;79(6):933–41.
29. Maeda H, Arai Y, Aoki Y, Okubo K, Okada T, Ueda Y. Leuprolide causes pure red cell aplasia. J Urol 1998;160(2):501.
30. van Hooren HG, Fischl F, Aboulghar MA, Nicollet B, Behre HM, Van der Ven H, Simon A, Kilani Z, Barri PN, Haberle M, Braat DD, Lambalk N; European and Middle East Orgalutran Study Group. Comparable clinical outcome using the GnRH antagonist ganirelix or a long protocol of the GnRH agonist triptorelin for the prevention of premature LH surges in women undergoing ovarian stimulation. Hum Reprod 2001;16(4):644–51.
31. Fluker M, Grifo J, Leader A, Levy M, Meldrum D, Muasher SJ, Rinehart J, Rosenwaks Z, Scott RT Jr, Schoolcraft W, Shapiro DB; North American Ganirelix Study Group. Efficacy and safety of ganirelix acetate versus leuprolide acetate in women undergoing controlled ovarian hyperstimulation. Fertil Steril 2001;75(1):38–45.
32. Kono T, Ishii M, Taniguchi S. Intranasal buserelin acetate-induced pigmented roseola-like eruption. Br J Dermatol 2000;143(3):658–9.
33. Hirashima N, Shinogi T, Sakashita N, Narisawa Y. A case of cutaneous injury induced by the subcutaneous injection of leuprolide acetate. Nishinihon J Dermatol 2001;63:384–6.
34. Fogelman I. Gonadotropin-releasing hormone agonists and the skeleton. Fertil Steril 1992;57(4):715–24.
35. Stoch SA, Parker RA, Chen L, Bubley G, Ko YJ, Vincelette A, Greenspan SL. Bone loss in men with prostate cancer treated with gonadotropin-releasing hormone agonists. J Clin Endocrinol Metab 2001;86(6):2787–91.
36. Kiratli BJ, Srinivas S, Perkash I, Terris MK. Progressive decrease in bone density over 10 years of androgen deprivation therapy in patients with prostate cancer. Urology 2001;57(1):127–32.
37. Smith MR, McGovern FJ, Zietman AL, Fallon MA, Hayden DL, Schoenfeld DA, Kantoff PW, Finkelstein JS. Pamidronate to prevent bone loss during androgen-deprivation therapy for prostate cancer. N Engl J Med 2001;345(13):948–55.
38. Diamond TH, Winters J, Smith A, De Souza P, Kersley JH, Lynch WJ, Bryant C. The antiosteoporotic efficacy of intravenous pamidronate in men with prostate carcinoma receiving combined androgen blockade: a double blind, randomized, placebo-controlled crossover study. Cancer 2001;92(6):1444–50.
39. Toussirot E, Wendling D. Fibromyalgia developed after administration of gonadotrophin-releasing hormone analogue. Clin Rheumatol 2001;20(2):150–2.
40. van der Sluis IM, Boot AM, Krenning EP, Drop SL, de Muinck Keizer-Schrama SM. Longitudinal follow-up of bone density and body composition in children with precocious or early puberty before, during and after cessation of GnRH agonist therapy. J Clin Endocrinol Metab 2002;87(2):506–12.
41. Paoletti AM, Serra GG, Cagnacci A, Vacca AM, Guerriero S, Solla E, Melis GB. Spontaneous reversibility of bone loss induced by gonadotropin-releasing hormone analogue treatment. Fertil Steril 1996;65(4):707–10.
42. Wei JT, Gross M, Jaffe CA, Gravlin K, Lahaie M, Faerber GJ, Cooney KA. Androgen deprivation therapy for prostate cancer results in significant loss of bone density. Urology 1999;54(4):607–11.
43. Daniell HW, Dunn SR, Ferguson DW, Lomas G, Niazi Z, Stratte PT. Progressive osteoporosis during androgen deprivation therapy for prostate cancer. J Urol 2000;163(1):181–6.
44. Pierce SJ, Gazvani MR, Farquharson RG. Long-term use of gonadotropin-releasing hormone analogues and hormone replacement therapy in the management of endometriosis: a randomized trial with a 6-year follow-up. Fertil Steril 2000;74(5):964–8.
45. Van Gerpen JA, McKinley KL. Leuprolide-induced myopathy. J Am Geriatr Soc 2002;50(10):1746.
46. Pope JE, Joneja M, Hong P. Anti-androgen treatment of prostatic carcinoma may be a risk factor for development of rheumatoid arthritis. J Rheumatol 2002;29(11):2459–62.
47. Whelan JG 3rd, Vlahos NF. The ovarian hyperstimulation syndrome. Fertil Steril 2000;73(5):883–96.
48. Mancini A, Milardi D, Di Pietro ML, Giacchi E, Spagnolo AG, Di Donna V, De Marinis L, Jensen L. A case of forearm amputation after ovarian stimulation for in vitro fertilization–embryo transfer. Fertil Steril 2001;76(1):198–200.
49. Beerendonk CC, van Dop PA, Braat DD, Merkus JM. Ovarian hyperstimulation syndrome: facts and fallacies. Obstet Gynecol Surv 1998;53(7):439–49.
50. Chillik C, Young E, Gogorza S, Estofan D, Neuspiller N, Antunes N Jr, Borges E Jr, Vantman D, Fabres C, Montoya JM, Madero JI, Gutierrez-Najar A, Bronfenmajer S, Kovacs A, Kroeze S; Out HJ. Latin-American Puregon IVF Study Group. A double-blind clinical trial comparing a fixed daily dose of 150 and 250 IU of recombinant follicle-stimulating hormone in women undergoing in vitro fertilization. Fertil Steril 2001;76(5):950–6.
51. Abramov Y, Elchalal U, Schenker JG. Febrile morbidity in severe and critical ovarian hyperstimulation syndrome: a multicentre study. Hum Reprod 1998;13(11):3128–31.
52. Uhler ML, Budinger GR, Gabram SG, Zinaman MJ. Perforated duodenal ulcer associated with ovarian hyperstimulation syndrome: Case Report. Hum Reprod 2001;16(1):174–6.
53. Jirecek S, Nagele F, Huber JC, Wenzl R. Ovarian hyperstimulation syndrome caused by GnRH-analogue treatment without gonadotropin therapy in a patient with polycystic ovarian syndrome. Acta Obstet Gynecol Scand 1998;77(9):940–1.
54. Castelbaum AJ, Bigdeli H, Post KD, Freedman MF, Snyder PJ. Exacerbation of ovarian hyperstimulation by leuprolide reveals a gonadotroph adenoma. Fertil Steril 2002;78(6):1311–13.
55. Lesny P, Maguiness SD, Hay DM, Robinson J, Clarke CE, Killick SR. Ovarian hyperstimulation syndrome and benign intracranial hypertension in pregnancy after in-vitro fertilization and embryo transfer: case report. Hum Reprod 1999;14(8):1953–5.
56. Ludwig M, Katalinic A, Diedrich K. Use of GnRH antagonists in ovarian stimulation for assisted reproductive technologies compared to the long protocol. Meta-analysis. Arch Gynecol Obstet 2001;265(4):175–82.

57. Ludwig M, Tolg R, Richardt G, Katus HA, Diedrich K. Myocardial infarction associated with ovarian hyperstimulation syndrome. JAMA 1999;282(7):632–3.
58. Belaen B, Geerinckx K, Vergauwe P, Thys J. Internal jugular vein thrombosis after ovarian stimulation. Hum Reprod 2001;16(3):510–12.
59. Loret de Mola JR, Kiwi R, Austin C, Goldfarb JM. Subclavian deep vein thrombosis associated with the use of recombinant follicle-stimulating hormone (Gonal-F) complicating mild ovarian hyperstimulation syndrome. Fertil Steril 2000;73(6):1253–6.
60. Yoshii F, Ooki N, Shinohara Y, Uehara K, Mochimaru F. Multiple cerebral infarctions associated with ovarian hyperstimulation syndrome. Neurology 1999;53(1):225–7.
61. Worrell GA, Wijdicks EF, Eggers SD, Phan T, Damario MA, Mullany CJ. Ovarian hyperstimulation syndrome with ischemic stroke due to an intracardiac thrombus. Neurology 2001;57(7):1342–4.
62. Stewart JA, Hamilton PJ, Murdoch AP. Thromboembolic disease associated with ovarian stimulation and assisted conception techniques. Hum Reprod 1997;12(10):2167–73.
63. Schofield RS, Hill JA, McGinn CJ, Aranda JM. Hormone therapy in men and risk of cardiac allograft rejection. J Heart Lung Transplant 2002;21(4):493–5.
64. Casoli P, Tumiati B, La Sala G. Fatal exacerbation of systemic lupus erythematosus after induction of ovulation. J Rheumatol 1997;24(8):1639–40.
65. Mahler C. Is disease flare a problem? Cancer 1993;72(Suppl 12):3799–802.
66. Taylor CW, Green S, Dalton WS, Martino S, Rector D, Ingle JN, Robert NJ, Budd GT, Paradelo JC, Natale RB, Bearden JD, Mailliard JA, Osborne CK. Multicenter randomized clinical trial of goserelin versus surgical ovariectomy in premenopausal patients with receptor-positive metastatic breast cancer: an intergroup study. J Clin Oncol 1998;16(3):994–9.
67. Jimenez-Gordo AM, Espinosa E, Zamora P, Feliu J, Rodriguez-Salas N, Gonzalez-Baron M. Pregnancy in a breast cancer patient treated with a LHRH analogue at ablative doses. Breast 2000;9(2):110–12.
68. Pazos F, Escobar-Morreale HF, Balsa J, Sancho JM, Varela C. Prospective randomized study comparing the long-acting gonadotropin-releasing hormone agonist triptorelin, flutamide, and cyproterone acetate, used in combination with an oral contraceptive, in the treatment of hirsutism. Fertil Steril 1999;71(1):122–8.

Gonadorelin antagonists

General Information

The gonadorelin antagonists include abarelix, cetrorelix, degarelix, detirelix, ganirelix, iturelix, prazarelix, ramorelix, and teverelix (all rINNs).

Gonadorelin agonists suppress the release of gonadotropin after an initial surge: pituitary suppression takes up to 2 weeks to develop. Competitive antagonists at gonadorelin receptors cause immediate inhibition of gonadotropin secretion without down-regulating the receptor. This class of agents would therefore be preferable to gonadorelin agonists when a rapid clinical effect is desired, for example in controlled ovarian stimulation.

Early gonadorelin antagonists were of low potency and tended to cause histamine release (1). However, ganirelix and cetrorelix are better tolerated (1,2). They do not share the lipophilic and histamine-releasing properties of earlier generation gonadorelin antagonists and neither do they lead to depot formation. There appears to be a narrow therapeutic margin in ovarian stimulation protocols. Ganirelix concentrations correlate with body weight, and it has been suggested that the dose should be adjusted to weight to maximize pregnancy rates (3). The adverse effects of ganirelix are usually mild and include minor injection site reactions, mild nausea, and malaise (1).

Organs and Systems

Endocrine

In a small, controlled study of 10 healthy men, cetrorelix increased concentrations of insulin, leptin, and apolipoprotein A-I compared with placebo (4). The clinical significance of these findings has yet to be determined.

Skin

Local injection reactions are common and probably dose-related. In an open study of cetrorelix in its lowest effective dose of 0.25 mg/day, 3 of 346 women described local reactions (5). In another study of 154 women, 115 of whom were randomized to one 3 mg dose of cetrorelix, 25% had transitory redness or itching at the injection site (2). In a multicenter European study of 463 women randomized to ganirelix and 238 to buserelin, 17% of those given ganirelix had moderate skin redness, bruising, pain, or itching 1 hour after subcutaneous injection; this had mostly disappeared after 4 hours (6).

Five of 168 men with prostate cancer treated with abarelix had urticaria and pruritus, which resolved without treatment (7).

Reproductive system

Ovarian hyperstimulation syndrome is far less common with gonadorelin receptor antagonists than agonists in induction of ovulation (2,5). Hot flushes are rare, in contrast to gonadorelin receptor agonists: in a prospective, uncontrolled study of 346 women given cetrorelix, there was only one case of hot flushes (5).

References

1. Gillies PS, Faulds D, Balfour JA, Perry CM. Ganirelix. Drugs 2000;59(1):107–11.
2. Olivennes F, Belaisch-Allart J, Emperaire JC, Dechaud H, Alvarez S, Moreau L, Nicollet B, Zorn JR, Bouchard P, Frydman R. Prospective, randomized, controlled study of in vitro fertilization-embryo transfer with a single dose of a luteinizing hormone-releasing hormone (LH-RH) antagonist (cetrorelix) or a depot formula of an LH-RH agonist (triptorelin). Fertil Steril 2000;73(2):314–20.
3. Trew GH. Optimizing gonadotrophin-releasing hormone antagonist protocols. Hum Fertil (Camb) 2002;5(1):G13–16.
4. Buchter D, Behre HM, Kliesch S, Chirazi A, Nieschlag E, Assmann G, von Eckardstein A. Effects of testosterone suppression in young men by the gonadotropin releasing hormone antagonist cetrorelix on plasma lipids, lipolytic

enzymes, lipid transfer proteins, insulin, and leptin. Exp Clin Endocrinol Diabetes 1999;107(8):522–9.
5. Felberbaum RE, Albano C, Ludwig M, Riethmuller-Winzen H, Grigat M, Devroey P, Diedrich K. Ovarian stimulation for assisted reproduction with HMG and concomitant midcycle administration of the GnRH antagonist cetrorelix according to the multiple dose protocol: a prospective uncontrolled phase III study. Hum Reprod 2000;15(5):1015–20.
6. Borm G, Mannaerts B. Treatment with the gonadotrophin-releasing hormone antagonist ganirelix in women undergoing ovarian stimulation with recombinant follicle stimulating hormone is effective, safe and convenient: results of a controlled, randomized, multicentre trial. The European Orgalutran Study Group. Hum Reprod 2000; 15(7):1490–8.
7. Trachtenberg J, Gittleman M, Steidle C, Barzell W, Friedel W, Pessis D, Fotheringham N, Campion M, Garnick MB; Abarelix Study Group. A phase 3, multicenter, open label, randomized study of abarelix versus leuprolide plus daily antiandrogen in men with prostate cancer. J Urol 2002;167(4):1670–4.

Gonadotropins

General Information

Human chorionic gonadotropin (HCG, hCG), extracted from the urine of pregnant women, has mainly luteinizing hormone (LH) activity. Human menopausal gonadotropin (HMG, hMG) contains both follicle-stimulating hormone (FSH) and luteinizing hormone in about equal amounts. Where materials of natural origin are used, the relative amounts of follicle-stimulating hormone and luteinizing hormone in pituitary gonadotropin extracts vary with the extraction procedure used. However, in recent years, both pure recombinant versions of human FSH and human LH (rhFSH, rhLH) have become available and have increasingly replaced the natural products.

Luteinizing hormone-releasing hormone (LHRH) is used in the treatment of infertility (1). It induces pulsatile release of gonadotropin, and excessive stimulation can result. However, if used over a period of time, the receptors cease to respond and there can be a fall in the concentrations of luteinizing hormone and follicle-stimulating hormone and a fall in sex steroid concentrations to the castrato range.

Treatment schedules for induction of ovulation have been described in a number of papers, but individual sensitivity of the ovaries varies greatly. Complications are generally considered more likely when the dose is excessive compared with individual needs; their incidence varies greatly from clinic to clinic, apparently because of differences in formulations and the dosage schedule used. Problems include superovulation, multiple pregnancy, and the hyperstimulation syndrome, which consists of rapid ovarian enlargement with intraperitoneal effusion (2). Ascites and hydrothorax are occasionally seen, probably due to an increase in vascular permeability at high estrogen concentrations (3). Vascular accidents have been reported, namely thrombophlebitis (4) and obstruction of the basilar artery (SED-12, 1033) (5). Gonadotropins have also been stated, although with much less certainty, to cause cardiomyopathy and behavioral and intellectual disturbances (SED-12, 1033) (6,7).

Observational studies

The European Metrodin HP Study Group has assessed the efficacy and safety of a highly purified urinary FSH in combination with human chorionic gonadotropin in inducing spermatogenesis in 28 men with primary complete isolated hypogonadotrophic hypogonadism, of whom 25 achieved spermatogenesis (8). Mean testicular volume increased by about 7 ml during treatment. Adverse events considered to be related to human chorionic gonadotropin were acne ($n = 3$), weight gain ($n = 2$), and gynecomastia ($n = 1$). Acne can be attributed to increased testosterone. Gynecomastia is an adverse effect of human chorionic gonadotropin treatment (9), and it may be caused by raised serum estradiol concentrations.

In 71 women undergoing in vitro fertilization and embryo transfer using recombinant human follicle-stimulating hormone in doses sufficient to attain a pregnancy rate of 24% (10), the main adverse effect was mild pain at the site of injection (less than 20% of patients) but there were two cases of ovarian hyperstimulation syndrome. In less than 10% of patients, redness, swelling, or bruising was seen and one patient developed headache.

The efficacy of recombinant human luteinizing hormone (rhLH) for supporting follicular development induced by recombinant human follicle-stimulating hormone (rhFSH) has been investigated in hypogonadotropic hypogonadal women (11). A total of 42 adverse events were reported in 14 of the 53 cycles in this study. Of these, 32 adverse events occurred in 11 of the 42 cycles treated with rhLH, and 10 occurred in three of the 11 cycles not treated with rhLH. The most frequent adverse events were pelvic and abdominal pain, headache, breast pain, nausea, ovarian enlargement, and somnolence. These adverse events are similar to those reported during therapy with follicle-stimulating hormone alone (11).

Comparative studies

When recombinant and urinary versions of follicle-stimulating hormone were compared under double-blind conditions in an in vitro fertilization program in a randomized, multicenter study (12), the former was more potent. There were no clinically relevant differences in safety between the two products and no cases of ovarian hyperstimulation syndrome.

The efficacy and safety of recombinant human follicle-stimulating hormone (r-hFSH) has been compared with that of highly purified urinary follicle-stimulating hormone (u-hFSH HP) in women undergoing ovarian stimulation for in vitro fertilization, including intracytoplasmic sperm injection, in a prospective, randomized study in 278 patients, who were treated with gonadotropin-releasing hormone and then received one of the two formulations in doses of 150 IU/day subcutaneously for the first 6 days; on day 7 the dose was adjusted, if necessary, according to the ovarian response (13). Human chorionic gonadotropin (10 000 IU subcutaneously) was administered once there was more than one follicle 18 mm in diameter and two others of 16 mm or larger. Rr-hFSH was more effective than u-hFSH HP in inducing multiple follicular development. There were seven cases (5.0%) of ovarian hyperstimulation syndrome in those given r-hFSH and three (2.2%) in those given u-hFSH HP; this difference was not significant.

General adverse effects

The short- and long-term effects of ovulation induction have been reported (8). In the short term, clomiphene and gonadotropins cause ovarian hyperstimulation syndrome (ovarian enlargement, bloating, and nausea) and multiple pregnancies; gonadotropins also cause ectopic pregnancy. In the long term, clomiphene may cause an increased risk of ovarian cancer.

Recombinant human chorionic gonadotropin

Recombinant human luteinizing hormone has now very largely replaced the product prepared from the urine of pregnant women (uhCG). In an open, randomized trial in 297 ovulatory infertile women in 20 US infertility centers, recombinant hCG 250 micrograms and 500 micrograms was compared with urinary hCG 10 000 U USP in assisted reproduction (14). The women were treated for a single cycle with one or the other. The mean numbers of oocytes retrieved per treatment group were equivalent (13–14). Although the numbers of fertilized oocytes on day 1 after oocyte retrieval and of cleaved embryos on the day of embryo transfer were significantly higher with 500 micrograms of recombinant hCG than with 250 micrograms, the incidence of the anticipated adverse events also tended to be higher.

More exact data on the adverse effects and relative safety of the recombinant and urinary formulations have been provided in a similar investigation in 259 women (15). In terms of safety, rhCG was well tolerated at a dose of up to 30 000 IU. Moderate ovarian hyperstimulation syndrome was reported in 12% of patients who received uhCG and 12% of those who received two injections of rhCG. There were no moderate or severe complications in patients who received a single dose of rhCG up to 30 000 IU. The results seem to show that a single dose of rhCG is effective in inducing final follicular maturation and early luteinization in in vitro fertilization and embryo transfer patients and is comparable with uhCG 5000 IU. The dose of rhCG that gave the highest efficacy to safety ratio was 15 000–30 000 IU.

The recombinant and urinary forms of human chorionic gonadotropin have also been compared in an international multicenter study, with similar findings (16), but it was notable that significantly more patients who were given uhCG reported local reactions (particularly inflammation and pain), presumably because of the presence of biological impurities.

Organs and Systems

Hematologic

Resistance of activated protein C and deep calf vein thrombosis has been reported during controlled ovarian stimulation for in vitro fertilization (17). The thrombosis occurred on the eighth day of human menopausal gonadotropin use and before human chorionic gonadotropin was given.

Reproductive system

There is a risk of ovarian hyperstimulation when an ovulation-inducing drug is followed by rapid ovarian enlargement with peritoneal effusion. The incidence of these complications varies with the product and dosage schedule used; in experienced hands, the frequency of complications may be no more than about 4%.

- In an unusual case reported in detail from Saudi Arabia, a 28-year-old woman receiving gonadotropins developed acute respiratory distress, abdominal pain, and severe hyponatremia associated with the syndrome of inappropriate antidiuretic hormone secretion (SIADH) (18). A multiple pregnancy nevertheless resulted and three fetuses went to term successfully.

While it is possible that the gonadotropins themselves induced SIADH, it seems more likely that it was a secondary complication of ovarian hyperstimulation.

The dangers of ovarian hyperstimulation with gonadotropins should not be underestimated. Quite apart from the risks of abdominal complications and even myocardial infarction, it can cause marked changes in liver function tests (19). It has been suggested that ultrasonographic monitoring is a means of detecting impending ovarian hyperstimulation, so that treatment can be suspended in good time (20).

- A 33-year-old woman developed severe symptomatic ovarian hyperstimulation after being given 10 000 IU of urinary human chorionic gonadotropin for empty follicle syndrome (21).

Although it has generally been thought that ovarian hyperstimulation would not occur when treating cases of empty follicle syndrome, this suggests that even when dealing with such patients, particularly if there is any reason to think that they are at risk of ovarian hyperstimulation, it is wise to take the usual precautions, using a much lower dose of human chorionic gonadotropin and adding progesterone for luteal support.

Just how dangerous and even life-threatening such hyperstimulation can be is illustrated by a recent case (22).

- A 28-year-old woman who had undergone attempted hormonal induction of ovulation presented some days later with ascites, oliguria, and vomiting. Over 2 weeks she developed severe hypoalbuminemia, due to a combination of intractable vomiting, intravenous rehydration, paracentesis, hypercatabolism, and proteinuria, with gross edema and progressively worsening liver function. Her serum albumin dropped to 9 g/l with liver function abnormalities: aspartate transaminase

462 IU/l, alkaline phosphatase 706 IU/l, bilirubin 26 μmol/l, prothrombin time 19 seconds. Paracentesis and total parenteral nutrition coincided with rapid clinical improvement.

Other presenting signs of ovarian hyperstimulation include ascites, hydrothorax, thrombophlebitis, and, as in one recently reported case, acute dyspnea (23).

"Prolonged coasting" may offer possibilities as a means of preventing ovarian hyperstimulation syndrome where excessive doses of gonadotropins have been given (SEDA-20, 389); it involves temporarily withholding the gonadotropins and giving only a gonadotropin-releasing hormone agonist until the plasma estradiol concentration has fallen sufficiently; however, experience to date shows that it is not foolproof and that spontaneous abortions can result where pregnancies have already started.

In vitro maturation of immature oocytes represents a potential alternative for fertility treatment in patients who are likely to suffer hyperstimulation. In two patients considered to be at risk of hyperstimulation, because of polycystic ovaries, priming with hCG 10 000 IU (specified only as the IVF-C brand) was followed by removal of the oocytes 36 hours later (24). Oocytes considered to be mature at the time of collection were inseminated using in vitro fertilization or intracytoplasmic sperm injection (ICSI), and the resulting embryos were cultured to the blastocyst stage. Transfer of these blastocysts resulted in pregnancy in both patients. Immature oocytes were matured in a culture medium containing 30% human follicular fluid, recombinant follicle-stimulating hormone 1 IU/ml, hCG 10 IU/ml, and recombinant epidermal growth factor (rhEGF) 10 ng/ml. ICSI was then carried out. Two and five expanded blastocysts were obtained after 5 days of culture and were cryopreserved. The findings suggested that one can avoid the risk of ovarian hyperstimulation when using hCG in women with polycystic ovaries and that (at least when using mature oocytes) pregnancy can be established.

Immunologic

Gonadotropins of natural origin contain various allergens, which can give rise to hypersensitivity reactions. This was a serious problem with the "PMS" gonadotropin formulations formerly made from the serum of pregnant mares but now apparently obsolete; it was also described in the past with an FSH formulation of porcine origin. However hypersensitivity reactions can also occur to extracts of human material.

- A generalized allergic reaction to human menopausal gonadotropin (Pergonal) has been described during controlled ovarian hyperstimulation (25). In this case a desensitization protocol allowed the patient to complete her treatment cycle without further problems. Subsequently recombinant follicle stimulating hormone was used successfully and uneventfully.

On occasion, there have even been such reactions to highly purified human products, notably FSH; they can be managed by changing the treatment to intramuscular recombinant follicle stimulating hormone (26).

Long-Term Effects

Tumorigenicity

In a prospective study of 1200 infertile women in Israel, including a subgroup of women who developed breast cancer, there was no statistical association with the use of fertility-inducing drugs (27).

A subfertile man treated with human menopausal gonadotropin + human chorionic gonadotropin (hMG + hCG) developed a malignant teratoma of the testis; however, in view of his history a cause-and-effect relation was dubious (28).

Malignant melanoma

Concern that the drug treatment of female infertility might predispose the user to malignant melanoma was first engendered by a US study published in 1995 (29). Among women who had used clomiphene citrate for infertility the incidence of melanoma was higher (RR = 1.8; 95% CI = 0.8, 3.5) than among American women in general. However, in a case-cohort study of nearly 4000 infertile women there was a similar increase in the incidence of melanoma among those who had been treated with human chorionic gonadotropin compared with the rest; there was no association with the use of clomiphene.

Quite apart from the inherent discrepancy in these findings, several pieces of evidence have confused the debate. In the first place, the cohort of melanoma cases was small—barely a handful. In the second place, some earlier papers had suggested that infertility in women might of itself have an association with melanoma. The same impression came from various studies, in which the incidences of cancers in infertile women were examined (30–32). If that were true, it could affect the initial findings in either direction: a high spontaneous incidence might mask a real drug effect, or it might provide a predisposition to melanoma, which the drugs might then more readily trigger.

In the meantime, data from Australia have shown no greater incidence of melanoma among women who had used fertility drugs and undergone in vitro fertilization than in the country's general female population (33). Since then there has been one more significant paper, again from Australia, using data from a specialized fertility clinic in Queensland, relating to all women who attended the center over a decade (34). Whenever possible, the women were traced and their subsequent history noted. Originally intended as a retrospective case-cohort study using a subcohort, the approach had to be amended because no cases of melanoma were found in the subcohort. The work therefore proceeded as a matched case-control study; all the data were taken and set against publicly available figures on melanoma in Queensland. After some necessary exclusions, 3186 women were included; care was taken to minimize recall bias. Fourteen women developed melanoma after fertility treatment, eight cases being invasive. The expected incidence in the general population would have been 15.8 cases in the same period. The incidence actually observed was therefore only 0.89 of that anticipated (95% CI = 0.54, 1.48).

The numbers of women who had used clomiphene or human menopausal gonadotropin were too small to make more differentiated calculations, but the incidence of melanoma seemed to correspond to that in the general population.

On current evidence, there seems no reason to discourage fertility-promoting drug treatments because of any risk of melanoma; they may even reduce it to some extent. However, this does not alter the fact that the data are deficient in various ways. Quite apart from the small numbers of melanoma cases that have been recorded, all the work to date has been performed in relatively sunny parts of the world; it is not known what would happen in other climates. Within countries, there are sharp differences in melanoma figures; in the USA, where about 32 000 new cases of skin melanoma were projected for 1994 (35), the highest melanoma rates occur among light-skinned populations in areas of intense sunlight, for example Arizona; the same applies to Queensland, Australia. In the USA as a whole there is a melanoma incidence among whites of 12.4 per 100 000 (36), while mortality rates vary inversely with latitude (37). Furthermore, in whites there has been a recent increase in the incidence of melanoma, during the precise period that this type of treatment has become popular, but probably for entirely different reasons, which may be associated with lifestyles and holiday habits; the reported incidence in whites rose by no less than 102% from 1973 to 1991 (37). Finally, as the Australian authors themselves stressed, the fact that the Queensland clinic was a private institution specializing in IVF/GIFT therapy means that women with endocrine- or ovulation-associated infertility may not so readily have been referred to it.

All this makes it very difficult to find a baseline incidence for melanoma with which cases treated for infertility can be compared. It is to be hoped that data of this type will continue to arrive from other centers, so that a definitive judgement will become possible.

Ovarian cancer

The hypothesis that the use of fertility drugs, including human gonadotropins and clomiphene, which increase the endogenous secretion of gonadotropins, might increase the risk of ovarian cancer appears to have come first clearly into the open in 1996 (38). However one can distil similar suggestions from other work from 1992 onwards (39–41), and anecdotal reports of an association have accumulated. The hypothesis has emerged that the increased number of ovulations (or the high concentrations of estrogen and gonadotropin) induced by drugs given to treat infertility could promote the development of ovarian cancers.

Ovarian cancer is much less common in married women, and during the last 30 years a direct inverse association has been found between the number of pregnancies and the duration of use of oral contraception on the one hand and the occurrence of ovarian cancer on the other. In 1971 a Lancet reviewer suggested that incessant ovulation might be a causal factor for the development of cancer of the ovary, in that the repeated rupture of follicles involved a cycle of damage to the surface epithelium, alternating with repair involving mitogenic activity and thereby in turn a risk of mutations (42). On the other hand, as has been pointed out, no correlation has been found between the risk of ovarian cancer and the age at menarche and menopause, that is the length of the fertile period, which might be anticipated if the so-called "ovulation hypothesis" is correct.

An alternative suggestion has been that gonadotropins, by enhancing the transformation of ovarian epithelial cells, also increase the risk of malignant transformation in this tissue. This idea is compatible with the inverse relations between ovarian cancer and pregnancy or oral contraception, since the latter processes suppress the secretion of gonadotropins.

Both the hypothesis of ovarian injury and that of gonadotropic influence seem to provide tempting explanations for any relation that there may be between infertility treatment and ovarian cancer, since such treatment both induces further ovarian "injury" by ovulation (sometimes multiple) and increases circulating gonadotropin concentrations. However, the existence of a possible mechanism does not prove that there actually is an association.

The stumbling block in either proving or disproving a link between the drugs and the cancers is the fact that infertility itself proves to be a risk factor for ovarian cancer. Women who fail to become pregnant have a higher risk of ovarian malignancy than other women, irrespective of whether they are taking drugs or not. A study from Denmark in 1997 showed that among infertile women the overall risk of ovarian cancer was not influenced by the use (or otherwise) of treatment with anti-fertility drugs (43). There is also American work that shows that among infertile women with a high risk of ovarian cancer circulating gonadotropin concentrations are low, which is what one would expect in such a group, but which does not tally well with the theory of gonadotropic causation (44).

Given current evidence, and with anecdotal reports that add nothing to the discussion of a possible cause-and-effect relation, one can discern considerable polarization in the discussion. It is not irrelevant, nor is it uncharitable, to point out that whereas fully independent academic workers have been most vocal in expressing concern, the papers that seek to dismiss an association between the drugs and the cancers have tended to emerge from groups that acknowledge support from pharmaceutical companies that produce the drugs used in this field. That is natural, and it results in the sort of argument and counter-argument that may do something to promote the emergence of the truth. However, it is currently unhelpful to the physician who is treating women for infertility and who is anxious to know what to tell the concerned patient, as well as finding some way of reducing whatever risks treatment may carry. However, bearing in mind the fact that the use of high doses of fertility drugs certainly brings with it other risks (for example that of sometimes dangerous overstimulation), this could be a reason for applying some of the more restrained available dosage schemes, and for avoiding persisting with this inherently abrasive treatment when it has failed to produce results on two or more occasions.

Drug Administration

Drug formulations

The composition of different formulations of hCG is not entirely consistent, and could account for some discrepancies in clinical studies, as well as introducing risks. For example, previously, formulations of hCG have been shown to be toxic to Kaposi's sarcoma (KS) cells. However, clinical studies using commercial hCG formulations in the human sarcoma are highly contradictory (45). The apparent discrepancies between different studies may be because both pro- and anti-KS components are present in varying proportions in different hCG formulations. As certain hCG formulations may not only lack the ability to control Kaposi's sarcoma, but also contain contaminant KS growth factor(s), the authors suggested caution when using crude hCG for the treatment of Kaposi's sarcoma.

These findings point to the need to reconsider the international standards applicable to the standardization, formulation, and marketing of hCG products, whether of natural or recombinant origin.

Drug dosage regimens

The incidence of ovarian hyperstimulation is highly dependent on the therapeutic regimen. In one study (46) the following methods were compared:

- a conventional human menopausal gonadotropin + human chorionic gonadotropin (hMG + hCG) program;
- the hMG step-down method, in which the daily dose of hMG was reduced from 150 IU to 75 IU when the follicle diameter reached 11–13 mm;
- the sequential hMG + gonadotropin-releasing hormone (GnRH) method, in which hMG injection was switched to pulsatile GnRH administration (20 micrograms/120 minutes subcutaneously) when the follicle diameter reached 11–13 mm;
- a new, modified hMG + GnRH method, in which pulsatile GnRH was injected together with hMG; daily hMG was stopped and the GnRH dosage was changed from 10 to 20 micrograms when the follicle diameter reached 11–13 mm.

Initially, the established methods were used randomly to treat 34 cycles in 20 women; subsequently, five patients who failed to conceive after treatment with sequential hMG + GnRH were then treated by the new method. More than eight growing follicles and multiple pregnancies were observed during treatment by the conventional method. The incidence of ovarian hyperstimulation syndrome was 26% with the conventional method, 20% with the step-down method, and 0% with the sequential hMG + GnRH method; however, the rate of ovulation was only 50% with the sequential hMG + GnRH method. By contrast, with the new method fewer than three growing follicles occurred in 82% of patients, there was a 100% rate of ovulation, and there were no multiple pregnancies or ovarian hyperstimulation syndrome. Moreover, the new method induced pregnancy in three out of five patients. The authors considered their modified method suitable for the treatment of severe hypogonadotrophic amenorrhea. In view of the risks attached to ovarian hyperstimulation, this type of program certainly merits further evaluation.

References

1. Reissmann T, Felberbaum R, Diedrich K, Engel J, Comaru-Schally AM, Schally AV. Development and applications of luteinizing hormone-releasing hormone antagonists in the treatment of infertility: an overview. Hum Reprod 1995;10(8):1974–81.
2. Engel T, Jewelewicz R, Dyrenfurth I, Speroff L, Vande Wiele RL. Ovarian hyperstimulation syndrome. Report of a case with notes on pathogenesis and treatment. Am J Obstet Gynecol 1972;112(8):1052–60.
3. Mroueh A, Kase N. Acute ascites and hydrothorax after gonadotropin therapy. Report of a case. Obstet Gynecol 1967;30(3):346–9.
4. Nwosu UC, Corson SL, Bolognese RJ. Hyperstimulation and multiple side-effects of menotropin therapy: a case report. J Reprod Med 1974;12(3):117–20.
5. Humbert G, Delaunay P, Leroy J, Robert M, Schuhl JF, Poussin A, Augustin P. Accident vasculaire cérébral au cours d'un traitement par les gonadotrophines. [Cerebrovascular accident during treatment with gonadotropins.] Nouv Presse Méd 1973;2(1):28–30.
6. Lovel TW, Porter GD. Cardiomyopathy after gonadotrophin treatment. BMJ 1977;1(6059):511.
7. Servais JF, Mormont C, Bostem F, Legros JJ. Perturbations neuropsychiques graves chez un jeune adolescent soumis à une thérapeutique endocrinienne. [Severe neuropsychic disturbances in a young adolescent treated with an endocrine therapy.] Acta Psychiatr Belg 1976;76(1):97–106.
8. Vollenhoven BJ, Healy DL. Short- and long-term effects of ovulation induction. Endocrinol Metab Clin North Am 1998;27(4):903–14.
9. European Metrodin HP Study Group. Efficacy and safety of highly purified urinary follicle-stimulating hormone with human chorionic gonadotropin for treating men with isolated hypogonadotropic hypogonadism. Fertil Steril 1998;70(2):256–62.
10. Strowitzki T, Kentenich H, Kiesel L, Neulen J, Bilger W. Ovarian stimulation in women undergoing in-vitro fertilization and embryo transfer using recombinant human follicle stimulating hormone (Gonal-F) in non-down-regulated cycles. Hum Reprod 1995; 10(12):3097–101.
11. Loumaye E, Piazzi A, Warne D, Kalubi M, Cox P, Lancaster S, Rotere S, Sauvage M, Ursicino G, Baird D, et al. Recombinant human luteinizing hormone (LH) to support recombinant human follicle-stimulating hormone (FSH)-induced follicular development in LH- and FSH-deficient anovulatory women: a dose-finding study. The European Recombinant Human LH Study Group. J Clin Endocrinol Metab 1998;83(5):1507–14.
12. Out HJ, Mannaerts BM, Driessen SG, Coeling H, Bennink HJ. A prospective, randomized, assessor-blind, multicentre study comparing recombinant and urinary follicle stimulating hormone (Puregon versus Metrodin) in in-vitro fertilization. Hum Reprod 1995;10(10):2534–40.
13. Frydman R, Howles CM, Truong F. A double-blind, randomized study to compare recombinant human follicle stimulating hormone (FSH; Gonal-F) with highly

purified urinary FSH (Metrodin) HP) in women undergoing assisted reproductive techniques including intracytoplasmic sperm injection. The French Multicentre Trialists. Hum Reprod 2000;15(3):520–5.
14. Chang P, Kenley S, Burns T, Denton G, Currie K, DeVane G, O'Dea L. Recombinant human chorionic gonadotropin (rhCG) in assisted reproductive technology: results of a clinical trial comparing two doses of rhCG (Ovidrel) to urinary hCG (Profasi) for induction of final follicular maturation in in vitro fertilization–embryo transfer. Fertil Steril 2001;76(1):67–74.
15. Loumaye E; European Recombinant LH Study Group. Human recombinant luteinizing hormone is as effective as, but safer than, urinary human chorionic gonadotropin in inducing final follicular maturation and ovulation in in vitro fertilization procedures: results of a multicenter double-blind study. J Clin Endocrinol Metab 2001;86(6):2607–18.
16. Hugues JN; International Recombinant Human Chorionic Gonadotropin Study Group. Induction of ovulation in World Health Organization group II anovulatory women undergoing follicular stimulation with recombinant human follicle-stimulating hormone: a comparison of recombinant human chorionic gonadotropin (rhCG) and urinary hCG. Fertil Steril 2001;75(6):1111–18.
17. Ludwig M, Felberbaum RE, Diedrich K. Deep vein thrombosis during administration of HMG for ovarian stimulation. Arch Gynecol Obstet 2000;263(3):139–41.
18. Samman Y, Ghoneim H, Hashim IA. Syndrome of inappropriate ADH as a manifestation of severe ovarian hyperstimulation syndrome. J Obstet Gynaecol 2001; 21:201–3.
19. Borgaonkar MR, Marshall JK. Marked elevation of serum transaminases may be associated with ovarian hyperstimulation syndrome. Am J Gastroenterol 1999; 94(11):3373.
20. Grio R, Patriarca A, Ramondini L, Ferrara L, Curti A, Piacentino R. Il monitoraggio ecografico come metodo di prevenzione dei rischi da iperstimolazione ovarica in corso di trattamento farmacologico. [Ultrasonic monitoring as a method of preventing risks of ovarian hyperstimulation during drug therapy.] Minerva Ginecol 1999;51(1–2):15–17.
21. Evbuomwan IO, Fenwick JD, Shiels R, Herbert M, Murdoch AP. Severe ovarian hyperstimulation syndrome following salvage of empty follicle syndrome. Hum Reprod 1999;14(7):1707–9.
22. Davis AJ, Pandher GK, Masson GM, Sheron N. A severe case of ovarian hyperstimulation syndrome with liver dysfunction and malnutrition. Eur J Gastroenterol Hepatol 2002;14(7):779–82.
23. Garrett CW, Gaeta TJ. Ovarian hyperstimulation syndrome: acute onset dyspnea in a young woman. Am J Emerg Med 2002;20(1):63–4.
24. Son WY, Yoon SH, Lee SW, Ko Y, Yoon HG, Lim JH. Blastocyst development and pregnancies after IVF of mature oocytes retrieved from unstimulated patients with PCOS after in-vivo HCG priming. Hum Reprod 2002;17(1):134–6.
25. Harrison S, Wolf T, Abuzeid MI. Administration of recombinant follicle stimulating hormone in a woman with allergic reaction to menotropin: a case report. Gynecol Endocrinol 2000;14(3):149–52.
26. Battaglia C, Salvatori M, Regnani G, Primavera MR, Genazzani AR, Artini PG, Volpe A. Allergic reaction to a highly purified urinary follicle stimulating hormone preparation in controlled ovarian hyperstimulation for in vitro fertilization. Gynecol Endocrinol 2000;14(3):158–61.
27. Potashnik G, Lerner-Geva L, Genkin L, Chetrit A, Lunenfeld E, Porath A. Fertility drugs and the risk of breast and ovarian cancers: results of a long-term follow-up study. Fertil Steril 1999;71(5):853–9.
28. Rubin SO. Malignant teratoma of testis in a subfertile man treated with HCG and HMG. A case report. Scand J Urol Nephrol 1973;7(1):81–4.
29. Rossing MA, Daling JR, Weiss NS, Moore DE, Self SG. Risk of cutaneous melanoma in a cohort of infertile women. Melanoma Res 1995;5(2):123–7.
30. Ron E, Lunenfeld B, Menczer J, Blumstein T, Katz L, Oelsner G, Serr D. Cancer incidence in a cohort of infertile women. Am J Epidemiol 1987;125(5):780–90.
31. Brinton LA, Melton LJ 3rd, Malkasian GD. Jr., Bond A, Hoover R. Cancer risk after evaluation for infertility. Am J Epidemiol 1989;129(4):712–22.
32. Modan B, Ron E, Lerner-Geva L, Blumstein T, Menczer J, Rabinovici J, Oelsner G, Freedman L, Mashiach S, Lunenfeld B. Cancer incidence in a cohort of infertile women. Am J Epidemiol 1998;147(11):1038–42.
33. Venn A, Watson L, Lumley J, Giles G, King C, Healy D. Breast and ovarian cancer incidence after infertility and in vitro fertilisation. Lancet 1995;346(8981):995–1000.
34. Young P, Purdie D, Jackman L, Molloy D, Green A. A study of infertility treatment and melanoma. Melanoma Res 2001;11(5):535–41.
35. Boring CC, Squires TS, Tong T, Montgomery S. Cancer statistics, 1994. CA Cancer J Clin 1994;44(1):7–26.
36. Rees LAG, Eisner MP, Kosary CL, Hankey BF, Miller BA, Clegg L, Edwards BK, editors. SEER Cancer Statistics Review, 1973-1999. Bethesda MD: National Cancer Institute, 2002. http.//seer.cancer.gov/csr/1973-1999/37.
37. Glass AG, Hoover RN. The emerging epidemic of melanoma and squamous cell skin cancer. JAMA 1989; 262(15):2097–100.
38. Shushan A, Paltiel O, Iscovich J, Elchalal U, Peretz T, Schenker JG. Human menopausal gonadotropin and the risk of epithelial ovarian cancer. Fertil Steril 1996; 65(1):13–18.
39. Whittemore AS, Harris R, Itnyre J. Characteristics relating to ovarian cancer risk: collaborative analysis of 12 US case-control studies. II. Invasive epithelial ovarian cancers in white women. Collaborative Ovarian Cancer Group. Am J Epidemiol 1992;136(10):1184–203.
40. Banks E, Beral V, Reeves G. The epidemiology of epithelial ovarian cancer: a review. Int J Gynecol Cancer 1997;7:425–38.
41. Rossing MA, Daling JR, Weiss NS, Moore DE, Self SG. Ovarian tumors in a cohort of infertile women. N Engl J Med 1994;331(12):771–6.
42. Fathalla MF. Incessant ovulation—a factor in ovarian neoplasia? Lancet 1971;2(7716):163.
43. Mosgaard BJ, Lidegaard O, Kjaer SK, Schou G, Andersen AN. Infertility, fertility drugs, and invasive ovarian cancer: a case-control study. Fertil Steril 1997; 67(6):1005–12.
44. Helzlsouer KJ, Alberg AJ, Gordon GB, Longcope C, Bush TL, Hoffman SC, Comstock GW. Serum gonadotropins and steroid hormones and the development of ovarian cancer. JAMA 1995;274(24):1926–30.
45. Simonart T, Van Vooren JP, Meuris S. Treatment of Kaposi's sarcoma with human chorionic gonadotropin. Dermatology 2002;204(4):330–3.
46. Yokoi N, Uemura T, Murase M, Kondoh Y, Ishikawa M, Hirahara F. A modified hMG-GnRH method for the induction of ovulation in infertile women with severe hypogonadotropic amenorrhea. Endocr J 2002; 49(2):159–64.

Granulocyte colony-stimulating factor (G-CSF)

See also Myeloid colony stimulating factors

General Information

Granulocyte colony-stimulating factor (G-CSF) primarily increases the production and function of neutrophils by stimulating the proliferation of committed myeloid precursors, rather than pluripotential stem cells (1).

Recombinant human forms of G-CSF that have been developed include filgrastim (rINN), lenograstim (rINN), nartograstim (rINN), and pegfilgrastim (rINN) and pegnartograstim (rINN), which are pegylated derivatives of filgrastim and nartograstim.

Besides common therapeutic indications, G-CSF has also been used in severe chronic neutropenic diseases (congenital, cyclic, idiopathic), aplastic anemia, and neonatal neutropenia. G-CSF is sometimes used in healthy volunteers to mobilize blood progenitor cells or granulocytes before infusion into neutropenic patients.

Observational studies

In all clinical studies carried out to date, G-CSF has been well tolerated, whether given subcutaneously or intravenously. At the recommended doses (5–10 micrograms/kg), generalized musculoskeletal and transient bone pains, headache, and mild rash are the commonest adverse effects (2). No additional adverse effects or delayed consequences have been so far reported in neonates treated at birth for presumed bacterial sepsis (SEDA-20, 337). An increase in the size of the spleen has been reported (3,4). Transient rises in alkaline phosphatase, lactate dehydrogenase, and uric acid are considered to be normal physiological consequences of the rise in the neutrophil count (5). Long-term G-CSF administration in patients with severe congenital neutropenia has also been considered to be relatively safe, with discontinuation or temporary withdrawal in only seven of 44 patients (6).

Two reviews have examined the available data on the effects of hemopoietic growth factors on the duration of neutropenia and mortality in drug-induced agranulocytosis, which mostly consists of isolated case reports or small series of patients (7,8). The authors reached contrasting opinions, suggesting that hemopoietic growth factors might or might not be of interest in patients with severe drug-induced agranulocytosis. Adverse effects were noted in 13 of 118 case reports (7). Although most of them were benign, pulmonary toxicity or acute respiratory distress syndrome have been noted in a few patients.

Comparative studies

Few studies have directly compared the safety of the various available colony-stimulating factors. The frequency and severity of adverse effects associated with the prophylactic use of filgrastim (a bacterial cell-derived G-CSF) or sargramostim (a yeast cell-derived GM-CSF) have been assessed in a retrospective review of the medical records of 490 cancer patients from 10 centers (9). Sargramostim-treated patients had significantly more frequent non-infectious fever, fatigue, diarrhea, injection site reactions, edema, and dermatological adverse effects, whereas skeletal pain was more frequent with filgrastim. In addition, switching to the alternative treatment was more frequent in the sargramostim group (18% of patients) than in the filgrastim group (none of the patients). The authors tried to minimize selection bias, but the strength of the results was limited by the retrospective nature of the study.

The effects and the safety of a 5-day regimen of G-CSF ($n = 9$) or GM-CSF ($n = 8$) have been compared (10). Most patients complained of flu-like symptoms in both groups (six and seven respectively), but rash at the injection site was observed only in four patients treated with GM-CSF. In the G-CSF group, there was a fall in platelet count (below 150×10^9/l) in five patients, raised serum lactic dehydrogenase activity, and raised uric acid concentrations; three patients required transient treatment with allopurinol.

Use in healthy volunteers

The G-CSF is sometimes used in healthy volunteers to mobilize blood progenitor cells or granulocytes before infusion into neutropenic patients (11).

The safety of filgrastim in healthy donors has been evaluated in a large prospective multicenter study (12). The interim results, obtained from the first 150 enrolled donors aged 18–64 years who received either 10 or 16 micrograms/kg/day, have shown that 99 patients had at least one adverse effect graded as mild (grade I) in 35% of cases, moderate (grade II) in 62%, and severe (grade III) in 3%. Bone pain and headaches were the most common acute adverse events, and all the patients completely recovered after withdrawal of filgrastim. There were no apparent differences in the proportion, the severity, or the type of adverse effects according to the administered regimen.

That the use of G-CSF in healthy donors of peripheral blood progenitor cells is reasonably safe has been confirmed in an analysis of adverse effects in 737 evaluable patients included in three independent databases from Spain, the USA, and Japan (13–15). In one study, the overall incidence of adverse effects was 67%. The most common adverse effects were bone pain (71–90%), headache (17–54%), fatigue (6–33%), insomnia (up to 14%), nausea/vomiting (3–13%), and low-grade fever (6%). Although most adverse effects were rated as moderate, about two-thirds of the patients required analgesics for bone pain or headache. Other adverse events, such as non-cardiac chest pain, paresthesia, itching, or minor injection site reactions, were rare. Very few patients discontinued G-CSF because of clinical toxicity. Doses higher than 8.8 micrograms/kg/day, patients younger than 35 years of age, and female sex were significant risk factors for bone pain, headache, and nausea/vomiting respectively (15).

Moderate thrombocytopenia was common after apheresis; there was more severe but asymptomatic and promptly reversible thrombocytopenia (below 50×10^{12}/l) in up to 3.9% of patients (14,15). However, the respective contributions of apheresis and G-CSF in thrombocytopenia are difficult to assess. There was also a fall in the absolute neutrophil count to less than 1×10^9/l in 3% of patients 9–16 days after G-CSF withdrawal (15). Serum alkaline phosphatase and lactate dehydrogenase activities were increased about two-fold compared with pre-treatment, a finding that was explicable by G-CSF-induced neutrophilia (14,15). Symptoms of hypercoagulability have also been found in healthy donors.

However, more severe or unexpected consequences, including spontaneous splenic rupture, anaphylactoid reactions, deep necrotizing folliculitis, a psoriasiform eruption, acute gouty arthritis, iritis or episcleritis, and unexpectedly prolonged thrombocytopenia have been mentioned (SEDA-20, 337) (SEDA-21, 378) (SEDA-22, 407).

Among 90 healthy donors given 10 and 16 micrograms/kg/day of filgrastim for stem cell mobilization, severe adverse effects were mostly found in patients who had been given the higher dose (16), but one obese patient (body weight 170 kg) who received 10 micrograms/kg/day had a non-traumatic spleen rupture that resolved spontaneously.

Sufficient data on the potential long-term effects of G-CSF in healthy volunteers are still lacking. In one study, 101 healthy donors who had received filgrastim for a median of 6 days were questioned after a median of 43 (range 34–74) months to assess their current health; 70 donors also had a complete blood count (17). No unusual disease was detected and the blood counts were within the reference range. In 20 donors followed for 6–12 months after peripheral blood progenitor cell collection, there were no particular symptoms or hematological abnormalities (15).

The possible carcinogenic effects of G-CSF have also been discussed. There is as yet no indication of an increased risk of cancer, and no cases of acute or chronic leukemia were detected in a telephone interview study performed after a median of 39 months after peripheral blood progenitor cell donation in 281 donors (18).

Organs and Systems

Cardiovascular

Cardiovascular events have seldom been described in patients given colony-stimulating factors. However, possible excesses of cardiovascular events and unexpected deaths have been suggested (SED-13, 1115) (19), although the actual risk was not fully evaluated. In three isolated reports, acute arterial thrombosis or angina pectoris were deemed to have resulted from hypercoagulability with extreme leukocytosis and G-CSF-induced abnormalities in platelet aggregation (SEDA-20, 337) (SEDA-21, 377) (20). Increased platelet aggregation has also been found in healthy volunteers (21). Although the relevance of these findings is unclear, caution is warranted in patients predisposed to thromboembolic events.

- A 46-year-old donor denied pre-existing cardiac symptoms, but smoking and a family history of coronary artery disease were noted as possible risk factors (22). The pre-treatment electrocardiogram was normal. Six hours after the second and the third doses of G-CSF 10 micrograms/kg before peripheral blood progenitor cell collection, he developed symptoms and signs of cardiac ischemia, including palpitation, chest discomfort, trigeminy, and T wave inversion. However, troponin was unchanged. Cardiac catheterization showed severe coronary artery occlusion and he underwent percutaneous transluminal coronary angioplasty. He finally admitted mild exertional chest discomfort 2 weeks before the first dose of G-CSF.

Although not described during clinical trials, typical capillary leak syndrome has been anecdotally observed after G-CSF administration, illustrating the possible consequences of accelerated release of activated granulocytes (SEDA-22, 407) (23).

Microthrombotic necrotizing panniculitis has been reported (24).

- A 49-year-old woman received subcutaneous filgrastim 300 micrograms/day into the upper thighs for neutropenia prophylaxis after treatment of relapsing Hodgkin's disease with mitoguazone, etoposide, vinorelbine, and ifosfamide. After 3 days she suddenly developed fever, painful livedo, deeply infiltrated edema on the legs and thighs, and inflamed livedoid erythema on both soles. Deep biopsy specimens showed small vessel thrombosis with subcutaneous necrosis and hemorrhage. She recovered over the next 4 weeks after filgrastim withdrawal and prednisone treatment.

Although a causal relation was difficult to ascertain in the context of malignancy and cytotoxic chemotherapy, the short time to occurrence after G-CSF favored a causative role.

Respiratory

Pulmonary toxicity in patients receiving chemotherapy

Whether G-CSF can cause pulmonary toxicity or enhance chemotherapy-induced pulmonary toxicity is a matter of continuing debate (SED-13, 1115) (SEDA-21, 377). Some studies have suggested an increased risk of pulmonary complications in patients with hematological malignancies treated with various chemotherapeutic regimens who received G-CSF. In a review of 20 cases of interstitial pneumonia (including three that were fatal) observed during or within 10 days of G-CSF treatment, the chemotherapy regimen consisted of cyclophosphamide (95%), bleomycin (55%), methotrexate (25%), and etoposide (20%); most patients had non-Hodgkin's lymphoma (25). In another report, acute febrile interstitial pneumonitis occurred in five patients with non-Hodgkin's lymphoma who were receiving prophylactic G-CSF ($n = 3$) or GM-CSF ($n = 2$) within less than 48 hours after the second to fourth cycles of chemotherapy (doxorubicin, cyclophosphamide, bleomycin, methotrexate, plus methylprednisolone) (26). Lymphocytic alveolitis was confirmed in four of these patients, and all three patients tested had an increased number of CD8+ T cells. Even though all the patients received high-dose methylprednisolone, two died as a result of diffuse and extensive interstitial pulmonary fibrosis, identified at postmortem.

Several epidemiological studies have more accurately focused on this potential problem, but the results are conflicting. Unfortunately, most of them were retrospective and involved historical controls. Interstitial pneumonia was identified in eight of 40 patients treated with antineoplastic drugs (mostly methotrexate and bleomycin) plus G-CSF, while no such cases were found before the use of G-CSF among 35 historical controls (27). Severe pulmonary toxicity was observed in four of 12 patients treated with BACOP (bleomycin, doxorubicin, cyclophosphamide, vincristine, plus prednisone) plus G-CSF compared with one of 24 historical controls who did not receive G-CSF (28). Of 52 patients treated with CHOP (cyclophosphamide, doxorubicin, vincristine, plus prednisolone), pulmonary symptoms were found in six who received G-CSF compared with none of 49 patients treated before the availability of G-CSF (29). This last study also raised the possibility that the intensified schedule of CHOP administration (every 2 weeks instead of every 3 weeks) allowed in patients undergoing G-CSF is a possible explanation for increased pulmonary toxicity. In contrast, other investigators failed to confirm that G-CSF increases the pulmonary toxicity of antineoplastic drugs, at least bleomycin (SEDA-21, 377). This was particularly exemplified by French authors who were unable to find an increased incidence of pulmonary complications in an analysis of two randomized controlled trials in 278 patients who received a bleomycin-containing regimen plus G-CSF or placebo (30).

Other predisposing factors have been suggested in five of 310 patients who developed acute adult respiratory distress syndrome (ARDS) after receiving G-CSF after allogeneic bone marrow transplantation or conventional chemotherapy (31). All had also been exposed to drugs or procedures with significant pulmonary toxicity. Respiratory symptoms developed suddenly, in conjunction with rapid recovery of the white blood cell count. Retrospective investigations showed that all five patients had the HLA-B51 or HLA-B52 antigens. In addition, plasma concentrations of tumor necrosis factor alfa and interleukin-8 were high at the onset of the ARDS. These effects did not occur in 45 patients who did not develop ARDS. The authors suggested that the risk of G-CSF-induced ARDS increases when the white blood cell count rises rapidly in patients who have the following conditions: HLA-B51 or HLA-B52 antigens, treatment with drugs with pulmonary toxicity, and a concomitant infection before recovery from granulocytopenia.

Whatever the truth of the matter, G-CSF should be regarded as a possible cause of pulmonary complications. The abrupt increase in the number of activated neutrophils after G-CSF may account for exacerbation of latent chemotherapy-induced pulmonary damage. Endothelial damage subsequent to increased neutrophil activity (that is, enhanced superoxide release and increased adhesion molecule expression and adherence) or the release of cytokines (IL-1, IL-6, TNF) has been advanced as possible mechanisms. In addition, transient slight hypoxia was found in G-CSF users, although no relation with specific cytotoxic drug treatment or previous radiotherapy was identified (32). A sudden increase in neutrophil count, a rise in LDH and C reactive protein, and the occurrence of dyspnea or fever in G-CSF-treated patients were proposed as possible early signs of the subsequent development of interstitial pneumonia.

Pulmonary toxicity in patients not receiving chemotherapy

The G-CSF can cause severe pulmonary toxicity in patients who are not receiving concomitant chemotherapy. For example, several reports have suggested that G-CSF administration for drug-induced agranulocytosis can play a role in the development or worsening of the adult respiratory distress syndrome (ARDS) (33).

- Fatal non-cardiac pulmonary edema has been reported in a 59-year-old man with renal amyloidosis who received G-CSF for 3 days for stem cell mobilization (34).

The authors extensively reviewed the available experimental and clinical data on the pulmonary toxicity of growth factors.

Another case suggested that G-CSF alone can cause severe pulmonary toxicity (35).

- A 72-year-old man with a normal chest X-ray was unnecessarily treated with G-CSF (5 micrograms/kg/day) for very moderate cytopenia. Five days later, he complained of dyspnea and fatigue, but without fever. His chest X-ray showed diffuse bilateral alveolar opacities and he had a low oxygen saturation. Blood cultures were negative, and infectious pneumonitis (with *Mycobacterium tuberculosis*, *Pneumocystis jiroveci*, *Herpes simplex*, and cytomegalovirus) was ruled out. Despite glucocorticoid and antibiotic treatment, he required mechanical ventilation and died 12 days after the onset of symptoms.

Nervous system

There is no clear evidence of specific central nervous system adverse effects due to G-CSF. In one patient, neurological symptoms, such as blurred vision, weakness, and headache, were attributed to G-CSF-induced extreme hyperleukocytosis with subsequent hyperviscosity (SEDA-21, 377). Encephalopathy, cortical blindness and seizures have also been mentioned in single case report (SEDA-21, 377).

Sensory systems

Severe retinal hemorrhage with a slowly reversible loss of visual acuity, and massive vitreous hemorrhage recurring after further G-CSF treatment and resulting in irreversible loss of vision in the affected eye have each been reported in single patients (SEDA-21, 378) (SEDA-22, 408). Concomitant hyperleukocytosis was suggested as a possible cause in the first patient, whereas G-CSF-induced reactivation of primary ocular inflammation (probably infectious in origin) was advanced as an explanation in the second case.

- A 61-year-old healthy donor developed marginal keratitis with associated mild uveitis after being given injections of filgrastim and sargramostim for 3 days (36). Topical prednisolone and withdrawal of sargramostim produced improvement within 24 hours, while filgrastim injections were continued.

Iritis and episcleritis have also been mentioned in healthy donors of blood progenitor cells.

Endocrine

Several studies have suggested that single or short-term administration of G-CSF did not produce significant changes in the serum concentrations of cortisol, growth hormone, prolactin, follicle-stimulating hormone, luteinizing hormone, or thyrotropin (SEDA-20, 337) (SEDA-21, 378).

Thyroid function and thyroid antibodies were not modified in 20 breast cancer patients (37), and only one case of hypothyroidism with increased thyroid antibodies has been reported (SEDA-20, 337). G-CSF had no effect on thyroid function in 33 patients with cancer, even in patients with pre-existing antibodies (38). Subclinical and spontaneously reversible hyperthyroidism occurred in eight patients without thyroid antibodies and with normal thyroid function before treatment, but this was felt to be related to stressful procedures.

Metabolism

Reductions in serum cholesterol concentrations have been sometimes noted in patients receiving G-CSF (2).

Hematologic

Erythrocytes

In a healthy woman, G-CSF was suggested to have transiently reactivated an alloantibody to an erythrocyte antigen (anti-Jka antibody) (39). This antibody was apparently passively transferred to the transplant recipient, who developed a high-titer of anti-Jka antibody during the first month after transplantation. This report raised the possibility that transplant recipients may develop hemolytic reactions to G-CSF subsequent to erythrocyte transfusion.

Leukocytes

The transient and moderate rises in leukocyte alkaline phosphatase and uric acid serum concentrations that are often observed after G-CSF treatment are considered to arise from an increased neutrophil count (SEDA-17, 396). Similarly, serum lactate dehydrogenase and alkaline phosphatase activities are often increased, and this should be interpreted as the consequence of enzyme release after growth factor-induced leukocyte recovery (SED-13, 1115).

Eosinophilia can occur in patients receiving long-term G-CSF for congenital neutropenia (6). Patients with congenital neutropenia or Felty's syndrome may also be susceptible to anemia and/or thrombocytopenia (6,40).

Platelets and clotting factors

There have been isolated reports of arterial thrombosis in patients or donors treated with G-CSF. In one study, there was more frequent and significantly more severe thrombocytopenia in patients who received G-CSF until 2 days before chemotherapy compared with controls, who had post-chemotherapy G-CSF only (41). This suggests that administration of G-CSF before chemotherapy can increase the bone marrow toxicity of the latter, a potentially relevant finding in patients undergoing intensification of chemotherapy with shortening treatment intervals. Isolated cases of thrombocytopenia have been reported in HIV-infected patients (SEDA-20, 337), and a reduced platelet count, sometimes associated with coagulation abnormalities, was retrospectively identified in nine of 28 patients who received prolonged G-CSF with antiretroviral drugs (42). Emperipolesis of neutrophils within megakaryocytes, an unusual feature of thrombocytopenia, was also reported in one patient receiving high-dose G-CSF (43).

Although abnormalities in platelet aggregation have been described in healthy volunteers (21), coagulation disorders are not typical features in patients who receive G-CSF. Only one HIV-infected patient treated with zidovudine and increasing G-CSF doses had a disseminated intravascular coagulopathy (42).

Hemostatic changes due to G-CSF have been investigated in 22 healthy donors (44). The patients received G-CSF 5 micrograms/kg bd for 5 days and underwent a series of laboratory tests before and 96 hours after G-CSF administration, that is, immediately before leukapheresis. The results suggested possible hypercoagulability, including significant increases in Von Willebrand factor and factor VIII and evidence of thrombin generation. The clinical relevance of these findings and of the previously reported effects of G-CSF on platelet aggregation (SED-14, 1270) is unknown.

Treatment with G-CSF in 26 healthy donors for 5–7 days produced transient changes in endothelial cell and clotting activation markers (45). Although these abnormalities may indicate a risk of thrombotic complications, their clinical relevance to healthy donors is unknown.

- A 53-year-old man with aplastic anemia had clinically asymptomatic and reversible hypercoagulability after the transfusion of granulocytes obtained from G-CSF-stimulated donors (46).

The authors stressed the recurrence of the disorder after each of the three granulocyte transfusions that the patient had received and suggested that adverse effects might occur after transfusion performed with G-CSF-mobilized granulocytes, even though the patient has not been given G-CSF.

The differential effects of G-CSF and GM-CSF on several coagulation parameters have been compared in 34 patients who received the colony-stimulating factors after bone marrow transplantation (47). The data suggested activation of the coagulation system in patients treated with GM-CSF, which resulted in a tendency to more frequent veno-occlusive disease of the liver and a significantly higher incidence of hemorrhage.

Hemopoietic tissues

Asymptomatic but significant increases in spleen volume (up to 150%) concomitant with neutrophilia have been reported in about 25% of patients treated with G-CSF for severe chronic neutropenia (6,48).

Of 13 patients with glycogen storage disease type 1b and neutropenia or neutrophil dysfunction treated with G-CSF, all developed splenomegaly, usually after 3 months of treatment (49). Hypersplenism, as defined by moderate thrombocytopenia on at least two consecutive blood counts, was found in five patients, but none required specific interventions. In one carefully documented case, splenomegaly with extramedullary hemopoiesis was deemed to result from the mobilization of early hemopoietic progenitors from the marrow to the spleen (50). Experimental data suggested that reseeding of hemopoietic cells from the bone marrow may account for this phenomenon (51).

Splenic rupture has been reported in patients with cancer and in healthy donors, and should be anticipated by regular assessment of splenic size during prolonged treatment.

- Spontaneous splenic rupture, with histological evidence of massive extramedullary myelopoiesis after splenectomy, has been reported in a 33-year-old healthy donor who received G-CSF for 6 days (52).
- Life-threatening splenic rupture occurred in a 22-year-old woman with acute myeloid leukemia (53). The rupture was diagnosed in the presence of abdominal pain and signs of hypovolemic shock, 10 days after she started G-CSF treatment to support peripheral blood stem cell transplantation. Histology after splenectomy showed only small clusters of myeloblasts and no specific cause for the rupture. In particular, she was still pancytopenic at the time of splenic rupture.

One patient also had rapid and generalized lymph node enlargement and lymphopenia with recurrence of lymphadenopathy after a further course of G-CSF (54).

Liver

Clinical trials did not suggest G-CSF-induced hepatotoxicity, and very few cases of liver abnormalities have been reported (SED-13, 1116) (SEDA-19, 343). Although it may have been coincidental, the chronological features were in keeping with drug-induced hepatotoxicity in at least two patients, since increases in serum liver enzymes or acute hepatitis associated with pancreatitis recurred after renewed administration of G-CSF. One additional case of fatal fulminant hepatitis could have been due to alcohol abuse and the use of several concomitant drugs.

Urinary tract

No evidence of nephrotoxicity emerged from clinical trials, but a transient increase in serum creatinine concentration has been described (SEDA-20, 337).

- A 4-year-old girl was given filgrastim (30 micrograms/kg/day) for severe congenital neutropenia diagnosed at birth (55). Two months later she developed microscopic hematuria and recurrent episodes of macroscopic hematuria and proteinuria. Renal ultrasonography was normal and no obvious cause was found, but filgrastim was continued. Microscopic hematuria and multiple episodes of macroscopic hematuria with mild proteinuria persisted for 4 years. At this stage, she had an acute episode of macroscopic hematuria with more severe proteinuria and an increase in serum creatinine concentration (202 μmol/l). There were features of membranoproliferative glomerulonephritis type I on renal biopsy. Her renal function improved after filgrastim withdrawal and again deteriorated after reintroduction, with a persistent increase in serum creatinine concentration. Hematuria and proteinuria partially responded to glucocorticoids. Filgrastim was finally replaced by lenograstim when she was 13 years old, and this resulted in reduced proteinuria and improved renal function.

Although the girl also had hepatitis C virus infection during the course of her disease, renal dysfunction preceded this. The persistence of hematuria and proteinuria after the disappearance of hepatitis C virus RNA also argued against a role of hepatitis C infection.

Isolated and reversible hematuria was noted in several patients receiving long-term treatment for congenital neutropenia (6).

Although suggested in one report, G-CSF does not appear to increase the risk of renal allograft rejection (SEDA-20, 337).

Skin

A wide range of cutaneous reactions have been reported in patients receiving G-CSF. Most skin disorders were minor with a skin rash or itching in about 8% of patients (56).

Injection-site reactions

Localized cutaneous lesions were sometimes noted after subcutaneous injection and mimicked those described with GM-CSF. Injection-site subcutaneous nodules infiltrated by leukemic cells have been found in patients treated for acute leukemia (SEDA-19, 343), but in two other patients, inflammatory macrophages were misinterpreted as malignant cells (SEDA-20, 337).

The G-CSF can cause a lichenoid reaction at injection sites (57).

- A 40-year-old woman with metastatic breast cancer received cyclic subcutaneous G-CSF for chemotherapy-induced neutropenia. After 5 months she had a pruritic rash at injection sites. She did not change the injection sites and the lesions recurred after each injection. Biopsy showed a lichenoid reaction and the lesions healed with residual pigmentation after topical steroid application and G-CSF discontinuation. GM-CSF was well tolerated.
- Erythema exsudativum multiforme developed in a 40-year-old healthy donor 3 days after lenograstim was started for peripheral blood stem cell mobilization (58). The lesions were on the hips, apart from the site of lenograstim injection, and resolved 1 week after withdrawal.

Neutrophilic dermatitis

The possible role of G-CSF in inducing or exacerbating neutrophilic dermatitis (Sweet's syndrome) is in keeping with its stimulant effects on the production and functions of neutrophils. Although the ability of G-CSF to induce Sweet's syndrome (acute febrile neutrophilic dermatosis) is disputed, because the underlying malignant disease is a possible confounding factor, several reports of biopsy-proven Sweet's syndrome have been convincing; they have shown variously a close temporal relation between G-CSF treatment and the variations in neutrophil count or the recurrence of the lesions after G-CSF re-administration; one report concerned two patients with chronic neutropenia (SED-13, 1116) (SEDA-20, 338) (SEDA-21,

378). Localized Sweet's syndrome can also occur (SEDA-20, 338). The spectrum of forms of G-CSF-induced neutrophilic dermatitis is wide. In two children with painful erythematous lesions attributed to G-CSF, histology showed microscopic, sterile, neutrophilic abscesses in one and neutrophilic panniculitis in the other (59). Other forms of neutrophilic dermatitis mentioned in G-CSF-treated patients have included isolated cases of bullous pyoderma gangrenosum and neutrophilic eccrine hidradenitis (SEDA-21, 378) (SEDA-22, 408) (60). Sweet's syndrome has also been described in a case of hairy cell leukemia (61).

Other skin complications

Disseminated vesiculopustular lesions, generalized and indurated erythematous papules or plaques, severe exacerbation of acne, and lenograstim-induced erythema nodosum, with recurrence on filgrastim administration, were mentioned in isolated patients (SED-13, 1116) (SEDA-20, 337). Finally, several reports convincingly involved G-CSF in exacerbations of chronic psoriasis or psoriatic arthritis, suggesting that activated neutrophils play an important role in the occurrence and propagation of skin inflammation (SEDA-21, 378) (62).

Musculoskeletal

Transient bone and musculoskeletal pain preceding myeloid recovery by 2–3 days are the commonest adverse effects of G-CSF, and occur in up to 25% of patients. Bone pain usually disappears despite continued treatment, but severe, narcotic-resistant, generalized bone pain was attributed to bone marrow necrosis in one patient (63).

The G-CSF-induced exacerbation of pseudogout occurred in two patients (SEDA-20, 337) (SEDA-22, 408).

- A 69-year-old man with a non-small-cell lung cancer treated with paclitaxel and nedaplatin developed polyarthralgia and myalgia with rising fever after receiving G-CSF for 5 days (64). Similar symptoms recurred after the second cycle of chemotherapy and on retreatment with G-CSF. Synovial biopsy showed acute synovitis with a foreign body-type giant cell reaction.

Worsening of rheumatoid symptoms has been reported in patients receiving G-CSF, particularly in patients with neutropenia due to Felty's syndrome (SEDA-19, 344) (SEDA-20, 338). Although concern about the short-term safety of G-CSF has been raised in these patients, other investigators feel that G-CSF can be used for a prolonged period in most patients without a flare-up of rheumatoid symptoms (SEDA-22, 408). Similar conclusions were reached in patients with underlying rheumatoid arthritis (SEDA-21, 378). The mechanisms of rheumatological flare-up are unclear. G-CSF-induced localized neutrophil activation or G-CSF-mediated increases in local neutrophil responses to TNF-alfa have both been suggested as underlying processes.

Several investigators have diagnosed bone mineral loss, with features of osteopenia/osteoporosis on radiography, quantitative computed tomography, or absorptiometry, in patients receiving long-term G-CSF for severe congenital neutropenia (6,65). In one child there was significant improvement in bone mineral density with pamidronate (66). In another child, who had osteoporotic vertebral collapse, extensive investigations showed reduced bone mineral content, reduced concentrations of osteocalcin, and features of osteoporosis on bone biopsy (SEDA-19, 344). The role of G-CSF was unclear, because bone mineral loss is a possible complication of the underlying disease. Indeed, improvement or stabilization during G-CSF treatment was noted in several patients (6). Furthermore, there was no apparent effect on height, head circumference, or weight in patients under 18 years of age (6). In another study, there was bone mineral loss with features of osteopenia/osteoporosis in 15 of 30 patients treated with G-CSF for a mean of 5.8 years for severe chronic neutropenia (65). However, six of nine patients investigated before G-CSF treatment had evidence of osteopenia/osteoporosis.

These reports and the findings of G-CSF-induced mobilization of osteoclastic progenitors in healthy volunteers (67) support a possible role of G-CSF in bone changes.

Immunologic

Leukocytoclastic vasculitis is a well-described and confirmed adverse effect of G-CSF, as documented in several reports, with recurrence after renewed administration of G-CSF (SEDA-19, 343). Most cases were confined to the skin, and renal insufficiency with hematuria and proteinuria was noted in only very few patients. Based on 18 cases reported in the literature or to the manufacturers, vasculitis was thought to have occurred in 6% of patients with chronic benign neutropenia, but in only six of about 200 000 patients with malignant disease (68). Vasculitis usually developed when the neutrophil count rose above 800×10^6/l, suggesting that an increase in neutrophil count may play a role in necrotic vasculitis. Against this background, the occurrence of vasculitis is not considered as treatment-limiting and does not preclude further G-CSF administration if the absolute neutrophil count is lower than 1000×10^6/l.

Antibodies to rG-CSF have not so far been reported, even in patients on long-term treatment.

Exacerbation of lupus-like symptoms, with seizures, psychosis, and vasculitis, has been noted during three of 12 treatment courses in neutropenic patients with severe systemic lupus erythematosus (69).

Type I reactions

Although IgE-specific antibodies have not been yet detected, filgrastim is undoubtedly associated with type I allergic reactions. This has been illustrated in well-documented reports of anaphylactic reactions, urticaria, and angioedema, with positive intradermal tests in several patients (SEDA-20, 338) (70,71). However, anaphylaxis to G-CSF is supposedly rare and the manufacturer is aware of only two cases of anaphylactoid reactions among 20 000 patients treated with filgrastim (72). One report has suggested possible cross-reactivity between filgrastim and other products derived from *Escherichia coli* (73). Although one patient who developed an anaphylactic-like reaction, with dyspnea, hypotension, and a pruritic erythematous skin rash, within minutes of G-CSF injection, later tolerated GM-CSF uneventfully (74), possible cross-reactivity between G-CSF and GM-CSF has been reported in at least one patient (75).

Long-Term Effects

Tumorigenicity

G-CSF-induced leukemia and myelodysplasia in patients with aplastic anemia or congenital neutropenia

Concerns have arisen over the prolonged use of G-CSF in patients with aplastic anemia, congenital neutropenia, or similar disorders and a possible increased or accelerated risk of myelodysplasia or acute leukemia (SED-14, 1274). Several investigators have noted reversible increases in circulating blasts during G-CSF treatment, and isolated reports have indicated a shortened delay in the occurrence of myelodysplasia and/or acute myeloid leukemia in this setting (SED-13, 1117) (SEDA-20, 338) (76). An abnormal karyotype (mostly monosomy 7) was sometimes found, and in vitro proliferation of myeloblasts by G-CSF was obtained in several patients. In addition, the potential role of point mutations on the G-CSF receptor has been also discussed as regards four of 28 patients with congenital neutropenia, two of whom developed acute myeloid leukemia (77). Myelodysplastic syndrome with monosomy 7 was also associated with G-CSF in another patient, with a reduction in the number of monosomy 7 positive cells after G-CSF withdrawal and a further increase after readministration (78).

This has been analysed in a number of epidemiological studies, most of which involved historical controls. The underlying predisposition of patients with aplastic anemia to develop myeloid malignancy has usually confounded attempts to determine whether growth factors are contributing factors.

In a retrospective study of 72 adults with aplastic anemia, of whom 18 received G-CSF and 23 received ciclosporin, five developed myelodysplastic syndrome (79). Four of them had received G-CSF + ciclosporin and all four had monosomy 7. The hematological disease was diagnosed within 16–31 months after the diagnosis of aplastic anemia and 12–20 months after the start of G-CSF treatment. Two died from acute leukemia. The incidence of myelodysplastic syndrome in this subgroup of patients was therefore 8.3% after 2 years and 39% after 3 years, whereas no case was observed over a 20-year period in patients not receiving this combined treatment. Univariate analysis showed that G-CSF + ciclosporin and G-CSF alone for more than 1 year were the most significant risk factors for the short-term development of monosomy 7 myelodysplastic syndrome.

In a prospective, multicenter, cohort study of 113 patients with aplastic anemia under 18 years of age, 12 developed myelodysplastic syndrome after a median of 37 months after the diagnosis of aplastic anemia and four others developed other cytogenetic clonal changes, of which the most common abnormality was monosomy 7 (80). From a multivariate analysis, G-CSF treatment duration and non-response to immunosuppressive therapy at 6 months were statistically significant risk factors for the development of myelodysplastic syndrome. The risk increased in proportion to the duration of G-CSF treatment, and the relative risks of the myelodysplastic syndrome were respectively 4.4 and 8.7 times higher in patients who received G-CSF for more than 120 and 180 days, compared with those who received it for less.

In contrast, a number of other studies did not confirm that the G-CSF increases the risk of myelodysplasia or acute leukemia, but the authors did not rule out a possible leukemogenic effect. In a study of patients with severe aplastic anemia the frequencies of cytogenetic abnormalities and myelodysplasia or leukemia were similar in 87 patients treated with G-CSF in addition to immunosuppressive treatment compared with 57 patients who did not receive G-CSF (81). Although the authors stated that a leukemogenic effect of G-CSF was unlikely, they mentioned that the median interval of appearance of cytogenetic abnormalities was shorter in the G-CSF group.

In another study the data from an international register of patients with severe chronic neutropenia were analysed (82). Of 352 patients treated with G-CSF for congenital neutropenia and followed for a mean of 6 years (maximum 11 years), 31 developed myelodysplasia or leukemia, whereas there were no cases in 344 patients with idiopathic or cyclic neutropenia. Associated cytogenetic clonal changes consisted of partial or complete loss of chromosome seven in 18 patients and abnormalities in chromosome 21 in nine. Isolated cytogenetic abnormalities were also found in nine other patients. None of the patients had abnormal marrow cytogenetic changes before G-CSF therapy. A more complete analysis failed to identify any correlation between G-CSF dose and treatment duration in patients who developed myelodysplasia or leukemia compared with those who were not affected. Although this argues against a role of G-CSF in the conversion of congenital neutropenia to myelodysplasia or leukemia, the authors recognized that a direct leukemogenic role of G-CSF could not be completely ruled out.

After a median follow-up of 43 months in 123 children treated with G-CSF, there was no difference in the incidence of secondary myelodysplasia or acute myeloid leukemia, in patients with aplastic anemia who survived longer than 2 years compared with the expected rate calculated before the use of G-CSF (83). Similarly, there was no evidence of an increased risk of myelodysplasia or acute myeloid leukemia in 54 patients treated with G-CSF for 4–6 years for severe congenital neutropenia (6).

Finally, in a randomized study in 102 patients of the safety and efficacy of lenograstim (5 micrograms/kg/day for 14 weeks) combined with standard immunosuppressants, there were no differences between the groups in survival, hematological response, or the occurrence of secondary leukemia (one case of myelodysplastic syndrome in each group) at a median follow-up of 5 years (84).

The role of G-CSF in leukemic transformation therefore remains unproven, primarily because these patients might be otherwise predisposed or have a previous history of immunosuppressive therapy. Although the clinical benefits of G-CSF probably outweigh any hazard of leukemogenesis, the possibility of an increased risk of myelodysplastic syndrome or acute myeloid leukemia under the influence of G-CSF should be borne in mind.

Careful monitoring of morphological bone marrow changes and cytogenetic studies are therefore recommended, and large randomized trials with long-term follow-up are still awaited to clarify these findings.

Stimulation of tumors or leukemic cells in patients with cancer

Because growth factor receptors are found on several tumor cell lines, there has been great concern that G-CSF may stimulate tumor progression (SED-13, 1117) (SEDA-20, 338) (SEDA-21, 378), with some anecdotal evidence of a temporal relation between G-CSF administration and the development or acceleration of malignancies, such as gastric cancer or Hodgkin's diseaseodgkin's disease (SED-13, 1117) (85–87). However, early clinical data and the results of several randomized controlled trials in patients with various malignancies provided no evidence for increased relapse rates (88,89).

With the demonstration of growth factor receptors on leukemic cells, the question has also been raised of whether there could be stimulation of leukemic cell growth with promotion of malignancies, or acceleration in the progression of myelodysplastic syndromes to acute myeloid leukemias. Although there has been some reluctance to use G-CSF in acute myeloid leukemia, no clear evidence of disease acceleration or recurrence was found in several trials (SED-13, 1117) (SEDA-21, 379). Based on an analysis of available in vitro data and published clinical trials, the risk of significant stimulation of leukemia or leukemic clone with an increased incidence of leukemia regrowth is currently estimated to be very low (90). Although clinical benefits are still debated in this setting, growth factors are considered to be safe in reducing the duration of neutropenia in patients with acute myeloid leukemia.

Although G-CSF is not believed to stimulate malignant lymphoid cells, G-CSF receptors have been found in patients with T cell leukemia, and this was associated with a significant increase in T cell leukemia cells in several patients (SEDA-21, 379). Other uncommon consequences of G-CSF have included blast mobilization with a phenotype change from common acute lymphoblastic leukemia to biphenotypic leukemia in one patient (87).

The risk of secondary cancer has been assessed in 412 children treated with etoposide and anthracyclines for acute lymphoblastic leukemia, 99 of whom also received G-CSF and 58 of whom received cranial irradiation (91). Overall, 20 children developed myeloid leukemia and myelodysplastic syndrome at a median of 2.3 years after treatment. The 6-year cumulative incidence of these secondary cancers was 11% among patients who received G-CSF, close to that observed in those who received cranial irradiation (12%), but significantly higher than in those who received neither irradiation nor G-CSF (2.7%).

Acceleration of myelodysplastic syndrome

A reversible increase in circulating blasts has been noted during G-CSF treatment in several patients with myelodysplastic syndrome, and other reports have documented a reversible secondary myelodysplastic syndrome or accelerated progression of a previous myelodysplastic syndrome (SEDA-21, 379) (89). In other instances, pseudoleukemia features or transient leukoerythroblastosis were evidenced on bone marrow biopsy (SEDA-19, 344) (SEDA-20, 338). Although there was no increased incidence of acute myeloblastic leukemia in G-CSF-treated patients with myelodysplastic syndrome, it has been considered that patients whose bone marrow contains more than 20% of blast cells should be regarded as being at higher risk of leukemic transformation (89).

Myeloma

The safety of growth factors in patients with myeloma is also of concern, as they can stimulate the proliferation of myeloma cells through IL-6 expression. Only isolated case reports, including accounts of the mobilization of clonal myeloma cells into the peripheral circulation, rapid progression of a multiple myeloma, or the new onset of a monoclonal gammopathy, directly or indirectly support the view that caution should be exercised in patients with multiple myeloma (SED-13, 1118) (92).

Susceptibility Factors

Renal disease

A hemodialysis patient developed refractory pleural effusion with prolonged leukopenia and thrombocytopenia, and another developed sudden cyanotic dyspnea with subsequent death after G-CSF administration for drug-induced neutropenia (93). The authors suggested that hemodialysis patients receiving G-CSF may have an increased risk of adverse effects.

Drug Administration

Drug formulations

Pegfilgrastim was developed by adding a polyethylene glycol molecule to the *N*-terminus of filgrastim. In a phase III study in 301 patients with advanced breast cancer who underwent myelosuppressive chemotherapy a single injection of pegfilgrastim had similar efficacy and safety profile to repeated injections of filgrastim (94).

Drug–Drug Interactions

Theophylline

A 30% increase in theophylline clearance occurred after the administration of G-CSF or GM-CSF (SEDA-20, 338).

Vincristine

In one study there was a synergistic effect of GM-CSF or G-CSF and cumulative doses of vincristine in causing severe atypical neuropathy (SEDA-20, 339).

Interference with Diagnostic Tests

Blood glucose analysis

Artifactual hypoglycemia occurred in patients taking G-CSF when blood glucose was analysed on the Ektachem 700 analyser (SEDA-20, 339).

Hepatitis B surface antigen

A single dose of G-CSF in a healthy donor produced a false positive test for hepatitis B surface antigen using an enzyme immunoassay (95).

References

1. Lieschke GJ, Burgess AW. Granulocyte colony-stimulating factor and granulocyte-macrophage colony-stimulating factor. N Engl J Med 1992;327(2):99–106.
2. Vial T, Descotes J. Clinical toxicity of cytokines used as haemopoietic growth factors. Drug Saf 1995;13(6):371–406.
3. Kojima S, Fukuda M, Miyajima Y, Matsuyama T, Horibe K. Treatment of aplastic anemia in children with recombinant human granulocyte colony-stimulating factor. Blood 1991;77(5):937–41.
4. Sheridan WP, Morstyn G, Wolf M, Dodds A, Lusk J, Maher D, Layton JE, Green MD, Souza L, Fox RM. Granulocyte colony-stimulating factor and neutrophil recovery after high-dose chemotherapy and autologous bone marrow transplantation. Lancet 1989;2(8668):891–5.
5. Herrmann F. G-CSF: status quo and new indications. Infection 1992;20(4):183–8.
6. Bonilla MA, Dale D, Zeidler C, Last L, Reiter A, Ruggeiro M, Davis M, Koci B, Hammond W, Gillio A, et al. Long-term safety of treatment with recombinant human granulocyte colony-stimulating factor (r-metHuG-CSF) in patients with severe congenital neutropenias. Br J Haematol 1994;88(4):723–30.
7. Beauchesne MF, Shalansky SJ. Nonchemotherapy drug-induced agranulocytosis: a review of 118 patients treated with colony-stimulating factors. Pharmacotherapy 1999;19(3):299–305.
8. Vial T, Gallant C, Choquet-Kastylevsky G, Descotes J. Treatment of drug-induced agranulocytosis with haematopoietic growth factors. A review of the clinical experience. BioDrugs 1999;11:185–200.
9. Milkovich G, Moleski RJ, Reitan JF, Dunning DM, Gibson GA, Paivanas TA, Wyant S, Jacobs RJ. Comparative safety of filgrastim versus sargramostim in patients receiving myelosuppressive chemotherapy. Pharmacotherapy 2000;20(12):1432–40.
10. Fischmeister G, Kurz M, Haas OA, Micksche M, Buchinger P, Printz D, Ressmann G, Stroebel T, Peters C, Fritsch G, Gadner H. G-CSF versus GM-CSF for stimulation of peripheral blood progenitor cells (PBPC) and leukocytes in healthy volunteers: comparison of efficacy and tolerability. Ann Hematol 1999;78(3):117–23.
11. Anderlini P, Przepiorka D, Champlin R, Korbling M. Biologic and clinical effects of granulocyte colony-stimulating factor in normal individuals. Blood 1996;88(8):2819–25.
12. Beelen DW, Ottinger H, Kolbe K, Ponisch W, Sayer HG, Knauf W, Stockschlader M, Scheid C, Schaefer UW. Filgrastim mobilization and collection of allogeneic blood progenitor cells from adult family donors: first interim report of a prospective German multicenter study. Ann Hematol 2002;81(12):701–9.
13. Anderlini P, Donato M, Chan KW, Huh YO, Gee AP, Lauppe MJ, Champlin RE, Korbling M. Allogeneic blood progenitor cell collection in normal donors after mobilization with filgrastim: the M.D. Anderson Cancer Center experience. Transfusion 1999;39(6):555–60.
14. de la Rubia J, Martinez C, Solano C, Brunet S, Cascon P, Arrieta R, Alegre A, Bargay J, de Arriba F, Canizo C, Lopez J, Serrano D, Verdeguer A, Torrabadella M, Diaz MA, Insunza A, de la Serna J, Espigado I, Petit J, Martinez M, Benlloch L, Sanz M. Administration of recombinant human granulocyte colony-stimulating factor to normal donors: results of the Spanish National Donor Registry. Spanish Group of Allo-PBT. Bone Marrow Transplant 1999;24(7):723–8.
15. Murata M, Harada M, Kato S, Takahashi S, Ogawa H, Okamoto S, Tsuchiya S, Sakamaki H, Akiyama Y, Kodera Y. Peripheral blood stem cell mobilization and apheresis: analysis of adverse events in 94 normal donors. Bone Marrow Transplant 1999;24(10):1065–71.
16. Kroger N, Renges H, Sonnenberg S, Kruger W, Gutensohn K, Dielschneider T, Cortes-Dericks L, Zander AR. Stem cell mobilisation with 16 microg/kg vs 10 microg/kg of G-CSF for allogeneic transplantation in healthy donors. Bone Marrow Transplant 2002; 29(9):727–30.
17. Cavallaro AM, Lilleby K, Majolino I, Storb R, Appelbaum FR, Rowley SD, Bensinger WI. Three to six year follow-up of normal donors who received recombinant human granulocyte colony-stimulating factor. Bone Marrow Transplant 2000;25(1):85–9.
18. Anderlini P, Chan FA, Champlin RE, Korbling M, Strom SS. Long-term follow-up of normal peripheral blood progenitor cell donors treated with filgrastim: no evidence of increased risk of leukemia development. Bone Marrow Transplant 2002;30(10):661–3.
19. Lindemann A, Rumberger B. Vascular complications in patients treated with granulocyte colony-stimulating factor (G-CSF). Eur J Cancer 1993;29A(16):2338–9.
20. Conti JA, Scher HI. Acute arterial thrombosis after escalated-dose methotrexate, vinblastine, doxorubicin, and cisplatin chemotherapy with recombinant granulocyte colony-stimulating factor. A possible new recombinant granulocyte colony-stimulating factor toxicity. Cancer 1992;70(11):2699–702.
21. Kuroiwa M, Okamura T, Kanaji T, Okamura S, Harada M, Niho Y. Effects of granulocyte colony-stimulating factor on the hemostatic system in healthy volunteers. Int J Hematol 1996;63(4):311–16.
22. Vij R, Adkins DR, Brown RA, Khoury H, DiPersio JF, Goodnough T. Unstable angina in a peripheral blood stem and progenitor cell donor given granulocyte-colony-stimulating factor. Transfusion 1999;39(5):542–3.
23. Oeda E, Shinohara K, Kamei S, Nomiyama J, Inoue H. Capillary leak syndrome likely the result of granulocyte colony-stimulating factor after high-dose chemotherapy. Intern Med 1994;33(2):115–19.
24. Dereure O, Bessis D, Lavabre-Bertrand T, Exbrayat C, Fegueux N, Biron C, Guilhou JJ. Thrombotic and necrotizing panniculitis associated with recombinant human granulocyte colony-stimulating factor treatment. Br J Dermatol 2000; 142(4):834–6.
25. Niitsu N, Iki S, Muroi K, Motomura S, Murakami M, Takeyama H, Ohsaka A, Urabe A. Interstitial pneumonia in patients receiving granulocyte colony-stimulating factor during chemotherapy: survey in Japan 1991–96. Br J Cancer 1997;76(12):1661–6.
26. Couderc LJ, Stelianides S, Frachon I, Stern M, Epardeau B, Baumelou E, Caubarrere I, Hermine O. Pulmonary toxicity of chemotherapy and G/GM-CSF: a report of five cases. Respir Med 1999;93(1):65–8.
27. Iki S, Yoshinaga K, Ohbayashi Y, Urabe A. Cytotoxic drug-induced pneumonia and possible augmentation by G-CSF—clinical attention. Ann Hematol 1993; 66(4):217–18.
28. Lei KI, Leung WT, Johnson PJ. Serious pulmonary complications in patients receiving recombinant granulocyte colony-stimulating factor during BACOP chemotherapy for aggressive non-Hodgkin's lymphoma. Br J Cancer 1994;70(5):1009–13.

29. Yokose N, Ogata K, Tamura H, An E, Nakamura K, Kamikubo K, Kudoh S, Dan K, Nomura T. Pulmonary toxicity after granulocyte colony-stimulating factor-combined chemotherapy for non-Hodgkin's lymphoma. Br J Cancer 1998;77(12):2286–90.
30. Bastion Y, Reyes F, Bosly A, Gisselbrecht C, Yver A, Gilles E, Maral J, Coiffier B. Possible toxicity with the association of G-CSF and bleomycin. Lancet 1994;343(8907):1221–2.
31. Takatsuka H, Takemoto Y, Mori A, Okamoto T, Kanamaru A, Kakishita E. Common features in the onset of ARDS after administration of granulocyte colony-stimulating factor. Chest 2002;121(5):1716–20.
32. White K, Cebon J. Transient hypoxaemia during neutrophil recovery in febrile patients. Lancet 1995;345(8956):1022–4.
33. Demuynck H, Zachee P, Verhoef GE, Schetz M, Van den Berghe G, Lauwers P, Boogaerts MA. Risks of rhG-CSF treatment in drug-induced agranulocytosis. Ann Hematol 1995;70(3):143–7.
34. Gertz MA, Lacy MQ, Bjornsson J, Litzow MR. Fatal pulmonary toxicity related to the administration of granulocyte colony-stimulating factor in amyloidosis: a report and review of growth factor-induced pulmonary toxicity. J Hematother Stem Cell Res 2000;9(5):635–43.
35. Ruiz-Arguelles GJ, Arizpe-Bravo D, Sanchez-Sosa S, Rojas-Ortega S, Moreno-Ford V, Ruiz-Arguelles A. Fatal G-CSF-induced pulmonary toxicity. Am J Hematol 1999;60(1):82–3.
36. Esmaeli B, Ahmadi MA, Kim S, Onan H, Korbling M, Anderlini P. Marginal keratitis associated with administration of filgrastim and sargramostim in a healthy peripheral blood progenitor cell donor. Cornea 2002;21(6):621–2.
37. Van Hoef ME, Howell A. Risk of thyroid dysfunction during treatment with G-CSF. Lancet 1992;340(8828): 1169–70.
38. Duarte R, De Luis DA, Lopez-Jimenez J, Roy G, Garcia A. Thyroid function and autoimmunity during treatment with G-CSF. Clin Endocrinol (Oxf) 1999;51(1):133–4.
39. Norol F, Bonin P, Charpentier F, Bierling P, Beaujean F, Cartron JP, Bories D, Kuentz M. Apparent reactivation of a red cell alloantibody in a healthy individual after G-CSF administration. Br J Haematol 1998;103(1):256–8.
40. Wun T. The Felty syndrome and G-CSF-associated thrombocytopenia and severe anemia. Ann Intern Med 1993;118(4):318–19.
41. de Wit R, Verweij J, Bontenbal M, Kruit WH, Seynaeve C, Schmitz PI, Stoter G. Adverse effect on bone marrow protection of prechemotherapy granulocyte colony-stimulating factor support. J Natl Cancer Inst 1996;88(19):1393–8.
42. Mueller BU, Burt R, Gulick L, Jacobsen F, Pizzo PA, Horne M. Disseminated intravascular coagulation associated with granulocyte colony-stimulating factor therapy in a child with human immunodeficiency virus infection. J Pediatr 1995;126(5 Pt 1):749–52.
43. Migita M, Fukunaga Y, Watanabe A, Maruyama K, Ohta K, Kaneko K, Kaneda M, Kakinuma K, Yamatoto M. Emperipolesis of neutrophils by megakaryocytes and thrombocytopenia observed in a case of Kostmann's syndrome during intravenous administration of high-dose rhG-CSF. Br J Haematol 1992;80(3):413–15.
44. LeBlanc R, Roy J, Demers C, Vu L, Cantin G. A prospective study of G-CSF effects on hemostasis in allogeneic blood stem cell donors. Bone Marrow Transplant 1999;23(10):991–6.
45. Falanga A, Marchetti M, Evangelista V, Manarini S, Oldani E, Giovanelli S, Galbusera M, Cerletti C, Barbui T. Neutrophil activation and hemostatic changes in healthy donors receiving granulocyte colony-stimulating factor. Blood 1999;93(8):2506–14.
46. Mizuno S, Okamura T, Iwasaki H, Ohno Y, Akashi K, Inaba S, Niho Y. Hypercoagulable state following transfusions of granulocytes obtained from granulocyte colony-stimulating factor-stimulated donors. Int J Hematol 2000; 72(1):115–17.
47. Bonig H, Burdach S, Gobel U, Nurnberger W. Growth factors and hemostasis: differential effects of GM-CSF and G-CSF on coagulation activation—laboratory and clinical evidence. Ann Hematol 2001;80(9):525–30.
48. Dale DC, Bonilla MA, Davis MW, Nakanishi AM, Hammond WP, Kurtzberg J, Wang W, Jakubowski A, Winton E, Lalezari P, et al. A randomized controlled phase III trial of recombinant human granulocyte colony-stimulating factor (filgrastim) for treatment of severe chronic neutropenia. Blood 1993;81(10):2496–502.
49. Calderwood S, Kilpatrick L, Douglas SD, Freedman M, Smith-Whitley K, Rolland M, Kurtzberg J. Recombinant human granulocyte colony-stimulating factor therapy for patients with neutropenia and/or neutrophil dysfunction secondary to glycogen storage disease type 1b. Blood 2001;97(2):376–82.
50. Litam PP, Friedman HD, Loughran TP Jr. Splenic extramedullary hematopoiasis in a patient receiving intermittently administered granulocyte colony-stimulating factor. Ann Intern Med 1993;118(12):954–5.
51. Nakayama T, Kudo H, Suzuki S, Sassa S, Mano Y, Sakamoto S. Splenomegaly induced by recombinant human granulocyte-colony stimulating factor in rats. Life Sci 2001;69(13):1521–9.
52. Falzetti F, Aversa F, Minelli O, Tabilio A. Spontaneous rupture of spleen during peripheral blood stem-cell mobilisation in a healthy donor. Lancet 1999;353(9152):555.
53. Kasper C, Jones L, Fujita Y, Morgenstern GR, Scarffe JH, Chang J. Splenic rupture in a patient with acute myeloid leukemia undergoing peripheral blood stem cell transplantation. Ann Hematol 1999;78(2):91–2.
54. Kawachi Y, Ozaki S, Sakamoto Y, Uchida T, Mori M, Setsu K, Tani K, Asano S. Richter's syndrome showing pronounced lymphadenopathy in response to administration of granulocyte colony-stimulating factor. Leuk Lymphoma 1994;13(5–6):509–14.
55. Magen D, Mandel H, Berant M, Ben-Izhak O, Zelikovic I. MPGN type I induced by granulocyte colony stimulating factor. Pediatr Nephrol 2002;17(5):370–2.
56. Asnis LA, Gaspari AA. Cutaneous reactions to recombinant cytokine therapy. J Am Acad Dermatol 1995;33(3):393–410.
57. Viallard AM, Lavenue A, Balme B, Pincemaille B, Raudrant D, Thomas L. Lichenoid cutaneous drug reaction at injection sites of granulocyte colony-stimulating factor (filgrastim). Dermatology 1999;198(3):301–3.
58. Mori T, Sato N, Watanabe R, Okamoto S, Ikeda Y. Erythema exsudativum multiforme induced by granulocyte colony-stimulating factor in an allogeneic peripheral blood stem cell donor. Bone Marrow Transplant 2000; 26(2):239–40.
59. Prendiville J, Thiessen P, Mallory SB. Neutrophilic dermatoses in two children with idiopathic neutropenia: association with granulocyte colony-stimulating factor (G-CSF) therapy. Pediatr Dermatol 2001;18(5):417–21.
60. Johnson ML, Grimwood RE. Leukocyte colony-stimulating factors. A review of associated neutrophilic dermatoses and vasculitides. Arch Dermatol 1994;130(1):77–81.
61. Glaspy JA, Baldwin GC, Robertson PA, Souza L, Vincent M, Ambersley J, Golde DW. Therapy for neutropenia in hairy cell leukemia with recombinant human granulocyte colony-stimulating factor. Ann Intern Med 1988;109(10):789–95.
62. Couderc LJ, Philippe B, Franck N, Balloul-Delclaux E, Lessana-Leibowitch M. Necrotizing vasculitis and

exacerbation of psoriasis after granulocyte colony-stimulating factor for small cell lung carcinoma. Respir Med 1995; 89(3):237–8.

63. Katayama Y, Deguchi S, Shinagawa K, Teshima T, Notohara K, Taguchi K, Omoto E, Harada M. Bone marrow necrosis in a patient with acute myeloblastic leukemia during administration of G-CSF and rapid hematologic recovery after allotransplantation of peripheral blood stem cells. Am J Hematol 1998;57(3):238–40.
64. Tsukadaira A, Okubo Y, Takashi S, Kobayashi H, Kubo K. Repeated arthralgia associated with granulocyte colony stimulating factor administration. Ann Rheum Dis 2002;61(9):849–50.
65. Yakisan E, Schirg E, Zeidler C, Bishop NJ, Reiter A, Hirt A, Riehm H, Welte K. High incidence of significant bone loss in patients with severe congenital neutropenia (Kostmann's syndrome). J Pediatr 1997;131(4):592–7.
66. Sekhar RV, Culbert S, Hoots WK, Klein MJ, Zietz H, Vassilopoulou-Sellin R. Severe osteopenia in a young boy with Kostmann's congenital neutropenia treated with granulocyte colony-stimulating factor: suggested therapeutic approach. Pediatrics 2001;108(3):E54.
67. Purton LE, Lee MY, Torok-Storb B. Normal human peripheral blood mononuclear cells mobilized with granulocyte colony-stimulating factor have increased osteoclastogenic potential compared to nonmobilized blood. Blood 1996;87(5):1802–8.
68. Jain KK. Cutaneous vasculitis associated with granulocyte colony-stimulating factor. J Am Acad Dermatol 1994;31(2 Pt 1):213–15.
69. Euler HH, Harten P, Zeuner RA, Schwab UM. Recombinant human granulocyte colony stimulating factor in patients with systemic lupus erythematosus associated neutropenia and refractory infections. J Rheumatol 1997;24(11):2153–7.
70. Jaiyesimi I, Giralt SS, Wood J. Subcutaneous granulocyte colony-stimulating factor and acute anaphylaxis. N Engl J Med 1991;325(8):587.
71. Sasaki O, Yokoyama A, Uemura S, Fujino S, Inoue Y, Kohno N, Hiwada K. Drug eruption caused by recombinant human G-CSF. Intern Med 1994;33(10):641–3.
72. Brown SL, Hill E. Subcutaneous granulocyte colony-stimulating factor and acute anaphylaxis. N Engl J Med 1991;325:587.
73. Stone HD Jr, DiPiro C, Davis PC, Meyer CF, Wray BB. Hypersensitivity reactions to *Escherichia coli*-derived polyethylene glycolated-asparaginase associated with subsequent immediate skin test reactivity to *E. coli*-derived granulocyte colony-stimulating factor. J Allergy Clin Immunol 1998;101(3):429–31.
74. Keung YK, Suwanvecho S, Cobos E. Anaphylactoid reaction to granulocyte colony-stimulating factor used in mobilization of peripheral blood stem cell. Bone Marrow Transplant 1999;23(2):200–1.
75. Shahar E, Krivoy N, Pollack S. Effective acute desensitization for immediate-type hypersensitivity to human granulocyte–monocyte colony stimulating factor. Ann Allergy Asthma Immunol 1999;83(6 Pt 1):543–6.
76. Dantal J, Hourmant M, Cantarovich D, Giral M, Blancho G, Dreno B, Soulillou JP. Effect of long-term immunosuppression in kidney-graft recipients on cancer incidence: randomised comparison of two cyclosporin regimens. Lancet 1998;351(9103):623–8.
77. Tidow N, Pilz C, Teichmann B, Muller-Brechlin A, Germeshausen M, Kasper B, Rauprich P, Sykora KW, Welte K. Clinical relevance of point mutations in the cytoplasmic domain of the granulocyte colony-stimulating factor receptor gene in patients with severe congenital neutropenia. Blood 1997;89(7):2369–75.
78. Nishimura M, Yamada T, Andoh T, Tao T, Emoto M, Ohji T, Matsuda K, Kameda N, Satoh Y, Matsutani A, Azuno Y, Oka Y. Granulocyte colony-stimulating factor (G-CSF) dependent hematopoiesis with monosomy 7 in a patient with severe aplastic anemia after ATG/CsA/G-CSF combined therapy. Int J Hematol 1998;68(2):203–11.
79. Kaito K, Kobayashi M, Katayama T, Masuoka H, Shimada T, Nishiwaki K, Sekita T, Otsubo H, Ogasawara Y, Hosoya T. Long-term administration of G-CSF for aplastic anaemia is closely related to the early evolution of monosomy 7 MDS in adults. Br J Haematol 1998;103(2):297–303.
80. Kojima S, Ohara A, Tsuchida M, Kudoh T, Hanada R, Okimoto Y, Kaneko T, Takano T, Ikuta K, Tsukimoto I; Japan Childhood Aplastic Anemia Study Group. Risk factors for evolution of acquired aplastic anemia into myelodysplastic syndrome and acute myeloid leukemia after immunosuppressive therapy in children. Blood 2002; 100(3):786–90.
81. Locasciulli A, Arcese W, Locatelli F, Di Bona E, Bacigalupo A; Italian Aplastic Anaemia Study Group. Treatment of aplastic anaemia with granulocyte-colony stimulating factor and risk of malignancy. Italian Aplastic Anaemia Study Group. Lancet 2001;357(9249):43–4.
82. Freedman MH, Bonilla MA, Fier C, Bolyard AA, Scarlata D, Boxer LA, Brown S, Cham B, Kannourakis G, Kinsey SE, Mori PG, Cottle T, Welte K, Dale DC. Myelodysplasia syndrome and acute myeloid leukemia in patients with congenital neutropenia receiving G-CSF therapy. Blood 2000;96(2):429–36.
83. Imashuku S, Hibi S, Nakajima F, Mitsui T, Yokoyama S, Kojima S, Matsuyama T, Nakahata T, Ueda K, Tsukimoto I, et al. A review of 125 cases to determine the risk of myelodysplasia and leukemia in pediatric neutropenic patients after treatment with recombinant human granulocyte colony-stimulating factor. Blood 1994;84(7):2380–1.
84. Gluckman E, Rokicka-Milewska R, Hann I, Nikiforakis E, Tavakoli F, Cohen-Scali S, Bacigalupo A; European Group for Blood and Marrow Transplantation Working Party for Severe Aplastic Anemia. Results and follow-up of a phase III randomized study of recombinant human-granulocyte stimulating factor as support for immunosuppressive therapy in patients with severe aplastic anaemia. Br J Haematol 2002;119(4):1075–82.
85. Soutar RL. Acute myeloblastic leukemia and recombinant granulocyte colony stimulating factor. BMJ 1991; 303(6794):123–4.
86. Stathopoulos GP, Moschopoulos N, Apostolopoulou E, Papakostas P, Samelis GF. Acute non-lymphocytic leukaemia complicating gastric cancer treated with epipodophyllotoxin containing chemotherapy and G-CSF. Acta Oncol 1994;33(6):713–14.
87. Matsuzaki A, Ohga S, Ueda K, Okamuras. Induction of CD33-positive blasts by granulocyte colony-stimulating factor in a child with common acute lymphoblastic leukemia. Int J Ped Hematol Oncol 1994;1:339–41.
88. Vose JM, Armitage JO. Clinical applications of hematopoietic growth factors. J Clin Oncol 1995;13(4):1023–35.
89. Schriber JR, Negrin RS. Use and toxicity of the colony-stimulating factors. Drug Saf 1993;8(6):457–68.
90. Rowe JM, Liesveld JL. Hematopoietic growth factors in acute leukemia. Leukemia 1997;11(3):328–41.
91. Relling MV, Boyett JM, Blanco JG, Raimondi S, Behm FG, Sandlund JT, Rivera GK, Kun LE, Evans WE, Pui CH. Granulocyte colony-stimulating factor and the risk of secondary myeloid malignancy after etoposide treatment. Blood 2003;101(10):3862–7.
92. Kobbe G, Germing U, Soehngen D, Aul C, Heyll A. Massive extramedullary disease progression in a patient

with stable multiple myeloma during G-CSF priming for peripheral blood progenitor mobilization. Oncol Rep 1999;6(5):1151–2.

93. Nakamura M, Sakemi T, Fujisaki T, Matsuo S, Ikeda Y, Nishimoto A, Ohtsuka Y, Tomiyoshi Y. Sudden death or refractory pleural effusion following treatment with granulocyte colony-stimulating factor in two hemodialysis patients. Nephron 1999;83(2):178–9.
94. Holmes FA, O'Shaughnessy JA, Vukelja S, Jones SE, Shogan J, Savin M, Glaspy J, Moore M, Meza L, Wiznitzer I, Neumann TA, Hill LR, Liang BC. Blinded, randomized, multicenter study to evaluate single administration pegfilgrastim once per cycle versus daily filgrastim as an adjunct to chemotherapy in patients with high-risk stage II or stage III/IV breast cancer. J Clin Oncol 2002;20(3):727–31.
95. Warren K, Eastlund T. False-reactive test for hepatitis B surface antigen following administration of granulocyte-colony-stimulating factor. Vox Sang 2002;83(3):247–9.

Granulocyte–macrophage colony-stimulating factor (GM-CSF)

See also Myeloid colony stimulating factors

General Information

Granulocyte–macrophage colony-stimulating factor (GM-CSF) primarily increases the production and activity of neutrophils, and stimulates the proliferation of monocytes and eosinophils.

Recombinant human forms of GM-CSF that are in use include molgramostim and sargramostim. Based on a retrospective review and historical comparison, the safety of molgramostim has been thought to be less than that of sargramostim (1). However, there were no significant differences in the adverse effects profiles and severity of adverse effects with GM-CSF and G-CSF in 181 patients with cancers randomized to receive sargramostim (a yeast cell-derived GM-CSF) or filgrastim (a bacterial cell-derived G-CSF) for chemotherapy-induced myelosuppression (2).

Uses

The potential clinical applications of GM-CSF have been lengthily reviewed (3). It is used:

- to reduce chemotherapy-induced myelosuppression in patients with metastatic sarcoma, breast cancer, or melanoma.
- to facilitate the harvesting of peripheral blood stem cells for autologous bone marrow transplantation.
- in cyclic neutropenia.
- to aid recovery after high doses of ionizing radiation, and less successfully, for severe aplastic anemia.

GM-CSF has also been approved for the alleviation of neutropenia following myeloablative treatment with autologous bone marrow transplantation and ganciclovir-induced neutropenia in patients with AIDS (4).

General adverse effects

The adverse effects of GM-CSF are dose-related and have usually been tolerable. At the doses usually recommended, systemic adverse effects develop in 25–30% of patients, but they are rarely treatment-limiting (5). Doses over 250 micrograms/m^2 and the intravenous route are associated with more frequent adverse effects.

Bone pain and flu-like symptoms, with fever, myalgia, chills, and headache, are the most frequent adverse effects (5–7). These reactions occur in 40–60% of all treated patients (8) and are probably due to the activation of secondary cytokines (such as TNF-alfa and IL-1) (9). Other frequently reported adverse effects include erythematous eruptions at the injection site, thrombophlebitis, nausea, facial flushing, dyspnea, and gastrointestinal disorders with anorexia and weight loss. Severe fatigue and weakness are rare.

The first dose of GM-CSF can be followed within 3 hours by flushing, hypotension, tachycardia, dyspnea, musculoskeletal pain, and nausea and vomiting (6). At very high doses (generally over 16 micrograms/kg/day), erythroderma, weight gain, and edema with pleuropericardial effusions and ascites have been reported (10). Renal symptoms have also been described (11,12), as have various biochemical abnormalities, possibly due to secondary hyperaldosteronism (13–15).

Fever was observed in up to 50% of patients at doses over 3 micrograms/kg. The fact that the fever peaks at a constant time after GM-CSF injection, the lack of clinical and biological signs of infection, and a prompt response to paracetamol have been proposed as criteria to recognize GM-CSF-induced iatrogenic fever (16), but this concept is still disputed (17).

Organs and Systems

Cardiovascular

Mild local phlebitis sometimes occurs at intravenous sites of administration of GM-CSF. Central venous catheter site thrombosis, inferior vena cava thrombosis, and possible pulmonary embolism have sometimes been observed (5,18). Although chemotherapy for breast cancer is associated with a higher risk of developing vascular thrombosis, iliac artery thrombosis was attributed to GM-CSF in two patients (19).

Raynaud's phenomenon has been reported, but confounding factors including the use of high-dose antineoplastic drugs are possible (5).

A rapidly reversible first-dose syndrome (dyspnea, hypoxia, tachycardia, and hypotension) can occur within the first hour after the first continuous infusion in 15–30% of patients (5). A dose-limiting vascular leak syndrome was consistently described in patients receiving GM-CSF 30 micrograms/kg/day or more, but lower doses were also reported to induce a clinically relevant capillary leak syndrome (SEDA-22, 408) (20,21). Continuation of GM-CSF treatment at the same dose or lower and careful management was possible in some patients. Endothelial cell damage with an increase in the transcapillary escape rate of albumin and the possible role of IL-1 and TNF production by GM-CSF-activated monocytes were suggested as possible mechanisms. This was consistent with the observation of marked hypoalbuminemia in some instances associated with edema and ascites after GM-CSF in four of nine patients treated for myelodysplastic syndrome or aplastic anemia (22).

Respiratory

It has been suggested that, as in the case of G-CSF, GM-CSF can increase the pulmonary toxicity of bleomycin and facilitate the development of the adult respiratory distress syndrome (ARDS), but evidence is still very sparse (SED-13, 1112) (SEDA-19, 342).

Acute febrile interstitial pneumonitis occurred within less than 48 hours after the second to fourth cycles of chemotherapy (doxorubicin, cyclophosphamide, bleomycin, methotrexate, plus methylprednisolone) in five patients with non-Hodgkin's lymphoma who were receiving prophylactic G-CSF ($n = 3$) or GM-CSF ($n = 2$) (23). Lymphocytic alveolitis was confirmed in four of these patients and all three patients tested had an increased number of CD8+ T cells. Even though all the patients received high-dose methylprednisolone, two died as a result of diffuse and extensive interstitial pulmonary fibrosis, demonstrated at postmortem. Although both G-CSF and GM-CSF can cause acute pneumonitis in patients with cancers, it is still unknown to what extent hemopoietic growth factors are involved in this complication.

In one patient, interstitial pulmonary edema with pulmonary failure was supposedly a first-dose reaction (24). Reversible eosinophilic pneumonia has also been reported (SEDA-19, 342).

One patient had acute bronchospasm after a subcutaneous injection of GM-CSF around a lower limb ulcer (25).

Nervous system

Very few neurological adverse effects have been associated with GM-CSF.

- Mania occurred in a 41-year-old woman taking GM-CSF who had previously tolerated G-CSF (SEDA-20, 339).
- A 49-year-old woman with chronic hepatitis C received filgrastim (G-CSF) for interferon-alfa-induced leukopenia (26). Filgrastim was withdrawn after 3 months, because of leg cramps and back pain. She later received sargramostim (GM-CSF) 500 micrograms twice weekly and she noticed gait unsteadiness and headaches within 2 weeks. During the next 3 months, she developed progressive confusion, forgetfulness, and lethargy, and both interferon alfa and sargramostim were withdrawn. She rapidly deteriorated and died from central hypoventilation 6 days later. Autopsy showed atypical, perivascular, lymphoid infiltrates in the white matter, basal ganglia, hypothalamus, brain stem, cerebellum, and spinal cord. Serum hepatitis C virus DNA sequences were not detected.

This case of fulminant perivascular lymphocytic proliferation suggests that some of the effects of GM-CSF on white blood cell proliferation can sometimes produce unexpected adverse effects.

Endocrine

Three patients with positive thyroid antibodies before GM-CSF treatment developed hypothyroidism or biphasic thyroiditis (27,28), whereas no similar thyroid dysfunction has been observed in patients without pre-existing thyroid antibodies (27). Based on these reports, GM-CSF has been thought to exacerbate underlying autoimmune thyroiditis.

Metabolism

Serum cholesterol concentrations have reportedly fallen in patients given GM-CSF (29).

Electrolyte balance

Severe symptomatic hypokalemia was thought to have resulted from increased intracellular potassium uptake linked to massive leukocytosis after GM-CSF (15).

Hematologic

Acute exacerbation of autoimmune thrombocytopenia (30) or hemolytic anemia has been linked to macrophage activation (31), and it has been suggested that patients with previous autoimmune blood disorders are at increased risk of hematological toxicity from GM-CSF.

A transient, moderate, and reversible rise in leukocyte alkaline phosphatase, lactate dehydrogenase (LDH) and serum uric acid concentrations is usually observed in cancer patients receiving supportive treatment with GM-CSF or G-CSF. Serum LDH increased from 37 to 85% and there was a linear relation between increased leukocyte production and the rise in serum LDH (32). Increases in serum LDH activity should therefore not be interpreted as indicative of disease progression, unless LDH activity remains high after growth factor withdrawal.

Erythrocytes

A typical vaso-occlusive crisis with increased hemolysis was noted within minutes after intracutaneous injection of GM-CSF in a patient with stable sickle cell disease (SEDA-19, 342). Topical GM-CSF was later uneventful.

Leukocytes

Dose-related and sometimes marked eosinophilia has been noted after GM-CSF (33). Although usually not associated with symptoms, excessive eosinophilia with fatal necrotizing pneumonia and Loeffler's endocarditis has been described (34).

Clotting factors

A marked reduction in vitamin K-dependent coagulation factors, which was prevented by vitamin K administration, has been described in patients with acute myeloid leukemia who were given GM-CSF (SEDA-19, 342).

The differential effects of G-CSF and GM-CSF on several coagulation parameters have been compared in 34 patients who received the colony-stimulating factors after bone marrow transplantation (35). The data suggested activation of the coagulation system in patients treated with GM-CSF, which resulted in a tendency to more frequent veno-occlusive disease of the liver and a significantly higher incidence of hemorrhage.

Hemopoietic tissues
Although GM-CSF acts primarily on neutrophils, stimulating effects on the myeloid lineage and other cells or cytokines of the immune system can be associated with deleterious consequences, as illustrated in several case reports. Splenomegaly with histologically documented splenic extramedullary hemopoiesis of all three lineages and histiocytic bone marrow proliferation have been described (36–38). More severe outcomes have been described, such as reactive hemophagic histiocytosis resulting in fatal pancytopenia in two bone marrow transplant patients (39). Extensive and persistent bone marrow histiocytosis was considered the likely cause of delayed bone marrow engraftment and subsequent death in both patients. These effects may have been the consequences of GM-CSF-induced proliferation and activation of the monocyte/macrophage system.

Liver

A moderate increase in serum transaminase activities sometimes occurs in patients receiving GM-CSF. More severe hepatotoxicity has been briefly reported in patients who received GM-CSF after autologous bone marrow transplantation (SEDA-19, 342). Hyperbilirubinemia was also found in 8% of bone marrow transplant patients and considered as possible ground for molgramostim withdrawal (1).

Urinary tract

There was no evidence of nephrotoxicity secondary to GM-CSF during clinical trials, but the possible occurrence of transient renal insufficiency has been discussed (1).

Skin

Cutaneous reactions to GM-CSF occur in about 50% of patients and have been reviewed (40); there is concern that autoimmune skin diseases, psoriasis, and other dermatoses might be exacerbated.

GM-CSF often causes erythema and itching at subcutaneous injection sites, with a particularly high incidence of relapsing macular pruritic infiltrates at sites of injection in patients with inflammatory breast cancer (SEDA-20, 339). Based on a retrospective review, molgramostim-induced rash was the most common treatment-limiting adverse event in bone marrow transplant patients, but further administration of sargramostim may be well tolerated (1).

Cutaneous reactions in 57 cancer patients given GM-CSF have been described in detail. They included localized immediate angioedema (8%), generalized cutaneous reactions (21%), or both (16%) (41). Generalized reactions consisted mostly of maculopapular, exfoliative, and urticarial eruptions, which resolved after topical treatment, dosage reduction, or treatment withdrawal. There was usually hyperkeratosis, mild spongiosis, lymphocytic exocytosis, and perivascular infiltration by lymphocytes, neutrophils, and eosinophils. Eosinophil activation was supposedly involved in the pathogenesis of these lesions, as was also suggested in the report of atopic dermatitis-like eruptions in two patients (42) or the acute revelation of an underlying epidermolysis bullosa acquisita in a previously asymptomatic patient (43).

As with G-CSF, GM-CSF-induced activation of neutrophils can play a critical role in the occurrence of neutrophilic dermatoses and other skin disorders. Other reports have described acute exacerbation of previous pyoderma gangrenosum (44) and subcorneal pustular dermatosis around injection sites (SEDA-19, 342).

Additional isolated reports suggesting an immunological response or inappropriate cytokine secretion subsequent to GM-CSF administration include accounts of erythema multiforme (SEDA-19, 342) and acutely generalized exacerbation of pre-existing psoriasis (45). The latter report is in keeping with the finding that GM-CSF is sometimes raised in patients with psoriasis.

Musculoskeletal

Transient bone pain is common with GM-CSF. Prompt reactivation or worsening of rheumatoid symptoms has been observed in several patients with Felty's syndrome and in one seropositive rheumatoid arthritic patient (SED-13, 1113) (46,47). GM-CSF-induced acute IL-6 release and an increase in acute phase proteins were thought to be involved.

Immunologic

Hypersensitivity reactions
Although anaphylactic reactions without any documented immune-mediated mechanism have been reported in about 8% of patients with testicular cancer given GM-CSF (48), GM-CSF has only otherwise rarely been associated with allergic reactions. Of two patients who had possible immune-mediated reactions (SEDA-19, 342) one had an immediate recurrent local reaction followed by systemic hypersensitivity reaction after sargramostim, and the other had a maculopapular pruritic eruption after molgramostim. Cross-reaction between the two recombinant forms of GM-CSF was suggested by the results of skin prick tests in one patient, but both patients thereafter tolerated filgrastim uneventfully.

However, cross-sensitivity and possible desensitization have been documented.

- A 42-year-old woman with defective immunological function had generalized pruritus, flushing, shortness of breath, and general discomfort within 30 minutes of her 16th intravenous injection of molgramostim (49). Her symptoms resolved with adrenaline, hydrocortisone, and promethazine. Despite the prophylactic use of glucocorticoids and antihistamines, she developed a similar reaction after molgramostim readministration and 4 hours after the fourth injection of filgrastim. Positive skin prick tests to molgramostim and filgrastim suggested IgE-mediated hypersensitivity. An acute desensitization protocol starting with molgramostim 0.0008 micrograms increasing to 320 micrograms was successful, and molgramostim was later continued uneventfully.

Vasculitis
GM-CSF can cause or exacerbate cutaneous leukocytoclastic vasculitis with possible renal or pulmonary involvement (SED-13, 1113). This adverse effect was substantiated by the prompt recurrence of vasculitis

after drug re-administration in several patients or the report of relapsing necrotizing vasculitis at all GM-CSF injection sites.

Antibodies to GM-CSF
Formation of antibodies to recombinant GM-CSF has been detected in 31% of patients treated with sargramostim and in 95% of patients treated with molgramostim derived from *Escherichia coli* (50,51). Although the clinical relevance of this is uncertain, a significant modification of exogenous GM-CSF pharmacokinetics, a reduction in the rise in leukocyte count, and a reduction in the frequency of GM-CSF-associated adverse effects have been suggested as possible consequences. Use of the subcutaneous route and repeated administration were deemed to increase the likelihood of antibody occurrence (51). However, the fact that most patients receiving growth factors are already likely to be immunocompromised as a result of intensive chemotherapy might also account for discrepancies between the widespread use of growth factors and the paucity of reports on antibodies against growth factors. In fact only one of eight potentially immunocompromised patients had anti-GM-CSF antibody titers and they were very low (51). Antibodies to GM-CSF have not been found after prolonged use in patients with AIDS (52).

Death

There were more frequent adverse effects and an increased death rate due to pulmonary complications, sepsis, or arterial thrombosis in lung cancer patients treated with chemotherapy plus radiotherapy and GM-CSF (SEDA-20, 339).

Long-Term Effects

Tumorigenicity

Previous fears that GM-CSF might give rise to progression of pre-leukemic conditions have not been substantiated (53).

The possibility that growth factors can stimulate the growth of malignant and leukemic cells, or accelerate the progression of myelodysplastic syndrome to acute myeloid leukemia has been discussed in the monograph on G-CSF section. At the moment, there is no indication from clinical trials that GM-CSF actually increases the risk of tumor growth or the relapse rate in patients with various malignancies (29,54–56). Isolated reports have referred to delayed occurrence of B cell non-Hodgkin's lymphoma after GM-CSF treatment for aplastic anemia and de novo occurrence of diffuse oligoclonal plasmocytosis after both GM-CSF and G-CSF for high-grade glioma (SEDA-19, 342).

Although reversible increases in circulating blasts during GM-CSF treatment are sometimes noted and have raised concern on the possible accelerated occurrence of acute leukemia, the progression of myelodysplastic syndromes to acute myeloid leukemia has been only anecdotally reported (SEDA-19, 342) (57). There was no evidence of significant leukemic cell proliferation in patients with acute myeloid leukemia, and no increased risk of graft failure, leukemogenesis, relapse, or death after a median follow-up of 36 months in 128 patients who underwent autologous bone marrow transplantation for lymphoid malignancies (29,58). Finally, one report has suggested that a GM-CSF-induced abrupt rise in peripheral blasts may have caused diffuse infiltration and proliferation of leukemic blast cells in the spleen, and subsequent fatal hemorrhagic spleen rupture (59).

Susceptibility Factors

Age

In a large, randomized, placebo-controlled trial in 264 very low birth weight neonates, treatment with GM-CSF for 28 days was not associated with specific toxic effects, but the incidence of nosocomial infections was not reduced (60).

Other features of the patient

Bone marrow transplantation
Because the production of cytokines (for example IL-1 or TNF-alfa) involved in the stimulation of cells responsible for graft-versus-host disease can be enhanced by hemopoietic growth factors, the use of growth factors after allogeneic transplantation is theoretically risky. However, in reviews of trials of G-CSF or GM-CSF in allogeneic bone marrow transplantation there were no increases in late engraftment failures, relapse rates, or exacerbation of graft-versus-host disease (54,61).

HIV infection
The safety and activity of subcutaneous GM-CSF (300 micrograms/day for 1 week and 150 micrograms twice weekly for 11 weeks) has been compared with no treatment in 244 leukopenic HIV-infected patients (62). Adverse effects were reported in most of the patients treated with GM-CSF and consisted of flu-like symptoms (98%), bone pain (42%), and injection site reactions (85%). There was a two-fold increase in serum transaminase and alkaline phosphatase activities in 5.7% of patients. There was a moderate, but not significant, increase in HIV p24 antigen concentration. The few relevant clinical trials have provided no convincing evidence that GM-CSF enhances HIV replication or accelerates HIV-associated diseases (for example infections or neoplasms) in patients with AIDS (63). Only one patient with AIDS and ultrasonographic confirmation of enhanced Kaposi's sarcoma lesions temporally related to GM-CSF used for interferon- and zidovudine-related severe neutropenia has been reported (SEDA-19, 343).

Drug–Drug Interactions

Theophylline

A 30% increase in theophylline clearance occurred after the administration of G-CSF or GM-CSF (SEDA-20, 338).

Vincristine

In one study there was a synergistic effect of GM-CSF or G-CSF and cumulative doses of vincristine in causing severe atypical neuropathy (SEDA-20, 339).

References

1. Ippoliti C, Przepiorka D, Smith T, Maiese S, Giralt S, Andersson BS, Deisseroth AB, Champlin RE. Adverse effects of molgramostim in marrow transplant recipients. Clin Pharm 1993;12(7):520–5.
2. Beveridge RA, Miller JA, Kales AN, Binder RA, Robert NJ, Harvey JH, Windsor K, Gore I, Cantrell J, Thompson KA, Taylor WR, Barnes HM, Schiff SA, Shields JA, Cambareri RJ, Butler TP, Meister RJ, Feigert JM, Norgard MJ, Moraes MA, Helvie WW, Patton GA, Mundy LJ, Henry D, Sheridan MJ, et al. A comparison of efficacy of sargramostim (yeast-derived RhuGM-CSF) and filgrastim (bacteria-derived RhuG-CSF) in the therapeutic setting of chemotherapy-induced myelosuppression. Cancer Invest 1998;16(6):366–73.
3. Armitage JO. Emerging applications of recombinant human granulocyte–macrophage colony-stimulating factor. Blood 1998;92(12):4491–508.
4. Brito-Babapule F. Therapeutic applications of the myeloid haematopoietic growth factors. Transfus Sci 1991;12:25.
5. Vial T, Descotes J. Clinical toxicity of cytokines used as haemopoietic growth factors. Drug Saf 1995;13(6):371–406.
6. Neumanaitis J. Granulocyte–macrophage-colony-stimulating factor: a review from preclinical development to clinical application. Transfusion 1993;33(1):70–83.
7. Devereux S, Linch DC. Granulocyte–macrophage colony-stimulating factor. Biotherapy 1990;2(4):305–13.
8. Klingemann HG, Shepherd JD, Eaves CJ, Eaves AC. The role of erythropoietin and other growth factors in transfusion medicine. Transfus Med Rev 1991;5(1):33–47.
9. Devereux S, Bull HA, Campos-Costa D, Saib R, Linch DC. Granulocyte macrophage colony stimulating factor induced changes in cellular adhesion molecule expression and adhesion to endothelium: in-vitro and in-vivo studies in man. Br J Haematol 1989;71(3):323–30.
10. Goldstone AH, Khwaja A. The role of haemopoietic growth factors in bone marrow transplantation. Leuk Res 1990;14(8):721–9.
11. Brandt SJ, Peters WP, Atwater SK, Kurtzberg J, Borowitz MJ, Jones RB, Shpall EJ, Bast RC Jr, Gilbert CJ, Oette DH. Effect of recombinant human granulocyte–macrophage colony-stimulating factor on hematopoietic reconstitution after high-dose chemotherapy and autologous bone marrow transplantation. N Engl J Med 1988;318(14):869–76.
12. Herrmann F, Lindemann Mertelsmann R. Polypeptides controlling hemopoietic blood cell development and activation. Blut 1987;58:173.
13. Kojima S, Fukuda M, Miyajima Y, Matsuyama T, Horibe K. Treatment of aplastic anemia in children with recombinant human granulocyte colony-stimulating factor. Blood 1991;77(5):937–41.
14. Potter MN, Mott MG, Oakhill A. Granulocyte–macrophage colony-stimulating factor (GM-CSF), hypocalcemia, and hypomagnesemia. Ann Intern Med 1990;112(9):715.
15. Viens P, Thyss A, Garnier G, Ayela P, Lagrange M, Schneider M. GM-CSF treatment and hypokalemia. Ann Intern Med 1989;111(3):263.
16. Gluck S, Gagnon A. Neutropenic fever in patients after high-dose chemotherapy followed by autologous haematopoietic progenitor cell transplantation and human recombinant granulocyte–macrophage colony stimulating factor. Bone Marrow Transplant 1994;14(6):989–90.
17. Khwaja A, Choppa R, Goldstone AH, Linch DC. Acute-phase response in patients given rhIL-3 after chemotherapy. Lancet 1992;339(8809):1617.
18. Stephens LC, Haire WD, Schmit-Pokorny K, Kessinger A, Kotulak G. Granulocyte macrophage colony stimulating factor: high incidence of apheresis catheter thrombosis during peripheral stem cell collection. Bone Marrow Transplant 1993;11(1):51–4.
19. Tolcher AW, Giusti RM, O'Shaughnessy JA, Cowan KH. Arterial thrombosis associated with granulocyte–macrophage colony-stimulating factor (GM-CSF) administration in breast cancer patients treated with dose-intensive chemotherapy: a report of two cases. Cancer Invest 1995;13(2):188–92.
20. Arning M, Kliche KO, Schneider W. GM-CSF therapy and capillary-leak syndrome. Ann Hematol 1991;62(2–3):83.
21. Emminger W, Emminger-Schmidmeier W, Peters C, Susani M, Hawliczek R, Hocker P, Gadner H. Capillary leak syndrome during low dose granulocyte–macrophage colony-stimulating factor (rh GM-CSF) treatment of a patient in a continuous febrile state. Blut 1990;61(4):219–21.
22. Kaczmarski RS, Mufti GJ. Hypoalbuminaemia after prolonged treatment with recombinant granulocyte macrophage colony stimulating factor. BMJ 1990; 301(6764):1312–3.
23. Couderc LJ, Stelianides S, Frachon I, Stern M, Epardeau B, Baumelou E, Caubarrere I, Hermine O. Pulmonary toxicity of chemotherapy and G/GM-CSF: a report of five cases. Respir Med 1999;93(1):65–8.
24. Miniero R, Madon E, Artesani L, Busca A, Sandri A, Aglietta M, Ramenghi U. Acute pulmonary failure after the first administration of recombinant human granulocyte–macrophage colony-stimulating factor. Leukemia 1992; 6(4):352–3.
25. Dupre D, Schoenlaub P, Coloigner M, Plantin P. Réaction anaphylactique après injection locale de GM-CSF au cours d'un ulcère veineux de jambe. [Anaphylactic reaction after local injection of GM-CSF in venous leg ulcer.] Ann Dermatol Venereol 1999;126(2):161.
26. Riggs JE, Mansmann PT, Cook LL, Schochet SS Jr, Hogg JP. Fulminant CNS perivascular lymphocytic proliferation: association with sargramostim, a hematopoietic growth factor. Clin Neuropharmacol 1999; 22(5):288–91.
27. Hoekman K, von Blomberg-van der Flier BM, Wagstaff J, Drexhage HA, Pinedo HM. Reversible thyroid dysfunction during treatment with GM-CSF. Lancet 1991;338(8766): 541–2.
28. Hansen PB, Johnsen HE, Hippe E. Autoimmune hypothyroidism and granulocyte–macrophage colony-stimulating factor. Eur J Haematol 1993;50(3):183–4.
29. Schriber JR, Negrin RS. Use and toxicity of the colony-stimulating factors. Drug Saf 1993;8(6):457–68.
30. Lieschke GJ, Maher D, Cebon J, O'Connor M, Green M, Sheridan W, Boyd A, Rallings M, Bonnem E, Metcalf D, et al. Effects of bacterially synthesized recombinant human granulocyte–macrophage colony-stimulating factor in patients with advanced malignancy. Ann Intern Med 1989;110(5):357–64.
31. Nathan FE, Besa EC. GM-CSF and accelerated hemolysis. N Engl J Med 1992;326(6):417.
32. Sarris AH, Majlis A, Dimopoulos MA, Younes A, Swann F, Rodriguez MA, McLaughlin P, Cabanillas F. Rising serum lactate dehydrogenase often caused by granulocyte- or granulocyte–macrophage colony stimulating factor and not tumor progression in patients with lymphoma or myeloma. Leuk Lymphoma 1995;17(5–6):473–7.

33. Gonzales-Chambers R, Rosenfeld C, Winkelstein A, Dameshek L. Eosinophilia resulting from administration of recombinant granulocyte–macrophage colony-stimulating factor (rhGM-CSF) in a patient with T-gamma lymphoproliferative disease. Am J Hematol 1991; 36(2):157–9.
34. Donhuijsen K, Haedicke C, Hattenberger S, Hauswaldt C, Freund M. Granulocyte–macrophage colony-stimulating factor-related eosinophilia and Loeffler's endocarditis. Blood 1992;79(10):2798.
35. Bonig H, Burdach S, Gobel U, Nurnberger W. Growth factors and hemostasis: differential effects of GM-CSF and G-CSF on coagulation activation—laboratory and clinical evidence. Ann Hematol 2001;80(9):525–30.
36. Lindemann A, Herrmann F, Mertelsmann R, Gamm H, Rumpelt HJ. Splenic hematopoiesis following GM-CSF therapy in a patient with hairy cell leukemia. Leukemia 1990;4(8):606–7.
37. Lang E, Cibull ML, Gallicchio VS, Henslee-Downey PJ, Davey DD, Messino MJ, Harder EJ. Proliferation of abnormal bone marrow histiocytes, an undesired effect of granulocyte macrophage-colony-stimulating factor therapy in a patient with Hurler's syndrome undergoing bone marrow transplantation. Am J Hematol 1992;41(4): 280–4.
38. Wilson PA, Ayscue LH, Jones GR, Bentley SA. Bone marrow histiocytic proliferation in association with colony-stimulating factor therapy. Am J Clin Pathol 1993; 99(3):311–3.
39. Al-Homaidhi A, Prince HM, Al-Zahrani H, Doucette D, Keating A. Granulocyte–macrophage colony-stimulating factor-associated histiocytosis and capillary-leak syndrome following autologous bone marrow transplantation: two case reports and a review of the literature. Bone Marrow Transplant 1998;21(2):209–14.
40. Wakefield PE, James WD, Samlaska CP, Meltzer MS. Colony-stimulating factors. J Am Acad Dermatol 1990; 23(5 Pt 1):903–12.
41. Mehregan DR, Fransway AF, Edmonson JH, Leiferman KM. Cutaneous reactions to granulocyte-monocyte colony-stimulating factor. Arch Dermatol 1992;128(8):1055–9.
42. Yamada H, Tubaki K, Ashida T, et al. Does recombinant granulocyte–macrophage colony-stimulating factor (GM-CSF) play a crucial role in the pathogenesis of atopic dermatitis after bone marrow transplantation (BMT). Med Science Res 1991;19:395.
43. Ward JC, Gitlin JB, Garry DJ, Jatoi A, Luikart SD, Zelickson BD, Dahl MV, Skubitz KM. Epidermolysis bullosa acquisita induced by GM-CSF: a role for eosinophils in treatment-related toxicity. Br J Haematol 1992;81(1): 27–32.
44. Perrot JL, Benoit F, Segault D, Jaubert J, Guyotat D, Claudy A. Pyoderma gangrenosum aggravé par administration de GM-CSF. [Pyoderma gangrenosum aggravated by GM-CSF administration.] Ann Dermatol Venereol 1992;119(11):846–8.
45. Kelly R, Marsden RA, Bevan D. Exacerbation of psoriasis with GM-CSF therapy. Br J Dermatol 1993; 128(4):468–9.
46. Hazenberg BP, Van Leeuwen MA, Van Rijswijk MH, Stern AC, Vellenga E. Correction of granulocytopenia in Felty's syndrome by granulocyte–macrophage colony-stimulating factor. Simultaneous induction of interleukin-6 release and flare-up of the arthritis. Blood 1989;74(8):2769–70.
47. de Vries EG, Willemse PH, Biesma B, Stern AC, Limburg PC, Vellenga E. Flare-up of rheumatoid arthritis during GM-CSF treatment after chemotherapy. Lancet 1991;338(8765):517–18.
48. Bokemeyer C, Schmoll HJ, Harstrick A. Side-effects of GM-CSF treatment in advanced testicular cancer. Eur J Cancer 1993;29A(6):924.
49. Shahar E, Krivoy N, Pollack S. Effective acute desensitization for immediate-type hypersensitivity to human granulocyte-monocyte colony stimulating factor. Ann Allergy Asthma Immunol 1999;83(6 Pt 1):543–6.
50. Gribben JG, Devereux S, Thomas NS, Keim M, Jones HM, Goldstone AH, Linch DC. Development of antibodies to unprotected glycosylation sites on recombinant human GM-CSF. Lancet 1990;335(8687):434–7.
51. Ragnhammar P, Friesen HJ, Frodin JE, Lefvert AK, Hassan M, Osterborg A, Mellstedt H. Induction of anti-recombinant human granulocyte–macrophage colony-stimulating factor (*Escherichia coli*-derived) antibodies and clinical effects in nonimmunocompromised patients. Blood 1994;84(12):4078–87.
52. Scadden DT, Agosti J. No antibodies to granulocyte macrophage colony-stimulating factor with prolonged use in AIDS. AIDS 1993;7(3):438.
53. Negrin RS, Haeuber DH, Nagler A, Olds LC, Donlon T, Souza LM, Greenberg PL. Treatment of myelodysplastic syndromes with recombinant human granulocyte colony-stimulating factor. A phase I-II trial. Ann Intern Med 1989;110(12):976–84.
54. Vose JM, Armitage JO. Clinical applications of hematopoietic growth factors. J Clin Oncol 1995; 13(4):1023–35.
55. Rowe JM, Liesveld JL. Hematopoietic growth factors in acute leukemia. Leukemia 1997;11(3):328–41.
56. Terpstra W, Lowenberg B. Application of myeloid growth factors in the treatment of acute myeloid leukemia. Leukemia 1997;11(3):315–27.
57. Yoshida Y, Nakahata T, Shibata A, Takahashi M, Moriyama Y, Kaku K, Masaoka T, Kaneko T, Miwa S. Effects of long-term treatment with recombinant human granulocyte–macrophage colony-stimulating factor in patients with myelodysplastic syndrome. Leuk Lymphoma 1995;18(5–6):457–63.
58. Estey EH. Use of colony-stimulating factors in the treatment of acute myeloid leukemia. Blood 1994;83(8): 2015–19.
59. Zimmer BM, Berdel WE, Ludwig WD, Notter M, Reufi B, Thiel E. Fatal spleen rupture during induction chemotherapy with rh GM-CSF priming for acute monocytic leukemia. Clinical case report and in vitro studies. Leuk Res 1993;17(3):277–83.
60. Cairo MS, Agosti J, Ellis R, Laver JJ, Puppala B, deLemos R, Givner L, Nesin M, Wheeler JG, Seth T, van de Ven C, Fanaroff A. A randomized, double-blind, placebo-controlled trial of prophylactic recombinant human granulocyte–macrophage colony-stimulating factor to reduce nosocomial infections in very low birth weight neonates. J Pediatr 1999;134(1):64–70.
61. Lazarus HM, Rowe JM. Clinical use of hematopoietic growth factors in allogeneic bone marrow transplantation. Blood Rev 1994;8(3):169–78.
62. Barbaro G, Di Lorenzo G, Grisorio B, Soldini M, Barbarini G. Effect of recombinant human granulocyte–macrophage colony-stimulating factor on HIV-related leukopenia: a randomized, controlled clinical study. AIDS 1997;11(12):1453–61.
63. Ross SD, DiGeorge A, Connelly JE, Whiting GW, McDonnell N. Safety of GM-CSF in patients with AIDS: a review of the literature. Pharmacotherapy 1998;18(6):1290–7.

Grepafloxacin

See also Fluoroquinolones

General Information

Grepafloxacin is a synthetic fluoroquinolone antibiotic with extensive tissue distribution and strong antibacterial activity in vivo (1,2). However, it was withdrawn in 1999 because of its adverse cardiovascular effects, which included dysrhythmias (3–5).

Observational studies

In phase II and III trials of grepafloxacin in a total of more than 3000 patients, the most common adverse events with grepafloxacin 400 or 600 mg were gastrointestinal, such as nausea, vomiting, and diarrhea. Significantly more patients reported a mild unpleasant metallic taste with grepafloxacin than with ciprofloxacin, but under 1% of patients withdrew because of this. Headache occurred significantly more often with ciprofloxacin than grepafloxacin. In a study of more than 9000 patients, only 2.3% reported adverse events (nausea 0.8%; gastrointestinal symptoms 0.4%; dizziness 0.3%; photosensitization 0.04%). Rarely, an unpleasant taste has been reported as an adverse event in spontaneous reports (6).

Organs and Systems

Nervous system

Headache was recorded in patients taking grepafloxacin, at rates similar to those reported with ciprofloxacin and ofloxacin (8–9%), during short-course treatment of urinary tract infections (7).

Gastrointestinal

With grepafloxacin 600 mg/day the rates of the following adverse events were noticeably higher than with 400 mg/day: nausea (15 versus 11%), vomiting (6 versus 1%), and diarrhea (4 versus 3%) (8).

References

1. Suzuki T, Kato Y, Sasabe H, Itose M, Miyamoto G, Sugiyama Y. Mechanism for the tissue distribution of grepafloxacin, a fluoroquinolone antibiotic, in rats. Drug Metab Dispos 2002;30(12):1393–9.
2. Yamamoto H, Koizumi T, Hirota M, Kaneki T, Ogasawara H, Yamazaki Y, Fujimoto K, Kubo K. Lung tissue distribution after intravenous administration of grepafloxacin: comparative study with levofloxacin. Jpn J Pharmacol 2002;88(1):63–8.
3. Gibaldi M. Grepafloxacin withdrawn from market. Drug Ther Topics Suppl 2000;29:6.
4. Carbon C. Comparison of side effects of levofloxacin versus other fluoroquinolones. Chemotherapy 2001;47(Suppl 3):9–14; discussion 44–8.
5. Zhanel GG, Ennis K, Vercaigne L, Walkty A, Gin AS, Embil J, Smith H, Hoban DJ. A critical review of the fluoroquinolones: focus on respiratory infections. Drugs 2002;62(1):13–59.
6. Goldblatt EL, Dohar J, Nozza RJ, Nielsen RW, Goldberg T, Sidman JD, Seidlin M. Topical ofloxacin versus systemic amoxicillin/clavulanate in purulent otorrhea in children with tympanostomy tubes. Int J Pediatr Otorhinolaryngol 1998;46(1–2):91–101.
7. Chodosh S, Lakshminarayan S, Swarz H, Breisch S. Efficacy and safety of a 10-day course of 400 or 600 milligrams of grepafloxacin once daily for treatment of acute bacterial exacerbations of chronic bronchitis: comparison with a 10-day course of 500 milligrams of ciprofloxacin twice daily. Antimicrob Agents Chemother 1998;42(1):114–20.
8. Stahlmann R, Schwabe R. Safety profile of grepafloxacin compared with other fluoroquinolones. J Antimicrob Chemother 1997;40(Suppl A):83–92.

Griseofulvin

General Information

Griseofulvin was originally isolated in 1939 as a natural product of *Penicillium griseofulvum* (1). It interferes with fungal microtubule formation, disrupting the cell's mitotic spindle formation and arresting the metaphase of cell division. Griseofulvin is a fungistatic compound and is active against *Trichophyton*, *Microsporon*, and *Epidermophyton* species (2). With the development of newer safer azoles and the introduction of terbinafine, all of which are easy to administer, the indications for griseofulvin have dwindled (3).

Pharmacokinetics

Griseofulvin is commercially available for oral administration as griseofulvin microsize (4 μm particle size) and griseofulvin ultramicrosize (1 μm particle size). The oral availability of the micronized formulation is variable, 25–70%; ultramicronized griseofulvin, in contrast, is almost completely absorbed (4–6). Peak plasma concentrations occur about 4 hours after dosing. Griseofulvin distributes to keratin precursor cells and is concentrated in skin, hair, nails, liver, adipose tissue, and skeletal muscle. In skin, a concentration gradient is established over time, with the highest concentrations in the outermost stratum corneum (7,8). However, within 48–72 hours after withdrawal, plasma concentrations of griseofulvin are markedly reduced and it is no longer detectable in the stratum corneum (4–6). The half-life of griseofulvin is 9–21 hours (9). It is oxidatively demethylated and conjugated with glucuronic acid, primarily in the liver; its major metabolite, 6-desmethylgriseofulvin, is microbiologically inactive (10). Within 5 days, about one-third of a single dose of micronized griseofulvin is excreted in the feces, and 50% in the urine, predominantly as glucuronidated 6-desmethylgriseofulvin (10,11). The slow penetration rate of griseofulvin into tissues may explain difficulties and delays in eradication of infection in nails (SED-12, 676) (12).

General adverse effects

The more common adverse effects of griseofulvin include headache and a variety of gastrointestinal symptoms. Griseofulvin can cause photosensitivity and exacerbate lupus and porphyria. Cases of erythema multiforme-like reactions, toxic epidermal necrolysis, and a reaction resembling serum sickness have been reported. Proteinuria, nephrosis, hepatotoxicity, leukopenia, menstrual irregularities, estrogen-like effects, and reversible impairment of hearing have been reported rarely (4–6,13). Griseofulvin is teratogenic in animals and has mutagenic and carcinogenic potential, but the significance of these observations for humans is unclear (13).

Organs and Systems

Nervous system

Headache is the most common adverse effect of griseofulvin (14). It occurs in about 50% of patients and can be severe. Drowsiness, dizziness, fatigue, confusion, depression, irritability, and insomnia have also been observed (14). Impaired co-ordination and unsteadiness while walking have been reported in some cases when there was confusion (15). Peripheral neuritis has been attributed to griseofulvin, but with little proof of a causal relation (16).

Sensory systems

Eyes
Blurring of vision has been reported with griseofulvin (17).

Taste
Griseofulvin can cause dysgeusia; both taste and smell disturbances may occur more frequently than has been realized (SED-12, 676)(18).

Psychological, psychiatric

The psychiatric effects of griseofulvin can be very disturbing and are aggravated by alcohol (SED-12, 676) (14).

Endocrine

An estrogen-type effect has been reported in children, affecting the genitals and the breasts (SED-11, 567)(19).

Griseofulvin interferes with porphyrin metabolism. In man, transient increases in erythrocyte protoporphyrin concentrations have been demonstrated, and the production and excretion of porphyrins is increased. Acute intermittent porphyria is an absolute contraindication to griseofulvin. In patients with other forms of porphyria it should also be avoided, in view of the many alternatives (20–25).

Hematologic

There is no evidence that griseofulvin can cause serious blood disorders. However, leukopenia, neutropenia, and monocytosis have been reported (14,26).

Gastrointestinal

Anorexia, a feeling of bloating, mild nausea, and mild diarrhea are common (17). Vomiting, abdominal cramps, and more severe diarrhea are rare. Black, furry tongue, glossodynia, angular stomatitis, and taste disturbances have been described (18).

Liver

While there have been anecdotal reports of hepatitis (14) and cholestasis (27), a causal relation has never been shown.

Skin

Dermatological adverse effects are not uncommon with griseofulvin and are of considerable variety. The following have been described: urticaria (28,29), photosensitivity eruptions (30), erythema multiforme (31), morbilliform rashes (32), serum sickness-like reactions (33), fixed drug eruption (29,34,35), Stevens–Johnson syndrome (36), vasculitis (37), toxic epidermal necrolysis (38,39), and lupus erythematosus (40,41).

- A 40-year-old woman had a burning sensation and erythema of the lips, buccal mucosa, palate, and vulva, which recurred within 4 hours of oral rechallenge with griseofulvin 125 mg (42).

The risk of serious skin disorders has been estimated in 61 858 users, aged 20–79 years, of oral antifungal drugs identified in the UK General Practice Research Database (43). They had received at least one prescription for oral fluconazole, griseofulvin, itraconazole, ketoconazole, or terbinafine. The background rate of serious cutaneous adverse reactions (corresponding to non-use of oral antifungal drugs) was 3.9 per 10 000 person-years (95% CI = 2.9, 5.2). Incidence rates for current use were 15 per 10 000 person-years (1.9, 56) for itraconazole, 11.1 (3.0, 29) for terbinafine, 10 (1.3, 38) for fluconazole, and 4.6 (0.1, 26) for griseofulvin. Cutaneous disorders associated with the use of oral antifungal drugs in this study were all mild.

Immunologic

The triggering of a lupus-like syndrome by griseofulvin, by way of an allergic reaction, has been described, but is rare (44).

Second-Generation Effects

Pregnancy

Embryotoxicity and mutagenicity have been shown in animal experiments with high doses of griseofulvin. Although for this reason most handbooks and drug formularies warn against the use of griseofulvin during pregnancy, there are no reports of any adverse effects on the human fetus, despite the fact that griseofulvin has been on the market since the early 1960s and has been used extensively and, no doubt, during many pregnancies (SED-12, 676) (19,45–47).

Susceptibility Factors

Patients with porphyria are at risk; acute intermittent porphyria is an absolute contraindication to griseofulvin.

Exposure to intense natural or artificial sunlight should be avoided during treatment with griseofulvin.

Patients with pre-existing systemic lupus erythematosus may be more susceptible to the development of skin manifestations from griseofulvin (48).

Drug–Drug Interactions

Alcohol

The effects of alcohol are potentiated by griseofulvin, and the use of alcohol increases the risk and severity of psychiatric disturbances.

Ciclosporin

Ciclosporin blood concentrations halved in a patient who took griseofulvin 500 mg/day, despite an increase in ciclosporin dose by 70% (49). When griseofulvin was withdrawn, the ciclosporin concentration rose. This interaction is attributable to induction of cytochrome P450 by griseofulvin.

Coumarin anticoagulants

Griseofulvin is a potent inducer of cytochrome P450 and has a significant effect on P450 expression in hepatocytes (SEDA-12, 236). It therefore increases the rate of metabolism of coumarin anticoagulants (50). However, both increases and decreases in prothrombin time have been reported (SED-12, 676) (18).

Oral contraceptives

The combination of griseofulvin with oral contraceptives can lead to oligomenorrhea, amenorrhea, and breakthrough bleeding; unintended pregnancies have been reported (51). In a case of oligomenorrhea after treatment with griseofulvin, the use of a higher estrogen oral contraceptive restored regularity of the menstrual cycle (SEDA-12, 237) (51). The fact that griseofulvin has an estrogen-like effect in children suggests that it may affect the rate of estrogen metabolism (SED-12, 676) (52).

Phenobarbital

The concomitant use of phenobarbital reduces griseofulvin concentrations, an effect that has been attributed to induction of liver enzymes by phenobarbital (53).

References

1. Oxford AE, Raistrick H, Simonart P. Studies in the biochemistry of microorganisms: Griseofulvin, C17H17O6Cl, a metabolic product of Penicillium griseofulvum. Biochem J 1939;33:240–8.
2. Gull K, Trinci AP. Griseofulvin inhibits fungal mitosis. Nature 1973;244(5414):292–4.
3. Graybill JR, Sharkey PK. Fungal infections and their management. Br J Clin Pract Suppl 1990;71:23–31.

4. Blumer JL. Pharmacologic basis for the treatment of tinea capitis. Pediatr Infect Dis J 1999;18(2):191–9.
5. Gupta AK, Sauder DN, Shear NH. Antifungal agents: an overview. Part I. J Am Acad Dermatol 1994;30(5 Pt 1):677–98.
6. Gupta AK, Sauder DN, Shear NH. Antifungal agents: an overview. Part II. J Am Acad Dermatol 1994;30(6):911–33.
7. Epstein WL, Shah VP, Riegelman S. Griseofulvin levels in stratum corneum. Study after oral administration in man. Arch Dermatol 1972;106(3):344–8.
8. Shah VP, Riegelman S, Epstein WL. Determination of griseofulvin in skin, plasma, and sweat. J Pharm Sci 1972;61(4):634–6.
9. Rowland M, Riegelman S, Epstein WL. Absorption kinetics of griseofulvin in man. J Pharm Sci 1968;57(6):984–9.
10. Lin CC, Magat J, Chang R, McGlotten J, Symchowicz S. Absorption, metabolism and excretion of 14C-griseofulvin in man. J Pharmacol Exp Ther 1973;187(2):415–22.
11. Lin C, Symchowicz S. Absorption, distribution, metabolism, and excretion of griseofulvin in man and animals. Drug Metab Rev 1975;4(1):75–95.
12. Shah VP, Riegelman S, Epstein WL. Griseofulvin absorption, metabolism and excretion. In: Robinson HM, editor. The Diagnosis and Treatment of Fungal Infections. Sprnigfield IL: Thomas, 1974:315.
13. Friedlander SF, Suarez S. Pediatric antifungal therapy. Dermatol Clin 1998;16(3):527–37.
14. Gotz H, Reichenberger M. Ergebnisse einer Fragebogenaktion bei 1670 Dermatologen der Bundesrepublik Deutschland uber Nebenwirkungen bei der Griseofulvin Therapie. [Results of questionnaires of 1670 dermatologists in West Germany concerning the side effects of griseofulvin therapy.] Hautarzt 1972; 23(11):485–92.
15. Hillstrom L, Kjellin A. Centralnervosa symtom som biverkning vid myjosbehandling med griseofulvin. [Central nervous symptoms as side effects of mycosis treatment with griseofulvin.] Lakartidningen 1974; 71(44):4310.
16. Livingood CS, Stewart RH, Webster SB. Cutaneous vasculitis caused by griseofulvin. Cutis (NY) 1970;6:1346.
17. Swartz JH. Infections caused by dermatophytes. N Engl J Med 1962;267:1359–61.
18. Cohen J. Antifungal chemotherapy. Lancet 1982; 2(8297):532–7.
19. Walter AM, Heilmeyer L. Antibiotika Fibel. In: Otten H, Siegenthaler W, editors. Antimykotica. Stuttgart: Georg Thieme Verlag, 1975:676.
20. Ziprkowski L, Szeinberg A, Crispin M, Krakowski A, Zaidman J. The effect of griseofulvin in hereditary porphyria cutanea tarda. Investigation of porphyrins and blood lipids. Arch Dermatol 1966;93(1):21–7.
21. Bickers DR. Environmental and drug factors in hepatic porphyria. Acta Dermatol Venereol Suppl (Stockh) 1982;100:29–41.
22. Shimoyama T, Nonaka S. Biochemical studies on griseofulvin-induced protoporphyria. Ann NY Acad Sci 1987; 514:160–9.
23. Knasmuller S, Parzefall W, Helma C, Kassie F, Ecker S, Schulte-Hermann R. Toxic effects of griseofulvin: disease models, mechanisms, and risk assessment. Crit Rev Toxicol 1997;27(5):495–537. Erratum in: Crit Rev Toxicol. 1998;28(1):102.
24. Felsher BF, Redeker AG. Acute intermittent porphyria: effect of diet and griseofulvin. Medicine (Baltimore) 1967;46(2):217–23.
25. Smith AG, De Matteis F. Drugs and the hepatic porphyrias. Clin Haematol 1980;9(2):399–425.
26. Weinstein L. In: Goodman L, Gilman A, editors. The Pharmacological Basis of Therapeutics, Antifungal

Agents. 4th ed. London: The MacMmillan Press Ld, 1970,1299–305.
27. Chiprut RO, Viteri A, Jamroz C, Dyck WP. Intrahepatic cholestasis after griseofulvin administration. Gastroenterology 1976;70(6):1141–3.
28. Ahrens J, Graybill JR, Craven PC, Taylor RL. Treatment of experimental murine candidiasis with liposome-associated amphotericin B. Sabouraudia 1984;22(2):163–6.
29. Feinstein A, Sofer E, Trau H, Schewach-Millet M. Urticaria and fixed drug eruption in a patient treated with griseofulvin. J Am Acad Dermatol 1984;10(5 Pt 2):915–17.
30. Kojima T, Hasegawa T, Ishida H, Fujita M, Okamoto S. Griseofulvin-induced photodermatitis—report of six cases. J Dermatol 1988;15(1):76–82.
31. Rustin MH, Bunker CB, Dowd PM, Robinson TW. Erythema multiforme due to griseofulvin. Br J Dermatol 1989;120(3):455–8.
32. Gaudin JL, Bancel B, Vial T, Bel A. Hepatite aiguë cytolytique et eruption morbiliforme imputables a la prise de griseofulvine. [Acute cytolytic hepatitis and morbilliform eruption caused by ingestion of griseofulvin.] Gastroenterol Clin Biol 1993;17(2):145–6.
33. Colton RL, Amir J, Mimouni M, Zeharia A. Serum sickness-like reaction associated with griseofulvin. Ann Pharmacother 2004;38(4):609–11.
34. Savage J. Fixed drug eruption to griseofulvin. Br J Dermatol 1977;97(1):107–8.
35. Thyagarajan K, Kamalam A, Thambiah AS. Fixed drug eruption to griseofulvin. Mykosen 1981;24(8):482–4.
36. Walinga H, van Beugen L. Syndroom van Stevens–Johnson na gebruik van griseofulvine. [Stevens–Johnson syndrome following administration of griseofulvin.] Ned Tijdschr Geneeskd 1981;125(19):759–60.
37. Amita DB, Danon YL, Garty BZ. Kawasaki-like syndrome associated with griseofulvin treatment. Clin Exp Dermatol 1993;18(4):389.
38. Taylor B, Duffill M. Toxic epidermal necrolysis from griseofulvin. J Am Acad Dermatol 1988;19(3):565–7.
39. Mion G, Verdon R, Le Gulluche Y, Carsin H, Garcia A, Guilbaud J. Fatal toxic epidermal necrolysis after griseofulvin. Lancet 1989;2(8675):1331.
40. Miyagawa S, Okuchi T, Shiomi Y, Sakamoto K. Subacute cutaneous lupus erythematosus lesions precipitated by griseofulvin. J Am Acad Dermatol 1989;21(2 Pt 2):343–6. Erratum in: J Am Acad Dermatol 1990;22(2 Pt 2):345.
41. Anderson WA, Torre D. Griseofulvin and lupus erythematosus. J Med Soc N J 1966;63(5):161–2.
42. Thami GP, Kaur S, Kanwar AJ. Erythema multiforme due to griseofulvin with positive re-exposure test. Dermatology 2001;203(1):84–5.
43. Castellsague J, Garcia-Rodriguez LA, Duque A, Perez S. Risk of serious skin disorders among users of oral antifungals: a population-based study. BMC Dermatol 2002;2(1):14.
44. Watsky MS, Lynfield YL. Lupus erythematosus exacerbated by griseofulvin. Cutis 1976;17(2):361–3.
45. Pohler H, Michalski H. Allergisches Exanthem nach Griseofulvin. [Allergic exanthema caused by griseofulvin.] Dermatol Monatsschr 1972;158(5):383–90.
46. Inoue H, Baba H, Awano K, Yoshikawa K. Genotoxic effect of griseofulvin in somatic cells of *Drosophila melanogaster*. Mutat Res 1995;343(4):229–34.
47. Marchetti F, Tiveron C, Bassani B, Pacchierotti F. Griseofulvin-induced aneuploidy and meiotic delay in female mouse germ cells. II. Cytogenetic analysis of one-cell zygotes. Mutat Res 1992;266(2):151–62.
48. Miyagawa S, Sakamoto K. Adverse reactions to griseofulvin in patients with circulating anti-SSA/Ro and SSB/La autoantibodies. Am J Med 1989;87(1):100–2.
49. Abu-Romeh SH, Rashed A. Cyclosporin A and griseofulvin: another drug interaction. Nephron 1991;58(2):237.
50. Okino K, Weibert RT. Warfarin–gniseofulrin interaction. Drug Intell Clin Pharm 1986;20(4):291–3.
51. McDaniel PA, Caldroney RD. Griseofulvin-oral contraceptive. Drug Intell Clin Pharm 1986;20:291.
52. Bickers DR. Antifungal therapy: potential interactions with other classes of drugs. J Am Acad Dermatol 1994;31(3 Pt 2):S87–90.
53. Riegelman S, Rowland M, Epstein WL. Griseofulvin-phenobarbital interaction in man JAMA 1970;213(3):426–31.

Guanethidine

General Information

Guanethidine, an adrenergic neuron blocking drug, which was once used to treat hypertension, is obsolete for oral use and this indication. However, it has been used as eye-drops in cases of glaucoma, chemical sympathectomy, ptosis, and eyelid retraction (SEDA-1, 366). The reduction in intraocular pressure is small. In general, tissues treated topically with guanethidine become sensitized to sympathomimetic acting drugs. This is useful in glaucoma, for which adrenaline can be administered in low dosage in combination with guanethidine. After instillation of guanethidine-containing eye-drops, conjunctival hyperemia, ocular pain, and stinging have been described (1,2).

References

1. Heilmann K. [Behavior of intraocular pressure during long-term treatment with a guanethidine-adrenaline combination.] Klin Monatsbl Augenheilkd 1983;183(1):17–21.
2. Havener WH. Ocular Pharmacology. 4th ed. Saint Louis: C.V. Mosby,, 1978.

Guar gum

General Information

Guar gum is a low-viscosity water-soluble dietary fiber that has been used to treat diabetes because it slows the absorption of glucose from the gut. However, adverse effects such as regurgitation, obstipation, abdominal cramps, diarrhea, and itching are common (1). Partially hydrolysed guar gum has been added to enteral formulas and food products as a source of dietary fiber; it can reduce laxative use, diarrhea in septic patients receiving total enteral nutrition, and symptoms of irritable bowel syndrome (2).

In a systematic review of 11 trials of the use of guar gum to treat obesity, the most common adverse events were abdominal pain, flatulence, diarrhea, and cramps; 11 patients (3%) dropped out owing to adverse events (3).

Organs and Systems

Gastrointestinal

Of 26 reports of suspected adverse reactions to a diet formulation containing guar gum (Cal-Ban 3000), there were 18 cases of esophageal obstruction and seven of small bowel obstruction (4). There were pre-existing esophageal or gastric disorders in 50% of those with esophageal obstruction, including peptic stricture, pyrosis, hiatus hernia, esophagitis, gastric stapling, Schatzki ring, and muscular dystrophy. Fourteen patients with esophageal obstruction were treated successfully by endoscopy, although the tenacious gel-like material was often difficult to remove. One patient who developed a pulmonary embolism after surgical repair of an intraoperative esophageal tear died.

Immunologic

Guar gum can cause occupational rhinitis (5) and asthma (6). Of 162 employees at a carpet-manufacturing plant where guar gum was used to adhere dye to the fiber, 37 (23%) had a history suggestive of occupational asthma and 59 (36%) occupational rhinitis (7). Eight (5%) had immediate skin reactivity to guar gum and 11 (8.3%) had serum IgE antibodies to guar gum.

An employee of a pet food plant developed a severe cough, rhinitis, and conjunctivitis, and skin tests confirmed guar allergy. The symptoms resulted in obstructive sleep apnea which resolved after absence from work and recurred after rechallenge with guar gum dust (8).

References

1. Chuang LM, Jou TS, Yang WS, Wu HP, Huang SH, Tai TY, Lin BJ. Therapeutic effect of guar gum in patients with non-insulin-dependent diabetes mellitus. J Formos Med Assoc 1992;91(1):15–19.
2. Slavin JL, Greenberg NA. Partially hydrolyzed guar gum: clinical nutrition uses. Nutrition 2003;19(6):549–52.
3. Pittler MH, Ernst E. Guar gum for body weight reduction: meta-analysis of randomized trials. Am J Med 2001; 110(9):724–30.
4. Lewis JH. Esophageal and small bowel obstruction from guar gum-containing "diet pills": analysis of 26 cases reported to the Food and Drug Administration. Am J Gastroenterol 1992;87(10):1424–8.
5. Kanerva L, Tupasela O, Jolanki R, Vaheri E, Estlander T, Keskinen H. Occupational allergic rhinitis from guar gum. Clin Allergy 1988;18(3):245–52.
6. Lagier F, Cartier A, Somer J, Dolovich J, Malo JL. Occupational asthma caused by guar gum. J Allergy Clin Immunol 1990;85(4):785–90.
7. Malo JL, Cartier A, L'Archeveque J, Ghezzo H, Soucy F, Somers J, Dolovich J. Prevalence of occupational asthma and immunologic sensitization to guar gum among employees at a carpet-manufacturing plant. J Allergy Clin Immunol 1990;86(4 Pt 1):562–9.
8. Leznoff A, Haight JS, Hoffstein V. Reversible obstructive sleep apnea caused by occupational exposure to guar gum dust. Am Rev Respir Dis 1986;133(5):935–6.

Gum resins

General Information

Gum resins comprise a diverse variety of substances, including asafoetida (*Ferula*), colophony, frankincense (*Boswellia*), and myrrh (*Commiphora*).

Colophony

Colophony, a natural unmodified gum resin from *Pinus* species (terebinth), used in cosmetics such as mascara, lipsticks, creams, and hair removal products, is a known contact allergen. Modifications have been made to colophonium, resulting in a variety of ester gums.

Frankincense

Preparations from the gum resin of *Boswellia serrata* have been used as traditional remedies in Ayurvedic medicine in India for inflammatory diseases (1). The gum contains substances that have anti-inflammatory properties; they are pentacyclic triterpenes related to boswellic acid, which inhibit leukotriene biosynthesis in neutrophilic granulocytes by inhibiting 5-lipoxygenase. Certain boswellic acids also inhibit elastase in leukocytes, inhibit proliferation, induce apoptosis, and inhibit topoisomerases in cancer cell lines.

Use in asthma

In a double-blind, placebo-controlled study in 40 patients aged 18–75 years with bronchial asthma who were given *Boswellia serrata* 300 mg tds for 6 weeks, 28 had improved dyspnea, a reduced number of attacks, increases in FEV_1, FVC, and peak flow, and reduced eosinophil counts and ESR (2). Of 40 patients, aged 14–58 years, given lactose 300 mg tds for 6 weeks, only 11 improved.

Use in colitis

In patients with ulcerative colitis, *Boswellia serrata* 350 mg tds for 6 weeks produced improvements in stool properties, histopathology of rectal biopsies, hemoglobin, serum iron, calcium, phosphorus, proteins, and total leukocyte and eosinophil counts, with remission in 82% of patients (3). The corresponding figure with sulfasalazine 1 g tds was 75%.

In 30 patients aged 18–48 years with chronic colitis, characterized by vague lower abdominal pain, rectal bleeding, diarrhea, and palpable tender descending and sigmoid colons, *Boswellia serrata* (900 mg/day for 6 weeks) produced remission in 14 of 20 patients, and sulfasalazine (3 g/day for 6 weeks) in 4 of 10 patients (4). There were few adverse effects.

Myrrh

Myrrh is an oleo gum resin obtained from the stem of *Commiphora molmol*, a tree that grows in north-east Africa and the Arabian Peninsula. In mice, myrrh showed no mutagenic effects and was a potent cytotoxic drug against solid tumor cells (5). The antitumor potential of *C. molmol* was comparable to that of cyclophosphamide. Studies in hamsters suggested an antischistosomal activity of myrrh (6).

Use in schistosomiasis

The efficacy and adverse effects of myrrh and the most effective dosage schedule have been studied in 204 (169 men and 35 women) patients with schistosomiasis, aged 12–68, years and 20 healthy non-infected age- and sex-matched volunteers (6). The patients were divided into two groups: 86 patients with schistosomal colitis and 118 with hepatosplenic schistosomiasis, the latter being further divided into two subgroups: 77 patients with compensated disease and 41 with decompensated disease. All but 12 had received one or more courses of praziquantel. The dosage of myrrh was 10 mg/kg/day for 3 days on an empty stomach 1 hour before breakfast. A second course of 10 mg/kg/day for 6 days was given to patients who still had living ova in rectal or colonic biopsy specimens. The response rate to a single course of myrrh was 92% in 187 patients. The cure rates were 91%, 94%, and 90% in patients with schistosomal colitis, compensated hepatosplenic schistosomiasis and decompensated hepatosplenic schistosomiasis respectively. The cure rate was less in patients who had previously taken praziquantel and in patients with impaired liver function. *Schistosoma hematobium* infection was the most responsive ($n = 4$, cure rate 100%), followed by mixed infections ($n = 29$, cure rate 93%). Those infected with *Schistosoma mansoni* had the lowest cure rate ($n = 171$, cure rate 91%). There was no impairment of liver function after treatment with myrrh. In contrast, liver function tests significantly improved in patients with impaired liver function. There were no significant effects of myrrh on the electrocardiogram. Adverse effects of myrrh were reported in 24 of the 204 patients. Giddiness, somnolence, and mild fatigue were the most common (2.5%), and all other adverse effects were minor and less frequent. None of the healthy volunteers reported any adverse effects, nor were there any significant changes in liver or kidney function. A second course of myrrh resulted in a cure in 13 of the 17 patients who did not respond to a single course.

Use in fascioliasis

The efficacy of myrrh has been studied in seven patients aged 10–41 years (five men, two women) with fascioliasis and 10 age- and sex-matched healthy volunteers (7). Myrrh was given orally in the morning on an empty stomach in a dosage of 12 mg/kg/day for 6 days. All the patients were passing *Fasciola* eggs in their stools (mean 36 eggs per gram of stool). The symptoms and signs of fascioliasis resolved during treatment with myrrh, and *Fasciola* eggs could not be demonstrated in the stools 3 weeks and 3 months after treatment. Anti-fasciola antibody titers became negative in six of the seven patients. There were no adverse effects.

Organs and Systems

Immunologic

In a retrospective study, 1270 patients with leg ulcers were tested for contact allergy with colophonium and the modified ester gum: 31 patients were positive to colophonium alone, 41 to the ester gum alone, and 33 to both colophonium and the ester gum (8). The authors recommended that the patch test tray for patients with leg ulcers should include both colophonium and the ester gum resin.

Two other patients with cheilitis due to contact allergy to a lipstick reacted positively to glyceryl hydrogenated rosinate, an ester gum, and the main component of the rosinate, glyceryl abietate (both patchtested at 20% in petrolatum) (9).

References

1. Ammon HP. Boswelliasauren (Inhaltsstoffe des Weihrauchs) als wirksame Prinzipien zur Behandlung chronisch entzundlicher Erkrankungen. [Boswellic acids (components of frankincense) as the active principle in treatment of chronic inflammatory diseases.] Wien Med Wochenschr 2002;152(15–16):373–8.
2. Gupta I, Gupta V, Parihar A, Gupta S, Ludtke R, Safayhi H, Ammon HP. Effects of *Boswellia serrata* gum resin in patients with bronchial asthma: results of a double-blind, placebo-controlled, 6-week clinical study. Eur J Med Res 1998;3(11):511–14.
3. Gupta I, Parihar A, Malhotra P, Singh GB, Ludtke R, Safayhi H, Ammon HP. Effects of *Boswellia serrata* gum resin in patients with ulcerative colitis. Eur J Med Res 1997;2(1):37–43.
4. Gupta I, Parihar A, Malhotra P, Gupta S, Ludtke R, Safayhi H, Ammon HP. Effects of gum resin of *Boswellia serrata* in patients with chronic colitis. Planta Med 2001;67(5):391–5.
5. al-Harbi MM, Qureshi S, Ahmed MM, Rafatullah S, Shah AH. Effect of *Commiphora molmol* (oleo-gum-resin) on the cytological and biochemical changes induced by cyclophosphamide in mice. Am J Chin Med 1994;22(1):77–82.
6. Sheir Z, Nasr AA, Massoud A, Salama O, Badra GA, El-Shennawy H, Hassan N, Hammad SM. A safe, effective, herbal antischistosomal therapy derived from myrrh. Am J Trop Med Hyg 2001;65(6):700–4.
7. Massoud A, El Sisi S, Salama O, Massoud A. Preliminary study of therapeutic efficacy of a new fasciolicidal drug derived from *Commiphora molmol* (myrrh). Am J Trop Med Hyg 2001;65(2):96–9.
8. Salim A, Shaw S. Recommendation to include ester gum resin when patch testing patients with leg ulcers. Contact Dermatitis 2001;44(1):34.
9. Bonamonte D, Foti C, Angelini G. Contact allergy to ester gums in cosmetics. Contact Dermatitis 2001;45(2):110–11.

Gusperimus

General Information

Gusperimus is a guanidine derivative with antitumor and immunosuppressive properties. Its mechanism of action is not well understood and may involve blockade of the maturation of B and T lymphocytes and monocytes, with inhibition of both cell-mediated and antibody-mediated immunity. In preliminary clinical trials in transplant patients, adverse effects at low doses included mild-to-moderate leukopenia, facial and perioral numbness, anorexia, gastrointestinal disturbances, facial flushing, and weakness (1–3). Bone marrow suppression has been observed at high doses.

References

1. Philip AT, Gerson B. Toxicology and adverse effects of drugs used for immunosuppression in organ transplantation. Clin Lab Med 1998;18(4):755–65.
2. First MR. An update on new immunosuppressive drugs undergoing preclinical and clinical trials: potential applications in organ transplantation. Am J Kidney Dis 1997;29(2):303–17.
3. Birck R, Warnatz K, Lorenz HM, Choi M, Haubitz M, Grunke M, Peter HH, Kalden JR, Gobel U, Drexler JM, Hotta O, Nowack R, Van Der Woude FJ. 15-Deoxyspergualin in patients with refractory ANCA-associated systemic vasculitis: a six-month open-label trial to evaluate safety and efficacy. J Am Soc Nephrol 2003;14(2):440–7.

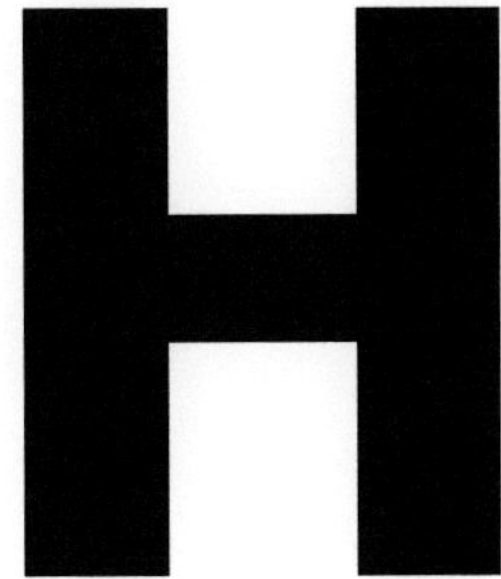

Haemophilus influenzae type b (Hib) vaccine

See also Vaccines

General Information

Haemophilus influenzae causes several infectious diseases in man, the most serious being meningitis. Most cases of *Haemophilus influenzae* infection are due to type b of the organism (Hib). Two types of Hib vaccines have been developed: Hib capsular polysaccharide (PRP) vaccines are first-generation Hib vaccines, while Hib conjugate vaccines are second-generation vaccines. The capsular polysaccharide vaccines do not protect infants and children under 18 months, whereas Hib conjugate vaccines have greater immunogenicity and induce a high rate of protection in children under 18 months. The latter have therefore completely replaced the first-generation polysaccharide vaccines.

Comparisons of adverse reactions to different vaccines are difficult, because vaccines are virtually always administered together with other vaccines. However, the general experience is that adverse reactions to Hib vaccine are mild. Most reactions develop when the vaccine is given simultaneously with DTP vaccine. There have been no deaths or permanent sequelae attributable to Hib immunization.

Four different types of conjugated vaccines are commercially available:

1. PRP-D Hib vaccine (a mutant polypeptide of diphtheria toxin covalently linked to PRP), for example ProHIBit (produced by Connaught Laboratories, Philadelphia).
2. HbOC vaccine (Hib oligosaccharides linked to the non-toxic diphtheria toxin variant CRM197), for example HibTITER (produced by Lederle-Praxis Biologicals, Pearl River, NY).
3. PRP-OMC (PRP conjugated to outer membrane protein of Neisseria meningitidis group B), for example PedvaxHIB (produced by Merck Sharp & Dohme Research Laboratories).
4. PRP-T Hib vaccine (tetanus toxoid linked to PRP), for example ActHIB or OmniHIB (produced by Pasteur Merieux, Lyon, France) and PRP-T (produced by Pasteur Mérieux Connaught and Glaxo SmithKline).

PRP-D-Hib has been almost completely replaced by different conjugated Hib vaccines (1–3). The four types of conjugated Hib vaccines have been reviewed (SED-12, 803) (SEDA-16, 377) (SEDA-17, 367) (SEDA-18, 330). More than 100 million doses of conjugated vaccines have now been administered worldwide, and no reports of deaths, anaphylaxis, or residual neurological damage have been causally connected with them.

In a study of the tolerability and immunogenicity of Hib vaccines, 30 volunteers aged 69–84 years were immunized with either Pedvax-Hib (a conjugate of Hib polysaccharide and an outer membrane protein complex of *Neisseria meningitidis*-PRP-OMP) or Hib TITER (a conjugate of Hib oligosaccharide and a non-toxic mutant diphtheria toxin, CRM 197-HbOC) (4). The volunteers received a pediatric dose. Before immunization, 40% of the volunteers had serum anti-PRP antibody concentrations below 1.0 μg/ml. Four weeks after immunization, all the volunteers had concentrations over 1.0 μg/ml, which is generally considered to be protective. Adverse effects of immunization were mild, except in one volunteer given HbOC, who developed extensive erythema and swelling at the injection site.

Different vaccines and immunization strategies have been evaluated in Denmark, Finland, Iceland, Norway, and Sweden (5). Few places outside Scandinavia have collected data on Hib immunization programs for so long (more than a decade has elapsed since universal Hib immunization was initiated in Scandinavia) and with similar accuracy. Phase 3 studies with PRP-D-Hib vaccine were done in Finland in the late 1980s, and PRP-D-Hib vaccine has been the only vaccine used in Iceland. HbOC vaccine was first compared with PRP-D-Hib vaccine in Finland and then reintroduced to the primary health-care system as the only Hib vaccine used. Finally, PRP-T-Hib vaccine was first temporarily used in Finland, and then as almost the only vaccine in Denmark, Norway, and Sweden. Besides the different conjugate vaccines, the immunization programs have differed in other aspects, such as immunization schedule and administration of vaccines (separate versus simultaneous administration with other vaccines, such as DT, DTP, DTaP, IPV, or MMR).

Experience with PRP-D derives from Finland and Iceland. In Finland, 14.1 adverse reactions per 100 000 doses were reported in all, consisting respectively of 5.3, 6.3, 4.4, and 2.9 per 100 000 doses of local reactions, fever, rash, and irritability. These rates probably underestimate the true rate. In Iceland, adverse effects have not been monitored, but no serious events have been reported. For PRP-CRM, there were 17.8 per 100 000 doses in all, of which 7.7 per 100 000 doses were due to local reactions, 8.9 to fever, and 8.3 to rash. PRP-T currently enjoys the largest use in Scandinavia, being the routine choice in three countries. Of 115 reactions reported in Denmark, none was of serious concern; most were local reactions, fever, or rash. In Norway, the incidence of systemic reactions was 1 in 550 doses; fever and other symptoms and signs similar to those after DTP vaccination were the most common complaints. However, two findings were characteristic of Norway, where local reactions were reported with an overall frequency of 1/1500 doses:

- immediate mild allergic reactions were more common than if DTP or IPV was given alone; their incidence was 1 in 35 000 doses of PRP-T;
- large swellings at the vaccination site, with edema and sometimes bluish or other discoloration of the legs, were reported in 18 children, suggesting an incidence of about 1 in 30 000 doses; this reaction developed within hours after vaccination and subsided within 24 hours; all the vaccinees recovered spontaneously without treatment or sequelae.

About 1.5 million doses of PRP-T have been used in Sweden. Similar concerns about adverse reactions have been raised as in Norway, and further elucidation has recently begun. In Finland (where PRP-T was used in

1990–93), there were 15.9 reports per 100 000 doses; 6.2 per 100 000 doses were local reactions, 5.9 fever, 2.8 rash, and 2.4 irritability (5).

Notwithstanding the different approaches taken in the various Scandinavian countries, the results are similar: before vaccination against invasive Hib diseases, first introduced in Finland in 1986, the incidence of cases in the five Scandinavian countries was 49 per 100 000 per year in 0- to 4-year olds and 3.5 per 100 000 overall. During the next decade, Hib conjugates given to young children had about 95% effectiveness, regardless of which conjugate was used, whether two or three primary doses were used, and at no matter what age in early infancy the first vaccination was given. Invasive diseases due to Hib have thus been nearly eliminated.

On the request of the French Drug Agency, the Regional Pharmacovigilance Center of Tours has analysed the adverse events that occurred in 1986–90 with the use of three different tetravalent DTwP-IPV vaccines produced by French vaccine manufacturers (6). The most frequent adverse events were local reactions (43% of the 631 events reported). Serious adverse events represented 25% of all reported events, including 23 reports of persistent crying, 12 febrile seizures, 14 apyretic seizures, and 3 reports of shock-like events.

Immunological interference, particularly to the Hib response, has been assessed in 135 infants at 2, 4, 6, and 18 months of age in studies of two different types of administration of DTaP and Hib vaccines: combined administration of the two vaccines mixed in the same syringe and simultaneous administration of separate injections at different sites (7). The vaccines were well tolerated and there were no differences in the rates of local and systemic reactions. Immune responses were also comparable between the two groups.

In 57 volunteers, 32 of whom had recently undergone splenectomy, who received Hib conjugate vaccine, antibodies to Hib were measured at 2, 6, 12, 24, and 36 months after immunization (8). All tolerated the vaccine well and reached protective antibody titers. The authors concluded that the vaccine is safe and protective in patients with thalassemia.

Combinations of vaccines

Since immunization against diphtheria, tetanus, and pertussis is recommended at the same age as immunization against *Haemophilus influenzae*, children must usually receive two intramuscular injections at separate sites during the same visit. Combined vaccines, for example DTP/Hib vaccines, requiring one injection, could be preferable and are commercially available. Results of clinical trials comparing the safety and efficacy of combined and simultaneously administrated vaccines (Hib, DTP, MMR, IPV) have been presented (SEDA-17, 369) (SEDA-18, 330). In general, the rates of local and systemic reactions and antibody responses did not differ significantly between the groups. The immunogenicity and safety of a diphtheria–tetanus–pertussis–Hib combination vaccine (tetanus-conjugated Hib vaccine) have been compared with those of the same combination obtained by the reconstitution of lyophilized Hib vaccine with liquid DTP vaccine in 262 healthy infants randomized to receive injections at 2, 4, and 6 months of age, a subgroup of 134 of whom received a booster dose at 12 months (9). Systemic and local reactions were generally mild and did not differ significantly between the two groups. With regard to Hib antibodies, the combination vaccine was at least as immunogenic as the lyophilized formulation.

Four-, five- and six-component combination vaccines based on DTaP or DTwP vaccine, and including other antigens such as hepatitis B or Hib or IPV, will play an important role in future worldwide immunization programs. The first hexavalent combination vaccines (DTaP-IPV-HB-Hib) were licensed in Germany; two hexavalent vaccines are available, manufactured by SmithKline Beecham and Aventis Pasteur.

The Hexavalent Study Group has compared the immunogenicity and safety of a new liquid hexavalent vaccine against diphtheria, tetanus, pertussis, poliomyelitis, hepatitis B, and Hib (DTP + IPV + HB + Hib vaccine, manufactured by Aventis Pasteur MSD, Lyon, France) with two reference vaccines, the pentavalent DTP + IPV + Hib vaccine and the monovalent hepatitis B vaccine, administrated separately at the same visit (10). Infants were randomized to receive either the hexavalent vaccine ($n = 423$) or (administered at different local sites) the pentavalent and the HB vaccine ($n = 425$) at 2, 4, and 6 months of age. The hexavalent vaccine was well tolerated (for details, see the monograph on Pertussis vaccines). At least one local reaction was reported in 20% of injections with hexavalent vaccine compared with 16% after the receipt of pentavalent vaccine or 3.8% after the receipt of hepatitis B vaccine. These reactions were generally mild and transient. At least one systemic reaction was reported in 46% of injections with hexavalent vaccine, whereas the respective rate for the recipients of pentavalent and HB vaccine was 42%. No vaccine-related serious adverse event occurred during the study. The hexavalent vaccine provided immune responses adequate for protection against the six diseases.

Regimens using different conjugated vaccines for primary series

Currently most advisory bodies for immunization practice recommend that the same Hib conjugate vaccine used to initiate a priming series should be continued for the entire series. However, interest in using different vaccines for sequential doses (mixed regimens) has been long-standing. Two- or three-dose mixed regimens of Hib conjugate vaccines have been compared in two randomized trials in 140 and 181 infants (11). In both trials, a group of infants received PRP-meningococcal protein conjugate vaccine (OMP, outer membrane protein) at 2 months of age, followed by either the same or another conjugate vaccine, oligosaccharide CRM197 Hib vaccine (HbOC, Hib oligosaccharides linked to the non-toxic diphtheria toxin variant CRM197) or PRP-tetanus toxoid Hib vaccine, either once (at 4 months of age) or twice (at 4 and 6 months of age). All the mixed regimens provided a mean anti-PRP antibody concentration that did not differ substantially compared with currently recommended regimens of proven or inferred efficacy. Recipients of a second dose of OMP vaccine had higher rates of swelling, erythema, and induration compared with the other recipients.

Organs and Systems

Nervous system

The neurological complications of conjugated Hib vaccines have been reviewed (12). A single convulsion occurred 12 hours after immunization in a 3-month-old child and a hyporesponsive episode occurred in another 3-month-old child.

Guillain–Barré syndrome has been reported after immunization with several different vaccines, including Hib conjugate vaccine (13,14). One patient had also received DTP and oral poliomyelitis vaccine.

Metabolism

The incidence of diabetes mellitus has been studied in Finnish children born between October 1983 and September 1985 compared with children born between October 1985 and 1987 (1). Of the children born in 1985–87, 50% received Hib vaccine (diphtheria conjugated PRP-D-Hib vaccine) at 3, 4, and 6 months as a primary course and a booster dose at 14–18 months; the other 50% received one dose of the same vaccine at the age of 24 months. Taking into account the documented increase in diabetes in Finnish children, the small difference between the incidence rate of diabetes in children born during the period 1985–87 and immunized at 18 months and the incidence rate of children born in 1983–85 and not immunized against Hib disease was expected, with a slightly higher non-significant incidence in immunized children. In children over 4 years of age primed during the first year of life the incidence rate of diabetes was also slightly but non-significantly higher than in children immunized at 18 months of age. The authors concluded that early PRP-D-Hib immunization does not increase the risk of diabetes during the first 10 years of life.

This study has been criticized on the grounds that the authors did not present data comparing the incidence rates of children born in 1985–87 and primed during the first year of life with children born in 1983–85 and not immunized (15). The critics presented significant differences in the incidence rate of diabetes between the two groups of children and concluded that immunization had increased the risk of diabetes. However, the relative risk of diabetes during the first 10 years of life in the immunized children born in 1985–87 was 1.19 compared with the non-immunized children born in 1983–85.

In another Finnish study, about 116 000 children born in Finland between 1 October 1985 and 31 August 1987 were randomized to receive four doses of Hib vaccine (PPR-D, Connaught) starting at 3 months of life or one dose starting after 24 months of life (16). A control cohort included all 128 500 children born in Finland in the 24 months before the study. The difference in cumulative incidence between those who received four doses of the vaccine and those who received none was 54 cases of diabetes per 100 000 at 7 years (relative risk = 1.26). Most of the extra cases of diabetes occurred in statistically significant clusters starting about 38 months after immunization and lasting about 6–8 months. The authors concluded that exposure to Hib immunization is associated with an increased risk of type 1 diabetes mellitus.

In 1997, US researchers suggested that immunization at 28 days after birth can cause type 1 diabetes mellitus in susceptible individuals. In May 1998, several institutions, including the National Institute of Allergy and Infectious Diseases, the Centers for Disease Control, the World Health Organization, and the UK's Department of Health, sponsored a workshop to assess the evidence of a possible link. Immunologists, diabetologists, epidemiologists, policymakers, and observers debated the available evidence and concluded that a causal link between immunization and type 1 diabetes is not supported. The results of a large, randomized, controlled trial of immunization against Hib carried out in Finland in 1985–87 (5) were also reanalysed and showed no association between the incidence of diabetes mellitus and the addition of another antigen to the schedule, irrespective of timing. Data reanalysis was made possible by prospective linking of individual information on exposure (in this case infant immunization or the administration of placebo) with the Finnish diabetes register (17).

Susceptibility Factors

Other features of the patient

Of 23 patients with Hodgkin's disease and splenectomy immunized with Hib conjugate vaccine, most responded, although the antibody response was significantly lower than in healthy people (18). There were adverse effects in three of the vaccinees: in one case nausea, vertigo, and weakness occurred 2–4 days after administration of the vaccine, myalgias occurred in another case, and fever and myalgias (after primary immunization, with milder symptoms after the booster) in a third.

References

1. Karvonen M, Cepaitis Z, Tuomilehto J. Association between type 1 diabetes and *Haemophilus influenzae* type b vaccination: birth cohort study. BMJ 1999;318(7192):1169–72.
2. Evans Geoffrey. Personal communication, 1999.
3. Dukes MNG, Swartz B. Responsibility for Drug-induced Injury. Amsterdam: Elsevier, 1988.
4. Kantor E, Luxenberg JS, Lucas AH, Granoff DM. Phase I study of the immunogenicity and safety of conjugated Hemophilus influenzae type b vaccines in the elderly. Vaccine 1997;15(2):129–32.
5. Peltola H, Aavitsland P, Hansen KG, Jonsdottir KE, Nokleby H, Romanus V. Perspective: a five-country analysis of the impact of four different *Haemophilus influenzae* type b conjugates and vaccination strategies in Scandinavia. J Infect Dis 1999;179(1):223–9.
6. Jonville-Bera AP, Autret-Leca E, Radal M. [Adverse effects of the vaccines Tetracoq, IPAD/DTCP and DTCP. A French study of regional drug monitoring centers.] Arch Pediatr 1999;6(5):510–15.
7. Lee CY, Thipphawong J, Huang LM, Lee PI, Chiu HH, Lin W, Debois H, Harrison D, Xie F, Barreto L. An evaluation of the safety and immunogenicity of a five-component acellular pertussis, diphtheria, and tetanus toxoid vaccine (DTaP) when combined with a *Haemophilus influenzae* type b–tetanus toxoid conjugate vaccine (PRP-T) in Taiwanese infants Pediatrics 1999;103(1):25–30.
8. Cimaz R, Mensi C, D'Angelo E, Fantola E, Milone V, Biasio LR, Carnelli V, Zanetti AR. Safety and

immunogenicity of a conjugate vaccine against *Haemophilus influenzae* type b in splenectomized and nonsplenectomized patients with Cooley anemia. J Infect Dis 2001;183(12):1819–21.
9. Amir J, Melamed R, Bader J, Ethevenaux C, Fritzell B, Cartier JR, Arminjon F, Dagan R. Immunogenicity and safety of a liquid combination of DTP-PRP-T vs lyophilized PRP-T reconstituted with DTP. Vaccine 1997;15(2): 149–54.
10. Mallet E, Fabre P, Pines E, Salomon H, Staub T, Schodel F, Mendelman P, Hessel L, Chryssomalis G, Vidor E, Hoffenbach A, Abeille A, Amar R, Arsene JP, Aurand JM, Azoulay L, Badescou E, Barrois S, Baudino N, Beal M, Beaude-Chervet V, Berlier P, Billard E, Billet L, Blanc B, Blanc JP, Bohu D, Bonardo C, Bossu C; Hexavalent Vaccine Trial Study Group. Immunogenicity and safety of a new liquid hexavalent combined vaccine compared with separate administration of reference licensed vaccines in infants. Pediatr Infect Dis J 2000;19(12):1119–27.
11. Bewley KM, Schwab JG, Ballanco GA, Daum RS. Interchangeability of *Haemophilus influenzae* type b vaccines in the primary series: evaluation of a two-dose mixed regimen. Pediatrics 1996;98(5):898–904.
12. Weinberg GA, Granoff DM. Polysaccharide–protein conjugate vaccines for the prevention of *Haemophilus influenzae* type b disease. J Pediatr 1988;113(4):621–31.
13. D'Cruz OF, Shapiro ED, Spiegelman KN, Leicher CR, Breningstall GN, Khatri BO, Dobyns WB. Acute inflammatory demyelinating polyradiculoneuropathy (Guillain–Barré syndrome) after immunization with *Haemophilus influenzae* type b conjugate vaccine. J Pediatr 1989;115(5 Pt 1):743–6.
14. Gervaix A, Caflisch M, Suter S, Haenggeli CA. Guillain–Barré syndrome following immunisation with *Haemophilus influenzae* type b conjugate vaccine. Eur J Pediatr 1993;152(7):613–14.
15. Classen JB, Classen DC. Association between type 1 diabetes and Hib vaccine. Causal relation is likely. BMJ 1999;319(7217):1133.
16. Classen JB, Classen DC. Clustering of cases of insulin dependent diabetes (IDDM) occurring three years after *Hemophilus influenza* B (HiB) immunization support causal relationship between immunization and IDDM. Autoimmunity 2002;35(4):247–53.
17. Jefferson T. Vaccination and its adverse effects: real or perceived. Society should think about means of linking exposure to potential long term effect. BMJ 1998;317(7152):159–60.
18. Jakacki R, Luery N, McVerry P, Lange B. *Haemophilus influenzae* diphtheria protein conjugate immunization after therapy in splenectomized patients with Hodgkin disease. Ann Intern Med 1990;112(2):143–4.

Hair dyes

General Information

Hair dyes (for example henna, paraphenylenediamine, and paratoluenediamine) have been reviewed (1). They have moderate to low acute toxicity. Poisoning is rare and occurs only after oral ingestion. Contact sensitization usually occurs from unprotected professional exposure, but the prevalence has stabilized or fallen over the years. In vitro genotoxicity tests of hair dye ingredients have often been positive, but the relation to in vivo carcinogenicity is not clear and there is no in vivo evidence of genotoxicity. Despite the results of various studies that have suggested an association between the use of hair dyes and bladder cancer, a number of studies, including prospective investigations in large populations and systematic reviews, have shown no convincing associations with bladder cancer and other cancers. The results of direct toxicity studies and epidemiological studies suggest that hair dyes and their ingredients do not cause adverse reproductive effects.

Organs and Systems

Immunologic

Allergic reactions to constituents of hair dyes are not uncommon and are generally due to delayed hypersensitivity. Immediate hypersensitivity reactions have been described, but they are rare and seldom life-threatening.

Contact allergy to the paraphenylene group of hair dyes is well established (2). To test for cross-reactivity between these oxidative dyes and the new generation of hair dyes, 40 hairdressers allergic to paraphenylenediamine were selected; none reacted to any of the four acid dyes, two FD&C dyes, or four D&C dyes, suggesting that these newer hair dyes are safe alternatives to the paraphenylene-based hair dyes (3).

There is a risk of sensitization from paraphenylenediamine when it is applied to the skin in combination with henna (4–6). This can result in contact allergic reactions as well as persistent contact leukoderma, as illustrated in five patients with paint-on henna tattoos (7). All were positive on patch-testing with paraphenylenediamine. One developed erythema multiforme 4 weeks after the last application and the authors found no other causes of erythema multiforme.

The use of the combination of henna and paraphenylenediamine in 20 cases over 2 years in Khartoum (Sudan) resulted in severe toxicity (SEDA-9, 142). The initial symptoms were those of angioedema, with massive edema of the face, lips, glottis, pharynx, neck, and bronchi. These occurred within hours of the application of the dye-mix to the skin. In some the symptoms progressed on the second day to anuria and acute renal insufficiency, with death on the third day. Dialysis helped some patients, but others died from renal tubular necrosis.

The oxidation product of paratoluenediamine has been identified as a rare cause of a life-threatening immediate hypersensitivity reaction (8).

- A 45-year-old woman developed extensive urticarial lesions 30 minutes after the application of a hair dye, starting on the scalp and face, followed by abdominal cramps, watery diarrhea, vomiting, dysphonia, and loss of consciousness. A prick test with a 1/128 dilution of the hair dye showed a positive reaction, but individual dye constituents did not. Prick testing with the oxidation products of the individual dye constituents showed a strongly positive reaction to oxidized paratoluenediamine, which was weaker after addition of an antioxidant to the mixture.

Ten healthy controls had negative prick tests with the oxidized paratoluenediamine.

Long-Term Effects

Tumorigenicity

In a review of cohort and case-control studies of occupational exposure to hair dyes among hairdressers, barbers, and beauticians, the relative risk of bladder cancer was 1.4 from cohort studies, and somewhat over 1.0 from case-control studies; however, there were confounding factors, particularly since allowance for smoking was lacking or inadequate in most studies (9). In five case-control studies of personal use of hair dyes, there was no evidence of an increased risk of bladder cancer. In nine cohort studies the relative risk of lymphoid neoplasms overall was 1.2 (1.5 for non-Hodgkin's lymphomas and 1.1 for multiple myeloma). Of five case-control studies, three reported some association with lymphoid neoplasms, but the estimates of relative risk were only moderately above 1.0 and there was insufficient allowance for potential confounding factors, including social class and greying hair, which could correlate with both hair dye use and lymphoid neoplasms. No other neoplasms, including those of breast, skin, and lung were related to the use of hair dyes. In another study there was an increased risk of Hodgkin's disease among women who reported the use of hair coloring products before 1980 (OR = 1.3; CI = 1, 1.8) (10).

Drug Administration

Drug overdose

In one case deliberate ingestion of paraphenylenediamine with suicidal intent caused severe oropharyngeal edema, rhabdomyolysis, and cardiac death after 4 hours despite full supportive treatment (11).

Myocarditis has been attributed to paraphenylenediamine poisoning (12).

- An 18-year-old woman developed asphyxia and rhabdomyolysis after taking paraphenylenediamine 5 g. An electrocardiogram showed ventricular extra beats and inverted T waves. The serum CK activity was 28 020 μkat/l. Transthoracic echocardiography showed left and right ventricular hypokinesis and a left ventricular apical thrombus. Anticoagulation treatment with heparin was initiated. A follow-up echocardiogram performed on the 15th day showed normalization of ventricular function and disappearance of the thrombus.

In two patients acute oliguric renal insufficiency due to acute tubular necrosis followed paraphenylenediamine intoxication; there was associated vomiting, angioedema, cyanosis, and intravascular hemolysis (13). One patient recovered and the other died with septicemia. In four other cases acute renal insufficiency was due to rhabdomyolysis.

References

1. Nohynek GJ, Fautz R, Benech-Kieffer F, Toutain H. Toxicity and human health risk of hair dyes. Food Chem Toxicol 2004;42(4):517–43.
2. Sosted H, Agner T, Andersen KE, Menne T. 55 cases of allergic reactions to hair dye: a descriptive, consumer complaint-based study. Contact Dermatitis 2002;47(5):299–303.
3. Fautz R, Fuchs A, van der Walle H, Henny V, Smits L. Hair dye-sensitized hairdressers: the cross-reaction pattern with new generation hair dyes. Contact Dermatitis 2002;46(6):319–24.
4. Tosti A, Pazzaglia M, Corazza M, Virgili A. Allergic contact dermatitis caused by mehindi. Contact Dermatitis 2000;42(6):356.
5. Mohamed M, Nixon R. Severe allergic contact dermatitis induced by paraphenylenediamine in paint-on temporary "tattoos". Australas J Dermatol 2000;41(3):168–71.
6. Lestringant GG, Bener A, Frossard PM. Cutaneous reactions to henna and associated additives. Br J Dermatol 1999;141(3):598–600.
7. Jappe U, Hausen BM, Petzoldt D. Erythema-multiforme-like eruption and depigmentation following allergic contact dermatitis from a paint-on henna tattoo, due to paraphenylenediamine contact hypersensitivity. Contact Dermatitis 2001;45(4):249–50.
8. Pasche-Koo F, French L, Piletta-Zanin PA, Hauser C. Contact urticaria and shock to hair dye. Allergy 1998;53(9):904–5.
9. La Vecchia C, Tavani A. Epidemiological evidence on hair dyes and the risk of cancer in humans. Eur J Cancer Prev 1995;4(1):31–43.
10. Zhang Y, Holford TR, Leaderer B, Boyle P, Zahm SH, Flynn S, Tallini G, Owens PH, Zheng T. Hair-coloring product use and risk of non-Hodgkin's lymphoma: a population-based case-control study in Connecticut. Am J Epidemiol 2004;159(2):148–54.
11. Ashraf W, Dawling S, Farrow LJ. Systemic paraphenylenediamine (PPD) poisoning: a case report and review. Hum Exp Toxicol 1994;13(3):167–70.
12. Zeggwagh AA, Abouqal R, Abidi K, Madani N, Zekraoui A, Kerkeb O. Thrombus ventriculaire gauche et myocardite toxique induite par la paraphenylene diamine. [Left ventricular thrombus and myocarditis induced by paraphenylenediamine poisoning.] Ann Fr Anesth Reanim 2003;22(7):639–41.
13. Bourquia A, Jabrane AJ, Ramdani B, Zaid D. Toxicite systemique de la paraphenylene diamine. Quatre observations. [Systemic toxicity of paraphenylenediamine. 4 cases.] Presse Méd 1988;17(35):1798–800.

Halofantrine

General Information

Halofantrine is a phenanthrene-methanol derivative of an aminoalcohol, active against multidrug-resistant *Plasmodium falciparum* malaria. Halofantrine was known during World War II but was little used at that time. It is slowly and incompletely absorbed with peak concentrations 3.5–6 hours after dosing. Its absorption in its original formulation was unpredictable (SEDA-13, 820).

Dose-finding studies with halofantrine showed treatment failures with a single dose but cures with two doses, one of 1000 mg and one of 500 mg. A regimen of 500 mg at 6-hourly intervals was also effective. Three doses of 500 mg at 6-hourly intervals were also used in a French study and treatment resulted in cure in semi-immune subjects. The dosage was insufficient in non-immune Caucasian patients.

Halofantrine is not indicated for prophylactic use. However, of 480 army personnel who took two doses of 1500 mg each on the third and the tenth days after they had returned to a non-malarial area, only one had *P. falciparum* malaria during the next 5 months (SEDA-13, 820) (1). There were no adverse effects, except for one case of morbilliform rash possibly due to the halofantrine.

General adverse effects

Adverse effects with the dosages originally recommended have in general been mild, no more than nausea, diarrhea, headache, and pruritus (SEDA-13, 820) (2–4). Pruritus occurred markedly less often with halofantrine than with chloroquine (SEDA-16, 306). A comparison between high-dose chloroquine (35 mg/kg total in three daily doses) and halofantrine in the standard dose (total 25 mg/kg given at 6-hour intervals) in patients 4–14 years old showed a fairly similar frequency of adverse effects. Itching was a common adverse effect of chloroquine (4).

Organs and Systems

Cardiovascular

In 1993, the sudden cardiac death of a 37-year-old woman after her ninth dose of halofantrine was reported. A subsequent prospective study showed that halofantrine was associated with a dose-related lengthening of the QT interval by more than 25% (SEDA-17, 328). Mefloquine did not cause such changes, but the combination of mefloquine with halofantrine had a more pronounced effect on the electrocardiogram. However, in the region where this investigation was carried out (on the Thai–Burmese border area) thiamine deficiency is common, and patients in this area have longer baseline QT intervals than are usually reported (SEDA-17, 328). Two patients, mother and son, both with congenital prolongation of the QT interval, suffered sustained episodes of torsade de pointes after a total dose of 1000 mg of halofantrine, and there have been other reports of dysrhythmias, including death in a patient who took mefloquine and halofantrine (SEDA-20, 260) (SEDA-21, 295). Dysrhythmias due to halofantrine may respond to propranolol (5).

African children who received halofantrine (three doses of 8 mg/kg 6-hourly) for uncomplicated *P. falciparum* malaria had increases in both the PR interval and the QT_c interval; out of 42 children in the study, two children developed first-degree heart block and one child second-degree heart block; the QT_c interval either increased by more than 125% of baseline value or by more than 0.44 seconds (an effect that persisted for at least 48 hours) (6).

There have been recent reports in the French medical press of cases of significant QT_c prolongation in children returning to France, and caution in its use has been urged (7). A small trial in non-immune adults in the Netherlands and France also showed increased QT_c dispersion with halofantrine but not artemether + lumefantrine (8).

- Death due to a dysrhythmia was reported in a woman who had taken halofantrine for malaria (9). She had a normal electrocardiogram before treatment and no family history of heart disease.

Prolongation of the QT interval occurred in 10 of 25 children treated with halofantrine (24 mg/kg oral suspension in three divided doses) for acute falciparum malaria (10).

Electrocardiographic monitoring is recommended for children and adults taking halofantrine.

Gastrointestinal

Gastrointestinal adverse effects are more common with halofantrine than with other antimalarial drugs (11).

Immunologic

Anaphylactic shock has been attributed to halofantrine (12).

Long-Term Effects

Drug tolerance

Early laboratory studies suggested cross-resistance of halofantrine with mefloquine. In rats, parasites that are resistant to mefloquine, quinine, chloroquine, and amodiaquine are also markedly resistant to halofantrine (13).

Susceptibility Factors

Pre-existing cardiac conduction abnormalities, including those induced by other drugs, are a definite risk. Due consideration should be given not only to the half-life of such drugs, but also to the tissue concentrations and total clearances of the agents involved.

Drug Administration

Drug formulations

Halofantrine is available in a micronized form. Early information suggested that this improved absorption, but two later studies provided conflicting evidence: there was a wide range of serum concentrations of halofantrine and its main metabolite *N*-desbutylhalofantrine after the administration of half of the standard dose (2) or the usual dose of 500 mg given three times with 6-hour intervals (3). In general, concentrations were similar to those obtained with the older formulation. Taking the drug with food is thought to increase absorption.

Food–Drug Interactions

Grapefruit juice

Since halofantrine is metabolized to *N*-debutyl-halofantrine by CYP3A4, grapefruit juice increases its systemic availability (14). Twelve healthy men and women took halofantrine 500 mg with water, orange juice, or grapefruit juice (250 ml/day for 3 days and once 12 hours before halofantrine) in a crossover study. Compared with water, grapefruit juice significantly increased halofantrine AUC and C_{max} 2.8-fold and 3.2-fold respectively; there was no significant change in half-life. Maximum QT_c interval prolongation increased significantly from 17 ms when halofantrine was taken with water to 31 ms when it was taken with grapefruit juice. Grapefruit juice should be avoided by patients taking halofantrine.

References

1. Baudon D, Bernard J, Moulia-Pelat JP, Martet G, Sarrouy J, Touze JE, Spiegel A, Lantrade P, Picq JJ. Halofantrine to prevent falciparum malaria on return from malarious areas. Lancet 1990;336(8711):377.
2. Fadat G, Louis FJ, Louis JP, Le Bras J. Efficacy of micronized halofantrine in semi-immune patients with acute uncomplicated falciparum malaria in Cameroon. Antimicrob Agents Chemother 1993;37(9):1955–7.
3. Bouchaud O, Basco LK, Gillotin C, Gimenez F, Ramiliarisoa O, Genissel B, Bouvet E, Farinotti R, Le Bras J, Coulaud JP. Clinical efficacy and pharmacokinetics of micronized halofantrine for the treatment of acute uncomplicated falciparum malaria in nonimmune patients. Am J Trop Med Hyg 1994;51(2):204–13.
4. Wildling E, Jenne L, Graninger W, Bienzle U, Kremsner PG. High dose chloroquine versus micronized halofantrine in chloroquine-resistant *Plasmodium falciparum* malaria. J Antimicrob Chemother 1994;33(4):871–5.
5. Toivonen L, Viitasalo M, Siikamaki H, Raatikka M, Pohjola-Sintonen S. Provocation of ventricular tachycardia by antimalarial drug halofantrine in congenital long QT syndrome. Clin Cardiol 1994;17(7):403–4.
6. Sowunmi A, Falade CO, Oduola AM, Ogundahunsi OA, Fehintola FA, Gbotosho GO, Larcier P, Salako LA. Cardiac effects of halofantrine in children suffering from acute uncomplicated falciparum malaria. Trans R Soc Trop Med Hyg 1998;92(4):446–8.
7. Olivier C, Rizk C, Zhang D, Jacqz-Aigrain E. Allongement de l'espace QT_c compliquant la prescription d'halofantrine chez deux enfants presentant un accès palustre a *plasmodium falciparum*. [Long QT_c interval complicating halofantrine therapy in 2 children with *Plasmodium falciparum* malaria.] Arch Pediatr 1999;6(9):966–70.
8. van Agtmael M, Bouchaud O, Malvy D, Delmont J, Danis M, Barette S, Gras C, Bernard J, Touze JE, Gathmann I, Mull R. The comparative efficacy and tolerability of CGP 56697 (artemether + lumefantrine) versus halofantrine in the treatment of uncomplicated falciparum malaria in travellers returning from the Tropics to The Netherlands and France. Int J Antimicrob Agents 1999;12(2):159–69.
9. Malvy D, Receveur MC, Ozon P, Djossou F, Le Metayer P, Touze JE, Longy-Boursier M, Le Bras M. Fatal cardiac incident after use of halofantrine. J Travel Med 2000;7(4):215–16.
10. Herranz U, Rusca A, Assandri A. Emedastine–ketoconazole: pharmacokinetic and pharmacodynamic interactions in healthy volunteers. Int J Clin Pharmacol Ther 2001;39(3):102–9.
11. Anabwani G, Canfield CJ, Hutchinson DB. Combination atovaquone and proguanil hydrochloride vs. halofantrine for treatment of acute *Plasmodium falciparum* malaria in children. Pediatr Infect Dis J 1999;18(5):456–61.
12. Fourcade L, Gachot B, De Pina JJ, Heno P, Laurent G, Touze JE. Choc anaphylactique associé au traitement du paludisme par halofantrine. [Anaphylactic shock related to the treatment of malaria with halofantrine.] Presse Méd 1997;26(12):559.
13. Peters W, Robinson BL, Ellis DS. The chemotherapy of rodent malaria. XLII. Halofantrine and halofantrine resistance. Ann Trop Med Parasitol 1987;81(5):639–46.
14. Charbit B, Becquemont L, Lepere B, Peytavin G, Funck-Brentano C. Pharmacokinetic and pharmacodynamic interaction between grapefruit juice and halofantrine. Clin Pharmacol Ther 2002;72(5):514–23.

Halogenated quinolines

General Information

The halogenated quinolines include clioquinol (iodochlorohydroxyquinoline), diiodohydroxyquinoline, broxyquinoline, and chlorquinaldol (all rINNs). Once regarded as a prophylactic and remedy for simple diarrhea, some of them remain in limited use for special purposes, notably for the treatment of amebiasis when no alternative is available.

A major epidemic of subacute myelo-optic neuropathy (SMON) in Japan during 1956–70 was identified as being due to clioquinol, which led to the withdrawal of halogenated quinolines in Japan itself and subsequently elsewhere. There is every reason to believe that the adverse effects seen with clioquinol can occur with the other hydroxyquinolines, but some of them are still sold freely in various parts of the world (1).

Organs and Systems

Nervous system

DoTS classification (BMJ 2003;327:1222–5)

Adverse reaction: subacute myelo-optic neuropathy
Dose-relation: collateral effect
Time-course: intermediate
Susceptibility factors: genetic (?Japanese more susceptible)

There was a major epidemic of subacute myelo-optic neuropathy (SMON) in Japan during 1956–70. In 1970 a clinical observation led to case-control and cohort studies, which identified clioquinol as the culprit. A few cases were also reported elsewhere in the world, in Australia (2), Denmark (3), the Netherlands (4), Sweden (5–7), Switzerland (8), the UK (9–11), and the USA (12); some cases involved halogenated quinolines other than clioquinol. Prolonged use of diiodohydroxyquinoline in high doses has been associated with loss of vision and optic atrophy (SED-11, 594) (13). Halogenated quinolines were withdrawn in Japan and the epidemic abated (14).

The main abdominal symptoms of SMON are diarrhea and abdominal pain, sometimes accompanied by nausea, vomiting, constipation, a bloated feeling in the abdomen, and meteorism. The neurological symptoms are acute or subacute in nature; sensory disturbances are characteristic and spread gradually from the feet up to the navel. Some 20–40% of cases have visual disturbances ranging from blurred vision to atrophy of the optic nerve and blindness. There is a wide range of mental symptoms.

The clearest proof of the cause-and-effect relation in Japan was the finding of clioquinol chelates in the green furring of the tongue and the greenish urine. There has been no clear explanation for the much higher incidence of cases in Japan than elsewhere, but several hypotheses have been suggested (15).

The risk is related to dose and duration of therapy (16):

- at a dose of 750 mg/day for less than 4 weeks there is little risk
- at a dose of 750–1500 mg/day for less than 2 weeks the risk is about 1%
- at a dose of 750–1500 mg/day for more than 2 weeks the risk is about 35%
- a dose of 1800 mg/day can cause symptoms within 5 days
- higher doses can cause symptoms within 24 hours.

The events in Japan, where the total of documented cases was some 10 000 (17), have been fully documented in earlier volumes from 1968 onwards (see for example SEDA-4, 253). Little further evidence has since accumulated, despite a major international conference at Kyoto, Japan, in April 1979 to examine the evidence. Since the withdrawal of such drugs in Japan descriptions of large numbers of new cases have ceased. The effect should now be largely of historical interest, but the condition continues to be reported very sporadically (SEDA-10, 326).

Endocrine

Diiodohydroxyquinoline can slightly enlarge the thyroid gland (18).

Hematologic

Thrombocytopenia has (unconvincingly) been ascribed to topical clioquinol (19).

Drug Administration

Drug administration route

Up to 40% of topically applied clioquinol can be absorbed percutaneously in man (20). Formulations that contain clioquinol are often used to treat diaper rash; in a child of 10 kg treated with 1 g of clioquinol 3% tds, the amount of drug applied would be 9 mg/kg/day. However, it is possible that in infants with diaper rashes the actual absorption of the drug would be over 40%, since absorption through inflamed skin occurs more readily than through intact skin, and infant skin is more permeable than adult skin (21).

In dogs treated with 5 g of a topical clioquinol 3% formulation twice daily over 28 days (about 17 mg/kg/day) there was significant toxicity (loss of weight, lethargy, paralysis, hepatotoxicity) (22).

References

1. Chetley A. Problem Drugs. London and Atlantic Highlands: Zed Books, 1995;62–8.
2. Selby G. Subacute myelo-optic neuropathy in Australia. Lancet 1972;1(7742):123–5.
3. Kjaersgaard K. Amnesia after clioquinol. Lancet 1971;2(7733):1086.
4. van Balen AT. Toxic damage to the optic nerve caused by iodochlorhydroxyquinoline (Enterovioform). Ophthalmologica 1971;163(1):8–9.
5. Osterman PO. Myelopathy after clioquinol treatment. Lancet 1971;2(7723):544.
6. Strandvik B, Zetterstrom R. Amaurosis after broxyquinoline. Lancet 1968;1(7548):922–3.
7. Berggren L, Hansson O. Absorption of intestinal antiseptics derived from 8-hydroxyquinolines. Clin Pharmacol Ther 1968;9(1):67–70.
8. Kaeser HE, Wuthrich R. Zur Frage der Neurotoxizität der Oxychinoline, [Possible neurotoxicity of oxyquinolines.] Dtsch Med Wochenschr 1970;95(33):1685–8.
9. Spillane JD. S.M.O.N. Lancet 1971;2(7738):1371–2.
10. McEwen LM. Neuropathy after clioquinol. BMJ 1971; 4(780):169–70.
11. McEwen LM, Constantinopoulos P. The use of a dietary and antibacterial regime in the management of intrinsic allergy. Ann Allergy 1970;28(6):256–66.
12. Gholz LM, Arons WL. Prophylaxis and therapy of amebiasis and shigellosis with iodochlorhydroxyquin. Am J Trop Med Hyg 1964;13:396–401.
13. Cook GC. Tropical medicine. Postgrad Med J 1991;67(791):798–822.
14. Kono R. Subacute myelo-optico-neuropathy, a new neurological disease prevailing in Japan. Jpn J Med Sci Biol 1971;24(4):195–216.
15. Dukes MNG. The paradox of clioquinol and SMON. In: D'Arcy PF, Griffin JP, editors. Iatrogenic Diseases, Update 1981. Oxford–New York–Toronto: Oxford University Press, 1981;105.
16. Oakley GP Jr. The neurotoxicity of the halogenated hydroxyquinolines. A commentary JAMA 1973;225(4):395–7.
17. Soda I, editor. Drug-Induced Sufferings: Medical, Pharmaceutical, and Legal Aspects. Proceedings of the Kyoto International Conference Against Drug-Induced Sufferings, Kyoto, 14–18 April 1979. Amsterdam: Excerpta Mexica, 1980.
18. Castenfors H, Allgoth AM. The effect of iodochlorohydroxyquinoline, diiodohydroxyquinoline and dichlorohydroxyquinaldine on the thyroid uptake of radio-iodine. Scand J Clin Lab Invest 1957;9(3):270–2.
19. Khaleeli AA. Quinaband-induced thrombocytopenic purpura in a patient with myxoedema coma. BMJ 1976;2(6035):562–3.
20. Stohs SJ, Ezzedeen FW, Anderson AK, Baldwin JN, Makoid MC. Percutaneous absorption of iodochlorhydroxyquin in humans. J Invest Dermatol 1984;82(2):195–8.
21. Public Citizen, Health Research Group. Clioquinol (Letter to FDA). Public Citizen, 1985.
22. Ezzedeen FW, Stohs SJ, Kilzer KL, Makoid MC, Ezzedeen NW. Percutaneous absorption and disposition of iodochlorhydroxyquin in dogs. J Pharm Sci 1984;73(10): 1369–72.

Haloperidol

See also Neuroleptic drugs

General Information

Haloperidol is a butyrophenone neuroleptic drug. The enzymes involved in its biotransformation include oxidative cytochrome P450 isozymes, carbonyl reductase, and uridine diphosphoglucose glucuronosyltransferase (1). It is mainly cleared by glucuronidation.

There has been a randomized, placebo-controlled comparison of haloperidol (mean dose 1.8 mg/day), trazodone (200 mg/day), and behavior management techniques in 149 patients with Alzheimer's disease (2). Although 34% of the subjects improved relative to baseline, there were no significant differences in outcomes among the four arms; there were significantly fewer cases of bradykinesia and parkinsonian gait in those given behavioral therapy. These results suggest that other treatments for agitation in dementia need to be considered and evaluated; likewise, they are consistent with the results of a meta-analysis (3) and a clinical trial (4).

Haloperidol 2–3 mg/day and 0.50–0.75 mg/day have been compared in 71 outpatients with Alzheimer's disease (5). After 12 weeks, there was a favorable therapeutic effect of haloperidol 2–3 mg/day, although 25% of the patients developed moderate to severe extrapyramidal signs.

A thorough review of the pharmacokinetics of haloperidol, with special emphasis on interactions, has been published (1).

Organs and Systems

Cardiovascular

Intravenous haloperidol is often prescribed to treat agitation, and torsade de pointes has on occasions occurred (SEDA-20, 36). In a cross-sectional cohort study QT_c intervals were measured before the intravenous administration of haloperidol plus flunitrazepam, and continuous electrocardiographic monitoring was performed for at least 8 hours after ($n = 34$) (6); patients who received only flunitrazepam served as controls. The mean QT_c interval after 8 hours in those who were given haloperidol was longer than in those who were given flunitrazepam alone; four patients given haloperidol had a QT_c interval of more than 500 ms after 8 hours. However, none developed ventricular tachydysrhythmias.

In a case-control study, haloperidol-induced QT_c prolongation was associated with torsade de pointes (7). The odds ratio of developing torsade de pointes in a patient with QT_c prolongation to over 550 ms compared with those with QT_c intervals shorter than 550 ms was 33 (95% CI = 6, 195). The sample consisted of all critically ill adult patients in medical, cardiac, and surgical intensive care units at a tertiary hospital who received intravenous haloperidol and had no metabolic, pharmacological, or neurological risk factors known to cause torsade de pointes, or if the dysrhythmia developed more than 24 hours after intravenous haloperidol. Of 223 patients who fulfilled the inclusion criteria, eight developed torsade de pointes. A group of 41 patients, randomly selected from the 215 without torsade de pointes, served as controls. The length of hospital stay after the development of haloperidol-associated torsade de pointes was significantly longer than that after the maximum dose of intravenous haloperidol in the control group. The overall incidence of torsade de pointes was 3.6% and 11% in patients who received intravenous haloperidol 35 mg or more over 24 hours.

Several cases of torsade de pointes have been reported with intravenous haloperidol used with low-dose oral haloperidol (8).

The effects of haloperidol dose and plasma concentration and CYP2D6 activity on the QT_c interval have been studied in 27 Caucasian patients taking oral haloperidol (aged 23–77 years, dosages 1.5–30 mg/day) (9). Three patients had a QT_c interval longer than 456 ms, which can be considered as the cut-off value for a risk of cardiac dysrhythmias. There was no correlation between QT_c interval and haloperidol dosage or plasma concentrations or CYP2D6 activity.

Asystolic cardiac arrest has been reported after intravenous haloperidol (10).

In one case, the use of carbamazepine and haloperidol led to prolongation of the QT_c interval and cardiac complications (11).

- A 75-year-old man developed ventricular fibrillation and cardiac arrest after intravenous haloperidol (12). His past history included coronary bypass surgery and coronary angioplasty. As he continued to have severe chest pain, emergency angioplasty was performed. On day 3 he received haloperidol by infusion 2 mg/hour, with 2 mg increments every 10 minutes (up to 20 mg in 6 hours) as needed for relief of agitation. Before haloperidol, his QT_c interval was normal; after haloperidol it increased to 570 ms. The next day he developed ventricular fibrillation. Subsequent electrocardiograms showed prolonged QT_c intervals of 579 and 615 ms, and haloperidol was withdrawn; the QT_c returned to normal.
- A 76-year-old man developed torsade de pointes while taking tiapride 300 mg/day; the QT_c interval 1 day after starting treatment was 600 ms; the dysrhythmia resolved when tiapride was withdrawn (13).
- A 39-year-old man died suddenly 1 hour after taking a single oral dose of haloperidol 5 mg (14). He had myasthenia, alcoholic hepatitis, and electrolyte abnormalities due to inadequate nutritional state. His electrocardiogram showed prolongation of the QT_c interval (460 ms). Autopsy showed a cardiomyopathy but no explanation for sudden death.

However, malignant dysrhythmias can occur without changes in the QT interval (SEDA-24, 54).

- A 64-year-old woman underwent coronary artery bypass surgery and was given intravenous haloperidol for agitation and to avoid postoperative delirium; she developed torsade de pointes (15).
- Asystolic cardiac arrest occurred in a 49-year-old woman after she had received haloperidol 10 mg intramuscularly for 2 days; no previous QT_c prolongation had been observed (16).

Respiratory

A single case of fatal pulmonary edema was reported in 1982 in association with haloperidol (17).

Nervous system

Three cases of radial nerve palsy were reported in demented elderly patients confined to wheelchairs who were treated with haloperidol. The combination of extrapyramidal and sedative adverse effects, added to wheelchair confinement, may have resulted in pressure on the upper arm with subsequent neuropathy (18).

Extrapyramidal effects

- A 28-year-old woman simultaneously developed four types of tardive extrapyramidal symptoms (dystonia, dyskinesia, choreoathetotic movements, and myoclonus) while taking haloperidol; the symptoms were subsequently relieved by the use of low-dose risperidone (3 mg/day) (19).

Akathisia

A nocturnal eating/drinking syndrome secondary to neuroleptic drug-induced restless legs syndrome has been attributed to low-dose haloperidol in a 51-year-old schizophrenic woman (20).

Neuroleptic malignant syndrome

Neuroleptic malignant syndrome has been reported with haloperidol (21).

- A 21-year-old Turkish man with succinic semialdehyde dehydrogenase deficiency and mental retardation developed neuroleptic malignant syndrome after a single dose of haloperidol 10 mg for anxiety and agitation, having never received a neuroleptic drug before.

Several reports have suggested a higher incidence and severity of extrapyramidal symptoms during haloperidol treatment in congenitally poor metabolizers of substrates of CYP2D6 and a patient with a poor metabolizer polymorphism of the CYP2D6 gene developed neuroleptic malignant syndrome after receiving haloperidol (22). All frequent polymorphisms of CYP2D6 were therefore investigated in the second patient, who was a carrier of the wild-type genotype CYP2D6 *1/ *1, which is common in subjects of Caucasian origin. The authors concluded that a genetic defect of haloperidol metabolism via CYP2D6 was unlikely as a reason for the neuroleptic malignant syndrome in this case.

Endocrine

The relation of prolactin concentrations and certain adverse events has been explored in large randomized, double-blind studies. In 813 women and 1912 men, haloperidol produced dose-related increases in plasma prolactin concentrations in men and women, but they were not correlated with adverse events such as amenorrhea, galactorrhea, or reduced libido in women or with erectile dysfunction, ejaculatory dysfunction, gynecomastia, or reduced libido in men (23).

No further rise in plasma prolactin concentration was observed with dosages of haloperidol over 100 mg/day, which was explained as being related to saturation of the pituitary dopamine receptors by a modest amount of haloperidol (24).

The time-course of the prolactin increase has been examined in 17 subjects whose prolactin concentrations rose during the first 6–9 days of treatment with haloperidol (25). The increase was followed by a plateau that persisted, with minor fluctuations, throughout the 18 days of observation. Patients whose prolactin concentrations increased above 77 ng/ml ($n = 2$) had hypothyroidism, and it is known that TRH (thyrotropin) stimulates the release of prolactin (26).

The effects of haloperidol and quetiapine on serum prolactin concentrations have been compared in 35 patients with schizophrenia during a drug-free period for at least 2 weeks in a randomized study (27). There was no significant difference in prolactin concentration between the groups at the start of the study; control prolactin concentrations were significantly lower with quetiapine than with haloperidol. Two patients taking haloperidol had galactorrhea related to hyperprolactinemia.

Metabolism

Glucose metabolism has been studied in 10 patients taking haloperidol; none had impaired glucose tolerance and only one had a glycemic peak delay (28).

Liver

Occasional reports of cholestatic jaundice with haloperidol have been published (29,30).

Urinary tract

Retroperitoneal fibrosis has been attributed to haloperidol; since this condition affects the kidney, it should be differentiated from other causes of obstructive uropathy (31).

Skin

Haloperidol has been reported to have caused skin rashes.

- A 41-year-old man who had been taking weekly methotrexate 15 mg for 10 months for psoriasis started to take haloperidol 1.5 mg bd for a psychotic illness, and 2 weeks later developed sudden redness and swelling of the face and hands accompanied by redness and watering of both eyes (32). He had diffuse erythema, edema, scaling, and erosions over his face, the anterior aspect of the neck, and the backs of both hands. A skin biopsy showed parakeratosis, acanthosis, spongiosis, focal epidermal cell degeneration, and dermal edema, accompanied by a moderate lymphomononuclear infiltrate, consistent with subacute dermatitis. A diagnosis of pellagra-like photosensitivity dermatitis, caused by combined deficiency of niacin, riboflavin, and other water-soluble vitamins, probably precipitated by haloperidol, was therefore considered. Haloperidol was withdrawn, vitamins were administered, and the condition resolved in the next 5 days.
- A 55-year-old man who had been treated for a manic-depressive disorder for about 5 years developed toxic epidermal necrolysis after being given carbamazepine and haloperidol (33).

Sexual function

Sexual dysfunction can occur with neuroleptic drugs (SED-14, 149) (SEDA-22, 54) (34,35).

- A 49-year-old man with bipolar disorder had erectile dysfunction shortly after starting to take haloperidol 50 mg/day and lithium 1500 mg/day (36). Before this he had had normal sexual function. After 2 months, the dosage of haloperidol was reduced to 20 mg/day, but the sexual dysfunction persisted and did not improve with sildenafil. He was then switched to olanzapine 10 mg/day and lithium 1200 mg/day and 1 week later his sexual dysfunction had disappeared.

Second-Generation Effects

Pregnancy

Although studies have failed to identify an increased rate of malformations with haloperidol, isolated cases have been reported (SED-14, 152) (37) (SEDA-22, 54) (38,39).

Teratogenicity

Several instances of limb reduction after the use of haloperidol during pregnancy suggest that it would be prudent not to use this drug during the first trimester, the period of limb development (37). There is also reason to argue that prenatally administered drugs of this class influence the offspring after the drug has been eliminated, and can produce behavioral teratogenicity; since neurotransmitter systems continue to develop long after birth, such drugs might influence behavior in an adverse way over a very long time (40).

Fetotoxicity

A neonate had severe hypothermia after antenatal exposure to haloperidol (41). He weighed 3710 g at birth and did not need resuscitation; his axillary temperature was 35°C and he had severe generalized hypotonia. His temperature rose to 36.5°C after 6 hours of rewarming with an overhead radiant heater.

Drug Administration

Drug additives

General allergic reactions have also been reported following injections of parabens-containing formulations of lidocaine and hydrocortisone and after oral use of barium sulfate contrast suspension, haloperidol syrup, and an antitussive syrup, all of which contained parabens (42).

Drug–Drug Interactions

General

Based on published data in humans, concomitant medications were classified as potential inhibitors (cimetidine, fluoxetine, levopromazine, paroxetine, and thioridazine) or inducers of haloperidol metabolism (carbamazepine, phenobarbital, and phenytoin).

Alcohol

Haloperidol increased blood alcohol concentrations (43).

Anticoagulants

Haloperidol has been reported to lower anticoagulant effectiveness through enzyme induction (44).

Buspirone

Buspirone increases haloperidol concentrations in some patients (SEDA-21, 39).

Carbamazepine

Haloperidol inhibits the metabolism of carbamazepine. In Japanese patients with schizophrenia, serum concentrations of carbamazepine were about 40% lower in the absence of haloperidol (45).

Chlorpromazine

- A 40-year-old man with schizophrenia developed a raised plasma concentration of haloperidol in combination with chlorpromazine and during overlap treatment with clozapine (46). Like haloperidol, chlorpromazine is a competitive inhibitor of CYP2D6; however, clozapine appears to be largely metabolized by CYP1A2.

Itraconazole

Adverse effects can result from increased plasma concentrations of haloperidol during itraconazole treatment. This has been observed in 13 schizophrenic patients treated with haloperidol 12 or 24 mg/day who took itraconazole 200 mg/day for 7 days (47). Plasma concentrations of haloperidol were significantly increased and neurological adverse effects were more common. Itraconazole is a potent inhibitor of CYP3A4.

Lithium

Persistent dysarthria with apraxia has been reported with a combination of lithium carbonate and haloperidol (48).

Lorazepam

Several cases of torsade de pointes have been reported with intravenous haloperidol used with lorazepam to treat delirium (SEDA-18, 30) (SEDA-18, 47). Acid mucopolysaccharide deposition may be associated with neuroleptic drug treatment as a possible mechanism contributing to rare cardiovascular adverse events (49).

Methyldopa

Dementia occurred when methyldopa was combined with haloperidol (50).

Nefazodone

Hepatic enzyme inhibition by nefazodone can significantly raise concentrations and toxicity of haloperidol (1).

Valproate

An interaction between valproate and haloperidol has been reported (51).

- A 30-year-old man with bipolar affective disorder was given intravenous sodium valproate 20 mg/kg/day without any major problem. Later, he was given oral haloperidol 10 mg bd for persistent aggressive behavior and manic symptoms. The next day he developed a sense of imbalance and started swaying. He was drowsy and had cerebellar ataxia. Haloperidol was withdrawn and within 1 day his ataxia had disappeared completely in spite of continuing valproate.

Food–Drug Interactions

Grapefruit inhibits CYP3A4, but in one study there was no interaction with haloperidol (52).

Smoking

The extent to which smoking, the genotype for CYP2D6, and the concomitant use of enzyme inducers or inhibitors can explain variations in steady-state plasma concentrations of haloperidol has been evaluated in 92 patients (53). Smokers were treated with higher doses of haloperidol than non-smokers, supporting the view that smokers require larger doses of neuroleptic drugs than non-smokers to achieve therapeutic effects. Poor metabolizers had higher concentrations of haloperidol metabolites, but not of haloperidol, than extensive metabolizers. Altogether, the patients took about 150 different drugs; compared with the rest of the group, there was a tendency for patients taking inducers to be treated with slightly higher doses of haloperidol on average and to have lower dose-normalized plasma concentrations of haloperidol, although the differences were not significant.

References

1. Kudo S, Ishizaki T. Pharmacokinetics of haloperidol: an update. Clin Pharmacokinet 1999;37(6):435–56.
2. Teri L, Logsdon RG, Peskind E, Raskind M, Weiner MF, Tractenberg RE, Foster NL, Schneider LS, Sano M, Whitehouse P, Tariot P, Mellow AM, Auchus AP, Grundman M, Thomas RG, Schafer K, Thal LJ. Alzheimer's Disease Cooperative Study. Treatment of agitation in AD: a randomized, placebo-controlled clinical trial. Neurology 2000;55(9):1271–8.
3. Schneider LS, Pollock VE, Lyness SA. A metaanalysis of controlled trials of neuroleptic treatment in dementia. J Am Geriatr Soc 1990;38(5):553–63.
4. Sultzer DL, Gray KF, Gunay I, Berisford MA, Mahler ME. A double-blind comparison of trazodone and haloperidol for treatment of agitation in patients with dementia. Am J Geriatr Psychiatry 1997;5(1):60–9.
5. Devanand DP, Marder K, Michaels KS, Sackeim HA, Bell K, Sullivan MA, Cooper TB, Pelton GH, Mayeux R. A randomized, placebo-controlled dose-comparison trial of haloperidol for psychosis and disruptive behaviors in Alzheimer's disease. Am J Psychiatry 1998;155(11):1512–20.
6. Hatta K, Takahashi T, Nakamura H, Yamashiro H, Asukai N, Matsuzaki I, Yonezawa Y. The association between intravenous haloperidol and prolonged QT interval. J Clin Psychopharmacol 2001;21(3):257–61.
7. Sharma ND, Rosman HS, Padhi ID, Tisdale JE. Torsades de pointes associated with intravenous haloperidol in critically ill patients. Am J Cardiol 1998;81(2):238–40.
8. Jackson T, Ditmanson L, Phibbs B. Torsade de pointes and low-dose oral haloperidol. Arch Intern Med 1997;157(17):2013–15.
9. LLerena A, Berecz R, de la Rubia A, Dorado P. QT_c interval lengthening and debrisoquine metabolic ratio in psychiatric patients treated with oral haloperidol monotherapy. Eur J Clin Pharmacol 2002;58(3):223–4.
10. Huyse F, van Schijndel RS. Haloperidol and cardiac arrest. Lancet 1988;2(8610):568–9.
11. Iwahashi K. Significantly higher plasma haloperidol level during cotreatment with carbamazepine may herald cardiac change. Clin Neuropharmacol 1996;19(3):267–70.
12. Douglas PH, Block PC. Corrected QT interval prolongation associated with intravenous haloperidol in acute coronary syndromes. Catheter Cardiovasc Interv 2000;50(3):352–5.
13. Iglesias E, Esteban E, Zabala S, Gascon A. Tiapride-induced torsade de pointes. Am J Med 2000;109(6):509.
14. Remijnse PL, Eeckhout AM, van Guldener C. Plotseling overlijden na eenmalige orale toediening van haloperidol. [Sudden death following a single oral administration of haloperidol.] Ned Tijdschr Geneeskd 2002;146(16):768–71.
15. Perrault LP, Denault AY, Carrier M, Cartier R, Belisle S. Torsades de pointes secondary to intravenous haloperidol after coronary bypass grafting surgery. Can J Anaesth 2000;47(3):251–4.
16. Johri S, Rashid H, Daniel PJ, Soni A. Cardiopulmonary arrest secondary to haloperidol. Am J Emerg Med 2000;18(7):839.
17. Mahutte CK, Nakasato SK, Light RW. Haloperidol and sudden death due to pulmonary edema. Arch Intern Med 1982;142(10):1951–2.
18. Sloane PD, McLeod MM. Radial nerve palsy in nursing home patients: association with immobility and haloperidol. J Am Geriatr Soc 1987;35(5):465–6.
19. Suenaga T, Tawara Y, Goto S, Kouhata SI, Kagaya A, Horiguchi J, Yamanaka Y, Yamawaki S. Risperidone treatment of neuroleptic-induced tardive extrapyramidal symptoms. Int J Psychiatry Clin Pract 2000;4:241–3.
20. Horiguchi J, Yamashita H, Mizuno S, Kuramoto Y, Kagaya A, Yamawaki S, Inami Y. Nocturnal eating/drinking syndrome and neuroleptic-induced restless legs syndrome. Int Clin Psychopharmacol 1999;14(1):33–6.
21. Neu P, Seyfert S, Brockmoller J, Dettling M, Marx P. Neuroleptic malignant syndrome in a patient with succinic semialdehyde dehydrogenase deficiency. Pharmacopsychiatry 2002;35(1):26–8.
22. Mihara K, Suzuki A, Kondo T, Yasui N, Furukori H, Nagashima U, Otani K, Kaneko S, Inoue Y. Effects of the CYP2D6*10 allele on the steady-state plasma concentrations of haloperidol and reduced haloperidol in Japanese patients with schizophrenia. Clin Pharmacol Ther 1999;65(3):291–4.
23. Kleinberg DL, Davis JM, de Coster R, Van Baelen B, Brecher M. Prolactin levels and adverse events in patients treated with risperidone. J Clin Psychopharmacol 1999;19(1):57–61.
24. Zarifian E, Scatton B, Bianchetti G, Cuche H, Loo H, Morselli PL. High doses of haloperidol in schizophrenia. A clinical, biochemical, and pharmacokinetic study. Arch Gen Psychiatry 1982;39(2):212–15.
25. Spitzer M, Sajjad R, Benjamin F. Pattern of development of hyperprolactinemia after initiation of haloperidol therapy. Obstet Gynecol 1998;91(5 Pt 1):693–5.
26. Feek CM, Sawers JS, Brown NS, Seth J, Irvine WJ, Toft AD. Influence of thyroid status on dopaminergic inhibition of thyrotropin and prolactin secretion: evidence for an additional feedback mechanism in the control of thyroid hormone secretion. J Clin Endocrinol Metab 1980;51(3):585–9.
27. Atmaca M, Kuloglu M, Tezcan E, Canatan H, Gecici O. Quetiapine is not associated with increase in prolactin secretion in contrast to haloperidol. Arch Med Res 2002;33(6):562–5.
28. Chae BJ, Kang BJ. The effect of clozapine on blood glucose metabolism. Hum Psychopharmacol 2001;16(3):265–71.
29. Ishak KG, Irey NS. Hepatic injury associated with the phenothiazines. Clinicopathologic and follow-up study of 36 patients. Arch Pathol 1972;93(4):283–304.

30. Dincsoy HP, Saelinger DA. Haloperidol-induced chronic cholestatic liver disease. Gastroenterology 1982;83(3):694–700.
31. Jeffries JJ, Lyall WA, Bezchlibnyk K, Papoff PM, Newman F. Retroperitoneal fibrosis and haloperidol. Am J Psychiatry 1982;139(11):1524–5.
32. Thami GP, Kaur S, Kanwar AJ. Delayed reactivation of haloperidol induced photosensitive dermatitis by methotrexate. Postgrad Med J 2002;78(916):116–17.
33. Arima Y, Iwata K, Hamasaki Y, Katayama I. A case of toxic epidermal necrolysis associated with two drugs. Nishinihon J Dermatol 2001;63:63–5.
34. Weiner DM, Lowe FC. Psychotropic drug-induced priapism: Incidence, mechanism and management. CNS Drugs 1998;9:371–9.
35. Michael A, Calloway SP. Priapism in twins. Pharmacopsychiatry 1999;32(4):157.
36. Tsai SJ, Hong CJ. Haloperidol-induced impotence improved by switching to olanzapine. Gen Hosp Psychiatry 2000;22(5):391–2.
37. Kopelman AE, McCullar FW, Heggeness L. Limb malformations following maternal use of haloperidol. JAMA 1975;231(1):62–4.
38. Austin MP, Mitchell PB. Psychotropic medications in pregnant women: treatment dilemmas. Med J Aust 1998;169(8):428–31.
39. Cohen LS, Rosenbaum JF. Psychotropic drug use during pregnancy: weighing the risks. J Clin Psychiatry 1998;59(Suppl 2):18–28.
40. Coyle I, Wayner MJ, Singer G. Behavioral teratogenesis: a critical evaluation. Pharmacol Biochem Behav 1976;4(2):191–200.
41. Mohan MS, Patole SK, Whitehall JS. Severe hypothermia in a neonate following antenatal exposure to haloperidol. J Paediatr Child Health 2000;36(4):412–13.
42. Kaminer Y, Apter A, Tyano S, Livni E, Wijsenbeek H. Delayed hypersensitivity reaction to orally administered methylparaben. Clin Pharm 1982;1(5):469–70.
43. Morselli PL. Further observations on the interaction between ethanol and psychotropic drugs. Arzneimittelforschung 1971;2:20.
44. Risch SC, Groom GP, Janowsky DS. The effects of psychotropic drugs on the cardiovascular system. J Clin Psychiatry 1982;43(5 Pt 2):16–31.
45. Iwahashi K, Miyatake R, Suwaki H, Hosokawa K, Ichikawa Y. The drug–drug interaction effects of haloperidol on plasma carbamazepine levels. Clin Neuropharmacol 1995;18(3):233–6.
46. Allen SA. Effect of chlorpromazine and clozapine on plasma concentrations of haloperidol in a patient with schizophrenia. J Clin Pharmacol 2000;40(11):1296–7.
47. Yasui N, Kondo T, Otani K, Furukori H, Mihara K, Suzuki A, Kaneko S, Inoue Y. Effects of itraconazole on the steady-state plasma concentrations of haloperidol and its reduced metabolite in schizophrenic patients: in vivo evidence of the involvement of CYP3A4 for haloperidol metabolism. J Clin Psychopharmacol 1999;19(2):149–54.
48. Bond WS, Carvalho M, Foulks EF. Persistent dysarthria with apraxia associated with a combination of lithium carbonate and haloperidol. J Clin Psychiatry 1982;43(6):256–7.
49. Ellman JP. Sudden death. Can J Psychiatry 1982;27(4):331–3.
50. Thornton WE. Dementia induced by methyldopa with haloperidol. N Engl J Med 1976;294(22):1222.
51. Ranjan S, Jagadheesan K, Nizamie SH. Cerebellar ataxia with intravenous valproate and haloperidol. Aust NZ J Psychiatry 2002;36(2):268.
52. Yasui N, Kondo T, Suzuki A, Otani K, Mihara K, Furukori H, Kaneko S, Inoue Y. Lack of significant pharmacokinetic interaction between haloperidol and grapefruit juice. Int Clin Psychopharmacol 1999;14(2):113–18.
53. Pan L, Vander Stichele R, Rosseel MT, Berlo JA, De Schepper N, Belpaire FM. Effects of smoking, CYP2D6 genotype, and concomitant drug intake on the steady state plasma concentrations of haloperidol and reduced haloperidol in schizophrenic inpatients. Ther Drug Monit 1999;21(5):489–97.

Halothane

See also General anesthetics

General Information

Halothane is a non-inflammable hydrocarbon that induces anesthesia, with little tendency to excitement. Contrary to earlier assumptions, halothane is metabolized, the consequences of which are discussed below (1,2).

Organs and Systems

Cardiovascular

Halothane, isoflurane, and sevoflurane are potent coronary vasodilators, able to produce some degree of coronary steal in ischemic regions. Despite this, halothane may preferentially dilate large coronary arteries and/or interfere with platelet aggregation. If these experimental effects are confirmed, halothane may be the anesthetic of choice in the non-failing ischemic heart (3).

Halothane has a mild depressive effect on cardiac performance (4). In human ventricular myocardium, halothane interacted with L-type calcium channels by interfering with the dihydropyridine binding site; this may, at least in part, explain its negative inotropic effect (5).

Halothane depressed cardiovascular function significantly more than isoflurane in younger adults, but the falls in systolic and diastolic blood pressures in elderly patients were significantly greater with isoflurane (6).

Cardiac dysrhythmias

Halothane produces bradycardia, but dysrhythmias, most often ventricular in origin, also occur during maintenance of anesthesia. They were noted in 53% of 679 patients (7). Concomitant administration of catecholamines increases the risk of dysrhythmias.

Bundle branch block and aberrant conduction were noted in children during halothane anesthesia (8).

In a double-blind, randomized, controlled study of 77 children undergoing halothane anesthesia for adenoidectomy, the effects of atropine 0.02 mg/kg, glycopyrrolate 0.04 mg/kg, and physiological saline were compared (9). There was no difference in the incidence of ventricular dysrhythmias. Atropine prevented bradycardia but was associated with sinus tachycardia in most patients. The bradycardias that occurred in the groups that received glycopyrrolate or placebo were short-lived and resolved spontaneously.

Pulsus alternans in association with hypercapnia occurred in a study of 120 patients who breathed spontaneously during halothane anesthesia (10). End-tidal carbon dioxide concentration was allowed to rise freely until pulsus alternans or other cardiac dysrhythmias occurred. Ten of the patients developed pulsus alternans, which was promptly relieved on institution of positive pressure ventilation and the return of end-tidal carbon dioxide concentration to normal. The mechanism and the significance of this phenomenon are not well understood.

Respiratory

Halothane is not irritant to the respiratory tract. Respiratory depression is a consequence only of high concentrations of halothane. A certain degree of bronchodilatation is observed, and may explain the fact that a beneficial effect of halothane was described in a 17-year-old woman with acute severe asthma who did not respond to conventional treatment (11).

Preterm infants can become apneic during the immediate postoperative period, even if the ventilatory response to CO_2 is not depressed after halothane anesthesia (12). In a prospective study in 167 preterm infants after inguinal herniorrhaphy with halothane/nitrous oxide anesthesia, only one had an episode of apnea up to 2 days postoperatively; however, the authors recommended careful monitoring until complete recovery from anesthesia has occurred (13).

Nervous system

In contrast to enflurane, cerebral irritability is very rare with halothane (14).

Halothane can cause an increase in intracranial pressure (15), as can other inhalational anesthetics, which can constitute a particular risk if the pressure is already raised before anesthesia. In neonates, the intracranial pressure may fall (16).

A child who underwent induction of anesthesia with halothane developed hiccups associated with pulmonary edema (17).

- An 8-year-old girl with a history of seizures and cerebral ischemic strokes secondary to moyamoya disease underwent anesthetic induction with halothane and 70% nitrous oxide. She had had three previous uneventful anesthetics. Hiccups started within seconds of induction of anesthesia and did not cease until 20 minutes later, when she was paralysed, intubated, and ventilated. During the next 20 minutes a period of hemodynamic instability ensued, with increasing oxygen requirements. The procedure was stopped and pulmonary edema was confirmed on chest X-ray. The child was transferred to the intensive care unit and ventilated overnight. Further recovery was uneventful.

Hiccups during anesthesia are often thought to be benign. Negative pressure pulmonary edema is usually associated with an obstructed airway, as occurs with laryngospasm, or other causes of upper airway obstruction, but was presumably the cause in this child.

The effect of increasing and decreasing concentrations of halothane on the cerebral circulation in 11 young children (aged 4 months to 3.5 years) undergoing minor urological surgery under general relaxant and caudal anesthesia has been studied (18). Cerebral blood flow velocity was measured in the middle cerebral artery using transcranial Doppler ultrasound. There was significantly increased cerebral blood flow velocity when the dose was increased from 0.5 to 1.0 minimum alveolar concentration (MAC) and from 0.5 to 1.5 MAC, but not when it was increased from 1.0 to 1.5 MAC. When the halothane concentration was reduced from 1.5 to 1.0 MAC, cerebral blood flow velocity fell significantly, whereas there was no effect when the concentration was reduced from 1.0 to 0.5 MAC. These results suggest that there is cerebrovascular hysteresis in response to increasing and decreasing concentrations of halothane.

Psychological, psychiatric

Slight depression of mood, lasting up to 30 days, along with a non-specific slowing of the electroencephalogram for 1–2 weeks, was observed after halothane. In 16 healthy young men, halothane anesthesia had negative effects on postoperative mood and intellectual function, the changes being greatest 2 days after anesthesia, with restoration of function after 8 days (19). In seven subjects, serial electroencephalography, serum bromide determinations, and psychological tests before and after halothane anesthesia showed that there was significant psychological impairment 2 days after anesthesia (20).

The effect of a single preoperative dose of the opioid oxycodone on emergence behavior has been studied in a randomized trial in 130 children (21). Oxycodone prophylaxis, compared with no premedication, significantly reduced the incidence of post-halothane agitation.

Mineral balance

Halothane can cause an increase in circulating concentrations of bromide and fluoride (20), which can be associated with impaired urine-concentrating ability in response to antidiuretic hormone (22).

Hematologic

Halothane produced inhibition of in vitro platelet aggregation and an increase in bleeding time (23).

Gastrointestinal

Postoperative nausea and vomiting can occur after halothane anesthesia (24). In one series, postoperative vomiting occurred in 13 of 29 patients who had received halothane for induction, but when dyxirazine was added during anesthesia the incidence of postoperative vomiting was significantly reduced (three of 29 patients) (25).

Liver

The greatest disadvantage of halothane is its ability to cause liver damage (26).

Incidence

The death rate due to halothane-induced liver damage was estimated in 1993 at one in 35 000 anesthetics (27), three times greater than the one in 110 000 incidence reported in 1976 (28). Both immune function and the metabolism of halothane play important roles in the pathophysiology of liver damage (29). Human hepatic microsomal carboxylesterase is a target antigen in halothane hepatitis, protein disulfide isomerase is an important factor in the mechanism of liver impairment, and an associated immune response may be involved (SEDA-18, 116). So-called halothane-induced liver antigens are novel antigens found in the livers of some individuals who have been exposed to halothane, but not in the livers of unexposed individuals (30).

A retrospective review of the case-notes of 44 patients with drug-induced hepatotoxicity diagnosed in 1978–96 found only one case attributable to halothane (31). Antibiotics, non-steroidal anti-inflammatory drugs, and psychotropic drugs accounted for 73% of the cases.

Mechanisms

The mechanisms by which halothane causes hepatic toxicity have been reviewed (32). Oxidative metabolism of halothane to trifluoroacetate occurs in the liver, probably via CYP2E1. In rats, trifluoroacetylated CYP2E1 has been identified after exposure to halothane, as has antibody formation to this antigen (33). Covalent binding of halothane (34), after its activation to the trifluoroacetyl halide, to proteins in human liver microsomes has also been shown (35). It has been suggested that some genetic factor determines the risk of developing halothane hepatitis (36). A report of halothane hepatitis in three pairs of closely related women (37) raised the possibility of a pharmacogenetic defect in these patients, with increased production of hepatotoxic metabolites.

Most recorded cases of liver disorders occurred after either repeated exposure (38) or prolonged exposure (39) to halothane. In one case, hepatitis developed 3 weeks after a single halothane anesthetic in a 37-year-old renal transplant recipient who had previously been exposed to isoflurane (40); this report suggests that previous exposure to isoflurane may predispose to subsequent halothane toxicity.

Halothane also reduces liver blood flow during anesthesia, and this could increase the release of potentially hepatotoxic halothane metabolites. The role of reduced halothane metabolites and inorganic fluoride, which may covalently link to liver macromolecules, has been stressed; in keeping with this hypothesis is the observation of halothane hepatitis in patients who simultaneously take enzyme-inducing agents, for example barbiturates (41) or rifampicin (42).

It is therefore tempting to suggest that patients with one or several predisposing factors, for example a pharmacogenetic trait, hepatic hypoxia, or enzyme induction, are likely to produce large amounts of hepatotoxic halothane metabolites that covalently bind to liver macromolecules, rendering them immunogenic. The finding that repeated administration increases the risk of halothane jaundice (43,44) supports this hypothesis.

Presentation

Two patterns of liver damage associated with halothane have been observed (45). One pattern is a mild derangement of liver enzymes, which occurs in about one in four anesthetics. The other pattern is rare but is associated with severe hepatitis, often resulting in fulminant liver failure. This severe form occurs more often in middle-aged, obese women, usually after multiple anesthetics, and is known as halothane hepatitis. It is defined as unexplained severe liver damage occurring within 28 days of halothane exposure in a person with a previously normal liver, and it occurs in 1:35 000 halothane exposures. With repeated exposure to halothane within 1 month, the frequency of acute liver failure increases to 1:3700. The overall incidence of halothane hepatitis is falling, owing to reduced use of halothane. Survival after liver transplantation in patients with fulminant hepatic failure is lower than that after liver transplantation for other reasons.

A case of halothane hepatitis has been reported in a child (46).

- A 6-year-old boy sustained pelvic injuries and a femoral fracture. The first anesthetic he received consisted of thiopental, suxamethonium, isoflurane, and nitrous oxide. He also received two units of blood. He subsequently underwent four halothane anesthetics over 6 weeks for dilatation of a urethral stricture. Two days after the last anesthetic he was noted to be jaundiced. He had a negative viral screen but was positive for antitrifluoroacetyl IgG antibodies. He developed fulminant hepatic failure with grade 2 hepatic encephalopathy and underwent an auxiliary liver transplantation 24 days after his last exposure to halothane. He died of septicemia 18 days later. Both at autopsy and on a previous hepatobiliary scan he was noted to have had extensive native liver regeneration.

Halothane hepatitis in children is rare, and occurs in 1:82 000 to 1:200 000 exposures. Children as young as 11 months are not exempt from the risk, contrary to what was once thought and there is a growing number of reports of halothane hepatitis in children (47). It has been noted that sevoflurane is not metabolized to trifluoroacetic acid and may prove to be a better alternative for repeated anesthesia in children (48).

A retrospective review of the case-notes of 44 patients with drug-induced hepatotoxicity diagnosed in 1978–96 found only one case attributable to halothane (31). Antibiotics, non-steroidal anti-inflammatory drugs, and psychotropic drugs accounted for 73% of the cases.

Urinary tract

Renal blood flow, glomerular filtration rate, and urinary volume are sometimes mildly and reversibly reduced. In contrast, repeated massive polyuria has been reported in a 46-year-old man after two anesthetics with halothane (49). Acute renal insufficiency has been described (50) but is rare.

Skin

A young nurse complained of a skin rash with edema of the eyelids after repeated professional exposure to halothane (51).

Immunologic

Halothane can suppress host defence mechanisms; the clinical consequences are unclear (SED-11, 210) (SEDA-3, 101) (SEDA-4, 77) (SEDA-5, 121) (SEDA-11, 109).

Body temperature

Halothane reduces body temperature and can cause shivering, although active thermoregulation does not occur until the core temperature is reduced by 2.5°C (52). The shivering can be attenuated by flumazenil, despite a lower core temperature (53).

Halothane in association with suxamethonium is the most frequent cause of malignant hyperthermia attributed to general anesthesia (54). Standard in vitro caffeine-halothane contracture testing was performed on 32 patients with a past history of malignant hyperthermia diagnosed on clinical grounds; they were compared with a matched control group of 120 subjects who were considered clinically to be at low risk of malignant hyperthermia (55). The sensitivity of the test was 97% and the specificity 78%.

Second-Generation Effects

Pregnancy

Halothane strongly reduces uterine contractility during labor (56).

Fetotoxicity

Halothane can be used as an anesthetic by maternal inhalation for fetal surgery and improves surgical exposure by relaxing the uterus. However, the effects of halothane on fetal cardiovascular homeostasis have been evaluated, and the authors concluded that halothane had a significant negative effect on the fetal heart and peripheral vasculature; it was therefore considered a poor anesthetic for this purpose (57).

Lactation

Halothane is readily excreted into breast milk (58).

Drug Administration

Drug administration route

In a randomized, double-blind, placebo-controlled comparison of intranasal and intramuscular atropine in 80 children, the intranasal route was equally effective at preventing halothane-induced bradycardia (59).

Drug overdose

Suicide attempts with halothane have sometimes succeeded, but in patients who recovered there was no residual damage. A 4-year-old boy was accidentally given halothane intravenously; he recovered fully within a few hours (60). Accidental intravenous injection and illicit inhalation have both caused pulmonary edema (61).

Drug–Drug Interactions

Disulfiram

Disulfiram is an inhibitor of CYP2E1. In 20 patients undergoing halothane-based maintenance of anesthesia at an end-tidal concentration of 1% for an average of 3 hours, disulfiram 500 mg taken the night before substantially attenuated trifluoroacetate production, as judged by its urinary excretion (62). It was suggested that a single dose of disulfiram may provide effective prophylaxis against halothane hepatitis.

Non-depolarizing muscle relaxants

Halothane potentiates the effects of non-depolarizing muscular relaxants (SED-11, 210) (63).

References

1. Weis KH, Engelhardt W. Is halothane obsolete? Two standards of judgement. Anaesthesia 1989;44(2):97–100.
2. Pedersen T, Johansen SH. Serious morbidity attributable to anaesthesia. Considerations for prevention. Anaesthesia 1989;44(6):504–8.
3. Merin RG. Physiology, pathophysiology and pharmacology of the coronary circulation with particular emphasis on anesthetics. Anaesthesiol Reanim 1992;17(1):5–26.
4. Maze M, Mason DM. Aetiology and treatment of halothane-induced arrhythmias. Clin Anaesthesiol 1983;1:301.
5. Schmidt U, Schwinger RH, Bohm S, Uberfuhr P, Kreuzer E, Reichart B, Meyer L, Erdmann E, Bohm M. Evidence for an interaction of halothane with the L-type Ca^{2+} channel in human myocardium. Anesthesiology 1993;79(2):332–9.
6. McKinney MS, Fee JP, Clarke RS. Cardiovascular effects of isoflurane and halothane in young and elderly adult patients. Br J Anaesth 1993;71(5):696–701.
7. Yokoyama K. Arrhythmias due to halothane anesthesia. Jpn J Anesthesiol 1978;27:64.
8. Lindgren L. E.C.G changes during halothane and enflurane anaesthesia for E.N.T. surgery in children. Br J Anaesth 1981;53(6):653–62.
9. Reinoso-Barbero F, Gutierrez-Marquez M, Diez-Labajo A. Prevention of halothane-induced bradycardia: is intranasal premedication indicated? Paediatr Anaesth 1998;8(3): 195–9.
10. Saghaei M, Mortazavian M. Pulsus alternans during general anesthesia with halothane: effects of permissive hypercapnia. Anesthesiology 2000;93(1):91–4.
11. Obata T, Masaki T, Nezu T, Iikura Y. Treatment of status asthmaticus with halothane: a case report. Iryo 1992;46: 204–10.
12. Palmisano BW, Setlock MA, Doyle MK, Rosner DR, Hoffman GM, Eckert JE. Ventilatory response to carbon dioxide in term infants after halothane and nitrous oxide anesthesia. Anesth Analg 1993;76(6):1234–7.
13. Haga S, Shima T, Momose K, Andoh K, Hoshi K, Hashimoto Y. [Postoperative apnea in preterm infants after inguinal herniorrhaphy.] Masui 1993;42(1):120–2.
14. Smith PA, Macdonald TR, Jones CS. Convulsions associated with halothane anaesthesia. Two case reports. Anaesthesia 1966;21(2):229–33.
15. Cunitz G, Danhauser I, Gruss P. Die Wirkung von Enflurane (Ethrane) im Vergleich zu Halothan auf den intracraniellen Druck. [Effect of enflurane (Ethrane) on intracranial pressure in comparison with halothane.] Anaesthesist 1976;25(7):323–30.
16. Friesen RH, Thieme RE, Honda AT, Morrison JE Jr. Changes in anterior fontanel pressure in preterm neonates receiving isoflurane, halothane, fentanyl, or ketamine. Anesth Analg 1987;66(5):431–4.

17. Stuth EA, Stucke AG, Berens RJ. Negative-pressure pulmonary edema in a child with hiccups during induction. Anesthesiology 2000;93(1):282–4.
18. Paut O, Bissonnette B. Effect of halothane on the cerebral circulation in young children: a hysteresis phenomenon. Anaesthesia 2001;56(4):360–5.
19. Davison LA, Steinhelber JC, Eger EI 2nd, Stevens WC. Psychological effects of halothane and isoflurane anesthesia. Anesthesiology 1975;43(3):313–24.
20. Bruchiel KJ, Stockard JJ, Calverley RK, Smith NT, Scholl ML, Mazze RI. Electroencephalographic abnormalities following halothane anesthesia. Anesth Analg 1978;57(2):244–51.
21. Neunteufl T, Berger R, Pacher R. Endothelin receptor antagonists in cardiology clinical trials. Expert Opin Investig Drugs 2002;11(3):431–43.
22. Mazze RI, Calverley RK, Smith NT. Inorganic fluoride nephrotoxicity: prolonged enflurane and halothane anesthesia in volunteers. Anesthesiology 1977;46(4):265–71.
23. Dalsgaard-Nielsen J, Risbo A, Simmelkjaer P, Gormsen J. Impaired platelet aggregation and increased bleeding time during general anaesthesia with halothane. Br J Anaesth 1981;53(10):1039–42.
24. Kenny GN. Risk factors for postoperative nausea and vomiting. Anaesthesia 1994;49(Suppl):6–10.
25. Karlsson E, Larsson LE, Nilsson K. The effects of prophylactic dixyrazine on postoperative vomiting after two different anaesthetic methods for squint surgery in children. Acta Anaesthesiol Scand 1993;37(1):45–8.
26. Feher J, Vasarhelyi B, Blazovics A. A halotan hepatitis. [Halothane hepatitis.] Orv Hetil 1993;134(33):1795–8.
27. Elliott RH, Strunin L. Hepatotoxicity of volatile anaesthetics. Br J Anaesth 1993;70(3):339–48.
28. Bottiger LE, Dalen E, Hallen B. Halothane-induced liver damage: an analysis of the material reported to the Swedish Adverse Drug Reaction Committee, 1966–1973. Acta Anaesthesiol Scand 1976;20(1):40–6.
29. Smith GC, Kenna JG, Harrison DJ, Tew D, Wolf CR. Autoantibodies to hepatic microsomal carboxylesterase in halothane hepatitis. Lancet 1993;342(8877):963–4.
30. Kenna JG, Knight TL, van Pelt FN. Immunity to halothane metabolite-modified proteins in halothane hepatitis. Ann NY Acad Sci 1993;685:646–61.
31. Aithal PG, Day CP. The natural history of histologically proved drug induced liver disease. Gut 1999;44(5):731–5.
32. Pumford NR, Halmes NC, Hinson JA. Covalent binding of xenobiotics to specific proteins in the liver. Drug Metab Rev 1997;29(1–2):39–57.
33. Eliasson E, Kenna JG. Cytochrome P450 2E1 is a cell surface autoantigen in halothane hepatitis. Mol Pharmacol 1996;50(3):573–82.
34. Nuscheler M, Conzen P, Schwender D, Peter K. Fluoridinduzierte Nephrotoxizität: Fakt oder Fiktion? [Fluoride-induced nephrotoxicity: factor fiction?] Anaesthesist 1996;45(Suppl 1):S32–40.
35. Madan A, Parkinson A. Characterization of the NADPH-dependent covalent binding of [^{14}C]halothane to human liver microsomes: a role for cytochrome P450 2E1 at low substrate concentrations. Drug Metab Dispos 1996;24(12):1307–13.
36. Ranek L, Dalhoff K, Poulsen HE, Brosen K, Flachs H, Loft S, Wantzin P. Drug metabolism and genetic polymorphism in subjects with previous halothane hepatitis. Scand J Gastroenterol 1993;28(8):677–80.
37. Hoft RH, Bunker JP, Goodman HI, Gregory PB. Halothane hepatitis in three pairs of closely related women. N Engl J Med 1981;304(17):1023–4.
38. Dahmash NS, Ayoola EA, Al-Nozha M. Halothane induced hepatotoxicity in a Saudi male. Ann Saudi Med 1993;13:314–16.
39. Shimizu H, Namba H, Ishima T. Liver dysfunction after halothane therapy in two cases with life threatening asthma. KoKyu 1993;12:229–32.
40. Slayter KL, Sketris IS, Gulanikar A. Halothane hepatitis in a renal transplant patient previously exposed to isoflurane. Ann Pharmacother 1993;27(1):101.
41. Bidard JM, Casio N, Gerolami A, et al.. Deux observations d'hépatite toxique par association d'halothane—un inducteur enzymatique. Nouv Presse Méd 1980;9:883.
42. Steiner F, Pottecher T, Bellocq JP. Ictère grave post opératoire: rôle de l'halothane et des tuberculostatiques. Cah Anesthesiol 1980;23:1019.
43. Fee JP, Black GW, Dundee JW, McIlroy PD, Johnston HM, Johnston SB, Black IH, McNeill HG, Neill DW, Doggart JR, Merrett JD, McDonald JR, Bradley DS, Haire M, McMillan SA. A prospective study of liver enzyme and other changes following repeat administration of halothane and enflurane. Br J Anaesth 1979;51(12):1133–41.
44. Schlippert W, Anuras S. Recurrent hepatitis following halothane exposures. Am J Med 1978;65(1):25–30.
45. Neuberger J. Halothane hepatitis. Eur J Gastroenterol Hepatol 1998;10(8):631–3.
46. Munro HM, Snider SJ, Magee JC. Halothane-associated hepatitis in a 6-year-old boy: evidence for native liver regeneration following failed treatment with auxiliary liver transplantation. Anesthesiology 1998;89(2):524–7.
47. Kenna JG, Neuberger J, Mieli-Vergani G, Mowat AP, Williams R. Halothane hepatitis in children. BMJ (Clin Res Ed) 1987;294(6581):1209–11.
48. Murat I. There is no longer a place for halothane in paediatric anaesthesia. Paediatr Anaesth 1998;8(2):184.
49. Dallera F, Caccialanza E, Segalini A, et al.. Un caso di poliuria probabilmente da fluotano. Acta Anaesthesiol Ital 1983;34:83.
50. Gelman ML, Lichtenstein NS. Halothane-induced nephrotoxicity. Urology 1981;17(4):323–7.
51. Bodman R. Skin sensitivity to halothane vapour. Br J Anaesth 1979;51(11):1092.
52. Sessler DI, Olofsson CI, Rubinstein EH, Beebe JJ. The thermoregulatory threshold in humans during halothane anesthesia. Anesthesiology 1988;68(6):836–42.
53. Weinbroum AA, Geller E. Flumazenil improves cognitive and neuromotor emergence and attenuates shivering after halothane-, enflurane- and isoflurane-based anesthesia. Can J Anaesth 2001;48(10):963–72.
54. Drury PM, Gilbertson AA. Malignant hyperpyrexia and anaesthesia. Two case reports. Br J Anaesth 1970;42(11): 1021–3.
55. Allen GC, Larach MG, Kunselman AR. The sensitivity and specificity of the caffeine-halothane contracture test: a report from the North American Malignant Hyperthermia Registry. The North American Malignant Hyperthermia Registry of MHAUS. Anesthesiology 1998;88(3):579–88.
56. Neumark J, Faller T. Halothan, Enfluran und ihr Einfluss auf die Uterusaktivität am Geburts-Termin. [The effects of halothane and enflurane on uterine activity during childbirth.] Prakt Anaesth 1978;13(1):7–12.
57. Sabik JF, Assad RS, Hanley FL. Halothane as an anesthetic for fetal surgery. J Pediatr Surg 1993;28(4):542–6.
58. Cote CJ, Kenepp NB, Reed SB, Strobel GE. Trace concentrations of halothane in human breast milk. Br J Anaesth 1976;48(6):541–3.
59. Annila P, Rorarius M, Reinikainen P, Oikkonen M, Baer G. Effect of pre-treatment with intravenous atropine or glycopyrrolate on cardiac arrhythmias during halothane anaesthesia for adenoidectomy in children. Br J Anaesth 1998;80(6):756–60.
60. Trombini Garcia R, Salomao JB, Benincasa SC, et al.. Instilagaio acidental de halotano em una crianca de quatro anos. J Pediatr 1984;56:323.

61. Martindale. The Extra Pharmacopoeia. London: Pharmaceutical Press, 1977.
62. Kharasch ED, Hankins D, Mautz D, Thummel KE. Identification of the enzyme responsible for oxidative halothane metabolism: implications for prevention of halothane hepatitis. Lancet 1996;347(9012):1367–71.
63. Hughes R, Payne JP. Interaction of halothane with non-depolarizing neuromuscular blocking drugs in man. BMJ 1979;2:1425.

Helicobacter pylori eradication regimens

General Information

Drugs and regimens for *Helicobacter pylori* eradication have been reviewed (1,2). The major factor in choosing an antibiotic regimen is the pattern of antibiotic resistance in the community. Generally two antimicrobial drugs plus bismuth or ranitidine or a proton pump inhibitor such as omeprazole are required to achieve a cure rate of over 90% and avoid the resistance that occurs when clarithromycin or metronidazole is the single antimicrobial used. In regions where metronidazole and clarithromycin resistance is common initial quadruple therapy with bismuth, metronidazole, tetracycline, and a proton pump inhibitor is recommended. In general, higher doses and longer duration of therapy are associated with better outcomes. Although therapy for 1 week has become accepted in first-line regimens, therapy for 2 weeks is better when treating nitroimidazole-resistant or clarithromycin-susceptible strains.

Adverse effects of these regimens are related to the individual drugs used.

Comparative studies

The MACH-2 study has assessed the role of omeprazole in triple therapy in 539 patients with duodenal ulcers associated with *H. pylori* (3). The addition of omeprazole resulted in significantly higher eradication rates (over 90%) than antibiotics alone (amoxicillin plus clarithromycin about 25%; clarithromycin plus metronidazole 70%), and reduced the impact of primary resistance to metronidazole. About one-third of the patients who took amoxicillin reported diarrhea/loose stools. The frequency of taste disturbance was dose-dependent with clarithromycin. Increased liver enzymes were more commonly reported in those taking metronidazole. The addition of omeprazole did not increase the frequency of reported adverse effects.

The DU-MACH study assessed the efficacy of two omeprazole-based triple therapies (omeprazole, amoxicillin, clarithromycin versus omeprazole, metronidazole, clarithromycin) given for 1 week to 149 patients for eradicating *H. pylori*, healing duodenal ulcers, and preventing ulcer relapse over 6 months after treatment (4). Both regimens achieved high eradication rates (about 90%) and were well tolerated. Adverse effects were similar in the two groups, and included diarrhea, taste disturbance, headache, nausea, and dyspepsia.

Ranitidine 300 mg bd and omeprazole 20 mg bd have been compared as components of triple therapies (combining them with either amoxicillin plus clarithromycin or amoxicillin plus metronidazole) in 320 patients with *H. pylori* (5). Omeprazole and ranitidine combined with two antibiotics for 1 week were equally effective in eradicating *H. pylori*. This result questions the role of profound acid suppression in eradication. There was no difference in the reported adverse effects, which included nausea, vomiting, diarrhea, metallic taste, skin rashes, and headache.

In a similar study in 221 patients with peptic ulcer disease associated with *H. pylori*, rabeprazole has been compared with omeprazole and lansoprazole (combining them with amoxicillin plus clarithromycin for 1 week) (6). Rabeprazole was as effective as omeprazole and lansoprazole in eradicating *H. pylori* (84–88% each). There were no differences in reported adverse events. Common adverse effects were soft stools, glossitis, taste disturbances, and skin rashes.

Dual therapy (omeprazole plus clarithromycin) for 2 weeks has been compared with triple therapy (omeprazole plus amoxicillin and clarithromycin) for 1 week in the eradication of *H. pylori* in 145 patients with duodenal ulcers (7). Triple therapy was significantly more effective in eradicating *H. pylori* (71 versus 48%). There were no significant differences in compliance or adverse effects. The most frequent adverse effects were metallic taste and nausea in the dual-therapy group and metallic taste, mild abdominal pain, and diarrhea in the triple-therapy group.

Quadruple therapy (omeprazole, amoxicillin, roxithromycin, and metronidazole for 1 week) has been studied in an open trial in 169 patients with *H. pylori* (8). This regimen achieved an eradication rate of 92%. It was also beneficial in patients infected with pretreatment resistant strains to the antibiotics, in which cases the eradication rates achieved (over 90%) were similar to eradication rates in patients infected with sensitive strains. Compliance was good and there was only one serious adverse effect, anaphylaxis, probably due to amoxicillin. Frequent adverse effects were abdominal distension (10%), glossitis (9%), and diarrhea (8%).

Sucralfate 1 g tds in combination with amoxicillin 500 mg tds and clarithromycin 400 mg bd for 2 weeks was as effective as a combination of lansoprazole 30 mg bd plus amoxicillin 500 mg tds and clarithromycin 400 mg bd for 2 weeks for *H. pylori* eradication in a randomized, multicenter trial in 150 patients (9). There was no significant difference in adverse effects between the two groups. Diarrhea, abdominal pain, glossitis, and taste disturbance were the adverse effects commonly reported.

In an open trial, 7-day triple therapy with omeprazole 30 mg bd, amoxicillin 500 mg tds, and clarithromycin 400 mg bd was safe and effective in eradicating *H. pylori* in 12 of 13 patients undergoing hemodialysis (10). There were adverse effects in two patients (compared with three of 27 patients not undergoing hemodialysis) and treatment had to be discontinued in one, owing to severe nausea and vomiting.

Placebo-controlled studies

The effect of eradicating *H. pylori* in 20 patients with chronic idiopathic urticaria has been assessed in a randomized, placebo-controlled trial (11). After 7 days of treatment with omeprazole 20 mg bd, amoxicillin 500 mg bd, and clarithromycin 500 mg bd *H. pylori* was eradicated in nine of 10 patients (compared with three of 10 in the placebo group) and there was a significant improvement in urticaria in four of these nine (compared with one of the seven in whom *H. pylori* was not eradicated). No serious adverse effects were reported in either treatment group.

In a randomized, controlled trial in 120 patients supplementation with inactivated *Lactobacillus acidophilus* tds significantly improved the efficacy of a standard 7-day regimen with rabeprazole 20 mg bd, clarithromycin 250 mg tds, and amoxicillin 500 mg tds (12). There was no significant difference in adverse effects between the two groups. Those reported were abdominal pain, nausea, and diarrhea.

In a randomized, placebo-controlled trial in 60 healthy, asymptomatic subjects who screened positive for *H. pylori*, supplementation with *Lactobacillus* GG twice daily for 14 days significantly reduced the adverse effects (diarrhea, nausea, taste disturbance) and improved the overall tolerability of a standard 7-day eradication regimen consisting of rabeprazole 20 mg bd, clarithromycin 500 mg bd, and tinidazole 500 mg bd (13).

Organs and Systems

Gastrointestinal

Pseudomembranous colitis has been reported in an 86-year-old woman with non-ulcer dyspepsia a few days after she had taken triple eradication therapy (omeprazole 20 mg bd, metronidazole 400 mg tds, and clarithromycin 500 mg bd); she recovered after treatment with oral vancomycin (14).

Susceptibility Factors

Age

The efficacy of triple therapy with bismuth plus amoxicillin and metronidazole has been assessed in an open trial in 26 children with duodenal ulcers associated with *H. pylori* (15). *Helicobacter pylori* was eradicated in 25 children and the ulcer was healed in 24. During a mean follow-up of nearly 2 years, the annual ulcer relapse rate was 9% (compared with 56% in historical controls, in whom the infection was not eradicated). Adverse events were reported by 13% of the children, and included diarrhea, dizziness, nausea, and vomiting.

Triple therapy with bismuth plus amoxicillin and metronidazole for 2 weeks has been compared with dual therapy with omeprazole plus amoxicillin for 2 weeks in 126 patients over the age of 60 years, who were *H. pylori* positive and had functional dyspepsia (16). Eradication rates were similar in the two groups 2 months after the end of therapy (66% with triple therapy and 64% with dual therapy), and there was a significant reduction in dyspeptic symptoms in patients in whom *H. pylori* was eradicated compared with those in whom infection persisted. Adverse effects were reported by 15% of patients who took triple therapy (nausea and metallic taste) compared with 4% of those who took dual therapy (nausea and headache). In all cases no adverse effect was severe enough to interrupt therapy.

Drug Administration

Drug dosage regimens

The effect of adding adherence-enhancing measures to triple therapy with omeprazole plus amoxicillin and metronidazole for 10 days has been studied in 119 Australian patients with *H. pylori* infection (17). The adherence-enhancing measures were:

- the provision of the medication in a dose-dispensing unit;
- the use of a medication chart;
- the provision of an information sheet about the treatment;
- a reminder by telephone 2 days after the start of therapy.

Ten days of triple therapy was effective for *H. pylori* eradication (85–90%) and patient adherence was excellent in both groups (97%). Attempts to improve adherence had no impact on outcome and adverse effects were common and were significantly associated with treatment failure and poor adherence to therapy in both groups. There were no significant differences in the adverse effects profiles. Female sex predicted more adverse effects. Two patients reported severe adverse effects, 19 reported moderate adverse effects, and 75 reported mild adverse effects. Common adverse effects included anorexia and nausea (35%), vomiting (7%), constipation (16%), diarrhea/flatulence (37%), abdominal pain/cramps (27%), a metallic taste (44%), headache/dizziness (48%), rash/itch (3%), lethargy/confusion (9%), and insomnia/agitation (4%). The authors attributed the unusually high prevalence of adverse effects to comprehensive reporting.

References

1. Goodwin CS. Antimicrobial treatment of *Helicobacter pylori* infection. Clin Infect Dis 1997;25(5):1023–6.
2. Nakajima S, Graham DY, Hattori T, Bamba T. Strategy for treatment of *Helicobacter pylori* infection in adults. II. Practical policy in 2000 Curr Pharm Des 2000;6(15): 1515–29.
3. Lind T, Megraud F, Unge P, Bayerdorffer E, O'morain C, Spiller R, Veldhuyzen Van Zanten S, Bardhan KD, Hellblom M, Wrangstadh M, Zeijlon L, Cederberg C. The MACH2 study: role of omeprazole in eradication of *Helicobacter pylori* with 1-week triple therapies. Gastroenterology 1999;116(2):248–53.
4. Zanten SJ, Bradette M, Farley A, Leddin D, Lind T, Unge P, Bayerdorffer E, Spiller RC, O'Morain C, Sipponen P, Wrangstadh M, Zeijlon L, Sinclair P. The DU-MACH study: eradication of *Helicobacter pylori* and ulcer healing in patients with acute duodenal ulcer using

omeprazole based triple therapy. Aliment Pharmacol Ther 1999;13(3):289–95.
5. Savarino V, Zentilin P, Bisso G, Pivari M, Mele MR, Mela GS, Mansi C, Vigneri S, Termini R, Celle G. Head-to-head comparison of 1-week triple regimens combining ranitidine or omeprazole with two antibiotics to eradicate *Helicobacter pylori.* Aliment Pharmacol Ther 1999;13(5):643–9.
6. Miwa H, Ohkura R, Murai T, Sato K, Nagahara A, Hirai S, Watanabe S, Sato N. Impact of rabeprazole, a new proton pump inhibitor, in triple therapy for *Helicobacter pylori* infection—comparison with omeprazole and lansoprazole. Aliment Pharmacol Ther 1999;13(6):741–6.
7. Calvet X, Lopez-Lorente M, Cubells M, Bare M, Galvez E, Molina E. Two-week dual vs. one-week triple therapy for cure of *Helicobacter pylori* infection in primary care: a multicentre, randomized trial. Aliment Pharmacol Ther 1999;13(6):781–6.
8. Okada M, Nishimura H, Kawashima M, Okabe N, Maeda K, Seo M, Ohkuma K, Takata T. A new quadruple therapy for *Helicobacter pylori*: influence of resistant strains on treatment outcome. Aliment Pharmacol Ther 1999;13(6):769–74.
9. Adachi K, Ishihara S, Hashimoto T, Hirakawa K, Niigaki M, Takashima T, Kaji T, Kawamura A, Sato H, Okuyama T, Watanabe M, Kinoshita Y. Efficacy of sucralfate for *Helicobacter pylori* eradication triple therapy in comparison with a lansoprazole-based regimen. Aliment Pharmacol Ther 2000;14(7):919–22.
10. Tsukada K, Miyazaki T, Katoh H, Masuda N, Ojima H, Fukai Y, Nakajima M, Manda R, Fukuchi M, Kuwano H, Tsukada O. Seven-day triple therapy with omeprazole, amoxycillin and clarithromycin for *Helicobacter pylori* infection in haemodialysis patients. Scand J Gastroenterol 2002;37(11):1265–8.
11. Gaig P, Garcia-Ortega P, Enrique E, Papo M, Quer JC, Richard C. Efficacy of the eradication of *Helicobacter pylori* infection in patients with chronic urticaria. A placebo-controlled double blind study. Allergol Immunopathol (Madr) 2002;30(5):255–8.
12. Canducci F, Armuzzi A, Cremonini F, Cammarota G, Bartolozzi F, Pola P, Gasbarrini G, Gasbarrini A. A lyophilized and inactivated culture of *Lactobacillus acidophilus* increases *Helicobacter pylori* eradication rates. Aliment Pharmacol Ther 2000;14(12):1625–9.
13. Armuzzi A, Cremonini F, Bartolozzi F, Canducci F, Candelli M, Ojetti V, Cammarota G, Anti M, De Lorenzo A, Pola P, Gasbarrini G, Gasbarrini A. The effect of oral administration of *Lactobacillus GG* on antibiotic-associated gastrointestinal side-effects during *Helicobacter pylori* eradication therapy. Aliment Pharmacol Ther 2001;15(2):163–9.
14. Harsch IA, Hahn EG, Konturek PC. Pseudomembranous colitis after eradication of *Helicobacter pylori* infection with a triple therapy. Med Sci Monit 2001;7(4):751–4.
15. Huang FC, Chang MH, Hsu HY, Lee PI, Shun CT. Long-term follow-up of duodenal ulcer in children before and after eradication of *Helicobacter pylori.* J Pediatr Gastroenterol Nutr 1999;28(1):76–80.
16. Catalano F, Branciforte G, Brogna A, Bentivegna C, Luca S, Terranova R, Michalos A, Dawson BK, Chodash HB. *Helicobacter pylori*-positive functional dyspepsia in elderly patients: comparison of two treatments. Dig Dis Sci 1999;44(5):863–7.
17. Henry A, Batey RG. Enhancing compliance not a prerequisite for effective eradication of *Helicobacter pylori*: the HelP Study. Am J Gastroenterol 1999;94(3):811–15.

Hemin and heme arginate

General Information

Hemin (hematin), an exogenous source of heme, is used to treat acute intermittent porphyria and other hepatic porphyrias. It is generally well tolerated in the recommended doses, although thrombophlebitis, coagulation defects, circulatory collapse, and occasional renal insufficiency have been reported (1).

Thrombophlebitis is seen in up to 10% of patients, and this effect, as well as effects on coagulation (prolongation of the prothrombin and thromboplastin times, increased fibrin degradation products, and thrombocytopenia), may be caused by degradation products of hemin (2). There is evidence that slower infusion rates reduce the risk of adverse effects (3).

Heme arginate is more stable than hemin, but it is still not established whether its adverse effects (thrombophlebitis, anaphylaxis, and psychosis) (4) are fewer and whether its therapeutic effect is better than that of hemin (5).

References

1. Khanderia U. Circulatory collapse associated with hemin therapy for acute intermittent porphyria. Clin Pharm 1986;5(8):690–2.
2. Mustajoki P, Tenhunen R, Pierach C, Volin L. Heme in the treatment of porphyrias and hematological disorders. Semin Hematol 1989;26(1):1–9.
3. Simionatto CS, Cabal R, Jones RL, Galbraith RA. Thrombophlebitis and disturbed hemostasis following administration of intravenous hematin in normal volunteers. Am J Med 1988;85(4):538–40.
4. Kostrzewska E, Gregor A, Tarczynska-Nosal S. Heme arginate (Normosang) in the treatment of attacks of acute hepatic porphyrias. Mater Med Pol 1991;23(4):259–62.
5. Herrick AL, McColl KE, Moore MR, Cook A, Goldberg A. Controlled trial of haem arginate in acute hepatic porphyria. Lancet 1989;1(8650):1295–7.

Hemostatic compounds, miscellaneous

General Information

A number of compounds that have, or supposedly have, hemostatic activity are reviewed here. Some of them are obsolete and are included largely for historical interest. Others, such as fibrin glue, are still in use.

Aminaphtone

Experiments in the 1970s with aminaphtone (2-hydroxy-3-methyl-1,4-naphthohydroquinone-2-*p*-aminobenzoate) suggested that it could significantly shorten the bleeding time in both normal and heparinized rabbits and mice (1). Subsequent clinical experiments showed no adverse effects and toxicological studies in animals showed no evidence of acute or long-term toxicity, even at quite high doses (1). No adverse effects were noted when patients who had initially been involved in an efficacy study of limited duration were treated with aminaphtone for a further year (2). No data are available on the absorption or metabolism of aminaphtone in humans. It has been claimed that aminaphtone may improve symptoms related to chronic venous insufficiency as well as lymphatic stasis (3).

Carbazochrome and carbazochrome salicylate

Adrenochrome, an oxidation product of adrenaline, is stabilized by binding to monosemicarbazone (adrenochrome monosemicarbazide). Its solubility is greatly enhanced by combination with sodium salicylate. The product, carbazochrome salicylate, can be given either by intramuscular injection or orally. The solution for intramuscular injection is hypertonic, and patients usually experience a brief stinging pain at the site of injection. Experiments in animals have shown a significant reduction in normal bleeding time when adrenochrome monosemicarbazide is given (4). This has been attributed to a direct effect on capillaries, as increased capillary resistance has been observed in experimental animals. Despite documentation of a transient reduction in bleeding time in humans in early experiments in the 1940s, subsequent double-blind controlled trials did not identify a useful reduction in blood loss after surgery (5–8). Despite the similarity to adrenaline, it is remarkably non-toxic and administration is not associated with the general systemic effects of sympathomimetic drugs (such as tachycardia, anxiety, or hypertension).

Fibrin glue

Fibrin glue is a topical biological adhesive, the effect of which imitates the final stages of coagulation. It contains two separate components, fibrinogen plus factor XIII, and thrombin plus calcium chloride. It is covered in a separate monograph.

5-Hydroxytryptamine creatinine sulfate

Platelets contain serotonin (5-hydroxytryptamine), which they take up from the plasma and store in dense granules. The serotonin is released when platelets are activated. Although serotonin was originally believed to play a vital part in platelet aggregation, it is now known that it does not, although it can contribute to local vasoconstriction. Treatment with reserpine induces depletion of serotonin in platelets, but this is not associated with any bleeding tendency (9). Nevertheless, belief in the importance of serotonin in hemostasis stimulated the search for analogues that might prove to be useful hemostatic agents, and 2-(5-hydroxy-3-indolyl) ethylamine creatinine sulfate was proposed as a hemostatic agent. However, subsequent clinical studies offered no evidence of benefit. Vertigo and tachycardia were reported in some patients who received the drug by rapid intravenous injection (10).

Naftazone

Naftazone (beta-naphthoquinone semicarbazone) is prepared by diazotization of sulfonic acid with beta-naphthol, and its properties are similar to those of adrenochrome. Naftazone significantly reduces the normal bleeding time as well as blood loss in rabbits and dogs. In many ways, this drug resembles adrenochrome, but it may in addition have certain effects at the cellular level. A double-blind, controlled study in patients undergoing prostatectomy reported significantly lower blood loss and transfusion requirements in the subjects receiving naftazone (11). No significant adverse effects were reported, but 4% of patients complained of transient and moderate nausea and gastric pain in a multicenter study of the efficacy and tolerance of naftazone in which two dosage regimens were compared (12).

Pectin

Pectin is a carbohydrate found in fruits, and is particularly rich in the rind of citrus fruits and in apples. It is a gelling agent and contributes to the solidification of jams. A formulation of pectin called Sangostop® was introduced as a hemostatic agent in 1935, and it was claimed that it could reduce bleeding in a variety of conditions. The active component consisted of colloidal polygalacturonic acid esters from apple pectin. It was given in a variety of ways: locally, orally, by subcutaneous or intravenous injection, or per rectum. The solution for local and oral use contained 5% pectin (3% for the preparation for intravenous administration). Several published reports from the 1930s claimed that pectin had a hemostatic effect, but these were based purely on subjective clinical judgement. Randomized controlled trials, with quantification of blood loss, have never been carried out.

It is clear that pectin, which has been given to a large number of patients in the past, rarely has adverse effects (13), although the toxicological investigations which would now be required by regulatory authorities have not been conducted. The largest study involved the use of Sangostop® in more than 400 patients undergoing surgery (14). Pectin was subsequently shown to have antifibrinolytic activity in vitro (15), which could explain its hemostatic effect. There has been one report of anaphylaxis in a patient given Sangostop® intravenously (16).

Sulfonaphtine

A number of claims were made in the 1950s that sodium 4-amino-1-naphthalene-1-sulphonate (sulfonaphtine glucoside, naphthionine glucoside) had hemostatic properties of clinical value. It was subjected to clinical evaluation because it is related to Congo Red dye, for which similar claims had been made in 1933. Thrombophlebitis was a common problem after intravenous administration of Congo Red, and so clinical trials with that dye were abandoned while other congeners were sought. Sulfonaphtine has been reported to enhance blood coagulation and to reduce the whole blood clotting time and bleeding time (17,18). However, no randomized, double-blinded clinical trials have been conducted. No adverse effects of sulfonaphtine, including thrombophlebitis, have been reported. It is no longer available commercially.

Thrombin and thromboplastin

Numerous tissue extracts, prepared from a variety of animal tissues, have been claimed to be effective hemostatic agents. Examples of tissue extracts that are no longer available include thrombin extracts (such as Thrombinar and Thrombostat) and thromboplastin extracts (such as Clauden, Fibraccel, and Tachostyptan). Others include Coagulen, Clauden, Coazimol, Manetol, Thrombocytine, and Frénovex.

Thrombin is prepared from bovine plasma by reacting thrombin with thromboplastin in the presence of calcium. Thromboplastin is prepared as a micellar suspension of at least six phospholipids extracted from porcine brain and mixed in fixed proportions. It is stable at +4°C for several years (19).

Thromboplastin accelerates in-vitro coagulation, but only at certain concentrations and has been given intravenously by injection or infusion. Infusion shortens the bleeding time and normalizes both thrombin generation and prothrombin consumption in vitro for up to 3 hours in a small group of uremic patients (20). It has been used to treat postoperative hemorrhage in the oral cavity (21) and biliary tract (22). There were no adverse effects involving circulatory or cardiac function in healthy human subjects after intravenous injection of 10 ml, but rapid injection can reduce the blood pressure (23).

References

1. Pepeu G. Toxicological and pharmacological investigations on aminonaphtone (2-hydroxy-2-methyl-14-naphtohydroquinone-2-amino-benzoate). Quad Coag 1975;1:19–25.
2. Jurgens J. Clinical practice in the bleeding prophylaxis of thrombocytogenic haemorrhagic diatheses using the haemostatic preparation "aminaphtone". Quad Coag 1970;14:1.
3. De Anna D, Mari F, Intini S, Gasbarro V, Sortini A, Pozza E, Marzola R, Taddeo U, Bresadola F, Donini I. Effetti della terapia con aminaftone sulla stasi venosa e linfatica cronica. [Effects of therapy with aminaftone on chronic venous and lymphatic stasis.] Minerva Cardioangiol 1989;37(5):251–4.
4. Klemm WR, Bolton GR. Comparative evaluation of systemic coagulants in dogs. Arzneimittelforschung 1967;17(12):1573–4.
5. Forman GH, Naylor MN. Haemostatic properties of adrenochrome monosemicarbazone in dental surgery. Br Dental J 1964;117:280.
6. Dykes ER, Anderson R. Carbazochrome salicylate as a systematic hemostatic agent in plastic operations. A clinical evaluation. JAMA 1961;177:716–17.
7. Marcus AJ, Spaet TH. Ineffectiveness of Adrenosem in pulmonary surgery. J Thorac Surg 1958;35(6):821–4.
8. Swan HT, Nutt AB, Jowett GH, Ferguson WJ, Blackburn EK. Monosemicarbazone of adrenochrome (Adrenoxyl) and cataract surgery. Effect on capillary resistance and incidence of hyphaema. Br J Ophthalmol 1961;45:415.
9. Haverback BJ, Dutcher TF, Shore PA, Tomich EG, Terry LL, Brodie BB. Serotonin changes in platelets and brain induced by small daily doses of reserpine; lack of effect of depletion of platelet serotonin on hemostatic mechanisms. N Engl J Med 1957;256(8):343–5.
10. Greco AS. Impiego del solfato doppio di 5-ossitriptamina e creatinina (Antemovis) in soggetti con emostasi normale operati di tonsillectomia. [Use of the double sulfate of 5-hydroxytryptamine and creatinine (Antemovis) in tonsillectomy patients with normal hemostasis.] Minerva Otorinolaringol 1957;7(1):26–7.
11. Charles O, Coolsaet B. Prevention des hémorraghies en chirurgie prostatique. A propos de l'étude de l'activité hémostatique dans la prostatectomie d'une nouvelle molecule: la mono-semicarbazone de la beta naphtoquinone (naftazone). [Prevention of hemorrhage in prostatic surgery. Apropos of the study of the hemostatic activity in prostatectomy of a new molecule: beta-naphthoquinone monosemicarbazone (naftazone).] Ann Urol (Paris) 1972;6(3):209–12.
12. Zicot M. Etude multicentrique de l'efficacité et de la tolérance de la naftazone (Mediaven 10 mg). Comparaison de deux schémas posologiques. [Multicenter study of the efficacy and tolerance of naftazone (Mediaven 10 mg). Comparison of 2 dosage schemes.] Rev Med Liege 1993;48(4):224–8.
13. Joseph GH. Medical literature on pectin and pectin pastes. Bulletin of the National Formulary Committee 1940;9:2.
14. Gohrbrandt E. The action of pectin as a blood coagulant. Dtsch Med Wochenschr 1936;62:1625.
15. Nilsson IM, Bjorkman SE, von Studnitz, Hallen A. Antifibrinolytic activity of certain pectins. Thromb Diath Haemorrh 1961;6:177–87.
16. Coeli L, Cuoghi I, Sandri G, Tagliapietra L. Un caso di grave shock anafilattico dopo somministrazione endovenosa di una soluzione di polisaccaridi a scopo emostatico (Sangostop). [Case of severe anaphylactic shock caused by intravenous administration of a solution of polysaccharides (Sangostop) for hemostasis.] Chir Ital 1969;21(1): 226–30.
17. Poller L. A study of naphthionin, a new haemostatic drug. J Clin Pathol 1955;8(4):331–3.
18. Poller L, More JR. A study of Naphtionin in the management of the bleeding defect in patients with thrombocytopenia. J Clin Pathol 1964;17:680–4.
19. Schoch A. Über die Entwicklung und Erprobung des Hämostyptikums Tachostyptan. [The development and testing of a hemostatic called Tachostyptan.] Ther Umsch 1955;12(2):26–32.
20. Schimpf K, Hanf-Hoppe HW, Immich H. Intravenous infusion of a standardised coagulation active phospholipid complex in uremic coagulation deficiency. Return to normal of thrombin generation and prothrombin consumption. Thromb Diath Haemorrh 1972;27(3):554–8.
21. Gerstmann W. Die Behandlung von Nachblutungen nach chirurgischen Eingriffen im Kieferbereich mit dem Haemostypticum Tachostyptan. [The treatment of postoperative hemorrhage in the oral cavity with the hemostyptic tachostyptan.] Zahnarztl Rundsch 1955;64(14):371–2.
22. Munte A, Krumpoch B, Eisenburg J. Symptom Hämobilie. Fallbericht bei primar biliarer Zirrhose. [The symptom hemobilia.] MMW Munch Med Wochenschr 1975; 117(42):1695–6.
23. Reichel H, Martini F, Bleichert A. Untersuchungen bei die Kreislaufwirkung eines neuen Haemostypticums. [Effect of a new hemostatic agent on blood circulation.] Arzneimittelforschung 1953;3(5):252–3.

Heparins

General Information

Heparins are mucopolysaccharides whose molecules are of varying lengths. Unfractionated (standard) heparin contains molecules of average molecular weight of 12 000–15 000 Da. Low molecular weight heparins contain molecules whose average molecular weight is below 5000 Da. Each formulation of a low molecular weight heparin contains a different range of sizes of molecules, but they have in common more activity against factor X than thrombin compared with standard heparin, a longer duration of action, and a lower risk of thrombocytopenia. They can be given subcutaneously once a day without the monitoring of activated partial thromboplastin time that is necessary for standard heparin. Low molecular weight heparins include bemiparin, certoparin, dalteparin, enoxaparin, nadroparin, reviparin, and tinzaparin.

Non-anticoagulant uses

A therapeutic role for heparin has been proposed in inflammatory bowel disease, particularly in ulcerative colitis (1). This beneficial response may result from mechanisms other than anticoagulation, including the restoration of high-affinity receptor binding by anti-ulcerogenic growth factors, such as basic fibroblast growth factor, that normally rely on the presence of heparian sulfate proteoglycans (2).

General adverse effects

The major adverse effect of heparin is bleeding. Thrombocytopenia occurs in some 5% of patients receiving standard heparin but is uncommon in those receiving low molecular weight heparins; bleeding as a result is rare. Long-term use can lead to osteoporosis. General vasospastic reactions have been reported and, exceptionally, skin necrosis can occur. Allergic reactions to heparin are well-known but rare. Tumor-inducing effects have not been described and the possibility of an anti-tumor effect has been raised.

Organs and Systems

Cardiovascular

Bolus administration of heparin causes vasodilatation and a fall in arterial blood pressure of 5–10 mmHg (3). Some convincing data have been reported concerning the role in these reactions of chlorbutol which has been used as a bactericidal and fungicidal ingredient in some heparin formulations (4).

Cardiogenic shock can occur in parallel with disseminated intravascular coagulation (5). In these circumstances heparin is thought to act as a hapten in a heparin–protein interaction that stimulates antibody production and an antigen–antibody reaction associated with release of platelet and vasoactive compounds.

General vasospastic reactions have been described in patients receiving heparin, exceptionally complicated by skin necrosis (6). Vasospastic reactions are probably part of the syndrome of thrombohemorrhagic complications considered above.

Nervous system

Effects of heparin on the nervous system, other than those due to bleeding, have not been reported.

Endocrine

Heparin-induced hypoaldosteronism is well documented, both in patients treated with standard heparin, even at low doses, and in patients treated with low molecular weight heparin (7,8). The most important mechanism of aldosterone inhibition appears to be a reduction in both the number and affinity of angiotensin II receptors in the zona glomerulosa (7). A direct effect of heparin on aldosterone synthesis, with inhibition of conversion of corticosterone to 18-hydroxycorticosterone, has also been suggested. This effect is believed to be responsible for the hyperkalemia that can occur in heparin-treated patients with impaired renal function and particularly in patients on chronic hemodialysis (9), or with diabetes mellitus, or who are taking other potentially hyperkalemic drugs.

Metabolism

Heparin has a strong clearing action on postprandial lipidemia by activating lipoprotein lipase. This has been thought to be associated with an increase in free fatty acid-induced dysrhythmias and death in patients with myocardial infarction.

- Substantial hypertriglyceridemia occurred in a pregnant woman who received long-term subcutaneous heparin treatment (10).

However, the risk of hyperlipidemia seems to have been exaggerated, since the extent of lipolysis is usually small (11).

Electrolyte balance

Hyperkalemia is an occasional complication of heparin therapy. It has been attributed to hypoaldosteronism, and fludrocortisone has been used to treat it (12). It has been suggested that marked hyperkalemia is only likely to occur in the presence of other factors that alter potassium balance (13).

Low molecular weight heparin is less likely to cause hyperkalemia than standard heparin. In 28 men, mean age 70 years, given low molecular weight heparin (40 mg subcutaneously every 12 hours) for deep venous thrombosis prophylaxis after an operation, the serum potassium concentration did not change significantly after 4 days of therapy (4.25 mmol/l before therapy and 4.35 mmol/l) (14).

However, in 85 patients enoxaparin therapy was associated with an increase in mean potassium concentration from 4.26 mmol/l at baseline to 4.43 mmol/l on the third day; potassium concentrations exceeded 5.0 mmol/l in 9% (15). There was no life-threatening or symptomatic hyperkalemia. Neither plasma renin activity nor aldosterone concentrations changed significantly and there was no correlation between the increase in potassium concentrations and the presence of diabetes mellitus or treatment with angiotensin converting enzymes inhibitors, angiotensin receptor blockers, beta-blockers, or potassium-wasting diuretics.

Hematologic

Hemorrhage

The major adverse effect of heparin is bleeding, and it can occur with low molecular weight heparins as well as with standard heparin (16).

DoTS classification (BMJ 2003;327:1222–5)
Dose-relation: toxic effect
Time-course: early
Susceptibility factors: treatment with antiplatelet drugs, sex, age, renal function

Frequency
An authoritative review of the relevant literature was published in 1993 and is still valid (17). Its authors concluded that the use of heparin in therapeutic dosages (over 15 000 IU/day) is typically marked by an average daily frequency of fatal, major, and major and minor bleeding episodes of 0.05, 0.8, and 2.0% respectively; these frequencies are about twice those expected without heparin therapy. In 2656 medical patients studied by the Boston Collaborative Drug Surveillance Program, the crude risk of bleeding from heparin (route unspecified) was 9% but varied with dose: 4.9% for doses below 50 IU/kg per dose, 8.1% for doses of 50–99 IU/kg per dose, and 17% for doses of 100 IU/kg per dose or more (18). The 7-day cumulative risk for any kind of bleeding was 9.1%. Melena, hematomas, and macrohematuria were the most frequent manifestations; intracranial bleeding and pulmonary bleeding were rare.

Presentation
In the Boston Collaborative Drug Surveillance Program study mentioned above (18), the localization of bleeding, expressed in percentages and broadly classified as major/minor, was as follows:

- gastrointestinal hemorrhage 49/11
- vaginal hemorrhage 11/8 (1/3 postpartum)
- bleeding from wounds and accidental soft-tissue trauma 11/28
- retroperitoneal bleeding 6/0
- genitourinary bleeding other than vaginal 6/35
- intracranial hemorrhage 5/0
- epistaxis 4/10
- other forms of blood loss 8/8.

An FDA Health Advisory warning was issued in December 1997 after 30 cases of spinal hematoma had been reported in patients undergoing spinal or epidural anesthesia while receiving low molecular weight heparin perioperatively. In the European literature, the risk of spinal hematoma in patients receiving low molecular weight heparin was not considered clinically significant. In Europe, low molecular weight heparin is given once a day and at a smaller total daily dose; this enables the placement (and removal) of needles and catheters during periods of reduced low molecular weight heparin activity. Identification of further risk factors is difficult, owing to the rarity of spinal hematoma. However, several possible risk factors have been suggested: about 75% of the patients were elderly women, in 22 patients an epidural catheter was used, and in 17 patients the first dose of low molecular weight heparin was administered while the catheter was indwelling; 12 patients received antiplatelet drugs and/or warfarin in addition to low molecular weight heparin (19). The authors formulated recommendations for minimizing the risk of spinal hematoma, including using the smallest effective dose of low molecular weight heparin perioperatively, delaying heparin therapy as long as possible postoperatively, and removing catheters when anticoagulant activity is low. Furthermore, they warned against combining low molecular weight heparin with antiplatelet drugs or oral anticoagulants.

Relation to dose
Subgroup analyses of randomized trials and prospective cohort studies point to an association, as one would expect, between the incidence of bleeding and the anticoagulant response as measured by a test of blood coagulation, for example the activated partial thromboplastin time (APTT). For instance, there were five major bleeding episodes in 10 patients whose APTT was prolonged to more than twice the upper limit of their therapeutic range but only one episode in 40 patients whose APTT remained in the therapeutic range (relative risk 20) (20). Furthermore, there is an increased rate of major bleeding with intermittent intravenous use compared with continuous intravenous heparin infusion. No differences in major bleeding are generally detected between continuous intravenous and subcutaneous heparin (21).

Time-course
In the Boston Collaborative Drug Surveillance Program study mentioned above, the peak incidence of bleeding was on the third day after the start of heparin therapy, which suggests a relatively safe initial 48-hour period in systemic heparinization (18). However, bleeding can be expected at any time during therapy, if the dosage becomes excessive or if susceptibility factors, such as trauma, intervene.

Susceptibility factors
In the Boston Collaborative Drug Surveillance Program study mentioned above, bleeding correlated with aspirin treatment, with sex, and probably with age and renal function (18). A meta-analysis of randomized trials reported that those aged over 70 are associated with the risk of major bleeding (22). Recent surgery or trauma also increase the risk.

Low molecular weight heparin
Because of its reduced activity on overall clotting, low molecular weight heparin is expected to cause less bleeding than standard heparin. However, several meta-analyses of randomized comparisons of low molecular weight heparin with standard heparin in the prevention of postoperative deep venous thrombosis showed no difference in the incidence of major bleeding (23,24). For low molecular weight heparin, the rates of major bleeding ranged from 0 to 3% and fatal bleeding from 0 to 0.8% (21). A later meta-analysis of randomized comparisons in the initial curative treatment of deep venous thrombosis showed a 35% reduction in major bleeding in patients treated with low molecular weight heparin, but this result was not significant (25).

Thrombocytopenia
Thrombocytopenia (100×10^9/l or lower) occurs in about 3–7% of patients, independent of the mode of administration or the dose and type of heparin (26,27). The incidence varies largely among published series, but the overall average may be some 5% (28). There was a higher incidence in some older studies (29), but this may have

been due to the presence of impurities in the heparin then available, and some of the studies clearly included cases of thrombocytopenia not attributable to heparin. Even the current incidence is to some extent uncertain, because of differences in methods of diagnosis and in the definitions used (30,31). Low molecular weight heparin is significantly less likely to cause thrombocytopenia than unfractionated heparin (27).

Two types of heparin-induced thrombocytopenia have been defined. Type I (mild) occurs within the first few days of heparin administration, while type II (severe), which is less common, is generally seen after a week or more of treatment and is often complicated by the recurrence of thromboembolic events.

A third variety, so-called "delayed-onset heparin-induced thrombocytopenia" has also been described in several reports. In 12 patients, recruited from secondary and tertiary care hospitals, thrombocytopenia and associated thrombosis occurred at a mean of 9.2 (range 5–19) days after the withdrawal of heparin; nine received additional heparin, with further falls in platelet counts (32). In a retrospective case series, 14 patients, seen over a 3-year period, developed thromboembolic complications a median of 14 days after treatment with heparin (33). The emboli were venous ($n = 10$), or arterial ($n = 2$), or both ($n = 2$); of the 12 patients with venous embolism, 7 had pulmonary embolism. Platelet counts were mildly reduced in all but two patients at the time of the second presentation. On readmission, 11 patients received therapeutic heparin, which worsened their clinical condition and further reduced the platelet count.

- A 44-year-old woman developed delayed-onset thrombocytopenia and cerebral thrombosis 7 days after a single dose of standard heparin 5000 units (34).

Type I heparin-induced thrombocytopenia

DoTS classification (BMJ 2003;327:1222–5)

Dose-relation: toxic effect
Time-course: early
Susceptibility factors: not known

Type I heparin-induced thrombocytopenia is common and is characterized by a mild transient thrombocytopenia (with platelet counts that usually do not fall below 50×10^9/l); the thrombocytopenia occurs on the first few days of heparin administration (usually 1–5 days) and requires careful monitoring but not usually withdrawal of heparin. Type I thrombocytopenia is generally harmless and very probably results from direct heparin-induced platelet aggregation. Thrombocytopenia is most common when large doses of heparin are used, or in some particular circumstances, such as after thrombolytic therapy (35) or in the early orthopedic postoperative period (36); it can abate in spite of continued therapy. Type I thrombocytopenia is a non-immune reaction, probably due to a direct activating effect of heparin on platelets.

Type II heparin-induced thrombocytopenia

DoTS classification (BMJ 2003;327:1222–5)

Dose-relation: hypersusceptibility effect
Time-course: delayed
Susceptibility factors: previous heparin therapy, co-administration of antiplatelet drugs or oral anticoagulants

Type II heparin-induced thrombocytopenia is less common than Type I but is often associated with severe thrombocytopenia. It is generally accepted that heparin-induced thrombocytopenia refers to platelet counts of less than 150×10^9/l or a reduction in platelet count of 30–50% to a previous count. In some cases, platelet counts that have fallen to 50% from a high normal previous count would remain apparently normal but should be considered as potentially heparin-induced thrombocytopenia.

Mechanism

Type II thrombocytopenia is probably an immune-mediated phenomenon, a fact that has been the subject of much specific investigation (27,37–42). It has been proposed that the diagnosis should depend on two criteria: the association of one or more clinical events and laboratory evidence of a heparin-dependent immunoglobulin (36).

Diagnosis

Laboratory diagnosis of heparin-induced thrombocytopenia can be made either using functional tests (demonstration of platelet activation of normal donor platelets in vitro by the patient's serum in the presence of heparin) or by screening for antibodies (27,43). The duration of the antibody response can vary from weeks to months up to 1 year. The two types of tests are complementary; both should be used when the reported results of either are inconsistent with the clinical problem.

Susceptibility factors

The risk of thrombocytopenia is increased in patients with a history of previous heparin therapy (44). Thrombocytopenia and/or thromboembolic complications can occur sooner in patients with a history of previous exposure to heparin, suggesting an anamnestic response (28,43).

The results of some prospective studies, including mainly transient benign thrombocytopenia (type I heparin-induced thrombocytopenia), have suggested that thrombocytopenia is more common in patients who have received the bovine lung type of heparin than in those who have received the porcine intestinal mucosa type (45–47). Type II thrombocytopenia is certainly more common in patients treated with standard heparin than in those treated with low molecular weight heparin (36), but there is usually cross-reactivity between standard heparin and low molecular weight heparin.

Heparin-coated catheters can sustain the thrombocytopenia in patients with heparin-associated antiplatelet antibodies (48,49) and therefore have to be removed from such patients.

Presentation

Heparin-induced thrombocytopenia usually occurs with a delayed onset (a week or more) and is often complicated by paradoxical recurrence of thromboembolic events, leading to life-threatening complications. The general term "heparin-induced thrombocytopenia" is as a rule used to designate this phenomenon.

Thrombosis can occur before the onset of overt thrombocytopenia (36). In some cases dramatic thrombotic events occur in association with antibodies without significant fall in platelet count (43). Thrombotic complications include new or recurrent arterial thromboembolism, often localized in the distal aorta and legs or presenting as myocardial infarction and hemiplegia (50), but also in the brachial artery (51), often requiring surgical treatment. In older reports there was a higher incidence of arterial than of venous thrombosis, but later reports documented that venous thrombosis is four times more common than arterial thrombosis (52). Heparin-induced thrombocytopenia can be associated with deep venous thrombosis and pulmonary embolism, but unusual forms of thrombosis, such as adrenal hemorrhagic infarction due to adrenal vein thrombosis, a complication that must be considered in patients who develop abdominal pain or unexplained hypotension during heparin therapy, are not uncommon.

Venous limb gangrene due to heparin-induced thrombocytopenia is characterized by distal tissue losses, with extensive venous thrombosis involving large veins and small venules (53). This reaction seems to be related to acquired deficiency of protein C induced by concomitant oral anticoagulants.

Patients with heparin-induced thrombocytopenia have a reported mortality of 25–30% and amputation rates of up to 25% (54). The development of the syndrome is not related to the dose of heparin in the therapeutic range (that is it is a hypersusceptibility reaction). This has been confirmed by the fact that thrombocytopenia with thromboembolic complications sometimes occurs after the limited exposure that is involved in "flushing" with heparin and saline to maintain the patency of venous catheters (55).

Management

In view of the severity of the Type II syndrome, it has been recommended that heparin therapy be monitored by twice-weekly platelet counts (56).

Heparin-induced thrombocytopenia demands immediate withdrawal of heparin (43), after which platelet counts usually return to normal within 2–3 days, that is much faster than after early-onset thrombocytopenia. Rechallenge with heparin leads to an abrupt fall in the number of platelets and to reappearance of the clinical signs and symptoms, sometimes leading to sudden death (57).

From the therapeutic point of view, prophylaxis of thrombosis must be continued after withdrawal of heparin, since even when there is no evidence of thrombosis in association with heparin-induced thrombocytopenia, thrombosis can follow after some days (52). Because of cross-reactivity, low molecular weight heparin should not be used when heparin has been withdrawn because of heparin-induced thrombocytopenia; nor should warfarin be used, because of the risk of venous gangrene, at least until the thrombocytopenia has resolved. Patients with life-threatening or limb-threatening thrombosis can be treated with thrombolytic drugs. Current views are that two antithrombotic drugs should be used, for example danaparoid plus lepirudin (58).

Eosinophilia

Eosinophilia has rarely been attributed to heparin, with positive rechallenge (52,59).

Liver

Minor increases in serum transaminases without evidence of liver dysfunction are common in patients receiving standard heparin or low molecular weight heparin given therapeutically or prophylactically (60,61). This rise is more pronounced for alanine transaminase than for aspartate transaminase and occurs after 5–10 days of heparin treatment (61). The source of heparin has no relation to the development of raised transaminases. After withdrawal of heparin and sometimes even in spite of continued treatment (60,61), the transaminases return to normal (62,63). The mechanism of these increases has not been elucidated. A concomitant increase in gamma-glutamyl transpeptidase activity has been described in some patients (64).

In one study of patients receiving heparin, the isoenzyme pattern of lactate dehydrogenase was studied; all had rises in the hepatic form of the enzyme, suggesting hepatocellular damage as the most likely source (60).

Heparin-associated hepatotoxicity has not been reported.

Skin

Erythematous nodules or infiltrated and sometimes eczema-like plaques at the site of injection are common adverse effects of subcutaneous standard heparin 3–21 days after starting heparin treatment. They are probably delayed-type hypersensitivity reactions and are also seen with low molecular weight heparin (65–69). There can be cross-reactivity between standard heparin and low molecular weight heparin (69).

Erythromelalgia has been described with enoxaparin (70).

In cases of local reactions, skin tests should not be performed, since they are rarely helpful in detecting potential cross-reactivity between low molecular weight heparin and heparin (65,71).

Two renal transplant recipients developed calcinosis cutis (tender erythematous subcutaneous nodules with induration, ulceration, and necrosis), confirmed by bone scan and biopsies, at the site of subcutaneous administration of nadroparin (72). Both had secondary hyperparathyroidism and a raised calcium-phosphate product at the time of administration. The authors suggested that the high concentration of calcium in nadroparin (220 mmol/l) had been an important factor, since in the same patients subcutaneous injections of nicomorphine or dalteparin did not cause subcutaneous nodules. Three more cases were found after retrospective examination of all 51 adult patients who underwent a renal transplantation in the same hospital during 7 months, and there were no other cases of calcinosis cutis at the injection sites of low molecular weight heparins after nadroparin was replaced by dalteparin.

Skin necrosis

Heparin-induced skin necrosis was first described in 1973 (73) and was later observed in patients with the thrombohemorrhagic syndrome (74,75). The skin pathology develops 6–9 days after the start of subcutaneous heparin treatment and usually develops at the site of subcutaneous injection. However, it can also occur at sites distant from the site of injection (76) or after intravenous therapy (77). Vasculitis is likely to be present, perhaps with fever (78). There is an increased risk of thrombocytopenia and thrombotic complications in patients who have had previous heparin-associated skin necrosis episodes (79).

Various physiopathological mechanisms have been suggested (80), particularly heparin-induced thrombocytopenia, vasculitis caused by a type III hypersensitivity reaction, local trauma at the site of injection, and poor vascularization of adipose tissue resulting in reduced absorption of heparin, as seen in diabetic lipodystrophy. This form of skin necrosis must be distinguished from vasospastic skin necrosis and from skin necrosis induced by cholesterol embolization. Ergotism will be a differential diagnosis in patients who are receiving prophylaxis with the combination of low dose heparin and dihydroergotamine (81). In evaluating any necrotic skin reaction, one must always consider its infectious origin (particularly *Escherichia coli* or *Pseudomonas*) related to unsterile injections (82).

Several patients with heparin-induced skin necrosis were positive for HIT-IgG using the platelet ^{14}C-serotonin release assay, even though they did not develop thrombocytopenia (83). Skin necrosis has been particularly reported in patients receiving standard heparin but also occasionally with low molecular weight heparins, such as dalteparin (84) or enoxaparin (79).

The clinical and histological pictures of heparin-induced skin necrosis are similar to those found in so-called "coumarin necrosis." Laboratory examinations show inflammatory changes, with anemia, leukocytosis, eosinophilia, a raised erythrocyte sedimentation rate, and a positive capillary fragility test. The vasculitis can lead to organ involvement, such as glomerulonephritis (85).

Heparin-induced skin necrosis can be associated with high morbidity and occasional mortality. Heparin should be withdrawn when it occurs. The risk of recurrence if heparin is given again later is not known (86).

Musculoskeletal

Heparin-associated osteoporosis is observed with both standard heparin and low molecular weight heparin, although it is far less pronounced with the latter. The incidence of heparin-associated osteoporosis is not known, but it is probably less than 5% with standard heparin. The highest estimates are derived from studies of pregnant patients and should be interpreted cautiously, since pregnancy, even in the absence of heparin therapy, is sometimes itself associated with osteoporosis. Overall, it appears that osteoporosis can occur in patients given heparin for longer than 10 weeks and usually for a minimum of 4 months. The effect is rarely complicated by fractures. It has been suggested that during long-term heparin therapy, calcium supplements be given (87).

The processes involved are bone resorption and inhibition of bone deposition. Standard heparin may affect both phenomena, whereas low molecular weight heparin seems to affect only the rate of bone formation. Heparin-associated osteoporosis has been attributed to enhancement of collagenolysis or to enzyme inhibition by heparin. Other authors have stressed the resemblance to hyperparathyroid osteopathy. Further possibilities include deficiency of vitamin D analogues (88) and ascorbic acid deprivation at the site of osteoblast activity. Heparin-induced osteolysis may explain the metastatic calcification that can occur in patients with end-stage renal insufficiency treated by hemodialysis, which is sometimes associated with calcified subcutaneous nodules (89).

Sexual function

Heparin has been associated with priapism (90). The frequency and severity of iatrogenic priapism as a result of heparin therapy seems to be greater than with any other type of medical treatment (91). However, it is uncertain whether it is heparin or the underlying thrombotic condition that causes the complication.

Immunologic

A wide range of allergic reactions have been described in patients receiving heparin, including urticaria, conjunctivitis, rhinitis, asthma, cyanosis, tachypnea, a feeling of oppression, fever, chills, angioedema, and anaphylactic shock.

- A patient with end-stage renal disease developed recurrent anaphylaxis after receiving heparin during hemodialysis (92). There were raised concentrations of total and mature tryptase at 1 hour, but although the latter returned to normal by 24 hours the former did not. Prick tests were negative with heparin, enoxaparin, and danaparoid, but intradermal skin tests were positive with heparin and enoxaparin. Danaparoid was used as an anticoagulant during dialysis for the next 3 years without any adverse effects.

In some cases of allergy to a heparin formulation, the precipitating agent will prove to be a preservative, such as chlorocresol (93) or chlorbutol (94), rather than heparin itself.

Second-Generation Effects

Pregnancy

The maternal rate of bleeding complications during heparin treatment is about 2%. This is consistent with the reported rates of bleeding associated with heparin therapy in non-pregnant women, and in warfarin therapy when used for the treatment of venous thrombosis (95). Subcutaneous heparin given just before labor can also cause a persistent anticoagulant effect at the time of delivery; the mechanism of this prolonged effect is unclear (96).

Another pregnancy-associated hazard of long-term heparin administration is maternal osteoporosis, as clearly illustrated by several reports of pregnant women who developed severe osteoporosis after having received heparin, in some cases complicated by multiple vertebral fractures (97,98). Long-term heparin therapy during pregnancy results in changes in calcium homeostasis, which may be dose-related in the therapeutic range of doses (99). The incidence of osteoporotic fractures was 2.2% (four patients) in 184 women receiving long-term subcutaneous prophylaxis with twice-daily heparin during pregnancy (100). In another study, the incidence of osteopenia in 70 pregnant women on long-term heparin was 17%; there was also a regression in the degree of osteopenia postpartum (101). It is difficult to distinguish between the mean bone loss that occurs in normal pregnancy and the additive effect on bone demineralization that results from heparin therapy; further prospective studies on bone demineralization during pregnancy are needed to clarify this point.

Fetotoxicity

An adverse fetal outcome occurs in about one-third of pregnancies after either oral anticoagulant or heparin treatment (102). However, the high rate of adverse fetal outcomes associated with heparin during pregnancy is in part a reflection of the severity of pre-existing maternal diseases (103). Moreover, some studies have suggested that unfractioned heparin is relatively safe for the fetus and is the anticoagulant therapy of choice during pregnancy, whereas oral anticoagulants may not be, particularly during the first trimester (95,104). Heparin does not cross the placenta, and therefore does not have the potential to cause fetal bleeding or teratogenicity (105). Low molecular weight heparins and heparinoids similarly do not cross the placenta (106,107).

Lactation

Heparin is not secreted into breast milk and can be given safely to nursing mothers (108).

Drug–Drug Interactions

Benzodiazepines

In healthy non-fasting subjects, 100–1000 IU of heparin given intravenously caused a rapid increase in the unbound fractions of diazepam, chlordiazepoxide, and oxazepam (109,110), but no change in the case of lorazepam (109). The clinical implications of this finding are not known.

Digitoxin

Reduced plasma protein binding of digitoxin has been reported after the administration of heparin (111). In 10 hemodialysed patients taking maintenance digitoxin therapy, there was reduced binding in vitro because of heparin-induced lipolysis, and not as a consequence of in vivo binding of digitoxin to plasma proteins.

Dobutamine hydrochloride

Dobutamine hydrochloride and heparin should not be mixed or infused through the same intravenous line, as this causes precipitation (112).

Glyceryl trinitrate

Resistance to heparin has been observed in patients in coronary care units receiving intravenous glyceryl trinitrate. Although this has been imputed to propylene glycol in glyceryl trinitrate formulations (113), resistance has also been described with propylene glycol-free formulations. The underlying mechanism might be a qualitative abnormality of antithrombin III induced by glyceryl trinitrate (114). It has also been reported that heparin concentrations can be markedly reduced by glyceryl trinitrate (115).

Interference with Diagnostic Tests

Acid phosphatase activity

Concentrations of heparin as low as 1 IU/ml give 80% inhibition of acid phosphatase activity in leukocytes (116).

Aminoglycosides

Heparin can interfere with the determination of aminoglycosides by enzyme-multiplied immunoassays, resulting in lower values than with the use of other assays (117,118). In the case of gentamicin, the lower values may be due to direct binding of gentamicin to heparin, as well as a more complex interaction involving heparin, gentamicin, and proteins (117). Blood samples for the determination of aminoglycosides by enzyme immunoassays should not be collected in heparinized tubes or from indwelling lines (118).

Arterial blood gases

Heparin can affect the analysis of arterial blood gases (119). Addition of excess heparin and acid mucopolysaccharide to the syringe can alter the Henderson–Hasselbalch equation, simulating metabolic acidosis. It is advisable to coat the syringe with heparin and remove all excess heparin before blood sampling.

Calcium

Pseudo-hypocalcemia can occur in hemodialysis patients, particularly in those who have chylomicronemia before administration of heparin (120). This spurious hypocalcemia is thought to result from lipolytic activity in vitro, sufficient to produce calcium soaps of fatty acid. This can be detected and eliminated by the analysis of blood samples immediately after venepuncture. During hemodialysis, there is a significant fall in plasma ionized calcium after intravenous administration of heparin (an average reduction of 0.03 mmol/l after 10 000 IU) (121).

Chromogenic lysate assay for endotoxin

Heparin has a dose-related inhibitory effect on the chromogenic lysate assay for endotoxin (122). There was a 90% reduction in detectable endotoxin at concentrations of heparin as low as 30 U/ml.

Ciclosporin

Measured ciclosporin concentrations differ according to the use of heparin or EDTA as anticoagulant (123).

Propranolol

Interference by heparin with the measurement of propranolol when the blood is collected from a heparinized cannula is well documented (124). There is no in vivo interaction, since the beta-blockade is unchanged (125).

Thyroid function tests

Artefactual increases of as much as 50% in total thyroxine, estimated by a competitive protein-binding assay, and of as much as 30% in triiodothyronine resin uptake are probably due to rapid and continuing lipolytic hydrolysis of triglycerides after blood has been drawn (126). Thyroid function tests should therefore always be performed on blood samples taken before (or a sufficient time after) heparin treatment (127). An increase in serum-free thyroxine concentrations has also been reported after low molecular weight heparin, by up to 171% in specimens taken 2–6 hours after injection. When specimens were obtained 10 hours after injection, the effects were smaller, but with concentrations still up to 40% above normal the results can still cause errors of interpretation (128).

References

1. Brazier F, Yzet T, Boruchowicz A, Columbel JC, Duchmann JC, Dupas JL. Treatment of ulcerative colitis with heparin. Gastroenterology 1996;110:A872.
2. Day R, Forbes A. Heparin, cell adhesion, and pathogenesis of inflammatory bowel disease. Lancet 1999;354(9172):62–5.
3. Bjoraker DG, Ketcham TR. Hemodynamic and platelet response to the bolus intravenous administration of porcine heparin. Thromb Haemost 1983;49(1):1–4.
4. Bowler GM, Galloway DW, Meiklejohn BH, Macintyre CC. Sharp fall in blood pressure after injection of heparin containing chlorbutol. Lancet 1986;1(8485):848–9.
5. Schimpf K, Barth P. Heparinshock mit Verbrauchsreaktion des Blutgerinnungssystems? [Heparin shock with consumption reaction of the blood coagulation system?] Klin Wochenschr 1966;44(10):544–7.
6. Gayer W. Seltene Beobachtungen von Heparin-Unvertreglichkeit. [Unusual case of heparin intolerance.] Gynaecologia 1968;166(1):25.
7. Oster JR, Singer I, Fishman LM. Heparin-induced aldosterone suppression and hyperkalemia. Am J Med 1995;98(6):575–86.
8. Levesque H, Cailleux N, Noblet C, Gancel A, Moore N, Courtois H. Hypoaldosteronisme induit par les héparines de bas poids moleculaire. [Hypoaldosteronism induced by low molecular weight heparins.] Presse Méd 1991;20(1):35.
9. Hottelart C, Achard JM, Moriniere P, Zoghbi F, Dieval J, Fournier A. Heparin-induced hyperkalemia in chronic hemodialysis patients: comparison of low molecular weight and unfractionated heparin. Artif Organs 1998;22(7):614–17.
10. Watts GF, Cameron J, Henderson A, Richmond W. Lipoprotein lipase deficiency due to long-term heparinization presenting as severe hypertriglyceridaemia in pregnancy. Postgrad Med J 1991;67(794):1062–4.
11. Wolf R, Beck OA, Hochrein H. Der Einfluss von Heparin auf die Haufigkeit von Rhythmusstorungen beim akuten Myokardinfarkt. [The effect of heparin on the incidence of arrhythmias after acute myocardial infarction.] Dtsch Med Wochenschr 1974;99(30):1549–53.
12. Sherman DS, Kass CL, Fish DN. Fludrocortisone for the treatment of heparin-induced hyperkalemia. Ann Pharmacother 2000;34(5):606–10.
13. Canova CR, Fischler MP, Reinhart WH. Effect of low-molecular-weight heparin on serum potassium. Lancet 1997;349(9063):1447–8.
14. Abdel-Raheem MM, Potti A, Tadros S, Koka V, Hanekom D, Fraiman G, Danielson BD. Effect of low-molecular-weight heparin on potassium homeostasis. Pathophysiol Haemost Thromb 2002;32(3):107–10.
15. Koren-Michowitz M, Avni B, Michowitz Y, Moravski G, Efrati S, Golik A. Early onset of hyperkalemia in patients treated with low molecular weight heparin: a prospective study. Pharmacoepidemiol Drug Saf 2004;13(5):299–302.
16. Pachter HL, Riles TS. Low dose heparin: bleeding and wound complications in the surgical patient. A prospective randomized study. Ann Surg 1977;186(6):669–74.
17. Landefeld CS, Beyth RJ. Anticoagulant-related bleeding: clinical epidemiology, prediction, and prevention. Am J Med 1993;95(3):315–28.
18. Walker AM, Jick H. Predictors of bleeding during heparin therapy. JAMA 1980;244(11):1209–12.
19. Horlocker TT, Wedel DJ. Spinal and epidural blockade and perioperative low molecular weight heparin: smooth sailing on the Titanic. Anesth Analg 1998;86(6):1153–6.
20. Norman CS, Provan JL. Control and complications of intermittent heparin therapy. Surg Gynecol Obstet 1977;145(3):338–42.
21. Levine MN, Raskob G, Landefeld S, Kearon C. Hemorrhagic complications of anticoagulant treatment. Chest 2001;119(1 Suppl):S108–21.
22. Campbell NR, Hull RD, Brant R, Hogan DB, Pineo GF, Raskob GE. Aging and heparin-related bleeding. Arch Intern Med 1996;156(8):857–60.
23. Leizorovicz A, Haugh MC, Chapuis FR, Samama MM, Boissel JP. Low molecular weight heparin in prevention of perioperative thrombosis. BMJ 1992;305(6859):913–20.
24. Nurmohamed MT, Rosendaal FR, Buller HR, Dekker E, Hommes DW, Vandenbroucke JP, Briet E. Low-molecular-weight heparin versus standard heparin in general and orthopaedic surgery: a meta-analysis Lancet 1992;340(8812):152–6.
25. Leizorovicz A, Simonneau G, Decousus H, Boissel JP. Comparison of efficacy and safety of low molecular weight heparins and unfractionated heparin in initial treatment of deep venous thrombosis: a meta-analysis. BMJ 1994;309(6950):299–304.
26. Scott BD. Heparin-induced thrombocytopenia. A common but controllable condition. Postgrad Med 1989;86(5):153–5, 158.
27. Warkentin TE, Chong BH, Greinacher A. Heparin-induced thrombocytopenia: towards consensus. Thromb Haemost 1998;79(1):1–7.
28. Kelton JG. Heparin-induced thrombocytopenia. Haemostasis 1986;16(2):173–86.
29. Bell WR, Tomasulo PA, Alving BM, Duffy TP. Thrombocytopenia occurring during the administration of heparin. A prospective study in 52 patients. Ann Intern Med 1976;85(2):155–60.
30. Kahl K, Heidrich H. The incidence of heparin-induced thrombocytopenias. Int J Angiol 1998;7(3):255–7.
31. Yamamoto S, Koide M, Matsuo M, Suzuki S, Ohtaka M, Saika S, Matsuo T. Heparin-induced thrombocytopenia in hemodialysis patients. Am J Kidney Dis 1996;28(1):82–5.
32. Warkentin TE, Kelton JG. Delayed-onset heparin-induced thrombocytopenia and thrombosis. Ann Intern Med 2001;135(7):502–6.
33. Rice L, Attisha WK, Drexler A, Francis JL. Delayed-onset heparin-induced thrombocytopenia. Ann Intern Med 2002;136(3):210–15.
34. Warkentin TE, Bernstein RA. Delayed-onset heparin-induced thrombocytopenia and cerebral thrombosis after a single administration of unfractionated heparin. N Engl J Med 2003;348(11):1067–9.
35. Balduini CL, Noris P, Bertolino G, Previtali M. Heparin modifies platelet count and function in patients who have undergone thrombolytic therapy for acute myocardial infarction. Thromb Haemost 1993;69(5):522–3.

36. Warkentin TE, Levine MN, Hirsh J, Horsewood P, Roberts RS, Gent M, Kelton JG. Heparin-induced thrombocytopenia in patients treated with low-molecular-weight heparin or unfractionated heparin. N Engl J Med 1995;332(20):1330–5.
37. Chong BH, Fawaz I, Chesterman CN, Berndt MC. Heparin-induced thrombocytopenia: mechanism of interaction of the heparin-dependent antibody with platelets. Br J Haematol 1989;73(2):235–40.
38. Burgess JK, Lindeman R, Chesterman CN, Chong BH. Single amino acid mutation of Fc gamma receptor is associated with the development of heparin-induced thrombocytopenia. Br J Haematol 1995;91(3):761–6.
39. Brandt JT, Isenhart CE, Osborne JM, Ahmed A, Anderson CL. On the role of platelet Fc gamma RIIa phenotype in heparin-induced thrombocytopenia. Thromb Haemost 1995;74(6):1564–72.
40. Carlsson LE, Santoso S, Baurichter G, Kroll H, Papenberg S, Eichler P, Westerdaal NA, Kiefel V, van de Winkel JG, Greinacher A. Heparin-induced thrombocytopenia: new insights into the impact of the FcgammaRIIa-R-H131 polymorphism. Blood 1998;92(5):1526–31.
41. Barrowcliffe TW, Johnson EA, Thomas D. Antithrombin III and heparin. Br Med Bull 1978;34(2):143–50.
42. Boshkov LK, Warkentin TE, Hayward CP, Andrew M, Kelton JG. Heparin-induced thrombocytopenia and thrombosis: clinical and laboratory studies. Br J Haematol 1993;84(2):322–8.
43. Warkentin TE. Heparin-induced thrombocytopenia. Pathogenesis, frequency, avoidance and management. Drug Saf 1997;17(5):325–41.
44. Kakkasseril JS, Cranley JJ, Panke T, Grannan K. Heparin-induced thrombocytopenia: a prospective study of 142 patients. J Vasc Surg 1985;2(3):382–4.
45. Bell WR, Royall RM. Heparin-associated thrombocytopenia: a comparison of three heparin preparations. N Engl J Med 1980;303(16):902–7.
46. Green D, Martin GJ, Shoichet SH, DeBacker N, Bomalaski JS, Lind RN. Thrombocytopenia in a prospective, randomized, double-blind trial of bovine and porcine heparin. Am J Med Sci 1984;288(2):60–4.
47. Rao AK, White GC, Sherman L, Colman R, Lan G, Ball AP. Low incidence of thrombocytopenia with porcine mucosal heparin. A prospective multicenter study. Arch Intern Med 1989;149(6):1285–8.
48. Laster J, Silver D. Heparin-coated catheters and heparin-induced thrombocytopenia. J Vasc Surg 1988;7(5):667–72.
49. Pelouze GA, Coste B, Rassam T, Valat JD. Thrombopénie immunoallergique déclenche par le revêtement héparine d'un catheter. [Immunoallergic thrombopenia caused by heparin coating of a catheter.] Presse Méd 1989;18(30):1481.
50. Cimo PL, Moake JL, Weinger RS, Ben-Menachem YB, Khalil KG. Heparin-induced thrombocytopenia: association with a platelet aggregating factor and arterial thromboses. Am J Hematol 1979;6(2):125–33.
51. Moore JR, Weiland AJ. Heparin-induced thromboembolism: a case report. J Hand Surg [Am] 1979;4(4):382–5.
52. Warkentin TE, Kelton JG. A 14-year study of heparin-induced thrombocytopenia. Am J Med 1996;101(5): 502–7.
53. Warkentin TE, Elavathil LJ, Hayward CP, Johnston MA, Russett JI, Kelton JG. The pathogenesis of venous limb gangrene associated with heparin-induced thrombocytopenia. Ann Intern Med 1997;127(9):804–12.
54. Wallis DE, Lewis BE, Pifarre R, Scanlon PJ. Active surveillance for heparin induced thrombocytopenia or thromboembolism. Chest 1994;106:120.
55. Rizzoni WE, Miller K, Rick M, Lotze MT. Heparin-induced thrombocytopenia and thromboembolism in the postoperative period. Surgery 1988;103(4):470–6.
56. Godal HC. Report of the International Committee on Thrombosis and Haemostasis. Thrombocytopenia and heparin. Thromb Haemost 1980;43(3):222–4.
57. Becker PS, Miller VT. Heparin-induced thrombocytopenia. Stroke 1989;20(11):1449–59.
58. Hirsh J, Warkentin TE, Raschke R, Granger C, Ohman EM, Dalen JE. Heparin and low-molecular-weight heparin: mechanisms of action, pharmacokinetics, dosing considerations, monitoring, efficacy, and safety. Chest 1998;114(Suppl 5):S489–510.
59. Bircher AJ, Itin PH, Buchner SA. Skin lesions, hypereosinophilia, and subcutaneous heparin. Lancet 1994;343(8901):861.
60. Dukes GE Jr, Sanders SW, Russo J Jr, Swenson E, Burnakis TG, Saffle JR, Warden GD. Transaminase elevations in patients receiving bovine or porcine heparin. Ann Intern Med 1984;100(5):646–50.
61. Toulemonde F, Kher A. Heparine et transaminases: une énigme sans importance en 1994? Therapie 1994;49:355.
62. Carlson MK, Gleason PP, Sen S. Elevation of hepatic transaminases after enoxaparin use: case report and review of unfractionated and low-molecular-weight heparin-induced hepatotoxicity. Pharmacotherapy 2001;21(1):108–13.
63. Hui CK, Yuen MF, Ng IO, Tsang KW, Fong GC, Lai CL. Low molecular weight heparin-induced liver toxicity. J Clin Pharmacol 2001;41(6):691–4.
64. Lambert M, Laterre PF, Leroy C, Lavenne E, Coche E, Moriau M. Modifications of liver enzymes during heparin therapy. Acta Clin Belg 1986;41(5):307–10.
65. Phillips JK, Majumdar G, Hunt BJ, Savidge GF. Heparin-induced skin reaction due to two different preparations of low molecular weight heparin (LMWH). Br J Haematol 1993;84(2):349–50.
66. Moreau A, Dompmartin A, Esnault P, Michel M, Leroy D. Delayed hypersensitivity at the injection sites of a low-molecular-weight heparin. Contact Dermatitis 1996;34(1):31–4.
67. Valdes F, Vidal C, Fernandez-Redondo V, Peteiro C, Toribio J. Eczema-like plaques to enoxaparin. Allergy 1998;53(6):625–6.
68. Mendez J, Sanchis ME, de la Fuente R, Stolle R, Vega JM, Martinez C, Armentia A, Sanchez P, Fernandez A. Delayed-type hypersensitivity to subcutaneous enoxaparin. Allergy 1998;53(10):999–1003.
69. Koch P, Hindi S, Landwehr D. Delayed allergic skin reactions due to subcutaneous heparin-calcium, enoxaparin-sodium, pentosan polysulfate and acute skin lesions from systemic sodium-heparin. Contact Dermatitis 1996;34(2):156–8.
70. Conri CL, Azoulai P, Constans J, Sebban A, Le Mouroux A, Midy D, Baste JC. Erythromélalgie et héparine de bas poids moléculaire. [Erythromelalgia and low molecular weight heparin.] Therapie 1994;49(6):518–19.
71. Wutschert R, Piletta P, Bounameaux H. Adverse skin reactions to low molecular weight heparins: frequency, management and prevention. Drug Saf 1999;20(6):515–25.
72. van Haren FM, Ruiter DJ, Hilbrands LB. Nadroparin-induced calcinosis cutis in renal transplant recipients. Nephron 2001;87(3):279–82.
73. O'Toole RD. Heparin: adverse reaction. Ann Intern Med 1973;79(5):759.
74. Fried M, Kahanovich S, Dagan R. Enoxaparin-induced skin necrosis. Ann Intern Med 1996;125(6):521–2.
75. White PW, Sadd JR, Nensel RE. Thrombotic complications of heparin therapy: including six cases of heparin-induced skin necrosis. Ann Surg 1979;190(5):595–608.
76. Levine LE, Bernstein JE, Soltani K, Medenica MM, Yung CW. Heparin-induced cutaneous necrosis unrelated to injection sites. A sign of potentially lethal complications. Arch Dermatol 1983;119(5):400–3.

77. Kelly RA, Gelfand JA, Pincus SH. Cutaneous necrosis caused by systemically administered heparin. JAMA 1981;246(14):1582–3.
78. Stavorovsky M, Lichtenstein D, Nissim F. Skin petechiae and ecchymoses (vasculitis) due to anticoagulant therapy. Dermatologica 1979;158(6):451–61.
79. Fowlie J, Stanton PD, Anderson JR. Heparin-associated skin necrosis. Postgrad Med J 1990;66(777):573–5.
80. Vanderweidt P. Necroses cutanées étendues et multiples sous HBPM. Nouv Dermatol 1996;15:450.
81. Schlag G, Poigenfurst J, Gaudernak T. Risk/benefit of heparin–dihydroergotamine thromboembolic prophylaxis. Lancet 1986;2(8521–22):1465.
82. Kumar PD. Heparin-induced skin necrosis. N Engl J Med 1997;336(8):588–9.
83. Warkentin TE. Heparin-induced skin lesions. Br J Haematol 1996;92(2):494–7.
84. Santamaria A, Romani J, Souto JC, Lopez A, Mateo J, Fontcuberta J. Skin necrosis at the injection site induced by low-molecular-weight heparin: case report and review. Dermatology 1998;196(2):264–5.
85. Jones BF, Epstein MT. Cutaneous heparin necrosis associated with glomerulonephritis. Australas J Dermatol 1987;28(3):117–18.
86. Sallah S, Thomas DP, Roberts HR. Warfarin and heparin-induced skin necrosis and the purple toe syndrome: infrequent complications of anticoagulant treatment. Thromb Haemost 1997;78(2):785–90.
87. Chigot P, De Gennes C, Samama MM. Ostéoporose induite soit par l'héparine non fractionée soit par l'héparine de bas poids moleculaire. [Osteoporosis induced either by unfractionated heparin or by low molecular weight heparin.] J Mal Vasc 1996;21(3):121–5.
88. Dahlman T, Lindvall N, Hellgren M. Osteopenia in pregnancy during long-term heparin treatment: a radiological study post partum. Br J Obstet Gynaecol 1990;97(3): 221–8.
89. Fox JG, Walli RK, Jaffray B, Simpson HK. Calcified subcutaneous nodules due to calcium heparin injections in a patient with chronic renal failure. Nephrol Dial Transplant 1994;9(2):187–8.
90. Clark SK, Tremann JA, Sennewald FR, Donaldson JA. Priapism: an unusual complication of heparin therapy for sudden deafness. Am J Otolaryngol 1981;2(1):69–72.
91. Adjiman S, Fava P, Bitker MO, Chatelain C. Priapisme induit par l'héparine: un pronostic plus sombre? [Priapism induced by heparin. A more serious prognosis?] Ann Urol (Paris) 1988;22(2):125–8.
92. Berkun Y, Haviv YS, Schwartz LB, Shalit M. Heparin-induced recurrent anaphylaxis. Clin Exp Allergy 2004;34(12):1916–18.
93. Ainley EJ, Mackie IG, Macarthur D. Adverse reaction to chlorocresol-preserved heparin. Lancet 1977;1(8013): 705.
94. Dux S, Pitlik S, Perry G, Rosenfeld JB. Hypersensitivity reaction to chlorbutol-preserved heparin. Lancet 1981;1(8212):149.
95. Ginsberg JS, Hirsh J. Use of antithrombotic agents during pregnancy. Chest 1992;102(Suppl 4):S385–90.
96. Anderson DR, Ginsberg JS, Burrows R, Brill-Edwards P. Subcutaneous heparin therapy during pregnancy: a need for concern at the time of delivery. Thromb Haemost 1991;65(3):248–50.
97. de Swiet M, Ward PD, Fidler J, Horsman A, Katz D, Letsky E, Peacock M, Wise PH. Prolonged heparin therapy in pregnancy causes bone demineralization. Br J Obstet Gynaecol 1983;90(12):1129–34.
98. Douketis JD, Ginsberg JS, Burrows RF, Duku EK, Webber CE, Brill-Edwards P. The effects of long-term heparin therapy during pregnancy on bone density. A prospective matched cohort study. Thromb Haemost 1996;75(2):254–7.
99. Dahlman T, Sjoberg HE, Hellgren M, Bucht E. Calcium homeostasis in pregnancy during long-term heparin treatment. Br J Obstet Gynaecol 1992;99(5):412–16.
100. Dahlman TC. Osteoporotic fractures and the recurrence of thromboembolism during pregnancy and the puerperium in 184 women undergoing thromboprophylaxis with heparin. Am J Obstet Gynecol 1993;168(4):1265–70.
101. Nelson-Piercy C, Letsky EA, de Swiet M. Low-molecular-weight heparin for obstetric thromboprophylaxis: experience of sixty-nine pregnancies in sixty-one women at high risk. Am J Obstet Gynecol 1997;176(5):1062–8.
102. Hall JG, Pauli RM, Wilson KM. Maternal and fetal sequelae of anticoagulation during pregnancy. Am J Med 1980;68(1):122–40.
103. Ginsberg JS, Kowalchuk G, Hirsh J, Brill-Edwards P, Burrows R. Heparin therapy during pregnancy. Risks to the fetus and mother. Arch Intern Med 1989;149(10): 2233–6.
104. Ginsberg JS, Hirsh J. Use of antithrombotic agents during pregnancy. Chest 1995;108(Suppl 4):S305–11.
105. Flessa HC, Kapstrom AB, Glueck HI, Will JJ. Placental transport of heparin. Am J Obstet Gynecol 1965;93(4):570–3.
106. Forestier F, Daffos F, Capella-Pavlovsky M. Low molecular weight heparin (PK 10169) does not cross the placenta during the second trimester of pregnancy study by direct fetal blood sampling under ultrasound. Thromb Res 1984;34(6):557–60.
107. Omri A, Delaloye JF, Andersen H, Bachmann F. Low molecular weight heparin Novo (LHN-1) does not cross the placenta during the second trimester of pregnancy. Thromb Haemost 1989;61(1):55–6.
108. O'Reilly R. Anticoagulant, Antithrombotic and Thrombolytic Drugs. New York: MacMillan, 1980;1347.
109. Desmond PV, Roberts RK, Wood AJ, Dunn GD, Wilkinson GR, Schenker S. Effect of heparin administration on plasma binding of benzodiazepines. Br J Clin Pharmacol 1980;9(2):171–5.
110. Routledge PA, Kitchell BB, Bjornsson TD, Skinner T, Linnoila M, Shand DG. Diazepam and N-desmethyldiazepam redistribution after heparin. Clin Pharmacol Ther 1980;27(4):528–32.
111. Lohman JJ, Hooymans PM, Koten ML, Verhey MT, Merkus FW. Effect of heparin on digitoxin protein binding. Clin Pharmacol Ther 1985;37(1):55–60.
112. Hasegawa GR, Eder JF. Dobutamine–heparin mixture inadvisable. Am J Hosp Pharm 1984;41(12):2588, 2590.
113. Col J, Col-Debeys C, Lavenne-Pardonge E, Meert P, Hericks L, Broze MC, Moriau M. Propylene glycol-induced heparin resistance during nitroglycerin infusion. Am Heart J 1985;110(1 Pt 1):171–3.
114. Becker RC, Corrao JM, Bovill EG, Gore JM, Baker SP, Miller ML, Lucas FV, Alpert JA. Intravenous nitroglycerin-induced heparin resistance: a qualitative antithrombin III abnormality Am Heart J 1990;119(6):1254–61.
115. Brack MJ, Gershlick AM. Nitrate infusion even in lower dose decreases the anticoagulant effect of heparin through a direct effect on heparin levels. Eur Heart J 1991;12:80.
116. DeChatelet LR, McCall CE, Cooper MR, Shirley PS. Inhibition of leukocyte acid phosphatase by heparin. Clin Chem 1972;18(12):1532–4.
117. Walters MI, Roberts WH. Gentamicin/heparin interactions: effects on two immunoassays and on protein binding. Ther Drug Monit 1984;6(2):199–202.
118. Krogstad DJ, Granich GG, Murray PR, Pfaller MA, Valdes R. Heparin interferes with the radioenzymatic

and homogeneous enzyme immunoassays for aminoglycosides. Clin Chem 1982;28(7):1517–21.
119. Ordog GJ, Wasserberger J, Balasubramaniam S. Effect of heparin on arterial blood gases. Ann Emerg Med 1985;14(3):233–8.
120. Godolphin W, Cameron EC, Frohlich J, Price JD. Spurious hypocalcemia in hemodialysis patients after heparinization. In-vitro formation of calcium soaps. Am J Clin Pathol 1979;71(2):215–18.
121. Biswas CK, Ramos JM, Kerr DN. Heparin effect on ionised calcium concentration. Clin Chim Acta 1981;116(3):343–7.
122. McConnell JS, Cohen J. Effect of anticoagulants on the chromogenic *Limulus* lysate assay for endotoxin. J Clin Pathol 1985;38(4):430–2.
123. Prasad R, Maddux MS, Mozes MF, Biskup NS, Maturen A. A significant difference in cyclosporine blood and plasma concentrations with heparin or EDTA anticoagulant. Transplantation 1985;39(6):667–9.
124. Wood M, Shand DG, Wood AJ. Altered drug binding due to the use of indwelling heparinized cannulas (heparin lock) for sampling. Clin Pharmacol Ther 1979;25(1):103–7.
125. De Leveld, Piafasky KM. Lack of heparin effect on propranolol-induced beta adrenoreceptor blockade. Clin Pharmacol Ther 1982;31:216.
126. Thompson JE, Baird SG, Thomson JA. Effect of i.v. heparin on serum free triiodothyronine levels. Br J Clin Pharmacol 1977;4:701.
127. Wilkins TA, Midgley JE, Giles AF. Treatment with heparin and results for free thyroxin: an in vivo or an in vitro effect? Clin Chem 1982;28(12):2441–3.
128. Stevenson HP, Archbold GP, Johnston P, Young IS, Sheridan B. Misleading serum free thyroxine results during low molecular weight heparin treatment. Clin Chem 1998;44(5):1002–7.

Hepatitis vaccines

See also Vaccines

General Information

Hepatitis A

The successful propagation of hepatitis A virus in cell culture made the development of hepatitis A vaccines a realistic possibility. Various experimental hepatitis A vaccines have been tested in clinical trials. In December 1991, the first hepatitis A vaccine was licensed in Western European countries. Currently, two different hepatitis vaccines (prepared using different inactivation process) as well as vaccines for children (containing 720 enzyme-linked immunosorbent assay units per dose) and adults (containing 1440 units per dose) are commercially available and further products are under development. The results of safety and immunogenicity testing of hepatitis A vaccines developed by SmithKline-Beecham and by Merck Research Laboratories have been reviewed (SEDA-16, 384) (SEDA-17, 373) (SEDA-18, 333) (SEDA-21, 331). These vaccines were highly immunogenic. There were mild transient reactions at injection sites, but systemic reactions were minor and uncommon.

In a paper dealing mainly with indications for the use of hepatitis vaccine, the data on the hepatitis A vaccines most widely used, HAVRIX (manufactured by Glaxo SmithKline) and VAQTA (manufactured by Merck), have been summarized (1). The data are based on prelicensure clinical trials and worldwide follow-up reports. No serious adverse effects have been attributed to hepatitis A vaccines. In children who received HAVRIX, soreness (15%) and induration (4%) at the injection site, feeding problems (8%), and headaches (4%) have been the most frequently observed adverse effects. In children who received VAQTA, the most common adverse effects were pain (19%), tenderness (17%), and warmth (9%) at the injection site. The reported frequencies were similar to the frequencies reported with hepatitis B vaccines.

Hepatitis B

Two types of hepatitis B vaccine are commercially available: plasma-derived hepatitis B vaccine and yeast recombinant hepatitis B virus vaccine. The two vaccines are equally immunogenic, protective, and safe. However, in most countries the recombinant vaccine is considered the vaccine of choice.

Plasma-derived hepatitis B virus vaccine

Plasma-derived hepatitis B virus vaccine is prepared from the plasma of chronic HBsAg carriers, and consists of purified, inactivated 20-nm HBsAg particles adsorbed on to an aluminium adjuvant. The use of a vaccine produced with plasma derived from infected individuals represented a major departure from conventional approaches, and safety testing has therefore been designed to cover all possibilities of risk and to ensure freedom from transmission of residual HBV and other blood-borne agents. Various clinical trials (SEDA-10, 289) (SEDA-11, 289) have confirmed the safety of plasma-derived hepatitis B virus vaccines produced by different manufacturers. Fears that plasma-derived vaccine may transmit AIDS can be considered unfounded.

Subsequent to the identification of HIV and the growing knowledge of its relatively easy inactivation with procedures such as heat or triple-step chemical inactivation, the complete safety and suitability of plasma-derived vaccines that meet WHO requirements has now been generally accepted and their safety demonstrated (SEDA-12, 279). This type of hepatitis B vaccine is generally well tolerated. The most common adverse effect has been local soreness at the injection site. Less common local reactions include erythema, swelling, and induration; all usually subside within 48 hours. Transient low-grade fever has occurred occasionally; but malaise, fatigue, vomiting, dizziness, myalgia, and arthralgia have been infrequent. Individual reports of more severe suspected adverse effects (erythema multiforme, hepatitis-like changes in liver function, hypersensitivity, lichen planus, menstrual abnormality, myasthenia gravis, neurological disorders including transverse myelitis and Guillain–Barré syndrome, reactive arthritis, Takayasu's arteritis, urticaria, uveitis) are very rare and are no more than could be expected by chance (SED-12, 804) (SEDA-16, 384) (SEDA-17, 373) (SEDA-18, 334). In one reported case with neurological symptoms, a preceding viral illness was the likely cause and in the patient with hepatitis-like symptoms mentioned above, the possibility of other causes was not excluded. In a case with urticaria, patch tests revealed a hypersensitivity to thiomersal, the preservative in the vaccine.

By 1988 it was possible to summarize the adverse effects reported after the distribution of over 1.8 million doses of plasma-derived hepatitis B vaccine (Table 1) (2). From 1982 onwards, the Centers for Disease Control, the Food and Drug Administration, and the manufacturers, Merck Sharp & Dohme, had supported a special surveillance system to monitor spontaneous reports of reactions to plasma-derived hepatitis vaccine. During the first 3 years, about 850 000 persons were immunized. In all, 41 reports were received for one of the following neurological adverse events: convulsion ($n = 5$), Bell's palsy ($n = 10$), Guillain–Barré syndrome ($n = 9$), lumbar radiculopathy ($n = 5$), brachial plexus neuropathy ($n = 3$), optic neuritis ($n = 5$), and transverse myelitis ($n = 4$). Half of these events occurred after the first vaccine dose. However, no conclusive causal association could be made between any neurological adverse event and the vaccine (3).

Yeast-derived recombinant hepatitis B vaccine

The yeast-derived recombinant vaccines first licensed in 1986 represented the first vaccine of any kind manufactured by recombinant technology. The vaccines are prepared using antigen produced by recombinant technology in yeast (*Saccharomyces cerevisiae*). The recombinant vaccine produced by Merck, Sharp & Dohme was as immunogenic and protective against hepatitis B as plasma-derived vaccine (4). Clinical reactions in this series were mild and transient. About 17% of all recipients had pain, soreness, and tenderness at the injection site. A smaller proportion reported headache, weakness, nausea, or malaise. Between February 1984 and August 1986, 33 investigators in 19 countries carried out clinical trials with the yeast-derived recombinant hepatitis B vaccine produced by SmithKline Biologicals. Among other risk groups, neonates, patients with thalassemia and sickle cell anemia, and hemodialysis patients have been vaccinated. All the results point to the safety and acceptability of a yeast-derived vaccine. The incidence of reported reactions varied widely in different studies depending on the scrupulousness with which minor signs were reported. No serious, severe, or anaphylactic reactions occurred. The incidence of local and systemic reactions reported in each study tended to decrease after successive doses, suggesting that immunization did not induce hypersensitivity (SEDA-12, 280).

Reports of studies of the efficacy and safety of recombinant hepatitis vaccines have been published (SED-12, 805) (SEDA-14, 282) (SEDA-15, 351) (SEDA-16, 385) (SEDA-17, 373) (SEDA-18, 334). Table 1 shows the adverse effects reported after the distribution of 205 000 doses of recombinant vaccine.

Third-generation hepatitis B vaccines

Between 5 and 15% of healthy immunocompetent individuals do not seroconvert after receipt of the currently licensed hepatitis B vaccines containing only the major surface protein HbsAg without pre-S epitopes. In a study of a hepatitis B vaccine containing pre-S1, pre-S2, and antigenic components of both viral subtypes adw and ayw, all three antigenic components were produced in a continuous mammalian cell line, after transfection of the cells with recombinant hepatitis B surface antigen DNA (5). The vaccine was manufactured as an aluminium hydroxide adjuvant formulation. The new vaccine (5, 10, 20, or 50 μg) was given to 68 individuals with HBs antibody titers below 10 IU/l. Seroconversion rates in the four groups were 60, 76, 64, and 80%. There were local or systemic reactions in 15%. No dose-related incidence was seen.

Surveillance of hepatitis B adverse events in the USA and Australia

Adverse events after hepatitis B vaccine reported between 1 January 1991 and 31 May 1995 to the US Vaccine Adverse Events Reporting System have been reviewed (6). The patients included 58 neonates and 192 infants who were immunized with hepatitis B

Table 1 Adverse effects after immunization with recombinant and plasma-derived hepatitis B vaccine

Adverse effect	Recombinant vaccine[a]		Plasma-derived vaccine[b]	
	Number of adverse effects	Rate per dose	Number of adverse effects	Rate per dose
Pruritus	2	1:103 000	38	1:48 000
Urticaria	2	1:103 000	23	1:79 000
Exanthems	6	1:103 000	58	1:30 000
Angioedema	–	–	8	1:228 000
Facial edema	1	1:205 000	10	1:182 000
Eczema	–	–	2	1:912 000
Nodule formation	–	–	3	1:608 000
Erythema nodosum	1	1:205 000	1	1:1 823 000
Total	12	1:17 000	99	1:18 000

[a] Over 200 000 doses distributed (August 1986–April 1987).
[b] Over 1.8 million doses distributed (July 1982–December 1987).

vaccine alone and 1469 infants who had received hepatitis B vaccine in combination with DTP vaccine. The serious adverse events reported in neonates and infants included fever, agitation, and apnea. The events reported for infants who received hepatitis B vaccine and DTP vaccine simultaneously were compared with the events reported for infants who received either DTP vaccine or hepatitis B vaccine alone. The reports filed for the infants who received DTP vaccine alone or in combination with hepatitis B vaccine differed from the reports filed for infants who received hepatitis B vaccine alone, suggesting that these events may have been associated with the DTP vaccine. The reviewers concluded that no unexpected adverse events had occurred in neonates and infants given hepatitis B vaccine, despite the administration of at least 12 million doses.

Between 1988 and 1996, the Australian Drug Evaluation Committee received some 600 reports of suspected adverse events after hepatitis B immunization. There were no serious events, and the overwhelming majority were well-known mild-to-moderate local or systemic reactions (7). Musculoskeletal symptoms, such as arthralgia, arthritis, and myalgia, were mentioned in 106 reports.

General adverse effects

The reports of major adverse reactions that have been published since the introduction of recombinant hepatitis B vaccine have been reviewed (8). In the clinical trials with hepatitis B vaccine, the most frequent adverse effects were soreness at the injection site, sometimes accompanied by erythema (3–29%), fatigue (15%), headache (9%), and a temperature increase higher than 37.7°C. The postmarketing surveillance literature (4.5 million doses) showed an overall rate of one adverse effect per 15 500 doses. Of these, local reactions were reported at a rate of 1 in 85 000 doses. Systemic reactions included nausea, rash, headache, fever, malaise, fatigue, flu-like symptoms, diarrhea, urticaria, paresthesia, and somnolence, all of which resolved, generally within 24–48 hours of vaccine administration. Reactions were less frequent with subsequent doses. Major adverse effects have been published as case reports: anaphylaxis; urticaria, erythema nodosum, lichen planus; arthritis, Reiter's syndrome; pulmonary and cutaneous vasculitis; systemic lupus erythematosus; glomerulonephritis; Evan's syndrome, thrombocytopenic purpura; acute posterior multifocal placoid pigment epitheliopathy; Guillain–Barré syndrome, transverse myelitis, multiple sclerosis, acute cerebellar ataxia; chronic fatigue syndrome. Table 2 summarizes the reports. Discussing the cause of the reported major adverse effects and a possible causal relation with vaccine administration, the authors considered that apart from anaphylaxis and urticaria, most of the reactions described were not allergic in nature and that the symptoms were those of immune-complex disease due to autoimmune mechanisms. Because of the extreme rarity of such serious adverse events, coincidence seems the

Table 2 Summary of important adverse effects after recombinant hepatitis B vaccination

Adverse effect	Sex	Age (years)	Number	Time after immunization	Duration of symptoms
Nervous system					
Cerebellar ataxia	F	25	2	10 days	4 months
Demyelination	F	26	3	6 weeks	3 weeks
Demyelination	F	28	2	6 weeks	3 months
Multiple sclerosis	F	43	1	7–10 weeks	4 weeks
Transverse myelitis	M	40	1	2 weeks	6 weeks
Hematologic					
Evans' syndrome	M	33	2	2 days	2 months
Thrombocytopenic purpura	F	15	3	4 weeks	4 months
Thrombocytopenic purpura	F	21	2	3 weeks	2 months+
Skin					
Erythema nodosum	F	43	1	4 days	Several weeks
Lichen planus	F	19	2	2 months	Not reported
Lichen planus	M	50	2	1 month	3 months
Acute posterior multifocal placoid pigment epitheliopathy	M	31	4	3 days	9 months
Urticaria	F	24	1	30 minutes	30 minutes
Musculoskeletal					
Polyarthritis + erythema nodosum	M	31	1	1 day	6 weeks
Polyarthritis	F	41	1	2 weeks	7 months
Reiter's syndrome	M	29	2	4 weeks	4 months
Rheumatoid arthritis	F	49	1	24 hours	Not reported
Immunologic					
Pulmonary and cutaneous vasculitis	F	45	1	2 days	1 week
Systemic lupus erythematosus	F	43	1	2 weeks	Not reported
Median		31		14 days	8 weeks
Average		32		19 days	11 weeks

simplest explanation, but an immune-complex mediated pathogenesis should not be excluded, given the close temporal relation between immunization and the onset of disease. Apart from immune-complex mechanisms, there may be reactions to other components of the vaccine, such as thiomersal, aluminium, or small quantities of yeast proteins.

Hexavalent immunization, including hepatitis B

The Hexavalent Study Group has compared the immunogenicity and safety of a new liquid hexavalent vaccine against diphtheria, tetanus, pertussis, poliomyelitis, hepatitis B, and *Haemophilus influenzae* type b (DTP + IPV + HB + Hib vaccine, manufactured by Aventis Pasteur MSD, Lyon, France) with two reference vaccines, the pentavalent DTP + IPV + Hib vaccine and the monovalent hepatitis B vaccine, administrated separately at the same visit (9). Infants were randomized to receive either the hexavalent vaccine ($n = 423$) or (administered at different local sites) the pentavalent and the HB vaccine ($n = 425$) at 2, 4, and 6 months of age. The hexavalent vaccine was well tolerated (for details, see the monograph Pertussis vaccines). At least one local reaction was reported in 20% of injections with hexavalent vaccine compared with 16% after the receipt of pentavalent vaccine or 3.8% after the receipt of hepatitis B vaccine. These reactions were generally mild and transient. At least one systemic reaction was reported in 46% of injections with hexavalent vaccine, whereas the respective rate for the recipients of pentavalent and HB vaccine was 42%. No vaccine-related serious adverse event occurred during the study. The hexavalent vaccine provided immune responses adequate for protection against the six diseases.

Hepatitis E

Hepatitis E is an important cause of morbidity and mortality in young adults in developing countries, and is particularly dangerous in pregnant women. Through recombinant technology a hepatitis E vaccine has been developed; in its first clinical trials the vaccine was found to be safe and immunogenic (10).

Organs and Systems

Nervous system

Hepatitis A

Probable posthepatitis A immunization encephalopathy has been reported (11).

Hepatitis B

Neuralgic amyotrophy (12), febrile convulsions (13), and Guillain–Barré syndrome (14) have been attributed to hepatitis B vaccine. Fatal inflammatory polyradiculoneuropathy has been reported in temporal relation to hepatitis B administration (15).

Demyelination

Two patients developed neurological symptoms and signs of central nervous system demyelination 6 weeks after administration of recombinant hepatitis B vaccine (16). One was a known case of pre-existent multiple sclerosis but the other had no history of neurological diseases. Both had HLA haplotype DR2 and B7, which are associated with multiple sclerosis. A causal link between immunization and demyelination cannot be established from these two case reports, but the time interval would fit a proposed immunological mechanism. In addition, the Centers for Disease Control (CDC) in Atlanta, Georgia, received reports on four cases of "chronic demyelinating disease." Several other reports describe related conditions or other forms of neurological disorder.

- Acute myelitis occurred in a 56-year-old man 3 weeks after hepatitis B immunization (17).
- Optic neuritis has been attributed to hepatitis B vaccine (18).
- Transverse myelitis developed 3 weeks after the first dose of hepatitis B vaccine in an 11-year-old girl (19).

Guillain–Barré syndrome occurred in a 7-year-old girl after the administration of recombinant hepatitis vaccine (20). The author noted that several other such incidents had been reported after the use of recombinant vaccines, two involving optic neuritis and one Guillain–Barré syndrome.

Multiple sclerosis

Eight cases of nervous system diseases suspected to be either recurrent disseminated encephalitis or multiple sclerosis after hepatitis B immunization have been reported (21). Symptoms started in four cases at 4–14 days after vaccination, and in the other four cases 42–70 days after vaccination. There was a family history of multiple sclerosis in two patients, one of whom had had symptoms compatible with optic neuritis before immunization. In a third patient, there was a history of an episode compatible with Lhermitte's sign. The authors concluded that the risk of demyelinating diseases is unknown. They recommended avoiding hepatitis B immunization in individuals with a personal or familial history of symptoms suggestive of an inflammatory or demyelinating disease.

- A 45-year-old woman with a history of epilepsy developed a lumbosacral acute demyelinating polyneuropathy 1 month after her second hepatitis B immunization (22). She had an uncommon syndrome that combined demyelinating and axonal features confined to the lumbosacral roots whose relation to Guillain–Barré syndrome was unclear. Viral or bacterial causes of the disease could not be found.

The authors concluded that a relation between immunization and disease could not be excluded.

- A 44-year-old female health worker developed bilateral optic neuritis 7 days after immunization against poliomyelitis (OPV) and hepatitis B (23). All hematological, biochemical, bacterial, and virological investigations were normal, and there was no evidence of demyelination on MRI scanning.

Although the current hepatitis B vaccine seems to be one of the safest ever produced, concerns are still sometimes expressed (SEDA-22, 346) (24), particularly since 1996 when a French neurologist announced that he had seen several cases of multiple sclerosis or demyelinating disease in women who had received hepatitis B vaccine. This report was taken up by the media and anti-immunization groups, resulting in further inquiry. In 1998 the French Health Authorities invited leading experts in the fields of immunization and possible adverse effects to meet in Paris and discuss scientific studies carried out in France on the possible relation between hepatitis B vaccine and multiple sclerosis. The conclusion of the meeting was that there was no evidence of a causal link between multiple sclerosis and hepatitis B vaccine. Nevertheless, the Minister of Health decided to stop hepatitis B immunization of schoolchildren aged 11–12 years, but to continue immunizing infants and adults at high risk. The rationale for this decision was the limited opportunity for the full discussion needed to attain informed consent during immunization sessions carried out in schools. It was recommended that immunization of school children and adolescents would in future be performed by general practitioners, who have a better opportunity to discuss the benefits and risks of immunization on an individual basis and to obtain informed consent.

The impact of this decision, or any other to curtail an immunization program, should not be underestimated. It raises concerns not only about the safety of the hepatitis B vaccine, but also about the safety of vaccines in general. In view of this, the WHO took strong action, and its Global Program on Immunization issued a statement in 1997 (after the French media had taken up the issue) that there was no evidence that hepatitis B vaccine causes multiple sclerosis (25). This conclusion was based on the following considerations:

- A comparison of the geographical incidence and prevalence of hepatitis B with that of multiple sclerosis, which shows large differences: Scandinavia and Northern Europe have the highest rates of multiple sclerosis and the lowest rates of hepatitis B infection, whereas in Africa and in Asia there are very low rates of multiple sclerosis and the highest rates of hepatitis B infection. If the virus does not cause multiple sclerosis, it is unlikely that the vaccine can do so.
- None of the postmarketing surveillance studies from the different vaccine manufacturers in North America showed any evidence of an increased risk of multiple sclerosis.
- Reanalysis by the WHO of the French data showed that the notification rate of demyelinating diseases following the administration of the hepatitis B vaccine was 0.6 cases/100 000 vaccinees, which is a lower rate than the expected incidence in the same population (estimated in France to be 1–3 cases/100 000 vaccinees).

The data and analyses were examined once more at a scientific conference organized by the Viral Hepatitis Prevention Board in collaboration with WHO, assisted by experts from many disciplines. Their final conclusion, published in a press release, was that the available scientific data did not demonstrate a causal association between hepatitis B vaccine and central nervous system diseases, including multiple sclerosis (26). It was pointed out moreover that since 1981 more than a billion doses of hepatitis B vaccine had been used worldwide, with an outstanding record of safety and efficacy. The WHO also warned of the consequences of stopping any immunization program on the basis of unfounded concerns, as had happened with pertussis vaccine in the UK, leading to major epidemics of natural pertussis in that country.

The National Multiple Sclerosis Society in the USA made a statement referring to anecdotal reports suggesting that immunization against hepatitis B may increase the risk of multiple sclerosis (27). They noted that:

- such reports had not been confirmed by any statistically significant scientific studies to date;
- because of the potential for public concern about this issue, further studies of the possibility of association of hepatitis B vaccine and demyelinating disease, including multiple sclerosis, were already under way in the USA and Europe;
- hepatitis B infection could result in serious, sometimes fatal, disease and immunization was effective in its prevention.

The official French position on hepatitis B immunization, expressed in January 1999, was that children should be vaccinated against hepatitis B, that adolescents should receive a dose of hepatitis B vaccine if they have not been vaccinated earlier, that adults at risk should be similarly vaccinated, and that the obligation is maintained for health professionals to be vaccinated against hepatitis B. The steps taken in 1998 had sought only to ensure that informed consent could be attained before children were vaccinated.

All available data that may throw light on the hypothesis that hepatitis B vaccine is causally linked to multiple sclerosis have been carefully reviewed (28). The authors concluded that the most plausible explanation for the observed temporal association between immunization and multiple sclerosis is coincidence.

A statement from the Viral Hepatitis Prevention Board (8 June 2000), working closely together with the WHO, is worth repeating: the data available to date do not show a causal association between hepatitis B immunization and central nervous system demyelinating disease, including multiple sclerosis. No evidence presented indicates a need to change public health policies with respect to hepatitis B immunization. Therefore, based on demonstrated important benefits (including prevention of liver cirrhosis and primary liver cancer) and a purely hypothetical risk, the Viral Hepatitis Prevention Board supports the recommendation of the WHO that all countries should have universal infant and/or adolescent immunization programs and should continue to immunize adults at increased risk of hepatitis B infection as appropriate (29).

However, the French Ministry of Health has already compensated 14 patients on the basis of a link between hepatitis B vaccine and neurological effects (multiple sclerosis, retrobulbar neuritis) or rheumatological symptoms. According to a press release from the French Ministry of Health, the decision was taken in the interest of the patients, and despite the fact that even the experts from the Agence française de securité sanitaire des produits, who were charged with regularly re-evaluating the safety profile of hepatitis B vaccine, have not yet been able to conclude whether there is an actual association between the vaccine and the development of multiple sclerosis or autoimmune disorders. It also stated that the decision in no way challenges the benefit:harm evaluation of hepatitis B vaccine and recommendations with respect to national immunization policies (30).

In the USA, following public discussions on the safety of hepatitis B vaccine, health officials, testifying in 1999 before the Government Reform Subcommittee on Criminal Justice, Drug Policy, and Human Resources, said that use of the vaccine has been monitored for 15 years, that it has not been proven to be the cause of deaths, and is only rarely linked to serious adverse effects (31).

Further studies have confirmed that there is no scientific evidence of a causal link between hepatitis B vaccine and multiple sclerosis (32–35). A European-wide study should be particularly mentioned. In 643 patients in various European countries during 1993–97, 15% of whom received various immunizations within 1 year before relapse, there was no increase in the risk in immunized patients compared with patients who did not receive any vaccine (36).

The results of a hospital-based case-control study in 121 patients with a first episode of central nervous demyelination occurring within 180 days after either hepatitis B vaccine or other vaccines have been reported (37). The results were compared with age- and sex-matched controls seen during the same period. No conclusion regarding a causal relation between hepatitis B vaccine and a first MS episode could be drawn, but the authors were not able to exclude such an association with certainty.

In summary the international consensus is that hepatitis B vaccine is still among the safest and most powerful vaccines in immunization programs and that it should be used worldwide.

Leukoencephalitis

Two episodes of leukoencephalitis occurred in a previously healthy patient after a second dose of HB vaccine and rechallenge with a third dose (38).

- A 39-year-old woman developed a complete right homonymous hemianopia and severe dyslexia 4 weeks after receiving a second dose of HB vaccine. Brain MRI showed a large lesion that occupied most of the left occipital lobe and extended into the splenium of the corpus callosum. Histological examination with immunoperoxidase staining, although not pathognomonic, was consistent with demyelinating disease. She underwent surgery and 1 week later there was marked improvement in her condition. Three months later (4.5 months after the second dose), she received a third dose of HB vaccine and 11 days later developed a left hemiparesis and acute progressive deterioration in vision. Brain MRI showed a new large lesion in the right parieto-occipital region, with the characteristics associated with the previous lesion. In comparison with previous findings, there was significant improvement in the left occipital lobe, in which there remained a proencephalic cyst. She was treated with dexamethasone and markedly improved. At 1 year and 2.5 years after the first episode she had residual dyslexia and a complete right homonymous hemianopia. An MRI scan showed almost complete resolution of the previous findings, with the exception of the proencephalic cyst.

The authors considered that acute leukoencephalitis is a rare but possible complication of HB vaccine.

Sensory systems

Eyes

Three days after recombinant hepatitis B booster immunization, a 31-year-old man developed acute posterior multifocal placoid pigment epitheliopathy (visual loss) and eosinophilia (39,40).

Papillitis (41) and retinal vein occlusion (42) have been attributed to hepatitis B vaccine.

Optic neuritis has been attributed to immunization with hepatitis A and B (43).

- A 21-year-old woman developed acute irreversible loss of vision to 0.05 and a nasal visual field defect in the left eye 2 weeks after immunization with hepatitis A and B and yellow fever vaccine. An MRI scan showed hyperintense thickening of the optic nerve, and a diagnosis of optic neuritis was made. Vision acuity did not recover but the scotoma disappeared within 6 weeks.

Ears

Two cases of hearing loss have been reported in patients given hepatitis B immunization (39). Acute tinnitus with permanent audiovestibular damage has been reported in temporal relation to hepatitis B administration (44).

Hematologic

There have been reports of individual cases of thrombocytopenia purpura (45) and pancytopenia (46) in temporal relation with hepatitis B vaccination.

- A healthy 7-year-old girl developed thrombocytopenic purpura after hepatitis B immunization, three doses of vaccine every month followed by a booster (47).

Pancytopenia has been reported in temporal relation to hepatitis B administration (48).

Mouth

Oral lichenoid lesions have been reported in temporal relation to hepatitis B administration (49).

Urinary tract

Acute glomerulonephritis (50) and minimal-change nephrotic syndrome (51) have been attributed to hepatitis B vaccine.

Skin

Erythema multiforme (52) and pityriasis rosea (53) have been reported after hepatitis B vaccination.

Alopecia (54), anetoderma (a disorder characterized by loss of dermal substance clinically and loss of elastic substance histologically) (55), lichen planus (56), urticaria (57), and white dot syndrome (58) have been attributed to hepatitis B vaccine.

Four cases of urticaria and one case of angioedema have been reported after hepatitis B immunization (59). The results emphasize that urticaria can be due to sensitization to the hepatitis Bs antigen itself, hyperimmunization, or a non-allergic reaction.

The first case of erythermalgia (paroxysmal attacks of bilateral pain in the extremities, with an acute increase in local heat in the affected parts, the production and aggravation of the distress by heat, relieved by cold) probably caused by hepatitis B vaccine has been reported (60).

- A 17-year-old boy developed the symptoms of erythermalgia two days after a third dose of hepatitis B vaccine. He was severely ill and recovered only 2 months after treatment with immunoglobulin and hypnotherapy. During hospitalization it was learned that he had had transient moderate pain of both feet for 3 nights after the second dose of vaccine.

The disease that followed the third dose of hepatitis B vaccine therefore met the criteria for positive rechallenge.

Musculoskeletal

In 31 cases of suspected chronic fatigue syndrome associated with hepatitis B immunization, no causal relation was determined (61).

Juvenile chronic polyarthropathy (62) and reactive arthritis (63) have been attributed to hepatitis B vaccine. Erythema nodosum and polyarthritis occurred the day after Engerix-B vaccine administration (64). The authors referred to reports of three other cases of polyarthritis in the literature.

Immunologic

Hepatitis A

Vasculitis suspected to be caused by the first dose of hepatitis A vaccine has been reported (SEDA-21, 331).

Hepatitis B

Polyarteritis nodosa (53), Sjögren's syndrome (65), lymphocytic vasculitis (66), vasculitis (67), and systemic lupus erythematosus (68) have been attributed to hepatitis B vaccine.

- After hepatitis B immunization, three doses of vaccine every month followed by a booster, a healthy 24-year-old woman lost weight and developed migratory arthralgia (47). Acute disseminated lupus erythematosus was diagnosed.

The authors discussed the possibility that immunization could have introduced an antigen that may have provoked an autoimmune reaction in genetically predisposed family members.

Churg–Strauss vasculitis (allergic angiitis and granulomatosis) has been attributed to hepatitis B immunization (69).

- A 20-year-old woman developed chronic rhinitis 1 month after the last dose of hepatitis B, followed about 1 year later by severe asthma, nasal polyposis, and petechial purpura in her fingernail beds and on her feet. A skin biopsy from the left leg showed infiltrates consistent with leukocytoclastic vasculitis.

The interval between immunization and the development of the vasculitis made it very difficult to establish a causal relation in this case.

Large artery vasculitis (two cases) (70) and polyarteritis nodosa (71) have been reported in temporal relation to hepatitis B administration.

A case of arthritis (72) and three cases of vasculitis (73) have been described 7–20 days after immunization with hepatitis B. A causal relation in such very rare cases is unclear, and probably they do not occur more than could be expected by chance.

Second-Generation Effects

Teratogenicity

In the children of 10 women who had received hepatitis B vaccine during the first trimester of pregnancy there were no congenital abnormalities; at 2–12 months the infants were physically and developmentally normal for their ages (74).

Drug Administration

Drug additives

To increase immunogenicity, the hepatitis A vaccines commercially available are coupled to adjuvant aluminium phosphate or aluminium hydroxide. However, alum precipitates provoke inflammatory responses at the injection site. Immunostimulating reconstituted influenza virosomes have therefore been used as an alternative adjuvant. In 1994, a hepatitis A vaccine using the new adjuvant was licensed in Switzerland, and it was later approved for use in other countries: the vaccine was well tolerated and highly immunogenic (SEDA-20, 290) (SEDA-22, 344). Nine people with a history of ocular sensitivity were immunized with hepatitis B, without untoward reactions. However, this result in such a small series should not be overestimated (75). There have been reports of three cases of inflammatory nodular reactions after hepatitis B immunization; aluminium allergy was confirmed (76–78).

Four cases of reactions to thiomersal in hepatitis B vaccines (both plasma-derived and recombinant) have been reported from two centers (79,80). Although thiomersal is present in these vaccines at a concentration of only 1:20 000, it can cause severe cutaneous reactions of the delayed hypersensitivity type, and sometimes the reactions can be very long lasting.

To interpret strictly the package insert for hepatitis B vaccines would preclude its administration to persons with a history of ocular sensitivity to thiomersal.

Drug dosage regimens

Revaccination is sometimes necessary because only 50–70% of immunocompromised persons, especially dialysis patients, develop antibodies, and the anti-HBs titers in these cases are low. In revaccinated non-responders to primary hepatitis immunization using either 20 μg of plasma-derived vaccine or 10 μg of recombinant vaccine, depending on the vaccine used for previous doses, the revaccinations were well tolerated (81,82). Only 6.6% of the vaccinees reported slight irritation at the injection site, tenderness, minimal pain, or swelling lasting for a few hours up to 2 days.

Drug administration route

Aiming at cost reduction of hepatitis B immunization programs, the administration of low doses (2 micrograms) of vaccine given intradermally had by 1987 been evaluated in clinical trials in health-care workers (83) and children (84). The resulting seroconversion rates were 96 and over 90%, respectively. A minimum of local side effects occurred. In a comparison of antibody responses and adverse effects after intradermal or subcutaneous administration of 2 micrograms of a plasma-derived hepatitis B vaccine and intramuscular administration of 20 μg, the intradermal and intramuscular routes gave the highest seroconversion rates (100 and 96%, respectively) and the highest mean titers of anti-HBs (85). The aluminium adjuvant in the vaccine was assumed to cause a substantial number of local reactions (37% discoloration, 17% itching, and 13% nodule formation) after intradermal administration; other routes of administration showed adverse effects only rarely. Correct intradermal deposition of the vaccine is crucial.

Drug–Drug Interactions

Other vaccines

When recombinant hepatitis B vaccine was given together with DTP vaccine and oral poliomyelitis vaccine, there was no evidence of increased reactogenicity after simultaneous administration compared with hepatitis B vaccine alone (86).

In 40 children born to HBsAg-positive mothers who had received second and third doses of hepatitis B vaccine simultaneously with DTP vaccine and inactivated poliomyelitis vaccine, immunogenicity and reactogenicity were comparable with non-simultaneous administration of the different vaccines (87).

References

1. Rosenthal P. Hepatitis A vaccine: current indications. J Pediatr Gastroenterol Nutr 1998;27(1):111–13.
2. Quast U, Freiburg K. Zur Verträglichkeit gentechnisch hergestellter Impfstoffe. Die gelben Hefte. Immunbiol Inform 1988;28(1):41.
3. Shaw FE Jr, Graham DJ, Guess HA, Milstien JB, Johnson JM, Schatz GC, Hadler SC, Kuritsky JN, Hiner EE, Bregman DJ, et al.. Postmarketing surveillance for neurologic adverse events reported after hepatitis B vaccination. Experience of the first three years. Am J Epidemiol 1988;127(2):337–52.
4. Hilleman MR. Yeast recombinant hepatitis B vaccine. Infection 1987;15(1):3–7.
5. Zuckerman JN. Hepatitis B third-generation vaccines: improved response and conventional vaccine non-response—third generation pre-S/S vaccines overcome non-response. J Viral Hepat 1998;5(Suppl 2):13–15.
6. Niu MT, Davis DM, Ellenberg S. Recombinant hepatitis B vaccination of neonates and infants: emerging safety data from the Vaccine Adverse Event Reporting System. Pediatr Infect Dis J 1996;15(9):771–6.
7. Anonymous. Adverse events following hepatitis B immunization. Aust Adv Drug React Bull 1996;15:6.
8. Grotto I, Mandel Y, Ephros M, Ashkenazi I, Shemer J. Major adverse reactions to yeast-derived hepatitis B vaccines—a review. Vaccine 1998;16(4):329–34.
9. Mallet E, Fabre P, Pines E, Salomon H, Staub T, Schodel F, Mendelman P, Hessel L, Chryssomalis G, Vidor E, Hoffenbach A, Abeille A, Amar R, Arsene JP, Aurand JM, Azoulay L, Badescou E, Barrois S, Baudino N, Beal M, Beaude-Chervet V, Berlier P, Billard E, Billet L, Blanc B, Blanc JP, Bohu D, Bonardo C, Bossu C; Hexavalent Vaccine Trial Study Group. Immunogenicity and safety of a new liquid hexavalent combined vaccine compared with separate administration of reference licensed vaccines in infants. Pediatr Infect Dis J 2000;19(12):1119–27.
10. Safary A. Perspectives of vaccination against hepatitis E. Intervirology 2001;44(2–3):162–6.
11. Hughes PJ, Saadeh IK, Cox JP, Illis LS. Probable post-hepatitis A vaccination encephalopathy. Lancet 1993;342(8866):302.
12. Reutens DC, Dunne JW, Leather H. Neuralgic amyotrophy following recombinant DNA hepatitis B vaccination. Muscle Nerve 1990;13(5):461.
13. Hartman S. Convulsion associated with fever following hepatitis B vaccination. J Paediatr Child Health 1990;26(1):65.
14. Sinsawaiwong S, Thampanitchawong P. Guillain–Barré syndrome following recombinant hepatitis B vaccine and literature review. J Med Assoc Thai 2000;83(9):1124–6.
15. Sindern E, Schroder JM, Krismann M, Malin JP. Inflammatory polyradiculoneuropathy with spinal cord involvement and lethal outcome after hepatitis B vaccination. J Neurol Sci 2001;186(1–2):81–5.
16. Herroelen L, de Keyser J, Ebinger G. Central-nervous-system demyelination after immunisation with recombinant hepatitis B vaccine. Lancet 1991;338(8776):1174–5.
17. Mahassin F, Algayres JP, Valmary J, Bili H, Coutant G, Bequet D, Daly JP. Myelite aiguë après vaccination contre l'hépatite B. [Acute myelitis after vaccination against hepatitis B.] Presse Méd 1993;22(40):1997–8.
18. Albitar S, Bourgeon B, Genin R, Fen-Chong M, N'Guyen P, Serveaux MO, Atchia H, Schohn D. Bilateral retrobulbar optic neuritis with hepatitis B vaccination. Nephrol Dial Transplant 1997;12(10):2169–70.
19. Trevisani F, Gattinara GC, Caraceni P, Bernardi M, Albertoni F, D'Alessandro R, Elia L, Gasbarrini G. Transverse myelitis following hepatitis B vaccination. J Hepatol 1993;19(2):317–18.
20. Tuohy PG. Guillain-Barre syndrome following immunisation with synthetic hepatitis B vaccine. NZ Med J 1989;102(863):114–15.
21. Tourbah A, Gout O, Liblau R, Lyon-Caen O, Bougniot C, Iba-Zizen MT, Cabanis EA. Encephalitis after hepatitis B vaccination: recurrent disseminated encephalitis or MS? Neurology 1999;53(2):396–401.
22. Creange A, Temam G, Lefaucheur JP. Lumbosacral acute demyelinating polyneuropathy following hepatitis B vaccination. Autoimmunity 1999;30(3):143–6.
23. Stewart O, Chang B, Bradbury J. Simultaneous administration of hepatitis B and polio vaccines associated with bilateral optic neuritis. Br J Ophthalmol 1999;83(10):1200–1.
24. Marshall E. A shadow falls on hepatitis B vaccination effort. Science 1998;281(5377):630–1.
25. Expanded programme on immunization (EPI). Lack of evidence that hepatitis B vaccine causes multiple sclerosis. Wkly Epidemiol Rec 1997;72(21):149–52.
26. World Health Organization. Press Release. WHO/67, 2 October 1998.
27. Medical Advisory Board of the National Multiple Sclerosis Society: Statement from 14 August 1998. National Multiple

Sclerosis Society: News Desk Research Bulletins, 3 September 1998.

28. Monteyne P, Andre FE. Is there a causal link between hepatitis B vaccination and multiple sclerosis? Vaccine 2000;18(19):1994–2001.
29. WHO. Press release. Hepatitis B and multiple sclerosis. Geneva, 8 June 2000. http://www.who.int/vaccines-diseases/safety/hottop/hepb.htm (accessed 20 August 2000).
30. French Ministry of Health. Press release, 23 May 2000. Compensation for hepatitis B vaccination. http:www.who.int/vaccines-diseases/safety/hottop/hepb.htm (accessed 2 August 2000).
31. Associated Press. Press release, 15 April 1999. Hepatitis vaccine safety questioned in the United States. http://www.who.int/vaccines-diseases/safety/hottop/HBV_Press.html (accessed 2 August 2000).
32. Hostetler L. Vaccinations and multiple sclerosis. N Engl J Med 2001;344(23):1795.
33. Gellin BG, Schaffner W. The risk of vaccination—the importance of "negative" studies. N Engl J Med 2001;344(5):372–3.
34. Ascherio A, Zhang SM, Hernan MA, Olek MJ, Coplan PM, Brodovicz K, Walker AM. Hepatitis B vaccination and the risk of multiple sclerosis. N Engl J Med 2001;344(5):327–32.
35. Soubeyrand B, Boisnard F, Bruel M, Debois H, Delattre D, Gauthier A, Soum S, Thebault C. Pathologies démyélinisantes du système nerveux central rapportées après vaccination hépatite B par GenHevac B (1989–1998). [Central nervous system demyelinating disease following hepatitis B vaccination with GenHevac B. Review of ten years of spontaneous notifications (1989–1998).] Presse Méd 2000;29(14):775–80.
36. Confavreux C, Suissa S, Saddier P, Bourdes V, Vukusic S; Vaccines in Multiple Sclerosis Study Group. Vaccinations and the risk of relapse in multiple sclerosis. Vaccines in Multiple Sclerosis Study Group. N Engl J Med 2001;344(5):319–26.
37. Touze E, Gout O, Verdier-Taillefer MH, Lyon-Caen O, Alperovitch A. Premier épisode de démyelinisation du système nerveux central et vaccination contre l'hépatite B. [The first episode of central nervous system demyelinization and hepatitis B virus vaccination.] Rev Neurol (Paris) 2000;156(3):242–6.
38. Konstantinou D, Paschalis C, Maraziotis T, Dimopoulos P, Bassaris H, Skoutelis A. Two episodes of leukoencephalitis associated with recombinant hepatitis B vaccination in a single patient. Clin Infect Dis 2001;33(10):1772–3.
39. Brezin A, Lautier-Frau M, Hamedani M, Rogeaux O, Hoang PL. Visual loss and eosinophilia after recombinant hepatitis B vaccine. Lancet 1993;342(8870):563–4.
40. Biacabe B, Erminy M, Bonfils P. A case report of fluctuant sensorineural hearing loss after hepatitis B vaccination. Auris Nasus Larynx 1997;24(4):357–60.
41. Berkman N, Benzarti T, Dhaoui R, Mouly P. Neuro-papillite bilaterale au decours d'une vaccination contre l'hépatite B. [Bilateral neuro-papillitis after hepatitis B vaccination.] Presse Méd 1996;25(28):1301.
42. Devin F, Roques G, Disdier P, Rodor F, Weiller PJ. Occlusion of central retinal vein after hepatitis B vaccination. Lancet 1996;347(9015):1626.
43. Voigt U, Baum U, Behrendt W, Hegemann S, Terborg C, Strobel J. Optikusneuritis nach Impfung gegen Hepatitis A, B und Gelbfieber mit irreversiblem Visusverlust. [Neuritis of the optic nerve after vaccinations against hepatitis A, hepatitis B and yellow fever.] Klin Monatsbl Augenheilkd 2001;218(10):688–90.
44. DeJonckere PH, de Surgeres GG. Acute tinnitus and permanent audiovestibular damage after hepatitis B vaccination. Int Tinnitus J 2001;7(1):59–61.
45. Maezono R, Escobar AM. Purpura trombocitopenico apos vacina de hepatite B. [Thrombocytopenic purpura after hepatitis B vaccine.] J Pediatr (Rio J) 2000; 76(5):395–8.
46. Viallard JF, Boiron JM, Parrens M, Moreau JF, Ranchin V, Reiffers J, Leng B, Pellegrin JL. Severe pancytopenia triggered by recombinant hepatitis B vaccine. Br J Haematol 2000;110(1):230–3.
47. Finielz P, Lam-Kam-Sang LF, Guiserix J. Systemic lupus erythematosus and thrombocytopenic purpura in two members of the same family following hepatitis B vaccine. Nephrol Dial Transplant 1998;13(9):2420–1.
48. Ashok Shenoy K, Prabha Adhikari MR, Chakrapani M, Shenoy D, Pillai A. Pancytopenia after recombinant hepatitis B vaccine—an Indian case report. Br J Haematol 2001;114(4):955.
49. Anonymous. Cutaneous drug reaction case reports: from the world literature. Am J Clin Dermatol 2001;2:49–56.
50. Carmeli Y, Oren R. Hepatitis B vaccine side-effect. Lancet 1993;341(8839):250–1.
51. Islek I, Cengiz K, Cakir M, Kucukoduk S. Nephrotic syndrome following hepatitis B vaccination. Pediatr Nephrol 2000;14(1):89–90.
52. Loche F, Schwarze HP, Thedenat B, Carriere M, Bazex J. Erythema multiforme associated with hepatitis B immunization. Clin Exp Dermatol 2000;25(2):167–8.
53. De Keyser F, Naeyaert JM, Hindryckx P, Elewaut D, Verplancke P, Peene I, Praet M, Veys E. Immune-mediated pathology following hepatitis B vaccination. Two cases of polyarteritis nodosa and one case of pityriasis rosea-like drug eruption. Clin Exp Rheumatol 2000;18(1):81–5.
54. Wise RP, Kiminyo KP, Salive ME. Hair loss after routine immunizations. JAMA 1997;278(14):1176–8.
55. Daoud MS, Dicken CH. Anetoderma after hepatitis B immunization in two siblings. J Am Acad Dermatol 1997;36(5 Pt 1):779–80.
56. Trevisan G, Stinco G. HBV vaccination and lichen planus. G Ital Dermatol Venereol 1993;128:545–8.
57. Hudson TJ, Newkirk M, Gervais F, Shuster J. Adverse reaction to the recombinant hepatitis B vaccine. J Allergy Clin Immunol 1991;88(5):821–2.
58. Baglivo E, Safran AB, Borruat FX. Multiple evanescent white dot syndrome after hepatitis B vaccine. Am J Ophthalmol 1996;122(3):431–2.
59. Barbaud A, Trechot P, Reichert-Penetrat S, Weber M, Schmutz JL. Allergic mechanisms and urticaria/angioedema after hepatitis B immunization. Br J Dermatol 1998;139(5):925–6.
60. Rabaud C, Barbaud A, Trechot P. First case of erythermalgia related to hepatitis B vaccination. J Rheumatol 1999;26(1):233–4.
61. Anonymous. Alleged link between hepatitis B vaccine and chronic fatigue syndrome. CMAJ 1992;146(1):37–8.
62. Bracci M, Zoppini A. Polyarthritis associated with hepatitis B vaccination. Br J Rheumatol 1997;36(2):300–1.
63. Biasi D, De Sandre G, Bambara LM, Carletto A, Caramaschi P, Zanoni G, Tridente G. A new case of reactive arthritis after hepatitis B vaccination. Clin Exp Rheumatol 1993;11(2):215.
64. Rogerson SJ, Nye FJ. Hepatitis B vaccine associated with erythema nodosum and polyarthritis. BMJ 1990;301(6747):345.
65. Toussirot E, Lohse A, Wendling D, Mougin C. Sjogren's syndrome occurring after hepatitis B vaccination. Arthritis Rheum 2000;43(9):2139–40.
66. Drucker Y, Prayson RA, Bagg A, Calabrese LH. Lymphocytic vasculitis presenting as diffuse subcutaneous edema after hepatitis B virus vaccine. J Clin Rheumatol 1997;3:158–61.

67. Mathieu E, Fain O, Krivitzky A. Cryoglobulinemia after hepatitis B vaccination. N Engl J Med 1996;335(5):355.
68. Tudela P, Marti S, Bonal J. Systemic lupus erythematosus and vaccination against hepatitis B. Nephron 1992;62(2):236.
69. Vanoli M, Gambini D, Scorza R. A case of Churg–Strauss vasculitis after hepatitis B vaccination. Ann Rheum Dis 1998;57(4):256–7.
70. Zaas A, Scheel P, Venbrux A, Hellmann DB. Large artery vasculitis following recombinant hepatitis B vaccination: 2 cases. J Rheumatol 2001;28(5):1116–20.
71. Saadoun D, Cacoub P, Mahoux D, Sbai A, Piette JC. Vascularites postvaccinales: à propos de trois observations. [Postvaccine vasculitis: a report of three cases.] Rev Med Interne 2001;22(2):172–6.
72. Casals JL, Vazguez MA. Artritis inducida por vacunacion antihepatitis B. [Arthritis induced by antihepatitis B vaccine.] An Med Interna 1999;16(11):601–2.
73. Le Hello C, Cohen P, Bousser MG, Letellier P, Guillevin L. Suspected hepatitis B vaccination related vasculitis. J Rheumatol 1999;26(1):191–4.
74. Levy M, Koren G. Hepatitis B vaccine in pregnancy: maternal and fetal safety. Am J Perinatol 1991;8(3):227–32.
75. Kirkland LR. Ocular sensitivity to thimerosal: a problem with hepatitis B vaccine? South Med J 1990;83(5):497–9.
76. Cosnes A, Flechet ML, Revuz J. Inflammatory nodular reactions after hepatitis B vaccination due to aluminium sensitization. Contact Dermatitis 1990;23(2):65–7.
77. Hutteroth TH, Quast U. Aluminiumhydroxid-Granulome nach Hepatitis-B-Impfung (Fragen aus der Praxis). [Aluminum hydroxide granuloma following hepatitis B vaccination.] Dtsch Med Wochenschr 1990;115(12):476.
78. Skowron F, Grezard P, Berard F, Balme B, Perrot H. Persistent nodules at sites of hepatitis B vaccination due to aluminium sensitization. Contact Dermatitis 1998;39(3):135–6.
79. Rietschel RL, Adams RM. Reactions to thimerosal in hepatitis B vaccines. Dermatol Clin 1990;8(1):161–4.
80. Jungkunz G, Kohler P, Holbach M, Schweisfurth H. Kasuistik: Zwei Fälle mit heftiger lokaler Reaktion nach aktiver Hepatitis-B-Impfung bei Sensibilisierung auf Thiomersal. Hyg Med 1990;15:418–20.
81. Jilg W, Schmidt M, Deinhardt F. Immune response to hepatitis B revaccination. J Med Virol 1988;24(4):377–84.
82. Jilg W, Schmidt M, Weinel B, Kuttler T, Brass H, Bommer J, Muller R, Schulte B, Schwarzbeck A, Deinhardt F. Immunogenicity of recombinant hepatitis B vaccine in dialysis patients. J Hepatol 1986;3(2):190–5.
83. Safary A, Andre F. Clinical development of a new recombinant DNA hepatitis B vaccine. Postgrad Med J 1987;63(Suppl 2):105–7.
84. Wiedermann G, Ambrosch F, Kremsner P, Kunz C, Hauser P, Simoen E, Andre F, Safary A. Reactogenicity and immunogenicity of different lots of a yeast-derived hepatitis B vaccine. Postgrad Med J 1987;63(Suppl 2):109–13.
85. Wahl M, Hermodsson S. Intradermal, subcutaneous or intramuscular administration of hepatitis B vaccine: side effects and antibody response. Scand J Infect Dis 1987;19(6):617–21.
86. Giammanco G, Li Volti S, Mauro L, Bilancia GG, Salemi I, Barone P, Musumeci S. Immune response to simultaneous administration of a recombinant DNA hepatitis B vaccine and multiple compulsory vaccines in infancy. Vaccine 1991;9(10):747–50.
87. Torres JM, Bruguera M, Vidal J, Artigas N. Immune response, efficacy and reactogenicity of hepatitis B vaccine administered simultaneously with DTP and poliomyelitis vaccine. Gastroenterol Hepatol 1993;16:470–3.

Herbal medicines

See also Individual plant genera

General Information

In principle, herbal medicines have the potential to elicit the same types of adverse reactions as synthetic drugs; the body has no way of distinguishing between "natural" and man-made compounds. Herbal medicines consist of whole extracts of plant parts (for example roots, leaves) and contain numerous potentially active molecules. Synergy is normally assumed to play a part in the medicinal effects of plant extracts, and medical herbalists have always claimed that whole plant extracts have superior effects over single isolated constituents. Similarly, it is also claimed that combinations of herbs have synergistic effects. There is in vitro and/or in vivo evidence to support the occurrence of synergism between constituents in certain herbal extracts (1,2); however, clinical evidence is lacking, and it is in any case uncertain how far the principle extends. Synergy is also taken to mean an attenuation of undesirable effects, another key tenet of herbalism being that the toxicity of plant extracts is less than that of a single isolated constituent. However, theoretically, plant constituents could also interact to render a herbal preparation more toxic than a single chemical constituent. Virtually no evidence is available to substantiate either hypothesis. It is also important to determine whether herbal treatments that have been shown to be as effective as conventional drugs have a better safety profile. Contrary to the belief of most herbalists, long-standing experience is by no means a reliable yardstick when it comes to judging the risk of adverse reactions (3).

Herbal medicine continues to be a growth area. In the UK, retail sales of complementary medicines (licensed herbal medicines, homoeopathic remedies, essential oils used in aromatherapy) were estimated to be £72 million in 1996, an increase of 36% in real terms since 1991 (4). This, however, is likely to be a gross underestimate as popular products sold as food supplements, including *Ginkgo biloba* and garlic, were not included. According to a detailed analysis of the herbal medicines market in Germany and France, total sales of herbal products in those countries in 1997 were US$1.8 billion and US$1.1 billion respectively (5). In 1994, annual retail sales of botanical medicines in the USA were estimated to be around US$1.6 billion; in 1998, the figure was closer to US$4 billion (6).

Some of the most useful data on trends in the use of herbal medicines come from two surveys of US adults carried out in 1991 and 1997/98, which involved over 1500 and over 2000 individuals respectively (7,8). The use of at least one form of complementary therapy in the 12 months preceding the survey increased significantly from 34% in 1990 to 42% in 1997. Herbal medicine was one of the therapies showing the most increase over this time period: there was a statistically significant increase in self-medication with herbal medicine from 2.5% of the sample in 1990 to 13% in 1997 (8). Disclosure rates to physicians of complementary medicine use were below 40% in both surveys (8). Furthermore, 18% of prescription medicine users took prescription medicines concurrently with herbal remedies and/or high-dose vitamins. These aspects of user behaviour clearly have implications for safety.

A hospital-based study from Oman has suggested that 15% of all cases of self-poisoning seen in this setting are with traditional medicines (9). A case series from Thailand has suggested that in patients with oral squamous cell carcinoma the use of herbal medicines before the first consultation with a healthcare professional increases the risk of an advanced stage almost six-fold (10) and survey data from the USA have suggested that herb–drug interactions may be a significant problem in a sizeable proportion of patients (11).

Several herbal medicines pose serious problems for surgical patients, for example through an increased bleeding tendency (12,13). Vulnerable populations also include children (14), and too few safety data are available to recommend herbal medicines during pregnancy or lactation (15). Several investigators have pointed out the potential of herbal medicines to harm certain organs, for example the liver (16) or the skin (17). Laxatives are often based on herbal extracts, and the risks of herbal laxatives have been emphasized (18). Many authors have reviewed the risks of herbal medicines in general terms (19,20).

The reasons for the popularity of herbal medicine are many and diverse. It appears that complementary medicine is not usually used because of an outright rejection of conventional medicine, but more because users desire to control their own health (5) and because they find complementary medicine to be more congruent with their own values, beliefs, and philosophical orientations toward health and life (21). Also, users may consult different practitioners for different reasons (5). An important reason for the increase in use is that consumers (often motivated by the lay press) consider complementary medicine to be "natural" and assume it is "safe". However, this notion is dangerously misleading; adverse effects have been associated with the use of complementary therapies (22). Furthermore, complementary therapies may not only be directly harmful (for example adverse effects of a herbal formulation), but like other medical treatments have the potential to be indirectly harmful (for example through being applied incompetently, by delaying appropriate effective treatment, or by causing needless expense) (23).

Incidence of adverse effects

Most of the data on adverse effects associated with herbal medicines is anecdotal, and assessment and classification of causality is often not possible. Likewise, there have been few attempts to determine systematically the incidence of adverse effects of non-orthodox therapies.

Of 1701 patients admitted to two general wards of a Hong Kong hospital, 3 (0.2%) had adverse reactions to Chinese herbal drugs; two of the three were serious (24). In a retrospective study of all 2695 patients admitted to a Taiwan department of medicine during 10 months 4% were admitted because of drug-related problems, and herbal remedies ranked third amongst the categories of medicines responsible (25). In an active surveillance adverse drug reaction reporting program conducted in a family medicine ward of the National Taiwan University Hospital, Chinese crude drugs were responsible for five hospital admissions (22% of the total) or 12% of all adverse reactions observed in the study (26). This is a part of the world where the herbal tradition is particularly strong; the figures do not apply elsewhere.

The incidence of contact sensitization associated with topical formulations containing plant extracts was significant when evaluated in 1032 consecutive or randomly selected patients visiting patch test clinics in The Netherlands (27).

In a 5-year toxicological study of traditional remedies and food supplements carried out by the Medical Toxicology Unit at Guy's and St. Thomas' Hospital, London, 1297 symptomatic enquiries by medical professionals were evaluated (28). Of these, an association was considered to have been confirmed, probable, or possible in 12, 35, and 738 cases respectively. Ten of the confirmed cases were related to Chinese or Indian herbal remedies. As a result of these findings, in October 1996 the UK Committee on Safety of Medicines extended its yellow card scheme for adverse drug reaction reporting to include unlicensed herbal remedies, which are marketed mostly as food supplements in the UK (the scheme had always applied to licensed herbal medicines) (29,30). This was an important milestone in herbal pharmacovigilance.

A report from the Uppsala Monitoring Centre of the WHO has summarized all suspected adverse reactions to herbal medicaments reported from 55 countries worldwide over 20 years (31). A total of 8985 case reports were on record. Most originated from Germany (20%), followed by France (17%), the USA (17%), and the UK (12%). Allergic reactions were the most frequent serious adverse events and there were 21 deaths. The authors pointed out that adverse reactions to herbal medicaments constitute only about 0.5% of all adverse reactions on record.

General adverse effects

Several reviews have focused on herbal medicines and have covered:

- the toxicity of medicinal plants (32–34);
- the safety of herbal products in general (35–46);
- adverse effects in specific countries, for example the USA (47) and Malaysia (48);
- adverse effects on specific organs (49), such as the cardiovascular system (50), the liver (51,52), and the skin (53,54);
- the safety of herbal medicines in vulnerable populations: elderly patients (55), pregnant women (56), and surgical patients (57,58);
- carcinogenicity (59);
- the adverse effects of herbal antidepressants (60);
- the adverse effects of Chinese herbal medicaments (61,62);
- the adverse effects of Ayurvedic medicines (63);
- herb–drug interactions (64–75);
- pharmacovigilance of herbal medicines (76).

Direct effects associated with herbal medicines can occur in several ways:

- hypersusceptibility reactions
- collateral reactions
- toxic reactions
- drug interactions
- contamination

- false authentication
- lack of quality control.

Some of these effects relate to product quality. While there are some data on certain of these aspects, information on other aspects is almost entirely lacking. For example, there are isolated case reports of interactions between conventional medicines and complementary (usually herbal) remedies (23,77,78), although further information is largely theoretical (79).

Even a perfectly safe remedy (mainstream or unorthodox) can become unsafe when used incompetently. Medical competence can be defined as doing everything in the best interest of the patient according to the best available evidence. There are numerous circumstances, both in orthodox and complementary medicine, when competence is jeopardized:

- missed diagnosis
- misdiagnosis
- disregarding contraindications
- preventing/delaying more effective treatments (for example misinformation about effective therapies; loss of herd immunity through a negative attitude toward immunization)
- clinical deterioration not diagnosed
- adverse reaction not diagnosed
- discontinuation of prescribed drugs
- self-medication.

The attitude of consumers toward herbal medicines can also constitute a risk. When 515 users of herbal remedies were interviewed about their behavior vis a vis adverse effects of herbal versus synthetic over-the-counter drugs, a clear difference emerged. While 26% would consult their doctor for a serious adverse effect of a synthetic medication, only 0.8% would do the same in relation to herbal remedies (80).

The only way to minimize incompetence is by proper education and training, combined with responsible regulatory control. While training and control are self-evident features of mainstream medicine they are often not fully incorporated in complementary medicine. Thus the issue of indirect health risk is particularly pertinent to complementary medicine. Whenever complementary practitioners take full responsibility for a patient, this should be matched with full medical competence; if on the other hand, competence is not demonstrably complete, the practitioner in question should not assume full responsibility (81).

Asian herbalism

Most reports of adverse effects associated with herbal remedies relate to Chinese herbal medicines (82). This is an issue of growing concern, particularly because in many Western countries the popularity of Chinese herbalism is increasing. This is happening in the almost complete absence of governmental control (83) or of systematic research into the potential hazards of Chinese herbal formulations (84).

There have been several reports of adverse effects associated with Asian herbal formulations (85–105). Most of the serious adverse effects of Chinese herbal remedies are associated with formulations containing aconitine, anticholinergic compounds, aristolochic acid, or podophyllin, contaminating substances (106). Problems with Chinese herbal formulations are intensified because of nomenclature, since common, botanical, and Chinese names exist side by side, making confusion likely.

In a German hospital specializing in Chinese herbalism of 145 patients who had been treated within 1 year 53% reported having had at least one adverse effect attributable to Chinese herbal medicines (107). Nausea, vomiting, and diarrhea were the most common complaints. It should be noted that causality in these cases can only be suspected and not proven. In the same institution about 1% of 1507 consecutive patients treated with Chinese herbal mixtures had clinically relevant rises in liver enzymes (108,109). *Glycyrrhiza* radix and *Atractylodis macrocephalae* rhizome were most consistently associated with such problems. In most of these cases there were no associated clinical signs and the abnormalities tended to normalize without specific therapy and in spite of continued treatment with the Chinese herbal mixtures.

When 1100 Australian practitioners of traditional Chinese medicine were asked to complete questionnaires about the adverse effects of Chinese herbal mixtures, they reported 860 adverse events, including 19 deaths (110). It was calculated that each practitioner had encountered an average of 1.4 adverse events during each year of full-time practice.

A physician prospectively monitored all 1265 patients taking traditional Chinese medicines at his clinic during 33 months (111). Liver enzymes were measured before the start of therapy and 3 and 10 weeks later. Alanine transaminase activity was raised in 107 patients (8.5%) who initially had normal values. Of these patients, about 25% reported symptoms such as abdominal discomfort, looseness of bowels, loss of appetite, or fatigue.

A retrospective analysis of all adverse events related to herbal medicines and dietary supplements reported to the California Poison Control System has given data on the risks of the adverse effects of herbal medicines (112). Between January 1997 and June 1998, 918 calls relating to such supplements were received. Exposures resulting in adverse reactions occurred most often at recommended doses. There were 233 adverse events, of which 29% occurred in children. The products most frequently implicated were zinc (38%), *Echinacea* (8%), witch hazel (6%), and chromium picolinate (6%). Most of the adverse events were not severe and required no treatment; hospitalization was required in only three cases.

Quality control and purity of herbal products

Quality control for herbal medicaments that are sold as dietary supplements in most countries is poor (113,114). Thus, considerable variations in the contents of active ingredients have been reported, with lot-to-lot variations of up to 1000% (115). In most countries, the sale and supply of herbal remedies is to a large extent uncontrolled and unregulated; most herbal remedies are sold as unlicensed food supplements and their safety, efficacy, and quality have therefore not been assessed by licensing authorities. Adulteration and contamination of herbal remedies with other plant material and conventional drugs have been documented (25,116) (Table 1).

Table 1 Potential adulterants that should be taken into account in the quality control of herbal medicines

Type of adulterant	Examples
Allopathic drugs	Analgesic and anti-inflammatory agents (for example aminophenazone, indometacin, phenylbutazone), benzodiazepines, glucocorticoids, sulfonylureas, thiazide diuretics, thyroid hormones
Botanicals	*Atropa belladonna*, *Digitalis* species, *Colchicum*, *Rauwolfia serpentina*, pyrrolizidine-containing plants (see separate monograph on pyrrolizidines)
Fumigation agents	Ethylene oxide, methyl bromide, phosphine
Heavy metals	Arsenic, cadmium, lead, mercury
Micro-organisms	*Escherichia coli* (certain strains), *Pseudomonas aeruginosa*, *Salmonella*, *Shigella*, *Staphylococcus aureus*
Microbial toxins	Aflatoxins, bacterial endotoxins
Pesticides	Carbamate insecticides and herbicides, chlorinated pesticides (for example aldrin, dieldrin, heptachlor, DDT, DDE, HCB, HCH isomers), dithiocarbamate fungicides, organic phosphates, triazine herbicides
Radionuclides	^{134}Cs, ^{137}Cs, ^{103}Ru, ^{131}I, ^{90}Sr

The authors of a survey of German importers of Chinese herbs concluded that "only rarely" had herbal drugs to be returned because of contamination (117). The authors also stated that "a 100% check for all possible contaminants is not possible." However, there have been many reports of adulteration and contamination relate to Chinese herbal remedies (118). Instances include adulteration/contamination with conventional drugs (119,120), heavy metals (121–127), and other substances (128,129).

When 27 samples of commercially available camomile formulations were tested in Brazil, it was found that all of them contained adulterants and only 50% had the essential oils needed to produce anti-inflammatory activity (130).

Concerns about the quality and safety of herbal remedies are justified, and there have been repeated calls for greater control and regulation (28,131,132).

Adulteration with allopathic drugs

Barbiturates

Phenobarbital has been reported as a contaminant in a Chinese patent medicine (133).

- A 10-year-old boy developed respiratory depression and became comatose after taking the Chinese patent medicine "Diankexing" for 6 months. His urine phenobarbital concentration was 95 μg/ml (target range 20–40 μg/ml). The remedy was withdrawn and he was successfully treated with activated charcoal.

Benzodiazepines

The Botanical Lab in the USA has manufactured the herbal medicines PC-SPES and SPES (134). These two products are marketed as "herbal dietary supplements" for "prostate health" and for "strengthening the immune system" respectively. They are sold through the internet, by mail order, by phone order, and through various distributors and health care professionals. An analytical report from the California Department of Health in 2002 showed that samples of PC-SPES and SPES have been contaminated with alprazolam and warfarin. The Canadian Medicines Regulatory Authority also reported similar contaminations. In view of these reports Health Canada, the Irish Medicines Board, and the State Health Director of California all warned consumers to stop using these two products immediately and to consult their healthcare practitioners. Botanic Lab also informed consumers of these laboratory findings and issued a product recall of all lots of PC-SPES, pending further reports from additional testing of PC-SPES in both commercial and academic laboratories.

In 2001 the California State Health Director warned consumers to stop using the herbal product Anso Comfort capsules immediately, because the product contains the undeclared prescription drug chlordiazepoxide. Chlordiazepoxide is a benzodiazepine that is used for anxiety and as a sedative and can be dangerous if not taken under medical supervision (135). Anso Comfort capsules, available by mail or telephone order from the distributor in 60-capsule bottles, were clear with dark green powder inside. The label was yellow with green English printing and a picture of a plant. An investigation by the California Department of Health Services Food and Drug Branch and Food and Drug Laboratory showed that the product contained chlordiazepoxide. The ingredients for the product were imported from China and the capsules were manufactured in California. Advertising for the product claimed that the capsules were useful for the treatment of a wide variety of illnesses, including high blood pressure and high cholesterol, in addition to claims that it was a natural herbal dietary supplement. The advertising also claimed that the product contained only Chinese herbal ingredients and that consumers could reduce or stop their need for prescribed medicines. No clear medical evidence supported any of these claims. The distributor, NuMeridian (formerly known as Top Line Project), voluntarily recalled the product nationwide.

A San Francisco woman with a history of diabetes and high blood pressure was hospitalized in January 2001 with life-threatening hypoglycemia after she consumed Anso Comfort capsules. This may have been due to an interaction of chlordiazepoxide with other unspecified medications that she was taking.

Glucocorticoids

Wau Wa cream is marketed in several countries as a herbal cream for eczema. After repeatedly observing surprising therapeutic successes, UK doctors analysed three samples of this cream given to them by three patients (136). The samples contained 0.013% clobetasol propionate, a powerful glucocorticoid that does not occur naturally.

Betamethasone, 0.1–0.3 mg per capsule, has been detected in Cheng Kum and Shen Loon, two herbal medicines that are popular for their benefits in joint pain, skin problems, colds, menopausal symptoms, and dysmenorrhea (137). Over-exposure to betamethasone can result in typical signs of glucocorticoid excess, such as moon face, hypertension, easy bruising, purple abdominal striae, truncal obesity, and hirsutism. The recommended daily adult dose of Cheng Kum is 1–3 capsules per day, and there have been reports of glucocorticoid-induced adverse effects in patients taking Cheng Kum and Shen Loon, even in the absence of other exogenous corticosteroid consumption.

- Two patients, a 29-year-old woman and a 10-year-old girl, developed Cushingoid features after taking Shen Loon for 4 and 5 months respectively (138). Their morning plasma cortisol concentrations were increased and adrenal suppression was confirmed by a short Synacthen test. Both recovered after withdrawal of the remedy and treatment with prednisone.

The New Zealand Medicines and Medical Devices Safety Authority (Medsafe) has notified that the further importation of these herbal products into New Zealand will be stopped at Customs. However, because of the risk of adrenal suppression from glucocorticoid, consumers have been sent a letter advising them against abruptly discontinuing these products. They should continue with the treatment and see their general practitioner as soon as possible for instructions on how they can be safely weaned off the product. Medsafe has issued a letter to doctors advising them to determine whether patients taking Cheng Kum or Shen Loon are at risk of adrenal suppression by estimating the potential total dose of glucocorticoid (from Cheng Kum or Shen Loon plus any exogenous steroids) and the duration of use, by examining the patient for signs of glucocorticoid excess, and by ascertaining if other risk factors for adrenal suppression are present (such as Addison's disease and AIDS).

Hypoglycemic drugs

Herbal medicines, particularly Chinese ones, are sometimes contaminated with conventional synthetic drugs (139). In 2000 the California Department of Health Services Food and Drug Branch issued a warning to consumers that they should immediately stop using five herbal products because they contained two prescription drugs that were not listed as ingredients and that are unsafe without monitoring by a physician (140). The products were Diabetes Hypoglucose Capsules, Pearl Hypoglycemic Capsules, Tongyi Tang Diabetes Angel Pearl Hypoglycemic Capsules, Tongyi Tang Diabetes Angel Hypoglycemic Capsules, and Zhen Qi Capsules. The products were available by mail order and could be purchased by telephone or via the Internet. Their manufacturers claimed that they contained only natural Chinese herbal ingredients. However, after a diabetic patient in Northern California had had several episodes of hypoglycemia after taking Diabetes Hypoglucose Capsules, an investigation by the Department showed that they contain the antidiabetic drugs glibenclamide (glyburide) and phenformin.

Penicillamine

Penicillamine unexpectedly caused myasthenia gravis when present as an unrecognized additive in Chinese herbs (141).

Various

A systematic review included 18 case reports, two case series, and four analytical studies showing adulteration with various allopathic drugs (142). The adulterants included phenazone (aminopyrine), clobetasol propionate and other glucocorticoids, diazepam, diclofenac, glibenclamide, hydrochlorothiazide, indometacin, mefenamic acid, methylsalicylate, phenacetin, phenylbutazone, and phenytoin.

In 2002 the Medicines Safety Authority of the Ministry of Health in New Zealand (Medsafe) ordered the withdrawal of several traditional Chinese medicines sold as herbal remedies, since they contained scheduled medicines and toxic substances (143). The products included the following allopathic drugs:

- Wei Ge Wang tablets, which contained sildenafil
- Sang Ju Gan Mao Pian tablets, which contained diclofenac and chlorphenamine
- Yen Qiao Jie Du Pian capsules, which contained chlorphenamine, diclofenac, and paracetamol
- Xiaoke Wan pills, which contained glibenclamide
- Shuen Feng cream, which contained ketoconazole
- Dezhong Rhinitis drops, which contained ephedrine hydrochloride.

The New Zealand Director General of Health issued a Public Statement asking people to stop taking these products and to seek medical advice. Medsafe asked all importers and distributors of traditional Chinese medicines to cease all distribution and sale of these products, to withdraw them from retail outlets, and to ensure that other products they sell do not contain scheduled medicines.

Adulteration with botanicals

Two cases have been reported of contamination of plantain (a plant of the genus *Plantago*) by *Digitalis lanata* (144). Both patients suffered from serious overdose of cardiac glycosides with toxic serum digoxin concentrations as a result.

Adulteration with heavy metals

In 2002 the Medicines Safety Authority of the Ministry of Health in New Zealand (Medsafe) ordered the withdrawal of several traditional Chinese medicines sold as herbal remedies, since they contained scheduled medicines and toxic substances (143). The products included Niu Huang Jie Du Pian tablets, which contain 4% arsenic.

In Taipei, 319 children aged 1–7 years were screened for increased blood lead concentrations (145). The consumption of Chinese herbal medicines was significantly correlated with blood lead concentrations. In 2803 subjects from Taipei a history of herbal drug taking proved to be a major risk factor for increased blood lead concentrations (146).

- A 56-year-old woman developed the signs and symptoms of lead poisoning after taking an Indian herbal medicine for many years (147). Her blood and urine lead concentrations were 1530 ng/ml and 4785 μg/day. She also had raised liver enzymes. After withdrawal of the remedy and treatment with penicillamine, she made a full recovery.
- Czech doctors reported the case of a 26-year-old woman who had taken an Ayurvedic remedy (Astrum FE Femikalp) for sterility (148). It contained lead 113 mg/kg. Her blood lead concentration was raised and

normalized 1 month after withdrawal of the remedy. Lead poisoning was also confirmed by hair analysis.

Of 260 Asian patent medicines available in California, 7% contained undeclared pharmaceuticals. When 251 samples were tested for heavy metals, 24 products contained at least 10 parts per million of lead, 36 contained arsenic, and 35 contained mercury (149).

Three Singapore patients with chronic arsenic poisoning with characteristic skin changes had taken Chinese herbal remedies for many years to treat their asthma; two had cancers likely to be due to arsenic (150).

Cases of adulteration with the heavy metals mercury (151) and lead (152) have been reported.

- A 5-year-old Chinese boy developed motor and vocal tics. His parents had given him a Chinese herbal spray to treat mouth ulcers. The spray contained mercury 878 ppm. Mercury poisoning was confirmed by the blood mercury concentration (183 nmol/l, normal value for adults under 50 nmol/l).
- A 5-year-old boy of Indian origin with encephalopathy, seizures, and developmental delay developed persistent anemia. The more obvious causes were ruled out and his blood lead concentration was high (860 ng/ml). He was treated with chelation therapy and his blood lead concentration fell. For the previous 4 years his parents had given him "Tibetan Herbal Vitamins," produced in India, which contained large amounts of lead. The investigators calculated that over that time he had ingested around 63 g of lead.

A total of 54 samples of Asian remedies, purchased in Vietnam, Hong Kong, Florida, New York, and New Jersey, were analysed for heavy metal adulteration (153). They contained concentrations of arsenic, lead, and mercury that ranged from merely exceeding published guidelines (74%) to toxic (49%).

Ayurvedic medicines have also been reportedly adulterated and contaminated (154). For example, they have repeatedly been associated with arsenic poisoning, including hyperpigmentation and hyperkeratosis (155). Of 70 unique Ayurvedic products manufactured in India or Pakistan and sold in Boston, mostly for gastrointestinal disorders, 14 contained lead, mercury, and/or arsenic, in concentrations up to about 100 mg/g (156).

Adulteration with inorganic chemicals

There is a practice among urbanized South African blacks to replace traditional herbal ingredients of purgative enemas with sodium or potassium dichromate. This switch can result in serious toxicity, characterized by acute renal insufficiency, gastrointestinal hemorrhage, and hepatocellular dysfunction (157,158).

Contamination with micro-organisms

When 62 samples of medicinal plant material and 11 samples of herbal tea were examined in Croatia, fungal contamination was found to be abundant (159). *Aspergillus flavus*, a known producer of aflatoxins was present in 11 and one sample respectively. Mycotoxins were found in seven of the samples analysed.

Kombucha "mushroom" is a symbiotic yeast/bacteria aggregate surrounded by a permeable membrane. An outbreak of skin lesions affecting 20 patients from a village near Tehran has been reported (160). The lesions were painless and had a central black necrotic area, marginal erythema, and severe peripheral edema. These clinical signs led to the suspicion of anthrax infection. It turned out that all patients had applied Kombucha mushroom locally as a painkiller. The skin lesions had developed 5–7 days after the application of the material. Cultures from the skin lesions confirmed the presence of *Bacillus anthracis*. Cultures of the Kombucha mushrooms were inconclusive, owing to multiple bacterial contamination and overgrowth, but it was shown that anthrax would grow on uncontaminated material. The patients all recovered with antibiotic therapy.

Contamination with pesticides

Some herbal medicaments are contaminated with pesticides (161).

Drug overdose

In a retrospective study of 2764 poisoning cases admitted to eight urban hospitals in Zimbabwe between 1998 and 1999, 7% of all cases and 13% of all deaths were related to traditional medicines (162). The authors noted that these figures were markedly lower than those from a similar survey 10 years earlier.

Susceptibility factors

Owing to extensive modifications of drug formulations and chemical extracts from an expanding range of natural products, herbal formulations may contain ingredients that are particularly harmful to individuals with glucose-6-phosphate dehydrogenase (G6PD) deficiency. Extra vigilance is therefore required when herbal medicinal formulations, including topical applications, are used by patients with G6PD deficiency and even their carers (163).

Thallophytes

Liver damage has been attributed to *Spirulina*, a type of blue–green algae.

- A 52-year-old Japanese man was admitted with signs and symptoms consistent with toxic liver damage (164). His medical history relevant to liver disease was unremarkable; in particular, his liver enzymes had been normal. It turned out that 5 weeks before admission he had started taking a remedy containing *Spirulina*. A lymphocyte stimulation test for *Spirulina* was positive and infectious hepatitis was excluded. Liver biopsy was consistent with toxic liver injury. After withdrawal of *Spirulina* all his liver enzymes quickly returned to normal.

Proprietary herbal mixtures

Numerous herbal mixtures are promoted worldwide, for example through the Internet. In many cases their herbal ingredients are not disclosed.

Copaltra

Copaltra is a herbal tea sold in France as an adjuvant therapy for diabetes. It contains *Coutarea latiflora* (50 g) and *Centaurium erythreae* (50 g).

- A 49-year-old black woman was admitted with jaundice and raised liver enzymes 4 months after starting to take

Copaltra (165). She also took fenofibrate, polyunsaturated fatty acids, metformin, benfluorex, and veralipride. Liver biopsy confirmed the diagnosis of acute, severe, cytolytic hepatitis, most likely drug-induced. She made a full recovery after withdrawal of Copaltra.

The authors mentioned that five similar cases of Copaltra-induced hepatitis have been reported to the French authorities.

Essiac

Essiac is a Canadian herbal mixture promoted as a cancer cure. It has been reported to have caused fever (166).

- A 46-year-old woman with a squamous cell carcinoma of the cervix developed neutropenic fever during radiation therapy, 10 days after taking Essiac. The fever resolved after antibiotic therapy, but it delayed her radiation therapy for 9 days and required 4 days of hospitalization.

The authors felt that Essiac had caused this problem, but causality was uncertain, not least because she also took four other herbal medicaments.

Herbalife

Herbalife is a complex herbal formula that is promoted for weight loss. Acute mania has been attributed to it (167).

- A 39-year-old man developed classic symptoms of mania within 4–72 hours of taking Herbalife. He continued to take it and after several days became psychotic, paranoid, and out of control, culminating in a high-speed car chase with the police. Bipolar disorder was diagnosed and treated, including withdrawal of the Herbalife, and he remained free of symptoms 3 months later.

The author thought it likely that the herbal mixture had caused the psychotic illness in a man who had no previous history of mental disturbance.

Iberogast

Iberogast contains extracts of bitter candy tuft, chamomile flower, peppermint leaves, caraway fruit, licorice root, lemon balm leaves, angelica root, celandine, and milk thistle fruit, and has been used to treat dyspepsia (168). In a systematic review, adverse events were rare and similar to those found with placebo (169).

Isabgol

Isabgol is an Italian herbal mixture that is promoted for constipation.

- Syncytial giant cell hepatitis occurred in a 26-year-old woman who used Isabgol (170). Autoimmune disease and viral infections were excluded.

The authors felt that the causative role of the Isabgol was supported by the spontaneous and dramatic clinical, biochemical, and histological improvement that followed the withdrawal of Isabgol without any further therapy.

Jai Wey Guo Sao

- A 36-year-old woman was admitted to hospital because of general malaise (171). She had lost 5 kg within 6 months. She was found to have interstitial renal fibrosis and irreversible renal insufficiency. She had taken a Chinese herbal mixture Jai wey guo sao to treat irregular menses. The formulation contained *Angelica sinensis* root, *Rhemanniae* root and rhizome, *Ligustici* rhizome, *Paeoniae lactiflore* root, ginseng root, *Eucommiae* cortex, and honey.

The causative agent in this case could not be identified beyond doubt.

Kampo medicines

All admission records of patients suspected of having liver problems related to Kampo medicines between 1979 and 1999 in a Japanese Department of Oriental Medicine were reviewed (172). There were 30 cases that were suspected of being caused by Kampo medicines. On closer examination, nine seemed to be definitely unrelated, six were probably unrelated, nine were possibly related, and six were definitely or probably related to Kampo medicines. There were no deaths on record.

Sho-saiko-to is a so-called kampo medicine, a mixture of herbs, including Chinese date, ginger root, and licorice root. It is reportedly contraindicated in patients taking interferons, patients with liver cirrhosis or hepatoma, and patients with chronic hepatitis and a platelet count of $100 \times 10^9/l$ (http://www.kamponews.com). Sho-saiko-to has repeatedly been implicated in interstitial or eosinophilic pneumonias.

- A 45-year-old woman developed a high fever, a non-productive cough, and severe dyspnea (173). Her chest X-ray showed bilateral alveolar infiltrates. Treatment with antibiotics was not successful and her condition deteriorated. She was finally put on mechanical ventilation and subsequently improved dramatically. It turned out that she had previously taken sho-saiko-to for liver dysfunction of unknown cause.

Based on a positive lymphocyte stimulation test, the authors were confident that this herbal remedy had caused pulmonary edema.

Corneal opacities causing photophobia have been attributed to a Kampo medicine (174).

- A 30-year-old Japanese woman developed bilateral photophobia. There were dust-like opacities in both corneae. She had a superficial keratectomy, and electron microscopy identified the opacities as lipid-like particles. She had intermittently taken a Kampo medicine composed of 18 different herbal ingredients. Her photophobia coincided with episodes of taking this medicine. The remedy was withdrawn and her symptoms subsequently subsided. She then abstained from the Kampo medicine without recurrence.

Severe liver damage has been attributed to a Kampo medicine (175).

- A 50-year-old Japanese woman with a 20-year history of asthma was taking steroids and bronchodilators when she started self-medicating with a Kampo mixture called Saiko-Keishi-Kankyo-To. Two months later, she developed acute severe liver damage. The Kampo mixture was withdrawn and she promptly recovered.

The authors attributed the liver damage to one ingredient of the mixture, *Trichosanthes* radix, a Chinese medicament that is prepared from the root of *Trichosanthes kirilowii maxim* (Tian-hua-fen).

Lipokinetix

The slimming aid "LipoKinetix" contains norephedrine hydrochloride, sodium usinate, 3,5-diiodothyronine, yohimbine hydrochloride, and caffeine. Seven patients all had the signs and symptoms of acute toxic hepatitis after taking this dietary supplement (176). Three patients had taken no other concomitant medications. All recovered spontaneously after "LipoKinetix" was withdrawn.

Rio Hair Naturalizer System

Rio Hair Naturalizer System is a complex mixture of metallic salts and botanical extracts promoted to straighten curled hair. The product has been popular with African Americans in the USA. A survey of 464 individuals who had complained to the FDA about this remedy showed that 95% had experienced hair breakage and hair loss (177). Three-quarters of those who had hair loss had lost 40% or more; regrowth took 8 months on average.

Ting kung teng

Cholinergic poisoning has been attributed to a Chinese herbal mixture, Ting kung teng.

- A 73-year-old man developed a cholinergic syndrome, with dizziness, sweating, chills, lacrimation, salivation, rhinorrhea, nausea, and vomiting after taking the Chinese patent medicine Ting kung teng for arthritis (178). The herbal mixture contained tropane alkaloids with cholinergic activity. After withdrawal of the remedy he made a swift and complete recovery.

Tsumura

Tsumura, a Japanese herbal mixture has been associated with hepatotoxicity (179).

- A 49-year-old Japanese woman had taken oral Tsumura for about 6 weeks to treat internal hemorrhoids when she felt unwell. Her liver enzymes were raised and a diagnosis of drug-induced hepatic damage caused by *Angelica radix* and *Bupleuri* radix contained in the mixture was made. The liver function tests normalized 4 months after withdrawal.

Monographs on herbal products

Each of the monographs on herbal products in this encyclopedia has the following structure:

- Family: each monograph is organized under a family of plants (for example Liliaceae).
- Genera: the various genera that are included under the family name are tabulated (for example the family Liliaceae contains 94 genera); the major source of information on families and genera is the Plants National Database (http://plants.usda.gov/index.html).
- Species: in each monograph some species are dealt with separately. For example, in the monograph on Liliaceae, four species are included under their Latin names and major common names—*Sassafras albidum* (sassafras), *Allium sativum* (garlic), *Colchicum autumnale* (autumn crocus), and *Ruscus aculeatus* (butcher's broom).

Each monograph includes the following information in varying amounts:

- Alternative common names; the major sources of this information are *A Modern Herbal* by Mrs M Grieve (1931; http://www.botanical.com/botanical/mgmh/mgmh.html) and *The Desktop Guide to Complementary and Alternative Medicine: an Evidence-Based Approach* by E Ernst, MH Pittler, C Stevenson, and A White (Mosby, 2001).
- Active ingredients; the major source of this information is the *Dictionary of Plants Containing Secondary Metabolites* by John S Glasby (Taylor & Francis, 1991).
- Uses, including traditional and modern uses.
- Adverse effects.

The families of plants and their species that are the subjects of monographs are listed in Table 2 by alphabetical order of family. The same data are listed in Table 3 by alphabetical order of species. Other monographs cover the Basidiomycetes (*Lentinus edodes*, shiitake) and algae. Table 4 gives the Latin equivalents of the common names. To locate a plant by its common name, convert the common name into the Latin name using Table 4 and then find out to which family it belongs by consulting Table 3.

Table 2 Families of plants and their species that are the subjects of monographs in this encyclopedia (by alphabetical order of family)

Family (common name)	Species (common name)
Acoraceae (calamus)	*Acorus calamus* (calamus root)
Aloeaceae (aloe)	*Aloe capensis* (aloe)
	Aloe vera (aloe)
Amaranthaceae (amaranth)	*Pfaffia paniculata* (Brazilian ginseng)
Anacardiaceae (sumac)	*Rhus species* (sumac)
Apiaceae (carrot)	*Ammi majus* (bishop's weed)
	Ammi visnaga (toothpick weed)
	Angelica sinensis (dong quai)
	Conium maculatum (hemlock)
	Coriandrum sativum (coriander)
	Ferula assa-foetida (asafetida)
Apocynaceae (dogbane)	*Rauwolfia serpentina* (snakeroot)
Araliaceae (ginseng)	*Eleutherococcus senticosus* (Siberian ginseng)
	Panax ginseng (Asian ginseng)
Arecaceae (palm)	*Areca catechu* (areca, betel)
	Serenoa repens (saw palmetto)
Aristolochiaceae (birthwort)	*Aristolochia* species (Dutchman's pipe)
	Asarum heterotropoides (Xu xin)
Asclepiadaceae (milkweed)	*Asclepias tuberosa* (pleurisy root)
	Xysmalobium undulatum (xysmalobium)

Family (common name)	Species (common name)
Asteraceae (aster)	*Achillea millefolium* (yarrow)
	Anthemis species *and Matricaria recutita* (chamomile)
	Arnica montana (arnica)
	Artemisia absinthium (wormwood)
	Artemisea annua (Qinghaosu)
	Artemisia cina (wormseed)
	Artemisia vulgaris (common wormwood)
	Calendula officinalis (marigold)
	Callilepis laureola (impila, ox-eye daisy)
	Chrysanthemum vulgaris (common tansy)
	Cynara scolymus (artichoke)
	Echinacea species (coneflower)
	Eupatorium species (thoroughwort)
	Inula helenium (elecampane)
	Petasites species (butterbur)
	Senecio species (ragwort)
	Silybum marianum (milk thistle)
	Tanacetum parthenium (feverfew)
	Tussilago farfara (coltsfoot)
Berberidaceae (barberry)	*Berberis vulgaris* (European barberry)
	Caulophyllum thalictroides (blue cohosh)
	Dysosma pleianthum (bajiaolian)
	Mahonia species (barberry)
Boraginaceae (borage)	*Cynoglossum officinale* (hound's tongue)
	Symphytum officinale (black wort)
	Heliotropium species (heliotrope)
Brassicaceae (mustard)	*Armoracia rusticana* (horseradish)
	Brassica nigra (black mustard)
	Raphanus sativus var. niger (black radish)
	Sinapis species (mustard)
Campanulaceae (bellflower)	*Lobelia inflata* (Indian tobacco)
Cannabaceae	*Humulus lupulus* (hop)
Capparaceae (caper)	*Capparis spinosa* (caper plant)
Celastraceae (bittersweet)	*Catha edulis* (khat, qat)
	Euonymus europaeus (spindle tree)
	Tripterygium wilfordii (Lei gong teng)
Chenopodiaceae (goosefoot)	*Chenopodium ambrosioides* (American wormseed)
Clusiaceae (mangosteen)	*Hypericum perforatum* (St John's wort)
Convolvulaceae (morning glory)	*Convolvulus scammonia* (Mexican scammony)
	Ipomoea purga (jalap)
Coriariaceae	*Coriaria arborea* (tutu)
Cucurbitaceae (cucumber)	*Bryonia alba* (white bryony)
	Citrullus colocynthis (colocynth)
	Ecballium elaterium (squirting cucumber)
	Momordica charantia (karela fruit, bitter melon)
	Sechium edule (chayote)
Cupressaceae (cypress)	*Juniperus communis* (juniper)
Cycadaceae (cycad)	*Cycas circinalis* (false sago palm)
Droseraceae (sundew)	*Dionaea muscipula* (Venus flytrap)
Dryopteraceae (wood fern)	*Dryopteris filix-mas* (male fern)
Ericaceae (heath)	*Arctostaphylos uva-ursi* (bearberry)
	Gaultheria procumbens (wintergreen)
	Ledum palustre (marsh Labrador tea)
	Vaccinium macrocarpon (cranberry)
Euphorbiaceae (spurge)	*Breynia officinalis* (Chi R Yun)
	Croton tiglium (croton)
	Ricinus communis (castor oil plant)
Fabaceae (pea)	*Cassia* species (senna)
	Crotalaria species (rattlebox)
	Cyamopsis tetragonoloba (cluster bean)
	Cytisus scoparius (Scotch broom)
	Dipteryx species (tonka beans)
	Genista tinctoria (dyer's broom)
	Glycyrrhiza glabra (liquorice)
	Lupinus species (lupin)
	Medicago sativa (alfalfa)
	Melilotus officinalis (sweet clover)
	Myroxylon species (balsam of Peru)
	Pithecollobium jiringa (jering fruit)
	Sophora falvescens (Ku shen)
	Trifolium pratense (red clover)
Gentianaceae (gentian)	*Gentiana* species (gentian)
	Swertia species (felwort)
Ginkgoaceae	*Ginkgo biloba* (maidenhair)
Hippocastanaceae (horse chestnut)	*Aesculus hippocastanum* (horse chestnut)
	Illicium species (star anise)
Illiciaceae (star anise)	*Crocus sativus* (Indian saffron)
Iridaceae (iris)	*Juglans regia* (English walnut)
Juglandaceae (walnut)	*Krameria* species (ratany)
Krameriaceae (Krameria)	*Hedeoma pulegoides* (pennyroyal)
Lamiaceae (mint)	*Lavandula angustifolia* (lavender)
	Mentha piperita (peppermint)
	Mentha pulegium (pennyroyal)
	Salvia miltiorrhiza (danshen)
	Salvia officinalis (sage)
	Scutellaria species (skullcap)
	Teucrium species (germander)
Lauraceae (laurel)	*Cinnamonum camphora* (camphor tree)
	Laurus nobilis (laurel)
	Sassafras albidum (sassafras)
Liliaceae (lily)	*Allium sativum* (garlic)
	Colchicum autumnale (autumn crocus)
	Ruscus aculeatus (butcher's broom)
	Veratrum species (hellebore)
Loganiaceae (Logania)	*Strychnos nux-vomica* (nux vomica)
Lycopodiaceae (club moss)	*Lycopodium serratum* (clubmoss)
Malvaceae (mallow)	*Gossypium* species (cotton)
	Psoralea corylifolia (bakuchi)
Meliaceae (mahogany)	*Azadirachta indica* (bead tree)
Menispermaceae (moonseed)	*Stephania* species (Jin bu huan)
Myristicaceae (nutmeg)	*Myristica fragrans* (nutmeg)
Myrtaceae (myrtle)	*Eucalyptus* species (eucalyptus)
	Melaleuca alternifolia (tea tree)
Onagraceae (evening primrose)	*Oenothera biennis* (evening primrose)
	Chelidonium majus (celandine)

Continued

Table 2 Continued

Family (common name)	Species (common name)
Papaveraceae (poppy)	*Papaver somniferum* (opium poppy)
	Passiflora incarnata (passion flower)
Passifloraceae (passion flower)	*Harpagophytum procumbens* (devil's claw)
Pedaliaceae (sesame)	*Phytolacca americana* (pokeweed)
Phytolaccaceae (pokeweed)	*Piper methysticum* (kava kava)
Piperaceae (pepper)	*Plantago* species (plantain)
Plantaginaceae (plantain)	*Anthoxanthum odoratum* (sweet vernal grass)
Poaceae (grass)	*Polygonum* (knotweed)
Polygonaceae (buckwheat)	*Rheum palmatum* (rhubarb)
	Aconitum napellus (monkshood)
Ranunculaceae (buttercup)	*Cimicifuga racemosa* (black cohosh)
	Delphinium species (delphinium)
	Hydrastis canadensis (golden seal)
	Pulsatilla species (pasque flower)
	Ranunculus damascenus (buttercup)
	Rhamnus purshianus (cascara sagrada)
Rhamnaceae (buckthorn)	*Ziziphus jujuba* (dazao)
	Crataegus species (hawthorn)
Rosaceae (rose)	*Prunus* species (plum)
	Zingiber officinale (ginger)
	Asperula odorata (sweet woodruff)
Rubiaceae (madder)	*Cephaelis ipecacuanha* (ipecac)
	Hintonia latiflora (copalchi bark)
	Morinda citrifolia (noni)
	Rubia tinctorum (madder)
	Uncaria tomentosa (cat's claw)
	Agathosma betulina (buchu)
Rutaceae (rue)	*Citrus auranticum* (bergamot)
	Citrus paradisi (grapefruit)
	Dictamnus dasycarpus (densefruit pittany)
	Pilocarpus species (pilocarpus)
	Ruta graveolens (rue)
	Salix species (willow)
Salicaceae (willow)	*Blighia sapida* (akee)
Sapindaceae (soapberry)	*Paullinia cupana* (guaraná)
	Selaginella doederleinii (spike moss)
Selaginellaceae (spike moss)	*Anisodus tanguticus* (Zangqie)
Solanaceae (potato)	*Capsicum annum* (chili pepper)
	Datura candida (angel's trumpet)
	Datura stramonium (Jimson weed)
	Datura suaveolens (angel's trumpet)
	Lycium barbarum (Chinese wolfberry)
	Mandragora species (mandrake)
	Nicotiana tabacum (tobacco)
	Scopolia species (scopola)
	Sterculia species (sterculia)
Sterculiaceae (cacao)	*Taxus* species (yew)
Taxaceae (yew)	*Camellia sinensis* (green tea)
Theaceae (tea)	*Urtica dioica* (stinging nettle)
Urticaceae (nettle)	*Valeriana* (valerian)
Valerianaceae (valerian)	*Vitex agnus-castus* (chaste tree)
Verbenaceae (verbena)	*Phoradendron flavescens* (American mistletoe)
Viscaceae (Christmas mistletoe)	*Viscum album* (mistletoe)

Table 3 Families of plants and their genera or species that are the subjects of monographs in this encyclopedia (by alphabetical order of genus or species)

Genus or species (common name)	Family (common name)
Achillea millefolium (yarrow)	Asteraceae (aster)
Aconitum napellus (monkshood)	Ranunculaceae (buttercup)
Acorus calamus (calamus root)	Acoraceae (calamus)
Aesculus hippocastanum (horse chestnut)	Hippocastanaceae (horse chestnut)
Agathosma betulina (buchu)	Rutaceae (rue)
Allium sativum (garlic)	Liliaceae (lily)
Aloe capensis (aloe)	Aloeaceae (aloe)
Aloe vera (aloe)	Aloeaceae (aloe)
Ammi majus (bishop's weed)	Apiaceae (carrot)
Ammi visnaga (toothpick weed)	Apiaceae (carrot)
Angelica sinensis (dong quai)	Apiaceae (carrot)
Anisodus tanguticus (zangqie),	Solanaceae (potato)
Anthemis species (chamomile)	Asteraceae (aster)
Anthoxanthum odoratum (sweet vernal grass)	Poaceae (grass)
Arctostaphylos uva-ursi (bearberry)	Ericaceae (heath)
Areca catechu (areca, betel)	Arecaceae (palm)
Aristolochia species (Dutchman's pipe)	Aristolochiaceae (birthwort)
Armoracia rusticana (horseradish)	Brassicaceae (mustard)
Arnica montana (arnica)	Asteraceae (aster)
Artemisea annua (qinghaosu)	Asteraceae (aster)
Artemisia absinthium (wormwood)	Asteraceae (aster)
Artemisia cina (wormseed)	Asteraceae (aster)
Artemisia vulgaris (common wormwood)	Asteraceae (aster)
Asarum heterotropoides (xu xin)	Aristolochiaceae (birthwort)
Asclepias tuberosa (pleurisy root)	Asclepiadaceae (milkweed)
Asperula odorata (sweet woodruff)	Rubiaceae (madder)
Azadirachta indica (bead tree)	Meliaceae (mahogany)
Berberis vulgaris (European barberry)	Berberidaceae (barberry)
Blighia sapida (akee)	Sapindaceae (soapberry)
Brassica nigra (black mustard)	Brassicaceae (mustard)
Breynia officinalis (chi r yun)	Euphorbiaceae (spurge)
Bryonia alba (white bryony)	Cucurbitaceae (cucumber)
Calendula officinalis (marigold)	Asteraceae (aster)
Callilepis laureola (impila, ox-eye daisy)	Asteraceae (aster)
Camellia sinensis (green tea)	Theaceae (tea)
Capparis spinosa (caper plant)	Capparaceae (caper)
Capsicum annum (chili pepper)	Solanaceae (potato)
Cassia species (senna)	Fabaceae (pea)
Catha edulis (khat, qat)	Celastraceae (bittersweet)
Caulophyllum thalictroides (blue cohosh)	Berberidaceae (barberry)
Cephaelis ipecacuanha (ipecac)	Rubiaceae (madder)
Chelidonium majus (celandine)	Papaveraceae (poppy)
Chenopodium ambrosioides (American wormseed)	Chenopodiaceae (goosefoot)
Chrysanthemum vulgaris (common tansy)	Asteraceae (aster)
Cimicifuga racemosa (black cohosh)	Ranunculaceae (buttercup)

Genus or species (common name)	Family (common name)
Cinnamonum camphora (camphor tree)	Lauraceae (laurel)
Citrullus colocynthis (colocynth)	Cucurbitaceae (cucumber)
Citrus auranticum (bergamot)	Rutaceae (rue)
Citrus paradisi (grapefruit)	Rutaceae (rue)
Colchicum autumnale (autumn crocus)	Liliaceae (lily)
Conium maculatum (hemlock)	Apiaceae (carrot)
Convolvulus scammonia (Mexican scammony)	Convolvulaceae (morning glory)
Coriandrum sativum (coriander)	Apiaceae (carrot)
Coriaria arborea (tutu)	Coriariaceae
Crataegus species (hawthorn)	Rosaceae (rose)
Crocus sativus (Indian saffron)	Iridaceae (iris)
Crotalaria species (rattlebox)	Fabaceae (pea)
Croton tiglium (croton)	Euphorbiaceae (spurge)
Cyamopsis tetragonoloba (cluster bean)	Fabaceae (pea)
Cycas circinalis (false sago palm)	Cycadaceae (cycad)
Cynara scolymus (artichoke)	Asteraceae (aster)
Cynoglossum officinale (hound's tongue)	Boraginaceae (borage)
Cytisus scoparius (Scotch broom)	Fabaceae (pea)
Datura candida (angel's trumpet)	Solanaceae (potato)
Datura stramonium (Jimson weed)	Solanaceae (potato)
Datura suaveolens (angel's trumpet)	Solanaceae (potato)
Delphinium species (delphinium)	Ranunculaceae (buttercup)
Dictamnus dasycarpus (densefruit pittany)	Rutaceae (rue)
Dionaea muscipula (Venus flytrap)	Droseraceae (sundew)
Dipteryx species (tonka beans)	Fabaceae (pea)
Dryopteris filix-mas (male fern)	Dryopteraceae (wood fern)
Dysosma pleianthum (bajiaolian)	Berberidaceae (barberry)
Ecballium elaterium (squirting cucumber)	Cucurbitaceae (cucumber)
Echinacea species (coneflower)	Asteraceae (aster)
Eleutherococcus senticosus (Siberian ginseng)	Araliaceae
Eucalyptus species (eucalyptus)	Myrtaceae (myrtle)
Euonymus europaeus (spindle tree)	Celastraceae (bittersweet)
Eupatorium species (thoroughwort)	Asteraceae (aster)
Ferula assa-foetida (asafetida)	Apiaceae (carrot)
Gaultheria procumbens (wintergreen)	Ericaceae (heath)
Genista tinctoria (dyer's broom)	Fabaceae (pea)
Gentiana species (gentian)	Gentianaceae (gentian)
Ginkgo biloba (maidenhair)	Ginkgoaceae
Glycyrrhiza glabra (liquorice)	Fabaceae (pea)
Gossypium (cotton)	Malvaceae (mallow)
Harpagophytum procumbens (devil's claw)	Pedaliaceae (sesame)
Hedeoma pulegoides (pennyroyal)	Lamiaceae (mint)
Heliotropium species (heliotrope)	Boraginaceae (borage)
Hintonia latiflora (copalchi bark)	Rubiaceae (madder)
Humulus lupulus (hop)	Cannabaceae
Hydrastis canadensis (golden seal)	Ranunculaceae (buttercup)
Hypericum perforatum (St John's wort)	Clusiaceae (mangosteen)

Genus or species (common name)	Family (common name)
Illicium species (star anise)	Illiciaceae (star anise)
Inula helenium (elecampane)	Asteraceae (aster)
Ipomoea purga (jalap)	Convolvulaceae (morning glory)
Juglans regia (English walnut)	Juglandaceae (walnut)
Juniperus communis (juniper)	Cupressaceae (cypress)
Krameria species (ratany)	Krameriaceae (Krameria)
Laurus nobilis (laurel)	Lauraceae (laurel)
Lavandula angustifolia (lavender)	Lamiaceae
Ledum palustre (marsh Labrador tea)	Ericaceae (heath)
Lobelia inflata (Indian tobacco)	Campanulaceae (bellflower)
Lupinus species (lupin)	Fabaceae (pea)
Lycium barbarum (Chinese wolfberry)	Solanaceae (potato)
Lycopodium serratum (clubmoss)	Lycopodiaceae (club moss)
Mahonia species (barberry)	Berberidaceae (barberry)
Mandragora species (mandrake)	Solanaceae (potato)
Matricaria recutita (chamomile)	Asteraceae (aster)
Medicago sativa (alfalfa)	Fabaceae (pea)
Melaleuca alternifolia (tea tree)	Myrtaceae (myrtle)
Melilotus officinalis (sweet clover)	Fabaceae (pea)
Mentha piperita (peppermint)	Lamiaceae
Mentha pulegium (pennyroyal)	Lamiaceae (mint)
Momordica charantia (karela fruit, bitter melon)	Cucurbitaceae (cucumber)
Morinda citrifolia (noni)	Rubiaceae (madder)
Myristica fragrans (nutmeg)	Myristicaceae (nutmeg)
Myroxylon species (balsam of Peru)	Fabaceae (pea)
Nicotiana tabacum (tobacco)	Solanaceae (potato)
Oenothera biennis (evening primrose)	Onagraceae (evening primrose)
Panax ginseng (Asian ginseng)	Araliaceae (ginseng)
Papaver somniferum (opium poppy)	Papaveraceae (poppy)
Passiflora incarnata (passion flower)	Passifloraceae (passion flower)
Paullinia cupana (guaraná)	Sapindaceae (soapberry)
Petasites species (butterbur)	Asteraceae (aster)
Pfaffia paniculata (Brazilian ginseng)	Amaranthaceae (amaranth)
Phoradendron flavescens (American mistletoe)	Viscaceae (Christmas mistletoe)
Phytolacca americana (pokeweed)	Phytolaccaceae (pokeweed)
Pilocarpus species (pilocarpus)	Rutaceae (rue)
Piper methysticum (kava kava)	Piperaceae (pepper)
Pithecollobium jiringa (jering fruit)	Fabaceae (pea)
Plantago species (plantain)	Plantaginaceae (plantain)
Polygonum (knotweed)	Polygonaceae (buckwheat)
Prunus species (plum)	Rosaceae (rose)
Psoralea corylifolia (bakuchi)	Malvaceae (mallow)
Pulsatilla species (pasque flower)	Ranunculaceae (buttercup)
Ranunculus damascenus (buttercup)	Ranunculaceae (buttercup)
Raphanus sativus var. niger (black radish)	Brassicaceae (mustard)
Rauwolfia serpentina (snakeroot)	Apocynaceae (dogbane)
Rhamnus purshianus (cascara sagrada)	Rhamnaceae (buckthorn)

Continued

Table 3 Continued

Genus or species (common name)	Family (common name)
Rheum palmatum (rhubarb)	Polygonaceae (buckwheat)
Rhus species (sumac)	Anacardiaceae (sumac)
Ricinus communis (castor oil plant)	Euphorbiaceae (spurge)
Rubia tinctorum (madder)	Rubiaceae (madder)
Ruscus aculeatus (butcher's broom)	Liliaceae (lily)
Ruta graveolens (rue)	Rutaceae (rue)
Salix species (willow)	Salicaceae (willow)
Salvia miltiorrhiza (danshen)	Lamiaceae (mint)
Salvia officinalis (sage)	Lamiaceae (mint)
Sassafras albidum (sassafras)	Lauraceae (laurel)
Scopolia species (scopola)	Solanaceae (potato)
Scutellaria species (skullcap)	Lamiaceae (mint)
Sechium edule (chayote)	Cucurbitaceae (cucumber)
Selaginella doederleinii (spike moss)	Selaginellaceae (spike moss)
Senecio species (ragwort)	Asteraceae (aster)
Serenoa repens (saw palmetto)	Arecaceae (palm)
Silybum marianum (milk thistle)	Asteraceae (aster)
Sinapis species (mustard)	Brassicaceae (mustard)
Sophora falvescens (ku shen)	Fabaceae (pea)
Stephania species (jin bu huan)	Menispermaceae (moonseed)
Sterculia species (sterculia)	Sterculiaceae (cacao)
Strychnos nux-vomica (nux vomica)	Loganiaceae (Logania)
Swertia species (felwort)	Gentianaceae (gentian)
Symphytum officinale (black wort)	Boraginaceae (borage)
Tanacetum parthenium (feverfew)	Asteraceae (aster)
Taxus species (yew)	Taxaceae (yew)
Teucrium species (germander)	Lamiaceae (mint)
Trifolium pratense (red clover)	Fabaceae
Tripterygium wilfordii (lei gong teng)	Celastraceae (bittersweet)
Tussilago farfara (coltsfoot)	Asteraceae (aster)
Uncaria tomentosa (cat's claw)	Rubiaceae (madder)
Urtica dioica (stinging nettle)	Urticaceae (nettle)
Vaccinium macrocarpon (cranberry)	Ericaceae (heath)
Valeriana (valerian)	Valerianaceae (valerian)
Veratrum species (hellebore)	Liliaceae (lily)
Viscum album (mistletoe)	Viscaceae (Christmas mistletoe)
Vitex agnus-castus (chaste tree)	Verbenaceae (verbena)
Xysmalobium undulatum (xysmalobium)	Asclepiadaceae (milkweed)
Zingiber officinale (ginger)	Rosaceae
Ziziphus jujuba (dazao)	Rhamnaceae (buckthorn)

Table 4 Conversion of common names of plants to Latin names

Common name	Latin name (genus or species)
Akee	*Blighia sapida*
Alfalfa	*Medicago sativa*
Aloe	*Aloe capensis*
Aloe	*Aloe vera*
American mistletoe	*Phoradendron flavescens*
American wormseed	*Chenopodium ambrosioides*
Angel's trumpet	*Datura candida*
Angel's trumpet	*Datura suaveolens*
Areca, betel	*Areca catechu*
Arnica	*Arnica montana*
Artichoke	*Cynara scolymus*
Asafetida	*Ferula assa-foetida*
Asian ginseng	*Panax ginseng*
Autumn crocus	*Colchicum autumnale*
Bajiaolian	*Dysosma pleianthum*
Bakuchi	*Psoralea corylifolia*
Balsam of Peru	*Myroxylon* species
Barberry	*Mahonia* species
Bead tree	*Azadirachta indica*
Bearberry	*Arctostaphylos uva-ursi*
Bergamot	*Citrus auranticum*
Bishop's weed	*Ammi majus*
Black cohosh	*Cimicifuga racemosa*
Black mustard	*Brassica nigra*
Black radish	*Raphanus sativus* var. niger
Black wort	*Symphytum officinale*
Blue cohosh	*Caulophyllum thalictroides*
Brazilian ginseng	*Pfaffia paniculata*
Buchu	*Agathosma betulina*
Butcher's broom	*Ruscus aculeatus*
Butterbur	*Petasites* species
Buttercup	*Ranunculus damascenus*
Calamus root	*Acorus calamus*
Camphor tree	*Cinnamonum camphora*
Caper plant	*Capparis spinosa*
Cascara sagrada	*Rhamnus purshianus*
Castor oil plant	*Ricinus communis*
Cat's claw	*Uncaria tomentosa*
Celandine	*Chelidonium majus*
Chamomile	*Anthemis* species
Chamomile	*Matricaria recutita*
Chaste tree	*Vitex agnus-castus*
Chayote	*Sechium edule*
Chi r yun	*Breynia officinalis*
Chili pepper	*Capsicum annum*
Chinese wolfberry	*Lycium barbarum*
Clubmoss	*Lycopodium serratum*
Cluster bean	*Cyamopsis tetragonoloba*
Colocynth	*Citrullus colocynthis*
Coltsfoot	*Tussilago farfara*
Common tansy	*Chrysanthemum vulgaris*
Common wormwood	*Artemisia vulgaris*
Coneflower	*Echinacea* species
Copalchi bark	*Hintonia latiflora*
Coriander	*Coriandrum sativum*
Cotton	*Gossypium* species
Cranberry	*Vaccinium macrocarpon*
Croton	*Croton tiglium*
Danshen	*Salvia miltiorrhiza*
Dazao	*Ziziphus jujuba*
Delphinium	*Delphinium* species
Densefruit pittany	*Dictamnus dasycarpus*
Devil's claw	*Harpagophytum procumbens*
Dong quai	*Angelica sinensis*
Dutchman's pipe	*Aristolochia* species
Dyer's broom	*Genista tinctoria*
Elecampane	*Inula helenium*
English walnut	*Juglans regia*
Eucalyptus	*Eucalyptus* species
European barberry	*Berberis vulgaris*
Evening primrose	*Oenothera biennis*
False sago palm	*Cycas circinalis*
Felwort	*Swertia* species
Feverfew	*Tanacetum parthenium*
Garlic	*Allium sativum*

Common name	Latin name (genus or species)
Gentian	*Gentiana* species
Germander	*Teucrium* species
Ginger	*Zingiber officinale*
Golden seal	*Hydrastis canadensis*
Grapefruit	*Citrus paradisi*
Green tea	*Camellia sinensis*
Guaraná	*Paullinia cupana*
Guar gum	*Cyamopsis tetragonoloba*
Hawthorn	*Crataegus* species
Heliotrope	*Heliotropium* species
Hellebore	*Veratrum* species
Hemlock	*Conium maculatum*
Hop	*Humulus lupulus*
Horse chestnut	*Aesculus hippocastanum*
Horseradish	*Armoracia rusticana*
Hound's tongue	*Cynoglossum officinale*
Impila, ox-eye daisy	*Callilepis laureola*
Indian saffron	*Crocus sativus*
Indian tobacco	*Lobelia inflata*
Ipecac	*Cephaelis ipecacuanha*
Jalap	*Ipomoea purga*
Jering fruit	*Pithecollobium jiringa*
Jimson weed	*Datura stramonium*
Jin bu huan	*Stephania* species
Juniper	*Juniperus communis*
Karela fruit, bitter melon	*Momordica charantia*
Kava kava	*Piper methysticum*
Khat, qat	*Catha edulis*
Knotweed	*Polygonum*
Ku shen	*Sophora falvescens*
Laurel	*Laurus nobilis*
Lavender	*Lavandula angustifolia*
Lei gong teng	*Tripterygium wilfordii*
Liquorice	*Glycyrrhiza glabra*
Lupin	*Lupinus* species
Madder	*Rubia tinctorum*
Maidenhair	*Ginkgo biloba*
Male fern	*Dryopteris filix-mas*
Mandrake	*Mandragora* species
Marigold	*Calendula officinalis*
Marsh Labrador tea	*Ledum palustre*
Mexican scammony	*Convolvulus scammonia*
Milk thistle	*Silybum marianum*
Mistletoe	*Viscum album*
Monkshood	*Aconitum napellus*
Mustard	*Sinapis* species
Noni	*Morinda citrifolia*
Nutmeg	*Myristica fragrans*
Nux vomica	*Strychnos nux-vomica*
Opium poppy	*Papaver somniferum*
Pasque flower	*Pulsatilla* species
Passion flower	*Passiflora incarnata*
Pennyroyal	*Hedeoma pulegoides*
Pennyroyal	*Mentha pulegium*
Peppermint	*Mentha piperita*
Pilocarpus	*Pilocarpus* species
Plantain	*Plantago* species
Pleurisy root	*Asclepias tuberosa*
Plum	*Prunus* species
Pokeweed	*Phytolacca americana*
Qinghaosu	*Artemisea annua*
Ragwort	*Senecio* species
Ratany	*Krameria* species
Rattlebox	*Crotalaria* species
Red clover	*Trifolium pratense*
Rhubarb	*Rheum palmatum*
Rue	*Ruta graveolens*
Sage	*Salvia officinalis*
Sassafras	*Sassafras albidum*
Saw palmetto	*Serenoa repens*
Scopola	*Scopolia* species
Scotch broom	*Cytisus scoparius*
Senna	*Cassia* species
Siberian ginseng	*Eleutherococcus senticosus*
Skullcap	*Scutellaria* species
Snakeroot	*Rauwolfia serpentina*
Spike moss	*Selaginella doederleinii*
Spindle tree	*Euonymus europaeus*
Squirting cucumber	*Ecballium elaterium*
St John's wort	*Hypericum perforatum*
Star anise	*Illicium* species
Sterculia	*Sterculia* species
Stinging nettle	*Urtica dioica*
Sumac	*Rhus* species
Sweet clover	*Melilotus officinalis*
Sweet vernal grass	*Anthoxanthum odoratum*
Sweet woodruff	*Asperula odorata*
Tea tree	*Melaleuca alternifolia*
Thoroughwort	*Eupatorium* species
Tobacco	*Nicotiana tabacum*
Tonka beans	*Dipteryx* species
Toothpick weed	*Ammi visnaga*
Tutu	*Coriaria arborea*
Valerian	*Valeriana*
Venus flytrap	*Dionaea muscipula*
White bryony	*Bryonia alba*
Willow	*Salix* species
Wintergreen	*Gaultheria procumbens*
Wormseed	*Artemisia cina*
Wormwood	*Artemisia absinthium*
Xu xin	*Asarum heterotropoides*
Xysmalobium	*Xysmalobium undulatum*
Yarrow	*Achillea millefolium*
Yew	*Taxus* species
Zang qie	*Anisodus tanguticus*

References

1. Phillipson JD. Traditional medicine treatment for eczema: experience as a basis for scientific acceptance. Eur Phytotelegram 1994;6:33–40.
2. Barnes J. A close look at synergy and polyvalent action in medicinal plants. Inpharma 1999;1185:3–4.
3. Ernst E, De Smet PA, Shaw D, Murray V. Traditional remedies and the "test of time". Eur J Clin Pharmacol 1998;54(2):99–100.
4. Anonymous. Complementary Medicines. London: Mintel International Group, 1997:13.
5. Institute of Medical Statistics Self-Medication International. Herbals in Europe. London: IMS Self-Medication International, 1998.
6. Brevoort P. The booming US botanical market. A new overview. Herbalgram 1998;44:33–46.
7. Eisenberg DM, Kessler RC, Foster C, Norlock FE, Calkins DR, Delbanco TL. Unconventional medicine in the United States. Prevalence, costs, and patterns of use. N Engl J Med 1993;328(4):246–52.
8. Eisenberg DM, Davis RB, Ettner SL, Appel S, Wilkey S, Van Rompay M, Kessler RC. Trends in alternative medicine use in the United States, 1990–1997: results of a follow-up national survey. JAMA 1998;280(18):1569–75.

9. Hanssens Y, Deleu D, Taqi A. Etiologic and demographic characteristics of poisoning: a prospective hospital-based study in Oman. J Toxicol Clin Toxicol 2001;39(4):371–80.
10. Kerdpon D, Sriplung H. Factors related to advanced stage oral squamous cell carcinoma in southern Thailand. Oral Oncol 2001;37(3):216–21.
11. Rogers EA, Gough JE, Brewer KL. Are emergency department patients at risk for herb–drug interactions? Acad Emerg Med 2001;8(9):932–4.
12. Ang-Lee MK, Moss J, Yuan CS. Herbal medicines and perioperative care. JAMA 2001;286(2):208–16.
13. Ernst E. Use of herbal medications before surgery. JAMA 2001;286(20):2542–3.
14. Tomassoni AJ, Simone K. Herbal medicines for children: an illusion of safety? Curr Opin Pediatr 2001;13(2):162–9.
15. Ernst E, Pittler MH, Stevinson C, White AR, Eisenberg D. The Desktop Guide to Complementary and Alternative Medicine. Edinburgh: Mosby, 2001.
16. Seeff LB, Lindsay KL, Bacon BR, Kresina TF, Hoofnagle JH. Complementary and alternative medicine in chronic liver disease. Hepatology 2001;34(3):595–603.
17. Mantle D, Gok MA, Lennard TW. Adverse and beneficial effects of plant extracts on skin and skin disorders. Adverse Drug React Toxicol Rev 2001;20(2):89–103.
18. Xing JH, Soffer EE. Adverse effects of laxatives. Dis Colon Rectum 2001;44(8):1201–9.
19. Elvin-Lewis M. Should we be concerned about herbal remedies. J Ethnopharmacol 2001;75(2–3):141–64.
20. Ko R. Adverse reactions to watch for in patients using herbal remedies. West J Med 1999;171(3):181–6.
21. Astin JA. Why patients use alternative medicine: results of a national study. JAMA 1998;279(19):1548–53.
22. Abbot NC, White AR, Ernst E. Complementary medicine. Nature 1996;381(6581):361.
23. De Smet PA. Health risks of herbal remedies. Drug Saf 1995;13(2):81–93.
24. Chan TY, Chan AY, Critchley JA. Hospital admissions due to adverse reactions to Chinese herbal medicines. J Trop Med Hyg 1992;95(4):296–8.
25. Lin SH, Lin MS. A survey on drug-related hospitalization in a community teaching hospital. Int J Clin Pharmacol Ther Toxicol 1993;31(2):66–9.
26. Wu FL, Yang CC, Shen LJ, Chen CY. Adverse drug reactions in a medical ward. J Formos Med Assoc 1996;95(3):241–6.
27. Bruynzeel DP, van Ketel WG, Young E, van Joost T, Smeenk G. Contact sensitization by alternative topical medicaments containing plant extracts. The Dutch Contact Dermatoses Group. Contact Dermatitis 1992;27(4):278–9.
28. Shaw D, Leon C, Kolev S, Murray V. Traditional remedies and food supplements. A 5-year toxicological study (1991–1995). Drug Saf 1997;17(5):342–56.
29. Anonymous. Extension of the Yellow Card scheme to unlicensed herbal remedies. Curr Prob Pharmacovig 1996;22:10.
30. Yamey G. Government launches green paper on mental health. BMJ 1999;319(7221):1322.
31. Farah MH, Edwards R, Lindquist M, Leon C, Shaw D. International monitoring of adverse health effects associated with herbal medicines. Pharmacoepidemiol Drug Saf 2000;9:105–12.
32. Winslow LC, Kroll DJ. Herbs as medicines. Arch Intern Med 1998;158(20):2192–9.
33. Miller LG. Herbal medicinals: selected clinical considerations focusing on known or potential drug–herb interactions. Arch Intern Med 1998;158(20):2200–11.
34. Mashour NH, Lin GI, Frishman WH. Herbal medicine for the treatment of cardiovascular disease: clinical considerations. Arch Intern Med 1998;158(20):2225–34.
35. Saller R, Reichling J, Kristof O. Phytotherapie-Behandlung ohne Nebenwirkungen? [Phytotherapy—treatment without side effects?] Dtsch Med Wochenschr 1998;123(3):58–62.
36. Bateman J, Chapman RD, Simpson D. Possible toxicity of herbal remedies. Scott Med J 1998;43(1):7–15.
37. Ernst E. Harmless herbs? A review of the recent literature. Am J Med 1998;104(2):170–8.
38. Shaw D. Risks or remedies? Safety aspects of herbal remedies in the UK. J R Soc Med 1998;91(6):294–6.
39. Marrone CM. Safety issues with herbal products. Ann Pharmacother 1999;33(12):1359–62.
40. Ko RJ. Causes, epidemiology, and clinical evaluation of suspected herbal poisoning. J Toxicol Clin Toxicol 1999;37(6):697–708.
41. Ernst E. Phytotherapeutika. Wie harmlos sind sie wirklich? Dtsch Arzteblatt 1999;48:3107–8.
42. Calixto JB. Efficacy, safety, quality control, marketing and regulatory guidelines for herbal medicines (phytotherapeutic agents). Braz J Med Biol Res 2000;33(2):179–89.
43. De Smet PA. Herbal remedies. N Engl J Med 2002;347(25):2046–56.
44. Ernst E, Pittler MH. Risks associated with herbal medicinal products Wien Med Wochenschr 2002;152(7–8): 183–9.
45. Ali MS, Uzair SS. Natural organic toxins. Hamdard Medicus 2002;XLIV:86–93.
46. Gee BC, Wilson P, Morris AD, Emerson RM. Herbal is not synonymous with safe. Arch Dermatol 2002;138(12): 1613.
47. Matthews HB, Lucier GW, Fisher KD. Medicinal herbs in the United States: research needs. Environ Health Perspect 1999;107(10):773–8.
48. Hussain SH. Potential risks of health supplements—self-medication practices and the need for public health education. Int J Risk Saf Med 1999;12:167–71.
49. Fontana RJ. Acute liver failure. Curr Opin Gastroenterol 1999;15:270–7.
50. Valli G, Giardina EG. Benefits, adverse effects and drug interactions of herbal therapies with cardiovascular effects. J Am Coll Cardiol 2002;39(7):1083–95.
51. Chitturi S, Farrell GC. Herbal hepatotoxicity: an expanding but poorly defined problem. J Gastroenterol Hepatol 2000;15(10):1093–9.
52. Haller CA, Dyer JE, Ko R, Olson KR. Making a diagnosis of herbal-related toxic hepatitis. West J Med 2002; 176(1):39–44.
53. Ernst E. Adverse effects of herbal drugs in dermatology. Br J Dermatol 2000;143(5):923–9.
54. Holsen DS. Flora og efflorescenser—om planter som arsak til hudsykdom. [Plants and plant produce—about plants as cause of diseases.] Tidsskr Nor Laegeforen 2002;122(17): 1665–9.
55. Ernst E. Adverse effects of unconventional therapies in the elderly: a systematic review of the recent literature. J Am Aging Assoc 2002;25:11–20.
56. Ernst E. Herbal medicinal products during pregnancy: are they safe? BJOG 2002;109(3):227–35.
57. Hodges PJ, Kam PC. The peri-operative implications of herbal medicines. Anaesthesia 2002;57(9):889–99.
58. Cheng B, Hung CT, Chiu W. Herbal medicine and anaesthesia. Hong Kong Med J 2002;8(2):123–30.
59. Bartsch H. Gefahrliche Naturprodukte: sind Karzinogene im Kräutertee? [Hazardous natural products. Are there carcinogens in herbal teas?] MMW Fortschr Med 2002;144(41):14.
60. Pies R. Adverse neuropsychiatric reactions to herbal and over-the-counter "antidepressants". J Clin Psychiatry 2000;61(11):815–20.

61. Tomlinson B, Chan TY, Chan JC, Critchley JA, But PP. Toxicity of complementary therapies: an eastern perspective. J Clin Pharmacol 2000;40(5):451–6.
62. Bensoussan A, Myers SP, Drew AK, Whyte IM, Dawson AH. Development of a Chinese herbal medicine toxicology database. J Toxicol Clin Toxicol 2002; 40(2):159–67.
63. Ernst E. Ayurvedic medicines. Pharmacoepidemiol Drug Saf 2002;11(6):455–6.
64. Boullata JI, Nace AM. Safety issues with herbal medicine. Pharmacotherapy 2000;20(3):257–69.
65. Shapiro R. Safety assessment of botanicals. Nutraceuticals World 2000; July/August 52–63.
66. Saller R, Iten F, Reichling J. Unerwünschte Wirkungen und Wechselwirkungen von Phytotherapeutika. Erfahrungsheilkunde 2000;6:369–76.
67. Pennachio DL. Drug–herb interactions: how vigilant should you be? Patient Care 2000;19:41–68.
68. Ernst E. Possible interactions between synthetic and herbal medicinal products. Part 1: a systematic review of the indirect evidence. Perfusion 2000;13:4–6, 8.
69. Ernst E. Interactions between synthetic and herbal medicinal products. Part 2: a systematic review of the direct evidence. Perfusion 2000;13:60–70.
70. Blumenthal M. Interactions between herbs and conventional drugs: introductory considerations. Herbal Gram 2000;49:52–63.
71. Ernst E. Herb–drug interactions: potentially important but woefully under-researched. Eur J Clin Pharmacol 2000;56(8):523–4.
72. De Smet PAGM, Touw DJ. Sint-janskruid op de balans van werking en interacties. Pharm Weekbl 2000;135:455–62.
73. Abebe W. Herbal medication: potential for adverse interactions with analgesic drugs. J Clin Pharm Ther 2002;27(6):391–401.
74. Mason P. Food–drug interactions: nutritional supplements and drugs. Pharm J 2002;269:609–11.
75. Scott GN, Elmer GW. Update on natural product—drug interactions. Am J Health Syst Pharm 2002;59(4):339–47.
76. Rahman SZ, Singhal KC. Problems in pharmacovigilance of medicinal products of herbal origin and means to minimize them. Uppsala Rep 2002;17:1–4.
77. De Smet PAGM, D'Arcy PF. Drug interactions with herbal and other non-orthodox drugs. In: D'Arcy PF, McElnay JC, Welling PG, editors. Mechanisms of Drug Interactions. Heidelberg: Springer Verlag, in press.
78. Stockley I. Drug Interactions. 4th ed. London: The Pharmaceutical Press, 1996.
79. Newall CA, Anderson LA, Phillipson JD. Herbal medicines. A guide for health-care professionals. London: The Pharmaceutical Press, 1996.
80. Barnes J, Mills SY, Abbot NC, Willoughby M, Ernst E. Different standards for reporting ADRs to herbal remedies and conventional OTC medicines: face-to-face interviews with 515 users of herbal remedies. Br J Clin Pharmacol 1998;45(5):496–500.
81. Ernst E. Competence in complementary medicine. Comp Ther Med 1995;3:6–8.
82. Bensoussan A, Myers SP. Towards a safer choice. The practice of traditional Chinese medicine in Australia. Campbelltown: University of Western Sydney Macarthur, 1996.
83. Aslam M. Asian medicine and its practice in Britain. In: Evans WC, editor. Trease and Evans' Pharmacognosy. 14th ed. London: WB Saunders, 1996:488–504.
84. Zhu DY, Bai DL, Tang XC. Recent studies on traditional Chinese medicinal plants. Drug Dev Res 1996;39:147–57.
85. Sanders D, Kennedy N, McKendrick MW. Monitoring the safety of herbal remedies. Herbal remedies have a heterogeneous nature. BMJ 1995;311(7019):1569.
86. Itoh S, Marutani K, Nishijima T, Matsuo S, Itabashi M. Liver injuries induced by herbal medicine, syo-saiko-to (xiao-chai-hu-tang). Dig Dis Sci 1995;40(8):1845–8.
87. Perharic L, Shaw D, Leon C, De Smet PA, Murray VS. Possible association of liver damage with the use of Chinese herbal medicine for skin disease. Vet Hum Toxicol 1995;37(6):562–6.
88. Okuda T, Umezawa Y, Ichikawa M, Hirata M, Oh-i T, Koga M. A case of drug eruption caused by the crude drug Boi (Sinomenium stem/Sinomeni caulis et Rhizoma). J Dermatol 1995;22(10):795–800.
89. Homma M, Oka K, Ikeshima K, Takahashi N, Niitsuma T, Fukuda T, Itoh H. Different effects of traditional Chinese medicines containing similar herbal constituents on prednisolone pharmacokinetics. J Pharm Pharmacol 1995;47(8):687–92.
90. Centers for Disease Control and Prevention (CDC). Adverse events associated with ephedrine-containing products—Texas, December 1993–September 1995. MMWR Morb Mortal Wkly Rep 1996;45(32):689–93.
91. Doyle H, Kargin M. Herbal stimulant containing ephedrine has also caused psychosis. BMJ 1996;313(7059):756.
92. Nadir A, Agrawal S, King PD, Marshall JB. Acute hepatitis associated with the use of a Chinese herbal product, ma-huang. Am J Gastroenterol 1996;91(7):1436–8.
93. Tojima H, Yamazaki T, Tokudome T. [Two cases of pneumonia caused by Sho-saiko-to.] Nihon Kyobu Shikkan Gakkai Zasshi 1996;34(8):904–10.
94. Ishizaki T, Sasaki F, Ameshima S, Shiozaki K, Takahashi H, Abe Y, Ito S, Kuriyama M, Nakai T, Kitagawa M. Pneumonitis during interferon and/or herbal drug therapy in patients with chronic active hepatitis. Eur Respir J 1996;9(12):2691–6.
95. Doi Y, Uchida K, Tamura N, et al. A case of Sho-Saiko-To induced pneumonitis followed up by DLST testing BALF (bronchoalveolar lavage fluid) findings. Jpn J Chest Dis 1996;55:147–51.
96. Pena JM, Borras M, Ramos J, Montoliu J. Rapidly progressive interstitial renal fibrosis due to a chronic intake of a herb (*Aristolochia pistolochia*) infusion. Nephrol Dial Transplant 1996;11(7):1359–60.
97. Schmeiser HH, Bieler CA, Wiessler M, van Ypersele de Strihou C, Cosyns JP. Detection of DNA adducts formed by aristolochic acid in renal tissue from patients with Chinese herbs nephropathy. Cancer Res 1996;56(9): 2025–8.
98. Vanherweghem JL, Abramowicz D, Tielemans C, Depierreux M. Effects of steroids on the progression of renal failure in chronic interstitial renal fibrosis: a pilot study in Chinese herbs nephropathy. Am J Kidney Dis 1996;27(2):209–15.
99. Lai RS, Chiang AA, Wu MT, Wang JS, Lai NS, Lu JY, Ger LP, Roggli V. Outbreak of bronchiolitis obliterans associated with consumption of *Sauropus androgynus* in Taiwan. Lancet 1996;348(9020):83–5.
100. Horowitz RS, Feldhaus K, Dart RC, Stermitz FR, Beck JJ. The clinical spectrum of Jin Bu Huan toxicity. Arch Intern Med 1996;156(8):899–903.
101. Kobayashi Y, Hasegawa T, Sato M, Suzuki E, Arakawa M. [Pneumonia due to the Chinese medicine Pien Tze Huang.] Nihon Kyobu Shikkan Gakkai Zasshi 1996;34(7):810–15.
102. Nakada T, Kawai B, Nagayama K, Tanaka T. A case of hepatic injury induced by Sai-rei-to. Acta Hepatol Jap 1996;37:233–8.
103. Shiota Y, Wilson JG, Matsumoto H, Munemasa M, Okamura M, Hiyama J, Marukawa M, Ono T, Taniyama K, Mashiba H. Adult respiratory distress

syndrome induced by a Chinese medicine, Kamisyoyo-san. Intern Med 1996;35(6):494–6.

104. Yoshida EM, McLean CA, Cheng ES, Blanc PD, Somberg KA, Ferrell LD, Lake JR. Chinese herbal medicine, fulminant hepatitis, and liver transplantation. Am J Gastroenterol 1996;91(12):2647–8.
105. Yeo KL, Tan VCC. Severe hyperbilirubinemia associated with Chinese herbs. A case report. Singapore Paediatr J 1996;38:180–2.
106. Chan TY, Critchley JA. Usage and adverse effects of Chinese herbal medicines. Hum Exp Toxicol 1996;15(1): 5–12.
107. Melchart D, Hager S, Weidenhammer W, Liao JZ, Sollner C, Linde K. Tolerance of and compliance with traditional drug therapy among patients in a hospital for Chinese medicine in Germany. Int J Risk Saf Med 1998;11:61–4.
108. Melchart D, Linde K, Weidenhammer W, Hager S, Shaw D, Bauer R. Liver enzyme elevations in patients treated with traditional Chinese medicine. JAMA 1999;282(1):28–9.
109. Melchart D, Linde K, Hager S, Kaesmayr J, Shaw D, Bauer R, Weidenhammer W. Monitoring of liver enzymes in patients treated with traditional Chinese drugs. Complement Ther Med 1999;7(4):208–16.
110. Bensoussan A, Myers SP, Carlton AL. Risks associated with the practice of traditional Chinese medicine: an Australian study. Arch Fam Med 2000;9(10):1071–8.
111. Al-Khafaji M. Monitoring of liver enzymes in patients on Chinese medicine. J Chin Med 2000;62:6–10.
112. Yang S, Dennehy CE, Tsourounis C. Characterizing adverse events reported to the California Poison Control System on herbal remedies and dietary supplements: a pilot study. J Herb Pharmacother 2002;2(3):1–11.
113. Murch SJ, KrishnaRaj S, Saxena PK. Phytopharmaceuticals: problems, limitations, and solutions. Sci Rev Altern Med 2000;4:33–7.
114. Tyler VE. Product definition deficiencies in clinical studies of herbal medicines. Sci Rev Altern Med 2000;4:17–21.
115. Gurley BJ, Gardner SF, Hubbard MA. Content versus label claims in *Ephedra*-containing dietary supplements. Am J Health Syst Pharm 2000;57(10):963–9.
116. De Smet PAGM. Toxicological outlook on the quality assurance of herbal remedies. In: De Smet PAGM, Keller K, Hansel R, Chandler RF, editors. Adverse Effects of Herbal Drugs. 1. Heidelberg: Springer-Verlag, 1992:1–72.
117. Wrobel A. Umfrage zu Kräutern und Kräuterprodukten bezüglich Pestizid- und Schadstoff-belastungen. Akupunktur 2002;30:38–40.
118. Huang WF, Wen KC, Hsiao ML. Adulteration by synthetic therapeutic substances of traditional Chinese medicines in Taiwan. J Clin Pharmacol 1997;37(4):344–50.
119. Abt AB, Oh JY, Huntington RA, Burkhart KK. Chinese herbal medicine induced acute renal failure. Arch Intern Med 1995;155(2):211–12.
120. Gertner E, Marshall PS, Filandrinos D, Potek AS, Smith TM. Complications resulting from the use of Chinese herbal medications containing undeclared prescription drugs. Arthritis Rheum 1995;38(5):614–17.
121. Bayly GR, Braithwaite RA, Sheehan TM, Dyer NH, Grimley C, Ferner RE. Lead poisoning from Asian traditional remedies in the West Midlands—report of a series of five cases. Hum Exp Toxicol 1995;14(1):24–8.
122. Espinoza EO, Mann MJ, Bleasdell B. Arsenic and mercury in traditional Chinese herbal balls. N Engl J Med 1995;333(12):803–4.
123. Worthing MA, Sutherland HH, al-Riyami K. New information on the composition of Bint al Dhahab, a mixed lead monoxide used as a traditional medicine in Oman and the United Arab Emirates. J Trop Pediatr 1995;41(4):246–7.
124. Wu MS, Hong JJ, Lin JL, Yang CW, Chien HC. Multiple tubular dysfunction induced by mixed Chinese herbal medicines containing cadmium. Nephrol Dial Transplant 1996;11(5):867–70.
125. Centers for Disease Control and Prevention (CDC). Mercury poisoning associated with beauty cream—Texas, New Mexico, and California, 1995–1996. MMWR Morb Mortal Wkly Rep 1996;45(19):400–3.
126. Wu TN, Yang KC, Wang CM, Lai JS, Ko KN, Chang PY, Liou SH. Lead poisoning caused by contaminated Cordyceps, a Chinese herbal medicine: two case reports. Sci Total Environ 1996;182(1–3):193–5.
127. Prpic-Majic D, Pizent A, Jurasovic J, Pongracic J, Restek-Samarzija N. Lead poisoning associated with the use of Ayurvedic metal-mineral tonics. J Toxicol Clin Toxicol 1996;34(4):417–23.
128. Lana-Moliner F, Sanchez-Cubas S. Fetal abnormalities and use of substances sold in 'herbal remedies' shops. Drug Saf 1996;14(1):68.
129. Oliver MR, Van Voorhis WC, Boeckh M, Mattson D, Bowden RA. Hepatic mucormycosis in a bone marrow transplant recipient who ingested naturopathic medicine. Clin Infect Dis 1996;22(3):521–4.
130. Brandao MGL, Freire N, Vianna-Soares CD. Vigilância de fitoterápicos em Minas Gerais. Verificação da qualidade de diferentes amostras comerciais de camomila. Cad Saude Publica Rio de Janeiro 1998;14:613–16.
131. Chan TY. Monitoring the safety of herbal medicines. Drug Saf 1997;17(4):209–15.
132. Sheerin NS, Monk PN, Aslam M, Thurston H. Simultaneous exposure to lead, arsenic and mercury from Indian ethnic remedies. Br J Clin Pract 1994;48(6):332–3.
133. Boyer EW, Kearney S, Shannon MW, Quang L, Woolf A, Kemper K. Poisoning from a dietary supplement administered during hospitalization. Pediatrics 2002;109(3):E49. http://www.pediatrics.org (Pediatrics Electronic Pages), 2002.
134. Anonymous. Herbal dietary supplements (PC-SPES and SPES). Adulteration with prescription only medicines precipitates regulatory action. WHO Pharmaceuticals Newslett 2002;2:1–2.
135. Anonymous. Herbal medicine. Warning: found to contain chlordiazepoxide. WHO Pharm Newslett 2001;1:2–3.
136. Daniels J, Shaw D, Atherton D. Use of Wau Wa in dermatitis patients. Lancet 2002;360(9338):1025.
137. Anonymous. Traditional medicines. Adulterants/undeclared ingredients pose safety concerns. WHO Pharmaceuticals Newslett 2002;1:11–12.
138. Florkowski CM, Elder PA, Lewis JG, Hunt PJ, Munns PL, Hunter W, Baldwin D. Two cases of adrenal suppression following a Chinese herbal remedy: a cause for concern? NZ Med J 2002;115(1153):223–4.
139. Lau KK, Lai CK, Chan AW. Phenytoin poisoning after using Chinese proprietary medicines. Hum Exp Toxicol 2000;19(7):385–6.
140. Anonymous. Herbal medicines. Warning: found to contain antidiabetics. WHO Newslett 2000;2:4–5.
141. Raynauld JP, Lee YS, Kornfeld P, Fries JF. Unilateral ptosis as an initial manifestation of D-penicillamine induced myasthenia gravis. J Rheumatol 1993;20(9):1592–3.
142. Ernst E. Adulteration of Chinese herbal medicines with synthetic drugs: a systematic review. J Intern Med 2002;252(2):107–13.
143. Anonymous. Traditional medicines. Several Chinese medicines withdrawn due to presence of prescription and pharmacy-only components. WHO Pharmaceuticals Newslett 2003;1:2–3.

144. Slifman NR, Obermeyer WR, Aloi BK, Musser SM, Correll WA Jr, Cichowicz SM, Betz JM, Love LA. Contamination of botanical dietary supplements by Digitalis lanata. N Engl J Med 1998;339(12):806–11.
145. Cheng TJ, Wong RH, Lin YP, Hwang YH, Horng JJ, Wang JD. Chinese herbal medicine, sibship, and blood lead in children. Occup Environ Med 1998;55(8):573–6.
146. Chu NF, Liou SH, Wu TN, Ko KN, Chang PY. Risk factors for high blood lead levels among the general population in Taiwan. Eur J Epidemiol 1998;14(8):775–81.
147. Ibrahim AS, Latif AH. Adult lead poisoning from a herbal medicine. Saudi Med J 2002;23(5):591–3.
148. Senft V, Kaderabkova A. [Herbal concentrates Astrum—health or intoxication with heavy metals?] Prakt Lek 2002;82:551–3.
149. Ko RJ. Adulterants in Asian patent medicines. N Engl J Med 1998;339(12):847.
150. Wong ST, Chan HL, Teo SK. The spectrum of cutaneous and internal malignancies in chronic arsenic toxicity. Singapore Med J 1998;39(4):171–3.
151. Li AM, Chan MH, Leung TF, Cheung RC, Lam CW, Fok TF. Mercury intoxication presenting with tics. Arch Dis Child 2000;83(2):174–5.
152. Moore C, Adler R. Herbal vitamins: lead toxicity and developmental delay. Pediatrics 2000;106(3):600–2.
153. Garvey GJ, Hahn G, Lee RV, Harbison RD. Heavy metal hazards of Asian traditional remedies. Int J Environ Health Res 2001;11(1):63–71.
154. Fletcher J, Aslam M. Possible dangers of Ayurvedic herbal remedies. Pharm J 1991;247:456.
155. Treleaven J, Meller S, Farmer P, Birchall D, Goldman J, Piller G. Arsenic and Ayurveda. Leuk Lymphoma 1993;10(4–5):343–5.
156. Saper RB, Kales SN, Paquin J, Burns MJ, Eisenberg DM, Davis RB, Phillips RS. Heavy metal content of Ayurvedic herbal medicine products. JAMA 2004;292(23):2868–73.
157. Wood R, Mills PB, Knobel GJ, Hurlow WE, Stokol JM. Acute dichromate poisoning after use of traditional purgatives. A report of 7 cases. S Afr Med J 1990;77(12):640–2.
158. Dunn JP, Krige JE, Wood R, Bornman PC, Terblanche J. Colonic complications after toxic tribal enemas. Br J Surg 1991;78(5):545–8.
159. Halt M. Moulds and mycotoxins in herb tea and medicinal plants. Eur J Epidemiol 1998;14(3):269–74.
160. Sadjadi J. Cutaneous anthrax associated with the Kombucha "mushroom" in Iran. JAMA 1998;280(18):1567–8.
161. Zuin VG, Vilegas JH. Pesticide residues in medicinal plants and phytomedicines. Phytother Res 2000;14(2):73–88.
162. Tagwireyi D, Ball DE, Nhachi CF. Poisoning in Zimbabwe: a survey of eight major referral hospitals. J Appl Toxicol 2002;22(2):99–105.
163. Li AM, Hui J, Chik KW, Li CK, Fok TF. Topical herbal medicine causing haemolysis in glucose-6-phosphate dehydrogenase deficiency. Acta Paediatr 2002;91(9):1012.
164. Iwasa M, Yamamoto M, Tanaka Y, Kaito M, Adachi Y. *Spirulina*-associated hepatotoxicity. Am J Gastroenterol 2002;97(12):3212–13.
165. Wurtz AS, Vial T, Isoard B, Saillard E. Possible hepatotoxicity from Copaltra, an herbal medicine. Ann Pharmacother 2002;36(5):941–2.
166. von Gruenigen VE, Hopkins MP. Alternative medicine in gynecologic oncology: A case report. Gynecol Oncol 2000;77(1):190–2.
167. Katz JL. A psychotic manic state induced by an herbal preparation. Psychosomatics 2000;41(1):73–4.
168. Madisch A, Melderis H, Mayr G, Sassin I, Hotz J. Ein Phytotherapeutikum und seine modifizierte Rezeptur bei funktioneller Dyspepsie. Ergebnisse einer doppelblinden plazebokontrollierten Vergleichsstudie. [A plant extract and its modified preparation in functional dyspepsia. Results of a double-blind placebo controlled comparative study.] Z Gastroenterol 2001;39(7):511–17.
169. Saller R, Pfister-Hotz G, Iten F, Melzer J, Reichling J. Iberogast: Eine moderne phytotherapeutische Arznmittelkombination zur Behandung funktioneller Erkrankungen des Magen-Darm-Trakts (Dyspepsie, Colon irritable)—von der Pflanzenheilkunde zur "Evidence Based Phytotherapy". [Iberogast: a modern phytotherapeutic combined herbal drug for the treatment of functional disorders of the gastrointestinal tract (dyspepsia, irritable bowel syndrome)—from phytomedicine to "evidence based phytotherapy." A systematic review.] Forsch Komplementarmed Klass Naturheilkd 2002;9(Suppl 1):1–20.
170. Fraquelli M, Colli A, Cocciolo M, Conte D. Adult syncytial giant cell chronic hepatitis due to herbal remedy. J Hepatol 2000;33(3):505–8.
171. Ng YY, Yu S, Chen TW, Wu SC, Yang AH, Yang WC. Interstitial renal fibrosis in a young woman: association with a Chinese preparation given for irregular menses. Nephrol Dial Transplant 1998;13(8):2115–17.
172. Mantani N, Kogure T, Sakai S, Goto H, Shibahara N, Kita T, Shimada Y, Terasawa K. Incidence and clinical features of liver injury related to Kampo (Japanese herbal) medicine in 2,496 cases between 1979 and 1999: problems of the lymphocyte transformation test as a diagnostic method. Phytomedicine 2002;9(4):280–7.
173. Miyazaki E, Ando M, Ih K, Matsumoto T, Kaneda K, Tsuda T. [Pulmonary edema associated with the Chinese medicine shosaikoto.] Nihon Kokyuki Gakkai Zasshi 1998;36(9):776–80.
174. Akatsu T, Santo RM, Nakayasu K, Kanai A. Oriental herbal medicine induced epithelial keratopathy. Br J Ophthalmol 2000;84(8):934.
175. Hanawa T. A case of bronchial asthma with liver dysfunction caused by Kampo medicine, Saiko-keisi-kankyo-to, and recovered smoothly in general through natural course. Phytomed 2000;SII:123.
176. Favreau JT, Ryu ML, Braunstein G, Orshansky G, Park SS, Coody GL, Love LA, Fong TL. Severe hepatotoxicity associated with the dietary supplement LipoKinetix. Ann Intern Med 2002;136(8):590–5.
177. Swee W, Klontz KC, Lambert LA. A nationwide outbreak of alopecia associated with the use of a hair-relaxing formulation. Arch Dermatol 2000;136(9):1104–8.
178. Lin CC, Chen JC. Medicinal herb Erycibe Henri Prain ("Ting Kung Teng") resulting in acute cholinergic syndrome. J Toxicol Clin Toxicol 2002;40(2):185–7.
179. Nagai K, Hosaka H, Ishii K, Shinohara M, Sumino Y, Nonaka H, Akima M, Yamamuro W. A case report: acute hepatic injury induced by Formula secundarius-haemorrhoica. J Med Soc Toho Univ 1999;46:311–17.

Hexacarbacholine

General Information

Hexacarbacholine is obsolete. Accounts of its adverse effects will be found in earlier volumes in this series (SED-10, 213) (SEDA-6, 131).

Hexachloroparaxylene

General Information

Hexachloroparaxylene has been used in China and Russia as an antihelminthic drug, principally to treat the liver fluke infections (clonorchiasis due to *Clonorchis sinensis*, schistosomiasis due to *Schistosoma japonicum*, and opisthorchiasis due to *Opisthorchiidae* (1,2). However, other treatments are preferred. It is also used very extensively in the veterinary field in Russia.

Hexachloroparaxylene causes gastrointestinal reactions, cardiac dysrhythmias (perhaps in over 50% of cases), and nephrotoxicity. Hemolysis can occur both early and late, and death can occur from the hemolytic–uremic syndrome (SEDA-4, 219). Late-onset hemolysis after treatment is associated with beta-thalassemia, while early-onset hemolysis is associated with hemoglobin H disease.

References

1. Wan ZR. [Preliminary clinical observations on the treatment of clonorchiasis sinensis with hexachloroparaxylene.] Zhonghua Nei Ke Za Zhi 1979;18(6):406–8.
2. Plotnikov NN, Karnaukov VK, Zal'nova NS, Alekseeva MI, Borisov IA, Stromskaia TF. Lechenie fastsioleza u cheloveka khloksilom (geksakhlorparaksilol). [Treatment of human fascioliasis with chloxyle (hexachloroparaxylene).] Med Parazitol (Mosk) 1965;34(6):725–9.

Hexachlorophene

See also Disinfectants and antiseptics

General Information

Hexachlorophene has been extensively used as an ingredient of innumerable kinds of consumer goods and medical formulations. Since 1961, when it was reported that daily bathing of newborn infants with a 3% hexachlorophene suspension prevented colonization of the skin by coagulase-positive staphylococci, hexachlorophene has been widely used in hospital nurseries.

However, hexachlorophene readily penetrates excoriated or otherwise damaged skin and absorption through intact skin has also been described. The most dramatic complication reported was due to accidental use in talcum powder in neonates, with neurological and other features and many deaths (1). Since then there has been reticence to use hexachlorophene in young infants at all, and certainly the customary 3% emulsion is too strong (2).

As a result of investigations of the toxicity of hexachlorophene in animals and reports of accidental intoxication in France, the FDA in 1972 banned all non-prescription uses of this drug, restricting hexachlorophene to prescription use only, as a surgical scrub and hand-wash product for health-care personnel. Hexachlorophene was excluded from cosmetics, except as a preservative in concentrations not exceeding 0.1%. Other countries followed suit. An extensive critical review of hexachlorophene is given by Delcour-Firquet (3).

Organs and Systems

Respiratory

- Occupational asthma occurred in a pediatric nurse who had worked with hexachlorophene for 15 years (4). The initial symptom was rhinitis but at the time of diagnosis she was also suffering from attacks of asthma.

Nervous system

Neurotoxicity has been observed after dermal application of hexachlorophene to large areas of burned or otherwise excoriated skin, after accidental application of extremely high concentrations on intact skin, and after ingestion. If hexachlorophene is applied in high concentrations or at frequent intervals to the intact skin, excoriation will result, increasing the risk of systemic effects.

In animals, there is a clear relation between dosage, blood concentrations, duration of treatment, and morphological and functional disturbances of the nervous system. In the lower dose range, there is unequivocal histological evidence of neurotoxicity, but without symptoms of neurotoxicity (SEDA-9, 397) (SEDA-11, 486).

Five Chinese patients aged 14–39 years were treated for *Conorchiasis sinensis* infection with oral hexachlorophene 20 mg/kg for 5–6 days (5). They developed nausea, vomiting, diarrhea, abdominal pain, general muscle weakness, and soreness in the eyeballs and legs. Of eight children treated similarly, one became comatose on the fourth day, with temporary loss of light reflex, alternating dilatation and contraction of the pupils, and positive cerebrospinal tract signs (6). The fundus showed papillary edema. Recovery followed symptomatic treatment.

In experimental animals, hexachlorophene can cause cerebral edema (7), and occasional cases have also been reported in humans (8). It affects exclusively the white matter of the brain and spinal cord and produces a spongiform encephalopathy, transforming the white matter into an extensive network of cystic spaces lined by fragments of myelin. Electron microscopy shows intramyelinic edema, with splitting and separation of the myelin lamellae. Nerve damage due to hexachlorophene appears to be reversible, although it takes many weeks for all the holes in the white matter to disappear. However, extensive edema occurring within a rigid structure such as the spinal canal can result in infarction of nervous tissue. In one study of all premature infants who weighed under 1400 g at birth and who survived at least 4 days, there was a significant association between repeated whole-body bathing in 3% hexachlorophene soap (undiluted pHisoHex) and a vacuolar encephalopathy of the brainstem reticular formation (9).

Sensory systems

Optic atrophy has been described after oral or topical use of hexachlorophene (10).

Second-Generation Effects

Teratogenicity

Teratogenicity has been reported (11), but was not confirmed in an expert review (12). In a 1977 study of Swedish medical personnel it was suggested that repeated handwashing with hexachlorophene-containing detergents during the first trimester of pregnancy could be associated with a greatly increased incidence of both major and minor birth defects in the offspring (11). This publication was the subject of extensive discussion, but it had several serious methodological deficiencies, and the hypothesis that hexachlorophene was teratogenic has never been further examined or confirmed. One reason why it was initially taken seriously was the fact that hexachlorophene crosses the placenta and accumulates in fetal neural tissue in mice and rats; the administration of toxic doses in these species is associated with birth defects, including cleft palate, hydrocephalus, anophthalmia, and microphthalmia in rats.

Topical exposure of male neonatal rats to a commercial hexachlorophene formulation produced significantly reduced fertility, resulting in inability to ejaculate. It was possibly caused by dioxin, an "androgenic" contaminant of hexachlorophene, responsible for permanent disruption of the integrated ejaculatory reflex. However, in subneurotoxic concentrations, hexachlorophene did not seem to cause significant impairment of spermatogenesis in rats or dogs.

Lactation

Hexachlorophene is secreted into breast milk (13).

Susceptibility Factors

Age

The blood concentrations of hexachlorophene, determined during newborn skin care with hexachlorophene bathing, cover a range that varies between studies (14–17) but are similar to the concentrations associated with neurotoxicity in monkeys (18), rats (19), and mice (SEDA-9, 397). In interpreting hexachlorophene plasma concentrations, it must be remembered that most of the hexachlorophene is probably distributed very rapidly into lipophilic tissues and that low plasma concentrations may correspond to high tissue concentrations.

A critical review of the available data on the risk of hexachlorophene bathing or other kinds of hexachlorophene use in neonatal skin care has suggested that there is ample evidence of the toxic potential of this disinfectant. It is absolutely contraindicated in infants with a low birth weight (under 2000 g), excoriated areas of the skin, and raised serum bilirubin. The use of a dusting powder with a maximal concentration of 0.3–0.5% seems to be connected with a lower risk of toxicity, but there was marked absorption of hexachlorophene after the application of 0.33% hexachlorophene dusting powder (20) and further information is needed about the pharmacokinetics of hexachlorophene in neonates.

The view that a small degree of edematous change in the central nervous system caused by hexachlorophene use in neonates should be reversible and is very probably without influence on the further development of the child cannot be accepted, because these changes are certainly the first signs of central nervous system toxicity.

- In a neonate treated with a 3% hexachlorophene lotion which had not been rinsed off, the skin became excoriated 4 days later and there was muscular twitching, which progressed to convulsions (21). Four days after withdrawal of hexachlorophene, the convulsions disappeared; recovery was complete.

In assessing the use of hexachlorophene in the nursery, one also has to consider the fact that infections with highly infective strains of staphylococci, producing serious life-threatening diseases, do not appear to be prevented or aborted by hexachlorophene bathing, and the problem that reduced staphylococcal colonization of infants by hexachlorophene may lead to an increased number of infections with Gram-negative bacteria.

Other features of the patient

Owing to the high absorption rate of hexachlorophene through damaged skin and the risk of fatal intoxication, the use of hexachlorophene in the treatment of burns or on otherwise excoriated skin is strongly contraindicated.

- A 10-year-old boy who had sustained 25% first-degree and second-degree burns and was treated with frequent daily applications of a 3% hexachlorophene emulsion (diluted and undiluted) developed a fatal encephalopathy (7).

In six of eight burned children, including four with a history of convulsive seizures after hexachlorophene use, serum concentrations of hexachlorophene were 4–74 ng/ml (approximately equivalent to blood concentrations of 2–37 ng/ml) (22).

In 1972, six deaths related to the use of hexachlorophene in patients with burns were reported to the FDA (23).

In four children, two of whom were being treated with 3% hexachlorophene baths for burns and two for severe congenital ichthyosis, the interval between exposure and symptoms ranged from 6 hours to 10 days (24). All showed severe vacuolation of the white matter in different areas of the cerebrum and cerebellum.

Drug Administration

Drug administration route

Hexachlorophene in vaginal lubricants is variably absorbed from the vaginal mucosa, and hexachlorophene can be identified in maternal and cord serum in an appreciable number of women in whom vaginal examinations during labor were carried out with a hexachlorophene-containing antiseptic lubricant (25). Because of the potential for neonatal hexachlorophene toxicity, the use of alternative lubricants for pelvic examinations is recommended.

Drug overdose

In France, in 1972, 6% hexachlorophene was accidentally included in certain batches of a baby talcum powder. French law prohibited publication of the detailed report on the consequences of this contamination, until litigation was concluded. In 1977, a detailed report of 18 children involved in this accidental poisoning appeared (26) and in 1982 a report described 204 children (SEDA-10, 433) (1). Follow-up investigations of 14 surviving children have also appeared (26). There were no obvious cerebral sequelae, but follow-up was not long enough to exclude the possibility of more subtle damage, which may be manifest by learning difficulties or behavior disorders.

In four cases of accidental ingestion of hexachlorophene in human subjects, anorexia, nausea, vomiting, abdominal cramps, and diarrhea occurred (27). No neurological symptoms were reported.

- Bilateral atrophy of the optic nerve occurred in a 31-year-old woman who had ingested 10–15 ml of a 3% hexachlorophene emulsion orally each day for 10–11 months. She had also applied large amounts of hexachlorophene solution to her face every day as self-treatment for pimples. She was depressed during this period, noted no headache, diplopia, or dizziness, but may have had intermittent numbness of the left foot.
- Acute bilateral optic nerve necrosis occurred in a 7-year-old boy who accidentally received 3% hexachlorophene emulsion (about 12 g) over 52 hours. After the last dose he complained of intermittent blindness. Peritoneal dialysis was ineffective, and he died 98 hours after the last dose.

References

1. Martin-Bouyer G, Lebreton R, Toga M, Stolley PD, Lockhart J. Outbreak of accidental hexachlorophene poisoning in France. Lancet 1982;1(8263):91–5.
2. Garcia-Bunuel L. Toxicity of hexachlorophene. Lancet 1982;1(8282):1190.
3. Delcour-Firquet MP. La toxicité de l'hexachlorophène. [Toxicity of hexachlorophene.] Arch Belg Med Soc 1980;38(1):1–43.
4. Nagy L, Orosz M. Occupational asthma due to hexachlorophene. Thorax 1984;39(8):630–1.
5. Chung HL, Tsao WC, Hsue HC, Kuo CH, Ko HY, Mo PS, Chang HY, Chuo HT, Chou WH. Hexachlorophene (G-11) as a new specific drug against clonorchiasis sinensis; its efficacy and toxicity in experimental and human infection. Chin Med J (Engl) 1963;82:691–701.
6. John L, Wang CN, Yue JH, Wang MN, Chang CF, Chens S. Hexachlorophene in the treatment of clonorchiasis sinensis. Chin Med J (Engl) 1963;82:702–11.
7. Kinoshita Y, Matsumura H, Igisu H, Yokota A. Hexachlorophene-induced brain edema in rat observed by proton magnetic resonance. Brain Res 2000;873(1):127–30.
8. Chilcote R, Curley A, Loughlin HH, Jupin JA. Hexachlorophene storage in a burn patient associated with encephalopathy. Pediatrics 1977;59(3):457–9.
9. Shuman RM, Leech RW, Alvord EC Jr. Neurotoxicity of hexachlorophene in humans. II. A clinicopathological study of 46 premature infants. Arch Neurol 1975;32(5):320–5.
10. Slamovits TL, Burde RM, Klingele TG. Bilateral optic atrophy caused by chronic oral ingestion and topical application of hexachlorophene. Am J Ophthalmol 1980;89(5):676–9.
11. Halling H. Suspected link between exposure to hexachlorophene and malformed infants. Ann NY Acad Sci 1979;320:426–35.
12. Baltzar B, Ericson A, Kallen B. Delivery outcome in women employed in medical occupations in Sweden. J Occup Med 1979;21(8):543–8.
13. West RW, Wilson DJ, Schaffner W. Hexachlorophene concentrations in human milk. Bull Environ Contam Toxicol 1975;13(2):167–9.
14. Curley A, Kimbrough RD, Hawk RE, Nathenson G, Finberg L. Dermal absorption of hexochlorophane in infants. Lancet 1971;2(7719):296–7.
15. Alder VG, Burman D, Corner BD, Gillespie WA. Absorption of hexachlorophane from infants' skin. Lancet 1972;2(7773):384–5.
16. Plueckhahn VD. Hexachlorophane and skin care of newborn infants. Drugs 1973;5(2):97–107.
17. Tyrala EE, Hillman LS, Hillman RE, Dodson WE. Clinical pharmacology of hexachlorophene in newborn infants. J Pediatr 1977;91(3):481–6.
18. Bressler R, Walson PD, Fulginitti VA. Hexachlorophene in the newborn nursery. A risk-benefit analysis and review. Clin Pediatr (Phila) 1977;16(4):342–51.
19. Kennedy GL Jr, Dressler IA, Richter WR, Keplinger ML, Calandra JC. Effects of hexachlorophene in the rat and their reversibility. Toxicol Appl Pharmacol 1976;35(1):137–45.
20. Alder VG, Burman D, Simpson RA, Fysh J, Gillespie WA. Comparison of hexachlorophane and chlorhexidine powders in prevention of neonatal infection. Arch Dis Child 1980;55(4):277–80.
21. Herter WB. Hexachlorophene poisoning. Kaiser Found Med Bull 1959;7:228.
22. Larson DL. Studies show hexachlorophene causes burn syndrome. Hospitals 1968;42(24):63–4.
23. Lockart JD. How toxic is hexachlorophene? Pediatrics 1972;50:229.
24. Mullick FG. Hexachlorophene toxicity. Human experience at the Armed Forces Institute of Pathology. Pediatrics 1973;51(2):395–9.
25. Strickland DM, Leonard RG, Stavchansky S, Benoit T, Wilson RT. Vaginal absorption of hexachlorophene during labor. Am J Obstet Gynecol 1983;147(7):769–72.
26. Goutieres F, Aicardi J. Accidental percutaneous hexachlorophane intoxication in children. BMJ 1977;2(6088):663–5.
27. Wear JB Jr, Shanahan R, Ratliff RK. Toxicity of ingested hexachlorophene. JAMA 1962;181:587–9.

Hexanetriol

General Information

1,2,6-hexanetriol is used as a humectant, solvent, and viscosity-controlling agent in medicaments and cosmetics.

Organs and Systems

Immunologic

- A 35-year-old woman had a 3-week history of pruritic erythema, edema, and linear vesiculation of the upper arms where she had applied fluocinonide cream (1). Patch tests with the cream were positive, but the active ingredient fluocinonide (0.05% in petrolatum) was negative, while 1,2,6-hexanetriol 5% showed strong positive reactions on days 3 and 7.

Reference

1. Miura Y, Hata M, Yuge M, Numano K, Iwakiri K. Allergic contact dermatitis from 1,2,6-hexanetriol in fluocinonide cream. Contact Dermatitis 1999;41(2):118–19.

Hexetidine

See also Disinfectants and antiseptics

General Information

Hexetidine has been used as an oral cavity antiseptic. At the concentration normally used (1 mg/ml), it is effective in vitro against Gram-positive bacteria and *Candida albicans*, but insufficiently active against most Gram-negative bacteria. However, the duration of the reduction in germ count is not longer than 1 hour. When applied to mucosae it also appears to have a mild local anesthetic property. Very little critical work on hexetidine has been published (SEDA-11, 482).

Organs and Systems

Sensory systems

Of 61 patients in whom hexetidine was used as a buccal and pharyngeal antiseptic, a minority, generally those who had just undergone tonsillectomy, complained of a burning sensation and a salty taste (1).

Skin

Allergic contact dermatitis has been reported (SEDA-11, 482) (2).

Drug Administration

Drug administration route

It is not clear whether the use of hexetidine as a spray, of which some will certainly be inhaled, affects its clinical tolerance. Adverse effects were not recorded in 81 patients treated in this way, but the report was not sufficiently detailed for a full assessment (3).

References

1. Platt P, Otten E. Untersuchungen über die Wirksamkeit von Hexidine bei akuten Erkrankungen des Rachens und der Mundhöhle sowie nach Tonsillektomie. Therapiewoche 1969;19:1565.
2. Merk H, Ebert L, Goerz G. Allergic contact dermatitis due to the fungicide hexetidine. Contact Dermatitis 1982; 8(3):216.
3. Mann HJ, Wagner B. Klinische Erfahrugen bei der Behandlung der Tonsilitis acuta und der Pharyngitis acuta mit Hexoral Spray. Therapiewoche 1972;22:4316.

Hippocastanaceae

See also Herbal medicines

General Information

The family of Hippocastanaceae contains the single genus *Aesculus* (buckeye, horse chestnut).

Aesculus species

Aescin is a complex mixture of triterpene saponins prepared from the seeds of the horse chestnut, *Aesculus hippocastanum*. It consists of a water-soluble fraction (alpha-aescin) and a water-insoluble fraction (beta-aescin).

Adverse effects

A systematic review of randomized trials of extracts of horse chestnut in chronic venous insufficiency showed that adverse effects are usually mild, for example pruritus, nausea, headache, dizziness, and gastrointestinal symptoms (1).

Urinary tract

Beta-aescin has been repeatedly associated with acute renal insufficiency when given intravenously in massive doses. Whether such effects can also occur after oral administration is unclear, as animal studies have shown poor absorption of beta-aescin from the gastrointestinal tract. (SEDA-3, 181) (SEDA-9, 190).

Skin

Contact dermatitis has been ascribed to aescin (2), as has contact urticaria (3).

Drug interactions

Beta-aescin can precipitate renal insufficiency when combined with aminoglycoside antibiotics (SEDA-3, 181) (SEDA-9, 190).

References

1. Pittler MH, Ernst E. Horse-chestnut seed extract for chronic venous insufficiency. A criteria-based systematic review. Arch Dermatol 1998;134(11):1356–60.
2. Comaish JS, Kersey PJ. Contact dermatitis to extract of horse chestnut (esculin). Contact Dermatitis 1980;6(2):150–1.
3. Escribano MM, Munoz-Bellido FJ, Velazquez E, Delgado J, Serrano P, Guardia J, Conde J. Contact urticaria due to aescin. Contact Dermatitis 1997;37(5):233.

Histamine H_2 receptor antagonists

See also Individual agents

General Information

The histamine H_2 receptor antagonists are selective antagonists at histamine receptors in the stomach, reducing gastric acid secretion.

The overall safety record of the currently marketed agents, particularly cimetidine and ranitidine, which have had extensive worldwide use, is excellent, and in practice safety issues seldom affect drug choice (1), except perhaps when it is necessary to avoid interactions with phenytoin, theophylline, or warfarin. Surveillance studies, which have been going on for a quarter of a century (including 10-year studies in many patients, mainly involving cimetidine and ranitidine), have failed to detect any serious adverse effects other than those recognized by 1980, or any adverse effect on mortality (2).

The H_2 receptor antagonists do not prevent gastroduodenal ulceration by non-steroidal anti-inflammatory drugs, but they do prevent stress-induced ulceration and bleeding. In intensive care units there is evidence of a beneficial effect, but in patients with hematemesis and melena there is little evidence that H_2 receptor antagonists reduce rates of transfusion, surgical intervention, or mortality (SEDA-19, 326).

Observational studies

The use, efficacy, and adverse effects of non-prescription H_2 receptor antagonists and alginate-containing formulations obtained from community pharmacies have been evaluated in 767 customers with dyspepsia (3). Most obtained some or complete symptom relief (75%) and were completely satisfied with the product (78%). H_2 receptor antagonists were more likely to produce complete relief of symptoms than alginate-containing formulations. Only 3% reported adverse effects: diarrhea, constipation, bloating, and flatulence from alginate formulations, and dry mouth, altered bowel habit, diarrhea, and constipation from H_2 receptor antagonists.

Changes in healthcare utilization resulting from a formulary switch from nizatidine to cimetidine have been studied in 704 patients (4). There was no evidence of increased healthcare utilization during the 6 months after the formulary switch, which led to considerable pharmaceutical savings. During this period only four (0.004%) adverse drug reactions associated with cimetidine were reported; urticaria, nausea and vomiting, leg cramps, and impotence.

Comparative studies

Several treatments are available for promoting the healing of gastric and duodenal ulcers associated with the use of non-steroidal anti-inflammatory drugs (NSAIDs). They include histamine receptor antagonists, proton pump inhibitors, and prostaglandin analogues. Two large randomized, double-blind, multicenter trials in a total of 1456 patients have compared the efficacy of ranitidine 150 mg bd with omeprazole 20 or 40 mg/day (ASTRONAUT study) (5) and omeprazole 20 or 40 mg/day with misoprostol 200 micrograms qds (OMNIUM study) (6) in the treatment of NSAID-induced ulcers. The proportions of the patients with treatment success at 8 weeks were 77% with both doses of omeprazole, 63% with ranitidine, and 71% with misoprostol. The most frequent adverse effects were diarrhea in 11% and abdominal pain in 8% of patients taking misoprostol. Both these adverse effects were 2–4 times more frequent with misoprostol than with omeprazole. Withdrawal from the study owing to adverse effects was also more frequent in the misoprostol arm of the OMNIUM study.

Placebo-controlled studies

The effects of ranitidine 75 mg, famotidine 10 mg, and placebo, given 1 hour after a standard lunch, on intragastric acidity have been compared in 24 healthy volunteers (7). Low-dose ranitidine and famotidine reduced acidity significantly more than placebo during the daytime and nighttime. The effect of ranitidine was significantly greater than famotidine during the first 2.5 hours after dosing.

Organs and Systems

Cardiovascular

Rapid intravenous administration of ranitidine, cimetidine, or famotidine can precipitate cardiovascular complications, notably bradycardia, hypotension, and dysrhythmias (SEDA-20, 317).

Hematologic

H_2 receptor antagonists cause a significant reduction in the absorption of vitamin B_{12} from food. This is thought to be due to impaired release of the vitamin from food protein, which requires gastric acid and pepsin as the initial step in the absorption process. This can be sufficient to cause vitamin deficiency and anemia, notably in patients who have low body stores of vitamin B_{12} and are taking an H_2 receptor antagonist over a long period (8).

- Vitamin B_{12} deficiency has been reported in a 78-year-old non-vegetarian white woman with gastro-esophageal reflux who had taken H_2 receptor antagonists and omeprazole for 4.5 years (9).

Pancreas

The risk of acute pancreatitis associated with the use of acid-suppressing drugs has been assessed in a retrospective cohort study with a nested case-control design within the General Practice Research Database in the UK (10). The study included 180 178 people aged 20–74 years who had received at least one prescription for cimetidine, famotidine, nizatidine, ranitidine, lansoprazole, or omeprazole from January 1992 to September 1997, and who did not have major risk factors for pancreatic diseases. There were no cases of pancreatitis among users of famotidine, lansoprazole, or nizatidine. The relative risk compared with non-use, corrected for age, sex, calendar year, and use of medication known to be associated with pancreatitis was 1.3 (95% CI = 0.4, 4.1) for ranitidine, 2.1 (0.6,7.2) for cimetidine, and 1.1 (0.3,4.6) for omeprazole. The results do not support an association between acute pancreatitis and acid-suppressing drugs.

Musculoskeletal

In 33 patients taking cimetidine, ranitidine, or famotidine for more than 2 years there was little effect on the degree of bone mineral density (11).

Immunologic

Early studies suggested an increased risk of nosocomial pneumonia associated with H_2 receptor antagonists in critically ill patients. To investigate this further, two randomized studies have been performed. One compared ranitidine (0.25 mg/kg/hour intravenously) with sucralfate (1 g every 6 hours via nasogastric tube) for prophylaxis against stress-induced gastritis in 96 severely injured patients (12). Ranitidine was associated with a 1.5 times increased risk of developing any infection compared with sucralfate. Furthermore, of the 49 patients who received ranitidine, 14 developed 26 separate episodes of pneumonia, while of the 47 patients who received sucralfate, 10 developed 14 episodes of pneumonia. The other study, placebo-controlled, compared intravenous ranitidine (50 mg tds) and pirenzepine (10 mg tds) in 158 patients who were being mechanically ventilated; the pneumonia rates were similar in the three groups (13).

In another study of stress ulcer prophylaxis, 53 critically ill patients were randomized to receive sucralfate 1 g 6-hourly, cimetidine 300 mg 8-hourly, or cimetidine 900 mg/day by continuous intravenous infusion (14). Although bacterial colonization was increasingly likely in patients with a persistent alkaline gastric environment, gastric luminal pH and the degree of bacterial colonization of the stomach were similar in the three groups.

Long-Term Effects

Tumorigenicity

Tumor-inducing effects have been much discussed ever since the introduction of the H_2 receptor antagonists but their existence has not been clearly established. The discussion was seeded by:

- findings of intestinal metaplasia of the gastric epithelium in rats used for chronic toxicity studies, though only at extraordinarily high doses, followed by the appearance of intramucosal carcinomas in the pyloric region after 11 months of study;
- reports of patients taking cimetidine in whom gastric carcinoma was diagnosed; however, the drug has been widely (and sometimes without careful prior diagnosis) used in patients with a range of gastric disorders, and some of these are believed to have had early carcinomas at the time when cimetidine was started (15);
- the fact that cimetidine can undergo nitrosylation to form a mutagen;
- the structural resemblance of cimetidine to tiotidine, which can cause gastric carcinoma in animals.

In a retrospective case-control assessment of medical records of 56 patients who died of cardio-esophageal adenocarcinoma and 56 age- and sex-matched controls who died of myocardial infarction, subjects who died of cardio-esophageal adenocarcinoma were more likely to have consumed H_2 receptor antagonists (RR = 7.5; 95% CI = 1.3,42) (16).

However, there is still no valid reason for considering the H_2 receptor antagonists to be tumorigenic, and when studies have detected some excess incidence of gastric cancer in long-term users of H_2 receptor antagonists this was attributable to selection bias (17). The fact that drugs of this type have now been released for self-medication in many countries seems very likely to lead to an increase in the incidence of cases in which an H_2 receptor antagonist is used without prior exclusion of premalignant or malignant change, thus confusing the situation further.

Second-Generation Effects

Teratogenicity

In 178 women who took H_2 receptor antagonists during the first 3 months of pregnancy and 178 pregnant controls there was no evidence of teratogenicity (SEDA-21, 362).

Susceptibility Factors

Renal disease

In patients with renal insufficiency the elimination of H_2 receptor antagonists is subject to significant and clinically relevant alterations (18). Doses should be reduced, and ranitidine bismuth citrate should be avoided altogether in severe renal insufficiency.

Dialysis has no major effect on dosage schedules, because only negligible amounts of H_2 receptor antagonists are removed by this route (SEDA-19, 326).

Drug–Drug Interactions

Alcohol

A meta-analysis of 24 studies showed that cimetidine and ranitidine, but not famotidine or nizatidine, caused small increases in blood alcohol concentrations (19). The mechanism is unclear, but one possibility is inhibition of gastric alcohol dehydrogenase. However, relative to accepted legal definitions of intoxication the effect of any histamine receptor antagonist on blood alcohol concentrations is unlikely to be clinically significant.

References

1. Feldman M, Burton ME. Histamine2-receptor antagonists. Standard therapy for acid-peptic diseases. 1. N Engl J Med 1990;323(24):1672–80.
2. Colin-Jones DG, Langman MJ, Lawson DH, Logan RF, Paterson KR, Vessey MP. Postmarketing surveillance of the safety of cimetidine: 10 year mortality report. Gut 1992;33(9):1280–4.
3. Krska J, John DN, Hansford D, Kennedy EJ. Drug utilization evaluation of nonprescription H2-receptor antagonists and alginate-containing preparations for dyspepsia. Br J Clin Pharmacol 2000;49(4):363–8.
4. Good CB, Fultz SL, Trilli L, Etchason J. Therapeutic substitution of cimetidine for nizatidine was not associated with an increase in healthcare utilization. Am J Manag Care 2000;6(10):1141–6.
5. Yeomans ND, Tulassay Z, Juhasz L, Racz I, Howard JM, van Rensburg CJ, Swannell AJ, Hawkey CJ. A comparison of omeprazole with ranitidine for ulcers associated with nonsteroidal antiinflammatory drugs. Acid Suppression Trial: Ranitidine versus Omeprazole for

NSAID-Associated Ulcer Treatment (ASTRONAUT) Study Group. N Engl J Med 1998;338(11):719–26.
6. Hawkey CJ, Karrasch JA, Szczepanski L, Walker DG, Barkun A, Swannell AJ, Yeomans ND. Omeprazole compared with misoprostol for ulcers associated with nonsteroidal antiinflammatory drugs. Omeprazole versus Misoprostol for NSAID-induced Ulcer Management (OMNIUM) Study Group. N Engl J Med 1998;338(11):727–34.
7. Hamilton MI, Sercombe J, Pounder RE. Control of intragastric acidity with over-the-counter doses of ranitidine or famotidine. Aliment Pharmacol Ther 2001;15(10):1579–83.
8. Force RW, Nahata MC. Effect of histamine H2-receptor antagonists on vitamin B12 absorption. Ann Pharmacother 1992;26(10):1283–6.
9. Ruscin JM, Page RL 2nd, Valuck RJ. Vitamin B(12) deficiency associated with histamine(2)-receptor antagonists and a proton-pump inhibitor. Ann Pharmacother 2002;36(5):812–16.
10. Eland IA, Alvarez CH, Stricker BH, Rodriguez LA. The risk of acute pancreatitis associated with acid-suppressing drugs. Br J Clin Pharmacol 2000;49(5):473–8.
11. Adachi Y, Shiota E, Matsumata T, Iso Y, Yoh R, Kitano S. Bone mineral density in patients taking H2-receptor antagonist. Calcif Tissue Int 1998;62(4):283–5.
12. O'Keefe GE, Gentilello LM, Maier RV. Incidence of infectious complications associated with the use of histamine2-receptor antagonists in critically ill trauma patients. Ann Surg 1998;227(1):120–5.
13. Hanisch EW, Encke A, Naujoks F, Windolf J. A randomized, double-blind trial for stress ulcer prophylaxis shows no evidence of increased pneumonia. Am J Surg 1998;176(5):453–7.
14. Ortiz JE, Sottile FD, Sigel P, Nasraway SA. Gastric colonization as a consequence of stress ulcer prophylaxis: a prospective, randomized trial. Pharmacotherapy 1998;18(3):486–91.
15. Colin-Jones DG, Langman MJ, Lawson DH, Vessey MP. Cimetidine and gastric cancer: preliminary report from post-marketing surveillance study. BMJ (Clin Res Ed) 1982;285(6351):1311–13.
16. Suleiman UL, Harrison M, Britton A, McPherson K, Bates T. H2-receptor antagonists may increase the risk of cardio-oesophageal adenocarcinoma: a case-control study. Eur J Cancer Prev 2000;9(3):185–91.
17. Moller H, Nissen A, Mosbech J. Use of cimetidine and other peptic ulcer drugs in Denmark 1977–1990 with analysis of the risk of gastric cancer among cimetidine users. Gut 1992;33(9):1166–9.
18. Gladziwa U, Koltz U. Pharmacokinetic optimisation of the treatment of peptic ulcer in patients with renal failure. Clin Pharmacokinet 1994;27(5):393–408.
19. Weinberg DS, Burnham D, Berlin JA. Effect of histamine-2 receptor antagonists on blood alcohol levels: a meta-analysis. J Gen Intern Med 1998;13(9):594–9.

HMG coenzyme-A reductase inhibitors

See also Individual agents

General Information

Statins inhibit HMG-CoA reductase and reduce cellular cholesterol synthesis (1). Lower intracellular cholesterol concentrations cause over-expression of the LDL receptor in the plasma membrane of hepatocytes. This overexpression increases the clearance of circulating LDL, reducing plasma concentrations of LDL cholesterol.

The statins include atorvastatin, bervastatin, cerivastatin, crilvastatin, dalvastatin, fluvastatin, glenvastatin, lovastatin, mevastatin, pitavastatin, pravastatin, rosuvastatin, simvastatin, and tenivastatin (all rINNs). Atorvastatin, cerivastatin, fluvastatin, lovastatin, pravastatin, and simvastatin are covered in separate monographs.

The adverse effects of the statins are mostly limited to slight increases in liver and muscle enzymes in the blood. Hypersensitivity reactions are very rare. There is no evidence of tumor-inducing effects. Second-generation effects are suspected, and statins should not be used during pregnancy.

Organs and Systems

Nervous system

Ratings on a depression scale rose in four out of six men given cholesterol-lowering drugs, in two of them to a degree that met the criteria for mild clinical depression (2).

Statins interfere with the production of isoprene which is somehow connected with sleep, but there have been neither changes in sleep EEG measures relevant to insomnia nor changes in the quality of sleep (SEDA-13, 1327) (3). However, there has been a report of sleep disturbances (4).

- Three months after starting to take metoprolol 100 mg bd and simvastatin 10 mg/day, a 55-year-old man reported restless nights and nightmares, which he had not previously experienced. The dose of metoprolol was reduced to 50 mg bd, with no observable benefit. Simvastatin was withdrawn 2 weeks later and pravastatin 20 mg/day was prescribed, with substantial improvement in the quality of sleep; however, some unpleasant nightmares still occurred. Four weeks later, metoprolol was also withdrawn and atenolol 100 mg/day was prescribed. Thereafter, the quality of sleep was significantly improved, and 6 months later the patient did not report any nightmares. Sleep disturbances recurred after a later attempt to reintroduce simvastatin in place of pravastatin. The same effect occurred when, during treatment with pravastatin, substitution of atenolol with metoprolol was attempted.

In this case, the statins may have interacted with metoprolol, and it may have been relevant that metoprolol is more lipid-soluble than atenolol.

Peripheral neuropathy occurs with statins, and perhaps with all cholesterol-lowering drugs, and may be related to reduced production of ubiquinone, as suggested in a review (5). Moreover, it appears that once a statin produces a neuropathy, rechallenge with any other statin is likely to cause a recurrence. This is reported to occur 1–3 weeks after rechallenge, whereas the resolution takes 4–6 weeks after withdrawal (5).

In a series of seven cases of neuropathy, all were axonal peripheral neuropathies and both thick and thin nerve fibers were affected (6). No cause of peripheral neuropathy other than statin treatment could be identified. In this series at least four of the cases were irreversible, probably due to long exposure to statins (4–7 years versus 1–2 years in previous reports). Besides an effect on ubiquinone, interference with cholesterol synthesis may alter nerve membrane function, since cholesterol is a ubiquitous component of human cell membranes. Neuropathy has not been observed in extensive long-term trials of lipid-lowering drugs. It could be due to patient selection, a low frequency of the adverse effect, or lack of attention to symptoms of peripheral neuropathy. The observed association may also not be causal.

In a case-control study of 166 cases of idiopathic polyneuropathy, of which 35 had a definite diagnosis, the odds ratio for neuropathy was 14 for statin users compared with non-users (7).

With the current level of information, it is prudent to consider withdrawal of statins in patients with symptoms compatible with polyneuropathy.

Sensory systems

One should be alert to the possibility of color blindness due to statins (8), although the risk is uncertain.

Owing to the high cholesterol content of the human lens, ocular changes have been looked for during trials with statins. It has been concluded that cataract does not occur. Although the degree of lens opacities increases during treatment, the incidence does not differ from that seen in an untreated control population (9). With fenofibrate serving as control, lovastatin or simvastatin did not reduce visual acuity during treatment for 2 years (SEDA-13, 1328) (10). According to a review, there is no danger during long-term treatment and there should be no requirement for regular ophthalmological examination (11).

Psychological, psychiatric

Animal and cross-sectional studies have suggested that serum lipid concentrations can cause altered cognitive function, mood, and behavior (11).

Metabolism

Although the statins seem to be similar in their ability to lower LDL, there are also dissimilarities. For instance, simvastatin increases HDL cholesterol with increasing doses, whereas atorvastatin does not (12). The clinical significance of this is unknown.

Hematologic

Hematological adverse effects can occur during treatment with both simvastatin and atorvastatin, according to a brief review (13). They include thrombotic thrombocytopenic purpura and severe thrombocytopenic purpura.

Liver

HMG CoA reductase inhibitors can be associated with small rises in alanine transaminase activity, but have not been definitely associated with severe morbidity involving altered hepatic function. All cases of acute liver failure related to the use of lovastatin have been reviewed, and probably the frequency is similar to the background rate. This suggests that periodic monitoring of alanine transaminase in these patients would be burdensome and expensive (14).

The term "transaminitis" has been coined to describe a rise in the activities of serum transaminases without clinical symptoms. One author has suggested that in such cases one should switch from one statin to another, thereby preventing unnecessary withdrawal of statin treatment in dyslipidemic patients at high cardiovascular risk (15).

A return to normal or only slightly increased values of transaminases is often seen after a short period. The overall probability of having an increase in transaminase activity more than three times the top of the reference range is 0.7% (16). The probability may be increased in patients with pre-existing minor hepatic changes, as has been seen in one patient with systemic lupus erythematosus (17). There seems to be no difference between the various drugs in this respect (11), but when simvastatin and atorvastatin, each at a dose of 80 mg/day, were compared in 826 hypercholesterolemic patients there were fewer drug-related gastrointestinal symptoms and clinically significant transaminase rises with simvastatin (18). Frank hepatitis is rare. A cholestatic picture has also been reported (19). The mechanisms of these reactions are not known.

In one series, the frequency of liver toxicity was similar in patients taking pravastatin or simvastatin (20), while in another study there was a difference 6 months after the start of the study when the simvastatin group showed increases in liver enzymes (SEDA-13, 1327) (21).

In a comparison of atorvastatin with pravastatin, of 224 patients taking atorvastatin, two had clinically significant increases in alanine transaminase activity (22). They recovered during the next 4 months, one after withdrawal of atorvastatin and the other after a dosage reduction. Withdrawals due to adverse effects were similar in the two groups. One patient developed hepatitis while taking atorvastatin, but was able to tolerate simvastatin (23). The authors concluded that this adverse effect was not a class effect. Eosinophils in a liver-biopsy specimen pointed to an immunological mechanism.

Pancreas

Pancreatitis has been observed during treatment with simvastatin (q.v.).

- A 77-year-old woman taking rosuvastatin developed acute pancreatitis, which resolved on withdrawal (24). No other cause for the pancreatitis was found. She had had a similar episode 1 year before precipitated by atorvastatin, which resolved on withdrawal.

The authors suggested that pancreatitis may be a class effect of the statins.

Skin

Adverse effects of statins on the skin are rare, although statins can affect cutaneous lipid content. A series of skin reactions have been described in patients using statins (25).

Musculoskeletal

Rhabdomyolysis is a problem with several lipid-lowering drugs (SEDA-13, 1325) (SEDA-13, 1328) (SEDA-13,

1330) (SEDA-19, 409), especially when they are used in combination (26). In individuals with pre-existing renal insufficiency this can lead to an earlier need for chronic dialysis (27). Interactions between various hypolipidemic drugs and other drugs also sometimes cause rhabdomyolysis (SEDA-18, 426). For instance, itraconazole markedly increases plasma concentrations of lovastatin, and in one subject plasma creatine kinase was increased 10-fold within 24 hours of administration of this combination (28).

In four patients with muscle symptoms while taking statins, creatine kinase activity was normal, but they were subsequently able to distinguish from their symptoms whether they were taking drug or placebo; muscle biopsies showed evidence of mitochondrial dysfunction (29).

Hypothyroidism predisposes to rhabdomyolysis and screening thyroid function has been advocated before starting hypolipidemic drugs (SEDA-21, 458).

Myopathic symptoms, predominantly stiffness and tenderness of proximal limb muscles and difficulty in rising from a low chair, can develop within a month of starting therapy and most cases develop within 3 months. Most patients recover after withdrawal. Sometimes a glucocorticoid is needed to reverse the myopathy. In one patient, histological investigation of muscle biopsies suggested that the myopathy was due, at least in part, to an inflammatory reaction (30). The serum coenzyme Q concentration is reduced by about 30% during statin treatment, because the enzyme is carried by LDL particles, although the concentrations during long-term treatment are equal to those in healthy controls (SEDA-13, 1328) (31,32). Ubiquinone (coenzyme-Q) is part of the oxidative respiratory pathway generating ATP, and deficiency could impede the function of myocytes, leading to an increase in serum creatine kinase and even cell destruction, with release of myoglobin, which in its turn can block kidney tubules and thereby produce anuria.

- Simvastatin 5 mg/day caused rhabdomyolysis in a 61-year-old man who was not taking concomitant interacting drugs (33).
- An elderly lady with chronic renal insufficiency developed rhabdomyolysis during simvastatin therapy (34). Her symptoms of muscle pain, fatigue, myoglobulinuria, oliguria, and pulmonary edema occurred 48 hours after the first dose of simvastatin. Simvastatin was immediately withdrawn, and she was dialysed for 1 week.

Myopathy, defined as muscle symptoms with a rise in creatine kinase greater than 10 times the upper limit of the reference range, was found in one study in only one patient who was taking 40 mg od and in four patients taking 80 mg/day, out of a total of 8245 patients. The number of patients with rhabdomyolysis was, according to postmarketing reporting from the first million individuals taking lovastatin, 24 in all. Seventeen of those had taken other medications that are known to increase the risk (35). There is some evidence that patients with other concomitant illnesses may be at greater risk of myopathy than would be anticipated from experience in controlled trials.

Diplopia may be an early sign of generalized drug-induced muscle dysfunction. Altogether, 71 cases of diplopia, possibly related to various HMG-CoA inhibitors, have been collected from adverse drug reactions-reporting databases. The information was mostly too scanty to judge a causal relation, but improvement occurred in 33 on withdrawal, and two patients had positive rechallenge data (36).

- A 67-year-old woman had ocular myasthenia while taking various statins and also bezafibrate (37). Atorvastatin had the smallest effect.

The authors suggested that this was a variant of a generalized myopathy and was due to a low co-enzyme Q10 concentration.

Exercise-induced muscle pain, without myopathy and a rise in creatine kinase activity, can probably be caused by statins. This has been described in seven patients with heterozygous familial hypercholesterolemia and consisted of pain during exercise and cramps in the following hours (38).

Symptomatic rises in creatine kinase activity to over 10 times the upper end of the reference range occurred in 0, 1, and 0.9% of patients taking placebo, cerivastatin 0.4 mg, or cerivastatin 0.8 mg respectively (39), and rhabdomyolysis has been described in patients taking cerivastatin (40,41). However, in a review of the pharmacological properties and therapeutic efficacy of cerivastatin in hypercholesterolemia, it was stated that cerivastatin only infrequently causes rhabdomyolysis when given alone (42).

Four cases of tendinopathy have been reported in three men and one woman taking statins (43). The diagnoses were extensor tenosynovitis in the hands, tenosynovitis of the tibialis anterior tendon, and Achilles tendinopathy. Two patients were taking simvastatin and two atorvastatin. The tendinopathy developed 1–2 months after the start of treatment. The outcome was consistently favorable within 1–2 months after drug withdrawal.

Sexual function

Erectile dysfunction has been reported in 12% of 339 men treated with fibrate derivatives or statins, compared with 5.6% of similar patients not taking these drugs (44). The mechanism is unknown and should be confirmed in randomized studies. A class effect has been suggested by the case of a 57-year-old man who had impotence after taking lovastatin for 2 weeks and also when he later tried pravastatin (45).

Immunologic

Lupus-like symptoms have been reported in patients taking statins (46).

Long-Term Effects

Tumorigenicity

It has been suspected that low concentrations of serum cholesterol might be associated with an increased risk of cancer or overall mortality. All fibrates and statins cause cancer in rodents, but the relevance of this finding to man has been questioned (47). In an epidemiological study these risks were almost non-existent after adjusting for confounding factors. However, in the CARE study, breast cancer occurred in one patient in the control group and 12 in the pravastatin group (48). The incidence of cancers, both during clinical studies and up to 9 years after, has been reassuring (49).

Drug–Drug Interactions

General

Many statins are metabolized by CYP3A4, and this and other mechanisms of drug interactions involving statins have been reviewed (50). Other drugs metabolized by CYP3A4 can greatly increase statin concentrations in the body and precipitate rhabdomyolysis. Although the statins are similar in their ability to lower cholesterol concentrations, there are dissimilarities in their interactions with other drugs.

With the exception of fluvastatin and pravastatin, the statins are metabolized by CYP3A4. Selective inhibition of CYP3A4 or of P-glycoprotein (50) in the small intestine probably increases the systemic availability of CYP3A4 substrates. Some drugs that are metabolized by this enzyme, such as the macrolide antibiotics and the antidepressant nefazodone, can greatly enhance the concentrations of statins in the body and thereby precipitate rhabdomyolysis. However, other drugs that are metabolized by CYP3A4, such as cimetidine, have not been reported to have this effect.

Antifungal azoles

The antifungal azoles inhibit CYP isozymes and can therefore interact with some statins.

Fluconazole
In a randomized, double-blind, crossover study in 12 healthy volunteers, fluconazole increased the plasma concentrations of fluvastatin and prolonged its elimination; the mechanism was probably inhibition of the CYP2C9-mediated metabolism of fluvastatin (51). Care should be taken if fluconazole or other potent inhibitors of CYP2C9 are given to patients using fluvastatin.

Itraconazole
The effects of itraconazole, a potent inhibitor of CYP3A4, on the pharmacokinetics of atorvastatin, cerivastatin, and pravastatin have been evaluated in an open, randomized, crossover study in 18 healthy subjects who took single doses of atorvastatin 20 mg, cerivastatin 0.8 mg, or pravastatin 40 mg, with and without itraconazole 200 mg (52). Itraconazole markedly raised atorvastatin plasma concentrations (2.5-fold) and produced modest rises in the plasma concentrations of cerivastatin (1.3-fold) and pravastatin (1.5-fold). These results suggest that in patients taking itraconazole, cerivastatin or pravastatin may be preferable to atorvastatin.

Physicians should check for lipid-lowering drugs before treating elderly individuals with itraconazole (53). Susceptibility to this interaction varies from statin to statin, in that simvastatin is more affected than pravastatin (54). Concomitant use of simvastatin with itraconazole should be avoided, and the same holds true for atorvastatin (55). In another study, the blood concentration of fluvastatin was not significantly increased, whereas that of lovastatin was (56).

Ketoconazole
Ketoconazole can also cause rhabdomyolysis when taken with both lovastatin and simvastatin (57).

Chlorzoxazone

- A 73-year-old woman had rhabdomyolysis, cholestatic hepatitis, and mild renal insufficiency 14 days after she started to take the centrally acting muscle relaxant chlorzoxazone while also taking simvastatin (58). Withdrawal of the causal medication and conservative therapy with volume substitution and forced diuresis was followed by almost complete resolution of the symptoms.

The authors believed that either the two drugs had interacted by metabolism through the same hepatic enzyme, or that chlorzoxazone had caused cholestasis which then increased the blood concentration of simvastatin.

Ciclosporin

Most drug interactions associated with rhabdomyolysis occur when ciclosporin is combined with simvastatin or lovastatin. It has been suggested that if a statin is to be combined with ciclosporin, pravastatin or fluvastatin should be chosen instead (59).

Coumarin anticoagulants

Interactions of statins with warfarin, resulting in an increased bleeding tendency, have been reported (35), including interactions of anticoagulants with both lovastatin (35) and fluvastatin (60).

Three patients taking fluvastatin 20 mg/day had raised international normalized ratios (INRs), with a risk of bleeding (61).

- A 67-year-old man receiving a stable maintenance dosage of warfarin experienced an increased INR without bleeding when his atorvastatin therapy was switched to fluvastatin. His warfarin dosage was reduced and his INR stabilized. The fluvastatin was switched back to atorvastatin, and the warfarin dosage was increased to maintain the patient's goal INR (62).

In 46 adults taking warfarin, a change from pravastatin to simvastatin caused a significant increase in INR from 2.42 to 2.74 without an overall change in the dose of warfarin; there were no unusual episodes of bleeding (63).

In three patients taking stable warfarin dosages with INRs in the target range, the INRs increased when fluvastatin was added (60). Although none had a bleeding episode, they did require a reduction in their weekly warfarin dosage to achieve an appropriate degree of anticoagulation.

In contrast, in 12 patients chronically maintained on warfarin, atorvastatin 80 mg/day for 2 weeks had no important effect on mean prothrombin time (63).

In 21 healthy men, cerivastatin 300 micrograms did not alter the pharmacokinetics of *R*- and *S*-warfarin, or the pharmacodynamics of a single oral dose of warfarin 25 mg (64).

In a patient given the anticoagulant acenocoumarol, the INR increased from the target range (2–3.5) to 9.0, 3 weeks after starting simvastatin 20 mg/day. It is conceivable either that the two drugs competed for hepatic metabolism or that the oral anticoagulant was displaced from plasma albumin by simvastatin (65). The former mechanism is supported by the observation that pravastatin, which is only bound 50% to albumin, interacted with the anticoagulant fluindione and raised the INR (66).

Diltiazem

Diltiazem interacts with lovastatin but not with pravastatin (67). In 10 healthy volunteers given lovastatin orally with or without intravenous diltiazem in a randomized, two-way, crossover design, the interaction of diltiazem with lovastatin was primarily a first-pass effect, due to inhibition of CYP3A4 (68). Thus, drug interactions with diltiazem may become evident when a patient is switched from intravenous to oral dosing.

Fibrates

In a retrospective series, 4 (5%) out of 80 subjects taking lovastatin and gemfibrozil developed a myopathy. Based on this and on reports to US Food and Drug Administration the combined use of the two drugs is discouraged, especially in patients with compromised renal and/or hepatic function. Elderly women may be at special risk (69,70).

Some investigators have concluded that rare drug-induced reversible hepatotoxicity calls for close monitoring of liver enzymes in long-term treatment with statin-fibrate combinations (71).

Combination therapy with fluvastatin and bezafibrate 400 mg/day in 71 patients with persistent hypertriglyceridemia resulted in no significant increase in creatine kinase activity or in the frequency of myalgia (72).

- In contrast, although in vitro studies have not shown any evidence of pharmacokinetic interactions between cerivastatin and gemfibrozil (42), there was myalgia and a marked increase in creatine kinase in a 74-year-old woman with normal renal function who took gemfibrozil 1200 mg/day 3 weeks after she started to take cerivastatin 0.3 mg/day (41).

Since then several other cases have been described:

- a 64-year-old woman (73)
- a 63-year-old man with diabetes mellitus (74)
- a 75-year-old man (75)
- a 68-year-old man (76).

The last patient fared well on a combination of gemfibrozil and cerivastatin until he received influenza vaccination. Rhabdomyolysis has been reported with various viruses, including influenza A and B and inactivation of the virus does not totally prevent this.

Gemfibrozil also increased plasma concentrations of simvastatin and its active form, simvastatin acid, in a randomized, double-blind, crossover study in 10 healthy volunteers given gemfibrozil or placebo orally for 3 days before a single dose of simvastatin (77). This suggests that the increased risk of myopathy in combination treatment is at least partly pharmacokinetic in origin. Because gemfibrozil does not inhibit CYP3A4 in vitro, the mechanism of the pharmacokinetic interaction is probably inhibition of non-CYP3A4-mediated metabolism of simvastatin acid.

Grapefruit juice

Grapefruit juice inhibits CYP3A4, and serum concentrations of atorvastatin, but not of pravastatin, increased after administration of double-strength grapefruit juice 200 ml tds for 2 days (78).

When 10 healthy volunteers took simvastatin 24 hours after a large amount of grapefruit juice in a non-randomized, crossover study, the effect on the AUC of simvastatin was only about 10% of the effect observed when grapefruit juice and simvastatin were taken together (79). The interaction potential of even large amounts of grapefruit juice with CYP3A4 substrates dissipates within 3–7 days after ingestion of the last dose.

HIV protease inhibitors

Healthy volunteers were given protease inhibitors and statins, and the authors concluded that simvastatin should be avoided and that atorvastatin could be used with caution in people taking ritonavir and saquinavir (80). Dosage adjustment of pravastatin may be necessary with co-administration of ritonavir and saquinavir. Pravastatin does not alter the pharmacokinetics of nelfinavir, and thus appears to be safe for co-administration.

Macrolides

The macrolide antibiotic erythromycin together with statins enhances the risk of rhabdomyolysis (SED-13, 1328) (81), as do clarithromycin and azithromycin (82).

Nefazodone

The antidepressant nefazodone increases the risk of rhabdomyolysis from statins (83).

Red yeast rice

Rhabdomyolysis in a stable renal transplant recipient was attributed to the presence of red yeast rice (*Monascus purpureus*) in a herbal mixture (84). The condition resolved when he stopped taking the product. Rice fermented with red yeast contains several types of mevinic acids, including monacolin-K, which is identical to lovastatin. The authors postulated that the interaction of ciclosporin with these compounds through cytochrome P450 had resulted in the adverse effect. Transplant recipients must be cautioned against using herbal products to lower their lipid concentrations, in order to prevent such complications.

St John's wort

St John's wort induces CYP3A4 and reduces blood concentrations of CYP3A4 substrates. In one study, St John's wort reduced plasma concentrations of simvastatin but not pravastatin (85).

Troglitazone

When troglitazone was added in four men with diabetes using insulin and taking atorvastatin, serum LDL cholesterol and triglycerides increased by 23 and 21%

respectively (86). This suggests a drug interaction, but further studies are warranted to substantiate this.

References

1. Duriez P. Mécanismes d'action des statines et des fibrates. [Mechanisms of actions of statins and fibrates.] Therapie 2003;58(1):5–14.
2. Davidson KW, Reddy S, McGrath P, Zitner D, MacKeen W. Increases in depression after cholesterol-lowering drug treatment. Behav Med 1996;22(2):82–4.
3. Eckernas SA, Roos BE, Kvidal P, Eriksson LO, Block GA, Neafus RP, Haigh JR. The effects of simvastatin and pravastatin on objective and subjective measures of nocturnal sleep: a comparison of two structurally different HMG CoA reductase inhibitors in patients with primary moderate hypercholesterolaemia. Br J Clin Pharmacol 1993;35(3):284–9.
4. Boriani G, Biffi M, Strocchi E, Branzi A. Nightmares and sleep disturbances with simvastatin and metoprolol. Ann Pharmacother 2001;35(10):1292.
5. Ziajka PE, Wehmeier T. Peripheral neuropathy and lipid-lowering therapy. South Med J 1998;91(7):667–8.
6. Jeppesen U, Gaist D, Smith T, Sindrup SH. Statins and peripheral neuropathy. Eur J Clin Pharmacol 1999; 54(11):835–8.
7. Gaist D, Jeppesen U, Andersen M, Garcia Rodriguez LA, Hallas J, Sindrup SH. Statins and risk of polyneuropathy: a case-control study. Neurology 2002;58(9):1333–7.
8. Lintott CJ, Scott RS, Nye ER, Robertson MC, Sutherland WH. Simvastatin (MK 733): an effective treatment for hypercholesterolemia. Aust NZ J Med 1989;19(4):317–20.
9. Laties AM, Shear CL, Lippa EA, Gould AL, Taylor HR, Hurley DP, Stephenson WP, Keates EU, Tupy-Visich MA, Chremos AN. Expanded clinical evaluation of lovastatin (EXCEL) study results. II. Assessment of the human lens after 48 weeks of treatment with lovastatin. Am J Cardiol 1991;67(6):447–53.
10. Schmidt J, Schmitt C, Hockwin O, Paulus U, von Bergmann K. Ocular drug safety and HMG-CoA-reductase inhibitors. Ophthalmic Res 1994;26(6):352–60.
11. Farmer JA, Torre-Amione G. Comparative tolerability of the HMG-CoA reductase inhibitors. Drug Saf 2000;23(3):197–213.
12. Mikhailidis DP, Wierzbicki AS. HDL-cholesterol and the treatment of coronary heart disease: contrasting effects of atorvastatin and simvastatin. Curr Med Res Opin 2000;16(2):139–46.
13. Groneberg DA, Barkhuizen A, Jeha T. Simvastatin-induced thrombocytopenia. Am J Hematol 2001;67(4):277.
14. Tolman KG. The liver and lovastatin. Am J Cardiol 2002;89(12):1374–80.
15. Dujovne CA. Side effects of statins: hepatitis versus "transaminitis"-myositis versus "CPKitis". Am J Cardiol 2002;89(12):1411–13.
16. Black DM, Bakker-Arkema RG, Nawrocki JW. An overview of the clinical safety profile of atorvastatin (Lipitor), a new HMG-CoA reductase inhibitor. Arch Intern Med 1998;158(6):577–84.
17. Jimenez-Alonso J, Osorio JM, Gutierrez-Cabello F, Lopez de la Osa A, Leon L, Mediavilla Garcia JD. Atorvastatin-induced cholestatic hepatitis in a young woman with systemic lupus erythematosus. Grupo Lupus Virgen de las Nieves. Arch Intern Med 1999;159(15):1811–12.
18. Illingworth DR, Crouse JR 3rd, Hunninghake DB, Davidson MH, Escobar ID, Stalenhoef AF, Paragh G, Ma PT, Liu M, Melino MR, O'Grady L, Mercuri M, Mitchel YB; Simvastatin Atorvastatin HDL Study Group. A comparison of simvastatin and atorvastatin up to maximal recommended doses in a large multicenter randomized clinical trial. Curr Med Res Opin 2001;17(1):43–50.
19. Spreckelsen U, Kirchhoff R, Haacke H. Cholestatischer Iikterus Wahrend Lovastatin-Einnahme. [Cholestatic jaundice during lovastatin medication.] Dtsch Med Wochenschr 1991;116(19):739–40.
20. Ballare M, Campanini M, Catania E, Bordin G, Zaccala G, Monteverde A. Acute cholestatic hepatitis during simvastatin administration. Recenti Prog Med 1991;82(4):233–5.
21. Muggeo M, Travia D, Querena M, Zenti MG, Bagnani M, Branzi P, et al.. Long term treatment with pravastatin, simvastatin and gemfibrozil in patients with primary hypercholesterolaemia, a controlled study. Drug Invest 1992;4:376–85.
22. Assmann G, Huwel D, Schussman KM, Smilde JG, Kosling M, Withagen AJ, Wunderlich J, Stoel I, Van Dormaal JJ, Neuss J, et al.. Efficacy and safety of atorvastatin and pravastatin in patients with hypercholesterolemia Eur J Intern Med 1999;10:33–9.
23. Nakad A, Bataille L, Hamoir V, Sempoux C, Horsmans Y. Atorvastatin-induced acute hepatitis with absence of cross-toxicity with simvastatin. Lancet 1999;353(9166):1763–4.
24. Singh S, Nautiyal A, Dolan JG. Recurrent acute pancreatitis possibly induced by atorvastatin and rosuvastatin. Is statin induced pancreatitis a class effect? JOP 2004;5(6):502–4.
25. Adcock BB, Hornsby LB, Jenkins K. Dermographism: an adverse effect of atorvastatin. J Am Board Fam Pract 2001;14(2):148–51.
26. van Puijenbroek EP, Du Buf-Vereijken PW, Spooren PF, van Doormaal JJ. Possible increased risk of rhabdomyolysis during concomitant use of simvastatin and gemfibrozil. J Intern Med 1996;240(6):403–4.
27. Biesenbach G, Janko O, Stuby U, Zazgornik J. Terminales myoglobinurisches Niereneversagen unter Lovastatintherapie bei praexistenter chronischer Nierenfunktionsstorungo. [Terminal myoglobinuric renal failure in lovastatin therapy with pre-existing chronic renal insufficiency.] Wien Klin Wochenschr 1996;108(11):334–7.
28. Neuvonen PJ, Jalava KM. Itraconazole drastically increases plasma concentrations of lovastatin and lovastatin acid. Clin Pharmacol Ther 1996;60(1):54–61.
29. Phillips PS, Haas RH, Bannykh S, Hathaway S, Gray NL, Kimura BJ, Vladutiu GD, England JD; Scripps Mercy Clinical Research Center. Statin-associated myopathy with normal creatine kinase levels. Ann Intern Med 2002;137(7):581–5.
30. Giordano N, Senesi M, Mattii G, Battisti E, Villanova M, Gennari C. Polymyositis associated with simvastatin. Lancet 1997;349(9065):1600–1.
31. Laaksonen R, Ojala JP, Tikkanen MJ, Himberg JJ. Serum ubiquinone concentrations after short- and long-term treatment with HMG-CoA reductase inhibitors. Eur J Clin Pharmacol 1994;46(4):313–17.
32. Laaksonen R, Jokelainen K, Sahi T, Tikkanen MJ, Himberg JJ. Decreases in serum ubiquinone concentrations do not result in reduced levels in muscle tissue during short-term simvastatin treatment in humans. Clin Pharmacol Ther 1995;57(1):62–6.
33. Pershad A, Cardello FP. Simvastatin and rhabdomyolysis—a case report and brief review. J Pharm Technol 1999;15:88–9.
34. Al Shohaib S. Simvastatin-induced rhabdomyolysis in a patient with chronic renal failure. Am J Nephrol 2000;20(3):212–13.
35. Mantell G, Burke MT, Staggers J. Extended clinical safety profile of lovastatin. Am J Cardiol 1990;66(8):B11–15.
36. Fraunfelder FW, Fraunfelder FT, Edwards R. Diplopia and HMG-CoA reductase inhibitors. J Toxicol Cutaneous Ocul Toxicol 1999;18:287–9.
37. Parmar B, Francis PJ, Ragge NK. Statins, fibrates, and ocular myasthenia. Lancet 2002;360(9334):717.

38. Sinzinger H, Schmid P, O'Grady J. Two different types of exercise-induced muscle pain without myopathy and CK-elevation during HMG-Co-enzyme-A-reductase inhibitor treatment. Atherosclerosis 1999;143(2):459–60.
39. Insull W Jr, Isaacsohn J, Kwiterovich P, Ra P, Brazg R, Dujovne C, Shan M, Shugrue-Crowley E, Ripa S, Tota R. Efficacy and safety of cerivastatin 0.8 mg in patients with hypercholesterolaemia: the pivotal placebo-controlled clinical trial. Cerivastatin Study Group. J Int Med Res 2000;28(2):47–68.
40. Rodriguez ML, Mora C, Navarro JF. Cerivastatin-induced rhabdomyolysis. Ann Intern Med 2000;132(7):598.
41. Pogson GW, Kindred LH, Carper BG. Rhabdomyolysis and renal failure associated with cerivastatin–gemfibrozil combination therapy. Am J Cardiol 1999;83(7):1146.
42. Plosker GL, Dunn CI, Figgitt DP. Cerivastatin: a review of its pharmacological properties and therapeutic efficacy in the management of hypercholesterolaemia. Drugs 2000; 60(5):1179–206.
43. Chazerain P, Hayem G, Hamza S, Best C, Ziza JM. Four cases of tendinopathy in patients on statin therapy. Joint Bone Spine 2001;68(5):430–3.
44. Bruckert E, Giral P, Heshmati HM, Turpin G. Men treated with hypolipidaemic drugs complain more frequently of erectile dysfunction. J Clin Pharm Ther 1996;21(2):89–94.
45. Halkin A, Lossos IS, Mevorach D. HMG-CoA reductase inhibitor-induced impotence. Ann Pharmacother 1996; 30(2):192.
46. Antonov D, Kazandjieva J, Etugov D, Gospodinov D, Tsankov N. Drug-induced lupus erythematosus. Clin Dermatol 2004;22(2):157–66.
47. Cattley RC. Carcinogenicity of lipid-lowering drugs. JAMA 1996;275(19):1479.
48. Sacks FM, Pfeffer MA, Moye LA, Rouleau JL, Rutherford JD, Cole TG, Brown L, Warnica JW, Arnold JM, Wun CC, Davis BR, Braunwald E. The effect of pravastatin on coronary events after myocardial infarction in patients with average cholesterol levels. Cholesterol and Recurrent Events Trial investigators. N Engl J Med 1996;335(14):1001–9.
49. Dalen JE, Dalton WS. Does lowering cholesterol cause cancer? JAMA 1996;275(1):67–9.
50. Horsmans Y. Differential metabolism of statins: importance in drug–drug interactions. Eur Heart J Suppl 1999;1(Suppl T):T7–12.
51. Kantola T, Backman JT, Niemi M, Kivisto KT, Neuvonen PJ. Effect of fluconazole on plasma fluvastatin and pravastatin concentrations. Eur J Clin Pharmacol 2000;56(3):225–9.
52. Mazzu AL, Lasseter KC, Shamblen EC, Agarwal V, Lettieri J, Sundaresen P. Itraconazole alters the pharmacokinetics of atorvastatin to a greater extent than either cerivastatin or pravastatin. Clin Pharmacol Ther 2000;68(4):391–400.
53. Horn M. Coadministration of itraconazole with hypolipidemic agents may induce rhabdomyolysis in healthy individuals. Arch Dermatol 1996;132(10):1254.
54. Neuvonen PJ, Kantola T, Kivisto KT. Simvastatin but not pravastatin is very susceptible to interaction with the CYP3A4 inhibitor itraconazole. Clin Pharmacol Ther 1998;63(3):332–41.
55. Kantola T, Kivisto KT, Neuvonen PJ. Effect of itraconazole on the pharmacokinetics of atorvastatin. Clin Pharmacol Ther 1998;64(1):58–65.
56. Kivisto KT, Kantola T, Neuvonen PJ. Different effects of itraconazole on the pharmacokinetics of fluvastatin and lovastatin. Br J Clin Pharmacol 1998;46(1):49–53.
57. Gilad R, Lampl Y. Rhabdomyolysis induced by simvastatin and ketoconazole treatment. Clin Neuropharmacol 1999;22(5):295–7.
58. Bielecki JW, Schraner C, Briner V, Kuhn M. Rhabdomyolyse und cholestatische Hepatitis unter der Behandlung mit Simvastatin und Chlorzoxazon. [Rhabdomyolysis and cholestatic hepatitis under treatment with simvastatin and chlorzoxazone.] Schweiz Med Wochenschr 1999;129(13):514–18.
59. Stirling CM, Isles CG. Rhabdomyolysis due to simvastatin in a transplant patient: Are some statins safer than others? Nephrol Dial Transplant 2001;16(4):873–4.
60. Trilli LE, Kelley CL, Aspinall SL, Kroner BA. Potential interaction between warfarin and fluvastatin. Ann Pharmacother 1996;30(12):1399–402.
61. Kline SS, Harrell CC. Potential warfarin–fluvastatin interaction. Ann Pharmacother 1997;31(6):790.
62. Andrus MR. Oral anticoagulant drug interactions with statins: case report of fluvastatin and review of the literature. Pharmacotherapy 2004;24(2):285–90.
63. Stern R, Abel R, Gibson GL, Besserer J. Atorvastatin does not alter the anticoagulant activity of warfarin. J Clin Pharmacol 1997;37(11):1062–4.
64. Schall R, Muller FO, Hundt HK, Ritter W, Duursema L, Groenewoud G, Middle MV. No pharmacokinetic or pharmacodynamic interaction between rivastatin and warfarin. J Clin Pharmacol 1995;35(3):306–13.
65. Grau E, Perella M, Pastor E. Simvastatin–oral anticoagulant interaction. Lancet 1996;347(8998):405–6.
66. Trenque T, Choisy H, Germain ML. Pravastatin: interaction with oral anticoagulant? BMJ 1996;312(7035):886.
67. Azie NE, Brater DC, Becker PA, Jones DR, Hall SD. The interaction of diltiazem with lovastatin and pravastatin. Clin Pharmacol Ther 1998;64(4):369–77.
68. Masica AL, Azie NE, Brater DC, Hall SD, Jones DR. Intravenous diltiazem and CYP3A-mediated metabolism. Br J Clin Pharmacol 2000;50(3):273–6.
69. Goldstein MR. Myopathy and rhabdomyolysis with lovastatin taken with gemfibrozil. JAMA 1990;264(23):2991–2.
70. Kogan AD, Orenstein S. Lovastatin-induced acute rhabdomyolysis. Postgrad Med J 1990;66(774):294–6.
71. Athyros VG, Papageorgiou AA, Hatzikonstandinou HA, Didangelos TP, Carina MV, Kranitsas DF, Kontopoulos AG. Safety and efficacy of long-term statin–fibrate combinations in patients with refractory familial combined hyperlipidemia. Am J Cardiol 1997;80(5):608–13.
72. Spieker LE, Noll G, Hannak M, Luscher TF. Efficacy and tolerability of fluvastatin and bezafibrate in patients with hyperlipidemia and persistently high triglyceride levels. J Cardiovasc Pharmacol 2000;35(3):361–5.
73. Bermingham RP, Whitsitt TB, Smart ML, Nowak DP, Scalley RD. Rhabdomyolysis in a patient receiving the combination of cerivastatin and gemfibrozil. Am J Health Syst Pharm 2000;57(5):461–4.
74. Ozdemir O, Boran M, Gokce V, Uzun Y, Kocak B, Korkmaz S. A case with severe rhabdomyolysis and renal failure associated with cerivastatin–gemfibrozil combination therapy—a case report. Angiology 2000;51(8):695–7.
75. Alexandridis G, Pappas GA, Elisaf MS. Rhabdomyolysis due to combination therapy with cerivastatin and gemfibrozil. Am J Med 2000;109(3):261–2.
76. Plotkin E, Bernheim J, Ben-Chetrit S, Mor A, Korzets Z. Influenza vaccine—a possible trigger of rhabdomyolysis induced acute renal failure due to the combined use of cerivastatin and bezafibrate. Nephrol Dial Transplant 2000;15(5):740–1.
77. Backman JT, Kyrklund C, Kivisto KT, Wang JS, Neuvonen PJ. Plasma concentrations of active simvastatin acid are increased by gemfibrozil. Clin Pharmacol Ther 2000;68(2):122–9.
78. Lilja JJ, Kivisto KT, Neuvonen PJ. Grapefruit juice increases serum concentrations of atorvastatin and has no effect on pravastatin. Clin Pharmacol Ther 1999;66(2):118–27.

79. Lilja JJ, Kivisto KT, Neuvonen PJ. Duration of effect of grapefruit juice on the pharmacokinetics of the CYP3A4 substrate simvastatin. Clin Pharmacol Ther 2000;68(4):384–90.
80. Fichtenbaum CJ, Gerber JG, Rosenkranz SL, Segal Y, Aberg JA, Blaschke T, Alston B, Fang F, Kosel B, Aweeka F; NIAID AIDS Clinical Trials Group. Pharmacokinetic interactions between protease inhibitors and statins in HIV seronegative volunteers: ACTG Study A5047. AIDS 2002;16(4):569–77.
81. Spach DH, Bauwens JE, Clark CD, Burke WG. Rhabdomyolysis associated with lovastatin and erythromycin use. West J Med 1991;154(2):213–15.
82. Grunden JW, Fisher KA. Lovastatin-induced rhabdomyolysis possibly associated with clarithromycin and azithromycin. Ann Pharmacother 1997;31(7–8):859–63.
83. Jacobson RH, Wang P, Glueck CJ. Myositis and rhabdomyolysis associated with concurrent use of simvastatin and nefazodone. JAMA 1997;277(4):296–7.
84. Prasad GV, Wong T, Meliton G, Bhaloo S. Rhabdomyolysis due to red yeast rice (*Monascus purpureus*) in a renal transplant recipient. Transplantation 2002;74(8):1200–1.
85. Sugimoto K, Ohmori M, Tsuruoka S, Nishiki K, Kawaguchi A, Harada K, Arakawa M, Sakamoto K, Masada M, Miyamori I, Fujimura A. Different effects of St John's wort on the pharmacokinetics of simvastatin and pravastatin. Clin Pharmacol Ther 2001;70(6):518–24.
86. DiTusa L, Luzier AB. Potential interaction between troglitazone and atorvastatin. J Clin Pharm Ther 2000;25(4):279–82.

Hormonal contraceptives—emergency contraception

See also Estrogens

General Information

For a complete account of the adverse effects of estrogens, readers should consult the following monographs as well as this one:

- Diethylstilbestrol
- Estrogens
- Hormonal contraceptives—oral
- Hormone replacement therapy—estrogens
- Hormone replacement therapy—estrogens + androgens
- Hormone replacement therapy—estrogens + progestogens

A review of the English language literature has shown that in the USA, the source of most of the evidence, the two most commonly used forms of emergency contraception are the Yuzpe regimen (high-dose ethinylestradiol + high-dose levonorgestrel) and "Plan B" (high-dose levonorgestrel alone) (1). Although both methods sometimes stop ovulation, they may also act by reducing the probability of implantation, through an effect on the endometrium (the "post-fertilization effect"). The available evidence for the latter mechanism is moderately strong. If this is the manner in which development of a zygote is prevented one would anticipate a certain proportion of failures, with the possibility of second-generation injury. This finding also has potential implications in such areas as informed consent, emergency department protocols, and conscience clauses, since it is more in the character of abortion than true contraception, making the term "emergency contraception" or "post-coital contraception" a slight misnomer.

Estrogens

Various estrogens and estrogen + progestogen combinations have been used in post-coital contraception. Courses of high-dose oral diethylstilbestrol, ethinylestradiol, conjugated estrogens, or combinations of estrogen and progestogen for 4–6 days are all effective. Estrogens are postovulatory rather than postcoital contraceptives, and so it is necessary to know the exact time of unprotected intercourse in relation to a woman's menstrual cycle (2). Depending on the frequency and timing of intercourse, a 5-day course of post-coital estrogen, introduced within 72 hours, gives a pregnancy rate of 0.03–0.3%.

Diethylstilbestrol has been widely used as a post-coital contraceptive. However, it is no longer in use in many countries for this purpose, because of the possible adverse effect on the development of a surviving fetus (see separate monograph).

Ethinylestradiol has been used in the past as a postcoital contraceptive, with a daily dose of 5 mg/day for 5 days. This method has a high incidence of adverse reactions, nausea, vomiting, and breast tenderness being the most frequent (3); the first menstrual cycle after treatment is likely to be abnormal.

Progestogens

Clinical trials of desogestrel implants showed that they were effective, but with bleeding irregularities and ovarian cysts as the primary adverse effects (4).

The "morning after" method of suppressing pregnancy is usually less well tolerated than normal hormonal contraception, and variants on the dosage schedule continue to be studied in an attempt to improve tolerability without undermining the reliability of the method.

Two regimens for emergency contraception started within 72 hours of unprotected coitus have been studied: (a) the progestogen levonorgestrel in two separate doses each of 0.75 mg; (b) the Yuzpe regimen of combined oral contraceptives—ethinylestradiol 100 micrograms + levonorgestrel 0.5 mg repeated 12 hours later (5). The relative risk of pregnancy for levonorgestrel compared with the Yuzpe regimen was 0.36 (95% C1 = 0.18, 0.70). Nausea and vomiting were significantly less frequent with the levonorgestrel regimen. Adverse effects of both regimens were nausea, vomiting, dizziness, fatigue, headache, breast tenderness, and low abdominal pain. However, all of these adverse effects were less frequent with levonorgestrel.

Estrogen + progestogen combinations

In recent years it has become common to use a combination of estrogen and progestogen for post-coital contraception. For example, a tablet containing ethinylestradiol 100 micrograms and levonorgestrel

0.5 mg (or norgestrel 1 mg) taken twice with an interval of 12 hours has been used (6). This treatment must begin within 72 hours of unprotected intercourse. The approach seems to be as effective as ethinylestradiol alone, while producing somewhat less nausea and vomiting (7). Apart from this the adverse effects most commonly experienced are as with estrogen alone. Overall failure rates are about 2–3%, with perhaps twice this failure rate when taken at mid-cycle. However, bearing in mind the rate of pregnancy after unprotected intercourse, the protective effect is not impressive; the chance of pregnancy is probably only halved.

It is probably impossible to define an ideal dose for this purpose. Essentially the aim is to provide a sufficient hormonal jolt to derange nidation and the development of the zygote, and this might be attained in various ways; the most acceptable dosage schemes will be those that are best tolerated. Because oral contraceptives are generally more readily available than specially formulated products, they have sometimes been used for this purpose in deliberate overdose. Even low-dose oral contraceptives, if taken in sufficient quantities, will prove effective post-coital contraception (8); progestogen-only tablets are also effective in a single dose, for example levonorgestrel 0.6 mg taken within 12 hours, but irregular bleeding, nausea, and dizziness are common adverse effects (SEDA-16, 466).

The FDA has approved a marketing application for the Prevent Emergency Contraceptive Kit (Gynetics), which contains tablets for post-coital emergency contraception, packaged with a urinary pregnancy test. The application is based on a regimen that consists of two tablets containing ethinylestradiol and levonorgestrel to be taken within 72 hours of unprotected intercourse and two tablets to be taken 12 hours later. This regimen is about 75% effective in preventing pregnancy. The most common adverse effects are nausea, vomiting, menstrual irregularities, breast tenderness, headache, abdominal pain and cramps, and dizziness (9).

Androgens

The synthetic androgen danazol has also been evaluated for post-coital use, but with inconsistent results (8); doses of twice 400 mg or twice 600 mg seem to be reliable while a single dose of 600 mg seems to be insufficient. A 10% incidence of vomiting, headache, and breast tenderness has been reported and a lower incidence (1–2%) of vomiting (10).

Antiprogesterones

The antiprogesterone mifepristone, almost exclusively used as an abortifacient, has also been tried as a post-coital contraceptive (11). In one randomized comparative trial, a single dose of mifepristone 600 mg was at least as effective as the usual hormonal method (12). Women who took mifepristone had lower rates of adverse effects, particularly nausea and vomiting, but their next menstrual period was more likely to be delayed. In another randomized trial, both methods were equally effective (SEDA-16, 466). The use of an estrogen + a progestogen had a higher total incidence of adverse effects, but mifepristone was associated with the greatest cycle disruption. If mifepristone was given in the follicular phase, 52% of women had a delay of 4 days or more in the onset of their next menstrual period (indicating that ovulation had been inhibited); when it was given in the luteal phase, 84% of women menstruated on time.

Physical methods

A non-hormonal approach to emergency contraception is insertion of an intrauterine contraceptive device up to 7 days after ovulation in a cycle during which unprotected intercourse has occurred (13).

Comparison of methods

The combined estradiol + levonorgestrel (Yuzpe regimen), the levonorgestrel-only regimen, and post-coital copper intrauterine devices have been compared by the Clinical Practice Gynaecology and Social and Sexual Issues Committees of the Society of Obstetricians and Gynaecologists of Canada. Sponsor: The Society of Obstetricians and Gynaecologists of Canada (13) and the following recommendations made:

1. Women who have had unprotected intercourse and want to prevent pregnancy should be offered hormonal emergency contraception up to 5 days after intercourse.
2. A copper IUCD can be used up to 7 days after intercourse in women who have no contraindications.
3. Women should be advised that the levonorgestrel regimen is more effective and causes fewer adverse effects than the Yuzpe regimen.
4. Either one double dose of the levonorgestrel regimen (1.5 mg) or the regular two-dose levonorgestrel regimen (0.75 mg each dose) can be used, as they have similar efficacy with no difference in adverse effects.
5. Hormonal emergency contraception should be started as soon as possible after unprotected sexual intercourse.
6. Women of reproductive age should be provided with a prescription for hormonal emergency contraception in advance of need.
7. The woman should be evaluated for pregnancy if menses have not begun within 21 days after emergency contraception.
8. A pelvic examination is not indicated for the provision of hormonal emergency contraception.

Second-Generation Effects

Pregnancy

In pregnancies that occur after failure of progestogen-only emergency oral contraception, the possibility of ectopic pregnancy should be considered, according to a Prescriber Update article recently posted on the New Zealand Medsafe website (14). This may occur by the same mechanism by which pregnancies in women using daily progestogen-only oral contraceptives are more likely to be ectopic than pregnancies in users of other contraceptive methods. The Centre for

Adverse Reaction Monitoring has received three reports of ectopic pregnancies after the use of progestogen-only emergency oral contraceptives, and prescribers are reminded to advise women about the possibility of ectopic pregnancy after failure of progestogen-only emergency oral contraceptives. Women should seek prompt medical attention if, after using a progestogen-only emergency oral contraceptive, amenorrhea or any other symptoms suggestive of pregnancy occur.

Susceptibility Factors

Post-coital contraception should not be used when there are absolute contraindications to estrogen; these include pregnancy, unstable angina, transient ischemic attacks, liver disease, undiagnosed genital bleeding, or a history of thromboembolism. Some absolute contraindications to long-term use, such as breast cancer and arterial disease, are not contraindications to short-term use (15).

References

1. Kahlenborn C, Stanford JB, Larimore WL. Postfertilization effect of hormonal emergency contraception. Ann Pharmacother 2002;36(3):465–70.
2. Notelovitz M. Estrogens and postcoital contraception. Female Patient 1981;6(7):36–8.
3. Haspels AA, Van Santen MR. Post coital contraception. J Gynaecol Endocrinol 1986;2(1–2):17–24.
4. Diaz S, Pavez M, Moo-Young AJ, Bardin CW, Croxatto HB. Clinical trial with 3-keto-desogestrel subdermal implants. Contraception 1991;44(4):393–408.
5. Grimes D, Von Hertzen H, Piaggio G, Van Look PFA. Randomised controlled trial of levonorgestrel versus the Yuzpe regimen of combined oral contraceptives for emergency contraception. Task Force on Postovulatory Methods of Fertility Regulation. Lancet 1998;352(9126):428–33.
6. Anonymous. Norsk Legemiddelhaåndbok 1998, 1999 for Helsepersonell. Oslo: Norsk Legemiddelhaåndbok, 1998.
7. Haspels AA, Van Santen MR. Postcoital contraception. Pediatr Adolesc Gynecol 1984;2:63.
8. Trussell J, Stewart F, Guest F, Hatcher RA. Emergency contraceptive pills: a simple proposal to reduce unintended pregnancies. Fam Plann Perspect 1992;24(6):269–73.
9. Anonymous. Oral contraceptives—approved for emergency use. WHO Newslett 1998;9/10:12.
10. Anzen B, Zetterstrom J. Post-coital Contraception. Workshop on Contraceptive Methods. Uppsala: Swedish Medical Products Agency, 1994:2.
11. Glasier A, Thong KJ, Dewar M, Mackie M, Baird DT. Postcoital contraception with mifepristone. Lancet 1991;337(8754):1414–15.
12. Glasier A, Thong KJ, Dewar M, Mackie M, Baird DT. Mifepristone (RU 486) compared with high-dose estrogen and progestogen for emergency postcoital contraception. N Engl J Med 1992;327(15):1041–4.
13. Dunn S, Guilbert E, Lefebvre G, Allaire C, Arneja J, Birch C, Fortier M, Jeffrey J, Vilos G, Wagner MS, Grant L, Beaudoin F, Cherniak D, Pellizzari R, Sadownik L, Saraf-Dhar R, Turnbull V; Clinical Practice Gynaecology and Social Sexual Issues Committees, Society of Obstetricians and Gynaecologists of Canada (SOGC). Emergency contraception. J Obstet Gynaecol Can 2003;25(8):673–87.
14. Anonymous. Oral contraceptives. Ectopic pregnancy following emergency oral contraceptive failure. WHO Pharmaceuticals Newslett 2002;4:10.
15. Reader FC. Emergency contraception. BMJ 1991;302(6780):801.

Hormonal contraceptives—intracervical and intravaginal

See also Progestogens

General Information

The intracervical and intravaginal methods of contraception have not come into regular use, and experience with them has therefore been limited.

For a complete account of the adverse effects of progestogens, readers should consult the following monographs as well as this one:

- Hormonal contraceptives—progestogen implants
- Hormonal contraceptives—progestogen injections
- Hormonal contraceptives—oral
- Hormone replacement therapy—estrogens + progestogens
- Medroxyprogesterone
- Progestogens.

Intracervical contraceptives

When an intracervical device releasing levonorgestrel 20 mg/day was studied in 198 women over 2 years of use, a total of seven pregnancies occurred (1). All began during the first year and six occurred after the unnoticed expulsion of the device. One pregnancy occurred in an epileptic woman taking carbamazepine, while the intracervical device remained in place. In three cases the device was removed because of infection, in all three instances during the first year of use; in one case *Neisseria gonorrhoeae* was found and in another *Chlamydia trachomatis*. During the study, mean body weight increased, but remarkably there was a statistically significant reduction in the mean diastolic and systolic blood pressures after 1 and 2 years of use compared with the pre-insertion values.

Intravaginal contraceptives

As early as 1978, the vaginal administration of steroids for contraceptive purposes was attempted, at that time using vaginal rings containing medroxyprogesterone acetate or both norgestrel and estradiol. It was later found that complete inhibition of ovulation could as a rule be attained by the daily intravaginal application of a product containing norethisterone 1 mg and mestranol 50 micrograms (2).

Progestogen-only vaginal rings

Vaginal administration of steroid-containing polymer rings has been studied for at least 25 years as a means of contraception, without gaining wide acceptance. In a large multicenter WHO trial with a levonorgestrel ring, releasing 20 micrograms/day, the 1-year pregnancy rate was 4.5% (3). The main reason for discontinuation was menstrual disturbances (17%), followed by frequent expulsion of the ring and vaginal symptoms.

The finding of erythematous lesions in the vagina in some women has led to the development of a more flexible device. The Population Council has also developed a vaginal ring containing Nestorone progestin (16-methylene-17α-acetoxy-19-norpregn-4-ene-3,20-dione) for 6 months of continuous use (4). Ovulation inhibition was achieved in over 97% of the segments studied, with rings releasing 50, 75, or 100 micrograms/day. No pregnancies occurred in women who used the low-dose ring, while one pregnancy each occurred with the intermediate-dose and high-dose rings, for 6-month cumulative pregnancy rates of 0.0, 1.9, and 2.1% respectively; it is not clear why the reported pregnancy rates were higher with the higher doses. However, bleeding irregularities were common, and this form of contraception still demands further development work.

A low-dose levonorgestrel vaginal ring has also been studied. Women using vaginal rings releasing levonorgestrel 20 mg/day had more bleeding or spotting days than women using other hormonal contraceptives, with menstrual patterns similar to those of progestogen-only tablet users (5). Irregular and infrequent bleeding was also recorded by some women. Analysis of menstrual calendar data from WHO phase III clinical trials showed that the percentage of women who experience bleeding patterns defined as "acceptable" increases steadily from 39% in the first 3 months to 56% during months 10–12 (6). Frequent and irregular bleeding were the most common problems. In another study in 108 women there were four pregnancies during 1 year of investigation, with a discontinuation rate of 71%. Menstrual disturbances were the main adverse effects and also the most common reason for discontinuation, occurring in 45% of cycles during the first month (7).

References

1. Ratsula K. Clinical performance of a levonorgestrel-releasing intracervical contraceptive device during the first two years of use. Contraception 1989;39(2):187–93.
2. Coutinho EM, Silva AR, Carreira C, Barbosa I. Ovulation inhibition following vaginal administration of pills containing norethindrone and mestranol. Contraception 1984;29(2):197–202.
3. Brache V, Alvarez-Sanchez F, Faundes A, Jackanicz T, Mishell DR Jr, Lahteenmaki P. Progestin-only contraceptive rings. Steroids 2000;65(10–11):687–91.
4. British National Formulary. 2001;September:624.
5. Belsey EM. Vaginal bleeding patterns among women using one natural and eight hormonal methods of contraception. Contraception 1988;38(2):181–206.
6. Fraser IS. Vaginal bleeding patterns in women using once-a-month injectable contraceptives. Contraception 1994;49(4):399–420.
7. Gao J, Sun HZ, Song GY, Ma LY. Clinical investigation of a low-dose levonorgestrel-releasing vaginal ring. Fertil Steril 1986;46(4):626–30.

Hormonal contraceptives—male

General Information

The notion that an oral contraceptive closely similar to that used in women might be developed for men has been discussed for about 45 years, but the concept has not yet found wide acceptance. Delays in putting the concept into practice have related variously to difficulties in finding an effective combination, complaints of reduced libido or potency, and the long delay between the start of treatment and the attainment of azoospermia.

Of the many possible formulations tested all have proved to have unacceptable facets, generally including a very slow onset of action, uncertain reliability, and undesirable effects on biochemistry, body weight, or sexual function. However, some progress has been made with the combination of oral desogestrel and intramuscular testosterone.

In a study of the effects of various combinations of desogestrel and testosterone, including a sequential pattern, the optimal dosage to induce azoospermia seemed to be desogestrel 300 micrograms/day by mouth and testosterone enantate 50 mg weekly by intramuscular injection (1). Among 24 subjects, there were no withdrawals clearly related to the treatment. During weeks 1–3, adverse effects were reduced sex drive ($n = 4$), tiredness ($n = 1$), and a sensation of depression ($n = 1$); during weeks 4–24 they included mild acne ($n = 10$), increased sexual interest ($n = 3$), emotional lability ($n = 2$), tiredness ($n = 2$), night sweats ($n = 1$), and headache ($n = 1$). However, laboratory studies showed that desogestrel had clear effects on lipid metabolism in dosages of 150 micrograms/day or more, with reductions in HDL cholesterol, apolipoprotein, A1 lipoprotein, sex hormone binding globulin, and to some extent total cholesterol and LDL cholesterol. If this approach can be developed to provide a more convenient dosage scheme, these biochemical changes will be among those that need to be followed carefully.

A combination of oral desogestrel 150 or 300 micrograms + intramuscular testosterone 50 or 100 mg has been tested in 24 young men and compared with historical data from studies on a combination of oral levonorgestrel + intramuscular testosterone (2). All the doses tested achieved azoospermia. All the groups tended to gain weight compared with their baseline, but the weight gain was greatest (and statistically significant) in men who received the higher dose of testosterone. Adverse effects were acceptably low; acne occurred in occasional cases, but no one developed gynecomastia.

In a similar study limited to 8 weeks, the various formulations rapidly suppressed LH and FSH to a similar extent, irrespective of dosage, while testosterone concentrations fell slightly during treatment, with evidence of a linear dose-response relation (3). There were minor changes in plasma concentrations of inhibin B, but in seminal fluid it was suppressed, becoming undetectable in all the men who took desogestrel 300 micrograms/day. There were no significant changes in lipoproteins, fibrinogen, or sexual behavior during treatment, and only minor falls in hematocrit and hemoglobin concentration.

References

1. Wu FC, Balasubramanian R, Mulders TM, Coelingh-Bennink HJ. Oral progestogen combined with testosterone as a potential male contraceptive: additive effects between desogestrel and testosterone enanthate in suppression of spermatogenesis, pituitary-testicular axis, and lipid metabolism. J Clin Endocrinol Metab 1999;84(1):112–22.
2. Anawalt BD, Herbst KL, Matsumoto AM, Mulders TM, Coelingh-Bennink HJ, Bremner WJ. Desogestrel plus testosterone effectively suppresses spermatogenesis but also causes modest weight gain and high-density lipoprotein suppression. Fertil Steril 2000;74(4):707–14.
3. Martin CW, Riley SC, Everington D, Groome NP, Riemersma RA, Baird DT, Anderson RA. Dose-finding study of oral desogestrel with testosterone pellets for suppression of the pituitary-testicular axis in normal men. Hum Reprod 2000;15(7):1515–24.

Hormonal contraceptives—oral

General Information

For a complete account of the adverse effects of estrogens, readers should consult the following monographs as well as this one:

- Diethylstilbestrol
- Estrogens
- Hormonal contraceptives—emergency contraception
- Hormone replacement therapy—estrogens
- Hormone replacement therapy—estrogens + androgens
- Hormone replacement therapy—estrogens + progestogens.

For a complete account of the adverse effects of progestogens, readers should consult the following monographs as well as this one:

- Hormonal contraceptives—implants
- Hormonal contraceptives—progestogen injections
- Hormonal contraceptives—intracervical and intravaginal
- Hormone replacement therapy—estrogens + progestogens
- Medroxyprogesterone
- Progestogens.

Hormonal contraception relies on the actions of estrogens and progestogens, of which oral contraceptives contain a mixture. The adverse effects of the separate components are discussed in other monographs.

The commonly available combinations of oral contraceptives include (estrogen first):

- ethinylestradiol + desogestrel
- ethinylestradiol + levonorgestrel
- ethinylestradiol + norethisterone
- ethinylestradiol + norgestimate
- mestranol + norethisterone.

Other forms of administration include:

- implantation
- intracervical administration
- intramuscular injection
- intravaginal administration
- transdermal administration.

These forms of contraception are covered in other monographs.

Efficacy

Hormonal contraceptives based on combinations of estrogen + progestogen, administered cyclically each month, are among the most effective forms of contraception. During typical use, only some 3% of women using combined oral contraceptives become pregnant in the first year of use, despite the failures of compliance that inevitably occur (1). The pregnancy rate for progestogen-only oral contraceptives is somewhat higher, about 5% (2). Compared with the original high-dose combination products, the lower dosages now in current use offer a smaller margin for error if tablets are missed; the efficacy of progestogen-only contraceptives is even more dependent on correct use. The accidental pregnancy rates for injectable and implanted hormonal contraceptives are lower than for the oral products, primarily because they do not depend on the daily taking of a tablet. The 1-year pregnancy rate for depot medroxyprogesterone acetate (injectable) is 0.3% and for levonorgestrel implants 0.09%.

Mechanisms of action

Estrogen and progestogen together inhibit gonadotropin secretion and thus prevent ovulation. Estrogen also stabilizes the endometrium and potentiates the action of the progestogen. In addition, the progestogen has contraceptive effects on the cervical mucus (thickening the mucus to make it hostile to sperm penetration), the endometrium (interfering with implantation), and the fallopian tubes (altering ovum transport). The original fixed-dose combinations have given way to formulations that contain lower doses, as well as to variants on the principle. The estrogen dosage, originally 150 micrograms or more, today normally lies in the range of 30–35 micrograms ethinylestradiol; even lower doses have been investigated, but these result in an unsatisfactory bleeding pattern and have little effect on ovulation. Doses of progestogens have fallen from the 5 mg (or even 10 mg) originally in use in 1960 to 1 mg or less today. To calculate the dose of progestogen that offers the highest benefit-to-harm balance is not easy, particularly since the relative potency of any progestogen can be expressed in various ways (for example in terms of its effect on the human endometrium, its androgenic or corticosteroid potency, or its ability to inhibit ovulation); these do not run parallel to one another and it is not at all clear which of these activities are relevant to the various long-term safety issues.

Progestogen-only products do not have inhibition of ovulation as their main effect; up to half of all cycles are ovulatory, and the contraceptive potential relates largely to changes in the consistency of the cervical mucus and the creation of a hostile environment for the sperm, as well as changes in tubal motility and ovum transport; after a period of treatment, endometrial atrophy occurs, rendering nidation unlikely.

Unusual combinations

Ethinylestradiol + chlormadinone acetate

In 19 650 women who had received six cycles of treatment with chlormadinone acetate 2 mg and ethinylestradiol 30 micrograms, cycle control was good, with beneficial reductions in intracyclic bleeding, severe withdrawal bleeding, dysmenorrhea, and amenorrhea (3). At baseline, 70% of the women had androgen-related skin disorders. After six cycles of chlormadinone acetate 2 mg + ethinylestradiol 30 micrograms, these disorders were improved in 87% of patients, including 29% who had complete resolution. The incidence of greasy or very greasy hair fell from 47 to 17%. There were two cases of venous thromboembolism. Breast pain (3.6%) and migraine or headache (2.6%) were the most frequently reported adverse events, but these symptoms disappeared in most women (85 and 80%) who had had them before treatment.

Ethinylestradiol + drospirenone

The effects of a monophasic oral contraceptive containing drospirenone 3 mg and ethinylestradiol 30 micrograms on pre-existing premenstrual symptoms has been studied in 326 women during 13 menstrual cycles (4). There were beneficial effects on water retention and appetite. Concentration was not significantly affected, and assessments of undesired hair changes and feelings of well-being did not change appreciably. There were no adverse effects of note.

Cyproterone acetate + a progestogen

There has been a single report of autoimmune hepatitis with the combination of cyproterone acetate and a progestogen (5). Similar events have been described very occasionally with other oral contraceptives and with diethylstilbestrol; they are not unique to cyproterone.

General adverse effects

The incidence of common adverse reactions to oral contraceptives varies with population and product. Many users have some mild reactions during the initial months of treatment, which disappear entirely as use continues; a small proportion of users withdraw at an early phase, because of individual intolerance, and turn to other methods of contraception. Relatively common adverse effects of combined oral contraceptives include intermenstrual bleeding, nausea or vomiting, breast tenderness, and headaches, although reactions are highly individual and problems can often be overcome by changing to a formulation with a greater or lesser content of active substances. Some women develop mild fever. Occasionally, oral contraceptive users report depression (or more usually a vague sensation of malaise), reduced libido, acne, or weight gain. Women taking combined oral contraceptives are also at greater risk of *Chlamydia* infection and of modest impairments of glucose and lipid metabolism. The most serious complications attributable to oral contraceptives are cardiovascular diseases, but these are extremely rare and are even less common now, with lower-dose formulations, than in earlier decades; these much discussed risks are reviewed separately above. Hypersensitivity reactions have been observed, but only very rarely.

Tumor-inducing effects are discussed in the monograph on estrogens. The risks of epithelial ovarian and endometrial cancer are reduced by combined oral contraceptives. Effects on other cancers are slight.

Overall benefit-to-harm balance of combined oral contraceptives

A comprehensive analysis by The Alan Guttmacher Institute in the USA in 1991 evaluated the health risks of various contraceptive methods, as well as the health risks of a normal female reproductive life without contraceptives (6). Because combined oral contraceptives are highly effective, they prevent pregnancy-related deaths, particularly those associated with ectopic pregnancy. This factor more than offsets the small increased risk of cardiovascular disease related to current use, resulting in averted deaths at all ages (ranging from 3.9 per 100 000 current users at ages 15–19 up to 19 per 100 000 at ages 40–44 in the USA). They also prevent future deaths from ovarian and endometrial cancers (from 23 per 100 000 at ages 15–19 to 10 per 100 000 at ages 40–44). Current oral contraceptive use also prevents 1614 hospitalizations per 100 000 users annually. Most of these avoided hospital admissions are because of prevention of the complications of pregnancy, but they also include a reduced rate of hospitalization due to ovarian cysts, benign breast disease, upper genital tract infection, urinary tract infection, and invasive cancers of the ovary and endometrium. The conditions for which hospitalization rates may be slightly increased among combined oral contraceptive users include: myocardial infarction; stroke; venous thrombosis and embolism; invasive cancers of the breast, cervix, and liver; cervical intraepithelial neoplasia; and gallbladder disease.

Data from the classic Nurses' Health Study, followed up in 1994, reflected no difference in all-cause mortality between women who had ever used oral contraceptives and those who had never used them (7). There was also no increase in mortality associated with duration of use and no relation with time since first use or time since last use. Similarly, in the OFPA (Oxford) study, the overall 20-year mortality risk for oral contraceptive users compared with women using diaphragms or IUCDs was 0.9, suggesting no effect (8). Although the number of deaths from each cause was small, the pattern is consistent with the risks found in other studies. Oral contraceptive users had somewhat higher death rates from ischemic heart disease and cervical cancer, but lower rates of ovarian cancer mortality. Breast cancer mortality was similar for oral contraceptive users and non-users.

In developing countries, wherever there is a high maternal mortality rate, the risk of oral contraception is low in comparison (9). For all women in developing countries below the age of 40, oral contraceptive use is substantially safer than no method at all or traditional methods, about as safe as IUCDs, but not as safe as sterilization or as traditional methods backed by legal abortion performed by trained physicians.

Some of the risks have only become evaluable with much longer experience, for example those relating to the development of malignancies (covered in the monograph on estrogens). Data on these matters, too, seem reassuring; any cancer-promoting effect in one direction is at least counterbalanced by the reduction of risk in another.

Any consideration of major issues relating to the balance of benefit and harm, such as cancer or mortality rates, should be supplemented by a consideration of less prominent ones, for example, a reduction in disorders of the menstrual cycle (such as dysmenorrhea, menorrhagia, and the premenstrual syndrome) and the reduced risks of iron deficiency anemia, functional ovarian cysts, uterine fibroids, benign breast disease, pelvic inflammatory disease, and ectopic pregnancy (10,11).

Finally, since much of the work relates to high-dose products, it is important to stress that more recent work and reviews have confirmed the even greater relative safety of lower-dose products, although one must now express concern that the third-generation products may have increased certain risks once more. All the same, the broad picture of the safety of oral contraception is reassuring. Even at an earlier stage, such authoritative workers as Vessey and Doll (12) emphasized that the medical and social benefits of using oral contraceptives considerably outweighed the risks, while emphasizing the need to contain such risks as there are, that is by careful patient selection and supervision and by the use of oral contraceptives with the lowest possible dosages.

Progestogen-only oral contraceptives

Progestogen-only oral contraceptives are taken continuously and not cyclically. They not only lack the estrogen component of combined oral contraceptives but also have a lower dose of progestogen than even the current low-dose combined oral contraceptives. Progestogen-only contraceptives are therefore indicated for women who desire oral contraception but who have contraindications to or poor experience with the estrogen in combined oral contraceptives, who are breastfeeding, who are older (especially smokers), or who simply wish to keep their exogenous hormone doses to a minimum (11). The drawbacks of progestogen-only contraceptives are that menstrual irregularity is common and that careful compliance is necessary in order to achieve high efficacy.

The pharmacokinetics of progestogens in progestogen-only contraceptives are somewhat different from those in combined oral contraceptives, because of the interaction of estrogen and progestogen in the combination products. One of the major differences is that, as noted above, the plasma concentrations of progestogen rise over time in users of combined oral contraceptives; this does not happen in women taking progestogen-only contraceptives. The change is due in part to estrogen stimulation of serum hormone-binding globulin (SHBG) production, increased binding of progestogen to SHBG, and reduced progestogen clearance with combined oral contraceptives. In contrast, progestogen-only contraceptives cause reduced SHBG concentrations and modest falls in progestogen concentrations over time.

Organs and Systems

Cardiovascular

The cardiovascular complications of oral contraceptives include venous thrombosis and thromboembolism, arterial damage, and hypertension.

Venous thromboembolism

A central issue almost from the beginning of the oral contraceptive era has been the undoubted ability of these products to increase the risk of thromboembolic and allied complications. It was the dominant reason for the progressive reduction in hormonal content of these products during their first 20 years; it led at one point to a precipitate and poorly motivated replacement of mestranol by ethinylestradiol as the estrogenic component; and rightly or wrongly it has played a central role in the recent debate concerning modified products based on newer progestogens.

History

The fact that some women could develop thromboembolic complications as a result of taking oral contraceptives first emerged in 1961, although at that time the evidence was anecdotal and poorly quantified. The first reasonably quantified investigation conducted on a sufficient scale to merit conclusions was published in 1967 by the UK Medical Research Council (13). This and other large studies conducted during the early years (and considered in older volumes in this series) concluded that women using oral contraceptives ran a greater risk than non-users of developing deep venous thrombosis, pulmonary embolism, cerebral thrombosis, myocardial infarction, and retinal thrombosis. Later papers and case reports described deep venous thrombosis, portal venous thrombosis, and pulmonary embolism (14–16). The Boston Collaborative Drug Surveillance Program follow-up study of more than 65 000 healthy women in 1980–82 found a positive association between current oral contraceptive use and venous thromboembolism (rate ratio 2.8); there was also a positive association between current oral contraceptive use and stroke or myocardial infarction (17). A UK study using data from 1978, by which time lower-dose products were increasing in use, pointed to an approximate doubling of the risk of thromboembolism compared with controls (SEDA-7, 387). The early 1980s were nevertheless marked by a series of critical papers that sought to question the entire concept of there being a link.

Much of the work on both sides of the argument was less than watertight. Some studies failed to consider the confounding effects of other risk factors (notably smoking) or the likelihood of detection bias (particularly for venous thromboembolism, which is much more common in young women than myocardial infarction or stroke). The results of some studies were also confounded by uncertainties in the history of drug exposure. A landmark paper to resolve the issue concluded that the link with venous thromboembolism in subjects without predisposition had been consistently observed in case-control and cohort studies (18). However, the evidence regarding myocardial infarction, various types of stroke, and cardiovascular mortality was less consistent. By 1990, an international Consensus Development Meeting reached agreement on the following statement regarding the relation between oral contraceptive use and cardiovascular disease (19):

> The majority of epidemiological studies strongly suggest an association between current oral contraceptive use and certain cardiovascular deaths. Although the relative risk is increased, the absolute risk is small. Because the risk of myocardial infarction is apparent in current users, disappears on cessation of use, and is not associated with duration of use, there is no epidemiologic support for the hypothesis that risk of cardiovascular diseases is of atherogenic origin .... Whether particular formulations or progestogens have qualitative advantages or disadvantages merits further study. Estrogens and progestogens interact at many levels, and in epidemiologic studies of users of combined oral contraceptives it is difficult to assign a risk to either component separately. Moreover, it is physiologically unsound to do so .... Alterations in plasma lipid, carbohydrate, and hemostasis variables are of major importance for the development of cardiovascular diseases, and their concentrations can be influenced by sex steroids, including artificial steroids contained in oral contraceptives. The pharmacodynamic responses ... are dependent on not only the type and dosage of sex steroids, but also on intra- and interindividual variability in pharmacokinetics.

Frequency

It has been confirmed that the incidence and mortality rates of thrombotic diseases among young women are low (20). However, the risk is increased by oral contraceptives and there is variation in the degree of risk, depending on the accompanying progestogen. The spontaneous incidence of venous thromboembolism in healthy non-pregnant women (not taking any oral contraceptive) is about five cases per 100 000 women per year of use. The incidence in users of third-generation formulations is about 15 per 100 000 women per year. The incidence in users of third-generation formulations is about 25 per 100 000 women per year: this excess incidence has not been satisfactorily explained by bias or confounding. The risks of venous thromboembolism increase with age and is likely to be increased in women with other known factors for venous thromboembolism, such as obesity. The risk in pregnancy has been estimated at 60 cases per 100 000 pregnancies.

The Medicines Commission of the UK has reviewed all currently available relevant data and has confirmed that the incidence of venous thromboembolism is about 25 per 100 000 women per year of use (21). The incidence of venous thrombembolism in users of second-generation combined oral contraceptives is about 15 per 100 000 women per year of use. This indicates a small excess risk of about 100 000 women-years for women using third-generation combined oral contraceptives containing desogestrel or gestodene, which has not been satisfactorily explained by bias or confounding. However, the absolute risk of venous thromboembolism in women taking combined oral contraceptives containing desogestrel or gestodene is very small and is much less than the risk of venous thromboembolism in pregnancy.

The incidence of venous thromboembolic disease in about 540 000 women born between 1941 and 1981 and taking oral contraceptives was 4.1–4.2 cases per 10 000 woman-years (22).

In another study, the figures ranged from 1895 events per 100 000 women-years when norgestimate was used to 3969 per 100 000 women-years when desogestrel was used (23). Although the authors did not find the difference statistically significant, it runs parallel to findings from other work regarding a higher risk when third-generation progestogens are used.

In women aged 15–29 years who used oral contraceptives containing third-generation progestogens, venous thromboembolism was twice as common as arterial complications. In women aged 30–44 years of age the number of arterial complications exceeded the number of venous complications by about 50%. However, in women under 30 years, deaths from arterial complications were 3.5 times more common than deaths from venous complications and in women aged 30–44 years 8.5 times more common. Women over 30 years of age who take oral contraceptives containing third-generation progestogens may have a lower risk of thrombotic morbidity, disability, and mortality than users of second-generation progestogens. However, a weighted analysis such as this does not result in any consistent recommendation of a particular progestogen type.

Nevertheless, some groups continue to produce data from their own systems that fail to confirm this. Some of these studies, including unpublished data circulated to experts for purposes of special pleading, have used selected material, and one can only consider them flawed. On the other hand, Jick et al. may be entirely right in their finding that, insofar as the special risk of idiopathic cerebral hemorrhage is concerned, no material difference in risk has been demonstrated between products of the second generation and those of the third generation (24).

And in another study it was found that users of oral contraceptives with second-generation progestogens have 30% greater increased risk of thrombotic diseases, a 260% greater increased risk of thrombotic deaths, and a 220% greater increased risk of post-thrombotic disability than users of oral contraceptives with third-generation progestogens (20).

Effects of dosage and formulation

As noted above, the early recognition of thromboembolic complications had repercussions for the formulation of the oral contraceptives; the progestogen and estrogen contents were both progressively reduced, and in 1969/70 mestranol was replaced by ethinylestradiol, on the grounds that the dose could thereby be halved (although it is not at all certain that this reduced the estrogenic contribution to thromboembolic events). By the late 1980s, when a major cohort study based in Oxford examined the problem (8), products containing estrogen 50 micrograms accounted for about 70% of the woman-years of tablet use, most of the remainder being accounted for by lower doses.

By the mid-1990s it was reasonably well proven that progressive dose reduction had reduced the risk of thrombotic complications (25). Epidemiological studies showed that users of low-dose combined products had small, and often statistically non-significant, rises in the risks of myocardial infarction (SEDA-16, 465) (26,27), thrombotic stroke (28–30), venous thromboembolism (31), and subarachnoid hemorrhage (28,30,32). Several of these studies compared the risks presented by different doses and found somewhat higher rates for products containing more than 50 micrograms of estrogen but somewhat lower rates among women currently using the lower-dose formulations (26,28,29,33).

A group in The Netherlands has stressed the fact that even though the risk of venous thrombosis is small in absolute terms, oral contraceptives form the major cause of thrombotic disease in young women. The risk is higher during the first year of use (up to one per 1000 per year), among women with a prothrombotic predisposition, and with third-generation progestogens (34).

Presentation

The commonest presentation is deep venous thrombosis in the leg, which can lead to pulmonary embolism. Fatal pulmonary embolism has even been reported after intravenous injections of conjugated estrogens (35). Despite the improvement noted with reduced doses, incidental case reports of severe cardiovascular events during the use of low-dose products have continued to appear. They include incidents of cerebral venous thrombosis and subarachnoid hemorrhage, fatal central angiitis, sinus thrombosis, and cerebral ischemia. In one series of 22 cases of cerebral infarction involving either arteries or veins, all the oral contraceptives that had been used contained a low dose of ethinylestradiol (36). Thromboembolism in other veins, such as the hepatic vein, that is Budd–Chiari syndrome, has occasionally been reported (37); the first 10 such cases were reported as long ago as 1972 and the increasing number since then has at times raised some concern (SEDA-6, 344) (SEDA-7, 386). A case of renal vein thrombosis has also occurred (38). Incidental reports continue to appear of thrombotic incidents in relatively unusual forms, including a further case of mesenteric thrombosis leading to intestinal necrosis (39) and a report of fatal pulmonary embolism following intravenous injections of conjugated estrogens (35).

The incidence of hepatic veno-occlusive disease in 249 consecutive women treated with norethisterone who underwent allogenic hemopoietic stem cell transplantation was 27% compared with 3% in women without this treatment (40). One-year survival rates were 17% and 73% in patients with ($n = 24$) or without veno-occlusive disease ($n = 225$) respectively. Because of this adverse effect, norethisterone should not be used in patients undergoing bone-marrow transplantation. Heparin prophylaxis does not affect the risk of death from veno-occlusive disease.

Susceptibility factors

By 1980 it was considered clear that the risk of thromboembolic events was further increased under particular conditions. It was higher in smokers, in older women, and in the obese, and appropriate warnings were issued. The fact that these warnings to a large extent eliminated the high-risk individuals who had formed part of the early population of oral contraceptive users means that data from the early period cannot be used to provide a valid historical comparison with later findings (41,42).

Thrombotic diathesis

Early epidemiological data on the recurrence of thrombosis (43) indicated something of an inherited predisposition, and others found a low content of fibrinolytic activators in the vessel wall of women who 6–12 months earlier had experienced a thrombotic complication while using oral contraceptives (44); high doses of estrogen affected the concentrations of such activators (45). However, such lesions are apparently not exclusive to users of oral contraceptives (SEDA-8, 360) and examination of the vessel wall is not of predictive value in determining risk.

The risk of venous thrombosis among carriers of the factor V Leiden mutation is increased eight-fold overall and 30-fold among carriers who take an oral contraceptive (46,47). This mutation results in resistance to activated protein C and thereby potentiates the prothrombotic effect of oral contraceptives. Early work suggested a greater risk after major surgery (48,49). However, epidemiological studies of postoperative venous thromboembolism are limited and disputed (50). There is no documented excess risk of postoperative thrombosis associated with low-dose combined oral contraceptives among women without other risk factors (51). If it is correct that some effects on coagulation persist for several weeks, it is wise to withdraw these products a month before surgery (50). From a practical point of view, any decision regarding possible discontinuation of combined oral contraceptives before surgery should take into consideration the need for alternative and adequate contraception during the interim. If the woman chooses to stop taking combined oral contraceptives, progestogen-only formulations (as well as barrier methods) are deemed suitable (50). A recommended alternative to discontinuation of a combined oral contraceptive is heparin in low doses (51).

Age

The increase in risk with age is clear (6), although the underlying risk of cardiovascular disease also rises as age progresses. The US Food and Drug Administration has concluded that the benefits may outweigh the risks in healthy non-smoking women over age 40, and it has in most countries been common for over two decades to advise reticence in the use of oral contraceptives after the age of 35.

Obesity

Obesity has repeatedly been shown to play a role, and its relevance to particular types of complication has been demonstrated. The Oxford Family Planning Association's 1987 data showed that the risk of myocardial infarction or angina increased significantly with weight (52).

Smoking

Smoking has been very clearly incriminated as a susceptibility factor for thromboembolism and arterial thrombosis in women taking the oral contraceptive, and its apparently synergistic role has been well defined and quantified (53,54). The 1989 case-control analysis of the RCGP cohort study estimated the relative risk of myocardial infarct during current oral contraceptive use at only 0.9 for non-smokers, but at 3.5 for women smoking under 15 cigarettes per day, and as much as 21 for users of more than 15 cigarettes per day (55). Smoking increases not only the risk of myocardial infarction among oral contraceptive uses (27), but also the risk of angina pectoris (52), thrombotic stroke (28,29), and subarachnoid hemorrhage, and it can double or treble mortality (56–58). There has also been further confirmation that the effect is dose-related, light smokers having twice the risk of coronary heart disease and heavier smokers having up to four times the risk, compared with non-smokers; cessation of smoking is accompanied by a reduction in risk of coronary heart disease to the level prevalent among non-smokers within 3–5 years (54).

Smoking contributes to effects on the procoagulation process in young women (59). The effects of oral contraceptives on the coagulation system are much greater in smokers than non-smokers (44). Oral contraceptive users who were smokers generally have significantly lower fibrinolytic activity than non-smokers (60), but not consistently (61).

Others

Women of blood group O have less of a risk of thromboembolism (15). The risk of thromboembolic complications may be greater where there is a history of diabetes, hypertension, and pre-eclamptic toxemia. In some studies there has been an association with type II hyperlipoproteinemia, hypercholesterolemia, and atheroma (62–66). Hypertension may be an additional risk factor when considered in relation to oral contraceptive use.

Mechanisms

Study of the mechanisms that might underlie the link between oral contraceptives and thromboembolic events is of importance in developing safer formulations, but also in identifying, if possible, individuals at particular risk who should be advised to change to alternative contraceptive methods.

The 1990 international consensus statement cited above noted that: "Oral contraceptives induce alterations in hemostasis variables. There are changes in the concentrations of a large number of specific plasma components of the coagulation and fibrinolytic systems, although usually within the normal range .... It is conceivable that these effects are estrogen-mediated because they have not been demonstrated in progestogen-only preparations. There is a dose-dependent relationship in the case of estrogen, although in combination tablets, the progestogens might exert a modifying effect .... Further attention should be given to changes in factor VIIc and fibrinogen induced by oral contraceptives and also to the association between carbohydrate metabolism and fibrinolysis."

Quantification of coagulation factors is notoriously difficult, because of the interrelations among the various components of the coagulation cascade, the broad range of normal values, and considerable inter-laboratory variability (51). This variability is illustrated by a WHO study of users of combined oral contraceptives, conducted on several continents, which showed statistically significant differences among clinical centers in prothrombin time, fibrin plate lysis, plasminogen, and activated partial thromboplastin time (SEDA-16, 464). Effects also vary between different populations, users of different doses, users of different products, and tests performed at different periods of the medication cycle (61,67).

The term "hypercoagulability" has been used to describe a supposed pre-thrombotic state, identifiable by certain changes in the hemostatic system, but to date there is no broad-spectrum laboratory test for assessing the risk of thrombosis in a given individual, although coagulation changes in vitro have sometimes been regarded as proof of a thrombotic state. Deviations in laboratory data from patients with thromboses have often been interpreted as demonstrating the cause of the thrombosis, whereas they may simply be a consequence.

Despite the variations that are found, the overall conclusion is that oral contraceptives cause an increase in coagulation factors I (fibrinogen), II, VII, IX, X, and XII, and a reduction in antithrombin III concentrations, which would be expected to predispose to venous thromboembolism, especially if not counterbalanced by an increase either in fibrinolytic activity or of other inhibitory proteins of the coagulation, such as protein C (68).

There is also fairly strong evidence that immunological mechanisms play a role in thrombotic episodes associated with oral contraceptives, especially when they occur in the absence of risk factors for vascular disease (69), although this has been contested (70). In one series of reports on cerebral infarction, circulating immune complexes and/or specific antihormone antibodies were found in 15 of 20 patients (36). In a large series of women with venous or arterial thrombosis, anti-ethinylestradiol antibodies were absent in non-users but present in 72% of users; they were also present in 33% of healthy oral contraceptive users without thrombosis (SEDA-16, 465). In half of the cases there were both anti-ethinylestradiol antibodies and a history of smoking were found jointly in half of the cases.

There is a significant rise in fibrinogen concentrations during the early months of oral contraceptive use, and concentrations return to baseline after withdrawal (71). Prolonged use of oral contraception also seems to lower concentrations of antiaggregatory prostacyclin (72).

Some work that was considered to show severe acquired plasma resistance to activated protein C among users of third-generation (as opposed to second-generation) products has been re-examined by a French group (73). In their view the technical measures used to demonstrate the effect of activated protein C introduced a bias of interpretation and hence false results; they have further argued that such a test cannot demonstrate the presence of a raised thromboembolic risk in asymptomatic women taking these contraceptives, since it is non-specific and subject to changes in the plasma concentrations of many coagulation factors that are themselves increased or decreased by estrogens and progestogens. They point, for example, to protein S (74), changes in which account for the differential effect of oral contraceptives on Rosing's assay (75), but which are in their view irrelevant to issues of thromboembolic risk with oral contraceptives; the androgenic potential of the progestogen may further counteract the effect of estrogens in the test. More generally, in such a complex situation in which there is a "modification of the modification," there is no hemostasis-related test that provides a risk indicator for thrombosis. This argument is sound, but it naturally remains theoretical; the question of thromboembolism with the third-generation products must, as pointed out above, be resolved on the basis of epidemiological data, and certainly those data now strongly point to an increased risk.

Relative roles of estrogens and progestogens

The risk of thrombosis is closely associated with the estrogen component (76) for both arterial and venous events and with the progestogen for arterial events; however, if a particular progestogen is metabolized to estrogen or raises estrogen concentrations, it will make a contribution to venous complications. Estrogen alone has after all been incriminated as a cause of thromboembolism when given to men (77); the risk of puerperal thromboembolism after estrogen inhibition of lactation has been shown in several studies (78); non-contraceptive estrogens clearly increase the risk of acute myocardial infarction in women under 46 years of age (79). Changes in coagulation factors appear to be related to the estrogen dose (44,45,80,81). Progestogen-only formulations do not have any significant effect on the coagulation system.

Third-generation oral contraceptives and thromboembolism

There are now reasons to doubt whether the third-generation oral contraceptives are indeed safer than their predecessors in respect to thromboembolism and substantial grounds for believing that they present greater risks.

The first reason is theoretical. The demonstrated effects of the new substances and combinations on lipids and carbohydrates do not have any major relevance to the thromboembolic process. The latter is linked primarily to changes in the hemostatic system and blood coagulation, involving platelet aggregation, coagulation factors, fibrinogen concentrations, and blood viscosity.

The second reason is kinetic. It is true that the dose of estrogen (probably the main instrument in inducing thromboembolism) has been kept to a minimum, but the new progestogen gestodene tends to accumulate in the system with continued use, and the concentrations of ethinylestradiol increase simultaneously; this increase is due to the ability of gestodene to inhibit cytochrome P450 and therefore to inhibit the breakdown of estrogen, as well as its own metabolism (82). Similar findings emerged with desogestrel, although they were somewhat less marked (83).

The third reason is hematological. The third-generation contraceptives have greater adverse effects on the clotting system than those of the second generation. In particular, women using the third-generation products have a greater resistance to activated protein C (84), a shift that is associated with a higher risk of thrombosis.

The fourth reason is epidemiological. During the period 1987–88, when the third-generation products were relatively new, anecdotal reports of thromboembolic events appeared, including at least one death, and partly for this reason a series of large controlled studies were set up. The findings of three such studies (British, European, and global) became available to the drug control authorities late in 1995 and were subsequently published. The UK Committee on Safety of Medicines, considering all three, concluded that the risk of venous thromboembolic events in these third-generation oral contraceptives was about double that in users of the previous generation of products using the older progestogens (30 as opposed to 15 per 100 000 woman-years, the risk in healthy women being only five per 100 000). Despite the different populations studied, the individual studies produced broadly consistent results. The global study on four continents found a relative risk of 2.6 when comparing the desogestrel/gestodene products with the older variety, while the European study found a relative risk of 1.5–1.6. Various later papers pointed in the same direction. In Denmark, there was an increase in hospital admissions for primary venous thromboembolism in young women coinciding with the introduction of the third-generation products (85). Papers from The Netherlands have confirmed the main trend (86,87).

Authoritative reviews and editorials have further confirmed the correctness of the above findings. There has been some criticism of the individual studies on various points of detail, but it is difficult to see that this in any way undermines what is now very consistent evidence that the third-generation oral contraceptives increase the risk of thromboembolic events to a substantially greater degree than previous products. Some work that has been advanced as pointing to the safety of third-generation products (88) proves to relate primarily to the second-generation combinations, with only a few late entrants using the more recent oral contraceptives, and other work was performed on a very small scale.

As a rule, the study of adverse reactions must relate to current and emergent issues. However, now and again it can be instructive to look back into recent history. When a drug problem has been fairly clearly defined, and particularly when it has for a time been the subject of debate and even frank controversy, one can learn something from the processes involved. How did the facts become known? Why did the controversy emerge? And could the risk have been detected and eliminated earlier?

Since their appearance in the late 1950s, oral contraceptives have gone through several stages of development. What are now in retrospect referred to as first-generation oral contraceptives were high-dose combinations of progestogens (more particularly norethynodrel, norethisterone, and lynestrenol in doses of 2.5 mg or more) and the estrogen mestranol 75 micrograms. A decade later a second generation emerged, with substantially lower doses, commonly half of those used earlier and some new progestogens, notably the more potent levonorgestrel. Finally, in the early 1980s some manufacturers introduced so-called third-generation products, a particular characteristic of which was the use of entirely new, very potent progestogens, among them desogestrel and gestodene. Clinical studies of contraceptives that contained gestodene and desogestrel suggested that they are very similar to one another, although differences in dosage and potency could account for reports that products that contain gestodene provide better cycle control (89).

Almost from the earlier years, the risk of thromboembolic complications among users of "the pill" was recognized, and by the mid-1960s it was well documented (90,91). Progressive reductions in dosage, in particular that of the estrogenic component, during the period that first- and second-generation products held sway were widely regarded as having reduced this risk to manageable proportions, although it was not eliminated. The relative risk with first-generation products was highly variable (2–11), but the best work in the UK and the USA fairly consistently reached an estimate of 4–6 (92–94). With the second-generation products the relative risk of thromboembolic complications was again variously estimated, but a large cohort study published in 1991 set it at 1.5 with products containing the lowest doses of estrogen, and 1.7 with products containing intermediate doses of estrogen (33).

The fact that both prescribers and users of medicines are likely to anticipate that new drugs will be in some way better than those that have gone before means that both groups are in principle receptive to potentially spurious claims and suggestions. By the time the third-generation oral contraceptives were marketed, this type of contraception had been around for a quarter of a century; the risk of thromboembolism, the most widely publicized problem in the field, seemed by that time to have receded with progressive reductions in dosage. There was every reason to hope that it would recede further with the newest generation of products. That expectation was further nurtured by the even lower doses latterly attainable. It also seems to have been fostered by some of the suggestive promotion that appeared, although that in fact related as a rule merely to an improved lipid spectrum, which in turn raised the theoretical possibility, also discussed but not documented by some clinical investigators (95), that arterial and cardiac risks might be less.

What in fact happened was that by 1989 alarm bells began to ring in Germany, where the regulatory authorities were alerted to the submission of an unusually high number of spontaneous reports of thromboembolic complications thought to be associated with the new products. Cases continued to accumulate, long-term studies already begun were completed, and in 1995 Britain's Committee on Safety of Medicines made a public statement to the effect that the risk of thromboembolic complications among hitherto healthy users of third-generation products was approximately twice than that seen with second-generation products (SEDA-19, xix). The studies in question, including work by the World Health Organization and others (SED-14, 1410), were subsequently published and confirmed that conclusion, as did later work (96). It was further reinforced by others (97), who worked on a smaller scale but provided well-documented evidence that while a factor V Leiden mutation or a biased family history could increase the risk in individual cases, they did not explain the higher thrombosis risk seen with a product based on desogestrel than with contraceptives that incorporated levonorgestrel, norethisterone, or lynestrenol.

Currently one must ask why the particular risk of the third-generation contraceptives was identified so late. These third-generation products had been in development since the late 1970s and the first had been marketed in 1981–82, some 14 years before the Committee on Safety of Medicines issued its statement. Could society not have done better and thereby reduced the risks to which women were exposed? There are two principal answers, both of them at least partly in the affirmative.

The first is that products of this type could well have been entered at an earlier date into large studies of oral contraception and their effects. A series of university centers around the world, as well as bodies such as Britain's Royal College of Physicians and Royal College of General Practitioners, have throughout the oral contraceptive era either sponsored or participated in prolonged cohort and case-control studies of these products. Experience with data on thromboembolism suggests that significant data are likely to be obtainable in a cohort study of manageable size within some 5–7 years. The use of third-generation products may have been small in the early years, but they were aggressively promoted in major oral contraceptive markets to ensure rapid growth, in all probability sufficient to provide adequate recruitment. One would hesitate to argue that such studies should be a universal condition of the marketing of drugs, but when the products concerned have immense social significance and considerable potential for good and harm, as the oral contraceptives do, and when the compounds involved are entirely new, there is at least a sound medical reason for such work in every case. That work was performed with successive forms of the earlier oral contraceptive products, in which dosages were progressively reduced, and there was particular reason to set it in motion on the introduction of products that contained new chemical components with some significant structural and pharmacological differences from the older progestogens. A straightforward statistical calculation shows that an early cohort study involving some 30 000–50 000 women taking a third-generation product could within 2 years have shown the degree of increase in the thrombotic risk, which was actually not elicited until much later.

The second answer with respect to the earlier acquisition of risk data must come from the laboratory. Not from animal studies, which in this field are of very restricted value, but from biochemical and particularly hematological work. When during the 1990s various groups began to examine in detail the effects of the third-generation contraceptives on processes related to the clotting system, they identified a series of properties that could very well explain an increased incidence of thrombosis.

The first of these was an increase in circulating concentrations of factor VII produced by the desogestrel plus estrogen combination, which was some 20–30% higher than that seen with a second-generation product based on levonorgestrel (98). The methods used to carry out this work were available before 1988 (99), and it is not at all clear from the published material whether there was a failure to compare the two generations in this respect at an early date, or whether such work was performed and either overlooked or misinterpreted.

A second finding related to the effects of activated protein C on thrombin generation in low-platelet plasma via the intrinsic or extrinsic clotting pathways. Using a method developed on the basis of work first published in 1997 (100), a Dutch group in Maastricht found that all types of combined oral contraceptives induced acquired resistance to activated protein C. With the third-generation contraceptives, however, the effect was significantly more marked than with those of the second generation: in other words, these drugs significantly reduced the ability of activated protein C to down-regulate the formation of thrombin (84). However, this work only became feasible in the late 1990s.

A third underlying mechanism seems to involve a reduction in concentrations of free protein S, again more pronounced with third-generation products. When protein S falls, the antifibrinolytic effect of the so-called thrombin-activated fibrinolysis inhibitor is increased; in other words, fibrinolysis is impeded, with an increased risk of clotting problems (101). Again, however, these are recent methods, which were not available when the third-generation products were launched.

The laboratory findings therefore suggest that a greater thrombosis-inducing effect of the third-generation oral contraceptives can be explained and even anticipated on the basis of known mechanisms. Not all the relevant methods were available in the early years, but that relating to factor VII most certainly was. It is unfortunate, to say the least, that such work was either not performed or not properly interpreted.

All in all, had a combination of hematological methods and field studies been initiated sufficiently soon, the increased risk of thromboembolism with the third-generation oral contraceptives could have been detected some years earlier, sufficient for society to take decisions on the benefit-to-harm balance of these drugs before so much needless injury was incurred.

The third-generation oral contraceptives: a judicial assessment

It was extraordinary to find a major epidemiological dispute regarding drug safety being handled by the High Court in England in late July 2002, when the Court handed down its decision regarding thromboembolic events induced by the third-generation oral contraceptives (102). Essentially, a group of women who claimed to have been injured as a consequence of having using this latest version of "the pill," based on two new progestogens, had sought to reclaim extensive damages from the manufacturers, since in their view the product did not possess the degree of safety which, in the words of European law, the user was legitimately entitled to expect. Since the safety achieved with the widely used products of the second generation was so widely regarded as acceptable, the Court had to decide whether the newer products had significantly failed to meet that standard. Faced with a long procession of expert epidemiological witnesses from both sides, and with some flat contradictions, the judge was obliged to rule on their arguments.

However, that it was an English court in which the issue came to be debated was not surprising, for it was in England that the Committee on Safety of Medicines had written to prescribers in 1995 stating that three unpublished studies on the safety of combined oral contraceptives in relation to venous thromboembolism had indicated about "a two-fold increase in the risk of such conditions" compared with the preceding generation of products. This issue of a "two-fold increase" became crucial to the case. "For reasons of causation," as the Judge put it, the claimants had accepted the burden of proving that the increase in risk was not less than two-fold.

In fact, the English authorities, having rejected a vigorous defence of these products by the manufacturers, were by 1999 speaking more precisely of an increase in risk, as compared with the earlier products "of about 1.7–1.8 after adjustment," which was "not fully explained by bias or confounding"; appropriate label warnings were therefore imposed. These new warnings, summarized, said that an increased risk associated with combined oral contraceptives generally was well established, but was smaller than that associated with pregnancy (60 cases per 100 000 pregnancies). In healthy non-pregnant women who were not taking any combined contraceptive it was about five cases per 100 000 woman-years; in those taking the second-generation products it was about 15; and for third-generation products it was about 25. By September 2001, the European Union's Committee on Proprietary Pharmaceutical Products had formed its own view, and here too it was concluded that the "best estimate of the magnitude of the increased risk is in the range of 1.5–2.0."

In Court to support the claimants, Professor Alexander Walker assessed the relative risk of the third-generation products at 2.2, Dame Margaret Thorogood at 2.1, and Professor Klim McPherson at about 1.9. The experts for the defendants took the view that the relative risk was well below two, and could well be zero. As Mr Justice Mackay noted, having listened to these experts: " ... the debate between them has been unyielding, at times almost rancorous in tone, and with a few honourable exceptions ... devoid of willingness to countenance that there may be two sides to the question. So, science has failed to give women clear advice spoken with one voice."

There was also fundamental disagreement on confidence intervals when calculating relative risks in such matters: "The Defendants say that to establish causation in the individual, and therefore a relative risk which is greater than two, there must be seen not just a point estimate but also a lower confidence interval which is greater than two in order for the result to be significantly different from two."

The Court was faced with "a series of studies with different point estimates and largely overlapping confidence intervals. Time after time experts have had their attention drawn to point estimates from studies that appear, to the layman's eye, to be very different. Almost invariably they have dismissed those apparent differences by reference to the overlapping confidence intervals, saying that the figures are statistically compatible and there is no significant difference." Confronted with such material, the Court chose to set aside as inexact and theoretical much of the statistical rhetoric. Having done that, the Judge felt himself in a position to emerge "from that forest into broader more open country where the simpler concept of the balance of probabilities rules." Constructing his judgement in that way, Mr Justice Mackay advanced in the course of 100 pages to the conclusion that the claimants had failed to demonstrate a doubling of the risk. In his view, "the most likely figure to represent the relative risk is around 1.7."

This extraordinary and wise judgement merits most careful reading by anyone anxious to understand the safety issues surrounding oral contraceptives. First, because of the insight that it demonstrates into the manner—not always edifying—in which evidence in this vital matter has been adduced, interpreted, and argued over in the course of more than a decade. Secondly, because it arrives, through a process of tight reasoning, at what is for the moment the most reliable conclusion we have. It seems beyond all possible doubt that the third generation of oral contraceptives is primarily characterized by an increased risk of thromboembolic complications. Whether that risk is great enough to warrant financial compensation is a matter for lawyers to decide. But given the lack of any tangible benefit to the user, the risk is clearly significant in human terms, and it is hard to see that there is any valid reason at all for continuing to use these products.

Arterial complications

Arterial disease and acute arterial disorders and their links to oral contraception have long been a matter of concern, partly because of actual reported instances of apparent complications, but largely because of the metabolic changes caused by the oral contraceptives. In particular, it has been thought that the effects of these products in raising blood pressure, affecting clotting, or changing the circulating concentrations of blood lipids and carbohydrates could result in cardiac and arterial risks, including an earlier onset of atherosclerosis and the occurrence of myocardial infarction and stroke. Basilar artery occlusion secondary to thrombosis (103), cerebral infarction (104,105), retinal vascular complications (106), and encephalopathy with renovascular hypertension (107) and acute myocardial infarction (108,109) have all been reported. There have been over 40 reports of intestinal ischemia and infarction in oral contraceptive users, with a high mortality rate (39,110).

The initial question must be whether the clinical data point to the emergence of complications of this type. The 1990 International Consensus Meeting found an increase in acute cardiovascular accidents during use of oral contraceptives, but not persisting after they had been discontinued. There is also a great deal of anecdotal evidence, although in view of the massive scale on which oral contraceptives have been used over 40 years, coincidence alone would lead to the accumulation of many reports of adverse events. Other evidence suggesting an increase in arterial thrombotic events has been noted incidentally in the discussion of venous events above. There is also evidence that the chance of unexpected cardiovascular death is lower in oral contraceptive users who have been taking a product based on one of the new progestogens in particular. In over 300 000 women there was a cardiovascular death rate of 4.3 per 100 000 women-years among users of combined oral contraceptives containing levonorgestrel, 1.5 per 100 000 among users of those based on desogestrel, and 4.8 per 100 000 among users of oral contraceptives containing gestodene (111). The relative risk estimates compared with levonorgestrel were 0.4 (95% CI = 0.1, 2.1) and 1.4 (0.5, 4.5) for desogestrel and gestodene respectively. However, it should be added that this is precisely one of the studies that concluded that the new progestogens substantially increased the incidence of venous thromboembolism.

However, a fatal flaw of most such studies was their failure to provide an adequate analysis of co-existent risk factors other than oral contraception. In fact, there is not a great deal of evidence of appreciable risks of this type among oral contraceptive users, unless other risk factors are present. The 1989 case-control analysis of the Royal College of General Practitioners cohort study showed that current oral contraception increased the risk of acute myocardial infarction, but only among smokers. The large cohort study from the Oxford Family Planning Association (OFPA) similarly found no significantly increased risk of myocardial infarction or angina pectoris among either current or former use of oral contraceptives, but a strong dose-related effect of current smoking. In an analogous manner, many studies have shown that the risk of coronary heart disease in oral contraceptive users or other women increases directly with body weight (52,54) and with age (6), but not clearly with oral contraceptive use alone. Nor does one find any published evidence that the risk of late arterial disease, notably atherosclerosis, is higher among users of oral contraceptives, despite the fact that with some 40 years of experience one would expect any such trend to have become evident by the end of the 20th century.

Alongside this clinical material one is faced with the biochemical evidence of changes in the oral contraceptive user. However, various findings make it impossible to draw clear pathogenetic conclusions from these biochemical data. As far as lipids are concerned, there is no doubt that oral contraceptives as a group increase low-density lipoprotein and reduce high-density lipoprotein and cholesterol; this shift is usually regarded as inducing a propensity to atherosclerosis, but here its significance is not so simple to assess. HDL cholesterol, for example, can be divided into subfractions, of which HDL2 seems to be more responsive to estrogens and progestogens; the concentration of HDL2 has been thought to correlate better with a reduced risk of cardiovascular disease than does total HDL cholesterol (112). The picture is further complicated by the fact that when estrogens are used in postmenopausal women they can raise HDL, a change that might be considered to have a favorable effect (113–115). What is more, the effects of these products on lipids change with time, rendering short-term studies useless as a basis for risk assessment. It could be that the older oral contraceptives raise the risk in the short term, as suggested above, but actually lower it in the long term.

It is by no means impossible that the overall effect of oral contraceptives on the arterial system is exercised through a complex of different mechanisms. In this respect it is worth recalling the "insulin resistance syndrome" or "metabolic syndrome," which comprises a set of metabolic risk factors for cardiovascular disease (specifically coronary heart disease and arterial disease) (116). These interrelated risk factors include hyperinsulinemia and impaired glucose tolerance, hypertriglyceridemia, reduced high-density lipoprotein (HDL) concentrations, and hypertension, with insulin resistance as a potential underlying factor. Hormonal contraceptives can variously affect these metabolic conditions, and the effect depends in part on steroid type and dose. Lower doses and newer formulations do not change HDL concentrations or increase blood pressure, but insulin resistance and hypertriglyceridemia still occur. These latter changes are caused primarily by the estrogen component of combined oral contraceptives, but the progestogen component can also modify these effects. The formulations with the least unfavorable metabolic effects are those that contain norethindrone or that are based on the newer progestogens, such as desogestrel, gestodene, or norgestimate. However, as noted elsewhere, it has yet to be determined whether the metabolic changes confer any clinical benefit.

Finally, it is fair to set the possible adverse effects of these hormonal products, and particularly of estrogen, against the fact that estrogen also has certain favorable effects on the arterial wall. It has been suggested that estrogen has a calcium channel blocking effect that relaxes the vessel walls, thus increasing blood flow (117). Others have documented in monkeys the fact that estrogens dilate the coronary arteries, an effect unrelated to plasma lipid concentrations, blood pressure, or heart rate (SED-13, 1217) (118). They have also found evidence in their animal studies that estrogen + progestogen administration to hypercholesterolemic animals reduces both their HDL cholesterol concentrations and their arterial lesions.

Frequency

West German data over the period 1955–80 showed no community-wide increase in the incidence of ischemic heart disease, cerebral vascular embolism, or pulmonary embolism, despite the rapid growth in oral contraceptive use (and the prevalence of high-dose products) during much of that period (119). The Oxford Family Planning Association's 1989 paper on its cohort study, which had followed up more than 17 000 women for an average of nearly 16 years, found no significant overall effect of oral contraceptive use on mortality, with a relative risk of 0.9 (8). Mortality from diseases of the circulatory system had slightly increased; the relative risk of death from ischemic heart disease in current or past oral contraceptive users was 3.3 (95% CI = 0.9–17.9), while data on fatal cerebrovascular disease were too few to be interpreted.

Similarly, a massive Finnish mortality study, covering 1 585 000 women-years of oral contraceptive use and two million women-years of copper-bearing intrauterine device use, showed no increase in relative risk among oral contraceptive users for myocardial infarction or cerebral hemorrhage deaths; however, there might have been an increased risk of death from pulmonary embolism among users of oral contraceptives (42).

An analysis of the cardiovascular mortality risk associated with low-dose oral contraceptives (under 50 micrograms of ethinylestradiol) in the USA showed that among non-smokers and light smokers the mortality among current oral contraceptive users was likely to be lower than the mortality due to pregnancy (25). Only among heavier smokers over 30 years old did the risk of oral contraceptive use exceed the risk of pregnancy. The researchers noted that in countries with higher maternal mortality rates than the USA, even older women who are both heavy smokers and oral contraceptive users would have a lower mortality risk than that associated with pregnancy.

A 5-year case-control study involving all Danish hospitals has once more quantified the thromboembolic risks associated with oral contraceptives as a whole; the risk with third-generation products was some 30% higher than with second-generation products (RR = 1.3; CI = 1.0, 1.8) (120). However, data on cerebral thrombosis from the same study showed that with third-generation products the mean risk was some 40% lower than with second-generation products (RR = 0.6; CI = 0.4, 0.9) (121).

Susceptibility factors

The effect of smoking has been investigated on a large scale in Denmark, where the incidence of smoking among women is much higher than in many other countries (122). Evidence has emerged that the combination of smoking with oral contraceptive use may have a synergistic effect on the risks of acute myocardial infarction and cerebral thromboembolism (but not of venous thromboembolism), particularly among users of high doses (50 micrograms). The authors therefore suggested that the very low-dose products, which in Denmark contain 20 micrograms of ethinylestradiol, should be preferred in smokers. While this conclusion is clear and defensible, the situation is somewhat complicated by the fact that in Denmark the only products that contain this low dose of estrogen are those in which it is combined with either desogestrel or gestodene, that is third-generation progestogens. It could well be that the safest combined oral contraceptives for smokers will prove to be those in which the 20 micrograms dose of estrogen is combined with a more traditional progestogen.

For current or potential users of oral contraceptives the question arises whether it is not wise to examine the individual's possible predisposition to thromboembolism (thrombophilia) before deciding for or against this form of birth control. It has been suggested that in teenage users who might prove to be carriers of the Factor V Leiden mutation, routine screening would not be economically justified (123). It was instead the author's view that clinicians can use thoughtful screening questions to identify potentially high-risk patients for thrombophilia and consider testing for inherited risk factors case by case.

Estrogens versus progestogens

As far as the estrogens are concerned, the original estrogen, mestranol, was abruptly replaced by ethinylestradiol in most or all products after a wide-scale panic relating to the thrombosis issue in 1969. The motive lay entirely in the fact that the ethinylestradiol was about twice as potent, so that the dose could be halved. Whether this in fact led to any reduction in cardiovascular thromboembolic risk was never specifically examined. The choice of estrogen might still be relevant to the extent that (physiological) 17-β-estradiol in microcrystalline form later became available for oral use and in theory might prove safer in some respects than semisynthetic estrogens, since it seems to have less effect on the fibrinolytic system.

The question of the progestogens has come acutely to the fore as a result of the debate regarding the third-generation progestogens gestodene and desogestrel. At the time of marketing, no specific claim appears to have been made that they would present a lesser degree of risk of thromboembolism. However, emphasis was placed on experimental findings that might indicate a better cardiovascular prognosis. The older oral contraceptives produce an increase in low density lipoprotein and a reduction in high density lipoprotein and cholesterol; those changes may have some relevance to the occurrence of arterial disease. By avoiding them, and having the lowest possible estrogen content, the new combinations were expected to be safer, although this had in no sense been proven. However, the manner in which this information was presented could have introduced a degree of confusion in the minds of prescribers and users, and the belief appears to have arisen that these third-generation oral contraceptives might prove less likely than their predecessors to cause thromboembolic disorders. That this is not so in relation to venous thromboembolism is discussed above. The theoretical argument that the risk of atherosclerosis and its associated complications might in the long run be less is so far entirely unproven, and with the fall in use of these products following these unfavorable findings (124), it seems uncertain whether the data necessary to examine that hypothesis will ever be accumulated.

Persistence of risk after discontinuation

Most, but not all, studies have concluded that the effect of oral contraception on the risk of cardiovascular disorders disappears after withdrawal (6,41,54,125–127). The Nurses' Health Study found no differences in either incidence of or mortality from various cardiovascular diseases between never-users and past-users, regardless of the duration of use, or the time since last use (7). The nested case-control analysis of the RCGP study showed that, although stroke risk was higher among current oral contraceptive users regardless of smoking status, former users had an increased risk only if they were current smokers. Such conclusions are supported most strongly by a 1990 meta-analysis of published studies on the relation between past use of oral contraceptives and myocardial infarction, which produced an adjusted relative risk estimate of 1.01, suggesting no association (128). Thus, there does not appear to be a long-term mechanism at work, such as atherosclerosis, but rather an effect confined to current use, such as thrombosis (41,54). However, there have been only a few studies of stroke in relation to previous oral contraceptive use, and those studies have produced inconsistent results; thus, meta-analysis of stroke data is precluded.

With some of the newer drugs, the effects may (as seems to be the case with the older drugs) persist for a number of weeks and justify the withdrawal of these products some time before surgery or other risks. A study of changes in hemostasis after withdrawal of the newer combined oral contraceptives (ethinylestradiol 30 micrograms plus either desogestrel or gestodene) (41) showed that several weeks elapsed before plasma concentrations of fibrinogen, factor X, and antithrombin III returned to baseline.

It should be noted that a few studies have produced deviant conclusions, for reasons that are not clear. Some found that the risk of fatal myocardial infarction was similar for current and past users (26), whereas others actually reported a lower risk of cerebral thromboembolic attack in former users compared with never users (29).

In summary, the final chapter in the story of oral contraceptives and arterial lesions has not yet been written. However, in the light of long experience there is currently reason for optimism. There is no reasonable evidence that oral contraceptives, whatever their biochemical effects, actually do increase the risk of atherosclerosis; as to the occurrence of acute arterial events, these are explained largely or entirely by the presence of risk factors other than oral contraception.

Hypertension

The association between combined oral contraceptives and hypertension, noted and confirmed as early as 1961, has been explored in a multicenter clinical trial carried out by the WHO (129,130) and on a lesser scale in many other reports, yet the facts remain surprisingly puzzling. It has become clear that the use of oral contraceptives in any dose can cause a mean increase in blood pressure, the effect being much more marked in some individuals than others. With the current range of oral contraceptives a substantial proportion of users show some increase in blood pressure compared with their pre-treatment condition (131), but the rise is rarely of clinical significance. Clinical hypertension seems unlikely to occur in more than 1–5% of women (132). The incidence may have been higher with the older high-dose products, but that is not entirely clear. The figures have to be set against the incidence of hypertension in a population of otherwise healthy women of fertile age, which is about 2%. The rise in blood pressure can appear at any time during treatment and persists for at least as long as the drug is taken, sometimes for several months longer, but even then it generally returns to normal. In order to detect women who react poorly, blood pressure measurements should be an integral part of the follow-up care of all women taking oral contraceptives. Considerable research has shown no overall increase in blood pressure or in the prevalence of hypertension associated with use of progestogen-only contraceptives; nor does the available information point to any increase in other cardiovascular disorders.

It is not clear why many women remain normotensive while others have a rise in blood pressure. No confirmation has been obtained of early beliefs that hypertension during oral contraception was more likely to occur in black American women, or in women with a history of hypertension during pregnancy (56,133). However, there is clinical evidence that this can occur and that the women involved may have a defect in dopaminergic transmission affecting blood pressure and prolactin secretion (134); pre-existent abnormalities of platelet function and fibrinolysis have also been linked with this complication (SEDA-6, 348).

Published studies, in which various doses have been used, show that there is no clear relation between blood pressure and estrogen intake. The progestogens seem to be involved, but here too most specific studies fail to detect a dose–response relation (131). However, some do: in a 1977 analysis of data from the large prospective study by the Royal College of General Practitioners (RCGP), with oral contraceptives containing ethinylestradiol 50 micrograms and norethisterone acetate 1, 3, or 4 mg, the risk of hypertension increased with increasing progestogen dose (135).

The rise in blood pressure might reflect water retention caused by the mineralocorticoid effect of progestogens, but that is probably not the complete explanation. These drugs have an effect on the renin-angiotensin system, but there actually seems to be some fall in responsiveness to plasma renin activity. Other possible pathophysiological mechanisms discussed so far include insufficient adaptation to increased production of angiotensin and aldosterone, an increase in cardiac output, and changes in the metabolism of catecholamines. The estrogenic component of oral contraceptives has been stated to be the more important factor in producing abnormalities in the renin system, but the progestogen may also play a role. Some workers have found higher estrogen concentrations in oral contraceptive users who develop hypertension (136).

As might be expected, the few women with severe hypertension during oral contraceptive use, whether or not they were hypertensive before that time, run a somewhat greater risk of acute secondary complications due to hypertension, such as subarachnoid hemorrhage. If the hypertension is severe and persistent one might anticipate long-term effects on the cardiovascular system and kidneys. Nested case-control studies using data from the RCGP study showed that hypertension was an independent risk factor for both stroke (28) and myocardial infarction (55); after controlling for other variables, including oral contraceptive use, the odds ratios (or estimated relative risks) associated with hypertension were 2.8 for stroke and 2.4 for myocardial infarction. In that study, oral contraceptive use did not further increase the risk associated with either hypertension or a history of toxemia of pregnancy. Nevertheless, hypertensive women who take oral contraceptives should be monitored carefully.

Respiratory

Oral contraception is not considered to be relevant to the induction or aggravation of respiratory disorders, although the fact that a very few women have allergic reactions to these formulations could in theory be relevant to the occurrence of asthma.

Nervous system

Headache has long been reported as a reaction to oral contraceptives, just as it occurs unpredictably with many other forms of drug treatment; it is probable that women who are susceptible to headaches at certain phases of the menstrual cycle are more likely to react to oral contraceptives in this way. However, it does not seem to be in any sense consistent; in a placebo-controlled trial conducted as long ago as 1971, when doses of estrogens were high, headache was not found to be associated with use of combined oral contraceptives containing mestranol either 50 or 100 mg (137). In many other studies of the adverse effects of oral contraceptives, it is not possible to ascertain whether the prevalence of specific complaints, such as headache, is actually increased, because there is no appropriate comparison group.

Because migraine headaches are of vascular origin and are sometimes linked to the menstrual cycle, it is pertinent to consider whether hormonal contraception is appropriate in women suffering from this condition (138). No association of migraine headache with stroke has been demonstrated. However, some women with migraine have an increase in the severity and frequency of headache when they take combined oral contraceptives, just as some other migraine sufferers describe a relation to the menstrual cycle. As a precaution, women who have migraine headaches with focal neurological symptoms should not take combined oral contraceptives.

Despite initial concern (SEDA-6, 349), combined oral contraceptives do not appear to worsen seizure control in most women with epilepsy, although seizure frequency should be carefully monitored. The primary consideration in selecting a contraceptive method for an epileptic woman is the need for dependability, but antiepileptic drugs that are enzyme inducers reduce the effectiveness of hormonal contraceptives. Women who wish to take combined oral contraceptives, but for whom enzyme-inducing drugs provide the best seizure control, should be given combined oral contraceptives with a relatively high dose of estrogen (for example ethinylestradiol 50 micrograms). Fewer seizures occur during the luteal phase (low estrogen) of the menstrual cycle, suggesting that estrogens (or oral contraceptives) may be epileptogenic.

Reversible electroencephalographic changes, probably due to progestogenic effects (139), have been observed in 25–60% of oral contraceptive users.

There are various reports of chorea (140,141), hemichorea (142), and paraballism (143). In one case, chorea was the first sign of lupus erythematosus (144).

Acute abdominal symptoms in users of hormonal contraceptives suggest embolism or infarction at some site, but there can be unusual explanations.

- Right-sided lower abdominal pain occurred in a 15-year-old girl, and had been present throughout the 3 months that she had used the product but it had now become so severe as to demand emergency care. The problem was traced to cutaneous nerve entrapment in the abdominal wall (145).

It is not clear how this could have resulted from the treatment, but it might have entailed fluid redistribution in or around an old appendicectomy scar. It may be noted that nerve entrapment is recognized as a possible adverse effect of oral contraceptives in the carpal tunnel syndrome.

Results from the Oxford Family Planning Association Study showed no relation between oral contraceptive use and the incidence of multiple sclerosis (146). Conversely, multiple sclerosis is no longer considered to be a contraindication to hormonal contraceptive use.

Sensory systems

Eyes

It is still difficult to judge whether there is a correlation between ocular pathology and the use of oral contraceptives, with the exception of thromboembolic incidents that affect the retinal circulation. Oral contraceptives have several times been reported to reduce the tolerability to contact lenses, but in any case this abates in some people as the years pass. However, pregnancy itself may result in loss of contact lens tolerance both for scleral and corneal lenses, lenses often having to be refitted after pregnancy; a similar effect of oral contraceptives is thus not entirely unlikely (147), even though other workers have failed to detect any such change (148). Similar doubts relate to the induction of macular hole with retinal detachment, but in one study 20 of 24 women with this complication were using oral contraceptives (SEDA-6, 348). Finally, there is one case report of retinal migraine linked to the end of oral contraceptive treatment cycles (149).

Ears

Aggravation of existing otosclerosis has been observed several times; in one series of five cases, withdrawal of the medication stabilized four cases while the fifth improved (150). There is no reason to expect a reduction in hearing except in cases of otosclerosis; indeed, in a study of several thousand American women, hearing was generally found to be better among current oral contraceptive users than in never-users, and was intermediate in past users (151). A long-term study of chronic oral contraceptive users, which included otological, audiological, and vestibular examinations, found no impairment of the function of the healthy internal ear (152).

Psychological, psychiatric

Psychiatric symptoms have been described in women taking oral contraceptives in isolated case reports (153,154), probably reflecting non-specific effects in susceptible individuals. As to psychological effects, many physicians have found that certain women react to oral contraceptives by becoming morose or unhappy (155), but this does not necessarily mean that they meet the clinical criteria of true depression, the incidence of which has not been found to be increased (156). Several possible biological mechanisms for mood changes have been suggested; however, when nervousness and depression among combined oral contraceptive users are carefully evaluated over time, the pattern is so inconsistent that it is difficult to study. If one looks for anything like consistent depression one is unlikely to find it (137).

Many women who change to an oral contraceptive after unsatisfactory experience with other forms of contraception find greater sexual satisfaction (156) because of relief from worry about pregnancy.

Endocrine

Both long-term and short-term progestational therapy can suppress pituitary ACTH production to some extent, as studied with the metyrapone test. Medroxyprogesterone and chlormadinone suppress the reaction to metyrapone almost completely. Recovery was rapid after withdrawal of therapy. However, no conclusion was drawn as to the relative effect of the ethinylestradiol that was also given. The cortisol secretion rate is depressed in women taking norethindrone and mestranol, and the suggestion has been made that the gluconeogenic effect of glucocorticoids is markedly potentiated in subjects taking estrogens or estrogen-like substances. Adrenal cortical insufficiency has been related to the use of ethinylestradiol and dimethisterone taken during 1 year. The ascorbic acid content of the anterior pituitary is reduced in the presence of estrogen-induced adenohypophyseal hypertrophy.

Fasting growth hormone concentrations are higher in women using a contraceptive agent than in controls (157).

Oral contraceptives can cause an increase in total thyroxine (158) and a fall in the percentage of free thyroxine (159). The uptake of radioactive iodine in the thyroid is usually normal; total uptake of radioactive iodine may be reduced (159). The effect of progestogens on thyroxine-binding globulin may possibly counteract the estrogenic action. The net result will be a rise in protein-bound iodine and a fall in resin triiodothyronine uptake (160). It has been suggested that oral contraceptives may actually have some protective effect against thyroid disease.

Metabolism

Lipid metabolism

The 1990 report of the International Consensus Development Meeting stated the following regarding the effects of oral contraceptives on carbohydrate and lipid metabolism (19): "All currently used oral contraceptives can cause deterioration in glucose tolerance accompanied by hyperinsulinemia. There is no evidence that the use of combined oral contraceptives is accompanied by overt symptoms of diabetes .... The progestogen component is mainly responsible for the effects of oral contraceptives on carbohydrate metabolism, but the estrogen component may modulate the influence. The magnitude of the impact on glucose metabolism depends on the type of progestogen and also on the doses of a given steroid."

As has become clear since that time, these effects do not run parallel for all oral contraceptives; the third-generation products, which contain either desogestrel or gestodene, have rather different effects, the significance of which is unclear.

Lipid changes seen with the most widely used combined oral contraceptives comprise an increase in low density lipoprotein and reductions in high density lipoprotein and cholesterol. The third-generation products have these effects to a much smaller extent, leading to claims that they would be less likely to have long-term adverse cardiovascular effects related to atherosclerosis. However, such a claim reflects an all too readily adopted belief that the lipid changes produced by the more traditional combined oral contraceptives are in this respect capable of causing this type of (primarily arterial) cardiovascular disease. This is of itself far from certain.

Changes in lipid metabolism among users of progestogen-only contraceptives are minimal. Some studies have shown very small falls in HDL and HDL2 cholesterol, but no effect on other parameters of lipid metabolism. The androgenicity of progestogens parallels their effect on lipoprotein metabolism, but dosage must also be taken into account. For example, although levonorgestrel is more androgenic than norethindrone, its progestational potency is also greater, and levonorgestrel is therefore given in a lower dose for contraceptive purposes; the net result is that there is no clinical difference in lipid effects, as has been shown conclusively (161).

Adolescents with polycystic ovary syndrome are regarded as candidates for long-term combined hormonal treatment using a product of the oral contraceptive type, and there has been some concern about possible unfavorable late metabolic effects, notably on lipids. The risks with two combined products, one based on cyproterone acetate 2 mg and the other on desogestrel 0.15 mg, both with an estrogen, have been estimated in 24 women (95). After 12 months the hirsutism score was improved, but while triglycerides and HDL cholesterol were significantly increased by cyproterone, the only relevant effect of the desogestrel combination was a raised concentration of apolipoprotein A1. The authors concluded that the desogestrel combination was therefore to be preferred in such patients.

Carbohydrate metabolism

Carbohydrate metabolism was known at an early date to be affected by combined oral contraceptives. A mild to moderate degree of insulin resistance was found in some investigations (162,163). However, the considerably impaired glucose tolerance described in some users in the 1960s was directly dose-dependent. Although findings since then have not been entirely consistent (164), it is clear that the low-dose products introduced after the first decade of use had much less marked effects (165), as did the third-generation products based on newer progestogens. The clinical significance of these effects is limited. Even for the second-generation products, no difference was found across the board between ever users and never users in the incidence of diabetes mellitus. Prospective studies in England in 1979 and 1989 (166,167) showed no increased risk of diabetes in oral contraceptive users compared with controls or ex-users. These are, however, population-wide findings, and in some high-risk individuals, the effects on carbohydrate metabolism can be undesirable, with a significant deterioration in glucose tolerance (168); patients with serious or brittle diabetes should therefore not use these forms of contraception (169). It may also be wise to advise other contraceptive methods in women with a history of gestational diabetes, who might possibly be sensitive to these effects of the oral products (170). However, because of the increased risk of pregnancy complications in diabetic women, a highly effective contraceptive method such as the combined oral contraceptive is usually desirable, and it has been reasonably well demonstrated that there is no reason to avoid this type of formulation completely in a woman with stable and well-controlled diabetes. A clinical study of young women with insulin-dependent diabetes mellitus showed no significant differences between women using various combined oral contraceptives (containing up to 50 micrograms of ethinylestradiol) and non-users in hemoglobin A_{1c} concentrations, albumin excretion rates, and diabetic retinopathy (171). Possible very long-term consequences of changes in carbohydrate (and lipid) metabolism are considered further in this record and in connection with the cardiovascular system.

Most studies of carbohydrate metabolism have shown little effect of progestogen-only contraceptives, but there is a suggestion of slight deterioration in glucose tolerance and raised plasma insulin concentrations. Women with diabetes mellitus can generally take progestogen-only contraceptives without a change in insulin requirements.

Body weight

Body weight tends to increase in some women without a clear explanation, although it could be attributable in some individuals to improved appetite, water retention, or conceivably the anabolic effect of an androgenic progestogen. The increase is usually less than 2 kg and occurs during the first 6 months of use. Studies that record weight change over time have generally found similar fluctuations in oral contraceptive users and non-users (137). Cyclic weight gain purely due to fluid retention can also occur.

Nutrition

Alterations in plasma vitamin concentrations have been observed in oral contraceptive users, and attributed to reduced absorption and changes in plasma protein-binding capacity (172).

Vitamin A

While most vitamin concentrations in the blood fall (168), vitamin A concentrations increase, although carotene concentrations fall. Curiously, an isolated report of hypercarotenemia has been published (173).

Vitamin B_6

Alterations in vitamin B_6 metabolism have been discussed, particularly in connection with the suspicion that an oral contraceptive might cause depression. An additional daily intake of pyridoxine has long been suggested as a means of correcting the complex changes observed during use of oral contraceptives (174,175); there are no firm data proving that such medication has any useful effect in most women, but the approach may be tried empirically when mood changes are a problem (176).

Vitamin B_{12}

Vitamin B_{12} deficiency has been seen in healthy oral contraceptive users in whom serum vitamin B_{12} binding proteins were not altered.

Folate

Both sequential and non-sequential types of oral contraceptives impair the absorption of polyglutamic folate but not that of monoglutamic folate; the change can result in megaloblastic anemia in predisposed subjects, for example those with celiac disease or having a deficient diet (177).

Vitamin C

Some studies have suggested that ascorbic acid concentrations are lower in the leukocytes and platelets of oral contraceptive users (178); however, this has not been confirmed (179).

Vitamin D

Studies of the effects of oral contraceptives on serum concentrations of vitamin D derivatives have given variable results.

Wintertime concentrations of 25-hydroxycolecalciferol were measured in 66 young women aged 20–40 years who did and did not use oral contraceptives (180). The initial mean 25-hydroxycolecalciferol concentration in the 26 users was 41% higher than in the 40 non-users before adjustment for age and vitamin D intake (83 versus 59 nmol/l), and 39% higher after adjustment. In five women who stopped taking oral contraceptives during the year after the initial measurement the 25-hydroxycolecalciferol concentrations fell by an average of 26 nmol/l, whereas the concentrations in women whose use or non-use of oral contraceptives was constant did not change. The effect on 25-hydroxycolecalciferol concentrations was not related to the dosage of ethinylestradiol, the type of oral contraceptive, or the duration of use.

However, in another study there was no difference in the concentrations of 25-hydroxycolecalciferol between controls and women who took oral contraceptives containing ethinylestradiol 30–50 micrograms for more than 1 year (181).

The time of year and the point during the menstrual cycle during which vitamin D derivatives are measured may be important. In seven women there was a two-fold rise in the serum concentration of 1,25-dihydroxycolecalciferol on day 15 of the menstrual cycle compared with days 1 and 8, without a detectable change in the serum calcium concentration (182). This increase did not occur in five women taking oral contraceptives, and there was a small but significant fall in the serum calcium concentration.

Mineral balance

Users of oral contraceptives excrete significantly less calcium than non-users (183) and estrogen treatment prevents bone loss in postmenopausal women (184); it is thus likely that the diminished urinary calcium excretion observed in women using oral contraceptives results from suppression of bone resorption by exogenous estrogens. Long-term use of oral contraceptives may therefore affect skeletal bone stores and prevent the development of osteoporosis. In line with these findings is an investigation showing an increase in radio-opacities in the mandibles of women using oral contraceptives (185).

Metal metabolism

Sex hormones can cause changes in metal metabolism, including both increased and reduced plasma zinc concentrations and raised serum copper; however, serum magnesium is not affected (186). The clinical importance of these effects is not known.

Hematologic

Iron status is improved in most oral contraceptive users because of reduced menstrual blood loss; an important benefit of oral contraceptive use is therefore a reduction in the prevalence of iron deficiency anemia (187). Much of the relevant research has been with higher dosages than are currently used. However, a study of a low-dose combined oral contraceptive (ethinylestradiol 30 micrograms plus desogestrel 0.15 mg) documented significantly lower menstrual blood loss than at baseline (188). Most women had normal values of hemoglobin, hematocrit, erythrocyte index, and serum ferritin both before and during oral contraceptive administration, with no significant changes. However, two women who had menorrhagia (defined as menstrual blood loss greater than 80 ml) and low serum ferritin before oral contraceptive use experienced improvement in both of these parameters while taking oral contraceptives. The cyclic variation in serum iron during the menstrual cycle has also been found to be less pronounced during the use of anovulatory agents (189).

The binding capacity of serum proteins is altered by oral contraceptives (190) and leads to alterations in the serum concentrations of various substances, including thyroxine, cortisol, and serum iron (191), and in serum iron binding capacity, which are all increased.

Erythrocyte enzymopathies have rarely been observed during pregnancy and oral contraceptive treatment (192) and in these cases a cause and effect relation seems likely.

Hemostatic variables have been reviewed in women taking oral contraceptives containing desogestrel and gestodene in comparison with oral contraceptives containing levonorgestrel (193). The database of 17 comparative studies was homogeneous. There were no differential effects for coagulation and fibrinolysis parameters, except for factor VII, which was consistently increased by 20% among users of third-generation oral contraceptives than among users of second-generation oral contraceptives. Factor VII is not a risk marker for venous thrombotic disease.

Data from the Leiden Thrombophilia Study have been used to construct a case-control study, based on contraceptive users who had experienced a first episode of objectively proven deep vein thrombosis (97). Patients and controls were considered thrombophilic when they had protein C deficiency, protein S deficiency, antithrombin deficiency, factor V Leiden mutation, or a prothrombin 20210 A mutation. Among healthy women, the risk of developing deep vein thrombosis was trebled in the first 6 months and doubled in the first year of contraceptive use. Among women with thrombophilia, the risk of deep vein thrombosis was increased 19-fold during the first 6 months and 11-fold (95% CI = 2.1, 57) in the first year of use. Venous thrombosis during the first period of oral contraceptive use might actually point to the presence of an inherited clotting defect.

Coagulation factors in users of progestogen-only contraceptives have not been studied extensively using current laboratory methods, but there appears to be little effect. Perhaps the most informative study is a randomized clinical trial of two progestogen-only contraceptives (norethindrone 0.35 mg and levonorgestrel 0.03 mg) (161), which showed a reduction in several coagulation factors among women who switched from a combined oral contraceptive, but no change among women who had not previously been using a hormonal contraceptive. Thus progestogen-only contraceptives appear to be particularly suitable for women who desire oral contraception but who are at increased risk of thrombosis, including older women who are smokers.

Mouth and teeth

Gingivitis, of varying degrees of severity, is sometimes associated with oral contraceptive use, apparently because the steroids alter the microbial flora in the mouth (194). A case of gingival hyperplasia is described under "Reproductive system".

Even a low-dose oral contraceptive combination has an effect on the composition of saliva (195); although large individual variations were noted, protein, sialic acid, hexosamine, fucose, hydrogen ion concentration, and total electrolyte concentration fell, while the secretion rates increased. The sodium and hydrogen ion concentrations increased in parotid gland secretion and sodium in submandibular gland secretion. To what extent these changes might affect the dental status of the patient is unknown.

Oral pyogenic granulomata have been reported both in pregnant patients and in patients using oral contraceptives (196).

Progestogens, alone or together with estrogen, cause an increase in the width and tortuosity of peripheral blood vessels in the oral mucosa, which become more susceptible to local irritants and show increased permeability (197).

Gastrointestinal

Mild gastrointestinal complaints, such as nausea, vomiting and vague abdominal pain, were seen in 10–30% of patients in earlier studies when high-dose products were in use. A placebo-controlled clinical trial in 1971 documented a higher prevalence of nausea and vomiting among combined oral contraceptive users than among women taking either a placebo or a progestogen-only oral contraceptive; the prevalence was also higher for the combined oral contraceptive containing mestranol 100 micrograms than for the combination product containing mestranol 50 micrograms (137). Such effects are much less common with the low doses used today. Nausea, if it occurs, is associated with the estrogen component of combined oral contraceptives; its frequency and severity generally decline over time.

The relation between oral contraceptive use and inflammatory bowel disease was analysed in two case-control studies published in the 1990s (198,199). Both found a significantly increased risk among current users compared with never users for Crohn's disease, but only the former study detected an increased risk of ulcerative colitis; a dose–response effect was suggested for Crohn's disease. When the data were stratified by smoking status in the latter study, the increased risk was found only among current smokers.

Reversible ischemic colitis, an unusual condition in young people, has been described in 17 young women, with evidence for an association with oral contraceptives (200). Ischemic colitis occurs uncommonly in younger people. The median duration of illness was 2.1 days (range 1–4 days). All recovered with supportive care. Ten women (59%) were using low-dose estrogenic oral contraceptive agents, compared with the 1988 US average of 19% oral contraceptive users among women aged 15–44 years. The odds ratio showed a greater than 6-fold relative risk for the occurrence of ischemic colitis among oral contraceptive users.

Diarrhea, probably coincidental, is bound to occur on occasion in the very large population of oral contraceptive users; when it does so, the efficacy of the product is likely to be diminished and additional contraceptive methods may need to be used.

Liver

During the early years of oral contraception, with high-dose products in use, jaundice and other hepatic complications were a source of concern; with current products this is no longer the case. Most women experience no adverse effects on liver function, but occasional hepatic changes can occur, including intrahepatic cholestasis, cholelithiasis, vascular complications, and even tumors, which are discussed in the record on estrogens. It has been argued (37) that women with a history of liver disease whose liver function tests have returned to normal can take oral contraceptives with careful monitoring. However, it is widely considered that oral contraception should be avoided in women with a history of cholestatic jaundice of pregnancy; past or current benign or malignant hepatic tumors; active hepatitis; or familial defects of biliary excretion.

The most common change is a short-term rise in serum transaminases (201), which often abates if treatment is continued. An increase in serum alkaline phosphatase is usual, while serum transaminases can be normal to markedly increased (202). Long-term use leads to changes in hepatic ultrastructure, with involvement of the mitochondria, which develop crystalline inclusions. Furthermore, hypertrophy of the smooth endoplasmic reticulum and changes in the biliary canaliculi have been shown (203,204). These changes are not usually accompanied by any clinical symptoms. The Budd–Chiari syndrome can occur in connection with thromboembolism.

Benign liver tumors (hepatocellular adenoma and focal nodular hyperplasia) are extremely rare conditions that appear to be related to oral contraceptive use (205).

Jaundice as a result of oral contraceptive treatment has been repeatedly described. Whereas in the Swedish population figures between 1:100 and 1:4000 were published when the early high-dose formulations were still in use (206), the overall incidence was estimated in 1979 at about 1:10 000 (9), and the current incidence is certainly further reduced. When such hepatic symptoms occur, they usually do so within the first month of medication (207), and jaundice may be accompanied by anorexia, malaise, and pruritus. Very few cases arise after the third month of medication and those reported are regarded by some as unlikely to be due to oral contraceptives. Microscopic examination of the liver shows intrahepatic cholestasis. When medication is stopped, symptoms usually disappear rapidly and the reaction does not seem to leave any sequelae (208). Genetic components seem to be important for the development of the reaction; women who have experienced jaundice or severe pruritus in late pregnancy seem to be especially susceptible to jaundice or gallbladder disease when using oral contraceptives (209). Discussion of mechanisms has related mostly to estrogens (210), but cases have been described in individuals taking progestogens only (206); the explanation might be the conversion of the latter to estrogens in vivo (211). The cause of cholestasis is unknown, but animal data suggest that there is inhibition of bile flow and of the biliary excretion of bilirubin and bile salts.

Peliosis hepatis has been described in association with contraceptive-induced hepatic tumors and has sometimes developed in isolation, perhaps as a herald of more serious changes to follow, for example cirrhosis and portal hypertension; one such case ultimately required an orthotopic liver transplant (212).

Sinusoidal dilatation in the liver has been reported rarely.

- A 23-year-old woman developed an acute painful syndrome with cytolysis after 7 years of oral contraceptive use; she recovered promptly after oral contraceptive withdrawal (213).

Hepatic adenomatosis, which seems to have been reported only some 38 times, is a condition with a female preponderance; in earlier work it was noted that in 46% of the female patients oral contraception had been used. This means, however, that in the other 54% it had not, and it should be borne in mind that the condition can also occur in men.

- A 35-year-old woman, who had been fitted with Norplant 2 years before and had used oral contraceptives for some 20 years before that, developed epigastric and right upper quadrant abdominal pain (214). A liver mass was found and at surgery proved to consist of multiple adenomata; part of the liver had to be resected.

What is of potential concern is that in this case, as in a very few previously described, there was also evidence of hepatocellular dysplasia, which could be a pre-malignant condition. However, with widespread use of Norplant, some reported adverse events, such as this, may be purely coincidental.

Results in 1977 from the Boston Collaborative Drug Surveillance Program suggested that oral contraceptive users are more often diagnosed as having acute hepatitis than are non-users (215). There was no similar finding in the similarly early study by the UK Royal College of General Practitioners (135).

Biliary tract

The Boston Collaborative Drug Surveillance Program found in 1973 that of a large series of 212 patients with gallbladder disease 31% were using oral contraceptives, compared with only 20% of controls (216). In another study, the risk of gallbladder surgery was twice as high in oral contraceptive users as in non-users (217). A decade later, after dosages had fallen, a 1982 study from the UK Royal College of General Practitioners showed that there was no overall increased risk of gallbladder disease in the long term and that the previously demonstrated short-term increase in risk is due to acceleration of the onset of gallbladder disease in women already susceptible to it (135). The risk may also be age-related, the relative risk of gallstone disease being higher in young women using oral contraceptives than in older users (218–220).

- A 21-year-old woman developed increasing jaundice, with severe pruritus and weight loss, after a bout of dyspepsia (221). She had been taking contraceptives for 4 years (cyproterone acetate 2 mg, ethinylestradiol 0.035 mg). Laboratory tests at first suggested cholestatic hepatitis, but ultrasonography showed biliary sludge in the gallbladder and dilatation of the common bile duct and the smaller biliary passages. There was a space-occupying lesion near the papilla: it was not fixed and had no vascular supply. At endoscopic retrograde cholangiopancreatography the lesion was removed. It consisted of jelly-like viscous streaky bile without calculi. Within a few days the jaundice disappeared, the pruritus ceased, and liver function returned to normal.

A meta-analysis in 1993 of the relation between combined oral contraceptives and gallbladder disease yielded a small increased risk for women who had ever used oral contraceptives (pooled estimated RR = 1.38) (222). There was a dose-related effect in the therapeutic range of doses, suggesting that, although the risk is less with lower-dose combined oral contraceptives, there may still be a weak relation. The increased risk appears to be concentrated in the early years of oral contraceptive use, suggesting that oral contraceptives accelerate the development of the disease. On the other hand, the 1994 findings in the Nurses' Health Study II showed no substantial increase in risk associated with ever use of oral contraceptives, but relative risks of 1.6 for long-term use and for current use, after adjusting for body mass index and several other confounding variables (218). A 1994 report from the Oxford FPA study similarly suggested no relation with ever use of oral contraceptives (223).

The finding that oral contraceptive use causes an increase in the cholesterol concentration in bile and a shift in the chenodeoxycholic/cholic acid ratio suggests a biochemical basis for the increase in gallbladder disease among oral contraceptive users (224,225). Effects on gallstone formation may well be due to the estrogen content, for example since exogenous estrogens seem to increase the risk of gallbladder disease in men (226), while in women they can increase the cholesterol saturation of bile and hence the lithogenic index (227).

Pancreas

Acute pancreatitis has been reported as a very unusual complication of oral contraceptive treatment (228), as have increases in serum amylase (229).

Urinary tract

Over the years a few reports have suggested a higher incidence of urinary infections in users of oral contraceptives, but this probably reflected differing or altered patterns of sexual behavior.

Hemolytic–uremic syndrome seen in one very long-term user may have been due to antisteroid hormone antibodies (230).

Skin

Various types of skin reactions can occur during oral contraceptive treatment, but bearing in mind the vast number of women who take oral contraceptives, major skin reactions due to oral contraceptive treatment seem to be rare. The incidence, even including all minor complications, has been estimated at 5% (231), but field experience suggests that that is a generous figure. The figure includes chloasma, seborrhea, hirsutism, pruritus, herpes gestationis, porphyria cutanea tarda, and allergic reactions such as urticaria.

Low-dose combined oral contraceptive use generally results in improvement of acne, although occasionally a user has worsening of acne owing to the androgenic potency of the progestin used. Use of a less androgenic progestogen, for example norgestimate (232) or desogestrel or the antiandrogen cyproterone acetate (233,234), can have a favorable effect in patients with pre-existing acne, reducing the severity of the condition; an oral contraceptive in which cyproterone acetate replaces the progestogen has proved helpful in women with pre-existing acne.

The efficacy and adverse effects of oral cyproterone acetate 2 mg in combination with ethinylestradiol 35 micrograms in facial acne tarda have been studied in 890 women aged 15–50 years, of whom 96 withdrew prematurely from the study (235). Of these 96 women, only 30 withdrew because of adverse events: menstrual problems ($n = 11$), headache ($n = 10$), increased body weight ($n = 3$), and thrombophlebitis ($n = 1$). Five women withdrew because of poor efficacy. In all, 260 patients had adverse events during treatment. The incidence fell as the study progressed. Of those events that first occurred during treatment, the most frequently cited were breast tension (12%), headache (8.9%), nausea (5.8%), nervousness (4.0%), and dizziness (2.6%). There were no serious adverse events. There were no clinical significant changes in body weight or blood pressure.

There is a possible association of oral contraceptives with erythema nodosum, which has been linked to the use of either estrogens or progestogens or a combination of the two; however, probably neither hormone directly causes the condition but merely creates a fertile background for its generation by other antigens.

Pre-existing condyloma acuminata have been stated to increase during oral contraception, with regression after withdrawal (236).

Increased pigmentation of areas exposed to sunlight, as well as photosensitivity, has been incidentally observed in some users, and is probably analogous to the pigment changes that can occur in pregnancy.

In one case, pityriasis lichenoides disappeared after withdrawal of oral contraceptives (237).

Sweet's syndrome (acute febrile neutrophilic dermatosis) has been attributed to an oral contraceptive (238). However, bearing in mind that the syndrome has a variable presentation and is thought to represent a form of hypersensitivity reaction, it is not at all clear that there was a true cause-and-effect relation.

Hair

Contraceptives induce a condition of pseudopregnancy, and alopecia during treatment and after withdrawal has been seen. Of five women who developed diffuse alopecia while taking oral contraceptives, three had male pattern baldness while they were taking the treatment; two began to lose their hair after having stopped taking treatment, and these resembled postpartum baldness (239). One woman did not regain her hair 20 months after having stopped taking the oral contraceptive. However, the incidence of alopecia among users of oral contraceptives is very low, and the association may be coincidental, since there are also case reports of improvement in the quality of the hair (240).

Musculoskeletal

Although some studies have shown that combined oral contraceptives increase bone mineral density, the available evidence suggests that any beneficial effect is rather small (241), and is presumably related to the dosage of estrogen. The effects may depend in part on the age of women being studied, as normally bone mass density continues to increase until it peaks in women in their 20s and 30s, and then remains constant until the premenopausal period, when it begins to fall. For example, a study of young women (aged 19–22 years) showed that those taking very low-dose combined oral contraceptives (with as little as 20 micrograms of ethinylestradiol) had no change in bone density over 5 years, whereas non-users had a significant increase (242).

There were some early reports of localized mandibular osteitis in women using oral contraceptives subsequent to surgery of the mandibular molar teeth (SEDA-2, 316). It has been suggested that changes in the hemostasis could be the cause.

It appears that oral contraceptive use reduces the prevalence of severe disabling rheumatoid arthritis. Although studies of this have produced discrepant results, a meta-analysis of studies that met specific methodological criteria produced an overall adjusted pooled odds ratio of 0.73 (243). The authors suggested that oral contraceptives do not actually prevent rheumatoid arthritis, but modify the disease process to prevent progression to severe disease. Pregnancy has similar effects. It is unclear whether it is the estrogen or the progestogen component of oral contraceptives that is responsible.

Sexual function

Occasionally, women report reduced libido, which may have a hormonal basis. One study showed that users of oral contraceptives had no rise in female-initiated sexual activity at the time when ovulation should have occurred, whereas non-users did show such an increase in sexual activity (244).

Reproductive system

Tumor-inducing effects of hormonal contraceptives are dealt with in the record on estrogens.

Breasts

Breast tenderness or pain can occur in some women (245,246), especially with estrogen-dominant formulations, although it is notable that other women with a history of breast discomfort experience improvement when they begin to take oral contraceptives.

- A woman with Wilson's disease treated with penicillamine developed severe hirsutism (247). After treatment with oral contraceptives, her breasts enlarged rapidly, and she had cyclic mastodynia. Around the same time she also developed gingival hyperplasia.

Benign breast disease (including fibroadenoma and cystic change) is less common among users of combined oral contraceptive than in the general population (205).

Ovaries

Women currently taking oral contraceptives are less likely than non-users to have functional ovarian cysts. This protective effect appears to be more modest with lower dose monophasic formulations than with those containing 35 micrograms or more of estrogen (248,249). Functional ovarian cysts (or persistent ovarian follicles) occur more often in users of progestogen-only contraceptives than in combined oral contraceptive users or in women using no hormonal contraceptive method. Follicular development is delayed and the follicle continues to grow for a period of time, but these enlarged follicles usually regress spontaneously and are not of clinical significance.

Uterus

Effects on menstrual function depend on the dose used and the sensitivity of the individual user; they may be welcome or unwelcome (188,250). Menses generally become more regular and predictable, and dysmenorrhea is less common and less severe. The number of days of blood loss in each menstrual period is often reduced, as is the amount of menstrual flow; thus women who previously had iron deficiency anemia associated with menorrhagia have increased iron stores. A comparison of women who kept menstrual diary records as part of WHO trials has confirmed that users of combined oral contraceptives in adequate dosages have more regular menstrual cycles than do users of other hormonal methods (251). None of the combined oral contraceptive users in these studies had amenorrhea (defined as the absence of bleeding throughout a 90-day reference period), although shorter periods of amenorrhea have occasionally been reported in other studies, particularly with very low-dosage formulations and with longer-term use.

Intermenstrual bleeding (breakthrough bleeding or spotting) often occurs, especially during the first few cycles of treatment, and is often the reason that women choose to stop taking an oral contraceptive. When using products based on newer progestogens it seems that better control may be offered by formulations that contain gestodene compared with desogestrel and by levonorgestrel compared with norethindrone (252), but the absence of standardized methods makes such conclusions tentative. Research on triphasic formulations is too sparse to allow firm conclusions on this point. One study confirmed the long-standing experience that intermenstrual bleeding rates vary inversely with both estrogen and progestogen dose (253). However, one finds no evidence that breakthrough bleeding is an indication of reduced contraceptive efficacy, despite speculation regarding a possible relation.

Dysmenorrhea is less common and less severe among women who use oral contraceptives of any type, provided that ovulation is inhibited; this emerges both from experience and from prospective studies; the effect seems to be maintained as long as the oral contraceptive is continued. There seem to be no significant differences in this respect between monophasic products with low or high progestogen doses, those with high progestogen doses, or triphasic products (250).

Since post-treatment amenorrhea of more than 6 months duration was first suggested as an adverse reaction in around 1965, much work has been devoted to delineating the risk and prognosis of menstrual changes after the withdrawal of hormonal contraception. It is now recognized that post-treatment amenorrhea occurs in 0.7–0.8% of women, but this is no different from the background rate of spontaneous secondary amenorrhea. No cause and effect relation between oral contraceptive use and subsequent amenorrhea has been documented.

Menstrual irregularities are common among women taking progestogen-only contraceptives and are often the reason a user chooses to discontinue the method (254,255). Users of progestogen-only contraceptives are more likely than users of other hormonal contraceptive methods to have frequent bleeding (251). Infrequent bleeding, amenorrhea, and irregular bleeding among progestogen-only contraceptive users are more likely than among combined oral contraceptive users, but less prominent than among women using levonorgestrel-releasing vaginal rings or DMPA.

There has been concern at various times that prolonged oral contraception might cause permanent changes in the genital system. When high-dose products were in use, various studies showed condensation of the superficial cortical layers of the ovary (SEDA-8, 863). Severe atrophy of the endometrium after a period of oral contraception has been described (256), but the report usually quoted is one that dates from a period when high doses were in use, and the incidence is not known, since the endometrium is not usually examined. Certainly, the endometrium will go into a resting phase in women who have amenorrhea, but there is no reason to believe that it will become permanently unresponsive.

Epidemiological studies of the relation between oral contraceptive use and pelvic endometriosis have variously shown an increased risk, a reduced risk, and no effect (257). For example, an Italian study showed an increased risk among ever users of oral contraceptives, but this increase occurred only among former users, not current users (258). Furthermore, the authors noted that a similar pattern had been shown in several large cohort studies (OFPA, RCGP, and Walnut Creek). There was no association in the Italian study with recency, latency, or duration of use, suggesting that any relation to oral contraceptive use is not a true biological relation but instead the result of selection and other biases.

Pelvic inflammatory disease, often resulting in infertility, ectopic pregnancy, or chronic pelvic pain, is a well-known pathological state that actually occurs at a somewhat lower incidence in oral contraceptive users and also tends to be less severe in these women compared with non-users (259–261). The biological mechanism for this protective effect may be the changes in cervical mucus or reduced menstrual bleeding (and thus reduced retrograde menstrual blood in the uterus). On the other hand, the relevant reviews have concluded that combined oral contraceptives provide no protection against lower reproductive tract infection (particularly cervical infections with *Chlamydia* or gonococcus) and may even have an adverse effect. This possible increased risk appears to be the result of an increase in the area of cervical ectropion associated with the estrogen in combined oral contraceptives.

Candidiasis of the vagina in oral contraceptive users without evidence of diabetes mellitus has often been reported.

Immunologic

There is a sex difference in immune responsiveness, but little attention has been paid to the possible role played by sex hormones in its regulation. This lack of insight has led to the question of whether the use of oral contraceptives might affect the immune response, for better or for worse. An authoritative review of the immunological effects of estrogens and progestogens has concluded that, although understanding of any effect is incomplete, it is not likely that the low doses used in oral contraceptives would have negative effects on the immune system (262).

If that is the case, there must be another explanation for periodic reports that suggest an increased risk of systemic infections in oral contraceptive users. In a 1974 study by the British Royal College of General Practitioners oral contraceptive users had a higher than average incidence of certain infectious diseases (135).

Support for the concept that oral contraceptives might increase the risk of infection has been presented in other studies, and workers in the tropics have remarked that pregnant women appear to be unduly sensitive to malarial infestation (WHO, unpublished data).

The antibody response to tetanus toxoid in women is considerably lower in oral contraceptive users than in controls (263).

A depressed lymphocyte response to phytohemagglutinin has been observed in a series of women taking oral contraceptives (264); the reduction in phytohemagglutinin response reflects impaired T cell function, and this finding is of interest in view of the fact that a deficiency of T cell function is important in certain autoimmune diseases. Another consequence of prolonged impairment of T cell function would be an increased susceptibility to infectious diseases.

There have been several studies of the effect of sex hormones on serum immunoglobulin titers. In a study of the effect of four different oral contraceptives on the serum concentration of IgA, IgG, and IgM, the concentrations of all three immunoglobulins fell during the first course of treatment and returned to normal during subsequent cycles (265). There was some evidence that the steroid-induced reduction in immunoglobulins was predominantly caused by the estrogenic component. Subsequently, a study was conducted in which plasma from women currently taking combined oral contraceptives, past users of such products, women who had never used them, and non-users with a history of venous thrombosis was examined for the presence of immunoglobulin G (IgG) that showed specific binding of ethinylestradiol (266). There was no increase in "specific" IgG and no evidence of ethinylestradiol binding in oral contraceptive users compared with non-users. This study therefore provided no support for the hypothesis that a significant percentage of oral contraceptive users develop a specific IgG with high binding affinity for ethinylestradiol, which might be causally linked to the development of thrombotic phenomena in oral contraceptive users.

Numerous case reports have suggested that combined oral contraceptives can cause systemic lupus erythematosus (144,267). However, systematic examination of this issue in a 1994 case-control study showed no association (268).

Aggravation of bronchial asthma, eczema, rashes, angioedema, and vasomotor rhinitis have been incidentally observed, and cold urticaria has been reported in women taking oral contraceptives (269). It is not known whether in any particular individual the hypersensitivity reaction is due to the hormones themselves or to other ingredients in the tablet. Nasal provocation tests with suspensions of contraceptive steroids in patients with allergic rhinitis or pollinosis who had been taking these products showed a positive response in one-third of cases; the same patients also reacted to topical estrogens (270). Life-threatening anaphylaxis with a positive rechallenge test occurred in a young woman using oral contraceptives, but this must be extraordinarily rare (271).

The immunological effects of two contraceptive combinations, namely Valette (ethinylestradiol 0.03 mg + dienogest 2.0 mg) and Lovelle (ethinylestradiol 0.02 mg + desogestrel 0.15 mg), have been examined during one treatment cycle (272). The latter significantly increased the numbers of lymphocytes, monocytes, and granulocytes. Valette reduced the CD4 lymphocyte count after 10 days and Lovelle did the opposite. Lovelle increased CD19 and CD23 cell counts after 21 days. Phagocytic activity was unaffected by either treatment. After 10 days, both contraceptives reduced the serum concentrations of IgA, IgG, and IgM, which remained low at day 21 with Lovelle but returned to baseline with Valette. Secretory IgA was unaffected by either contraceptive. Neither treatment affected concentrations of interleukins, except for a significant difference between the treatment groups in interleukin-6 after 10 days, which resolved after 21 days. Concentrations of non-immunoglobulin serum components fluctuated; macroglobulin was increased by Valette. However, total protein and albumin concentrations were reduced more by Lovelle than Valette. Complement factors also fluctuated. There was no evidence of sustained immunosuppression with either Valette or Lovelle.

Infection risk

Data on the risk of infection with HIV (human immunodeficiency virus) with combined oral contraceptives are sparse; some studies suggest an adverse effect and others show no association (259,273).

Body temperature

Body temperature tends to rise slightly in some users of oral contraceptives (274,275) Progesterone has a mild thermogenic effect, reflected in changes in body temperature during the normal menstrual cycle. Mild pyrexia in users of oral contraceptives may reflect this, but the patient should always be examined to exclude infection.

Long-Term Effects

Drug abuse

Children under 6 years who have accidentally ingested oral contraceptives have experienced nausea and vomiting for 10–15 hours after ingestion (SEDA-1, 306). Occasionally, apathy, drowsiness, and slight increases in transaminase activities have been reported.

Drug withdrawal

Although it was originally believed that women who stopped taking oral contraceptives, particularly after a long period of use, were more likely to have amenorrhea, careful analysis has shown that that is not the case. The likelihood of conception is reduced during the first 1–2 months after discontinuation, but cumulative conception rates after several months are not affected.

Tumorigenicity

The carcinogenic effects of oral contraceptives are covered in the monograph on estrogens.

Second-Generation Effects

Fertility

The return of fertility after a period of oral contraception has been differently assessed at different times. Although there can be a delay of 1–2 months in the return of fertility after withdrawal of a combined oral contraceptive, within a few months conception rates are similar to those of women who stop using non-hormonal contraception (41,276,277). In 48 patients classified as having amenorrhea after oral contraceptive use the subsequent conception rate was no lower than in a control group not with amenorrhea (278). There appears to be a shorter delay with low-dose than high-dose products (279). Delay in the return of ovulation has on occasion led to the erroneous conclusion that the first pregnancy after oral contraceptive use might be unduly prolonged (SEDA-6, 351).

There does not appear to be any clinically significant delay in return of fertility after discontinuation of progestogen-only contraceptives. Although there have been no large studies, data from several small studies suggest no effect. Furthermore, because progestogen-only contraceptives prevent ovulation in only about half of cycles, and because the pregnancy prevention effects fall rapidly if a tablet is taken late, the normal reproductive physiology presumably returns quickly after tablet discontinuation.

Pregnancy

The likelihood of ectopic pregnancy in women taking oral contraceptives has to be set against the normal incidence in the population, taking care to use the same denominator; one can express it as the proportion of women who experience such an event, or as the proportion of pregnancies that occur and prove to be ectopic (280). The proportion of pregnancies that implant at an extrauterine site is 0.005 for both combined oral contraceptive users and women using no contraception, but, because oral contraceptive users are much less likely to conceive, their rate of ectopic pregnancy is much lower (0.005 per 1000 woman years, compared with 2.6 per 1000 woman years for women using no contraception). The incidence of ectopic pregnancies is also somewhat lower for combined oral contraceptives than for other contraceptive methods. In the past there was some concern about a possible increased risk of ectopic gestation after withdrawal of oral contraceptives (281), but this is no longer considered to be an issue.

Up to 10% of pregnancies among users of progestogen-only contraceptives implant outside the uterus; this is not greatly different to the ectopic pregnancy rate in unprotected women, but it is much higher than among users of adequate combined oral contraception (280). The reasons may relate to changes in tubal motility and delay in ovum transport.

Teratogenicity

Oral contraceptives are neither teratogenic nor mutagenic, and there is little concern about the risk of congenital anomalies if an oral contraceptive is accidentally taken during an early unrecognized pregnancy. The American College of Obstetrics and Gynecology concluded in 1993 that there was no causal link (282). Reviews have come to the same conclusion (283,284), as has a meta-analysis completed in 1995 (285). In theory the androgenicity of a progestogen could result in virilization, but it is most unlikely to be taken sufficiently late or in sufficiently high doses to have this effect.

Gene toxicity

The fear that oral contraceptives might prove to induce chromosomal abnormalities was expressed when they were relatively new, but has largely been laid to rest. When aborted fetuses from women who used oral contraceptives were compared with those from non-users, there was no difference in the frequency of abnormal karyotypes or in sex ratio between the two groups. Certainly, data have been presented showing a slightly raised frequency of minor chromosomal changes in children whose mothers had been exposed to oral contraceptives before pregnancy, but from a genetic point of view, these scattered findings are not alarming.

Sex of the offspring

There was early minor evidence that the use of oral contraceptives might result in a predominance of female births (286). However, later evidence has been indecisive (287,288). If there is any effect at all it must be extremely small.

Congenital anomalies

A number of early American studies appeared to show that children exposed in utero to oral contraceptives ran a slightly increased risk of being born with certain types of birth defects; in particular a syndrome was described comprising multiple malformations involving the vertebrae, anus, cardiac structures, trachea, esophagus, renal structures and limbs (abbreviated to VACTERL) (289). The entire VACTERL syndrome was in fact seldom or never encountered; clusters of defects falling within this group were seen, but the associations were very variable. Furthermore, virilization of the female fetus and some of the other elements in the VACTERL group have been described after exposure to certain progestogens, hormonal pregnancy tests, or (rarely) to oral contraceptives taken in error in early pregnancy.

In a 1983 retrospective study of 155 children with congenital limb reductions 18 mothers (12%) were found to have taken oral contraceptives inadvertently during early pregnancy compared with only one mother in a control group, a relative risk of 24; adjustment for smoking hardly altered the figure (289). However, other work has suggested that smoking carries a higher risk of malformations than the use of oral contraceptives (SED-12, 1022) (290).

The results of such studies have led some reviewers to conclude that oral contraceptives are slightly teratogenic, but caution is needed. The conclusion of the 1980 WHO report cited above that such an effect is slight or absent probably remains valid for all widely used oral contraceptives; naturally, newer products might have other effects.

Congenital malformations may occur after the use of hormonal (estrogen + progestogen) pregnancy tests, now obsolete, since these high doses of a hormonal combination represented aggressive interference with any early pregnancy. A 1967 report suggested some association with meningomyelocele or hydrocephalus, and later retrospective studies provided some evidence of cardiac defects or limb reduction anomalies. Such studies always raise methodological doubts, but it is not unthinkable that these tests were harmful, since they sometimes induced bleeding even in early pregnancy; they could thus impair embryonic nutrition.

Lactation

The effects of combined oral contraceptives on lactation have been examined carefully (291,292), since estrogens are well-known inhibitors of ovulation in large doses. Even products containing 30 micrograms of ethinylestradiol reduce the volume of milk (293); the composition of the milk is also slightly altered, but again one has the impression that the effect is not important, except in a very poorly nourished population. Both progestogens and estrogens are excreted in the milk, their proportions correlating with those in plasma, but the absolute concentrations are lower. The plasma/milk ratio varies from compound to compound, probably owing to variations in the degree of protein binding and (for progestogens) also to the variable amount of fat in the milk. The amount of steroid transferred in 600 ml of milk is estimated at 0.1% or less of the daily dose taken. Although newborn infants might be relatively sensitive to these hormonal substances, because of the immaturity of their detoxification systems, no adverse effects have been found when they were looked for systematically; nevertheless, isolated cases of gynecomastia have been noted in babies when their mothers were taking oral contraceptives during lactation.

In an 8-year follow-up of Swedish children whose mothers used combined oral contraceptives while breastfeeding, there were no negative effects on health, growth, or development (294). It should be realized that the hormonal content of natural human milk and cows' milk is not negligible. If hormonal contraception is to be used during lactation, it would be sensible to prefer low-dose progestogens rather than combinations with estrogens; they are not the most effective contraceptives, but probably sufficient to supplement the contraceptive effect of lactation itself and they are unlikely to inhibit lactation.

There is much evidence that progestogen-only contraceptives (including tablets, injectables, and implants) have no adverse effects on milk production (295); they reach the milk in negligible amounts and have no adverse effects on the breast-fed infant (296).

Susceptibility Factors

There are no hard and fast rules about prescribing oral contraceptives in women at risk of complications; the degree of risk resulting from a particular factor has to be considered from case to case.

Absolute contraindications

Combined oral contraceptives should not be used by women with the following absolute contraindications:

1. thrombophlebitis or venous thromboembolic disorders (current or past)
2. cerebrovascular disease (current or past)
3. coronary artery or ischemic heart disease (current or past)
4. breast cancer (current or past)
5. endometrial cancer or other estrogen-dependent neoplasia (current or past)
6. hepatic adenoma or carcinoma (current or past)
7. impaired liver function (current)
8. less than 2 weeks postpartum
9. breastfeeding and less than 6 weeks postpartum
10. known or suspected pregnancy
11. use of enzyme-inducing drugs, specifically the antimicrobial drugs rifampicin and griseofulvin and many anticonvulsants.

Relative contraindications

Combined oral contraceptives should be used only with caution and careful monitoring by women with the following relative contraindications:

1. aged over 35 years and/or obese and/or currently smoking 15 or more cigarettes per day; when all three factors are present this can be regarded as an absolute contraindication
2. migraine, particularly with focal neurological symptoms
3. hypertension (current, controlled)
4. diabetes, particularly with retinopathy, neuropathy, or vascular disease
5. familial hyperlipidemia or current treatment for hyperlipidemia
6. gallbladder disease (current)
7. cholestatic jaundice of pregnancy or with prior oral contraceptive use
8. unexplained abnormal vaginal bleeding
9. breastfeeding, particularly if less than 6 months postpartum
10. major surgery, with prolonged immobility.

Although sickle cell disease is sometimes listed as a contraindication to oral contraceptive use, it has been suggested that this may not be justified (297). Women with sickle cell disease need highly effective contraception, because pregnancy is associated with increased morbidity and mortality to both mother and fetus, as well as the increased likelihood that the infant will have sickle cell disease. Theoretically, combined oral contraceptives should be given with caution, because of the increased risk of thrombosis associated with both sickle cell disease and combined oral contraceptives, but the limited available evidence indicates no change in hematological parameters among women using hormonal contraceptives. Progestogen-only formulations may be preferred, not only to avoid the potential risk of thrombosis but also because studies suggest that sickle cell crises may be inhibited.

The Oxford Family Planning Association's continuing study has shown convincingly that death from all causes is more than doubled in oral contraceptive users who smoke 15 or more cigarettes daily (298).

Drug Administration

Drug formulations

Low-dose oral contraceptives based on the older progestogens are relatively well tolerated in the short term, better so than the products that preceded them and those that came later. Two placebo-controlled studies with the combination of levonorgestrel 100 micrograms and ethinylestradiol in 704 patients over six cycles showed no differences in unwanted effects compared with placebo; in particular there was no evidence of weight gain (299).

Drug dosage regimens

Different schemes of administration have been studied and compared with one another without identifying any pattern of use that is ideal for all women. Various sequential programs of use, intended to mimic more closely the physiological changes in hormone secretion during the normal cycle rather than using a fixed combination throughout, have given better cycle control in some women, but others react better to the traditional pattern, in which the same combination is used throughout the 20-day period of use. The normophasic formulations use a popular sequential scheme; in these products the seven first tablets contain only estrogen and the next 14 tablets both estrogen and progestogen, giving an endometrium of a more normal secretory phase type; this in turn leads to more pronounced withdrawal bleeding. A further development of this principle, the triphasic type of product, involves administering a three-step regimen, in which the change from estrogenic to progestogenic dominance is more gradual; it appears to be helpful in avoiding excessive intermenstrual bleeding when this has been a problem, and it is apparently less likely than monophasic products to cause an unwanted reduction in HDL cholesterol (300). However, there is evidence that triphasic formulations based on norgestrel could carry the same increased risk of thromboembolic disorders as that seen with the third-generation oral contraceptives, because of a higher resistance to activated protein C than with the corresponding monophasic products (301).

In the "estrophasic" form of administration, ethinylestradiol 20 micrograms is given on days 1–5 of the cycle, 30 micrograms on days 6–12, and 35 micrograms on days 13–21. Norethisterone acetate 1 mg is also given throughout this period. The literature to date has not shown that this regimen, although claimed to be more "physiological" in its composition, is in fact better tolerated than a comparable combination in which ethinylestradiol is given in a dose of 30 micrograms throughout (302). However, the reduction in what may at some phases of the cycle be an unnecessarily high estrogen dose, that is more than is needed to maintain cycle control, is a healthy step, and it may be useful to have a further alternative product for women who do not find any existing formulation fully satisfactory.

There is continued interest in natural 17-β-estradiol in a form suitable for oral use, in view of the likelihood that it will produce fewer adverse effects than the synthetic estrogens used in most oral contraceptives. The particular problem has been to secure adequate cycle control with 17-β-estradiol, which is rapidly metabolized to estrone in the intestinal wall and liver; the degradation process is actually accelerated by progestogens. One approach under development in Germany involves combining this estrogen with dienogest, a progestogen that is reported to have no antiestrogenic activity (303). Preliminary work suggests that this can be successful, but one must be cautious in assuming that the end-product will be safer in all respects. There is evidence of a lesser effect of the natural estrogen on fibrinolysis, liver function, and lipid metabolism, but one must bear in mind that the true incidence of thromboembolic and other complications of the existing oral contraceptives is only now emerging after many years of worldwide use.

Drug–Drug Interactions

General

Two categories of drug interactions have been reported with oral contraceptives (304).

Interactions in which other drugs influence the effects of contraceptive steroids

The best known interactions are those in which another drug impairs the effect of the contraceptive steroids, leading to breakthrough bleeding and even pregnancy; such interactions are due primarily (but not exclusively) to enzyme induction, resulting in accelerated breakdown of the contraceptive steroids (305). This is a greater problem today than it was when higher-dose contraceptives with a larger reserve of contraceptive potency were in use. Many reported interactions of this type are single cases, and in some such instances it is likely that contraceptive failure was in fact due to poor adherence to therapy, diarrhea, or vomiting, rather than a direct interaction (306). However, with at least the enzyme-inducing anticonvulsants and rifampicin there are well-established major interactions.

In a few cases the activity of oral contraceptives is enhanced by other drugs; this is less likely to cause problems, but if the effect is very marked or prolonged one might suffer the consequences of hyperestrogenicity (306).

Interactions in which oral contraceptives interfere with the metabolism of other drugs

Studies in animals and in vitro studies in human liver microsomes have shown that oral contraceptives can inhibit the metabolism of other drugs that undergo various forms of oxidative metabolism. In contrast, oral contraceptives seem to induce glucuronidation. For example, oral contraceptives reduce the clearance of aminophenazone (aminopyrine) (307), phenazone (antipyrine) (308,309), and pethidine (310). It has been suggested that the estrogenic component of oral contraceptives is necessary for inhibition of drug oxidation, since women taking progestogens alone had a normal clearance of phenazone, whereas those taking a combination tablet had impaired elimination of phenazone (311). However, such interactions are rarely of clinical significance.

Alcohol

Women taking oral contraceptives have a significant fall in the absolute elimination rate of ethanol (105 mg/kg/hour) compared with controls (121 mg/kg/hour). The percentage elimination rate of ethanol is also significantly reduced in women taking oral contraceptives (0.015% per hour) compared with control subjects (0.019% per hour). These results are consistent during the three phases of the menstrual cycle and when body leanness is taken into consideration (312).

Antacids

Antacids apparently do not affect the systemic availability of oral contraceptives, but since magnesium-containing antacids can cause diarrhea, they might reduce absorption of contraceptive steroids.

Anticoagulants

Oral contraceptives have been reported to reduce the effect of anticoagulants, probably because oral contraceptives have an antagonistic effect on certain clotting factors, although they potentiate the action of acenocoumarol (SEDA-5, 371).

One study showed a significant increase in the clearance of phenprocoumon, owing to accelerated glucuronidation. As phenprocoumon is metabolized by hydroxylation as well as by direct glucuronidation, the increased clearance may mean that induction of the latter process over-rides inhibition of the former (313).

Antiepileptic drugs

Enzyme inducers

Failure of contraceptive therapy and breakthrough bleeding have been noted repeatedly in patients concurrently taking various enzyme-inducing anticonvulsant drugs (305,314). These include phenytoin, primidone, ethosuximide, phenobarbital, and carbamazepine. The specific isozyme responsible for metabolic 2-hydroxylation of ethinylestradiol is CYP3A4, which is induced by anticonvulsants (304). However, in addition to enzyme induction, the anticonvulsants can increase the binding of sex hormone- binding globulin. Since sex steroids bind with high affinity to sex hormone-binding globulin and since phenobarbital increases sex hormone-binding globulin capacity, unbound active steroid concentrations will tend to fall during treatment with phenobarbital (315). In addition, in animals, phenobarbital increases steroid metabolism in both the gut wall and liver (316).

The newer anticonvulsants have not been studied as intensively as the older drugs, but felbamate, oxcarbazepine, and topiramate have enzyme-inducing activity and reduce plasma steroid concentrations (317).

Non-enzyme inducers

Valproic acid, which is not an enzyme inducer, has no detectable effect on the pharmacokinetics of progestogens and estrogens (318).

The newer anticonvulsants have not been studied as intensively as the older drugs as regards the possibility of interference with the effects of oral contraceptives. The available data suggest that women taking oral contraceptives can also take gabapentin, lamotrigine, tiagabine, and vigabatrin without significant pharmacokinetic interactions; the effect of zonisamide is uncertain (313).

Management

The use of an alternative contraceptive method has long been advised in women taking antiepileptic drugs, unless they can be treated with the traditional high-dose oral products, for example containing 80–100 micrograms of estradiol (314); for effective protection they may also need a shortened tablet-free interval. A fair test is to see whether a woman taking oral contraceptives and anticonvulsants has adequate cycle control; if not, for example if there is mid-cycle spotting, this is a sign of interference and an alternative method will certainly be advisable.

Ascorbic acid

Ascorbic acid (vitamin C) is extensively sulfated in the gastrointestinal mucosa and competes with ethinylestradiol, which is also extensively sulfated. Plasma ethinylestradiol concentrations are increased by ascorbic acid in women, both after a single dose of ethinylestradiol and during long-term oral contraceptive use, but the results are not consistent. On one occasion it was claimed that this effectively transformed a low-dose oral contraceptive into a high-dose formulation (319). It seems very dubious whether ascorbic acid in fact interferes significantly with the effects of oral contraceptives.

Benzodiazepines

Oral contraceptives alter the metabolism of some benzodiazepines that undergo oxidation (chlordiazepoxide, alprazolam, diazepam) or nitroreduction (nitrazepam) (320). Oral contraceptives inhibit enzyme activity and reduce the clearances of these drugs. There is nevertheless no evidence that these interactions are of clinical importance. For other benzodiazepines that undergo oxidative metabolism, such as bromazepam and clotiazepam, no change has ever been found in oral contraceptive users.

Some other benzodiazepines are metabolized by glucuronic acid conjugation. Of these, the clearance of temazepam was increased when oral contraceptives were administered concomitantly, but the clearance of lorazepam and oxazepam was not (321). Again, it is unlikely that these are interactions of clinical importance.

Beta-blockers

Oral contraceptives increase the AUC and plasma concentrations of metoprolol, oxprenolol, and propranolol, but statistical significance is reached only with metoprolol. The changes are consistent with inhibition of hydroxylating enzymes, but are unlikely to be of clinical relevance (322).

Broad-spectrum antibiotics

There are sporadic, but well documented, reports of women using oral contraceptive steroids who became pregnant while taking a variety of antibiotics (323). However, there is much interindividual variation, which may explain the fact that some studies have shown no interference between oral contraceptives and antibiotics. Current suspicion focuses primarily on the broad-spectrum antibiotics (324), including ampicillin and the tetracyclines. The purported mechanism is apparently not enzyme induction but interference with the enterohepatic circulation of ethinylestradiol. Ethinylestradiol can be conjugated with both sulfate and glucuronic acid; sulfation occurs primarily in the small intestinal mucosa, while glucuronidation occurs mainly in the liver. These conjugates are excreted in the bile and then reach the colon, where they may be hydrolysed by gut bacteria to liberate unchanged ethinylestradiol, which can be reabsorbed (304). Broad-spectrum antibiotics may suppress this bacterial effect, resulting in reduced plasma hormone concentrations. The antibiotics doxycycline (325) and tetracycline (246) have been shown to have no effect on serum concentrations of exogenous estrogens and progestogens in women taking combined oral contraceptives containing ethinylestradiol 35 micrograms; however, in one of these studies endogenous progesterone was also assessed and there was no mid-cycle rise suggestive of ovulation.

Ciclosporin

Several case reports have suggested that the elimination of ciclosporin can be impaired by oral contraceptives, resulting in increased plasma ciclosporin concentrations. Ciclosporin undergoes hydroxylation and *N*-demethylation, in which cytochrome P450 is involved, so competitive enzyme inhibition probably explains the interaction. Dosages of ciclosporin should be reviewed carefully (326).

Clofibric acid

Oral contraceptives increase the plasma clearance of clofibric acid, which is mainly metabolized by glucuronidation (327,328).

Fluconazole

The effect of fluconazole 150 mg on circulating ethinylestradiol concentrations has been studied on day 6 of one of two cycles in women taking oral contraceptives (329). The serum concentrations of ethinylestradiol (C_{max} and AUC) were significantly increased by fluconazole, but t_{max} was not affected. These findings suggest that there is a potential for a clinically significant interaction between fluconazole and ethinylestradiol, by inhibition of estrogen metabolism.

Since oral contraceptive users sometimes need to be treated for vaginal candidiasis, the question arises which of the available treatments can be used without risk of impairing contraception. In a crossover placebo-controlled study, fluconazole 300 mg weekly for two cycles has been studied in 21 healthy women using Ortho-Novum 7/7/7 as a contraceptive (330). Fluconazole in this dose, which is twice that ordinarily recommended, produced small but statistically significant increases in the AUC_{0-24} for both ethinylestradiol (mean 24% increase) and norethindrone (mean 13%). The C_{max} of ethinylestradiol was slightly, but just significantly, higher with fluconazole than placebo. The C_{max} for norethindrone was not different between the two groups. There were no adverse events related to fluconazole. These changes are such that one should not anticipate any increased risk of contraceptive failure when fluconazole is given simultaneously.

Glucocorticoids

In standard reference works, oral contraceptives are commonly listed as increasing the circulating concentrations of glucocorticoids (80), but variable effects have been reported with different glucocorticoids.

In oral contraceptive users there is a 30–50% reduction in the clearance of prednisolone and a prolonged half-life (331). These alterations result from changes in both protein binding, which is increased, presumably owing to increased concentrations of glucocorticoid-binding globulin, and unbound drug clearance, which is reduced, presumably owing to inhibition of metabolism. It has therefore been suggested that lower doses of prednisolone should be used in oral contraceptive users.

In 40 healthy women oral contraceptives had a greater effect on prednisolone than on budesonide (44). In oral contraceptive users, the average plasma concentration of simultaneously administered prednisolone was 131% higher than in a control group, whereas the average plasma concentration of budesonide was only 22% higher. Mean plasma cortisol concentrations were suppressed by 90% and 82% with prednisolone and by 22% and 28% with budesonide in oral contraceptive users and controls, respectively. Ethinylestradiol plasma concentrations were not affected by either glucocorticoid. The authors concluded that the oral contraceptive made no difference to the plasma concentrations of budesonide or cortisol suppression after the administration of budesonide capsules. These findings suggest that oral budesonide can be used in the usual doses without problems in women using oral contraceptives.

Griseofulvin

Griseofulvin modifies hepatic enzyme activity in mice, and although there is no good evidence of a major enzyme-inducing effect in humans, several case reports of pregnancies in women taking both oral contraceptives and griseofulvin suggest an interaction; the authorities in several countries have warned that the contraceptive effect may be diminished (332).

Methylxanthines

The clearances of both theophylline and caffeine are reduced in oral contraceptive users and half-lives are increased, probably because of inhibition of hepatic metabolism by cytochrome P450 (333). Caution in dosage is advisable.

Neuroleptic drugs

A single case of neuroleptic malignant syndrome has been described in a woman taking haloperidol and thioridazine, 12 hours after she started to take an oral contraceptive. The authors suggested that this could have been a pharmacodynamic interaction involving dopaminergic neurotransmission (334).

A kinetic study in which ziprasidone (40 mg/day) or placebo were co-administered with a second-generation oral contraceptive has provided evidence that ziprasidone is unlikely to interfere with oral contraception (335).

Opioid analgesics

Increased glucuronidation may explain the fact that oral contraceptives enhance morphine clearance (336).

Paracetamol

Paracetamol might have a similar effect to ascorbic acid, that is competition with ethinylestradiol for sulfation capacity in the gut. Paracetamol significantly reduced the AUC of ethinylestradiol sulfate but had no effect on plasma levonorgestrel concentrations

In six healthy women, a single dose of paracetamol 1 g significantly increased the AUC of ethinylestradiol by 22% and reduced the AUC of ethinylestradiol sulfate (337). Plasma concentrations of levonorgestrel were unaltered. This interaction could be of clinical significance in women taking oral contraceptives who take paracetamol regularly or suddenly stop taking it, but it is doubtful whether it has any practical repercussions.

The clearance of paracetamol was 22% greater in men than women, entirely because of increased glucuronidation, there being no sex-related differences in the sulfation or oxidative metabolism of paracetamol (338). Paracetamol clearance in women using oral contraceptive steroids was 49% greater than in the control women. Glucuronidation and oxidative metabolism were both induced in contraceptive users (by 78% and 36% respectively) but sulfation was not altered. Although sex-related differences in paracetamol metabolism are unlikely to be of clinical importance, induction of paracetamol metabolism by oral contraceptive steroids may have clinical and toxicological consequences.

Rifamycins

Increased intermenstrual or breakthrough bleeding and pregnancy have been reported in women taking rifampicin in conjunction with contraceptive steroids (339). There is evidence that rifampicin increases the rate of metabolism of both the estrogenic and progestogenic components of oral contraceptives through hepatic microsomal enzyme induction (340) involving the same CYP isozyme as that induced by anticonvulsants, CYP3A. A four-fold increase in the rate of steroid metabolism has been shown; it is therefore unwise for women taking rifampicin to rely on steroid contraception and an alternative method should be used.

Roxithromycin

Roxithromycin does not interfere with the pharmacokinetics of oral contraceptives (341).

Salicylates

In a small study, the degree of erythrocyte aggregation during oral contraception was, at least in the short term, partly reversed by treatment with acetylsalicylic acid 100 mg/day (342).

Salicylic acid clearance is higher in users of oral contraceptives, owing to increases in the glycine and glucuronic acid conjugation pathways. In eight men, eight women, and eight women taking oral contraceptive steroids, the clearance of salicylic acid after an oral dose of aspirin 900 mg was 61% higher in the men than in the control women, largely because of increased activity of the glycine conjugation pathway (salicyluric acid formation) (343). Salicylic acid clearance was 41% higher in contraceptive users than in the control women, because of increases in both the glycine and glucuronic acid conjugation pathways. These data confirm the importance of hormonal factors in the regulation of drug conjugation reactions and suggest that sex-related differences in the disposition of salicylic acid and aspirin may be of clinical importance.

Tricyclic antidepressants

Oral contraceptives reduce the clearance of imipramine, probably by reducing hepatic oxidation, and thus increase its half-life. Hydroxylation of amitriptyline is inhibited by contraceptive steroids. The clinical significance is uncertain, but there is at least anecdotal evidence of an increase in antidepressant adverse effects (344). Caution should be exercised when tricyclic antidepressants are used long term in women taking oral contraceptives.

Troleandomycin

There have been several reports of hepatic cholestasis in women taking both troleandomycin and oral contraceptives (345). Oxidation of troleandomycin by CYP3A4 produces a derivative (probably a nitrosylated derivative) that binds tightly to the enzyme and thereby causes inactivation. This inhibition is highly selective for CYP3A4, and hepatic accumulation of ethinylestradiol is possible.

Smoking

The polycyclic hydrocarbons in cigarette smoke are potent inducers of certain cytochrome P450 isozymes. There is a marked increase in the 2-hydroxylation of natural estradiol in smokers, but not of ethinylestradiol, suggesting that the two estrogens are metabolized by different P450 enzymes. There is thus probably no pharmacokinetic interaction between smoking and oral contraceptives, but women taking oral contraception should be encouraged to avoid heavy smoking because of the risks to the cardiovascular system.

References

1. Hatcher RA, Trussell J, Stewart F, Stewart OK, Kowal D, Guest F, Cates W Jr, Policar MS. Contraceptive Technology. 16th rev ed. New York: Irvington Publishers, 1994.
2. McCann MF, Potter LS. Progestin-only oral contraception: a comprehensive review Contraception 1994;50(6 Suppl 1): S1–195.
3. Schramm G, Steffens D. Contraceptive efficacy and tolerability of chlormadinone acetate 2 mg/ethinylestradiol 0.03 mg (Belara): results of a post-marketing surveillance study. Clin Drug Invest 2002;22:221–31.
4. Brown C, Ling F, Wan J. A new monophasic oral contraceptive containing drospirenone. Effect on premenstrual symptoms. J Reprod Med 2002;47(1):14–22.
5. Kacar S, Akdogan M, Kosar Y, Parlak E, Sasmaz N, Oguz P, Aydog G. Estrogen and cyproterone acetate combination-induced autoimmune hepatitis. J Clin Gastroenterol 2002;35(1):98–100.
6. Harlap S, Kost K, Forrest JD. Preventing Pregnancy, Protecting Health: a New Look at Birth Control Choices in the United States. New York: The Alan Guttmacher Institute, 1991.
7. Colditz GA. Oral contraceptive use and mortality during 12 years of follow-up: the Nurses' Health Study. Ann Intern Med 1994;120(10):821–6.
8. Vessey MP, Villard-Mackintosh L, McPherson K, Yeates D. Mortality among oral contraceptive users: 20 year follow up of women in a cohort study. BMJ 1989;299(6714):1487–91.
9. Population Information Program. Update on Usage, Safety and Side Effects. Population Reports, Oral Contraceptives, Ser. A, No. 5. Baltimore, MD: John Hopkins University, 1979.
10. DaVanzo J, Parnell AM, Foege WH. Health consequences of contraceptive use and reproductive patterns. Summary of a report from the US National Research Council. JAMA 1991;265(20):2692–6.
11. Szarewski A, Guillebaud J. Contraception. BMJ 1991;302(6787):1224–6.
12. Vessey MP, Doll R. Evaluation of existing techniques: is "the pill" safe enough to continue using? Proc R Soc Lond B Biol Sci 1976;195(1118):69–80.
13. A preliminary communication to the Medical Research Council by a Subcommittee. Risk of thromboembolic disease in women taking oral contraceptives. BMJ 1967;2(548):355–9.
14. Miwa LJ, Edmunds AL, Shaefer MS, Raynor SC. Idiopathic thromboembolism associated with triphasic oral contraceptives. DICP 1989;23(10):773–5.
15. Lamy AL, Roy PH, Morissette JJ, Cantin R. Intimal hyperplasia and thrombosis of the visceral arteries in a young woman: possible relation with oral contraceptives and smoking. Surgery 1988;103(6):706–10.
16. Scolding NJ, Gibby OM. Fatal pulmonary embolus in a patient treated with Marvelon. J R Coll Gen Pract 1988;38(317):568.
17. Porter JB, Hunter JR, Jick H, Stergachis A. Oral contraceptives and nonfatal vascular disease. Obstet Gynecol 1985;66(1):1–4.
18. Realini JP, Goldzieher JW. Oral contraceptives and cardiovascular disease: a critique of the epidemiologic studies. Am J Obstet Gynecol 1985;152(6 Pt 2):729–98.
19. Skouby SO, Committee Chairman. Consensus Development Meeting: Metabolic aspects of oral contraceptives of relevance for cardiovascular diseases. Am J Obstet Gynecol 1990;162:1335.
20. Lidegaard O. Thrombotic diseases in young women and the influence of oral contraceptives. Am J Obstet Gynecol 1998;179(3 Pt 2):S62–7.
21. Anonymous. Oral contraceptives containing gestodene or desogestrel-up-date: revised product information. WHO Pharm Newslett 1999;7/8:3.
22. Farmer RD, Lawrenson RA. Oral contraceptives and venous thromboembolic disease: the findings from database studies in the United Kingdom and Germany. Am J Obstet Gynecol 1998;179(3 Pt 2):S78–86.
23. Burnhill MS. The use of a large-scale surveillance system in Planned Parenthood Federation of America clinics to monitor cardiovascular events in users of combination oral contraceptives. Int J Fertil Womens Med 1999;44(1):19–30.
24. Jick SS, Myers MW, Jick H. Risk of idiopathic cerebral haemorrhage in women on oral contraceptives with differing progestagen components. Lancet 1999;354(9175):302–3.
25. Schwingl PJ, Ory HW, King TDN. Modeled estimates of cardiovascular mortality risks in the US associated with low dose oral contraceptives. Unpublished draft, 1995.
26. Thorogood M, Mann J, Murphy M, Vessey M. Is oral contraceptive use still associated with an increased risk of fatal myocardial infarction? Report of a case-control study. Br J Obstet Gynaecol 1991;98(12):1245–53.
27. Rosenberg L, Palmer JR, Shapiro S. Use of lower dose oral contraceptives and risk of myocardial infarction. Circulation 1991;83:723.
28. Hannaford PC, Croft PR, Kay CR. Oral contraception and stroke. Evidence from the Royal College of General Practitioners' Oral Contraception Study. Stroke 1994;25(5):935–42.
29. Lidegaard O. Oral contraception and risk of a cerebral thromboembolic attack: results of a case-control study. BMJ 1993;306(6883):956–63.
30. Thorogood M, Mann J, Murphy M, Vessey M. Fatal stroke and use of oral contraceptives: findings from a case-control study. Am J Epidemiol 1992;136(1):35–45.
31. Thorogood M, Mann J, Murphy M, Vessey M. Risk factors for fatal venous thromboembolism in young women: a case-control study. Int J Epidemiol 1992;21(1):48–52.
32. Longstreth WT, Nelson LM, Koepsell TD, van Belle G. Subarachnoid hemorrhage and hormonal factors in women. A population-based case-control study. Ann Intern Med 1994;121(3):168–73.
33. Gerstman BB, Piper JM, Tomita DK, Ferguson WJ, Stadel BV, Lundin FE. Oral contraceptive estrogen dose and the risk of deep venous thromboembolic disease. Am J Epidemiol 1991;133(1):32–7.
34. Rosendaal FR, Helmerhorst FM, Vandenbroucke JP. Oral contraceptives, hormone replacement therapy and thrombosis. Thromb Haemost 2001;86(1):112–23.
35. Zreik TG, Odunsi K, Cass I, Olive DL, Sarrel P. A case of fatal pulmonary thromboembolism associated with the use of intravenous estrogen therapy. Fertil Steril 1999;71(2):373–5.
36. Chopard JL, Moulin T, Bourrin JC, et al. Contraception orale et accident vasculaire cérébral ischémique. Semin Hop (Paris) 1988;64:2075.
37. Lindberg MC. Hepatobiliary complications of oral contraceptives. J Gen Intern Med 1992;7(2):199–209.
38. Bohler J, Hauenstein KH, Hasler K, Schollmeyer P. Renal vein thrombosis in a dehydrated patient on an oral contraceptive agent. Nephrol Dial Transplant 1989;4(11):993–5.
39. Hassan HA. Oral contraceptive-induced mesenteric venous thrombosis with resultant intestinal ischemia. J Clin Gastroenterol 1999;29(1):90–5.

40. Hagglund H, Remberger M, Klaesson S, Lonnqvist B, Ljungman P, Ringden O. Norethisterone treatment, a major risk-factor for veno-occlusive disease in the liver after allogeneic bone marrow transplantation. Blood 1998;92(12):4568–72.
41. Grimes DA. The safety of oral contraceptives: epidemiologic insights from the first 30 years. Am J Obstet Gynecol 1992;166(6 Pt 2):1950–4.
42. Hirvonen E, Idanpaan-Heikkila J. Cardiovascular death among women under 40 years of age using low-estrogen oral contraceptives and intrauterine devices in Finland from 1975 to 1984. Am J Obstet Gynecol 1990;163(1 Pt 2):281–4.
43. Cirkel U, Schweppe KW. Fettstoffwechsel und orale Kontrazeptiva. Arztl Kosmetol 1985;15:253.
44. Fruzzetti F, Ricci C, Fioretti P. Haemostasis profile in smoking and nonsmoking women taking low-dose oral contraceptives. Contraception 1994;49(6):579–92.
45. Thorogood M, Villard-Mackintosh L. Combined oral contraceptives: risks and benefits. Br Med Bull 1993;49(1):124–39.
46. Machin SJ, Mackie IJ, Guillebaud J. Factor V Leiden mutation, venous thromboembolism and combined oral contraceptive usage. Br J Fam Planning 1995;21:13–14.
47. Rosenberg L, Palmer JR, Sands MI, Grimes D, Bergman U, Daling J, Mills A. Modern oral contraceptives and cardiovascular disease. Am J Obstet Gynecol 1997;177(3):707–15.
48. Vessey MP, Doll R, Fairbairn AS, Glober G. Postoperative thromboembolism and the use of oral contraceptives. BMJ 1970;3(715):123–6.
49. Greene GR, Sartwell PE. Oral contraceptive use in patients with thromboembolism following surgery, trauma, or infection. Am J Public Health 1972;62(5):680–5.
50. Whitehead EM, Whitehead MI. The pill, HRT and postoperative thromboembolism: cause for concern? Anaesthesia 1991;46(7):521–2.
51. Beller FK. Cardiovascular system: coagulation, thrombosis, and contraceptive steroids is there a link? In: Goldzieher JW, Fotherby K, editors. Pharmacology of the Contraceptive Steroids. New York: Raven Press, 1994:309.
52. Mant D, Villard-Mackintosh L, Vessey MP, Yeates D. Myocardial infarction and angina pectoris in young women. J Epidemiol Community Health 1987;41(3):215–19.
53. Frederiksen H, Ravenholt RT. Thromboembolism, oral contraceptives, and cigarettes. Public Health Rep 1970;85(3):197–205.
54. Rich-Edwards JW, Manson JE, Hennekens CH, Buring JE. The primary prevention of coronary heart disease in women. N Engl J Med 1995;332(26):1758–66.
55. Croft P, Hannaford PC. Risk factors for acute myocardial infarction in women: evidence from the Royal College of General Practitioners' oral contraception study. BMJ 1989;298(6667):165–8.
56. Jain AK. Cigarette smoking, use of oral contraceptives, and myocardial infarction. Am J Obstet Gynecol 1976;126(3):301–7.
57. Beral V. Mortality among oral-contraceptive users. Royal College of General Practitioners' Oral Contraception Study. Lancet 1977;2(8041):727–31.
58. Petitti DB, Wingerd J. Use of oral contraceptives, cigarette smoking, and risk of subarachnoid haemorrhage. Lancet 1978;2(8083):234–5.
59. Bruni V, Rosati D, Bucciantini S, Verni A, Abbate R, Pinto S, Costanzo G, Costanzo M. Platelet and coagulation functions during triphasic oestrogen–progestogen treatment. Contraception 1986;33(1):39–46.
60. Kjaeldgaard A, Larsson B. Long-term treatment with combined oral contraceptives and cigarette smoking associated with impaired activity of tissue plasminogen activator. Acta Obstet Gynecol Scand 1986;65(3):219–22.
61. Von Hugo R, Briel RC, Schindler AE. Wirkung oraler Kontrazeptiva auf die Blutgerinnung bei rauchenden und nichtrauchenden Probandinnen. Aktuel Endokrinol Stoffwechsel 1989;10:6.
62. Inman WH, Vessey MP. Investigation of deaths from pulmonary, coronary, and cerebral thrombosis and embolism in women of child-bearing age. BMJ 1968;2(599):193–9.
63. Arthes FG, Masi AT. Myocardial infarction in younger women. Associated clinical features and relationship to use of oral contraceptive drugs. Chest 1976;70(5):574–83.
64. Koenig W, Gehring J, Mathes P. Orale Kontrazeptiva und Myokardinfarkt bei jungen Frauen. Herz Kreisl 1984;16:508.
65. Zatti M. Contraccettivi orali: alterazioni delle variabili fisiologiche. C Ital Chim Clin 1983;8:249.
66. Leone A, Lopez M. Rôle du tabac et de la contraception orale dans l'infarctus du myocarde de la femme: description d'un cas. [Role of tobacco and oral contraception in myocardial infarction in the female. Description of a case.] Pathologica 1984;76(1044):493–8.
67. Gevers Leuven JA, Kluft C, Bertina RM, Hessel LW. Effects of two low-dose oral contraceptives on circulating components of the coagulation and fibrinolytic systems. J Lab Clin Med 1987;109(6):631–6.
68. Poller L. Oral contraceptives, blood clotting and thrombosis. Br Med Bull 1978;34(2):151–6.
69. Plowright C, Adam SA, Thorogood M, Beaumont V, Beaumont JL, Mann JI. Immunogenicity and the vascular risk of oral contraceptives. Br Heart J 1985;53(5):556–61.
70. Syner FN, Moghissi KS, Agronow SJ. Study on the presence of abnormal proteins in the serum of oral contraceptive users. Fertil Steril 1983;40(2):202–9.
71. Ernst E. Oral contraceptives, fibrinogen and cardiovascular risk. Atherosclerosis 1992;93(1–2):1–5.
72. Ylikorkala O, Puolakka J, Viinikka L. Oestrogen containing oral contraceptives decrease prostacyclin production. Lancet 1981;1(8210):42.
73. Gris JC, Jamin C, Benifla JL, Quere I, Madelenat P, Mares P. APC resistance and third-generation oral contraceptives: acquired resistance to activated protein C, oral contraceptives and the risk of thromboembolic disease. Hum Reprod 2001;16(1):3–8.
74. Marque V, Alhenc-Gelas M, Plu-Bureau G, Oger E, Scarabin PY. The effects of transdermal and oral estrogen/progesterone regimens on free and total protein S in postmenopausal women. Thromb Haemost 2001;86(2):713–14.
75. Rosing J, Middeldorp S, Curvers J, Christella M, Thomassen LG, Nicolaes GA, Meijers JC, Bouma BN, Buller HR, Prins MH, Tans G. Low-dose oral contraceptives and acquired resistance to activated protein C: a randomised cross-over study. Lancet 1999;354(9195):2036–40.
76. Porter JB, Hunter JR, Danielson DA, Jick H, Stergachis A. Oral contraceptives and nonfatal vascular disease—recent experience. Obstet Gynecol 1982;59(3):299–302.
77. Bailar JC 3rd, Byar DP. Estrogen treatment for cancer of the prostate. Early results with 3 doses of diethylstilbestrol and placebo. Cancer 1970;26(2):257–61.
78. Badaracco MA, Vessey MP. Recurrence of venous thromboembolic disease and use of oral contraceptives. BMJ 1974;1(901):215–17.
79. Jick H, Dinan B, Herman R, Rothman KJ. Myocardial infarction and other vascular diseases in young women. Role of estrogens and other factors. JAMA 1978;240(23):2548–52.
80. Stadel BV. Oral contraceptives and cardiovascular disease (first of two parts). N Engl J Med 1981;305(11):612–18.

81. Bottiger LE, Boman G, Eklund G, Westerholm B. Oral contraceptives and thromboembolic disease: effects of lowering oestrogen content. Lancet 1980;1(8178):1097–101.
82. Jung-Hoffmann C, Kuhl H. Interaction with the pharmacokinetics of ethinylestradiol and progestogens contained in oral contraceptives. Contraception 1989;40(3):299–312.
83. Guengerich FP. Mechanism-based inactivation of human liver microsomal cytochrome P-450 IIIA4 by gestodene. Chem Res Toxicol 1990;3(4):363–71.
84. Rosing J, Tans G, Nicolaes GA, Thomassen MC, van Oerle R, van der Ploeg PM, Heijnen P, Hamulyak K, Hemker HC. Oral contraceptives and venous thrombosis: different sensitivities to activated protein C in women using second- and third-generation oral contraceptives. Br J Haematol 1997;97(1):233–8.
85. Mellemkjaer L, Sorensen HT, Dreyer L, Olsen J, Olsen JH. Admission for and mortality from primary venous thromboembolism in women of fertile age in Denmark, 1977–95. BMJ 1999;319(7213):820–1.
86. Vandenbroucke JP, Bloemenkamp KW, Helmerhorst FM, Rosendaal FR. Mortality from venous thromboembolism and myocardial infarction in young women in the Netherlands. Lancet 1996;348(9024):401–2.
87. Herings RM, Urquhart J, Leufkens HG. Venous thromboembolism among new users of different oral contraceptives. Lancet 1999;354(9173):127–8.
88. Hannaford PC, Kay CR. The risk of serious illness among oral contraceptive users: evidence from the RCGP's oral contraceptive study. Br J Gen Pract 1998;48(435):1657–62.
89. Bruni V, Croxatto H, De La Cruz J, Dhont M, Durlot F, Fernandes MT, Andrade RP, Weisberg E, Rhoa M. A comparison of cycle control and effect on well-being of monophasic gestodene-, triphasic gestodene- and monophasic desogestrel-containing oral contraceptives. Gestodene Study Group. Gynecol Endocrinol 2000;14(2):90–8.
90. Marks LV. Sexual chemistry. A history of the contraceptive pill. New Haven: Yale University Press, 2001;138–57.
91. Sartwell PE, et al.. Oral contraceptives and relative risk of death from venous and pulmonary thromboembolism in the United States; an epidemiologic case-control study. Am J Epidemiol 1969;90:365.
92. Royal College of General Practitioners. Oral contraception and thrombo-embolic disease. J R Coll Gen Pract 1967;13(3):267–79.
93. Vessey MP, Doll R. Investigation of relation between use of oral contraceptives and thromboembolic disease. BMJ 1968;2(599):199–205.
94. Vessey MP, Doll R. Investigation of relation between use of oral contraceptives and thromboembolic disease. A further report. BMJ 1969;2(658):651–7.
95. Creatsas G, Koliopoulos C, Mastorakos G. Combined oral contraceptive treatment of adolescent girls with polycystic ovary syndrome. Lipid profile. Ann NY Acad Sci 2000;900:245–52.
96. Jick H, Kaye JA, Vasilakis-Scaramozza C, Jick SS. Risk of venous thromboembolism among users of third generation oral contraceptives compared with users of oral contraceptives with levonorgestrel before and after 1995: cohort and case-control analysis. BMJ 2000;321(7270):1190–5.
97. Bloemenkamp KW, Rosendaal FR, Helmerhorst FM, Buller HR, Vandenbroucke JP. Enhancement by factor V Leiden mutation of risk of deep-vein thrombosis associated with oral contraceptives containing a third-generation progestagen. Lancet 1995;346(8990):1593–6.
98. Kemmeren JM, Algra A, Grobbee DE. Third generation oral contraceptives and risk of venous thrombosis: meta-analysis. BMJ 2001;323(7305):131–4.
99. Bonnar J, Daly L, Carroll E. Blood coagulation with a combination pill containing gestodene and ethinyl estradiol. Int J Fertil 1987;32(Suppl):21–8.
100. Nicolaes GA, Thomassen MC, Tans G, Rosing J, Hemker HC. Effect of activated protein C on thrombin generation and on the thrombin potential in plasma of normal and APC-resistant individuals. Blood Coagul Fibrinolysis 1997;8(1):28–38.
101. Meijers JC, Middeldorp S, Tekelenburg W, van den Ende AE, Tans G, Prins MH, Rosing J, Buller HR, Bouma BN. Increased fibrinolytic activity during use of oral contraceptives is counteracted by an enhanced factor XI-independent down regulation of fibrinolysis: a randomized cross-over study of two low-dose oral contraceptives. Thromb Haemost 2000;84(1):9–14.
102. High Court. XYZ and others (Claimants) versus (1) Schering Health Care Limited, (2) Organon Laboratories Limited and (3) John Wyeth & Brother Limited. Judgement by the Hon. Mr Justice Mackay. London, 29 July 2002. Case No: 0002638. Neutral Citation No: (2002) EWHC 1420 (QB).
103. Biller J, Haberland C, Toffol GJ, O'Reilly D, Tentler RL. Basilar artery occlusion in an adolescent girl: a risk of oral contraceptives? J Child Neurol 1986;1(4):347–50.
104. Iuliano G, Di Domenico G, Masullo C, et al. Terapia contracettiva trifasica et ictus cerebri. Riv Neurobiol 1985;85:231.
105. Sanchez-Guerra M, Valle N, Blanco LA, Combarros O, Pascual J. Brain infarction after postcoital contraception in a migraine patient. J Neurol 2002;249(6):774.
106. Lalive d'Epinai SP, Trub P. Retinale vaskuläre Komplikationen bei oralen Kontrazeptiva. Klin Mbl Augenheilkd 1986;188:394.
107. Bradley JR, Reynolds J, Williams PF, Appleton DS. Encephalopathy in renovascular hypertension associated with the use of oral contraceptives. Postgrad Med J 1986;62(733):1031–3.
108. Landau E, Lessing JB, Weintraub M, Michowitz M. Acute myocardial infarction in a young woman taking oral contraceptives. A case report. J Reprod Med 1986;31(10): 1008–10.
109. Janion M, Wojtacha P, Wozakowska-Kaplon B, Kurzawski J, Klank-Szafran M, Ciuraszkiewicz K. Myocardial infarction in a female patient using oral contraceptives—a case report. Kardiol Pol 2002;56:75–8.
110. Schneiderman DJ, Cello JP. Intestinal ischemia and infarction associated with oral contraceptives. West J Med 1986;145(3):350–5.
111. Jick H, Jick SS, Gurewich V, Myers MW, Vasilakis C. Risk of idiopathic cardiovascular death and nonfatal venous thromboembolism in women using oral contraceptives with differing progestagen components. Lancet 1995;346(8990):1589–93.
112. Fotherby K. Oral contraceptives and lipids. BMJ 1989;298(6680):1049–50.
113. Burch JC, Byrd BF Jr, Vaughn WK. The effects of long-term estrogen on hysterectomized women. Am J Obstet Gynecol 1974;118(6):778–82.
114. Gordon T, Kannel WB, Hjortland MC, McNamara PM. Menopause and coronary heart disease. The Framingham Study. Ann Intern Med 1978;89(2):157–61.
115. Hammond CB, Jelovsek FR, Lee KL, Creasman WT, Parker RT. Effects of long-term estrogen replacement therapy. I. Metabolic effects. Am J Obstet Gynecol 1979;133(5):525–36.
116. Godsland IF, Crook D. Update on the metabolic effects of steroidal contraceptives and their relationship to cardiovascular disease risk Am J Obstet Gynecol 1994;170(5 Pt 2): 1528–36.

117. Collins P, Rosano GM, Jiang C, Lindsay D, Sarrel PM, Poole-Wilson PA. Cardiovascular protection by oestrogen—a calcium antagonist effect? Lancet 1993;341(8855):1264–5.
118. Williams JK, Adams MR, Herrington DM, Clarkson TB. Short-term administration of estrogen and vascular responses of atherosclerotic coronary arteries. J Am Coll Cardiol 1992;20(2):452–7.
119. Detering K, Kallischnig G. The cardiovascular risk of oral contraception with special reference to German mortality statistics. New Trends Gynecol Obstet 1985;1:360.
120. Lidegaard O, Edstrom B, Kreiner S. Oral contraceptives and venous thromboembolism: a five-year national case-control study. Contraception 2002;65(3):187–96.
121. Lidegaard O, Kreiner S. Contraceptives and cerebral thrombosis: a five-year national case-control study. Contraception 2002;65(3):197–205.
122. Lidegaard O. Smoking and use of oral contraceptives: impact on thrombotic diseases. Am J Obstet Gynecol 1999;180(6 Pt 2):S357–63.
123. Sass AE, Neufeld EJ. Risk factors for thromboembolism in teens: when should I test? Curr Opin Pediatr 2002;14(4):370–8.
124. Skjeldestad FE. Pillesal, fødslar og svangerskapsavbrøt før og etter "Marvelon saken". [Sale of oral contraceptives, births and abortions prior to and after the "Marvelon issue".] Tidsskr Nor Laegeforen 2000;120(3):339–44.
125. Collaborative Group for the Study of Stroke in Young Women. Oral contraception and increased risk of cerebral ischemia or thrombosis. N Engl J Med 1973;288(17):871–8.
126. Inman WH. Oral contraceptives and fatal subarachnoid haemorrhage. BMJ 1979;2(6203):1468–70.
127. Helmrich SP, Rosenberg L, Kaufman DW, Strom B, Shapiro S. Venous thromboembolism in relation to oral contraceptive use. Obstet Gynecol 1987;69(1):91–5.
128. Stampfer MJ, Willett WC, Colditz GA, Speizer FE, Hennekens CH. Past use of oral contraceptives and cardiovascular disease: a meta-analysis in the context of the Nurses' Health Study. Am J Obstet Gynecol 1990;163 (1 Pt 2):285–91.
129. WHO Special Programme of Research, Development and Research Training in Human Reproduction. The WHO multicentre trial of the vasopressor effects of combined oral contraceptives: 1. Comparisons with IUD. Task Force on Oral Contraceptives. Contraception 1989;40(2):129–45.
130. WHO Special Programme of Research, Development and Research Training in Human Reproduction. The WHO multicentre trial of the vasopressor effects of combined oral contraceptives: 2. Lack of effect of estrogen. Task Force on Oral Contraceptives. Contraception 1989;40(2):147–56.
131. Woods JW. Oral contraceptives and hypertension. Hypertension 1988;11(3 Pt 2):II11–15.
132. Connell EB. Oral contraceptives. The current risk-benefit ratio. J Reprod Med 1984;29(Suppl 7):513–23.
133. Pritchard JA, Pritchard SA. Blood pressure response to estrogen–progestin oral contraceptive after pregnancy-induced hypertension. Am J Obstet Gynecol 1977;129(7):733–9.
134. Lehtovirta P, Ranta T, Seppala M. Elevated prolactin levels in oral contraceptive pill-related hypertension. Fertil Steril 1981;35(4):403–5.
135. Royal College of General Practitioners' Oral Contraception Study. Effect on hypertension and benign breast disease of progestagen component in combined oral contraceptives. Lancet 1977;1(8012):624.
136. Kaul L, Curry CL, Ahluwalia BS. Blood levels of ethynylestradiol, caffeine, aldosterone and desoxycorticosterone in hypertensive oral contraceptive users. Contraception 1981;23(6):643–51.
137. Goldzieher JW, Moses LE, Averkin E, Scheel C, Taber BZ. A placebo-controlled double-blind crossover investigation of the side effects attributed to oral contraceptives. Fertil Steril 1971;22(9):609–23.
138. Mattson RH, Rebar RW. Contraceptive methods for women with neurologic disorders. Am J Obstet Gynecol 1993;168(6 Pt 2):2027–32.
139. Lobo RA, Gibbons WE. The role of progestin therapy in breast disease and central nervous system function. J Reprod Med 1982;27(Suppl 8):515–21.
140. Asherson RA, Harris NE, Gharavi AE, Hughes GR. Systemic lupus erythematosus, antiphospholipid antibodies, chorea, and oral contraceptives. Arthritis Rheum 1986;29(12):1535–6.
141. Leys D, Destee A, Petit H, Warot P. Chorea associated with oral contraception. J Neurol 1987;235(1):46–8.
142. Buge A, Vincent D, Rancurel G, Cheron F. Hémichorée et contraceptifs oraux. [Hemichorea and oral contraceptives.] Rev Neurol (Paris) 1985;141(10):663–5.
143. Driesen JJ, Wolters EC. Oral contraceptive induced paraballism. Clin Neurol Neurosurg 1987;89(1):49–51.
144. Mathur AK, Gatter RA. Chorea as the initial presentation of oral contraceptive induced systemic lupus erythematosus. J Rheumatol 1988;15(6):1042–3.
145. Peleg R. Abdominal wall pain caused by cutaneous nerve entrapment in an adolescent girl taking oral contraceptive pills. J Adolesc Health 1999;24(1):45–7.
146. Villard-Mackintosh L, Vessey MP. Oral contraceptives and reproductive factors in multiple sclerosis incidence. Contraception 1993;47(2):161–8.
147. Soni PS. Effects of oral contraceptive steroids on the thickness of human cornea. Am J Optom Physiol Opt 1980;57(11):825–34.
148. De Vries Reilingh A, Reiners H, Van Bijsterveld OP. Contact lens tolerance and oral contraceptives. Ann Ophthalmol 1978;10(7):947–52.
149. Byrne E. Retinal migraine and the pill. Med J Aust 1979;2(12):659–60.
150. Jorge A, Schwartzman Y. Efectos de los anticonceptivos sobre la otosclerosis. Rev Bras Oto-Rino-Laringol 1975;41:46.
151. Loveland DB. Auditory levels according to use of oral contraceptives in 5449 women. J Am Aud Soc 1975;1:28.
152. Zanker K, Kessler L. Innenohrstörung durch orale hormonale Kontrazeptive? Z Klin Med 1985;40:1897.
153. Calanchini C. Die Auslösung eines Zwangssyndroms durch Ovulationshemmer. [Development of a compulsive syndrome by ovulation inhibitors.] Schweiz Arch Neurol Psychiatr 1986;137(4):25–31.
154. Van Winter JT, Miller KA. Breakthrough bleeding in a bulimic adolescent receiving oral contraceptives. Pediat Adolesc Gynecol 1986;4:39.
155. Chang AM, Chick P, Milburn S. Mood changes as reported by women taking the oral contraceptive pill. Aust NZ J Obstet Gynaecol 1982;22(2):78–83.
156. Fleming O, Seager CP. Incidence of depressive symptoms in users of the oral contraceptive. Br J Psychiatry 1978;132:431–40.
157. Jacobs AJ, Odom MJ, Word RA, Carr BR. Effect of oral contraceptives on adrenocorticotropin and growth hormone secretion following CRH and GHRH administration. Contraception 1989;40(6):691–9.
158. Walden CE, Knopp RH, Johnson JL, Heiss G, Wahl PW, Hoover JJ. Effect of estrogen/progestin potency on clinical chemistry measures. The Lipid Research Clinics Program Prevalence Study. Am J Epidemiol 1986;123(3):517–31.

159. Barsivala V, Virkar K. Thyroid functions of women taking oral contraceptives. Contraception 1974;9(3):305–14.
160. WHO Task Force on Oral Contraceptives. Oral and injectable hormonal contraceptive and signs and symptoms of vitamin deficiency and goitre: prevalence studies in five centres in the developing and developed world. WHO Bull 1983.
161. Ball MJ, Ashwell E, Gillmer MD. Progestagen-only oral contraceptives: comparison of the metabolic effects of levonorgestrel and norethisterone. Contraception 1991;44(3):223–33.
162. Ramamoorthy R, Saraswathi TP, Kanaka TS. Carbohydrate metabolic studies during twelve months of treatment with a low-dose combination oral contraceptive. Contraception 1989;40(5):563–9.
163. Simon D, Senan C, Garnier P, Saint-Paul M, Garat E, Thibult N, Papoz L. Effects of oral contraceptives on carbohydrate and lipid metabolisms in a healthy population: the Telecom study. Am J Obstet Gynecol 1990;163(1 Pt 2):382–7.
164. Spellacy WN. Carbohydrate metabolism during treatment with estrogen, progestogen, and low-dose oral contraceptives. Am J Obstet Gynecol 1982;142(6 Pt 2):732–4.
165. Elkind-Hirsch K, Goldzieher JW. Metabolism: carbohydrate metabolism. In: Goldzieher JW, Fotherby K, editors. Pharmacology of the Contraceptive Steroids. New York: Raven Press, 1994:345.
166. Wingrave SJ, Kay CR, Vessey MP. Oral contraceptives and diabetes mellitus. BMJ 1979;1(6155):23.
167. Hannaford PC, Kay CR. Oral contraceptives and diabetes mellitus. BMJ 1989;299(6711):1315–16.
168. World Health Organization. Oral Contraceptives: Technical and Safety Aspects. WHO Offset Publications, 64. Geneva: World Health Organization, 1982.
169. Gaspard U. Contraception orale, métabolisme glucidique et critères de surveillance. [Oral contraception, glucid metabolism and monitoring criteria.] Contracept Fertil Sex (Paris) 1988;16(2):113–18.
170. Speroff L, Darney PD. A Clinical Guide for Contraception. Baltimore, Maryland: Williams & Wilkins, 1992.
171. Garg SK, Chase HP, Marshall G, Hoops SL, Holmes DL, Jackson WE. Oral contraceptives and renal and retinal complications in young women with insulin-dependent diabetes mellitus. JAMA 1994;271(14):1099–102.
172. Amatayakul K. Metabolism: vitamins and trace elements. In: Goldzieher JW, Fotherby K, editors. Pharmacology of the Contraceptive Steroids. New York: Raven Press, 1994:363.
173. Malnick SD, Halperin M, Geltner D. Hypercarotenemia associated with an oral contraceptive. DICP 1989;23(10):811.
174. Rose DP. The influence of oestrogens on tryptophan metabolism in man. Clin Sci 1966;31(2):265–72.
175. Price SA, Toseland PA. Oral contraceptives and depression. Lancet 1969;2(7612):158–9.
176. Anonymous. Depression and oral contraceptives: the role of pyridoxine. Drug Ther Bull 1978;16(22):86–7.
177. Kornberg A, Segal R, Theitler J, Yona R, Kaufman S. Folic acid deficiency, megaloblastic anemia and peripheral polyneuropathy due to oral contraceptives. Isr J Med Sci 1989;25(3):142–5.
178. Rivers JM. Oral contraceptives and ascorbic acid. Am J Clin Nutr 1975;28(5):550–4.
179. Weininger J, King JC. Effect of oral contraceptives on ascorbic acid status of young women consuming a constant diet. Nutr Rep Int 1977;15(3):255–64.
180. Harris SS, Dawson-Hughes B. The association of oral contraceptive use with plasma 25-hydroxyvitamin D levels. J Am Coll Nutr 1998;17(3):282–4.
181. Schreurs WH, van Rijn HJ, van den Berg H. Serum 25-hydroxycholecalciferol levels in women using oral contraceptives. Contraception 1981;23(4):399–406.
182. Gray TK, McAdoo T, Hatley L, Lester GE, Thierry M. Fluctuation of serum concentration of 1,25-dihydroxyvitamin D3 during the menstrual cycle. Am J Obstet Gynecol 1982;144(8):880–4.
183. Goulding A, McChesney R. Diminished urinary calcium excretion by women using oral contraceptives. Aust NZ J Med 1976;6:251.
184. Recker RR, Saville PD, Heaney RP. Effect of estrogens and calcium carbonate on bone loss in postmenopausal women. Ann Intern Med 1977;87(6):649–55.
185. Darzenta NC, Giunta JL. Radiographic changes of the mandible related to oral contraceptives. Oral Surg Oral Med Oral Pathol 1977;43(3):478–81.
186. Prasad AS, Oberleas D, Moghissi KS, Lei KY, Stryker JC. Effect of oral contraceptive agents on nutrients: I. Minerals. Am J Clin Nutr 1975;28(4):377–84.
187. Amatayakul K. Metabolism: vitamins and trace elements. In: Goldzieher JW, Fotherby K, editors. Pharmacology of the Contraceptive Steroids. New York: Raven Press, 1994.
188. Larsson G, Milsom I, Lindstedt G, Rybo G. The influence of a low-dose combined oral contraceptive on menstrual blood loss and iron status. Contraception 1992;46(4):327–34.
189. Mardell M, Zilva JF. Effect of oral contraceptives on the variations in serum-iron during the menstrual cycle. Lancet 1967;2(7530):1323–5.
190. Lucis OJ, Lucis R. Oral contraceptives and endocrine changes. Bull World Health Organ 1972;46(4):443–50.
191. Rahman HA, et al. A report on the effect of oral contraceptives on blood picture, serum iron and TIBC in twenty cases of healthy Egyptian women. Bull Alexandr Fac Med 1982.
192. Kendall AG, Charlow GF. Red cell pyruvate kinase deficiency: adverse effect of oral contraceptives. Acta Haematol 1977;57(2):116–20.
193. Winkler UH. Effects on hemostatic variables of desogestrel- and gestodene-containing oral contraceptives in comparison with levonorgestrel-containing oral contraceptives: a review. Am J Obstet Gynecol 1998;179(3 Pt 2):S51–61.
194. Zachariasen RD. Ovarian hormones and gingivitis. J Dent Hyg 1991;65(3):146–50.
195. Magnusson I, Ericson T, Hugoson A. The effect of oral contraceptives on the concentration of some salivary substances in women. Arch Oral Biol 1975;20(2):119–26.
196. Mussalli NG, Hopps RM, Johnson NW. Oral pyogenic granuloma as a complication of pregnancy and the use of hormonal contraceptives. Int J Gynaecol Obstet 1976;14(2):187–91.
197. Delaunay P, Commissionat Y. Contraception orale et muqueuse buccale. [Oral contraception and oral mucosa.] Actual Odontostomatol (Paris) 1980;34(129):149–56.
198. Boyko EJ, Theis MK, Vaughan TL, Nicol-Blades B. Increased risk of inflammatory bowel disease associated with oral contraceptive use. Am J Epidemiol 1994;140(3):268–78.
199. Sandler RS, Wurzelmann JI, Lyles CM. Oral contraceptive use and the risk of inflammatory bowel disease. Epidemiology 1992;3(4):374–8.
200. Deana DG, Dean PJ. Reversible ischemic colitis in young women. Association with oral contraceptive use. Am J Surg Pathol 1995;19(4):454–62.
201. Hargreaves T. Oral contraceptives and liver function. J Clin Pathol 1970;23(Suppl):3.
202. Stoll BA, Andrews JT, Mofferam R. Liver damage from oral contraceptives. BMJ 1966;1:960.
203. Larsson-Cohn U, Stenram U. Liver ultrastructure and function in icteric and non-icteric women using oral contraceptive agents. Acta Med Scand 1967;181(3):257–64.
204. Perez V, Gorodisch S, De Martire J, Nicholson R, Di Paola G. Oral contraceptives: long-term use produces

fine structural changes in liver mitochondria. Science 1969;165:1805.
205. WHO Scientific Group. Oral contraceptives and neoplasia. World Health Organ Tech Rep Ser 1992;817:1–46.
206. Westerholm B. Oral contraceptives and jaundice: Swedish experience. In: Baker SB de C, Tripot J, editors. Proceedings, European Society for the Study of Drug Toxicity, Oxford, 1968. Amsterdam: Excerpta Medica, 1969:158–63.
207. Ockner RK, Davidson CS. Hepatic effects of oral contraceptives. N Engl J Med 1967;276(6):331–4.
208. Briggs MH, Briggs M. Metabolic effects of hormonal contraceptives. In: Chang CF, Griffin D, Woolman A, editors. Recent Advances in Fertility Regulation. Beijing, 1980;81;83–111
209. Dalen E, Westerholm B. Occurrence of hepatic impairment in women jaundiced by oral contraceptives and in their mothers and sisters. Acta Med Scand 1974;195(6):459–63.
210. Adlercreutz H, Tenhunen R. Some aspects of the interaction between natural and synthetic female sex hormones and the liver. Am J Med 1970;49:630–48.
211. Brown JB, Blair HAF. Urinary oestrogen metabolites of 17-norethisterone and esters. Proc R Soc Med 1960;53:433.
212. van Erpecum KJ, Janssens AR, Kreuning J, Ruiter DJ, Kroon HM, Grond AJ. Generalized peliosis hepatis and cirrhosis after long-term use of oral contraceptives. Am J Gastroenterol 1988;83(5):572–5.
213. Heresbach D, Deugnier Y, Brissot P, Bourel M. Dilatations sinusoi_dales et prise de contraceptifs oraux. A propos d'un cas avec revue de la litterature. [Sinusoid dilatation and the use of oral contraceptives. Apropos of a case with a review of the literature.] Ann Gastroenterol Hepatol (Paris) 1988;24(4):189–91.
214. Suarez AA, Brunt EM, Di Bisceglie AM. A 35-year-old woman with progesterone implant contraception and multiple liver masses. Semin Liver Dis 2001;21(3):453–9.
215. Morrison AS, Jick H, Ory HW. Oral contraceptives and hepatitis. A report from the Boston Collaborative Drug Surveillance Program, Boston University Medical Center. Lancet 1977;1(8022):1142–3.
216. Anonymous. Oral contraceptives and venous thromboembolic disease, surgically confirmed gallbladder disease, and breast tumours. Report from the Boston Collaborative Drug Surveillance Programme. Lancet 1973;1(7817):1399–404.
217. Stolley PD, Tonascia JA, Tockman MS, Sartwell PE, Rutledge AH, Jacobs MP. Thrombosis with low-estrogen oral contraceptives. Am J Epidemiol 1975;102(3):197–208.
218. Grodstein F, Colditz GA, Hunter DJ, Manson JE, Willett WC, Stampfer MJ. A prospective study of symptomatic gallstones in women: relation with oral contraceptives and other risk factors. Obstet Gynecol 1994;84(2):207–14.
219. Scragg RK, McMichael AJ, Seamark RF. Oral contraceptives, pregnancy, and endogenous oestrogen in gall stone disease—a case-control study. BMJ (Clin Res Ed) 1984;288(6433):1795–9.
220. Strom BL, Tamragouri RN, Morse ML, Lazar EL, West SL, Stolley PD, Jones JK. Oral contraceptives and other risk factors for gallbladder disease. Clin Pharmacol Ther 1986;39(3):335–41.
221. Riederer J. Verschlussikterus durch sludge im Ductus choledochus. [Obstructive jaundice due to sludge in the common bile duct.] Dtsch Med Wochenschr 2000;125(1–2):11–14.
222. Thijs C, Knipschild P. Oral contraceptives and the risk of gallbladder disease: a meta-analysis. Am J Public Health 1993;83(8):1113–20.
223. Vessey M, Painter R. Oral contraceptive use and benign gallbladder disease; revisited. Contraception 1994;50(2):167–73.
224. Bennion LJ, Ginsberg RL, Gernick MB, Bennett PH. Effects of oral contraceptives on the gallbladder bile of normal women. N Engl J Med 1976;294(4):189–92.
225. Tritapepe R, Di Padova C, Zuin M, Bellomi M, Podda M. Lithogenic bile after conjugated estrogen. N Engl J Med 1976;295(17):961–2.
226. Coronary Drug Project. Gallbladder disease as a side effect of drugs influencing lipid metabolism. N Engl J Med 1977;296(21):1185–90.
227. Kern F Jr, Everson GT, DeMark B, McKinley C, Showalter R, Braverman DZ, Szczepanik-Van Leeuwen P, Klein PD. Biliary lipids, bile acids, and gallbladder function in the human female: effects of contraceptive steroids. J Lab Clin Med 1982;99(6):798–805.
228. Mungall IP, Hague RV. Pancreatitis and the pill. Postgrad Med J 1975;51(602):855–7.
229. Burke M. Pregnancy, pancreatitis and the pill. BMJ 1972;4(839):551.
230. Schillinger F, Montagnac R, Birembaut P, Hopfner C. Syndrome hémolytique et urémique au décours d'une contraception orale. [Hemolytic–uremic syndrome during oral contraception.] Rev Fr Gynecol Obstet 1986;81(12):721–5.
231. Barrière H, Roubeix Y. Dermatoses et oestroprogestatifs. Gaz Med Fr 1977;84:1485.
232. Lucky AW, Henderson TA, Olson WH, Robisch DM, Lebwohl M, Swinyer LJ. Effectiveness of norgestimate and ethinyl estradiol in treating moderate acne vulgaris. J Am Acad Dermatol 1997;37(5 Pt 1):746–54.
233. Charoenvisal C, Thaipisuttikul Y, Pinjaroen S, Krisanapan O, Benjawang W, Koster A, Doesburg W. Effects on acne of two oral contraceptives containing desogestrel and cyproterone acetate. Int J Fertil Menopausal Stud 1996;41(4):423–9.
234. Wendler J, Siegert C, Schelhorn P, Klinger G, Gurr S, Kaufmann J, Aydinlik S, Braunschweig T. The influence of Microgynon and Diane-35, two sub-fifty ovulation inhibitors, on voice function in women. Contraception 1995;52(6):343–8.
235. Gollnick H, Albring M, Brill K. The efficacy of oral cyproterone acetate in combination with ethinylestradiol in acne tarda of the facial type. J Dermatol Treat 1998;9:71–9.
236. Mariotti F, Ruocco V. Oral contraceptives and sharpened condylomas. Riforma Med 1971;85:429.
237. Hollander A, Grots IA. Mucha–Habermann disease following estrogen–progesterone therapy. Arch Dermatol 1973;107(3):465.
238. Saez M, Garcia-Bustinduy M, Noda A, Guimera F, Dorta S, Escoda M, Fagundo E, Sanchez R, Martin-Herrera A, Garcia Montelongo R. Sweet's syndrome induced by oral contraceptive. Dermatology 2002;204(1):84.
239. Greenwald AE. Anovulatorios y alopecia. [Oral contraceptives and alopecia.] Dermatol Iber Lat Am 1970;12:29–36.
240. Schoberberger R, Husslein P, Kunze M. Akzeptanz und Befindlichkeit unter einer norgestimathaltigen Kombinationspille. [Acceptance and subjective well-being with a norgestimate combination pill.] Gynakol Rundsch 1991;31(2):65–76.
241. Fortney JA, Feldblum PJ, Talmage RV, Zhang J, Godwin SE. Bone mineral density and history of oral contraceptive use. J Reprod Med 1994;39(2):105–9.
242. Polatti F, Perotti F, Filippa N, Gallina D, Nappi RE. Bone mass and long-term monophasic oral contraceptive treatment in young women. Contraception 1995;51(4):221–4.
243. Spector TD, Hochberg MC. The protective effect of the oral contraceptive pill on rheumatoid arthritis: an overview of the analytic epidemiological studies using meta-analysis. J Clin Epidemiol 1990;43(11):1221–30.
244. Adams DB, Gold AR, Burt AD. Rise in female-initiated sexual activity at ovulation and its suppression by oral contraceptives. N Engl J Med 1978;299(21):1145–50.

245. Rozenbaum H. Petits problèmes de la contraception Mastodynies et contraceptifs oraux. [Little problems of contraception. Mastodynia and oral contraceptives.] Concours Med 1979;101(20):3341–2.
246. Mutti P, Cesarini R. Considerazioni sulle principali complicanze e controindicazioni dell'uso dei contraccettivi orali. [Principle complications and contraindications of the use of oral contraceptives.] Minerva Ginecol 1979;31(5):363–75.
247. Rose BI, LeMaire WJ, Jeffers LJ. Macromastia in a woman treated with penicillamine and oral contraceptives. A case report. J Reprod Med 1990;35(1):43–5.
248. Holt VL, Daling JR, McKnight B, Moore D, Stergachis A, Weiss NS. Functional ovarian cysts in relation to the use of monophasic and triphasic oral contraceptives. Obstet Gynecol 1992;79(4):529–33.
249. Lanes SF, Birmann B, Walker AM, Singer S. Oral contraceptive type and functional ovarian cysts. Am J Obstet Gynecol 1992;166(3):956–61.
250. Milsom I, Sundell G, Andersch B. The influence of different combined oral contraceptives on the prevalence and severity of dysmenorrhea. Contraception 1990;42(5):497–506.
251. Belsey EM. Vaginal bleeding patterns among women using one natural and eight hormonal methods of contraception. Contraception 1988;38(2):181–206.
252. Rosenberg MJ, Long SC. Oral contraceptives and cycle control: a critical review of the literature. Adv Contracept 1992;8(Suppl 1):35–45.
253. Saleh WA, Burkman RT, Zacur HA, Kimball AW, Kwiterovich P, Bell WK. A randomized trial of three oral contraceptives: comparison of bleeding patterns by contraceptive types and steroid levels. Am J Obstet Gynecol 1993;168(6 Pt 1):1740–5.
254. Mall-Haefeli M. Was bringt die Micropille? [What does the micropill bring?] Ther Umsch 1986;43(5):365–71.
255. Fraser IS. Menstrual changes associated with progestogen-only contraception. Acta Obstet Gynecol Scand Suppl 1986;134:21–7.
256. Toth F, Kerenyin T. Changes of endometrium during contraceptive treatment. Acta Morphol Acad Sci Hung 1973;14:114.
257. Vercellini P, Ragni G, Trespidi L, Oldani S, Crosignani PG. Does contraception modify the risk of endometriosis? Hum Reprod 1993;8(4):547–51.
258. Parazzini F, Ferraroni M, Bocciolone L, Tozzi L, Rubessa S, La Vecchia C. Contraceptive methods and risk of pelvic endometriosis. Contraception 1994;49(1):47–55.
259. Cates W Jr, Stone KM. Family planning, sexually transmitted diseases and contraceptive choice: a literature update—Part II. Fam Plann Perspect 1992;24(3):122–8.
260. Expert Committee on Pelvic Inflammatory Disease. Pelvic inflammatory disease. Research directions in the 1990s. Sex Transm Dis 1991;18(1):46–64.
261. McGregor JA, Hammill HA. Contraception and sexually transmitted diseases: interactions and opportunities. Am J Obstet Gynecol 1993;168(6 Pt 2):2033–41.
262. Schuurs AHWM, Geurts TBP, Goorissen EM. Immunologic effects of estrogens, progestins, and estrogen–progestin combinations. In: Goldzieher JW, Fotherby K, editors. Pharmacology of the Contraceptive Steroids. New York: Raven Press, 1994:379–99.
263. Joshi UM, Rao SS, Kora SJ, Dikshit SS, Virkar KD. Effect of steroidal contraceptives on antibody formation in the human female. Contraception 1971;3:327.
264. Hagen C, Froland A. Depressed lymphocyte response to P.H.A. in women taking oral contraceptives. Lancet 1972;1(7761):1185.
265. Klinger G, Schubert H, Stelzner A, Krause G, Carol W. Zum Verhalten der Serumimmunoglobulin Titer von IgA, IgG und IgM bei Kurz- und Langzeitapplikation verschiedener hormonaler Kontrazeptiva. [Serum immunoglobulin titer of IgA, IgG and IgM during short- and long-term administration of contraceptive hormones.] Dtsch Gesundheitsw 1978;33(23):1057–62.
266. Huang NH, Li C, Goldzieher JW. Absence of antibodies to ethinyl estradiol in users of oral contraceptive steroids. Fertil Steril 1984;41(4):587–92.
267. Kulisevsky Bojarski J, Rodriguez de la Serna A, Rovira Gols A, Roig Arnall C. Migraña acompañada como manifestaciôn del lupus eritematoso sistemicon: presentación de 2 casos. [Complicated migraine as a manifestation of systemic lupus erythematosus. Presentation of 2 cases.] Med Clin (Barc) 1986;87(3):112–14.
268. Strom BL, Reidenberg MM, West S, Snyder ES, Freundlich B, Stolley PD. Shingles, allergies, family medical history, oral contraceptives, and other potential risk factors for systemic lupus erythematosus. Am J Epidemiol 1994;140(7):632–42.
269. Burns MR, Schoch DR, Grayzel AI. Cold urticaria and an oral contraceptive. Ann Intern Med 1983;98(6):1025–6.
270. Pelikan Z. Possible immediate hypersensitivity reaction of the nasal mucosa to oral contraceptives. Ann Allergy 1978;40(3):211–19.
271. Scinto J, Enrione M, Bernstein D, Bernstein IL. In vitro leukocyte histamine release to progesterone and pregnanediol in a patient with recurrent anaphylaxis associated with exogenous administration of progesterone. J Allergy Clin Immunol 1990;85:228.
272. Klinger G, Graser T, Mellinger U, Moore C, Vogelsang H, Groh A, Latterman C, Klinger G. A comparative study of the effects of two oral contraceptives containing dienogest or desogestrel on the human immune system. Gynecol Endocrinol 2000;14(1):15–24.
273. Howe JE, Minkoff HL, Duerr AC. Contraceptives and HIV. AIDS 1994;8(7):861–71.
274. Anonymous. Verhoging lichaamstemperatuur bij orale anticonceptiva. Geneesmiddelenbulletin 1998;32:85–6.
275. Rogers SM, Baker MA. Thermoregulation during exercise in women who are taking oral contraceptives. Eur J Appl Physiol Occup Physiol 1997;75(1):34–8.
276. Vessey MP, Wright NH, McPherson K, Wiggins P. Fertility after stopping different methods of contraception. BMJ 1978;1(6108):265–7.
277. Harlap S, Davies AM. The Pill and Births: The Jerusalem Study, Final Report. US Department of Health, Education and Welfare, National Institute of Child Health and Development. Bethesda, MD: Center for Population Research, 1978:219.
278. Hull MG, Bromham DR, Savage PE, Jackson JA, Jacobs HS. Normal fertility in women with post-pill amenorrhoea. Lancet 1981;1(8234):1329–32.
279. Bracken MB, Hellenbrand KG, Holford TR. Conception delay after oral contraceptive use: the effect of estrogen dose. Fertil Steril 1990;53(1):21–7.
280. Franks AL, Beral V, Cates W Jr, Hogue CJ. Contraception and ectopic pregnancy risk. Am J Obstet Gynecol 1990;163(4 Pt 1):1120–3.
281. Weiss DB, Aboulafia Y, Milewidsky A. Ectopic pregnancy and the pill. Lancet 1976;2(7978):196–7.
282. American College of Obstetricians and Gynecologists (ACOG). Contraceptives and congenital anomalies. ACOG Committee Opinion: Committee on Gynecologic Practice. Number 124-July 1993. Int J Gynaecol Obstet 1993;42(3):316–17.
283. Bracken MB. Oral contraception and congenital malformations in offspring: a review and meta-analysis of the prospective studies. Obstet Gynecol 1990;76(3 Pt 2): 552–7.

284. Simpson JL, Phillips OP. Spermicides, hormonal contraception and congenital malformations. Adv Contracept 1990;6(3):141–67.
285. Raman-Wilms L, Tseng AL, Wighardt S, Einarson TR, Koren G. Fetal genital effects of first-trimester sex hormone exposure: a meta-analysis. Obstet Gynecol 1995;85(1):141–9.
286. Keseru TL, Maraz A, Szabo J. Oral contraception and sex ratio at birth. Lancet 1974;1(7853):369.
287. Rothman KJ, Liess J. Gender of offspring after oral-contraceptive use. N Engl J Med 1976;295(16):859–61.
288. Janerich DT, Piper JM. Sex of offspring after use of oral contraceptives. N Engl J Med 1977;296(23):1360–1.
289. McCredie J, Kricker A, Elliott J, Forrest J. Congenital limb defects and the pill. Lancet 1983;2(8350):623.
290. Nikschick S, Goretzlehner G, Boldt O, Leineweber B, Radzuweit H, Hagen A, Born B, Melzer H, Nowak M, Fischer R, et al. Fehlbildungshaufigkeit nach Anwendung hormonaler Kontrazeptiva. [Incidence of abnormalities following the use of hormonal contraceptives.] Zentralbl Gynakol 1989;111(17):1152–9.
291. Nilsson S, Nygren KG. Transfer of contraceptive steroids to human milk. Res Reprod 1979;11(1):1–2.
292. McCann MF, Liskin LS, Piotrow PT, Rinehard W, Fox G, editors. Breast-feeding, fertility, and family planning. Population Reports, Series J, No. 24. Baltimore, Maryland, Population Information Program, 1984.
293. World Health Organization (WHO) Task Force on Oral Contraceptives. Effects of hormonal contraceptives on breast milk composition and infant growth. Stud Fam Plann 1988;19(6 Pt 1):361–9.
294. Nilsson S, Mellbin T, Hofvander Y, Sundelin C, Valentin J, Nygren KG. Long-term follow-up of children breast-fed by mothers using oral contraceptives. Contraception 1986;34(5):443–57.
295. World Health Organization Task force for Epidemiological Research on Reproductive Health; Special Programme of Research, Development and Research Training in Human Reproduction. Progestogen-only contraceptives during lactation: I. Infant growth. Contraception 1994;50(1):35–53.
296. World Health Organization, Task Force for Epidemiological Research on Reproductive Health; Special Programme of Research, Development, and Research Training in Human Reproduction. Progestogen-only contraceptives during lactation: II. Infant development. Contraception 1994;50(1):55–68.
297. Howard RJ, Tuck SM. Haematological disorders and reproductive health. Br J Fam Plann 1993;19:147.
298. Vessey M, Painter R, Yeates D. Mortality in relation to oral contraceptive use and cigarette smoking. Lancet 2003;362(9379):185–91.
299. Coney P, Washenik K, Langley RG, DiGiovanna JJ, Harrison DD. Weight change and adverse event incidence with a low-dose oral contraceptive: two randomized, placebo-controlled trials. Contraception 2001;63(6):297–302.
300. Fotherby K, Caldwell AD. New progestogens in oral contraception. Contraception 1994;49(1):1–32.
301. Kluft C, de Maat MP, Heinemann LA, Spannagl M, Schramm W. Importance of levonorgestrel dose in oral contraceptives for effects on coagulation. Lancet 1999;354(9181):832–3.
302. Rowan JP. "Estrophasic" dosing: A new concept in oral contraceptive therapy. Am J Obstet Gynecol 1999;180(2 Pt 2):302–6.
303. Hoffmann H, Moore C, Kovacs L, Teichmann AT, Klinger G, Graser T, Oettel M. Alternatives for the replacement of ethinylestradiol by natural 17 beta-estradiol in dienogest-containing oral contraceptives. Drugs Today 1999;35(Suppl C):105–13.
304. Back DJ, Orme ML. Pharmacokinetic drug interactions with oral contraceptives. Clin Pharmacokinet 1990;18(6):472–84.
305. Back DJ, Orme MLE. Drug interactions. In: Goldzieher JW, Fotherby K, editors. Pharmacology of the Contraceptive Steroids. New York: Raven Press, 1994:407.
306. Shenfield GM, Griffin JM. Clinical pharmacokinetics of contraceptive steroids. An update. Clin Pharmacokinet 1991;20(1):15–37.
307. Sonnenberg A, Koelz HR, Herz R, Benes I, Blum AL. Limited usefulness of the breath test in evaluation of drug metabolism: a study in human oral contraceptive users treated with dimethylaminoantipyrine and diazepam. Hepatogastroenterology 1980;27(2):104–8.
308. Homeida M, Halliwell M, Branch RA. Effects of an oral contraceptive on hepatic size and antipyrine metabolism in premenopausal women. Clin Pharmacol Ther 1978;24(2):228–32.
309. Teunissen MW, Srivastava AK, Breimer DD. Influence of sex and oral contraceptive steroids on antipyrine metabolite formation. Clin Pharmacol Ther 1982;32(2):240–6.
310. Crawford JS, Rudofsky S. Some alterations in the pattern of drug metabolism aociated with pegnancy, oral contraceptives, and the newly-born. Br J Anaesth 1966;38(6):446–54.
311. Chambers DM, Jefferson GC, Chambers M, Loudon NB. Antipyrine elimination in saliva after low-dose combined or progestogen-only oral contraceptive steroids. Br J Clin Pharmacol 1982;13(2):229–32.
312. Jones MK, Jones BM. Ethanol metabolism in women taking oral contraceptives. Alcohol Clin Exp Res 1984;8(1):24–8.
313. Monig H, Baese C, Heidemann HT, Ohnhaus EE, Schulte HM. Effect of oral contraceptive steroids on the pharmacokinetics of phenprocoumon. Br J Clin Pharmacol 1990;30(1):115–18.
314. Crawford P, Chadwick DJ, Martin C, Tjia J, Back DJ, Orme M. The interaction of phenytoin and carbamazepine with combined oral contraceptive steroids. Br J Clin Pharmacol 1990;30(6):892–6.
315. Nilsson S, Victor A, Nygren KG. Plasma levels of d-norgestrel and sex hormone binding globulin during oral d-norgestrel medication immediately after delivery and legal abortion. Contraception 1977;15(1):87–92.
316. Back DJ, Breckenridge AM, Crawford FE, Orme ML, Rowe PH. Phenobarbitone interaction with oral contraceptive steroids in the rabbit and rat. Br J Pharmacol 1980;69(3):441–52.
317. Wilbur K, Ensom MH. Pharmacokinetic drug interactions between oral contraceptives and second-generation anticonvulsants. Clin Pharmacokinet 2000;38(4):355–65.
318. Crawford P, Chadwick D, Cleland P, Tjia J, Cowie A, Back DJ, Orme ML. The lack of effect of sodium valproate on the pharmacokinetics of oral contraceptive steroids. Contraception 1986;33(1):23–9.
319. Briggs MH. Megadose vitamin C and metabolic effects of the pill. BMJ (Clin Res Ed) 1981;283(6305):1547.
320. Jochemsen R, van der Graaff M, Boeijinga JK, Breimer DD. Influence of sex, menstrual cycle and oral contraception on the disposition of nitrazepam. Br J Clin Pharmacol 1982;13(3):319–24.
321. Patwardhan RV, Mitchell MC, Johnson RF, Schenker S. Differential effects of oral contraceptive steroids on the metabolism of benzodiazepines. Hepatology 1983;3(2):248–53.
322. Kendall MJ, Quarterman CP, Jack DB, Beeley L. Metoprolol pharmacokinetics and the oral contraceptive pill. Br J Clin Pharmacol 1982;14(1):120–2.
323. Hughes BR, Cunliffe WJ. Interactions between the oral contraceptive pill and antibiotics. Br J Dermatol 1990;122(5):717–18.

324. Friedman CI, Huneke AL, Kim MH, Powell J. The effect of ampicillin on oral contraceptive effectiveness. Obstet Gynecol 1980;55(1):33–7.
325. Neely JL, Abate M, Swinker M, D'Angio R. The effect of doxycycline on serum levels of ethinyl estradiol, norethindrone, and endogenous progesterone. Obstet Gynecol 1991;77(3):416–20.
326. Deray G, le Hoang P, Cacoub P, Assogba U, Grippon P, Baumelou A. Oral contraceptive interaction with cyclosporin. Lancet 1987;1(8525):158–9.
327. Liu HF, Magdalou J, Nicolas A, Lafaurie C, Siest G. Oral contraceptives stimulate the excretion of clofibric acid glucuronide in women and female rats. Gen Pharmacol 1991;22(2):393–7.
328. Miners JO, Robson RA, Birkett DJ. Gender and oral contraceptive steroids as determinants of drug glucuronidation: effects on clofibric acid elimination. Br J Clin Pharmacol 1984;18(2):240–3.
329. Sinofsky FE, Pasquale SA. The effect of fluconazole on circulating ethinyl estradiol levels in women taking oral contraceptives. Am J Obstet Gynecol 1998;178(2):300–4.
330. Hilbert J, Messig M, Kuye O, Friedman H. Evaluation of interaction between fluconazole and an oral contraceptive in healthy women. Obstet Gynecol 2001;98(2):218–23.
331. Legler UF, Benet LZ. Marked alterations in dose-dependent prednisolone kinetics in women taking oral contraceptives. Clin Pharmacol Ther 1986;39(4):425–9.
332. van Dijke CP, Weber JC. Interaction between oral contraceptives and griseofulvin. BMJ (Clin Res Ed) 1984;288(6424):1125–6.
333. Patwardhan RV, Desmond PV, Johnson RF, Schenker S. Impaired elimination of caffeine by oral contraceptive steroids. J Lab Clin Med 1980;95(4):603–8.
334. Rivera JM, Iriarte LM, Lozano F, Garcia-Bragado F, Salgado V, Grilo A. Possible estrogen-induced NMS. DICP 1989;23(10):811.
335. Muirhead GJ, Harness J, Holt PR, Oliver S, Anziano RJ. Ziprasidone and the pharmacokinetics of a combined oral contraceptive. Br J Clin Pharmacol 2000;49(Suppl 1):S49–56.
336. Watson KJR, Ghabrial H, Mashford ML, Harman PJ, Breen KJ, Desmond PV. The oral contraceptive pill increases morphine clearance but does not increase hepatic blood flow. Gastroenterology 1986;90:1779.
337. Rogers SM, Back DJ, Stevenson PJ, Grimmer SF, Orme ML. Paracetamol interaction with oral contraceptive steroids: increased plasma concentrations of ethinyloestradiol. Br J Clin Pharmacol 1987;23(6):721–5.
338. Miners JO, Attwood J, Birkett DJ. Influence of sex and oral contraceptive steroids on paracetamol metabolism. Br J Clin Pharmacol 1983;16(5):503–9.
339. Skolnick JL, Stoler BS, Katz DB, Anderson WH. Rifampin, oral contraceptives, and pregnancy. JAMA 1976;236(12):1382.
340. Bolt HM, Kappus H, Bolt M. Effect of rifampicin treatment on the metabolism of oestradiol and 17 alpha-ethinyloestradiol by human liver microsomes. Eur J Clin Pharmacol 1975;8(5):301–7.
341. Archer JS, Archer DF. Oral contraceptive efficacy and antibiotic interaction: a myth debunked. J Am Acad Dermatol 2002;46(6):917–23.
342. El Bouhmadi A, Laffargue F, Raspal N, Brun JF. 100 mg acetylsalicylic acid acutely decreases red cell aggregation in women taking oral contraceptives. Clin Hemorheol Microcirc 2000;22(2):99–106.
343. Miners JO, Grgurinovich N, Whitehead AG, Robson RA, Birkett DJ. Influence of gender and oral contraceptive steroids on the metabolism of salicylic acid and acetylsalicylic acid. Br J Clin Pharmacol 1986;22(2):135–42.
344. Krishnan KR, France RD, Ellinwood EH Jr. Tricyclic-induced akathisia in patients taking conjugated estrogens. Am J Psychiatry 1984;141(5):696–7.
345. Miguet JP, Vuitton D, Pessayre D, Allemand H, Metreau JM, Poupon R, Capron JP, Blanc F. Jaundice from troleandomycin and oral contraceptives. Ann Intern Med 1980;92(3):434.

Hormonal contraceptives—progestogen implants

See also Progestogens

General Information

Hormonal formulations for implantation contain progestogens, including the following:

- levonorgestrel
- etonogestrel
- desogestrel
- megestrol
- norethisterone.

For a complete account of the adverse effects of progestogens, readers are urged to consult the following monographs as well as this one:

- Hormonal contraceptives—progestogen injections
- Hormonal contraceptives—intracervical and intravaginal
- Hormonal contraceptives—oral
- Hormone replacement therapy—estrogens + progestogens
- Medroxyprogesterone
- Progestogens.

Levonorgestrel

Subdermal implanted silastic rods containing levonorgestrel (Norplant) have been widely studied and used with the support of the Population Council, but have fallen out of favor in a number of industrialized countries, because of complications. Six rods are inserted subdermally into the arm using a special device; each contains 35 mg of levonorgestrel, which is released into the circulation over 5 years. The total amount of levonorgestrel released daily during the first 500 days averages about 60 micrograms, falling to a plateau of 30 micrograms/day for the remainder of the 5-year period during which the product remains effective. It then has to be removed and replaced. The contraceptive effect of the implant does not seem to be caused primarily by ovulation inhibition, since after about the first year of use the hormone concentrations are too low to have this effect (1,2).

A product similar in approach to Norplant is the biodegradable subdermal capsular implant Capronor, which releases levonorgestrel over 12–18 months. Doses of 12 and 21.6 mg in capsules of differing size have been compared (3). Ovulation occurred in all cycles at the lower dose and in a quarter of cycles at the higher dose, so it is likely that the contraceptive effect results essentially from other progestogen-induced changes. Several users had local swelling or itching of the skin at the capsule insertion site, relieved by topical glucocorticoids.

The effectiveness, adverse events, and acceptability of the FDA-approved variant of levonorgestrel capsule implants in the USA over 5 years and the determinants of these outcomes have been studied (4). There were three pregnancies, yielding a 5-year cumulative rate of 1.3 per 100 users, an average annual rate of three per 1000 women. Ectopic pregnancy occurred at a rate of 0.6 per 1000 woman-years. There were no pregnancies in women who weighed less than 79 kg. Medical conditions that most often led to removal of the implant were prolonged or irregular menstrual bleeding, followed by headache, weight gain, and mood changes. Weight gain averaged 1 kg/year.

Etonogestrel

Implanon, which became available in 1999, is a subdermal implant that contains 68 mg of etonogestrel, the active metabolite of desogestrel. The product and field experience is therefore still limited. During the first 2 years after implantation, there is no ovulation; ovulation occurs occasionally in the third year, and it is recommended that the implant be removed after this time. As with Norplant, the principal problem is the occurrence of irregular bleeding (5), which leads some 25–30% of users to ask that the implant be removed. After some time, amenorrhea occurs in some 20% of users. There was a clinically significant increase in bodyweight in 20% of women carrying the implant (6). There may also be some local irritation from the implant, and minor scarring at the implantation site (7,8). In clinical trials the implant had no effect on coagulation measures, hemostasis, fat metabolism, or hepatic function, but according to the approved product information sheet the possibility of a slight increase in insulin resistance cannot be excluded.

Desogestrel

In clinical trials, implants containing desogestrel were effective, but with bleeding irregularities and ovarian cysts as the primary adverse effects (9).

Megestrol

Implants filled with megestrol acetate gave an unexpectedly high incidence of tubal pregnancies, while the absolute number of ectopic pregnancies was clearly greater than that expected for the general population (10). This finding reflects the same type of effect as has been described from time to time with oral progestogen-only products.

Norethisterone

A biodegradable delivery system using subcutaneous implants of fused pellets made from norethisterone and pure cholesterol has been tested (11).

General adverse effects

Generally speaking, the systemic effects of progestogen implants are very similar to those of low-dose oral progestogen-only contraception, except for variations due to the progressive change in the amount of hormone released. Many studies using various metabolic measures have shown no significant pattern of deviation from normal values (12,13), either during use of the implant or after removal (14).

Acceptability

As in the case of injectable depot contraceptives (SED-14, 1433) subdermal contraceptive implants are more likely to be used in developing countries, in order to overcome social and compliance problems, and that this can in principle involve risks to which underprivileged populations may be especially subject. All the same, acceptance is strikingly good (15). In a survey of data from eight developing countries, information was available on 7977 women starting Norplant, of whom 6625 used intrauterine devices and 1419 had been sterilized; most of the participants were followed for 5 years. All of the methods produced satisfactory degrees of contraception and, with a few exceptions, no characteristic morbidity was detected among Norplant users compared with the other groups. The two principal exceptions concerned gallbladder disease, which was 50% more common in women who used Norplant, and hypertension and borderline hypertension, the incidence of which was markedly raised in current implant users (RR = 1.81; 95% CI = 1.12, 2.92). Other unexpected findings were increased rates of respiratory disease and reduced risks of inflammatory disease of the genital tract in users of Norplant compared with sterilized women and those who used an intrauterine device (16).

In Burkina Faso, experience in 1660 women over 4 years has been critically reviewed (17). There were 247 withdrawals before the fourth year, for various reasons, including cycle disorders (60 withdrawals), unspecified medical reasons ($n = 53$), personal objections ($n = 47$), weight gain ($n = 14$), and contraceptive failure ($n = 2$). Menstrual disorders, including amenorrhea, spotting, and hypermenorrhea, occurred in 51% of the cases. The investigators stressed the need for a good information and sensitization campaign to reduce the number of implant withdrawals before the fourth year of use, since the product often seems to be withdrawn for insufficient reasons.

A study in Senegal produced similar findings over 5 years; the method was safe and effective, but dissatisfaction with cycle control was again a prominent reason for requesting removal of the implant (18).

A Thai study in 88 asymptomatic, young, HIV-1-positive women immediately after delivery has similarly confirmed the good acceptability of Norplant in a developing country, despite the high incidence of irregular bleeding and some instances of headache and hair loss (19).

In 10 718 women in China, Norplant was reliable and no serious or fatal effects were reported (20). When pregnancies did occur, only 3.1 per 100 were ectopic, which is higher than for the general population in Beijing but much lower than in US studies of Norplant (presumably because of lower rates of pelvic inflammatory disease in China). The 5-year continuation rate was 72 per 100 acceptors. Hemoglobin concentrations increased during the first year of use and remained high, presumably because of a reduction in menstrual blood loss. Although early findings suggested a reduction in platelet counts, follow-up work showed that in this population these were already low on admission to the study. Insertion-related complications necessitated removal in only 21 users.

In a study in Greece the method was well accepted by adolescents, although the study was small (13 subjects) (21). No significant problems arose during the 24-month follow-up period.

On the other hand, Norplant has been criticized in some Western countries, primarily because of adverse effects at the implantation site. An overview of adverse events reported to the FDA over 3 years, during which more than 700 000 implants were estimated to be in place, cited reports of 24 women hospitalized for infections at the insertion site and 14 who were either hospitalized or disabled because of difficulties associated with capsule removal (22). Fourteen women (two per 100 000) were reportedly hospitalized because of strokes. Three women developed thrombotic thrombocytopenic purpura and six developed thrombocytopenia. Finally, 39 Norplant users developed pseudotumor cerebri (benign intracranial hypertension), an incidence of 5.5 per 100 000; this condition is associated with obesity or recent weight gain, conditions that were present in most of the women for whom data were given. Although the rates of stroke and pseudotumor cerebri were slightly less than the expected rates in the general population of women of reproductive age, one has to take into account the well-known under-reporting of adverse events to agencies such as the FDA; the figures could therefore mean that Norplant users are actually at increased risk.

Reviewing the overall scene in Britain, Hannaford has pointed to the considerable difference in acceptance rates for Norplant in the industrialized world and developing countries and has stressed the fact that the adverse reaction incidence is, according to the best evidence, low (23).

Rapid rejection of implantable progestogen-based contraceptives by some users, because of discomfort and local complications (for example because of breakage or migration of the device, or less than expert placement and removal), has attracted much attention in past reviews.

Organs and Systems

Cardiovascular

Norplant does not alter the blood pressure (24).

Nervous system

Headache is fairly common in women using progestogen implants (25).

Psychological, psychiatric

Two cases of major depression and panic disorder, developing soon after insertion of Norplant and resolving after removal, have been reported, but a causal association was not proven (26).

Five women using the Norplant system developed major depression, two of whom also developed obsessive-compulsive disorder and one of whom also developed agoraphobia (27). They had no prior psychiatric history but developed major depression within 1–3 months after insertion of Norplant. The depression worsened over time and in all cases resolved within 1–2 months after removal of Norplant. There was no recurrence of depression after 7–8 months in four cases available for follow-up. In addition to major depression, obsessive-compulsive disorder developed in two women and symptoms of agoraphobia developed in one woman during Norplant treatment, which resolved after removal.

Metabolism

Norplant does not alter body weight (28).

Hematologic

Research on blood coagulation has produced inconsistent results, usually showing little effect, as one would expect from a progestogen-based method without an estrogen component (29).

During 1 year of observation of 23 healthy fertile African women, beginning at the time that a Norplant device was inserted, the mean packed cell volume rose slightly but significantly from 40.5 to 42.2, but the mean total leukocyte, neutrophil, and lymphocyte counts all fell significantly, as did the mean platelet count (30). In four patients, the platelet counts were only 50–80 $\times$ 10^9/l. The rise in packed cell volume might, according to the authors, help to counter anemia in people in developing countries. However, the fall in the platelet count is hard to explain.

Skin

Some women who use progestogen implants develop acne, because of the androgenic activity of levonorgestrel. Three women developed severe acne vulgaris within several weeks to a few months after either insertion of a levonorgestrel IUCD (two women, 27 and 33 years of age) or subcutaneous implantation of etonogestrel (a 26-year-old woman) (31).

Reproductive system

The most frequent adverse effect of progestogen implants is irregular menstrual bleeding (32), which in some countries has reduced the acceptability of the treatment (33). It is common during the first year of use but tends to become much less marked thereafter (12,28,34). In one study, the incidence of menstrual irregularity in Norplant users was 73% compared with only 5% in a comparable population using oral contraceptives (35). There is also a fairly high incidence of breakthrough bleeding or amenorrhea (36). The cause of the irregular bleeding is not fully understood, but there is evidence that an increase in endometrial vascular fragility might precipitate vessel breakdown and hence breakthrough bleeding (37).

It is not clear why some women are more susceptible to this complication than others. In a Thai study in a large number of Norplant users irregular bleeding was characterized by low estradiol concentrations, absence of luteal activity, and a thin hyperechoic pattern in the endometrium (38). The possible role of cellular apoptosis in the endometrial response to Norplant has been investigated using immunohistochemistry, but with negative results (39). However, among Norplant users the superficial endometrial blood vessels are more fragile than in controls and even more fragile than in untreated women with dysfunctional uterine bleeding (40).

An unusual approach to dealing with this irregular bleeding has been to give an antiprogestogen simultaneously. In 50 Chinese women with implants, mifepristone 50 mg once every 4 weeks has been compared with placebo (41). In all the women, regardless of treatment, the frequency of bleeding fell significantly over 1 year of observation, as it commonly does. However, women who took mifepristone had significantly shorter episodes of bleeding during treatment than during the 90 days before treatment started; the duration of bleeding episodes fell more gradually in the controls. Women who used mifepristone were more likely to find the treatment acceptable than the women who used placebo. Despite concerns that antiprogestogenic effects may jeopardize contraception, there were no pregnancies. In the view of the investigators, this approach may offer a useful strategy to relieve unwanted adverse effects of implants until bleeding patterns improve spontaneously with time.

A second unusual approach to the bleeding problem has been to give vitamin E. There is evidence that there is a poor angiogenic response in the endometrium of users of Norplant, and it has been hypothesized that this might be caused by an imbalance of pro-oxidant and antioxidant processes. A placebo-controlled study has suggested that vitamin E (200 mg/day for 10 days monthly) significantly reduces the number of monthly bleeding days (42). However, there was also some reduction in bleeding days with placebo, and this approach would need further study before the results could be accepted as clinically useful.

Amenorrhea is uncommon in women with progestogen implants, but the monthly blood loss is usually reduced rather than increased (43). Menstrual irregularity does not appear to be correlated with body mass index.

The appearance of enlarged ovarian follicles is a recognized complication of Norplant, but the reported incidence varies, probably because different methods are used to recognize them. Serial ultrasonography produces much higher figures than clinical methods and has led to exaggerated concern; the enlarged follicles are transient and do not require intervention (44).

Breast discharge has been reported in some women with progestogen implants (45).

Infection risk

Insertion-related complications include infection, hematoma formation, local irritation, scar formation, early implant expulsions, and allergic reactions to the dressing. A pooled analysis of insertion site complications in multicountry studies showed that 0.8% of women develop infection after insertion of Norplant, generally within the first week, but sometimes several months later (46). Implant expulsion occurred at some stage in 0.4% of users, often because of infection but sometimes because of poor placement. Two-thirds of expulsions were reported more than 2 months after insertion. The rates of such complications vary widely between practices and between countries.

Second-Generation Effects

Fertility

As with other progestogen-based contraceptive methods, the return of fertility after withdrawal is rapid: serum levonorgestrel concentrations are undetectable within a week after implant removal, and normal cycles usually resume during the first month.

Teratogenicity

Because the pregnancy rate among users of Norplant is quite low, the rate of ectopic pregnancy is also very low. There is no evidence that infants conceived during Norplant use are at higher risk of birth defects.

Lactation

One particular advantage of progestogen-only contraception is its suitability for use during breastfeeding, since there are no estrogens to impede lactation. The infant's intake of steroids is low and appears to be acceptable; its daily intake of steroids (estimated from concentrations in maternal milk during the first month of use) has been estimated to be 90–100 nanograms of levonorgestrel (Norplant), 75–120 nanograms of etonogestrel (Implanon), and 50 and 110 nanograms of nestorone (Nestorone and Elcometrine implants respectively) (47). However, it is still considered advisable to defer the implantation of these devices until 6 weeks after delivery, in view of the theoretical possibility of an adverse influence on the neonate.

Drug Administration

Drug formulations

The practical problems associated with Norplant have related to its physical form rather than its pharmacological profile. Practitioners specially trained in the insertion and removal of the device usually handle it without major problems, but without this special instruction it can be difficult to ensure that the rods are properly placed and that they are removed without scarring or other complications. Even given appropriate handling, the rods can cause problems as a result of migration or breakage in situ.

An implant can usually be removed in under a quarter of an hour under local anesthesia, but removal can be more difficult if the clinician is inexperienced, if the rods were not positioned properly at insertion, or if fibrous tissue has grown around them.

If removal is not expertly handled in problematic cases, considerable scarring can result, and some users have proceeded to litigation as a consequence of such complications. Complications in the removal of Norplant capsules have been evaluated in 3416 cases from 11 countries (48). Complications were reported in 4.5% of removals, usually attributable to implants being broken during removal (1.7%) or being embedded below the subdermal plane (1.2%). Logistic regression analysis showed that the most important risk factors for complicated removals were complications at insertion and an infection at the implant site (before or at the time or removal). For women without complications, the mean removal time was 12 minutes, but for those with complications the mean increased to 30 minutes. These results illustrate the necessity of proper insertion technique, under aseptic conditions. Capsules become surrounded by a fibrous sheath within 3 months after implantation; beyond a few months, there is no difference in complication rate by duration of use.

Modified Norplant

A modified system, Norplant-2, requires only two instead of six rods. In 140 women using the Norplant-2 contraceptive subdermal implant system there were no accidental pregnancies over 3 years (49). Adverse effects that caused withdrawal from the study were acne, headache, and pain at the implant site. The termination rate for these medical reasons in year 3 of the study was 4.6%. The other main reason for termination was prolonged menstrual flow; the 3-year cumulative termination rate for menstrual irregularities was 3.8%.

References

1. Alvarez F, Brache V, Tejada AS, Faundes A. Abnormal endocrine profile among women with confirmed or presumed ovulation during long-term Norplant use. Contraception 1986;33(2):111–19.
2. Sivin I, Diaz S, Holma P, Alvarez-Sanchez F, Robertson DN. A four-year clinical study of NORPLANT implants. Stud Fam Plann 1983;14(6–7):184–91.
3. Darney PD, Monroe SE, Klaisle CM, Alvarado A. Clinical evaluation of the Capronor contraceptive implant: preliminary report. Am J Obstet Gynecol 1989;160(5 Pt 2):1292–5.
4. Sivin I, Mishell DR Jr, Darney P, Wan L, Christ M. Levonorgestrel capsule implants in the United States: a 5-year study. Obstet Gynecol 1998;92(3):337–44.
5. Affandi B. An integrated analysis of vaginal bleeding patterns in clinical trials of Implanon. Contraception 1998;58(Suppl 6):S99–107.
6. Croxatto HB, Urbancsek J, Massai R, Coelingh Bennink H, van Beek A. A multicentre efficacy and safety study of the single contraceptive implant Implanon. Implanon Study Group. Hum Reprod 1999;14(4):976–81.
7. Anonymous. Etonorgestrel. Geneesmiddelenbulletin 1999;33:123–4.
8. Admiraal PJJ, Luers JFJ. Etonogestrel implantaat. Pharma Selecta 1999;15:152–5.
9. Diaz S, Pavez M, Moo-Young AJ, Bardin CW, Croxatto HB. Clinical trial with 3-keto-desogestrel subdermal implants. Contraception 1991;44(4):393–408.
10. Croxatto HD, Diaz S, Rosati S, Croxatto HB. Adnexal complications in women under treatment with progestogen implants. Contraception 1975;12(6):629–37.
11. Gupta G, Saxena BB, Landesman R, Ledger WJ. Preparation, properties, and release rate of norethindrone (NET) from subcutaneous implants. In: Zatuchni GI, Goldsmith A, Shelton JD, Seiarra JJ, editors. Long-Acting Contraceptive Delivery Systems. Philadelphia: Harper and Row, 1984,425
12. Croxatto HB. NORPLANT: levonorgestrel-releasing contraceptive implant. Ann Med 1993;25(2):155–60.
13. Singh K, Viegas OA, Loke D, Ratnam SS. Effect of Norplant-2 rods on liver, lipid and carbohydrate metabolism. Contraception 1992;45(5):463–72.
14. Singh K, Viegas OA, Loke DF, Ratnam SS. Evaluation of liver function and lipid metabolism following Norplant-2 rods removal. Adv Contracept 1993;9(3):233–9.
15. Glasier A. Implantable contraceptives for women: effectiveness, discontinuation rates, return of fertility, and outcome of pregnancies. Contraception 2002;65(1):29–37.
16. Meirik O, Farley TM, Sivin I. Safety and efficacy of levonorgestrel implant, intrauterine device, and sterilization. Obstet Gynecol 2001;97(4):539–47.
17. Kone B, Lankoande J, Ouedraogo CM, Ouedraogo A, Bonane B, Dao B, Sanou J. La Contraception par les implants sous-cutanes de lévonorgestral (Norplant). Experience africaine du Burkina Faso. [Contraception with levonorgestrel (Norplant) subcutaneous implants. African experience in Burkina Faso.] Contracept Fertil Sex 1999;27(2):162–3.
18. Ba MG, Moreau JC, Sokal D, Dunson R, Dao B, Kouedou D, Diadhiou F. A 5-year clinical evaluation of Norplant implants in Senegal. Contraception 1999;59(6):377–81.
19. Taneepanichskul S, Tanprasertkul C. Use of Norplant implants in the immediate postpartum period among asymptomatic HIV-1-positive mothers. contraception 2001;64(1):39–41.
20. Gu SJ, Du MK, Zhang LD, Liu YL, Wang SH, Sivin I. A 5-year evaluation of NORPLANT contraceptive implants in China. Obstet Gynecol 1994;83(5 Pt 1):673–8.
21. Cardamakis E, Georgopoulos A, Fotopoulos A, Sykiotis GP, Pappas AP, Lazaris D, Tzingounis VA. Clinical experience with Norplant subdermal implant system as long-term contraception during adolescence. Eur J Contracept Reprod Health Care 2002;7(1):36–40.
22. Wysowski DK, Green L. Serious adverse events in Norplant users reported to the Food and Drug Administration's MedWatch Spontaneous Reporting System. Obstet Gynecol 1995;85(4):538–42.
23. Hannaford P. Postmarketing surveillance study of Norplant in developing countries. Lancet 2001;357(9271):1815–16.
24. Davies GC, Newton JR. Subdermal contraceptive implants—a review: with special reference to Norplant. Br J Fam Plann 1991;17:4.
25. Population Council, Center for Biomedical Research, New York, New York 10021, USA. sivin@popcbr.rockefeller.edu.
26. Wagner KD, Berenson AB. Norplant-associated major depression and panic disorder. J Clin Psychiatry 1994;55(11):478–80.
27. Wagner KD. Major depression and anxiety disorders associated with Norplant. J Clin Psychiatry 1996;57(4):152–7.
28. Pasquale SA, Knuppel RA, Owens AG, Bachmann GA. Irregular bleeding, body mass index and coital frequency in Norplant contraceptive users. Contraception 1994;50(2):109–16.
29. Shaaban MM, Elwan SI, el-Kabsh MY, Farghaly SA, Thabet N. Effect of levonorgestrel contraceptive implants, Norplant, on blood coagulation. Contraception 1984;30(5):421–30.
30. Aisien AO, Sagay AS, Imade GE, Ujah IA, Nnana OU. Changes in menstrual and haematological indices among Norplant acceptors. Contraception 2000;61(4):283–6.

31. Cohen EB, Rossen NN. Acne vulgaris bij gebruik van progestagenen in een hormoonspiraal of een subcutaan implantaat. [Acne vulgaris in connection with the use of progestagens in a hormonal IUD or a subcutaneous implant.] Ned Tijdschr Geneeskd 2003;147(43):2137–9.
32. Singh K, Viegas OA, Liew D, Singh P, Ratnam SS. Norplant-2 rods: one year experience in Singapore. Contraception 1988;38(4):429–40.
33. Rehan N, Inayatullah A, Chaudhary I. Norplant: reasons for discontinuation and side-effects. Eur J Contracept Reprod Health Care 2000;5(2):113–18.
34. Shoupe D, Mishell DR Jr, Bopp BL, Fielding M. The significance of bleeding patterns in Norplant implant users. Obstet Gynecol 1991;77(2):256–60.
35. Berenson AB, Wiemann CM, Rickerr VI, McCombs SL. Contraceptive outcomes among adolescents prescribed Norplant implants versus oral contraceptives after one year of use. Am J Obstet Gynecol 1997;176(3):586–92.
36. Brache V, Faundes A, Alvarez F, Cochon L. Nonmenstrual adverse events during use of implantable contraceptives for women: data from clinical trials. Contraception 2002;65(1):63–74.
37. Hickey M, d'Arcangues C. Vaginal bleeding disturbances and implantable contraceptives. Contraception 2002;65(1):75–84.
38. Kaewrudee S, Taneepanichskul S. Norplant users with irregular bleeding. Ultrasonographic assessment and evaluation of serum concentrations of estradiol and progesterone. J Reprod Med 2000;45(12):983–6.
39. Rogers PA, Lederman F, Plunkett D, Affandi B. Bcl-2, Fas and caspase 3 expression in endometrium from levonorgestrel implant users with and without breakthrough bleeding. Hum Reprod 2000;15(Suppl 3):152–61.
40. Hickey M, Dwarte D, Fraser IS. Superficial endometrial vascular fragility in Norplant users and in women with ovulatory dysfunctional uterine bleeding. Hum Reprod 2000;15(7):1509–14.
41. Cheng L, Zhu H, Wang A, Ren F, Chen J, Glasier A. Once a month administration of mifepristone improves bleeding patterns in women using subdermal contraceptive implants releasing levonorgestrel. Hum Reprod 2000;15(9):1969–72.
42. Subakir SB, Setiadi E, Affandi B, Pringgoutomo S, Freisleben HJ. Benefits of vitamin E supplementation to Norplant users—in vitro and in vivo studies. Toxicology 2000;148(2–3):173–8.
43. Balogh SA, Klavon SL, Basnayake S, Puertollano N, Ramos RM, Grubb GS. Bleeding patterns and acceptability among Norplant users in two Asian countries. Contraception 1989;39(5):541–53.
44. Alvarez-Sanchez F, Brache V, de Oca VM, Cochon L, Faundes A. Prevalence of enlarged ovarian follicles among users of levonorgestrel subdermal contraceptive implants (Norplant). Am J Obstet Gynecol 2000;182(3):535–9.
45. Segal M. Norplant: Birth Control at Arm's Reach. FDA: Office of Women's Health Website. http://www.fda.gov/bbs/topics/CONSUMER/CON00009.html, 2001.
46. Klavon SL, Grubb GS. Insertion site complications during the first year of NORPLANT use. Contraception 1990;41(1):27–37.
47. Diaz S. Contraceptive implants and lactation. Contraception 2002;65(1):39–46.
48. Dunson TR, Amatya RN, Krueger SL. Complications and risk factors associated with the removal of Norplant implants. Obstet Gynecol 1995;85(4):543–8.
49. Chompootaweep S, Kochagarn E, Tang-Usaha J, Theppitaksak B, Dusitsin N. Experience of Thai women in Bangkok with Norplant-2 implants. Contraception 1998;58(4):221–5.

Hormonal contraceptives—progestogen injections

See also Progestogens

General Information

For a complete account of the adverse effects of progestogens, readers should consult the following monographs as well as this one:

- Hormonal contraceptives—intracervical and intravaginal
- Hormonal contraceptives—oral
- Hormonal contraceptives—progesterone implants
- Hormone replacement therapy—estrogens + progestogens
- Medroxyprogesterone
- Progestogens.

Injectable hormonal contraceptives, which are normally composed of long-acting esters of progestogens, have obvious practical advantages over oral products when user compliance is poor, for example in illiterate or mentally subnormal women or in some populations in developing countries. However, the fact that they are used in this type of patient has led to some social protest against their use, as if they were intended to undermine free will or provide cheap but unpleasant contraception for the underprivileged. This may in turn explain some unbalanced criticism of these products in terms of efficacy and safety. Their sometimes incomplete cycle control is indeed a practical disadvantage, but not a risk, and the fact that they contain no estrogen actually means that they are safer in those respects when risks of hormonal contraception are due mainly to estrogenic effects, particularly thromboembolic complications. All in all, the injectable hormonal contraceptives provide effective, reversible, and relatively safe contraception, which can well be used not only in the populations named above but also, for example, in some women who smoke or when an estrogen is contraindicated (1,2).

General adverse effects

The degree to which women tolerate the adverse effects of long-acting injectable contraceptives seems to vary from one population to another, and it can be important to examine the frequency and severity of complaints in different environments. Particularly in developed countries, these products are often stated to cause mood changes, weight gain, and demineralization, but in developing countries they are very widely used. A worldwide review has surveyed the incidence of these conditions in users and has compared some of the figures with those found with an implantable product (Norplant; see the monograph on Hormonal contraceptives–progestogen injections) (3). Perhaps surprisingly, a consensus seems to be emerging that depot medroxyprogesterone acetate implants do not in fact result in an increase in the incidence of depression or in the severity of pre-existing depression, even after 1 or 2 years, nor do they cause significant weight gain. Similarly, Norplant did not cause depression.

Subgroups of users of depot medroxyprogesterone acetate may have reduced spinal bone density, but this seems to be reversible after withdrawal, even after several years of drug exposure (4). Bone mineral density in one cross-sectional study was lower among users of depot medroxyprogesterone acetate, but withdrawal was followed by complete recovery of normal bone density (4). A current study in the USA is expected to provide further data on this matter in women who have used medroxyprogesterone acetate for as long as 10 years.

Norethisterone enantate

The adverse effects of norethisterone enantate when used as a 2-monthly injectable contraceptive have been compared in various populations with those of depot medroxyprogesterone acetate and were found to be closely similar (5,6).

The largest single trial conducted with norethisterone enantate, covering some 9000 women-months of use, provided a fair picture of its adverse effects. Menstrual irregularity (prolonged bleeding, spotting, or amenorrhea) was the main complaint. Other adverse effects were periodic abdominal bloating and tender breasts, both of which were thought to be due to water retention and were relieved by diuretics. There was no associated weight gain. More than 50 of the women had pre-existing hypertension, and in these users the injections did not significantly affect blood pressure, which generally remained below 140/90 mmHg. Blood clotting was also not affected. High density lipoprotein cholesterol concentrations in the women treated were significantly lower than in the controls. The results of glucose tolerance tests did not differ significantly (7).

Three studies carried out in Bangladesh (8), Pakistan (9), and China (10) showed similar adverse reactions patterns. In the Bangladeshi study, nine of 254 women had a rise in both systolic and diastolic blood pressures, but five had a reduction of the same magnitude. In the Chinese women there were no significant changes in blood pressure. However, five Chinese women developed abnormal liver function tests and three of these women had liver enlargement after treatment for more than 2 years.

Other compounds and combinations

Other progestogen-only injectables have been tested, but those examined so far appear to have similar properties to the formulations that are already available.

Combined estrogen + progestogen injectables have been the subject of much experimentation. Administered monthly, they were developed in order to provide more dependable patterns of vaginal bleeding. Many formulations have been evaluated, and two of these have undergone phase III clinical trials by the WHO: one contains medroxyprogesterone acetate 25 mg with estradiol cipionate 5 mg and the other norethisterone enantate 50 mg plus estradiol valerate 5 mg. Analysis of daily menstrual diary record cards for women using these methods, compared with several other contraceptive methods and no method, showed that bleeding patterns for women receiving monthly injections were more regular, but not entirely normal (11). Although the median experience was similar to that of women not using contraception, the range of menstrual patterns was much wider. The outcome in this respect was found to be acceptable in only 70% of cycles during the first year of use, but later this figure rose to 85–90%. Under 10% of women discontinued use during the first year because of bleeding irregularities or amenorrhea, a rate that is presumably related in part to thorough counselling.

References

1. DaVanzo J, Parnell AM, Foege WH. Health consequences of contraceptive use and reproductive patterns. Summary of a report from the US National Research Council. JAMA 1991;265(20):2692–6.
2. Szarewski A, Guillebaud J. Contraception. BMJ 1991;302(6787):1224–6.
3. Kaunitz AM. Long-acting hormonal contraception: assessing impact on bone density, weight, and mood. Int J Fertil Womens Med 1999;44(2):110–17.
4. Cundy T, Cornish J, Evans MC, Roberts H, Reid IR. Recovery of bone density in women who stop using medroxyprogesterone acetate. BMJ 1994;308(6923):247–8.
5. Salem HT, Salah M, Aly MY, Thabet AI, Shaaban MM, Fathalla MF. Acceptability of injectable contraceptives in Assiut, Egypt. Contraception 1988;38(6):697–710.
6. Kazi AI. Comparative evaluation of two once-a-month contraceptive injections. J Pak Med Assoc 1989;39(4):98–102.
7. Howard G, Blair M, Fotherby K, Elder MG, Bye P. Seven years clinical experience of the injectable contraceptive, norethisterone enanthate. Br J Fam Plann 1985;11:9.
8. Chowdhury TA. A clinical study on injectable contraceptive Noristerat. Bangladesh Med J 1985;14(2–3):28–35.
9. Kazi A, Holck SE, Diethelm P. Phase IV study of the injection Norigest in Pakistan. Contraception 1985;32(4):395–403.
10. Frederiksen H, Ravenholt RT. Thromboembolism, oral contraceptives, and cigarettes. Public Health Rep 1970;85(3):197–205.
11. Fraser IS. Menstrual changes associated with progestogen-only contraception. Acta Obstet Gynecol Scand Suppl 1986;134:21–7.

Hormonal replacement therapy—estrogens + androgens

See also Estrogens *and* Androgens

General Information

For a complete account of the adverse effects of estrogens, readers should consult the following monographs as well as this one:

- Diethylstilbestrol
- Estrogens
- Hormonal contraceptives—emergency contraception
- Hormonal contraceptives—oral
- Hormone replacement therapy—estrogens
- Hormone replacement therapy—estrogens + progestogens.

An estrogen + an androgen

This variant on the theme of estrogen replacement therapy has been propagated from various centers for different reasons (1,2).

The theoretical starting point is the observation that (particularly after oophorectomy) there are deficiencies of both testosterone and androstenedione (3) and from the observation that estrogens alone do not relieve all menopausal symptoms. While there may well be justification for androgen replacement after oophorectomy, it is not clear that most of the claims made for use of this approach following a natural menopause are sufficiently well founded to justify the risks involved.

Adding an androgen to estrogen replacement therapy in the menopause has been thought to provide supplementary benefit with respect to climacteric symptoms, fatigue, and impaired libido, as well as favorably affecting muscle mass, skin quality, and bone density. It is also stated that androgens improve relief of vasomotor symptoms and relieve depression and anxiety when they occur after the menopause in this group of patients. Some workers have concluded that in women who respond to conjugated estrogens with a rise in blood pressure (not a common response by any means), this effect could be avoided by the addition of an androgen. Yet others have asserted that when the hematocrit falls during estrogen therapy, the effect can be prevented by an androgen.

The main reason for caution with the use of androgens is the susceptibility of menopausal women to their virilizing effects, which can sometimes prove irreversible. Deepening of the voice, hirsutism, and acne can occur in many patients at an early stage of treatment and can prove distressing. There may be enlargement of the clitoris, although not consistently.

However, there are other reasons for caution. Statements with respect to the effect of estrogen + androgen combinations on blood lipids are, for example, contradictory, depending on the combinations used. If androgens are to be used, the effect on lipoproteins should at all events be monitored (1).

It is doubtful whether one can avoid unwanted androgenic effects by cautious dosing. For example, the published data seem to show that a desired effect on libido is only likely to occur at androgen doses sufficient to produce serum testosterone concentrations in the virilizing range (over 2 ng/ml), and that even after withdrawal of such doses virilizing concentrations of testosterone are maintained for many months.

Finally, androgens actually appear in some respects to counter the desired effects of estrogens in this patient group. Doppler flowmetry has been used to study the cardiovascular effects of adding an androgen to an estrogen in an open, randomized study in 40 patients over 8 months, all of whom were using transdermal estradiol (50 micrograms/day) and cyclic medroxyprogesterone acetate (10 mg/day) (4). Half of the subjects then received additional testosterone undecanoate (40 mg/day). The investigators concluded that while the androgen improved sexual desire and satisfaction and had no effect on endometrial thickness, it did in part counteract the beneficial effects of the estrogens on cerebral vascular activity and lipids. The most notable change was a significant increase in the pulsatility index of the middle cerebral artery. The androgen also resulted in a 10% reduction in HDL cholesterol concentration within 8 months. The authors therefore urged caution in using androgens, at least in the manner used in this study.

There are naturally some groups that have worked together with manufacturers to profile the supposed advantages of particular estrogen + androgen regimens, especially when these are available in the form of fixed combination formulations.

The adverse effects of estrogen + androgen therapy include mild hirsutism and acne (5). One group of workers, who examined the use of "Estratest" (an esterified combination of estrogen and methyltestosterone), concluded that in their experience under 5% of women developed acne or facial hirsutism, a frequency similar to that experienced when using conjugated estrogens 0.625 mg/day. Women had significantly less nausea with the estrogen + androgen treatment than with conjugated estrogen therapy. Cancers, cardiovascular disease, thromboembolism, and liver disease were stated to be rare among users of the combination. The only adverse events exceeding 4% of total reports were alopecia, acne, weight gain, and hirsutism (6). However, much higher rates of complications with such combinations have been reported from other centres (1).

The evident disadvantage of a fixed combination is that it renders it impossible to carry out any fine adjustment of dosages, such as might be called for in the light of the clinical response and adverse effects in a given individual.

All in all, it seems very doubtful whether any of the supposed benefits of androgen therapy justify the risks involved, except possibly as a transitional measure in those recently oophorectomized women who have acute symptoms of sudden androgen withdrawal.

An estrogen + an androgen + a progestogen

Another variant on hormone replacement therapy involves using all three types of sex steroid in parallel, starting from the argument that during the fertile period all three are synthesized by the ovary (7). A "natural" version of this therapy uses estradiol, testosterone (with or without dehydroepiandrosterone), and progesterone in an appropriate pharmaceutical form (for example micronized), so that absorption is attained without the need for 17-substitution. This approach naturally avoids some of the undesirable effects of the synthetic steroids, and has been stated to improve menopausal depression and anxiety. However, the adverse effects of all three types of component can be experienced.

References

1. Kaunitz AM. The role of androgens in menopausal hormonal replacement. Endocrinol Metab Clin North Am 1997;26(2):391–7.
2. Casson PR, Carson SA. Androgen replacement therapy in women: myths and realities. Int J Fertil Menopausal Stud 1996;41(4):412–22.
3. Davis S. Testosterone deficiency in women. J Reprod Med 2001;46(Suppl 3):291–6.
4. Penotti M, Sironi L, Cannata L, Vigano P, Casini A, Gabrielli L, Vignali M. Effects of androgen supplementation

of hormone replacement therapy on the vascular reactivity of cerebral arteries. Fertil Steril 2001;76(2):235–40.
5. Cameron DR, Braunstein GD. Androgen replacement therapy in women. Fertil Steril 2004;82(2):273–89.
6. Barrett-Connor E. Efficacy and safety of estrogen/androgen therapy. Menopausal symptoms, bone, and cardiovascular parameters. J Reprod Med 1998;43(Suppl 8):746–52.
7. Hargrove JT, Osteen KG. An alternative method of hormone replacement therapy using the natural sex steroids. Infert Reprod Med Clin North Am 1995;6:653–74.

Hormone replacement therapy—estrogens

See also Estrogens

General Information

For a complete account of the adverse effects of estrogens, readers should consult the following monographs as well as this one:

- Diethylstilbestrol
- Estrogens
- Hormonal contraceptives—emergency contraception
- Hormonal contraceptives—oral
- Hormone replacement therapy—estrogens + androgens
- Hormone replacement therapy—estrogens + progestogens.

Estrogen replacement therapy was until recently widely recommended for the prevention of osteoporosis in middle-aged and older women (1). Long-term estrogen therapy also reduces the incidence of ischemic heart disease in such women (2). However, it has always been difficult to know in which women such prophylactic use is likely to be needed, and this dilemma is compounded by the prospect of adverse reactions, which can include any of the acute effects listed in the estrogen monograph, but also in some cases long-term effects such as tumors.

The multiplicity of hormone replacement therapy regimens in use (involving one or two drugs, continuous or intermittent treatment, and various forms of administration) makes it difficult to express any general conclusion about the benefit-to-harm balance, and there has been a thoughtful review of the obstacles to assessing these matters objectively and scientifically, including questions of both ethics and trial design (3). Even the ultimate effect of hormone replacement therapy on the incidence of ischemic heart disease remains subject to dispute (4), and incidental reports of cardiac complications, sometimes in women with entirely healthy coronary vessels, continue to cause concern (5). For such reasons, much work has been devoted to determining the lowest effective dose of estrogen needed to achieve particular results.

An extraordinarily thorough review of all significant controlled studies of estrogen replacement therapy has been published by the Cochrane Collaboration (6). The participants totalled 2511 and the trials lasted 0.25–3 years. The primary purpose was to confirm efficacy, but data on adverse effects were also collected. Withdrawal because of adverse events, commonly breast tenderness, edema, joint pains, and psychological symptoms, was not significantly higher with HRT than placebo (OR = 1.38; 95% CI = 0.87, 2.21). Breast tenderness and withdrawal bleeding were the only significant problems in terms of frequency. The studies did not justify the conclusion that there are serious adverse effects, such as thrombosis and malignancies.

Carefully assessed data like these illustrate the delicacy of the balance in the debate regarding the benefit-to-harm balance of long-term HRT; extreme statements have been made in both directions, and clearly most are not justified. A reasoned critical review, stressing how inadequate many of the data still are on both efficacy and safety issues, has been published (7).

Observational studies

A Japanese study of the use of estriol 2 mg/day for 12 months in 68 postmenopausal women with climacteric symptoms showed a significant effect in relieving hot flushes, night sweats, and insomnia (8,9). There were significant falls in serum follicle stimulating hormone (FSH) and luteinizing hormone (LH) concentrations, but no effect on lipids, bone demineralization, or blood pressure. There was slight vaginal bleeding in 14% of women treated during a natural menopause, but histological and ultrasound evaluation showed no changes in the endometrium or breasts. It is evident, however, that higher doses might be needed when treating women of other races with a higher body weight. Other workers have found that when given with a progestogen over long periods, estriol 2.0 mg/day seems much less likely to cause undesirable lipid changes than are equine conjugated estrogens, which can cause increased HDL cholesterol and triglyceride concentrations (10).

Comparative studies

In a randomized, multicenter study in Denmark 376 perimenopausal women with climacteric symptoms were randomly allocated to oral sequential combined treatment with regimens based on estrogen plus either desogestrel or medroxyprogesterone acetate (11). Both treatments effectively alleviated menopausal complaints within 6 months and gave good cycle control. Bleeding pattern and mood disturbances were more favorably affected by desogestrel, but overall the differences in adverse effects (irregular bleeding and a slight tendency to hypotension) were not large. It should be noted, however, that with cyclic combined hormone replacement therapy treatment, the bleeding pattern alone does not seem to be a reliable means of distinguishing cases in which the endometrium is atrophic or inactive from those in which it is proliferative or hyperplastic (12).

Organs and Systems

Cardiovascular

One of the most serious aspects of the thromboembolic complications now widely acknowledged as being associated with HRT is that their emergence coincides with the development of the conclusion that the role of HRT in reducing the risk of coronary heart disease is at best unproven. A form of treatment that was originally viewed as potentially beneficial to the cardiovascular system is at present on balance perhaps harmful (13).

A US group examined potential risk factors for venous thromboembolic events in women assigned to HRT in the Postmenopausal Estrogen/Progestin Interventions (PEPI) study, a 3-year double-blind study in 875 postmenopausal women designed to assess the effects of HRT on heart disease risk factors (HDL cholesterol, fibrinogen, blood pressure, and insulin) (14). Women with a history of estrogen-associated venous thromboembolic events were excluded. Ten women, all assigned to HRT, had a venous thromboembolic event during the study. Only baseline fibrinogen varied significantly between those who had a venous thromboembolic event while assigned to HRT event (mean 2.49 g/l) and those who did not have an event (mean 2.81 g/l). Adjusting for covariates did not affect this finding. As the authors remarked, the lower fibrinogen concentrations among women who subsequently reported venous thromboembolic events may be a marker for a specific, but as yet undefined, coagulopathy that is magnified in the presence of exogenous hormones. However, larger studies are needed to confirm this hypothesis.

Since much of the evidence of thromboembolic complications with HRT relates to the use of conjugated equine estrogens, the degree of risk when natural 17-beta-estradiol was used instead has been examined in Norway in a population-based case-control study involving consecutive women, aged 44–70 years, discharged from a University Hospital between 1990 and 1996 with a diagnosis of deep venous thrombosis or pulmonary embolism (15). Women with cancer-associated thrombosis were excluded. Random controls were used. The material comprised 176 cases and 352 controls, that is two controls for each case. All the women who received HRT had been given estradiol. The frequency of HRT use was 28% (50/176) in cases and 26% (93/352) in controls. The estimated matched crude odds ratio was 1.13 (CI = 0.71, 1.78), which shows no significant association of overall use of estradiol-based HRT and thromboembolism. However, when the duration of exposure to HRT was taken into account by stratification, there was an increased risk of thromboembolism during the first year of use, with a crude odds ratio of 3.54 (CI = 1.54, 5.2). This effect was reduced by extended use to a crude odds ratio of 0.66 (CI = 0.39, 1.10) after the first year of use. The authors concluded that the use of estradiol for HRT was associated with a three-fold increase in the risk of venous thromboembolism, but that this increased risk was restricted to the first year of use. One is bound to wonder whether this shift in risk was genuine or reflects only the limitations of the study.

Among the less common forms of thromboembolism that have been reported is occlusion of the retinal vein, familiar with the oral contraceptives but unusual with HRT (16).

Ear, nose, throat

Visual hallucinations have been associated with estrogen in a patient with Charles Bonnet syndrome (17).

- An 84-year-old woman with poor visual acuity secondary to bilateral, non-exudative, age-related macular degeneration had non-threatening visual hallucinations 2 weeks after starting oral estrogen for osteoporosis. The estrogen was withdrawn and the hallucinations subsided. She was given estrogen twice more and each time the hallucinations recurred.

In this patient estrogen may have promoted release phenomena and triggered the hallucinatory episodes.

Nervous system

Over the years there have been reports that headache or classical migraine is either alleviated or exacerbated by HRT. This has been studied in 50 menopausal women with headaches who were randomized to either transdermal estradiol 50 micrograms for 7 days a month or oral conjugated estrogens 0.625 mg/day for 28 days, both regimens being supplemented with medroxyprogesterone acetate 10 mg/day during the latter half of each month (18). In patients with episodic tension headache there was no significant change in headache pattern. However, in women with migraine without aura the frequency and duration of the attacks increased significantly during HRT in the subgroup using the oral formulation; the transdermal formulation had no effect on the migraine pattern.

Sensory systems

The possibility that estrogen replacement therapy might cause dryness of the eyes has been reviewed in the light of data from the large Women's Health Study in the USA (19), and this work has been further reviewed (20). Questionnaires were sent to 25 665 participants. For every 3-year increase in the duration of replacement therapy there was a 15% increase in the incidence of dry eye syndrome. The risk was greater in women who used estrogen alone than in those who used combined estrogen + progestogen regimens. The evidence was not statistically strong, but it suggests that there is some correlation and that users and prescribers should be aware of it.

Metabolism

Lipids

Changes in lipids have been observed with both HRT and oral contraceptives and have sometimes been promoted as potentially advantageous, but it is not clear how significant such changes are, at least in biochemical terms. A review and pooled analysis of 248 prospective studies available up to the year 2000 has provided data on this issue in postmenopausal women (21). All estrogen-only regimens raised HDL cholesterol and lowered LDL and total cholesterol. Oral estrogens raised triglycerides. Transdermal 17-beta-estradiol lowered triglycerides.

Weight

Weight gain is widely believed to be a common consequence of HRT, and the desire to avoid obesity is a major reason why some women decline treatment. However, the potential effects of HRT need to be distinguished from effects that could be due to changing lifestyle or ageing. The effects of short-term hormone replacement and age on alterations in weight, body composition, and energy balance have therefore been studied in a prospective study in 18 healthy women aged 45–55 years and in 15 aged 70–80 years, with measurements at baseline, repeated after 1 month of transdermal estrogen (Estraderm 50 micrograms/day), and again after a further month of transdermal estrogen with vaginal progesterone (100 mg bd) added for the final 7 days (22). In neither age group did estrogen treatment correlate with anthropometric changes. Resting energy expenditure and activity were positively correlated with fat-free mass, while energy intake was not. Resting energy expenditure, energy intake, and activity were lower in older women when adjusted for fat-free mass. Changes in weight during treatment were not statistically significant. In addition, there was no difference between the groups in body mass index, fat mass, fat-free mass, total body water, or waist-to-hip ratio. This work has confirmed the reduction in energy expenditure that occurs with ageing, and it suggests that there is no effect of HRT on resting energy expenditure or body weight.

Hematologic

There has been a randomized, placebo-controlled study in 25 postmenopausal women to investigate the mechanisms that could underlie the induction of thrombosis by unopposed estrogens (23). Fasting and fat-load-stimulated plasma concentrations of clotting factor VII were measured after 8 weeks of oral 17-beta-estradiol (2 mg/day). Estradiol increased the mean fasting and postprandial plasma concentrations of total factor VII by 17 and 21% respectively, but did not affect the fasting and/or postprandial plasma concentrations of active factor VII. These findings argue against the idea that raised concentrations of total factor VII underlie the increased risk of arterial thromboembolism in these women.

It has been firmly concluded, in the light of prior evidence, that HRT increases the risk of venous thrombosis, this risk not being outweighed by any demonstrable benefit in terms of arterial cardiovascular disease (24). This conclusion is now being increasingly accepted, and the effects of postmenopausal HRT on blood coagulation have been intensively studied and documented over the years. However, the effects in older women, who have the highest risk of thromboembolism, are not well defined, and a US group has studied the association between HRT and concentrations of natural anticoagulant proteins in this subpopulation in a cross-sectional study in women of 65 years or older participating in the Cardiovascular Health Study (25). Protein C antigen and antithrombin were measured in HRT users (230 taking an unopposed estrogen and 60 taking an estrogen with a progestogen) and a comparison group of 196 non-users. Estrogen use was associated with significantly higher protein C concentrations (4.80 versus 4.30 micrograms/ml); the results were similar with estrogen/progestogen. In both user groups, antithrombin was significantly lower than in non-users (109% for each treatment group versus 115% in non-users). Adjustment for factors related to prescription of HRT and to anticoagulant protein concentrations had little impact on the results. For antithrombin, the association with HRT was larger for thinner Caucasian women and black women. The authors concluded that venous thrombosis from HRT may be partly mediated by alterations in antithrombin, but not by protein C concentrations.

Although the thrombogenic potential of oral estrogen in postmenopausal women is well documented, it has been argued that direct studies of the effect of estrogen replacement on hemostasis are largely lacking and not well known (26). A review of a series of randomized trials has shown that the treatment has no significant effect on concentrations of fibrinogen and factor VII. Plasma concentrations of antithrombin and protein S fell with oral estrogen but not with transdermal estrogen. No form of replacement affected protein C concentrations, but there was activation of coagulation in the presence of oral estrogen, as reflected by a rise in the concentration of prothrombin fragment 1 + 2. As far as fibrinolysis is concerned, oral estrogen reduces plasma PAI-1 and tPA, leading to an increase in fibrinolytic potential. The absence of an effect of transdermal estrogen on coagulation and fibrinolysis suggests that the route of estrogen administration is important, but it has not to date been convincingly shown that transdermal estrogen in equi-effective doses is less thrombogenic than the oral form.

Urinary tract

Since microalbuminuria can be regarded as being associated with renal and cardiovascular disease, evidence that the incidence of microalbuminuria is higher during treatment with oral contraceptives or hormone replacement therapy deserves to be taken seriously. A Dutch group has performed a case-control study of baseline and dispensing data relating to 4301 women participating in a study on the prevention of renal and vascular disease; the main outcome measure was microalbuminuria (30–300 mg/day) (27). After adjusting for age, hypertension, diabetes, obesity, hyperlipidemia, and smoking, the odds ratio for microalbuminuria was 1.90 (CI = 1.23, 2.93) for premenopausal oral contraceptive users and 2.05 (1.12, 3.77) for postmenopausal hormone replacement therapy users. The point estimate increased dose-dependently, albeit insignificantly, according to the estrogen content of the oral contraceptives (30–50 micrograms) and was greater in oral contraceptives with a second-generation progestogen (OR = 2.04) than those using a third-generation progestogen (OR = 1.39; CI = 0.63, 3.06). In the case of HRT, the odds ratio increased with the duration of HRT, that in women who had used the product for more than 5 years being double that in others.

Skin

- A 54-year-old woman developed melasma, macular hyperpigmentation associated with increased estrogen states, in atypical sites after starting to take HRT; on withdrawal it began to fade (28).

Musculoskeletal

Despite the evidence that estrogens can be of value in countering osteoporosis, some studies have suggested that women who use them are more likely to have back pain than those who do not; the possible causal link has remained unclear, and continues so despite recent confirmation of the phenomenon. Baseline information on estrogen replacement therapy, functional status, back pain and function, and other variables has been obtained in 7209 elderly white American women (mean age 71 years) enrolled in a study of osteoporotic fractures; X-rays were also taken at baseline and an average of 3.7 years later (29). A total of 1039 women were using estrogen replacement therapy at baseline, 2016 reported former use, and 4154 had never used estrogen replacement therapy. Compared with never-users, a significantly higher percentage of current estrogen users reported clinical back pain (53 versus 43%) and back impairment (12 versus 9.2%) at baseline and at the follow-up visit (pain 51 versus 41; impairment 16 versus 12%). This occurred despite a higher prevalence of vertebral fractures in never-users of estrogen at the baseline visit. The increased likelihood of back pain and impairment of function in current and former estrogen users remained in evidence, despite statistical adjustment for possibly interfering factors. The relative risks for impaired back function in former and current users at follow-up were 1.1 (0.9, 1.3) and 1.6 (1.3, 2.0) respectively (30).

Reproductive system

Breasts

Two doses of transdermal estrogen, 50 and 100 micrograms/day, have been compared with placebo in preventing bone loss in postmenopausal women over 24 months (31). Bone mineral density in the lumbar spine was only marginally better with the higher dose; the slightly better effect was largely offset by a higher incidence of breast pain, reported by 8% of women on placebo, by 6% of those who took 50 micrograms/day, and by 17% of women who took 100 micrograms/day.

Uterus

It has long been recognized that periodic or irregular uterine bleeding will occur in some women using HRT. While it is simple to dismiss this merely as a reactivation of endometrial proliferation and shedding, some workers have sought to examine the precise mechanism of this unwanted complication, particularly because it might prove to be the harbinger of more serious events involving the endometrium. From recent work in the UK it has been concluded that estrogen treatment appears to alter the endometrial expression of matrix metalloprotease 9 (MMP-9) and the tissue inhibitor of metalloproteases (TIMP-1) as well as the local balance between these molecules (32). This alteration may promote breakdown of the endometrial extracellular matrix and blood vessels and hence bleeding.

There could be fairly simple ways of screening for endometrial disorders in women using HRT. A study in 93 such women has confirmed the earlier finding that if a Papanicolaou smear is taken from the vagina the presence of endometrial cells in the smear gives some (non-specific) indication that there are endometrial changes, which may range from hyperplasia or polyps to endometrial carcinoma (33).

Immunologic

Two healthy young women took estrogen supplements for some 3 years and then developed classic Sjögren's syndrome (34). The syndrome was most severe in the woman who had taken the higher dose. These cases seem to have confirmed earlier reports that estrogens can play a role in the pathogenesis of Sjögren's syndrome in susceptible patients.

Long-Term Effects

Drug dependence

While the effects of estrogen treatment on mental function and mood are generally assessed as positive, work in Britain has raised the possibility of some form of psychological dependence. The starting point was the finding in various studies that a proportion of women in whom hormone replacement therapy was terminated had a return of psychological symptoms, such as low mood and tiredness, despite the fact that their circulating estrogen concentrations were high. A questionnaire-based study was therefore carried out in 600 women, mean age 46 years; in most of them, HRT with implants had been undertaken after hysterectomy, and the mean duration of use was 5 years. Among those with high circulating estradiol concentrations (more than 500 pmol/l) 40% reported a need to use top-up doses of HRT to cope with daily activities, 78% spoke of low mood and tiredness (apparently when estrogen concentrations were falling), 80% experienced a "buzz" (which was undefined) 1–2 weeks after receiving a new implant, and 75% claimed that life without an implant would be "terrible." These effects, interpreted as evidence of dependence, were almost absent in women with lower circulating estrogen concentrations. The authors were of the opinion that circulating concentrations of some 300 pmol/l, which are sufficient to maintain bone mass, should be the therapeutic aim, and that there will then be much less of a dependence problem than when higher concentrations are attained (35,36).

Mutagenicity

A finding that needs further study is that when estrogens are used for the treatment of osteoporosis they may have some genotoxic potential, as evidenced by their ability to cause an increased frequency of sister chromatid exchange (37).

Tumorigenicity

The associations between hormone replacement therapy and breast, endometrial, and ovarian cancers are discussed in the monograph on estrogens.

Susceptibility Factors

Age

When a young woman undergoes a surgical menopause it is clear that estrogen replacement treatment, if given at all, is likely to be needed for many years, and in the present state of knowledge this is probably justifiable, provided that the effects are monitored. The dilemma that the physician faces in such cases has been discussed in the light of a patient in whom gross obesity compounded the possible risk of thrombosis; the patient was nevertheless treated with an implant and remained well for 4 years (38).

Renal disease

Estrogen replacement therapy may have untoward effects in patients with renal disease, including an increased risk of thrombosis of dialysis access and potentially worsening of coronary artery disease, probably because the excretion of estrogens is impaired (39).

Drug Administration

Drug dosage regimens

The amount of estrogen taken during estrogen replacement is usually about one quarter of that found in oral contraceptives, and is intended to be sufficient to restore physiological amounts of endogenous estrogens. During the physiological cycle, menstrual discomfort of all types is at its mildest (and usually absent) during the mid-follicular phase when plasma estradiol concentrations are 60–150 pg/ml (40). In replacement therapy some workers seek to titrate the dose of estrogen individually in order to maintain this level, hoping thereby not only to avoid adverse effects associated with hyper- or hypo-estrogenicity but also to optimize the therapeutic effect. Strictly speaking this individualized treatment is called for because of the variability of estrogen clearance, but in normal women plasma levels are rarely measured, an approximate adaptation of dosage being undertaken purely on the basis of subjective reactions.

There is no benefit and sometimes a disadvantage to giving estrogen alone for only 25 days a month; in particular, estrogen withdrawal symptoms such as decreased well being, headaches, and hot flushes can occur each time the treatment is interrupted.

It is widely recommended that estrogen replacement therapy, if it is to be used at all, should be initiated at the time of menopause or within 3 years of it, since it is at this time that bone loss can be most severe. Many physicians go on to argue that once it has been started hormonal replacement therapy should continue for at least 20 years and perhaps indefinitely, in view of evidence that withdrawal may be followed by accelerated bone loss, at least comparable to that observed after the menopause. Later use of estrogen, once bone has already been lost, does not result in appreciable recovery of bone, although further loss can still be prevented. Large comparative studies have suggested that a series of alternative regimens for hormone replacement therapy should be available, so that for each individual woman the most appropriate form of treatment can be chosen; no one regimen is ideal for all, and finding the best approach for a given patient may be a matter of trial and error (41).

For the acute treatment of climacteric vasomotor symptoms it seems clear that micronized 17-beta-estradiol in a dose as low as 0.25 mg can be sufficient; however, a starting dose of 1 mg is advisable, with subsequent adjustments as necessary. At a dose of 2 mg the proportion of women who withdraw from treatment with the active product because of adverse effects was twice that seen with placebo (42). To provide longer-term protection against early postmenopausal bone loss, treatment with estradiol in a dose of 1 mg/day, balanced by a progestogen, is adequate (43). Most workers believe that the estrogen is best counterbalanced by a progestogen when used in the long term, but here there is still some disagreement about the doses needed.

Drug administration route

If it is indeed true that transdermal estrogens have certain advantages over oral estrogens in terms of safety, this needs to be better documented than hitherto; as in so many instances, the evidence is confusing, because of the multiplicity of products and doses. In 35 postmenopausal women who had been amenorrheic for at least 1 year, two consecutive 2-month courses of transdermal estrogen (estradiol patches 25 micrograms and 50 micrograms) were randomly followed by a 2-month course of treatment with either an estradiol patch 100 micrograms/day or an estradiol patch 50 micrograms/day combined with either progesterone 300 mg/day or medroxyprogesterone acetate 5 mg/day during the last 14 days (44). Neither transdermal estradiol alone nor transdermal estradiol plus progestogen altered the lipoprotein profile, LDL resistance to oxidation, or LDL particle size. However, all treatments similarly reduced myeloperoxidase protein concentrations.

In a case-control study 155 postmenopausal women who had had venous thromboembolism were compared with 381 matched controls (45). In all, 32 cases and 27 controls were current users of oral replacement therapy, whereas 30 cases and 93 controls were current users of transdermal products. After adjustment for potential confounding variables, the estimated risk ratio for venous thromboembolism in current users of the oral products compared with the transdermal users was 4.0 (1.9–8.3). This is strong evidence that the transdermal route was considerably safer. However, the conclusions of different studies continue to conflict with one another, no doubt in part because of variations in the formulations and patterns of use of the products.

Drug–Drug Interactions

Dexamfetamine

Preclinical studies (as well as anecdotal clinical reports in the course of the years) seem to show that estrogens, through their effects on the central nervous system, can affect behavioral responses to psychoactive drugs. In an unusual crossover study, the subjective and physiological effects of oral dexamfetamine 10 mg have been assessed after pretreatment with estradiol (46). One group of healthy young women used estradiol patches (Estraderm TTS, total dose 0.8 mg), which raised plasma estradiol concentrations to about 750 pg/ml, and a control group used placebo patches. Most of the subjective and physiological effects of dexamfetamine were not affected by acute estradiol treatment, but the estrogen did increase the magnitude of the effect of dexamfetamine on subjective ratings of "pleasant stimulation" and reduced ratings of "want more." Estradiol also produced some subjective effects when used alone, raising ratings of "feel drug," "energy and intellectual efficiency," and "pleasant stimulation."

References

1. Turner RT, Riggs BL, Spelsberg TC. Skeletal effects of estrogen. Endocr Rev 1994;15(3):275–300.
2. Grey AB, Cundy TF, Reid IR. Continuous combined oestrogen/progestin therapy is well tolerated and increases bone density at the hip and spine in post-menopausal osteoporosis. Clin Endocrinol (Oxf) 1994;40(5):671–7.
3. Ylikorkala O. Balancing between observational studies and randomized trials in prevention of coronary heart disease by estrogen replacement: HERS study was no revolution. Acta Obstet Gynecol Scand 2000;79(12):1029–36.
4. Lloyd G. Hormone replacement therapy and ischaemic heart disease: continuing questions but still no answers. Int J Clin Pract 2000;54(7):416–17.
5. Steiner MK, Clarkson PB, Lip GY. Myocardial infarction complicating hormone replacement therapy in a young woman with normal coronary arteries. Int J Clin Pract 2000;54(7):475–7.
6. MacLennan A, Lester S, Moore V. Oral estrogen replacement therapy versus placebo for hot flushes: a systematic review. Climacteric 2001;4(1):58–74.
7. Barrett-Connor E, Stuenkel CA. Hormone replacement therapy (HRT)—risks and benefits. Int J Epidemiol 2001;30(3):423–6.
8. Takahashi K, Manabe A, Okada M, Kurioka H, Kanasaki H, Miyazaki K. Efficacy and safety of oral estriol for managing postmenopausal symptoms. Maturitas 2000;34(2):169–77.
9. Takahashi K, Okada M, Ozaki T, Kurioka H, Manabe A, Kanasaki H, Miyazaki K. Safety and efficacy of oestriol for symptoms of natural or surgically induced menopause. Hum Reprod 2000;15(5):1028–36.
10. Itoi H, Minakami H, Iwasaki R, Sato I. Comparison of the long-term effects of oral estriol with the effects of conjugated estrogen on serum lipid profile in early menopausal women. Maturitas 2000;36(3):217–22.
11. Saure A, Planellas J, Poulsen HK, Jaszczak P. A double-blind, randomized, comparative study evaluating clinical effects of two sequential estradiol–progestogen combinations containing either desogestrel or medroxyprogesterone acetate in climacteric women. Maturitas 2000;34(2):133–42.
12. Burch D, Bieshuevel E, Smith S, Fox H. Can endometrial protection be inferred from the bleeding pattern on combined cyclical hormone replacement therapy. Maturitas 2000;34(2):155–60.
13. Rossouw JE. Hormone replacement therapy and cardiovascular disease. Curr Opin Lipidol 1999;10(5):429–34.
14. Whiteman MK, Cui Y, Flaws JA, Espeland M, Bush TL. Low fibrinogen level: A predisposing factor for venous thromboembolic events with hormone replacement therapy. Am J Hematol 1999;61(4):271–3.
15. Hoibraaten E, Abdelnoor M, Sandset PM. Hormone replacement therapy with estradiol and risk of venous thromboembolism—a population-based case-control study. Thromb Haemost 1999;82(4):1218–21.
16. Cahill M, O'Toole L, Acheson RW. Hormone replacement therapy and retinal vein occlusion. Eye 1999;13(Pt 6):798–800.
17. Fernandes LH, Scassellati-Sforzolini B, Spaide RF. Estrogen and visual hallucinations in a patient with Charles Bonnet syndrome. Am J Ophthalmol 2000;129(3):407.
18. Nappi RE, Cagnacci A, Granella F, Piccinini F, Polatti F, Facchinetti F. Course of primary headaches during hormone replacement therapy. Maturitas 2001;38(2):157–63.
19. Schaumberg DA, Buring JE, Sullivan DA, Dana MR. Hormone replacement therapy and dry eye syndrome. JAMA 2001;286(17):2114–19.
20. Barney NP. Can hormone replacement therapy cause dry eye? Arch Ophthalmol 2002;120(5):641–2.
21. Godsland IF. Effects of postmenopausal hormone replacement therapy on lipid, lipoprotein, and apolipoprotein (a) concentrations: analysis of studies published from 1974–2000. Fertil Steril 2001;75(5):898–915.
22. Anderson EJ, Lavoie HB, Strauss CC, Hubbard JL, Sharpless JL, Hall JE. Body composition and energy balance: lack of effect of short-term hormone replacement in postmenopausal women. Metabolism 2001;50(3):265–9.
23. de Valk-de Roo GW, Stehouwer CD, Emeis JJ, Nicolaas-Merkus A, Netelenbos C. Unopposed estrogen increases total plasma factor VII, but not active factor VII—a short-term placebo-controlled study in healthy postmenopausal women. Thromb Haemost 2000;84(6):968–72.
24. Rosendaal FR, Helmerhorst FM, Vandenbroucke JP. Oral contraceptives, hormone replacement therapy and thrombosis. Thromb Haemost 2001;86(1):112–23.
25. Cushman M, Psaty BM, Meilahn EN, Dobs AS, Kuller LH. Post-menopausal hormone therapy and concentrations of protein C and antithrombin in elderly women. Br J Haematol 2001;114(1):162–8.
26. Petit L, Alhenc-Gelas M, Aiach M, Scarabin PY. Hormone replacement therapy of the menopause and haemostasis. Sang Thromb Vaiss 2002;14:32–8.
27. Monster TB, Janssen WM, de Jong PE, de Jong-van den Berg LT; Prevention of Renal Vascular End Stage Disease Study Group. Oral contraceptive use and hormone replacement therapy are associated with microalbuminuria. Arch Intern Med 2001;161(16):2000–5.
28. Covic A, Goldsmith DJ, Segall L, Stoicescu C, Lungu S, Volovat C, Covic M. Rifampicin-induced acute renal failure: a series of 60 patients. Nephrol Dial Transplant 1998;13(4):924–9.
29. Musgrave DS, Vogt MT, Nevitt MC, Cauley JA. Back problems among postmenopausal women taking estrogen replacement therapy: the study of osteoporotic fractures. Spine 2001;26(14):1606–12.
30. Symmons DP, van Hemert AM, Vandenbroucke JP, Valkenburg HA. A longitudinal study of back pain and radiological changes in the lumbar spines of middle aged women. I. Clinical findings. Ann Rheum Dis 1991;50(3):158–61.
31. Arrenbrecht S, Boermans AJ. Effects of transdermal estradiol delivered by a matrix patch on bone density in hysterectomized, postmenopausal women: a 2-year placebo-controlled trial. Osteoporos Int 2002;13(2):176–83.
32. Hickey M, Higham J, Sullivan M, Miles L, Fraser IS. Endometrial bleeding in hormone replacement therapy users: preliminary findings regarding the role of matrix metalloproteinase 9 (MMP-9) and tissue inhibitors of MMPs. Fertil Steril 2001;75(2):288–96.
33. Montz FJ. Significance of "normal" endometrial cells in cervical cytology from asymptomatic postmenopausal women receiving hormone replacement therapy. Gynecol Oncol 2001;81(1):33–9.
34. Nagler RM, Pollack S. Sjögren's syndrome induced by estrogen therapy. Semin Arthritis Rheum 2000;30(3):209–14.
35. O'Leary A, Bowen-Simpkins P, Tejura H, Rajesh U. Are high levels of oestradiol after implants associated with features of dependence? Br J Obstet Gynaecol 1999;106(9):960–3.
36. Bewley S, Granleese J. Repeat oestradiol implants: features of dependence? J Obstet Gynaecol 1999;19(2):190–1.
37. Sahin FI, Sahin I, Ergun MA, Saracoglu OF. Effects of estrogen and alendronate on sister chromatid exchange (SCE) frequencies in postmenopausal osteoporosis patients. Int J Gynaecol Obstet 2000;71(1):49–52.

38. Ewies AAA, Olah KSJ. Endometrial adenocarcinoma treated by hysterectomy and bilateral salpingo-oophorectomy at age 22-the dilemma of long-term HRT. J Obstet Gynaecol 2000;20:639–40.
39. Mattix H, Singh AK. Estrogen replacement therapy: implications for postmenopausal women with end-stage renal disease. Curr Opin Nephrol Hypertens 2000;9(3):207–14.
40. de Lignieres B. Hormone replacement therapy: clinical benefits and side-effects. Maturitas 1996;23(Suppl):S31–6.
41. Heikkinen JE, Vaheri RT, Ahomaki SM, Kainulainen PM, Viitanen AT, Timonen UM. Optimizing continuous-combined hormone replacement therapy for postmenopausal women: a comparison of six different treatment regimens. Am J Obstet Gynecol 2000;182(3):560–7.
42. Notelovitz M, Lenihan JP, McDermott M, Kerber IJ, Nanavati N, Arce J. Initial 17beta-estradiol dose for treating vasomotor symptoms. Obstet Gynecol 2000;95(5):726–31.
43. Bjarnason NH, Byrjalsen I, Hassager C, Haarbo J, Christiansen C. Low doses of estradiol in combination with gestodene to prevent early postmenopausal bone loss. Am J Obstet Gynecol 2000;183(3):550–60.
44. Hermenegildo C, Garcia-Martinez MC, Valldecabres C, Tarin JJ, Cano A. Transdermal estradiol reduces plasma myeloperoxidase levels without affecting the LDL resistance to oxidation or the LDL particle size. Menopause 2002;9(2):102–9.
45. Scarabin PY, Oger E, Plu-Bureau G, EStrogen and THromboEmbolism Risk Study Group. Differential association of oral and transdermal oestrogen-replacement therapy with venous thromboembolism risk. Lancet 2003;362(9382):428–32.
46. Justice AJ, de Wit H. Acute effects of estradiol pretreatment on the response to d-amphetamine in women. Neuroendocrinology 2000;71(1):51–9.

Hormone replacement therapy—estrogens + progestogens

See also Estrogens *and* Progestogens

General Information

For a complete account of the adverse effects of estrogens, readers should consult the following monographs as well as this one:

- Diethylstilbestrol
- Estrogens
- Hormonal contraceptives—emergency contraception
- Hormonal contraceptives—oral
- Hormone replacement therapy—estrogens
- Hormone replacement therapy—estrogens + androgens.

For a complete account of the adverse effects of progestogens, readers should consult the following monographs as well as this one:

- Hormonal contraceptives—intracervical and intravaginal
- Hormonal contraceptives—oral
- Hormonal contraceptives—progestogen implants
- Hormonal contraceptives—progestogen injections
- Medroxyprogesterone
- Progestogens.

Two alternatives to long-term estrogen therapy have been proposed, because of the fear of certain risks (particularly malignancy) that might result in postmenopausal women:

- combined estrogen + progestogen regimens with a monthly interruption to allow for withdrawal bleeding
- long-term therapy with estrogens alone periodically interrupted by a cycle of combined treatment.

In those few countries in which hysterectomy is still endemic it has been argued that in the residual minority of women with an intact uterus combination therapy should be the normal form of HRT. Therapeutic benefits have also been claimed from using the combination. Unfortunately, some of the publications that have made claims for the therapeutic advantages of adding progestogens to estrogens in HRT have not provided exact comparative data, and the beneficial effects which are described are not clearly different from those claimed for estrogen alone.

The dispute about the benefit to harm balance of the various competing forms of HRT for use in the climacteric or postmenopausally is becoming increasingly intense, with a sharp division of opinion between protagonists and critics of the individual patterns of treatment. The view was often defended by earlier workers that, at least for certain classes of users, some form of combined estrogen + progestogen treatment is likely to be more appropriate and perhaps more physiological than estrogen replacement alone. Many variants have been used and none is likely to be ideal for all subjects. Some have argued that in the climacteric there are sound reasons for using estrogen with intermittent progestogen and that it is much underused, despite the fact that uterine bleeding and other adverse progestogenic effects are, with some combined formulations (but not all), major reasons for patient noncompliance and early withdrawal (1).

Observational studies

In 104 women with established postmenopausal osteoporosis, continuous estrogen + progestogen therapy resulted in increases in bone mineral density of the femoral neck and a fall in systolic blood pressure; the most common adverse effects were mastalgia (44%) and vaginal bleeding (29%) (2).

The combined use of estradiol and dydrogesterone reduce both diastolic and systolic blood pressures in postmenopausal women in whom the diastolic pressure had been raised (3). Evidence is also advanced from various quarters that adding a progestogen to adequate dosages of an estrogen promotes new bone formation, restores bone that has been lost and reduces the risk of carcinoma of the breast.

When 16 diabetic and hypertensive postmenopausal women aged 47–57 years were treated cyclically with estradiol plus norgestrel, existing proteinuria and even creatinine clearance often improved (4). The effects were unrelated to conventional risk factors for vascular complications, such as raised blood pressure, plasma glucose, or serum cholesterol.

General adverse effects

Of 206 postmenopausal women who took the oral combination of estradiol valerate plus norethisterone (5) eight withdrew because of bleeding during year 1; during years 2 and 3 there were no withdrawals because of bleeding. By the end of year 3, 133 patients had completed the study. There were serious adverse effects in 24, but there was no definite relation to therapy. The numbers of adverse events reported each year by the patients who completed the study are shown in Table 1. The authors concluded that this combination was effective in the majority of patients and was well tolerated.

Distinguishing adverse effects due to estrogens or progestogens

When patients have adverse effects during combined hormone replacement therapy it is necessary to determine whether the progestogen or the estrogen is causing the problem. If heavy bleeding or breast tenderness is the primary complaint, the estrogen component is probably the problem and therefore the dose should be reduced. If the patient complains of irritability, depression, water retention, or headaches, the problems are probably due to the progestogen component and the latter should in that case be changed or the dose adjusted; since several different progestogens are in use (particularly norethindrone, norethindrone acetate, medroxyprogesterone acetate, and micronized progesterone) there is a degree of choice.

Benefit to harm balance

With increasing concern over the long-term safety of hormone replacement therapy, the benefit to harm balance has to be continually reassessed, and conclusions as to its prophylactic or therapeutic value need to be adjusted as experience accumulates. Not all the promises held out for the benefits of this therapy have been confirmed. For example, while estrogens prevent peripheral bone loss they do not prevent vertebral fractures (6) and in a 2-year placebo-controlled, crossover study in 34 healthy postmenopausal women, treatment with transdermal estrogen alone (Menorest 50 micrograms/day) did not improve lipid profiles or any indices of arterial function (7).

It is remarkable that, despite decades of accumulated observational evidence, the balance of benefits and harms for hormone use in healthy postmenopausal women remains uncertain (8). Quite apart from the constantly changing spectrum of the available data, one explanation for the confusion is the relatively high proportion of poor-quality clinical work, particularly studies that are designed to promote particular commercialized forms of treatment from among the many alternatives available.

A study that cannot be faulted on that score is the Women's Health Initiative, a randomized, controlled, primary prevention trial (planned to last for 8.5 years), in which 16 608 postmenopausal women aged 50–79 years with an intact uterus at baseline were recruited at 40 US clinical centers over the period 1993–98 (9). In one part of this study, 8506 participants received conjugated equine estrogens 0.625 mg/day plus medroxyprogesterone acetate 2.5 mg/day; 8102 were given placebo. The primary desired outcome was reduction of coronary heart disease (non-fatal myocardial infarction and death), with invasive breast cancer as the primary anticipated adverse outcome. After a mean of 5.2 years, the data and safety monitoring board recommended stopping the trial of estrogen plus progestogen versus placebo because the test statistic for invasive breast cancer exceeded the stopping boundary for this adverse effect and the global index statistic supported harms exceeding benefits. The estimated hazard ratios (and 95% confidence intervals) were:

- coronary disease 1.29 (1.02, 1.63; $n = 286$)
- breast cancer 1.26 (1.00, 1.59; $n = 290$)
- stroke 1.41 (1.07, 1.85; $n = 212$)
- pulmonary embolism 2.13 (1.39, 3.25; $n = 101$)
- colorectal cancer 0.63 (0.43, 0.92; $n = 112$)
- endometrial cancer 0.83 (0.47, 1.47; $n = 47$)
- hip fracture 0.66 (0.45, 0.98; $n = 106$)
- death due to other causes 0.92 (0.74, 1.14; $n = 331$).

What the above amounts to is that the absolute excess risks per 10 000 woman-years attributable to the use of an estrogen plus a progestogen were seven more coronary heart disease events, eight more strokes, eight more pulmonary embolisms, and eight more invasive breast cancers, while the risk reductions per 10 000 woman-years were six fewer colorectal cancers and five fewer hip fractures. The absolute excess risk of events included in the global index was 19 per 10 000 woman-years. The overall harms in this study thus clearly exceeded the benefits. All-cause mortality was not affected.

Other published studies, many of which are of limited scope, do not run closely parallel to the above findings

Table 1 The numbers of adverse events in 3 successive years in patients taking estradiol valerate + norethisterone (5)

Adverse event	Year 1 ($n = 164$)	Year 2 ($n = 144$)	Year 3 ($n = 133$)
Cardiovascular			
Hypertension	5	3	—
Palpitation	4	4	3
Phlebitis	3	—	—
Respiratory			
Breathlessness	3	0	1
Metabolism			
Weight gain	10	5	2
Gastrointestinal			
Abdominal pain	2	2	—
Musculoskeletal			
Fractures	7	1	1
Joint/bone pain	6	3	6
Reproductive system			
Menopausal symptoms	4	1	5
Breast tenderness	63	4	3
Breast lumps	2	4	2
Bleeding/spotting	91	60	24
Abnormal smear	—	2	—
Ovarian cysts	1	1	4
Other adverse events	105	53	34
Total	306	143	85

from the Women's Health Initiative, and the data on cardiovascular effects remain particularly confusing. However, Beral and colleagues have pointed out optimistically that "substantial new data should soon be available from randomized trials of estrogen-alone hormonal replacement therapy versus placebo," although they added that "few additional trial data on combined hormone replacement therapy are expected for about a decade" (10). They also pointed out that existing randomized trials are too small to provide reliable evidence on some basic matters, including the relative risks of the various compounds in use.

Organs and Systems

Cardiovascular

Despite biologically plausible mechanisms whereby estrogens might be expected to confer cardioprotection in postmenopausal women, as well as observational data suggesting cardiovascular benefit, the literature continues to provide contradictory outcomes on this. Electrocardiographic work has suggested that not only the estrogen but also the progestogen component of HRT can have some impact on the electrophysiological properties of the heart (11), the clinical significance of which, if any, is not understood. The picture is further confused by evidence that a particular regimen may initially increase the risk, yet confer long-term benefit, as in the Heart and Estrogen/progestin Replacement Study (HERS), while in other well-planned work, such as the recent Estrogen Replacement and Atherosclerosis trial (ERA), there was no benefit (12).

There has been a randomized trial in 270 postmenopausal women to evaluate the effects on cardiovascular risk markers of two continuous combined estrogen + progestogen replacement products (17-beta-estradiol 1 mg with or without norethindrone acetate 0.25 or 0.5 mg) compared with unopposed estrogen or placebo (13). LDL cholesterol was reduced to a similar extent in all those who took the active treatment (10–14% from baseline). Compared with unopposed 17-beta-estradiol, 17-beta-estradiol plus norethindrone acetate 0.5 mg enhanced the reductions in total cholesterol and apolipoprotein B concentrations. The combination of 17-beta-estradiol plus norethindrone blunted or reversed the increases in concentrations of high-density lipoprotein cholesterol, apolipoprotein A-I, and triglycerides produced by 17-beta-estradiol alone. The effects of 17-beta-estradiol plus norethindrone on hemostatic variables were similar to those of 17-beta-estradiol alone, except for factor VII activity, which was significantly reduced by 17-beta-estradiol plus norethindrone acetate 0.25 and 0.5 mg. The combination of 17-beta-estradiol plus norethindrone blunted reductions in C peptide and insulin concentrations produced by unopposed 17-beta-estradiol, but did not affect them compared with placebo. The authors concluded that 17-beta-estradiol plus norethindrone produced favorable changes in most cardiovascular risk markers and had a profile distinct from that of unopposed estrogen.

The findings of the randomized HERS suggested that in women with clinically recognized heart disease, HRT might be associated with early harm but late benefit in terms of coronary events. The findings of that study seem in the meantime to have been confirmed by some further US work. In one study the histories and subsequent course of 981 postmenopausal women who had survived a first myocardial infarct and had thereafter used estrogen or estrogen + progestogen were examined (14). Relative to the risk in a parallel group of women not currently using hormones there was a suggestion of increased risk during the first 60 days after starting hormone therapy (RR = 2.16; CI = 0.94, 4.95) but of reduced risk with current hormone use for longer than 1 year (RR = 0.76), although the confidence intervals were wide.

However, in a second study, data on 1857 women from the Coumadin Aspirin Reinfarction Study were used to assess the incidence of cardiac deaths or unstable angina as related to the use of HRT. Of the population studied, 524 (28%) had used HRT at some point and 111 of the latter (21%) had started HRT after suffering a myocardial infarct ("new users"). Women who began HRT after their first myocardial infarct had a significantly higher subsequent incidence of unstable angina than women who had never used hormones (39 versus 20%); however, these new hormone users suffered death or recurrence of myocardial infarct at a much lower rate than never-users (4 versus 15%). These differences are striking. Prior/current users had no excess risk of the composite end-point after adjustment. Users of estrogen plus progestogen had a lower incidence of death, infarct, or unstable angina during follow-up than users of estrogen only (RR = 0.56) (15). As Grady and Hulley have commented in an editorial, current data seem to make it clear that "postmenopausal hormone therapy should not be used for the purpose of preventing coronary disease unless future data from well-designed randomized trials document such benefit" (16).

The thrombotic complications of combined HRT in a potentially high-risk group have been assessed in a randomized, multicenter study in the USA in 2763 women, average age 67 years (17). All had some degree of pre-existing coronary heart disease but no previous venous thromboembolism, and none had undergone hysterectomy. They took either conjugated equine estrogens 0.625 mg + medroxyprogesterone acetate 2.5 mg or a placebo. During an average 4.1 years of follow-up, 34 women in the hormone therapy group and 13 in the placebo group had venous thromboembolism (relative risk = 2.7, excess risk = 3.9 per 1000 woman-years). The mean risk for venous thromboembolism was increased among women who had leg fractures (RR = 18) or cancer (RR = 4) and it was also raised several-fold for 3 months after in-patient surgery or non-surgical hospitalization. The risk was approximately halved by the use of aspirin or statins.

Metabolism

Hyperlipidemic postmenopausal women taking combined sequential estrogen + progestogen replacement therapy have large fluctuations in lipid and lipoprotein concentrations. These fluctuations depend on the hormonal phase, that is estrogen alone or combined with progestogen. Progestogens blunt or even overwhelm the estrogenic effects on lipoproteins (18).

Progestogen has also been claimed to produce more favorable concentrations of HDL cholesterol (19), but this is a questionable conclusion; most work seems to show that whereas estrogen alone increases HDL concentrations (for example by some 7%), combined treatment weakens this favorable effect and actually can reduce HDL concentrations by some 16%.

Changes in lipids have been observed with both HRT and oral contraceptives and have sometimes been promoted as potentially advantageous, but it is not clear how significant such changes are, at least in biochemical terms. A review and pooled analysis of 248 prospective studies available up to the year 2000 has provided data on this issue in postmenopausal women (20). All estrogen-only regimens raised HDL cholesterol and lowered LDL and total cholesterol. Oral estrogens raised triglycerides. Transdermal 17-beta-estradiol lowered triglycerides. Progestogens had little effect on estrogen-induced reductions in LDL and total cholesterol. Estrogen-induced increases in HDL and triglycerides were opposed according to the type of progestogen in the following order (from least to greatest effect): dydrogesterone and medrogestone, progesterone, cyproterone acetate, medroxyprogesterone acetate, transdermal norethindrone acetate, norgestrel, and oral norethindrone acetate. Tibolone reduced HDL cholesterol and triglyceride concentrations. Raloxifene reduced LDL cholesterol concentrations. In 41 studies of 20 different formulations, HRT generally lowered lipoprotein (a). Thus, the route of estrogen administration and the type of progestogen used determine the effects of HRT on lipid and lipoprotein concentrations.

In another study an estrogen + progestogen combination produced no adverse effects on serum lipids or lipoproteins (21), but this again may depend very much on the exact combination and duration of treatment.

Whatever the truth, the question arises whether the modifications in lipid effects resulting from the addition of progestogen will not interfere with the favorable impact of estrogen on coronary artery disease; there has been some earlier evidence that the combined therapy is rather less effective than plain estrogen in preventing cardiac disorders (SEDA-16, 459).

Female sex hormones can also have effects on lipids when they are given transdermally, and this has been studied retrospectively in 159 women who used transdermal or oral replacement therapy (22). All used either transdermal estradiol 0.05 mg twice weekly or oral conjugated estrogen 0.625 mg/day, each combined with oral medroxyprogesterone acetate 2.5 mg/day. The mean increases in HDL cholesterol in the first year and second year averaged 10 and 31% with oral treatment, the corresponding figures for transdermal therapy being 14 and 34%. With oral therapy the mean reductions in total cholesterol in the first and second years were 2.9 and 15%, and with transdermal treatment 5.6 and 5.7%. With oral treatment, the mean falls in LDL cholesterol in the first and second years were 6.2 and 18% and with transdermal treatment 7.9 and 16% respectively. Transdermal treatment reduced triglyceride concentrations by 34%, whereas oral estrogen treatment increased them by 19% at the end of 2 years. Both treatments changed serum lipids favorably. Nevertheless, triglycerides were increased by oral estrogen but reduced by transdermal treatment at 2 years.

It has been hypothetically suggested that the use of HRT could slow the progression of atherosclerosis by an effect on lipids. In a 1-year study of 321 women with increased thickness of the carotid intima media who were using either various forms of HRT or none at all, there was no slowing in the progression of subclinical atherosclerosis and no unfavorable effect on the process (23). HRT significantly reduced LDL cholesterol, fibrinogen, and FSH.

Reproductive system

Adding a progestogen to estrogen therapy means that regular withdrawal bleeding occurs, probably in some 97% of users up to the age of 60 years. This could explain why such combinations, although increasingly advocated, have not been used on a wider scale; few women relish the prospect of regular "menstrual" bleeding persisting for many years after the menopause, and it might introduce new and unforeseen risks, particularly to the aging uterus. However, on theoretical and practical grounds, such combinations have been developed and used for relatively short periods of treatment during the climacteric itself to regularize bleeding and to relieve menopausal symptoms. The pattern of short-term adverse effects of these products is very similar to that of the combined oral contraceptives.

Some cases have underlined the need to use an estrogen in combination with a progestogen, rather than unopposed estrogen, when treating women who have undergone radical surgery (removal of both the ovaries and uterus) for endometriosis. If unopposed estrogen replacement is given, any residual area of endometriosis will rapidly expand (24).

Continuous administration of an estrogen + progestogen combination is effective in achieving amenorrhea with prolonged use (75% at 6 months). An adverse effect of such a regimen is a high incidence of unpredictable break-through bleeding, particularly during the initial months of treatment (25).

Mammary tension and mastodynia are adverse effects related to the action of estrogens (26). In postmenopausal women estrogen + progestogen replacement therapy can be associated with an increase in mammographic density and with the onset or worsening of mastodynia. Tibolone, a steroid with estrogenic, progestogenic, and some androgenic activity, does not seem to affect breasts of normal structure and can be considered a first-rate replacement therapy in women whose breasts are rather dense or who have benign mastopathy (26).

Various companies and investigational groups continue to examine the relative efficacy and safety of different forms of combined postmenopausal treatment. In a randomized, placebo-controlled trial 579 women were treated for 26 cycles with sequential combinations of 17-beta-estradiol 1 mg plus dydrogesterone 5 or 10 mg or 17-beta-estradiol 2 mg with dydrogesterone 10 or 20 mg (27). The effects of these treatments in the 442 women who underwent biopsy were considered satisfactory in terms of cycle control and endometrial response, but the 1 mg dose of 17-beta-estradiol was associated with more intermittent uterine bleeding than the 2 mg dose. Higher doses of dydrogesterone were associated with a higher incidence of cyclical bleeds and a later time of onset.

Long-Term Effects

Tumorigenicity

Breast cancer

The complexity of the relation between hormonal replacement therapy and breast cancer has been stressed in previous volumes (SED-14, 1454) (SEDA-22, 465), and much depends on the type of replacement therapy given and the class of tumor studied. This latter point has been underscored by a US study that provided evidence that the use of combined hormonal replacement therapy increases the risk of lobular, but not ductal, breast carcinoma in middle-aged women (28).

An American cohort study designed to determine whether increases in risk associated with an estrogen + progestogen regimen are greater than those associated with estrogen alone has been carried out based on follow-up data for 1980–1995 from the National Breast Cancer Detection Demonstration Project (29). From 46 355 postmenopausal women, mean age at the start of follow-up was 58 years, 2082 cases of breast cancer were identified. Increases in risk with estrogen only and estrogen + progestogen were restricted to use within the previous 4 years, the relative risks being 1.2 and 1.4 respectively. The relative risk increased by 0.01 with each year of estrogen use and by 0.08 with each year of estrogen + progestogen use. Among women with a BMI of 24.4 kg/m^2 or less, the mean increases in relative risk were 0.03 and 0.12 with each year of estrogen use and estrogen + progestogen use respectively. These associations were evident for the majority of invasive tumors with ductal histology and regardless of the extent of invasive disease. The risk in heavier women did not increase with the use of estrogen only or estrogen + progestogen. These data suggest that estrogen + progestogen increases the risk of breast cancer beyond that associated with estrogen alone.

Endometrial cancer

Because sequential combined hormone replacement therapy with estrogen + progestogen for 10–24 days per month can increase the risk of endometrial cancer in the long run, attention has been devoted to the possibility of giving the two types of hormone continuously. In one retrospective case-control study in the USA it was concluded that the risk of endometrial cancer among users of continuous combined treatment, relative to women who had never used hormone replacement therapy, was 0.6 (95% CI = 0.3, 1.3); the risk relative to women who used intermittent combined therapy was 0.4 (CI = 0.2, 1.1) (30). The authors' conclusions were cautious, since most continuous combined hormonal therapy had been fairly short-term (under 72 months), but the figures suggested that women taking continuous combined hormone replacement therapy for several years were not at an increased risk of endometrial cancer compared with women who had never taken hormone replacement therapy and might in fact be at reduced risk of endometrial cancer.

In the meantime, others have concluded that the risk of endometrial cancer is present, but is less with combined therapy than with unopposed estrogen. However, the picture is not simple; the contradictions could be explained by the fact that risks appear to vary both by usage patterns and by patient characteristics, such as body weight and a history of diabetes (31).

Susceptibility Factors

Genetic factors

In a population-based, case-control study in 232 postmenopausal women who had had a non-fatal myocardial infarct during the previous 3 years, a stratified random sample of 723 postmenopausal women without a history of infarction acted as controls (32). Among hypertensive women, the presence of the prothrombin 20210 G→A variant was a significant risk factor for infarct (OR = 4.32; 95% CI = 1.52, 12) and in this group there was also a significant interaction between the use of HRT and the presence of the prothrombin variant in increasing the risk of infarction. Compared with non-users of HRT with the wild-type genotype, women who were current users and who had the prothrombin variant ($n = 8$) had a nearly 11-fold increase in the risk of a non-fatal myocardial infarct. The interaction was absent among non-hypertensive women. No interaction with HRT was found for factor V Leiden in either hypertensive or non-hypertensive women. These findings suggest that screening for the prothrombin variant may allow a better assessment of the risks and benefits associated with HRT in individual postmenopausal women.

Other features of the patient

While the extent of vaginal bleeding when using estrogens plus progestogens varies somewhat with the exact formulation and dose, another determining factor is the pretreatment state of the endometrium: a thick endometrium at the start of treatment results in significantly more bleeding days than a thin endometrium (33). This might be a helpful predictor of the extent to which a particular woman will find this type of HRT acceptable.

Drug Administration

Drug formulations

The impact of a new formulation of low-dose micronized medroxyprogesterone plus 17-beta-estradiol on lipid profiles in menopausal women has been studied for 12 months. Total cholesterol concentrations fell 8.4%, low-density lipoprotein cholesterol fell 18%, and high-density lipoprotein cholesterol increased 6.9%; total triglycerides increased 12%. The most frequently reported adverse events were menorrhagia, breast tenderness, cervical polyps or cysts, bloating, fatigue or lethargy, influenza or a flu-like syndrome, back pain, headaches, irritability, and depression (34).

Drug dosage regimens

In 438 postmenopausal women, randomly assigned to either constant 17-beta-estradiol (1 mg/day) plus inter mittent norgestimate 90 micrograms (3 days off, 3 days on) or a fixed combination of 17-beta-estradiol (2 mg/day) with norethisterone acetate (1 mg), the two regimens had similar bleeding profiles and provided comparable relief from vasomotor symptoms (1). However, breast discomfort and edema were experienced by twice as many subjects who used the fixed combination. The intermittent regimen was notably free of endometrial hyperplasia.

Drug administration route

In an open, non-comparative study, the efficacy of a low dose transdermal estrogen (Oesclim 25 transdermal patches, releasing 17-beta-estradiol 25 micrograms/day) was tested in 60 women with postmenopausal symptoms over 8 weeks (35). The dosage could be doubled if required and sequential treatment with an oral progestogen was also given for 12 days or more each month in all non-hysterectomized women. Of the 60 patients, 53 reacted satisfactorily to the basic dose and all the various treatments were said to be well tolerated. One could cite a dozen similar papers from the recent past in which the findings were so amorphous that they have not made a serious contribution to the evolution of knowledge.

In two multicenter, double-blind, randomized, controlled trials of three once-a-week transdermal systems delivering continuous combined 17-beta-estradiol + levonorgestrel (estrogen 45 micrograms/day + progestogen 15, 30, or 40 micrograms/day) to treat vasomotor symptoms and prevent estrogen-induced endometrial hyperplasia in 1138 women, all were highly effective (36). Reactions at the site of application, vaginal hemorrhage, and breast pain were the most common adverse events, and the proportion of women with amenorrhea increased over time in all the treatment groups.

Drug–Drug Interactions

Statins

With growing interest in the use of statins in women, the question naturally arises whether hormonal replacement could have any effect on their efficacy or safety. Data from the HERS (conducted in women with cardiac disorders) seem to have shown that there is no interaction (37). Estrogen replacement itself resulted in a significant increase in the early risk of primary events in women who did not use statins but not in statin users. Adjustment for statin use after randomization showed no adverse effect of estrogen on the efficacy of statins, in terms of either cardiovascular events or mortality.

References

1. Rozenberg S, Caubel P, Lim PC. Constant estrogen, intermittent progestogen vs. continuous combined hormone replacement therapy: tolerability and effect on vasomotor symptoms. Int J Gynaecol Obstet 2001;72(3):235–43.
2. Grey AB, Cundy TF, Reid IR. Continuous combined oestrogen/progestin therapy is well tolerated and increases bone density at the hip and spine in post-menopausal osteoporosis. Clin Endocrinol (Oxf) 1994;40(5):671–7.
3. Foster RH, Balfour JA. Estradiol and dydrogesterone. A review of their combined use as hormone replacement therapy in postmenopausal women. Drugs Aging 1997;11(4):309–32.
4. Mattix H, Singh AK. Estrogen replacement therapy: implications for postmenopausal women with end-stage renal disease. Curr Opin Nephrol Hypertens 2000;9(3):207–14.
5. Perry W, Wiseman RA, Cullen NM. Combined oral estradiol valerate–norethisterone treatment over three years in postmenopausal women. 1. Clinical aspects and endometrial histology. Gynecol Endocrinol 1998;12(2):109–22.
6. Gutteridge DH, Stewart GO, Prince RL, Price RI, Retallack RW, Dhaliwal SS, Stuckey BG, Drury P, Jones CE, Faulkner DL, Kent GN, Bhagat CI, Nicholson GC, Jamrozik K. A randomized trial of sodium fluoride (60 mg) +/− estrogen in postmenopausal osteoporotic vertebral fractures: increased vertebral fractures and peripheral bone loss with sodium fluoride; concurrent estrogen prevents peripheral loss, but not vertebral fractures. Osteoporos Int 2002;13(2):158–70.
7. Teede HJ, Liang YL, Kotsopoulos D, Zoungas S, Craven R, McGrath BP. Placebo-controlled trial of transdermal estrogen therapy alone in postmenopausal women: effects on arterial compliance and endothelial function. Climacteric 2002;5(2):160–9.
8. Rossouw JE, Anderson GL, Prentice RL, LaCroix AZ, Kooperberg C, Stefanick ML, Jackson RD, Beresford SA, Howard BV, Johnson KC, Kotchen JM, Ockene J; Writing Group for the Women's Health Initiative Investigators. Risks and benefits of estrogen plus progestin in healthy postmenopausal women: principal results From the Women's Health Initiative randomized controlled trial. JAMA 2002;288(3):321–33.
9. Lanzone A. The puzzle of hormone replacement therapy (HRT) and cardiovascular disease (CVD). J Endocrinol Invest 2002;25(1):1–3.
10. Beral V, Banks E, Reeves G. Evidence from randomised trials on the long-term effects of hormone replacement therapy. Lancet 2002;360(9337):942–4.
11. Haseroth K, Seyffart K, Wehling M, Christ M. Effects of progestin–estrogen replacement therapy on QT-dispersion in postmenopausal women. Int J Cardiol 2000;75(2–3):161–5.
12. Wenger NK. Hormonal and nonhormonal therapies for the postmenopausal woman: what is the evidence for cardioprotection? Am J Geriatr Cardiol 2000;9(4):204–9.
13. Davidson MH, Maki KC, Marx P, Maki AC, Cyrowski MS, Nanavati N, Arce JC. Effects of continuous estrogen and estrogen-progestin replacement regimens on cardiovascular risk markers in postmenopausal women. Arch Intern Med 2000;160(21):3315–25.
14. Heckbert SR, Kaplan RC, Weiss NS, Psaty BM, Lin D, Furberg CD, Starr JR, Anderson GD, LaCroix AZ. Risk of recurrent coronary events in relation to use and recent initiation of postmenopausal hormone therapy. Arch Intern Med 2001;161(14):1709–13.
15. Alexander KP, Newby LK, Hellkamp AS, Harrington RA, Peterson ED, Kopecky S, Langer A, O'Gara P, O'Connor CM, Daly RN, Califf RM, Khan S, Fuster V. Initiation of hormone replacement therapy after acute myocardial infarction is associated with more cardiac events during follow-up. J Am Coll Cardiol 2001;38(1):1–7.

16. Grady D, Hulley SB. Postmenopausal hormones and heart disease. J Am Coll Cardiol 2001;38(1):8–10.
17. Grady D, Wenger NK, Herrington D, Khan S, Furberg C, Hunninghake D, Vittinghoff E, Hulley S. Postmenopausal hormone therapy increases risk for venous thromboembolic disease. The Heart and Estrogen/progestin Replacement Study. Ann Intern Med 2000;132(9):689–96.
18. Weintraub MS, Grosskopf I, Charach G, Eckstein N, Ringel Y, Maharshak N, Rotmensch HH, Rubinstein A. Fluctuations of lipid and lipoprotein levels in hyperlipidemic postmenopausal women receiving hormone replacement therapy. Arch Intern Med 1998;158(16): 1803–6.
19. Gambrell RD Jr. Progestogens in estrogen-replacement therapy. Clin Obstet Gynecol 1995;38(4):890–901.
20. Godsland IF. Effects of postmenopausal hormone replacement therapy on lipid, lipoprotein, and apolipoprotein (a) concentrations: analysis of studies published from 1974–2000. Fertil Steril 2001;75(5):898–915.
21. Jensen J, Christiansen C. Dose-response effects on serum lipids and lipoproteins following combined oestrogen-progestogen therapy in post-menopausal women. Maturitas 1987;9(3):259–66.
22. Erenus M, Karakoc B, Gurler A. Comparison of effects of continuous combined transdermal with oral estrogen and oral progestogen replacement therapies on serum lipoproteins and compliance. Climacteric 2001;4(3):228–34.
23. Angerer P, Stork S, Kothny W, Schmitt P, von Schacky C. Effect of oral postmenopausal hormone replacement on progression of atherosclerosis: a randomized, controlled trial. Arterioscler Thromb Vasc Biol 2001;21(2):262–8.
24. Taylor M, Bowen-Simpkins P, Barrington J. Complications of unopposed oestrogen following radical surgery for endometriosis. J Obstet Gynaecol 1999;19(6):647–8.
25. Cameron ST, Critchley HOD. Continuous oestrogen and interrupted progestogen in HRT bleed-free regimens. Contemp Rev Obstet Gynaecol 1998;10:151–5.
26. Colacurci N, Mele D, De Franciscis P, Costa V, Fortunato N, De Seta L. Effects of tibolone on the breast. Eur J Obstet Gynecol Reprod Biol 1998;80(2):235–8.
27. Ferenczy A, Gelfand MM, van de Weijer PH, Rioux JE. Endometrial safety and bleeding patterns during a 2-year study of 1 or 2 mg 17 beta-estradiol combined with sequential 5–20 mg dydrogesterone. Climacteric 2002;5(1):26–35.
28. Li CI, Weiss NS, Stanford JL, Daling JR. Hormone replacement therapy in relation to risk of lobular and ductal breast carcinoma in middle-aged women. Cancer 2000;88(11):2570–7.
29. Schairer C, Lubin J, Troisi R, Sturgeon S, Brinton L, Hoover R. Menopausal estrogen and estrogen-progestin replacement therapy and breast cancer risk. JAMA 2000;283(4):485–91.
30. Hill DA, Weiss NS, Beresford SA, Voigt LF, Daling JR, Stanford JL, Self S. Continuous combined hormone replacement therapy and risk of endometrial cancer. Am J Obstet Gynecol 2000;183(6):1456–61.
31. Jain MG, Rohan TE, Howe GR. Hormone replacement therapy and endometrial cancer in Ontario, Canada. J Clin Epidemiol 2000;53(4):385–91.
32. Psaty BM, Smith NL, Lemaitre RN, Vos HL, Heckbert SR, LaCroix AZ, Rosendaal FR. Hormone replacement therapy, prothrombotic mutations, and the risk of incident nonfatal myocardial infarction in postmenopausal women. JAMA 2001;285(7):906–13.
33. Odmark IS, Jonsson B, Backstrom T. Bleeding patterns in postmenopausal women using continuous combination hormone replacement therapy with conjugated estrogen and medroxyprogesterone acetate or with 17beta-estradiol and norethindrone acetate. Am J Obstet Gynecol 2001;184(6):1131–8.
34. Harrison RF, Magill P, Kilminster SG. Impact of a new formulation of low-dose micronised medroxyprogesterone and 17-beta estradiol, on lipid profiles in menopausal women. Clin Drug Invest 1998;16:93–9.
35. Gadomska H, Barcz E, Cyganek A, Leocmach Y, Chadha-Boreham H, Marianowski L. Efficacy and tolerability of low-dose transdermal estrogen (Oesclim) in the treatment of menopausal symptoms. Curr Med Res Opin 2002;18(2):97–102.
36. Shulman LP, Yankov V, Uhl K. Safety and efficacy of a continuous once-a-week 17beta-estradiol/levonorgestrel transdermal system and its effects on vasomotor symptoms and endometrial safety in postmenopausal women: the results of two multicenter, double-blind, randomized, controlled trials. Menopause 2002;9(3):195–207.
37. Herrington DM, Vittinghoff E, Lin F, Fong J, Harris F, Hunninghake D, Bittner V, Schrott HG, Blumenthal RS, Levy R; HERS Study Group. Statin therapy, cardiovascular events, and total mortality in the Heart and Estrogen/Progestin Replacement Study (HERS). Circulation 2002;105(25):2962–7.

Human immunodeficiency virus (HIV) vaccine

See also Vaccines

General Information

The difficult problems connected with clinical trials that have not been approved by independent authorities were highlighted in 1991 when Zagury published the first reports of immunization of humans using *Vaccinia* vaccine expressing HIV glycoprotein gp-160 (1,2). The first HIV vaccine approved for clinical trial status (1989) by the US Food and Drug Administration (FDA) was a recombinant gp-160 vaccine produced in a baculovirus-insect cell expression system by MicroGeneSys (3). Since then, various clinical trials using different HIV vaccines have been carried out. However, all HIV vaccines are still experimental. An overview of the current status of HIV vaccine development, with emphasis on efficacy and safety, has been provided by the AIDS Division of the National Institute of Allergy and Infectious Diseases (4).

References

1. Dorozynski A, Anderson A. Deaths in vaccine trials trigger French inquiry. Science 1991;252(5005):501–2.
2. Guillaume JC, Saiag P, Wechsler J, Lescs MC, Roujeau JC. Vaccinia from recombinant virus expressing HIV genes. Lancet 1991;337(8748):1034–5.
3. Midthun K, Garrison L, Gershman K. Cellular immunity in HIV-1 rgp 160 vaccines. In: Abstracts, V International Conference on AIDS, Montreal, 1989:544.
4. National Institute of Allergy and Infectious Diseases (NIAID), National Institutes of Health (NIH). HIV vaccines. http://www.niaid.nih.gov/daids/vaccine/default.htm, 20/06/2005.

Human papilloma virus (HPV) vaccine

See also Vaccines

General Information

Cervical cancer is the second most common cause of cancer deaths in women worldwide and the number one cause in the developing world. It is almost invariably associated with HPV infection. HPV type 16 is found in about 50% of cervical cancers. About 70% of cervical cancers are associated with HPV types 16, 18, and 8 other HPV types. Types 18, 31, and 45 account for 25% of HVP-positive tumors. HPV types 6 and 11 can cause genital warts. The development of a safe and effective HPV vaccine could prevent pre-malignant and malignant disease associated with HPV infection. Various HPV vaccines are under development or are undergoing clinical trials. Among others, GlaxoSmithKline (bivalent HPV types 16 and 18) and Merck (HPV types 6, 11, 16, 18) are both conducting expanded phase III trials and the researchers say the results so far have been promising. Merck plans to apply for approval to the US Food and Drug Administration in late 2005.

Clinical studies with a recombinant vaccine (using *Vaccinia* virus expressing HPV 16, 18, E6, and E7 proteins) in patients with preinvasive and invasive cancer have been reviewed (1).

Observational studies

There has been a trial of a papilloma (HPV-16) virus-like particle vaccine in 72 healthy volunteers, aged 18–27 years (2). The vaccine was well tolerated and highly immunogenic.

Placebo-controlled studies

In a double-blind study in 2392 young women (aged 16–23 years) randomly assigned to either three doses of placebo or HPV-16 vaccine at day 0, month 2, and month 6, the vaccine reduced the incidence of both HPV-16 infection (3.8 per 100 woman-years at risk in the placebo group versus 0 per 100 woman-years at risk in the vaccine group) and HPV-16-related cervical intraepithelial neoplasia (all nine cases of neoplasia occurred among the placebo recipients) (3).

References

1. Adams M, Borysiewicz L, Fiander A, Man S, Jasani B, Navabi H, Lipetz C, Evans AS, Mason M. Clinical studies of human papilloma vaccines in pre-invasive and invasive cancer. Vaccine 2001;19(17–19):2549–56.
2. Harro CD, Pang YY, Roden RB, Hildesheim A, Wang Z, Reynolds MJ, Mast TC, Robinson R, Murphy BR, Karron RA, Dillner J, Schiller JT, Lowy DR. Safety and immunogenicity trial in adult volunteers of a human papillomavirus 16 L1 virus-like particle vaccine. J Natl Cancer Inst 2001;93(4):284–92.

3. Koutsky LA, Ault KA, Wheeler CM, Brown DR, Barr E, Alvarez FB, Chiacchierini LM, Jansen KU; Proof of Principle Study Investigators. A controlled trial of a human papillomavirus type 16 vaccine. N Engl J Med 2002;347(21):1645–51.

Hyaluronic acid

General Information

Hyaluronic acid is a naturally occurring polysaccharide that is widely distributed in body tissues and intracellular fluids, including the aqueous and vitreous humour, synovial fluid, and in the ground substance that surrounds cells (1). It is a high-molecular weight substance originally developed for use as a vitreous replacement. Although 98% of the product consists of water, it is very viscoelastic.

Uses

Hyaluronic acid is considered to have low inflammatory and antigenic potential, and has been used in various intraocular procedures. In addition to filtration bleb formation, it has been used to protect the corneal endothelium during intraocular lens implantation and keratoplasty, to reform the anterior chamber, to push back a bulging vitreous face, and in retinal detachment surgery as a vitreous replacement.

Hyaluronate sodium is also combined with sodium chondroitin sulfate (in Viscoat) as a corneal transplant preservation medium. Sodium chondroitin sulfate and other viscoelastic substances protect the corneal endothelium during intraocular surgery.

Hyaluronic acid is used topically to promote wound healing. A film containing hyaluronate sodium and carmellose is used to prevent surgical adhesion. Hyaluronic acid is increasingly being used in cosmetic dermatology to treat wrinkles in patients who are sensitive to bovine collagen.

Intra-articular injections of hyaluronic acid formulations of different molecular weights have been used in patients with osteoarthritis and can provide short-term benefit (2).

General adverse effects

The major adverse effect associated with the use of viscoelastic substances, such as hyaluronate sodium, is a transient rise in intraocular pressure in the immediate postoperative period, attributed to its viscoelastic nature, resulting in coating and plugging of the trabecular meshwork. For this reason, it is advisable to dilute hyaluronate sodium at the end of the surgical procedure with a balanced salt solution. Chondroitin sulfate is relatively less likely to precipitate such extreme rises in intraocular pressure because it is cleared rapidly from the trabecular meshwork. However, with any technique or chemical used in surgery there is always the potential for an unexpected adverse effect, and the risks of Viscoat include subepithelial calcium deposition and keratopathy (3).

After intra-articular injection, sodium hyaluronate can cause hemarthrosis, increased joint effusion volume, and possibly phlebitis. Other adverse effects are joint pain, septic arthritis, acute pseudogout, and anaphylaxis (4,5). Adverse events of this route of administration reportedly occur in about 2–4% of patients (6).

Organs and Systems

Skin

- An exudative granulomatous reaction started 2 days after the injection of hyaluronic acid (Hylaform) (dose not stated) for perioral wrinkles (7). The eczematous papular skin changes disappeared completely within 6 weeks, and could be provoked by intracutaneous testing with Hylaform (dose not stated). Histological examination showed a foreign body granuloma.

Immunologic

Immediate and delayed hypersensitivity reactions have been reported with hyaluronic acid (8).

References

1. Goa KL, Benfield P. Hyaluronic acid. A review of its pharmacology and use as a surgical aid in ophthalmology, and its therapeutic potential in joint disease and wound healing. Drugs 1994;47(3):536–66.
2. Anonymous. Hyaluronan for osteoarthrosis of the knee. Med Lett 1998;40:69–70.
3. Coffman MR, Mann PM. Corneal subepithelial deposits after use of sodium chondroitin. Am J Ophthalmol 1986;102(2):279–80.
4. Maillefert JF, Hirschhorn P, Pascaud F, Piroth C, Tavernier C. Acute attack of chondrocalcinosis after an intraarticular injection of hyaluronan. Rev Rhum Engl Ed 1997;64(10):593–4.
5. Luzar MJ, Altawil B. Pseudogout following intraarticular injection of sodium hyaluronate. Arthritis Rheum 1998;41(5):939–40.
6. Adams ME, Lussier AJ, Peyron JG. A risk-benefit assessment of injections of hyaluronan and its derivatives in the treatment of osteoarthritis of the knee. Drug Saf 2000;23(2):115–30.
7. Raulin C, Greve B, Hartschuh W, Soegding K. Exudative granulomatous reaction to hyaluronic acid (Hylaform). Contact Dermatitis 2000;43(3):178–9.
8. Andre P. Evaluation of the safety of a non-animal stabilized hyaluronic acid (NASHA—Q-Medical, Sweden) in European countries: a retrospective study from 1997 to 2001. J Eur Acad Dermatol Venereol 2004;18(4):422–5.

Hycanthone

General Information

Hycanthone is a derivative of lucanthone, but has less gastrointestinal and nervous system toxicity. It is effective against both *Schistosoma hematobium* and *Schistosoma mansoni* and is given as a single intramuscular injection in doses of 1.0–2.5 mg/kg (1,2). However, it has largely been superseded in the treatment of schistosomiasis by more recent, less toxic compounds. The most common adverse reactions to hycanthone, which occur in up to half of all patients treated with higher-dose regimens, is nausea and vomiting (3), often associated with abdominal colic and diarrhea. There can be muscle pain, and electrocardiographic changes can occur (4).

Organs and Systems

Liver

Hepatotoxicity occurs with hycanthone; serum transaminases are often raised and less commonly there is overt jaundice (5,6). Hepatitis was the major complication with hycanthone in the treatment of schistosomiasis, sometimes associated with pancreatitis (7,8). Hycanthone has also been evaluated as a potential antitumor agent, being used as a radiosensitizer; here too, hepatitis was a dose-limiting effect, occurring in some patients with doses of 100 mg/m2 per day (3). The lowest dosage that caused hepatitis was 70 mg/m2/day. In several cases the hepatotoxicity proved fatal (SED-11, 597) (7–9).

Long-Term Effects

Mutagenicity

Experimentally, hycanthone has been reported to be mutagenic in *Salmonella typhimurium* and *Escherichia coli*, but no human data are available (10,11).

Tumorigenicity

Experimentally, hycanthone has been reported to be carcinogenic in mice (12,13), but no human data are available.

Second-Generation Effects

Teratogenicity

Experimentally, hycanthone has been reported to be teratogenic (14,15), although no human data are available.

References

1. Dennis EW, Kobus W. A review of the clinical pharmacology of hycanthone. Egypt J Bilharz 1974;1(1):35–53.
2. Farah A, Berberian DA, Davison C, Dennis EW, Donikian MA, Drobeck HP, Ferrari RA, Yarinsky A. Hycanthone: a review of its experimental chemotherapy, pharmacology and toxicology. Egypt J Bilharz 1974;1(2):181–95.
3. Kovach JS, Moertel CG, Schutt AJ, Eagan RT. Phase I study of hycanthone. Cancer Treat Rep 1979;63(11–12):1965–9.
4. Takaoka L, Baldy JL, Passos JD, Soares EC, Zeitune JM, Siqueira JE. Alteracoes eletrocardiograficas em pacientes com esquistossomose mansonica tratados com hicantone. [Electrocardiographic changes in patients with schistosomiasis mansoni treated with hycanthone.] Rev Inst Med Trop Sao Paulo 1976;18(5):378–86.
5. Oostburg BF. Clinical trial with hycanthone in schistosomiasis mansoni in Surinam. Trop Geogr Med 1972;24(2):148–51.

6. Farid Z, Smith JH, Bassily S, Sparks HA. Hepatotoxicity after treatment of schistosomiasis with hycanthone. BMJ 1972;2(805):88–9.
7. Buchanan N, Thatcher CJ, Cane RD, Bartolomeo B. Fatal hepatic necrosis in association with the use of hycanthone. A case report. S Afr Med J 1978;53(7):257–8.
8. Goncalves CS, Buaiz V, Zanandrea J, Zanotti WM, Boni ES, de Castro Filho AK, Pereira FE. Reacoes toxicas com o uso do hycanthone. [Toxic reactions with the use of hycanthone.] AMB Rev Assoc Med Bras 1977;23(9):305–8.
9. Mengistu M. Fatal liver toxicity due to hycanthone (Etrenol) in a patient with pre-existing liver disease: a case report. Ethiop Med J 1982;20(3):145–7.
10. Hartman PE. Early years of the *Salmonella* mutagen tester strains: lessons from hycanthone. Environ Mol Mutagen 1989;14(Suppl 16):39–45.
11. Cook TM, Goldman CK. Hycanthone and its congeners as bacterial mutagens. J Bacteriol 1975;122(2):549–56.
12. Botros SS. Effect of praziquantel versus hycanthone on deoxyribonucleic acid content of hepatocytes in murine schistosomiasis mansoni. Pharmacol Res 1990;22(2):219–29.
13. Bulay O, Urman H, Patil K, Clayson DB, Shubik P. Carcinogenic potential of hycanthone in mice and hamsters. Int J Cancer 1979;23(1):97–104.
14. Moore JA. Teratogenicity of hycanthone in mice. Nature 1972;239(5367):107–9.
15. Nishimura H, Tanimura T. Clinical Aspects of the Teratogenicity of Drugs. Amsterdam, Oxford: Excerpta Medica, 1976.

Hydralazine

General Information

Hydralazine is a direct vasodilator that acts on vascular smooth muscle to produce systemic vasodilatation. As a result there is baroreceptor-mediated activation of the sympathetic nervous system and the renin–angiotensin system.

Vasodilators (as monotherapy) are associated acutely with flushing, headache, dizziness, reflex tachycardia, and palpitation. Chronic treatment can be complicated by fluid retention.

Organs and Systems

Cardiovascular

Aggravation of angina, presumably as a result of reflex tachycardia, has been reported with hydralazine.

- Pericarditis has been attributed to hydralazine in a 75-year-old man who developed a full-blown hydralazine-induced autoimmune syndrome (1).

The authors referred to a similar previously published case of late pericarditis after hydralazine treatment.

Nervous system

Peripheral neuropathy has been described in association with deficiency of pyridoxine (vitamin B6) in slow acetylators (2).

Metabolism

Salt and water retention mediated by secondary hyperaldosteronism can complicate hydralazine treatment, leading to weight gain and peripheral edema, loss of blood pressure control, and rarely cardiac failure (SED-8, 474).

Gastrointestinal

Anorexia, nausea, and vomiting can complicate hydralazine treatment, particularly initially (SED-8, 474).

Liver

Acute hepatitis (usually with negative antinuclear antibodies) has been attributed to hydralazine (3–7).

Skin

- A 44-year-old man taking hydralazine (dose not stated) developed a pruritic rash, attributed to a drug-induced lichenoid eruption, based on biopsy findings (8). The hydralazine was withdrawn and the rash resolved in a few weeks.

Immunologic

The lupus-like syndrome (SED-9, 318) with hydralazine occurs particularly in slow acetylators (and only rarely in fast acetylators) and in patients with the HLA-DR4 antigen. Blood dyscrasias and necrotizing vasculitis are additional features.

Current knowledge about the possible mechanisms of drug-induced lupus-like syndrome has been reviewed (9). Three mechanisms seem most plausible. One involves a change, possibly caused by a reactive metabolite, in the way that antigens are processed and presented to T cells, leading to the presentation of cryptic antigens. Another possibility is that a reactive metabolite binds to the class II major histocompatibility antigen and induces an autoimmune reaction analogous to a graft-versus-host reaction. A third possibility is that hydralazine inhibits DNA methylation, leading to an increase in DNA transcription and a generalized activation of the immune system.

A variety of vasculitic diseases, including Wegener's granulomatosis, microscopic polyangiitis, Churg–Strauss syndrome, and crescentic glomerulonephritis, are associated with antineutrophil cytoplasmic antibodies (ANCA) or leukocytoclastic vasculitis. In drug-induced ANCA-positive vasculitis, antimyeloperoxidase antibodies are most often found; they produce a perinuclear pattern of staining by indirect immunofluorescence (pANCA), but antiproteinase 3 (anti-PR3) antibodies can also occur (cANCA).

The possible drug causes of ANCA-positive vasculitis with high titers of antimyeloperoxidase antibodies in 30 new patients have been reviewed (10). The findings illustrate that this type of vasculitis is a predominantly drug-induced disorder. Only 12 of the 30 cases were not related to a drug. The most frequently implicated drug was hydralazine (10 cases); the remainder involved propylthiouracil (3 cases), penicillamine (2 cases), allopurinol (2 cases), and sulfasalazine.

Second-Generation Effects

Fetotoxicity

Thrombocytopenia has been reported in infants whose mothers were taking hydralazine with no evidence of the lupus-like syndrome (11).

The administration of hydralazine 25 mg bd at 34 weeks to a hypertensive pregnant woman was associated, within 1 week, with atrial extra beats in the fetus. These subsided when hydralazine was withdrawn, and the rest of the pregnancy and delivery was uneventful (12).

- A 29-year-old woman, 26 weeks pregnant, was treated with hydralazine for toxemia of pregnancy. She developed arthralgia and dyspnea and was subsequently found to be antinuclear antibody-positive. Following an induced labor, a low-birth-weight infant was born but died aged 36 hours. At autopsy the neonate was found to have a pericardial effusion and tamponade (13).

Although hydralazine was implicated as the cause of a maternal and neonatal lupus-like syndrome, the toxemia and low birth weight of the child make interpretation of the case difficult.

References

1. Franssen CF, el Gamal MI, Gans RO, Hoorntje SJ. Hydralazine-induced constrictive pericarditis. Neth J Med 1996;48(5):193–7.
2. Raskin NH, Fishman RA. Pyridoxine-deficiency neuropathy due to hydralazine. N Engl J Med 1965;273(22):1182–5.
3. Bartoli E, Massarelli G, Solinas A, Faedda R, Chiandussi L. Acute hepatitis with bridging necrosis due to hydralazine intake. Report of a case. Arch Intern Med 1979;139(6):698–9.
4. Forster HS. Hepatitis from hydralazine. N Engl J Med 1980;302(24):1362.
5. Itoh S, Ichinoe A, Tsukada Y, Itoh Y. Hydralazine-induced hepatitis. Hepatogastroenterology 1981;28(1):13–16.
6. Itoh S, Yamaba Y, Ichinoe A, Tsukada Y. Hydralazine-induced liver injury. Dig Dis Sci 1980;25(11):884–7.
7. Barnett DB, Hudson SA, Golightly PW. Hydrallazine-induced hepatitis? BMJ 1980;280(6224):1165–6.
8. Bargout R, Malhotra A. A 44-year-old man with a pruritic skin rash. Cleve Clin J Med 2001;68(11):952–3.
9. Uetrecht JP. Drug induced lupus: possible mechanisms and their implications for prediction of which new drugs may induce lupus. Exp Opin Invest Drugs 1996;5:851–60.
10. Choi HK, Merkel PA, Walker AM, Niles JL. Drug-associated antineutrophil cytoplasmic antibody-positive vasculitis: prevalence among patients with high titers of antimyeloperoxidase antibodies. Arthritis Rheum 2000;43(2):405–13.
11. Widerlov E, Karlman I, Storsater J. Hydralazine-induced neonatal thrombocytopenia. N Engl J Med 1980;303(21):1235.
12. Lodeiro JG, Feinstein SJ, Lodeiro SB. Fetal premature atrial contractions associated with hydralazine. Am J Obstet Gynecol 1989;160(1):105–7.
13. Yemini M, Shoham Z, Dgani R, Lancet M, Mogilner BM, Nissim F, Bar-Khayim Y. Lupus-like syndrome in a mother and newborn following administration of hydralazine; a case report. Eur J Obstet Gynecol Reprod Biol 1989;30(2):193–7.

Hydrazine

General Information

Hydrazine sulfate is sometimes promoted as an alternative cancer cure.

Organs and Systems

Liver

Hydrazine has been reported to cause liver damage (1).

- A 55-year-old man with maxillary sinus cancer declined conventional therapy and opted to treat his condition with hydrazine sulfate obtained via the Internet. He had followed the recommended regimen for 4 months when he developed fulminant hepatorenal failure, hepatic encephalopathy, and profound coagulopathy. He died of severe gastrointestinal hemorrhage.

Reference

1. Hainer MI, Tsai N, Komura ST, Chiu CL. Fatal hepatorenal failure associated with hydrazine sulfate. Ann Intern Med 2000;133(11):877–80.

Hydrocodone

See also Opioid analgesics

General Information

Hydrocodone is a semisynthetic narcotic analgesic and a cough suppressant, similar to codeine. It is metabolized to the *O*- and *N*-demethylated products, hydromorphone and norhydrocodone (1).

Drug Administration

Drug administration route

Five patients who abused prescribed opioids intranasally have been described (2). All took hydrocodone bitartrate plus cocaine ($n = 2$), codeine phosphate ($n = 2$), oxycodone hydrochloride ($n = 2$), or methadone hydrochloride ($n = 1$). The symptoms included nasal obstruction and congestion, foul smelling nasal crusting and discharge, headaches and nasal pain, and in one case dysphagia with odynophagia. Physical findings included a perforated septum, soft palate erosion, and a mucopurulent exudate. All except one patient had positive fungal cultures and two had invasive rhinitis. Not only can intranasal opioids cause septal perforation, commonly associated with intranasal cocaine, but it is also possible that intranasal abuse of opioids, especially hydrocodone, can cause localized immunosuppression, supporting the growth of fungal organisms.

References

1. Hutchinson MR, Menelaou A, Foster DJ, Coller JK, Somogyi AA. CYP2D6 and CYP3A4 involvement in the primary oxidative metabolism of hydrocodone by human liver microsomes. Br J Clin Pharmacol 2004;57(3):287–97.
2. Yewell J, Haydon R, Archer S, Manaligod JM. Complications of intranasal prescription narcotic abuse. Ann Otol Rhinol Laryngol 2002;111(2):174–7.

Hydromorphone

See also Opioid analgesics

General Information

Intolerable adverse effects or inadequate analgesia occur in 10–15% of patients with chronic pain given continuous intrathecal morphine. Hydromorphone is a semisynthetic derivative of morphine used extensively in the management of cancer pain. It is more soluble than morphine, has a slightly shorter duration of action, and is about five times more potent when given systemically.

In a retrospective review of 37 patients with chronic non-malignant pain (mostly from failed lumbosacral spine surgery) treated with intrathecal hydromorphone there was an analgesic response in six of the 16 patients who were switched from morphine to hydromorphone because of poor pain relief (1). Opioid-related adverse effects, such as nausea, vomiting, pruritus, and sedation, were also reduced by hydromorphone in the 21 patients who were switched to hydromorphone because of morphine-related adverse effects, especially 1 month after use. These results should be treated cautiously, because of the limitations of a retrospective study that lacks strict inclusion criteria, with obvious population bias and under-reporting, and without standardized procedures for rotation to hydromorphone.

Three randomized, double-blind comparisons of morphine and hydromorphone have been reported. Modified-release hydromorphone hydrochloride 4 mg bd was compared with modified-release morphine sulfate 30 mg bd in 89 patients with cancer pain (2). In all, 88 adverse effects were thought to be directly related to the study medication. Other adverse events were related to the disease process, the re-emergence of pain, or not specified.

In a comparison of hydromorphone and morphine delivered by continuous subcutaneous infusion in 74 patients with severe cancer pain, the number of adverse effects was small and comparable in both groups (3).

When epidural morphine (Duramorph 10 micrograms/kg/hour) was compared with epidural fentanyl (1 microgram/kg/hour) and epidural hydromorphone (1 microgram/kg/hour) in 90 children undergoing orthopedic procedures, hydromorphone was considered to be safe and efficacious (4). The combined incidences of pruritus, nausea, and vomiting were 25, 20, and 10% respectively and for pruritus alone 35, 15, and 8% respectively.

Organs and Systems

Sensory systems

In a retrospective review in a specialized otological center, 12 patients were identified with rapidly progressive hearing loss and a concurrent history of hydrocodone overuse with paracetamol (5). These patients were helped by cochlear implantation.

Drug Administration

Drug administration route

The use of intrathecal hydromorphone in the management of chronic non-malignant pain has been described (1).

References

1. Yeh HM, Chen LK, Shyu MK, Lin CJ, Sun WZ, Wang MJ, Mok MS, Tsai SK. The addition of morphine prolongs fentanyl-bupivacaine spinal analgesia for the relief of labor pain. Anesth Analg 2001;92(3):665–8.
2. Moriarty M, McDonald CJ, Miller AJ. A randomised crossover comparison of controlled release hydromorphone tablets with controlled release morphine tablets in patients with cancer pain. J Clin Res 1999;2:1–8.
3. Miller MG, McCarthy N, O'Boyle CA, Kearney M. Continuous subcutaneous infusion of morphine vs. hydromorphone: a controlled trial. J Pain Symptom Manage 1999;18(1):9–16.
4. Goodarzi M. Comparison of epidural morphine, hydromorphone and fentanyl for postoperative pain control in children undergoing orthopaedic surgery. Paediatr Anaesth 1999;9(5):419–22.
5. Friedman RA, House JW, Luxford WM, Gherini S, Mills D. Profound hearing loss associated with hydrocodone/acetaminophen abuse. Am J Otol 2000;21(2):188–91.

Hydroxycarbamide

See also Cytostatic and immunosuppressant drugs

General Information

Hydroxycarbamide (hydroxyurea) is used to treat a variety of cancers, myeloproliferative disorders, and sickle cell disease, and has been studied in patients with HIV infection (1). It inhibits ribonucleotide reductase and increases concentrations of iron nitrosyl hemoglobin, nitrite, and nitrate, suggesting in vivo metabolism of hydroxycarbamide to nitric oxide (2).

Organs and Systems

Hematologic

Concern about the toxicity of hydroxycarbamide, expressed in a report from the AIDS Clinical Trials Group (ACTG 5025 report), has led to a retrospective study of the antiviral activity, immunological effects, and tolerability of hydroxycarbamide in combination with didanosine (3). Hematological adverse events were the most frequent and involved 37 of the 65 patients. Neutropenia was the commonest adverse event (26 patients) and it was occasionally accompanied by anemia or thrombocytopenia. However, these effects normalized spontaneously, despite continued therapy.

Of 16 children receiving hydroxycarbamide in combination with nucleoside analogues, 4 developed neutropenia (below 1.5×10^9/l) by weeks 2 or 4 (4). Hydroxycarbamide was temporarily withdrawn and then reintroduced without further ill effects after the neutrophil count had returned to normal.

Mouth and teeth

In a retrospective study of the antiviral activity, immunological effects, and tolerability of hydroxycarbamide in combination with didanosine, mouth ulceration was recorded in eight of the 65 patients and this led to discontinuation in one patient (3).

Pancreas

In a retrospective study of the antiviral activity, immunological effects, and tolerability of hydroxycarbamide in combination with didanosine, there was increased serum amylase activity in 15 of the 65 patients; although asymptomatic, it occasioned withdrawal of therapy in four patients (3).

Skin

The incidence of skin lesions in patients taking hydroxycarbamide is 10–35%. They usually occur after several years of maintenance therapy. However, one patient developed lichen planus-like dermatitis on his hands after just 15 days of treatment (5).

Hydroxycarbamide can cause hyperpigmentation of the nails and palmar creases and leg ulcers (6,7). Leg ulcers occurred in 41 patients taking hydroxycarbamide (8). They had a mean age of 67 years and mean therapy duration of 5 years, and none had any underlying vascular disease. There were megaloblastic erythrocytes trapped in the capillary beds, causing local tissue anoxia, and the authors postulated that the megaloblastic erythrocytes had resulted from hydroxycarbamide and that the ulcers were due to consequent impaired circulation and cutaneous atrophy; they also commented that there was no major vascular disease that could have accounted for the leg ulcers. The degeneration of lichen planus-like skin lesions into full-blown ulcers has been described in 14 patients who developed extremely painful leg ulcers, most commonly on the malleoli. The patients had been taking hydroxycarbamide for an average of 6 years and nine had multiple ulcers (9).

Acral erythema, dermatomyositis-like changes on the backs of the hands, squamous cell neoplasms on sun-exposed sites, and ulcers on the legs, genitalia, and oral mucosae have also been reported (10).

Immunologic

Hydroxycarbamide has been associated with Behçet's syndrome (11).

Body temperature

- A 64-year-old woman with essential thrombocythemia developed a fever after 3 weeks of treatment with hydroxycarbamide 1000 mg/day; the fever subsided on withdrawal and recurred on rechallenge (12).

Drug–Drug Interactions

Busulfan

During long-term follow-up of patients treated with busulfan and hydroxycarbamide for essential thrombocythemia, seven patients (13%) taking hydroxycarbamide developed secondary acute leukemia, myelodysplasia, or solid tumors, compared with only one of the control group; none of the 20 patients who had never been treated with chemotherapy developed secondary malignancies compared with three of the 77 given hydroxycarbamide only and five of the 15 given busulfan plus hydroxycarbamide. This suggests that the combination of busulfan plus hydroxycarbamide causes a significantly increased risk of secondary malignancies (13).

References

1. Gibbs MA, Sorensen SJ. Hydroxyurea in the treatment of HIV-1. Ann Pharmacother 2000;34(1):89–93.
2. King SB. The nitric oxide producing reactions of hydroxyurea. Curr Med Chem 2003;10(6):437–52.
3. Biron F, Ponceau B, Bouhour D, Boibieux A, Verrier B, Peyramond D. Long-term safety and antiretroviral activity of hydroxyurea and didanosine in HIV-infected patients. J Acquir Immune Defic Syndr 2000;25(4):329–36.
4. Kline MW, Calles NR, Simon C, Schwarzwald H. Pilot study of hydroxyurea in human immunodeficiency virus-infected children receiving didanosine and/or stavudine. Pediatr Infect Dis J 2000;19(11):1083–6.
5. Radaelli F, Calori R, Faccini P, Maiolo AT. Early cutaneous lesions secondary to hydroxyurea therapy. Am J Hematol 1998;58(1):82–3.
6. O'Branski EE, Ware RE, Prose NS, Kinney TR. Skin and nail changes in children with sickle cell anemia receiving hydroxyurea therapy. J Am Acad Dermatol 2001;44(5):859–61.
7. Chaine B, Neonato MG, Girot R, Aractingi S. Cutaneous adverse reactions to hydroxyurea in patients with sickle cell disease. Arch Dermatol 2001;137(4):467–70.
8. Sirieix ME, Debure C, Baudot N, Dubertret L, Roux ME, Morel P, Frances C, Loubeyres S, Beylot C, Lambert D, Humbert P, Gauthier O, Dandurand M, Guillot B, Vaillant L, Lorette G, Bonnetblanc JM, Lok C, Denoeux JP. Leg ulcers and hydroxyurea: forty-one cases. Arch Dermatol 1999;135(7):818–20.
9. Best PJ, Daoud MS, Pittelkow MR, Petitt RM. Hydroxyurea-induced leg ulceration in 14 patients. Ann Intern Med 1998;128(1):29–32.
10. Vassallo C, Passamonti F, Merante S, Ardigo M, Nolli G, Mangiacavalli S, Borroni G. Muco-cutaneous changes during long-term therapy with hydroxyurea in chronic myeloid leukaemia. Clin Exp Dermatol 2001;26(2):141–8.
11. Vaiopoulos G, Terpos E, Viniou N, Nodaros K, Rombos J, Loukopoulos D. Behçet's disease in a patient with chronic myelogenous leukemia under hydroxyurea treatment: a case report and review of the literature. Am J Hematol 2001;66(1):57–8.

12. Braester A, Quitt M. Hydroxyurea as a cause of drug fever. Acta Haematol 2000;104(1):50–1.
13. Finazzi G, Ruggeri M, Rodeghiero F, Barbui T. Second malignancies in patients with essential thrombocythaemia treated with busulphan and hydroxyurea: long-term follow-up of a randomized clinical trial. Br J Haematol 2000;110(3):577–83.

Hydroxyzine

See also Antihistamines

General Information

Hydroxyzine is a first-generation antihistamine, a piperazine derivative, with antimuscarinic and sedative properties.

Organs and Systems

Skin

Two cases of drug allergy have been reported in a 37-year-old woman and a 66-year-old man, who received hydroxyzine for premedication before anesthesia (1,2). In these patients immediate skin tests with the implicated drug were positive.

Second-Generation Effects

Fetotoxicity

Hydroxyzine used in a fairly high dose (600 mg/day) in pregnancy has been reported to produce a neonatal withdrawal syndrome after delivery; this was characterized primarily by hyperactivity and irritability (SEDA-2, 151).

References

1. Okuda T, Karasawa F, Satoh T. [A case of drug allergy to hydroxyzine used for premedication.] Masui 2000;49(7):759–61.
2. Urabe K, Fujii K, Tezuka M, Okuda Y, Kitajima T, Yamazaki T, Yamakage A. [A case of acute urticaria from hydroxyzine hydrochloride used for preanesthetic medication.] Masui 2000;49(8):890–2.

Hyoscine

See also Anticholinergic drugs

General Information

Hyoscine is an anticholinergic drug, a stereoisomer of atropine. It is available in different salts, hyoscine hydrobromide and hyoscine butylbromide.

When given parenterally hyoscine butylbromide is effective but very short-acting; when given by mouth it is virtually inactive, even in doses up to 1 g, since it is hardly absorbed.

Hyoscine hydrobromide is used primarily in motion sickness; doses of 0.6 mg appear to be effective, particularly in combination with drugs having a mild central stimulant effect such as ephedrine.

Organs and Systems

Nervous system

Despite being a stereoisomer of atropine, hyoscine tends to have central depressant effects in conditions where atropine might be expected to cause excitation; however, excitation can occur (1). Hyoscine hydrobromide produces somnolence and dryness of the mouth in a high proportion of patients, and when ephedrine is not given the somnolence is likely to be present in the majority; some individuals also have headache, giddiness, and blurred vision.

Transdermal hyoscine is used by some anesthetists to minimize postoperative nausea and vomiting. The safety and efficacy of this form of treatment has been reviewed in an analysis of data from 23 trials involving 979 patients treated with hyoscine and 984 with placebo (2). The authors concluded that of 100 patients who are treated with hyoscine, 17 will escape postoperative nausea and vomiting that would otherwise have occurred; however, 18 will have visual disturbances, 8 will complain of dry mouth, 2 of dizziness, and 1 will become agitated. Although these are not necessarily prohibitive problems, they certainly do need to be considered when choosing a drug for this indication.

Psychological, psychiatric

In one study hyoscine premedication had detrimental effects on memory and on motor tasks compared with placebo, while atropine did not (3), although the difference is unlikely to be absolute. In view of certain of these effects, hyoscine hydrobromide is not a suitable antiemetic for those likely to drive vehicles before the effect has worn off, for example air passengers.

Immunologic

An isolated case of angioedema has been described during the use of hyoscine butylbromide (SEDA-8, 148).

Second-Generation Effects

Pregnancy

Two Japanese primigravidae, aged 25 and 28 years, developed the HELLP syndrome, a severe variant of pre-eclampsia in which there is Hemolysis, Elevated Liver enzymes, and a Low Platelet count (4). They were given parenteral hyoscine butylbromide for abdominal pain and had seizures 60–90 minutes later. One died from intracerebral hemorrhage some days later and the other survived after a cesarean section soon afterward. The authors speculated that anticholinergic drugs may enhance sympathetic nervous system activity, and in particular vasoconstriction, and should be avoided in pre-eclampsia. It is not clear how widespread their use is in other countries in managing abdominal pain in these circumstances.

Drug Administration

Drug administration route

A transdermal delivery system has been developed for prevention of motion sickness and vomiting, using an adhesive patch for postauricular application; the drug is released at a uniform rate for 72 hours. The adverse effects of this formulation are qualitatively typical of those reported for the oral and parenteral formulations of hyoscine and its congeners, although comparative studies suggest that the incidence is reduced with transdermal administration. Nevertheless, adverse effects involving the central nervous system, vision, bladder, and skin have been described, as have withdrawal symptoms after the patch is removed.

Dry mouth occurs in about 67% of subjects and drowsiness in about 16%. Transient effects on ocular accommodation, including blurred vision and mydriasis, have also been observed, in some cases possibly due to finger-to-eye contamination. Adverse effects on the central nervous system, including toxic psychosis (5) and hallucinations, have been reported only occasionally, as have other adverse reactions, such as dry, itchy eyes, difficulty in urinating, rashes, and erythema (6).

Attention has been drawn to potentially confusing clinical signs that can occur if a patch is applied for its antiemetic effect before general anesthesia; in one case the patient developed a right fixed pupil and became uncooperative; intravenous physostigmine had to be administered (SEDA-22, 157).

References

1. Ullman KC, Groh RH, Wolff FW. Treatment of scopolamine-induced delirium. Lancet 1970;1(7640):252.
2. Kranke P, Morin AM, Roewer N, Wulf H, Eberhart LH. The efficacy and safety of transdermal scopolamine for the prevention of postoperative nausea and vomiting: a quantitative systematic review. Anesth Analg 2002;95(1):133–43.
3. Anderson S, McGuire R, McKeown D. Comparison of the cognitive effects of premedication with hyoscine and atropine. Br J Anaesth 1985;57(2):169–73.
4. Kobayashi T, Sugimura M, Tokunaga N, Naruse H, Nishiguchi T, Kanayama N, Terao T. Anticholinergics induce eclamptic seizures. Semin Thromb Hemost 2002;28(6):511–14.
5. Rozzini R, Inzoli M, Trabucchi M. Delirium from transdermal scopolamine in an elderly woman. JAMA 1988;260(4):478.
6. Clissold SP, Heel RC. Transdermal hyoscine (Scopolamine). A preliminary review of its pharmacodynamic properties and therapeutic efficacy. Drugs 1985;29(3):189–207.

Ibopamine

General Information

Ibopamine is an orally active dopamine derivative that has been studied in patients with congestive heart failure (1). In theory, most, if not all, of the reported adverse effects can be considered to result from the drug's known pharmacological actions. Its gastrointestinal effects can be interpreted as being dopaminergic in nature, the occasional dizziness, flushing, and tremor as $beta_2$-adrenoceptor agonist effects, the tachycardia as an effect of $beta_1$-adrenoceptor stimulation or a reflex response to $beta_2$-adrenoceptor agonism. A reversible leukopenia has been described, but the relation to the drug was uncertain (2).

References

1. Nausieda PA. Sinemet "abusers". Clin Neuropharmacol 1985;8(4):318–27.
2. Said SA, Bucx JJ, Dankbaar H, Huizing G, van Gilst WH. Ibopamine-induced reversible leukopenia during treatment for congestive heart failure. Eur Heart J 1993;14(7):999–1001.

Ibritumomab

See also Monoclonal antibodies

General Information

Ibritumomab is a murine IgG_1 anti-CD20 antibody, the parent of the engineered chimeric antibody rituximab, a monoclonal antibody with mouse variable and human constant regions. It induces apoptosis and has antiproliferative effects. Ibritumomab tiuxetan (Zevalin) is composed of the monoclonal antibody ibritumomab, the linking chelator tiuxetan, and the radioisotope ^{90}yttrium (1).

General adverse effects

A wide range of adverse effects of ibritumomab has been reported. Most were hematological, thrombocytopenia being the most common, followed by a low hemoglobin and leukopenia. The most common non-hematological events were related to infusion and were similar to those reported with rituximab; they included weakness (54%), nausea (35%), chills (15%), and fever (21%) (2,3). Infectious complications during treatment with ibritumomab are rare, pneumonia being the most common. There is no obvious hepatotoxicity.

Organs and Systems

Immunologic

There has been one report of an anti-antibody response to ibritumomab (2).

Long-Term Effects

Tumorigenicity

Acute myelogenous leukemia has been attributed to ibritumomab (4).

- An 80-year-old woman with a small B cell extranodal lymphoma was initially given chlorambucil for 10 months, with complete remission for 2 years. When she developed recurrent lymph node swelling she was given ibritumomab tiuxetan, with near-complete remission. When she developed progressive disease 14 months later, she received cyclophosphamide, vincristine, and prednisone for one cycle. She had persistent pancytopenia, and a bone marrow biopsy showed extensive infiltration by acute myelogenous leukemia.

This seems to be the first case of drug-related acute myelogenous leukemia. Fluorescent in-situ hybridization studies on the bone marrow showed a signal consistent with rearrangement of the mixed myeloid leukemia (MLL) gene on chromosome 11. This abnormality was not present before treatment.

References

1. Krasner C, Joyce RM. Zevalin: ^{90}Yttrium labeled anti-CD20 (ibritumomab tiuxetan), a new treatment for non-Hodgkin's lymphoma. Curr Pharm Biotechnol 2001;2(4):341–9.
2. Witzig TE, White CA, Wiseman GA, Gordon LI, Emmanouilides C, Raubitschek A, Janakiraman N, Gutheil J, Schilder RJ, Spies S, Silverman DH, Parker E, Grillo-Lopez AJ. Phase I/II trial of IDEC-Y2B8 radioimmunotherapy for treatment of relapsed or refractory CD20(+) B cell non-Hodgkin's lymphoma. J Clin Oncol 1999; 17(12):3793–803.
3. Witzig TE, Flinn IW, Gordon LI, Emmanouilides C, Czuczman MS, Saleh MN, Cripe L, Wiseman G, Olejnik T, Multani PS, White CA. Treatment with ibritumomab tiuxetan radioimmunotherapy in patients with rituximab-refractory follicular non-Hodgkin's lymphoma. J Clin Oncol 2002;20(15):3262–9.
4. Nabhan C, Peterson LA, Kent SA, Tallman MS, Dewald G, Multani P, Gordon LI. Secondary acute myelogenous leukemia with MLL gene rearrangement following radioimmunotherapy (RAIT) for non-Hodgkin's lymphoma. Leuk Lymphoma 2002;43(11):2145–9.

Ibuprofen

See also Non-steroidal anti-inflammatory drugs

General Information

Like other NSAIDs, ibuprofen is a potent inhibitor of prostaglandin synthesis, and many or all of its therapeutic and toxic effects are linked to this characteristic. The general impression is that it is less potent and thus less toxic than indometacin in usual doses, but it has often been used in the past in relatively low doses. In a comparative, double-blind, crossover study of ibuprofen, naproxen, fenoprofen, and tolmetin in patients with rheumatoid arthritis, ibuprofen in equieffective doses was the best tolerated; however, patients and physicians preferred naproxen (1).

There are few data on the long-term safety of NSAIDs in the treatment of juvenile rheumatoid arthritis. In a study of the adverse reactions of patients treated with long-term ibuprofen, gastrotoxicity was directly correlated with dosage and 5% withdrew early because they had gastrointestinal bleeding, vomiting, severe rash, hearing loss, and abnormalities of liver function tests (SEDA-16, 110).

High dosages of ibuprofen for 4 years were used in 41 patients with cystic fibrosis to slow progression of lung disease and only two adverse effects (conjunctivitis and epistaxis) were drug-related (SEDA-20, 93).

General adverse reactions

Gastrointestinal adverse effects are the most frequent. They occur in up to 30% of patients and range from abdominal discomfort to serious bleeding or activation of peptic ulcer. Nervous system effects, with headache and dizziness, are very common. Severe renal impairment has not been noted. Blood dyscrasias can occur when high dosage treatment is prolonged. There is no significant general hepatotoxicity, but both the liver and the central nervous system (meningitis) can be affected as part of a hypersensitivity reaction.

Hypersensitivity reactions are uncommon, but they can be severe. Aseptic meningitis, hypotension, fever, conjunctivitis, arthralgias, and leukopenia were reported in a woman with systemic lupus erythematosus (2). Other similar patients have experienced fever with rashes, abdominal pain, headache, nausea and vomiting, signs of liver damage, and meningitis. This type of reaction seems to occur especially (but not exclusively) in patients with connective tissue diseases (SEDA-5, 105) (SEDA-10, 84) and it can be difficult to differentiate between a hypersensitivity reaction and a flare-up of the disease. Ibuprofen can provoke bronchospasm and anaphylaxis in asthmatics (SEDA-22, 116).

Tumor-inducing effects have not been reported.

Organs and Systems

Cardiovascular

Apart from the consequences of salt and water retention, ibuprofen does not affect myocardial or vascular function. Congestive heart failure has rarely been reported (3).

In a small comparison of ibuprofen and indometacin in preterm infants with patent ductus arteriosus there was no apparent difference in the rate of patent ductus arteriosus closure; ibuprofen did not impair cerebral hemodynamics or oxygenation, while indometacin impaired cerebral oxygen delivery (4).

Respiratory

Ibuprofen rarely provokes attacks of asthma in predisposed individuals. There is probably cross-sensitivity with aspirin; a death was reported after an asthmatic patient with no history of aspirin sensitivity took two ibuprofen tablets (SEDA-12, 86).

Pulmonary infiltrates with eosinophilia have been described with ibuprofen (SEDA-18, 104).

Two episodes of acute pulmonary edema and progressive pulmonary infiltrates without eosinophilia have been reported in a man with HIV infection after ibuprofen (SEDA-18, 104).

Nervous system

Headache, vertigo, tinnitus, and insomnia are the most frequent nervous system effects, but are rarely severe. Depression and other psychotic reactions have been reported. Some nervous system reactions (meningism and meningitis, lethargy, and irritability) are thought to result from hypersensitivity (SEDA-9, 91) (SEDA-18, 104) (5). This has been confirmed by a report of aseptic meningitis with increased intrathecal IgG synthesis and evidence of immune complexes in the cerebrospinal fluid (SEDA-16, 110).

Analgesic-induced headache, not uncommon in adults, has also been described in children. One report (6) described 12 children, aged 6–16 years, who gave a history of headaches on at least 4 days a week, for 3 months to 10 years. Eleven of the children had been taking paracetamol, six in combination with codeine, and one was taking ibuprofen alone. They were taking at least one dose of an analgesic for each headache and eight were taking analgesics every day. The headaches presented with increasing frequency and were related to overuse of analgesics, a typical finding in analgesic-induced headache. The analgesics were withdrawn; in six children the headaches resolved completely, another five children experienced a reduced frequency of headaches, and one resumed analgesic abuse.

The second report (7) was a retrospective study of patients seen in a pediatric headache clinic. During 8 months 98 patients were seen for headache; 46 of them suffered from daily or near daily headache and 30 were consuming analgesics daily. Follow-up information was available in 25. The average number of doses of analgesics per week they consumed was 26. The most commonly used medications were paracetamol and ibuprofen. In addition, a minority were taking combinations that contained aspirin, codeine, caffeine, propoxyphene, or butalbital, or other NSAIDs. Abrupt withdrawal of all analgesics concomitant with the use of amitriptyline 10 mg/day (in 22 patients) prompted a significant reduction in the frequency and severity of headache.

Sensory systems

Ocular reactions described to date are reversible and not severe. They include blurred vision, changes in color perception, and toxic amblyopia (8).

Ibuprofen significantly correlated with high-altitude retinal hemorrhages (SEDA-17, 110).

Vortex keratopathy has been described in a woman taking oral ibuprofen (SEDA-21, 105).

Metabolism

An increase in serum concentrations of uric acid has been described with ibuprofen (9).

Hematologic

Ibuprofen prolongs bleeding time, although less than aspirin (10). There are reports that a daily dose of less than 1 g does not affect the bleeding time (11).

Blood dyscrasias, ranging from thrombocytopenia and granulocytopenia to agranulocytosis and fatal pancytopenia, have been reported. (SED-9, 150). Reversible pure white cell aplasia with bone marrow plasmacytosis and complement-dependent IgG antibody has been observed in one patient (12).

Fatal autoimmune hemolytic anemia has been attributed to ibuprofen in a patient who was taking other drugs (13). Reversible hemolytic anemia has been described during ibuprofen treatment, but tartrazine, the orange dye in the coating of the brand used (Motrin 400), may have been responsible (14).

Gastrointestinal blood loss due to ibuprofen can cause iron deficiency anemia.

Gastrointestinal

When ibuprofen was first introduced, its gastrointestinal tolerance was regarded as better than with other NSAIDs, especially aspirin and indometacin. However, with the use of higher doses, which were probably equipotent with the usual doses of older agents, there seemed to be no significant differences. As with other NSAIDs there is a close correlation between efficacy and adverse effects. Gastrointestinal adverse effects include a variety of symptoms, such as irritation, nausea, anorexia, vomiting, dyspepsia, heartburn, abdominal discomfort, bleeding, hematemesis, and activation of peptic ulcer; 10–30% of patients taking prescription doses (for example for rheumatic conditions) develop these adverse effects (SED-9, 150) (15). It is not possible to give a reliable estimate of the frequency when the drug is used as a self-medication analgesic in lower doses, since exact information on the complications of self-medication is rarely available and there is always likely to be a proportion of misuse (for example ingestion of higher or lower doses than recommended).

Bleeding from a Meckel's diverticulum has been described with oral ibuprofen (SEDA-17, 110).

Irritation of the rectal mucosa after ibuprofen suppositories has also been reported (16). Ulcerative proctitis has been reported in a patient with systemic lupus erythematosus (SEDA-14, 94).

Liver

Ibuprofen is not directly hepatotoxic, but the liver can be damaged as part of a generalized hypersensitivity reaction. Toxic hepatitis with Stevens–Johnson syndrome has been described (17).

Ibuprofen has been rarely thought responsible for liver damage. A recent report has described three patients, 33–44 years old, with chronic hepatitis C infection who developed more than five-fold increases in serum liver transaminases after taking ibuprofen for musculoskeletal pain. In all three there were no associated symptoms of hepatitis, and serum transaminases normalized after ibuprofen was withdrawn (18).

Biliary tract

The vanishing bile duct syndrome has been associated with the use of ibuprofen in an atopic man, but the causal relation was not certain (19).

Urinary tract

Ibuprofen can cause renal impairment, ranging from an insignificant reduction to an acute fall in creatinine clearance associated with a general hypersensitivity reaction, especially in patients with systemic lupus erythematosus or acute tubular necrosis (20). The nephrotic syndrome without renal insufficiency and acute interstitial nephritis without the nephrotic syndrome have been described after self-administration of over-the-counter ibuprofen (SEDA-12, 86).

Irreversible renal insufficiency due to acute cortical necrosis triggered by severe renal hypoperfusion has been reported (SEDA-12, 86). A pharmacokinetic study showed that conversion of inactive *R*-ibuprofen to active *S*-ibuprofen was greater in patients with renal impairment than in healthy controls; this may aggravate renal insufficiency (21).

Acute deterioration in renal function can occur also in other at-risk patients, such as those with renal transplants (22,23).

Skin

Skin rashes usually occur during general hypersensitivity. Urticarial, purpuric, and erythematous changes with pruritus have been reported (15). Bullous pemphigoid has been described after 6 months of treatment and was observed in two other patients on ibuprofen (SEDA-14, 94). Photosensitization has been attributed to ibuprofen (SEDA-17, 110). The association between ibuprofen and dermatological superinfection in children with recent *Varicella* infection has not been demonstrated in a retrospective cohort study (SEDA-22, 116).

Ibuprofen exacerbates psoriasis (SEDA-12, 86) (SEDA-7, 108) (SEDA-8, 102).

Hair

Alopecia has been described in black women; normal hair growth returned after therapy was stopped (SED-11, 183) (24).

Immunologic

Anaphylaxis after ibuprofen was reported in a patient with asthma who was also taking zafirlukast, a leukotriene receptor antagonist (SEDA-22, 116).

Susceptibility Factors

Age

The controversy over the use of ibuprofen as an antipyretic or analgesic is still open and the question of whether it is safer than paracetamol in children has not been answered (SEDA-16, 110) (SEDA-17, 110) (SEDA-19, 96).

Other features of the patient

In patients with a history of peptic ulcer or systemic lupus erythematosus the benefit-to-harm balance must be evaluated before prescribing ibuprofen. The first group is in danger of ulcer exacerbation and the second of a severe generalized hypersensitivity reaction.

Drug Administration

Drug formulations

Modified-release formulations seem to cause the same adverse effects as conventionally formulated ibuprofen (25), and four-times-daily treatment is better tolerated than twice-daily (SEDA-12, 86).

Ibuprofen lysine is more rapidly absorbed than ibuprofen free acid, but the comparative tolerability of the two formulations is not known (SEDA-20, 93).

Drug overdose

In spite of the large number of prescriptions and over-the-counter sales, acute intoxication is rare. Symptoms are usually limited to nausea and vomiting, but more severe cases of coma, acidosis, mild hypothermia, renal insufficiency, and acute papillary necrosis have been described (SEDA-12, 86) (SEDA-22, 116). Treatment is supportive (SEDA-9, 81).

Drug–Drug Interactions

Aminoglycoside antibiotics

High-dose ibuprofen can slow the progression of lung disease in patients with cystic fibrosis and is usually well tolerated (SEDA-20, 93). However, transient renal insufficiency developed in four children with cystic fibrosis who were taking maintenance ibuprofen when an intravenous aminoglycoside was added to their regimen to treat an exacerbation of lung disease (26). Ibuprofen should probably be stopped during intravenous aminoglycoside therapy.

Antihypertensive agents

Ibuprofen interacts with antihypertensive agents, reducing their efficacy (27).

Aspirin

Patients with arthritis and vascular disease sometimes take both low-dose aspirin and other NSAIDs. However, concomitant treatment with ibuprofen can limit the cardioprotective effects of aspirin, according to the results of a study of the effects of ibuprofen, diclofenac, coxibs, and paracetamol on the antiplatelet activity of aspirin (28). The following combinations of drugs were used: aspirin (81 mg every morning) 2 hours before ibuprofen (400 mg every morning) or in the reverse order; aspirin 2 hours before rofecoxib (25 mg every morning or in the reverse order); enteric-coated aspirin 2 hours before ibuprofen (400 mg tds); and enteric-coated aspirin 2 hours before modified-release diclofenac (75 mg bd). Inhibition of the formation of serum thromboxane B2 (an index of COX-1 activity in platelets) and platelet aggregation by aspirin was blocked when a single daily dose of ibuprofen was given before aspirin, as well as when multiple daily doses of ibuprofen were given. Diclofenac, paracetamol, and rofecoxib did not affect the pharmacodynamics of aspirin. These results suggest that ibuprofen, but not diclofenac, paracetamol, or rofecoxib, antagonizes the irreversible inhibition of platelet COX-1 by aspirin and can therefore limit the cardioprotective effects of aspirin.

This hypothesis has now been supported in a study of over 7000 patients who were discharged after a first admission for cardiovascular disease between 1989 and 1997 and who took low-dose aspirin and survived for at least 1 month (29). The adjusted hazard ratios for all-cause mortality (HR = 1.93; 95% CI = 1.30, 287) and for cardiovascular mortality (HR = 1.73; CI = 1.05, 2.84) were significantly raised in patients who took ibuprofen (mean dose 1210 mg/day) in addition to the aspirin. There was no increase in hazard in patients who combined aspirin with diclofenac, which is consistent with the in vitro data. However, this study had many limitations (30), and further epidemiological studies are needed to address this potentially important interaction. In the meantime, when patients taking low-dose aspirin for cardioprotection also require long-term treatment with an NSAID, diclofenac would be preferable to ibuprofen.

Lithium

Ibuprofen can increase the serum lithium concentration (SEDA-13, 81).

Methotrexate

Ibuprofen can potentiate methotrexate-induced renal toxicity (31).

Pancreatic enzymes

An interaction between ibuprofen and pancreatic enzymes causing serious gastrointestinal damage has been described in animals (SEDA-21, 105).

Phenytoin

Ibuprofen inhibits the metabolism of phenytoin (32).

Sulfonylureas

Ibuprofen (150 mg, 3 doses) for arthralgias was associated with hypoglycemia in a 72-year-old man who was taking glibenclamide 2.5 mg/day for type 2 diabetes mellitus; after the last dose he lost consciousness, and his blood glucose concentration was under 2.2 mmol/l (33).

Tacrolimus

Acute renal insufficiency has been described in concomitant treatment with tacrolimus in two liver transplant recipients (SEDA-18, 104).

References

1. Gall EP, Caperton EM, McComb JE, Messner R, Multz CV, O'Hanlan M, Willkens RF. Clinical comparison of ibuprofen, fenoprofen calcium, naproxen and tolmetin sodium in rheumatoid arthritis. J Rheumatol 1982;9(3):402–7.
2. Mandell BF, Raps EC. Severe systemic hypersensitivity reaction to ibuprofen occurring after prolonged therapy. Am J Med 1987;82(4):817–20.
3. Schooley RT, Wagley PF, Lietman PS. Edema associated with ibuprofen therapy. JAMA 1977;237(16):1716–17.
4. Patel J, Marks KA, Roberts I, Azzopardi D, Edwards AD. Ibuprofen treatment of patent ductus arteriosus. Lancet 1995;346(8969):255.

5. Samuelson CO Jr, Williams HJ. Ibuprofen-associated aseptic meningitis in systemic lupus erythematosus. West J Med 1979;131(1):57–9.
6. Symon DN. Twelve cases of analgesic headache. Arch Dis Child 1998;78(6):555–6.
7. Vasconcellos E, Pina-Garza JE, Millan EJ, Warner JS. Analgesic rebound headache in children and adolescents. J Child Neurol 1998;13(9):443–7.
8. Williamson J, Sturrock RD. An ophthalmic study of ibuprofen in rheumatoid conditions. Curr Med Res Opin 1976;4(2):128–31.
9. Chalmers TM. Clinical experience with ibuprofen in rheumatoid arthritis. Schweiz Med Wochenschr 1971;101(8):280–2.
10. McIntyre BA, Philp RB, Inwood MJ. Effect of ibuprofen on platelet function in normal subjects and hemophiliac patients. Clin Pharmacol Ther 1978;24(5):616–21.
11. Thilo D, Nyman D, Duckert F. A study of the effect of the antirheumatic drug ibuprofen (Brufen) on patients being treated with the oral anti-coagulant phenprocoumon (Marcoumar). J Int Med Res 1974;2:276.
12. Mamus SW, Burton JD, Groat JD, Schulte DA, Lobell M, Zanjani ED. Ibuprofen-associated pure white-cell aplasia. N Engl J Med 1986;314(10):624–5.
13. Guidry JB, Ogburn CL Jr, Griffin FM Jr. Fatal autoimmune hemolytic anemia associated with ibuprofen. JAMA 1979;242(1):68–9.
14. Law IP, Wickman CJ, Harrison BR. Coombs'-positive hemolytic anemia and ibuprofen. South Med J 1979;72(6):707–10.
15. Davies EF, Avery GS. Ibuprofen: a review of its pharmacological properties and therapeutic efficacy in rheumatic disorders. Drugs 1971;2(5):416–46.
16. Caro H, Conture B, Pethilaz R, Royar JC. Etude clinique sur l'ibuprofen sous forme suppositoires. Gaz Med Fr 1976;83:372.
17. Sternlieb P, Robinson RM. Stevens–Johnson syndrome plus toxic hepatitis due to ibuprofen. NY State J Med 1978;78(8):1239–43.
18. Riley TR 3rd, Smith JP. Ibuprofen-induced hepatotoxicity in patients with chronic hepatitis C: a case series. Am J Gastroenterol 1998;93(9):1563–5.
19. Alam I, Ferrell LD, Bass NM. Vanishing bile duct syndrome temporally associated with ibuprofen use. Am J Gastroenterol 1996;91(8):1626–30.
20. Fong HJ, Cohen AH. Ibuprofen-induced acute renal failure with acute tubular necrosis. Am J Nephrol 1982;2(1):28–31.
21. Chen CY, Chen CS. Stereoselective disposition of ibuprofen in patients with renal dysfunction. J Pharmacol Exp Ther 1994;268(2):590–4.
22. Moghal NE, Hulton SA, Milford DV. Care in the use of ibuprofen as an antipyretic in children. Clin Nephrol 1998;49(5):293–5.
23. Stoves J, Rosenberg K, Harnden P, Turney JH. Acute interstitial nephritis due to over-the-counter ibuprofen in a renal transplant recipient. Nephrol Dial Transplant 1998;13(1):227–8.
24. Meyer HC. Alopecia associated with ibuprofen. JAMA 1979;242(2):142.
25. Fernandez L, Jacoby RK, Smith PJ, et al. Comparative trial of standard and sustained release formulations of ibuprofen in patients with osteoarthritis. Curr Med Res Opin 1982;7:610.
26. Kovesi TA, Swartz R, MacDonald N. Transient renal failure due to simultaneous ibuprofen and aminoglycoside therapy in children with cystic fibrosis. N Engl J Med 1998;338(1):65–6.
27. Radack KL, Deck CC, Bloomfield SS. Ibuprofen interferes with the efficacy of antihypertensive drugs. A randomized, double-blind, placebo-controlled trial of ibuprofen compared with acetaminophen. Ann Intern Med 1987;107(5):628–35.
28. Catella-Lawson F, Reilly MP, Kapoor SC, Cucchiara AJ, DeMarco S, Tournier B, Vyas SN, FitzGerald GA. Cyclooxygenase inhibitors and the antiplatelet effects of aspirin. N Engl J Med 2001;345(25):1809–17.
29. MacDonald TM, Wei L. Effect of ibuprofen on cardioprotective effect of aspirin. Lancet 2003;361(9357):573–4.
30. FitzGerald GA. Parsing an enigma: the pharmacodynamics of aspirin resistance. Lancet 2003;361(9357):542–4.
31. Cassano WF. Serious methotrexate toxicity caused by interaction with ibuprofen. Am J Pediatr Hematol Oncol 1989;11(4):481–2.
32. Sandyk R. Phenytoin toxicity induced by interaction with ibuprofen. S Afr Med J 1982;62(17):592.
33. Sone H, Takahashi A, Yamada N. Ibuprofen-related hypoglycemia in a patient receiving sulfonylurea. Ann Intern Med 2001;134(4):344.

Ibuproxam

See also Non-steroidal anti-inflammatory drugs

General Information

Ibuproxam is an NSAID that causes similar adverse effects to other NSAIDs.

Organs and Systems

Gastrointestinal

Gastrointestinal adverse effects have been reported with ibuproxam, including nausea, vomiting, occult gastrointestinal blood loss, and rectal pain (1).

Skin

Skin rashes have been reported with ibuproxam (1).

Reference

1. Scaranelli M, Delli Gatti I, Menegale G, et al. Casi di artrite reumatoide resistent al trattamento con farmaci antiflogistici non-steroidei: uso di dosi piu elevate di ibuproxam. Gaz Med Ital 1981;140:27.

Idoxuridine

General Information

Idoxuridine, which is active against *Herpes simplex* and *Varicella zoster*, has only been used in topical antiherpetic solutions. Idoxuridine has been used to treat superficial keratitis, but with poor results in deep stromal diseases because of poor solubility. However, idoxuridine is unstable and cannot eliminate the virus from the eye. Drug allergy and toxicity occur in 5–8% of patients.

Drug Administration

Drug administration route

Idoxuridine eye-drops are locally toxic, especially in patients with dry eyes, because of increased concentrations (or reduced tear secretion), and is topically sensitizing. Lacrimal punctum stenosis, lacrimation, follicular conjunctivitis, narrowing of meibomian gland orifices, inhibition of keratocyte mitosis and corneal stromal repair, and reductions in the strength of healing corneal wounds and the rate of epithelial regeneration are observed (1). After prolonged administration many changes in the conjunctival and corneal epithelium can occur, such as conjunctival cicatrization, punctate keratitis, subepithelial and intra-epithelial edema, and corneal opacities. Idoxuridine can also induce the emergence of resistant virus strains (2).

References

1. Havener WH. Ocular Pharmacology. . 4th ed. St Louis: CV Mosby, 1978.
2. Lass JH, Thoft RA, Dohlman CH. Idoxuridine-induced conjunctival cicatrization. Arch Ophthalmol 1983; 101(5):747–50.

Ifosfamide

See also Cytostatic and immunosuppressant drugs

General Information

Ifosfamide is an alkylating agent belonging to the group of oxazaphosphorines. It is used to treat a variety of solid tumors in children, including rhabdomyosarcoma, soft tissue sarcomas, Wilms' tumor, bone sarcomas, and neuroblastoma, and leukemias and lymphomas in adults. It is also sometimes used in combination with other drugs, such as doxorubicin or cisplatin and etoposide.

Organs and Systems

Cardiovascular

Atrial fibrillation has been attributed to ifosfamide after a dose of only 1800 mg/m^2, with mesna, in a regimen for metastatic breast cancer (1).

Nervous system

Convulsions, severe facial spasms, and trismus occurred 7 hours after an infusion of ifosfamide in a dose of 7 g/m^2, having not occurred at a dose of 5 g/m^2, during a phase II study in patients with solid tumors (2).

Severe encephalopathy has been noted in children treated with ifosfamide (1.8 g/m^2) alone. There were no susceptibility factors, such as impaired renal function or lowered albumin. Electroencephalographic abnormalities and seizures were reversible, despite prolonged coma (3).

In an evaluation of ifosfamide in 57 children with malignant solid tumors, all received 1.6 g/m^2/day for 5 days followed by mesna 400 mg/m^2 at 0.25, 4, and 6 hours after ifosfamide (4). Neurological toxicity occurred in 13 patients. The usual symptoms were somnolence and general weakness followed by confusion, tremors, ataxia, aphasia, urinary incontinence, and cranial nerve paralysis. The symptoms of neurotoxicity disappeared spontaneously within 72 hours of completion of the 5-day course. Some patients had recurrent neurotoxicity on rechallenge. In an analysis of the incidence and features of electroencephalographic changes associated with Ifosfamide/mesna therapy there was no significant association between the electroencephalographic record before and during treatment; electroencephalographic changes developed 12–24 hours before clinical toxicity. Discriminant analysis identified low serum albumin, high serum creatinine concentrations, and pelvic involvement by the underlying malignant disease as susceptibility factors for severe encephalopathy (5).

In 12 of 52 patients treated with ifosfamide there was neurocortical toxicity greater than grade 2 (6). They were successfully treated with intravenous methylthioninium chloride (methylene blue) 50 mg 3-hourly, which was also prophylactic in three patients.

Vitamin B_1 (thiamine) has also been suggested to be beneficial in treating ifosfamide-associated neurotoxicity (7).

Urinary tract

It has been thought that the metabolism of ifosfamide to chloroacetaldehyde is the mechanism whereby ifosfamide causes renal damage. However, this was not confirmed in a study of repeated doses of 6–9 g/m^2 in 15 children, in whom there was no correlation between the pharmacokinetics of ifosfamide or its metabolites and either acute renal toxicity or chronic renal toxicity at either 1 or 6 months after treatment (8). However, there were changes in the metabolism of ifosfamide with time, particularly a reduction in dechloroethylation, which correlated with the risk of chronic nephrotoxicity.

Children and adolescents given cumulative doses of 32–112 g/m^2 had only transient disturbances in renal function (9). In five children with renal tubular Fanconi syndrome caused by ifosfamide, all went on to develop rickets in the face of declining renal function. None had had pre-existing tubular damage and the syndrome developed at cumulative doses of ifosfamide of 39–99 g/m^2. There were low serum bicarbonate and phosphate concentrations, and supplementation of these resulted in bone healing but not renal recovery (10).

The susceptibility factors associated with chronic ifosfamide nephrotoxicity up to 28 months after treatment have been studied in 23 children. The authors concluded that cumulative doses of 100 g/m^2 or higher should be avoided in children with cancers (11).

Like cyclophosphamide, ifosfamide causes a hemorrhagic cystitis in a high proportion of patients, with an occasionally fatal outcome. The damage to urinary bladder epithelium is caused by acrolein, a metabolite that is excreted in the urine. In bone marrow transplant recipients, prior administration of busulfan, which itself causes hemorrhagic cystitis, can increase this risk of oxazaphosphorines (12). Mesna (sodium mercaptoethanesulfonate) is used to prevent this adverse effect. It is excreted by the kidney, and it binds and detoxifies acrolein in the urine; mesna also prevents the breakdown of acrolein precursors.

The phosphate disturbance that leads to Fanconi syndrome is well documented with ifosfamide. Of 43 children who received ifosfamide 3.5 g/m^2/day for 5 days for metastatic osteosarcoma, three developed the syndrome (13).

Second-Generation Effects

Fetotoxicity

The effects of second-trimester or third-trimester exposure to ifosfamide are poorly documented, although normal children have been described (14). In a 17-year-old pregnant woman with Ewing's sarcoma doxorubicin and ifosfamide during the 25th to 30th weeks of gestation did not affect the child, which was delivered at 32 weeks (15).

Drug Administration

Drug dosage regimens

There is a higher incidence of ifosfamide encephalopathy associated with the oral form compared with the intravenous form of ifosfamide; this has been attributed to metabolic differences between the two (16).

Drug–Drug Interactions

Cisplatin

Ifosfamide is associated with a peripheral neuropathy when it is given in combination with cisplatin (17). These symptoms improved within a few days after treatment with haloperidol.

References

1. Ingle JN, Krook JE, Mailliard JA, Hartmann LC, Wieand HS. Evaluation of ifosfamide plus mesna as first-line chemotherapy in women with metastatic breast cancer. Am J Clin Oncol 1995;18(6):498–501.
2. Pinkerton CR, Pritchard J. A phase II study of ifosfamide in paediatric solid tumours. Cancer Chemother Pharmacol 1989;24(Suppl 1):S13–15.
3. Gieron MA, Barak LS, Estrada J. Severe encephalopathy associated with ifosfamide administration in two children with metastatic tumors. J Neurooncol 1988;6(1):29–30.
4. Pratt CB, Horowitz ME, Meyer WH, Etcubanas E, Thompson EI, Douglass EC, Wilimas JA, Hayes FA, Green AA. Phase II trial of ifosfamide in children with malignant solid tumors. Cancer Treat Rep 1987;71(2):131–5.
5. Meanwell CA, Blake AE, Kelly KA, Honigsberger L, Blackledge G. Prediction of ifosfamide/mesna associated encephalopathy. Eur J Cancer Clin Oncol 1986;22(7):815–19.
6. Pelgrims J, De Vos F, Van den Brande J, Schrijvers D, Prove A, Vermorken JB. Methylene blue in the treatment and prevention of ifosfamide-induced encephalopathy: report of 12 cases and a review of the literature. Br J Cancer 2000;82(2):291–4.
7. Buesa JM, Garcia-Teijido P, Losa R, Fra J. Treatment of ifosfamide encephalopathy with intravenous thiamin. Clin Cancer Res 2003;9(12):4636–7.
8. Boddy AV, English M, Pearson AD, Idle JR, Skinner R. Ifosfamide nephrotoxicity: limited influence of metabolism and mode of administration during repeated therapy in paediatrics. Eur J Cancer 1996;32A(7):1179–84.
9. Goren MP, Pratt CB, Viar MJ. Tubular nephrotoxicity during long-term ifosfamide and mesna therapy. Cancer Chemother Pharmacol 1989;25(1):70–2.
10. Burk CD, Restaino I, Kaplan BS, Meadows AT. Ifosfamide-induced renal tubular dysfunction and rickets in children with Wilms tumor. J Pediatr 1990;117(2 Pt 1):331–5.
11. Skinner R, Pearson AD, English MW, Price L, Wyllie RA, Coulthard MG, Craft AW. Risk factors for ifosfamide nephrotoxicity in children. Lancet 1996;348(9027):578–80.
12. Thomas AE, Patterson J, Prentice HG, Brenner MK, Ganczakowski M, Hancock JF, Pattinson JK, Blacklock HA, Hopewell JP. Haemorrhagic cystitis in bone marrow transplantation patients: possible increased risk associated with prior busulphan therapy. Bone Marrow Transplant 1987;1(4):347–55.
13. Goorin AM, Harris MB, Bernstein M, Ferguson W, Devidas M, Siegal GP, Gebhardt MC, Schwartz CL, Link M, Grier HE. Phase II/III trial of etoposide and high-dose ifosfamide in newly diagnosed metastatic osteosarcoma: a pediatric oncology group trial. J Clin Oncol 2002;20(2):426–33.
14. Merimsky O, Le Chevalier T, Missenard G, Lepechoux C, Cojean-Zelek I, Mesurolle B, Le Cesne A. Management of cancer in pregnancy: a case of Ewing's sarcoma of the pelvis in the third trimester. Ann Oncol 1999;10(3):345–50.
15. Nakajima W, Ishida A, Takahashi M, Hirayama M, Washino N, Ogawa M, Takahashi S, Okada K. Good outcome for infant of mother treated with chemotherapy for Ewing sarcoma at 25 to 30 weeks' gestation. J Pediatr Hematol Oncol 2004;26(5):308–11.
16. Lind MJ, Margison JM, Cerny T, Thatcher N, Wilkinson PM. Comparative pharmacokinetics and alkylating activity of fractionated intravenous and oral ifosfamide in patients with bronchogenic carcinoma. Cancer Res 1989;49(3):753–7.
17. Drings P, Abel U, Bulzebruck H, Stiefel P, Kleckow M, Manke HG. Experience with ifosfamide combinations (etoposide or DDP) in non-small cell lung cancer. Cancer Chemother Pharmacol 1986;18(Suppl 2):S34–9.

Illiciaceae

See also Herbal medicines

General Information

The family of Illiciaceae contains a single genus, *Illicium*, the star anise species.

Illicium species

Illicium anisatum contains sesquiterpenoids, such as anisatin, anisotin, neoanisatin, and pseudoanisatin. *Illicium religiosum* (Japanese star anise) contains shikimic acid, anisatin and neoanisatin. *Illicium verum* (Chinese star anise) contains the monoterpenoid transanethole. Chinese star anise has been used to treat infant colic, but can be confused with Japanese star anise, which contains the neurotoxin anisatin.

Safrole is a mutagenic and animal carcinogenic monoterpenoid. It is the major component of oil of sassafras, and lesser quantities occur in essential oils from cinnamon, mace, nutmeg, and star anise. Some of its known or possible metabolites have mutagenic activity in bacteria and it has weak hepatocarcinogenic effects in rodents. Experiments in mice have suggested the possibility of transplacental and lactational carcinogenesis.

Adverse effects

When Japanese star anise was mixed into a commercially sold herbal tea, perhaps inadvertently consumption of the tea was associated with adverse events in 63 Dutch consumers (1). Their symptoms occurred 2–4 hours after they drank the tea and included general malaise, nausea, and vomiting. In 22 cases hospitalization was required, and 16 had generalized tonic-clonic seizures. All made a full recovery after withdrawal of the herbal tea. Anisatin is a non-competitive GABA receptor antagonist, which causes nervous system hyperactivity, and the authors believed that this mechanism explained the high rate of seizures in these patients.

- A 1-month-old girl developed status epilepticus after being given a large amount of star anis for colic (2).
- Two infants whose parents gave them star anise herbal tea developed tremors or spasms, hypertonia, hyperexcitability with crying, nystagmus, and vomiting (3). The Chinese star anise tea had been contaminated with Japanese star anise.

From February to September 2001, a matched case-control study was performed in infants aged under 3 months admitted to the pediatric emergency departments of two hospitals in Madrid (4). There were 23 cases, whose symptoms and signs were irritability, abnormal movements, vomiting, and nystagmus. The odds ratio for anise consumption was 18.0 (CI = 2.03, 631). Laboratory analyses showed contamination of *I. verum* by *I. anisatum*.

References

1. Johanns ES, van der Kolk LE, van Gemert HM, Sijben AE, Peters PW, de Vries I. Een epidemie van epileptische aanvallen na drinken van kruidenthee. [An epidemic of epileptic seizures after consumption of herbal tea.] Ned Tijdschr Geneeskd 2002;146(17):813–16.
2. Gil Campos M, Perez Navero JL, Ibarra De La Rosa I. Crisis convulsiva secundaria a intoxicacion por anis estrellado en un lactante. [Convulsive status secondary to star anise poisoning in a neonate.] An Esp Pediatr 2002;57(4):366–8.
3. Minodier P, Pommier P, Moulene E, Retornaz K, Prost N, Deharo L. Intoxication aiguë par la badiane chez le nourrisson. [Star anise poisoning in infants.] Arch Pediatr 2003;10(7):619–21.
4. Garzo Fernandez C, Gomez Pintado P, Barrasa Blanco A, Martinez Arrieta R, Ramirez Fernandez R, Ramon Rosa F, Grupo de Trabajo del Anis Estrellado. Casos de enfermedad de sintomatologia neurologica asociados al consumo de anis estrellado empleado como carminativo. [Cases of neurological symptoms associated with star anise consumption used as a carminative.] An Esp Pediatr 2002;57(4):290–4.

Iloprost

See also Prostaglandins

General Information

Iloprost is an analogue of prostacyclin (PGI_2), the pharmacodynamic properties of which it mimics, namely inhibition of platelet aggregation, vasodilatation, and cytoprotection (as yet ill-defined). Iloprost has greater chemical stability than prostacyclin, which facilitates its clinical use (1).

Iloprost is mainly used in patients with chronic critical leg ischemia due to atherosclerosis or Buerger's disease. Episodic digital ischemia in patients with systemic sclerosis or related disorders is another use. The most frequently observed adverse effects, facial flushing and headache, are caused by profound vasodilatation.

Most clinical experience with iloprost has been gained in patients with critical leg ischemia. An intermittent intravenous infusion of up to 2 nanograms/kg/minute for 2–4 weeks reduced rest pain and improved ulcer healing in roughly half of the patients with critical leg ischemia, including diabetics. Compared with placebo, the improvement obtained with iloprost was significant in most but not all individual clinical trials. In addition, a meta-analysis showed a 15% reduction in major amputation rate compared with placebo (2).

Observational studies

The use of iloprost has been proposed in patients with systemic sclerosis, a disease that is often characterized by pulmonary hypertension and Raynaud's phenomenon. Three patients with systemic sclerosis who were treated with iloprost developed acute thrombotic events (3). In one case, intestinal infarction occurred 1 day after infusion of iloprost. In another patient the left kidney was not perfused 22 days after the last infusion of iloprost because of thrombosis of the left renal artery. The last patient, 9 months after the start of treatment with iloprost, and 5 days after the last infusion, had an anterolateral myocardial infarction. The authors commented that their observations did not allow them to conclude that there is a direct relation between infusion of iloprost and thrombotic events. However, they said that this possibility should be considered, and they suggested that risk factors for thromboembolism should be carefully evaluated in each patient with systemic sclerosis who is receiving iloprost.

Inhalation of aerosolized iloprost is being tested in patients with severe primary or secondary pulmonary hypertension refractory to conventional therapy. The aim is to produce predominantly pulmonary vasodilatation without significant systemic effects. In an uncontrolled series of 19 patients, the most common adverse effects of inhaled iloprost were coughing, nausea, edema, and thoracic pain (4). In most patients, these effects were transient and rarely required a change in therapy.

Placebo-controlled studies

A multicenter, randomized, parallel-group comparison of two different doses of oral iloprost and placebo has been conducted, to identify the optimal dose of oral iloprost on the basis of efficacy and tolerability in patients with Raynaud's phenomenon secondary to systemic sclerosis (5). A total of 103 patients were given total daily doses of iloprost of 100 micrograms ($n = 33$) or 200 micrograms ($n = 35$) or placebo ($n = 35$) for 6 weeks. The mean percentage reductions in the frequency, total daily duration, and severity of attacks of Raynaud's phenomenon were greater in the iloprost groups at the end of treatment and at the end of follow-up. Adverse effects were reported by 80% of patients taking placebo, 85% taking oral iloprost 100 micrograms/day, and 97% taking oral iloprost 100 micrograms/day. There were significant differences in the frequency of five types of adverse events. Headache, flushing, nausea, and trismus were all more common with increasing iloprost dose, while flu-like illnesses were most commonly reported in the placebo group. Treatment was prematurely discontinued in 9, 30, and 51% respectively, and discontinuation was precipitated by adverse events in 6, 27, and 51%.

Comparative studies

In a randomized, controlled study of cyclic iloprost or nifedipine in 46 patients with systemic sclerosis, the predictable adverse effects of iloprost (headache, nausea and vomiting, and diarrhea) were common but quickly resolved after the end of the infusion (6). They rarely required a temporary dose reduction. Hypotension occurred less often than with nifedipine.

General adverse effects

The adverse effects of iloprost occur within or above the usual dosage range and are predictable from its pharmacological effects. Minor vascular reactions during infusion (characterized by facial flushing and headache) are so common as to make double-blind trials impossible. Gastrointestinal effects become more prevalent at higher dosages, and include nausea, vomiting, abdominal cramps, and diarrhea. Less common adverse effects include restlessness, sweating, local erythema along the infusion line, wheals, fatigue, and muscle pain. Clinically significant hypotension is rare with the doses tested. The untoward effects resolve rapidly after the infusion is discontinued.

Therapy with iloprost is usually started with a dosage of 0.5 nanogram/kg/minute and increased in increments until either minor vascular reactions occur or a dosage of 2 nanograms/kg/minute has been reached. The optimal total dose remains to be established.

Organs and Systems

Cardiovascular

Myocardial ischemia is unusual during infusion of iloprost. It mainly occurs in patients with pre-existing coronary disease, when it is ascribed to a steal phenomenon detrimental to the subendocardial tissue. As a rule it is transient and exceptionally proceeds to infarction. However, such an event has now been reported in a patient with systemic sclerosis (7).

- A 57-year-old man with a 1-year history of systemic sclerosis and ischemia of several digits received a first infusion of iloprost using the recommended stepwise increasing dosage scheme; he developed sudden chest pain, with inferior ST segment elevation. Emergency coronary angiography showed an occlusion of the circumflex coronary artery, for which a stent was inserted. At angiography 3 years earlier his coronary arteries had been normal. He died 5 months later from cardiogenic pulmonary edema.

Musculoskeletal

Four women with CREST syndrome or systemic sclerosis had pain and eventually contracture of the masseter muscles during infusion of iloprost for severe attacks of Raynaud's phenomenon (8). The adverse effect was quickly reversed by reducing the infusion rate. There were no electrocardiographic or cardiac enzyme changes. The mechanism of this effect is obscure.

Drug Administration

Drug administration route

An oral formulation has been investigated in patients with Raynaud's phenomenon secondary to systemic sclerosis and in patients with severe ischemia due to Buerger's disease or to atherosclerosis. The first reports were not particularly encouraging in terms of efficacy. Tolerance is acceptable: 6% of patients discontinued iloprost compared with 2% with placebo (9,10).

References

1. England MJ, Tjallinks A, Hofmeyr J, Harber J. Suppression of lactation. A comparison of bromocriptine and prostaglandin E2. J Reprod Med 1988;33(7):630–2.
2. Lee JB. Cardiovascular-renal effects of prostaglandins: the antihypertensive, natriuretic renal "endocrine" function. Arch Intern Med 1974;133(1):56–76.
3. Tedeschi A, Meroni PL, Del Papa N, Salmaso C, Boschetti C, Miadonna A. Thrombotic events in patients with systemic sclerosis treated with iloprost. Arthritis Rheum 1998;41(3):559–60.
4. Olschewski H, Ghofrani HA, Schmehl T, Winkler J, Wilkens H, Hoper MM, Behr J, Kleber FX, Seeger W. Inhaled iloprost to treat severe pulmonary hypertension. An uncontrolled trial. German PPH Study Group. Ann Intern Med 2000;132(6):435–43.
5. Black CM, Halkier-Sorensen L, Belch JJ, Ullman S, Madhok R, Smit AJ, Banga JD, Watson HR. Oral iloprost in Raynaud's phenomenon secondary to systemic sclerosis: a multicentre, placebo-controlled, dose-comparison study. Br J Rheumatol 1998;37(9):952–60.
6. Pfeiffer N, Grierson I, Goldsmith H, Hochgesand D, Winkgen-Bohres A, Appleton P. Histological effects in the iris after 3 months of latanoprost therapy: the Mainz 1 study. Arch Ophthalmol 2001;119(2):191–6.
7. Marroun I, Fialip J, Deleveaux I, Andre M, Lamaison D, Cabane J, Piette JC, Eschalier A, Aumaitre O. Infarctus du myocarde sous iloprost chez un patient atteint de sclérodermie. [Myocardial infarction and iloprost in a patient with scleroderma.] Therapie 2001;56(5):630–2.
8. Boubakri C, Bouchou K, Guy C, Roy M, Cathebras P. Douleurs masseterines: un effet indésirable méconnu de l'iloprost. [Masseter pain: aé little known, undesirable effect of iloprost.] Presse Méd 2000;29(35):1935–6.

9. Olsson AG, Carlson LA. Clinical, hemodynamic and metabolic effects of intraarterial infusions of prostaglandin E1 in patients with peripheral vascular disease. Adv Prostaglandin Thromboxane Res 1976;1:429–32.
10. Bugiardini R, Galvani M, Ferrini D, Gridelli C, Tollemeto D, Mari L, Puddu P, Lenzi S. Myocardial ischemia induced by prostacyclin and iloprost. Clin Pharmacol Ther 1985;38(1):101–8.

Imidapril

See also Angiotensin converting enzyme inhibitors

General Information

Imidapril is a long-acting, non-sulfhydryl ACE inhibitor that has been used in patients with hypertension, congestive heart failure, acute myocardial infarction, and diabetic nephropathy. It is a prodrug, rapidly converted in the liver to its active metabolite imidaprilat, which has a half-life of about 15 hours. Imidapril and its metabolites are mainly excreted in the urine.

Organs and Systems

Respiratory

The incidences of cough with imidapril and enalapril have been compared in a poorly designed open study in 489 hypertensive patients (1). The authors claimed a significantly smaller incidence of cough with imidapril. However, because of important methodological flaws, this result cannot be trusted.

Mineral balance

Hyperkalemia is a well-known adverse effect of ACE inhibitors and can sometimes be severe (2).

- An 85-year-old woman with diabetes mellitus and a prior myocardial infarction, who was taking ioxoprofen and imidapril, lost consciousness owing to marked bradycardia caused by hyperkalemia (7.4 mmol/l). An electrocardiogram showed T wave changes compatible with hyperkalemia. After right ventricular pacing she promptly recovered consciousness. She was given glucose and insulin and her plasma potassium fell to 4.1 mmol/l within 3 hours. Simultaneously her heart rate became normal.

References

1. Saruta T, Arakawa K, Iimura O, Abe K, Matsuoka H, Nakano T, Nakagawa M, Ogihara T, Kajiyama G, Hiwada K, Fujishima M, Nakajima M. Difference in the incidence of cough induced by angiotensin converting enzyme inhibitors: a comparative study using imidapril hydrochloride and enalapril maleate. Hypertens Res 1999;22(3):197–202.
2. Kurata C, Uehara A, Sugi T, Yamazaki K. Syncope caused by nonsteroidal anti-inflammatory drugs and angiotensin-converting enzyme inhibitors. Jpn Circ J 1999;63(12):1002–3.

Imipraminoxide

See also Tricyclic antidepressants

General Information

Imipraminoxide is an imipramine metabolite. In a comparison with the parent drug, efficacy was identical; adverse effects were of the same type but possibly less frequent (1).

Reference

1. Rapp W, Noren MB, Pedersen F. Comparative trial of imipramine N-oxide and imipramine in the treatment of out-patients with depressive syndromes. Acta Psychiatr Scand 1973;49(1):77–90.

Imiquimod

General Information

Imiquimod is an immune response enhancer that induces production of interferon and several other cytokines. It is used, in formulations containing 5%, to treat external genital and perianal warts/condylomata acuminata in adults (1). As imiquimod-treated warts regress, serum concentrations of interferon-alfa, interferon-beta, interferon-gamma, and tumor necrosis factor rise (2). Trials of imiquimod have failed to identify any particular systemic or laboratory abnormalities.

In one study, there was no deleterious effect on disease progression in HIV-infected patients, and the incidence of local adverse events with imiquimod (5% three times a week) for the treatment of anogenital warts was lower than has previously been reported in healthy individuals (3). In an uncontrolled trial of topical imiquimod 5% for the treatment of common warts and molluscum contagiosum in otherwise healthy patients, fever, healing with scarring, and healing with hyperpigmentation were each reported by one participant (4).

Organs and Systems

Skin

In randomized, double-blind studies, the most common adverse effects were inflammatory reactions at the injection site (mostly erythema and itching), which usually occurred after 2–5 weeks of treatment (5–7). These local reactions included erythema, erosions, excoriation, flaking, edema, scabbing, and induration, and were rarely severe enough to warrant withdrawal. Mild to moderate irritation has to be expected in up to 70% of patients if a 5% imiquimod cream is applied three times per week (6).

References

1. Czelusta AJ, Evans T, Arany I, Tyring SK. A guide to immunotherapy of genital warts. Focus on interferon and imiquimod. BioDrugs 1999;11:319–32.
2. Tyring SK, Arany I, Stanley MA, Tomai MA, Miller RL, Smith MH, McDermott DJ, Slade HB. A randomized, controlled, molecular study of condylomata acuminata clearance during treatment with imiquimod. J Infect Dis 1998; 178(2):551–5.
3. Gilson RJ, Shupack JL, Friedman-Kien AE, Conant MA, Weber JN, Nayagam AT, Swann RV, Pietig DC, Smith MH, Owens ML. A randomized, controlled, safety study using imiquimod for the topical treatment of anogenital warts in HIV-infected patients. Imiquimod Study Group. AIDS 1999;13(17):2397–404.
4. Hengge UR, Esser S, Schultewolter T, Behrendt C, Meyer T, Stockfleth E, Goos M. Self-administered topical 5% imiquimod for the treatment of common warts and molluscum contagiosum. Br J Dermatol 2000; 143(5):1026–31.
5. Beutner KR, Tyring SK, Trofatter KF Jr, Douglas JM Jr, Spruance S, Owens ML, Fox TL, Hougham AJ, Schmitt KA. Imiquimod, a patient-applied immune-response modifier for treatment of external genital warts. Antimicrob Agents Chemother 1998;42(4):789–94.
6. Ferenczy A. Immune response modifiers: imiquimod. J Obstet Gynaecol 1998;18(Suppl 2):76–8.
7. Syed TA, Ahmadpour OA, Ahmad SA, Ahmad SH. Management of female genital warts with an analogue of imiquimod 2% in cream: a randomized, double-blind, placebo-controlled study. J Dermatol 1998;25(7):429–33.

Immunoglobulins

General Information

Immunoglobulin preparations are concentrated protein solutions derived from the pooled plasma of adults or animals. They contain specific antibodies in proportion to the infectious and immunization experience of the population from whose plasma they are prepared (1). Large numbers of donors (at least 1000 donors per lot of final product) are used, in order to ensure inclusion of a broad spectrum of antibodies. Intravenous immunoglobulin is also derived from the pooled plasma of adults, but the alcohol-fractionation procedure is modified to a product suitable for intravenous use. The use of intravenous immunoglobulins in selected immunodeficiency and autoimmune diseases has been reviewed (2).

Specific immunoglobulins, termed "hyperimmune globulins," are derived from human donors known to have high titers of the desired antibody. Specific immunoglobulin preparations for use in infectious disease prevention include hepatitis B, rabies, tetanus, *Varicella zoster*, vaccinia, and cytomegalovirus immunoglobulin.

Specific immunoglobulins of animal origin still currently in use in some countries include antirabies immunoglobulin, diphtheria antitoxin, botulinum antitoxin, antivenins, antilymphocyte globulin, and antithymocyte globulin. Horse antisera against diphtheria (and subsequently against tetanus as well) were produced and used in therapy from about the beginning of the 20th century. Antidiphtheria and antitetanus immunoglobulins are now produced almost exclusively as fractions of plasma of human origin. There are, however, a few cases in which xenogeneic antisera are still used, despite their many and often serious adverse effects.

Uses

Preparations of human immunoglobulins given by intramuscular/subcutaneous administration are mainly given to prevent or treat specific diseases, such as rhesus disease (anti-D) or certain viral infections, for example measles, hepatitis A, hepatitis B, rabies, and cytomegalovirus. Polyclonal antilymphocyte preparations (for example antilymphocyte globulin and antithymocyte globulin) have been developed because of evidence that T cells are primarily responsible for rejection of transplants. Indications for treatment with, for example, horse antilymphocyte globulin and/or antithymocyte globulin are very much the same as the indications for the mouse monoclonal anti-CD3 (muromonab), namely acute rejection of transplants, and aplastic anemia (3,4).

Preparations for intravenous administration are mainly used in patients with general immune deficiency states (primary or secondary) or diseases like idiopathic thrombocytopenic purpura (ITP) and autoimmune diseases (5,6). Neurological disorders (for example Guillain–Barré syndrome and chronic demyelinating polyneuropathy) have been treated with intravenous immunoglobulin (7–9).

The efficacy and safety of intravenous immunoglobulin have been reported in primary and secondary immunodeficiency, as well as in some immune disorders such as idiopathic thrombocytopenic purpura, Kawasaki disease, and Guillain–Barré syndrome (10–15). Intravenous immunoglobulin is also used empirically in a variety of several autoimmune diseases (16). Higher dosages of intravenous immunoglobulin are used for autoimmune indications (400–2000 mg/kg) than in immunodeficiency diseases (100–400 mg/kg). Minor adverse effects, such as headache, myalgia, chest discomfort, and fever, occur in 10% of patients (17). The efficacy of intravenous immunoglobulin has been reported in patients with membranous and membranoproliferative lupus nephritis (16). High-dose intravenous immunoglobulin has also been beneficial in myasthenia gravis, multiple sclerosis, and multifocal motor neuropathy (18,19) and in patients with pemphigus vulgaris and bullous pemphigoid unresponsive to conventional immunosuppressive drugs (20,21).

Intravenous immunoglobulin administered to allogeneic bone marrow transplant recipients modifies graft-versus-host disease and prevents interstitial pneumonia and infections (14).

The use of intravenous immunoglobulins in selected immunodeficiency and autoimmune diseases has been reviewed (2).

Mechanisms of action

The effect of immunoglobulin therapy is either protection against microorganisms (antibody substitution, passive immunization), or immunomodulation, or both. The mechanism of the response in non-infectious diseases is still not clear, but in idiopathic thrombocytopenic purpura an early fall in platelet-associated IgG and IgM may be a primary event, due to interference with antibody binding by platelets (22). Several other mechanisms of action of intravenous immunoglobulin in autoimmune diseases have been suggested, such as enhanced suppressor activity, Fc receptor blockade on neutrophils and macrophages (23), inhibition of complement activation and modulation of anti-idiotype responses (24), cytokine modification, neutralization of superantigens, and regulation of T cells and the idiotypic network (16,25). The suppression of polyclonal immunoglobulin biosynthesis induced by high-dose immunoglobulin infusions has also been suggested as a possible mechanism (26).

General adverse effects

Specific immunoglobulins

When administering different lots of the same product of equine rabies immunoglobulin, significant differences in adverse reactions, reflecting differences in production or purification processes and protein content, have been observed (27). It has been concluded in the past that the incidence of reactions to antirabies immunoglobulin is particularly high, but any of these immunoglobulins can cause severe reactions. The WHO has recommended that animal immunoglobulins should be used only after tests to rule out hypersensitivity.

A review of the discovery of antitoxins, the development of antibody formulations, and possible adverse effects has appeared (28).

Intramuscular immunoglobulin

Allerglobuline is a human gammaglobulin formulation, given intramuscularly, that has been reported to have a protective effect against type I allergic diseases and chronic infections of the upper respiratory tract in both adults and children. In 64 patients given allerglobuline, pain and inflammation at the injection site were the most common adverse effects (29). Fever, drowsiness, headache, nausea, back pain, and conjunctivitis occurred in only few patients. One patient had a rash and myalgia after the third injection; when the rash occurred again after the fourth injection, the patient was withdrawn.

Intravenous immunoglobulin

Adverse effects of intravenous immunoglobulin are generally mild and self-limiting (25). Although more common during the first two infusions, reactions appear to be primarily related to the speed of infusion. When infusions are given over a 1–3-hour period, the incidence of reactions is less than 5% and they occur during the transfusion; when infusions are given rapidly, the reactions may appear soon after completing the infusion. In about 10% of cases they occur 30–60 minutes after the start of the infusion.

Reactions include flushing, myalgia, headache, fever, chills and shaking, low backache, nausea and vomiting, diarrhea, chest tightness and shortness of breath, wheezing, changes in blood pressure, tachycardia, and rashes (30,31). Most of the adverse effects are related to the rate of administration and can be attenuated by slowing the rate of the infusion (32) or by prior administration of hydrocortisone and/or an antihistamine. When infusions are given over a 1–3-hour period, the incidence of reactions is less than 5% and they occur during the transfusion; when infusions are given rapidly the reactions may appear soon after completing the infusion. The current high dosage of 0.8–1.0 g/kg intravenous immunoglobulin for 1–2 days (instead of the original dosage regimen of 0.4 g/kg for 5 days) for patients with idiopathic thrombocytopenic purpura is probably associated with an increased risk of adverse effects (33).

The rate of adverse effects associated with intravenous immunoglobulin varies among different studies, which has been attributed to factors such as the indication, the dosage, the infusion rate, and the patient's age (12). In one study, headache and chills were related to a higher dosage.

Of 37 patients with primary hypogammaglobulinemia who received 1235 immunoglobulin infusions, 10 had adverse reactions during 34 infusions (2.8% of all infusions), but only five reactions were moderately severe. The reactions are related to the rate of administration (34); a rate of 5 mg/kg/minute was well tolerated.

Of 56 patients with autoimmune diseases who received high dosages of intravenous immunoglobulin, 20 had at least one adverse effect after one or more courses of treatment (12). The most frequently reported adverse effects were low-grade fever, headache, and chills. The authors concluded that the occurrence of adverse effects with intravenous immunoglobulin was not related to the clinical response to treatment. However, patients who developed adverse effects during the first course of treatment were more at risk of adverse effects during subsequent courses.

Patients with thrombocytopenia generally tolerate intravenous immunoglobulin well (35). In 16 young patients aged 9 months to 22 years with immune-mediated hemocytopenias (13 with childhood immune thrombocytopenic purpura), who received a total of 210 infusions, minimal adverse effects (transient headaches) were experienced during only four infusions, and later infusions were problem-free in three of the four patients (36).

The most frequent adverse effects of intravenous immunoglobulin (Sandoz) for the treatment of various disorders (affecting 1–3% of patients in all) were headache, nausea, vomiting, and fever. Some other mild symptoms have an incidence below 1%, including abdominal pain, diarrhea, fatigue, malaise, dizziness, myalgia, and chest tightness.

Allerglobuline is an intravenous human gammaglobulin formulation that has been reported to have a protective effect against type I allergic diseases and chronic infections of the upper respiratory tract in both adults and children. In 64 patients given allerglobuline, pain and inflammation at the injection site were the most common adverse effects (29). Fever, drowsiness, headache, nausea, back pain, and conjunctivitis occurred in only few patients. One patient had a rash and myalgia after the third injection; when the rash occurred again after the fourth injection, the patient was withdrawn.

Polyclonal antilymphocyte immunoglobulins

Short-term toxicity from polyclonal antilymphocyte immunoglobulins has been particularly marked in patients treated with combined antilymphocyte/antithymocyte globulin preparations from immunized horses (37). Immediate adverse effects include leukopenia and thrombocytopenia, fever, arthralgia, rash, urticaria, hepatotoxicity, hyperglycemia, hypertension, and diarrhea (38). A later adverse effect is serum sickness. Many of the effects may be due to an increase in tumor necrosis factor (39).

The longer-term effects of immunosuppression, and in particular the residual hematological and immunological abnormalities in patients with aplastic anemia treated with antilymphocyte globulin, have been documented: there is toxicity to hemopoietic cells, eventually leading to clonal marrow diseases years after treatment (37). Paroxysmal nocturnal hemoglobinuria, refractory sideroblastic anemia, chronic myelomonocytic leukemia, or acute leukemia can develop 4–10 years after treatment (40).

Organs and Systems

Cardiovascular

Intravenous immunoglobulin expands the plasma volume and increases blood viscosity, which can lead to volume overload in patients with cardiac insufficiency (41). Stroke, thromboembolic events, and myocardial infarction have been reported after high-dose treatment with intravenous immunoglobulin, which increases plasma viscosity (41–43).

Thrombosis in elderly patients with an increased risk of thrombosis, such as those with hypertension or previous episodes of infarction, has been described (44). A few cases of thrombosis subsequent to intravenous immunoglobulin have been reported, including myocardial infarction in five patients, stroke in four cases, and spinal cord ischemia in one (45). It has been postulated that these events are induced by platelet activation and increased plasma viscosity (12).

Several cases of thrombosis have been reported after administration of intravenous immunoglobulin (31).

- A 75-year-old man with idiopathic thrombocytopenia purpura who was treated with intravenous immunoglobulin developed recurrent myocardial ischemia (46).
- A 54-year-old woman with idiopathic thrombocytopenic purpura received intravenous immunoglobulin 1 g/kg/day for 2 days and had an ischemic stroke with hemiparesis; 3 days later she had a deep vein thrombosis (47).
- A 33-year-old woman with Evans' syndrome received intravenous immunoglobulin 400 mg/kg/day and developed a deep vein thrombosis after 1 week (47). She was treated with warfarin, and 6 months later received an additional course of intravenous immunoglobulin for recurrent hemolytic anemia; 1 day later she died of pulmonary thromboembolism.
- A 70-year-old woman with polycythemia rubra vera and Guillain–Barré syndrome, but no known risk factors for thrombosis, had a cerebral infarction 10 days after receiving intravenous immunoglobulin; the authors wondered whether there was a relation to the polycythemia vera (48).

In a randomized, controlled study in 56 patients with untreated autoimmune thrombocytopenic purpura, who were treated with intravenous immunoglobulin 0.7 g/kg/day for 3 days, one had a deep vein thrombosis complicated by pulmonary embolism (49). One of 10 children with toxic epidermal necrolysis, for which they were given intravenous immunoglobulin 0.5 g/kg/day, developed a deep vein thrombosis requiring heparin (50). Of the 10 children, this child was the only one who received intravenous immunoglobulin for 7 days instead of the standard 4-day course.

- Transient hypertension occurred in a patient with dermatomyositis during therapy with intravenous immunoglobulin (51). In the past, his diastolic blood pressure had been 104–106 mm Hg, but he was normotensive with antihypertensive drug medication.

Several mechanisms for this transient hypertension were postulated, for example stimulation of the vascular endothelium to secrete endothelin to inhibit nitric oxide synthesis.

It has been recommended that patients with cardiac diseases should be monitored during intravenous immunoglobulin therapy, because hypertension and cardiac failure have occurred, presumably as a result of fluid overload or electrolyte shifts (52).

Respiratory

- A 35-year-old woman with idiopathic thrombocytopenic purpura treated with high dosages of intravenous immunoglobulin developed a recurrent lymphocytic pleural effusion (53).
- In a patient with Guillain–Barré syndrome, and a history of ischemic heart disease, intravenous immunoglobulin 400 mg/kg for 5 consecutive days caused severe bronchospasm and hypercapnia after a dose of 12.5 g had been given (15). The complaints disappeared after withdrawal of the intravenous immunoglobulin.

Nervous system

Headache occurred in 25% of all patients who received an infusion of intravenous immunoglobulin, probably related to larger volumes and fluid shifts, protein loads, and infusion rates (54). Intravenous immunoglobulin caused severe headache in 56% of patients without a history of migraine (55). The pathogenesis of this headache is unknown.

Severe headache has also been reported in children with idiopathic thrombocytopenic purpura using intravenous immunoglobulins (33). In a randomized, controlled study of patients with myasthenia gravis, two of six patients who received intravenous immunoglobulin developed severe headache after the initial dose of 2 g/kg (56).

In 14 patients with primary immunodeficiency disease, progressive neurodegeneration occurred and a possible relation to immunoglobulin therapy could not be ruled out (57).

Aseptic meningitis

Aseptic meningitis is characterized by headache, photophobia, nausea, vomiting, and meningism, and is confirmed by cerebrospinal fluid pleocytosis with 10–90%

polymorphonuclear cells, increased concentrations of several proteins, and negative cultures (SEDA-22, 344) (54,58,59). It has been described in 1–15% of patients receiving high dosages of intravenous immunoglobulin (60,61) and especially in subjects with a history of migraine (25,43,60). However, aseptic meningitis has also been reported after a low dose of intravenous immunoglobulin.

- A 50-year-old man developed aseptic meningitis after a low dose of intravenous immunoglobulin (3.5 g) (60). A few weeks after the first infusion, he received a second infusion and again developed symptoms of aseptic meningitis.

The authors thought it unlikely that aseptic meningitis had been caused by an allergic reaction. They proposed that the mechanism of aseptic meningitis involved the entry of immunoglobulin molecules into the cerebrospinal fluid, causing an inflammatory reaction.

It has also been suggested that release of histamine, serotonin, and prostaglandins affects the meningeal microvasculature (31).

- Two children with idiopathic thrombocytopenic purpura developed aseptic meningitis after receiving intravenous immunoglobulin 1 g/kg/day, with unusual large numbers of leukocytes in the cerebrospinal fluid (62).

To prevent aseptic meningitis, it has been advised that intravenous immunoglobulin should be infused at a slow rate and that diluted immunoglobulin solutions should be used (58). Aseptic meningitis can be prevented by the administration of propranolol (41,58). In addition, prehydration and an antihistamine have been helpful in some patients (41,58).

Possible mechanisms of aseptic meningitis include hypersensitivity reactions, stabilizing products, cytokines, cerebrovascular sensitivity, and direct meningeal irritation. It has been suggested that it is caused by aggregated immunoglobulin, antibody–antigen complex formation with subsequent complement activation, or stabilizing carbohydrates used during manufacture (30,59).

Cerebrovascular disease

Stroke and ischemic encephalopathy, probably caused by cerebral vasospasm after intravenous immunoglobulin, have been reported as possible complications of intravenous immunoglobulin (63).

- Hemiplegia occurred on the third day of intravenous immunoglobulin therapy in a 58-year-old man with graft-versus-host disease after transfusion of non-leukocyte-depleted erythrocytes (64). The hemiplegia resolved one day after withdrawal of intravenous immunoglobulin.
- Hemiplegia occurred in a child given intravenous immunoglobulin for idiopathic thrombocytopenic purpura (65).

The authors of both reports suggested that the hemiplegia had been caused either by transient hyperviscosity or by vasospasm.

Cerebral vasospasm, cerebral vasculitis, and serum hyperviscosity have been implicated in the pathogenesis of cerebral infarction after intravenous immunoglobulin (66).

Metabolism

Blood glucose should be monitored in patients with diabetes mellitus who receive glucose-containing intravenous immunoglobulin (41).

Hematologic

It has been recommended that the blood count be monitored during intravenous immunoglobulin therapy if there is evidence of mild leukopenia, neutropenia, or thrombocytopenia before the first infusion (18).

Erythrocytes

Severe acute hemolysis due to acquisition of red cell alloantibodies from donor serum has been reported (67–69). In other cases, the suggested mechanism of hemolytic anemia after high dosages of intravenous immunoglobulin was the presence of anti-A and/or anti-B antibodies in the plasma product (70).

Various immunoglobulin products contain IgG of molecular weight of a dimer or greater (over 300 kDa), which in the presence of serum can mimic immune complexes and bind to erythrocytes via CR1 (71). Especially in young adults, the immune complex-like moieties in intravenous immunoglobulin bind to erythrocytes and serve as opsonins in the mediation of erythrocyte sequestration, resulting in significant drops in hematocrit and hemoglobin concentrations (71). It has been suggested that the presence of immune complex-like moieties bound to erythrocyte CR1 after intravenous immunoglobulin treatment is correlated with in vivo hemolysis.

- Severe hemolytic anemia after high doses of intravenous immunoglobulin occurred in a 23-year-old woman with polymyositis (72).

This adverse reaction was probably due to the presence of allohemagglutinins A and B and high molecular weight IgG complexes in the formulation. Specifications in pharmacopeial monographs and product licenses require that intravenous immunoglobulin be free of significant titers of anti-A anti-B antibodies (SEDA-24, 385).

Leukocytes

High-dose immunoglobulin has been reported to cause neutropenia (31,73,74), disseminated intravascular coagulation and serum sickness (75). Neutropenia after intravenous immunoglobulin is frequent and seems to be transient and self-limiting (76). Neutropenia is not dose-related in the therapeutic range of doses.

It has been suggested that transient neutropenia can be induced by the presence of antineutrophil antibodies present in intravenous immunoglobulin. However, the possibility that immunoglobulin-mediated neutrophil agglutination causes pseudoleukopenia has also been raised (74). Increased leukocyte aggregation in the circulating pool of peripheral blood, induced by intravenous immunoglobulin, is particularly observed in people with hyperfibrinogenemia (74). It has been suggested that leukopenia detected by electronic counting is not necessarily associated with a real reduction in the absolute number of white blood cells in the peripheral blood, but is artefactual (74).

Platelets

In elderly patients, thrombotic events have been described in up to 10% in patients aged over 60, some of them fatal. Thrombotic events may be related to a rapid rise in numbers of circulating platelets (44,77).

Several cases of intravenous immunoglobulin-related thrombosis have been reported (78,79). It can be either venous or arterial (80). It has been suggested that thrombosis can be caused by platelet activation and increased plasma viscosity (79). In patients with vascular risk factors, such as old age, hypertension, and a history of stroke or coronary artery disease, complications, such as myocardial infarction, pulmonary embolism, stroke, and acute spinal cord events, have been described (80). Intravenous immunoglobulin enhances platelet aggregation and the release of adenosine triphosphate in human platelets in vitro. In addition, there is a dose-related increase in plasma viscosity with increasing plasma immunoglobulin concentration (79,80).

Liver

Although transient rises in liver enzymes have been documented, they are not considered to be serious (68).

Fatal hepatic veno-occlusive disease, characterized by hyperbilirubinemia, hepatomegaly, ascites, and weight gain, has been associated with intravenous immunoglobulin administered prophylactically to prevent transplant-related infections (79). To avoid such thrombotic complications, intravenous immunoglobulin should be infused at a slower rate in patients at risk, and high dosages (400–1000 mg/kg) should not be infused.

Urinary tract

Renal insufficiency after high dosages of intravenous immunoglobulin has been observed, mostly in patients with pre-existing renal disease (81). Acute renal insufficiency occurred within 7 days after the administration of intravenous immunoglobulin, with a peak at 5 days. About 40% of patients needed dialysis and 15% died despite treatment (all with severe underlying diseases); the mean time to recovery in survivors was about 10 days (82).

The US FDA has issued recommendations on safety precautions that physicians should take to reduce the potential risk of acute renal insufficiency, which appears to be uncommonly associated with infusion of intravenous immunoglobulin products (83,84). Since 1981, the FDA has received over 114 reports of renal dysfunction and/or acute renal insufficiency in patients given immunoglobulin, and a total of 17 deaths have been reported (32). As the problems have been associated with the use of specific immunoglobulin products, the FDA advises, that "physicians should carefully weigh the potential benefits of administering sucrose-containing intravenous immunoglobulin products against the risks of causing renal damage." Other cases of acute renal insufficiency have been described after the intravenous infusion of immunoglobulin (SEDA-22, 345) (73).

The pathophysiology of acute renal insufficiency due to immunoglobulins is probably related to hyperosmolar renal damage, due to sucrose present in 50 ml intravenous formulations (13,43,85–87). Acute renal insufficiency has also been attributed to sucrose in a kidney allograft recipient treated with intravenous immunoglobulin (88). The high solute load in the kidney can cause osmotic damage (32,82). The histopathology of renal tissue shows osmotic tubular injury, tubular vacuolization, and tubulointerstitial infiltrates (89,82). Cytological findings in the urine included the presence of macrophage-like tubular epithelial cells with multivacuolated cytoplasm (90). Formulations of intravenous immunoglobulin with sucrose as a stabilizer should not be used in patients with renal disease (31,81,91).

In a retrospective study of a heterogeneous group of 119 patients receiving intravenous immunoglobulin, two developed irreversible renal insufficiency and six had a rise in serum creatinine. These patients had received high dosages of two different formulations of intravenous immunoglobulin, one containing sucrose 1.76 g per gram of intravenous immunoglobulin; the other 0.5 g per gram. There was no relation between the amount of sucrose in the intravenous immunoglobulin and the development of renal insufficiency (82).

Studies in rats have suggested that after pinocytosis by renal tubular cells, sucrose is incorporated into phagolysosomes (32). The intracellular accumulation of sucrose leads to vacuole formation and cellular swelling. On withdrawal, renal insufficiency resolves in most cases. However, sometimes hemodialysis is necessary (69,89).

Risk factors for this adverse effect are pre-existing renal disease, age over 65 years, dehydration, diabetes mellitus, hypertension, and a high infusion rate (SEDA-22, 345) (10,13,32,43,86,92). To minimize the risk of renal insufficiency, it has been suggested that immunoglobulin should be diluted with hypotonic fluid, that the infusion rate should be reduced, and that dosing intervals should be increased (89). Patients should be adequately hydrated and potent diuretics should be avoided (10).

In most cases the acute renal insufficiency is reversible and recovery occurs after 7–15 days (10).

It has been suggested that kidney function should be monitored during intravenous immunoglobulin therapy if it is abnormal before the first infusion (18). In addition, these patients should be adequately hydrated during treatment with intravenous immunoglobulin (52).

Skin

Skin reactions to intravenous immunoglobulin are rare (52,93–95). Other reported reactions include urticaria, maculopapular rashes, petechiae, eczema, and erythema multiforme (31,96).

Pompholyx has been observed 5–7 days from the last day of therapy in three of 23 neurological patients treated with intravenous immunoglobulin (17,97). Pompholyx occurs on the palms of the hands and is characterized by small papules, subdermal vesicles, desquamation, and crusting.

Cutaneous vasculitis has been attributed to intravenous immunoglobulin (96)

- In a patient with type II mixed cryoglobulinemia, intravenous immunoglobulin caused severe cutaneous vasculitis accompanied by an increased cryocrit (98).

A simple method of mixing the patient's serum in vitro with intravenous immunoglobulin could probably predict this.

Hair

There have been a few cases of alopecia after the concomitant administration of intravenous immunoglobulin and steroid (49,99–102).

Immunologic

The administration of equine or other immunoglobulins is associated with a considerable risk of adverse effects and can produce virtually any type of early or late hypersensitivity reaction, ranging from asthma and urticaria to serum sickness and fatal anaphylaxis (103–106). Encephalitis (107), myocarditis (108), nephritis (109), and uveitis (110) can all be manifestations of such reactions. In one case, leukocytoclastic vasculitis was attributed to human immunoglobulin (96).

Of systemic reactions to immunoglobulins, those of an inflammatory nature are thought to be due to the presence of small complexes or microaggregates, probably leading to activation of the complement system. The symptoms are usually mild and influenza-like, and generally respond to slowing down or temporary interruption of the infusion. They include headache, hypotension, sweating, chills, fever, nausea, and vasomotor reactions. The frequency of such adverse reactions has fallen, probably because of the improved quality of the preparations. In 1978, the frequency of adverse reactions was as high as 55% in those receiving intravenous preparations containing 10–13% polymeric immunoglobulin, whereas by 2000, intravenous immunoglobulin preparations caused adverse reactions in only 3–4% (5). The more severe reactions may also be complement-mediated and may be due to a spontaneous activation of the complement system by the immunoglobulin preparation concerned; immunoglobulin aggregates may again be involved. The symptoms may be similar to those of inflammatory reactions, though they can be more severe. Such serious effects, including rare reactions of an anaphylactic type, may occur in as few as one in 6000 cases (111).

IgA deficiency is one of the more commonly encountered genetic disorders, and homozygotic deficiency is present in 0.3–0.03% of Caucasian populations. Such individuals may develop anti-IgA antibodies and have serum-sickness-like symptoms after the first administration of immunoglobulins, sometimes experiencing more severe reactions after repeated injections (112–114). A mild reaction due to sensitization to genetic IgA variants can also occur. Selective IgA deficiency is a contraindication to intravenous immunoglobulin, because of the risk of anaphylactic shock in patients with IgA deficiency and IgE or IgG antibodies against IgA, which react with IgA in intravenous immunoglobulin (13,17,30,31,41,52,61,94).

Some reports suggest that anaphylaxis due to intravenous immunoglobulin infusion occurs most often in patients with primary hypogammaglobulinemia (115,116). However, anaphylactic reactions have been seen in two atopic patients with idiopathic thrombocytopenic purpura, and the authors warned that children with atopic disease should not receive intravenous immunoglobulin (117).

In recipients of left ventricular assist devices awaiting cardiac transplantation treated with intravenous immunoglobulin, clinical manifestations of immune complex disease occurred during four of 27 (15%) monthly courses (118). The immune complex disease was characterized by fever, arthralgia, and maculopapular rashes.

Intravascular hemolysis is a rare adverse effect of immunoglobulins, due to the presence of anti-blood group antibodies (119–123).

Body temperature

Intravenous immunoglobulin can cause malaise and fever in patients with infections, probably through a temporarily increased titer of antibodies against different pathogenic microorganisms (124).

Multiorgan failure

Multiorgan failure has been described after intravenous infusion of immunoglobulin (125).

- A 3-year-old mentally retarded girl was given intravenous sulfonated immunoglobulin for prophylaxis of measles. After infusion of about 100 mg, she became cyanotic, confused, and tachycardic. Despite hydrocortisone she developed hypotensive shock. Multiorgan failure developed, with symptoms of disseminated intravascular coagulation, acute renal insufficiency, hepatic dysfunction, respiratory distress syndrome, and rhabdomyolysis. After plasma exchange and continuous hemofiltration she recovered without sequelae. The drug-induced lymphocyte stimulation test using gammaglobulin was negative. In addition, serum concentrations of IgA and IgG were normal. However, concentrations of cytokines, such as interleukin-6, TNF-α, and soluble interleukin-2 receptor, were very high. Complement C3, C4, and CH50 were reduced, but C3a was raised.

The authors suggested that an unknown mechanism associated with intravenous immunoglobulin infusion had caused non-specific activation of complement systems accompanied by fulminant hypercytokinemia.

Second-Generation Effects

Teratogenicity

Intravenous immunoglobulin is indicated for idiopathic thrombocytopenic purpura in pregnancy. No fetal abnormalities have been reported (101).

Susceptibility Factors

Because of reports of severe adverse effects, the presence of rheumatoid factor in patients with B cell neoplasia may constitute a contraindication to intravenous immunoglobulin (83).

Autoimmune disease

The risk of reactions to antilymphocyte globulin is increased in patients with autoimmune disease (126). Fever and chills, sometimes with extreme hyperpyrexia, nausea and vomiting, urticaria, and reduced platelet and granulocyte counts were reported after the administration of horse antithymocyte globulin.

Infusion of intravenous immunoglobulin 0.14 g/kg in 17 patients with autoimmune diseases, in whom circulating immunoglobulins had been depleted, was associated with a high incidence of serious adverse effects (94). Treatment was terminated in four patients because of adverse effects, including urticaria, severe hypotension, arthralgia, and chest discomfort.

In two reviews of intravenous immunoglobulin in systemic lupus erythematosus, there was worsening proteinuria and/or a rise in serum creatinine (127,128), whereas others treating similar patients did not detect deterioration (117,129).

Transplant recipients

The adverse effects of rabbit antithymocyte globulin in transplant recipients were pain and erythema at the injection site and in one instance polyarthritis with urticaria (130). Four cases in which malignant lymphoma developed in renal transplant recipients treated with antithymocyte globulin of animal origin have been reported (131).

Drug Administration

Drug contamination

Specifications in pharmacopeial monographs and product licences require intravenous immunoglobulin products to be free from significant amounts of anti-A and anti-B antibodies (132). It has been advised that a specification be adopted that will prevent the use of batches of intravenous immunoglobulin with abnormally high anti-D titers (over 1:64) (132).

Coagulation factors

Activated factor XIa has been demonstrated in samples of reconstituted intravenous immunoglobulin from eight different manufacturers (11). The degree of factor XIa contamination in intravenous immunoglobulin correlated with the manufacturer, suggesting that the purification process can affect residual factor XI concentration. Factor XIa can activate factor IX to factor IXa, and it can be hypothesized that there is a direct correlation between the presence of factor XI in intravenous immunoglobulin products and an increased risk of thrombotic complications.

Transmission of infection

The transmission of viral infections by immunoglobulins has occasionally been suspected. However, intravenous immunoglobulin preparations are considered relatively safe, and there are no reports of transmission of HIV or hepatitis B (44,101). This is probably because of the high degree of viral inactivation of the cold ethanol fractionation and the screening of every donation for several viruses, such as HIV and hepatitis B and C (85). Of 56 patients with autoimmune diseases who received 167 infusions of intravenous immunoglobulin, none developed antibodies to human immunodeficiency virus and hepatitis C virus or hepatitis B surface antigen (12).

In 1994, several cases of hepatitis C were reported, all traceable to a specific product (Gammagard®) (133). However, since the introduction of additional viral inactivation steps, such as solvent detergent, intravenous immunoglobulin is not considered to pose an infectious risk (69,101,134).

There has been some concern about possible transmission of hepatitis G. However, hepatitis G is an enveloped flavivirus with homology to hepatitis C and is probably also inactivated by the current procedures (58).

Although transmission of Creutzfeldt–Jakob disease through blood components and plasma products has never been documented, the FDA has suggested that there is a theoretical possibility that blood products may carry the responsible agent (135).

Transmission of hepatitis B and HIV after infusion of intravenous immunoglobulin has never been reported.

Life-threatening fulminant hepatitis due to transmission of human parvovirus B19 by intravenous immunoglobulin has been reported (136). The manufacturing process of this intravenous immunoglobulin product includes pasteurization (60°C for 10 hours), treatment with polyethylene glycol, ethanol fractionation, and nanofiltration. Removal of the small, non-lipid-enveloped parvovirus B19, which is highly resistant to different virus-reducing and inactivating steps, requires 15 nm nanofiltration.

A novel DNA virus, TT virus, has been implicated as a cause of post-transfusion hepatitis. A high prevalence of TT virus infection has been found in patients who received blood or blood components, such as factor VIII and IX concentrates. However, the PCR for TT virus DNA was negative in all 17 patients with immunodeficiency, who were treated prophylactically with intravenous immunoglobulin, as well as in 15 tested immunoglobulin formulations (137).

Drug administration route

Intramuscular, subcutaneous

Adverse effects associated with intramuscular or subcutaneous administration of immunoglobulin are extremely rare, and are usually related to IgA deficiency in the patient or to additives in the preparation (for example preservatives). Adverse effects associated with intravenous immunoglobulin are more frequently seen and may be either local or systemic (138,139). Local reactions are essentially attributable to the technique used and are not specific to the intravenous immunoglobulin.

Intravenous

Intravenous immunoglobulin is approved for the following indications: primary immune deficiencies, immune-mediated thrombocytopenia, Kawasaki disease, bone marrow transplantation, chronic B cell lymphocytic leukemia, and pediatric HIV infection (135). In addition, intravenous immunoglobulin is a promising immunomodulatory therapy for several neurological diseases, such as Guillain–Barré syndrome, chronic inflammatory demyelinating polyneuropathy, and multifocal motor neuropathy (41). Intravenous immunoglobulin has also been used in the treatment of several other antibody-mediated diseases, such as dermatomyositis, autoimmune neutropenia, pemphigus vulgaris, and pemphigus foliaceus (140–142).

Mild adverse effects of intravenous immunoglobulin, such as headache, chills, nausea, backache, and flushing, occur at a rate of 5–10% (101,135). Most of these reactions are self-limiting and associated with over-rapid infusion (41). In patients with adverse reactions to intravenous immunoglobulin there was a significant rise in plasma IL-6 and thromboxane B_2 (143).

Drug–Drug Interactions

Contrast media

Acute renal insufficiency after intravenous immunoglobulin therapy has been reported in association with the injection of iodinated radiocontrast agents (144). Contrast media and intravenous immunoglobulin formulations containing maltose or sucrose both have toxic effects on renal cells.

Interference with Diagnostic Tests

Serum sodium measurement

Pseudohyponatremia, a laboratory artefact due to hyperproteinemia, has been observed during intravenous immunoglobulin treatment (145).

- In a 38-year-old man with end-stage renal insufficiency and thrombocytopenia secondary to systemic lupus erythematosus, pseudohyponatremia occurred after treatment with intravenous immunoglobulin 1 g/kg for 2 days (146).

This phenomenon is explained by the fact that intravenous immunoglobulin increases the non-aqueous phase of the plasma, resulting in a relative loss of plasma water volume. Sodium is virtually restricted to serum water, so each volume of plasma measured will contain less sodium and be interpreted as hyponatremia. Using a direct ion-selective electrode avoids this problem.

References

1. Committee on Infectious Diseases. In: Red Book. 2003 Report of the Committee on Infectious Diseases. 26th ed. Elk Grove Village, IL: American Academy of Pediatrics, 2003:53–66.
2. Pirofsky B, Kinzey DM. Intravenous immune globulins. A review of their uses in selected immunodeficiency and autoimmune diseases. Drugs 1992;43(1):6–14.
3. Clark KR, Forsythe JL, Shenton BK, Lennard TW, Proud G, Taylor RM. Administration of ATG according to the absolute T lymphocyte count during therapy for steroid-resistant rejection. Transpl Int 1993;6(1):18–21.
4. Moore MA, Castro-Malaspina H. Immunosuppression in aplastic anemia—postponing the inevitable? N Engl J Med 1991;324(19):1358–60.
5. Bjorkander J. Antibody Deficiency Syndromes. Thesis. Sweden: University of Göteborg, 1985.
6. Hopkins SJ. Sandoglobulin. Drugs Today 1985;21:277.
7. Bril V, Ilse WK, Pearce R, Dhanani A, Sutton D, Kong K. Pilot trial of immunoglobulin versus plasma exchange in patients with Guillain–Barré syndrome. Neurology 1996;46(1):100–3.
8. Otten A, Vermeulen M, Bossuyt PM, Otten A. Intravenous immunoglobulin treatment in neurological diseases. J Neurol Neurosurg Psychiatry 1996;60(4):359–61.
9. van Dijk GW, Notermans NC, Franssen H, Oey PL, Wokke JH. Response to intravenous immunoglobulin treatment in chronic inflammatory demyelinating polyneuropathy with only sensory symptoms. J Neurol 1996;243(4):318–22.
10. Gras V, Andrejak M, Decocq G. Acute renal failure associated with intravenous immunoglobulins. Pharmacoepidemiol Drug Saf 1999;8(Suppl 1):S73–8.
11. Wolberg AS, Kon RH, Monroe DM, Hoffman M. Coagulation factor XI is a contaminant in intravenous immunoglobulin preparations. Am J Hematol 2000;65(1):30–4.
12. Sherer Y, Levy Y, Langevitz P, Rauova L, Fabrizzi F, Shoenfeld Y. Adverse effects of intravenous immunoglobulin therapy in 56 patients with autoimmune diseases. Pharmacology 2001;62(3):133–7.
13. Gupta N, Ahmed I, Nissel-Horowitz S, Patel D, Mehrotra B. Intravenous gammglobulin-associated acute renal failure. Am J Hematol 2001;66(2):151–2.
14. Winston DJ, Antin JH, Wolff SN, Bierer BE, Small T, Miller KB, Linker C, Kaizer H, Lazarus HM, Petersen FB, Cowan MJ, Ho WG, Wingard JR, Schiller GJ, Territo MC, Jiao J, Petrarca MA, Tonetta SA. A multicenter, randomized, double-blind comparison of different doses of intravenous immunoglobulin for prevention of graft-versus-host disease and infection after allogeneic bone marrow transplantation. Bone Marrow Transplant 2001;28(2):187–96.
15. Raphael JC, Chevret S, Harboun M, Jars-Guincestre MC; French Guillain–Barré Syndrome Cooperative Group. Intravenous immune globulins in patients with Guillain–Barré syndrome and contraindications to plasma exchange: 3 days versus 6 days. J Neurol Neurosurg Psychiatry 2001;71(2):235–8.
16. Levy Y, Sherer Y, George J, Rovensky J, Lukac J, Rauova L, Poprac P, Langevitz P, Fabbrizzi F, Shoenfeld Y. Intravenous immunoglobulin treatment of lupus nephritis. Semin Arthritis Rheum 2000;29(5):321–7.
17. Iannaccone S, Sferrazza B, Quattrini A, Smirne S, Ferini-Strambi L. Pompholyx (vesicular eczema) after i.v. immunoglobulin therapy for neurologic disease Neurology 1999;53(5):1154–5.
18. Bajaj NP, Henderson N, Bahl R, Stott K, Clifford-Jones RE. Call for guidelines for monitoring renal function and haematological variables during intravenous infusion of immunoglobulin in neurological patients. J Neurol Neurosurg Psychiatry 2001;71(4):562–3.
19. Hilkevich O, Drory VE, Chapman J, Korczyn AD. The use of intravenous immunoglobulin as maintenance therapy in myasthenia gravis. Clin Neuropharmacol 2001;24(3):173–6.
20. Ahmed AR. Intravenous immunoglobulin therapy for patients with bullous pemphigoid unresponsive to conventional immunosuppressive treatment. J Am Acad Dermatol 2001;45(6):825–35.
21. Ahmed AR. Intravenous immunoglobulin therapy in the treatment of patients with pemphigus vulgaris unresponsive to conventional immunosuppressive treatment. J Am Acad Dermatol 2001;45(5):679–90.
22. Ball S, Zuiable A, Roter BL, Hegde UM. Changes in platelet immunoprotein levels during therapy in adult immune thrombocytopenia. Br J Haematol 1985; 60(4):631–3.
23. Yu Z, Lennon VA. Mechanism of intravenous immune globulin therapy in antibody-mediated autoimmune diseases. N Engl J Med 1999;340(3):227–8.
24. Mouthon L, Kaveri SV, Spalter SH, Lacroix-Desmazes S, Lefranc C, Desai R, Kazatchkine MD. Mechanisms of action of intravenous immune globulin in immune-mediated diseases. Clin Exp Immunol 1996;104(Suppl 1):3–9.
25. Boulton-Jones R, Clark P. Intravenous immunoglobulin and sepsis. CPD Infection 2001;2:48–52.

26. Dammacco F, Iodice G, Campobasso N. Treatment of adult patients with idiopathic thrombocytopenic purpura with intravenous immunoglobulin: effects on circulating T cell subsets and PWM-induced antibody synthesis in vitro. Br J Haematol 1986;62(1):125–35.
27. Wilde H, Chomchey P, Prakongsri S, Puyaratabandhu P, Chutivongse S. Adverse effects of equine rabies immune gobulin. Vaccine 1989;7(1):10–11.
28. Gronski P, Seiler FR, Schwick HG. Discovery of antitoxins and development of antibody preparations for clinical uses from 1890 to 1990. Mol Immunol 1991;28(12):1321–32.
29. Bunnag C, Dhorranintra B, Jareoncharsri P. Effect of allerglobuline injection on serum immunoglobulin levels in ENT patients. Asian Pac J Allergy Immunol 1991;9(1):45–50.
30. Jolles S, Hughes J, Rustin M. The treatment of atopic dermatitis with adjunctive high-dose intravenous immunoglobulin: a report of three patients and review of the literature. Br J Dermatol 2000;142(3):551–4.
31. Wiles CM, Brown P, Chapel H, Guerrini R, Hughes RA, Martin TD, McCrone P, Newsom-Davis J, Palace J, Rees JH, Rose MR, Scolding N, Webster AD. Intravenous immunoglobulin in neurological disease: a specialist review. J Neurol Neurosurg Psychiatry 2002;72(4):440–8.
32. Haskin JA, Warner DJ, Blank DU. Acute renal failure after large doses of intravenous immune globulin. Ann Pharmacother 1999;33(7–8):800–3.
33. Bolton-Maggs PH. The management of immune thrombocytopenic purpura. Curr Paediatr 2002;12:298–303.
34. Leen CL, Yap PL, Williams PE, McClelland DB. Tolerance of Scottish National Blood Transfusion Service intravenous immunoglobulin in patients with primary hypogammaglobulinaemia: report of 1235 infusions. Scott Med J 1988;33(4):303–6.
35. Imbach P, Barandun S, d'Apuzzo V, Baumgartner C, Hirt A, Morell A, Rossi E, Schoni M, Vest M, Wagner HP. High-dose intravenous gammaglobulin for idiopathic thrombocytopenic purpura in childhood. Lancet 1981;1(8232):1228–31.
36. Kurtzberg J, Friedman HS, Chaffee S, Falletta JM, Kinney TR, Kurlander R, Matthews TJ, Schwartz RS. Efficacy of intravenous gamma globulin in autoimmune-mediated pediatric blood dyscratias. AM J Med 1987;83(4A):4–9.
37. Kawano Y, Nissen C, Gratwohl A, Wursch A, Speck B. Cytotoxic and stimulatory effects of antilymphocyte globulin (ALG) on hematopoiesis. Blut 1990;60(5): 297–300.
38. Frickhofen N, Kaltwasser JP, Schrezenmeier H, Raghavachar A, Vogt HG, Herrmann F, Freund M, Meusers P, Salama A, Heimpel H. Treatment of aplastic anemia with antilymphocyte globulin and methylprednisolone with or without cyclosporine. The German Aplastic Anemia Study Group. N Engl J Med 1991;324(19):1297–304.
39. Debets JM, Leunissen KM, van Hooff HJ, van der Linden CJ, Buurman WA. Evidence of involvement of tumor necrosis factor in adverse reactions during treatment of kidney allograft rejection with antithymocyte globulin. Transplantation 1989;47(3):487–92.
40. de Planque MM, Brand A, Kluin-Nelemans HC, Eernisse JG, van der Burgh F, Natarajan AT, Beverstock GC, Zwaan FE, Willemze R, van Rood JJ. Haematopoietic and immunologic abnormalities in severe aplastic anaemia patients treated with anti-thymocyte globulin. Br J Haematol 1989;71(3):421–30.
41. Stangel M, Hartung HP, Marx P, Gold R. Intravenous immunoglobulin treatment of neurological autoimmune diseases. J Neurol Sci 1998;153(2):203–14.
42. Reinhart WH, Berchtold PE. Effect of high-dose intravenous immunoglobulin therapy on blood rheology. Lancet 1992;339(8794):662–4.
43. Machkhas H, Harati Y. Side effects of immunosuppressant therapies used in neurology. Neurol Clin 1998;16(1):171–88.
44. Woodruff RK, Grigg AP, Firkin FC, Smith IL. Fatal thrombotic events during treatment of autoimmune thrombocytopenia with intravenous immunoglobulin in elderly patients. Lancet 1986;2(8500):217–18.
45. Alliot C, Rapin JP, Besson M, Bedjaoui F, Messouak D. Pulmonary embolism after intravenous immunoglobulin. J R Soc Med 2001;94(4):187–8.
46. Crouch ED, Watson LE. Intravenous immunoglobulin-related acute coronary syndrome and coronary angiography in idiopathic thrombocytopenic purpura—a case report and literature review. Angiology 2002;53(1):113–17.
47. Emerson GG, Herndon CN, Sreih AG. Thrombotic complications after intravenous immunoglobulin therapy in two patients. Pharmacotherapy 2002;22(12):1638–41.
48. Byrne NP, Henry JC, Herrmann DN, Abdelhalim AN, Shrier DA, Francis CW, Powers JM. Neuropathologic findings in a Guillain–Barré patient with strokes after IVIg therapy. Neurology 2002;59(3):458–61.
49. Godeau B, Chevret S, Varet B, Lefrere F, Zini JM, Bassompierre F, Cheze S, Legouffe E, Hulin C, Grange MJ, Fain O, Bierling P; French ATIP Study Group. Intravenous immunoglobulin or high-dose methylprednisolone, with or without oral prednisone, for adults with untreated severe autoimmune thrombocytopenic purpura: a randomised, multicentre trial. Lancet 2002;359(9300):23–9.
50. Tristani-Firouzi P, Petersen MJ, Saffle JR, Morris SE, Zone JJ. Treatment of toxic epidermal necrolysis with intravenous immunoglobulin in children. J Am Acad Dermatol 2002;47(4):548–52.
51. Keohane SG, Kavanagh GM, Gordon PM, Hunter JAA. Transient hypertension during infusion of intravenous gammaglobulin for dermatomyositis. J Dermatol Treat 1999;10:287–8.
52. Dahl MV, Bridges AG. Intravenous immune globulin: fighting antibodies with antibodies. J Am Acad Dermatol 2001;45(5):775–83.
53. Bolanos-Meade J, Keung YK, Cobos E. Recurrent lymphocytic pleural effusion after intravenous immunoglobulin. Am J Hematol 1999;60(3):248–9.
54. Kishiyama JL, Valacer D, Cunningham-Rundles C, Sperber K, Richmond GW, Abramson S, Glovsky M, Stiehm R, Stocks J, Rosenberg L, Shames RS, Corn B, Shearer WT, Bacot B, DiMaio M, Tonetta S, Adelman DC. A multicenter, randomized, double-blind, placebo-controlled trial of high-dose intravenous immunoglobulin for oral corticosteroid-dependent asthma. Clin Immunol 1999;91(2):126–33.
55. Finkel AG, Howard JF Jr, Mann JD. Successful treatment of headache related to intravenous immunoglobulin with antimigraine medications. Headache 1998;38(4):317–21.
56. Wolfe GI, Barohn RJ, Foster BM, Jackson CE, Kissel JT, Day JW, Thornton CA, Nations SP, Bryan WW, Amato AA, Freimer ML, Parry GJ; Myasthenia Gravis-IVIG Study Group. Randomized, controlled trial of intravenous immunoglobulin in myasthenia gravis. Muscle Nerve 2002;26(4):549–52.
57. Ziegner UH, Kobayashi RH, Cunningham-Rundles C, Espanol T, Fasth A, Huttenlocher A, Krogstad P, Marthinsen L, Notarangelo LD, Pasic S, Rieger CH, Rudge P, Sankar R, Shigeoka AO, Stiehm ER, Sullivan KE, Webster AD, Ochs HD. Progressive neurodegeneration in patients with primary immunodeficiency disease on IVIG treatment Clin Immunol 2002;102(1): 19–24.

58. Jolles S, Hill H. Management of aseptic meningitis secondary to intravenous immunoglobulin. BMJ 1998; 316(7135):936.
59. Wittstock M, Benecke R, Zettl UK. Therapie mit intravenös applizierten Immunglobulinen (IVIg). Indikationen und Nebenwirkungen. Neurol Rehabil 2000;6:121–4.
60. Attout H, Mallet H, Desmurs H, Berthier S, Gil H, de Wazieres B, Dupond JL. Méningite aseptique au course d'un traitement par immunoglobulines intraveineuses a très faibles doses. [Aseptic meningitis during treatment with very low doses of intravenous immunoglobulins.] Rev Med Interne 1998;19(2):140–1.
61. Al-Ghamdi H, Mustafa MM, Al-Fawaz I, Al-Dowaish A. Acute aseptic meningitis associated with administration of immunoglobulin in children: a case of report and review of the literature. Ann Saudi Med 1999;19:362–4.
62. Obando I, Duran I, Martin-Rosa L, Cano JM, Garcia-Martin FJ. Aseptic meningitis due to administration of intravenous immunoglobulin with an unusually high number of leukocytes in cerebrospinal fluid. Pediatr Emerg Care 2002;18(6):429–32.
63. Sztajzel R, Le Floch-Rohr J, Eggimann P. High-dose intravenous immunoglobulin treatment and cerebral vasospasm: A possible mechanism of ischemic encephalopathy? Eur Neurol 1999;41(3):153–8.
64. Hazouard E, Sauvagnac X, Corcia P, Legras A, Dequin PF, Ginies G. Accident vasculaire transitoire possiblement lié aux immunoglobulines intraveineuses. [Transient vascular accident, possibly related to intravenous immunoglobulins.] Presse Méd 1998;27(4):161.
65. Tsiouris J, Tsiouris N. Hemiplegia as a complication of treatment of childhood immune thrombocytopenic purpura with intravenously administered immunoglobulin. J Pediatr 1998;133(5):717.
66. Turner B, Wills AJ. Cerebral infarction complicating intravenous immunoglobulin therapy in a patient with Miller Fisher syndrome. J Neurol Neurosurg Psychiatry 2000;68(6):790–1.
67. Choudhry VP, Mahapatra M, Kashyap R. Immunoglobulin therapy in immunohematological disorders. Indian J Pediatr 1998;65(5):681–90.
68. Stangel M, Muller M, Marx P. Adverse events during treatment with high-dose intravenous immunoglobulins for neurological disorders. Eur Neurol 1998;40(3):173–4.
69. Wills AJ, Unsworth DJ. A practical approach to the use of intravenous immunoglobulin in neurological disease. Eur Neurol 1998;39(1):3–8.
70. Nakagawa M, Watanabe N, Okuno M, Kondo M, Okagawa H, Taga T. Severe hemolytic anemia following high-dose intravenous immunoglobulin administration in a patient with Kawasaki disease. Am J Hematol 2000;63(3):160–1.
71. Kessary-Shoham H, Levy Y, Shoenfeld Y, Lorber M, Gershon H. In vivo administration of intravenous immunoglobulin (IVIg) can lead to enhanced erythrocyte sequestration. J Autoimmun 1999;13(1):129–35.
72. Ballot-Brossier C, Mortelecque R, Sinegre M, Marceau A, Dauriat G, Courtois F. Poursuite du traitement d'une polymyosite par les immunoglobulines intraveineuses polyvalentes malgré la survenue d'une anémie hémolytique sévère. [Insisting on intravenous polyvalent immunoglobulin therapy in polymyositis in spite of the occurrence of sever hemolytic anemia.] Transfus Clin Biol 2001;8(2):94–9.
73. Lee YC, Woodfield DG, Douglas R. Clinical usage of intravenous immunoglobulins in Auckland. NZ Med J 1998;111(1060):48–50.
74. Zelster D, Fusman R, Chapman J, Rotstein R, Shapira I, Elkayam O, Eldor A, Arber N, Berliner S. Increased leukocyte aggregation induced by gamma-globulin: a clue to the presence of pseudoleukopenia. Am J Med Sci 2000;320(3):177–82.
75. Comenzo RL, Malachowski ME, Meissner HC, Fulton DR, Berkman EM. Immune hemolysis, disseminated intravascular coagulation, and serum sickness after large doses of immune globulin given intravenously for Kawasaki disease. J Pediatr 1992;120(6):926–8.
76. Berkovitch M, Dolinski G, Tauber T, Aladjem M, Kaplinsky C. Neutropenia as a complication of intravenous immunoglobulin (IVIG) therapy in children with immune thrombocytopenic purpura: common and non-alarming. Int J Immunopharmacol 1999;21(6):411–15.
77. Frame WD, Crawford RJ. Thrombotic events after intravenous immunoglobulin. Lancet 1986;2(8504):468.
78. Go RS, Call TG. Deep venous thrombosis of the arm after intravenous immunoglobulin infusion: case report and literature review of intravenous immunoglobulin-related thrombotic complications. Mayo Clin Proc 2000; 75(1):83–5.
79. Elkayam O, Paran D, Milo R, Davidovitz Y, Almoznino-Sarafian D, Zeltser D, Yaron M, Caspi D. Acute myocardial infarction associated with high dose intravenous immunoglobulin infusion for autoimmune disorders. A study of four cases. Ann Rheum Dis 2000;59(1):77–80.
80. Paran D, Herishanu Y, Elkayam O, Shopin L, Ben-Ami R. Venous and arterial thrombosis following administration of intravenous immunoglobulins. Blood Coagul Fibrinolysis 2005;16(5):313–8.
81. Dilhuydy MS, Delclaux C, De Precigout V, Haramburu F, Roger I, Deminiere C, Mercie P, Pellegrin JL, Aparicio M. Insufficance rénale aiguë après cure d'immunoglobulines polyvalentes. [Acute renal failure after polyvalent immunoglobulin therapy.] Presse Méd 2000;29(17):942–3.
82. Levy JB, Pusey CD. Nephrotoxicity of intravenous immunoglobulin. QJM 2000;93(11):751–5.
83. Barton JC, Herrera GA, Galla JH, Bertoli LF, Work J, Koopman WJ. Acute cryoglobulinemic renal failure after intravenous infusion of gamma globulin. Am J Med 1987;82(3 Spec No):624–9.
84. Pasatiempo AM, Kroser JA, Rudnick M, Hoffman BI. Acute renal failure after intravenous immunoglobulin therapy. J Rheumatol 1994;21(2):347–9.
85. Jolles S, Hughes J, Whittaker S. Dermatological uses of high-dose intravenous immunoglobulin. Arch Dermatol 1998;134(1):80–6.
86. Stahl M, Schifferli JA. The renal risks of high-dose intravenous immunoglobulin treatment. Nephrol Dial Transplant 1998;13(9):2182–5.
87. Laidlaw S, Bainton R, Wilkie M, Makris M. Acute renal failure in acquired haemophilia following the use of high dose intravenous immunoglobulin. Haemophilia 1999;5(4):270–2.
88. Tsinalis D, Dickenmann M, Brunner F, Gurke L, Mihatsch M, Nickeleit V. Acute renal failure in a renal allograft recipient treated with intravenous immunoglobulin. Am J Kidney Dis 2002;40(3):667–70.
89. Ahsan N. Intravenous immunoglobulin induced-nephropathy: a complication of IVIG therapy. J Nephrol 1998;11(3):157–61.
90. Khalil M, Shin HJ, Tan A, DuBose TD Jr, Ordonez N, Katz RL. Macrophage like vacuolated renal tubular cells in the urine of a male with osmotic nephrosis associated with intravenous immunoglobulin therapy. A case report. Acta Cytol 2000;44(1):86–90.
91. Sokos DR, Berger M, Lazarus HM. Intravenous immunoglobulin: appropriate indications and uses in hematopoietic stem cell transplantation. Biol Blood Marrow Transplant 2002;8(3):117–30.
92. Sati HI, Ahya R, Watson HG. Incidence and associations of acute renal failure complicating high-dose intravenous immunoglobulin therapy. Br J Haematol 2001;113(2):556–7.

93. Noseworthy JH, O'Brien PC, Weinshenker BG, Weis JA, Petterson TM, Erickson BJ, Windebank AJ, Whisnant JP, Stolp-Smith KA, Harper CM Jr, Low PA, Romme LJ, Johnson M, An KN, Rodriguez M. IV immunoglobulin does not reverse established weakness in MS. Neurology 2000;55(8):1135–43.
94. Schmaldienst S, Mullner M, Goldammer A, Spitzauer S, Banyai S, Horl WH, Derfler K. Intravenous immunoglobulin application following immunoadsorption: benefit or risk in patients with autoimmune diseases? Rheumatology (Oxford) 2001;40(5):513–21.
95. Morikawa M, Yamada H, Kato EH, Shimada S, Kishi T, Yamada T, Kobashi G, Fujimoto S. Massive intravenous immunoglobulin treatment in women with four or more recurrent spontaneous abortions of unexplained etiology: down-regulation of NK cell activity and subsets. Am J Reprod Immunol 2001;46(6):399–404.
96. Howse M, Bindoff L, Carmichael A. Facial vasculitic rash associated with intravenous immunoglobulin. BMJ 1998;317(7168):1291.
97. Peker S, Kuwert C, Paus R, Moll I. Palmar lokalisierte vesikuläre läsionen nach der intravenösen applikation van immunglobulinen. H G Z Hautkr 2000;75:7–8.
98. Yebra M, Barrios Y, Rincon J, Sanjuan I, Diaz-Espada F. Severe cutaneous vasculitis following intravenous infusion of gammaglobulin in a patient with type II mixed cryoglobulinemia. Clin Exp Rheumatol 2002;20(2): 225–7.
99. Ballow M. Mechanisms of action of intravenous immunoglobulin therapy and potential use in autoimmune connective tissue diseases. Cancer 1991;68(Suppl 6):1430–6.
100. Chan-Lam D, Fitzsimons EJ, Douglas WS. Alopecia after immunoglobulin infusion. Lancet 1987;1(8547):1436.
101. Silver RM. Management of idiopathic thrombocytopenic purpura in pregnancy. Clin Obstet Gynecol 1998; 41(2):436–48.
102. Leclech C, Maillard H, Penisson-Besnier I, Laine-Cessac P, Verret JL. Réaction cutanée inhabituelle après perfusion intraveineuse d'immunoglobulines polyvalentes. [Unusual skin reaction after intravenous infusion of polyvalent immunoglobulins: 3 case reports.] Presse Méd 1999;28(10):531.
103. Ducluceau R. Les accidents de la sérothérapie antitétanique. Bull Med Leg Toxicol Med 1971;14:26.
104. Charpin J, Louchet E, Gratecos LA. Subsiste-t-il encore des réactions allergiques de la sérothérapie? [Does an allergic reaction to serotherapy still occur?] Mars Med 1969;106(3):223–6.
105. Bianchi R, Dappen U, Hoigné R. Der anaphylaktische Schock des Menschen auf artfremdes Serum. Symptomatologie, Prophylaxe und Therapie. [Anaphylactic shock of humans towards foreign species serum. Symptomatology, prevention and therapy.] Helv Chir Acta 1967;34(3):257–73.
106. World Health Organization. The collection, fractionation, quality control, and uses of blood and blood products. Geneva: WHO, 1981.
107. Delwaide PJ, Radermecker M, Boverie J. Deux cas de neuropathies multiples d'origine sérothérapique avec paralysie phrénique. [Two cases of multiple neuropathies of a serotherapeutic origin with phrenic paralysis.] Acta Neurol Psychiatr Belg 1967;67(6):452–62.
108. Czirner J, Besznyak G. Myokardinfarkt-ähnliches Bild als seltene Komplikation nach Applikation von Tetanus-Antitoxin. [Myocardial infarct-like clinical picture as a rare complication following the application of tetanus antitoxin.] Z Gesamte Inn Med 1969;24(4):119–21.
109. Humphrey JH, White RG. Reactions due to antigen-antibody complexes (nephritis in man). Immunology for Students of Medicine. 3rd ed. Oxford: Blackwell Scientific Publications, 1970:458.
110. Suarez-Lopez J, Sanchez-Salorio M, Sanchez-Lado J. Uveitis exudativa de caracter sero-anafiláctico. Arch Soc Oftalmol Hisp-Am 1965;25:499.
111. Williams PE, Yap PL, Gillon J, Crawford RJ, Galea G, Cuthbertson B. Non-A, non-B hepatitis transmission by intravenous immunoglobulin. Lancet 1988;2(8609):501.
112. Avoy DR. Delayed serum sickness-like transfusion reactions in a multiply transfused patient. Vox Sang 1981;41(4):239–44.
113. Liblau R, Morel E, Bach JF. Autoimmune diseases, IgA deficiency, and intravenous immunoglobulin treatment. Am J Med 1992;93(1):114–15.
114. Nydegger UE. Intravenous immunoglobulin in combination with other prophylactic and therapeutic measures. Transfusion 1992;32(1):72–82.
115. Hachimi-Idrissi S, de Schepper J, de Waele M, Dab I, Otten J. Type III allergic reaction after infusion of immunoglobulins. Lancet 1990;336(8706):55.
116. McCluskey DR, Boyd NA. Anaphylaxis with intravenous gammaglobulin. Lancet 1990;336(8719):874.
117. Myer I, Andler W. Die Behandlung der idiopathischen thrombozytopenischen Purpura. Krankenhausarzt 1987;60:105.
118. John R, Lietz K, Burke E, Ankersmit J, Mancini D, Suciu-Foca N, Edwards N, Rose E, Oz M, Itescu S. Intravenous immunoglobulin reduces anti-HLA alloreactivity and shortens waiting time to cardiac transplantation in highly sensitized left ventricular assist device recipients. Circulation 1999;100(Suppl 19):II229–35.
119. Brox AG, Cournoyer D, Sternbach M, Spurll G. Hemolytic anemia following intravenous gamma globulin administration. Am J Med 1987;82(3 Spec No):633–5.
120. Chapman JF, Murphy MF, Berney SI, Ord J, Metcalfe P, Amess JA, Waters AH. Post-transfusion purpura associated with anti-Baka and anti-PIA2 platelet antibodies and delayed haemolytic transfusion reaction. Vox Sang 1987;52(4):313–7.
121. Lucas GS, Jobbins K, Bloom AL. Intravenous immunoglobulin and blood group antibodies. Lancet 1987;2(8561):742.
122. Ovesen H, Taaning E, Christensen BA. Posttransfusionel purpura (PTP) forarsaget af anti-Zwb (P1P2). [Posttransfusion purpura caused by ant-Zw b (P1(A2)).] Ugeskr Laeger 1986;148(43):2769–70.
123. Slichter SJ. Post-transfusion purpura: response to steroids and association with red blood cell and lymphocytotoxic antibodies. Br J Haematol 1982;50(4):599–605.
124. Teeling JL, Bleeker WK, Hack CE, Kuijpers TW. Nieuwe inzichten in het ontstaan van bijwerkingen van intraveneuze immunoglobuline (IVIG)-preparaten. Ned Tijdschr Allergie 2001;1:20–5.
125. Ikeda M, Hamasaki Y, Hataya H, Honda M, Sugai K. Multiorgan failure induced by intravenous immunoglobulin. Acta Paediatr 2000;89(11):1393.
126. Seiffert J, Brendel W, Lob G, et al. Improvement of the compatibility of ALG. Behring Inst Mitt 1972;51:255.
127. Schifferli J, Leski M, Favre H, Imbach P, Nydegger U, Davies K. High-dose intravenous IgG treatment and renal function. Lancet 1991;337(8739):457–8.
128. Woodruff RK, Grigg AP, Firkin FC, Smith IL. Fatal thrombotic events during treatment of autoimmune thrombocytopenia with intravenous immunoglobulin in elderly patients. Lancet 1986;2(8500):217–18.
129. Jayne DR, Davies MJ, Fox CJ, Black CM, Lockwood CM. Treatment of systemic vasculitis with pooled intravenous immunoglobulin. Lancet 1991;337(8750):1137–9.
130. Doney KC, Weiden PL, Storb R, Thomas ED. Treatment of graft-versus-host disease in human allogeneic marrow graft recipients: a randomized trial comparing

antithymocyte globulin and corticosteroids. Am J Hematol 1981;11(1):1–8.
131. Kheirbek AO, Molnar ZV, Choudhury A, Geis WP, Daugirdas JT, Hano JE, Ing TS. Malignant lymphoma in a renal transplant recipient treated with antithymocyte globulin. Transplantation 1983;35(3):267–8.
132. Turner CE, Thorpe SJ, Brasher MD, Thorpe R. Anti-Rh D activity of commercial intravenous immunoglobulin preparations. Vox Sang 1999;76(1):55–8.
133. Yap PL. Intravenous immunoglobulin and hepatitis C virus: an overview of transmission episodes with emphasis on manufacturing data. Clin Ther 1996;18(Suppl B):43–58.
134. Chidwick K, Matejtschuk P, Gascoigne E, Briggs N, More JE, Dash CH. Clinical experience with a new solvent detergent-treated intravenous immunoglobulin free of hypotensive effects. Vox Sang 1999;77(4):204–9.
135. Milgrom H. Shortage of intravenous immunoglobulin. Ann Allergy Asthma Immunol 1998;81(2):97–100.
136. Hayakawa F, Imada K, Towatari M, Saito H. Life-threatening human parvovirus B19 infection transmitted by intravenous immune globulin. Br J Haematol 2002;118(4):1187–9.
137. Azzari C, Resti M, Moriondo M, Gambineri E, Rossi ME, Novembre E, Vierucci A. Lack of transmission of TT virus through immunoglobulins. Transfusion 2001;41(12):1505–8.
138. Misbah SA, Chapel HM. Adverse effects of intravenous immunoglobulin. Drug Saf 1993;9(4):254–62.
139. Nydegger UE. Safety and side effects of i.v. immunoglobulin therapy. Clin Exp Rheumatol 1996;14(Suppl 15):S53–7.
140. Hern S, Harman K, Bhogal BS, Black MM. A severe persistent case of pemphigoid gestationis treated with intravenous immunoglobulins and cyclosporin. Clin Exp Dermatol 1998;23(4):185–8.
141. Enk AH, Knop J. Adjuvante Therapie von Pemphigus vulgaris und Pemphigus foliaceus mit intravenösen Immunoglobulinen. [Adjuvant therapy of pemphigus vulgaris and pemphigus foliaceus with intravenous immunoglobulins.] Hautarzt 1998;49(10):774–6.
142. Colonna L, Cianchini G, Frezzolini A, De Pita O, Di Lella G, Puddu P. Intravenous immunoglobulins for pemphigus vulgaris: adjuvant or first choice therapy? Br J Dermatol 1998;138(6):1102–3.
143. Bagdasarian A, Tonetta S, Harel W, Mamidi R, Uemura Y. IVIG adverse reactions: potential role of cytokines and vasoactive substances. Vox Sang 1998;74(2):74–82.
144. Bassilios N, Mercadal L, Deray G. Immunoglobulin as a risk factor for contrast media nephrotoxicity. Nephrol Dial Transplant 2001;16(7):1513–14.
145. Lawn N, Wijdicks EF, Burritt MF. Intravenous immune globulin and pseudohyponatremia. N Engl J Med 1998;339(9):632.
146. Ng SK. Intravenous immunoglobulin infusion causing pseudohyponatremia. Lupus 1999;8(6):488–90.

Immunotherapy

General Information

Desensitization is used in the treatment of IgE-mediated disease. Increasing doses of an allergen are injected subcutaneously over a varying time span. The aim of the treatment is to decrease sensitivity to the allergen and prevent the clinical symptoms caused by exposure to the allergen. Following immunotherapy, there can be an initial rise in specific serum IgE to the allergen, followed by a fall in specific IgE and a rise in specific IgG (blocking antibody). Immunotherapy also leads to reduced mediator release from mast cells in vitro, altered lymphocyte subsets, and down-regulation of cytokine secretion (interleukins 2, 4, and 5) by T cells (1).

It has been estimated that 60 million patients receive this treatment annually (2). Bearing in mind that about 40% of the population have atopy and that about half of these develop clinical disease ranging from rhinitis to life-threatening asthma, the scope for an effective and safe programme of desensitization is very large. However, there is no consensus on which extracts should be used, how often therapy should be given, and how long it should be continued if there is clinical improvement.

Efficacy

As far as the efficacy of immunotherapeutic desensitization is concerned, the merits of the treatment must be judged on the basis of:

1. Relief of symptoms and signs—a reduction in the response of a target organ to the specific allergen. In pollen rhinoconjunctivitis, a reduced response to the instillation of pollen into the conjunctival sac would be relevant. A reduction in the skin reaction to the specific allergen, especially a reduction in the late phase skin response (IgE-mediated), may be demonstrated. In asthma, a reduction in the specific bronchial response to inhaled allergen with an associated reduction in non-specific reactivity (measured by histamine or methacholine provocation) would indicate a response to treatment.
2. A reduction in or elimination of drug treatment.

Risks of desensitization

The risks of desensitization have to be set against the chance of benefits. The dominant risk is that of an allergic reaction. Subcutaneous injection of allergenic extracts can lead variously to:

- a transient wheal and flare at the injection site
- a localized delayed subcutaneous swelling with itching
- a systemic reaction in which urticaria, asthma, and hypotension may occur, the reaction not being severe enough to be classified as anaphylaxis
- anaphylaxis.

Large local reactions should be managed by a temporary reduction in the dose of the allergen, the use of antihistamines if needed, and ice applied to the injection site. Systemic reactions may resolve spontaneously or after one injection of adrenaline.

Anaphylaxis can be fatal and requires immediate treatment and measures to prevent recurrence. The Committee on Safety of Medicines, in a report cited below, recommended that allergenic products should only be given when facilities for full cardiopulmonary resuscitation are immediately available and that patients should be kept under medical observation for at least 2 hours after receiving an injection (3).

There is at present no evidence of any undesirable long-term adverse effect of repeated courses of allergenic extracts, although non-allergic individuals may develop hypersensitivity, particularly when they receive extracts that contain aluminium. An isolated case of extensive subcutaneous inflammation and fibrosis with overlying skin changes was seen in a patient after 5 months of maintenance therapy (SEDA-17, 207).

The extent and timing of the risk has been delineated in some individual studies. In 419 patients treated with extracts of grass pollen or house dust mite adsorbed on to aluminium hydroxide, local reactions occurred in 10.5% and systemic reactions in 4.8% (4). In a survey of 27 806 injections there were 143 (0.51%) systemic reactions, of which 83% were mild and 17% (that is five reactions) needed treatment with adrenaline (5).

In a 10-year review (1981–91) of the reactions caused by subcutaneous immunotherapy, when 192 505 injections were given to 2206 outpatients, there were 115 systemic reactions, with no deaths. The most frequent reaction (67% of the total) was asthma with urticaria, while asthma alone occurred in 22%. Systemic reactions were much more frequent in asthmatic patients, although one-third of patients with reactions had never previously suffered from asthma. Most systemic reactions occurred during maintenance therapy. Almost always a reaction occurred within 30 minutes of the injection and was promptly controlled by routine therapy (SEDA-21, 189).

Improved formulations

It has been suggested that tyrosine-absorbed formulations with relatively short half-lives may be more dangerous in terms of immediate anaphylaxis. The alumpyridine formulation Allpyral has a long half-life, and in the UK over 4 million injections have been given with no deaths reported. Most allergen extracts are today in fact alum-precipitated, thus slowing absorption of the allergen, providing sustained immune stimulation and reducing the risk of serious anaphylaxis. Further modifications of standard allergens have been tried. Interaction between formaldehyde and allergen extract causes changes in the net charge of the allergen proteins and their tertiary structure. This reduces allergenicity/IgE-binding activity but retains immunogenicity, allowing more "allergoid" than untreated allergen to be injected before anaphylactic symptoms occur. At the higher doses tolerated a higher specific IgG concentration results. The adsorption of the allergoid on to aluminium hydroxide results in a depot formulation.

Enzyme-potentiated allergen is formed when low doses of allergen are mixed with beta-glucuronidase. It has been claimed that this formulation of allergen results in minimal or no adverse effects (6).

An alternative to injection treatment is oral immunotherapy. Gastric protein degradation prevents the use of orally administered peptide immunotherapy, but an oral delivery system using enteric-protected antigen protopolysaccharide microspheres has been developed. These formulations have been assessed in clinical trials, but to date the patient numbers have been too small to allow any useful conclusions about efficacy or the risk of adverse effects (SEDA-21, 189) (SEDA-21, 190) (SEDA-22, 196).

Benefit to harm balance

The benefit to harm balance in desensitization treatment was examined in a meta-analysis published in 1995, covering 20 randomized, placebo-controlled, double-blind trials of allergen immunotherapy for asthma. Systemic reactions occurred in a mean of 32% (20–44%) of patients, but anaphylaxis was reported on only four occasions. It was concluded that immunotherapy was a treatment option in highly selected patients with extrinsic allergic asthma where a clinically relevant and unavoidable allergen is identified (7).

The US Food and Drug Administration appointed a panel of experts to review desensitization therapy in 1974. The panel concluded that extracts used in accordance with generally accepted principles are associated with a minimal and acceptable risk of immediate reaction.

The Committee on Safety of Medicines reviewed the UK experience with desensitization in 1986, weighing efficacy against risk. They considered the evidence for efficacy and found it convincing for ragweed pollen, bee and wasp venom, and some antibiotics, but thought the evidence for grass pollen and house-dust mite less convincing. The Committee warned of the dangers of anaphylaxis and bronchospasm and noted that 26 patients had died since 1957, 5 in the preceding 18 months. With different products the risk of death varied from one in 8000 to one in 321 750 with no deaths recorded with some formulations. Anaphylaxis and bronchospasm had been reported with all formulations, the incidence varying from one in 300 to one in 14 998 (3).

The Committee on Allergen Standardization of the American Academy of Allergy and Immunology investigated 46 fatalities that occurred during immunotherapy or skin testing. They noted that the nature and severity of the initial symptoms did not appear to predict the fatal outcome or indicate the cause of death (SEDA-13, 136). In the 5 years from 1985 to 1989, 17 deaths due to allergen immunotherapy were reported, of which 16 were in patients with asthma. None occurred with skin testing. Unstable asthma or accidental overdoses were major contributory factors. The annual fatality rate in the USA from administration of allergenic extracts is low, at one fatality per 2 million doses (8).

Risk management

Some circumstances of special risk can be identified and avoided (9). The frequency of systemic reaction varies from less than 1% in patients receiving conventional immunotherapy to more than 36% in patients receiving rush immunotherapy. Common risk factors for a fatal or systemic reaction include a history of asthma, increasing allergen dose, high allergen sensitivity, a previous systemic reaction and injection during the active allergen season.

The Canadian Society of Allergy and Clinical Immunology have published guidelines for the use of allergen immunotherapy and these are similar to those developed by the American Academy of Allergy, Asthma, and Immunology. They recommend therapy with specific, standardized allergenic materials, administered in high-dose schedules, to patients with allergy to insect stings or allergic rhinoconjunctivitis, and in some patients with asthma. The latter should be correctly diagnosed by a meticulous history, confirmed by positive skin tests and be insufficiently controlled by allergen avoidance and appropriate drug treatment (10).

The Thoracic Society of Australia and New Zealand and the Australasian Society of Immunology and Allergy have published guidelines for the use of specific allergen immunotherapy in the treatment of asthma patients (2). These should be read by practitioners who are considering immunotherapy for patients, especially those with asthma, who have a higher risk of a serious systemic reaction.

Specific allergens

Dermatophagoides farinae

The incidence of adverse systemic reactions during immunotherapy for perennial allergic rhinitis using standardized extracts of *Dermatophagoides farinae* has been estimated in 386 patients who received 22 722 injections. The incidence of systemic reactions was 6.22% per patient and 0.12% per injection. Systemic reactions began 3–30 minutes after an injection (average 11 minutes). Asthma, atopic dermatitis, and a high concentration of IgE (but not specific IgE) in serum were identified as important risk factors for severe systemic reactions. Systemic reactions occurred in 12 of 18 patients who had an IgE concentration over 100 U/ml and asthma and/or atopic dermatitis. In patients who had none of these risk factors the incidence of systemic reaction was 1.64% per patient. The authors estimated that the rate of systemic reactions could be reduced by 75% if patients with identified risk factors were strictly excluded from immunotherapy for allergic rhinitis (11).

Insect venoms

The efficacy of desensitization using subcutaneous maintenance venom immunotherapy is well established and is usually considered in patients with severe systemic allergic reactions to both yellow jacket and bee venom (grade III or IV according to Mueller).

Among 160 patients who were mostly allergic to bee venom and who were assessed for systemic allergic reactions to sting challenges while increasing the intervals of maintenance venom immunotherapy from 4–6 weeks to 3 months there were no serious adverse events (12). Two of 44 patients, who were deliberately stung during the 3-monthly maintenance therapy, had a mild systemic reaction. After withdrawal of venom immunotherapy, 22 patients allergic to bee venom were sting-challenged; one had a mild systemic reaction. In conclusion, the conventional 4–6 week maintenance interval can be safely extended to 3 months in most patients without any adverse events.

In 36 patients with a history of systemic reactions (grade III or IV according to Mueller) after exposure to a wasp sting, who were given immunotherapy with aluminium hydroxide-adsorbed wasp venom extract in an open retrospective study, a maintenance monthly depot of 50 000 SQU (50 micrograms) of venom was used (13). After the first year, the dose was injected every other month. Desensitization therapy was well tolerated. There were few mild local adverse events. Thirteen patients were exposed to stings during maintenance immunotherapy and four after withdrawal at the end of the 5-year treatment period. Field stings only provoked local skin reactions.

Near-fatal anaphylaxis, a rare complication of immunotherapy, has been reported (14).

- A 55-year-old man was stung by a *Polistes* wasp and had an anaphylactic reaction. Intradermal skin tests with wasp venoms were negative. Intradermal honeybee venom 1.0 microgram/ml and *Polistes* wasp venom 0.1 microgram/ml produced induration and erythema. Venom immunotherapy was given using the protocol of the Bayer Corporation: monthly maintenance injections of Bayer honeybee venom and *Polistes* wasp venom, 100 micrograms of each for 13 months without incident. Because of a national shortage of *Polistes* wasp venom manufactured by Bayer, *Polistes* wasp venom manufactured by ALK was substituted. Within minutes of receiving injections of 100 micrograms of Bayer honeybee venom and ALK *Polistes* wasp venom (both from new vials) he became light-headed and developed syncope. He recovered consciousness but remained hypotensive (74/0 mmHg). In a serum sample 2 hours after the start of the reaction serum tryptase was raised at 38 micrograms/ml (reference range 5.6–14 micrograms/ml) and IgE anti-honeybee venom and IgE anti-*Polistes* wasp venom concentrations were 3 and 10 ng/ml respectively.

The authors performed RAST inhibition to measure the relative potencies of the different venom extracts using the patient's serum as a source of IgE anti-venom. Although they initially suspected the new source of *Polistes* wasp venom, the relative potency tests showed greater variation in the honeybee venom. The IgG concentrations were consistent with this finding. This report emphasizes the care that must be taken with the preparation of each injection, especially when using a new batch of antigen.

Serum sickness has been described as a result of immunotherapy for wasp venom hypersensitivity. The illness was severe and treatment with glucocorticoids and seven plasma exchanges was required to induce a remission. There were two further relapses requiring the same treatment before recovery (SEDA-22, 197).

A follow-up of patients for 5 years after stopping venom immunotherapy has been reported. The authors concluded that the residual risk of a systemic reaction to a sting was 5–10% in adults. No severe or life-threatening reactions occurred with 270 challenge stings in 74 patients after 1–5 years without venom immunotherapy. The authors have extended these observations to 5–10 years and attempted to identify patients at greater risk of a reaction. Patients were surveyed for 3 consecutive years to determine the frequency of systemic reactions to field stings and the course of venom sensitivity. The patients included the original 74 (group 1) and 51 other patients followed after stopping venom immunotherapy (group 2). Eleven of the 74 patients in group 1 had field stings again after 3–7 years without venom immunotherapy. One systemic reaction (dyspnea) was reported. Of the 51 patients in group 2, 15 were stung, of whom 4 (26%) had systemic reactions, including respiratory symptoms necessitating the use of adrenaline. Six of the 13 patients (groups 1 and 2) with a systemic reaction to a sting after stopping venom immunotherapy had had a systemic reaction during venom immunotherapy (to an injection or a sting). Only six of 76 patients who had no reaction during venom immunotherapy had a systemic reaction when stung after cessation of venom immunotherapy. Other risk factors were persistent strongly positive skin test sensitivity and the severity of the pretreatment reaction (15).

References

1. van Bever HP, Vereecke IF, Bridts CH, De Clerck LS, Stevens WJ. Comparison between the in vitro cytokine production of mononuclear cells of young asthmatics with and without immunotherapy (IT). Clin Exp Allergy 1998;28(8):943–9.
2. Position Statement. Specific allergen immunotherapy for asthma. A position paper of the Thoracic Society of Australia and New Zealand and the Australasian Society of Clinical Immunology and Allergy. Med J Aust 1997;167(10):540–4.
3. CSM. Update. Desensitising vaccines. BMJ (Clin Res Ed) 1986;293:948.
4. Tabar AI, Garcia BE, Rodriguez A, Olaguibel JM, Muro MD, Quirce S. A prospective safety-monitoring study of immunotherapy with biologically standardized extracts. Allergy 1993;48(6):450–3.
5. Matloff SM, Bailit IW, Parks P, Madden N, Greineder DK. Systemic reactions to immunotherapy. Allergy Proc 1993;14(5):347–50.
6. Astarita C, Scala G, Sproviero S, Franzese A. Effects of enzyme-potentiated desensitization in the treatment of pollinosis: a double-blind placebo-controlled trial. J Investig Allergol Clin Immunol 1996;6(4):248–55.
7. Abramson MJ, Puy RM, Weiner JM. Is allergen immunotherapy effective in asthma? A meta-analysis of randomized controlled trials. Am J Respir Crit Care Med 1995;151(4):969–74.
8. Reid MJ, Lockey RF, Turkeltaub PC, Platts-Mills TA. Survey of fatalities from skin testing and immunotherapy 1985–1989. J Allergy Clin Immunol 1993;92(1 Pt 1):6–15.
9. Greineder DK. Risk management in allergen immunotherapy. J Allergy Clin Immunol 1996;98(6 Pt 3):S330–4.
10. Anonymous. Guidelines for the use of allergen immunotherapy. Canadian Society of Allergy and Clinical Immunology. CMAJ 1995;152(9):1413–19.
11. Ohashi Y, Nakai Y, Tanaka A, Kakinoki Y, Washio Y, Ohno Y, Yamada K, Nasako Y. Risk factors for adverse systemic reactions occurring during immunotherapy with standardized *Dermatophagoides farinae* extracts Acta Otolaryngol Suppl 1998;538:113–17.
12. Tattersfield AE, Town GI, Johnell O, Picado C, Aubier M, Braillon P, Karlstrom R. Bone mineral density in subjects with mild asthma randomised to treatment with inhaled corticosteroids or non-corticosteroid treatment for two years. Thorax 2001;56(4):272–8.
13. Harris M, Hauser S, Nguyen TV, Kelly PJ, Rodda C, Morton J, Freezer N, Strauss BJ, Eisman JA, Walker JL. Bone mineral density in prepubertal asthmatics receiving corticosteroid treatment. J Paediatr Child Health 2001;37(1):67–71.
14. Wolf BL, Hamilton RG. Near-fatal anaphylaxis after *Hymenoptera* venom immunotherapy J Allergy Clin Immunol 1998;102(3):527–8.
15. Golden DB, Kwiterovich KA, Kagey-Sobotka A, Lichtenstein LM. Discontinuing venom immunotherapy: extended observations. J Allergy Clin Immunol 1998;101(3):298–305.

Indanediones

General Information

Indanediones have the same anti-vitamin K action as the coumarins. However they are generally more toxic than the coumarins, and can cause allergic reactions capable of involving many organs and sometimes resulting in death (1). These reactions are mainly observed with phenindione and are very rare with other indanediones, such as fluindione.

In an MRC trial (2), a 2.25% incidence of reactions necessitated withdrawal of phenindione.

Organs and Systems

Cardiovascular

As with the coumarins, the main complication of the indanediones is bleeding. The incidence of hemorrhage varies, depending on the age of the patient, the intensity of treatment, and the indication for using an anticoagulant. Hematuria, bruising, and gastrointestinal bleeding are the commonest signs. The most common site of fatal hemorrhage is intracranial (3).

Hematologic

Agranulocytosis can occur during the first month of treatment with phenindione (4). Anemia, thrombocytopenia (5), and leukemoid reactions (6) have also been described.

Liver

Hepatitis can rarely occur during indanedione treatment, most often with phenindione, although occasionally with fluindione (7,8). The mechanism is probably allergic. Resistance to treatment may be associated with the appearance of this reaction (8).

Urinary tract

Phenindione can cause renal insufficiency and the nephrotic syndrome, usually preceded by fever and skin reactions. In such cases, renal biopsy shows interstitial edema with infiltration by eosinophils and plasma cells. Tubular necrosis has also been observed(9).

Skin

Skin reactions are the commonest manifestations of allergic reactions. They generally occur during the first month of treatment and include erythematous, scarlatiniform, papular, and urticarial rashes, sometimes accompanied by fever. Severe exfoliative dermatitis has been reported (10,11).

Skin necrosis can occur during therapy with phenindione (12), as it does with the coumarin congeners.

Second-Generation Effects

Lactation

Massive neonatal scrotal hematoma occurred while the breast-feeding mother was taking phenindione (13).

References

1. Perkins J. Phenindione sensitivity. Lancet 1962;1:127–30.
2. Report of the Working Party on Anticoagulant Therapy in Coronary Thrombosis to the Medical Research Council. Assessment of short-anticoagulant administration after cardiac infarction. BMJ 1969;1(640):335–42.
3. Lacroix P, Portefaix O, Boucher M, Ramiandrisoa H, Dumas M, Ravon R, Christides C, Laskar M. Condition de survenue des accidents hémorragiques intracraniens des antivitamines K. [The causes of intracranial hemorrhagic complications induced by antivitamins K.] Arch Mal Coeur Vaiss 1994;87(12):1715–19.
4. Ager JA, Ingram GI. Agranulocytosis during phenindione therapy. BMJ 1957;(5027):1102–3.
5. Farwell C. Thrombocytopenia due to phenindione (Hedulin) sensitivity; report of a case. Med Ann Dist Columbia 1959;28(2):82.
6. Wright JS. Phenindione sensitivity with leukaemoid reaction and hépato-renal damage. Postgrad Med J 1970;46(537):452–5.
7. Biour M, Davy JM, Poynard T, Levy VG. La fluindione est-elle hepatotoxique? [Is fluindione hepatotoxic?] Gastroenterol Clin Biol 1990;14(10):782.
8. Penot JP, Fontenelle P, Dorleac D. Hépatite aiguë cytolytique asymptomatique à la fluindione s'accompagnant d'une resistance au traitement. A propos d'un cas. Revue de la litterature. [Asymptomatic acute cytolytic hepatitis due to fluindione and associated with resistance to treatment: a case report and review of the literature.] Arch Mal Coeur Vaiss 1998;91(2):267–70.
9. Smith K. Acute renal failure in phenindione sensitivity. BMJ 1965;5452:24–6.
10. Hollman A, Wong HO. Phenindione sensitivity. BMJ 1964;5411:730–2.
11. Copeman PW. Phenindione toxicity. BMJ 1965;5456:305.
12. Eldon K, Lindahl F. Hudnekroser efter behandling med fenindion (Dindevan). [Skin necrosis after treatment with phenindione (Dindevan).] Ugeskr Laeger 1980; 142(15):965.
13. Eckstein HB, Jack B. Breast-feeding and anticoagulant therapy. Lancet 1970;1(7648):672–3.

Indapamide

See also Diuretics

General Information

Indapamide is a thiazide-like diuretic. Although it was introduced as a specific antihypertensive drug without appreciable diuretic action, the effects of indapamide are no different from those of bendroflumethiazide.

Organs and Systems

Sensory systems

Transient myopia associated with diffuse choroidal thickening has been described in a 38-year-old white man who had taken indapamide for hypertension; it resolved after withdrawal (1).

Metabolism

The metabolic effects of indapamide appear to be as common as those of thiazides (SEDA-14, 185) (SEDA-15, 216). The metabolic effects of hydrochlorothiazide 25 mg/day and indapamide 2.5 mg/day for 6 months have been compared in a randomized, double-blind study in 44 patients with mild to moderate hypertension (2). There was little difference between the effects of the drugs on a wide range of lipid parameters, glucose, and potassium. The purported metabolic differences with indapamide are unlikely to be of sufficient magnitude to warrant its preferential use in hyperlipidemia.

Electrolyte balance

Cases of severe indapamide-induced hypokalemia have been reported (SED-11, 424) (SEDA-15, 213).

Liver

Severe acute hepatitis associated with indapamide has been reported (3). Serum bilirubin and liver enzymes were greatly raised. All normalized over 6 months after withdrawal of indapamide.

Urinary tract

Interstitial nephritis leading to acute renal insufficiency has been reported with indapamide (4).

Skin

Hypersensitivity to indapamide can provoke serious adverse skin reactions (SEDA-17, 260) (SEDA-18, 234).

One patient had several episodes of fixed drug eruption during treatment with indapamide (5). The diagnosis was confirmed by positive controlled oral challenge.

Pemphigus foliaceus has been described in relation to indapamide (6).

Drug–Drug Interactions

Sulfamethoxazole

The possibility of cross-reactivity with other sulfonamide derivatives was investigated by controlled oral challenge tests with sulfamethoxazole, sulfadiazine, and furosemide. The test with sulfamethoxazole was positive.

References

1. Blain P, Paques M, Massin P, Erginay A, Santiago P, Gaudric A. Acute transient myopia induced by indapamide. Am J Ophthalmol 2000;129(4):538–40.
2. Spence JD, Huff M, Barnett PA. Effects of indapamide versus hydrochlorothiazide on plasma lipids and

lipoproteins in hypertensive patients: a direct comparison. Can J Clin Pharmacol 2000;7(1):32–7.
3. Safer L, Ben Mimoun H, Brahem A, Hanza J, Harzallah S, Abdellati S, Bdioui F, Saffar H. Severe acute hepatitis induced by indapamide. Report of a case. Sem Hop Paris 1998;74:1274.
4. Newstead CG, Moore RH, Barnes AJ. Interstitial nephritis associated with indapamide. BMJ 1990;300(6735):1344.
5. De Barrio M, Tornero P, Zubeldia JM, Sierra Z, Matheu V, Herrero T. Fixed drug eruption induced by indapamide. Cross-reactivity with sulfonamides. J Investig Allergol Clin Immunol 1998;8(4):253–5.
6. Bayramgurler D, Ercin C, Apaydin R, Unal G. Indapamide-induced pemphigus foliaceus. J Dermatol Treat 2001;12(3):175–7.

Indinavir

See also Protease inhibitors

General Information

Indinavir is an HIV protease inhibitor.

Organs and Systems

Cardiovascular

A hypertensive crisis caused a secondary reversible posterior leukoencephalopathy in a patient taking indinavir-containing antiretroviral therapy (1).

- A 40-year-old man, who had taken stavudine 30 mg bd, lamivudine 150 mg bd, and indinavir 800 mg qds, developed an occipital headache, nausea, and vomiting. His blood pressure was 220/140 mmHg and he had bilateral papilledema. His blood pressure was controlled and his symptoms disappeared. An MRI scan of the brain showed lesions in the periventricular white matter; the nuclei semiovale and occipital asta were most severely affected. Indinavir was withdrawn and replaced by nelfinavir; his blood pressure returned to normal and the MRI white matter lesions disappeared.

In a retrospective analysis of 198 normotensive patients in a protease inhibitor comparison study, 30% of those who took indinavir developed stage I or worse hypertension, compared with none of the patients who took nelfinavir, ritonavir, or saquinavir (2).

Respiratory

Shock and respiratory failure have been attributed to indinavir (3).

- A 36-year-old HIV-positive man had started to take zidovudine and zalcitabine 9 months earlier together with co-trimoxazole as primary prophylaxis against *Pneumocystis jiroveci*, but switched to indinavir, stavudine, and lamivudine. Two hours after the first dose of indinavir he developed a high fever, generalized myalgia, and malaise and started to vomit. After the second dose he developed shock and cyanosis. A chest X-ray was compatible with adult respiratory distress syndrome. All cultures were negative for bacterial, viral, mycobacterial, and fungal pathogens. He recovered in 6 days and antiretroviral treatment without indinavir was reintroduced without recurrent problems.

The authors suggested that the severe shock and respiratory distress syndrome had been due to an idiosyncratic reaction to indinavir.

Nervous system

There has been a report of painful neuropathy in two patients who took ritonavir and indinavir respectively (4).

Paraparesis due to epidural lipomatosis has been attributed to indinavir (5).

- A 35-year-old man, who had taken indinavir 2400 mg/day, lamivudine 300 mg/day, and stavudine 80 mg/day for 10 months, developed a slowly progressive paraparesis, with sensory disturbances in the legs. An MRI scan was consistent with epidural lipomatosis. On withdrawal of indinavir, the symptoms gradually resolved.

Although indinavir can cause abnormal fat accumulation, this is thought to have been the first report of epidural lipomatosis.

Metabolism

Protease inhibitors are associated with hyperglycemia and possible diabetes mellitus. In a prospective study in 12 patients indinavir caused hyperglycemia and reduced insulin sensitivity (6).

Hematologic

Indinavir has been associated with severe hemolytic anemia (7).

- A 32-year-old Caucasian, who was taking lamivudine, stavudine, and indinavir for HIV infection, presented with pallor following a period of fatigue and headache (8). His hemoglobin was 8.2 g/dl and there were no clinical findings to suggest bleeding. The reticulocyte count was 3.5% and a direct Coombs' test was negative. A diagnosis of hemolytic anemia secondary to indinavir was made, the indinavir was stopped, and he was transfused with concentrated erythrocytes. The other antiretroviral drugs were continued, saquinavir was added, and a normal hemoglobin concentration was maintained.

Indinavir has been associated with thrombocytopenia (9).

Liver

Indinavir has been compared with abacavir in a randomized equivalence trial in 562 patients who were also taking lamivudine and zidovudine (10). The only significant difference in adverse effects was that there was hyperbilirubinemia in 8% of those taking indinavir and 2% of those taking abacavir. It has been postulated that indinavir-induced hyperbilirubinemia is due to inhibition of bilirubin UDP glucuronyl transferase activity, since it is more common in individuals with Gilbert's syndrome (11).

Urinary tract

Indinavir causes nephrolithiasis as a result of precipitation of indinavir crystals in the urinary tract (12,13). It is dose-related and can be prevented by adequate hydration. In 615 patients (18 864 person-years of follow-up) who did not have risk factors for nephrolithiasis, the incidence was 8.6 episodes per 1000 person-years (14).

Several reports have suggested that patients using indinavir may also develop a syndrome consisting of back or flank pain, accompanied by crystalluria, renal function abnormalities, and evidence of tubulointerstitial nephritis on renal biopsy, but without obvious renal calculus formation (15–17).

In a French analysis of 22 510 urinary calculi performed by infrared spectroscopy, drug-induced urolithiasis was divided into two categories: first, stones with drugs physically embedded ($n = 238$; 1.0%), notably indinavir monohydrate ($n = 126$; 53%), followed by triamterene ($n = 43$; 18%), sulfonamides ($n = 29$; 12%), and amorphous silica ($n = 24$; 10%); secondly, metabolic nephrolithiasis induced by drugs ($n = 140$; 0.6%), involving mainly calcium + vitamin D supplementation ($n = 56$; 40%) and carbonic anhydrase inhibitors ($n = 33$; 24%) (18). Drug-induced stones are responsible for about 1.6% of all calculi in France. Physical analysis and a thorough drug history are important elements in the diagnosis.

The incidence of urolithiasis with indinavir has been estimated at 9% (19) but, according to some, may be as high as 20%. Indinavir calculi are often radiolucent and may be missed on CT scan rather than by using a contrast medium (which is itself not without risk) (20,21). It may therefore be that in some cases in which other renal complications with indinavir have been described there was in fact undetected renal stone formation. Any patient taking indinavir who develops renal colic should be suspected of having renal stones (22).

In two cases long-term use of indinavir appeared to have been responsible for renal atrophy (23), and again one wonders whether crystals may have been present but radiologically invisible.

Reversible renal insufficiency (which again could have been due to crystalluria) has been reported with indinavir (24).

- A 38-year-old man developed renal insufficiency while taking indinavir. His serum creatinine increased over a period of about 1 year, but urinalysis was persistently normal. A renal biopsy showed marked tubular crystal deposition. The indinavir was withdrawn, and after 2 months his serum creatinine returned to normal.

Since the basic problem in many such cases is probably crystalluria, it should be possible to treat it with rehydration, perhaps supplemented by brief interruption of therapy; this has been the conclusion of a study in which the unwanted renal effects of indinavir were prominent (25). Of 74 individuals infected with HIV-1 and taking indinavir 2.4 g/day orally, 15 had indinavir-related urological adverse effects (19 episodes), most commonly dull flank pain and dysuria. Microhematuria occurred in 16 of the 19 episodes. Four patients had urinary tract distension on ultrasonography as a possible indirect sign of urolithiasis and one passed a stone. In 4 patients treatment had to be stopped permanently, but in the other 11 it was continued. Some patients required dosage reduction and/or interruption of treatment: only conservative therapeutic measures were required, consisting of rehydration (fluid intake of at least 1.5 l/day) and analgesics.

Of 23 indinavir-treated patients with persistent pyuria, four had interstitial nephritis, seven had urothelial inflammation, 10 had both interstitial nephritis and urothelial inflammation, and two had non-specific urinary tract inflammation (26). In all, 21 patients had multinucleated histiocytes identified by cytological testing of urine specimens. Urine abnormalities resolved in all 20 patients who stopped taking indinavir, and pyuria persisted in the other 3. Six patients had raised serum creatinine concentrations, which returned to baseline when indinavir was withdrawn.

Skin

HIV-positive/AIDS patients using indinavir develop rashes early in treatment, a finding that is familiar with various other drugs used in this condition. This problem has been quantified in a study using data from postmarketing surveillance (27). Of 110 HIV/AIDS patients with a rash, 67% reported that it had occurred within 2 weeks of the start of indinavir therapy. The rash was initially localized in all cases, but in the majority it went on to spread to other body areas, involving all parts of the body in no less than 44%. It was usually pruritic but not accompanied by fever. Relief was often obtained by use of topical antihistamines or oral or topical glucocorticoids. More than half the patients decided to continue therapy despite the rash.

However, cutaneous toxicity can have a major influence on adherence to treatment and can impact adversely on the quality of life. Of 84 patients taking indinavir plus two nucleoside reverse transcriptase inhibitors for 20 months, 48 developed cheilitis, 34 had skin dryness and pruritus, 10 developed asteatotic dermatitis on the trunk, arms, and thighs, and 10 complained of scalp defluvium (28). Severe alopecia was observed in one patient, while six reported that their body hair had become fairer and thinner and shed considerably. Multiple pyogenic granulomas were observed in the toenails of five patients and softening of the nail plate was noted in five. The temporal relation between starting indinavir and the onset of these effects was striking and regression occurred on withdrawal.

Suggested mechanisms for these adverse effects include:

- retinoid-like effects due to homologies of the amino acid sequences of the HIV-1 protease and cytoplasmic retinoic-acid binding protein type 1 (CRABP-1)
- inhibition of CYP3A by indinavir, resulting in reduced oxidation of retinoic acid and hence augmentation of its biological effects.

Hair

Alopecia has been attributed to indinavir in 10 men (29). Of 337 patients who were given indinavir as part of combination antiretroviral therapy with nucleoside analogues, five (1.5%) developed severe alopecia a median of 50 days after starting indinavir. Three had diffuse shedding of hair involving the entire scalp, and two were initially aware of circumscribed circular areas of alopecia resulting in complete severe hair loss. Although indinavir was discontinued in all five cases, there was no regrowth a median of 30 days later (30).

Nails

Paronychia associated with indinavir has been reported (31,32). In 288 patients in a retrospective cohort study, paronychia was associated with indinavir, with a hazard ratio of 4.7 (33).

Musculoskeletal

Increased bone mineral density has been documented in patients taking indinavir (34) although in another study protease inhibitor-containing regimens caused accelerated loss of bone density (35).

- Widespread osteosclerosis, accompanied by increased serum concentrations of osteocalcin and C telopeptide, developed in a 56-year-old man who took indinavir 800 mg tds for 27 months (36).

This patient had been taking vitamin A 1 mg/day for 20 years and the authors proposed that the indinavir had also had a vitamin A-like effect.

Frozen shoulder has been attributed to indinavir (SEDA-24, 347) (37). In one case it was associated with Dupuytren's contracture and in one case each with arthralgias and tendinitis (38). An adhesive capsulitis seems to be present.

The results of a questionnaire survey of 878 people with HIV infection treated with antiretroviral drugs confirmed the risk of arthralgias in patients taking indinavir. The authors suggested that crystal deposition in joints, analogous to the crystalluria with nephrolithiasis that indinavir and other protease inhibitors can cause, might be responsible.

Susceptibility Factors

Sex

The pharmacokinetics of indinavir in 220 women and 94 men have been compared; there was no difference (39).

Drug–Drug Interactions

Cannabinoids

The effects of smoked marijuana (3.95% tetrahydrocannabinol; up to three cigarettes per day) and oral dronabinol (2.5 mg tds) on the pharmacokinetics of indinavir 800 mg 8-hourly ($n = 28$) have been evaluated in a randomized, placebo-controlled study in HIV-infected patients (40). On day 14, marijuana reduced the 8-hour AUC of indinavir by 15%, the C_{max} by 14%, and the C_{min} by 34%. However, only the change in C_{max} was significant. Dronabinol had no effects.

Carbamazepine

Failure of combination therapy including indinavir has been attributed to an interaction of indinavir with carbamazepine (41).

- A 48-year-old HIV-positive man taking indinavir, zidovudine, and lamivudine developed *Herpes zoster* infection, which was treated with famciclovir. Postherpetic neuralgia was treated with carbamazepine, and his plasma indinavir concentration fell substantially. The carbamazepine was withdrawn after 2.5 months and 2 weeks later HIV-RNA was detectable in his plasma (6×10^3/ml). His circulating virus was resistant to lamivudine. With a further increase in viral load, his therapy was changed to nevirapine, didanosine, and stavudine.

This treatment failure, and possibly the resistance to lamivudine, was attributed to induction of drug metabolism by carbamazepine.

Didanosine

The absorption of indinavir was not affected by co-administration of didanosine in an encapsulated enteric bead formulation in 24 patients (42).

Levothyroxine

Inhibition of glucuronyl transferase activity by indinavir has been blamed for an interaction of indinavir with levothyroxine, causing hyperthyroidism (43).

- A 36-year-old woman, who had taken levothyroxine for several years, took stavudine, lamivudine, and indinavir for 1 month and developed nervousness, palpitation, restlessness, weakness, and weight loss. She had an undetectable serum TSH concentration and raised unbound serum T4 and T3. The dose of levothyroxine was reduced to one-third and then to one-sixth of the previous dose, and the thyroid function tests returned to normal.

Phenylpropanolamine

In one case the use of phenylpropanolamine with triple drug therapy for HIV prophylaxis led to a hypertensive crisis (44). As the patient had previously tolerated phenylpropanolamine well, one must suspect that one or more of the anti-HIV drugs (probably indinavir) had interfered with the metabolic breakdown of the phenylpropanolamine.

Ritonavir

Using ritonavir as a booster may allow indinavir to be given twice daily and with food. In a cohort survey of 100 patients the combination of indinavir plus ritonavir (400 mg/400 mg or 800 mg/100 mg bd) was a safe and effective option to reduce the tablet burden and improve adherence (45).

Sildenafil

There is good evidence that indinavir can substantially increase plasma concentrations of sildenafil (46). Since HIV infection commonly leads to erectile dysfunction, the drugs may well be used together and it will then be prudent to use a lower dose of sildenafil.

Silybum marianum (milk thistle)

The pharmacokinetics of indinavir 800 mg 8-hourly have been studied in the presence and absence of milk thistle 175 mg (containing silymarin 153 mg) tds for 3 weeks in an open study in 10 healthy volunteers; milk thistle had no significant effect except a small reduction in $C_{min.ss}$ (47).

Venlafaxine

Venlafaxine 50 mg 8-hourly reduced the AUC of a single dose of indinavir 800 mg by 28% in nine healthy subjects (48).

Diagnosis of Adverse Drug Reactions

The adverse effects of indinavir have been retrospectively evaluated and correlated with indinavir trough concentration in 63 patients taking indinavir + ritonavir 800/100 mg bd (49). The median indinavir trough concentration of 1446 ng/ml was associated with 60% of measured toxicity. Of 49 patients with an indinavir trough concentration over 500 ng/ml, 46 had at least one dosage adjustment; the main reason for dosage adjustment was toxicity ($n = 43$). The common adverse effects affected the skin (vitamin A-like reactions; $n = 39$), kidneys (renal colic, nephrolithiasis, renal insufficiency; $n = 35$), gastrointestinal tract (nausea, vomiting, and diarrhea; $n = 32$), and liver ($n = 14$). After dosage adjustment, the median indinavir trough concentration was 459 ng/ml, which was associated with 8% of toxicity. Trough concentrations over 500 ng/ml correlated with increased toxicity. The authors concluded that indinavir trough concentrations below 500 ng/ml are safe, and that an optimal concentration range for indinavir trough concentration could be 150–500 ng/ml in patients taking twice daily indinavir + ritonavir.

References

1. Giner V, Fernandez C, Esteban MJ, Galindo MJ, Forner MJ, Guix J, Redon J. Reversible posterior leukoencephalopathy secondary to indinavir-induced hypertensive crisis: a case report. Am J Hypertens 2002;15(5):465–7.
2. Cattelan AM, Trevenzoli M, Sasset L, Rinaldi L, Balasso V, Cadrobbi P. Indinavir and systemic hypertension. AIDS 2001;15(6):805–7.
3. Dieleman JP, in 't Veld B, Borleffs JC, Schreij G. Acute respiratory failure associated with the human immunodeficiency virus (HIV) protease inhibitor indinavir in an HIV-infected patient. Clin Infect Dis 1998;26(4):1012–13.
4. Colebunders R, De Droogh E, Pelgrom Y, Depraetere K, De Jonghe P. Painful hyperaesthesia caused by protease inhibitors? Infection 1998;26(4):250–1.
5. Cersosimo MG, Lasala B, Folgar S, Micheli F. Epidural lipomatosis secondary to indinavir in an HIV-positive patient. Clin Neuropharmacol 2002;25(1):51–4.
6. Dube MP, Edmondson-Melancon H, Qian D, Aqeel R, Johnson D, Buchanan TA. Prospective evaluation of the effect of initiating indinavir-based therapy on insulin sensitivity and B cell function in HIV-infected patients. J Acquir Immune Defic Syndr 2001;27(2):130–4.
7. Morrison-Griffiths S, Newman M, O'Mahony C, Pirmohamed M. Haemolytic anaemia associated with indinavir. Postgrad Med J 1999;75(883):313–15.
8. Watson A. Reversible acute haemolysis associated with indinavir. AIDS 2000;14(4):465–6.
9. Durand JM. Indinavir and thrombocytopenia. AIDS 1999;13(1):148–9.
10. Staszewski S, Keiser P, Montaner J, Raffi F, Gathe J, Brotas V, Hicks C, Hammer SM, Cooper D, Johnson M, Tortell S, Cutrell A, Thorborn D, Isaacs R, Hetherington S, Steel H, Spreen W; CNAAB3005 International Study Team. Abacavir–lamivudine–zidovudine vs indinavir–lamivudine–zidovudine in antiretroviral-naive HIV-infected adults: A randomized equivalence trial. JAMA 2001;285(9):1155–63.
11. Sen S, Jalan R. Is "Gilbert's" the culprit in indinavir-induced hyperbilirubinemia? Hepatology 2002;35(5):1269–70.
12. Pietroski NA. Treating HIV with protease inhibitors. Drug efficacy, tolerability, and dosing. Am Druggist 1996;213:50–7.
13. Tsao JW, Kogan SC. Images in clinical medicine. Indinavir crystalluria. N Engl J Med 1999;340(17):1329.
14. Dworkin MS, Wan PT. Indinavir, zidovudine, lamivudine: 3-year follow-up. Ann Intern Med 2001;134(2):165.
15. Kopp JB, Miller KD, Mican JA, Feuerstein IM, Vaughan E, Baker C, Pannell LK, Falloon J. Crystalluria and urinary tract abnormalities associated with indinavir. Ann Intern Med 1997;127(2):119–25.
16. Tashima KT, Horowitz JD, Rosen S. Indinavir nephropathy. N Engl J Med 1997;336(2):138–40.
17. Chen SC, Nankivell BJ, Dwyer DE. Indinavir-induced renal failure. AIDS 1998;12(4):440–1.
18. Cohen-Solal F, Abdelmoula J, Hoarau MP, Jungers P, Lacour B, Daudon M. Les lithiases urinaires d'origine médicamenteuse. [Urinary lithiasis of medical origin.] Therapie 2001;56(6):743–50.
19. Hermieu J, Prevot M, Ravery V, Sauty L, Moulinier F, Delmas V, Bouvet E, Boccon-Gibod L. Urolithiasis and the protease inhibitor indinavir. Eur Urol 1999;35(3):239–41.
20. Schwartz BF, Schenkman N, Armenakas NA, Stoller ML. Imaging characteristics of indinavir calculi. J Urol 1999;161(4):1085–7.
21. Sundaram CP, Saltzman B. Urolithiasis associated with protease inhibitors. J Endourol 1999;13(4):309–12.
22. Kohan AD, Armenakas NA, Fracchia JA. Indinavir urolithiasis: an emerging cause of renal colic in patients with human immunodeficiency virus. J Urol 1999;161(6):1765–8.
23. Hanabusa H, Tagami H, Hataya H. Renal atrophy associated with long-term treatment with indinavir. N Engl J Med 1999;340(5):392–3.
24. Grabe DW, Eisele G, Miller C, Singh J, Stein D. Indinavir-induced nephropathy. Clin Nephrol 1999;51(3):181–3.
25. Hug B, Naef M, Bucher HC, Sponagel L, Lehmann K, Battegay M. Treatment for human immunodeficiency virus with indinavir may cause relevant urological side-effects, effectively treatable by rehydration. BJU Int 1999;84(6):610–14.
26. Sokal E. Lamivudine for the treatment of chronic hepatitis B. Expert Opin Pharmacother 2002;3(3):329–39.
27. Gajewski LK, Grimone AJ, Melbourne KM, Vanscoy GJ. Characterization of rash with indinavir in a national patient cohort. Ann Pharmacother 1999;33(1):17–21.
28. Calista D, Boschini A. Cutaneous side effects induced by indinavir. Eur J Dermatol 2000;10(4):292–6.
29. Bouscarat F, Prevot MH, Matheron S. Alopecia associated with indinavir therapy. N Engl J Med 1999;341(8):618.
30. d'Arminio Monforte A, Testa L, Gianotto M, Gori A, Franzetti F, Sollima S, Bini T, Moroni M. Indinavir-related alopecia. AIDS 1998;12(3):328.

31. Dauden E, Pascual-Lopez M, Martinez-Garcia C, Garcia-Diez A. Paronychia and excess granulation tissue of the toes and finger in a patient treated with indinavir. Br J Dermatol 2000;142(5):1063–4.
32. Sass JO, Jakob-Solder B, Heitger A, Tzimas G, Sarcletti M. Paronychia with pyogenic granuloma in a child treated with indinavir: the retinoid-mediated side effect theory revisited. Dermatology 2000;200(1):40–2.
33. Colson AE, Sax PE, Keller MJ, Turk BK, Pettus PT, Platt R, Choo PW. Paronychia in association with indinavir treatment. Clin Infect Dis 2001;32(1):140–3.
34. Nolan D, Upton R, McKinnon E, John M, James I, Adler B, Roff G, Vasikaran S, Mallal S. Stable or increasing bone mineral density in HIV-infected patients treated with nelfinavir or indinavir. AIDS 2001;15(10): 1275–80.
35. Tebas P, Powderly WG, Claxton S, Marin D, Tantisiriwat W, Teitelbaum SL, Yarasheski KE. Accelerated bone mineral loss in HIV-infected patients receiving potent antiretroviral therapy. AIDS 2000;14(4):F63–7.
36. Begovac J, Bayer K, Krpan D, Kusec V. Osteosclerosis and periostal new bone formation during indinavir therapy. AIDS 2002;16(5):803–4.
37. Peyriere H, Mauboussin JM, Rouanet I, Rouveroux P, Hillaire-Buys D, Balmes P. Frozen shoulder in HIV patients treated with indinavir: report of three cases. AIDS 1999;13(16):2305–6.
38. Cooper CL, Parbhakar MA, Angel JB. Hepatotoxicity associated with antiretroviral therapy containing dual versus single protease inhibitors in individuals coinfected with hepatitis C virus and human immunodeficiency virus. Clin Infect Dis 2002;34(9):1259–63.
39. Burger DM, Siebers MC, Hugen PW, Aarnoutse RE, Hekster YA, Koopmans PP. Pharmacokinetic variability caused by gender: do women have higher indinavir exposure than men? J Acquir Immune Defic Syndr 2002;29(1):101–2.
40. Kosel BW, Aweeka FT, Benowitz NL, Shade SB, Hilton JF, Lizak PS, Abrams DI. The effects of cannabinoids on the pharmacokinetics of indinavir and nelfinavir. AIDS 2002;16(4):543–50.
41. Hugen PW, Burger DM, Brinkman K, ter Hofstede HJ, Schuurman R, Koopmans PP, Hekster YA. Carbamazepine–indinavir interaction causes antiretroviral therapy failure. Ann Pharmacother 2000;34(4):465–70.
42. Damle BD, Mummaneni V, Kaul S, Knupp C. Lack of effect of simultaneously administered didanosine encapsulated enteric bead formulation (Videx EC) on oral absorption of indinavir, ketoconazole, or ciprofloxacin. Antimicrob Agents Chemother 2002;46(2):385–91.
43. Lanzafame M, Trevenzoli M, Faggian F, Marcati P, Gatti F, Carolo G, Concia E. Interaction between levothyroxine and indinavir in a patient with HIV infection. Infection 2002;30(1):54–5.
44. Khurana V, de la Fuente M, Bradley TP. Hypertensive crisis secondary to phenylpropanolamine interacting with triple-drug therapy for HIV prophylaxis. Am J Med 1999;106(1):118–19.
45. Burger DM, Hugen PW, Aarnoutse RE, Dieleman JP, Prins JM, van der Poll T, ten Veen JH, Mulder JW, Meenhorst PL, Blok WL, van der Meer JT, Reiss P, Lange JM. A retrospective, cohort-based survey of patients using twice-daily indinavir + ritonavir combinations: pharmacokinetics, safety, and efficacy J Acquir Immune Defic Syndr 2001;26(3):218–24.
46. Merry C, Barry MG, Ryan M, Tjia JF, Hennessy M, Eagling VA, Mulcahy F, Back DJ. Interaction of sildenafil and indinavir when co-administered to HIV-positive patients. AIDS 1999;13(15):F101–7.
47. Piscitelli SC, Formentini E, Burstein AH, Alfaro R, Jagannatha S, Falloon J. Effect of milk thistle on the pharmacokinetics of indinavir in healthy volunteers. Pharmacotherapy 2002;22(5):551–6.
48. Levin GM, Nelson LA, DeVane CL, Preston SL, Eisele G, Carson SW. A pharmacokinetic drug–drug interaction study of venlafaxine and indinavir. Psychopharmacol Bull 2001;35(2):62–71.
49. Solas C, Basso S, Poizot-Martin I, Ravaux I, Gallais H, Gastaut JA, Durand A, Lacarelle B. High indinavir Cmin is associated with higher toxicity in patients on indinavir–ritonavir 800/100 mg twice-daily regimen. J Acquir Immune Defic Syndr 2002;29(4):374–7.

Indometacin

See also Non-steroidal anti-inflammatory drugs

General Information

Indometacin is the best-known and most thoroughly tested indoleacetic acid derivative. It is one of the most effective NSAIDs, and most of its toxic and therapeutic effects appear to be due to marked inhibition of prostaglandin synthesis. Because of its potency, its clinical efficacy is comparable, if not superior, to any other NSAID, but for precisely the same reason its adverse effects on the gastrointestinal tract and the nervous system inevitably limit its use. However, patients who tolerate it reasonably well are naturally not anxious to exchange it for any newer drugs with fewer problems but less potency. A meta-analysis of patients' preference in 37 crossover comparisons of indometacin with newer NSAIDs did not provide evidence of a trend to replace indometacin with newer NSAIDs (1).

Tropesin is the tropic acid ester of indometacin, and its adverse effects profile is similar to that of indometacin (SEDA-17, 113).

General adverse reactions

Adverse effects, in up to 60% of patients, are closely related to indometacin's strong anti-inflammatory potency. Gastric irritation, including ulcers, bleeding, and perforation, predominates. Nervous system complications are related to cerebral edema. Headache is common. Hematological effects are infrequently reported. Nephrotoxicity is exacerbated by pre-existing renal impairment. Ocular toxicity can follow long-term use.

Cross-reactivity with aspirin has been reported (2). The hazards of administering topical indometacin to asthmatic patients should be widely known (3).

Tumor-induced effects have not been demonstrated.

Organs and Systems

Cardiovascular

Clinical experience and reports have provided little evidence that indometacin precipitates angina or myocardial infarction. However, an individual angina-provoking effect has been documented (4), and there are grounds for believing that it can happen.

Intravenous administration of indometacin increases blood pressure, coronary vascular resistance, and myocardial oxygen demands, decreasing coronary flow. A controlled short-term study showed that indometacin increased blood pressure in patients with mild untreated essential hypertension (SEDA-17, 108). In view of the increasing use of parenteral administration, the acute hemodynamic effects of indometacin may now occur more often, especially in the elderly (5). The mechanism is poorly understood, but apparently a direct action is exerted on the resistance vessels in various regions. This is probably independent of indometacin's action on prostaglandin formation. The clinical relevance is largely unknown, but other NSAIDs should probably be prescribed for patients with occlusive vascular diseases affecting the cerebral and/or coronary vessels.

Other systemic cardiovascular adverse effects are due to salt and fluid retention and also to a reduction in the vasodilator action of circulating prostaglandins E_2 and I_2 (6).

Unlike other NSAIDs, indometacin acts as a cerebral vasoconstrictor. It reduces cerebral flow by up to 35% and the response to hypercapnia disappears (SEDA-10, 79). It also reduces blood flow in the splanchnic vascular bed, by increasing local vascular resistance, but does not impair circulation in the forearm and leg muscles.

Respiratory

Inhibition of prostaglandin synthesis explains indometacin's ability to provoke or aggravate asthma in hypersensitive patients (7). Indometacin in ophthalmic solution reportedly caused such deterioration in asthmatic patients as to require mechanical ventilation (3,8). Cross-sensitivity between indometacin and aspirin has been observed.

Nervous system

Adverse reactions to indometacin involving the central nervous system are frequent and come second in importance only to gastrointestinal effects. They are attributed to salt and water retention. Up to 60% of patients experience headache (often migraine-like), frontal throbbing, and vertigo. Vomiting, tinnitus, ataxia, tremor, dizziness, and insomnia follow. Somnolence, confusion, hallucinations (especially in the elderly), and psychotic symptoms have been described. Coma, clonic seizures, and myoclonic spasms (SEDA-18, 101) can develop. Muscle weakness and paresthesia, that is, peripheral neuropathy, may develop in elderly patients, but recede after withdrawal (9,10).

Indometacin is used for non-invasive closure of symptomatic ductus arteriosus in the preterm infant. Intravenous administration causes an instant reduction in cerebral blood flow, increasing cerebral vascular resistance. The clinical significance for the nervous system of these hemodynamic changes is unknown (11,12), but they seem to be linked to the effects seen in the central nervous system. Advantage has been taken of this effect for reducing intracranial hypertension in patients with severe head injury (SEDA-15, 99).

Indometacin is also used in preterm infants as prophylaxis against intraventricular hemorrhage. In a prospective, randomised, placebo-controlled trial in 431 preterm neonates, low-dose indometacin prevented intraventricular hemorrhage without adverse cognitive or motor outcomes at 36 months (13).

Low-dose indometacin (0.1 mg/kg), begun in the first 24 hours of life and given every 24 hours for 6 doses, was not associated with adverse neurodevelopmental outcome at 36 months corrected age (14).

Sensory systems

Prolonged therapy can cause a number of adverse reactions in the eyes. Trivial effects are ocular discomfort, conjunctival pain, and increased ocular tension, but mydriasis, photophobia, blurred vision, diplopia, amblyopia, and loss of vision can occur. The most serious complications are retinopathy with reduced retinal sensitivity, and corneal and retinal pigmentation. They are reversible, but improvement is slow. A report on indometacin retinopathy has added more doubt than certainty to the question of the frequency and severity of retinal toxicity (SEDA-14, 93). Patients taking prolonged therapy should have regular ophthalmic examinations.

Metabolism

Indometacin reduces the area under the corticotropin (ACTH) plasma concentration–time curve after insulin in normal men, possibly because of the role of prostaglandins in the control of ACTH secretion (15).

One report has described low plasma ascorbic acid concentrations during indometacin treatment, and a case of hyperglycemia has been reported (16).

Electrolyte balance

Hyperkalemia has been reported in patients with preexisting renal disease treated with indometacin (SEDA-4, 65) (SEDA-5, 90) (SEDA-6, 93) and in a patient with Bartter's syndrome receiving concomitant oral potassium chloride (SEDA-11, 92) (17). Indometacin caused a high serum potassium concentration in a young athlete (SEDA-14, 93).

Mineral balance

During indometacin therapy, urinary excretion of zinc and calcium can increase significantly (18). The clinical relevance is not known.

Fluid balance

Salt and fluid retention is an adverse effect of indometacin, although it is less important than with the pyrazolone derivatives. Indometacin can antagonize antihypertensive agents, including beta-adrenoceptor antagonists (19,20). The effect on blood pressure in normotensive patients has not been adequately studied.

Severe water intoxication caused by inappropriate ADH secretion has been described in an elderly woman taking indometacin (SEDA-17, 108).

Hematologic

Anemia caused by repetitive gastrointestinal bleeding is a relatively frequent, although indirect, hematological adverse effect.

Blood dyscrasias, sometimes fatal aplastic anemia (21), isolated granulocytopenia, and agranulocytosis have been reported (22). The International Agranulocytosis and Aplastic Anemia study showed that indometacin was significantly associated with agranulocytosis and aplastic anemia (23).

Since indometacin is an inhibitor of platelet aggregation, impairment of thrombocyte function is frequent, but thrombocytopenia is rare. Severe clotting defects due to inhibition of platelet aggregation in premature infants have been described (24). Postoperative bleeding is significantly more frequent in indometacin-treated patients. Indometacin should probably not be used postoperatively in patients at increased risk of bleeding (SEDA-8, 103).

Gastrointestinal

Gastrotoxicity is the main adverse effect of indometacin, and symptoms range from abdominal discomfort to ulcer penetration and perforation (25). The phenomenon of gastric mucosal adaptation has been evoked to explain the relatively low incidence of severe adverse effects, compared with the acute gastric damage that occurs in short-term studies. In healthy volunteers, indometacin produced acute gastroduodenal damage in all cases, but resolved in almost all, despite continuing administration. The author hypothesized that the severity of mucosal damage depends on the reduction in mucosal blood flow (SEDA-16, 108) (SEDA-17, 108).

Small bowel ulceration with thickening of the bowel wall and stricture formation in the terminal ileum and the ileocecal junction occurred in a patient with rheumatoid arthritis taking long-term indometacin (SEDA-12, 84). This is one reason why prolonged courses of indometacin should be avoided whenever possible, especially in elderly women.

Osmosin, a formulation that contains potassium bicarbonate and releases indometacin osmotically, was withdrawn because of reports of intestinal irritation, bleeding, perforation, and even death. These adverse effects were most probably caused by the very high local concentrations of indometacin and potassium in the lower part of the gastrointestinal tract produced by the tablet, which shifted the adverse reactions from the stomach to the intestine (SEDA-8, 103) (26).

Like other NSAIDs, a diaphragm-like right-sided colonic stricture has been described in a woman taking indometacin suppositories (27). Perforation of colonic diverticula has been described (28).

The use of indometacin suppositories can be associated with rectal irritation, mucosal inflammation, or necrosis with bleeding (29). The local effect on the gastric mucosa is less important than the systemic one, and suppositories do not cause fewer gastric lesions than oral formulations (30).

Liver

Despite reversible changes in liver enzyme tests (31) and a fatal case of acute hepatocellular necrosis, which may have been related to indometacin, the drug is rarely hepatotoxic (32). Indometacin-associated cholestatic liver injury has been described. The reaction was not severe and recovery was rapid and uneventful (33).

Urinary tract

Indometacin nephrotoxicity is rare in patients with normal renal function, but indometacin can aggravate preexisting renal impairment, as has been observed in patients with glomerulonephritis, nephrotic syndrome, systemic lupus erythematosus, and cirrhosis complicated by ascites (SED-8, 219) (SEDA-4, 65) (SEDA-7, 108) (SEDA-11, 85). Severe but reversible loss of renal function in patients with systemic lupus erythematosus in the absence of active renal disease suggests that mesangial contraction in the glomerulus could significantly reduce the capillary surface area available for filtration and hence reduce the glomerular filtration rate (34,35). There is a significant reduction in the glomerular filtration rate and a concomitant drop in renal excretion of sodium and water in patients with compensated cirrhosis without ascites treated with indometacin (SEDA-18, 101).

Probable indometacin-induced renal papillary necrosis has been described in two patients with chronic juvenile arthritis (SEDA-8, 103).

Reversible acute renal insufficiency with eosinophilia has been described (36).

The harmful effect of indometacin on renal function has been used therapeutically to induce medical nephrectomy (SEDA-7, 108).

Skin

Reactions to indometacin range from urticaria and pruritus to fixed rashes, purpura, and maculopapular and morbilliform eruptions. Toxic epidermal necrolysis has also been described (37). The frequency of skin reactions is lower than with pyrazolone derivatives. There is cross-sensitivity with aspirin.

Whether indometacin exacerbates psoriasis is not certain, but one report (38) suggests that it can.

Indometacin can exacerbate dermatitis herpetiformis (SEDA-10, 81).

Musculoskeletal

Progressive destruction of large weight-bearing hip joints was first observed during long-term indometacin therapy more than 25 years ago (SEDA-11, 87) (39). In one comparison of the effects of azapropazone and indometacin, the osteoarthritic process in the hip progressed more quickly in patients treated with indometacin, no doubt a further indication of its powerful inhibitory effect on prostaglandin synthesis (40). The mechanisms responsible for the harmful effect of NSAIDs on osteoarthritic joints have been reviewed (SEDA-11, 87).

Sexual function

Inhibition of prostaglandin synthesis can cause impotence. A healthy man became impotent while taking short-term indometacin 150 mg/day (SEDA-5, 101).

Immunologic

Masking of infection and abnormal immune reactions have been reported (41). It is not clear whether this has any clinical significance.

Second-Generation Effects

Fertility

Ovulation was inhibited by indometacin at high doses in the preovulatory period (SEDA-16, 109).

Pregnancy

The use of indometacin in late pregnancy has been much debated. Because of its ability to inhibit prostaglandin synthesis it can be used to arrest premature labor for a short time, although there is no evidence that it reduces the incidence of premature delivery. The hazards of using it as a tocolytic agent seem to outweigh any theoretical advantage, since there are many reports of serious adverse neonatal effects after the treatment of preterm labor with indometacin. They include premature closure of the ductus arteriosus, pulmonary hypertension with persistent fetal circulation, fetal anuria, severe oligohydramnios, necrotizing enterocolitis, perinatal death, and severe respiratory distress syndrome resulting in oxygen dependence for several days (SED-11, 179) (42–44) (SEDA-5, 101) (SEDA-6, 93) (SEDA-7, 108) (SEDA-8, 102) (SEDA-9, 88) (SEDA-12, 84) (SEDA-15, 99) (SEDA-16, 109) (SEDA-17, 108). The risks might be linked to the duration of use, but one study provided evidence that short-term indometacin can cause closure of the ductus arteriosus, even if several weeks elapse between treatment and delivery (45).

The risks involved in longer-term use are multiple, as several studies have shown. The use of indometacin and ibuprofen for more than 72 hours in 67 women in preterm labor was significantly associated with more oligohydramnios than either ritodrine or magnesium sulfate. Oligohydramnios developed in 70% of 37 women treated with indometacin, in 27% treated with ibuprofen, and in 2 controls (46).

Pregnant women taking beta-blockers for hypertension in pregnancy should not be given indometacin, as it can raise the blood pressure (47).

Teratogenicity

Indometacin in pregnancy is probably safe, provided its use is limited to the first 32 weeks of gestation. However, a possible teratogenic effect has been ascribed to it (48).

Cerebral ischemia has been described in premature twins following maternal use of indometacin (49).

The incidence and type of cerebral lesions were studied by ultrasound in 159 preterm infants: 76 fetuses were exposed to indometacin used as a tocolytic agent; in the other 83 pregnancies, tocolysis was either not started or limited to fenoterol. The incidence of periventricular leukomalacia was increased in infants exposed to any tocolytic agent; cystic lesions occurred more often in those exposed to indometacin (50).

Oligohydramnios and renal dysgenesis developed in one identical twin exposed to early prolonged high-dose indometacin. As indometacin causes oligohydramnios and renal dysgenesis in fetal monkeys, it may also have caused the abnormalities in this patient (51).

Antenatal indometacin therapy has been extensively reviewed (SEDA-18, 102). Data from a retrospective cohort study of 57 premature infants, born between the 24th and 30th weeks of gestation, whose mothers had been treated unsuccessfully with indometacin for preterm labor, confirmed several fetal and neonatal complications (52). However, the overall results provided inconclusive or contradictory data on the benefit to harm balance of indometacin as a tocolytic agent or as treatment for hydramnios (SEDA-18, 102).

Fetotoxicity

The possible association of indometacin tocolysis with neonatal necrotizing enterocolitis has been the subject of a case-control study (53). All cases of proven necrotizing enterocolitis were ascertained and four controls for each case were randomly identified. During 18 months there were 24 cases of necrotizing enterocolitis. Indometacin as a single tocolytic agent was not associated with necrotizing enterocolitis (OR = 1.0, 95% CI = 0.2, 4.8).

Lactation

The effects of indometacin during lactation are unclear. Convulsions in a breast-fed infant were linked to indometacin in the milk (54).

Susceptibility Factors

Age

Children

Pharmacokinetic factors (slow metabolism) may underlie the marked effect of indometacin on platelet aggregation in premature infants and small children. The use of indometacin in children with patent ductus arteriosus can be followed by a severe general reaction. Nephrotoxicity, abdominal distension, hemorrhagic enteritis, and necrotizing enterocolitis have been observed (SEDA-10, 81) (24,55). No retrospective study has shown that indometacin-treated infants have a higher incidence of retrolental hyperplasia or visual problems (56). Reopening of the ductus after indometacin-induced occlusion has been described (SEDA-18, 101), but the risks of using intravenous indometacin are few and it is more efficacious and safer than ligation.

Elderly people

Elderly patients are susceptible to the adverse effects of NSAIDs on the nervous system. A psychotic reaction has been described in one elderly man taking indometacin (57) and behavioral changes in another (58).

Gastrotoxicity is more frequent in this age group. Of 125 516 residents of US nursing homes during 1992–1996, patients who received at least one prescription for aspirin (n = 19 101) or NSAIDs (n = 9777) were identified (59). NSAID exposure increased the overall gastrointestinal-event-related hospitalization rate. The rates were highest in those taking sulindac, naproxen, or indometacin.

Other features of the patient

Patients with asthma or allergic rhinitis may be hypersensitive to indometacin and can develop severe general allergic reactions, especially if they are allergic to aspirin.

Indometacin should probably not be used postoperatively in patients with an increased risk of bleeding (SEDA-8, 103), because of its anti-platelet activity.

In athletes in training for a marathon, the use of indometacin may be dangerous, since it can provoke hyperkalemia and there is a risk of serious dysrhythmias (SEDA-14, 93).

Drug Administration

Drug formulations

Indometacin in eye-drop form can cause burning sensations, pruritus, local congestion and irritation, corneal epithelial changes, and edema of the eyelids (60).

Osmosin (Indosmos)

Osmosin (Indosmos) was an osmotic pump version of indometacin, which after a brief career, was withdrawn from the market in the summer of 1982. Indometacin, as a potent NSAID, found itself at the beginning of the 1980s facing heavy competition from a series of newer drugs that were about to be introduced; all were under patent, whereas some of the indometacin patents were about to expire, which could lead to a substantial fall in prices; some of the newer drugs (notably benoxaprofen, itself soon withdrawn, and piroxicam) were suitable for use as a single daily oral dose, which provided at least a marketing advantage; several were claimed, rightly or wrongly, to be relatively well-tolerated by the stomach. One possible answer to these problems seemed to be offered by developing an osmotic pump form of indometacin; in this form, the drug could be released relatively slowly, perhaps prolonging its duration of action and improving its gastric tolerability.

In fact, the question as to whether this form of indometacin really had these advantages has never been satisfactorily settled. The literature (61–64) does not appear to have shown a reduction in gastric adverse effects, at least not if one assesses the papers in question with the critical eye that must be brought to bear on claims of this type. On the other hand, it is clear that if a drug that has a potentially irritant action on the gastrointestinal tract is put into a modified-releasing form, tolerability problems may be displaced from the stomach to the lower parts of the gastrointestinal tract.

In the course of 1982, serious suspicions arose that this was indeed happening. In August, the UK's Committee on Safety of Medicines (CSM) stated that it had received 200 reports of adverse reactions to the product, which was considered a relatively high reporting level for a new drug, though more than 400 000 prescriptions had been issued over the previous 7 months. Many of the reports were of effects traditionally associated with indometacin (such as headache and gastrointestinal problems) and these did not seem to be less frequent with the new system. Two of the reports were of intestinal perforation distal to the duodenum, an unusual site for damage by NSAIDs. The CSM remarked that the release characteristics of the system might expose certain areas of the bowel to higher concentrations of indometacin than usual. It was also noted that the formulation contained potassium bicarbonate, a known bowel irritant (26).

It subsequently became clear that a fair number of cases of intestinal irritation, bleeding, perforation, and probably even death were attributable to the new formulation, leading to the product's withdrawal in countries where it had already been introduced.

The proposed mechanism of small bowel damage due to Osmosin is that the tablets adhered to the intestinal wall (or became lodged in diverticula), resulting in much higher local concentrations of indometacin and potassium than usual.

Indometacin-farnesil

Limited early experiences with indometacin-farnesil, a lipid-soluble indometacin derivative esterified with farnesol, suggested an adverse-effects profile similar to the indometacin, even though the compound was synthesized to reduce gastrotoxicity (SEDA-17, 109).

Drug administration route

Intravenous administration (in the treatment of ureteric colic) is effective and well tolerated. However, in 90% of patients who receive slow (5 minutes) intravenous injection, hypertension, nausea, vertigo, vomiting, and peptic ulcer symptoms have been documented (65). Intravenous administration should be avoided in patients with heart failure.

Intramuscular indometacin causes few adverse effects at the site of injection (redness, pain, induration) (SEDA-8, 102) and seems to have better systemic tolerability than intravenous indometacin: 26% of 388 patients treated with indometacin 100 mg/day developed an adverse effect (gastrointestinal or nervous system-related) and 4.6% interrupted treatment (66).

Drug–Drug Interactions

ACE inhibitors

Although lisinopril in association with indometacin reduced proteinuria in a small group of patients with nephritic syndrome, the combination also caused impairment of renal function and hyperkalemia in many patients (SEDA-16, 109).

Anti-platelet drugs

Indometacin potentiates the effect of anti-platelet drugs and anticoagulants (67).

Aspirin

Indometacin reduces the absorption of aspirin (68).

Beta-blockers

Attenuation of the hypotensive effect of propranolol and thiazide diuretics by indometacin was shown several years ago in a double-blind, placebo-controlled study of patients with essential hypertension (SEDA-6, 94).

Two women with pre-eclampsia treated with pindolol and propranolol became extremely hypertensive when indometacin was added for premature contractions (47). Pregnant women taking beta-blockers for hypertension in pregnancy should not be given indometacin, as it can raise the blood pressure (47).

Cyclophosphamide

Synergy between indometacin and cyclophosphamide has been advanced as the cause of a life-threatening acute water intoxication and severe hyponatremia observed in a patient with multiple myeloma and normal renal function (SEDA-15, 99).

Dipyridamole

Marked water retention has been observed during acute administration of dipyridamole in combination with indometacin (SEDA-13, 79).

Diuretics

Indometacin reduces the effect of diuretics (69). Combination of indometacin with Moduretic (co-amilozide; amiloride + hydrochlorothiazide) results in hyperkalemia (70).

Metformin

Renal insufficiency and severe metabolic acidosis developed in a patient with diabetes mellitus taking metformin after recent treatment with indometacin (SEDA-22, 118).

Muronomab

The interaction of indometacin with the immunosuppressive agent muromonab, a monoclonal antibody to CD3, is characterized by an increased risk of encephalopathic or psychotic features (71).

Probenecid

Probenecid inhibits the tubular secretion of indometacin (SEDA-4, 66).

References

1. Gotzsche PC. Patients' preference in indomethacin trials: an overview. Lancet 1989;1(8629):88–91.
2. Smith AP. Response of aspirin-allergic patients to challenge by some analgesics in common use. BMJ 1971;2(760):494–6.
3. Sheehan GJ, Kutzner MR, Chin WD. Acute asthma attack due to ophthalmic indomethacin. Ann Intern Med 1989;111(4):337–8.
4. Golding D. Angina and indomethacin. BMJ 1970;4(735):622.
5. Wennmalm A, Carlsson I, Edlund A, Eriksson S, Kaijser L, Nowak J. Central and peripheral haemodynamic effects of non-steroidal anti-inflammatory drugs in man. Arch Toxicol Suppl 1984;7:350–9.
6. Dzau VJ, Packer M, Lilly LS, Swartz SL, Hollenberg NK, Williams GH. Prostaglandins in severe congestive heart failure. Relation to activation of the renin–angiotensin system and hyponatremia. N Engl J Med 1984;310(6):347–52.
7. Szczeklik A, Gryglewski RJ, Czerniawska-Mysik G. Participation of prostaglandins in pathogenesis of aspirin-sensitive asthma. Naunyn Schmiedebergs Arch Pharmacol 1977;297(Suppl 1):S99–110.
8. Polachek J, Shvartzman P. Acute bronchial asthma associated with the administration of ophthalmic indomethacin. Isr J Med Sci 1996;32(11):1107–9.
9. Eade OE, Acheson ED, Cuthbert MF, Hawkes CH. Peripheral neuropathy and indomethacin. BMJ 1975;2(5962):66–7.
10. Rothermich NO. Deafness and hand tremor with indometacin. JAMA 1973;226:1471.
11. Van Bel F, Van de Bor M, Stijnen T, Baan J, Ruys JH. Cerebral blood flow velocity changes in preterm infants after a single dose of indomethacin: duration of its effect. Pediatrics 1989;84(5):802–7.
12. Edwards AD, Wyatt JS, Richardson C, Potter A, Cope M, Delpy DT, Reynolds EO. Effects of indomethacin on cerebral haemodynamics in very preterm infants. Lancet 1990;335(8704):1491–5.
13. Ment LR, Vohr B, Oh W, Scott DT, Allan WC, Westerveld M, Duncan CC, Ehrenkranz RA, Katz KH, Schneider KC, Makuch RW. Neurodevelopmental outcome at 36 months' corrected age of preterm infants in the Multicenter Indomethacin Intraventricular Hemorrhage Prevention Trial. Pediatrics 1996;98(4 Pt 1):714–18.
14. Couser RJ, Hoekstra RE, Ferrara TB, Wright GB, Cabalka AK, Connett JE. Neurodevelopmental follow-up at 36 months' corrected age of preterm infants treated with prophylactic indomethacin. Arch Pediatr Adolesc Med 2000;154(6):598–602.
15. Beirne J, Jubiz W. Effect of indomethacin on the hypothalamic–pituitary–adrenal axis in man. J Clin Endocrinol Metab 1978;47(4):713–16.
16. Thack JR, Bozeman MT. Indometacin induced hyperglycemia. J Am Acad Dermatol 1982;7:502.
17. Akbarpour F, Afrasiabi A, Vaziri ND. Severe hyperkalemia caused by indomethacin and potassium supplementation. South Med J 1985;78(6):756–7.
18. Ambanelli U, Ferraccioli GF, Serventi G, Vaona GL. Changes in serum and urinary zinc induced by ASA and indomethacin. Scand J Rheumatol 1982;11(1):63–4.
19. Durao V, Prata MM, Goncalves LM. Modification of antihypertensive effect of beta-adrenoceptor-blocking agents by inhibition of endogenous prostaglandin synthesis. Lancet 1977;2(8046):1005–7.
20. Watkins J, Abbott EC, Hensby CN, Webster J, Dollery CT. Attenuation of hypotensive effect of propranolol and thiazide diuretics by indomethacin. BMJ 1980;281(6242):702–5.
21. Menkes E, Kutas GJ. Fatal aplastic anemia following indomethacin ingestion. Can Med Assoc J 1977;117(2):118.
22. Cuthbert MF. Adverse reactions to non-steroidal antirheumatic drugs. Curr Med Res Opin 1974;2(9):600–10.
23. The International Agranulocytosis and Aplastic Anemia Study. Risks of agranulocytosis and aplastic anemia. A first report of their relation to drug use with special reference to analgesics. JAMA 1986;256(13):1749–57.
24. Friedman Z, Whitman V, Maisels MJ, Berman W Jr, Marks KH, Vesell ES. Indomethacin disposition and indomethacin-induced platelet dysfunction in premature infants. J Clin Pharmacol 1978;18(5-6):272–9.
25. Maclaurin BP, Richards DA, Heads D. Indomethacin-associated peptic ulceration. NZ Med J 1978;88(625): 439–41.
26. Anonymous. "Osmosin" may not reduce indometacin's side effects. Scrip 1983;82:1.
27. Hooker GD, Gregor JC, Ponich TP, McLarty TD. Diaphragm-like strictures of the right colon induced by indomethacin suppositories: evidence of a systemic effect. Gastrointest Endosc 1996;44(2):199–202.
28. Coutrot S, Roland D, Barbier J, Van Der Marcq P, Alcalay M, Matuchansky C. Acute perforation of colonic

diverticula associated with short-term indomethacin. Lancet 1978;2(8098):1055–6.

29. Levy N, Gaspar E. Letter: Rectal bleeding and indomethacin suppositories. Lancet 1975;1(7906):577.
30. Hansen TM, Matzen P, Madsen P. Endoscopic evaluation of the effect of indomethacin capsules and suppositories on the gastric mucosa in rheumatic patients. J Rheumatol 1984;11(4):484–7.
31. Fenech FF, Bannister WH, Grech JL. Hepatitis with biliverdinaemia in association with indomethacin therapy. BMJ 1967;3(558):155–6.
32. de Kraker-Sangster M, Bronkhorst FB, Brandt KH, Boersma JW. Massale Levercelnecrose na toediening van indometacine in combinatie met aminofenazon. [Massive liver cell necrosis following administration of indomethacin in combination with aminophenzone.] Ned Tijdschr Geneeskd 1981;125(45):1828–31.
33. Cappell MS, Kozicky O, Competiello LS. Indomethacin-associated cholestasis. J Clin Gastroenterol 1988;10(4):445–7.
34. ter Borg EJ, de Jong PE, Meyer S, van Rijswijk MH, Kallenberg CG. Indomethacin and ibuprofen-induced reversible acute renal failure in a patient with systemic lupus erythematosus. Neth J Med 1987;30(3-4):181–6.
35. ter Borg EJ, de Jong PE, Meijer S, Kallenberg CG. Renal effects of indomethacin in patients with systemic lupus erythematosus. Nephron 1989;53(3):238–43.
36. Fawaz-Estrup F, Ho G Jr. Reversible acute renal failure induced by indomethacin. Arch Intern Med 1981;141(12):1670–1.
37. O'Sullivan M, Hanly JG, Molloy M. A case of toxic epidermal necrolysis secondary to indomethacin. Br J Rheumatol 1983;22(1):47–9.
38. Katayama H, Kawada A. Exacerbation of psoriasis induced by indomethacin. J Dermatol 1981;8(4):323–7.
39. Rubens-Duval A, Villiaumey J, Kaplan G, Bailly D. Surmenage et detérioration rapide de coxo-fémorales arthrosiques au cours de thérapeutiques anti-inflammatoires non corticoides. [Overworking and fast deterioration of arthrosic hips during non-steroid anti-inflammatory treatment.] Rev Rhum Mal Osteoartic 1970;37(8):535–41.
40. Rashad S, Revell P, Hemingway A, Low F, Rainsford K, Walker F. Effect of non-steroidal anti-inflammatory drugs on the course of osteoarthritis. Lancet 1989;2(8662):519–22.
41. Romanowska-Gorecka B, Oleszczak B. Maskukacy wplyw indocydu na przebieg ropnych procesow zapalnych. [Masking effect of indocin on the course of purulent inflammatory processes.] Pol Tyg Lek 1969;24(52):2019–20.
42. Grella P, Zanor P. Premature labor and indomethacin. Prostaglandins 1978;16(6):1007–17.
43. Manchester D, Margolis HS, Sheldon RE. Possible association between maternal indomethacin therapy and primary pulmonary hypertension of the newborn. Am J Obstet Gynecol 1976;126(4):467–9.
44. Levin DL, Fixler DE, Morriss FC, Tyson J. Morphologic analysis of the pulmonary vascular bed in infants exposed in utero to prostaglandin synthetase inhibitors. J Pediatr 1978;92(3):478–83.
45. Moise KJ Jr, Huhta JC, Sharif DS, Ou CN, Kirshon B, Wasserstrum N, Cano L. Indomethacin in the treatment of premature labor. Effects on the fetal ductus arteriosus. N Engl J Med 1988;319(6):327–31.
46. Hendricks SK, Smith JR, Moore DE, Brown ZA. Oligohydramnios associated with prostaglandin synthetase inhibitors in preterm labour. Br J Obstet Gynaecol 1990;97(4):312–16.
47. Schoenfeld A, Freedman S, Hod M, Ovadia Y. Antagonism of antihypertensive drug therapy in pregnancy by indomethacin? Am J Obstet Gynecol 1989;161(5):1204–5.
48. Di Battista C, Laudizi L, Tamborino G. Focomelia ed agenesia del pene in neonato. Possible ruolo teratogeno di un farmaco assunto dalla madre in gravidanza. [Phocomelia and agenesis of the penis in a newborn infant. Possible teratogenic role of a drug taken by the mother during pregnancy.] Minerva Pediatr 1975;27(11):675–9.
49. Haddad J, Messer J, Casanova R, Simeoni U, Willard D. Indomethacin and ischemic brain injury in neonates. J Pediatr 1990;116(5):839–40.
50. Baerts W, Fetter WP, Hop WC, Wallenburg HC, Spritzer R, Sauer PJ. Cerebral lesions in preterm infants after tocolytic indomethacin. Dev Med Child Neurol 1990;32(10):910–18.
51. Restaino I, Kaplan BS, Kaplan P, Rosenberg HK, Witzleben C, Roberts N. Renal dysgenesis in a monozygotic twin: association with in utero exposure to indomethacin. Am J Med Genet 1991;39(3):252–7.
52. Norton ME, Merrill J, Cooper BA, Kuller JA, Clyman RI. Neonatal complications after the administration of indomethacin for preterm labor. N Engl J Med 1993;329(22):1602–7.
53. Parilla BV, Grobman WA, Holtzman RB, Thomas HA, Dooley SL. Indomethacin tocolysis and risk of necrotizing enterocolitis. Obstet Gynecol 2000;96(1):120–3.
54. Eeg-Olofsson O, Malmros I, Elwin CE, Steen B. Convulsions in a breast-fed infant after maternal indomethacin. Lancet 1978;2(8082):215.
55. Harinck E, van Ertbruggen I, Senders RC, Moulaert AJ. Problems with indomethacin for ductus closure. Lancet 1977;2(8031):245.
56. Merritt TA, Bejar R, Coraza M, et al. Clinical trials of intravenous indometacin for closure of the patent ductus arteriosus. Pediatr Cardiol 1983;4(Suppl 2):71.
57. Tharumaratnam D, Bashford S, Khan SA. Indomethacin induced psychosis. Postgrad Med J 2000;76(901):736–7.
58. Mallet L, Kuyumjian J. Indomethacin-induced behavioral changes in an elderly patient with dementia. Ann Pharmacother 1998;32(2):201–3.
59. Lapane KL, Spooner JJ, Mucha L, Straus WL. Effect of nonsteroidal anti-inflammatory drug use on the rate of gastrointestinal hospitalizations among people living in long-term care. J Am Geriatr Soc 2001;49(5):577–84.
60. Pichon P, Moreau PG. Complications cornéennes par usage de collyre a l'indométacine. [Corneal complications caused by indomethacin eyedrop.] Bull Soc Ophtalmol Fr 1990;90(4):449–51.
61. Young JH, Currie WJ. "Osmosin" in general practice: preliminary report of a double-blind study in the treatment of osteoarthritis. Curr Med Res Opin 1983;8 (Suppl 2):99–108.
62. Gallacchi G, Strolz F. Clinical evaluation of "Osmosin" versus piroxicam. Curr Med Res Opin 1983;8(Suppl 2):83–9.
63. Rhymer AR, Sromovsky JA, Dicenta C, Hart CB. "Osmosin": a multi-centre evaluation of a technological advance in the treatment of osteoarthritis. Curr Med Res Opin 1983;8(Suppl 2):62–71.
64. Bobrove AM, Calin A. Efficacy and tolerance of a novel precision-dose formulation of indomethacin: double-blind trials in rheumatoid arthritis and osteoarthritis. Curr Med Res Opin 1983;8(Suppl 2):55–61.
65. Galassi P, Vicentini C, Scapellato F, Laurenti C. L'impiego dell'indometacina e del metamizolo per via endovenosa nella colica renale. [Use of indomethacin and metamizole administered intravenously in renal colic. Comparative study.] Minerva Urol 1983;35(4):295–300.
66. Vincent G, Vincent H. Indocid 50 mg injectable dans la pathologie disco-vertebrale Sem Hop 1986;62:2189.
67. Chan TY, Lui SF, Chung SY, Luk S, Critchley JA. Adverse interaction between warfarin and indomethacin. Drug Saf 1994;10(3):267–9.

68. Jeremy R, Towson J. Interaction between aspirin and indomethacin in the treatment of rheumatoid arthritis. Med J Aust 1970;2(3):127–9.
69. Allan SG, Knox J, Kerr F. Interaction between diuretics and indomethacin. BMJ (Clin Res Ed) 1981;283(6306):1611.
70. Mor R, Pitlik S, Rosenfeld JB. Indomethacin- and Moduretic–induced hyperkalemia. Isr J Med Sci 1983;19(6):535–7.
71. Mignat C. Clinically significant drug interactions with new immunosuppressive agents. Drug Saf 1997;16(4):267–78.

Indoprofen

See also Non-steroidal anti-inflammatory drugs

General Information

Indoprofen is one of several NSAIDs that have been withdrawn because of adverse effects. The UK Licensing Authority suspended the product licence on grounds of safety in 1983, and in 1984 the Italian manufacturers decided to withdraw it from the world market. The UK decision was taken because there was a high rate of adverse drug reactions in a voluntary postmarketing surveillance study and the spontaneous adverse reaction reporting system had noted 217 serious adverse effects, mainly gastrointestinal bleeding and perforation. According to the manufacturers, the adverse effects profile in the UK did not emerge in other countries (1). A survey of adverse reactions in 6764 patients, mostly treated for 1 month or less, showed that life-threatening events were rare. A postmarketing surveillance study in 3823 osteoarthritic patients showed that serious adverse reactions were even less frequent (2).

Organs and Systems

Hematologic

The fact that indoprofen prolongs bleeding time and reduces platelet aggregation could result in indirect interactions with anticoagulants (3).

Gastrointestinal

When the UK Licensing Authority suspended the product licence the spontaneous adverse reaction reporting system had received 217 reports of serious adverse effects, mainly gastrointestinal bleeding and perforation.

Death

There were 46 deaths associated with indoprofen in three countries (UK 34, Italy 7, Germany 5), but only 11 were judged to be probably or possibly drug-related. Nine of these deaths were caused by gastrointestinal reactions.

Long-Term Effects

Tumorigenicity

The manufacturers' ultimate reason for worldwide withdrawal was the finding of carcinogenicity in long-term animal studies. To what extent the clinical events actually played a role in their decision is not clear.

References

1. Anonymous. Flosin hearing. Scrip 1984;883:14.
2. Emanueli A, Caso P, Gualtieri S, et al. Postmarketing surveillance of indoprofen. In: Proceedings, Scientific Symposium on Indoprofen in Inflammatory and Painful Conditions, Venice, 1982:95.
3. Jacono A, Caso P, Gualtieri S, Raucci D, Bianchi A, Vigorito C, Bergamini N, Iadevaia V. Clinical study of possible interactions between indoprofen and oral anticoagulants. Eur J Rheumatol Inflamm 1981;4(1):32–5.

Indoramin

See also Alpha-adrenoceptor antagonists

General Information

Indoramin is a postsynaptic selective alpha$_1$-adrenoceptor antagonist that is chemically distinct from the quinazolines. Unlike some other alpha-blockers, indoramin lowers blood pressure without a resulting reflex tachycardia or postural hypotension (1). However, it has largely been supplanted by more modern drugs, such as doxazosin, prazosin, and terazosin.

Organs and Systems

Nervous system

Indoramin penetrates the nervous system significantly and is reported to have a relatively high incidence of adverse effects, including sedation, dizziness, depression, headache, palpitation, dry mouth, and constipation (2). In a comparison with prazosin, prazosin produced a lower incidence of sedation, which is the most common adverse effect of indoramin, usually transient, in about 19% of cases (1). Other adverse effects that have sometimes led to withdrawal of indoramin have been dry mouth, dizziness, and failure of ejaculation. These adverse effects can be reduced by starting therapy with small doses and titrating gradually.

Drug–Drug Interactions

Alcohol

The sedative effect of indoramin is enhanced by alcohol (3).

References

1. Holmes B, Sorkin EM. Indoramin. A review of its pharmacodynamic and pharmacokinetic properties, and therapeutic efficacy in hypertension and related vascular, cardiovascular and airway diseases. Drugs 1986;31(6):67–99. Erratum in: Drugs 1986;32(4):preceding 291.
2. Marshall AJ, Kettle MA, Barritt DW. Evaluation of indoramin added to oxprenolol and bendrofluazide as a third agent in severe hypertension. Br J Clin Pharmacol 1980;10(3):217–21.
3. Abrams SM, Pierce DM, Johnston A, Hedges A, Franklin RA, Turner P. Pharmacokinetic interaction between indoramin and ethanol. Hum Toxicol 1989;8(3):237–41.

Infliximab

See also Monoclonal antibodies

General Information

Infliximab, a monoclonal chimeric human/murine antibody directed against tumor necrosis alfa, has been used in the treatment of severe active Crohn's disease (1,2), rheumatoid arthritis (3), and ankylosing spondylitis (4). From the available data submitted for Crohn's disease to the US and European regulatory agencies, the most significant acute adverse reactions were infusion reactions, defined as symptoms within 2 hours after intravenous infusion. The symptoms consisted of fever, chills, urticaria, dyspnea, chest pain, or hypotension, and occurred in 16% of infliximab-treated patients versus 6–7% of placebo-treated patients. Several adverse effects, such as upper respiratory tract infections, headaches, rash, or cough, were more common than with placebo, but severe adverse effects were only slightly more frequent (3.6 versus 2.6%). Clinical trials also showed an increase in the prevalence of antinuclear antibodies or the development of double-stranded DNA antibodies (9% of patients). Although there were clinical features suggestive of the lupus-like syndrome in only very few patients, this issue needs to be further investigated. Also of great concern is the report in several patients of lymphoma (5) or severe opportunistic infections (6). Patients taking concomitant immunosuppressive drugs should be carefully observed for such complications.

Organs and Systems

Cardiovascular

The preliminary results of a phase II trial in patients with moderate to severe congestive heart failure showed a higher incidence of worsening congestive heart failure and death in patients treated with infliximab compared with placebo (7). This led to warnings from regulatory agencies and to the limited use of infliximab in patients with congestive heart failure.

Death due to worsening of cardiac insufficiency in patients with congestive heart failure has been reported (SEDA-26, 401).

Respiratory

Allergic granulomatosis of the lung has been described after a second infusion of infliximab in one of 35 patients with active ankylosing spondylitis (8). The clinical and radiological symptoms resolved 8 weeks after withdrawal, but no other details were given.

- A 32-year-old man with Crohn's disease developed an eosinophilic pleural effusion soon after a second infusion of infliximab (9). He recovered within 8 weeks, but the effusion recurred after infliximab re-treatment 1 year later.

Nervous system

Features of aseptic meningitis have been reported after multiple infliximab injections (10).

- A 53-year-old man with severe rheumatoid arthritis and mixed type III cryoglobulinemia received his first four injections of infliximab uneventfully, but 4 hours after the fifth injection had severe muscle pain in the lower limbs, which required morphine and abated within 3 days. Similar symptoms were observed after the sixth injection. There were no signs of meningitis, the cerebrospinal fluid contained lymphocytes and increased concentrations of protein and IgG. Cultures were negative and MRI scans of the brain and the spine were normal. The CSF was normal 1 month later.

The authors speculated that the most likely explanation for these observations was linked to the lack of transfer of high-molecular weight soluble receptors and IgG across the blood–brain barrier, implying that control of brain tumor necrosis factor alfa cannot be obtained with monoclonal antibodies. They thought that neurological complications in diseases other than multiple sclerosis might be related to control of tumor necrosis factor alfa in the periphery, resulting in an enhanced contribution of brain-derived tumor necrosis factor alfa or other cytokines, such as interleukin-1.

Neurological events suggestive of demyelinating disorders in patients treated with tumor necrosis factor alfa antagonists and reported to the FDA's Adverse Events Reporting System have been reviewed (11). These included 17 cases temporarily associated with etanercept and two with infliximab, but complete information was lacking in a number of cases. The various hypothetical mechanisms by which tumor necrosis factor alfa antagonists might produce demyelinating events have been discussed (12). Briefly, they cause an increase in peripheral T cell autoreactivity, and their inability to cross the blood–brain barrier may account for exacerbation of central demyelinating disorders.

Sensory systems

Optic neuropathy has been described in patients with rheumatoid arthritis taking infliximab. In three patients aged 54–62 years, blurred vision or visual field loss in one or both eyes occurred after the third dose (13).

Ophthalmic examination showed anterior optic neuropathy in all three patients and MRI scanning ruled out demyelinating optic neuritis. In one patient an additional infusion of infliximab produced similar symptoms in the previously unaffected eye; vision failed to improve despite infliximab withdrawal and steroid treatment.

- Retrobulbar optic neuritis was diagnosed after the ninth dose of infliximab in a 55-year-old woman (14). MRI scanning showed demyelination of the left optic nerve and the visual field defect improved after treatment with prednisone.

Hematologic

The possible role of infliximab in the development of hypercoagulability disorders has been discussed in the context of a case of arterial thrombosis (15).

- A 72-year-old woman with refractory sarcoidosis developed venous thrombosis at a catheter site and extensive multiple thromboses in small arteries in her legs after receiving a third dose of infliximab for severe enteropathy. Anticardiolipin antibodies were detected, but antinuclear and anti-double-stranded DNA antibodies were negative.

Although infliximab has been associated with autoantibody production, it is not known whether it contributed to hypercoagulability in this patient.

Liver

Acute hepatitis with infliximab has been described (16).

- A 44-year-old woman, who had used oral contraceptives for many years and had taken mesalazine, mercaptopurine, and prednisone for Crohn's disease for 7 years, developed clinical and biological signs of acute mixed hepatitis 19 days after a single dose of infliximab 5 mg/kg. There were no symptoms suggestive of hypersensitivity and liver histology showed cholestasis without inflammation or eosinophilia. Other causes, such as a recent viral infection (hepatitis A, B, C, cytomegalovirus, *Herpes simplex*) or gallstones, were ruled out. Among various autoantibodies, only antinuclear antibody titers were slightly raised. Complete normalization was observed 2 months later.

Although the patient took other potentially hepatotoxic drugs, the time-course suggested that infliximab was the cause.

Skin

Skin reactions, including erythema multiforme in three patients and a lichenoid eruption in one, were attributed to infliximab (17). One patient had similar lesions after etanercept. Patch tests with infliximab in three patients were negative, but produced a flare-up of lesions in one patient and recurrence of malaise and nausea in another patient, suggesting that infliximab is well absorbed percutaneously.

- A 72-year-old man developed bullous skin lesions the day after receiving his fourth dose of infliximab for rheumatoid arthritis (18). Human antichimeric antibodies were positive, as were antinuclear antibodies, and he completely recovered after treatment with prednisone.

In three patients with severe Crohn's disease who required digestive surgery, infliximab before or immediately after surgery was discussed as an additional possible cause of postoperative poor wound healing with serious complications (19).

Patients with congestive heart failure has been reported (SEDA-26, 401).

Immunologic

Antibodies to infliximab

Treatment with infliximab can be associated with the formation of human antichimeric antibodies. Such antibodies were rarely detected in patients with rheumatoid arthritis who were also taking methotrexate, and low titers were detected in about 13% of patients with Crohn's disease. Their clinical relevance is unclear, although their presence has sometimes been associated with an increased risk of infusion reactions, the occurrence of serum sickness-like reactions after delayed re-treatment, and a shorter duration of response.

In a randomized, placebo-controlled trial in 573 patients with Crohn's disease, who responded to an initial infusion of infliximab and were then given repeated infusions, antibodies to infliximab were found in 14%; there was a trend toward a lower incidence of antibodies in patients taking concurrent glucocorticoids and immunosuppressive drugs (20). The incidence of infusion reactions was also higher in patients positive for antibodies to infliximab compared with patients without antibodies (16 versus 8%) and lower in patients who were taking both glucocorticoids and immunosuppressants compared with patients who were receiving neither (8 versus 32%).

The clinical significance of antibodies to infliximab has also been explored in 125 patients with Crohn's disease who were given infliximab, of whom 61% had antibodies after the fifth infusion; however, there was no further increase in incidence after subsequent treatment (21). The presence of antibodies was associated with a 2.4-fold increase in the risk of infusion reactions, lower serum infliximab concentrations, and a shorter duration of clinical response, compared with patients with no infliximab antibodies. Patients who received concomitant immunosuppressive therapy had a lower incidence of infliximab antibodies, higher infliximab serum concentrations, and a longer duration of clinical response. Pretreatment with glucocorticoids may reduce the risk of antibody formation, but it is not known whether a pretreatment test for human antichimeric antibodies has a predictive value for adverse reactions (22). However, there were technical issues relating to the antibody assay and definition of clinically relevant antibody titers in this study.

Autoantibodies and autoimmunity

Infliximab may increase the risk of autoimmunity, but the presence of antibodies did not predict the risk of lupus-like syndrome. In trials, the incidence of infliximab-induced anti-double-stranded DNA antibodies ranged from 5 to 34% of patients, depending on the assay method used and the duration of exposure (20–24). However, these abnormalities were rarely associated with clinical manifestations. In two large randomized trials in more than 900 infliximab-treated patients, only three developed a lupus-like syndrome, with no evidence of systemic organ involvement (20–24). However, since then, several reports have detailed infliximab-induced, lupus-like syndrome in patients with Crohn's colitis or rheumatoid arthritis, with improvement on withdrawal of infliximab (25,26).

Of 40 patients who had received multiple doses of an investigational liquid formulation of infliximab 2–4 years before, 10 had a severe delayed hypersensitivity reaction within 3–12 days after the first or the second re-infusion (27). This reaction mostly included myalgia, rash, fever, polyarthralgia, and pruritus. Although the six patients tested were negative for antibodies to infliximab before re-infusion, these antibodies were consistently raised after the reaction.

Infliximab binds to tumor necrosis factor alfa on cell surfaces and produces apoptotic cell death, releasing the nucleosomal autoantigens that induce autoantibody formation (28).

- A 69-year-old woman with a 5-year history of rheumatoid arthritis developed drug-induced lupus after receiving infliximab for 23 weeks. She had initially been given methotrexate and prednisone for 4 years. Then, because of lack of efficacy, infliximab was introduced. After three infusions of infliximab and only partial remission the dose was increased to 5 mg/kg, with success. However, before the sixth infusion she developed fever, polyarthralgia, myalgia, and general malaise. Serology excluded viral infection. Autoantibody assessment was positive, confirming the diagnosis of drug-induced lupus.

Hypersensitivity reactions

Both acute and delayed hypersensitivity reactions to infliximab have been reported in clinical trials (SEDA-24, 439).

Immediate infusion reactions to infliximab are usually defined by any significant adverse effect that occurs during or within 1–2 hours after the infusion. The symptoms mostly consist of flushing, rash, shortness of breath, wheeze, hotness, chest pain, vomiting, and abdominal pain.

Delayed reactions are defined by the occurrence of arthralgia and joint stiffness (that is a serum sickness-like reaction) in the days after infliximab administration; they have mostly been observed in patients with Crohn's disease who have received episodic treatment. In one patient the complication was associated with acute respiratory distress syndrome, which only became evident 10 days after re-treatment (22).

Incidence

Immediate hypersensitivity reactions to infliximab occur in 6–19% of adults.

In a retrospective evaluation of 165 patients (479 infliximab infusions) with Crohn's disease, the overall incidence of infusion reactions was 6.1% (29 episodes) (29). Acute infusion reactions within 24 hours of infusion were the most frequent (26 episodes) and delayed infusion reactions from 1 to 14 days after treatment were noted in three instances only. Prophylaxis with diphenhydramine and paracetamol and the use of a test dose of infliximab allowed additional infusions without consequences in patients with mild or moderate previous acute infusion reactions. Three of the four patients who had acute severe reactions received the same prophylaxis plus corticosteroids before re-treatment: one had a similar severe acute reaction, while the other two had no recurrences. This study also suggested that acute infusion reactions are probably not IgE-mediated, as tryptase and IgE serum concentrations were not raised.

Of 86 patients with Crohn's disease receiving infliximab 14% of patients experienced severe systemic reactions, with a significant difference between adults (21%) and children (3%), the reason for which was unclear (30).

There were severe infusion reactions, defined by any significant change in vital signs or the development of chest pain, wheeze, dyspnea, vomiting, abdominal pain, or rash, in 16 of 100 patients with refractory Crohn's disease (31). Half of them occurred during the first infusion, and the rate of infusion reactions was similar in patients taking concurrent immunosuppressants or glucocorticoids compared with those who were not. One patient had anaphylactic shock, five had significant hypotension, six had acute pulmonary symptoms, two had pruritus, flushing, or rash, and one had vomiting. The final patient, who had a previous history of chronic pancreatitis, had acute pancreatitis within 1 hour of treatment.

Immediate hypersensitivity reactions

Acute hypersensitivity reactions can mimic an anaphylactic reaction, but specific IgE antibodies have not so far been identified. A dose-escalation protocol has been proposed to desensitize patients who have had acute systemic reactions (32), but this has not always been successful (33). Although most reported anaphylactic reactions to infliximab have been mild, severe reactions can occur.

- A 36-year-old man with Crohn's disease became refractory to standard anti-inflammatory treatment (glucocorticoids, mercaptopurine, methotrexate, ciclosporin, tacrolimus) (33). Remission over 8 months was achieved with a single infusion of infliximab. With the onset of relapse he was given another infusion of infliximab and had an anaphylactic-like reaction within 1 minute.
- A 35-year-old woman with known hypersensitivity to mesalazine had severe symptoms, namely chest pain, dyspnea, productive cough, skin rash, and hypotension, during a third infusion of infliximab, and died 6 hours later from refractory hypotension and respiratory failure (34). Specific IgE or human antichimeric antibodies were not checked.
- A 33-year-old man with a 3-year history of Crohn's disease had previously received a well-tolerated single infusion of infliximab. When, 14 months later, he received a second infusion for exacerbation of the disease he had no immediate adverse effects, but complained of myalgia, arthralgia, nausea, and vomiting 7 days later and received diphenhydramine. After 3 days he had dyspnea, fever, and chills. An open lung biopsy showed features of eosinophilic pneumonia and no

infections or other obvious causes were found. He subsequently worsened and required intubation and mechanical ventilation for 13 days. He was given glucocorticoids and quadruple antituberculosis drug therapy and recovered completely within 2 months. Human antichimeric antibodies were raised (13 times normal).
- A 73-year-old woman had three separate episodes of vascular purpura (with leukocytoclastic vasculitis during the third episode) during each sequence of treatment with etanercept; she later developed similar cutaneous lesions after a third injection of infliximab (35).

Delayed hypersensitivity reactions
Delayed hypersensitivity reactions were mostly observed in patients with Crohn's disease who received episodic treatment. In one patient, this complication was associated with acute respiratory distress syndrome, which became evident only 10 days after retreatment (22).

Susceptibility factors
Susceptibility factors for the development of severe systemic reactions after infliximab retreatment have been analysed in 52 adults and 34 children with Crohn's disease (30). Acute severe systemic reactions were defined by symptoms of anaphylactic reactions that required pharmacological treatment, and delayed severe systemic reactions were defined by the occurrence of arthralgia and joint stiffness (that is serum sickness-like symptoms) requiring glucocorticoids in the days after infliximab retreatment. According to these definitions, severe systemic reactions developed in 14% of patients (four acute and eight delayed) during retreatment. They were significantly more frequent in adults than in children (21 versus 3%), and delayed systemic reactions were observed exclusively in adults. These reactions mostly occurred during the second infusion of infliximab, and particularly when retreatment was distant from the first infusion, that is beyond a 20-week interval. This suggested a higher potential for delayed hypersensitivity reactions when repeated doses are given within a longer time interval, and led the authors to recommend multiple early infusions if future infliximab retreatment is anticipated.

In a retrospective review of 361 infliximab infusions in 57 children with inflammatory bowel disease there were 35 episodes of infusion reactions (36). Female sex, previous episodes of infusion reactions, and the use of immunosuppressive therapy for less than 4 months were significant predictors of subsequent infusion reactions.

Infection risk

Infliximab can increase the susceptibility of patients to severe infections, and in particular opportunistic infections (SEDA-26, 402). In patients who received repeated infusions of infliximab, infections requiring antimicrobial treatment occurred in about 30% of patients and severe infections in 4% (20).

Bacterial infections
Blockade of tumor necrosis factor alfa impairs resistance to infections with intracellular pathogens such as mycobacteria, *Pneumocystis jiroveci*, *Listeria monocytogenes*, and *Legionella pneumophila* (37,38). Severe streptococcal and staphylococcal infections have also been observed. Case reports with very severe or fatal outcomes have usually been reported in patients taking concomitant immunosuppressants and have included:

- necrotizing fasciitis due to streptococcal infection (39)
- septicemia due to *Staphylococcus aureus* (40)
- *Listeria monocytogenes* infection (41)
- disseminated tuberculosis (42)
- listeriosis (37).

The safety and efficacy of infliximab have been assessed in 40 patients with severe active spondylarthropathy in a double-blind, randomized, placebo-controlled trial (43). One 65-year-old patient improved but 3 weeks after the third infusion developed a systemic illness. He had enlarged mediastinal lymph nodes and nodular lesion of the liver and spleen. Biopsy of the mediastinal lymph nodes showed tuberculosis, which was confirmed by culture. He was treated and recovered slowly.

Reactivation of latent tuberculosis is a major concern with infliximab (SEDA-26, 402), and accounts for about one-third of infections in these patients. According to data from the manufacturers, 130 cases of active tuberculosis were notified up to October 2001. Many of the cases were disseminated or extrapulmonary tuberculosis, and several patients died. Several case reports have provided detailed information in at least seven other patients, including three who developed miliary tuberculosis and one who developed *Mycobacterium tuberculosis* enteritis (44–48). A detailed analysis of 70 cases of tuberculosis reported to the FDA has been published (49). Two-thirds of the cases were noted after three or fewer infusions and 57% of the patients had extrapulmonary disease. There were 64 cases from countries with a low incidence of tuberculosis. From these reports and the number of patients treated with infliximab, the estimated rate of tuberculosis in patients with rheumatoid arthritis treated with infliximab was four times higher than the background rate. Patients with evidence of active infection should not receive infliximab until the infection is under control; all should be screened for tuberculosis before starting infliximab (50). From these and other data it has been estimated that the risk of tuberculosis in the first year of infliximab treatment is 0.035 in US citizens and 0.2% in non-US citizens. Further investigations, such as a chest X-ray and a Mantoux test, and prophylactic treatment with isoniazid, will show whether the incidence can be reduced in patients taking anti-TNF treatment (51).

In a multicenter trial in 70 patients with ankylosing spondylitis given infliximab, treatment had to be withdrawn in three patients because of systemic tuberculosis, allergic granulomatosis of the lung, or mild leukopenia; after withdrawal all three recovered (8). However, the allergic granulomatosis of the lung was probably due to a hypersensitivity reaction.

- An 11-year-old boy with Crohn's disease received infliximab and 3 days later developed fever, signs of cardiac failure, and *S. aureus* sepsis (52). At surgery an intramyocardial para-aortic abscess with destruction of the aortic valve was found, suggesting chronic infection, possibly activated by the use of infliximab.

Crohn's disease can lead to vasculitic changes of the aorta, which may have favored the development of the intramyocardial abscess in this case. The size of the abscess suggested persistence for several weeks.

Severe necrotizing fasciitis has been reported in a patient who was given infliximab (39).

- A 54-year-old man with rheumatoid arthritis for 12 years was given infliximab, with remission. He then developed a painful, confluent, erythematous, pustular rash over his trunk and limbs. Skin biopsy showed an acute pustular dermatitis. Five hours later he collapsed with a tachycardia (140/minute) and a blood pressure of 120/70 mmHg. He was apyrexial. His left leg was very tense, painful, and swollen, and he had a disseminated intravascular coagulopathy. There was marked necrosis of his adductor compartment and fascia of his left thigh and necrotic muscles were debrided. Blood cultures and skin swabs grew group A hemolytic streptococci. He then became unstable and died, despite efforts at resuscitation.

Viral infections

Infliximab can compromise antiviral defence mechanisms. There have been detailed reports of cytomegalovirus retinitis (53) and life-threatening disseminated cytomegalovirus infection (54). Most of these patients were taking concomitant immunosuppressants at the time of diagnosis.

- A 67-year-old woman with a 5-year history of rheumatoid arthritis, who had taken prednisone and methotrexate, was given infliximab (55). Her rheumatoid arthritis improved, but she developed multiple bilateral lesions of molluscum contagiosum on the upper and lower eyelids, despite normal CD4 and CD8 counts. She had had similar lesions during a previous course of infliximab. Excision biopsy confirmed the diagnosis.

Protozoal infections

There has been a detailed report of *P. jiroveci* pneumonia (56).

Fungal infections

In a review of 10 cases of histoplasmosis in patients treated with infliximab ($n = 9$) or etanercept ($n = 1$) the infection occurred within 1 week to 6 months after the first dose (57). Of these 10 patients, nine required treatment in an intensive care unit and one died. All lived in regions in which histoplasmosis was endemic. It was not possible to determine which patients had new infections or reactivation of previous infections.

In 41 patients with rheumatic disease who received a total of 300 infusions of infliximab over 9 months there were severe adverse effects in 15%, one of which was a case of histoplasmosis (58).

- A 28-year-old woman with unresponsive rheumatic disease developed histoplasmosis after a second infusion of infliximab. She had pet birds, and the authors thought that she had had reactivation of an infection rather than a new infection.

There have been other reports of histoplasmosis (59), invasive pulmonary aspergillosis (60), and extensive pulmonary coccidioidomycosis (61).

Death

- A 64-year-old man without heart failure was found dead 18 hours after a single infusion of infliximab for rheumatoid arthritis (62). No obvious cause was found at autopsy, except that the patient was known to have had frequent intervention by a pacemaker that had been implanted for several years.

Long-Term Effects

Tumorigenicity

There is great concern about the potential development of malignancy after blockade of tumor necrosis factor alfa, and it is biologically plausible. However, it is unclear whether this is a drug-related or a disease-related phenomenon.

There have been several cases of lymphoproliferative disease (B cell non-Hodgkin's lymphoma and nodular sclerosing Hodgkin's disease) in the 9 months after infliximab infusion in patients with Crohn's disease (63). The FDA received reports of 26 cases of lymphoproliferative disorders in patients treated with etanercept ($n = 18$) or infliximab ($n = 8$) over 20 months (64). Although this reporting rate does not exceed the age-adjusted incidence of lymphomas in the USA, spontaneous reporting underestimates the true incidence. In addition, several findings were similar to those reported in patients taking immunosuppressive drugs after transplantation. For example, 81% of the reported cases were non-Hodgkin's lymphomas. Also, the median time to occurrence after the start of anti-TNF-alfa treatment was only 8 weeks. Finally, lymphoma regressed in two patients after withdrawal and without specific cytotoxic therapy. Although the actual incidence of neoplasia was low, additional long-term data that take into account concomitant or previous immunosuppressive treatment are needed before firm conclusions can be reached.

References

1. Bell S, Kamm MA. Antibodies to tumour necrosis factor alpha as treatment for Crohn's disease. Lancet 2000;355(9207):858–60.
2. Wall GC, Heyneman C, Pfanner TP. Medical options for treating Crohn's disease in adults: focus on antitumor necrosis factor-alpha chimeric monoclonal antibody. Pharmacotherapy 1999;19(10):1138–52.
3. Maini R, St Clair EW, Breedveld F, Furst D, Kalden J, Weisman M, Smolen J, Emery P, Harriman G, Feldmann M, Lipsky P. Infliximab (chimeric anti-tumour necrosis factor alpha monoclonal antibody) versus placebo in rheumatoid arthritis patients receiving concomitant methotrexate: a randomised phase III trial. ATTRACT Study Group. Lancet 1999;354(9194):1932–9.
4. Keeling S, Oswald A, Russell AS, Maksymowych WP. Prospective observational analysis of the efficacy and safety of low-dose (3 mg/kg) infliximab in ankylosing spondylitis: 4-year follow up. J Rheumatol 2006;33(3):558–61.
5. Bickston SJ, Lichtenstein GR, Arseneau KO, Cohen RB, Cominelli F. The relationship between infliximab treatment

and lymphoma in Crohn's disease. Gastroenterology 1999;117(6):1433–7.
6. Morelli J, Wilson FA. Does administration of infliximab increase susceptibility to listeriosis? Am J Gastroenterol 2000;95(3):841–2.
7. Weisman MH. What are the risks of biologic therapy in rheumatoid arthritis? An update on safety. J Rheumatol Suppl 2002;65:33–8.
8. Braun J, Brandt J, Listing J, Zink A, Alten R, Golder W, Gromnica-Ihle E, Kellner H, Krause A, Schneider M, Sorensen H, Zeidler H, Thriene W, Sieper J. Treatment of active ankylosing spondylitis with infliximab: a randomised controlled multicentre trial. Lancet 2002;359(9313):1187–93.
9. Baig I, Storch I, Katz S. Infliximab induced eosinophilic pleural effusion in inflammatory bowel disease. Am J Gastroenterol 2002;97(Suppl):177.
10. Marotte H, Charrin JE, Miossec P. Infliximab-induced aseptic meningitis. Lancet 2001;358(9295):1784.
11. Mohan N, Edwards ET, Cupps TR, Oliverio PJ, Sandberg G, Crayton H, Richert JR, Siegel JN. Demyelination occurring during anti-tumor necrosis factor alpha therapy for inflammatory arthritides. Arthritis Rheum 2001;44(12):2862–9.
12. Robinson WH, Genovese MC, Moreland LW. Demyelinating and neurologic events reported in association with tumor necrosis factor alpha antagonism: by what mechanisms could tumor necrosis factor alpha antagonists improve rheumatoid arthritis but exacerbate multiple sclerosis? Arthritis Rheum 2001;44(9):1977–83.
13. ten Tusscher MP, Jacobs PJ, Busch MJ, de Graaf L, Diemont WL. Bilateral anterior toxic optic neuropathy and the use of infliximab. BMJ 2003;326(7389):579.
14. Foroozan R, Buono LM, Sergott RC, Savino PJ. Retrobulbar optic neuritis associated with infliximab. Arch Ophthalmol 2002;120(7):985–7.
15. Yee AM, Pochapin MB. Treatment of complicated sarcoidosis with infliximab anti-tumor necrosis factor-alpha therapy. Ann Intern Med 2001;135(1):27–31.
16. Menghini VV, Arora AS. Infliximab-associated reversible cholestatic liver disease. Mayo Clin Proc 2001;76(1):84–6.
17. Vergara G, Silvestre JF, Betlloch I, Vela P, Albares MP, Pascual JC. Cutaneous drug eruption to infliximab: report of 4 cases with an interface dermatitis pattern. Arch Dermatol 2002;138(9):1258–9.
18. Kent PD, Davis JM 3rd, Davis MD, Matteson EL. Bullous skin lesions following infliximab infusion in a patient with rheumatoid arthritis. Arthritis Rheum 2002;46(8):2257–8.
19. Griffin SP, Selby WS. Poor wound healing following surgery in three patients who received infliximab for Crohn's disease. J Gastroenterol Hepatol 2000;15(Suppl):78.
20. Hanauer SB, Feagan BG, Lichtenstein GR, Mayer LF, Schreiber S, Colombel JF, Rachmilewitz D, Wolf DC, Olson A, Bao W, Rutgeerts P; ACCENT I Study Group. Maintenance infliximab for Crohn's disease: the ACCENT I randomised trial. Lancet 2002;359(9317):1541–9.
21. Baert F, Noman M, Vermeire S, Van Assche G, D' Haens G, Carbonez A, Rutgeerts P. Influence of immunogenicity on the long-term efficacy of infliximab in Crohn's disease. N Engl J Med 2003;348(7):601–8.
22. Riegert-Johnson DL, Godfrey JA, Myers JL, Hubmayr RD, Sandborn WJ, Loftus EV Jr. Delayed hypersensitivity reaction and acute respiratory distress syndrome following infliximab infusion. Inflamm Bowel Dis 2002;8(3):186–91.
23. Charles PJ, Smeenk RJ, De Jong J, Feldmann M, Maini RN. Assessment of antibodies to double-stranded DNA induced in rheumatoid arthritis patients following treatment with infliximab, a monoclonal antibody to tumor necrosis factor alpha: findings in open-label and randomized placebo-controlled trials. Arthritis Rheum 2000;43(11):2383–90.
24. Mikuls TR, Moreland LW. Benefit-risk assessment of infliximab in the treatment of rheumatoid arthritis. Drug Saf 2003;26(1):23–32.
25. Ali Y, Shah S. Infliximab-induced systemic lupus erythematosus. Ann Intern Med 2002;137(7):625–6.
26. Klapman JB, Ene-Stroescu D, Becker MA, Hanauer SB. A lupus-like syndrome associated with infliximab therapy. Inflamm Bowel Dis 2003;9(3):176–8.
27. Hanauer SB, Rutgeerts PJ, D'Haens G, Targan SR, Kam L, Present DH, Wagner C, LaSorda J, Sands B, Livingstone RA. Delayed hypersensitivity to infliximab (Remicade) re-infusion after a 2-4 year interval without treatment. Gastroenterology 1999;116:A731.
28. Favalli EG, Sinigaglia L, Varenna M, Arnoldi C. Drug-induced lupus following treatment with infliximab in rheumatoid arthritis. Lupus 2002;11(11):753–5.
29. Cheifetz A, Smedley M, Martin S, Reiter M, Leone G, Mayer L, Plevy S. The incidence and management of infusion reactions to infliximab: a large center experience. Am J Gastroenterol 2003;98(6):1315–24.
30. Kugathasan S, Levy MB, Saeian K, Vasilopoulos S, Kim JP, Prajapati D, Emmons J, Martinez A, Kelly KJ, Binion DG. Infliximab retreatment in adults and children with Crohn's disease: risk factors for the development of delayed severe systemic reaction. Am J Gastroenterol 2002;97(6):1408–14.
31. Farrell RJ, Shah SA, Lodhavia PJ, Alsahli M, Falchuk KR, Michetti P, Peppercorn MA. Clinical experience with infliximab therapy in 100 patients with Crohn's disease. Am J Gastroenterol 2000;95(12):3490–7.
32. Puchner TC, Kugathasan S, Kelly KJ, Binion DG. Successful desensitization and therapeutic use of infliximab in adult and pediatric Crohn's disease patients with prior anaphylactic reaction. Inflamm Bowel Dis 2001;7(1):34–7.
33. O'Connor M, Buchman A, Marshall G. Anaphylaxis-like reaction to infliximab in a patient with Crohn's disease. Dig Dis Sci 2002;47(6):1323–5.
34. Lankarani KB. Mortality associated with infliximab. J Clin Gastroenterol 2001;33(3):255–6.
35. McCain ME, Quinet RJ, Davis WE. Etanercept and infliximab associated with cutaneous vasculitis. Rheumatology (Oxford) 2002;41(1):116–17.
36. Crandall WV, Mackner LM. Infusion reactions to infliximab in children and adolescents: frequency, outcome and a predictive model. Aliment Pharmacol Ther 2003;17(1): 75–84.
37. Kamath BM, Mamula P, Baldassano RN, Markowitz JE. *Listeria* meningitis after treatment with infliximab. J Pediatr Gastroenterol Nutr 2002;34(4):410–12.
38. Shanahan JC, St Clair W. Tumor necrosis factor-alpha blockade: a novel therapy for rheumatic disease. Clin Immunol 2002;103(3 Pt 1):231–42.
39. Chan AT, Cleeve V, Daymond TJ. Necrotising fasciitis in a patient receiving infliximab for rheumatoid arthritis. Postgrad Med J 2002;78(915):47–8.
40. Matzkies FG, Manger B, Schmitt-Haendle M, Nagel T, Kraetsch HG, Kalden JR, Schulze-Koops H. Severe septicaemia in a patient with polychondritis and Sweet's syndrome after initiation of treatment with infliximab. Ann Rheum Dis 2003;62(1):81–2.
41. Gluck T, Linde HJ, Scholmerich J, Muller-Ladner U, Fiehn C, Bohland P. Anti-tumor necrosis factor therapy and *Listeria monocytogenes* infection: report of two cases. Arthritis Rheum 2002;46(8):2255–7.
42. Liberopoulos EN, Drosos AA, Elisaf MS. Exacerbation of tuberculosis enteritis after treatment with infliximab. Am J Med 2002;113(7):615.
43. Van Den Bosch F, Kruithof E, Baeten D, Herssens A, de Keyser F, Mielants H, Veys EM. Randomized double-blind comparison of chimeric monoclonal antibody to

tumor necrosis factor alpha (infliximab) versus placebo in active spondylarthropathy. Arthritis Rheum 2002;46(3): 755–65.
44. Mayordomo L, Marenco JL, Gomez-Mateos J, Rejon E. Pulmonary miliary tuberculosis in a patient with anti-TNF-alpha treatment. Scand J Rheumatol 2002;31(1):44–5.
45. Nunez Martinez O, Ripoll Noiseux C, Carneros Martin JA, Gonzalez Lara V, Gregorio Maranon HG. Reactivation tuberculosis in a patient with anti-TNF-alpha treatment. Am J Gastroenterol 2001;96(5):1665–6.
46. Roth S, Delmont E, Heudier P, Kaphan R, Cua E, Castela J, Verdier JM, Chichmanian RM, Fuzibet JG. Anticorps anti-TNF alpha (infliximab) et tuberculose: à propos de 3 cas. Rev Med Interne 2002;23(3):312–16.
47. Rovere Querini P, Vecellio M, Sabbadini MG, Ciboddo G. Miliary tuberculosis after biological therapy for rheumatoid arthritis. Rheumatology 2002;41(2):231.
48. Wagner TE, Huseby ES, Huseby JS. Exacerbation of *Mycobacterium tuberculosis* enteritis masquerading as Crohn's disease after treatment with a tumor necrosis factor-alpha inhibitor. Am J Med 2002;112(1):67–9.
49. Keane J, Gershon S, Wise RP, Mirabile-Levens E, Kasznica J, Schwieterman WD, Siegel JN, Braun MM. Tuberculosis associated with infliximab, a tumor necrosis factor alpha-neutralizing agent. N Engl J Med 2001;345(15):1098–104.
50. Sandborn WJ, Hanauer SB. Infliximab in the treatment of Crohn's disease: a user's guide for clinicians. Am J Gastroenterol 2002;97(12):2962–72.
51. Antoni C, Braun J. Side effects of anti-TNF therapy: current knowledge. Clin Exp Rheumatol 2002;20(6 Suppl 28):S152–7.
52. Reichardt P, Dahnert I, Tiller G, Hausler HJ. Possible activation of an intramyocardial inflammatory process (*Staphylococcus aureus*) after treatment with infliximab in a boy with Crohn disease. Eur J Pediatr 2002;161(5): 281–3.
53. Haerter G, Manfras B, Schmitt M, Wendland T, Moch B. Severe CMV retinitis in a patient with HLA-B27 associated spondylarthropathy following immunosuppressive therapy with anti-TNF alpha (infliximab). Infection 2003;31(Suppl 1):150.
54. Helbling D, Breitbach TH, Krause M. Disseminated cytomegalovirus infection in Crohn's disease following anti-tumour necrosis factor therapy. Eur J Gastroenterol Hepatol 2002;14(12):1393–5.
55. Cursiefen C, Grunke M, Dechant C, Antoni C, Junemann A, Holbach LM. Multiple bilateral eyelid molluscum contagiosum lesions associated with TNFalpha-antibody and methotrexate therapy. Am J Ophthalmol 2002;134(2):270–1.
56. Tai TL, O'Rourke KP, McWeeney M, Burke CM, Sheehan K, Barry M. *Pneumocystis carinii* pneumonia following a second infusion of infliximab. Rheumatology (Oxford) 2002;41(8):951–2.
57. Lee JH, Slifman NR, Gershon SK, Edwards ET, Schwieterman WD, Siegel JN, Wise RP, Brown SL, Udall JN Jr, Braun MM. Life-threatening histoplasmosis complicating immunotherapy with tumor necrosis factor alpha antagonists infliximab and etanercept. Arthritis Rheum 2002;46(10):2565–70.
58. Fitzcharles MA, Clayton D, Menard HA. The use of infliximab in academic rheumatology practice: an audit of early clinical experience. J Rheumatol 2002;29(12):2525–30.
59. Nakelchik M, Mangino JE. Reactivation of histoplasmosis after treatment with infliximab. Am J Med 2002;112(1):78.
60. Warris A, Bjorneklett A, Gaustad P. Invasive pulmonary aspergillosis associated with infliximab therapy. N Engl J Med 2001;344(14):1099–100.
61. Ramzan NN, Shapiro MS, Robinson E, Smilack JD. Use of infliximab leading to extensive pulmonary coccidioidomycosis. Am J Gastroenterol 2002;97(Suppl):157.
62. de' Clari F, Salani I, Safwan E, Giannacco A. Sudden death in a patient without heart failure after a single infusion of 200 mg infliximab: does TNF-alpha have protective effects on the failing heart, or does infliximab have direct harmful cardiovascular effects? Circulation 2002;105(21):E183.
63. Drewe E, Powell RJ. Clinically useful monoclonal antibodies in treatment. J Clin Pathol 2002;55(2):81–5.
64. Brown SL, Greene MH, Gershon SK, Edwards ET, Braun MM. Tumor necrosis factor antagonist therapy and lymphoma development: twenty-six cases reported to the Food and Drug Administration. Arthritis Rheum 2002;46(12):3151–8.

Influenza vaccine

See also Vaccines

General Information

Influenza vaccine viruses are propagated in embryonated chicken eggs. The virus-containing extra-embryonic fluid is harvested, purified, and inactivated with formalin. Inactivated flu vaccine is produced either as whole virus vaccine or ether-disrupted split or subunit preparations. However, many other new or modified influenza vaccines are already available or are expected to appear in the near future, for example vaccines containing new adjuvants, live attenuated vaccines, and vaccines administered by alternative routes.

Comparisons of reactogenicity (and immunogenicity) of different vaccine types have been provided (SEDA-8, 299) (SEDA-10, 290) (SEDA-11, 290) (SEDA-12, 282) (SEDA-13, 286) (SEDA-14, 284) (SEDA-15, 351) (SEDA-16, 386) (SEDA-17, 375) (SEDA-18, 335) (1). In most of these trials the investigators found little difference in reactogenicity between the various vaccines.

The safety and immunogenicity of an inactivated subunit influenza vaccine containing MF59 (oil-in-water emulsion, squalene, and Tween 80 and sorbitan trioleate as stabilizers) as an adjuvant has been described in two studies of 92 and 211 elderly persons (65 years of age and over) (2,3). Investigations were carried out during three consecutive influenza seasons. Compared with a commercial non-adjuvant subunit vaccine containing the same influenza strains recommended by the World Health Organization, geometric mean titers and seroconversion rates were higher after the use of the newly developed vaccine. The adjuvant vaccine caused more local reactions than the conventional vaccine. However, the reactions were mild and limited to the first 2–3 days after immunization. Systemic reactions were not significantly different, except for mild transient malaise. Considering the better immunogenicity of the adjuvant vaccine, the authors recommended it particularly for elderly people, who are at greatest risk of developing severe influenza disease. The vaccine manufactured by Chiron Behring has been already licensed for persons of 65 years of age and over in Italy and Germany.

The results of several clinical trials with a liposomal influenza vaccine have been reviewed (4). This trivalent liposomal influenza vaccine consists of purified influenza hemagglutinin inserted into a membrane of phosphatidylcholine and phosphatidyl-ethanolamine; it contains 15 micrograms of hemagglutinin per viral strain per dose. The trials included two randomized studies (in 126 healthy nursing home residents aged 63–102 years and 72 elderly individuals aged 60–98 years) and four double-blind studies (in a total of 831 elderly persons aged 67–71 years and younger adults aged 28–38 years); further studies included 24 children and adults with cystic fibrosis and 49 children at high risk of influenza. In all of these studies, the liposomal vaccine was compared with commercially available whole and subunit influenza virus vaccines. In general, seroconversion rates were significantly higher with the liposomal vaccine than with the commercially available vaccines. Local adverse reactions, such as pain at the injection site (up to 62% of children and up to 11% of adults), local induration and swelling (33% of all vaccine recipients), or redness (5% of adults and 20% of children) were transient and usually mild. One child with cystic fibrosis and two elderly persons had severe pain. Between 68 and 100% of children with cystic fibrosis reported at least one systemic reaction (fatigue, cough, coryza, headache) after the liposomal vaccine compared with 23–50% after the commercially available subunit vaccine. Fatigue (up to 19%), malaise (up to 14%), headache (up to 10%), and cough (up to 8%) were the most common systemic reactions reported by young adults and elderly people. There were single cases of severe fatigue, cough, and diarrhea in children with cystic fibrosis, young adults, and elderly people. Liposomal influenza vaccine did not induce a mean antiphospholipid antibody response in the elderly volunteers.

In a randomized, double-blind study, trivalent, live, attenuated, cold-adapted intranasal influenza vaccine (FluMist) has been compared with intranasal placebo plus a trivalent injected inactivated influenza vaccine (5). The 200 patients were aged 65 years and over and had chronic cardiovascular or pulmonary conditions or diabetes mellitus. During the 7 days after immunization, sore throat was reported on at least one day by significantly more of the FluMist recipients (15 versus 2%). The increased frequency of sore throat may have been attributable to direct or indirect effects of vaccine virus replication. No other symptom was associated with FluMist. These findings were consistent with evaluations of other live, attenuated, cold-adapted influenza vaccine formulations in older adults. However, further studies of the safety of FluMist are warranted.

The immunogenicity and safety of inactivated intranasal influenza vaccine have been reviewed (6). The author concluded that the vaccine is highly immunogenic and well tolerated by most vaccinees, in terms of both local nasal symptoms and possible vaccine-mediated systemic symptoms. The symptoms were primarily mild, occasionally moderate, and in a few cases more severe; in most cases they lasted for only 1–2 days.

In 1997, an avian influenza A/Hongkong/97 (H5N1) virus emerged as a pandemic threat. A non-pathogenic variant influenza A/duck/Singapore/97 (H5N3) was identified as a leading vaccine candidate, but the non-adjuvanted antibody response was poor; however, the addition of the adjuvant MF59 (oil-in-water suspension) boosted the antibody responses to protective levels. In 65 volunteers who received either the non-adjuvanted or the adjuvanted vaccine, both vaccines were well tolerated and did not differ significantly. There was pain at the injection site of varying intensity in nine of the 32 volunteers who received the adjuvanted vaccine, and in none of the volunteers who received the non-adjuvanted vaccine (7).

General adverse effects

Local adverse reactions after flu immunization are few and infrequent. Slight to moderate tenderness, erythema, and induration at the injection site lasting 1–2 days occur in 15–30% of recipients. Fever, malaise, myalgia, and other symptoms of toxicity are rare (about 2%) and most often affect persons with no prior exposure to the flu antigens in the vaccine, for example young children. These reactions usually begin 6–12 hours after immunization and can last 1 or 2 days. They have been attributed to the vaccine, although the virus is inactivated. On the other hand, cases of respiratory diseases among vaccinees are coincidental. Although current flu vaccines are highly purified, they can cause hypersensitivity reactions such as hives or angioedema, perhaps due to residual egg protein (8,9). Notwithstanding the fact that the egg protein content is small, asthma or anaphylactic reactions with vascular purpura and encephalopathy can occur in those who are sensitive to the material (10,11).

Incidence

A nationwide surveillance system covering illness after flu immunization in the USA in 1976–77 among over 48 million persons immunized in 1976 with A/New Jersey/76 influenza vaccine (swine flu vaccine) resulted in a total of 4733 reports of illness, including reports of 223 deaths (12). Since most of the deaths occurred within 48 hours of immunization, the figures for deaths per 100 000 vaccinees (by diagnosis) were compared with the expected death rate (by the same diagnosis) per 100 000 population for a 2-day period. In general, the crude expected death rate was much higher than the death rate among vaccinees. Other than Guillain–Barré syndrome and rare cases of anaphylaxis, no serious illnesses seemed to be causally associated with flu immunization. However, widespread under-reporting of illness and death in the passive phase of this surveillance system impaired the validity of the study. Allergic skin reactions were reported at a rate of 0.3 per 100000 vaccinees and severe anaphylaxis at a rate of 0.024 per 100000. There was a cluster of four cases of encephalitis within 1 week of vaccine administration in one state. There were three deaths from cardiovascular disease in chronically ill persons over 70 years of age immunized in one clinic. It was not possible to establish a causative link between immunization and death. Persons immunized in the clinic died at rate of 5 per 100000 per day, in contrast to the expected rate of 17 per 100000 per day for people aged 65 years and older in the respective state.

Case reports of complications temporarily connected with the administration of flu vaccine have been published. They include reports of acute disseminated encephalitis (13), acute thrombocytopenic purpura (14), acute transverse myelitis (15), aseptic meningitis (16), bullous pemphigoid (SEDA-21, 334), encephalopathy (17), erythromelalgia (18), optic neuritis (19) with reversible blindness (SEDA-4, 226) (SEDA-21, 334), optic atrophy (SEDA-6, 287), pericarditis (SEDA-7, 324), polymyalgia rheumatica (20), microscopic polyangiitis involving the skin and joints (21), acute symmetrical polyarthropathy with orbital myositis and posterior scleritis (22), systemic vasculitis (23), a trigeminal neuralgia-like symptoms (24), and vascular purpura with histological features of cutaneous necrotizing vasculitis (25).

The current status of adjuvanted influenza vaccines has been reviewed (26). The authors concluded that the vaccine produces a higher titer of antibodies than non-adjuvanted or virosomal vaccines. Local reactions occur more often, but are mild and transient. The results of a trial with two doses of an intranasally administered inactivated virosome-formulated influenza vaccine containing *Escherichia coli* heat-labile toxin as a mucosal adjuvant in 106 volunteers aged 33–63 years have been reported (27). About 50% of vaccinees had local adverse reactions (44% after the first dose and 54% after the second dose) or systemic adverse reactions (48 and 46%) after administration of the vaccine. Rhinorrhea, sneezing, and headache were the most common reactions; they were mild and transient and resolved within 24–48 hours. No febrile reactions were associated with immunization. Between 77 and 92% of vaccinees developed protective hemagglutination inhibition antibody titers against the two influenzae A strains of the vaccine, whereas protective antibody titers against the B strain of the vaccine were achieved in only 49–58%.

Organs and Systems

Cardiovascular

Influenza infection has been a significant problem in cardiac transplant patients; immunization of such patients could therefore be beneficial. However, its use has been limited by concern that stimulation of the immune system might in principle cause an increased risk of cardiac rejection. In the renal transplant experience, influenza infection itself can trigger an immunological response to cause graft rejection, as well as predisposing to other infections. Another concern is whether an immunosuppressed cardiac transplant recipient could seroconvert sufficiently. In a case-control study in 18 cardiac transplant recipients and 18 control patients 6 months or more beyond transplant surgery, there were no differences in the incidence of cardiac rejection or immune responses (28).

There have been reports of pericarditis (29,30) in temporal relation to influenza vaccine.

Respiratory

Of 109 children with asthma aged 6 months to 18 years immunized with trivalent subvirion influenza vaccine, 59 vaccinees had no asthma symptoms on the day of immunization, but 50 had an exacerbation requiring prednisone (31). Antibody responses were not different in the two groups. Adverse effects, including local swelling at the injection site, fever, rash, and headache, were not different in the two groups.

Nervous system

Adverse effects of flu immunization on the nervous system range from polyneuropathy to meningoencephalitis and Guillain–Barré syndrome (32).

Examination of new cases of multiple sclerosis among the 45 million swine flu vaccine recipients indicated no excess over the expected frequencies. Inactivated swine flu vaccine did not influence the onset or exacerbation of the disease (33).

Guillain–Barré syndrome

Guillain–Barré syndrome was observed during the 1976/7 mass immunization campaign in the USA. The vaccine then used was A/New Jersey/76 (H1N1) flu vaccine (swine influenza). The overall incidence of cases of Guillain–Barré syndrome attributed to the use of vaccine at that time was 4.9–5.9 per million vaccinees (34). Various authors tried to settle the question of a cause and effect relation. Detailed reports have been published (SEDA-10, 289) (SEDA-11, 290) and the resulting litigation has been reviewed (35). In an analysis of computerized summaries of 1300 cases, immunized cases with extensive paresis or paralysis occurred in a characteristic epidemiological pattern, suggesting a causal relation between immunization and Guillain–Barré syndrome (34). Cases with limited motor involvement showed no such pattern. Unlike the 1976 swine flu vaccine, vaccines used subsequently have not been associated with an increased frequency of Guillain–Barré syndrome. It has been calculated that the risk of polyneuropathy following immunization is one in 200 000, compared with a population incidence of spontaneous Guillain–Barré syndrome of one in 1 000 000 (36).

The original Centers for Disease Control study of the relation between A/New Jersey/876 (swine flu) vaccine and Guillain–Barré syndrome showed a statistically significant association and suggested a causal association between the two events. In an evaluation of the medical records of all previously reported adult patients with Guillain–Barré syndrome in Michigan and Minnesota from 1 October 1976 to 31 January 1977, the relative risk during the 6 weeks after flu immunization in adults was 7.10 (excess cases attributed to the vaccine: 8.6 per million vaccinees in Michigan and 9.7 per million vaccinees in Minnesota), comparable to the relative risk of 7.60 found in the original study (37). There was no increase in the relative risk of Guillain–Barré syndrome beyond 6 weeks after immunization.

A retrospective study (1980–88) conducted to determine if the US Army's mass influenza immunization program was associated with an increased incidence of Guillain–Barré syndrome found no temporally related increase (38).

The number of reports of influenza vaccine-associated Guillain–Barré syndrome to the US Vaccine Adverse Event Reporting System increased from 37 in 1992–93 to 74 in 1993–94, raising concerns about a possible increase in vaccine-associated risk. Detailed data analyses showed that the relative risk of Guillain–Barré syndrome associated with influenza immunization, adjusted for age, sex, and vaccine season, was 2.0 for the 1992–93 season and 1.5 for the 1993–94 season. For the two seasons combined, the adjusted relative risk of 1.7 suggested that there was slightly more than one additional case of Guillain–Barré syndrome per million vaccinees. An accompanying editorial also referred to the occurrence of Guillain–Barré syndrome during the swine flu immunization campaign in 1976. The authors considered the results of this study as epidemiological evidence that immunization against strains of influenza other than swine flu may increase the risk of Guillain–Barré syndrome, albeit minimally (39).

Sensory systems

Four patients with corneal transplants developed ocular manifestations (bilateral graft rejection in two cases, uveitis, and epithelial and stromal herpetic kerato-uveitis) at 3 days to 6 weeks after the receipt of inactivated influenza vaccine (40). Whereas case reports of ocular manifestations after influenza immunization are known, this is perhaps the first report of vaccine-related herpetic recurrence. The authors advised caution when influenza immunization is considered for patients who have had a corneal transplant.

Urinary tract

There has been a report of minimal-change nephrotic syndrome (41) in temporal relation to influenza vaccine.

Skin

Influenza vaccine is one of at least 30 drugs believed to cause bullous pemphigoid or cicatricial pemphigoid (42).

- A 90-year-old woman developed a generalized bullous eruption resembling bullous pemphigoid 12 hours after influenza immunization (43).

Influenza vaccine can also cause pemphigus (44).

Musculoskeletal

There has been a report of rhabdomyolysis (45) in temporal relation to influenza vaccine.

Immunologic

Changes in the lymphocyte population similar to those observed during virus infections occurred within the first 2 weeks after immunization (46). There were no reports describing more severe courses of infectious diseases during this period.

The question of whether egg allergy is a justified contraindication to influenza immunization has been studied in 80 individuals with egg allergy and 124 control subjects, who received influenza vaccine containing ovalbumin/ovomucoid 0.02, 0.1, or 1.2 μg/ml (47). The individuals with egg allergy received the vaccine in two doses 30 minutes apart; the first dose was one-tenth and the second dose nine-tenths of the recommended dose. The patients with egg allergy, even those with significant allergic reactions after egg ingestion, safely received influenza vaccine in this two-dose protocol with vaccine containing no more than 1.2 μg/ml of egg protein.

There have been reports of individual cases of giant cell arteritis (48) and polymyalgia rheumatica (49,50) in temporal relation to influenza vaccine.

- A 70-year-old man, previously healthy, developed giant cell arteritis 5 days after influenza immunization (51).

The authors mentioned another case reported in 1976.

Drug Administration

Drug dosage regimens

Current recommendations for the use of influenza vaccine in adults are based on a single injection. This may not be valid in case of a new pandemic caused by an antigenic shift of the influenza virus. Currently, the only group for whom a second dose is recommended comprises children who have never been immunized. However, when two-dose regimens in adults have been studied, the second dose of vaccine has not been associated with higher rates of reactions than the first. People who have a stronger local reaction after a first injection are more likely to have another such reaction after a second injection (31).

Drug administration route

The intranasal administration of influenza vaccines has been reviewed (52). Trivalent cold-adapted intranasal influenza vaccine was used to immunize 1602 healthy children aged 15–71 months in a randomized, double-blind, placebo-controlled trial (53). One year later 1358 were reimmunized. The vaccine provided efficacy of 92% during 2 years against virologically confirmed influenza. Transient, minor symptoms of respiratory illness (rhinorrhea, nasal congestion, low-grade fever) were reported more often in vaccinees than in controls; no significant differences were noted after dose 1 and dose 2.

Drug–Drug Interactions

Anticoagulants

In a prospective study of the effect of flu immunization on the prothrombin time in eight patients taking long-term anticoagulant treatment the prothrombin time was prolonged by 40%. In healthy subjects there was no significant effect on warfarin metabolism (SEDA-10, 289).

- An 81-year-old patient who had been well controlled by anticoagulants for 12 years had an episode of gastrointestinal bleeding associated with influenza immunization (54).

However, others did not confirm this effect (55), and the lack of a clinical interaction with warfarin has also been confirmed by a report of the US Immunization Practices Advisory Committee (9).

Anticonvulsants

In a study of serum concentrations of the anticonvulsants phenytoin, phenobarbital, and carbamazepine, before and after mentally retarded patients received flu vaccine, the authors concluded that serum concentrations of these drugs may increase as a result of flu immunization and that dosage adjustments may be necessary (56).

Benzodiazepines

The metabolism of lorazepam and chlordiazepoxide was not altered by flu immunization (57).

Theophylline

After influenza immunization there was a reduction in blood theophylline concentrations in patients and healthy volunteers (58). The authors concluded that flu vaccine may influence the pharmacokinetics of several drugs, and a second group found that theophylline oxidation was significantly reduced at 1 day, but not at 7 days, after immunization (57). However, others did not confirm these effects (55,59). The lack of a clinical interaction with theophylline has also been confirmed by a report of the US Immunization Practices Advisory Committee (9).

References

1. Palache AM. Influenza vaccines. A reappraisal of their use. Drugs 1997;54(6):841–56.
2. Minutello M, Senatore F, Cecchinelli G, Bianchi M, Andreani T, Podda A, Crovari P. Safety and immunogenicity of an inactivated subunit influenza virus vaccine combined with MF59 adjuvant emulsion in elderly subjects, immunized for three consecutive influenza seasons. Vaccine 1999;17(2):99–104.
3. De Donato S, Granoff D, Minutello M, Lecchi G, Faccini M, Agnello M, Senatore F, Verweij P, Fritzell B, Podda A. Safety and immunogenicity of MF59-adjuvanted influenza vaccine in the elderly. Vaccine 1999;17(23–24):3094–101.
4. Holm KJ, Goa KL, Oxford JS, McElhaney JE. Liposomal influenza vaccine. Biodrugs 1999;11:137–46.
5. Jackson LA, Holmes SJ, Mendelman PM, Huggins L, Cho I, Rhorer J. Safety of a trivalent live attenuated intranasal influenza vaccine, FluMist, administered in addition to parenteral trivalent inactivated influenza vaccine to seniors with chronic medical conditions. Vaccine 1999;17(15–16):1905–9.
6. Glueck R. Review of intranasal influenza vaccine. Adv Drug Deliv Rev 2001;51(1–3):203–11.
7. Nicholson KG, Colegate AE, Podda A, Stephenson I, Wood J, Ypma E, Zambon MC. Safety and antigenicity of non-adjuvanted and MF59-adjuvanted influenza A/Duck/Singapore/97 (H5N3) vaccine: a randomised trial of two potential vaccines against H5N1 influenza. Lancet 2001;357(9272):1937–43.
8. Committee on Immunization. In: Guide for adult immunization. Philadelphia: American College of Physicians, 1985;58.
9. Centers for Disease Control (CDC). Prevention and control of influenza. MMWR Morb Mortal Wkly Rep 1987;36(24):373–80, 385–7.
10. Stefanini M, Piomelli S, Mele R, Ostroski JT, Colpoys WP. Acute vascular purpura following immunization with Asiatic-influenza vaccine. N Engl J Med 1958;259(1):9–12.
11. Yahr MD, Lobo-Antunes J. Relapsing encephalomyelitis following the use of influenza vaccine. Arch Neurol 1972;27(2):182–3.
12. Retailliau HF, Curtis AC, Storr G, Caesar G, Eddins DL, Hattwick MA. Illness after influenza vaccination reported through a nationwide surveillance system, 1976–1977. Am J Epidemiol 1980;111(3):270–8.
13. Nagano T, Mizuguchi M, Kurihara E, Mizuno Y, Tamagawa K, Komiya K. [A case of acute disseminated encephalomyelitis with convulsion, gait disturbance, facial palsy and multifocal CT lesions.] No To Hattatsu 1988;20(4):325–9.
14. Casoli P, Tumiati B. Porpora trombocitopenica idiopatica acuta dopo vaccinacione antinfluenzale. [Acute idiopathic thrombocytopenic purpura after anti-influenza vaccination.] Medicina (Firenze) 1989;9(4):417–18.
15. Bakshi R, Mazziotta JC. Acute transverse myelitis after influenza vaccination: magnetic resonance imaging findings. J Neuroimaging 1996;6(4):248–50.
16. Ichikawa N, Takase S, Kogure K. [Recurrent aseptic meningitis following influenza vaccination in a case of systemic lupus erythematosus.] Rinsho Shinkeigaku 1983;23(7):570–6.
17. Morimoto T, Oguni H, Awaya Y, Hayakawa T, Fukuyama Y. A case of a rapidly progressive central nervous system disorder manifesting as a pallidal posture and ocular motor apraxia. Brain Dev 1985;7(4):449–53.
18. Confino I, Passwell JH, Padeh S. Erythromelalgia following influenza vaccine in a child. Clin Exp Rheumatol 1997;15(1):111–13.
19. Hull TP, Bates JH. Optic neuritis after influenza vaccination. Am J Ophthalmol 1997;124(5):703–4.
20. Beijer WE, Sprenger MJ, Masurel N. Polymyalgia rheumatica und Grippa–Schutzimptung. [Polymyalgia rheumatica and influenza vaccination.] Dtsch Med Wochenschr 1993;118(5):164–5.
21. Kelsall JT, Chalmers A, Sherlock CH, Tron VA, Kelsall AC. Microscopic polyangiitis after influenza vaccination. J Rheumatol 1997;24(6):1198–202.
22. Thurairajan G, Hope-Ross MW, Situnayake RD, Murray PI. Polyarthropathy, orbital myositis and posterior scleritis: an unusual adverse reaction to influenza vaccine. Br J Rheumatol 1997;36(1):120–3.
23. Mader R, Narendran A, Lewtas J, Bykerk V, Goodman RC, Dickson JR, Keystone EC. Systemic vasculitis following influenza vaccination—report of 3 cases and literature review. J Rheumatol 1993;20(8):1429–31.
24. Demmler M, Heidel G. Trigeminus-Affektion nach Influenza-Schutzimpfung. [Trigeminal involvement following preventive influenza vaccination.] Psychiatr Neurol Med Psychol (Leipz) 1985;37(7):428–33.
25. Vidal E, Gaches F, Berdah JF, Nadalon S, Lavignac C, Mitrea L, Loustaud-Ratti V, Liozon F. Vasculitis after influenza vaccination. Rev Med Intern 1993;14:1173.
26. Dooley M, Goa KL. Adjuvanted influenza vaccine. Biodrugs 2000;14:61–9.
27. Gluck R, Mischler R, Durrer P, Furer E, Lang AB, Herzog C, Cryz SJ Jr. Safety and immunogenicity of intranasally administered inactivated trivalent virosome-formulated influenza vaccine containing *Escherichia coli* heat-labile toxin as a mucosal adjuvant J Infect Dis 2000;181(3):1129–32.
28. Kobashigawa JA, Warner-Stevenson L, Johnson BL, Moriguchi JD, Kawata N, Drinkwater DC, Laks H. Influenza vaccine does not cause rejection after cardiac transplantation. Transplant Proc 1993;25(4):2738–9.
29. Medearis DN Jr, Neill CA, Markowitz M. Influenza and cardiopulmonary disease. II. Med Concepts Cardiovasc Dis 1963;32:813–16.
30. Zanettini MT, Zanettini JO, Zanettini JP. Pericarditis. Series of 84 consecutive cases. Arquivos Brasileiros de Cardiologia 2004;82(4):360–9.
31. Park CL, Frank AL, Sullivan M, Jindal P, Baxter BD. Influenza vaccination of children during acute asthma exacerbation and concurrent prednisone therapy. Pediatrics 1996;98(2 Pt 1):196–200.

32. Hayase Y, Tobita K. Influenza virus and neurological diseases. Psychiatry Clin Neurosci 1997;51(4):181–4.
33. Kurland LT, Molgaard CA, Kurland EM, Wiederholt WC, Kirkpatrick JW. Swine flu vaccine and multiple sclerosis. JAMA 1984;251(20):2672–5.
34. Langmuir AD, Bregman DJ, Kurland LT, Nathanson N, Victor M. An epidemiologic and clinical evaluation of Guillain–Barré syndrome reported in association with the administration of swine influenza vaccines. Am J Epidemiol 1984;119(6):841–79.
35. Dukes MNG, Swartz B. Responsibility for Drug-induced Injury. Amsterdam: Elsevier, 1988.
36. Feschank R, Kunzel U, Quast U. Das Guillain–Barré syndrome-eine Impfkomplikation? Z Allg Med 1986;62:71.
37. Safranek TJ, Lawrence DN, Kurland LT, Culver DH, Wiederholt WC, Hayner NS, Osterholm MT, O'Brien P, Hughes JM. Reassessment of the association between Guillain–Barré syndrome and receipt of swine influenza vaccine in 1976–1977: results of a two-state study. Expert Neurology Group. Am J Epidemiol 1991;133(9):940–51.
38. Roscelli JD, Bass JW, Pang L. Guillain–Barré syndrome and influenza vaccination in the US Army, 1980–1988. Am J Epidemiol 1991;133(9):952–5.
39. Lasky T, Terracciano GJ, Magder L, Koski CL, Ballesteros M, Nash D, Clark S, Haber P, Stolley PD, Schonberger LB, Chen RT. The Guillain–Barré syndrome and the 1992–1993 and 1993–1994 influenza vaccines. N Engl J Med 1998;339(25):1797–802.
40. Solomon A, Siganos CS, Frucht-Pery J. Adverse ocular effects following influenza vaccination. Eye 1999;13(Pt 3a):381–2.
41. Kielstein JT, Termuhlen L, Sohn J, Kliem V. Minimal change nephrotic syndrome in a 65-year-old patient following influenza vaccination. Clin Nephrol 2000;54(3):246–8.
42. Vassileva S. Drug-induced pemphigoid: bullous and cicatricial. Clin Dermatol 1998;16(3):379–87.
43. Garcia-Doval I, Roson E, Feal C, De la Torre C, Rodriguez T, Cruces MJ. Generalized bullous fixed drug eruption after influenza vaccination, simulating bullous pemphigoid. Acta Dermatol Venereol 2001;81(6):450–1.
44. Mignogna MD, Lo Muzio L, Ruocco E. Pemphigus induction by influenza vaccination. Int J Dermatol 2000;39(10):800.
45. Plotkin E, Bernheim J, Ben-Chetrit S, Mor A, Korzets Z. Influenza vaccine—a possible trigger of rhabdomyolysis induced acute renal failure due to the combined use of cerivastatin and bezafibrate. Nephrol Dial Transplant 2000;15(5):740–1.
46. Gerth HG. Grippeschutzimpfung. Dtsch Med Wochenschr 1989;114:180.
47. James JM, Zeiger RS, Lester MR, Fasano MB, Gern JE, Mansfield LE, Schwartz HJ, Sampson HA, Windom HH, Machtinger SB, Lensing S. Safe administration of influenza vaccine to patients with egg allergy. J Pediatr 1998;133(5):624–8.
48. Perez C, Loza E, Tinture T. Giant cell arteritis after influenza vaccination. Arch Intern Med 2000;160(17):2677.
49. Liozon E, Ittig R, Vogt N, Michel JP, Gold G. Polymyalgia rheumatica following influenza vaccination. J Am Geriatr Soc 2000;48(11):1533–4.
50. Perez C, Maravi E. Polymyalgia rheumatica following influenza vaccination. Muscle Nerve 2000;23(5):824–5.
51. Finsterer J, Artner C, Kladosek A, Kalchmayr R, Redtenbacher S. Cavernous sinus syndrome due to vaccination-induced giant cell arteritis. Arch Intern Med 2001;161(7):1008–9.
52. Eyles JE, Williamson ED, Alpar HO. Intranasal administration of influenza vaccines: current status. Biodrugs 2000;13:35–59.
53. Belshe RB, Gruber WC. Prevention of otitis media in children with live attenuated influenza vaccine given intranasally. Pediatr Infect Dis J 2000;19(Suppl 5):S66–71.
54. Kramer P, Tsuru M, Cook CE, McClain CJ, Holtzman JL. Effect of influenza vaccine on warfarin anticoagulation. Clin Pharmacol Ther 1984;35(3):416–18.
55. Gomolin IH, Chapron DJ, Luhan PA. Lack of effect of influenza vaccine on theophylline levels and warfarin anticoagulation in the elderly. J Am Geriatr Soc 1985;33(4):269–72.
56. Jann MW, Fidone GS. Effect of influenza vaccine on serum anticonvulsant concentrations. Clin Pharm 1986;5(10):817–20.
57. Meredith CG, Christian CD, Johnson RF, Troxell R, Davis GL, Schenker S. Effects of influenza virus vaccine on hepatic drug metabolism. Clin Pharmacol Ther 1985;37(4):396–401.
58. Kramer P, McClain CJ. Depression of aminopyrine metabolism by influenza vaccination. N Engl J Med 1981;305(21):1262–4.
59. Grabowski N, May JJ, Pratt DS, Richtsmeier WJ, Bertino JS Jr. The effect of split virus influenza vaccination on theophylline pharmacokinetics. Am Rev Respir Dis 1985;131(6):934–8.

Inhaler propellants

General Information

Pulmonary delivery of drugs is the administration route of choice in respiratory diseases such as chronic obstructive pulmonary disease and asthma. Different devices are available, including metered-dose inhalers, dry powder inhalers, and nebulizers, and nearly 80% of asthmatic patients worldwide use metered dose inhalers (1). Chlorofluorocarbons have been used as an aerosol propellant in metered-dose inhalers; however, they deplete the ozone layer and are being replaced by more environment-friendly propellants, even though the contribution of aerosols of this type to the total global burden of chlorofluorocarbons is less than 0.5%. The first chlorofluorocarbon-free metered-dose inhaler for asthma treatment was approved by the FDA in 1996 (2) and the European Union has set 2005 as a target date for the withdrawal of all chlorofluorocarbon-based inhalers (1). In the USA, prescriptions for chlorofluorocarbon-free medications rose from 16.4 million in 1996 to 33.8 million in 2000 (2). Most of the chlorofluorocarbon-free medications were steroids for nasal use (27.2 million). However, chlorofluorocarbon-containing medications still represented two-thirds of all prescriptions and increased from 63.0 to 67.6 million dispensed (2).

Specific propellants

Freons (chlorofluorocarbons)

The multidose pressurized aerosols using chlorofluorocarbon propellants have been widely used.

In animal experiments, plasma concentrations of Freon 11 and Freon 12 of 20–35 μg/ml sensitized the heart to adrenaline and exercise. Severely ill asthmatic subjects (mean oxygen tension=55 mmHg, range 50–80) were studied following therapeutic doses of a beta$_2$-adrenoceptor agonist pressurized aerosol. Plasma concentrations of

Freon 11 up to 4.53 μg/ml and of Freon 12 up to 4.73 μg/ml were measured after two inhalations. It was concluded that a toxic concentration could only be reached if the aerosol was taken on every breath for over 12 consecutive breaths (3).

Other excipients

The effects of other constituents present in multidose pressurized aerosols have been investigated in 11 850 asthmatic patients. Three aerosols were compared. Two placebo multidose pressurized aerosols contained the same chlorofluorocarbons but different dispersing chemicals, oleic acid (MDI-OA) and lecithin NF (MDI-L). Another contained salmeterol xinafoate (0.025 mg) plus lecithin NF (MDI-S). Peak expiratory flow rate was measured before and 5 minutes after inhalation. A 20% fall in peak expiratory flow rate was defined as clinically significant bronchoconstriction. A total of 180 (1.5%) patients developed bronchoconstriction, 43 in the MDI-S group, 67 in the MDI-L group, and 70 in the MDI-OA group. Bronchoconstriction was significantly less with the salmeterol aerosol. It was suggested that one of the inert constituents is the likely irritant causing occasional acute bronchoconstriction. The risk of this effect increased with age and decreasing pretreatment peak expiratory flow rate (4).

Preservatives

Inhalation of distilled water will cause bronchoconstriction in 60% of infants with a history of wheeze (SEDA-17, 212). If nebulizer solutions are hypotonic or hypertonic or contain preservatives (such as benzalkonium chloride, edetic acid, sulfites and metabisulfite) they can cause paradoxical bronchoconstriction. It has been recommended that all nebulizer solutions should be isotonic and free of preservatives (SEDA-13, 132). Unit dose vials are available in which the drug solution is isotonic and preservative-free. However, multidose formulations are still available and are widely used, as the cost per dose is less.

Benzalkonium chloride at concentrations greater than 0.005 mg/ml causes histamine release from mast cells in vitro. At a concentration of 0.03 mg/ml an excess of 90% of the histamine content is released (5). This is in the range of the minimum concentration of benzalkonium chloride recommended as a disinfectant (0.025 mg/ml). Inhalation of benzalkonium chloride nebulizer solution causes concentration-related falls in FEV_1 in patients with asthma (6). Benzalkonium chloride 0.3 mg also causes a temporary increase in airway reactivity to histamine. This amount of benzalkonium chloride is similar to that in a 2.5 mg dose from a multidose vial of salbutamol (7). Ipratropium containing benzalkonium chloride 0.25 mg/ml causes bronchoconstriction in a proportion of patients with asthma. Bronchodilatation is seen when 2 ml (0.5 mg) of preservative-free ipratropium bromide solution is inhaled (8). Benzalkonium chloride 0.1 mg/ml does not alter the bronchodilator effect of salbutamol. The difference between salbutamol and ipratropium may be the lower concentration of benzalkonium chloride in the salbutamol solution (0.1 versus 0.25 mg/ml) and the greater potency and more rapid onset of the bronchodilator response to salbutamol (9). Individual case reports suggest that multiple doses of nebulized salbutamol (containing benzalkonium chloride) can cause serious deterioration in severe asthma. This can be reversed by changing to a benzalkonium chloride-free formulation (10).

EDTA (edetate) is also used as a preservative in nebulizer preparations and produces a concentration-related bronchoconstriction (11).

Hydrofluoroalkanes

The search for ozone-friendly propellants has concentrated on two hydrofluoroalkanes with physicochemical properties similar to the chlorofluorocarbons: hydrofluoroalkane 134a and hydrofluoroalkane 227 (1). A new generation of chlorofluorocarbon-free metered dose inhalers has been designed by the pharmaceutical industry to be equivalent to the currently marketed chlorofluorocarbon-containing inhalers in terms of efficacy, safety, and dose delivery. This goal was achieved by using the Modulite technology, by dissolving the drug in the propellant with the aid of a glycerol-like co-solvent (12).

Beta$_2$-adrenoceptor agonists

The therapeutic effects of salbutamol and salmeterol were unaffected by hydrofluoroalkane 134a, and there were no clinically significant differences in safety parameters (13,14). The safety of the hydrofluoroalkane 134a salbutamol sulfate inhaler, Airomir, has been evaluated in a postmarketing surveillance study (15). A non-randomized study has been performed in 6614 patients with obstructive airways disease taking metered doses of salbutamol delivered by inhalers using either hydrofluoroalkane or chlorofluorocarbon as the propellant. There were no significant differences between the groups in the rate of hospital admissions for the condition for which salbutamol was prescribed, in visits to accident and emergency departments, or in unscheduled home visits. There were adverse events in 25% of patients in both groups. The most common adverse events were infection, bronchospasm, and upper respiratory tract infection. Adverse events attributed to the medication occurred in 3.1% of the patients who used the hydrofluoroalkane propellant and 0.7% of those who used the chlorofluorocarbon. This difference was significant (OR = 4.34; 95% CI = 2.22, 8.52). In contrast, serious adverse events occurred more often with the chlorofluorocarbon (3.7%) than with the hydrofluoroalkane (2.7%), but this difference was not significant.

More patients using the hydrofluoroalkane (18%) withdrew from the study than patients using the chlorofluorocarbon (4.8%). Most of the withdrawals in both groups were unrelated to safety (9 and 3.2% respectively). The reasons for withdrawal included intercurrent illness, loss to follow-up, and inadvertent prescription errors. More patients using the hydrofluoroalkane withdrew because of an adverse event or because of the taste of the inhaler, 3.8 versus 0.9% and 3.1 versus 0.2% respectively. The authors concluded that the data supported the evidence already obtained in clinical trials that reformulation of salbutamol in a hydrofluoroalkane propellant does not result in changes in safety compared with a chlorofluorocarbon formulation.

Hydrofluoroalkane 134a and chlorofluorocarbon have been compared in two randomized, double-blind, placebo-controlled studies with salbutamol. Salbutamol 180 μg in hydrofluoroalkane 134a given 30 minutes before an exercise challenge was as safe and effective as 180 μg in chlorofluorocarbon in 24 patients with documented exercise-induced bronchospasm (16). In 63 patients with mild to moderate asthma salbutamol in hydrofluoroalkane 134a or chlorofluorocarbon were of comparable efficacy without any difference in the incidence of adverse events (17).

Glucocorticoids

Beclomethasone dipropionate and budesonide Modulite formulations have been compared with equivalent chlorofluorocarbon products in small groups of healthy volunteers and asthmatic patients (18): there was no significant difference in morning serum cortisol or urinary cortisol excretion, suggesting that the systemic availability of the inhaled corticosteroids with different propellants is similar. Moreover, plasma profiles of beclomethasone dipropionate and B17MP were similar after inhalation of beclomethasone dipropionate Modulite and beclomethasone dipropionate-chlorofluorocarbon, suggesting that pulmonary delivery to the lung is comparable with the two propellants (18).

There have been three randomized, double-blind studies in adult asthmatics of the efficacy and safety of a beclomethasone dipropionate-hydrofluoroalkane 134a formulation, equivalent in dose per actuation to the currently marketed beclomethasone dipropionate chlorofluorocarbon products (19–21). Daily doses of beclomethasone dipropionate hydrofluoroalkane 134a 1000 μg over 12 weeks given by metered-dose inhaler (19) or a spacer jet device (20) were equivalent in terms of safety and efficacy compared with beclomethasone dipropionate chlorofluorocarbon 1000 μg. The same was true for doses of 400 μg (21).

In another study, different doses of flunisolide hydrofluoroalkane were tested in 21 healthy adult volunteers for 4.5 days (170, 340, and 680 μg); there was a dose-related response after both single- and multiple-dose administration (22). There was no accumulation of flunisolide with repeated dosing, suggesting that the systemic availability of flunisolide hydrofluoroalkane is low. A randomized, double-blind, placebo-controlled study with daily doses of 80 and 160 μg over 12 weeks in 353 asthmatic children gave similar results (23).

These results suggest that the transition from chlorofluorocarbon-containing to chlorofluorocarbon-free metered-dose inhalers is possible without concerns about safety and efficacy.

Infection risk

Certain problems are peculiar to the use of wet nebulization inhalation devices. There is a risk of contamination of the airways with bacterial flora, which increases when treatment is given in a hospital (SEDA-2, 154). In one series of 41 patients in an intensive care unit who were being ventilated and were receiving nebulized salbutamol, all developed respiratory tract infections due to *Burkholderia* (*Pseudomonas*). The same organism (confirmed by molecular fingerprinting) was isolated from nebulizers and a multiple-dose bottle of salbutamol used for several of the patients. Appropriate infection control measures resolved the problem (SEDA-20, 185).

References

1. Bousquet J. Introduction. Modulite: simplifying the changeover. Respir Med 2002;96(Suppl D):S1–2.
2. Wysowski DK, Swann J. Use of inhalant medications with and without chlorofluorocarbon propellants in the United States, 1996–2000. J Allergy Clin Immunol 2002;110(1):51–3.
3. Dollery CT, Williams FM, Draffan GH, Wise G, Sahyoun H, Paterson JW, Walker SR. Arterial blood levels of fluorocarbons in asthmatic patients following use of pressurized aerosols. Clin Pharmacol Ther 1974;15(1):59–66.
4. Shaheen MZ, Ayres JG, Benincasa C. Incidence of acute decreases in peak expiratory flow following the use of metered-dose inhalers in asthmatic patients. Eur Respir J 1994;7(12):2160–4.
5. Read GW, Kiefer EF. Benzalkonium chloride: selective inhibitor of histamine release induced by compound 48/80 and other polyamines. J Pharmacol Exp Ther 1979;211(3):711–15.
6. Miszkiel KA, Beasley R, Rafferty P, Holgate ST. The contribution of histamine release to bronchoconstriction provoked by inhaled benzalkonium chloride in asthma. Br J Clin Pharmacol 1988;25(2):157–63.
7. Zhang YG, Wright WJ, Tam WK, Nguyen-Dang TH, Salome CM, Woolcock AJ. Effect of inhaled preservatives on asthmatic subjects. II. Benzalkonium chloride. Am Rev Respir Dis 1990;141(6):1405–8.
8. Rafferty P, Beasley R, Holgate ST. Comparison of the efficacy of preservative free ipratropium bromide and Atrovent nebuliser solution. Thorax 1988;43(6):446–50.
9. Kwong T, Flatt A, Crane J, Beasley R. The effect of benzalkonium chloride on the bronchodilator response to salbutamol nebuliser solution. NZ Med J 1990;103(898):457.
10. Beasley R, Fishwick D, Miles JF, Hendeles L. Preservatives in nebulizer solutions: risks without benefit. Pharmacotherapy 1998;18(1):130–9.
11. Beasley CR, Rafferty P, Holgate ST. Bronchoconstrictor properties of preservatives in ipratropium bromide (Atrovent) nebuliser solution. BMJ (Clin Res Ed) 1987;294(6581):1197–8.
12. Ganderton D, Lewis D, Davies R, Meakin B, Brambilla G, Church T. Modulite: a means of designing the aerosols generated by pressurized metered dose inhalers. Respir Med 2002;96(Suppl D):S3–8.
13. Kirby SM, Smith J, Ventresca GP. Salmeterol inhaler using a non-chlorinated propellant, HFA134a: systemic pharmacodynamic activity in healthy volunteers. Thorax 1995;50(6):679–81.
14. Donnell D, Harrison LI, Ward S, Klinger NM, Ekholm BP, Cooper KM, Porietis I, McEwen J. Acute safety of the CFC-free propellant HFA-134a from a pressurized metered dose inhaler. Eur J Clin Pharmacol 1995;48(6):473–7.
15. Ayres JG, Frost CD, Holmes WF, Williams DR, Ward SM. Postmarketing surveillance study of a non-chlorofluorocarbon inhaler according to the safety assessment of marketed medicines guidelines BMJ 1998;317(7163):926–30.
16. Hawksworth RJ, Sykes AP, Faris M, Mant T, Lee TH. Albuterol HFA is as effective as albuterol CFC in preventing exercise-induced bronchoconstriction. Ann Allergy Asthma Immunol 2002;88(5):473–7.
17. Langley SJ, Sykes AP, Batty EP, Masterson CM, Woodcock A. A comparison of the efficacy and tolerability of single doses of HFA 134a albuterol and CFC albuterol in mild-to-moderate asthmatic patients. Ann Allergy Asthma Immunol 2002;88(5):488–93.
18. Woodcock A, Acerbi D, Poli G. Modulite technology: pharmacodynamic and pharmacokinetic implications. Respir Med 2002;96(Suppl D):S9–15.
19. Anderson PB, Langley SJ, Mooney P, Jones J, Addlestone R, Rossetti A, Cantini L. Equivalent efficacy

and safety of a new HFA-134a formulation of BDP compared with the conventional CFC in adult asthmatics. J Investig Allergol Clin Immunol 2002;12(2):107–13.
20. Vondra V, Sladek K, Kotasova J, Terl M, Rossetti A, Cantini L. A new HFA-134a propellant in the administration of inhaled BDP via the Jet spacer: controlled clinical trial vs the conventional CFC. Respir Med 2002;96(10):784–9.
21. Woodcock A, Williams A, Batty L, Masterson C, Rossetti A, Cantini L. Effects on lung function, symptoms, and bronchial hyperreactivity of low-dose inhaled beclomethasone dipropionate given with HFA-134a or CFC propellant. J Aerosol Med 2002;15(4):407–14.
22. Nolting A, Abramowitz W. Multiple-dose proportionality study of flunisolide hydrofluoroalkane. Allergy Asthma Proc 2002;23(5):311–18.
23. Nayak A, Lanier R, Weinstein S, Stampone P, Welch M. Efficacy and safety of beclomethasone dipropionate extrafine aerosol in childhood asthma: a 12-week, randomized, double-blind, placebo-controlled study. Chest 2002;122(6):1956–65.

Inosine pranobex

General Information

Inosine pranobex is a synthetic product, also known as isoprinosine or inosine dimepranol acedobene, with antiviral properties that are assumed to be related to its effect on T cell-mediated immunity rather than to direct antiviral activity. It has been tried in a wide range of viral diseases and also in rheumatoid arthritis (1), multiple sclerosis (2), and alopecia (3). However, clinical trials have mostly shown only modest therapeutic benefit or none at all (1,4), and no specific adverse effects, except for an increase in serum uric acid concentrations (5), reflecting the metabolic pathways of purines (6).

Organs and Systems

Immunologic

Anecdotal reports have attributed aggravation of polymyositis (7) and generalized *Herpes zoster* virus infection to inosine pranobex (8).

Drug–Drug Interactions

Zidovudine

Inosine pranobex increased zidovudine plasma concentrations and half-life (9).

References

1. Brzeski M, Madhok R, Hunter JA, Capell HA. Randomised, double blind, placebo controlled trial of inosine pranobex in rheumatoid arthritis. Ann Rheum Dis 1990;49(5):293–5.
2. Milligan NM, Miller DH, Compston DA. A placebo-controlled trial of isoprinosine in patients with multiple sclerosis. J Neurol Neurosurg Psychiatry 1994;57(2):164–8.
3. Galbraith GM, Thiers BH, Jensen J, Hoehler F. A randomized double-blind study of inosiplex (isoprinosine) therapy in patients with alopecia totalis. J Am Acad Dermatol 1987;16(5 Pt 1):977–83.
4. Kinghorn GR, Woolley PD, Thin RN, De Maubeuge J, Foidart JM, Engst R. Acyclovir vs isoprinosine (immunovir) for suppression of recurrent genital *Herpes simplex* infection Genitourin Med 1992;68(5):312–16.
5. Sarciron ME, Delabre I, Walbaum S, Raynaud G, Petavy AF. Effects of multiple doses of isoprinosine on *Echinococcus multilocularis* metacestodes Antimicrob Agents Chemother 1992;36(1):191–4.
6. Thorsen S, Pedersen C, Sandstrom E, Petersen CS, Norkrans G, Gerstoft J, Karlsson A, Christensen KC, Hakansson C, Pehrson PO, et al. One-year follow-up on the safety and efficacy of isoprinosine for human immunodeficiency virus infection. Scandinavian Isoprinosine Study Group. J Intern Med 1992;231(6):607–15.
7. Chuck AJ, Lloyd Jones JK, Dunn NA. Is inosine pranobex contraindicated in autoimmune disease? BMJ (Clin Res Ed) 1988;296(6622):646.
8. Revuz J, Guillaume JC, Roujeau JC, Perroud AM. Généralisation d'un zona chez un sujet non immunodéprime recevant de l'isoprinosine et de la rifamycine S. V. [Generalization of zona in a nonimmunosuppressed patient receiving isoprinosine and rifamycin SV.] Ann Dermatol Venereol 1983;110(6–7):563.
9. De Simone C, Famularo G, Tzantzoglou S, Moretti S, Jirillo E. Inosine pranobex in the treatment of HIV infection: a review. Int J Immunopharmacol 1991;13(Suppl 1): 19–27.

Insulin

General Information

Insulin is used for substitution therapy in patients with an absolute or relative deficiency of insulin. Most of the insulins now prescribed are either human or highly purified insulins of animal origin or synthetic insulins closely related to human insulin. The use of insulin of lesser purity is declining, but it is still used in considerable quantities in Eastern and Central Europe and in less developed countries. In some countries, both highly purified insulins of Western origin in concentrations of 100 U/ml, and locally produced less pure insulins in concentrations of 20, 40, or 80 U/ml are available at the same time, creating confusion. Patients have to realize that the syringe used for injection has to be concordant with the specific strength of insulin for which it has been made. The manner and the site of administration, the variation in duration of action of the various insulin formulations, the grade of purification, and differences in concentration cause specific problems.

The effects of insulin are modified by various factors. The speed and extent of absorption of insulin depends, for example, on the site of injection (1), the depth of the subcutaneous injection, skin temperature (2), the presence of lipodystrophy, and variation in the extent of inactivation of injected insulin. The disposal of insulin depends on many factors. Exercise and hard work lower the blood glucose and thereby increase the effect of insulin. Infections and obesity reduce its effect. The timing of food intake and the composition of meals are also related to the action of insulin. A thin layer of fat, as sometimes occurs in the upper arm or in the thighs of thin men, can result in intramuscular injection, leading to faster absorption of long-acting insulins. This can reduce the absorption time by half (3). The major factors that affect the fate of injected insulin (and thereby also its risks) are listed in Table 1 (4).

Insulin has a half-life of only a few minutes when injected intravenously. It is therefore prepared in different formulations for subcutaneous injection, with different half-lives of absorption, giving different durations of action. The main formulations, with their approximate durations of action are given in Table 2.

An alternative method of altering the duration of action of insulin is to use analogues in which there are amino acid substitutions. Analogues are listed in Table 3. Insulin aspart, insulin detemir, insulin glargine, and insulin lispro are all covered in separate monographs.

General adverse effects

The major adverse effect of insulin is hypoglycemia, which is specifically dangerous when the patient's awareness of hypoglycemia is reduced or when long-acting formulations are used. Allergic reactions, although less common with newer formulations, regularly occur (5).

Table 1 The major factors that affect the fate of injected insulin

Variable	Clinical relevance
Insulin formulation	Ultra-short-acting insulin (half-life 0.5–2 hours) Regular insulin (half-life 2–4 hours) Intermediate-acting insulin (half-life 16–20 hours) Prolonged-acting insulin (half-life 36 hours and over) Intraindividual variation in absorption up to 50% Interindividual variation from day-to-day up to 25%
Insulin species	Of minimal importance
Injection technique	Contributes to variance
Injected region	Absorption faster from abdominal region than from femoral and gluteal regions; exercising the injected limb speeds up absorption (applies especially to regular insulin)
Subcutaneous blood flow	A major determinant of absorption rate and clinically significant for regular insulin (influenced by smoking, ambient temperature, exercise, and local massage)
Subcutaneous degradation of insulin	Usually of no clinical significance; in rare cases after insulin need exceeds 120 IU/day it might explain brittleness
Insulin antibodies	Increase unpredictably the circulating fraction of insulin and prolong its half-life; a rare cause of insulin resistance

Table 2 Formulations of human insulin (all rINNs) and their durations of action

Type of insulin	Onset of action (hours)	Maximum action (hours)	Duration of action (hours)
Ultra-short-acting			
Insulin aspart, insulin lispro	0.05–2	0.5–1.5	4
Short-acting			
Neutral insulin injection	0.3–0.5	1–3	5–8
Intermediate-acting			
Insulin zinc suspension (amorphous) (semilente)	1–2	6–10	12–16
Isophane insulin (Neutral Protamine Hagedorn, NPH)	1–2	4–6	11–20
Globin zinc insulin suspension	1–2	6–10	10–18
Compound insulin zinc suspension (lente)	2–4	3–12	14–24
Long-acting			
Protamine zinc insulin injection	4–6	16–24	24–36
Insulin zinc suspension (crystalline) (ultralente)	4–6	16–24	24–36
Insulin glargine, insulin detemir	0.5–1	1–24	22–28
Combined formulations			
Diphasic insulin injection	0.7–1	3–18	12–24

Rare complications are lipoatrophy or hypertrophy and insulin edema. Insulin has to be given by injection, with pumps or specific devices for intensive therapy, which all generate specific problems. Other ways of administrating insulin are still experimental.

Additives introduced as preservatives or to change the duration of action of insulin can also cause adverse effects.

Table 3 Insulin analogues

Analogue	Comments
Insulin aspart	Rapid-acting, short-acting; the proline at site 28 of the B chain is replaced by aspartate (B28Asp)
Insulin defalan	Prepared from insulin by removal of the terminal phenylalanine
Insulin detemir	Long-acting; the threonine is deleted at B30 and the lysine at B28 is acylated with a miristoyl side-chain (B29Lys (ϵ-tetradecanoyl)desB30)
Insulin glargine	Long-acting; the asparagine at A21 is replaced by glycine and two arginines are added to the C terminus of the B chain (A21Gly,B31Arg,B32Arg)
Insulin glulisine	Rapid-acting, short-acting; the asparagine at B3 is replaced by lysine and the lysine at B29 is replaced by glutamic acid (B3Lys,B29Glu)
Insulin lispro	Rapid-acting, short-acting (2–4 hours); the lysine at site 29 and the proline at site 28 of the B chain are interchanged (B28Lys,B29Pro)

Organs and Systems

Nervous system

Cerebral edema has been described during therapy of diabetic ketoacidosis with a large volume of fluid, resulting in rapid changes in plasma osmolality, mostly in young patients (SEDA-26, 462). However, in 10 adults with ketoacidosis, no signs of cerebral edema (supported by CT scans) were found (6).

Susceptibility factors for cerebral edema during ketoacidosis in children have been investigated in 61 cases of cerebral edema during 6977 hospital admissions (7). They were matched with two types of controls for each case: three children with ketoacidosis randomly selected and three children matched for age (within 2 years), onset of diabetes, blood pH, and serum glucose at entry. The results suggested that high initial serum urea concentrations and a low $PaCO_2$ are associated with an increased probability of cerebral edema. Children with these abnormalities should be monitored for signs of neurological deterioration, and hyperosmolar therapy should be immediately available. Treatment with bicarbonate was associated with an increased risk and should be avoided. In an accompanying editorial it was stated that high doses of insulin, hypotonic fluids, and bicarbonate are often seen as culprits, but it is also possible that it is an idiosyncratic response to diabetic ketoacidosis; there is no proof of either theory (8).

Metabolism

Hypoglycemia

The most frequent complication of insulin therapy is inadvertent hypoglycemia (9–11). Over 5% of deaths in diabetes can be attributed to hypoglycemia. The frequency increases with rigorous maintenance of normoglycemia (12,13). In the Diabetes Control and Complications Trial (DCCT) (14) the frequency of serious hypoglycemia was more than three times increased in the intensively treated group, and the frequency of the attacks was related to the concentration of HbA_{1c} (15). The UK Prospective Diabetes Study in patients with type 2 diabetes also showed an increased risk of hypoglycemia with more intensive treatment (16).

Attacks of hypoglycemia are often preceded by less marked attacks, which are unnoticed or not reported to the family or physician. Attacks can be caused by reduced resistance to insulin or switch to a type of insulin with a different duration of action. The reasons for hypoglycemia can be inaccurate or excessive insulin injections, heavy physical exercise, or omission of meals. The action of highly purified insulins and some new analogues, even when in long-acting form, is somewhat faster and shorter compared with less pure formulations. Errors in injection techniques, such as superficial subcutaneous injections, forming nodules or causing bleeding, can introduce variation in the absorption of insulin, resulting in an increase in the mean administered dose and in inadvertent hypoglycemia. Twice-daily isophane insulin for 6 months has been compared with once-daily ultralente insulin in 60 patients (17). Isophane was associated with fewer attacks of hypoglycemia, lower HbA_{1c}, lower evening glucose concentrations, and greater patient satisfaction.

The Somogyi effect, unnoticed hypoglycemia during sleep, causes a rebound increase in morning blood glucose with accompanying glycosuria. When, in response to this, the evening dose of long-acting insulin is increased, the risk of nocturnal hypoglycemia also increases, creating a vicious cycle. Blood glucose monitoring late at night helps to establish the diagnosis. Of 39 poorly controlled patients with insulin-treated diabetes aged 9–66 years, 22 had recurrent nocturnal hypoglycaemia, the best clinical clue to which was intermittent symptoms, however mild and infrequent they appeared to be (18).

Hypoglycemia can also be induced by concomitant diseases, for example renal disease, hepatic disease (cirrhosis), hypopituitarism, hypoadrenocorticalism, hypoglucagonism, hypothyroidism, malnutrition, anorexia nervosa, pregnancy, termination of pregnancy, recovery from infections, operations, or stress.

Frequency

In a review of 102 consecutive drug-induced, hospital-related cases of coma, 23 were caused by insulin only, 14 by insulin + glibenclamide, and 3 by insulin + metformin (19). The likelihood of readmission for hypoglycemia after a previous admission was 2.9 times greater.

Of 546 Spanish diabetic children and teenagers, 14% had one period of hypoglycemia and 21% had more than one episode (20). The highest incidence was in the morning, possibly related to the frugal Spanish breakfast and abundant food intake in the evening.

Hypoglycemia was retrospectively monitored in 1055 patients who had had type 2 diabetes for more than 2 months, and who visited the clinic at least twice in 6 months (21). They all received aggressive treatment to reach near-normal blood glucose concentrations. Symptoms of hypoglycemia were mentioned by 12% of those treated with diet alone, 16% of those using oral agents, and 30% of those using any form of insulin. In only five patients, all using insulin, was there severe hypoglycemia. A low HbA_{1c} concentration at follow-up, symptoms of hypoglycemia at the initial visit, and younger age were independently associated with an increased incidence of symptoms.

During 12 months, 244 episodes of severe hypoglycemia in 166 patients were recorded in a district with a population of 367 051 people (8655 with diabetes); there were 69 (7.1%) episodes in people with type 1 diabetes, 66 (7.3%) in people with type 2 diabetes using insulin, and 23 (0.8%) in those taking a sulfonylurea. Age, duration of diabetes, and lower social class were risk factors. The total cost of emergency treatment was estimated to be no more than $92 078 per year (22). In a German study in a comparable group of 200 000 people, there were 92 cases in those with type 1 diabetes and 146 cases in those with type 2 diabetes during 3 years (23). The estimated costs were lower: $88 676 per year for type 2 diabetes and $16 258 for type 1 diabetes.

In 28 children aged 3.1–8.3 years using twice- or thrice-daily insulin, blood glucose was measured with a subcutaneous continuous glucose monitoring system on 3 consecutive days and nights (24). Hypoglycemia was defined as a blood glucose concentration below 3.3 mmol/l for longer than 15 minutes. The prevalence of hypoglycemia was 10% and it was more common at night than during the day (19 versus 4.4%). Hypoglycemia at night had a longer duration (median 3.3 hours) and was asymptomatic in 91% of the episodes. The highest prevalence occurred at between 04.00 and 07.30. On a thrice-daily insulin injection regimen, nightly hypoglycemia was less frequent, but the frequency was higher on the following morning. With increasing age there was less hypoglycemia.

Mechanisms

The concentrations of the counter-regulatory hormones adrenaline and glucagon were higher before treatment of coma in insulin-treated persons admitted to hospital for hypoglycemia than in the fasting state. However, concentrations of adrenaline, glucagon, cortisol, and growth hormone are lower during a hypoglycemic episode in a diabetic than when these hormones are measured during induced hypoglycemia in non-diabetics (25). There was an inverse correlation between glucose and adrenaline in hypoglycemia, but no direct relation between the other hormones and blood glucose concentrations. The addition of intramuscular glucagon during intravenous glucose therapy did not result in different glucose concentrations at any time (25). In type 2 diabetes counter-regulatory hormones are reduced compared with controls, but the patients release the hormones at higher blood glucose concentrations than type 1 diabetics, and the glucagon response is not blunted (26,27).

- Low responses of counter-regulatory hormones during induced hypoglycemia in a 27-year-old woman with poorly controlled diabetes (HbA_{1c} 11%), with frequent hypoglycemic instances of which she was not aware, improved dramatically after 3 months of good regulation (28); only growth hormone showed no reaction.

Hypoglycemia increased beta-adrenoceptor sensitivity in healthy subjects but reduced it in type 1 diabetes (29).

In 20 insulin-treated diabetic patients with episodes of severe hypoglycemia in 1982–84, re-evaluated in 1992–94, emergency visits were reduced from 1.05/year to 0.42/year between 1984 and 1994 (30). There were no cases of fatal hypoglycemia. There was no association with HbA_{1c}. Multiple daily insulin doses reduced the frequency of hypoglycemia to one-third. In 1984, unawareness was a predisposing factor and most of the patients had deficient counter-regulation (adrenaline). Most patients had a long history of insulin injections (mean 29 years). In 1994, six patients were partly and eight patients totally retested and compared with 10 matched control patients with type 1 diabetes. When hypoglycemia was induced by insulin the patients with frequent hypoglycemia reached values under 3.0 mmol much faster, and in six patients the test had to be stopped before the normal duration of 3 hours for hypoglycemia; this never happened in the control patients. Counter-regulation was deficient in both 1984 and 1994, indicating that reduced counter-regulation can be permanent and does not only depend on specific circumstances.

In 86 intensively treated patients with type 1 diabetes aged 7–18 years, the incidence of severe hypoglycemia correlated with the serum activity of acetylcholine esterase. Patients with acetylcholine esterase activity at the median or above reported 3.0 events/year and those with acetylcholine esterase activity below the median reported 0.5 events/year, suggesting that a genetic factor may play a role in the emergence of severe hypoglycemia (31).

Presentation

Symptoms of hypoglycemia have to be expected when the blood glucose concentration is below 2.6 mmol/l. The effects of hypoglycemia vary from patient to patient and can vary in the same patient. The symptoms and signs are of two types: adrenergic effects, due to release of catecholamines, and neuroglycopenic effects, due to the effects of hypoglycemia on the nervous system.

- *Adrenergic effects* Hunger, restlessness, profuse sweating, palor, tachycardia, and palpitation.
- *Neuroglycopenic effects* Headache, confusion, drowsiness, fatigue, difficulties in finding words, frequent yawning, anxiety, blurred vision, diplopia, and numbness of the nose, lip, and fingers.

Some patients do not experience the noradrenergic symptoms of hypoglycemia. They are taken by surprise, may lose consciousness and have hypoglycemic blood glucose concentrations without any preceding symptoms. After frequent episodes of hypoglycemia, there is altered awareness of hypoglycemia (18,32,33). It is difficult to substantiate altered awareness. Neuroendocrine responses and symptoms of hypoglycemia, but not cognitive dysfunction, are shifted to lower plasma glucose concentrations after recent hypoglycemia (34). Repeated episodes of hypoglycemia reduce the awareness of symptoms of hypoglycemia. This is accompanied by a lower blood glucose concentration, to elicit the response of counter-regulatory hormones (35). Beta-blockers also suppress the adrenergic symptoms, apart from sweating, which is mediated by sympathetic cholinergic transmission. Training increases awareness (36). Intensively treated patients may have reduced preservation of higher brain functions (37). Some groups, mainly in the UK, have suggested that transfer from animal to human insulin increases unawareness (SEDA-15, 452) (38), but this was not substantiated in other studies (39–41).

Every patient treated with insulin (or with hypoglycemic agents) who develops a neurological or psychiatric disorder has to be considered to be hypoglycemic until proven otherwise.

A rapid fall in blood glucose in a diabetic patient can cause symptoms of hypoglycemia, even when blood glucose concentrations are still normal or above normal. Experience with pumps has shown that many patients continue to feel hypoglycemic for a long time after normoglycemia has been restored. After an attack of hypoglycemia, patients often felt less well for a period of up to 48 hours. Headache, tiredness, and lack of initiative may disappear only gradually. These symptoms in the morning may indicate unnoticed hypoglycemic periods during sleep. Wet pyjamas or sheets may also indicate unnoticed hypoglycemia. During anesthesia, profuse sweating may indicate hypoglycemia.

A rise in C reactive protein has been observed during spontaneous attacks of hypoglycemia in diabetics and after experimental hypoglycemia in healthy controls (42).

Cardiovascular effects of hypoglycemia

The cardiovascular effects of hypoglycemia include angina pectoris, dysrhythmias, electrocardiographic changes, and coronary thrombosis. Raised concentrations of catecholamines and reduced concentrations of potassium contribute to cardiac damage during hypoglycemia.

Respiratory effects of hypoglycemia

- A 19-year-old woman with diabetes developed hypoglycemia with pulmonary edema (43). This has previously been seen as a complication of insulin shock therapy for psychiatric illnesses.

Nervous system effects of hypoglycemia

When hypoglycemia does not resolve spontaneously or is not terminated, cerebral dysfunction becomes manifest as confusion or reduced consciousness. Lethargy and depression or obstructive behavior develop and are accompanied by loss of consciousness, snoring, deep respiration, and facial paralysis. Neurological involvement can appear as cramps, paralysis, hemiplegia, or paraplegia. Epileptic seizures can accompany attacks of hypoglycemia. In deep coma the pupils are dilated, but they may react to light. Coma can develop very rapidly.

In a teaching hospital in Edinburgh, 56 admissions of 51 patients for hypoglycemia were registered during 12 months; 41 patients had diabetes mellitus and 33 were using insulin (44). There was a high incidence of neurological effects. Psychiatric illness or alcoholism was common. Four patients died but only one as a direct consequence of hypoglycemia. A further six patients died within 15 months, not related to hypoglycemia.

In 37 drivers with type 1 diabetes, fewer corrective actions were taken when the blood glucose was below 2.8 mmol/l (45). This was related to increased neuroglycopenic symptoms and increased electroencephalographic theta-wave activity. The authors suggested that diabetics should not begin to drive when the blood glucose concentration is in the 4.0–4.5 mmol/l range. In two editorials, the possibility of further restricting driving licenses in people with diabetes has been discussed (46,47). However, there is no evidence of higher accident rates in drivers with diabetes.

A retrospective questionnaire was sent to 195 consecutive patients addressing questions of severe hypoglycemia, coma, awareness of hypoglycemia, and fear of hypoglycemia (48). The mean duration of diabetes was 20 years and 82% had received intensive therapy. Coma was reported in 19% and severe hypoglycemia in 41%. Coma was independently related to neuropathy, beta-blockers, and alcohol.

In reaction to a report of pulmonary edema and hypoglycemia (SEDA-24, 488) it has been noted that in many cases, one or more seizures precede pulmonary edema (acute respiratory distress syndrome), suggesting a neurogenic mechanism (49).

In 304 insulin-treated patients, 8.2% of those with type 1 diabetes and 2.2% of those with type 2 diabetes had blood glucose concentrations below 4 mmol/l on arrival in the clinic (50). None had complained of symptoms of hypoglycemia or had taken glucose, but when questioned, 59% had autonomic symptoms and 12% had neuroglycopenic symptoms; 29% were asymptomatic.

Autonomic failure can occur as a result of hypoglycemia, since antecedent hypoglycemia causes both defective glucose counter-regulation and lack of awareness of hypoglycemia. The role of the brain in lack of awareness of hypoglycemia and the question of whether the brain is the primary site for sensing hypoglycemia has been discussed (51). In older people, markedly fewer autonomic symptoms are reported and there is greater slowing of psychomotor performance. In young children, hypoglycemia can lead to more mood and behavioral disturbances than in adults, although they also occur in the latter. It may be that the cortical responses to recurrent hypoglycemia are less plastic and reversible than the hypothalamic and glucose-sensing functions (52).

Psychological and psychiatric effects of hypoglycemia

Using evidence from auditory-evoked brain potentials and hypoglycemic clamps, it has been argued that antecedent hypoglycemia not only reduces awareness, but also that several aspects of cognitive function are attenuated during subsequent hypoglycemia 18–24 hours later (53). However, there were no effects of repeated hypoglycemia on cognitive function in patients included in the DCCT, a large American study that included more than 1400 patients, which showed that normalization of blood glucose prevents or delays the development of secondary (microvascular) complications in type 1 diabetes (54).

Nevertheless, long periods of hypoglycemia can cause permanent brain damage. There is concern that frequent attacks of hypoglycemia impair brain function but there are few hard data.

Hypoglycemic coma due to insulin with extensive mental changes has been reported, including a review of six comparable cases in patients aged 37–56 years, whose coma lasted from 36 hours to 31 days (55).

- A 37-year-old man could not be wakened in the morning. He had injected insulin without eating. His blood glucose was 1.5 mmol/l and he did not improve with intravenous glucose 16 g. In hospital he remained unconscious with a blood glucose of 12.2 mmol/l. There was no alcohol in the blood, his pH was 7.35, and he had a normal anion gap (18 mmol/l). His serum creatinine concentration was 288 μmol/l and his creatine kinase activity was high, suggesting rhabdomyolysis. A brain CT scan was normal and repeated electroencephalography showed slow waves with reduced voltages but no focal changes or irritation. He gradually recovered and was discharged after 6 days. Because of the dissociation between physical and mental improvement he was checked after 6 months and still had antegrade memory loss and problems with memory, complaining that he needed reminders on paper, and had less vitality and reduced emotionality.

Of the six reviewed patients, two died in coma; the other four had neuropsychological problems that did not improve after 6 months and up to 2 years. They had comparable electroencephalographic changes. During coma there was hypokalemia and hypocalcemia combined with increased lipolysis; this may have accounted for the permanent cerebral changes.

Of 20 patients with severe hypoglycemic coma and 20 with no or light coma, those with hypoglycemia had chronic depression and anxiety and performed persistently more poorly in several cognitive tests (56).

In 42 patients with at least two episodes of severe hypoglycemia in the previous 2 years and 51 patients with no episodes, low blood glucose, hypoglycemia-impaired ability to do mental subtractions, and awareness of neuroglycopenia and hypoglycemia predicted future severe attacks of hypoglycemia (57). In another study, blood glucose awareness training increased adrenaline responses to hypoglycemia (58). However, in a reanalysis of data from the Diabetes Control and Complications Study, a large study relating the development of secondary complications to less strict control of blood glucose (14), there was no effect of repeated hypoglycemia (54).

The effect of hypoglycemia on cognitive function has been investigated in 142 children aged 6–15 years with type 1 diabetes intensively treated for 18 months; 58 had 111 periods of treatment. There were no effects on cognitive functions (59). In 29 prepubertal children, with diabetes for at least 12 months and using twice-daily mixed insulin, observed for two nights, asymptomatic hypoglycemia occurred in 13 children on the first night and in 11 children on the second night; cognitive performance was not altered, but mood was reduced (60).

In healthy volunteers hypoglycemia caused significant deterioration in short-term attention, whereas sustained attention and intelligence scores did not deteriorate (61).

Sensory effects of hypoglycemia

Temporary blindness after severe coma (62,63) and retinal damage by gazing in the sun during hypoglycemia (64) have been reported.

Differential diagnosis

When a patient does not react rapidly to sufficient therapy, other diagnoses have to be considered during suspected attacks of hypoglycemia.

Alcohol can confuse the diagnosis of hypoglycemia (SEDA-5, 386). Alcohol inhibits gluconeogenesis. It makes the patient more susceptible to hypoglycemia and can even cause hypoglycemia in healthy individuals. The symptoms of alcohol abuse and hypoglycemia are almost identical. If hypoglycemia is predominant, glucose administration will help. In attacks of hypoglycemia, the symptoms disappear rapidly after glucose intake.

Vascular episodes in older diabetics can mimic attacks of hypoglycemia. True epilepsy or strokes can cause comparable symptoms or accompany hypoglycemia.

Differentiation of hypoglycemia from hyperglycemic coma is usually not difficult. The development of hyperglycemic coma takes a longer time and the blood glucose concentration is high. However, urine testing may show positive glycosuria, if urine produced before the hypoglycemic period is still in the bladder. Even ketonuria may be present if a patient has been fasting for a long period.

Timing

The emergence of attacks of hypoglycemia depends on the times and amounts of food eaten and the duration of action of the insulin used (see Table 2). When only one type of insulin is used, the symptoms of hypoglycemia mostly occur at the end of the period of maximal insulin activity. Modern insulin therapy involves using a combination of long-acting and short-acting insulins. Long-acting insulins are given once or twice a day in combination with and/or in addition to short-acting insulins, which are given 2–4 times a day. Hypoglycemia can then develop at times when the combined effects are most prominent. Hypoglycemia in the mid-morning can be a consequence of the action of the long-acting insulin of the previous day and the short-acting insulin given earlier in the same morning. Hypoglycemia during the night or in the early morning can be caused by too much long-acting insulin or by short-acting insulin late at night without sufficient food. Repeated symptoms of hypoglycemia at the same time of the day indicate that the timing of the insulin injection or the relative proportions of long-acting and short-acting insulins have to be changed. If the interval between insulin injection and the subsequent meal is very short, the effective insulin concentration in the blood will still be low when glucose is absorbed from the gut. This will cause very high postprandial glucose concentrations. An increase in the dose of insulin will then cause hypoglycemia at a later time. It is therefore advisable to try first to increase the interval between the injection and start of the meal. New synthetic insulins, like lispro insulin, give a more rapid increase and fall of insulin concentrations than regular insulin; in that case, postprandial hypoglycemia can occur 1–3 hours after the injection (65).

Susceptibility factors

Hypoglycemia is an important problem in children (66–68). Children do not always establish the connection between the symptoms of threatening hypoglycemia and the danger involved. Overdosage of insulin is relatively common (SEDA-7, 406).

Older patients are particularly susceptible to hypoglycemia (69). Factors such as cerebral blood flow, blood PO_2 and PCO_2, permeability of the blood–brain barrier, and the presence of underlying neurological defects influence the hypoglycemic effects.

Hypoglycemic periods are often seen in "brittle diabetics," many of whom are overtreated with insulin. Changes in the insulin regimen (reduced use of long-acting insulin, frequent small injections of short-acting insulin) or the use of continuous infusion pumps can often lead to better results, but not everyone with brittle diabetes responds in that way (SEDA-7, 405). Apparently brittle diabetes may in fact be due to factitious hypoglycemia, the hypoglycemic periods of which are caused by surreptitious self-injection of insulin, Munchausen syndrome by proxy (SEDA-18, 413), or manipulation of the prescribed doses. In factitious hypoglycemia, low blood glucose concentrations are accompanied by high insulin concentrations but low concentrations of C peptide (70). Suicide attempts with insulin may be less uncommon than is often thought. A Medline search between 1966 and 1999 identified 46 papers containing 69 cases of factitious hypoglycemia; 46 were women, 52 were not diabetic, 29 had no close links with diabetes in their environment (71). In 47 the hypoglycemia was induced by insulin. Two patients died and one had severe impairment of intellectual function and short-term memory. In 32 cases unnecessary surgical procedures were performed.

Impaired hypoglycemic awareness was associated with an increased rate of severe hypoglycemia in 130 children and adolescents (aged 3–17 years) (72). One-third of the severe episodes developed without warning symptoms. Impaired awareness, young age, and recent attacks of hypoglycemia were independent susceptibility factors.

The authors of a systematic review of whether there is a difference in the frequency and awareness of hypoglycemia induced by human or animal insulins identified 52 randomized, controlled trials; 37 were double-blind (73). They found no support for the supposition that human insulin per se affects the frequency, severity, or symptoms of hypoglycemia. In a few studies, mainly of less rigorous design, there was an effect when people were transferred from animal to human insulin, indicating increased frequency or reduced awareness of hypoglycemia.

A questionnaire about the prevalence of severe hypoglycemia in relation to susceptibility factors was answered by 387 patients in 1984 and by 641 patients in 1998; 178 patients answered both questionnaires (74). The following changed significantly from 1984 to 1998: multiple injection therapy increased from 71 to 98%, daily self-monitoring from 17 to 48%, episodes of nocturnal hypoglycemia from 76 to 83%, and lack of awareness from 40 to 55%; HbA_{1c} fell from 7.6 to 7.4%.

Awareness of hypoglycemia

Avoidance of hypoglycemia for 3 months can improve hypoglycemic awareness for a period of over 3 years (75). In contrast, supervised induction of brief hypoglycemia twice weekly reduced clinical awareness of hypoglycemia by 33% and reduced the important adrenaline response, so reducing the behavioral and physiological defences against hypoglycemia (76).

Management

Patients have to be instructed to have a rapidly absorbed form of carbohydrate (for example dextrose tablets) available at all times and to use it when the first symptoms of hypoglycemia are felt. Often they fail to do so (77). If patients are used to self-monitoring, it is advisable that they monitor blood glucose first, although they should be told that a rapid drop in blood glucose concentration without reaching hypoglycemic values can cause a hypoglycemic reaction. Hypoglycemic reactions are sometimes difficult to discriminate from other feelings of malaise. Carbohydrate will always give rapid relief if the diagnosis is hypoglycemia and it is always safe to try taking it.

The conscious patient should take oral glucose at once. The treatment of choice in hypoglycemic coma is immediate intravenous injection of 20–50 g of dextrose. The patient may try to resist the injection, and help with the immobilization of the arm may therefore be needed. Injection of concentrated glucose solution outside a blood vessel leads to inflammatory and necrotic reactions. If intravenous injection of glucose is impossible, 1 mg of glucagon can be injected subcutaneously. However, in patients with residual insulin secretion (type 2 diabetes) glucagon may elicit extra insulin secretion and perpetuate hypoglycemia (78). The Epipen (a pen filled with a solution of adrenaline) is not a good substitute for the glucagon pen (in which glucagon must be dissolved before it can be used) in the treatment of hypoglycemia (79).

When the patient has taken high doses of long-acting insulin, hypoglycemia may relapse after a single dose of glucose has provided temporary relief, and monitoring should continue for a longer period. After hypoglycemic reactions elicited by long-acting insulins or oral hypoglycemic drugs the patient should be observed for possible recurrence during the next few days (80). The longer the duration of coma, the poorer the prognosis. Persistent posthypoglycemic coma can be due to cerebral edema. Fever can accompany this severe form of coma, which requires treatment with intravenous mannitol and glucocorticoids. Severe coma can last for several days and require intensive management. Encephalopathy with neurological symptoms can be the consequence.

Infusion of too much glucose over an extended period in the treatment of hypoglycemia is dangerous (81). Glucose utilization in the postabsorptive state is 2 mg/kg/minute and can increase, if insulin concentrations are high, to 6 mg/kg/minute (about 600 g/day in a 70 kg individual). It is better to infuse glucose in concentrations of 10 or 20% rather than 40%.

The opinion of experts about when and how to treat asymptomatic hypoglycemia in children varies greatly (82). Hypoglycemia in children is often undetected. Using a subcutaneous continuous glucose monitoring system (83) or the non-invasive Glucowatch biographer (84), hypoglycemic periods were more frequent and prolonged than when only fingerprick testing was available. For treating hypoglycemia in children, small doses of glucagon are suggested. The contents of a 1 mg/ml ampoule can be drawn into a 1 ml U100 syringe. For children under 2 years, 20 micrograms should be given initially; 10 micrograms is added for every year, up to 150 micrograms at age 15. When the effect is insufficient, the dose can be repeated once or twice (85).

Fat metabolism

- A 14-year-old adolescent girl, who had only used regular insulin developed lipoatrophy (86). Histology showed lipoblastoma-like cells, a possible sign of dedifferentiation. Skin tests showed no signs of allergy. The concentrations of immunoglobulins and TNF-alfa were normal.

Body weight

The DCCT Research Group has reported that patients in the intensive treatment group had substantial excess weight gain (87). In the first 9 months a group of patients who received intensive treatment gained 3.3 kg, compared with 1.2 kg in the control group; the percentage of people who gained more than 5 kg/m^2 was consistently higher with intensive therapy. This weight gain was related to both lean body mass and fat.

Fluid balance

Insulin edema is a rare complication, more often seen in the earlier years of insulin therapy (SEDA-11, 364). It is mostly seen when dysregulated patients with progressive weight loss are treated with relatively high amounts of insulin. Reduced sodium excretion (88), sodium reabsorption, and water retention by a possible direct action of insulin on the kidney may be involved (89). The role of aldosterone or of inhibition of the renin–angiotensin–aldosterone system in insulin edema is unclear. Insulin edema is a specific adverse effect, but it can aggravate pulmonary edema, congestive heart failure, and hypertension. Treatment consists of reduction of the insulin dose, after which the edema resolves within 3–4 days.

Insulin edema has been described in children with newly discovered diabetes (90).

- A 13-year-old girl with diabetes was given insulin 2 U/kg/day. She developed generalized edema and gained 20 kg over 2 weeks. With less insulin, furosemide, and later ephedrine the edema disappeared within 1 month.
- A 14-year-old girl with diabetes was given insulin up to 1.5 U/kg/day and gradually developed edema and gained 8.5 kg over 9 days. With furosemide, the edema gradually disappeared in 1 month.

Both of these children received rather high doses of insulin and they lacked the extreme acidosis that often occurs in young people when diabetes first appears.

Liver

Hepatic damage by regular human insulin has been reported (91).

- A 45-year-old man, who drank alcohol 60 g/day until diabetes was diagnosed, had mild liver function test abnormalities 6 months earlier, but only the gamma-glutamyl transpeptidase was raised (167 IU/l). When insulin was given, the transaminases also increased. Liver function normalized after withdrawal of insulin. Reinstitution of insulin and a switch to another human insulin formulation again increased the liver enzymes. He was managed with glibenclamide and liver biopsy was not performed. Lymphocyte stimulation tests gave negative results to all insulin formulations. All hepatitis-related virus markers were negative.

As the changes in this case were seen with different types of insulin, it is improbable that additions to the formulation were responsible. It is possible that the use of alcohol made the liver more sensitive to the damaging effects of exogenous insulin.

Skin

Hypertrophy of the subcutaneous tissues after insulin injections leads to delayed and variable insulin absorption. Of 282 children (160 boys and 122 girls, median age 12 years) prospectively evaluated for 3 months, 29% had mild skin hypertrophy and 18% had massive hypertrophy (92). The latter had higher HbA_{1c} concentrations and longer durations of diabetes and required more daily injections. There was no relation to the length of the needles used.

Amyloid-like deposition in the skin has been reported in a patient using porcine insulin (93).

- A 34-year-old man with a 17-year history of type 1 diabetes developed a 7 cm firm mass, distinct from adjacent areas of lipohypertrophy, and numerous smaller lesions of the same consistency. The lump consisted of acellular waxy material that appeared to be amyloid, formed by insulin. He had used porcine insulin for a long time.

This complication has been described before (SEDA-14, 373).

Musculoskeletal

A specific complication of the use of large amounts of insulin during hyperosmolar diabetic coma is rhabdomyolysis (94). Low intramuscular phosphate and potassium concentrations, often masked by relatively high blood glucose concentrations, may be important contributory factors.

Immunologic

Insulin allergy is quite common (SEDA-7, 403) (95–97). Allergy has been reported to human insulin and protamine (98) and to human insulin (99,100).

- A 41-year-old woman became allergic to all types of insulin (beef, pork, human, lente, etc.). She had used insulin for the first time during pregnancy and was intermittently treated unsatisfactorily with oral agents. She used lispro insulin for more than 6 months without an allergic reaction.
- A 54-year-old woman with gestational diabetes was later found to be allergic to chromium, pollen, dust, penicillin, acarbose, and metformin (101). She was treated with diet and glibenclamide, but later required insulin. With Humulin N insulin she developed a wheal of 15 mm immediately after the injection, which resolved in a few hours. However, a painful itchy induration appeared 2–3 hours after the injection and lasted a few days. She had an immediate reaction to isophane insulin, with induration, but insulin lispro was well-tolerated.
- A 5-year-old child with diabetes, Pierre Robin syndrome, cleft palate, allergic rhinitis, recurrent sinusitis, and obstructive sleep apnea, who had previously had skin rashes after penicillin, sulfonamides, and clindamycin, was given soluble and isophane human insulins (102). Three years later she developed local reactions, 2–5 cm areas, 30–120 minutes after injection. Skin-prick tests were negative for the diluent, isophane, and soluble insulin, but intradermal testing was positive with

both insulins. Cetirizine and dexamethasone added to the insulin gave temporary relief. She was then given insulin lispro by pump. After about 8 months, she started to develop local reactions again but with cetirizine and the pump her reactions were manageable.

- A 6-year-old boy developed recurrent generalized urticaria 1 year after he started to use human Mixtard insulin (103). The rash started 10 minutes after injections in the arms, thighs, and buttocks, at sites where earlier injections had been given, and disappeared within 12 hours. When he was changed to insulin lispro he had three urticarial reactions in the first 2 weeks and then sporadically. The reactions were treated with chlorphenamine for 2 years.

Presentation

Although serious systemic reactions are rare, local reactions at the site of injection are not infrequent. They appear as reddening, swelling, heat, burning, and itching, with or without frankly painful sensations. They can set in immediately or after some hours. The lesion can extend gradually and persist for variable periods. Some immediate reactions are related to IgE (or IgE/IgG) concentrations (104), but a direct relation between allergic reactions and a specific IgG fraction cannot be established (105).

- A 45-year-old woman who had used insulin for 4 years had a biphasic hypersensitivity reaction to human insulin (or another component of the injection fluid) (106). Within 20 minutes after the injection a swelling developed and in a later phase papular lesions with lichenoid features and post-inflammatory hyperpigmentation emerged. Histologically, there was neutrophilic infiltration with erythrocyte extravasation and eosinophilic amorphous material, surrounded by neutrophilic infiltrate. Saline injection did not elicit an effect. IgE anti-insulin antibodies were not found. There was no Arthus reaction (type IV allergy).

Other reactions are of the tuberculin granulomatous type or of the local vasculitis Arthus type. The local reactions can be accompanied, preceded, or followed by a generalized reaction, such as urticaria, nausea, vomiting, diarrhea, angioedema, wheezing, or anaphylactic shock. The last of these is rare, but sometimes fatal.

Insulin can induce local, painful lumps at injection sites. Sclerosing granulomata are occasionally seen (107) perhaps due to zinc (108). Such reactions are most commonly a consequence of an incorrect injection technique, generally the use of too short a needle or too superficial an injection. General edema (SEDA-11, 364) or abscesses (SEDA-7, 406) generated by insulin injections are extremely rare.

Lipodystrophy, lipoatrophy, or lipohypertrophy can be a consequence of chronic local insulin reactions that can be elicited by less pure as well as by highly purified preparations (109), but such reactions can also develop at sites distant to the injection.

Leukocytoclastic vasculitis has been attributed to human insulin.

- A 48-year-old woman with type 1 diabetes developed tender induration within 2–6 hours and persisting for 1–3 days after injection of both isophane and regular insulins (110). This was followed by intense itching and redness, but no wheal-and-flare reaction. Switching to semisynthetic insulin and other insulin analogues or continuous subcutaneous insulin infusion had no effect. After 3 years the condition became incapacitating. Humalog 5–6 times a day, including an injection at 0300 hours was the best tolerated regimen. Intradermal tests showed allergy to human, porcine, and bovine insulins, but no reaction to protamine or other additives. Skin biopsies showed a leukocytoclastic vasculitis. Prednisolone 10 mg/day plus azathioprine 50 mg/day, later replaced by methotrexate 7–15 mg/week, produced complete resolution within 8 weeks.

Pathogenesis

Allergic reactions to insulin were originally thought to be caused by impurities present in the formulation. However, after the introduction of monocomponent insulins and human synthetic insulins, these reactions continued to be seen, even in patients without a history of treatment with other insulins (111). Switching from animal to human insulin can paradoxically cause allergic reactions, which subside when treatment with animal insulin is re-introduced (112). In patients who have never used other types of insulin, allergic reactions can be seen when human insulin is used and anti-insulin antibodies can be demonstrated (113). Antibodies against human insulin have also been found in sera collected from patients before human insulin was available (114). However, insulin antibodies can be found during or before the emergence of type 1 diabetes. Circulating insulin-binding antibodies can increase insulin resistance (115) and extend insulin action by slowing release. The titers of antibodies fall when purified insulins or human insulin are used, but they can be demonstrated even when modern insulins of high purity have been used exclusively. Anti-receptor antibodies are seldom seen.

In India, insulin antibodies have been investigated in 25 patients with type 1 diabetes, 19 patients with so-called malnutrition-related diabetes, and eight patients with fibrocalculous pancreatopathy, who used bovine insulin because it was cheaper (116). Antibodies appeared within 3 months of treatment. The development of antibodies was not related to the type of diabetes. There was a fall in antibody titer with increased duration of treatment. There was no correlation between daily insulin requirement and antibody titers.

Allergic reactions can also be elicited by excipients in insulin formulations, such as Surfen (aminoquinuride) (117), zinc (118), and protamine (119,120). Remnants of fluids used for cleansing the skin can be co-injected in micro-amounts and elicit allergic reactions (121). Allergy to latex in vial tops or syringes can become manifest during insulin treatment (122). In excised (infected) lumps, amyloid fibrils, proteins containing intact insulin, were demonstrable (123). Plastic syringes can release silicone particles, which can diminish the effect of insulin (124) or themselves induce granulomatous reactions (125).

It has been suggested that increased concentrations of corticotropin-releasing hormone, which has an immunomodulatory effect and causes vasodilatation and mast cell degranulation, could play a role in urticaria that develops during hypoglycemic periods in type 1 diabetes (SEDA-13, 381). Adrenal hyperandrogenemia is found in many diseases with hypersensitivity (126).

Susceptibility factors

Intermittent insulin administration seems to favor the development of allergic reactions to insulin (SEDA-6, 369).

Continuous intraperitoneal infusion of insulin causes increased insulin immunogenicity, but it is not known if this is accompanied by an increased frequency of autoimmune diseases. Antibodies against insulin, thyroglobulin, thyroperoxidase, gastric parietal cells, smooth muscle, mitochondria, liver and kidney microsomes, endomysium, and gliadin, and antinuclear antibodies were determined before and yearly after transfer to continuous intraperitoneal infusion of insulin in 28 patients; 19 remained negative for all investigated antibodies and in the other 9 the anti-insulin titer increased but other antibody titers remained constant or fluctuated (127). The authors concluded that during continuous intraperitoneal infusion of insulin in type 1 diabetes the frequency of other autoimmune diseases like hyperthyroidism was not increased. However, this conclusion was criticized, as the small numbers did not allow a positive or negative conclusion (128).

Treatment

In 95% of cases the local reactions disappear spontaneously. A switch to less immunogenic, highly purified insulin, or insulin lispro (129), is necessary if the reactions persist. For local allergic reactions, antihistamines or the addition of hydrocortisone 2 mg along with the insulin are seldom needed. Hydrocortisone suppresses local allergic reactions. For generalized reactions, skin testing is often necessary to establish allergic desensitization. One should start with low intradermal doses and, if necessary, add hydrocortisone.

For therapy of local lumps, extravasation, etc., one should first seek to improve the injection technique. Substitution with highly purified insulin is recommended. Injection with purified insulin into the affected area may speed up resorption of the lumps. Lipodystrophy or lipoatrophy improve after switching to highly purified human or insulin lispro. Lipohypertrophy, on the other hand, often fails to respond to changes in the insulin regimen (130). Varying the injection site may help, but differences in absorption rate then have to be taken into account.

Insulin resistance is said to be present when more than 200 U/day have to be injected; it is generally due to insulin antibodies. In general, antibody titers fall when highly purified insulins are used, but they sometimes persist after the switch. Some diseases, such as infections, endocrine hyperfunctional states (acromegaly, Cushing's syndrome, thyrotoxicosis), leukemia, or stress, can contribute to insulin resistance. Recombinant IGF-I (insulin-like growth factor I), which has a structure comparable to insulin, may help to overcome insulin resistance (131); adverse effects are burning at the injection site, hypoglycemia, fluid retention, facial edema, increased heart rate, arthralgia, myalgia, parotid gland tenderness, and dyspnea.

Continuous subcutaneous insulin infusion with fast-acting insulin has been used in two cases.

- A 43-year-old man with type 1 diabetes developed local pruritus, redness, and swelling 4–5 times a week, 15–20 minutes after an injection, subsiding within 1–2 hours (132). Later he had a generalized urticarial reaction 5 minutes after an injection. Insulin lispro did not help. When checked for allergens, he was positive for all types of insulin and negative for additives. With oral mizolastine the local reactions abated for a week, but then reappeared with every injection. Generalized urticaria recurred later. With continuous subcutaneous insulin infusion the local reactions immediately disappeared and metabolic control was improved.
- A 79-year-old man used mixed insulin for 2 months and developed swelling at injection sites, lasting 48 hours (133). The lesions persisted despite switching to various types of insulin. He was allergic to insulin, as shown by a raised eosinophil count, a markedly increased IgE concentration, and antibodies to human, bovine, and porcine insulins in the RAST test. He was not allergic to needles or additives. With subcutaneous bolus doses of insulin lispro and Humulin he developed induration and wheal-and-flare reactions. When hydrocortisone 10 mg was added to each injection, the allergic reactions disappeared, but they recurred after 2 months. With continuous subcutaneous insulin infusion there were no allergic responses for 3 months. His raised IgE concentrations fell.

Long-Term Effects

Drug tolerance

Insulin resistance has been reported with continuous subcutaneous infusion.

- Diabetes mellitus in a 36-year-old man with acute pancreatitis could not be controlled with continuous subcutaneous insulin infusion, even with doses up to 1800 U/day, because of insulin resistance (134). Intravenous insulin by pump had to be stopped because of a catheter infection. The continuous subcutaneous infusion of freeze-dried insulin and the addition of aprotinin, a protease inhibitor, soluble dexamethasone or prednisolone, and intravenous immunoglobulin was ineffective. An implantable pump for intraperitoneal delivery established good regulation at a dosage of 30 U/day.
- A 23-year-old diabetic woman had severe subcutaneous insulin resistance for 11 years (135). Continuous subcutaneous insulin infusion with regular or insulin lispro did not prevent periods of fluctuating responses to insulin. The addition of heparin to insulin lispro in the pump improved serum insulin concentrations and metabolic control. The addition of heparin to regular insulin gave no improvement.

Heparin may improve the transport of insulin lispro but not of regular insulin.

Second-Generation Effects

Pregnancy

In a longitudinal cohort survey of 278 pregnant women with type 1 diabetes, the frequency of severe hypoglycemia increased two to three times compared with the last 4 months before pregnancy (25%, including 9% with hypoglycemic coma, before pregnancy and 41%, including 19% with coma, during pregnancy) (136). A history of severe hypoglycemia before pregnancy, a longer duration of diabetes, an HbA_{1c} concentration of 6.5% or less, and a daily insulin dose of over 0.1 U/kg were indicators of increased risk.

Continuous subcutaneous insulin infusion in pregnancy has been studied retrospectively in a nested case-control study (137). Those who used the pump had higher fasting blood glucose concentrations at the start, came sooner to the pregnancy clinic, used more insulin, put on more weight, and were more likely to have the baby admitted to the special baby care unit. Birth weights and neonatal hypoglycemia were similar.

- A 37-year-old nurse with type 1 diabetes was adequately treated with lispro and isophane insulin during her first pregnancy (138). In her second pregnancy, 3 years later, she had frequent episodes of hypoglycemia with the same regimen, for which she sometimes needed an injection of glucagon during the night. When the isophane in the evening was changed to glargine she had no more serious episodes of hypoglycemia.

Teratogenicity

In animals, teratogenicity of insulin during pregnancy has been observed (SEDA-8, 908) (139). No proof has been given that this also holds good in humans. A statistical significant relation found between insulin use for or during pregnancy and musculoskeletal anomalies (140) may also be caused by increased blood glucose or other to diabetes related factors.

Susceptibility Factors

Age

In 3805 children and adolescents with type 1 diabetes in 21 pediatric centers in 17 countries, feedback was given on the overall mean HbA_{1c} concentration in all the centers (141). After 3 years insulin therapy was more intensive, but glycemic control improved in only three centers. The relative risk of severe hypoglycemia was lowest in the center with the best glycemic control.

Drug Administration

Drug formulations

The formulation of insulin differs in various countries. A strength of 100 U/ml (U100) is increasingly used in many countries, but in other countries strengths of 20, 40, or 80 U/ml (U20, U40, and U80) are still in use. The increased frequency of travelling and tourism has increased the importance of the problem. In some countries in various parts of the world, both U40 insulin of variable purity and highly purified U100 insulin are available at the same time. U100 insulin used in U40 syringes causes severe unexpected hypoglycemia and the reverse induces apparent insulin resistance (SEDA-6, 367).

Drug contamination

A skin reaction to latex in rubber associated with an insulin formulation has been reported (142).

- In a 35-year-old woman, pruritic, erythematous, urticated plaques occurred at insulin injection sites, and persisted for 48 hours, after the use of a prefilled cartridge pen containing Humulin (Lilly) and Human Monotard (Novo Nordisk) aspirated from a punctured vial, but not when the insulin was taken directly from the vial. She had positive skin-prick tests to latex solutions. Both the cartridge bungs and the vial bungs contain butyl rubber with added natural rubber latex. Switching to latex-free vials alleviated the problem.

Drug administration route

The American Diabetes Association has published revised guidelines on insulin administration, including storage of insulin, use and reuse of needles, alternatives to syringes, injection techniques, and patient management related to dosing of insulin, self-monitoring, and hypoglycemia (143).

Developments in the administration of insulin through the skin, the mouth, the nose, and the lung have been reviewed (144). Methods of absorption other than subcutaneous, such as nasal insulin, buccal insulin, rectal insulin, and insulin in enteric-coated capsules, are still experimental. A problem in nasal administration is still how to get a daily reproducible dose (145). The frequency of hypoglycemia is comparable to the frequency with subcutaneous insulin (146). Nasal irritation, sometimes with congestion, and dyspnea (147) can occur. Pulmonary insulin, delivered by aerosol inhalation, is another experimental method. No lung obstruction was reported, but the uptake varied considerably (148).

Insulin syringes

Disposable syringes can release silicon particles into the insulin vials, reducing the effectiveness of insulin (149). This can happen when insulin is injected back into the vial, during correction for the desired dose, and is specifically seen when low doses are used for long periods. Flocculation of insulin, found before the expiry date, may be related to this problem (SEDA-12, 360).

Insulin pens

Insulin pens are being increasingly used for intensive insulin therapy. For low doses, pens are more accurate than syringes (150). In 48 children and adolescents pen devices were more accurate than syringes when under 5 U of insulin had to be injected; for higher doses pens and syringes were comparable (151).

Long-acting isophane insulin in pens can be insufficiently resuspended before an injection, resulting in a great variation in the dose of insulin per injection; in one study isophane content ranged from 5 to 214% (151). Only 10% of 109 patients tipped and rolled the pen more than 10 times. There was no relation between inadequate suspension and the number of attacks of hypoglycemia. It was mechanically proven that 20 cycles are necessary for good suspension. After education, suspension errors were less common in 80% of the patients. They had fewer attacks of hypoglycemia, but HbA_{1c} did not change.

A warning has been given that over 0.3 μl of blood (and viruses) can reflux in insulin cartridges in pen-like injectors. Reflux was measured using a rubber tube containing a dye solution. A questionnaire study in 193 patients using cartridges showed that 20 patients sometimes noted a reddish cartridge and that two patients shared their cartridges with other patients (152).

After injecting insulin, the pen has to be kept in place for some time. Many pens leak from the tip of the needle when the pen is removed from the injection site 7 seconds after the injection is finished. In one study only the Novopen 1.5 ml and Novolet 1.5 ml showed no leakage; eight of twenty 3 ml BD pens and Novo pens, 16 of 20 Novolets 3 ml and 19 of 20 Saline pens 3 ml (Lilly) leaked 4.0, 4.7, 5.9, and 9.2 mg respectively (153). It is necessary to keep the needle in place for 10–30 seconds after injection. Measured by ultrasonography, 86% of injections with needles of 12.7 mm and 38% of injections with needles of 8 mm in diabetic children with a BMI below the 60 percentile were intramuscular instead of subcutaneous (154). The injection changed from intramuscular to subcutaneous in half of the injections in the arm and in two-thirds of injections in the thigh when 8 mm needles were used. Nowadays, 6 mm needles are available in many countries.

In general, intensive therapy produces lower blood glucose concentrations and HbA_{1c} concentrations. This may result in worsening of proliferative retinopathy (155), or weight gain M14.42.9]. Pens can develop inaccuracies in rare instances, which may be unnoticed by the patient (156). Clogging of the system is often the cause. The result is diabetic coma or ketoacidosis, but this is not more frequent than with other systems. When needles are not regularly renewed, infections may emerge.

Insulin pumps

The usefulness of devices for constant subcutaneous, intravenous, or intraperitoneal insulin administration is well established. To establish feedback systems reliable, constantly functioning insulin sensors are essential, but they have been in a developmental phase for more than 25 years, and no long-acting glucose sensors for non-experimental use are yet available (157). Experience with pumps in large groups of patients has been reported (158–160). When starting intensive therapy, temporary worsening of secondary complications, mostly retinopathy, but sometimes nephropathy, has been reported (SEDA-14, 374). Weight gain is also a complication. The major candidates for insulin pump therapy include patients with type 1 diabetes, pregnant women, some types of brittle diabetics, patients wanting to become pregnant, and children.

Most pumps deliver insulin subcutaneously. Implantable pumps delivering insulin intraperitoneally with remote control devices are increasingly used (161,162). Pumps provide signals to alert users to malfunction, but leakage of connections often does not activate the alarm. Since the patient has no natural reserve of insulin, breakdown of the pump, leakage, or intercurrent infection without adjustment of the dose rapidly leads to ketoacidosis. The sudden release of insulin from a "runaway" pump is an exceptional event. Hypoglycemic deaths, infections (for example with *Mycobacterium fortuitum*) (163), local allergic reactions and infections, thrombosis in intravenous systems, allergy to nickel in needles (164), skin infections (165), needle breakage (SEDA-13, 382), problems with bad batteries, breakdown of the pump, leakage in delivery systems, or wrong insertion of the needle have all been described (SEDA-7, 405) (166). Pumps with sealed reservoirs (waterproof) can expel more insulin when used at high altitudes (skiing, mountaineering, pressurized cabins in airplanes) inducing serious hypoglycemia (SEDA-16, 486) (167); adapters that allow pressure equilibrium obviate this. Pumps that deliver insulin intravenously are almost obsolete, since they can cause thrombosis, vasculitis, and septicemia.

Efficacy

Continuous subcutaneous insulin infusion has been reviewed (168,169). Probably more than 100 000 patients in the USA are using it. Some studies have shown no difference in mean glucose concentration or HbA_{1c} compared with intensive treatment, but most have shown a slight difference favoring continuous subcutaneous infusion. With fast-acting analogues the postprandial glucose peaks are lower. In one study, when insulin delivery was intentionally interrupted, the increase in glucose concentrations or the development of ketonuria was later with regular insulin, but in another study there was no difference in the development of hyperglycemia or beta-hydroxybutyric acid between fast-acting analogues and regular insulin. Patients preferred to continue treatment with pumps.

Insulin delivery by a pump may be superior to glargine insulin. Continuous subcutaneous insulin infusion was compared with intensive therapy with insulin glargine plus insulin lispro in 19 patients (170). The patients who received insulin glargine were exposed to glucose concentrations under 3.9 mmol/l overnight for three times as long as those who used continuous subcutaneous insulin infusion.

In a meta-analysis of the metabolic and psychosocial impact of pumps, 52 studies were found; 22 were published before 1987 and 13 after 1993, the year in which the results of the DCCT were published (171). The authors stated that therefore conclusions about efficacy are not definitive. All pump malfunctions were reported before 1988. All types of changes were reported when the frequency and severity of hypoglycemia were compared with prepump times. Infection and skin irritation were expressed in different ways in the various studies. The risk of diabetic ketoacidosis fell after 1993. Most users preferred to continue pump treatment, mainly because of more flexibility, greater freedom, and improved glycemic control.

When continuous subcutaneous insulin infusion and sulfonylureas were compared in nine normolipidemic patients with type 2 diabetes, HbA_{1c} was not different but triglycerides and small LDL particles were reduced by the continuous infusion (172).

Continuous subcutaneous insulin infusion treatment is feasible in obese patients (BMI over 30 kg/m^2) with type 2 diabetes and severe insulin resistance, as has been shown in a study in 10 patients over 40 weeks (173). HbA_{1c} improved from 12 to 9.6% and weight was reduced by 2.5 kg. There were no adverse effects.

Use in children

In a randomized, crossover study in 10 children aged 7–10 years who used subcutaneous insulin pumps only in the evening and at nighttime, fasting, and 0300 hours, concentrations of blood glucose and fructosamine were improved (174). There was a better quality of life and a reduced fear of hypoglycemia. Children of this age may not be capable of handling a pump during the day.

In 95 patients aged 4–18 years with a median follow-up of 28 months, continuous subcutaneous insulin infusion produced no change in medical complications (diabetic ketoacidosis, visit to the emergency department), but there was a reduction in the number of episodes of hypoglycemia (175). HbA_{1c} was significantly lower than prepump values, but gradually increased in the first year and then remained stable.

In 118 children aged 1.5–18 years treated with continuous subcutaneous insulin infusion, HbA_{1c} in preschool children fell from 7.1 to 6.5%, in school children from 7.8 to 7.3%, and in adolescents from 8.1 to 7.4% (176). Daily insulin consumption did not increase and the frequency of severe episodes of hypoglycemia fell.

General adverse effects

Continuous intraperitoneal insulin infusion with implantable pumps has been assessed in 34 patients with poorly controlled diabetes (177). In two patients, the pump was explanted: in one patient with Werner's syndrome (no subcutaneous fat) the pump was explanted because of infection in the pocket, and one pump was explanted because the patient had local complaints and psychological problems. One patient refused to be included. Patients were followed for 58 months. HbA_{1c} fell from 10.0 to 9.0% in the first year and remained there. Median days in hospital fell from 45 to 13 after 1 year. The quality of life was relatively low and many had psychiatric problems. Although long-term glycemic control improved and lengths of hospital stay were reduced, normal glucose control and normal quality of life could not be achieved.

Local adverse effects

Implantable insulin infusion pumps have been reviewed (178,179), as has the use of pumps in children (180). In 31 centers, 914 pumps were implanted, representing 2121 patient-years. Some commonly reported pump complications were (178):

- hematoma or seroma, usually resolved by needle aspiration;
- pump migration, the frequency lessening with experience; surgical intervention is necessary;
- rare pump pocket infections; the causes were difficult to determine, but in two patients, coagulase-negative staphylococci were found, suggesting contamination with skin flora during refill;
- progressive thinning of the skin, 1–30 months after implantation in 2 per 100 patient-years; pain and skin erosion often followed; the cause is unclear; only a correlation with physical activity could be found.

Catheter malfunction was the most frequent event (obstruction, total occlusion, and peritoneal adhesions: 13, 10, and 3.1 events per 100 patient-years respectively). Flushing sometimes prevented occlusion. Better tip design had a big effect. Adhesion formation decreased with daily injections of heparin. The frequency of ketoacidosis was comparable to that reported with continuous subcutaneous insulin infusion and was usually related to catheter obstruction. It diminished during the review period. Episodes of severe hypoglycemia were fewer than during intensive subcutaneous therapy.

The tendency of insulin molecules to aggregate in concentrated solutions sometimes requires specific insulin or insulin lispro for pumps. There is a difference of opinion about whether insulin absorption kinetics change (improve) during placement of the catheter (SEDA-16, 488) (SEDA-18, 412). Changing the injection site and renewing the infusion system every 2–4 days is important in preventing clogging, local allergy, and infection at the insertion site.

In implanted pumps, catheters for continuous intraperitoneal insulin infusion can be obstructed by deposits of fibrin on the catheter tip. They mostly reappear after the plug is blown out, necessitating replacement (181). Hematoma, skin erosions, infections (182), pain, pump migration, and pocket complications are not rare (SEDA-20, 397) (183). Erosion of the cecum, mimicking appendicitis, is reported (184). During the start of pump therapy, some patients feel as if they are constantly hypoglycemic, even though low blood glucose concentrations cannot be objectified.

There was no macrophage activation in 10 patients with obstructed ($n = 3$) or non-obstructed ($n = 7$) catheters in implantable pumps (185).

When insulin delivery stops during continuous subcutaneous insulin infusion, ketoacidosis can develop rapidly, but it can be easily corrected if ketoacidosis has developed recently, although exceptions occur (186).

- A 32-year-old woman with well-regulated diabetes, using about 35 U/day of insulin by continuous subcutaneous infusion, tried a sauna for the first time when her blood glucose was 7 mmol/l. She stayed for about 45 minutes and the temperature reached 70°C for 10 minutes. The blood glucose concentration rose to 11 and 17 mmol/l, despite a bolus of insulin 6 units. She felt sick and vomited during the night; the next morning her blood glucose was 21 mmol/l and she had ketonuria, abdominal cramps, and extreme fatigue. Insulin 25 units by pump produced no improvement, but after opening a new vial, the situation improved; within 6 hours she was normoglycemic, and her ketonuria disappeared within 16 hours.

It is not clear in this case whether insulin had formed aggregates and fibrils due to the high temperature or if the action of counter-regulatory hormones induced by hyperthermia was increased, or both.

Problems with insulin delivery in implanted pumps are difficult to correct. A change in Hoechst 21 pH-neutral semisynthetic insulin 400 U/ml in accordance with regulations of the European Pharmacopoeia (SEDA-20, 397) resulted in more frequent clogging when this insulin was used in the Minimed 2001 implantable pump (MIP 2001). From October 1995 to October 1996, 17 pumps were implanted (187). The refilling period was reduced from 90 to 30–45 days and the reservoirs were washed with insulin-free buffer before each refill. Backflow was seen in 13 pumps after a mean period of 7.2 months. Modification of the manufacturing process produced 21PH ETP insulin (human semisynthetic insulin, Genapol-stabilized) 400 U/ml, Hoechst, with improved stability since July 1997. All pumps were specifically cleaned before the new insulin was used for refill. The refill period was increased from 38 to 78 days. In 16 pumps, only one backflow was seen after 14 months. The incidence of catheter blockage did not change. The better stability of this insulin for implantable pumps has been confirmed in a study in which 88 pumps were refilled every 45 days and 108 pumps every 90 days (188).

Pump failure

Almost all pumps are programmable and pump failure is rare (2 per 100 patient-years) (178).

Risk of hypoglycemia

Continuous subcutaneous insulin infusion in 75 youths aged 12–20 years has been compared with multiple daily injections over 12 months (189). HbA_{1c} was lower, and the number of attacks of hypoglycemia in the pump group was 50% less. Ketoacidosis seldom occurred: once during intensive therapy and twice during pump therapy. Weight increased more during pump treatment. Coping with diabetes was less difficult with pump therapy.

In 103 patients who used continuous subcutaneous insulin infusion for 2 years, the incidence of severe hypoglycemia fell from 0.70 cases/patient/year before treatment to 0.06 cases/patient/year during treatment, and HbA_{1c} improved from 7.7 to 7.2% (190). The incidence of abscesses was 0.1 cases/patient/year and of ketoacidosis 0.01 cases/patient/year. The patients with HbA_{1c} concentrations above 8.5% had a higher incidence of serious hypoglycemia and abscesses. Quality of life assessments showed great improvements. The reasons for continuous subcutaneous insulin infusion were optimization of metabolic control, greater flexibility, or prevention of severe hypoglycemia.

In 138 patients treated with continuous subcutaneous insulin infusion for 7 years, there was a fall in the incidence of episodes of serious hypoglycemia (from 0.31 to 0.09 cases/patient/year) and ketoacidosis (from 0.41 to 0.11 cases/patient/year); the number of infections was unchanged (0.2 infections/patient/year) (191).

When continuous subcutaneous insulin infusion was instituted in patients with long-standing poor glycemic control during a crossover study in 79 patients for 32 weeks, 17 dropped out after the first crossover, making it impossible to use the second arm. HbA_{1c} and quality of life both improved. There were more episodes of mild hypoglycemia with continuous subcutaneous insulin infusion (192). The authors of an editorial concluded that continuous subcutaneous insulin infusion can anticipate changes in insulin need, which is important for diabetics with a variable lifestyle or an exaggerated dawn phenomenon (193). For a large group the increase in cost and the hassle of continuous subcutaneous insulin infusion do not offset that, and multiple daily injections with glargine as basal insulin (see below) can be equally effective.

Continuous subcutaneous insulin infusion was found to be feasible in 56 children and adolescents (aged 7–23 years) (194). HbA_{1c} improved in 36 and deteriorated in 6. The rate of severe attacks of hypoglycemia fell, but not significantly. Hypoglycemia and seizure frequency were less overall in the group, with better HbA_{1c} concentrations. One patient had a catheter infection and was treated with local antibiotics and a new infusion system at another site.

Suitable types of insulin

Short-acting neutral buffered insulin by pump is sometimes ineffective. Treatment with non-buffered insulin can make things worse, but short-acting acidified insulin can improve HbA_{1c}. This type of insulin is well tolerated for over 3 years. The acid insulin may contain more monomers than neutral insulin, which may act less rapidly, as it contains more polymers (195).

Insulin lispro is sometimes less beneficial in continuous subcutaneous insulin infusion (196).

- A 58-year-old man with diabetes and unawareness of hypoglycemia had 53 emergency hospital admissions in 2 years before he started regular continuous subcutaneous insulin infusion. His attacks of hypoglycemia were reduced to one every 2–3 weeks. His mean blood glucose was 7.0 mmol/l. When insulin lispro was introduced in the pump he had an attack every 2–3 days for 68 days and hospital admission was required seven times. The mean blood glucose was 6.3 mmol/l. After he used soluble insulin instead of insulin lispro, the number of attacks of hypoglycemia fell substantially. The mean blood glucose was 6.4 mmol/l.

It may be that the more rapid diffusion and absorption of insulin lispro in diabetics who achieve tight metabolic control and have hypoglycemia unawareness destabilizes glycemic control.

Continuous subcutaneous insulin infusion with insulin lispro has been reported to give variable control (197).

- A 12-year-old boy with type 1 diabetes had problems with insulin lispro in his pump. After multiple daily injections, he started continuous subcutaneous insulin infusion with insulin lispro and could freely adjust his eating schedule; he had fewer episodes of hypoglycemia and his HbA_{1c} was 5.4%. Later, he developed a pattern of variable responsiveness to insulin, starting with increased responsiveness on the day on which he changed his subcutaneous needle, followed by reduced sensitivity and hyperglycemia on the third day. The infusion site was changed and Velosulin was added to insulin lispro, making it possible for him to use his injection site for 3 days consistently; the HbA_{1c} was 7.2%. After 2.5 years he started using insulin aspart. It then became possible to change the infusion site every 4–5 days, when the cartridge was empty. The HbA_{1c} fell to 6.2%.

Continuous subcutaneous insulin infusion has been compared with short-acting insulins plus glargine or isophane as long-acting insulins for 1 year in 32 patients with poor control (198). Four of them had serious attacks of hypoglycemia. There were no differences in HbA_{1c} or other metabolic parameters (including lipids). In those treated with continuous subcutaneous insulin infusion, the reduction in the amount of insulin required was larger.

Hoechst 21 pH-neutral insulin in intraperitoneal pumps increases the production of antibodies to insulin, in contrast to the same insulin in subcutaneous pumps (199). It is not clear whether the intraperitoneal route or modification of insulin during storage in the implanted reservoir causes greater antigenicity. When a newly designed side-port catheter on the Minimed pump was used in 40 patients for 450 days per patient, there was one catheter encapsulation, one clogging, and six cases of catheter/pump related underdelivery (200). This was comparable to the position before 1994, when the formula of the Hoechst 21 pH-neutral insulin was changed for the first time.

Other devices

Other devices, such as long-term subcutaneous catheters (201,202), which have to be renewed every 4 days (203), or intraperitoneal catheters (204) for pumps, pose the same types of problems as subcutaneous catheters for pumps, except that the catheters are indwelling for longer periods. The jet-stream injector, introduced as an alternative for people who are afraid of injections, has given problems with delayed pain and bleeding. The advantages of these methods are questionable.

Oral administration

Metabolism of insulin and the lack of a specific carrier to transport insulin through the gut made the oral route impossible (144).

Inhaled insulin

In the lungs, insulin has to be absorbed from the alveoli (144). Enhancers to give the particles the right size and constituency to reach the alveoli improve systemic availability (205). The relative potency of inhaled insulin is about 10%, which means that a 10-fold increase in dose is necessary. The effects of inhaled insulin are comparable to those of injected regular or fast-acting insulins or even faster. However, it is difficult to get a good action profile. The anatomy of the pharynx affects the transport of the particles. In smokers, the permeability of the lung epithelium is much greater and absorption from the alveoli is faster and higher than in non-smokers; during actual smoking, uptake is reduced. In the short term the excipients in the sprays have no adverse effects. More participants in a study of inhaled human insulin were satisfied with inhaled insulin than they were with subcutaneous insulin (206).

Ten severely hyperglycemic patients with type 2 diabetes taking oral agents were treated at random with two injections of isophane daily or with lyophilized nasal insulin before each meal, with an added injection of subcutaneous isophane when necessary (207). The periods were separated by 2 months. Nasal insulin produced control of diabetes comparable to isophane, except in three patients. Adverse effects included transient pruritus, sneezing and rhinorrhea, and chronic nasal crusts. One patient was withdrawn because of cough and dizziness after each nasal dose.

Inhaled insulin has been studied in 72 patients in an open, parallel-group, randomized trial for 12 weeks; 35 used inhaled insulin (152). The inhaled insulin was given three times before meals with isophane insulin at bedtime. Controls used their regular insulin two or three times a day with a long-acting insulin at bedtime. HbA_{1c} did not differ between the groups and there was no difference in the frequency or severity of attacks of hypoglycemia. Pulmonary function tests were stable and showed no differences between the groups. There were no serious or major adverse effects.

The dose of inhaled insulin is about 10 times higher than the subcutaneous dose that produces the same hypoglycemic effect. In an open, randomized, crossover study subcutaneous insulin was compared with a 10 times higher dose of inhaled insulin in 15 non-smoking patients with type 2 diabetes (208). The peak action of inhaled insulin was earlier. Apart from that, the effects were similar. There were no differences in FEV_1 at baseline or at 4 or 8 hours after treatment. Absorption of inhaled insulin is significantly higher in smokers (209). In non-diabetics, absorption is reduced in asthma (210). Inhaled insulin may increase the titer of insulin antibodies (211).

Nasal administration

Insulin is rapidly absorbed after nasal administration, but even with absorption enhancers its systemic availability is low and its metabolic effect very short (144).

Gelified nasal insulin has been compared with twice daily isophane insulin and three times daily subcutaneous regular insulin in 16 patients with type 1 diabetes (207). Three patients had to withdraw because of nasal burning and one because of persistent sinusitis. One patient had purulent sinusitis after 6 months. The efficacy of gelified insulin was comparable to that of regular insulin.

Transdermal administration

Application to the skin, a highly efficient general barrier, did not result in sufficient and reproducible absorption (144).

Drug overdose

- Insulin overdose has been reported in patients without diabetes (212) and in a 25-year-old man with Munchausen's syndrome (213).
- Suicide by insulin has been reported in a 68-year-old, non-diabetic physician who had also taken metoprolol and alcohol. The blood metoprolol concentration was 0.4 microgram/ml (usual target range 0.035–0.5 microgram/ml) and alcohol 122 mg/dl (27 mmol/l). C-peptide could not be detected, serum insulin was 1849 μU/ml (normal fasting concentration below 16 μU/ml) (214).

Hypokalemia, hypophosphatemia, and hypomagnesemia can occur after insulin overdose (215).

- A 47-year-old man with type 2 diabetes attempted suicide by taking a bottle of wine, triazolam 2 mg, zoplicone 75 mg, and subcutaneous insulin (soluble 300 U and isophane 1800 U). His blood glucose was 1.5 mmol/l, potassium 2.4 mmol/l, phosphate 0.74 mmol/l, and magnesium 1.06 mmol/l. After 80 ml of 50% glucose and gastric lavage he needed a glucose infusion 6.6 mg/kg/minute for 24 hours to keep his blood glucose at 5.5–11.1 mmol/l. There was no brain damage on neurological examination or CT scan.

Acute liver damage has been attributed to insulin overdose followed by excessive glucose administration (79).

- In a suicide attempt, a 48-year-old woman took clomipramine 225 mg, diazepam 50 mg, oxazepam 150 mg, flurazepam 120 mg, and aspirin 10 g and injected insulin subcutaneously (1000 U short-acting and 1000 U long-acting). Her blood glucose was undetectable. She was intubated and given 40% glucose 20 ml and an infusion of 20% glucose (total 100 g over 2 hours). She continued to receive intravenous glucose 40% with potassium chloride for 36 hours (total 4430 g) in spite of high glucose concentrations. Her aspartate and alanine transaminase activities rose to 420 and 610 U/l respectively, the total bilirubin to 147 μmol/l (mainly unconjugated), the alkaline phosphatase to 178 U/l, and the serum lactate to 6.8 mmol/l. An ultrasound scan of the liver was normal. When the glucose infusion was stopped, everything normalized rapidly.

Acute steatosis of the liver may have explained this presentation. In insulin overdose, the combination of greatly increased hepatic production of triglycerides from glucose and reduced production of apolipoprotein B 100 results in an insufficient increase in the transport of triglycerides in VLDL particles from liver to muscle and adipose tissue and contributes to the steatosis.

Drug–Drug Interactions

ACE inhibitors

Whether ACE inhibitors aggravate or generate hypoglycemia is debated (216). In a case-control study of 404 cases and 1375 controls, the risk of hypoglycemia was 5.5 times greater (95% CI = 4.0, 7.6) in insulin versus sulfonylurea users and was not influenced by use of ACE inhibitors overall (217). However, the use of enalapril was associated with an increased risk of hypoglycemia (OR = 2.4; 95% CI = 1.1, 5.3).

Beta-blockers

Beta-blockers have various effects on glucose metabolism, but these are usually too small to be of clinical significance (217,218). However, beta-blockers can block the adrenergic symptoms of hypoglycemia.

- A 68-year-old woman with diabetes and hypertension using 42 units of isophane insulin and propranolol 20 mg qds died with a blood glucose concentration below 1.4 mmol/l without any symptoms of hypoglycemia (219).

Clozapine

Severe insulin resistance with ketoacidosis (pH 6.9) has been reported with clozapine (220). After withdrawal, insulin requirements fell. Reinstitution of clozapine induced an identical increase in insulin need.

Glucocorticoids

Glucocorticoids are counter-regulatory and can cause increased insulin requirements. Conversely, reducing the dose of a glucocorticoid, without changing the dosage of insulin, can cause hypoglycemia.

Maprotiline

- Maprotiline, a tetracyclic antidepressant, repeatedly induced hypoglycemia in a 39-year-old woman with type 1 diabetes, even when the insulin dosage was reduced from 20 U/day to 4–10 U/day. Maprotiline seems to prolong the half-life of insulin. A glucagon stimulation test showed a maximum C-peptide concentration of only 0.22 nmol/l (221).

Olanzapine

Olanzapine has been reported to have precipitated diabetes (222).

- A 31-year-old man with a treatment-refractory psychiatric disorder without prior diabetes was given olanzapine 10 mg/day. After 3 months he developed hyperglycemia and an acidosis (pH 7.11). After treatment he needed at least 64 U/day of insulin, but 15 days after stopping olanzapine his insulin requirements fell and 15 days later insulin was withdrawn.

Interference with Diagnostic Tests

Blood glucose measurement

Three diabetic patients on chronic ambulatory peritoneal dialysis (CAPD) had symptoms of hypoglycemia when glucose readings on strips were higher than 4 mmol/l (223). Venous testing showed glucose concentrations as low as 1.8 mmol/l. Large amounts of glucose are used in CAPD, which not only affects the regulation of diabetes but can also affect the peritoneal wall. Since 1999, icodextrin has been used in dialysis fluids. Icodextrin is glucose-free and reduces the need for insulin. However, it is also absorbed systematically and can be metabolized to maltose and maltotriose. Paper systems that use either glucose oxidase or glucose dehydrogenase overestimate glucose readings when icodextrin is used, and patients and their carers are not able to measure low blood glucose concentrations. Another factor is that during end-stage renal insufficiency, insulin catabolism is reduced. This contributes to the problems when CAPD is changed to automated (overnight) peritoneal dialysis, in which daytime hypoglycemia can be prevented by reducing the amount of insulin used during the day.

Monitoring Therapy

Frequent self-control by pricking the fingertips can cause anemia (224) or pyoderma gangrenosum and fingertip ulceration (225).

Problems with the use of blood glucose measurement systems are reported from time to time. For example, it is easy to read glucose meters wrongly (SEDA-25, 508). Hypoglycemia was missed when a patient inadvertently switched the glucose meter from mmol/l to mg/dl and read 266 mg/dl as 26.6 mmol/l and 158 mg/dl as 15.8 mmol/l (226).

- An 89-year-old man wrongly read the glucose concentrations in his home glucose meter (227). The meter read 561 mg/dl and 591 mg/dl but testing in the clinic 2 hours later showed concentrations of 175 mg/dl and 188 mg/dl. He had read the digital display upside down: 591 instead of 165 and 561 instead of 195.

Patients should be instructed about the correct orientation of digital meters.

In Raynaud's phenomenon, blood glucose concentrations measured by finger prick are often lower than the real values (50). The arm reacts more slowly to rapid changes in glucose concentrations. When glucose is monitored in the arm, changes in glucose concentrations are later seen than when monitored by finger prick (228). Rubbing the arm reduces the differences (229).

The development of glucose sensor systems has been reviewed (230). An automated device for sampling in the arm (231) and a microdialysis-based glucose sensor system (232) have been developed.

References

1. Koivisto VA, Felig P. Alterations in insulin absorption and in blood glucose control associated with varying insulin injection sites in diabetic patients. Ann Intern Med 1980;92(1):59–61.
2. Sindelka G, Heinemann L, Berger M, Frenck W, Chantelau E. Effect of insulin concentration, subcutaneous fat thickness and skin temperature on subcutaneous insulin absorption in healthy subjects. Diabetologia 1994;37(4):377–80.
3. Vaag A, Handberg A, Lauritzen M, Henriksen JE, Pedersen KD, Beck-Nielsen H. Variation in absorption of NPH insulin due to intramuscular injection. Diabetes Care 1990;13(1):74–6.
4. Binder C, Lauritzen T, Faber O, Pramming S. Insulin pharmacokinetics. Diabetes Care 1984;7(2):188–99.
5. Burge MR, Schade DS. Insulins. Endocrinol Metab Clin North Am 1997;26(3):575–98.
6. Azzopardi J, Gatt A, Zammit A, Alberti G. Lack of evidence of cerebral oedema in adults treated for diabetic ketoacidosis with fluids of different tonicity. Diabetes Res Clin Pract 2002;57(2):87–92.
7. Glaser N, Barnett P, McCaslin I, Nelson D, Trainor J, Louie J, Kaufman F, Quayle K, Roback M, Malley R, Kuppermann N; Pediatric Emergency Medicine Collaborative Research Committee of the American Academy of Pediatrics. Risk factors for cerebral edema in children with diabetic ketoacidosis. The Pediatric Emergency Medicine Collaborative Research Committee of the American Academy of Pediatrics. N Engl J Med 2001;344(4):264–9.
8. Dunger DB, Edge JA. Predicting cerebral edema during diabetic ketoacidosis. N Engl J Med 2001;344(4):302–3.
9. Auzepy P, Caquet R. Hypoglycémies graves dues a l'insuline. Risques et accidents des médicaments antidiabétiques. [Severe hypoglycemia due to insulin. Risks and adverse effects of antidiabetic drugs.] Sem Hop 1983;59(10): 697–705.
10. Seltzer HS. Severe drug-induced hypoglycemia: a review. Compr Ther 1979;5(4):21–9.
11. McAulay V, Deary IJ, Frier BM. Symptoms of hypoglycaemia in people with diabetes. Diabet Med 2001;18(9):690–705.
12. Gold AE, Deary IJ, Frier BM. Recurrent severe hypoglycaemia and cognitive function in type 1 diabetes. Diabet Med 1993;10(6):503–8.
13. Egger M, Davey Smith G, Stettler C, Diem P. Risk of adverse effects of intensified treatment in insulin-dependent diabetes mellitus: a meta-analysis Diabet Med 1997;14(11):919–28.
14. The Diabetes Control and Complications Trial Research Group. The effect of intensive treatment of diabetes on the development and progression of long-term complications in insulin-dependent diabetes mellitus. N Engl J Med 1993;329(14):977–86.
15. The Diabetes Control and Complications Trial Research Group. Hypoglycemia in the Diabetes Control and Complications Trial. Diabetes 1997;46(2):271–86.
16. UK Prospective Diabetes Study (UKPDS) Group. Intensive blood-glucose control with sulphonylureas or insulin compared with conventional treatment and risk of complications in patients with type 2 diabetes (UKPDS 33). Lancet 1998;352(9131):837–53.
17. Taylor R, Davies R, Fox C, Sampson M, Weaver JU, Wood L. Appropriate insulin regimes for type 2 diabetes: a multicenter randomized crossover study. Diabetes Care 2000;23(11):1612–18.
18. Gale EA, Tattersall RB. Unrecognised nocturnal hypoglycaemia in insulin-treated diabetics. Lancet 1979;1(8125):1049–52.
19. Ben-Ami H, Nagachandran P, Mendelson A, Edoute Y. Drug-induced hypoglycemic coma in 102 diabetic patients. Arch Intern Med 1999;159(3):281–4.
20. Lopez MJ, Oyarzabal M, Rodriguez M, Barrio R, Hermoso F, Blasco L. Severe hypoglycemia in Spanish diabetic children and adolescents. Study Group of Infantile Diabetes of the Spanish Paediatric Endocrinology Society. J Pediatr Endocrinol Metab 1999;12(1):85–7.
21. Miller CD, Phillips LS, Ziemer DC, Gallina DL, Cook CB, El-Kebbi IM. Hypoglycemia in patients with type 2 diabetes mellitus. Arch Intern Med 2001;161(13): 1653–9.
22. Leese GP, Wang J, Broomhall J, Kelly P, Marsden A, Morrison W, Frier BM, Morris AD. DARTS/MEMO Collaboration. Frequency of severe hypoglycemia requiring emergency treatment in type 1 and type 2 diabetes: a population-based study of health service resource use. Diabetes Care 2003;26(4):1176–80.
23. Holstein A, Plaschke A, Egberts EH. Incidence and costs of severe hypoglycemia. Diabetes Care 2002;25(11):2109–10.
24. Amin R, Ross K, Acerini CL, Edge JA, Warner J, Dunger DB. Hypoglycemia prevalence in prepubertal children with type 1 diabetes on standard insulin regimen: use of continuous glucose monitoring system. Diabetes Care 2003;26(3):662–7.
25. Hvidberg A, Christensen NJ, Hilsted J. Counterregulatory hormones in insulin-treated diabetic patients admitted to an accident and emergency department with hypoglycaemia. Diabet Med 1998;15(3):199–204.

26. Levy CJ, Kinsley BT, Bajaj M, Simonson DC. Effect of glycemic control on glucose counterregulation during hypoglycemia in NIDDM. Diabetes Care 1998;21(8): 1330–8.
27. Burge MR, Schmitz-Fiorentino K, Fischette C, Qualls CR, Schade DS. A prospective trial of risk factors for sulfonylurea-induced hypoglycemia in type 2 diabetes mellitus. JAMA 1998;279(2):137–43.
28. Kaneto H, Ikeda M, Kishimoto M, Iida M, Hoshi A, Watarai T, Kubota M, Kajimoto Y, Yamasaki Y, Hori M. Dramatic recovery of counter-regulatory hormone response to hypoglycaemia after intensive insulin therapy in poorly controlled type I diabetes mellitus. Diabetologia 1998;41(8):982–3.
29. Fritsche A, Stumvoll M, Grub M, Sieslack S, Renn W, Schmulling RM, Haring HU, Gerich JE. Effect of hypoglycemia on beta-adrenergic sensitivity in normal and type 1 diabetic subjects. Diabetes Care 1998; 21(9):1505–10.
30. Oskarsson P, Adamson U, Sjobom NC, Lins PE. Long-term follow-up of insulin-dependent diabetes mellitus patients with recurrent episodes of severe hypoglycaemia. Diabetes Res Clin Pract 1999;44(3):165–74.
31. Nordfeldt S, Samuelsson U. Serum ACE predicts severe hypoglycemia in children and adolescents with type 1 diabetes. Diabetes Care 2003;26(2):274–8.
32. Gerich JE, Mokan M, Veneman T, Korytkowski M, Mitrakou A. Hypoglycemia unawareness. Endocr Rev 1991;12(4):356–71.
33. Amiel SA. R.D. Lawrence Lecture 1994. Limits of normality: the mechanisms of hypoglycaemia unawareness. Diabet Med 1994;11(10):918–24.
34. Hvidberg A, Fanelli CG, Hershey T, Terkamp C, Craft S, Cryer PE. Impact of recent antecedent hypoglycemia on hypoglycemic cognitive dysfunction in nondiabetic humans. Diabetes 1996;45(8):1030–6.
35. Hepburn DA, MacLeod KM, Frier BM. Physiological, symptomatic and hormonal responses to acute hypoglycaemia in type 1 diabetic patients with autonomic neuropathy. Diabet Med 1993;10(10):940–9.
36. Pohl J, Frohnau G, Kerner W, Fehm-Wolfsdorf G. Symptom awareness is affected by the subjects' expectations during insulin-induced hypoglycemia. Diabetes Care 1997;20(5):796–802.
37. Maran A, Lomas J, Macdonald IA, Amiel SA. Lack of preservation of higher brain function during hypoglycaemia in patients with intensively-treated IDDM. Diabetologia 1995;38(12):1412–18.
38. Teuscher A, Berger WG. Hypoglycaemia unawareness in diabetics transferred from beef/porcine insulin to human insulin. Lancet 1987;2(8555):382–5.
39. Colagiuri S, Miller JJ, Petocz P. Double-blind crossover comparison of human and porcine insulins in patients reporting lack of hypoglycaemia awareness. Lancet 1992;339(8807):1432–5.
40. George E, Bedford C, Peacey SR, Hardisty CA, Heller SR. Further evidence for a high incidence of nocturnal hypoglycaemia in IDDM: no effect of dose for dose transfer between human and porcine insulins. Diabet Med 1997;14(6):442–8.
41. Klein BE, Klein R, Moss SE. Risk of hypoglycemia in users of human insulin. The Wisconsin Epidemiologic study of Diabetic Retinopathy. Diabetes Care 1997;20(3):336–9.
42. Galloway PJ, Thomson GA, Fisher BM, Semple CG. Insulin-induced hypoglycemia induces a rise in C-reactive protein. Diabetes Care 2000;23(6):861–2.
43. Ortega E, Wagner A, Caixas A, Barcons M, Corcoy R. Hypoglycemia and pulmonary edema: a forgotten association. Diabetes Care 2000;23(7):1023–4.
44. Hart SP, Frier BM. Causes, management and morbidity of acute hypoglycaemia in adults requiring hospital admission. QJM 1998;91(7):505–10.
45. Cox DJ, Gonder-Frederick LA, Kovatchev BP, Julian DM, Clarke WL. Progressive hypoglycemia's impact on driving simulation performance. Occurrence, awareness and correction. Diabetes Care 2000;23(2):163–70.
46. Marrero D, Edelman S. Hypoglycemia and driving performance: a flashing yellow light? Diabetes Care 2000;23(2):146–7.
47. Frier BM. Hypoglycemia and driving performance. Diabetes Care 2000;23(2):148–50.
48. ter Braak EW, Appelman AM, van de Laak M, Stolk RP, van Haeften TW, Erkelens DW. Clinical characteristics of type 1 diabetic patients with and without severe hypoglycemia. Diabetes Care 2000;23(10):1467–71.
49. Matz R. Hypoglycemia, seizures, and pulmonary edema. Diabetes Care 2000;23(11):1715.
50. Bradley KJ, Paton RC. Silent hypoglycaemia at the diabetic clinic. Diabet Med 2001;18(5):425–6.
51. Cryer PE. Hypoglycaemia: the limiting factor in the glycaemic management of Type I and Type II diabetes. Diabetologia 2002;45(7):937–48.
52. Smith D, Amiel SA. Hypoglycaemia unawareness and the brain. Diabetologia 2002;45(7):949–58.
53. Fruehwald-Schultes B, Born J, Kern W, Peters A, Fehm HL. Adaptation of cognitive function to hypoglycemia in healthy men. Diabetes Care 2000;23(8):1059–66.
54. Austin EJ, Deary IJ. Effects of repeated hypoglycemia on cognitive function: a psychometrically validated reanalysis of the Diabetes Control and Complications Trial data. Diabetes Care 1999;22(8):1273–7.
55. Berger A, Croisier M, Jacot E, Kehtari R. Coma hypoglycémique de longue durée. [Hypoglycemic coma of long duration.] Rev Med Suisse Romande 1999;119(1): 49–53.
56. Strachan MW, Deary IJ, Ewing FM, Frier BM. Recovery of cognitive function and mood after severe hypoglycemia in adults with insulin-treated diabetes. Diabetes Care 2000;23(3):305–12.
57. Cox DJ, Gonder-Frederick LA, Kovatchev BP, Young-Hyman DL, Donner TW, Julian DM, Clarke WL. Biopsychobehavioral model of severe hypoglycemia. II. Understanding the risk of severe hypoglycemia. Diabetes Care 1999;22(12):2018–25.
58. Kinsley BT, Weinger K, Bajaj M, Levy CJ, Simonson DC, Quigley M, Cox DJ, Jacobson AM. Blood glucose awareness training and epinephrine responses to hypoglycemia during intensive treatment in type 1 diabetes. Diabetes Care 1999;22(7):1022–8.
59. Wysocki T, Harris MA, Mauras N, Fox L, Taylor A, Jackson SC, White NH. Absence of adverse effects of severe hypoglycemia on cognitive function in school-aged children with diabetes over 18 months. Diabetes Care 2003;26(4):1100–5.
60. Matyka KA, Wigg L, Pramming S, Stores G, Dunger DB. Cognitive function and mood after profound nocturnal hypoglycaemia in prepubertal children with conventional insulin treatment for diabetes. Arch Dis Child 1999;81(2):138–42.
61. McAulay V, Deary IJ, Ferguson SC, Frier BM. Acute hypoglycemia in humans causes attentional dysfunction while nonverbal intelligence is preserved. Diabetes Care 2001;24(10):1745–50.
62. Gold AE, Marshall SM. Cortical blindness and cerebral infarction associated with severe hypoglycemia. Diabetes Care 1996;19(9):1001–3.
63. Odeh M, Oliven A. Hypoglycemia and bilateral cortical blindness. Diabetes Care 1996;19(3):272–3.

64. Aiello LP, Arrigg PG, Shah ST, Murtha TJ, Aiello LM. Solar retinopathy associated with hypoglycemic insulin reaction. Arch Ophthalmol 1994;112(7):982–3.
65. Burge MR, Castillo KR, Schade DS. Meal composition is a determinant of lispro-induced hypoglycemia in IDDM. Diabetes Care 1997;20(2):152–5.
66. Daneman D, Frank M, Perlman K, Tamm J, Ehrlich R. Severe hypoglycemia in children with insulin-dependent diabetes mellitus: frequency and predisposing factors. J Pediatr 1989;115(5 Pt 1):681–5.
67. Amiel SA. Studies in hypoglycaemia in children with insulin-dependent diabetes mellitus. Horm Res 1996; 45(6):285–90.
68. Tupola S, Rajantie J. Documented symptomatic hypoglycaemia in children and adolescents using multiple daily insulin injection therapy. Diabet Med 1998; 15(6):492–6.
69. Jaap AJ, Jones GC, McCrimmon RJ, Deary IJ, Frier BM. Perceived symptoms of hypoglycaemia in elderly type 2 diabetic patients treated with insulin. Diabet Med 1998;15(5):398–401.
70. Arem R, Zoghbi W. Insulin overdose in eight patients: insulin pharmacokinetics and review of the literature. Medicine (Baltimore) 1985;64(5):323–32.
71. Charlton R, Smith G, Day A. Munchausen's syndrome manifesting as factitious hypoglycaemia. Diabetologia 2001;44(6):784–5.
72. Barkai L, Vamosi I, Lukacs K. Prospective assessment of severe hypoglycaemia in diabetic children and adolescents with impaired and normal awareness of hypoglycaemia. Diabetologia 1998;41(8):898–903.
73. Airey CM, Williams DR, Martin PG, Bennett CM, Spoor PA. Hypoglycaemia induced by exogenous insulin—"human" and animal insulin compared. Diabet Med 2000;17(6):416–32.
74. Bragd J, Adamson U, Lins PE, Wredling R, Oskarsson P. A repeated cross-sectional survey of severe hypoglycaemia in 178 Type 1 diabetes mellitus patients performed in 1984 and 1998. Diabet Med 2003;20(3):216–19.
75. Dagogo-Jack S, Fanelli CG, Cryer PE. Durable reversal of hypoglycemia unawareness in type 1 diabetes. Diabetes Care 1999;22(5):866–7.
76. Ovalle F, Fanelli CG, Paramore DS, Hershey T, Craft S, Cryer PE. Brief twice-weekly episodes of hypoglycemia reduce detection of clinical hypoglycemia in type 1 diabetes mellitus. Diabetes 1998;47(9):1472–9.
77. Clarke B, Ward JD, Enoch BA. Hypoglycaemia in insulin-dependent diabetic drivers. BMJ 1980;281(6240):586.
78. Thoma ME, Glauser J, Genuth S. Persistent hypoglycemia and hyperinsulinemia: caution in using glucagon. Am J Emerg Med 1996;14(1):99–101.
79. Monsod TP, Tamborlane WV, Coraluzzi L, Bronson M, Yong-Zhan T, Ahern JA. Epipen as an alternative to glucagon in the treatment of hypoglycemia in children with diabetes. Diabetes Care 2001;24(4):701–4.
80. Torres Marti A, Font J, Cano F, Rodriguez de Castro L, Camp J, Borras A, Milla J. Estudio epidemiologico del sindrome hipoglucemico en un servicio de urgencias. Analisis sobre 71 cases. [Epidemiologic study of hypoglycemic syndrome in an emergency unit. Study of 71 cases.] Med Clin (Barc) 1981;77(10):405–9.
81. Jolliet P, Leverve X, Pichard C. Acute hepatic steatosis complicating massive insulin overdose and excessive glucose administration. Intensive Care Med 2001;27(1): 313–6.
82. Tupola S, Sipila I, Huttunen NP, Salo S, Nuuja A, Akerblom HK. Management of asymptomatic hypoglycaemia in children and adolescents with Type 1 diabetes mellitus. Diabet Med 2000;17(10):752–3.
83. Deiss D, Kordonouri O, Meyer K, Danne T. Long hypoglycaemic periods detected by subcutaneous continuous glucose monitoring in toddlers and pre-school children with diabetes mellitus. Diabet Med 2001;18(4): 337–8.
84. Pitzer KR, Desai S, Dunn T, Edelman S, Jayalakshmi Y, Kennedy J, Tamada JA, Potts RO. Detection of hypoglycemia with the GlucoWatch biographer. Diabetes Care 2001;24(5):881–5.
85. Haymond MW, Schreiner B. Mini-dose glucagon rescue for hypoglycemia in children with type 1 diabetes. Diabetes Care 2001;24(4):643–5.
86. Jermendy G, Nadas J, Sapi Z. "Lipoblastoma-like" lipoatrophy induced by human insulin: morphological evidence for local dedifferentiation of adipocytes? Diabetologia 2000;43(7):955–6.
87. The Diabetes Control and Complications Trial Research Group. Influence of intensive diabetes treatment on body weight and composition of adults with type 1 diabetes in the Diabetes Control and Complications Trial. Diabetes Care 2001;24(10):1711–21.
88. Saule H. Insulin-induzierte Ödeme bei Adoleszenten mit Diabetes mellitus Typ I. [Insulin-induced edema in adolescents with type 1 diabetes mellitus.] Dtsch Med Wochenschr 1991;116(31–32):1191–4.
89. DeFronzo RA. The effect of insulin on renal sodium metabolism. A review with clinical implications. Diabetologia 1981;21(3):165–71.
90. Juliusson PB, Bjerknes R, Sovik O, Kvistad PH. Generaliserte odemer ved insulinbehandling av nyoppdaget diabetes mellitus. [Generalized edema following insulin treatment of newly diagnosed diabetes mellitus.] Tidsskr Nor Laegeforen 2001;121(8):919–20.
91. Tawata M, Ikeda M, Kodama Y, Aida K, Onaya T. A type 2 diabetic patient with liver dysfunction due to human insulin. Diabetes Res Clin Pract 2000;49(1):17–21.
92. Kordonouri O, Lauterborn R, Deiss D. Lipohypertrophy in young patients with type 1 diabetes. Diabetes Care 2002;25(3):634.
93. Swift B. Examination of insulin injection sites: an unexpected finding of localized amyloidosis. Diabet Med 2002;19(10):881–2.
94. Singhal PC, Abramovici M, Venkatesan J. Rhabdomyolysis in the hyperosmolal state. Am J Med 1990;88(1):9–12.
95. Kahn CR, Rosenthal AS. Immunologic reactions to insulin: insulin allergy, insulin resistance, and the autoimmune insulin syndrome. Diabetes Care 1979;2(3):283–95.
96. deShazo RD, Boehm TM, Kumar D, Galloway JA, Dvorak HF. Dermal hypersensitivity reactions to insulin: correlations of three patterns to their histopathology. J Allergy Clin Immunol 1982;69(2):229–37.
97. Ross JM. Allergy to insulin. Pediatr Clin North Am 1984;31(3):675–87.
98. Yoshino K, Takeda N, Muramatsu M, Morita H, Mune T, Ishizuka T, Yasuda K. [A case of generalized allergy to both human insulin and protamine in insulin preparation]. J Jpn Diabetes Soc 1999;42:927–30.
99. Warita E, Shimuzi H, Ubukata T, Mori M. [A case of human insulin allergy.] J Jpn Diabetes Soc 1999;42: 1013–15.
100. Abraham MR, al-Sharafi BA, Saavedra GA, Khardori R. Lispro in the treatment of insulin allergy. Diabetes Care 1999;22(11):1916–17.
101. Panczel P, Hosszufalusi N, Horvath MM, Horvath A. Advantage of insulin lispro in suspected insulin allergy. Allergy 2000;55(4):409–10.
102. Eapen SS, Connor EL, Gern JE. Insulin desensitization with insulin lispro and an insulin pump in a

5-year-old child. Ann Allergy Asthma Immunol 2000;85(5): 395–7.
103. Sackey AH. Recurrent generalised urticaria at insulin injection sites. BMJ 2000;321(7274):1449.
104. Kumar D. Insulin allergy: differences in the binding of porcine, bovine, and human insulins with anti-insulin IgE. Diabetes Care 1981;4(1):104–7.
105. Soto-Aguilar MC, deShazo RD, Morgan JE, Mather P, Ibrahim G, Frentz JM, Lauritano AA. Total IgG and IgG subclass specific antibody responses to insulin in diabetic patients. Ann Allergy 1991;67(5):499–503.
106. Al-Sheik OA. Unusual local cutaneous reactions to insulin injections: a case report. Saudi Med J 1998;19: 199–201.
107. Elte JW, van der Schroeff JG, van Leeuwen AW, Radder JK. Sclerosing granuloma after short-term administration of depot-insulin Hoechst. Case report and a review of the literature. Klin Wochenschr 1982; 60(23):1461–4.
108. Jordaan HF, Sandler M. Zinc-induced granuloma—a unique complication of insulin therapy. Clin Exp Dermatol 1989;14(3):227–9.
109. Young RJ, Steel JM, Frier BM, Duncan LJ. Insulin injection sites in diabetes—a neglected area? BMJ (Clin Res Ed) 1981;283(6287):349.
110. Mandrup-Poulsen T, Molvig J, Pildal J, Rasmussen AK, Andersen L, Skov BG, Petersen J. Leukocytoclastic vasculitis induced by subcutaneous injection of human insulin in a patient with type 1 diabetes and essential thrombocytemia. Diabetes Care 2002; 25(1):242–3.
111. Jones GR, Statham B, Owens DR, Jones MK, Hayes TM. Lipoatrophy and monocomponent porcine insulin. BMJ (Clin Res Ed) 1981;282(6259):190.
112. Silverstone P. Generalised allergic reaction to human insulin. BMJ (Clin Res Ed) 1986;292(6525):933–4.
113. Ganz MA, Unterman T, Roberts M, Uy R, Sahgal S, Samter M, Grammer LC. Resistance and allergy to recombinant human insulin. J Allergy Clin Immunol 1990;86(1):45–51.
114. Patterson R, Roberts M, Grammer LC. Insulin allergy: re-evaluation after two decades. Ann Allergy 1990;64(5): 459–62.
115. Kurtz AB, Nabarro JD. Circulating insulin-binding antibodies. Diabetologia 1980;19(4):329–34.
116. Goswami R, Jaleel A, Kochupillai NP. Insulin antibody response to bovine insulin therapy: functional significance among insulin requiring young diabetics in India. Diabetes Res Clin Pract 2000;49(1):7–15.
117. Goerz G, Ruzicka T, Hofmann N, Drost H, Gruneklee D. Granulomatöse allergische Reaktion vom verzögerten Typ auf Surfen. [Granulomatous allergic reaction of the delayed type to Surfen.] Hautarzt 1981;32(4):187–90.
118. Feinglos MN, Jegasothy BV. "Insulin" allergy due to zinc. Lancet 1979;1(8108):122–4.
119. Bruni S, Barolo P, Gamba S, Grassi G, Blatto A. Case of generalized allergy due to zinc and protamine in insulin preparation. Diabetes Care 1986;9(5):552.
120. Gin H, Aubertin J. Generalized allergy due to zinc and protamine in insulin preparation treated with insulin pump. Diabetes Care 1987;10(6):789–90.
121. Diem P. Allergy to insulin. BMJ 1980;281(6247):1068–9.
122. MacCracken J, Stenger P, Jackson T. Latex allergy in diabetic patients: a call for latex-free insulin tops. Diabetes Care 1996;19(2):184.
123. Dische FE, Wernstedt C, Westermark GT, Westermark P, Pepys MB, Rennie JA, Gilbey SG, Watkins PJ. Insulin as an amyloid–fibril protein at sites of repeated insulin injections in a diabetic patient. Diabetologia 1988;31(3):158–61.
124. Chantelau EA, Berger M. Pollution of insulin with silicone oil, a hazard of disposable plastic syringes. Lancet 1985;1(8443):1459.
125. Lapiere CM, Pierard GE, Hermanns JF, Lefebvre P. Unusual extensive granulomatosis after long-term use of plastic syringes for insulin injections. Dermatologica 1982;165(6):580–90.
126. Sacerdote AS. Hypoglycemic urticaria revisited. Diabetes Care 1999;22(5):861.
127. Lassmann-Vague V, SanMarco M, LeJeune PJ, Alessis C, Vague P, Belicar P. Autoimmunity and intraperitoneal insulin treatment by programmable pumps: lack of relationship. Diabetes Care 1998;21(11):2041–4.
128. Charles MA. Autoimmunity and intraperitoneal insulin. Diabetes Care 1998;21:2043–4.
129. Frigerio C, Aubry M, Gomez F, Graf L, Dayer E, de Kalbermatten N, Gaillard RC, Spertini F. Desensitization-resistant insulin allergy. Allergy 1997;52(2):238–9.
130. Valenta LJ, Elias AN. Insulin-induced lipodystrophy in diabetic patients resolved by treatment with human insulin. Ann Intern Med 1985;102(6):790–1.
131. Cusi K, DeFronzo RA. Treatment of NIDDM IDDM, and other insulin-resistant states with IGF-I. Diabetes Rev 1995;3:206–36.
132. Naf S, Esmatjes E, Recasens M, Valero A, Halperin I, Levy I, Gomis R. Continuous subcutaneous insulin infusion to resolve an allergy to human insulin. Diabetes Care 2002;25(3):634–5.
133. Pratt EJ, Miles P, Kerr D. Localized insulin allergy treated with continuous subcutaneous insulin. Diabet Med 2001;18(6):515–16.
134. Riveline JP, Capeau J, Robert JJ, Varroud-Vial M, Cerf-Baron I, Deburge A, Charpentier G. Extreme subcutaneous insulin resistance successfully treated by an implantable pump. Diabetes Care 2001;24(12):2155–6.
135. Tokuyama Y, Nozaki O, Kanatsuka A. A patient with subcutaneous-insulin resistance treated by insulin lispro plus heparin. Diabetes Res Clin Pract 2001;54(3):209–12.
136. Evers IM, ter Braak EW, de Valk HW, van Der Schoot B, Janssen N, Visser GH. Risk indicators predictive for severe hypoglycemia during the first trimester of type 1 diabetic pregnancy. Diabetes Care 2002;25(3): 554–9.
137. Simmons D, Thompson CF, Conroy C, Scott DJ. Use of insulin pumps in pregnancies complicated by type 2 diabetes and gestational diabetes in a multiethnic community. Diabetes Care 2001;24(12):2078–82.
138. Devlin JT, Hothersall L, Wilkis JL. Use of insulin glargine during pregnancy in a type 1 diabetic woman. Diabetes Care 2002;25(6):1095–6.
139. Landauer W. Is insulin a teratogen? Teratology 1972;5(2):129–35.
140. Queisser-Luft A, Eggers I, Stolz G, Kieninger-Baum D, Schlaefer K. Serial examination of 20,248 newborn fetuses and infants: correlations between drug exposure and major malformations. Am J Med Genet 1996;63(1): 268–76.
141. Danne T, Mortensen HB, Hougaard P, Lynggaard H, Aanstoot HJ, Chiarelli F, Daneman D, Dorchy H, Garandeau P, Greene SA, Hoey H, Holl RW, Kaprio EA, Kocova M, Martul P, Matsuura N, Robertson KJ, Schoenle EJ, Sovik O, Swift PG, Tsou RM, Vanelli M, Aman J; For the Hvidore Study Group on Childhood Diabetes. Persistent differences among centers over 3 years in glycemic control and hypoglycemia in a study of 3,805 children and adolescents with

type 1 diabetes from the Hvidore Study Group. Diabetes Care 2001;24(8):1342–7.

142. Roest MA, Shaw S, Orton DI. Insulin-injection-site reactions associated with type I latex allergy. N Engl J Med 2003;348(3):265–6.
143. American Diabetes Association. Insulin administration. Diabetes Care 2001;24(11):1984–7.
144. Heinemann L, Pfutzner A, Heise T. Alternative routes of administration as an approach to improve insulin therapy: update on dermal, oral, nasal and pulmonary insulin delivery. Curr Pharm Des 2001;7(14):1327–51.
145. Gizurarson S, Bechgaard E. Intranasal administration of insulin to humans. Diabetes Res Clin Pract 1991;12(2): 71–84.
146. Hilsted J, Madsbad S, Hvidberg A, Rasmussen MH, Krarup T, Ipsen H, Hansen B, Pedersen M, Djurup R, Oxenboll B. Intranasal insulin therapy: the clinical realities. Diabetologia 1995;38(6):680–4.
147. Heinemann L, Traut T, Heise T. Time-action profile of inhaled insulin. Diabet Med 1997;14(1):63–72.
148. Laube BL, Georgopoulos A, Adams GK 3rd. Preliminary study of the efficacy of insulin aerosol delivered by oral inhalation in diabetic patients. JAMA 1993;269(16):2106–9.
149. Chantelau E, Berger M, Bohlken B. Silicone oil released from disposable insulin syringes. Diabetes Care 1986;9(6):672–3.
150. Lteif AN, Schwenk WF. Accuracy of pen injectors versus insulin syringes in children with type 1 diabetes. Diabetes Care 1999;22(1):137–40.
151. Jehle PM, Micheler C, Jehle DR, Breitig D, Boehm BO. Inadequate suspension of neutral protamine Hagendorn (NPH) insulin in pens. Lancet 1999;354(9190):1604–7.
152. Skyler JS, Cefalu WT, Kourides IA, Landschulz WH, Balagtas CC, Cheng SL, Gelfand RA. Efficacy of inhaled human insulin in type 1 diabetes mellitus: a randomised proof-of-concept study. Lancet 2001; 357(9253):331–5.
153. Annersten M, Frid A. Insulin pens dribble from the tip of the needle after injection. Pract Diabetes Int 2000;17:109–11.
154. Tubiana-Rufi N, Belarbi N, Du Pasquier-Fediaevsky L, Polak M, Kakou B, Leridon L, Hassan M, Czernichow P. Short needles (8 mm) reduce the risk of intramuscular injections in children with type 1 diabetes. Diabetes Care 1999;22(10):1621–5.
155. Rosenlund EF, Haakens K, Brinchmann-Hansen O, Dahl-Jorgensen K, Hanssen KF. Transient proliferative diabetic retinopathy during intensified insulin treatment. Am J Ophthalmol 1988;105(6):618–25.
156. Hardy K, Gill G. Bubble ketoacidosis. Lancet 1988;1(8598):1336–7.
157. Fischer U. Fundamentals of glucose sensors. Diabet Med 1991;8(4):309–21.
158. Mecklenburg RS, Benson EA, Benson JW Jr, Blumenstein BA, Fredlund PN, Guinn TS, Metz RJ, Nielsen RL. Long-term metabolic control with insulin pump therapy. Report of experience with 127 patients. N Engl J Med 1985;313(8):465–8.
159. Mecklenburg RS, Guinn TS, Sannar CA, Blumenstein BA. Malfunction of continuous subcutaneous insulin infusion systems: a one-year prospective study of 127 patients. Diabetes Care 1986;9(4):351–5.
160. Chantelau E, Spraul M, Muhlhauser I, Gause R, Berger M. Long-term safety, efficacy and side-effects of continuous subcutaneous insulin infusion treatment for type 1 (insulin-dependent) diabetes mellitus: a one centre experience. Diabetologia 1989;32(7):421–6.
161. Saudek CD. Implantable insulin pumps: a current look. Diabetes Res Clin Pract 1990;10(2):109–14.
162. Belicar P, Lassmann-Vague V. Local adverse events associated with long-term treatment by implantable insulin pumps. The French EVADIAC Study Group experience. Evaluation dans le Diabete du Traitement par Implants Actifs. Diabétes Care 1998;21(2):325–6.
163. Toth EL, Boychuk LR, Kirkland PA. Recurrent infection of continuous subcutaneous insulin infusion sites with *Mycobacterium fortuitum*. Diabetes Care 1995;18(9): 1284–5.
164. Morton C. Nickel allergy: a complication of CSII. Pract Diabetes 1990;7:179.
165. Chantelau E, Lange G, Sonnenberg GE, Berger M. Acute cutaneous complications and catheter needle colonization during insulin-pump treatment. Diabetes Care 1987;10(4):478–82.
166. Fishman V, Fishman M. Practical problems with insulin pumps. N Engl J Med 1982;306(22):1369–70.
167. Wredling R, Lin PE, Adamson U. Pump "run-away" causing severe hypoglycaemia. Lancet 1989;2(8657):273.
168. Zinman B. Insulin pump therapy and rapid acting insulin: what have we learned? Int J Clin Pract Suppl 2001;(123):47–50.
169. Pickup J, Keen H. Continuous subcutaneous insulin infusion at 25 years: evidence base for the expanding use of insulin pump therapy in type 1 diabetes. Diabetes Care 2002;25(3):593–8.
170. King AB, Armstrong D. A comparison of basal insulin delivery: continuous subcutaneous insulin infusion versus glargine. Diabetes Care 2003;26(4):1322.
171. Weissberg-Benchell J, Antisdel-Lomaglio J, Seshadri R. Insulin pump therapy: a meta-analysis. Diabetes Care 2003;26(4):1079–87.
172. Rivellese AA, Patti L, Romano G, Innelli F, Di Marino L, Annuzzi G, Iavicoli M, Coronel GA, Riccardi G. Effect of insulin and sulfonylurea therapy, at the same level of blood glucose control, on low density lipoprotein subfractions in type 2 diabetic patients. J Clin Endocrinol Metab 2000;85(11):4188–92.
173. Wainstein J, Metzger M, Wexler ID, Cohen J, Raz I. The use of continuous insulin delivery systems in severely insulin-resistant patients. Diabetes Care 2001;24(7):1299.
174. Kaufman FR, Halvorson M, Kim C, Pitukcheewanont P. Use of insulin pump therapy at nighttime only for children 7–10 years of age with type 1 diabetes. Diabetes Care 2000;23(5):579–82.
175. Plotnick LP, Clark LM, Brancati FL, Erlinger T. Safety and effectiveness of insulin pump therapy in children and adolescents with type 1 diabetes. Diabetes Care 2003;26(4):1142–6.
176. Ahern JA, Boland EA, Doane R, Ahern JJ, Rose P, Vincent M, Tamborlane WV. Insulin pump therapy in pediatrics: a therapeutic alternative to safely lower HbA1c levels across all age groups. Pediatr Diabetes 2002;3(1):10–15.
177. DeVries JH, Eskes SA, Snoek FJ, Pouwer F, Van Ballegooie E, Spijker AJ, Kostense PJ, Seubert M, Heine RJ. Continuous intraperitoneal insulin infusion in patients with "brittle" diabetes: favourable effects on glycaemic control and hospital stay. Diabet Med 2002;19(6):496–501.
178. Pinget M, Jeandidier N. Long term safety and efficacy of intraperitoneal insulin infusion by means of implantable pumps. Horm Metab Res 1998;30(8):475–86.
179. Jeandidier N, Boivin S. Current status and future prospects of parenteral insulin regimens, strategies and delivery systems for diabetes treatment. Adv Drug Deliv Rev 1999;35(2–3):179–98.
180. Kaufman FR, Halvorson M, Miller D, Mackenzie M, Fisher LK, Pitukcheewanont P. Insulin pump therapy in type 1 pediatric patients: now and into the year 2000. Diabetes Metab Res Rev 1999;15(5):338–52.
181. Bousquet-Rouaud R, Castex F, Costalat G, Bastide M, Hedon B, Bouanani M, Jouvert S, Mirouze J. Factors

involved in catheter obstruction during long-term peritoneal insulin infusion. Diabetes Care 1993;16(5):801–5.
182. Levy RP, Borchelt MD, Kremer RM, Francis SJ, O'Connor CA. *Hemophilus influenza* infection of an implantable insulin-pump pocket. Diabetes Care 1992;15(11):1449–50.
183. Scavini M, Cristallo M, Sarmiento M, Dunn FL. Pump-pocket complications during long-term insulin delivery using an implanted programmable pump. Diabetes Care 1996;19(4):384–5.
184. Renard E, Taourel P, Quenet F, Domergue J, Bruel JM, Bringer J. Cecum erosion: unusual but serious complication of an implanted catheter for peritoneal insulin delivery. Diabetes Care 1995;18(3):408–9.
185. Kessler L, Tritschler S, Bohbot A, Sigrist S, Karsten V, Boivin S, Dufour P, Belcourt A, Pinget M. Macrophage activation in type 1 diabetic patients with catheter obstruction during peritoneal insulin delivery with an implantable pump. Diabetes Care 2001;24(2):302–7.
186. Bienvenu B, Timsit J. Sauna-induced diabetic ketoacidosis. Diabetes Care 1999;22(9):1584.
187. Renard E, Souche C, Jacques-Apostol D, Lauton D, Gibert-Boulet F, Costalat G, Bringer J, Jaffiol C. Improved stability of insulin delivery from implanted pumps using a new preparation process for infused insulin. Diabetes Care 1999;22(8):1371–2.
188. Boivin S, Belicar P, Melki V. Assessment of in vivo stability of a new insulin preparation for implantable insulin pumps. A randomized multicenter prospective trial. EVADIAC Group. Evaluation Dans le Diabéte du Traitement par Implants Actifs. Diabetes Care 1999;22(12):2089–90.
189. Boland EA, Grey M, Oesterle A, Fredrickson L, Tamborlane WV. Continuous subcutaneous insulin infusion. A new way to lower risk of severe hypoglycemia, improve metabolic control, and enhance coping in adolescents with type 1 diabetes. Diabetes Care 1999;22(11):1779–84.
190. Linkeschova R, Raoul M, Bott U, Berger M, Spraul M. Less severe hypoglycaemia, better metabolic control, and improved quality of life in type 1 diabetes mellitus with continuous subcutaneous insulin infusion (CSII) therapy; an observational study of 100 consecutive patients followed for a mean of 2 years. Diabet Med 2002;19(9):746–51.
191. Bruttomesso D, Pianta A, Crazzolara D, Scaldaferri E, Lora L, Guarneri G, Mongillo A, Gennaro R, Miola M, Moretti M, Confortin L, Beltramello GP, Pais M, Baritussio A, Casiglia E, Tiengo A. Continuous subcutaneous insulin infusion (CSII) in the Veneto region: efficacy, acceptability and quality of life. Diabet Med 2002;19(8):628–34.
192. DeVries JH, Snoek FJ, Kostense PJ, Masurel N, Heine RJ; Dutch Insulin Pump Study Group. A randomized trial of continuous subcutaneous insulin infusion and intensive injection therapy in type 1 diabetes for patients with long-standing poor glycemic control. Diabetes Care 2002;25(11):2074–80.
193. Schade DS, Valentine V. To pump or not to pump. Diabetes Care 2002;25(11):2100–2.
194. Maniatis AK, Klingensmith GJ, Slover RH, Mowry CJ, Chase HP. Continuous subcutaneous insulin infusion therapy for children and adolescents: an option for routine diabetes care. Pediatrics 2001;107(2):351–6.
195. Kamoi K, Sasaki H, Kobayashi T. Effect on glycemic control of short-acting acidified insulin administered three years in patients treated by continuous subcutaneous insulin infusion. J Jpn Diabetes Soc 2000;43:847–52.
196. Ooi C, Mullen P, Williams G. Insulin lispro: the ideal pump insulin for patients with severe hypoglycemic unawareness? Diabetes Care 1999;22(9):1598–9.
197. Becker DI. Pediatric use of insulin pumps: longer infusion site lifetime with NovoLog. Diabetes Care 2002;25(9):1663.
198. Lepore G, Dodesini AR, Nosari I, Trevisan R. Both continuous subcutaneous insulin infusion and a multiple daily insulin injection regimen with glargine as basal insulin are equally better than traditional multiple daily insulin injection treatment. Diabetes Care 2003;26(4):1321–2.
199. Jeandidier N, Boullu S, Busch-Brafin MS, Chabrier G, Sapin R, Gasser F, Pinget M. Comparison of antigenicity of Hoechst 21PH insulin using either implantable intraperitoneal pump or subcutaneous external pump infusion in type 1 diabetic patients. Diabetes Care 2002;25(1):84–8.
200. Gin H, Melki V, Guerci B, Catargi B; Evaluation dans le Diabéte du Traitement par Implants Actifs Study Group. Clinical evaluation of a newly designed compliant side port catheter for an insulin implantable pump: the EVADIAC experience. Evaluation dans le Diabéte du Traitement par Implants Actifs. Diabetes Care 2001;24(1):175.
201. Hanas R, Ludvigsson J. Side effects and indwelling times of subcutaneous catheters for insulin injections: a new device for injecting insulin with a minimum of pain in the treatment of insulin-dependent diabetes mellitus. Diabetes Res Clin Pract 1990;10(1):73–83.
202. Käär ML, Mäenpää J, Knip M. Insulin administration via a subcutaneous catheter. Effects on absorption. Diabetes Care 1993;16(10):1412–13.
203. Hanas SR, Carlsson S, Frid A, Ludvigsson J. Unchanged insulin absorption after 4 days' use of subcutaneous indwelling catheters for insulin injections. Diabetes Care 1997;20(4):487–90.
204. Wredling R, Adamson U, Lins PE, Backman L, Lundgren D. Experience of long-term intraperitoneal insulin treatment using a new percutaneous access device. Diabet Med 1991;8(6):597–600.
205. Heinemann L, Klappoth W, Rave K, Hompesch B, Linkeschowa R, Heise T. Intra-individual variability of the metabolic effect of inhaled insulin together with an absorption enhancer. Diabetes Care 2000;23(9):1343–7.
206. Gerber RA, Cappelleri JC, Kourides IA, Gelfand RA. Treatment satisfaction with inhaled insulin in patients with type 1 diabetes: a randomized controlled trial. Diabetes Care 2001;24(9):1556–9.
207. Lalej-Bennis D, Boillot J, Bardin C, Zirinis P, Coste A, Escudier E, Chast F, Peynegre R, Selam JL, Slama G. Efficacy and tolerance of intranasal insulin administered during 4 months in severely hyperglycaemic Type 2 diabetic patients with oral drug failure: a cross-over study. Diabet Med 2001;18(8):614–18.
208. Perera AD, Kapitza C, Nosek L, Fishman RS, Shapiro DA, Heise T, Heinemann L. Absorption and metabolic effect of inhaled insulin: intrapatient variability after inhalation via the Aerodose insulin inhaler in patients with type 2 diabetes. Diabetes Care 2002;25(12):2276–81.
209. Himmelmann A, Jendle J, Mellen A, Petersen AH, Dahl UL, Wollmer P. The impact of smoking on inhaled insulin. Diabetes Care 2003;26(3):677–82.
210. Henry RR, Mudaliar SR, Howland WC 3rd, Chu N, Kim D, An B, Reinhardt RR. Inhaled insulin using the AERx Insulin Diabetes Management System in healthy and asthmatic subjects. Diabetes Care 2003; 26(3):764–9.
211. Stoever JA, Palmer JP. Inhaled insulin and insulin antibodies: a new twist to an old debate. Diabetes Technol Ther 2002;4(2):157–61.
212. Winston DC. Suicide via insulin overdose in nondiabetics: the New Mexico experience. Am J Forensic Med Pathol 2000;21(3):237–40.

213. Bretz SW, Richards JR. Munchausen syndrome presenting acutely in the emergency department. J Emerg Med 2000;18(4):417–20.
214. Junge M, Tsokos M, Puschel K. Suicide by insulin injection in combination with beta-blocker application. Forensic Sci Int 2000;113(1–3):457–60.
215. Matsumura M, Nakashima A, Tofuku Y. Electrolyte disorders following massive insulin overdose in a patient with type 2 diabetes. Intern Med 2000;39(1):55–7.
216. Morris AD, Boyle DI, McMahon AD, Pearce H, Evans JM, Newton RW, Jung RT, MacDonald TM. ACE inhibitor use is associated with hospitalization for severe hypoglycemia in patients with diabetes. DARTS/MEMO Collaboration. Diabetes Audit and Research in Tayside, Scotland. Medicines Monitoring Unit. Diabetes Care 1997;20(9):1363–7.
217. Thamer M, Ray NF, Taylor T. Association between antihypertensive drug use and hypoglycemia: a case-control study of diabetic users of insulin or sulfonylureas. Clin Ther 1999;21(8):1387–400.
218. Wicklmayr M, Rett K, Dietze G, Mehnert H. Effects of beta-blocking agents on insulin secretion and glucose disposal. Horm Metab Res Suppl 1990;22:29–33.
219. Cooper JW. Fatal asymptomatic hypoglycemia in an elderly insulin-dependent diabetic patient taking an oral beta-blocking medication. Diabetes Care 1998;21(12): 2197–8.
220. Colli A, Cocciolo M, Francobandiera F, Rogantin F, Cattalini N. Diabetic ketoacidosis associated with clozapine treatment. Diabetes Care 1999;22(1):176–7.
221. Isotani H, Kameoka K. Hypoglycemia associated with maprotiline in a patient with type 1 diabetes. Diabetes Care 1999;22(5):862–3.
222. Gatta B, Rigalleau V, Gin H. Diabetic ketoacidosis with olanzapine treatment. Diabetes Care 1999;22(6):1002–3.
223. Mehmet S, Quan G, Thomas S, Goldsmith D. Important causes of hypoglycaemia in patients with diabetes on peritoneal dialysis. Diabet Med 2001;18(8):679–82.
224. Cordray JP, Merceron RE, Guillerd X, Nys P. Baisse du fer sérique due à l'auto-surveillance glycémique chez le diabétique. [Low serum iron level caused by self-monitoring of blood glucose in the diabetic patient.] Presse Méd 1991;20(7):310.
225. Cox NH, Dufton PA. Pyoderma gangrenosum and fingertip ulceration in a diabetic patient. Pract Diabetes 1987;4:236.
226. Prakash PK, Banerjee M, Harlow J, Hanna FW. An unusual case of hypoglycaemia. Diabet Med 2001;18(9):769–70.
227. Steward DE, Khardori R. An avoidable cause of false home glucose measurements. Diabetes Care 2001;24(4):794.
228. Jungheim K, Koschinsky T. Risky delay of hypoglycemia detection by glucose monitoring at the arm. Diabetes Care 2001;24(7):1303–6.
229. McGarraugh G. Glucose monitoring at the arm. Diabetes Care 2001;24:1304–6.
230. Koschinsky T, Heinemann L. Sensors for glucose monitoring: technical and clinical aspects. Diabetes Metab Res Rev 2001;17(2):113–23.
231. Fineberg SE, Bergenstal RM, Bernstein RM, Laffel LM, Schwartz SL. Use of an automated device for alternative site blood glucose monitoring. Diabetes Care 2001;24(7):1217–20.
232. Jungheim K, Wientjes KJ, Heinemann L, Lodwig V, Koschinsky T, Schoonen AJ; Glucose Monitoring Study Group. Subcutaneous continuous glucose monitoring: feasibility of a new microdialysis-based glucose sensor system. Diabetes Care 2001;24(9):1696–7.

Insulin aspart

See also Insulin

General Information

Insulin aspart is a rapid-acting synthetic insulin in which proline is replaced by aspartate at position 28 in the B chain. Insulin aspart has been reviewed (1). Its adverse effects do not differ from those of soluble human insulin and it has a similar effect on the blood glucose concentration (2).

A new development is the binding of two 9-fluorenylmethoxy-carbonyl moieties to two amino acids in the structure of aspart insulin, phenylalanine and lysine (3). This compound has no biological activity but gradually releases its groups and keeps diabetic animals in a good metabolic state over 2–3 days. Experiments in humans have not yet been reported.

Aspart insulin and biphasic insulin aspart (30% soluble rapid-acting insulin and 70% protamine-bound aspart insulin) have been reviewed (4).

Comparative studies

In a double-blind, crossover study of insulin aspart or soluble human insulin before meals and protamine zinc insulin before bedtime, 90 of 104 patients with type 1 diabetes completed the trial (5). Insulin aspart improved postprandial control by reducing hyperglycemic and hypoglycemic variations, but night-time control was inferior. There were 547 hypoglycemic episodes in the aspart period compared with 615 in the regular insulin period (no significant difference). However, there were only 20 major hypoglycemic events in 16 patients using aspart versus 44 events in 24 patients using human insulin. One patient was withdrawn with fatigue and anorexia during aspart. Convulsions during hypoglycemia occurred once in each group.

Insulin aspart had an increased maximal effect compared with regular insulin in euglycemic clamps in nondiabetics (6).

In an open comparison of insulin aspart and regular human insulin for 6 months in 882 patients with type 1 diabetes and extended to 714 patients for another 6 months, postprandial glucose concentrations were lower with insulin aspart (7). HbA_{1c} was slightly but significantly lower (7.78 versus 7.93%). There were no differences in hypoglycemic periods or adverse events.

Insulin aspart has been compared with regular insulin in 1065 patients for 26 weeks (8). HbA_{1c} improved significantly with aspart. The number of major attacks of hypoglycemia fell in the aspart group from 11 to 8%; there were no other differences.

Insulin aspart has been compared with buffered regular insulin by continuous subcutaneous infusion (9). There was some crystal formation with both formulations, but less with insulin aspart. Patients who used aspart required a slightly higher basal dose of insulin but had fewer unexplained attacks of hypoglycemia.

Frequent addition of isophane to a regimen of insulin aspart is unnecessary, as has been shown in a multicenter, multinational, randomized, open study in 368 patients followed for 64 weeks (10). Frequent addition of isophane up to four times daily to insulin aspart did not improve HbA_{1c} or change the number of episodes of hypoglycemia compared with regular insulin combined with isophane. Only postprandial blood glucose concentrations were reduced.

When insulin lispro and insulin aspart were compared in a single-blind, randomized, crossover study in 14 patients with type 1 diabetes, insulin lispro had a faster onset of action but a shorter duration (11). However, in another study the pharmacokinetic and the pharmacodynamic profiles of insulin aspart compared with human insulin were the same in 24 healthy Japanese as in non-Japanese (12). Insulin aspart and insulin lispro were equally effective in another 24 patients with type 1 diabetes (13).

Combination with long-acting insulin

In a multinational study for 6 months in 448 patients with type 1 diabetes, two-thirds were given the long-acting insulin detemir and one-third received isophane, both in addition to premeal rapid-acting insulin aspart (14). HbA_{1c} concentrations were comparable, but in the detemir group the risk of hypoglycemia was 22% less and the risk of nocturnal hypoglycemia was 34% lower. There were two cases of severe hypoglycemia with detemir and one with isophane. Three patients who used detemir developed reactions at the injection site (pain, myalgia, redness, or lipodystrophy) compared with one who used isophane (itching). One potentially allergic reaction was possibly related to detemir.

The new, short-acting insulins can be bound to protamine, allowing the preparation of mixed formulations. In an open, randomized, single-dose, three-way, crossover trial biphasic insulin aspart 30 (30% aspart plus 70% protaminated aspart, BIAsp 30), biphasic insulin lispro 25 (25% lispro plus 75% protaminated lispro, Mix 25), and biphasic human insulin 30 (30% regular plus 70% isophane insulin, BHI 30) were compared in 45 patients (15). Biphasic insulin aspart improved postprandial control better. There were 23 episodes of hypoglycemia with BIAsp 30, 19 with Mix 25, and 11 with BHI 30; two episodes with BIAsp 30, five with Mix 25, and two with BHI 30 required third-party intervention.

When 30% insulin aspart plus 70% protamine aspart was compared with the same mixture of regular plus isophane insulins, both injected twice-daily for 12 weeks, in 294 patients with type 1 and type 2 diabetes, control was better with the aspart mixture (16). There were fewer episodes of major hypoglycemia (20 versus 42) but the same number of minor episodes (362) with aspart.

Placebo-controlled studies

In a double-blind, crossover study with insulin aspart and human insulin in type 1 diabetes, human insulin was given 30 minutes before a meal with placebo immediately before the meal, or placebo was given 30 minutes before the meal with aspart insulin or human insulin immediately before the meal (17). On average, insulin aspart was absorbed twice as fast as human insulin. Postprandial glucose control improved on aspart. There were no episodes of serious hypoglycemia.

Organs and Systems

Immunologic

When short-acting insulins are given to patients who are allergic to regular insulin the allergic reactions can disappear. Although the short-acting insulins often have the same immunogenic epitopes, rapid dissociation of the fast-acting insulins into monomers can reduce their antigenic effects. Insulin lispro is known to be beneficial, and this has also been reported for aspart insulin (18).

- A 45-year-old man with type 2 diabetes treated with glibenclamide and metformin received combined chemotherapy for non-Hodgkin's lymphoma and was given premixed insulin. He developed local wheal-and-flare reactions immediately after the injections. Skin prick tests were positive for various types of insulin but weakly positive for lispro and negative for insulin aspart. He tolerated aspart insulin without any allergic reactions.

A few patients treated with insulin aspart developed antibodies, which cross-reacted with antibodies against human insulin and fell after 3 months (19). In lipodystrophy with lipoatrophic diabetes high insulin resistance is often found, for which leptin deficiency is one contributory factor.

Allergic reactions have been described with insulin aspart.

- A 53-year-old woman had type 2 diabetes that was not well controlled with diet and oral hypoglycemic drugs (20). She took intermediate-acting insulins, and after 2 months noticed redness and itching at injection sites. When she used insulin aspart and insulin lispro successively, the local reactions continued. She had a high serum concentration of total IgE (748 IU/ml; reference range below 400) and insulin-specific IgE (20 IU/ml; reference range below 0.34), positive insulin antibodies, and positive prick tests for insulin lispro, insulin aspart, human insulin, porcine insulin, and protamine. With intensive nutrition therapy and oral drugs her HbA_{1c} fell to 5.5%.
- A 29-year-old woman with raised insulin concentrations during therapy had lipodystrophy and high insulin antibody titers with high binding capacity and high affinity (21).

Insulin antibodies are rarely found in patients with lipodystrophy.

References

1. Lindholm A, Jacobsen LV. Clinical pharmacokinetics and pharmacodynamics of insulin aspart. Clin Pharmacokinet 2001;40(9):641–59.
2. Heinemann L, Weyer C, Rauhaus M, Heinrichs S, Heise T. Variability of the metabolic effect of soluble insulin and the rapid-acting insulin analogue insulin aspart. Diabetes Care 1998;21(11):1910–14.
3. Gershonov E, Shechter Y, Fridkin M. New concept for long-acting insulin: spontaneous conversion of an inactive modified insulin to the active hormone in circulation: 9-fluorenylmethoxycarbonyl derivative of insulin. Diabetes 1999;48(7):1437–42.

4. Chapman TM, Noble S, Goa KL. Insulin aspart: a review of its use in the management of type 1 and 2 diabetes mellitus. Drugs 2002;62(13):1945–81.
5. Home PD, Lindholm A, Hylleberg B, Round P. Improved glycemic control with insulin aspart: a multicenter randomized double-blind crossover trial in type 1 diabetic patients. UK Insulin Aspart Study Group. Diabetes Care 1998;21(11):1904–9.
6. Mudaliar SR, Lindberg FA, Joyce M, Beerdsen P, Strange P, Lin A, Henry RR. Insulin aspart (B28 asp-insulin): a fast-acting analogue of human insulin: absorption kinetics and action profile compared with regular human insulin in healthy nondiabetic subjects. Diabetes Care 1999;22(9):1501–6.
7. Raskin P, Guthrie RA, Leiter L, Riis A, Jovanovic L. Use of insulin aspart, a fast-acting insulin analogue, as the mealtime insulin in the management of patients with type 1 diabetes. Diabetes Care 2000;23(5):583–8.
8. Home PD, Lindholm A, Riis A; European Insulin Aspart Study Group. Insulin aspart vs. human insulin in the management of long-term blood glucose control in type 1 diabetes mellitus: a randomized controlled trial. Diabet Med 2000;17(11):762–70.
9. Bode BW, Strange P. Efficacy, safety, and pump compatibility of insulin aspart used in continuous subcutaneous insulin infusion therapy in patients with type 1 diabetes. Diabetes Care 2001;24(1):69–72.
10. DeVries JH, Lindholm A, Jacobsen JL, Heine RJ, Home PD; Tri-Continental Insulin Aspart Study Group. A randomized trial of insulin aspart with intensified basal NPH insulin supplementation in people with Type 1 diabetes. Diabet Med 2003;20(4):312–18.
11. Hedman CA, Lindstrom T, Arnqvist HJ. Direct comparison of insulin lispro and aspart shows small differences in plasma insulin profiles after subcutaneous injection in type 1 diabetes. Diabetes Care 2001;24(6):1120–1.
12. Kaku K, Matsuda M, Urae A, Irie S. Pharmacokinetics and pharmacodynamics of insulin aspart, a rapid-acting analogue of human insulin, in healthy Japanese volunteers. Diabetes Res Clin Pract 2000;49(2-3):119–26.
13. Plank J, Wutte A, Brunner G, Siebenhofer A, Semlitsch B, Sommer R, Hirschberger S, Pieber TR. A direct comparison of insulin aspart and insulin lispro in patients with type 1 diabetes. Diabetes Care 2002;25(11):2053–7.
14. Vague P, Selam JL, Skeie S, De Leeuw I, Elte JW, Haahr H, Kristensen A, Draeger E. Insulin detemir is associated with more predictable glycemic control and reduced risk of hypoglycemia than NPH insulin in patients with type 1 diabetes on a basal-bolus regimen with premeal insulin aspart. Diabetes Care 2003;26(3):590–6.
15. Hermansen K, Colombo M, Storgaard H, O'Stergaard A, Kolendorf K, Madsbad S. Improved postprandial glycemic control with biphasic insulin aspart relative to biphasic insulin lispro and biphasic human insulin in patients with type 2 diabetes. Diabetes Care 2002;25(5):883–8.
16. Boehm BO, Home PD, Behrend C, Kamp NM, Lindholm A. Premixed insulin aspart 30 vs. premixed human insulin 30/70 twice daily: a randomized trial in Type 1 and Type 2 diabetic patients. Diabet Med 2002;19(5):393–9.
17. Lindholm A, McEwen J, Riis AP. Improved postprandial glycemic control with insulin aspart. A randomized double-blind cross-over trial in type 1 diabetes. Diabetes Care 1999;22(5):801–5.
18. Airaghi L, Lorini M, Tedeschi A. The insulin analogue aspart: a safe alternative in insulin allergy. Diabetes Care 2001;24(11):2000.
19. Lindholm A, Jensen LB, Home PD, Raskin P, Boehm BO, Rastam J. Immune responses to insulin aspart and biphasic insulin aspart in people with type 1 and type 2 diabetes. Diabetes Care 2002;25(5):876–82.
20. Takata H, Kumon Y, Osaki F, Kumagai C, Arii K, Ikeda Y, Suehiro T, Hashimoto K. The human insulin analogue aspart is not the almighty solution for insulin allergy. Diabetes Care 2003;26(1):253–4.
21. Usui H, Makino H, Shikata K, Sugimoto T, Wada J, Yamana J, Matsuda M, Yoneda M, Koshima I. A case of congenital generalized lipodystrophy with lipoatrophic diabetes developing anti-insulin antibodies. Diabet Med 2002;19(9):794–5.

Insulin detemir

See also Insulin

General Information

Insulin detemir is a long-acting insulin analogue that lacks threonine at the B30 position and is acylated with a 14-carbon myristoyl fatty acid side-chain at the epsilon-amino group of the lysine in the B28 position. This stimulates binding to albumin and increases the half-life, extending its duration of action.

Comparative studies

In healthy volunteers, there was a dose-related increase in blood insulin concentrations after the administration of insulin detemir (1). However, there was no clear dose-response metabolic effect and individual variability was high.

Insulin detemir has been compared with protamine zinc insulin in 59 patients with type 1 diabetes (2). All used insulin detemir for 6 weeks and protamine zinc insulin for 6 weeks in a randomized order. About 2.35 times higher doses of detemir were necessary than protamine zinc insulin. Fasting blood glucose concentrations were lower at the end of the detemir period and there were fewer attacks of hypoglycemia.

In a 6-month, multinational, open, parallel-group comparison of insulin detemir and protamine zinc insulin in 448 patients with type 1 diabetes, the two treatments produced comparable HbA_{1c} concentrations and fasting plasma glucose concentrations with less within-subject variation in fasting blood glucose with insulin detemir (3). The risk of hypoglycemia was 22% lower with insulin detemir and 34% lower for nocturnal hypoglycemia.

Combination with short-acting insulin

In a multinational study for 6 months in 448 patients with type 1 diabetes, two-thirds were given insulin detemir and one-third received isophane, both in addition to premeal rapid-acting insulin aspart (3). HbA_{1c} concentrations were comparable, but in the detemir group the risk of hypoglycemia was 22% less and the risk of nocturnal hypoglycemia was 34% lower. There were two cases of severe hypoglycemia with detemir and one with isophane. Three patients who used detemir developed reactions at the injection site (pain, myalgia, redness, or lipodystrophy) compared with one who used isophane (itching). One potentially allergic reaction was possibly related to detemir.

Organs and Systems

Immunologic

An unspecified allergic reaction to insulin detemir has been reported (3).

References

1. Heinemann L, Sinha K, Weyer C, Loftager M, Hirschberger S, Heise T. Time-action profile of the soluble, fatty acid acylated, long-acting insulin analogue NN304. Diabet Med 1999;16(4):332–8.
2. Hermansen K, Madsbad S, Perrild H, Kristensen A, Axelsen M. Comparison of the soluble basal insulin analogue insulin detemir with NPH insulin: a randomized open crossover trial in type 1 diabetic subjects on basal-bolus therapy. Diabetes Care 2001;24(2):296–301.
3. Vague P, Selam JL, Skeie S, De Leeuw I, Elte JW, Haahr H, Kristensen A, Draeger E. Insulin detemir is associated with more predictable glycemic control and reduced risk of hypoglycemia than NPH insulin in patients with type 1 diabetes on a basal-bolus regimen with premeal insulin aspart. Diabetes Care 2003;26(3):590–6.

Insulin glargine

See also Insulin

General Information

Insulin glargine is a new long-acting human insulin analogue, in which phenylalanine is removed from site 30 of the C terminal of the B chain and two arginine molecules replace it, adding two positive charges; asparagine on site 21 of the A chain is replaced by the more stable glycine to avoid deamination. Older long-acting insulins, such as protamine zinc insulin and insulin zinc suspension (crystalline) (ultralente), had a maximal hypoglycemic effect after about 20 hours (in the middle of the night), and the glucose-lowering action then abated gradually. The newer analogues have a more constant profile of action (1–3).

The binding of insulin analogues to insulin and IGF-I receptors and their metabolic and mitogenic properties have been evaluated in vitro (4). In general the metabolic potencies correlated with insulin receptor binding and the mitogenic properties correlated with IGF-I receptor binding. The rapid-acting analogues resembled insulin, except that the binding of insulin lispro to the IGF-I receptor was slightly increased. Insulin glargine had a 6- to 8-fold greater affinity for IGF-I and mitogenic potency than human insulin (suggesting greater growth-stimulating potential). In insulin detemir the balance between the metabolic and mitogenic potency was not changed, but receptor affinity was reduced, which may explain its lower efficacy on a molar base in humans.

Insulin glargine has been reviewed (5,6). The general conclusion was that it is an effective long-acting insulin with no pronounced peaks of action. Patients using insulin glargine have a reduced risk of hypoglycemia. Insulin glargine, which is metabolically active for at least 24 hours, could have an overlapping effect after a second injection. However, there was no evidence of accumulation when insulin glargine, mean dose 24 U/day, was used in combination with insulin lispro for 11 days (7). In reaction to comments, and discussing whether fluctuations in insulin concentrations still occur during the administration of insulin glargine, the authors agreed that the dose should be constant for at least 2 days before a change is made. It is also not clear whether higher doses of insulin glargine could accumulate because of slower inactivation (8).

Comparative studies

The absorption of insulin glargine was delayed compared with protamine zinc insulin in a study using radioactive tracers (9).

In single-dose, double-blind, euglycemic clamp studies, insulin glargine had a smoother metabolic effect with a peakless profile of action starting at 2–4 hours and continuing over 24 hours than protamine zinc insulin, whose peak occurred at 4 hours and whose activity subsequently fell (10).

In a randomized, parallel-group study, there were fewer episodes of nocturnal and serious hypoglycemia when insulin glargine was compared with once- or twice-daily protamine zinc insulin (11,12). Other adverse reactions and reactions at the injection sites were identical.

Insulin glargine did not cause a peak in blood insulin concentration, compared with protamine zinc insulin and crystalline insulin zinc suspension (ultralente); the effect lasted 24 hours, almost comparable to continuous subcutaneous infusion of a short-acting insulin (13).

In general, one daily injection of insulin glargine gives more constant insulin concentrations and fewer nightly attacks of hypoglycemia than protamine zinc insulin. Treatment satisfaction was constantly better with insulin glargine in 517 patients (14). There was a consistent mean reduction in the perceived frequency of attacks of hypoglycemia. Other adverse effects were not mentioned.

- A 60-year-old man with type 2 diabetes received radiation therapy for a carcinoma of the esophagus and needed continuous enteric tube feeding (15). One daily injection of glargine controlled his diabetes well: his HbA_{1c} concentration was 6.1% and he had no episodes of hypoglycemia for almost 4 months. This made continuous infusion of a short-acting insulin unnecessary.

However, control can be inadequate with a once-daily injection.

- A 53-year-old man with type 1 diabetes needed tube feeding after a stroke and received glargine insulin once daily (16). He had marked hyperglycemia after 22 hours and when the dose was divided into two equal doses every 12 hours, the hyperglycemia was reduced.

Insulin glargine and protamine zinc insulin have been compared in 349 children and adolescents in a multicenter, open, randomized study (17). Besides the usual thrice-daily regimen of regular insulin they took either insulin glargine at bedtime or protamine zinc insulin at bedtime or twice daily. HbA_{1c} did not differ. The target for fasting blood glucose was 4.4–8.8 mmol/l, and 5% more patients who used insulin glargine reached the target (44% compared with 39% of the patients who used protamine zinc insulin). Symptomatic hypoglycemia was similar with the two treatments.

Six children were treated with insulin glargine and six with protamine zinc insulin as the long-acting insulin component (18). After 3 months, unbound insulin concentrations were lower during the night with insulin glargine. There were three cases of hypoglycemia with protamine zinc insulin and one with insulin glargine.

Combination with short-acting insulin

Insulin glargine plus a short-acting insulin has been compared with isophane insulin for 4 weeks in a double-blind study in 256 patients with type 1 diabetes (19). The patients were all taking once- or twice-daily isophane insulin and continued to do so or switched to insulin glargine with added zinc 30 or 80 micrograms/ml at bedtime. The patients who used insulin glargine had more attacks of hypoglycemia at the start of the study than those who used isophane insulin, but this tended to equalize during the 4 weeks. Fasting plasma glucose was lower in those who used insulin glargine. HbA_{1c} concentrations were not reported.

The combinations insulin lispro + insulin glargine and regular + isophane have been compared in a randomized, crossover study for 32 weeks in 25 patients (20). HbA_{1c} was not different, but the total insulin dose was lower with insulin lispro + insulin glargine and there were fewer episodes of nocturnal hypoglycemia.

Organs and Systems

Metabolism

In 619 patients with type 1 diabetes treated with protamine zinc insulin and insulin lispro, randomized to once-daily insulin glargine or to once-daily or twice-daily protamine zinc insulin for 16 weeks in an open study, there was no difference in the frequency of hypoglycemic episodes, severe hypoglycemia, or HbA_{1c} (21). Fasting plasma glucose concentrations were lower with insulin glargine.

In 518 patients with type 2 diabetes using protamine zinc insulin, with or without short-acting insulin, randomized to insulin glargine or protamine zinc insulin, there was less nocturnal hypoglycemia with insulin glargine (22). HbA_{1c} and mild symptomatic hypoglycemia was the same in both groups.

In 426 patients with type 2 diabetes poorly controlled with oral therapy, randomized to protamine zinc insulin or insulin glargine, glucose concentrations after dinner were lower with insulin glargine and there were significantly fewer attacks of hypoglycemia (23). HbA_{1c} was 8.2 and 8.1% with insulin glargine and protamine zinc insulin respectively.

Immunologic

Insulin glargine solved a problem in a man with type 1 diabetes after pork, beef, and human insulins had elicited allergic reactions (24). Antihistamines ameliorated the reactions but did not resolve them. Insulin glargine elicited no reactions, even when regular insulin was given. This case suggests that the A chain, which is modified in insulin glargine, is part of the allergic epitope. Tolerance to insulin glargine appeared to suppress allergy to regular insulin.

Drug Administration

Drug formulations

In contrast to most medium- and long-acting formulations, insulin glargine is a clear solution. In two cases, patients gave themselves rapid-acting insulin instead of glargine.

- A 25-year-old woman and a 52-year-old woman injected lispro instead of insulin glargine (25). The first realized her mistake and managed to prevent severe hypoglycemia by eating continuously, despite a fall in blood glucose to 3.7 mmol/l. The other had a blood glucose of 3.1 mmol/l and recovered after intravenous dextrose.

Four other mistakes have been reported (26,27). The authors advised the use of pens for injection of short-acting insulins, as all the mistakes were made by patients who used vials and syringes to administer both types of insulin.

References

1. Bolli GB, Di Marchi RD, Park GD, Pramming S, Koivisto VA. Insulin analogues and their potential in the management of diabetes mellitus. Diabetologia 1999; 42(10):1151–67.
2. Bolli GB, Owens DR. Insulin glargine. Lancet 2000;356(9228):443–5.
3. McKeage K, Goa KL. Insulin glargine: a review of its therapeutic use as a long-acting agent for the management of type 1 and 2 diabetes mellitus. Drugs 2001;61(11):1599–624.
4. Kurtzhals P, Schaffer L, Sorensen A, Kristensen C, Jonassen I, Schmid C, Trub T. Correlations of receptor binding and metabolic and mitogenic potencies of insulin analogues designed for clinical use. Diabetes 2000;49(6):999–1005.
5. Campbell RK, White JR, Levien T, Baker D. Insulin glargine. Clin Ther 2001;23(12):1938–57.
6. Home PD, Ashwell SG. An overview of insulin glargine. Diabetes Metab Res Rev 2002;18(Suppl 3):S57–63.
7. Heise T, Bott S, Rave K, Dressler A, Rosskamp R, Heinemann L. No evidence for accumulation of insulin glargine (LANTUS): a multiple injection study in patients with Type 1 diabetes. Diabet Med 2002;19(6):490–5.
8. Biermann E. No evidence for accumulation of insulin glargine (LANTUS). Diabet Med 2003;20(4):333–5.
9. Owens DR, Coates PA, Luzio SD, Tinbergen JP, Kurzhals R. Pharmacokinetics of ^{125}I-labeled insulin glargine (HOE 901) in healthy men: comparison with NPH insulin and the influence of different subcutaneous injection sites. Diabetes Care 2000;23(6):813–19.

10. Heinemann L, Linkeschova R, Rave K, Hompesch B, Sedlak M, Heise T. Time-action profile of the long-acting insulin analogue insulin glargine (HOE901) in comparison with those of NPH insulin and placebo. Diabetes Care 2000;23(5):644–9.
11. Pieber TR, Eugene-Jolchine I, Derobert E. Efficacy and safety of HOE 901 versus NPH insulin in patients with type 1 diabetes. The European Study Group of HOE 901 in type 1 diabetes. Diabetes Care 2000;23(2):157–62.
12. Ratner RE, Hirsch IB, Neifing JL, Garg SK, Mecca TE, Wilson CA. Less hypoglycemia with insulin glargine in intensive insulin therapy for type 1 diabetes. U.S. Study Group of Insulin Glargine in Type 1 Diabetes. Diabetes Care 2000;23(5):639–43.
13. Lepore M, Pampanelli S, Fanelli C, Porcellati F, Bartocci L, Di Vincenzo A, Cordoni C, Costa E, Brunetti P, Bolli GB. Pharmacokinetics and pharmacodynamics of subcutaneous injection of long-acting human insulin analogue glargine, NPH insulin, and ultralente human insulin and continuous subcutaneous infusion of insulin lispro. Diabetes 2000;49(12):2142–8.
14. Ooi C, Mullen P, Williams G. Insulin lispro: the ideal pump insulin for patients with severe hypoglycemic unawareness? Diabetes Care 1999;22(9):1598–9.
15. Putz D, Kabadi UM. Insulin glargine in continuous enteric tube feeding. Diabetes Care 2002;25(10):1889–90.
16. Clement S, Bowen-Wright H. Twenty-four hour action of insulin glargine (Lantus) may be too short for once-daily dosing: a case report. Diabetes Care 2002;25(8):1479–80.
17. Schober E, Schoenle E, Van Dyk J, Wernicke-Panten K; Pediatric Study Group of Insulin Glargine. Comparative trial between insulin glargine and NPH insulin in children and adolescents with type 1 diabetes. Diabetes Care 2001;24(11):2005–6.
18. Mohn A, Strang S, Wernicke-Panten K, Lang AM, Edge JA, Dunger DB. Nocturnal glucose control and free insulin levels in children with type 1 diabetes by use of the long-acting insulin HOE 901 as part of a three-injection regimen. Diabetes Care 2000;23(4):557–9.
19. Rosenstock J, Park G, Zimmerman J; U.S. Insulin Glargine (HOE 901) Type 1 Diabetes Investigator Group. Basal insulin glargine (HOE 901) versus NPH insulin in patients with type 1 diabetes on multiple daily insulin regimens. U.S. Insulin Glargine (HOE 901) Type 1 Diabetes Investigator Group. Diabetes Care 2000;23(8):1137–42.
20. Murphy NP, Keane SM, Ong KK, Ford-Adams M, Edge JA, Acerini CL, Dunger DB. Randomized cross-over trial of insulin glargine plus lispro or NPH insulin plus regular human insulin in adolescents with type 1 diabetes on intensive insulin regimens. Diabetes Care 2003;26(3):799–804.
21. Raskin P, Klaff L, Bergenstal R, Halle JP, Donley D, Mecca T. A 16-week comparison of the novel insulin analogue insulin glargine (HOE 901) and NPH human insulin used with insulin lispro in patients with type 1 diabetes. Diabetes Care 2000;23(11):1666–71.
22. Rosenstock J, Schwartz SL, Clark CM Jr, Park GD, Donley DW, Edwards MB. Basal insulin therapy in type 2 diabetes: 28-week comparison of insulin glargine (HOE 901) and NPH insulin. Diabetes Care 2001;24(4):631–6.
23. Yki-Jarvinen H, Dressler A, Ziemen M; HOE 901/300s Study Group. Less nocturnal hypoglycemia and better post-dinner glucose control with bedtime insulin glargine compared with bedtime NPH insulin during insulin combination therapy in type 2 diabetes. HOE 901/3002 Study Group. Diabetes Care 2000;23(8):1130–6.
24. Moriyama H, Nagata M, Fujihira K, Yamada K, Chowdhury SA, Chakrabarty S, Jin Z, Yasuda H, Ueda H, Yokono K. Treatment with human analogue (GlyA21, ArgB31, ArgB32) insulin glargine (HOE901) resolves a generalized allergy to human insulin in type 1 diabetes. Diabetes Care 2001;24(2):411–12.
25. Adlersberg MA, Fernando S, Spollett GR, Inzucchi SE. Glargine and lispro: two cases of mistaken identity. Diabetes Care 2002;25(2):404–5.
26. Schutta MH. Reducing mistakes in patient administration of glargine and lispro. Diabetes Care 2002;25(6):1098–9.
27. Phillips W, Lando H. Insulin confusion: an observation. Diabetes Care 2002;25(6):1103–4.

Insulin lispro

See also Insulin

General Information

Insulin lispro induces more rapid and constant release of insulin from the injection site, since it consists of monomeric insulin. The change of one or more amino acids in the insulin molecule prevents insulin from forming dimers or hexamers. More rapid absorption, rapid availability, and rapid inactivation make the action better than that of endogenously secreted insulin. When the interval between meals is long, the premeal blood glucose concentration increases rapidly.

After the administration of insulin lispro it is not necessary to delay a meal until sufficient insulin is absorbed. Insulin lispro can be given immediately before or during a meal and can be used when rapid action is important, as in outpatient treatment of ketonuria (1) or in continuous subcutaneous insulin infusion (2). Insulin lispro can be successful in patients with subcutaneous insulin resistance (3).

Observational studies

During Ramadan, insulin lispro reduced the number of attacks of hypoglycemia and reduced postprandial blood glucose (4). It also reduced post-snack raised blood glucose concentrations when sugar-rich snacks were used (5).

Combination with long-acting insulin

The combinations insulin lispro + insulin glargine and regular + NPH have been compared in a randomized, crossover study for 32 weeks in 25 patients (6). HbA_{1c} was not different, but the total insulin dose was lower with insulin lispro + insulin glargine and there were fewer episodes of nocturnal hypoglycemia.

The new short-acting insulins can be bound to protamine, allowing the preparation of mixed formulations. In a randomized, open, crossover study for 24 weeks, a 50% mixture of insulin lispro and protamine lispro injected immediately before each meal plus NPH in the evening gave a comparable profile to regular insulin injected 30 minutes before each meal plus NPH in the evening (7). There were no differences in HbA_{1c} or episodes of hypoglycemia. When Mix25TM (25% insulin lispro plus 75% protamine lispro) was compared with 30/70 human insulin in an open, randomized, crossover study during Ramadan, the daily average blood glucose concentration was better with the insulin lispro combination. The number of hypoglycemic episodes was the same with the two formulations (8).

In an open, randomized, single-dose, three-way, crossover trial, biphasic insulin aspart 30 (30% aspart plus 70% protaminated aspart, BIAsp 30), biphasic insulin lispro 25 (25% lispro plus 75% protaminated lispro, Mix 25), and biphasic human insulin 30 (30% regular plus 70% NPH insulin, BHI 30) were compared in 45 patients (9). Biphasic insulin aspart improved postprandial control better. There were 23 episodes of hypoglycemia with BIAsp 30, 19 with Mix 25, and 11 with BHI 30; two episodes with BIAsp 30, five with Mix 25, and two with BHI 30 required third-party intervention.

Comparative studies

In an open, randomized, crossover study, 113 patients with at least 6 months of continuous subcutaneous insulin infusion before the study were treated with regular insulin or insulin lispro (2). Postprandial blood glucose was lower and HbA_{1c} fell more with insulin lispro. There were no differences in catheter obstruction, hypoglycemic episodes, or other adverse effects. Satisfaction with treatment was better with insulin lispro.

There were no differences between human protamine zinc insulin and human ultralente insulin when either was added once or twice daily to insulin lispro (10).

When either insulin lispro or regular insulin was given during the evening meal in a randomized, double-blind study in insulin-using adolescents, insulin lispro reduced the number of hypoglycemic episodes at night but redistribution of evening carbohydrate might be necessary to reduce postprandial hypoglycemia (11).

Premeal hyperglycemia is common. The short action of insulin lispro can then be extended by the addition of protamine zinc insulin. In a 3-month study in addition to a once-daily injection of protamine zinc insulin, at each meal insulin lispro or insulin lispro + protamine zinc insulin was injected; the postprandial blood glucose concentration was lower, but the post-absorptive glucose concentration was higher in the insulin lispro-only group; there was no difference in HbA_{1c}. The addition of protamine zinc insulin (30% at breakfast, 40% at lunch, and 10% at dinner) improved post-absorptive glucose and HbA_{1c} (12).

Insulin Mix 25 (25% insulin lispro and 75% neutral protamine zinc insulin) reduced the glucose response to a standardized breakfast meal better than premixed 30% regular + 70% protamine zinc insulin when 22 patients with type 2 diabetes were studied three times in a double-blind fashion (13). Protamine zinc insulin mixed with insulin lispro has the same action profile of insulin lispro, with the continuing action of the long-acting component (14). The same mixture given three or four times daily provides acceptable control (15), but gives no possibility of adjusting the short-acting insulin regularly. Protamine zinc insulin must be mixed with insulin lispro in the syringe immediately before the meal (16). The mixture is not stable for longer as there is partial exchange of the rapid-acting analogue and the protamine-bound human insulin. Instant mixing is no solution when pens are used.

The use of insulin lispro instead of regular insulin reduced the frequency of nocturnal attacks of hypoglycemia but did not change HbA_{1c} (17). This was confirmed by the UK Prospective Diabetes Study (18), which also found a fall in postprandial glucose with an increase in fasting and preprandial glucose.

In an open, crossover, randomized study in 33 patients with type 1 diabetes who used regular or insulin lispro, the latter was associated with a lower incidence of severe hypoglycemia, mostly due to reduced nocturnal hypoglycemia; HbA_{1c} was not different (19).

A crossover comparison of regular insulin + protamine zinc insulin at bedtime with insulin lispro + multiple protamine zinc insulin showed no effect on overall hypoglycemia but there was less frequent severe hypoglycemia with the second treatment (20). The reduction in HbA_{1c} was small and not significant. Insulin doses were the same. Patients preferred the second treatment.

In an open, randomized, multicenter study, 33 women with type 1 diabetes for at least 2 years were randomized to preprandial lispro or regular insulin in week 15 of their pregnancy; both groups used NPH insulin as well (21). HbA_{1c} concentrations fell at the same rate. One patient in the regular group had one episode of severe hypoglycemia and one had three episodes. Biochemical hypoglycemia (under 3.0 mmol/l) was significantly more frequent in the lispro group (5.5 versus 3.9%). Retinopathy progressed during pregnancy in three of the 16 who used lispro and six of the 17 who used regular insulin; retinal aneurysms were seen at the beginning of the study in 10/16 and 5/17 patients respectively. There were no differences in the neonates.

When insulin lispro and insulin aspart were compared in a single-blind, randomized crossover study in 14 patients with type 1 diabetes, insulin lispro had a faster onset of action but a shorter duration (22). However, in another study, the pharmacokinetic and pharmacodynamic profiles of insulin aspart compared with human insulin in 24 healthy Japanese were the same as those in non-Japanese subjects (23).

Insulin aspart, insulin lispro, and buffered regular insulin in continuous subcutaneous insulin infusion have been compared in an open, randomized, parallel-group study in 146 patients (24). HbA_{1c}, hypoglycemic episodes, and blockages of pumps or infusion sets did not differ.

Insulin lispro and insulin aspart were equally effective in 24 patients with type 1 diabetes (25).

Insulin lispro and repaglinide were given to seven patients with diabetes related to cystic fibrosis (26). They had normal fasting blood glucose and insulin concentrations, but postprandial glucose concentrations were substantially raised. Insulin lispro had a larger and more sustained effect in lowering postprandial glucose than repaglinide. However, the doses of insulin lispro (0.1 U/kg) and repaglinide (1 mg) may not have been comparable.

Organs and Systems

Metabolism

Hypoglycemic events in 24 controlled trials of rapid-acting insulin analogues have been analysed (27). In 22 trials, insulin lispro was used, 19 studies were open and unblinded, and five were double-blind. In five of 22 studies there was a significant reduction in mild hypoglycemia, but there were no changes in the frequency of severe hypoglycemia in 10 of 12 studies that reported these events; there was a fall in nocturnal hypoglycemia in 6 studies, but in 18 studies there was no fall. The author stated that rapid-acting insulins are only appropriate in intensive therapy, which involves well-educated and well-motivated patients.

Lipoatrophy is rare with human recombinant insulin. Two cases of lipoatrophy induced by insulin lispro during continuous subcutaneous insulin infusion have been reported (28).

- An 8-year-old girl was switched to continuous subcutaneous insulin infusion using insulin lispro for better regulation after 4 years of diabetes. After 12 months she developed lipoatrophy of the abdominal wall, which progressed during the next months. When she changed to neutral buffered regular human insulin, no further lipoatrophy developed, but the existing atrophy did not improve either.
- A 51-year-old woman started to use continuous subcutaneous insulin and after 2 years the insulin was changed to insulin lispro. She developed lipoatrophy in the abdomen and buttocks 1 year later and there was an increase in the time before the bolus started to peak. Buffered regular human insulin stopped progression of the lipoatrophy.

Skin

Insulin lispro can cause lipoatrophy, but it was less extensive in a case in which it had occurred with regular insulin, perhaps because of the greater solubility of insulin lispro.

- Several combinations of regular and NPH insulin reduced the risk of hypoglycemia and optimized blood glucose in a 29-year-old woman who had had type 1 diabetes for 6 years (29). Continuous subcutaneous insulin infusion with regular insulin reduced the risk of hypoglycemia, but after 7 months she developed lipoatrophy. Changing the site of the cannula did not help. She was given insulin lispro instead and after 11 months a new, less extensive area of lipoatrophy emerged, which did not disappear.

Immunologic

The long-term antigenicity of insulin lispro and cross-reactivity with human insulin antibodies over 4 years has been investigated in 1221 patients with both type 1 and type 2 diabetes, either insulin-naïve or with prior insulin treatment, in a multicenter combination of controlled and non-controlled open studies (30). Like recombinant human insulin, insulin lispro elicited a low immunogenic response. The reversal of amino acids in B28 and B29 is in a relatively non-immunogenic area. Moreover, antigenicity often correlates with residence of insulin in subcutaneous tissues, and insulin lispro has a short residence time. The patients did not develop increased dosage requirements. Intermittent treatment did not increase specific or cross-reactive responses. The antibody responses were slightly higher in type 1 than in type 2 diabetes. In lipodystrophy with lipoatrophic diabetes, high insulin resistance is often found, for which leptin deficiency is one contributory factor.

Second-Generation Effects

Pregnancy

Rapid improvement of regulation by insulin lispro during pregnancy causes proliferative diabetic retinopathy more often. In 14 patients treated with insulin lispro to improve control before or at the beginning of pregnancy, six of the 10 patients with normal optic fundi remained negative. However, three patients developed bilateral progressive retinopathy with marked vision impairment, in two cases with vitreous hemorrhage; one patient with a negative examination 6 months before pregnancy, but with minimal lesions 18 months earlier, developed progressive retinopathy with vitreous hemorrhages in spite of multiple coagulations (31). The authors advised care when starting insulin lispro in patients with a history of retinal lesions and to look for those at risk by performing fluorescein angiography, which distinguishes incipient changes better.

In a comparison of premeal regular insulin and premeal insulin lispro in gestational diabetes there were fewer attacks of hypoglycemia, but fasting glucose, postprandial glucose, and HbA_{1c} were similar in the two groups (32). There were no fetal or neonatal abnormalities.

Susceptibility Factors

Age

The newer insulins are not registered for use in children in many countries. A report of the use of postprandial insulin lispro versus preprandial regular insulin in an open, crossover, randomized study in 24 prepubertal children showed no large differences (33). Fasting blood glucose was higher with insulin lispro. The number of hypoglycemic episodes was almost the same with both insulins. There was one case of severe hypoglycemia.

Renal disease

The pharmacodynamic and pharmacokinetic properties of regular soluble insulin and insulin lispro have been investigated in 12 patients with and without nephropathy in a double-blind, crossover study with euglycemic glucose clamping (34). Insulin clearance was reduced by 30–40% in patients with nephropathy, but in both groups the time to reach the maximal effect was shorter with insulin lispro. The overall metabolic effect of regular soluble insulin, but not of insulin lispro, was lower in nephropathy, in which a 50% higher dose of regular insulin may be necessary.

Drug Administration

Drug administration route

Insulin lispro by repeated injection has been compared with insulin lispro by continuous subcutaneous infusion in 41 patients who were C-peptide negative (35). HbA_{1c}, mean blood glucose concentrations, and mean insulin doses were significantly lower during continuous subcutaneous infusion; the frequency of attacks of hypoglycemia was the same.

References

1. Travaglini MT, Garg SK, Chase HP. Use of insulin lispro in the outpatient management of ketonuria. Arch Pediatr Adolesc Med 1998;152(7):672–5.
2. Renner R, Pfutzner A, Trautmann M, Harzer O, Sauter K, Landgraf R. Use of insulin lispro in continuous subcutaneous insulin infusion treatment. Results of a multicenter trial. German Humalog-CSII Study Group. Diabetes Care 1999;22(5):784–8.
3. Darmon P, Curtillet C, Boullu S, Laugier A, Dutour A, Oliver C. Insulin analogue lispro decreases insulin resistance and improves glycemic control in an obese patient with insulin-requiring type 2 diabetes. Diabetes Care 1998;21(9):1575.
4. Akram J, De Verga V. Insulin lispro (Lys(B28), Pro(B29) in the treatment of diabetes during the fasting month of Ramadan. Ramadan Study Group. Diabet Med 1999;16(10):861–6.
5. Kong N, Kitchen MM, Ryder RE. The use of lispro for high sugar content snacks between meals in intensive insulin regimens. Diabet Med 2000;17(4):331–2.
6. Murphy NP, Keane SM, Ong KK, Ford-Adams M, Edge JA, Acerini CL, Dunger DB. Randomized cross-over trial of insulin glargine plus lispro or NPH insulin plus regular human insulin in adolescents with type 1 diabetes on intensive insulin regimens. Diabetes Care 2003;26(3):799–804.
7. Herz M, Arora V, Sun B, Ferguson SC, Bolli GB, Frier BM. Basal-bolus insulin therapy in Type 1 diabetes: comparative study of pre-meal administration of a fixed mixture of insulin lispro (50%) and neutral protamine lispro (50%) with human soluble insulin. Diabet Med 2002;19(11):917–23.
8. Mattoo V, Milicevic Z, Malone JK, Schwarzenhofer M, Ekangaki A, Levitt LK, Liong LH, Rais N, Tounsi H; Ramadan Study Group. A comparison of insulin lispro Mix25 and human insulin 30/70 in the treatment of type 2 diabetes during Ramadan. Diabetes Res Clin Pract 2003;59(2):137–43.
9. Hermansen K, Colombo M, Storgaard H, OStergaard A, Kolendorf K, Madsbad S. Improved postprandial glycemic control with biphasic insulin aspart relative to biphasic insulin lispro and biphasic human insulin in patients with type 2 diabetes. Diabetes Care 2002;25(5):883–8.
10. Zinman B, Ross S, Campos RV, Strack T. Effectiveness of human ultralente versus NPH insulin in providing basal insulin replacement for an insulin lispro multiple daily injection regimen. A double-blind randomized prospective trial. The Canadian Lispro Study Group. Diabetes Care 1999;22(4):603–8.
11. Mohn A, Matyka KA, Harris DA, Ross KM, Edge JA, Dunger DB. Lispro or regular insulin for multiple injection therapy in adolescence. Differences in free insulin and glucose levels overnight. Diabetes Care 1999;22(1):27–32.
12. Ciofetta M, Lalli C, Del Sindaco P, Torlone E, Pampanelli S, Mauro L, Chiara DL, Brunetti P, Bolli GB. Contribution of postprandial versus interprandial blood glucose to HbA1c in type 1 diabetes on physiologic intensive therapy with lispro insulin at mealtime. Diabetes Care 1999;22(5):795–800.
13. Koivisto VA, Tuominen JA, Ebeling P. Lispro Mix25 insulin as premeal therapy in type 2 diabetic patients. Diabetes Care 1999;22(3):459–62.
14. Rave K, Heinemann L, Puhl L, Gudat U, Woodworth JR, Weyer C, Heise T. Premixed formulations of insulin lispro. Activity profiles in type 1 diabetic patients. Diabetes Care 1999;22(5):865–6.
15. Lalli C, Ciofetta M, Del Sindaco P, Torlone E, Pampanelli S, Compagnucci P, Cartechini MG, Bartocci L, Brunetti P, Bolli GB. Long-term intensive treatment of type 1 diabetes with the short-acting insulin analogue lispro in variable combination with NPH insulin at mealtime. Diabetes Care 1999;22(3):468–77.
16. Joseph SE, Korzon-Burakowska A, Woodworth JR, Evans M, Hopkins D, Janes JM, Amiel SA. The action profile of lispro is not blunted by mixing in the syringe with NPH insulin. Diabetes Care 1998;21(12):2098–102.
17. Heller SR, Amiel SA, Mansell P. Effect of the fast-acting insulin analogue lispro on the risk of nocturnal hypoglycemia during intensified insulin therapy. U.K. Lispro Study Group. Diabetes Care 1999;22(10):1607–11.
18. Gale EA. A randomized, controlled trial comparing insulin lispro with human soluble insulin in patients with Type 1 diabetes on intensified insulin therapy. The UK Trial Group. Diabet Med 2000;17(3):209–14.
19. Ferguson SC, Strachan MW, Janes JM, Frier BM. Severe hypoglycaemia in patients with type 1 diabetes and impaired awareness of hypoglycaemia: a comparative study of insulin lispro and regular human insulin. Diabetes Metab Res Rev 2001;17(4):285–91.
20. Colombel A, Murat A, Krempf M, Kuchly-Anton B, Charbonnel B. Improvement of blood glucose control in Type 1 diabetic patients treated with lispro and multiple NPH injections. Diabet Med 1999;16(4):319–24.
21. Persson B, Swahn ML, Hjertberg R, Hanson U, Nord E, Nordlander E, Hansson LO. Insulin lispro therapy in pregnancies complicated by type 1 diabetes mellitus. Diabetes Res Clin Pract 2002;58(2):115–21.
22. Hedman CA, Lindstrom T, Arnqvist HJ. Direct comparison of insulin lispro and aspart shows small differences in plasma insulin profiles after subcutaneous injection in type 1 diabetes. Diabetes Care 2001;24(6):1120–1.
23. Kaku K, Matsuda M, Urae A, Irie S. Pharmacokinetics and pharmacodynamics of insulin aspart, a rapid-acting analogue of human insulin, in healthy Japanese volunteers. Diabetes Res Clin Pract 2000;49(2–3):119–26.
24. Bode B, Weinstein R, Bell D, McGill J, Nadeau D, Raskin P, Davidson J, Henry R, Huang WC, Reinhardt RR. Comparison of insulin aspart with buffered regular insulin and insulin lispro in continuous subcutaneous insulin infusion: a randomized study in type 1 diabetes. Diabetes Care 2002;25(3):439–44.
25. Plank J, Wutte A, Brunner G, Siebenhofer A, Semlitsch B, Sommer R, Hirschberger S, Pieber TR. A direct comparison of insulin aspart and insulin lispro in patients with type 1 diabetes. Diabetes Care 2002;25(11):2053–7.
26. Moran A, Phillips J, Milla C. Insulin and glucose excursion following premeal insulin lispro or repaglinide in cystic fibrosis-related diabetes. Diabetes Care 2001; 24(10):1706–10.
27. Heinemann L. Hypoglycemia and insulin analogues: is there a reduction in the incidence? J Diabetes Complications 1999;13(2):105–14.

28. Griffin ME, Feder A, Tamborlane WV. Lipoatrophy associated with lispro insulin in insulin pump therapy: an old complication, a new cause? Diabetes Care 2001;24(1):174.
29. Ampudia-Blasco FJ, Hasbum B, Carmena R. A new case of lipoatrophy with lispro insulin in insulin pump therapy: is there any insulin preparation free of complications? Diabetes Care 2003;26(3):953–4.
30. Fineberg SE, Huang J, Brunelle R, Gulliya KS, Anderson JH Jr. Effect of long-term exposure to insulin lispro on the induction of antibody response in patients with type 1 or type 2 diabetes. Diabetes Care 2003;26(1):89–96.
31. Kitzmiller JL, Main E, Ward B, Theiss T, Peterson DL. Insulin lispro and the development of proliferative diabetic retinopathy during pregnancy. Diabetes Care 1999;22(5):874–6.
32. Jovanovic L, Ilic S, Pettitt DJ, Hugo K, Gutierrez M, Bowsher RR, Bastyr EJ 3rd. Metabolic and immunologic effects of insulin lispro in gestational diabetes. Diabetes Care 1999;22(9):1422–7.
33. Tupola S, Komulainen J, Jaaskelainen J, Sipila I. Postprandial insulin lispro vs. human regular insulin in prepubertal children with Type 1 diabetes mellitus. Diabet Med 2001;18(8):654–8.
34. Rave K, Heise T, Pfutzner A, Heinemann L, Sawicki PT. Impact of diabetic nephropathy on pharmacodynamic and Pharmacokinetic properties of insulin in type 1 diabetic patients. Diabetes Care 2001;24(5):886–90.
35. Hanaire-Broutin H, Melki V, Bessieres-Lacombe S, Tauber JP. Comparison of continuous subcutaneous insulin infusion and multiple daily injection regimens using insulin lispro in type 1 diabetic patients on intensified treatment: a randomized study. The Study Group for the Development of Pump Therapy in Diabetes. Diabetes Care 2000;23(9):1232–5.

Insulin-like growth factor (IGF-I)

General Information

Insulin growth factor (IGF) and the IGF-I receptor are structurally comparable to insulin and the insulin receptor. Recombinant human IGF-I has 54% identity to proinsulin. Insulin and IGF-I can bind to both receptors, but insulin can only transfer 1% of the IGF message on the IGF receptor and IGF-I only 1% of the insulin message on the insulin receptor.

Recombinant human IGF-I is used as an adjunct to insulin therapy in patients with large daily variations in insulin effect. It is sometimes given in insulin resistance syndromes caused by changes in the insulin receptor or in type B insulin resistance syndrome caused by antibodies to the insulin receptor.

In 14 adolescents, the addition of IGF-I to diabetic treatment for 12 weeks did not change leptin concentrations (1).

IGF-I was given as co-therapy with insulin in 223 patients for 12 weeks twice-daily (2). The doses of IGF-I were 40/40, 80/40, or 80/60 micrograms/kg. Patients who received co-therapy were able to reduce their daily doses of insulin. The number of episodes of hypoglycemia was the same, but glucose regulation was tighter during IGF-I co-therapy. The fall in HbA_{1c} concentration was greater with co-therapy (–1.2%) than with intensive therapy only (–0.7%). The dosage regimen of 40/40 micrograms/kg was well tolerated. Higher doses had no greater effect but were associated with edema, jaw pain, headache, palpitation, tachycardia, syncope, or early worsening of retinopathy.

Organs and Systems

Sensory systems

Of 199 patients, 16 developed significant worsening of retinopathy, including neovascularization, over 12 weeks; 12 of the 16 had optic disc swelling, which necessitated laser therapy in three of them (3). This was mostly seen in patients using a high dose of IGF-I, but a long-term effect of low-dose IGF-I could not be excluded either.

Immunologic

IGF-I can cause allergic reactions (4).

- A 75-year-old man with glucose intolerance, severe hyperinsulinemia, and extreme insulin resistance with anti-insulin receptor antibodies had immunosuppressive therapy and plasmapheresis to remove the antibodies, without lasting success. Treatment with hrIGF-I, 0.4 mg/kg/day, reduced HbA_{1c} from 13.8% to 8.0%. After 5 months he developed a generalized skin eruption 20 minutes after the injection. When IGF-I was withdrawn the HbA_{1c} rose again. After careful desensitization with hrIGF-I, 0.1 mg three times a week, IGF-I was continued, with good effect on HbA_{1c}.

Long-Term Effects

Tumorigenicity

A non-Hodgkin's lymphoma developed in the right femur of a 58-year-old man who had used IGF-I 40 micrograms bd (5) in a study of the effect of adding IGF to insulin therapy (SEDA-23, 457).

References

1. Thrailkill KM, Fowlkes JL, Hyde JF, Litton JC. The effects of co-therapy with recombinant human insulin-like growth factor I and insulin on serum leptin levels in adolescents with type 1 diabetes mellitus. Pediatr Diabetes 2001;2(1):25–9.
2. Thrailkill KM, Quattrin T, Baker L, Kuntze JE, Compton PG, Martha PM Jr. Cotherapy with recombinant human insulin-like growth factor I and insulin improves glycemic control in type 1 diabetes. RhIGF-I in IDDM Study Group. Diabetes Care 1999;22(4):585–92.
3. Lanzetta P, Malara C. Cotherapy with recombinant human IGF-I and insulin improves glycemic control in type 1 diabetes. Diabetes Care 2000;23(3):436–7.
4. Yamamoto T, Sato T, Mori T, Yamakita T, Hasegawa T, Miyamoto M, Hosoi M, Ishii T, Yoshioka K, Tanaka S, Fujii S. Clinical efficacy of insulin-like growth factor-1 in a patient with autoantibodies to insulin receptors: a case report. Diabetes Res Clin Pract 2000;49(1):65–9.
5. Mayer-Davis EJ. Cancer in a patient receiving IGF-I therapy. Diabetes Care 2000;23:433–4.

Interferon alfa

See also Interferons

General Information

Interferon alfa is used as purified natural leukocyte or lymphoblastoid human interferon, or as a recombinant DNA preparation. Work to assign the most frequently observed amino acids at each position has led to a so-called consensus interferon alfa (1). Relatively low doses (3–10 MU three times a week) are now being used in most indications, except in AIDS-related Kaposi's sarcoma (up to 30 MU/day). Although the half-life is only 4–5 hours, its biological effects persist for 2–3 days.

Observational studies

Considerable efforts have been made to improve the efficacy of interferon alfa in patients with chronic hepatitis C. Currently used regimens, including long-term interferon alfa alone or in combination with ribavirin, produce a sustained response rate of 40–50%. Other possibly effective strategies include a longer duration of treatment, higher fixed doses, and high-dose induction (2). A longer duration of treatment has been evaluated in patients with chronic hepatitis B. In 118 patients, treatment for 32 rather than 16 weeks enhanced the virological response to hepatitis B without increasing the severity of adverse effects, except for hair loss, which was more frequent during prolonged therapy (3).

A wide range of persistent symptoms has been reported during interferon alfa treatment for chronic hepatitis C. An analysis of 222 patients from the USA and France, enrolled in a multicenter trial, suggested that pretreatment symptoms were an important predictor of moderate or severe (defined as debilitating) adverse effects during treatment with interferon alfa (4). Compared with baseline, the incidences of moderate and severe fatigue, myalgia, arthralgia, headache, dry eyes, and dry mouth increased significantly after 6 months. In each case, the development of these debilitating adverse effects was associated with the presence of that symptom at baseline. They were more often reported in patients who received interferon alfa daily than three times weekly, and in US than French patients, suggesting possible differences in cultural attitudes toward illness. There was also increased use of antidepressants during the 6-month survey.

Low daily doses of interferon alfa have been used with small doses of cytarabine in the treatment of early chronic myelogenous leukemia (5). With doses sufficient to obtain a good cytogenetic response (for example 3.7 MU/m^2/day plus cytarabine 7.5 mg/day) toxicity was considered acceptable. There was significant fatigue in 43% of cases, significant neurological changes in 27%, weight loss in 19%, and oral ulcers in 4%.

Comparative studies

Interferon alfa, in combination with ribavirin, is currently first-line therapy for patients with chronic hepatitis C and compensated liver disease, and its use has been extensively reviewed (6). A meta-analysis of trials in patients who were previously non-responsive to interferon alfa alone showed that treatment withdrawal for an adverse event was more frequent in patients who received combination therapy (8.8%) compared with interferon alfa monotherapy (4%) (7). However, treatment withdrawal is more frequent in practice. In a retrospective analysis of 441 consecutive patients treated with interferon alfa and ribavirin, 25% of patients discontinued treatment because of adverse effects (8). The study identified female sex, a dose of interferon alfa above 15 MU/week, and naive patients as independent susceptibility factors for premature withdrawal.

Comparisons of different forms of interferon alfa

In a randomized comparison of recombinant interferon alfa-2b and interferon alfa n-3 (9 MU/week for 1 year) in 168 naive patients with chronic hepatitis C, there was no significant difference in clinical outcomes and the incidence or type of adverse effects between the groups (9). There was a non-significant trend toward more severe leukopenia and a higher incidence of severe thyroid disorders in patients who received recombinant interferon alfa-2b.

Pegylated interferon alfa-2a is a modified form of interferon alfa; it produces higher serum concentrations and has greater efficacy. In 1530 patients with chronic hepatitis C, pegylated interferon alfa-2b had a similar profile of adverse effects to unmodified interferon alfa-2b, but with more frequent dose-limiting neutropenia (10). Two other studies have shown that peginterferon alfa-2a once weekly is more effective than unmodified interferon alfa-2a three times weekly in patients with chronic hepatitis C (11,12). The frequency and severity of adverse effects with the two treatments were very similar and were consistent with the known adverse effects of interferon alfa. In one study, a neutrophil count below 0.5×10^9/l was more frequent with peginterferon alfa than with unmodified interferon alfa (12/265 versus 4/261), but none of these patients required treatment withdrawal or had serious infections in relation to neutropenia (12). In the other study, the proportion of patients who required dosage modification because of thrombocytopenia was also higher with peginterferon alfa (18 versus 6%), but no patients had clinically significant bleeding disorders (11). Taken together, these studies suggest that pegylated interferon alfa may produce more frequent or more severe hemotoxic effects than unmodified interferon alfa.

In 1530 patients with chronic hepatitis C, pegylated interferon alfa-2b had a similar profile of adverse effects to unmodified interferon alfa-2b, but with more frequent dose-limiting neutropenia (10). No particular adverse effect has emerged since the use of this new formulation.

General adverse effects

The adverse effects of interferon alfa have mostly been reported after systemic administration, as intranasal use was not associated with more frequent adverse effects than placebo (13). Almost all patients treated with interferon alfa have experienced adverse effects, most of which are mild to moderate in intensity and easily manageable without withdrawal of treatment (14). The incidence and profile of adverse effects reported with the available types of interferon alfa are very similar (SEDA-21, 369) (SEDA-22, 399), but they differ with the dose, schedule of administration, and the disease. At least 4–5% of patients with chronic hepatitis C had to discontinue treatment because of adverse effects, and dosage reduction was required in 9–22% of those receiving 9–15 MU/week (15). In a large retrospective evaluation of 11 241 patients with chronic viral hepatitis, the incidence of fatal or life-threatening adverse effects related to interferon alfa was one in 1000; events included irreversible liver failure, severe bone marrow depression, and attempted suicide (16). Overall, severe adverse effects were observed in 1% of patients, and comprised mostly thyroid disorders, neuropsychiatric manifestations, and cutaneous adverse effects. In other studies in patients with chronic hepatitis, the incidence of major adverse effects was 25% in 659 patients (17); in Japan, dosage reduction or withdrawal was necessary in 31% of 987 patients receiving relatively high dosages of interferon alfa (18–70 MU weekly) (18). The safety of interferon alfa in children appears to be similar to that in adults (19). The pathogenesis of most adverse effects observed with interferon alfa is poorly understood, but two main mechanisms are commonly postulated, namely a direct toxic effect or an indirect immune-mediated effect.

During the first days of treatment, virtually all patients have a flu-like syndrome with fever, chills, tachycardia, malaise, headache, arthralgias and myalgias, but tachyphylaxis usually develops after 1–2 weeks of treatment (20). Late febrile reactions are rarely noted (21). Although the severity increases with the dose, the flu-like syndrome is rarely treatment-limiting and it can be partly prevented by the prophylactic administration of paracetamol (acetaminophen). The acute release of fever-promoting factors, for example the eicosanoids, IL-1, and TNF alfa, secondary to interferon alfa is the suggested mechanism.

Although the adverse effects profiles of the currently available formulations of interferon alfa are very similar, patients who have adverse effects with one formulation can be successfully re-treated with another type of interferon alfa. This has been shown in 22 patients in whom lymphoblastoid interferon alfa was withdrawn because of severe adverse effects (leukopenia, thrombocytopenia, thyroid disorders, and psychiatric disturbances) and were successfully re-treated with similar dosages of leukocyte interferon alfa (22). Only one of these patients had severe leukopenia again.

Organs and Systems

Cardiovascular

Hypotension or hypertension, benign sinus or supraventricular tachycardia, and rarely distal cyanosis, have been reported within the first days of treatment in 5–15% of patients receiving high-dose interferon alfa (20). These adverse effects are usually benign, except in high-risk patients with a previous history of dysrhythmias, coronary disease, or cardiac dysfunction.

Cardiac complications

Severe or life-threatening cardiotoxicity is infrequent and mostly reported in the form of a subacute complication in patients with cancer, and in those with pre-existing heart disease or receiving high-dose interferon alfa. Atrioventricular block, life-threatening ventricular dysrhythmias, pericarditis, dilated cardiomyopathy, cardiogenic shock, asymptomatic or symptomatic myocardial ischemia or even infarction, and sudden death have been observed (SED-13, 1091) (SEDA-20, 326) (SEDA-22, 369) (23). The combination of high-dose interleukin-2 (IL-2) with interferon alfa enhanced cardiovascular complications, namely cardiac ischemia and ventricular dysfunction (24).

Cardiomyopathy has been attributed to interferon alfa in an infant (25).

- A 3-month-old boy was given interferon alfa (2.5–5.5 MU/m^2) for chronic myelogenous leukemia. After 7.5 months he developed progressive respiratory distress, with anorexia, irritability, and nocturnal sweating. A chest X-ray showed cardiomegaly, an echocardiogram showed a markedly dilated left ventricle, and an electrocardiogram showed left ventricular hypertrophy with abnormal repolarization. Viral cultures and serology for cytomegalovirus, parvovirus B19, and enterovirus were negative. Infectious diseases and metabolic disturbances were excluded. Interferon alfa was withdrawn and digoxin, furosemide, and an angiotensin-converting enzyme inhibitor were given. One year later, he was asymptomatic without further cardiac treatment.

Similar, but anecdotal reports were also described in patients without evidence of previous cardiac disease and receiving low-dose interferon alfa (SEDA-20, 326). In chronic viral hepatitis, only seven of 11 241 patients had severe cardiac adverse effects (16). The exact risk of such cardiovascular adverse effects is unknown. In patients with chronic viral hepatitis, cardiovascular test results were not modified when patients were re-examined after at least 6 months of treatment, even where there was an earlier cardiac history (26), but there was a potentially critical reversible reduction in left ventricular ejection of more than 10% in another prospective study (27).

Myocardial dysfunction can completely reverse after withdrawal of interferon alfa and does not exclude further treatment with lower doses (28).

- A 47-year-old man with renal cancer and no previous history of cardiovascular disease developed gradually worsening exertional dyspnea after he had received interferon alfa in a total dose of 990 MU over 5 years. Echocardiography and a myocardial CT scan confirmed a dilated cardiomyopathy, with left ventricle dilatation and diffuse heterogeneous perfusion at rest. He improved after interferon alfa withdrawal and treatment with furosemide, quinapril, and digoxin. Myocardial scintigraphy confirmed normal perfusion. He restarted low-dose interferon alfa (6 MU/week) 1 year later and had no recurrence of congestive heart failure after a 1-year follow-up period.

Patients with pre-existing cardiac disease are more likely to develop cardiovascular toxicity while receiving interferon alfa, but these complications are rare. Among 89 patients with chronic hepatitis C, 12-lead electrocardiography monthly during a 12-month treatment period and follow-up for 6-months showed only minimal and nonspecific abnormalities in five patients (two had right bundle branch block, one left anterior hemiblock, and two unifocal ventricular extra beats) (29). None of these disorders required treatment withdrawal, and complete noninvasive cardiovascular assessment was normal. Overall, the role of interferon alfa was uncertain and the 5.6% incidence of electrocardiographic abnormalities was suggested to be similar to that expected in the general population. Nevertheless, severe cardiac dysrhythmias are still possible in isolated cases, as illustrated by the development of third-degree atrioventricular block, reversible on withdrawal, in a 57-year-old man with lower limb arteritis but no other cardiovascular disorder (30).

Peripheral vascular complications

Raynaud's phenomenon

Raynaud's phenomenon can occur, particularly in patients with chronic myelogenous leukemia (SEDA-20, 326) (31), and severe cases were complicated by digital necrosis (SEDA-20, 326) (SEDA-21, 369).

In 24 cases of Raynaud's syndrome, interferon alfa was the causative agent in 14, interferon beta in 3, and interferon gamma in 5 (32). There was no consistent delay in onset and the duration of treatment before the occurrence of symptoms ranged from 2 weeks to more than 4 years. The most severe cases were complicated by digital artery occlusion and necrosis requiring amputation. Few patients had other ischemic symptoms, such as myocardial, ophthalmic, central nervous system, or muscular manifestations. Severe Raynaud's phenomenon was also reported in a 5-year-old girl with hepatitis C (33).

Cryoglobulinemia

Although most patients with mild-to-moderate clinical manifestations of hepatitis C virus-associated mixed cryoglobulinemia improved during treatment with interferon alfa, acute worsening of ischemic lesions has been reported in three patients who had prominent cryoglobulinemia-related ischemic manifestations (34). All three had acute progression of pre-existing peripheral ischemia or leg ulcers within the first month of treatment, and transmetatarsal or right toe amputations were required in two. The lesions healed after interferon alfa withdrawal. It was therefore suggested that the anti-angiogenic activity of interferon alfa may also impair revascularization and healing of ischemic lesions in patients with initially severe ischemic manifestations.

Venous thrombosis

Whereas clinically insignificant coagulation abnormalities have been documented in patients receiving high-dose continuous interferon alfa (35), isolated cases of venous thrombosis have been observed (SEDA-20, 329) (36). Interferon alfa can also induce the production of antiphospholipid antibodies (SEDA-20, 329) (SEDA-21, 371). In one study, antiphospholipid antibodies were found in five of 12 patients with melanoma treated with interferon alfa alone or with interferon alfa plus interleukin-2; deep venous thrombosis occurred in four patients with antiphospholipid antibodies (37). Although the underlying neoplasia undoubtedly played a role in the further development of venous thrombosis, the causative role of interferon alfa was suggested by the absence of antiphospholipid antibodies and venous thrombosis in eight patients treated with interleukin-2 alone.

Other vascular complications

Other anecdotal reports included acrocyanosis and peripheral arterial occlusion (SED-13, 1095) (SEDA-22, 400). Although the causal relation is unclear, interferon alfa was considered as a possible cause in the triggering of acute cerebrovascular hemorrhage or ischemic neurological symptoms in few patients (SEDA-21, 370) (SEDA-22, 400). The pathogenic mechanisms of these vascular effects are still unclear; vasculitis, hypercoagulability, vasospasm, a paradoxical anginal effect of interferon alfa, or an underlying cardiovascular disease have all been suggested as underlying processes.

Respiratory

The respiratory adverse effects of interferon alfa include interstitial pneumonitis (38), which is rare. Since the first description of interstitial pneumonitis associated with interferon alfa in Japanese patients who also used the popular "Sho-saiko-t" herbal formulation, similar cases have been described in Western patients, suggesting that interferon alfa can be the sole cause in some patients (SED-13, 1091) (SEDA-20, 326) (SEDA-21, 370) (39,40).

Interferon alfa was also suspected to be involved in one case of biopsy-proven bronchiolitis obliterans-organizing pneumonia (41). Clinical symptoms of pneumonitis appeared 3–12 weeks after the onset of interferon alfa therapy, and after withdrawal of treatment they usually completely resolved, either spontaneously or after a short course of glucocorticoid treatment. Immune-mediated pulmonary toxicity involving the activation of T cells was considered as a likely mechanism. The uncommon features of bronchiolitis obliterans-organizing pneumonia have been reported in three other patients who received interferon alfa together with ribavirin or cytosine arabinoside (42,43).

In four patients with hematological malignancies who developed symptoms suggestive of pneumonitis (that is a dry cough and dyspnea) after 1 week to 38 months of interferon alfa treatment, there was a marked reduction in carbon monoxide diffusion capacity in all cases, whereas there were pathological findings in ordinary chest X-rays in only two (44). What the authors called ultracardiography and high-resolution CT scanning were suggested to have higher sensitivity in evaluating pulmonary symptoms. In three patients, complete reversal was obtained after interferon alfa withdrawal, either spontaneously or after corticosteroid treatment, although one patient required long-term glucocorticoid treatment.

In a retrospective review of 70 patients with hepatitis C enrolled in four clinical trials, there were four cases of significant pulmonary toxicity (two of bronchiolitis obliterans and two of interstitial pneumonitis) (45). Three recovered completely, but one still required glucocorticoids for exertional dyspnea that persisted 17 months after interferon alfa withdrawal. The authors suggested that there was an increased risk with high-dose interferon, because three of these patients received high doses (5 MU/day) or pegylated interferon alfa. In contrast, they were unaware of any significant pulmonary toxicity in any of their approximately 500 patients with hepatitis C.

Interferon alfa can cause exacerbation of asthma (SED-14, 1248).

- Acute exacerbation of asthma has been reported in two men aged 27 and 57 years with a previous history of mild asthma (46). They developed progressive aggravation of asthma within 8–10 weeks of treatment for chronic hepatitis C, and finally required emergency treatment with systemic glucocorticoids and inhaled $beta_2$ adrenoceptor agonists. Severe asthma recurred 2–3 weeks after interferon alfa rechallenge in both patients.

Although these cases are anecdotal, they strongly suggest that interferon alfa should be regarded as a possible cause of asthma exacerbation in predisposed patients.

- Sustained and isolated dry cough has been attributed to interferon alfa in a 49-year-old woman (47). The symptoms disappeared after withdrawal, recurred on readministration, and again resolved after withdrawal. No other cause was found after thorough investigation.

Pleural effusion has been attributed to interferon alfa (48).

- A 54-year-old man received interferon alfa-2a, 9 MU/day, for chronic hepatitis C. He developed an asymptomatic right pleural effusion after 14 days. Although his serum titer of antinuclear antibodies was slightly increased, a more complete screening for autoimmune disease was negative. An infectious origin was also ruled out. The pleural effusion spontaneously disappeared after interferon alfa withdrawal and did not recur.

Although the mechanism of this adverse effect was purely speculative, it was suggested that interferon alfa might have induced a reaction similar to the immunopathological mechanism involved in serositis associated with systemic lupus erythematosus.

Pulmonary artery hypertension has been attributed to interferon alfa (49).

- A 23-year-old man taking hydroxycarbamide 1.5 g/day and interferon alfa-2b (less than 10 MU/day) for chronic lymphocytic leukemia had progressive dyspnea and a non-productive cough after about 5 months. The electrocardiogram showed right-axis deviation, incomplete right bundle-branch block, and right ventricular hypertrophy. The estimated pulmonary artery pressure by echocardiography was 80 mmHg and there were signs of right heart failure. Respiratory function tests showed a restrictive defect, and the chest X-ray showed pulmonary congestion without infiltrates. The patient's clinical status and respiratory function tests improved rapidly after withdrawal of interferon alfa while hydroxycarbamide was continued, and a mean pulmonary artery pressure of 34 mmHg was measured by right heart catheterization 1 month later. At 6 months, the systolic pulmonary artery pressure estimated by echocardiography had fallen to 35 mmHg and the electrocardiogram returned to normal after 1 year.

The authors mentioned that intravenous interferon alfa in sheep had caused an increase in pulmonary artery pressure.

Nervous system

Peripheral neuropathy

Dose-related distal paresthesia occurred in as many as 7% of patients (20), but new onset or worsening of neuropathy has rarely been attributed to interferon alfa. A sensorimotor polyneuropathy was the most frequent presentation (50). The symptoms usually developed after 2–28 weeks of treatment. Such reports were mostly described in patients who received high cumulative doses of interferon alfa, but induction or exacerbation of peripheral sensorimotor axonal neuropathy, particularly in patients with chronic hepatitis C and mixed cryoglobulinemia, was also observed after long-term or low-dose treatment (SED-13, 1092) (SEDA-20, 327) (SEDA-21, 370) (51). Nerve biopsy showed necrotizing vasculitis or axonal degeneration. Most patients stabilized or improved slowly over several months after interferon alfa withdrawal and/or treatment with corticosteroids. Several patients also required plasmapheresis or cyclophosphamide. Although several authors have suggested an autoimmune process, the underlying pathogenic mechanism is unclear.

Other rare forms of neuropathy (SED-13, 1092) include mononeuropathy multiplex (52), acute axonal polyneuropathy (53), anterior ischemic optic neuropathy (54), trigeminal sensory neuropathy (55), bilateral neuralgic amyotrophy (56), brachial plexopathy (57), and symptoms suggestive of leukoencephalopathy (58).

Cranial nerve palsies

There have been reports of interferon alfa-induced cranial nerve palsies, including Bell's palsy.

Two patients, one of whom also received ribavirin, had facial nerve palsy after 5 and 8 months of interferon alfa therapy (59). The palsy resolved completely in one patient after withdrawal and the administration of prednisolone; however, in the other case, the palsy resolved without drug withdrawal, suggesting coincidence.

Two other cases of Bell's palsy, which reversed after interferon alfa withdrawal, have been reported (60). Although the delay in onset (7.5 and 8 weeks) suggested that interferon alfa might be the cause, one patient had no recurrence after rechallenge. A coincidental adverse event cannot therefore be completely ruled out.

Demyelination

Various forms of interferon alfa-induced neuropathy have been reported (SED-14, 1249), but chronic inflammatory demyelinating polyneuropathy has seldom been described (61,62).

- In two patients with chronic hepatitis C or malignant melanoma, paresthesia and tiredness occurred after 6 weeks and 9 months of treatment respectively. Despite withdrawal of interferon alfa, the neurological symptoms worsened initially and a diagnosis of chronic inflammatory demyelinating polyneuropathy was finally confirmed several weeks later. One patient improved after an extended course of plasma exchange and the other required immunoglobulins and prednisolone. Mild to moderate neurological abnormalities persisted at follow-up in both patients.

Multiple sclerosis has been attributed to interferon alfa (63).

- A 29-year-old woman received interferon alfa-2b (6–10 MU/day) for chronic myeloid leukemia, and about 3 years later developed headaches, back pain, progressive visual disturbance, and a sensory deficit in the legs. MRI scans of the brain and spinal cord suggested a first episode of multiple sclerosis. In addition, the myelin basic protein concentration was slightly raised, and perimetry showed bilateral optic neuritis. Most of her neurological symptoms, except central vision impairment, improved after interferon alfa withdrawal and treatment with high-dose methylprednisolone. As a major partial cytogenetic response had been obtained with interferon, she was given natural interferon alfa (3 MU/day) 2 months later. After 2 days of treatment, she complained of transient but severe pain in the back and the legs, and developed acute paraplegia and loss of micturition desire. Again, interferon was withdrawn and she was given high-dose methylprednisolone. There was no further neurological deterioration at follow-up.

This account is reminiscent of the various autoimmune diseases that can be unmasked or exacerbated by interferon alfa.

Extrapyramidal effects

Extrapyramidal effects have been occasionally reported as a manifestation of persistent neurotoxicity induced by interferon alfa. This issue has been addressed in a report of severe refractory akathisia (64).

- A 28-year-old man received interferon alfa (5 MU/day for 28 days) for chronic hepatitis B. At the end of treatment he developed a slight parkinsonian gait, and 8 days later had a fever with vomiting, insomnia, restlessness, and raised serum creatine kinase activity (4946 IU/l). He had severe akathisia with psychomotor excitement and parkinsonism. Despite treatment with clonazepam, thioridazine, propranolol, trihexyphenidyl, and bromocriptine, his condition progressively worsened. He was finally given intravenous levodopa for 8 days and recovered dramatically within the next few days.

This report, together with previous experimental data, suggests that levodopa might be useful in alleviating some of the manifestations of persistent interferon alfa-induced neurotoxicity.

In two other patients, akathisia occurred shortly after they had started to take interferon alfa; one improved after the frequency of injections was reduced (65). Unfortunately, this report did not provide sufficient convincing evidence for a causal relation; the development of akathisia may have been coincidental.

Chorea is a very rare manifestation of interferon alfa neurotoxicity (SEDA-20, 327).

- A 68-year-old woman developed progressive personality changes and 2 months later permanent choreic movements of the four limbs (66). She had taken interferon alfa-2b (3 MU/day) and hydroxyurea 50 mg/kg/day for chronic myeloid leukemia for 2 years and had no history of psychiatric disorders. Neuropsychological testing showed frontal subcortical dysfunction. There were no abnormalities in the Huntington disease gene. She progressively worsened over the next 6 months. The electroencephalogram was disorganized, with diffuse slow waves, and she was bedridden. Interferon alfa was withdrawn. The chorea ceased 1 month later and she completely recovered cognitive function. Electroencephalography was normal 6 and 12 months later.

The authors attributed these events to antidopaminergic effects of interferon alfa.

Seizures

Although generalized tonic-clonic seizures have occasionally been described during trials of high doses of interferon alfa, they have also been reported after the use of intermediate or even low doses (67–69). There was a 1.3% incidence of generalized seizures in a retrospective study of 311 patients treated with low doses for chronic viral hepatitis (70). In another study, tonic-clonic seizures were identified in 4% of children treated for chronic hepatitis B (71). As seizures occurred only in children under 5 years of age with fever or potential perinatal nervous system injury, immaturity of the nervous system was suggested to be an additional factor for interferon alfa-induced neurotoxicity in children.

- In three patients, seizures occurred after a cumulative dose of 266–900 MU (72,73). Two were retreated with a lower dose and remained free of seizures, so that the strength of the causal relation was debatable (72). However, a dose-related effect was still possible.
- Another patient with a history of bipolar mood disorder experienced had his first four episodes of seizures with a prolonged delirious state 1 week after withdrawal of interferon alfa (73).

Reversible photosensitive seizures have also been reported (74).

- A 62-year-old man without a personal or family history of epilepsy received interferon alfa (3 MU three times a week) for 2 years for multiple myeloma. He had frequent episodes of myoclonic jerks in the face, especially when the sun was shining while driving his car. He also had one generalized seizure. Electroencephalography showed a paroxysmal response to intermittent photic stimulation and magnetic resonance imaging was normal. The seizures disappeared and his electroencephalogram normalized after interferon alfa withdrawal.

In this case, the possible role of interferon alfa was suspected only late during treatment, indicating that patients should be regularly questioned about neurological symptoms, because more severe complications might have occurred.

In a prospective study of the effect of interferon alfa (56 MU/day for 4 weeks then 27 MU/week for 20 weeks) in 56 patients with chronic hepatitis C, there was diffuse electroencephalographic slowing at 2 and 4 weeks of treatment, suggesting mild encephalopathy (75). These changes completely reversed after withdrawal. However, the dosage used in this Japanese study was relatively high compared with the dosages currently used in Western countries. In addition, the clinical relevance of these electroencephalographic changes was not investigated.

Neuromuscular function

A number of reports have confirmed that interferon alfa can induce or unmask underlying silent myasthenia gravis (SED-13, 1097) (SEDA-20, 327) (SEDA-21, 370). The diagnostic criteria for myasthenia gravis were clearly fulfilled in these reports, and an autoimmune reaction was the most likely mechanism, as each patient had positive serum anti-acetylcholine receptor antibodies and required permanent anticholinesterase drugs long after interferon alfa withdrawal. Myasthenia gravis developed in two patients treated with interferon alfa-2b for chronic hepatitis C, one of whom also took ribavirin (76,77). Both had an increase in acetylcholine receptor antibody titers and required permanent pyridostigmine and immunosuppressant treatment. These findings suggest that interferon alfa does not cause myasthenia gravis but unmasks it.

Sensory systems

Eyes

Ophthalmic disorders can occur during interferon alfa treatment (78–84) and some of the literature has been reviewed (85). Retinopathy consisting of cotton-wool spots and/or superficial retinal hemorrhages has been reported with a variable incidence (18–86%), and the available data suggest that the increased incidence can be influenced by an initial high dose of interferon alfa. Whereas diabetes mellitus and systemic hypertension have been identified as possible susceptibility factors, the incidence of retinopathy was not significantly increased in 19 patients with chronic renal insufficiency, compared with 17 patients without chronic renal insufficiency (86). However, it was felt that renal insufficiency may be associated with the most severe cases, that is those requiring dosage reductions.

In one study, in which prospective ophthalmic examinations were made before and at regular 2-week intervals after the beginning and end of treatment, 28 of 81 patients who received a uniform total dose of natural interferon alfa (478 MU) for chronic hepatitis C developed the typical findings of interferon-induced asymptomatic retinopathy (cotton-wool spots and/or retinal hemorrhages) (84). In contrast, there were no lesions in the 25 patients with chronic hepatitis C who did not receive interferon alfa or in the 20 with diabetes mellitus and/or hypertension but without chronic hepatitis C. Most of the cases were observed within 4 months of treatment, and the lesions always abated after withdrawal or even despite continuation, suggesting that treatment can be continued unless patients develop symptoms. Indeed, most patients with retinopathy associated with interferon alfa remained asymptomatic.

The pathogenesis of retinopathy associated with interferon alfa is unclear. In 45 patients with chronic hepatitis C (25 treated with interferon) there was an association between retinal hemorrhages caused by interferon alfa (six patients) and a concomitant significant increase in plasma-activated complement (C5a), compared with baseline C5a serum concentrations (87). However, the signification and contribution of raised C5a concentrations in the pathogenesis of ocular complications needs to be clarified, although it has been suggested that retinal hemorrhage could be predicted on the basis of raised C5a concentrations (88).

Although most patients with interferon alfa retinopathy remain asymptomatic, ocular complications, such as reduced vision or complete visual loss due to occlusive vasculitis, central retinal artery occlusion, or anterior ischemic optic neuropathy, continue to be reported in a very few patients (SED-13, 1096) (82,85,89–93). However, subclinical but eventually long-lasting or even irreversible abnormally long visual evoked responses have been identified in 24% of patients (SEDA-22, 403). Regular ophthalmological monitoring to detect retinal changes, even though the patient is still asymptomatic, is therefore strongly recommended in patients receiving interferon alfa.

Other isolated reports of ophthalmic abnormalities refer to optic neuritis with blurring of vision, cortical blindness with fatal encephalopathy, mononeural abducent nerve paralysis, and complete but reversible bilateral oculomotor nerve paralysis (SED-13, 1096) (94–97).

- A 60-year-old smoker was treated with interferon alfa (100 MU/week for 2 months and 9 MU/week for 15 weeks) for cutaneous melanoma. Ocular examination was normal before treatment, but he developed acute loss of peripheral vision in his left eye after 23 weeks. Examination was consistent with anterior ischemic optic neuropathy, and there was optic disc edema, a pupillary defect, and circular visual field constriction in the left eye. There was renal artery constriction in both eyes. Despite treatment with aspirin, high-dose dexamethasone, heparin, and finally withdrawal of interferon alfa, loss of visual function progressed and affected both eyes. Ciclosporin was started, but he was considered to have irreversible loss of visual function.

This report shows that interferon alfa can be a potent precipitator of extremely severe ocular disorders and also argues for careful ocular surveillance in patients receiving adjuvant interferon alfa for high-risk resected melanoma.

Of 57 patients treated with interferon for renal cell carcinoma, two developed multiple retinal exudates associated with visual disturbance; both had taken vinblastine concurrently. The precise role of interferon in this reaction is unknown (98).

Ears

In 49 patients, there was reversible otological impairment with tinnitus, mild-to-moderate hearing loss or both in respectively 8, 16, and 20% of patients after interferon alfa or interferon beta administration (SEDA-19, 336). These disorders tended to occur more frequently in patients on high cumulative doses, but led to withdrawal of treatment in only two patients. Complete but reversible hearing loss, and acute unilateral vestibular dysfunction with spontaneous vertigo and nystagmus have each been reported in one patient receiving interferon alfa (SEDA-21, 372).

Sudden hearing loss has been reported (SEDA-21, 372) and in one case of promptly reversible hearing loss on interferon alfa withdrawal, the presence of anti-endothelial cell antibodies was suggested to have played a role in the development of autoimmune microvascular damage (99).

Smell

Patients treated with interferon alfa sometimes complain of transient taste or smell alterations, but anosmia has been reported (SEDA-22, 403) (100).

- A 37-year-old man received interferon alfa for chronic hepatitis C. After 2 weeks he complained of smelling difficulties and subsequently developed complete anosmia. There were no other neurological symptoms and complete neurological examination was normal. Anosmia still persisted 13 months after drug withdrawal.
- In both patients, the persistence of anosmia late after interferon alfa was resumed indicates that a causal relation to treatment is purely speculative.

Psychological, psychiatric

Neuropsychiatric complications of interferon alfa were recognized in the early 1980s and represent one of the most disturbing adverse effects of interferon alfa (SED-13, 1091) (SEDA-20, 327) (SEDA-22, 400). Reviews have provided comprehensive analysis of the large amount of experimental and clinical data that have accumulated since 1979 (101,102).

DoTS classification (BMJ 2003; 327:1222–5)
Dose-relation: collateral effect
Time-course: intermediate or delayed
Susceptibility factors: pre-existing psychiatric disorders, organic brain injury, or addictive behavior

Presentation

Within a large spectrum of symptoms, complications are classified as acute, subacute, or chronic.

Acute neuropsychological disturbances are usually associated with the flu-like syndrome and include headache, fatigue, and weakness, drowsiness, somnolence, subtle impairment of memory or concentration, and lack of initiative (20). This pattern of cognitive impairment is similar to changes observed during influenza and has also been described in healthy patients who have received a single dose of interferon alfa (103). More severe acute manifestations (for example, marked somnolence or lethargy, frank encephalopathy with visual hallucinations, dementia or delirium, and sometimes coma) have been almost exclusively described in patients receiving more than 20–50 MU (20); vertigo, cramps, apraxia, tremor and dizziness were also reported.

The subacute or chronic neuropsychiatric effects of long-term therapy are usually non-specific, with cognitive impairment (for example visuospatial disorientation, attentional deficits, memory disturbances, slurred speech, difficulties in reading and writing), changes in emotion, mood, and behavior (for example psychomotor slowing, hypersomnia, loss of interest, affective disorders, irritability, agitation, delirium, paranoia, aggressiveness, and murderous impulses). Post-traumatic stress symptoms have also been reported (SEDA-22, 400). As a result, severe psychic distress can be observed during long-lasting treatment or in patients who are otherwise not severely affected (20,104). The most severe psychiatric complications of interferon alfa include rare cases of homicidal ideation, suicidal ideation, and attempted suicide (105).

The clinical features of mania have been described in four patients with malignant melanoma, with a detailed review of nine other published cases (106). Although seven suffered from depression during treatment, the onset of mania or hypomania was often associated with interferon alfa dosage fluctuation (withdrawal or dose reduction) or introduction of an antidepressant for interferon alfa-induced depression. In these patients, the risk of mood fluctuations persisted for several months after interferon alfa withdrawal, and low-dose gabapentin was considered useful in treating manic disorders and in preventing mood fluctuations. Interferon alfa was suggested as a possible cause of persistent manic-depressive illness for more than 4 years in a 40-year-old man (107). Although the manic episodes may have been coincidental, the negative history and the age of onset are in keeping with a possible role of interferon alfa treatment.

The clinical features, management, and prognosis of psychiatric symptoms in patients with chronic hepatitis C have been reviewed using data from 943 patients treated with interferon alfa (85%) or interferon beta (15%) for 24 weeks (108). Interferon-induced psychiatric symptoms were identified in 40 patients (4.2%) of those referred for psychiatric examination. They were classified in three groups according to the clinical profile: 13 cases of generalized anxiety disorder (group A), 21 cases of mood disorders with depressive features (group B), and six cases of other psychiatric disorders, including psychotic disorders with delusions/hallucinations ($n = 4$), mood disorders with manic features ($n = 1$), and delirium ($n = 1$) (group C). The time to onset of the symptoms differed significantly between the three groups: 2 weeks in group A, 5 weeks in group B, and 11 weeks in group C. Women were more often affected than men. There was no difference in the incidence or nature of the disorder according to the type of interferon used. Whereas most patients who required psychotropic drugs were able to complete treatment, 10 had to discontinue interferon treatment because of severe psychiatric symptoms, 5 from group B and five from group C. Twelve patients still required psychiatric treatment for more than 6 months after interferon withdrawal. In addition, residual symptoms (anxiety, insomnia, and mild hypothymia) were still present at the end of the survey in seven patients. Delayed recovery was mostly observed in patients in group C and in patients treated with interferon beta. Although several patients with a previous history of psychiatric disorders are sometimes successfully treated with interferon alfa, severe decompensation with persistent psychosis should be regarded as a major possible complication (109).

The neuropsychological adverse effects of long-term treatment have been assessed in 14 patients with myeloproliferative disorders using a battery of psychometric and electroneurological tests before and after 3, 6, 9, and 12 months of treatment (median dose 25 MU/week) (110). In contrast to several previous studies, there was no significant impairment of neurological function, and attention and short-term memory improved during treatment. Despite the small number of patients, these results suggest that prolonged interferon alfa treatment did not cause severe cognitive dysfunction, at least in patients with cancer.

Diagnosis

Electroencephalographic (EEG) findings show reversible cerebral changes with slowing of dominant alpha wave activity, and occasional appearance of one and two activity in the frontal lobes, suggesting a direct effect on fronto-subcortical functions. Marked electroencephalographic abnormalities are sometimes observed in asymptomatic patients. The pattern of changes is identical whatever the dose, but the severity of symptoms is dose- and schedule-related. Most patients improve or recover after dosage reduction or withdrawal, and protracted toxicity, with impaired memory, deficits in motor coordination, persistent frontal lobe executive functions, Parkinson-like tremor, and mild dementia, have been occasionally reported (111).

In a study of 67 patients with chronic viral hepatitis, the self-administered Minnesota Multiphasic Personality Inventory (MMPI), which determines the patient's psychological profile, significantly correlated with the clinical evaluation and was a sensitive and reliable tool for identifying patients at risk of depressive symptoms before the start of interferon alfa therapy (112). It was also successfully used to monitor patients during treatment.

Frequency

The most typical psychiatric symptoms reported by patients taking interferon alfa are depressive symptoms, at rates of 10–40% in most studies (113–116). In four clinical studies in a total of 210 patients with chronic hepatitis C, the rate of major depressive disorders during interferon alfa treatment was 23–41% (117–120).

Suicidal ideation or suicidal attempts have been reported in 1.3–1.4% of patients during interferon alfa treatment for chronic viral hepatitis or even within the 6 months after withdrawal (121,122), but the excess risk related to interferon alfa is not known.

Time-course

Subacute or chronic neuropsychiatric manifestations are more typically identified after several weeks of treatment and are among the most frequent treatment-limiting adverse effects (104,115,123–125). The onset can be insidious in patients treated with low doses, or subacute in those who receive high doses. Most patients develop severe depressive symptoms within the first 3 months of treatment (117–120).

Although psychiatric manifestations usually appear during interferon alfa therapy, delayed reactions can occur.

- A 37-year-old man without a previous psychiatric history developed major depression with severe psychotic features within days after the discontinuation of a 1-year course of interferon alfa-2b (126).

In 10 patients with melanoma and no previous psychiatric disorders, depression scores measured on the Montgomery-Asberg Depression Rating Scale were significantly increased after 4 weeks of high-dose interferon alfa (127). Patients whose scores were higher before treatment developed the worst symptoms of depression during treatment. This positive correlation provides striking evidence that baseline and regular assessment of mood and cognitive functions are necessary to detect disorders as early as possible.

Mechanisms

Although very few studies have specifically investigated the role of the underlying disease, the findings of significant neuropsychiatric deterioration during interferon alfa treatment compared with placebo or no treatment in chronic hepatitis C, chronic myelogenous leukemia, or amyotrophic lateral disease strongly suggested a causal role of interferon alfa (128–130).

The mechanism by which the systemic administration of interferon alfa produces neurotoxicity is unclear, and might result from a complex of direct and indirect effects involving the brain vasculature, neuroendocrine system, neurotransmitters and the secondary cytokine cascade with cytokines which exert effects on the nervous system, for example interleukin-1, interleukin-2, or tumor necrosis factor alfa (131). Whether a clinical effect is directly mediated through the action of a given cytokine or results from a secondary pathway through the induction of other cytokines or second messengers is difficult to determine.

A study in 18 patients treated with interferon alfa for chronic hepatitis C has given insights into the possible pathophysiological mechanism of depression (132). Depression rating scales, plasma tryptophan concentrations, and serum kynurenine and serotonin concentrations were measured at baseline and after 2, 4, 16, and 24 weeks of treatment with interferon alfa 3–6 MU 3–6 times weekly. During treatment, tryptophan and serotonin concentrations fell significantly, while kynurenine concentrations rose significantly. Depression rating scales also rose from baseline after the first month of treatment, with continued increases thereafter. In addition, there was a relation between increased scores of depression and changes in serum kynurenine and serotonin concentrations. These changes suggested a predominant role of the serotonergic system in the pathophysiological mechanisms of interferon alfa-associated depression. Accordingly, 35 of 42 patients included in three open trials of antidepressant treatment responded to a selective serotonin reuptake inhibitor drug, such as citalopram or paroxetine, and were able to complete interferon treatment (119,133,134).

Susceptibility factors

Various possible susceptibility factors have been analysed in several studies (118–120,135). Sex, the dose or type of interferon alfa (natural or recombinant), a prior personal history of psychiatric disease, substance abuse, the extent of education, the duration and severity of the underlying chronic hepatitis, and scores of depression before interferon alfa treatment were not significantly different between patients with and without interferon alfa-induced depression. Advanced age was suggested to be a risk factor in only one study (120). Although a worsening of psychiatric symptoms was noted during treatment in 11 patients receiving psychiatric treatment before starting interferon, only one was unable to complete the expected 6-month course of interferon alfa and ribavirin therapy (118).

Of 91 patients treated with interferon alfa-2b and low-dose cytarabine for chronic myelogenous leukemia, 22 developed severe neuropsychiatric toxicity (136). Their symptoms consisted mostly of severe depression or psychotic behavior, which resolved on withdrawal in all patients. The time to toxicity ranged from as early as 2 weeks to as long as 184 weeks after the start of treatment. Five of six patients had recurrent or worse symptoms after re-administration of both drugs. Several baseline factors were analysed, but only a pretreatment history of neurological or psychiatric disorders was considered to be a reliable risk factor. Severe neuropsychiatric toxicity developed during treatment in 63% of patients with previous neuropsychiatric disorders compared with 10% in patients without. It is unlikely that the combination of interferon alfa-2b with low-dose cytarabine potentiated the neuropsychiatric adverse effects of interferon alfa in this study. Indeed, previous experience with this combination, but after exclusion of patients with a psychiatric history, was not associated with such a high incidence of neuropsychiatric toxicity or any significant difference in toxicity between interferon alfa alone and interferon alfa plus low-dose cytarabine.

Patients receiving high doses of interferon alfa or long-term treatment are more likely to develop pronounced symptoms (123). A previous history of psychiatric disorders, organic brain injury, or addictive behavior are among potential susceptibility factors, but worsening of an underlying psychiatric disease is not the rule, provided that strict psychiatric surveillance and continuation of psychotropic drugs are maintained (137). Other putative susceptibility factors include the intraventricular administration of interferon alfa, previous or concomitant cranial irradiation, asymptomatic brain metastases, and pre-existing intracerebral ateriosclerosis (SED-13, 1092) (115,138–142). Despite early findings, co-infection with HIV has not been confirmed to be a susceptibility factor (SEDA-20, 327).

The occurrence of psychiatric disorders has been prospectively investigated in 63 patients who received a 6-month course of interferon alfa (9 MU/week) for hepatitis C (143). All were assessed at baseline with the Structured Clinical Interview for DSM-III-R (SCID) and monitored monthly with the Hopkins Symptoms Checklist (SCL-90). Most had a history of alcohol or polysubstance dependence, and 12 had a lifetime diagnosis of major depression. There were no significant changes in the SCL-90 scores during the 6-month period of survey in the 49 patients who completed the study, even in those who had a lifetime history of major depression. At 6 months, there was probable minor depression in eight patients and major depression in one; none had attempted suicide.

In a prospective study, 50 patients with chronic hepatitis B or C who received 18–30 MU/week of natural or recombinant interferon alfa were followed for 12 months (144). The SCID before starting interferon alfa identified 16 patients with a current psychiatric diagnosis and eight with a previous psychiatric disorder; 26 patients free of any psychiatric history constituted the control group. Psychiatric manifestations during treatment occurred in 11 patients (five from the control group), major depression in five, depressive disorders in three, severe dysphoria in two, and generalized anxiety disorder in one. Most of them were successfully treated with psychological support and drug therapy. Overall, 20 patients interrupted interferon alfa (10 in each group), including three for psychiatric adverse effects, but patients with a pre-existing or recent psychiatric diagnosis were no more likely to withdraw from treatment than the controls.

Of 33 patients with chronic hepatitis C treated with interferon alfa, 9 MU/week for 3–12 months, prospectively evaluated using the Montgomery-Asberg Depression Rating Scale (MADRS) before and after 12 weeks of treatment, eight developed depressive symptoms, of whom four had major depression without a previous psychiatric history (145). All four recovered after treatment with antidepressants. This study confirmed that a high baseline MADRS is significantly associated with the occurrence of depressive symptoms.

These studies have confirmed that previous psychiatric disorders are not necessarily a contraindication to a potentially effective treatment. However, patients with depressive symptoms immediately before treatment are still regarded at risk of severe psychiatric deterioration with treatment (113).

Management

The management of the psychiatric complications of interferon alfa has not been carefully investigated, but multiple approaches are theoretically possible. Various pharmacological and non-pharmacological interventions have been discussed (146), and prompt intervention should be carefully considered in every patient who develops significant neuropsychiatric adverse effects while receiving interferon alfa. Depending on the clinical manifestations, proposed treatment options include antidepressants, psychostimulants, or antipsychotic drugs.

Based on a possible reduction in central dopaminergic activity mediated by the binding of interferon alfa to opioid receptors, naltrexone has been proposed as a means of improving cognitive dysfunction (123).

Selective serotonin re-uptake inhibitors have been advocated as the drugs of choice to allow completion of interferon alfa treatment (113), but that was based on very limited experience and the unproven assumption that SSRIs are safe in patients with underlying liver disease. The preliminary results of a double-blind, placebo-controlled study showed that 2 weeks of pretreatment with paroxetine significantly reduced the occurrence of major depression in 16 patients on high-dose interferon alfa for malignant melanoma (147). In a placebo-controlled trial, the preventive effects of paroxetine (mean maximal dose of 31 mg) were studied in 40 patients with high-risk malignant melanoma and interferon alfa-induced depression (148). Treatment started 2 weeks before adjuvant high-dose interferon alfa. Paroxetine significantly reduced the incidence of major depression (45% in the placebo group and 11% in the paroxetine group) and the rate of interferon alfa withdrawal (35 versus 5%). Although the number of patients was small and the duration of the survey short (12 weeks), this suggests that paroxetine effectively prevents the risk of depressive disorders in patients eligible for high-dose interferon alfa. However, these results are limited, because patients with melanoma who receive adjuvant high-dose interferon alfa are particularly likely to develop depression. The safety of prophylaxis with paroxetine also requires additional data, because three patients taking paroxetine developed retinal hemorrhages, including one with irreversible loss of vision.

- In contrast to this study, a 31-year-old woman with major depressive disorder, which responded to paroxetine and trazodone, had progressive recurrence of mood disorders after the introduction of interferon alfa for essential thrombocythemia (149).

This suggests that interferon alfa can also reverse the response to antidepressants.

Endocrine

Pituitary

Interferon alfa can stimulate the hypothalamic–pituitary–adrenal axis, with a marked increase in cortisol and adrenocorticotrophic hormone secretion after acute administration (SED-13, 1093). No further stimulation was observed after several weeks of treatment, pointing to possible down-regulation of the ACTH secretory system. As a result, long-term treatment with interferon alfa is not thought to influence pituitary hormones significantly, and the concentration of several hormones, for example calcitonin, LH, FSH, prolactin, growth hormone, ACTH, cortisol, testosterone, and estradiol, were not modified by prolonged interferon alfa treatment (150,151). No clinical endocrinopathies attributable to such disorders in the regulation of these hormones have yet been reported.

Although the rate of growth was significantly lower than predicted in 35% of children receiving long-term treatment for recurrent respiratory papillomatosis (152), only one case of growth retardation has been reported in other settings (SEDA-19, 335). A significant reduction in weight and nutritional status was observed during treatment with interferon alfa for 6 months for chronic viral hepatitis in children aged 4–16 years, but this was transient and not associated with growth impairment (153).

Reversible hypopituitarism with antibodies to pituitary GH3 cells and exacerbation of Sheehan's syndrome have been reported (SED-13, 1093) (SEDA-21, 371).

A syndrome resembling inappropriate antidiuretic hormone secretion has been described in a few patients receiving high-dose interferon alfa (SED-13, 1093) (154).

Thyroid

Since the original 1988 report of hypothyroidism in patients with breast cancer receiving leukocyte-derived interferon alfa (155), numerous investigators have provided clear clinical and biological data on thyroid disorders induced by different forms of interferon in patients with various diseases (21,156–159). Two of these reports also mentioned associated adverse effects that developed concomitantly, namely myelosuppression and severe proximal myopathy (Hoffmann's syndrome).

Presentation and outcomes

The spectrum of interferon alfa-induced thyroid disorders ranges from asymptomatic appearance or increase in antithyroid autoantibody titers to moderate or severe clinical features of hypothyroidism, hyperthyroidism, and acute biphasic thyroiditis. Antithyroid hormone antibodies have also been found in one patient, and this could have been the cause of erroneously raised thyroid hormone concentrations (160).

The clinical, biochemical, and thyroid imaging characteristics of thyrotoxicosis resulting from interferon alfa treatment have been retrospectively analysed from data on 10 of 321 patients with chronic hepatitis (75 with chronic hepatitis B and 246 with chronic hepatitis C) who developed biochemical thyrotoxicosis (161). Seven patients had symptomatic disorders, but none had ocular symptoms or a palpable goiter. Six had features of Graves' disease that required interferon alfa withdrawal in four and prolonged treatment with antithyroid drugs in all six. Three presented with transient thyrotoxicosis that subsequently progressed to hypothyroidism and required interferon withdrawal in one and thyroxine treatment in all three.

Although much work on thyroid autoimmunity associated with interferon alfa has accumulated, little is known about the very long-term outcome of this disorder. In 114 patients with chronic hepatitis C and no previous thyroid disease who were treated with interferon alfa-2a for 12 months, data on thyroid status were retrospectively obtained at the end of treatment, 6 months after withdrawal, and after a median of 6.2 years (162). Among 36 patients who had thyroid autoantibodies at the end of treatment, the authors identified three groups according to the long-term outcome: 16 had persistent thyroiditis, 10 had remitting/relapsing thyroiditis (that is antibodies became negative after 6 months of therapy and were again positive thereafter), and 10 had transient thyroiditis. Therefore, 72% of these patients had chronic thyroid autoimmunity at the end of follow-up and 12 developed subclinical hypothyroidism. In contrast, only one of 78 patients negative for thyroid autoantibodies developed thyroid autoantibodies. Although none of the patients had clinical thyroid dysfunction, this study suggests that long-term surveillance of thyroid disorders is useful in patients who have high autoantibody titers at the end of treatment with interferon alfa.

Although thyroid disorders in patients treated with interferon alfa generally follows a benign course after interferon alfa withdrawal or specific treatment, severe long-lasting ophthalmopathy resulting from Graves' disease has been described in a 49-year-old woman (163).

Time-course

Clinical symptoms usually occur after 2–6 months of treatment and occasionally after interferon alfa withdrawal.

- A middle-aged woman developed subacute thyroiditis by the sixth month of treatment with interferon alfa (164). She also had the classic symptoms of hyperthyroidism, although it is clear that these could easily have been mistaken for adverse effects of interferon alfa itself, for example weakness, weight loss, and palpitation.

After 6 months of treatment, 12% of patients with chronic hepatitis C had thyroid disorders, compared with 3% of patients with chronic hepatitis B. This study also suggested a possible relation between low free triiodothyronine serum concentrations before treatment and the subsequent occurrence of thyroid dysfunction. After a follow-up of 6 months after the end of interferon alfa treatment, 60% of affected patients with chronic hepatitis C still had persistent thyroid dysfunction; all had been positive for thyroid peroxidase antibodies before treatment. Long-term surveillance is therefore needed in these patients.

Frequency

In a prospective study, the overall incidence of biochemical thyroid disorders was 12% in 254 patients with chronic hepatitis C randomized to receive ribavirin plus high-dose interferon alfa (6 MU/day for 4 weeks then 9 MU/week for 22 weeks) or conventional treatment (9 MU/week for 26 weeks) (165). There was no difference in the incidence or the time to occurrence of thyroid disorders between the groups. Of the 30 affected patients, 11 (37%) had positive thyroid peroxidase autoantibodies (compared with 1% of patients without thyroid dysfunction), nine developed symptomatic thyroid dysfunction, and only three had to discontinue treatment. There was no correlation between the viral response and the occurrence of thyroid disorders, and only female sex and Asian origin were independent predictors of thyroid disorders.

Data on the incidence of thyroid disorders in interferon alfa-treated patients vary, largely because the follow-up duration, the nature of the study (prospective or retrospective), biological monitoring, diagnostic criteria, and the underlying disease differ from study to study (156). The incidence of clinical or subclinical thyroid abnormalities is generally 5–12% in large prospective studies in patients with chronic hepatitis C treated for 6–12 months, but it reached 34% in one study (21,166). The incidence was far lower in patients with chronic hepatitis B, at 1–3%. A wider range in incidence was found in patients with cancer, with no clinical thyroid disorders in 54 patients treated during a mean of 16 months for hematological malignancies (167), whereas in many other studies there was a 10–45% incidence (156). Even more impressive was the escalating incidence of thyroid disorders in patients with cancer receiving both interferon alfa and interleukin-2 (qv).

Mechanisms

Possible mechanisms need to be clarified. Since thyroid autoantibodies are detected in most patients who develop thyroid disorders, the induction or exacerbation of pre-existing latent thyroid autoimmunity is the most attractive hypothesis. This is in accordance with the relatively frequent occurrence of other autoantibodies or clinical autoimmune disorders in patients who develop thyroid disorders (168). However, 20–30% of patients who develop thyroid diseases have no thyroid antibodies, and it is thus not yet proven that autoimmunity is the universal or primary mechanism. In fact, there were subtle and reversible defects in the intrathyroidal organification of iodine in 22% of antithyroid antibody-negative patients treated with interferon alfa (169). In addition, the acute systemic administration of interferon alfa in volunteers or chronic hepatitis patients reduces TSH concentrations (SED-13, 1093) (170), and in vitro studies have suggested that interferon alfa directly inhibits thyrocyte function (SED-13, 1093) (171). Finally, the thyroid autoantibody pattern in patients who developed thyroid dysfunction during cytokine treatment was not different from that of patients without thyroid dysfunction, but differed significantly from that of patients suffering from various forms of spontaneous autoimmune thyroid disease (172).

Susceptibility factors

In addition to the underlying disease, there are many potential susceptibility factors (21,173). There is as yet no definitive evidence that age, sex, dose, and duration of treatment play an important role in the development of thyroid disorders. However, patients with previous thyroid abnormalities are predisposed to develop more severe thyroid disease (SEDA-20, 328). The incidence of thyroid disease was not different between natural and recombinant interferon alfa. Although this should be taken into account, a previous familial or personal history of thyroid disease was generally not considered a major risk factor. Finally, only pre-treatment positivity or the development of thyroid antibodies during treatment seem to be strongly associated with the occurrence of thyroid dysfunction.

In 175 patients with hepatitis B or C virus infections, women with chronic hepatitis C and patients with previously high titers of antithyroid autoantibodies were more likely to develop thyroid disorders (174).

The immunological predisposition to thyroid disorders has been studied in 17 of 439 Japanese patients who had symptomatic autoimmune thyroid disorders during interferon alfa treatment (175). There was a significantly higher incidence of the human leukocyte antigen (HLA)-A2 haplotype compared with the general Japanese population (88 versus 41%), suggesting that HLA-A2 is a possible additional risk factor for the development of interferon alfa-induced autoimmune thyroid disease.

Among other potential predisposing factors, treatment with iodine for 2 months in 21 patients with chronic hepatitis C receiving interferon alfa did not increase the likelihood of thyroid abnormalities compared with eight patients who received iodine alone, but abnormal thyroid tests were more frequent compared with 27 patients who received interferon alfa alone (176). This suggests that excess iodine had no synergistic effects on the occurrence of thyroid dysfunction induced by interferon alfa.

The occurrence of thyroid dysfunction in 72 patients treated with interferon alfa plus ribavirin (1.0–1.2 g/day) has been compared with that of 75 age- and sex-matched patients treated with interferon alfa alone for chronic hepatitis C (177). Of the former, 42 patients, and of the latter, 40 patients had received previous treatment with interferon alfa alone. There was no difference in the rate of thyroid autoimmunity (antithyroglobulin, antithyroid peroxidase, and thyroid-stimulating hormone receptor antibodies) between the two groups, but the patients who received interferon alfa plus ribavirin developed subclinical or overt hypothyroidism more often (15 versus 4%). Similarly, the incidence of hypothyroidism increased to 19% in patients who underwent a second treatment with interferon alfa plus ribavirin compared with 4.8% after the first treatment with interferon alfa alone, while the incidence remained essentially the same in patients who had two consecutive treatments with interferon alfa alone

(4.7 and 7.1% respectively). Furthermore, there was no higher incidence of thyroid autoimmunity or clinical disorders after a second course of interferon alfa whether alone or combined with ribavirin in patients who had no thyroid autoantibodies at the end of a first course of interferon alfa alone, suggesting that these patients are relatively protected against the development of thyroid autoimmunity.

Management

The management of clinical thyroid dysfunction depends on the expected benefit of interferon alfa. Assay of thyroid antibodies before treatment, and regular assessment of TSH concentrations in treated patients, even after interferon alfa withdrawal, are useful as a means of predicting and detecting the risk of thyroid disorders. Complete recovery of normal thyroid function is usually observed after thyroxine replacement but sometimes requires interferon alfa withdrawal. Sustained hypothyroidism requiring long-term substitution treatment has occasionally been observed (SED-13, 1092) (178), and is more likely in patients with initially severe hypothyroidism and raised thyroid antibody titers (179). By contrast, hyperthyroidism generally requires the prompt withdrawal of interferon alfa, and severe forms may require radical radioiodine therapy. Although not enough data are available on the long-term consequences of interferon alfa-induced thyroid dysfunction, the recurrence of thyroid abnormalities after the administration of pharmacological doses of iodine should be borne in mind (180).

Parathyroid

Exacerbation of secondary hyperparathyroidism occurred in a 20-year-old renal transplant patient who also developed psoriasis during interferon alfa treatment (181). Both disorders resolved after withdrawal.

Adrenal

Of 62 initially autoantibody-negative patients treated with interferon alfa for chronic hepatitis C for a mean of 8 months, three developed antibodies to 21b-hydroxylase, a sensitive assay of adrenocortical autoimmunity (182). However, there were no cases of Addison's disease or subclinical adrenal insufficiency. This study suggested that the adrenal cortex is another potential target organ of autoimmune effects of interferon alfa, along with thyroid and pancreatic islet cells.

Metabolism

Diabetes mellitus

The development or worsening of insulin-dependent diabetes mellitus is limited to isolated case reports in patients treated with interferon alfa or interferon alfa plus interleukin-2 (SEDA-20, 328) (SEDA-21, 371). In chronic hepatitis, diabetes mellitus was noted in only 10 of 11 241 treated patients (16). Although a relation between chronic hepatitis C and the occurrence of glucose metabolism disorders is possible (183), reports of diabetes mellitus in patients treated with interferon alfa were probably more than coincidental. Indeed, there have been reports of prompt amelioration or complete recovery after interferon alfa withdrawal (SED-13, 1092) (184–186) and of successive episodes of diabetes after each course of interferon alfa (SEDA-21, 371).

- In three middle-aged patients, diabetes was diagnosed after 3–7 months of treatment with interferon alfa-2b and ribavirin, and two presented with severe ketoacidosis (187,188). There was a family history of diabetes in one patient and two had high titers of glutamic acid decarboxylase antibodies before treatment. One patient never had diabetes-related serum autoantibodies before or after interferon alfa therapy. All three required permanent insulin treatment despite withdrawal of interferon alfa.
- Insulin-dependent diabetes mellitus has been reported after 2 weeks to 6 months of treatment with interferon alfa in four patients with chronic hepatitis C (189). All discontinued interferon alfa, and one woman who restarted treatment had a subsequent increase in insulin requirements.

A 75 g oral glucose tolerance test was performed before and after 3 months of interferon alfa treatment in 32 patients with chronic hepatitis C, of whom 15 also had an intravenous glucose test (190). Baseline evaluation showed that five patients had mild diabetes mellitus, three had impaired glucose tolerance, and 24 were normal. After 3 months of treatment, two patients with diabetes mellitus shifted to impaired glucose tolerance, and all patients with impaired glucose tolerance had normal glucose tolerance. Only three initially normal patients developed impaired glucose tolerance and none had newly diagnosed diabetes mellitus. From these results, and in contrast to previous reports (SED-14, 1250), it appears that interferon alfa did not have any adverse effects on insulin sensitivity and glucose tolerance after 3 months of treatment.

Interferon alfa may produce more severe changes than interferon beta (191).

- A 39-year-old man with diabetes, stabilized with insulin 22 U/day for 13 years, received interferon beta (6 MU/day) for chronic hepatitis C. His diabetes progressively worsened, necessitating insulin 50 U/day. After 4 weeks, interferon beta was replaced by interferon alfa (10 MU/day). Shortly afterwards he developed severe diabetic ketoacidosis and shock, which reversed after hemodynamic support and continuous hemodiafiltration.

Mechanisms

Autoimmunity was suggested as a likely mechanism, with HLA-DR4 haplotype and/or islet cell antibody (ICA) positivity at the time of diagnosis in several patients. Because the induction of ICA antibodies in patients treated with interferon alfa has never been otherwise demonstrated (21), the triggering, rather than the induction, of a latent autoimmune phenomenon in patients with a genetic susceptibility is probable (192).

More direct interference with glucose metabolism cannot be excluded. Interferon alfa can reduce the sensitivity of peripheral tissues or liver to insulin and accelerate the destruction of stimulated pancreatic beta-cells (193,194); this could be a possible mechanism in patients not exhibiting islet cell antibodies. This is also in keeping with rare instances of induction or exacerbation of type II non-insulin dependent diabetes mellitus (SEDA-19, 335).

Insulin antibodies were also found in six of 58 patients treated for chronic viral hepatitis (195) and that was associated with signs of insulin allergy in one patient (SEDA-19, 335).

Susceptibility factors

Patients with obesity and a family or previous history of glucose intolerance should be considered more predisposed to interferon alfa-induced diabetes, but the association is not consistently found (SEDA-20, 328).

Dyslipidemia

Interferon alfa often affects lipid metabolism and produces a reversible reduction in cholesterol and, more consistently, increases in triglyceride concentrations (SEDA-20, 328) (SEDA-21, 371). Meticulous blood lipid investigation showed a significant rise in serum triglyceride and lipoprotein(a) concentrations and reductions in total cholesterol, HDL cholesterol, LDL cholesterol, and apoprotein A1.

Marked hypertriglyceridemia (10–20 μg/ml), which abates when treatment is withdrawn, has sometimes been observed (SED-13, 1093) (196,197). Inhibitory effects of interferon alfa on lipoprotein lipase and triglyceride lipase or increased hepatic lipogenesis have been suggested (198,199). Diet and lipid-lowering drugs have been proposed as means of maintaining acceptable triglyceride concentrations during long-term interferon alfa therapy. Although the possibility of pancreatic or cardiovascular complications should be borne in mind, no secondary clinical consequences of interferon alfa-induced blood lipid disorders have been so far reported.

In a prospective study of lipid changes in 36 patients with chronic hepatitis C treated with interferon alfa for 6 months, the most prominent findings included increases in triglycerides, VLDL cholesterol, and apolipoprotein B, and falls in HLD cholesterol and apolipoprotein A1 (200). Three patients also developed chylomicronemia and two of those had severe hypertriglyceridemia. All three patients had triglycerides over 2 μg/ml before treatment, suggesting that patients with abnormal serum triglyceride concentrations at baseline are more likely to develop marked hypertriglyceridemia.

Porphyria

- A severe acute flare of porphyria cutanea tarda has been reported in a 61-year-old man after 4 months of treatment with interferon alfa-2b plus ribavirin for chronic hepatitis C (201). No further relapse was observed after chloroquine treatment, despite continuation of the antiviral drugs.

This patient had previously had episodes of small blisters that spontaneously resolved, and hereditary porphyria cutanea tarda was demonstrated by chromatographic and mutation analysis.

Hematologic

Hematological toxicity due to interferon alfa commonly includes dose-related leukopenia, neutropenia, and thrombocytopenia, whereas anemia is rare and usually moderate (202).

Reductions in platelet count and leukocyte count were usually in the range of 30–50% compared with baseline, but severe and reversible thrombocytopenia (<49 × 10^9/l) or neutropenia (<0.9 × 10^9/l) were noted in 10 and 20% of patients (203). However, life-threatening neutropenia or thrombocytopenia were reported in only six of 11 241 patients with chronic viral hepatitis (16), and reports of Coombs'-negative hemolytic anemia or complete agranulocytosis are sparse (SED-13, 1094) (SEDA-20, 329).

In a retrospective study of 158 patients with chronic viral hepatitis treated for 6–12 months, lymphoblastoid interferon alfa produced the largest fall in leukocyte and platelet counts (−38 and −32% versus baseline values), recombinant interferon alfa was associated with intermediate toxicity (−32 and −26%), and leukocyte interferon alfa produced the smallest reduction (−27 and −22%) (204). The lowest mean values were observed after an average of 4–5 months. However, the clinical relevance of these differences is probably minimal, because the overall reduction in leukocyte and platelet numbers was small, and no patients developed clinical symptoms of cytopenia.

Mechanisms

Interferon alfa has direct myelosuppressive effects and can also cause hematological disorders by immune blood cell destruction, as suggested by reports of immune-mediated thrombocytopenia, immune hemolytic anemia (205,206), or a positive direct Coombs' test, with or without hemolysis (207–209).

The kinetics of the hemotoxic effects of interferon alfa have been studied in 76 patients with chronic hepatitis C (210). There were significant falls in white blood cell count and platelet count within 12 hours after the first injection, and a second fall in platelet count after 2 weeks, but not further thereafter. This rapid time-course suggests that liver or spleen sequestration of blood cells, rather than direct bone marrow suppression or immune-mediated hematological toxicity, is the most likely explanation for this acute hemotoxic effect, which does not preclude continuation of treatment.

Susceptibility factors

Susceptibility factors for severe hematological toxicity include cirrhosis and hypersplenism.

Prior interferon alfa treatment lasting for more than 6 months and withdrawn for 2–3 months was also one of the most significant factors to explain a reduced yield of peripheral blood stem cells in 88 previously autografted patients with myeloma undergoing G-CSF stimulation for future autotransplantation (211). As suggested by this study, the myelosuppressive effects of interferon alfa may be prolonged to such an extent that a minimum delay of more than 2–3 months after interferon alfa withdrawal should be considered before harvesting bone marrow cells.

Pancytopenia or aplasia, sometimes fatal, have been reported only in patients who had received previous chemotherapy, as has severe and even fatal erythrocytosis in patients with hairy cell leukemia (SED-13, 1094) (212–216).

Anemia

Isolated anemia is not a common feature of the hemotoxic effects of interferon alfa, and pure red cell aplasia has been reported in two patients with chronic leukemia for several months (217,218). Both patients improved progressively after replacement of interferon alfa by hydroxyurea. However, one required erythrocyte transfusions for 14 months.

- Pernicious anemia with a low vitamin B_{12} concentration and positive intrinsic factor antibodies has been reported in a 54-year-old woman who was receiving interferon alfa as a maintenance treatment for relapsing chronic hepatitis C (219).

Rapid exacerbation (1–21 days) or delayed (3–38 months) de novo appearance of immune hemolytic anemia has been reported after initiation of interferon alfa treatment in nine patients with lymphoproliferative disorders (220). However, this rare event was identified in only 1% of 581 patients receiving interferon alfa alone or as part of a chemotherapeutic regimen for chronic myelogenous leukemia (221). A mechanism close to that observed with alpha-methyldopa has been thought to be involved (208). The direct antiglobulin test was positive in 32% of 28 chronic myeloid leukemia patients after a median of 1 year of treatment with interferon alfa (222).

Interferon alfa can also induce multiple antibody formation to transfused blood cell antigens, with subsequent massive hemolysis (223).

- A 33-year-old man developed a delayed hemolytic reaction 7 days after red cell transfusion (224). Additional investigations showed the presence of an anti-M antibody, the production of which was supposedly caused by chemoimmunotherapy (interferon alfa, interleukin-2, and 5-fluorouracil) which was begun 24 hours after transfusion.

Leukopenia

The dose of interferon alfa is usually halved when the neutrophil count falls below 0.75×10^9/l or the drug is permanently withdrawn when it falls below 0.5×10^9/l. However, this issue has recently been challenged by a retrospective analysis of 11 patients with compensated cirrhosis, four of whom had severe neutropenia (that is 0.4 to 0.67×10^9/l) during the first 2 months of treatment (225). They remained asymptomatic and the neutropenia spontaneously reversed despite continued treatment.

In one study in 119 patients treated with interferon alfa and ribavirin for chronic hepatitis C, in whom neutropenia was not considered as a cause for exclusion or dosage modification, the neutrophil count fell by an average of 34% (31–74%) (226). During the course of treatment, 32 patients had at least one neutrophil count below 1×10^9/l, 11 had a neutrophil count below 0.75×10^9/l, and 2 had a neutrophil count below 0.5×10^9/l; however, none of these patients required dosage modification because of neutropenia. None of the 22 patients who developed documented or suspected bacterial infections during or immediately after treatment withdrawal had concomitant neutropenia. The three black patients with constitutional neutropenia (pretreatment neutrophil counts below 1.5×10^9/l) had only minimal changes in their neutrophil counts during treatment and no infection, suggesting that these patients can be safely treated.

Thrombocytopenia

Although inhibition of stem-cell proliferation is the most likely mechanism of hematological toxicity, increased platelet hepatic uptake has been suggested to account for thrombocytopenia (227). Raised serum thrombopoietin concentrations were found in patients with interferon alfa-induced thrombocytopenia (228). However, there is evidence that serum thrombopoietin concentrations in patients who have had thrombocytopenia during interferon alfa treatment for chronic viral hepatitis C either do not increase (in patients with compensated cirrhosis) or increase only moderately and less than expected (in non-cirrhotic patients) (229). The authors proposed that interferon alfa impairs liver production of thrombopoietin, raising the possibility of testing thrombopoietin administration in patients with severe thrombocytopenia before or during treatment with interferon alfa (230).

- In a 45-year-old man treated with pegylated interferon alfa-2b for relapsing chronic hepatitis C, thrombocytopenia recovered over 2 months, despite initial treatment with glucocorticoids and immunoglobulin (231).

Interferon alfa-induced immune-mediated thrombocytopenia shares many features with idiopathic thrombocytopenic purpuras and may be therefore coincidental (SED-13, 1094) (SEDA-20, 328) (SEDA-21, 371), but recurrence of thrombocytopenia on interferon alfa readministration strongly supports a causal role of interferon alfa (232). Cross reaction with interferon beta was not found in an isolated report (SEDA-20, 329). Even though severe and even fatal worsening of idiopathic thrombocytopenic purpura has been observed after administration of interferon alfa (SED-13, 1094) (SEDA-20, 328), interferon alfa was not considered harmful in patients with chronic hepatitis C who were previously positive for platelet-associated immunoglobulin G (233).

Thrombotic thrombocytopenic purpura is a possible complication of interferon alfa in patients with chronic myelogenous leukemia, and can develop even after a successful prolonged (2–3 years) treatment (234). Complete recovery is expected after prompt medical management with plasma exchange and glucocorticoids.

Platelet aggregation

The effects of interferon alfa-2b on platelet aggregation have been studied in 29 patients with melanoma who received a low-dose regimen (9 MU/week in five patients) or a high-dose regimen (100 MU/m^2/week intravenously for 4 weeks, then 30 MU/m^2/week subcutaneously for 48 weeks in 24 patients) (235). Compared with pretreatment values and healthy controls, there was significant inhibition of platelet aggregation in the high-dose group, while the effects were minimal in the low-dose group. In the high-dose group, the inhibition was more prominent during the subcutaneous maintenance dose and was still detectable 8 weeks after interferon alfa withdrawal in 60% of the tested samples. An increased risk of bleeding should therefore be anticipated in patients who receive high-dose interferon alfa.

Clotting factors

Clotting disorders due to interferon alfa have rarely been reported.

- Asymptomatic prolongation of the activated partial thromboplastin time associated with lupus anticoagulant and a reduction in the coagulation activity of factors IX, XI, and XII occurred after 10 weeks of interferon alfa-2b and ribavirin in a 60-year-old woman with chronic hepatitis C (236). There were no arguments in favor of an antiphospholipid syndrome, and all the abnormalities normalized after withdrawal.

Interferon alfa was suspected of having induced the development of anti-factor VIII autoantibodies in one patient with hemophilia who survived and one without hemophilia who subsequently died from acute hemorrhage (SED-13, 1094) (237,238).

- There was significant bleeding with hematomas in association with an inhibitor of factor VIII in a 58-year-old man who took interferon alfa for 1 year for chronic myelogenous leukemia (239). The factor VIII inhibitor, which was markedly raised, disappeared within 6 weeks of interferon alfa withdrawal and prednisone treatment.

By contrast, in a small uncontrolled study, there was no increase in antifactor VIII antibodies in patients with hemophilia A treated with interferon alfa (240).

Gastrointestinal

Mild and transient gastrointestinal disorders, namely nausea, vomiting, diarrhea or anorexia, were observed in 30–40% of patients, and their severity is typically dose-related (20). Dryness or inflammation of the oropharynx, and moderate stomatitis were sometimes noted, but severe painful oral ulcers recurring after interferon alfa re-administration have been reported (241). More severe forms of digestive disease have been described in isolated case histories with microscopic colitis and the occurrence or the exacerbation of ulcerative colitis (SED-13, 1094) (SEDA-21, 372).

Celiac disease

Celiac disease was observed after 2–3 months of interferon alfa treatment in two patients with chronic hepatitis C aged 34 and 38 years (242). Both had total villous atrophy on distal duodenal biopsy, were positive for antiendomysial antibodies, and responded to a gluten-free diet. Three other cases were reported after 1–5 months of treatment for chronic hepatitis C (37,243). The diagnosis was confirmed in all three patients, based on the presence of total villous atrophy on distal duodenal biopsy, positivity of antiendomysial antibodies, and recovery with a gluten-free diet. Pretreatment antiendomysial antibodies were positive in the two patients tested. As suggested in one patient, interferon alfa can be safely continued providing that a gluten-free diet is strictly respected.

Enteritis

Eosinophilic enteritis has been attributed to interferon alfa (244).

- A 23-year-old man with no previous history of digestive disorders took interferon alfa for chronic hepatitis C. After 2 weeks of treatment, he had severe abdominal pain and diarrhea. The absolute eosinophil count was 7.5×10^9/l, with 40% eosinophils on bone marrow aspiration and a markedly high IgE concentration. Radiological examination showed diffuse jejunal and ileal wall thickening and gross ascites with numerous eosinophils. Complete resolution was obtained after interferon alfa withdrawal and prednisolone treatment. There was no recurrence after prednisolone was withdrawn.
- A 23-year-old man with no previous history of digestive disorders took interferon alfa for chronic hepatitis C. After 2 weeks of treatment, he had severe abdominal pain and diarrhea. The absolute eosinophil count was 7.5×10^9/l, with 40% eosinophils on bone marrow aspiration and a markedly high IgE concentration. Radiological examination showed diffuse jejunal and ileal wall thickening and gross ascites with numerous eosinophils. Complete resolution was obtained after interferon alfa withdrawal and prednisolone treatment. There was no recurrence after prednisolone was withdrawn.

Colitis

Microscopic colitis and new or worsened ulcerative colitis have been attributed to interferon alfa (SED-13, 1094) (SEDA-21, 372). Ischemic colitis has been reported in two of 280 patients treated for chronic hepatitis C (245).

Liver

Asymptomatic and reversible rises in serum transaminases have been reported in 25–30% of patients receiving high-dose interferon alfa (20). Although direct hepatotoxicity has been suspected in isolated and unexplained cases of severe liver failure (SED-13, 1094), most data favored exacerbation of chronic viral hepatitis or latent autoimmuine hepatitis.

Exacerbation of chronic viral hepatitis

In the treatment of chronic hepatitis B, HBe seroconversion was sometimes preceded by transient and moderate worsening of serum transaminases, but severe exacerbation of chronic hepatitis B infection and fatal liver failure can occur. Such fatalities were reported in under 0.5% of patients with hepatitis B (246). Patients with active cirrhosis or a previous history of decompensated cirrhosis are particularly susceptible to these complications (247).

Acute exacerbation of hepatitis is an extremely rare complication of chronic hepatitis C treatment. An exaggerated immune response to hepatitis virus was supposedly the cause of acute icteric hepatitis in two patients (SEDA-21, 372) (248).

- A 43-year-old man had a moderate rise in hepatic transaminase activities after 4 weeks of interferon alfa treatment. His liver tests normalized after withdrawal, but the aspartate transaminase activity increased dramatically shortly after treatment was restarted. His condition rapidly deteriorated, with a diagnosis of hepatorenal failure, and he finally required liver transplantation. Histological examination of the liver showed advanced micronodular cirrhosis, a feature not found on pretreatment liver biopsy.

In another study, only four of 11 241 patients treated with interferon alfa died of fulminant liver failure (16).

Autoimmune hepatitis

More disturbing are reports of interferon alfa-induced acute exacerbation of latent autoimmune hepatitis (SED-13, 1094) (249–256). Further analysis showed that these patients were initially misdiagnosed as having hepatitis C, and autoimmune hepatitis reversible by glucocorticoid treatment was later proven to be the correct diagnosis. It was later found that latent chronic autoimmune hepatitis can be present in patients with unequivocal serological evidence of chronic hepatitis C (249,257). The co-existence of serological markers of autoimmune hepatitis and confirmed hepatitis C before treatment with interferon alfa in the same patient is very disturbing, because the distinction cannot readily be made on the basis of biological and histological data. As glucocorticoids can increase the extent of viremia, and since in addition interferon alfa can acutely exacerbate latent autoimmune liver disease, this has raised the question of how to deal with these patients. In those without serological markers of autoimmune liver disease, only close monitoring of liver function to detect any sudden increase in alanine transaminase activity is helpful, because the systematic detection of autoantibodies proves unable to predict the risk of overt autoimmune hepatitis (257). In those with both hepatitis C virus and autoantibodies, there is as yet no consensus on the therapeutic management. Glucocorticoids may actually increase the extent of viremia, while interferon alfa may exacerbate autoimmune hepatitis. As a result, controversies have emerged, with several investigators advocating glucocorticoids as first line treatment and providing a safe option in patients with high antibody titers, whereas others have found interferon alfa to be more appropriate (SED-13, 1094) (SEDA-20, 329) (SEDA-21, 372).

De novo induction rather than exacerbation of autoimmune hepatitis is still possible, as indicated by anecdotal reports in patients with cancer or chronic viral hepatitis (SED-13, 1094) (SEDA-22, 402). Such a very rare event is in keeping with the usual absence of autoantibody specific for autoimmune liver disease after interferon alfa treatment.

Positive serological markers of autoimmune hepatitis before treatment in patients with concomitant chronic hepatitis C are sometimes associated with further exacerbation of an underlying autoimmune liver disease during interferon alfa treatment. Of three patients with raised antimitochondrial antibodies (over 1:160), only the two patients with M2 (with or without M4 or M8) subtypes had biochemical exacerbation of cholestasis and an unfavorable response to interferon alfa (255). Although very few patients were investigated, determination of antibodies against submitochondrial particles may help to identify patients who are likely to have no benefit and even exacerbation of liver disease with interferon alfa.

In 25 children with chronic hepatitis C, pretreatment positivity for liver/kidney microsomal type 1 (LKM-1) antibodies was associated with more frequent treatment-limiting increases in serum alanine transaminase activity (256). Withdrawal of interferon alfa-2b because of hypertransaminasemia was required in three of four LKM-1 positive children compared with two of the 21 LKM-1 negative children. Although none developed features of autoimmune hepatitis, careful surveillance of hepatic function is recommended in LKM-1-positive patients.

Other complications

Interferon alfa-associated macrovesicular steatosis has been reported (258).

- A 50-year-old woman without a history of liver disease, dyslipidemia, diabetes, obesity, or alcoholism started taking interferon alfa (7.5 MU/day) for chronic myelogenous leukemia together with allopurinol and hydroxyurea for 2 weeks. Her liver tests were normal before treatment but transaminase activities were greatly increased after 2 weeks. Serological tests for hepatitis B and C and HIV were negative, as was screening for serum antitissue antibodies. Liver biopsy showed severe macrovesicular steatosis (80% of hepatocytes) without steatohepatitis. Liver tests completely normalized on interferon alfa withdrawal. A few weeks after interferon alfa was restarted in a lower dose (3–5 MU/day), she again had a rise in liver enzymes, and a second liver biopsy showed unchanged findings. Liver tests remained stable despite treatment continuation.

Other adverse liver effects reported with interferon alfa include primary biliary cirrhosis (SEDA-20, 329) and granulomatous hepatitis (SEDA-20, 329) (SEDA-21, 372) (259).

Pancreas

Asymptomatic rises in pancreatic enzymes and reversible acute pancreatitis have been reported in isolated patients, with no mention of hypertriglyceridemia (SEDA-19, 336).

- A 54-year-old man developed abdominal pain from the beginning of interferon alfa treatment (260). Two weeks later his serum amylase and lipase peaked at about three times the upper limit of normal. Careful radiological investigations ruled out pancreatic calcification and biliary or pancreatic lithiasis and showed only pancreatic enlargement. Complete improvement occurred after treatment withdrawal. As in the very few previous cases, there was no hypertriglyceridemia in this patient.

A definite case of pancreatitis proven by positive rechallenge was also briefly cited in a review of drug-associated pancreatitis spontaneously reported to the Dutch adverse drug reactions system (261).

Two cases of interferon alfa-induced acute pancreatitis in patients with chronic hepatitis C were particularly convincing, because other causes were carefully ruled out and clinical symptoms or biological abnormalities recurred after rechallenge in both patients (262). Although one patient also took ribavirin, recurrence was observed after re-administration of interferon alfa alone. Lipid disorders were not found in these patients, confirming that interferon alfa-induced pancreatitis is not due to hypertriglyceridemia.

Urinary tract

Mild and usually asymptomatic proteinuria, leukocyturia, microscopic hematuria, or moderate increases in serum creatinine were observed in 15–25% of patients (20). There was moderate deterioration of glomerular and tubular renal function in most interferon alfa-treated patients assessed prospectively with a number of renal function markers (263).

In patients receiving high-dose interferon alfa, severe proteinuria and nephrotic syndrome have sometimes been noted (264).

- A 57-year-old woman developed severe nephrotic syndrome after 3 months of interferon alfa re-treatment, and renal biopsy showed minimal change nephrotic syndrome with T cell-predominant interstitial nephritis (265). Proteinuria persisted despite interferon alfa withdrawal and resolved only after glucocorticoid treatment.
- A 55-year-old woman was treated with interferon alfa and ribavirin for 1 year and developed asymptomatic nephrotic syndrome with focal segmental glomerulosclerosis on renal biopsy (266). Proteinuria slowly improved over the next 21 months.

Interferon alfa-induced acute renal insufficiency is rare and has mostly been reported in patients with underlying renal disease, in those receiving high dosages, or in those with varied malignancies (SED-13; 1095) (SEDA-20, 329) (SEDA-21, 372) (267,268). Very few cases have been described in patients with chronic hepatitis (SEDA-21, 372) (SEDA-22, 402). It has also been reported after intravesical administration (SEDA-21, 372). When available, pathological findings have pointed variously to nephrotic syndrome with minimal-change nephropathy and acute tubulointerstitial nephritis, nephrotic syndrome with severe glomerular changes, membranoproliferative glomerulonephritis, extracapillary glomerulonephritis with crescents, focal segmental glomerulosclerosis, and acute tubular necrosis. Renal dysfunction usually resolves after withdrawal of interferon alfa, but irreversible alteration or incomplete resolution of renal function have occasionally been noted.

A review of 15 other available reports of renal insufficiency and proteinuria in patients with chronic myeloid leukemia or other malignancies confirmed that the histological spectrum of renal lesions associated with interferon alfa is varied, and includes membranous glomerulonephritis, minimal change glomerulonephritis, acute interstitial nephritis, hemolytic–uremic syndrome, and thrombotic microangiopathy. Renal complications were reversible in nine patients; three patients had persistent proteinuria, and four had persistent renal dysfunction, of whom three required chronic hemodialysis. Two-thirds of the patients developed renal complications within 1 month of treatment with interferon alfa, and one-third had received a relatively low dosage of interferon alfa (9–15 MU/week).

The mechanism of interferon alfa nephrotoxicity is probably multifactorial and may involve a direct nephrotoxic effect with a possible additive effect of concomitant NSAID therapy, a T cell-mediated immune effect, immune-complex renal disease, or an autoimmune etiology (SED-13, 1095) (269–274).

Acute renal insufficiency has also occurred as a consequence of interferon alfa-induced hemolytic–uremic syndrome, thrombotic thrombocytopenic purpura, or renal thrombotic microangiopathy (SED-13, 1095) (234,275–278). The diagnosis was made after 7 months to 10 years of treatment (median 50 months) with weekly doses of 15–70 MU. This rare but extremely severe complication has almost exclusively been reported in patients treated for chronic myelogenous leukemia, so that the respective roles of interferon alfa and the underlying hematological malignancy are undetermined. However, at least one case has been reported in a patient with hepatitis C (SEDA-22, 402). From a total of 15 cases, renal prognosis was poor, with early deaths in four patients, chronic hemodialysis in eight, and chronic renal insufficiency in three.

To determine the characteristics of thrombotic microangiopathy associated with interferon alfa, data from eight patients were carefully examined (279). All had chronic myeloid leukemia and had received high-dose interferon alfa (mean 39 MU/week) for a long time (mean 32 months) before diagnosis. Severe arterial hypertension was the most common sign before diagnosis. Five patients had distal ischemic lesions that required amputation in one, and all had typical lesions of renal thrombotic microangiopathy involving both glomeruli and small arterioles. After interferon alfa withdrawal, two recovered normal renal function, three had persistent renal insufficiency, one relapsed 17 months after treatment withdrawal, and two required chronic dialysis. One patient had already had reversible renal insufficiency during a previous course of interferon alfa. From a review of 21 other previously published similar cases, the authors confirmed that interferon alfa-induced thrombotic microangiopathy mostly occurred in patients with chronic myeloid leukemia, whereas only two cases were reported in patients with chronic hepatitis C and one in a patient with hairy cell leukemia. The delayed occurrence of renal toxicity was also suggested to be highly predictive of histological thrombotic microangiopathy.

Possible deleterious effects of interferon alfa on renal graft function are repeatedly reported (280).

- A 43-year-old man with stable renal graft function, taking ciclosporin, methylprednisolone, and azathioprine, developed chronic myelogenous leukemia and received interferon alfa (3 MU/day). Seven weeks later, he became tired and had increased proteinuria and a raised serum creatinine concentration (574 μmol/l). Interferon alfa was withdrawn and he received high-dose methylprednisolone for suspected acute graft rejection. This was unsuccessful and a first renal biopsy showed widespread interstitial edema that could not be correctly interpreted. Hemodialysis was restarted, and he finally developed a catheter infection and died from sepsis. Histology of the explanted renal graft showed severe, predominantly acute, vascular rejection.

The rapid occurrence of renal dysfunction after interferon alfa in this case suggested a causal relation.

Skin

A wide range of skin lesions has been reported, and most include skin dryness, rash, diffuse erythema, or urticaria, occurring in 5–12% of patients (20,281). However, severe dermatological complications are rare. In a prospective survey of 120 patients treated during 6–18 months for chronic viral hepatitis, only three developed lichen planus and one relapsing aphthous stomatitis (282).

Injection site reactions

Subcutaneous interferon alfa sometimes causes local erythema and skin induration, which can be prevented by regularly changing the site of injection. Isolated reports have described more severe local reactions, with inflammatory painful nodules, purpuric papules and vasculitis, local ulceration, and injection site necrosis (SED-13; 1095) (SEDA-20, 330) (SEDA-21, 372) (SEDA-22, 402). Despite previous findings, even patients receiving low-dose interferon alfa can have severe injection site reactions. A localized intradermal bullous eruption, which recurred following each interferon alfa injection, was also reported (283).

Severe injection site reactions have been extensively detailed in six patients who had local cutaneous necrosis or indurated erythema after 1–10 months of treatment with low-dose interferon alfa (284). Four patients had concomitant risk factors known to reduce microcirculation, that is beta-blockers, dihydroergotamine, and cigarette smoking. The lesions healed after medical treatment in five patients, but one required surgical excision. The ulcers healed slowly and full recovery occurred only after a mean of 16 weeks after drug withdrawal. The lesions did not recur after interferon alfa re-administration at the other injection sites.

As with interferon alfa, pegylated interferon alfa has been associated with injection site skin necrosis (285). Severe local reactions after subcutaneous injections mostly consist of ulceration and skin necrosis, but a variety of reactions have been described. Prominent suppuration and granulomatous dermatitis at the injection sites of interferon alfa have been reported in two patients (286). Three patients who had severe rashes while receiving pegylated interferon alfa-2a or 2b had positive intracutaneous tests to both pegylated forms of interferon alfa but not to standard interferon alfa-2a or 2b (287). One of these patients subsequently tolerated standard interferon alfa. Cutaneous ulcers have also been reported in patients treated with peginterferon alfa-2b (288,289). In the latter case, the lesions healed under local therapy and the same dose of interferon was maintained.

Lichen planus

The new occurrence or exacerbation of lichen planus is a well-known complication of interferon alfa, but this has been a source of a considerable debate (SED-13, 1095) (SEDA-20, 330) (SEDA-22, 402). Indeed, most patients have received interferon alfa for chronic hepatitis C, an underlying disease that is controversially thought to be associated with a spontaneously higher incidence of lichen planus (290). In addition, complete reversibility of previous lichen planus was sometimes observed in patients treated with interferon alfa (SEDA-20, 330). Whatever the truth of the matter, the recurrence of lesions after interferon alfa re-administration or reports of lichen planus in patients with cancer (291–293) argues strongly for a direct causal link with interferon alfa. Local treatment and PUVA were sometimes sufficient to alleviate symptoms, but withdrawal of interferon alfa was required in the most severe cases (SED-13, 1095).

Pemphigus and pemphigoid

Bullous pemphigus and pemphigoid with circulating pemphigus-like autoantibodies, pemphigus foliaceus with anti-intercellular IgG antibodies, and paraneoplastic pemphigus due to interferon alfa have rarely been reported (SED-13, 1095), as has extensive oral pemphigus (294).

- A 28-year-old woman developed oral ulcers after a 5-month course of interferon alfa-2a for chronic hepatitis C. She had multiple erosions on both lips, the tongue, the floor of the mouth, the soft palate, the pharyngeal walls, and the laryngeal mucosa, but there were no skin or genital lesions. Raised double-stranded DNA antibody titers were found. Histology showed pemphigus vulgaris, and complete resolution was obtained by withdrawal of interferon alfa and immunosuppressive and local treatment.

This case was thought to have been due to the immunomodulatory effects of interferon alfa.

Psoriasis

The first reports of psoriasis in cancer patients treated with high-dose interferon alfa were followed by a controversial debate (295,296). However, numerous cases have confirmed that interferon alfa can either induce typical psoriasis or worsen pre-existing psoriasis (SED-13, 1095) (297), an observation that is compatible with interferon alfa-induced imbalance toward an increased Th1 response. This was particularly exemplified by the reversibility of the lesions after withdrawal of treatment and the prompt recurrence of symptoms after interferon alfa re-administration. Exacerbation of psoriasis usually occurred within the first month, whereas a minimum of 2–3 months of treatment was required in patients without a past history of psoriasis (297). Psoriatic lesions at the sites of injection were suggested to be potential indicators for further generalization of psoriasis. In more severe cases, there was concomitant development of monoarticular or polyarticular joint symptoms (SED-13, 1095) (SEDA-21, 372). Pustular psoriasis with balanitis and erosive monoarthritis, suggesting incomplete Reiter's syndrome, was also reported in one patient with HLA-B27 (298).

Vitiligo

Vitiligo has sometimes been reported in patients with malignant melanoma, for example in 17–25% of patients receiving interferon alfa alone (SEDA-21, 372). There have also been a few reports of vitiligo in patients with chronic hepatitis C (SEDA-20, 330), and one patient had both scleroderma and vitiligo (SEDA-19, 336).

Other complications

A spectrum of cutaneous lesions has been described distant from sites of interferon alfa injection. The clinical and histological characteristics of inflammatory skin lesions that occurred away from injection sites have been investigated in 20 patients treated with interferon alfa-2a or 2b plus ribavirin for chronic hepatitis C (299). Cutaneous lesions developed between 2 weeks and 4 months and consisted of pruritic papular erythematous eruptions with occasional vesicles. These eczema-like skin lesions predominated on the distal limbs, the head, and the neck. Photosensitivity was also noted in four patients and mucous lesions in two. Skin biopsy mostly showed non-specific mononuclear infiltrates. The skin lesions were promptly reversible in 10 patients who required treatment withdrawal, while others improved after symptomatic treatment. Two of the three patients who again received the same or another type of interferon alfa had recurrence of their lesions. Skin tests performed in six patients were negative, including the two patients who relapsed after rechallenge with interferon alfa, and were therefore considered unhelpful.

- Radiation recall dermatitis developed in a 29-year-old woman after high-dose intravenous interferon alfa-2b was given 5 days after the completion of radiotherapy for malignant melanoma (300).

The authors suggested that interferon alfa can trigger an inflammatory reaction in patients whose inflammatory response threshold has been lowered by irradiation.

- A 46-year-old woman developed transient facial erythema with telangiectasia after each injection of interferon alfa, resolving within 1–2 days, and completely disappearing after definitive withdrawal of treatment 7 months later (301).
- Two patients treated with pegylated interferon alfa-2b and ribavirin developed cutaneous thrombotic microangiopathy (302).
- A 54-year-old woman had small bullous lesions mainly on the backs of her hands and feet after 6 months of treatment with pegylated interferon alfa-2b plus ribavirin for chronic hepatitis C. The lesions lasted 48 hours and healed rapidly after rupture of the bullae.
- A 62-year-old woman developed generalized pruritus and excoriated lesions after 5 months of treatment with pegylated interferon alfa-2b plus ribavirin. The lesions were maximal on the backs of her hands and feet after 8 months of treatment, but there were no bullae.

Skin biopsies in the last two patients showed microthrombi of the dermal capillaries and a necrotic epidermis. Immunofluorescence showed only fibrinogen. Some bullous lesions were still present 1 month after withdrawal in the first patient, while the second patient responded to local corticosteroids and a reduced dose of pegylated interferon alfa, but continued to have episodes of severe pruritus.

Other dermatological complications have in most instances been reported as single case histories, so that any causal relation with interferon alfa awaits confirmation. These reports have included worsening of lichen myxedematosus, injection site pyoderma gangrenosum, a polymorphous light eruption (SEDA-22, 372), and a fatal case of histiocytic cytophagic panniculitis (SEDA-20, 330).

- Meyerson's phenomenon, multiple focal and transient eczematous eruptions around melanocytic nevi, has been reported in a 24-year-old man when the dosage of interferon alfa for Behçet's disease was doubled (303).
- Bullous lesions with specific infiltrates of mycosis fungoides have been reported in a 67-year-old woman who took interferon alfa for 2 months for mycosis fungoides (304).

Although in the second case the syndrome could not be definitely attributed to interferon alfa, the authors noted that bullous mycosis fungoides is an extremely rare variant of this disease and withdrawal of interferon alfa led to healing of the blisters without further recurrence.

Hair

Moderate and reversible alopecia secondary to telogen effluvium is common (7–30%), and sometimes recedes despite continued treatment (305). Alopecia areata has very occasionally been described (306).

- Injection-site alopecia has been reported in three patients, affecting the thighs in two patients and the abdomen in one (307). A reversible focal telogen effluvium secondary to high local concentrations of interferon alfa was the most likely cause, indicating that rotating injection sites are needed to prevent this adverse effect.
- Alopecia areata after 7 months of interferon alfa, slowly reversible on withdrawal, has also been reported in a 36-year-old woman (308).

In two patients with previously natural curly hairs, the combination of interferon alfa plus ribavirin was suggested to have triggered a rapid change in hair texture, with diffuse straightening hairs, eyelashes, and eyebrow hypertrichosis (309). In one patient, a causal role of treatment was supported by the spontaneous recovery of hair abnormalities after withdrawal and the recurrence of similar abnormalities on rechallenge.

Excessive growth of eyelashes and nail damage due *to Tinea unguium* have been occasionally reported in patients receiving interferon alfa (SED-13, 1095) (SEDA-21, 372). Hypertrichosis of the eyelashes (trichomegaly) developed in two of 36 patients with chronic viral hepatitis who were examined for ocular complications during treatment with high-dose interferon alfa (18–30 MU/week) (86). These two patients had received the highest dose of interferon alfa.

Musculoskeletal

Arthralgia, myalgias, and muscle weakness are typically observed during the early influenza-like reaction (20). Direct muscle toxicity of interferon alfa can result in acute rhabdomyolysis, in some cases fatal after the dose of interferon alfa was increased (SEDA-19, 330) (SEDA-21, 372).

- A 26-year-old man with a malignant melanoma had two episodes of acute severe rhabdomyolysis after each exposure to a chemotherapy regimen containing interferon alfa and dacarbazine (310). As a few cases of rhabdomyolysis have been previously reported after interferon alfa alone (SEDA-19, 336) (SEDA-20, 330) (SEDA-22, 403), interferon alfa was suggested as the most likely cause.

- Acute rhabdomyolysis occurred in a 34-year-old woman with a melanoma treated with interferon alfa 20 $MU/m^2/$ day (311). There was no recurrence on retreatment with a lower dose (down to 6.6 MU/m^2/day), suggesting that this was a dose-related complication.
- A 34-year-old man with scleromyxedema had flu-like symptoms and muscle pain after the first injection of interferon alfa 6 MU (312). After three additional injections at 2-day intervals, his muscle symptoms worsened and were associated with mild quadriparesis, reduced deep tendon reflexes, dark urine, confusion, and agitation. Biological findings were consistent with acute rhabdomyolysis, and electromyography showed rare denervation potentials. His symptoms resolved and the laboratory findings normalized within 15 days.

Delayed muscular adverse effects have been occasionally reported including the clinical exacerbation of a latent myopathy (SEDA-19, 336), delayed and severe myopathic changes (313), myositis, polymyositis, and a Lambert–Eaton-like syndrome (SEDA-19, 336) (SEDA-20, 330) (SEDA-22, 403).

- Three patients developed unilateral or bilateral avascular necrosis of the femoral head after 3–54 months of treatment with interferon alfa for chronic myelogenous leukemia (314). One required bilateral hip replacement and two significantly improved after interferon alfa withdrawal. One patient received further interferon alfa without exacerbation.

Although there were risk factors for avascular necrosis in two of the patients (a short course of methylprednisolone and moderate alcohol consumption), the authors did not consider them to be significant. They identified seven other reported cases of avascular necrosis in patients with chronic myeloid leukemia, including two patients who were taking interferon alfa at the time of the complication. One patient with pre-existing avascular necrosis had an acute exacerbation within 1 month of interferon alfa and required hip replacement. Although any causal relation with treatment remains purely speculative, the authors argued that the known antiangiogenic effects of interferon alfa could have predisposed patients to avascular necrosis.

Sexual function

Sexual complaints attributed to interferon alfa, namely decreased libido, impotence, or erectile failure, are usually concomitant to other neuropsychiatric symptoms, and cases of reversible impotence are anecdotal (315). The mechanisms accounting for these adverse effects are unclear, and changes in sex hormone concentrations have not been consistently reported. In one study in healthy women, interferon alfa produced falls in serum progesterone and estradiol concentrations (316), but neither impairment of libido nor impairment of fertility has apparently been reported in women. No evidence of gonadal toxicity or sexual dysfunction was found in 43 men with hairy cell leukemia who received interferon alfa for 2–12 months compared with 33 patients who received no systemic therapy (317). Finally, sexual complaints reported during interferon alfa treatment of chronic hepatitis C were presumably related to fatigue, anxiety, or psychological disorders rather than to endocrinological changes (SEDA-21, 373).

Immunologic

Hypersensitivity reactions

No IgE-mediated immediate-type allergic reactions to interferon alfa have ever been conclusively documented. A recurrent non-IgE-mediated anaphylactic reaction, possibly due to mast cell degranulation, has been described in a patient with mastocytosis (318).

- A 64-year-old man with no history of allergy had progressive fatigue, loss of appetite, and facial edema after 6 months of interferon alfa-2b treatment for chronic hepatitis C (319). Angioedema was diagnosed and it resolved after withdrawal of interferon alfa and a short course of prednisolone. Serum immunoglobulin E and plasma bradykinin concentrations were raised, but the C1 esterase inhibitor and serum complement concentrations were normal.
- A 47-year-old man, who had previously received a 2-month course of interferon alfacon-1 for chronic hepatitis C, started interferon alfa-2b 8 months later (320). He developed mild generalized pruritus the day after the second injection, and dyspnea with diffuse urticaria within a few hours after the third injection. Skin tests were not performed, and IgG but not IgE antibodies to interferon alfa were found.

These cases do not formally show a causal relation with interferon alfa, and at best they suggest that an IgE-mediated reaction is probably not the cause of hypersensitivity reactions to interferon alfa. In the first case, the mechanism may have been similar to that observed with angiotensin-converting enzyme inhibitors.

Cases of contact dermatitis have suggested that interferon alfa-2c can cause cell-mediated delayed hypersensitivity (321,322).

Interferon alfa antibodies

Both binding and neutralizing antibodies to interferon alfa can be detected in interferon alfa-treated patients, and the incidence or clinical significance of these antibodies is the subject of continuous controversy, which has been addressed in a number of studies or general reviews (SED-13, 1096) (SEDA-20, 330) (SEDA-21, 373) (156,323–325).

In various studies, the incidence of antibody formation has ranged from zero to more than 50% of patients. However, any comparison between studies is difficult, because the underlying treated disease, the type of interferon used, the route of administration, the dosage regimen, the schedule of treatment, and the method of assay have differed from one investigation to another. Antibodies to interferon alfa have been reported to be more frequent in patients receiving long-term, instead of short-term, treatment, in patients receiving subcutaneous rather than intravenous interferon alfa, and in patients receiving low rather than high doses (156). Complete disappearance of interferon alfa antibodies was usually observed after withdrawal. Interferon alfa formulations also differ in antigenicity. Using the same anti-interferon alfa antibody assay, a higher frequency of antibodies to recombinant interferon alfa-2a has repeatedly been reported compared with other recombinant or natural interferon alfa formulations in patients treated by the same route and with the same treatment schedule. In 296 patients with chronic hepatitis, binding and neutralizing antibodies were found in 45 and 20% respectively of patients receiving recombinant interferon alfa-2a compared with 15 and 6.9% of those receiving recombinant interferon alfa-2b, and 9.4 and 1.2% of those receiving interferon alfa-n1 (326,327). There were similar differences in the immunogenic potential of the two recombinant interferon alfa formulations in 159 patients with chronic myelogenous leukemia (328). Overall, the incidence of binding antibodies is in the range of 20–50% for recombinant interferon alfa-2a, 6–10% for recombinant interferon alfa-2b, and 1–6% for interferon alfa-n1 (324).

The clinical significance of binding antibodies appears to be limited to a possible change in interferon alfa pharmacokinetics. By contrast, neutralizing antibodies, which are usually detected within 2–4 months of treatment, can theoretically reduce the clinical response to interferon alfa and cause interpatient variability in response to treatment, but this is still debated (323–325). Although several studies have failed to detect any loss of therapeutic response, response failure or the reversal of an initial clinical response, simultaneously with (or soon after) the appearance of neutralizing antibodies, have been reported. In large-scale studies, the clinical response to recombinant interferon alfa was significantly less in patients with neutralizing antibodies, and it has therefore been suggested that the appearance of neutralizing antibodies provides the prime explanation for those instances in which there is a relapse or a breakthrough of the disease before the completion of treatment (329–335). In addition, in patients who cease to respond therapeutically after recombinant interferon alfa antibody formation, a change to natural interferon alfa has proved successful in restoring the response in some cases (335–338). This has led to the suggestion that the formation of neutralizing antibodies represents a specific immune response to the recombinant preparations, and that natural interferon alfa can overcome the neutralizing activity of antibodies to recombinant interferon alfa. On the other hand, neutralizing antibodies were not associated with immune complex-associated diseases or hypersensitivity reactions, and exerted no influence on interferon alfa-associated adverse effects. They can even be accompanied by improvement in the flu-like syndrome.

Autoantibodies

Collectively, several antibodies (mostly antinuclear, antithyroid, parietal cell, liver/kidney microsome, and smooth muscle antibodies, and rheumatoid factor) can be detected before interferon alfa treatment in about one-third of patients. Increased titers or the occurrence of various autoantibodies were observed in 4–30% of previously autoantibody-negative patients (21,156). These autoantibodies do not affect the response to interferon alfa treatment (339–341). Although it was initially felt that interferon alfa might facilitate the development of autoimmune disease in patients previously positive for non-organ-specific autoantibodies, the evidence is still limited and the clinical consequences of such autoantibodies are unclear. Except for thyroiditis, large studies in patients with chronic viral hepatitis C receiving interferon alfa did not show a significant increase in overt autoimmune diseases, despite the pre-existence or further positivity of several autoantibodies (SED-13, 1096) (SEDA-20, 330) (SEDA-21, 373) (SEDA-22, 405). However, in 83 patients with chronic hepatitis C there were one or more pre-existing autoantibodies (mostly low-titer antinuclear antibodies) in 35 patients (group I), of whom seven had clinical evidence of immune-mediated disorders, whereas five of 48 patients without pre-existing autoantibodies (group II) had similar disorders (342). After 12–48 weeks of treatment with interferon alfa in 44 patients, there were new immune-mediated disorders in six of the 20 patients in group I (thyroid disorders in three, arthropathy in two, and psoriasis in one), but none in the 24 patients in group II. Patients who are positive for autoantibodies before interferon alfa may therefore be much more likely to develop autoimmune diseases, particularly thyroid disorders, during interferon alfa treatment.

As a result, there is no clear consensus about the management of patients previously positive for non-organ specific autoantibodies, but it is usually considered that low autoantibody titers or the absence of concomitant symptoms suggestive of autoimmune disease is not a contraindication to treatment.

Autoimmune disorders

The possibility of autoimmune disorders during interferon alfa treatment has been addressed by many authors. The spectrum of interferon alfa-induced immune diseases includes organ-specific and systemic autoimmune diseases, such as thyroiditis, diabetes, hematological disorders, systemic lupus erythematosus, rheumatoid arthritis, dermatological disease, and myasthenia gravis (156). Several have been discussed in appropriate sections elsewhere in this monograph. The exact role of interferon alfa is usually difficult to ascertain, because the underlying disease, that is chronic hepatitis C, can also be associated with immune-mediated disease.

Two studies have provided insights into the incidence and risk factors of the immune-mediated complications of interferon alfa in patients with chronic myeloid leukemia. In the first study, 13 of 46 patients had autoimmune manifestations consisting of a combination of autoimmune thyroiditis in four, a direct antiglobulin test without hemolysis in eight, cryoagglutinins in one, Raynaud's phenomenon in two, and chronic autoimmune hepatitis in one (343). Overall, six patients had clinically symptomatic manifestations after a median of 15 months of treatment. In the second study, there were autoimmune diseases in seven of 76 patients after a median of 19 months of treatment, including hypothyroidism in one, immune-mediated hemolysis in two, systemic lupus erythematosus in two, Raynaud's phenomenon in one, and mixed connective tissue disease in one (344). In both studies there was a strong association with female sex and it was confirmed that patients who developed clinical autoimmune complications had had relatively long exposures to interferon alfa.

The management of patients with chronic hepatitis C and associated features of autoimmune disease carries the risk of exacerbating the underlying disease. Different treatment strategies, including interferon alfa alone or combined with ribavirin or glucocorticoids, or no treatment, have been discussed (345).

Behçet's disease

Characteristic features of Behçet's disease or isolated positive skin tests were found in one study of patients with chronic myelogenous leukemia treated with interferon alfa (346). No other reports confirmed these findings.

Dermatomyositis

Occasional reports have suggested that interferon alfa can cause dermatomyositis (347).

- A 57-year-old woman received adjuvant high-dose interferon alfa 16 months after removal of a malignant melanoma. About 6 weeks later, she developed hand swelling, fatigue, myalgia, arthralgia, and weakness. Interferon alfa was withdrawn. She had multiple joint involvement, and radiological imaging showed bilateral interstitial pulmonary infiltrates. Anti-Jo antibodies were positive but other autoantibodies were negative. She also had violet eyelid discoloration with edema, tenderness in various muscle groups, and reduced strength in the shoulders. The muscle biopsy showed scattered necrotic fibers and basophilic regenerative fibers. She gradually recovered with methotrexate and corticosteroids, and the titer of anti-Jo antibodies fell dramatically.

Polyarteritis nodosa

Severe polyarteritis nodosa-like systemic vasculitis has been reported (SEDA-20, 330) and cutaneous polyarteritis nodosa has been attributed to interferon alfa (348).

- A 50-year-old woman was given interferon alfa for chronic hepatitis C and primary biliary cirrhosis, and within 2 months became febrile and developed a diffuse nodular erythematous rash. The skin biopsy showed typical features of necrotizing angiitis, and cutaneous periarteritis nodosa was diagnosed. Full recovery was obtained after interferon alfa withdrawal and prednisolone treatment.

According to the authors, it is not known whether this complication was directly due to interferon alfa, represented the triggering of latent periarteritis nodosa in a patient with primary biliary cirrhosis, or whether it was a coincidental adverse event.

Polymyositis

- Polymyositis has very rarely been associated with interferon alfa, but has been reported together with autoimmune thyroiditis in a 48-year-old woman after treatment for 5 months for malignant melanoma (349).

There have been two reports of polymyositis in association with interferon alfa treatment for hematological malignancies (123,350). In both cases, clinical and/or electrophysiological recovery occurred after drug withdrawal, spontaneously or after a short course of glucocorticoids.

Sarcoidosis

The early impression that interferon alfa, alone or in combination with ribavirin, could reactivate or cause new subcutaneous sarcoid nodules and pulmonary or generalized sarcoidosis, has been confirmed by several reports, with prompt recovery after interferon alfa withdrawal (SED-13, 1097) (SEDA-20, 330) (SEDA-22, 404). The incidence may have been underestimated; in one series, 3 patients out of 60 who received interferon alfa alone or combined with ribavirin developed pulmonary sarcoidosis (351). In a review of 27 cases, the time to onset was 15 days to 30 months, and there were dermatological signs in 50% (352). Five patients had also taken ribavirin, but an enhanced T cell immune reaction from the combination of interferon alfa plus ribavirin is speculative. However. the association of cutaneous or systemic sarcoidosis with interferon alfa, alone or in association with ribavirin, has been exemplified by various reports (353,354), including one patient whose sarcoidosis resolved with prednisone despite continued interferon alfa treatment (355).

- A 60-year-old woman receiving interferon alfa developed cutaneous sarcoid foreign body granulomas at the sites of a previously childhood skin injury (356).

This suggests that interferon alfa may facilitate the development of cutaneous sarcoid granuloma from particulate foreign matter.

De novo sarcoidosis has been reported in six patients (357–361) and reactivation of pre-existing disease in one (362). One of these patients had chronic hepatitis B, suggesting that interferon alfa treatment rather than the underlying disease was the most probable triggering factor. Remission was observed in all patients after withdrawal, either spontaneously or after glucocorticoid treatment.

Sjögren's syndrome

One report of Sjögren's syndrome in a patient taking interferon alfa should be regarded with caution (SEDA-20, 330).

Systemic lupus erythematosus and rheumatoid arthritis

The possible role of interferon alfa in the development of rheumatoid arthritis or systemic lupus erythematosus has been described in isolated cases (363,364), and confirmed cases of systemic lupus erythematosus have very occasionally been reported (SED-13, 1096) (SEDA-20, 330). In most of these cases, the predominance of young patients and female sex, the presence of renal or skin involvement, the findings of positive antibodies to double-stranded DNA, and the rapid onset after the start of treatment, as well as persistence of symptoms after interferon alfa withdrawal, are more in keeping with unmasking by interferon alfa of idiopathic lupus rather than with a new drug-induced illness. The reactivation or appearance of inflammatory rheumatological disorders consistent with rheumatoid arthritis or lupus-like polyarthritis were also consistently reported (SEDA-20, 330) (365,366). In a review of 37 published cases of interferon alfa-induced arthritis, symmetrical polyarthritis was the most common feature, and antinuclear antibodies or rheumatoid factor were found in 72 and 34%, respectively (367). Although spontaneous improvement was sometimes observed after withdrawal of interferon alfa, more severe cases required anti-inflammatory, antimalarial, or immunosuppressive drugs. In five of eight patients rechallenged with interferon alfa, there was recurrence of arthritis.

There was an unexpectedly high incidence of rheumatoid and lupus-like symptoms (27 of 137 patients), namely arthralgia, arthritis, myalgia, and Raynaud's phenomenon, in patients with myeloproliferative disorders taking interferon alfa alone or combined with interferon gamma (365). However, only a minority of affected patients fulfilled the diagnostic criteria for systemic lupus erythematosus. By contrast, systemic autoimmune diseases appeared to be genuine but very rare complications of interferon alfa in chronic hepatitis C, with only one case of lupus-like syndrome and two cases of polyarthritis in a survey of 677 patients (18).

Other reports included seronegative polyarthritis, acute seronegative monoarthritis of the hip, and seropositive monoarthritis of the metatarsophalangeal of the right foot (SED-13, 1097).

Systemic lupus erythematosus has been reported in two patients given interferon alfa for chronic hepatitis C (363,368). However, it is not known whether this complication was coincidental or treatment-related.

Systemic sclerosis

Systemic sclerosis has been attributed to interferon alfa-2a (369).

- A 52-year-old woman received interferon alfa-2a for chronic myeloid leukemia and after about 2 years developed fever, dyspnea, and limb edema. The erythrocyte sedimentation rate was 50 mm/hour and pulmonary imaging showed pulmonary vascular congestion. She improved after interferon alfa withdrawal and administration of diuretics, but similar symptoms recurred 3 months later. She also had progressive thickening of the skin on the hands and wrists. There was diffuse parenchymal and interstitial fibrosis of the lungs, absence of peristalsis on esophagogastroduodenoscopy, renal impairment, and positive antisclero-70 antibodies. Capillaroscopy showed typical features of scleroderma. Based on these findings, a diagnosis of systemic sclerosis was suggested and she slowly improved over the next months with cyclophosphamide, prednisone, iloprost, and hydroxyurea.

This patient had the HLA-DR11 haplotype, which is associated with systemic sclerosis, and this suggests that interferon alfa may have triggered the autoimmune phenomenon.

Vasculitis with cryoglobulinemia

Interferon alfa can sometimes aggravate hepatitis C-related cryoglobulinemia.

- A fatal exacerbation of hepatitis C-related cryoglobulinemia, preceded by rapid deterioration of neurological status, massive upper gastrointestinal bleeding, and diffuse hemorrhagic gastritis with vasculitic changes on gastroscopy, has been reported within the first 3 weeks of interferon alfa treatment in a 51-year-old woman (370).

However, cryoglobulin-associated vasculitis is a recognized manifestation of hepatitis C infection. Reports of vasculitis in interferon alfa-treated patients should therefore be interpreted with caution (SED-13, 1095) (371). In addition, several isolated reports suggested that exacerbation of cryoglobulinemia might also be the result of interferon alfa treatment (SEDA-19, 337).

Interferon alfa and transplantation

A possibly deleterious effect of pre- or post-transplant interferon alfa therapy in transplant recipients has been emphasized by several studies and case reports. These point to a higher incidence or greater severity of graft-versus-host reactions in patients who have received an allogeneic bone marrow transplant (SED-13, 1097) (372,373), significant deterioration of renal function or an increased risk of glucocorticoid-resistant rejection in renal transplant patients (SED-13, 1097) (374), and a possibly increased risk of acute or chronic rejection in liver transplant patients (375,376). These findings are still the subject of debate, as the available data consist mainly of retrospective or poorly controlled studies with a limited number of patients (377,378). In addition, several other investigators have failed to identify any deleterious influence of interferon alfa treatment in transplant recipients (SEDA-21, 373) (SEDA-22, 403). This issue warrants further large scale, prospective, controlled studies.

Immunosuppressive effects

Isolated reports of *Candida* esophagitis or *Pneumocystis jiroveci* (*Pneumocystis carinii*) infections in immunocompetent patients and the possible decrease in CD4+ T cells with or without opportunistic infections in several HIV-infected patients (SED-13, 1097) (379) suggest that unexpected immunosuppressive effects of interferon alfa can occur. An autoimmune destruction of CD4 cells in patients with a particular HLA haplotype has been proposed as a possible mechanism (380). One patient also had an acute and fatal acute precipitation of infection with *Entamoeba histolytica* (SEDA-22, 403). However, the available evidence is still very limited and no firm conclusion can be drawn on a possible association between interferon alfa treatment and a fall in CD4 cell count or an immunosuppressive effect.

Two patients aged 38 and 54 years with hemodialysis-dependent end-stage renal insufficiency developed severe bacterial infections, osteomyelitis, and prostatitis, within 3 months of interferon alfa-2b treatment for hepatitis C virus infection (381).

Possible exacerbation of latent parasitic infection by interferon alfa has been reported (SEDA-22, 403).

- Two patients receiving interferon alfa plus ribavirin for chronic hepatitis C developed symptomatic strongyloidiasis within 2–3 weeks of treatment (382).

Because both drugs have immunomodulatory effects, it was not determined which one was the more likely cause.

Graft-versus-host disease

There are still uncertainties about the possible relation between interferon alfa and an increased incidence or severity of acute graft-versus-host disease after bone marrow transplantation. Late-onset, severe, atypical chronic graft-versus-host disease has been attributed to interferon alfa (383).

- A 44-year-old woman received interferon alfa 6 MU/day for relapse of chronic myeloid leukemia 7 years after successful bone marrow transplantation. About 2 years later, interferon alfa was withdrawn because of diffuse erythematous skin lesions with discoid lupus erythematosus on skin biopsy and severe dysphagia with esophagitis and pseudomembranes at endoscopy. Fever, bilateral pulmonary infiltrates, and respiratory distress syndrome subsequently developed, and she required mechanical ventilation. An open lung biopsy showed features of chronic pulmonary graft-versus-host disease. All her symptoms completely resolved with ciclosporin and corticosteroids. An infectious cause was ruled out.

In this case, the clinical presentation was compatible with typical chronic graft-versus-host disease. Whether interferon alfa induced or aggravated chronic graft-versus-host disease in this patient was an open question.

Death

There is a debate as to whether previous interferon alfa adversely affects the outcome of bone marrow transplantation in chronic myelogenous leukemia.

In a retrospective study of 153 patients who underwent bone-marrow transplantation for chronic myelogenous leukemia, pretransplant interferon alfa treatment for more than 12 months was associated with a significant increase in transplant-related mortality during the first 2 years when compared with patients who received pretransplant interferon alfa for less than 12 months (28 of 46 patients versus nine of 38) (384). This adverse outcome was also more frequent in patients who discontinued treatment less than 3 months before transplantation.

Of eight studies, five showed no harmful effect and three suggested an increased risk of post-transplant complications or mortality (SEDA-22, 403) (SEDA-23, 395).

The outcome of bone marrow transplantation in 152 patients (86 on interferon alfa, 66 on chemotherapy) included in two consecutive randomized trials, has been analysed prospectively (385). Whereas the duration of interferon alfa treatment did not influence the outcome of transplantation, there was a significant reduction in survival: the 5-year survival was 45% in the 50 patients who were still receiving interferon alfa within 3 months before bone marrow transplantation and 71% in the 36 patients who were not. According to the authors, interferon alfa should not be prescribed in patients who are likely candidates for early bone marrow transplantation.

Long-Term Effects

Tumorigenicity

Compared with untreated patients and patients treated with busulfan or hydroxyurea, interferon alfa produced a significantly higher frequency of clonal aberrant cytogenetic abnormalities and chronic clonal evolution in patients with chronic myeloid leukemia (386). However, the possible role of interferon alfa in the secondary occurrence of hematological malignancies is purely speculative. Only isolated cases of myeloproliferative syndrome, leukemia, or lymphoma have been attributed to interferon alfa (SED-13, 1098) (SEDA-20, 331) (SEDA-21, 373). There was no increased incidence of second cancers in patients treated for hairy cell leukemia (SEDA-20, 331).

Second-Generation Effects

Teratogenicity

In experimental models there has been no evidence of mutagenic or teratogenic effects of interferon alfa, and placental transfer is unlikely or very low (387). Immediately after delivery, interferon alfa concentrations in the breast milk or in the sera of two newborns were very low compared with maternal serum concentrations (388). Uncomplicated and successful pregnancies have been detailed in several patients treated for hematological malignancies or chronic hepatitis C, with interferon alfa exposure during the first trimester or even the whole of pregnancy (SED-13, 1098) (SEDA-20, 331) (389–392). In only three cases have premature delivery or moderate intrauterine growth retardation been observed, and any direct causal relation to interferon alfa treatment is doubtful. One report mentioned transient and moderate thrombocytopenia in a neonate born to a woman who had received interferon alfa throughout pregnancy (391).

Although no long-term follow-up is as yet available, clinical examination performed up to 2–3 years after delivery in at least seven babies has proved normal. Despite these reassuring data, the safety of interferon alfa during pregnancy still awaits further documentation, and it is advisable to delay therapy of non-life-threatening disease in pregnant women, especially during the first trimester.

Susceptibility Factors

Age

There is little information on the use of interferon alfa in children with chronic hepatitis C. In a review of 19 studies published between 1990 and 2000, there were data on only 366 treated children (105 untreated) and they suggested a higher rate of sustained response than in adults (393). Besides flu-like symptoms, reversible weight loss, neutropenia, and alopecia were the most commonly reported adverse events, but adverse events were not systematically recorded in these studies.

Although the anti-angiogenic effects of interferon alfa have been successfully used to treat severe hemangiomas in infants, the possibility of spastic diplegia is a matter of concern (SEDA-22, 404). Spastic diplegia developed in five of 26 infants during treatment, with possibly significant functional sequelae (394), and in one of 53 infants treated for a median of 51 weeks (395). Persistent, severe, spastic diplegia occurred after 1 year of treatment in a 5-month-old boy (396). Because the immature central nervous system of infants may be more susceptible to interferon alfa toxicity, it has been stressed that this treatment should be reserved for infants with life-threatening hemangiomas (397). That interferon alfa can play a role in the occurrence of this acute neurological complication has been further substantiated by the finding of abnormally high interferon serum concentrations in 45% of neonates with spontaneous cerebral palsy compared with control children (398).

Renal disease

High daily dosage or serum concentrations of interferon alfa may be associated with more frequent and more severe adverse effects during the treatment of chronic hepatitis C in hemodialysis patients. In one study, three of 10 hemodialysis patients had severe neurological adverse effects (generalized seizures or posterior leukoencephalopathy) (399). In another study, three of six patients receiving daily injections had to discontinue treatment because of depression, loss of consciousness, and persistent high-grade fever, while no serious adverse effects were reported in three other patients who received interferon alfa three times a week (400). In both studies, there were significant changes in interferon alfa pharmacokinetics (higher C_{max}, AUC, and half-life) in hemodialysis patients compared with patients with normal renal function, consistent with altered clearance of interferon alfa.

Drug Administration

Drug formulations

The FDA has expanded the indications for a combination product to include patients with chronic hepatitis C who have not been treated with interferon alfa. This product, Rebetron Combination Therapy (Schering), contains recombinant interferon alfa-2b for injection (Intron A) plus ribavirin (Rebetol) in capsules, and was previously only approved for patients who had relapsed after treatment with interferon alone (401). Serious adverse effects, such as depression, suicidal ideation, and suicide, have occurred with this regimen and patients should be closely monitored.

Drug administration route

The use of intraspinal interferon alfa (1 MU three times a week for 4 weeks) in 22 patients with neoplastic meningitis was associated with frequent adverse effects that mostly manifested as chronic fatigue syndrome in 91% of patients (severe in 45%) and arachnoiditis in 73% (severe in 9%) (402). Interferon alfa-induced immune dysregulation in an immunologically predisposed patient was suggested to account for this complication.

Drug–Drug Interactions

Alcohol

Even moderate but continuing alcohol consumption needs to be taken seriously in patients receiving interferon alfa, and exacerbation of previous acute alcohol hepatitis has been reported in two patients with chronic hepatitis C, despite reduced alcohol consumption (403). Liver transaminases subsequently normalized after withdrawal of interferon alfa in both patients.

Angiotensin-converting enzyme inhibitors

An increased risk of severe and early but reversible neutropenia has been found in patients taking angiotensin-converting enzyme inhibitors (enalapril and captopril) with interferon alfa (404).

Carmustine

Owing to its antineoplastic properties, interferon alfa is sometimes used with cytostatic drugs. In 275 patients randomized to receive radiation and carmustine either alone or with interferon alfa for high-grade glioma, there was no significant improvement in the overall survival and time to disease progression in those given interferon alfa, but a higher incidence of adverse effects, namely fever, chills, myalgia, lethargy, headache, and seizures (405).

13-Cisretinoic acid

The combination of interferon alfa with 13-*cis*-retinoic acid may have potentiated the occurrence of fatal radiation pneumonitis (SEDA-21, 374).

Clozapine

Agranulocytosis was observed when interferon alfa was given to a patient taking long-term clozapine (SEDA-22, 404), but this is a known risk of the latter.

Coumarin anticoagulants

There have been two reports of increased prothrombin time in patients taking warfarin or acenocoumarol (SEDA-19, 337) (SEDA-22, 374).

Cyclophosphamide

Depending on the timing of exposure, interferon alfa may adversely affect the pharmacokinetic and hematological effects of cyclophosphamide. In 10 patients with multiple myeloma, interferon alfa given 2 hours before cyclophosphamide infusion significantly reduced cyclophosphamide clearance and produced less exposure to its metabolite 4-hydroxycyclophosphamide compared with interferon administration 24 hours after cyclophosphamide (406). This resulted in a significantly greater fall in white blood cell count in patients who received interferon alfa after cyclophosphamide.

Erythropoietin

Reduced efficacy of human erythropoietin, requiring increased erythropoietin dosages, has been clearly documented in several patients receiving interferon alfa

(407–409), an effect that is probably mediated by interferon alfa-induced suppression of erythropoiesis.

5-Fluorouracil

One would expect drugs with myelosuppressive effects to exacerbate the hematological toxicity of interferon alfa. However, even though interferon alfa is increasingly used with other cytotoxic drugs, no specific and unexpected adverse effects have been reported, except for the combination of interferon alfa with 5-fluorouracil, which produced increased serum concentrations of fluorouracil and a significantly higher incidence of severe adverse effects, namely gastrointestinal and myelosuppressive adverse effects (410,411).

Melphalan

Interferon-induced fever has been thought to increase the cytotoxicity of melphalan (412).

Oral hypoglycemic drugs

There has been one report of hypoglycemia in a patient treated with metformin and chlorpropamide (SEDA-21, 374).

Paroxetine

It has been suggested that concomitant treatment with paroxetine may be a susceptibility factor for retinal damage by interferon alfa (82).

Phenazone (antipyrine)

Interferon alfa inhibits several hepatic microsomal cytochrome P_{450} enzymes in vitro and in vivo (SED-13, 1099) (20,413). However, repeated injections of interferon alfa produced conflicting results, with no change in salivary phenazone clearance (SED-13, 1099) (414).

Ribavirin

The combination of interferon alfa with ribavirin is one of the most promising treatments for chronic hepatitis C. However, two patients developed rapid and particularly severe anemia within 4 and 6 weeks of combined treatment (415). One patient required erythrocyte transfusions, and both recovered after withdrawal. The combination of pure red cell aplasia due to interferon alfa and hemolytic anemia due to ribavirin was suggested to have accounted for this possible interaction.

There was an increased incidence of adverse skin effects, mostly eczema, malar erythema, and lichenoid eruptions, in 33 patients who received combination of interferon alfa with ribavirin compared with 35 patients treated with interferon alfa alone (416).

Thalidomide

In 13 patients with metastatic renal cell carcinoma, the combination of interferon alfa-2a (27 MU/week) and thalidomide produced severe neurological toxicity in four patients, an incidence that was considered to be far greater than would be expected with either drug alone (417).

Theophylline

Interferon alfa inhibits several hepatic microsomal cytochrome P_{450} enzymes in vitro and in vivo (20) and reduces theophylline clearance (SED-13, 1099) (418–420).

Zidovudine

Synergistic hemotoxicity has sometimes resulted from the combination of interferon alfa with zidovudine in AIDS-associated Kaposi's sarcoma, but this regimen is considered to be relatively safe (421,422).

References

1. Keeffe EB, Hollinger FB. Therapy of hepatitis C: consensus interferon trials. Consensus Interferon Study Group. Hepatology 1997;26(3 Suppl 1):S101–7.
2. Davis GL. New schedules of interferon for chronic hepatitis C. J Hepatol 1999;31(Suppl 1):227–31.
3. Janssen HL, Gerken G, Carreno V, Marcellin P, Naoumov NV, Craxi A, Ring-Larsen H, Kitis G, van Hattum J, de Vries RA, Michielsen PP, ten Kate FJ, Hop WC, Heijtink RA, Honkoop P, Schalm SW. Interferon alfa for chronic hepatitis B infection: increased efficacy of prolonged treatment. The European Concerted Action on Viral Hepatitis (EUROHEP). Hepatology 1999;30(1):238–43.
4. Cotler SJ, Wartelle CF, Larson AM, Gretch DR, Jensen DM, Carithers RL Jr. Pretreatment symptoms and dosing regimen predict side-effects of interferon therapy for hepatitis C. J Viral Hepat 2000;7(3):211–17.
5. Kantarjian HM, O'Brien S, Smith TL, Rios MB, Cortes J, Beran M, Koller C, Giles FJ, Andreeff M, Kornblau S, Giralt S, Keating MJ, Talpaz M. Treatment of Philadelphia chromosome-positive early chronic phase chronic myelogenous leukemia with daily doses of interferon alpha and low-dose cytarabine. J Clin Oncol 1999;17(1):284–92.
6. Scott LJ, Perry CM. Interferon-alpha-2b plus ribavirin: a review of its use in the management of chronic hepatitis C. Drugs 2002;62(3):507–56.
7. San Miguel R, Guillen F, Cabases JM, Buti M. Meta-analysis: combination therapy with interferon-alpha 2a/2b and ribavirin for patients with chronic hepatitis C previously non-responsive to interferon. Aliment Pharmacol Ther 2002;16(9):1611–21.
8. Gaeta GB, Precone DF, Felaco FM, Bruno R, Spadaro A, Stornaiuolo G, Stanzione M, Ascione T, De Sena R, Campanone A, Filice G, Piccinino F. Premature discontinuation of interferon plus ribavirin for adverse effects: a multicentre survey in "real world" patients with chronic hepatitis C. Aliment Pharmacol Ther 2002;16(9):1633–9.
9. Ascione A, De Luca M, Di Costanzo GG, Picciotto FP, Lanza AG, Canestrini C, Morisco F, Tuccillo C, Caporaso N. Incidence of side effects during therapy with different types of alpha interferon: a randomised controlled trial comparing recombinant alpha 2b versus leukocyte interferon in the therapy of naive patients with chronic hepatitis C. Curr Pharm Des 2002;8(11):977–80.
10. Manns MP, McHutchison JG, Gordon SC, Rustgi VK, Shiffman M, Reindollar R, Goodman ZD, Koury K, Ling M, Albrecht JK. Peginterferon alfa-2b plus ribavirin compared with interferon alfa-2b plus ribavirin for initial treatment of chronic hepatitis C: a randomised trial. Lancet 2001;358(9286):958–65.
11. Heathcote EJ, Shiffman ML, Cooksley WG, Dusheiko GM, Lee SS, Balart L, Reindollar R, Reddy RK, Wright TL,

Lin A, Hoffman J, De Pamphilis J. Peginterferon alfa-2a in patients with chronic hepatitis C and cirrhosis. N Engl J Med 2000;343(23):1673–80.

12. Zeuzem S, Feinman SV, Rasenack J, Heathcote EJ, Lai MY, Gane E, O'Grady J, Reichen J, Diago M, Lin A, Hoffman J, Brunda MJ. Peginterferon alfa-2a in patients with chronic hepatitis C. N Engl J Med 2000;343(23):1666–72.
13. Wiselka MJ, Nicholson KG, Kent J, Cookson JB, Tyrrell DA. Prophylactic intranasal alpha 2 interferon and viral exacerbations of chronic respiratory disease. Thorax 1991;46(10):706–11.
14. Saracco G, Rizzetto M. A practical guide to the use of interferons in the management of hepatitis virus infections. Drugs 1997;53(1):74–85.
15. Poynard T, Leroy V, Cohard M, Thevenot T, Mathurin P, Opolon P, Zarski JP. Meta-analysis of interferon randomized trials in the treatment of viral hepatitis C: effects of dose and duration. Hepatology 1996;24(4):778–89.
16. Fattovich G, Giustina G, Favarato S, Ruol A. A survey of adverse events in 11,241 patients with chronic viral hepatitis treated with alfa interferon. J Hepatol 1996;24(1):38–47.
17. De Sanctis GM, D'Errico DAF, Leonetti G, et al. Occurrence of major side effects in patients with chronic viral liver disease treated with interferons. Mediter J Infect Parasit Dis 1995;10:225–30.
18. Okanoue T, Sakamoto S, Itoh Y, Minami M, Yasui K, Sakamoto M, Nishioji K, Katagishi T, Nakagawa Y, Tada H, Sawa Y, Mizuno M, Kagawa K, Kashima K. Side effects of high-dose interferon therapy for chronic hepatitis C. J Hepatol 1996;25(3):283–91.
19. Iorio R, Pensati P, Botta S, Moschella S, Impagliazzo N, Vajro P, Vegnente A. Side effects of alpha-interferon therapy and impact on health-related quality of life in children with chronic viral hepatitis. Pediatr Infect Dis J 1997;16(10):984–90.
20. Vial T, Descotes J. Clinical toxicity of the interferons. Drug Saf 1994;10(2):115–50.
21. Vial T, Bailly F, Descotes J, Trepo C. Effets secondaires de l'interféron alpha. [Side effects of interferon-alpha.] Gastroenterol Clin Biol 1996;20(5):462–89.
22. Cacopardo B, Benanti F, Brancati G, Romano F, Nunnari A. Leucocyte interferon-alpha retreatment for chronic hepatitis C patients previously intolerant to other interferons. J Viral Hepat 1998;5(5):333–9.
23. Sonnenblick M, Rosin A. Cardiotoxicity of interferon. A review of 44 cases. Chest 1991;99(3):557–61.
24. Kruit WH, Punt KJ, Goey SH, de Mulder PH, van Hoogenhuyze DC, Henzen-Logmans SC, Stoter G. Cardiotoxicity as a dose-limiting factor in a schedule of high dose bolus therapy with interleukin-2 and alpha-interferon. An unexpectedly frequent complication. Cancer 1994;74(10):2850–6.
25. Angulo MP, Navajas A, Galdeano JM, Astigarraga I, Fernandez-Teijeiro A. Reversible cardiomyopathy secondary to alpha-interferon in an infant. Pediatr Cardiol 1999;20(4):293–4.
26. Kadayifci A, Aytemir K, Arslan M, Aksoyek S, Sivri B, Kabakci G. Interferon-alpha does not cause significant cardiac dysfunction in patients with chronic active hepatitis. Liver 1997;17(2):99–102.
27. Sartori M, Andorno S, La Terra G, Pozzoli G, Rudoni M, Sacchetti GM, Inglese E, Aglietta M. Assessment of interferon cardiotoxicity with quantitative radionuclide angiocardiography. Eur J Clin Invest 1995;25(1):68–70.
28. Kuwata A, Ohashi M, Sugiyama M, Ueda R, Dohi Y. A case of reversible dilated cardiomyopathy after alpha-interferon therapy in a patient with renal cell carcinoma. Am J Med Sci 2002;324(6):331–4.
29. Colivicchi F, Magnanimi S, Sebastiani F, Silvestri R, Magnanimi R. Incidence of electrocardiographic abnormalities during treatment with human leukocyte interferon-alfa in patients with chronic hepatitis C but without pre-existing cardiovascular disease. Curr Ther Res Clin Exp 1998;59:692–6.
30. Parrens E, Chevalier JM, Rougier M, Douard H, Labbe L, Quiniou G, Broustet A, Broustet JP. Apparition d'un bloc auriculo-ventriculaire du troisième degré sous interféron alpha: à propos d'un cas. [Third degree atrio-ventricular block induced by interferon alpha. Report of a case.] Arch Mal Coeur Vaiss 1999;92(1):53–6.
31. Creutzig A, Caspary L, Freund M. The Raynaud phenomenon and interferon therapy. Ann Intern Med 1996;125(5):423.
32. Schapira D, Nahir AM, Hadad N. Interferon-induced Raynaud's syndrome. Semin Arthritis Rheum 2002;32(3):157–62.
33. Iorio R, Spagnuolo MI, Sepe A, Zoccali S, Alessio M, Vegnente A. Severe Raynaud's phenomenon with chronic hepatis C disease treated with interferon. Pediatr Infect Dis J 2003;22(2):195–7.
34. Cid MC, Hernandez-Rodriguez J, Robert J, del Rio A, Casademont J, Coll-Vinent B, Grau JM, Kleinman HK, Urbano-Marquez A, Cardellach F. Interferon-alpha may exacerbate cryoblobulinemia-related ischemic manifestations: an adverse effect potentially related to its anti-angiogenic activity. Arthritis Rheum 1999;42(5):1051–5.
35. Mirro J Jr, Kalwinsky D, Whisnant J, Weck P, Chesney C, Murphy S. Coagulopathy induced by continuous infusion of high doses of human lymphoblastoid interferon. Cancer Treat Rep 1985;69(3):315–17.
36. Durand JM, Quiles N, Kaplanski G, Soubeyrand J. Thrombosis and recombinant interferon-alpha. Am J Med 1993;95(1):115–16.
37. Becker JC, Winkler B, Klingert S, Brocker EB. Antiphospholipid syndrome associated with immunotherapy for patients with melanoma. Cancer 1994;73(6): 1621–4.
38. Karim A, Ahmed S, Khan A, Steinberg H, Mattana J. Interstitial pneumonitis in a patient treated with alpha-interferon and ribavirin for hepatitis C infection. Am J Med Sci 2001;322(4):233–5.
39. Chin K, Tabata C, Sataka N, Nagai S, Moriyasu F, Kuno K. Pneumonitis associated with natural and recombinant interferon alfa therapy for chronic hepatitis C. Chest 1994;105(3):939–41.
40. Ishizaki T, Sasaki F, Ameshima S, Shiozaki K, Takahashi H, Abe Y, Ito S, Kuriyama M, Nakai T, Kitagawa M. Pneumonitis during interferon and/or herbal drug therapy in patients with chronic active hepatitis. Eur Respir J 1996;9(12):2691–6.
41. Ogata K, Koga T, Yagawa K. Interferon-related bronchiolitis obliterans organizing pneumonia. Chest 1994;106(2): 612–13.
42. Kumar AS, Russo MW, Esposito S, Borczuk A, Jacobson I, Brown M, Brown RS. Severe pulmonary toxicity of interferon and ribavirin therapy in chronic hepatitis C. Am J Gastroenterol 2001;96(Suppl):127.
43. Patel M, Ezzat W, Pauw KL, Lowsky R. Bronchiolitis obliterans organizing pneumonia in a patient with chronic myelogenous leukemia developing after initiation of interferon and cytosine arabinoside. Eur J Haematol 2001;67 (5–6): 318–21.
44. Anderson P, Hoglund M, Rodjer S. Pulmonary side effects of interferon-alpha therapy in patients with hematological malignancies. Am J Hematol 2003;73(1):54–8.
45. Kumar KS, Russo MW, Borczuk AC, Brown M, Esposito SP, Lobritto SJ, Jacobson IM, Brown RS Jr.

Significant pulmonary toxicity associated with interferon and ribavirin therapy for hepatitis C. Am J Gastroenterol 2002;97(9):2432–40.
46. Bini EJ, Weinshel EH. Severe exacerbation of asthma: a new side effect of interferon-alpha in patients with asthma and chronic hepatitis C. Mayo Clin Proc 1999;74(4):367–70.
47. Pileire G, Leclerc P, Hermant P, Meeus E, Camus P. Toux chronique isolée pendant un traitement par interféron. [Isolated chronic cough during interferon therapy.] Presse Méd 1999;28(17):913.
48. Takeda A, Ikegame K, Kimura Y, Ogawa H, Kanazawa S, Nakamura H. Pleural effusion during interferon treatment for chronic hepatitis C. Hepatogastroenterology 2000;47(35):1431–5.
49. Fruehauf S, Steiger S, Topaly J, Ho AD. Pulmonary artery hypertension during interferon-alpha therapy for chronic myelogenous leukemia. Ann Hematol 2001;80(5):308–10.
50. Boonyapisit K, Katirji B. Severe exacerbation of hepatitis C-associated vasculitic neuropathy following treatment with interferon alpha: a case report and literature review. Muscle Nerve 2002;25(6):909–13.
51. Tambini R, Quattrini A, Fracassetti O, Nemni R. Axonal neuropathy in a patient receiving interferon-alpha therapy for chronic hepatitis C. J Rheumatol 1997;24(8):1656–7.
52. Maeda M, Ohkoshi N, Hisahara S, Mizusawa H, Shoji S. [Mononeuropathy multiplex in a patient receiving interferon alpha therapy for chronic hepatitis C.] Rinsho Shinkeigaku 1995;35(9):1048–50.
53. Jaubert D, Hauteville D, Pelissier JF, Muzellec Y. Neuropathie periphérique au cours d'un traitement par interféron alpha. [Peripheral neuropathy during interferon alpha therapy.] Presse Méd 1991;20(5):221–2.
54. Purvin VA. Anterior ischemic optic neuropathy secondary to interferon alfa. Arch Ophthalmol 1995;113(8):1041–4.
55. Read SJ, Crawford DH, Pender MP. Trigeminal sensory neuropathy induced by interferon-alpha therapy. Aust NZ J Med 1995;25(1):54.
56. Bernsen PL, Wong Chung RE, Vingerhoets HM, Janssen JT. Bilateral neuralgic amyotrophy induced by interferon treatment. Arch Neurol 1988;45(4):449–51.
57. Loh FL, Herskovitz S, Berger AR, Swerdlow ML. Brachial plexopathy associated with interleukin-2 therapy. Neurology 1992;42(2):462–3.
58. Merimsky O, Reider I, Merimsky E, Chaitchik S. Interferon-related leukoencephalopathy in a patient with renal cell carcinoma. Tumori 1991;77(4):361–2.
59. Ogundipe O, Smith M. Bell's palsy during interferon therapy for chronic hepatitis C infection in patients with haemorrhagic disorders. Haemophilia 2000;6(2):110–12.
60. Hwang I, Calvit TB, Cash BD, Holtzmuller KC. Bell's palsy. A rare complication of interferon therapy for hepatitis C. Am J Gastroenterol 2002;87(Suppl):207–8.
61. Anthoney DA, Bone I, Evans TR. Inflammatory demyelinating polyneuropathy: a complication of immunotherapy in malignant melanoma. Ann Oncol 2000;11(9):1197–200.
62. Meriggioli MN, Rowin J. Chronic inflammatory demyelinating polyneuropathy after treatment with interferon-alpha. Muscle Nerve 2000;23(3):433–5.
63. Kataoka I, Shinagawa K, Shiro Y, Okamoto S, Watanabe R, Mori T, Ito D, Harada M. Multiple sclerosis associated with interferon-alpha therapy for chronic myelogenous leukemia. Am J Hematol 2002;70(2):149–53.
64. Sunami M, Nishikawa T, Yorogi A, Shimoda M. Intravenous administration of levodopa ameliorated a refractory akathisia case induced by interferon-alpha. Clin Neuropharmacol 2000;23(1):59–61.
65. Horikawa N, Yamazaki T, Sagawa M, Nagata T. A case of akathisia during interferon-alpha therapy for chronic hepatitis type C. Gen Hosp Psychiatry 1999;21(2):134–5.
66. Moulignier A, Allo S, Zittoun R, Gout O. Recombinant interferon-alpha-induced chorea and frontal subcortical dementia. Neurology 2002;58(2):328–30.
67. Hibi H, Itoh K, Kamiya T, Yamada Y, Shimoji T. [Grand mal like attack by interferon injection in case of renal cell carcinoma.] Hinyokika Kiyo 1991;37(1):69–72.
68. Janssen HL, Berk L, Vermeulen M, Schalm SW. Seizures associated with low-dose alpha-interferon. Lancet 1990;336(8730):1580.
69. Miller VS, Zwiener RJ, Fielman BA. Interferon-associated refractory status epilepticus. Pediatrics 1994;93(3):511–12.
70. Shakil AO, Di Bisceglie AM, Hoofnagle JH. Seizures during alpha interferon therapy. J Hepatol 1996;24(1):48–51.
71. Woynarowski M, Socha J. Seizures in children during interferon alpha therapy. J Hepatol 1997;26(4):956–7.
72. Ameen M, Russell-Jones R. Seizures associated with interferon-alpha treatment of cutaneous malignancies. Br J Dermatol 1999;141(2):386–7.
73. Seno H, Inagaki T, Itoga M, Miyaoka T, Ishino H. A case of seizures 1 week after the cessation of interferon-alpha therapy. Psychiatry Clin Neurosci 1999;53(3):417–20.
74. Brouwers PJ, Bosker RJ, Schaafsma MR, Wilts G, Neef C. Photosensitive seizures associated with interferon alfa-2a. Ann Pharmacother 1999;33(1):113–14.
75. Kamei S, Tanaka N, Mastuura M, Arakawa Y, Kojima T, Matsukawa Y, Takasu T, Moriyama M. Blinded, prospective, and serial evaluation by quantitative-EEG in interferon-alpha-treated hepatitis-C. Acta Neurol Scand 1999;100(1):25–33.
76. Borgia G, Reynaud L, Gentile I, Cerini R, Ciampi R, Dello Russo M, Piazza M. Myasthenia gravis during low-dose IFN-alpha therapy for chronic hepatitis C. J Interferon Cytokine Res 2001;21(7):469–70.
77. Weegink CJ, Chamuleau RA, Reesink HW, Molenaar DS. Development of myasthenia gravis during treatment of chronic hepatitis C with interferon-alpha and ribavirin. J Gastroenterol 2001;36(10):723–4.
78. Guyer DR, Tiedeman J, Yannuzzi LA, Slakter JS, Parke D, Kelley J, Tang RA, Marmor M, Abrams G, Miller JW, et al. Interferon-associated retinopathy. Arch Ophthalmol 1993;111(3):350–6.
79. Hayasaka S, Fujii M, Yamamoto Y, Noda S, Kurome H, Sasaki M. Retinopathy and subconjunctival haemorrhage in patients with chronic viral hepatitis receiving interferon alfa. Br J Ophthalmol 1995;79(2):150–2.
80. Kawano T, Shigehira M, Uto H, Nakama T, Kato J, Hayashi K, Maruyama T, Kuribayashi T, Chuman T, Futami T, Tsubouchi H. Retinal complications during interferon therapy for chronic hepatitis C. Am J Gastroenterol 1996;91(2):309–13.
81. Soushi S, Kobayashi F, Obazawa H, Kigasawa K, Shiraishi K, Itakura M, Matsuzaki S. [Evaluation of risk factors of interferon-associated retinopathy in patients with type C chronic active hepatitis.] Nippon Ganka Gakkai Zasshi 1996;100(1):69–76.
82. Hejny C, Sternberg P, Lawson DH, Greiner K, Aaberg TM Jr. Retinopathy associated with high-dose interferon alfa-2b therapy. Am J Ophthalmol 2001;131(6):782–7.
83. Jain K, Lam WC, Waheeb S, Thai Q, Heathcote J. Retinopathy in chronic hepatitis C patients during interferon treatment with ribavirin. Br J Ophthalmol 2001;85(10):1171–3.
84. Saito H, Ebinuma H, Nagata H, Inagaki Y, Saito Y, Wakabayashi K, Takagi T, Nakamura M, Katsura H, Oguchi Y, Ishii H. Interferon-associated retinopathy in a uniform regimen of natural interferon-alpha therapy for chronic hepatitis C. Liver 2001;21(3):192–7.
85. Hayasaka S, Nagaki Y, Matsumoto M, Sato S. Interferon associated retinopathy. Br J Ophthalmol 1998;82(3):323–5.

86. Kadayifcilar S, Boyacioglu S, Kart H, Gursoy M, Aydin P. Ocular complications with high-dose interferon alpha in chronic active hepatitis. Eye 1999;13(Pt 2):241–6.
87. Sugano S, Suzuki T, Watanabe M, Ohe K, Ishii K, Okajima T. Retinal complications and plasma C5a levels during interferon alpha therapy for chronic hepatitis C. Am J Gastroenterol 1998;93(12):2441–4.
88. Sugano S, Yanagimoto M, Suzuki T, Sato M, Onmura H, Aizawa H, Makino H. Retinal complications with elevated circulating plasma C5a associated with interferon-alpha therapy for chronic active hepatitis C. Am J Gastroenterol 1994;89(11):2054–6.
89. Ene L, Gehenot M, Horsmans Y, Detry-Morel M, Geubel AP. Transient blurred vision after interferon for chronic hepatitis C. Lancet 1994;344(8925):827–8.
90. Yamada H, Mizobuchi K, Isogai Y. Acute onset of ocular complications with interferon. Lancet 1994;343(8902): 914.
91. Lohmann CP, Kroher G, Bogenrieder T, Spiegel D, Preuner J. Severe loss of vision during adjuvant interferon alfa-2b treatment for malignant melanoma. Lancet 1999;353(9161):1326.
92. Perlemuter G, Bodaghi B, Le Hoang P, Izem C, Buffet C, Wechsler B, Piette JC, Cacoub P. Visual loss during interferon-alpha therapy in hepatitis C virus infection. J Hepatol 2002;37(5):701–2.
93. Gupta R, Singh S, Tang R, Blackwell TA, Schiffman JS. Anterior ischemic optic neuropathy caused by interferon alpha therapy. Am J Med 2002;112(8):683–4.
94. Manesis EK, Petrou C, Brouzas D, Hadziyannis S. Optic tract neuropathy complicating low-dose interferon treatment. J Hepatol 1994;21(3):474–7.
95. Merimsky O, Nisipeanu P, Loewenstein A, Reider-Groswasser I, Chaitchik S. Interferon-related cortical blindness. Cancer Chemother Pharmacol 1992;29(4):329–30.
96. Fukumoto Y, Shigemitsu T, Kajii N, Omura R, Harada T, Okita K. Abducent nerve paralysis during interferon alpha-2a therapy in a case of chronic active hepatitis C. Intern Med 1994;33(10):637–40.
97. Bauherz G, Soeur M, Lustman F. Oculomotor nerve paralysis induced by alpha II-interferon. Acta Neurol Belg 1990;90(2):111–14.
98. Fossa SD. Is interferon with or without vinblastine the "treatment of choice" in metastatic renal cell carcinoma? The Norwegian Radium Hospital's experience 1983–1986. Semin Surg Oncol 1988;4(3):178–83.
99. Cadoni G, Marinelli L, De Santis A, Romito A, Manna R, Ottaviani F. Sudden hearing loss in a patient hepatitis C virus (HCV) positive on therapy with alpha-interferon: a possible autoimmune-microvascular pathogenesis. J Laryngol Otol 1998;112(10):962–3.
100. Kraus I, Vitezic D. Anosmia induced with alpha interferon in a patient with chronic hepatitis C. Int J Clin Pharmacol Ther 2000;38(7):360–1.
101. Schaefer M, Engelbrecht MA, Gut O, Fiebich BL, Bauer J, Schmidt F, Grunze H, Lieb K. Interferon alpha (IFNalpha) and psychiatric syndromes: a review. Prog Neuropsychopharmacol Biol Psychiatry 2002;26(4):731–46.
102. Van Gool AR, Kruit WH, Engels FK, Stoter G, Bannink M, Eggermont AM. Neuropsychiatric side effects of interferon-alfa therapy. Pharm World Sci 2003;25(1):11–20.
103. Smith A, Tyrrell D, Coyle K, Higgins P. Effects of interferon alpha on performance in man: a preliminary report. Psychopharmacology (Berl) 1988;96(3):414–16.
104. Meyers CA, Valentine AD. Neurological and psychiatric adverse effects of immunological therapy. CNS Drugs 1995;3:56–68.
105. James CW, Savini CJ. Homicidal ideation secondary to interferon. Ann Pharmacother 2001;35(7–8):962–3.
106. Greenberg DB, Jonasch E, Gadd MA, Ryan BF, Everett JR, Sober AJ, Mihm MA, Tanabe KK, Ott M, Haluska FG. Adjuvant therapy of melanoma with interferon-alpha-2b is associated with mania and bipolar syndromes. Cancer 2000;89(2):356–62.
107. Monji A, Yoshida I, Tashiro K, Hayashi Y, Tashiro N. A case of persistent manic depressive illness induced by interferon-alfa in the treatment of chronic hepatitis C. Psychosomatics 1998;39(6):562–4.
108. Hosoda S, Takimura H, Shibayama M, Kanamura H, Ikeda K, Kumada H. Psychiatric symptoms related to interferon therapy for chronic hepatitis C: clinical features and prognosis. Psychiatry Clin Neurosci 2000;54(5): 565–72.
109. Schafer M, Boetsch T, Laakmann G. Psychosis in a methadone-substituted patient during interferon-alpha treatment of hepatitis C. Addiction 2000;95(7):1101–4.
110. Mayr N, Zeitlhofer J, Deecke L, Fritz E, Ludwig H, Gisslinger H. Neurological function during long-term therapy with recombinant interferon alpha. J Neuropsychiatry Clin Neurosci 1999;11(3):343–8.
111. Rohatiner AZ, Prior PF, Burton AC, Smith AT, Balkwill FR, Lister TA. Central nervous system toxicity of interferon. Br J Cancer 1983;47(3):419–22.
112. Scalori A, Apale P, Panizzuti F, Mascoli N, Pioltelli P, Pozzi M, Redaelli A, Roffi L, Mancia G. Depression during interferon therapy for chronic viral hepatitis: early identification of patients at risk by means of a computerized test. Eur J Gastroenterol Hepatol 2000;12(5):505–9.
113. Dieperink E, Willenbring M, Ho SB. Neuropsychiatric symptoms associated with hepatitis C and interferon alpha: A review. Am J Psychiatry 2000;157(6):867–76.
114. Zdilar D, Franco-Bronson K, Buchler N, Locala JA, Younossi ZM. Hepatitis C, interferon alfa, and depression. Hepatology 2000;31(6):1207–11.
115. Renault PF, Hoofnagle JH, Park Y, Mullen KD, Peters M, Jones DB, Rustgi V, Jones EA. Psychiatric complications of long-term interferon alfa therapy. Arch Intern Med 1987;147(9):1577–80.
116. Prasad S, Waters B, Hill PB, et al. Psychiatric side effects of interferon alpha-2b in patients treated for hepatitis C. Clin Res 1992;40:840A.
117. Bonaccorso S, Marino V, Biondi M, Grimaldi F, Ippoliti F, Maes M. Depression induced by treatment with interferon-alpha in patients affected by hepatitis C virus. J Affect Disord 2002;72(3):237–41.
118. Dieperink E, Ho SB, Thuras P, Willenbring ML. A prospective study of neuropsychiatric symptoms associated with interferon-alpha-2b and ribavirin therapy for patients with chronic hepatitis C. Psychosomatics 2003;44(2):104–12.
119. Hauser P, Khosla J, Aurora H, Laurin J, Kling MA, Hill J, Gulati M, Thornton AJ, Schultz RL, Valentine AD, Meyers CA, Howell CD. A prospective study of the incidence and open-label treatment of interferon-induced major depressive disorder in patients with hepatitis C. Mol Psychiatry 2002;7(9):942–7.
120. Horikawa N, Yamazaki T, Izumi N, Uchihara M. Incidence and clinical course of major depression in patients with chronic hepatitis type C undergoing interferon-alpha therapy: a prospective study. Gen Hosp Psychiatry 2003;25(1):34–8.
121. Janssen HL, Brouwer JT, van der Mast RC, Schalm SW. Suicide associated with alfa-interferon therapy for chronic viral hepatitis. J Hepatol 1994;21(2):241–3.
122. Rifflet H, Vuillemin E, Oberti F, Duverger P, Laine P, Garre JB, Cales P. Pulsions suicidaires chez des malades atteints d'hépatite chronique C au cours ou au décours du traitement par l'interféron alpha. [Suicidal impulses in

patients with chronic viral hepatitis C during or after therapy with interferon alpha.] Gastroenterol Clin Biol 1998;22(3):353–7.
123. Valentine AD, Meyers CA, Kling MA, Richelson E, Hauser P. Mood and cognitive side effects of interferon-alpha therapy. Semin Oncol 1998;25(1 Suppl 1):39–47.
124. Adams F, Quesada JR, Gutterman JU. Neuropsychiatric manifestations of human leukocyte interferon therapy in patients with cancer. JAMA 1984;252(7):938–41.
125. Bocci V. Central nervous system toxicity of interferons and other cytokines. J Biol Regul Homeost Agents 1988;2(3):107–18.
126. Prior TI, Chue PS. Psychotic depression occurring after stopping interferon-alpha. J Clin Psychopharmacol 1999;19(4):385–6.
127. Capuron L, Ravaud A. Prediction of the depressive effects of interferon alfa therapy by the patient's initial affective state. N Engl J Med 1999;340(17):1370.
128. McDonald EM, Mann AH, Thomas HC. Interferons as mediators of psychiatric morbidity. An investigation in a trial of recombinant alpha-interferon in hepatitis-B carriers. Lancet 1987;2(8569):1175–8.
129. Pavol MA, Meyers CA, Rexer JL, Valentine AD, Mattis PJ, Talpaz M. Pattern of neurobehavioral deficits associated with interferon alfa therapy for leukemia. Neurology 1995;45(5):947–50.
130. Poutiainen E, Hokkanen L, Niemi ML, Farkkila M. Reversible cognitive decline during high-dose alpha-interferon treatment. Pharmacol Biochem Behav 1994; 47(4):901–5.
131. Licinio J, Kling MA, Hauser P. Cytokines and brain function: relevance to interferon-alpha-induced mood and cognitive changes. Semin Oncol 1998;25(1 Suppl 1):30–8.
132. Bonaccorso S, Marino V, Puzella A, Pasquini M, Biondi M, Artini M, Almerighi C, Verkerk R, Meltzer H, Maes M. Increased depressive ratings in patients with hepatitis C receiving interferon-alpha-based immunotherapy are related to interferon-alpha-induced changes in the serotonergic system. J Clin Psychopharmacol 2002; 22(1):86–90.
133. Gleason OC, Yates WR, Isbell MD, Philipsen MA. An open-label trial of citalopram for major depression in patients with hepatitis C. J Clin Psychiatry 2002;63(3): 194–8.
134. Kraus MR, Schafer A, Faller H, Csef H, Scheurlen M. Paroxetine for the treatment of interferon-alpha-induced depression in chronic hepatitis C. Aliment Pharmacol Ther 2002;16(6):1091–9.
135. Pariante CM, Landau S, Carpiniello B; Cagliari Group. Interferon alfa-induced adverse effects in patients with a psychiatric diagnosis. N Engl J Med 2002; 347(2):148–9.
136. Hensley ML, Peterson B, Silver RT, Larson RA, Schiffer CA, Szatrowski TP. Risk factors for severe neuropsychiatric toxicity in patients receiving interferon alfa-2b and low-dose cytarabine for chronic myelogenous leukemia: analysis of Cancer and Leukemia Group B 9013. J Clin Oncol 2000;18(6):1301–8.
137. Van Thiel DH, Friedlander L, Molloy PJ, Fagiuoli S, Kania RJ, Caraceni P. Interferon-alpha can be used successfully in patients with hepatitis C virus-positive chronic hepatitis who have a psychiatric illness. Eur J Gastroenterol Hepatol 1995;7(2):165–8.
138. Adams F, Fernandez F, Mavligit G. Interferon-induced organic mental disorders associated with unsuspected pre-existing neurologic abnormalities. J Neurooncol 1988;6(4):355–9.
139. Meyers CA, Obbens EA, Scheibel RS, Moser RP. Neurotoxicity of intraventricularly administered alpha-interferon for leptomeningeal disease. Cancer 1991;68(1):88–92.
140. Hagberg H, Blomkvist E, Ponten U, Persson L, Muhr C, Eriksson B, Oberg K, Olsson Y, Lilja A. Does alpha-interferon in conjunction with radiotherapy increase the risk of complications in the central nervous system? Ann Oncol 1990;1(6):449.
141. Laaksonen R, Niiranen A, Iivanainen M, Mattson K, Holsti L, Farkkila M, Cantell K. Dementia-like, largely reversible syndrome after cranial irradiation and prolonged interferon treatment. Ann Clin Res 1988;20(3):201–3.
142. Mitsuyama Y, Hashiguchi H, Murayama T, Koono M, Nishi S. An autopsied case of interferon encephalopathy. Jpn J Psychiatry Neurol 1992;46(3):741–8.
143. Mulder RT, Ang M, Chapman B, Ross A, Stevens IF, Edgar C. Interferon treatment is not associated with a worsening of psychiatric symptoms in patients with hepatitis C. J Gastroenterol Hepatol 2000;15(3):300–3.
144. Pariante CM, Orru MG, Baita A, Farci MG, Carpiniello B. Treatment with interferon-alpha in patients with chronic hepatitis and mood or anxiety disorders. Lancet 1999;354(9173):131–2.
145. Castera L, Zigante F, Bastie A, Buffet C, Dhumeaux D, Hardy P. Incidence of interferon alfa-induced depression in patients with chronic hepatitis C. Hepatology 2002;35(4):978–9.
146. Valentine AD. Managing the neuropsychiatric adverse effects of interferon treatment. BioDrugs 1999;11:229–37.
147. Miller A, Musselman D, Pena S, Su C, Pearce B, Nemeroff C. Pretreatment with the antidepressant paroxetine, prevents cytokine-induced depression during IFN-alpha therapy for malignant melanoma. Neuroimmunomodulation 1999;6:237.
148. Musselman DL, Lawson DH, Gumnick JF, Manatunga AK, Penna S, Goodkin RS, Greiner K, Nemeroff CB, Miller AH. Paroxetine for the prevention of depression induced by high-dose interferon alfa. N Engl J Med 2001;344(13):961–6.
149. McAllister-Williams RH, Young AH, Menkes DB. Antidepressant response reversed by interferon. Br J Psychiatry 2000;176:93.
150. Del Monte P, Bernasconi D, De Conca V, Randazzo M, Meozzi M, Badaracco B, Mesiti S, Marugo M. Endocrine evaluation in patients treated with interferon-alpha for chronic hepatitis C. Horm Res 1995;44(3):105–9.
151. Muller H, Hiemke C, Hammes E, Hess G. Sub-acute effects of interferon-alpha 2 on adrenocorticotrophic hormone, cortisol, growth hormone and prolactin in humans. Psychoneuroendocrinology 1992;17(5):459–65.
152. Crockett DM, McCabe BF, Lusk RP, Mixon JH. Side effects and toxicity of interferon in the treatment of recurrent respiratory papillomatosis. Ann Otol Rhinol Laryngol 1987;96(5):601–7.
153. Gottrand F, Michaud L, Guimber D, Ategbo S, Dubar G, Turck D, Farriaux JP. Influence of recombinant interferon alpha on nutritional status and growth pattern in children with chronic viral hepatitis. Eur J Pediatr 1996;155(12):1031–4.
154. Farkkila AM, Iivanainen MV, Farkkila MA. Disturbance of the water and electrolyte balance during high-dose interferon treatment. J Interferon Res 1990;10(2):221–7.
155. Fentiman IS, Balkwill FR, Thomas BS, Russell MJ, Todd I, Bottazzo GF. An autoimmune aetiology for hypothyroidism following interferon therapy for breast cancer. Eur J Cancer Clin Oncol 1988;24(8):1299–303.
156. Vial T, Descotes J. Immune-mediated side-effects of cytokines in humans. Toxicology 1995;105(1):31–57.
157. Fortis A, Christopoulos C, Chrysadakou E, Anevlavis E. De Quervain's thyroiditis associated with interferon-

alpha-2b therapy for non-Hodgkin's lymphoma. Clin Drug Invest 1998;16:473–5.
158. Ghilardi G, Gonvers JJ, So A. Hypothyroid myopathy as a complication of interferon alpha therapy for chronic hepatitis C virus infection. Br J Rheumatol 1998;37(12):1349–51.
159. Schmitt K, Hompesch BC, Oeland K, von Staehr WG, Thurmann PA. Autoimmune thyroiditis and myelosuppression following treatment with interferon-alpha for hepatitis C. Int J Clin Pharmacol Ther 1999;37(4):165–7.
160. Papo T, Oksenhendler E, Izembart M, Leger A, Clauvel JP. Antithyroid hormone antibodies induced by interferon-alpha. J Clin Endocrinol Metab 1992;75(6): 1484–6.
161. Wong V, Fu AX, George J, Cheung NW. Thyrotoxicosis induced by alpha-interferon therapy in chronic viral hepatitis. Clin Endocrinol (Oxf) 2002;56(6):793–8.
162. Carella C, Mazziotti G, Morisco F, Manganella G, Rotondi M, Tuccillo C, Sorvillo F, Caporaso N, Amato G. Long-term outcome of interferon-alpha-induced thyroid autoimmunity and prognostic influence of thyroid autoantibody pattern at the end of treatment. J Clin Endocrinol Metab 2001;86(5):1925–9.
163. Binaghi M, Levy C, Douvin C, Guittard M, Soubrane G, Coscas G. Ophtalmopathie de Basedow sévère liée a l'interféron alpha. [Severe thyroid ophthalmopathy related to interferon alpha therapy.] J Fr Ophtalmol 2002;25(4): 412–15.
164. Sunbul M, Kahraman H, Eroglu C, Leblebicioglu H, Cinar T. Subacute thyroiditis in a patient with chronic hepatitis C during interferon treatment: a case report. Ondokuz Mayis Univ Tip Derg 1999;16:62–6.
165. Dalgard O, Bjoro K, Hellum K, Myrvang B, Bjoro T, Haug E, Bell H. Thyroid dysfunction during treatment of chronic hepatitis C with interferon alpha: no association with either interferon dosage or efficacy of therapy. J Intern Med 2002;251(5):400–6.
166. Preziati D, La Rosa L, Covini G, Marcelli R, Rescalli S, Persani L, Del Ninno E, Meroni PL, Colombo M, Beck-Peccoz P. Autoimmunity and thyroid function in patients with chronic active hepatitis treated with recombinant interferon alpha-2a. Eur J Endocrinol 1995;132(5):587–93.
167. Vallisa D, Cavanna L, Berte R, Merli F, Ghisoni F, Buscarini L. Autoimmune thyroid dysfunctions in hematologic malignancies treated with alpha-interferon. Acta Haematol 1995;93(1):31–5.
168. Marazuela M, Garcia-Buey L, Gonzalez-Fernandez B, Garcia-Monzon C, Arranz A, Borque MJ, Moreno-Otero R. Thyroid autoimmune disorders in patients with chronic hepatitis C before and during interferon-alpha therapy. Clin Endocrinol (Oxf) 1996;44(6):635–42.
169. Roti E, Minelli R, Giuberti T, Marchelli S, Schianchi C, Gardini E, Salvi M, Fiaccadori F, Ugolotti G, Neri TM, Braverman LE. Multiple changes in thyroid function in patients with chronic active HCV hepatitis treated with recombinant interferon-alpha. Am J Med 1996; 101(5):482–7.
170. Barreca T, Picciotto A, Franceschini R, et al. Effects of acute administration of recombinant interferon alpha 2b on pituitary hormone secretion in patients with chronic active hepatitis. Curr Ther Res 1992;52:695–701.
171. Yamazaki K, Kanaji Y, Shizume K, Yamakawa Y, Demura H, Kanaji Y, Obara T, Sato K. Reversible inhibition by interferons alpha and beta of ^{125}I incorporation and thyroid hormone release by human thyroid follicles in vitro. J Clin Endocrinol Metab 1993;77(5):1439–41.
172. Schuppert F, Rambusch E, Kirchner H, Atzpodien J, Kohn LD, von zur Muhlen A. Patients treated with interferon-alpha, interferon-beta, and interleukin-2 have a different thyroid autoantibody pattern than patients suffering from endogenous autoimmune thyroid disease. Thyroid 1997;7(6):837–42.
173. Watanabe U, Hashimoto E, Hisamitsu T, Obata H, Hayashi N. The risk factor for development of thyroid disease during interferon-alpha therapy for chronic hepatitis C. Am J Gastroenterol 1994;89(3):399–403.
174. Fernandez-Soto L, Gonzalez A, Escobar-Jimenez F, Vazquez R, Ocete E, Olea N, Salmeron J. Increased risk of autoimmune thyroid disease in hepatitis C vs hepatitis B before, during, and after discontinuing interferon therapy. Arch Intern Med 1998;158(13):1445–8.
175. Kakizaki S, Takagi H, Murakami M, Takayama H, Mori M. HLA antigens in patients with interferon-alpha-induced autoimmune thyroid disorders in chronic hepatitis C. J Hepatol 1999;30(5):794–800.
176. Minelli R, Braverman LE, Valli MA, Schianchi C, Pedrazzoni M, Fiaccadori F, Salvi M, Magotti MG, Roti E. Recombinant interferon alpha (rIFN-alpha) does not potentiate the effect of iodine excess on the development of thyroid abnormalities in patients with HCV chronic active hepatitis. Clin Endocrinol (Oxf) 1999;50(1):95–100.
177. Carella C, Mazziotti G, Morisco F, Rotondi M, Cioffi M, Tuccillo C, Sorvillo F, Caporaso N, Amato G. The addition of ribavirin to interferon-alpha therapy in patients with hepatitis C virus-related chronic hepatitis does not modify the thyroid autoantibody pattern but increases the risk of developing hypothyroidism. Eur J Endocrinol 2002;146(6):743–9.
178. Marcellin P, Pouteau M, Renard P, Grynblat JM, Colas Linhart N, Bardet P, Bok B, Benhamou JP. Sustained hypothyroidism induced by recombinant alpha interferon in patients with chronic hepatitis C. Gut 1992;33(6):855–6.
179. Mekkakia-Benhabib C, Marcellin P, Colas-Linhart N, Castel-Nau C, Buyck D, Erlinger S, Bok B. Histoire naturelle des dysthyroïdies survenant sous interféron dans le traitement des hépatites chroniques C. [Natural history of dysthyroidism during interferon treatment of chronic hepatitis C.] Ann Endocrinol (Paris) 1996;57(5):419–27.
180. Minelli R, Braverman LE, Giuberti T, Schianchi C, Gardini E, Salvi M, Fiaccadori F, Ugolotti G, Roti E. Effects of excess iodine administration on thyroid function in euthyroid patients with a previous episode of thyroid dysfunction induced by interferon-alpha treatment. Clin Endocrinol (Oxf) 1997;47(3):357–61.
181. Calvino J, Romero R, Suarez-Penaranda JM, Arcocha V, Lens XM, Mardaras J, Novoa D, Sanchez-Guisande D. Secondary hyperparathyroidism exacerbation: a rare side-effect of interferon-alpha? Clin Nephrol 1999;51(4):248–51.
182. Wesche B, Jaeckel E, Trautwein C, Wedemeyer H, Falorni A, Frank H, von zur Muhlen A, Manns MP, Brabant G. Induction of autoantibodies to the adrenal cortex and pancreatic islet cells by interferon alpha therapy for chronic hepatitis C. Gut 2001;48(3):378–83.
183. Fraser GM, Harman I, Meller N, Niv Y, Porath A. Diabetes mellitus is associated with chronic hepatitis C but not chronic hepatitis B infection. Isr J Med Sci 1996;32(7):526–30.
184. Gori A, Caredda F, Franzetti F, Ridolfo A, Rusconi S, Moroni M. Reversible diabetes in patient with AIDS-related Kaposi's sarcoma treated with interferon alpha-2a. Lancet 1995;345(8962):1438–9.
185. Guerci AP, Guerci B, Levy-Marchal C, Ongagna J, Ziegler O, Candiloros H, Guerci O, Drouin P. Onset of insulin-dependent diabetes mellitus after interferon-alfa therapy for hairy cell leukaemia. Lancet 1994;343(8906):1167–8.
186. Mathieu E, Fain O, Sitbon M, Thomas M. Diabète auto-immun après traitement par interféron alpha.

[Autoimmune diabetes after treatment with interferon-alpha.] Presse Méd 1995;24(4):238.
187. Eibl N, Gschwantler M, Ferenci P, Eibl MM, Weiss W, Schernthaner G. Development of insulin-dependent diabetes mellitus in a patient with chronic hepatitis C during therapy with interferon-alpha. Eur J Gastroenterol Hepatol 2001;13(3):295–8.
188. Recasens M, Aguilera E, Ampurdanes S, Sanchez Tapias JM, Simo O, Casamitjana R, Conget I. Abrupt onset of diabetes during interferon-alpha therapy in patients with chronic hepatitis C. Diabet Med 2001;18(9):764–7.
189. Mofredj A, Howaizi M, Grasset D, Licht H, Loison S, Devergie B, Demontis R, Cadranel JF. Diabetes mellitus during interferon therapy for chronic viral hepatitis. Dig Dis Sci 2002;47(7):1649–54.
190. Ito Y, Takeda N, Ishimori M, Akai A, Miura K, Yasuda K. Effects of long-term interferon-alpha treatment on glucose tolerance in patients with chronic hepatitis C. J Hepatol 1999;31(2):215–20.
191. Hayakawa M, Gando S, Morimoto Y, Kemmotsu O. Development of severe diabetic keto-acidosis with shock after changing interferon-beta into interferon-alpha for chronic hepatitis C. Intensive Care Med 2000;26(7):1008.
192. Fabris P, Betterle C, Greggio NA, Zanchetta R, Bosi E, Biasin MR, de Lalla F. Insulin-dependent diabetes mellitus during alpha-interferon therapy for chronic viral hepatitis. J Hepatol 1998;28(3):514–17.
193. Koivisto VA, Pelkonen R, Cantell K. Effect of interferon on glucose tolerance and insulin sensitivity. Diabetes 1989;38(5):641–7.
194. Imano E, Kanda T, Ishigami Y, Kubota M, Ikeda M, Matsuhisa M, Kawamori R, Yamasaki Y. Interferon induces insulin resistance in patients with chronic active hepatitis C. J Hepatol 1998;28(2):189–93.
195. di Cesare E, Previti M, Russo F, Brancatelli S, Ingemi MC, Scoglio R, Mazzu N, Cucinotta D, Raimondo G. Interferon-alpha therapy may induce insulin autoantibody development in patients with chronic viral hepatitis. Dig Dis Sci 1996;41(8):1672–7.
196. Elisaf M, Tsianos EV. Severe hypertriglyceridaemia in a non-diabetic patient after alpha-interferon. Eur J Gastroenterol Hepatol 1999;11(4):463.
197. Junghans V, Runger TM. Hypertriglyceridaemia following adjuvant interferon-alpha treatment in two patients with malignant melanoma. Br J Dermatol 1999;140(1):183–4.
198. Shinohara E, Yamashita S, Kihara S, Hirano K, Ishigami M, Arai T, Nozaki S, Kameda-Takemura K, Kawata S, Matsuzawa Y. Interferon alpha induces disorder of lipid metabolism by lowering postheparin lipases and cholesteryl ester transfer protein activities in patients with chronic hepatitis C. Hepatology 1997;25(6):1502–6.
199. Yamagishi S, Abe T, Sawada T. Human recombinant interferon alpha-2a (r IFN alpha-2a) therapy suppresses hepatic triglyceride lipase, leading to severe hypertriglyceridemia in a diabetic patient. Am J Gastroenterol 1994;89(12):2280.
200. Fernandez-Miranda C, Castellano G, Guijarro C, Fernandez I, Schoebel N, Larumbe S, Gomez-Izquierdo T, del Palacio A. Lipoprotein changes in patients with chronic hepatitis C treated with interferon-alpha. Am J Gastroenterol 1998;93(10):1901–4.
201. Jessner W, Der-Petrossian M, Christiansen L, Maier H, Steindl-Munda P, Gangl A, Ferenci P. Porphyria cutanea tarda during interferon/ribavirin therapy for chronic hepatitis C. Hepatology 2002;36(5):1301–2.
202. Ernstoff MS, Kirkwood JM. Changes in the bone marrow of cancer patients treated with recombinant interferon alpha-2. Am J Med 1984;76(4):593–6.
203. Poynard T, Bedossa P, Chevallier M, Mathurin P, Lemonnier C, Trepo C, Couzigou P, Payen JL, Sajus M, Costa JM. A comparison of three interferon alfa-2b regimens for the long-term treatment of chronic non-A, non-B hepatitis. Multicenter Study Group. N Engl J Med 1995;332(22):1457–62.
204. Toccaceli F, Rosati S, Scuderi M, Iacomi F, Picconi R, Laghi V. Leukocyte and platelet lowering by some interferon types during viral hepatitis treatment. Hepatogastroenterology 1998;45(23):1748–52.
205. de-la-Serna-Higuera C, Barcena-Marugan R, Sanz-de-Villalobos E. Hemolytic anemia secondary to alpha-interferon treatment in a patient with chronic C hepatitis. J Clin Gastroenterol 1999;28(4):358–9.
206. Landau A, Castera L, Buffet C, Tertian G, Tchernia G. Acute autoimmune hemolytic anemia during interferon-alpha therapy for chronic hepatitis C. Dig Dis Sci 1999;44(7):1366–7.
207. Akard LP, Hoffman R, Elias L, Saiers JH. Alpha-interferon and immune hemolytic anemia. Ann Intern Med 1986;105(2):306.
208. Barbolla L, Paniagua C, Outeirino J, Prieto E, Sanchez Fayos J. Haemolytic anaemia to the alpha-interferon treatment: a proposed mechanism. Vox Sang 1993;65(2):156–7.
209. Braathen LR, Stavem P. Autoimmune haemolytic anaemia associated with interferon alfa-2a in a patient with mycosis fungoides. BMJ 1989;298(6689):1713.
210. Dormann H, Krebs S, Muth-Selbach U, Brune K, Schuppan D, Hahn EG, Schneider HT. Rapid onset of hematotoxic effects after interferon alpha in hepatitis C. J Hepatol 2000;32(6):1041–2.
211. Singhal S, Mehta J, Desikan K, Siegel D, Singh J, Munshi N, Spoon D, Anaissie E, Ayers D, Barlogie B. Collection of peripheral blood stem cells after a preceding autograft: unfavorable effect of prior interferon-alpha therapy. Bone Marrow Transplant 1999;24(1):13–17.
212. Harousseau JL, Milpied N, Bourhis JH, Guimbretiere L, Talmant P. Aplasie fatale après traitement par interféron alpha d'une leucémie myéloïde chronique après greffe de moelle osseuse allogénique. [Lethal aplasia after treatment with alpha-interferon of recurrent chronic myeloid leukemia following allogeneic bone marrow graft.] Presse Méd 1988;17(2):80–1.
213. Hoffmann A, Kirn E, Krueger GR, Fischer R. Bone marrow hypoplasia and fibrosis following interferon treatment. In Vivo 1994;8(4):605–12.
214. Shepherd PC, Richards S, Allan NC. Severe cytopenias associated with the sequential use of busulphan and interferon-alpha in chronic myeloid leukaemia. Br J Haematol 1994;86(1):92–6.
215. Talpaz M, Kantarjian H, Kurzrock R, Gutterman JU. Bone marrow hypoplasia and aplasia complicating interferon therapy for chronic myelogenous leukemia. Cancer 1992;69(2):410–12.
216. Steis RG, VanderMolen LA, Lawrence J, Sing G, Ruscetti F, Smith JW 2nd, Urba WJ, Clark J, Longo DL. Erythrocytosis in hairy cell leukaemia following therapy with interferon alpha. Br J Haematol 1990;75(1):133–5.
217. Hirri HM, Green PJ. Pure red cell aplasia in a patient with chronic granulocytic leukaemia treated with interferon-alpha. Clin Lab Haematol 2000;22(1):53–4.
218. Tomita N, Motomura S, Ishigatsubo Y. Interferon-alpha-induced pure red cell aplasia following chronic myelogenous leukemia. Anticancer Drugs 2001;12(1):7–8.
219. Willson RA. Interferon alfa-induced pernicious anemia in chronic hepatitis C infection. J Clin Gastroenterol 2001;33(5):426–7.
220. Andriani A, Bibas M, Callea V, De Renzo A, Chiurazzi F, Marceno R, Musto P, Rotoli B. Autoimmune hemolytic anemia during alpha interferon treatment in nine

patients with hematological diseases. Haematologica 1996;81(3):258–60.

221. Sacchi S, Kantarjian H, O'Brien S, Cohen PR, Pierce S, Talpaz M. Immune-mediated and unusual complications during interferon alfa therapy in chronic myelogenous leukemia. J Clin Oncol 1995;13(9):2401–7.
222. Steegmann JL, Pinilla I, Requena MJ, de la Camara R, Granados E, Fernandez Villalta MJ, Fernandez-Ranada JM. The direct antiglobulin test is frequently positive in chronic myeloid leukemia patients treated with interferon-alpha. Transfusion 1997;37(4):446–7.
223. McNair ANB, Jacyna MR, Thomas HC. Severe haemolytic transfusion reaction occurring during alpha-interferon therapy for chronic hepatitis. Eur J Gastroenterol Hepatol 1991;3:193–4.
224. Parry-Jones N, Gore ME, Taylor J, Treleaven JG. Delayed haemolytic transfusion reaction caused by anti-M antibody in a patient receiving interleukin-2 and interferon for metastatic renal cell cancer. Clin Lab Haematol 1999;21(6):407–8.
225. Renou C, Harafa A, Bouabdallah R, Demattei C, Cummins C, Rifflet H, Muller P, Ville E, Bertrand J, Benderitter T, Halfon P. Severe neutropenia and post-hepatitis C cirrhosis treatment: is interferon dose adaptation at once necessary? Am J Gastroenterol 2002;97(5):1260–3.
226. Soza A, Everhart JE, Ghany MG, Doo E, Heller T, Promrat K, Park Y, Liang TJ, Hoofnagle JH. Neutropenia during combination therapy of interferon alfa and ribavirin for chronic hepatitis C. Hepatology 2002;36(5):1273–9.
227. Sata M, Yano Y, Yoshiyama Y, Ide T, Kumashiro R, Suzuki H, Tanikawa K. Mechanisms of thrombocytopenia induced by interferon therapy for chronic hepatitis B. J Gastroenterol 1997;32(2):206–10.
228. Shiota G, Okubo M, Kawasaki H, Tahara T. Interferon increases serum thrombopoietin in patients with chronic hepatitis C. Br J Haematol 1997;97(2):340–2.
229. Peck-Radosavljevic M, Wichlas M, Pidlich J, Sims P, Meng G, Zacherl J, Garg S, Datz C, Gangl A, Ferenci P. Blunted thrombopoietin response to interferon alfa-induced thrombocytopenia during treatment for hepatitis C. Hepatology 1998;28(5):1424–9.
230. Martin TG, Shuman MA. Interferon-induced thrombocytopenia: is it time for thrombopoietin. Hepatology 1998;28(5):1430–2.
231. Sagir A, Wettstein M, Heintges T, Haussinger D. Autoimmune thrombocytopenia induced by PEG-IFN-alpha2b plus ribavirin in hepatitis C. Dig Dis Sci 2002;47(3):562–3.
232. Zuffa E, Vianelli N, Martinelli G, Tazzari P, Cavo M, Tura S. Autoimmune mediated thrombocytopenia associated with the use of interferon-alpha in chronic myeloid leukemia. Haematologica 1996;81(6):533–5.
233. Taliani G, Duca F, Clementi C, De Bac C. Platelet-associated immunoglobulin G, thrombocytopenia and response to interferon treatment in chronic hepatitis C. J Hepatol 1996;25(6):999.
234. Rachmani R, Avigdor A, Youkla M, Raanani P, Zilber M, Ravid M, Ben-Bassat I. Thrombotic thrombocytopenic purpura complicating chronic myelogenous leukemia treated with interferon-alpha. A report of two successfully treated patients. Acta Haematol 1998;100(4):204–6.
235. Gutman H, Schachter J, Stopel E, Gutman R, Lahav J. Impaired platelet aggregation in melanoma patients treated with interferon-alpha-2b adjuvant therapy. Cancer 2002;94(3):780–5.
236. Carmona-Soria I, Jimenez-Saenz M, Gonzalez-Vilches J, Herrerias-Gutierrez JM. Development of lupic anticoagulant during combination therapy in a patient with chronic hepatitis C. J Hepatol 2001;34(6):965–7.
237. Castenskiold EC, Colvin BT, Kelsey SM. Acquired factor VIII inhibitor associated with chronic interferon-alpha therapy in a patient with haemophilia A. Br J Haematol 1994;87(2):434–6.
238. Stricker RB, Barlogie B, Kiprov DD. Acquired factor VIII inhibitor associated with chronic interferon-alpha therapy. J Rheumatol 1994;21(2):350–2.
239. English KE, Brien WF, Howson-Jan K, Kovacs MJ. Acquired factor VIII inhibitor in a patient with chronic myelogenous leukemia receiving interferon-alfa therapy. Ann Pharmacother 2000;34(6):737–9.
240. Mauser-Bunschoten EP, Damen M, Reesink HW, Roosendaal G, Chamuleau RA, van den Berg HM. Formation of antibodies to factor VIII in patients with hemophilia A who are treated with interferon for chronic hepatitis C. Ann Intern Med 1996;125(4):297–9.
241. Qaseem T, Jafri W, Abid S, Hamid S, Khan H. A case report of painful oral ulcerations associated with the use of alpha interferon in a patient with chronic hepatitis due to non-A non-B non-C virus. Mil Med 1993;158(2):126–7.
242. Bardella MT, Marino R, Meroni PL. Celiac disease during interferon treatment. Ann Intern Med 1999;131(2):157–8.
243. Cammarota G, Cuoco L, Cianci R, Pandolfi F, Gasbarrini G. Onset of coeliac disease during treatment with interferon for chronic hepatitis C. Lancet 2000;356(9240):1494–5.
244. Kakumitsu S, Shijo H, Akiyoshi N, Seo M, Okada M. Eosinophilic enteritis observed during alpha-interferon therapy for chronic hepatitis C. J Gastroenterol 2000;35(7):548–51.
245. Tada H, Saitoh S, Nakagawa Y, Hirana H, Morimoto M, Shima T, Shimamoto K, Okanoue T, Kashima K. Ischemic colitis during interferon-alpha treatment for chronic active hepatitis C. J Gastroenterol 1996;31(4):582–4.
246. Janssen HL, Brouwer JT, Nevens F, Sanchez-Tapias JM, Craxi A, Hadziyannis S. Fatal hepatic decompensation associated with interferon alfa. European concerted action on viral hepatitis (Eurohep). BMJ 1993; 306(6870):107–8.
247. Krogsgaard K, Marcellin P, Trepo C, Berthelot P, Sanchez-Tapias JM, Bassendine M, Tran A, Ouzan D, Ring-Larsen H, Lindberg J, Enriquez J, Benhamou JP, Bindslev N. Prednisolone withdrawal therapy enhances the effect of human lymphoblastoid interferon in chronic hepatitis B. INTERPRED Trial Group. J Hepatol 1996;25(6):803–13.
248. Lock G, Reng CM, Graeb C, Anthuber M, Wiedmann KH. Interferon-induced hepatic failure in a patient with hepatitis C. Am J Gastroenterol 1999;94(9):2570–1.
249. Farhat BA, Johnson PJ, Williams R. Hazards of interferon treatment in patients with autoimmune chronic active hepatitis. J Hepatol 1994;20(4):560–1.
250. Papo T, Marcellin P, Bernuau J, Durand F, Poynard T, Benhamou JP. Autoimmune chronic hepatitis exacerbated by alpha-interferon. Ann Intern Med 1992;116(1):51–3.
251. Payen JL, Rabbia I, Combis M, Voigt JJ, Vinel P, Pascal JP. Révélation d'une hépatite auto-immune par l'interféron. [Disclosure of autoimmune hepatitis by interferon.] Gastroenterol Clin Biol 1993;17(5):404–5.
252. Ruiz-Moreno M, Rua MJ, Carreno V, Quiroga JA, Manns M, Meyer zum Buschenfelde KH. Autoimmune chronic hepatitis type 2 manifested during interferon therapy in children. J Hepatol 1991;12(2):265–6.
253. Tran A, Beusnel C, Montoya ML, Lussiez V, Hebuterne X, Rampal P. Hépatite autoimmune de typ 1 révelée par un traitement par interféron. [Autoimmune

hepatitis type 1 revealed during treatment with interferon.] Gastroenterol Clin Biol 1992;16(8–9):722–3.
254. Vento S, Di Perri G, Garofano T, Cosco L, Concia E, Ferraro T, Bassetti D. Hazards of interferon therapy for HBV-seronegative chronic hepatitis. Lancet 1989;2(8668):926.
255. Garrido Palma G, Sanchez Cuenca JM, Olaso V, Pina R, Urquijo JJ, Lopez Viedma B, Bustamante M, Berenguer M, Berenguer J. Response to treatment with interferon-alfa in patients with chronic hepatitis C and high titers of -M2, -M4 and -M8 antimitochondrial antibodies. Rev Esp Enferm Dig 1999;91(3):168–81.
256. Iorio R, Giannattasio A, Vespere G, Vegnente A. LKM1 antibody and interferon therapy in children with chronic hepatitis C. J Hepatol 2001;35(5):685–7.
257. Garcia-Buey L, Garcia-Monzon C, Rodriguez S, Borque MJ, Garcia-Sanchez A, Iglesias R, DeCastro M, Mateos FG, Vicario JL, Balas A, et al. Latent autoimmune hepatitis triggered during interferon therapy in patients with chronic hepatitis C. Gastroenterology 1995; 108(6):1770–7.
258. Castera L, Kalinsky E, Bedossa P, Tertian G, Buffet C. Macrovesicular steatosis induced by interferon alfa therapy for chronic myelogenous leukaemia. Liver 1999;19(3):259–60.
259. Ryan BM, McDonald GS, Pilkington R, Kelleher D. The development of hepatic granulomas following interferon-alpha2b therapy for chronic hepatitis C infection. Eur J Gastroenterol Hepatol 1998;10(4):349–51.
260. Sevenet F, Sevenet C, Capron D, Descombes P. Pancréatite aiguë et interféron. [Acute pancreatitis and interferon.] Gastroenterol Clin Biol 1999;23(11):1256.
261. Eland IA, van Puijenbroek EP, Sturkenboom MJ, Wilson JH, Stricker BH. Drug-associated acute pancreatitis: twenty-one years of spontaneous reporting in The Netherlands. Am J Gastroenterol 1999;94(9):2417–22.
262. Eland IA, Rasch MC, Sturkenboom MJ, Bekkering FC, Brouwer JT, Delwaide J, Belaiche J, Houbiers G, Stricker BH. Acute pancreatitis attributed to the use of interferon alfa-2b. Gastroenterology 2000;119(1):230–3.
263. Kurschel E, Metz-Kurschel U, Niederle N, Aulbert E. Investigations on the subclinical and clinical nephrotoxicity of interferon alpha-2B in patients with myeloproliferative syndromes. Ren Fail 1991;13(2–3):87–93.
264. Selby P, Kohn J, Raymond J, Judson I, McElwain T. Nephrotic syndrome during treatment with interferon. BMJ (Clin Res Ed) 1985;290(6476):1180.
265. Nishimura S, Miura H, Yamada H, Shinoda T, Kitamura S, Miura Y. Acute onset of nephrotic syndrome during interferon-alpha retreatment for chronic active hepatitis C. J Gastroenterol 2002;37(10):854–8.
266. Willson RA. Nephrotoxicity of interferon alfa–ribavirin therapy for chronic hepatitis C. J Clin Gastroenterol 2002;35(1):89–92.
267. Nassar GM, Pedro P, Remmers RE, Mohanty LB, Smith W. Reversible renal failure in a patient with the hypereosinophilia syndrome during therapy with alpha interferon. Am J Kidney Dis 1998;31(1):121–6.
268. Dimitrov Y, Heibel F, Marcellin L, Chantrel F, Moulin B, Hannedouche T. Acute renal failure and nephrotic syndrome with alpha interferon therapy. Nephrol Dial Transplant 1997;12(1):200–3.
269. Averbuch SD, Austin HA 3rd, Sherwin SA, Antonovych T, Bunn PA Jr, Longo DL. Acute interstitial nephritis with the nephrotic syndrome following recombinant leukocyte a interferon therapy for mycosis fungoides. N Engl J Med 1984;310(1):32–5.
270. Kimmel PL, Abraham AA, Phillips TM. Membranoproliferative glomerulonephritis in a patient treated with interferon-alpha for human immunodeficiency virus infection. Am J Kidney Dis 1994;24(5):858–63.
271. Traynor A, Kuzel T, Samuelson E, Kanwar Y. Minimal-change glomerulopathy and glomerular visceral epithelial hyperplasia associated with alpha-interferon therapy for cutaneous T cell lymphoma. Nephron 1994;67(1):94–100.
272. Fahal IH, Murry N, Chu P, Bell GM. Acute renal failure during interferon treatment. BMJ 1993;306(6883):973.
273. Lederer E, Truong L. Unusual glomerular lesion in a patient receiving long-term interferon alpha. Am J Kidney Dis 1992;20(5):516–18.
274. Durand JM, Retornaz F, Cretel E, et al. Glomérulonéphrite extracapillaire au cours d'un traitement par interféron alpha. Rev Med Interne 1993;14:1138.
275. Jadoul M. Interferon-alpha-associated focal segmental glomerulosclerosis with massive proteinuria in patients with chronic myeloid leukemia following high dose chemotherapy. Cancer 1999;85(12):2669–70.
276. Honda K, Ando A, Endo M, Shimizu K, Higashihara M, Nitta K, Nihei H. Thrombotic microangiopathy associated with alpha-interferon therapy for chronic myelocytic leukemia. Am J Kidney Dis 1997;30(1):123–30.
277. Ravandi-Kashani F, Cortes J, Talpaz M, Kantarjian HM. Thrombotic microangiopathy associated with interferon therapy for patients with chronic myelogenous leukemia: coincidence or true side effect? Cancer 1999;85(12):2583–8.
278. Vacher-Coponat H, Opris A, Daniel L, Harle JR, Veit V, Olmer M. Thrombotic microangiopathy in a patient with chronic myelocytic leukaemia treated with alpha-interferon. Nephrol Dial Transplant 1999;14(10):2469–71.
279. Zuber J, Martinez F, Droz D, Oksenhendler E, Legendre C, Groupe D'Etude Des Nephrologues D'Ile-de-France (GENIF). Alpha-interferon-associated thrombotic microangiopathy: a clinicopathologic study of 8 patients and review of the literature. Medicine (Baltimore) 2002;81(4):321–31.
280. Bren A, Kandus A, Ferluga D. Rapidly progressive renal graft failure associated with interferon-alpha treatment in a patient with chronic myelogenous leukemia. Clin Nephrol 1998;50(4):266–7.
281. Asnis LA, Gaspari AA. Cutaneous reactions to recombinant cytokine therapy. J Am Acad Dermatol 1995;33(3):393–410.
282. Dalekos GN, Hatzis J, Tsianos EV. Dermatologic disease during interferon-alpha therapy for chronic viral hepatitis. Ann Intern Med 1998;128(5):409–10.
283. Andry P, Weber-Buisset MJ, Fraitag S, Brechot C, De Prost Y. Toxidermie bulleuse à l'Introna. [Bullous drug eruption caused by Introna.] Ann Dermatol Venereol 1993;120(11):843–5.
284. Sparsa A, Loustaud-Ratti V, Liozon E, Denes E, Soria P, Bouyssou-Gauthier ML, Le Brun V, Boulinguez S, Bedane C, Scribbe-Outtas M, Outtas O, Labrousse F, Bonnetblanc JM, Bordessoule D, Vidal E. Réactions cutanées ou nécrose à l'interféron alpha: peut-on reprendre l'interféron? A propos de six cas. [Cutaneous reactions or necrosis from interferon alpha: can interferon be reintroduced after healing? Six case reports.] Rev Med Interne 2000;21(9):756–63.
285. Kurzen H, Petzoldt D, Hartschuh W, Jappe U. Cutaneous necrosis after subcutaneous injection of polyethylene-glycol-modified interferon alpha. Acta Dermatol Venereol 2002;82(4):310–12.
286. Sanders S, Busam K, Tahan SR, Johnson RA, Sachs D. Granulomatous and suppurative dermatitis at interferon alfa injection sites: report of 2 cases. J Am Acad Dermatol 2002;46(4):611–16.
287. Jessner W, Kinaciyan T, Formann E, Steindl-Munda P, Ferenci P. Severe skin reactions during therapy for chronic

hepatitis C associated with delayed hypersensitivity to pegylated interferons. Hepatology 2002;36:361.

288. Heinzerling L, Dummer R, Wildberger H, Burg G. Cutaneous ulceration after injection of polyethylene-glycol-modified interferon alpha associated with visual disturbances in a melanoma patient. Dermatology 2000;201(2):154–7.

289. Bessis D, Charron A, Rouzier-Panis R, Blatiere V, Guilhou JJ, Reynes J. Necrotizing cutaneous lesions complicating treatment with pegylated-interferon alfa in an HIV-infected patient. Eur J Dermatol 2002;12(1):99–102.

290. Cribier B, Garnier C, Laustriat D, Heid E. Lichen planus and hepatitis C virus infection: an epidemiologic study. J Am Acad Dermatol 1994;31(6):1070–2.

291. Dupin N, Chosidow O, Frances C, et al. Lichen planus after alpha-interferon therapy for chronic hepatitis C. Eur J Dermatol 1994;4:535–6.

292. Strumia R, Venturini D, Boccia S, Gamberini S, Gullini S. UVA and interferon-alfa therapy in a patient with lichen planus and chronic hepatitis C. Int J Dermatol 1993;32(5):386.

293. Aubin F, Bourezane Y, Blanc D, Voltz JM, Faivre B, Humbert PH. Severe lichen planus-like eruption induced by interferon-alpha therapy. Eur J Dermatol 1995;5:296–9.

294. Marinho RT, Johnson NW, Fatela NM, Serejo FS, Gloria H, Raimundo MO, Velosa JF, Ramalho FJ, Moura MC. Oropharyngeal pemphigus in a patient with chronic hepatitis C during interferon alpha-2a therapy. Eur J Gastroenterol Hepatol 2001;13(7):869–72.

295. Quesada JR, Gutterman JU. Psoriasis and alpha-interferon. Lancet 1986;1(8496):1466–8.

296. Harrison PV, Peat MJ. Effect of interferon on psoriasis. Lancet 1986;2(8504):457–8.

297. Nguyen C, Misery L, Tigaud JD, Petiot A, Fiere D, Faure M, Claudy A. Psoriasis induit par l'interféron alpha. A propos d'une observation. [Psoriasis induced by interferon-alpha. Apropos of a case.] Ann Med Interne (Paris) 1996;147(7):519–21.

298. Cleveland MG, Mallory SB. Incomplete Reiter's syndrome induced by systemic interferon alpha treatment. J Am Acad Dermatol 1993;29(5 Pt 1):788–9.

299. Dereure O, Raison-Peyron N, Larrey D, Blanc F, Guilhou JJ. Diffuse inflammatory lesions in patients treated with interferon alfa and ribavirin for hepatitis C: a series of 20 patients. Br J Dermatol 2002;147(6):1142–6.

300. Thomas R, Stea B. Radiation recall dermatitis from high-dose interferon alfa-2b. J Clin Oncol 2002;20(1):355–7.

301. Tursen U, Kaya TI, Ikizoglu G. Interferon-alpha 2b induced facial erythema in a woman with chronic hepatitis C infection. J Eur Acad Dermatol Venereol 2002;16(3):285–6.

302. Creput C, Auffret N, Samuel D, Jian R, Hill G, Nochy D. Cutaneous thrombotic microangiopathy during treatment with alpha-interferon for chronic hepatitis C. J Hepatol 2002;37(6):871–2.

303. Krischer J, Pechere M, Salomon D, Harms M, Chavaz P, Saurat JH. Interferon alfa-2b-induced Meyerson's nevi in a patient with dysplastic nevus syndrome. J Am Acad Dermatol 1999;40(1):105–6.

304. Pfohler C, Ugurel S, Seiter S, Wagner A, Tilgen W, Reinhold U. Interferon-alpha-associated development of bullous lesions in mycosis fungoides. Dermatology 2000;200(1):51–3.

305. Tosti A, Misciali C, Bardazzi F, Fanti PA, Varotti C. Telogen effluvium due to recombinant interferon alpha-2b. Dermatology 1992;184(2):124–5.

306. Agesta N, Zabala R, Diaz-Perez JL. Alopecia areata during interferon alpha-2b/ribavirin therapy. Dermatology 2002;205(3):300–1.

307. Lang AM, Norland AM, Schuneman RL, Tope WD. Localized interferon alfa-2b-induced alopecia. Arch Dermatol 1999;135(9):1126–8.

308. Kernland KH, Hunziker T. Alopecia areata induced by interferon alpha? Dermatology 1999;198(4):418–19.

309. Bessis D, Luong MS, Blanc P, Chapoutot C, Larrey D, Guilhou JJ, Guillot B. Straight hair associated with interferon-alfa plus ribavirin in hepatitis C infection. Br J Dermatol 2002;147(2):392–3.

310. Hauschild A, Moller M, Lischner S, Christophers E. Repeatable acute rhabdomyolysis with multiple organ dysfunction because of interferon alpha and dacarbazine treatment in metastatic melanoma. Br J Dermatol 2001;144(1):215–16.

311. van Londen GJ, Mascarenhas B, Kirkwood JM. Rhabdomyolysis, when observed with high-dose interferon-alfa (HDI) therapy, does not always exclude resumption of HDI. J Clin Oncol 2001;19(17):3794.

312. Ozdag F, Akar A, Eroglu E, Erbil H. Acute rhabdomyolysis during the treatment of scleromyxedema with interferon alfa. J Dermatolog Treat 2001;12(3):167–9.

313. Dippel E, Zouboulis CC, Tebbe B, Orfanos CE. Myopathic syndrome associated with long-term recombinant interferon alfa treatment in 4 patients with skin disorders. Arch Dermatol 1998;134(7):880–1.

314. Kozuch P, Talpaz M, Faderl S, O'Brien S, Freireich EJ, Kantarjian H. Avascular necrosis of the femoral head in chronic myeloid leukemia patients treated with interferon-alpha: a synergistic correlation? Cancer 2000; 89(7):1482–9.

315. Alvarez JS, Sacristan JA, Alsar MJ. Interferon alpha-2a-induced impotence. Ann Pharmacother 1991;25:1397.

316. Kauppila A, Cantell K, Janne O, Kokko E, Vihko R. Serum sex steroid and peptide hormone concentrations, and endometrial estrogen and progestin receptor levels during administration of human leukocyte interferon. Int J Cancer 1982;29(3):291–4.

317. Schilsky RL, Davidson HS, Magid D, Daiter S, Golomb HM. Gonadal and sexual function in male patients with hairy cell leukemia: lack of adverse effects of recombinant alpha 2-interferon treatment. Cancer Treat Rep 1987;71(2):179–81.

318. Pardini S, Bosincu L, Bonfigli S, Dore F, Longinotti M. Anaphylactic-like syndrome in systemic mastocytosis treated with alpha-2-interferon. Acta Haematol 1991;85(4):220.

319. Ohmoto K, Yamamoto S. Angioedema after interferon therapy for chronic hepatitis C. Am J Gastroenterol 2001;96(4):1311–12.

320. Beckman DB, Mathisen TL, Harris KE, Boxer MB, Grammer LC. Hypersensitivity to IFN-alpha. Allergy 2001;56(8):806–7.

321. Detmar U, Agathos M, Nerl C. Allergy of delayed type to recombinant interferon alpha 2c. Contact Dermatitis 1989;20(2):149–50.

322. Pigatto PD, Bigardi A, Legori A, Altomare GF, Riboldi A. Allergic contact dermatitis from beta-interferon in eye-drops. Contact Dermatitis 1991;25(3):199–200.

323. Antonelli G. In vivo development of antibody to interferons: an update to 1996. J Interferon Cytokine Res 1997;17(Suppl 1):S39–46.

324. McKenna RM, Oberg KE. Antibodies to interferon-alpha in treated cancer patients: incidence and significance. J Interferon Cytokine Res 1997;17(3):141–3.

325. Bonino F, Baldi M, Negro F, Oliveri F, Colombatto P, Bellati G, Brunetto MR. Clinical relevance of anti-interferon antibodies in the serum of chronic hepatitis C patients treated with interferon-alpha. J Interferon Cytokine Res 1997;17(Suppl 1):S35–8.

326. Antonelli G, Currenti M, Turriziani O, Dianzani F. Neutralizing antibodies to interferon-alpha: relative frequency in patients treated with different interferon preparations. J Infect Dis 1991;163(4):882–5.
327. Antonelli G, Currenti M, Turriziani O, Riva E, Dianzani F. Relative frequency of nonneutralizing antibodies to interferon (IFN) in hepatitis patients treated with different IFN-alpha preparations. J Infect Dis 1992;165(3):593–4.
328. Von Wussow P, Hehlmann R, Hochhaus T, Jakschies D, Nolte KU, Prummer O, Ansari H, Hasford J, Heimpel H, Deicher H. Roferon (rIFN-alpha 2a) is more immunogenic than intron A (rIFN-alpha 2b) in patients with chronic myelogenous leukemia. J Interferon Res 1994;14(4):217–19.
329. Milella M, Antonelli G, Santantonio T, Currenti M, Monno L, Mariano N, Angarano G, Dianzani F, Pastore G. Neutralizing antibodies to recombinant alpha-interferon and response to therapy in chronic hepatitis C virus infection. Liver 1993;13(3):146–50.
330. Antonelli G, Giannelli G, Currenti M, Simeoni E, Del Vecchio S, Maggi F, Pistello M, Roffi L, Pastore G, Chemello L, Dianzani F. Antibodies to interferon (IFN) in hepatitis C patients relapsing while continuing recombinant IFN-alpha2 therapy. Clin Exp Immunol 1996;104(3):384–7.
331. Hanley JP, Jarvis LM, Simmonds P, Ludlam CA. Development of anti-interferon antibodies and breakthrough hepatitis during treatment for HCV infection in haemophiliacs. Br J Haematol 1996;94(3):551–6.
332. Roffi L, Mels GC, Antonelli G, Bellati G, Panizzuti F, Piperno A, Pozzi M, Ravizza D, Angeli G, Dianzani F, et al. Breakthrough during recombinant interferon alfa therapy in patients with chronic hepatitis C virus infection: prevalence, etiology, and management. Hepatology 1995;21(3):645–9.
333. Rajan GP, Seifert B, Prummer O, Joller-Jemelka HI, Burg G, Dummer R. Incidence and in-vivo relevance of anti-interferon antibodies during treatment of low-grade cutaneous T-cell lymphomas with interferon alpha-2a combined with acitretin or PUVA. Arch Dermatol Res 1996;288(9):543–8.
334. Tefferi A, Grendahl DC. Natural leukocyte interferon-alpha therapy in patients with chronic granulocytic leukemia who have antibody-mediated resistance to treatment with recombinant interferon-alpha. Am J Hematol 1996;52(3):231–3.
335. Russo D, Candoni A, Zuffa E, Minisini R, Silvestri F, Fanin R, Zaja F, Martinelli G, Tura S, Botta G, Baccarani M. Neutralizing anti-interferon-alpha antibodies and response to treatment in patients with Ph+ chronic myeloid leukaemia sequentially treated with recombinant (alpha 2a) and lymphoblastoid interferon-alpha. Br J Haematol 1996;94(2):300–5.
336. Milella M, Antonelli G, Santantonio T, Giannelli G, Currenti M, Monno L, Turriziani O, Pastore G, Dianzani F. Treatment with natural IFN of hepatitis C patients with or without antibodies to recombinant IFN. Hepatogastroenterology 1995;42(3):201–4.
337. Wussow PV, Jakschies D, Freund M, Hehlmann R, Brockhaus F, Hochkeppel H, Horisberger M, Deicher H. Treatment of anti-recombinant interferon-alpha 2 antibody positive CML patients with natural interferon-alpha. Br J Haematol 1991;78(2):210–16.
338. von Wussow P, Pralle H, Hochkeppel HK, Jakschies D, Sonnen S, Schmidt H, Muller-Rosenau D, Franke M, Haferlach T, Zwingers T, et al. Effective natural interferon-alpha therapy in recombinant interferon-alpha-resistant patients with hairy cell leukemia. Blood 1991;78(1):38–43.
339. Wada M, Kang KB, Kinugasa A, Shintani S, Sawada K, Nishigami T, Shimoyama T. Does the presence of serum autoantibodies influence the responsiveness to interferon-alpha 2a treatment in chronic hepatitis C? Intern Med 1997;36(4):248–54.
340. Cassani F, Cataleta M, Valentini P, Muratori P, Giostra F, Francesconi R, Muratori L, Lenzi M, Bianchi G, Zauli D, Bianchi FB. Serum autoantibodies in chronic hepatitis C: comparison with autoimmune hepatitis and impact on the disease profile. Hepatology 1997;26(3):561–6.
341. Noda K, Enomoto N, Arai K, Masuda E, Yamada Y, Suzuki K, Tanaka M, Yoshihara H. Induction of antinuclear antibody after interferon therapy in patients with type-C chronic hepatitis: its relation to the efficacy of therapy. Scand J Gastroenterol 1996;31(7):716–22.
342. Bell TM, Bansal AS, Shorthouse C, Sandford N, Powell EE. Low-titre auto-antibodies predict autoimmune disease during interferon-alpha treatment of chronic hepatitis C. J Gastroenterol Hepatol 1999;14(5):419–22.
343. Steegmann JL, Requena MJ, Martin-Regueira P, De La Camara R, Casado F, Salvanes FR, Fernandez Ranada JM. High incidence of autoimmune alterations in chronic myeloid leukemia patients treated with interferon-alpha. Am J Hematol 2003;72(3):170–6.
344. Tothova E, Kafkova A, Stecova N, Fricova M, Guman T, Svorcova E. Immune-mediated complications during interferon alpha therapy in chronic myelogenous leukemia. Neoplasma 2002;49(2):91–4.
345. Lunel F, Cacoub P. Treatment of autoimmune and extrahepatic manifestations of hepatitis C virus infection. J Hepatol 1999;31(Suppl 1):210–16.
346. Budak-Alpdogan T, Demircay Z, Alpdogan O, Direskeneli H, Ergun T, Bayik M, Akoglu T. Behçet's disease in patients with chronic myelogenous leukemia: possible role of interferon-alpha treatment in the occurrence of Behçet's symptoms. Ann Hematol 1997;74(1):45–8.
347. Dietrich LL, Bridges AJ, Albertini MR. Dermatomyositis after interferon alpha treatment. Med Oncol 2000;17(1):64–9.
348. Dohmen K, Miyamoto Y, Irie K, Takeshita T, Ishibashi H. Manifestation of cutaneous polyarteritis nodosa during interferon therapy for chronic hepatitis C associated with primary biliary cirrhosis. J Gastroenterol 2000;35(10):789–93.
349. Cirigliano G, Della Rossa A, Tavoni A, Viacava P, Bombardieri S. Polymyositis occurring during alpha-interferon treatment for malignant melanoma: a case report and review of the literature. Rheumatol Int 1999;19(1–2):65–7.
350. Hengstman GJ, Vogels OJ, ter Laak HJ, de Witte T, van Engelen BG. Myositis during long-term interferon-alpha treatment. Neurology 2000;54(11):2186.
351. Hoffmann RM, Jung MC, Motz R, Gossl C, Emslander HP, Zachoval R, Pape GR. Sarcoidosis associated with interferon-alpha therapy for chronic hepatitis C. J Hepatol 1998;28(6):1058–63.
352. Cogrel O, Doutre MS, Marliere V, Beylot-Barry M, Couzigou P, Beylot C. Cutaneous sarcoidosis during interferon alfa and ribavirin treatment of hepatitis C virus infection: two cases. Br J Dermatol 2002;146(2):320–4.
353. Savoye G, Goria O, Herve S, Riachi G, Noblesse I, Bastien L, Courville P, Lerebours E. Probable sarcoïdose cutanée après bi-thérapie associant ribavirine et interferon-alpha pour une hépatite chronique virale C. [Probable cutaneous sarcoidosis associated with combined ribavirin and interferon-alpha therapy for chronic hepatitis C.] Gastroenterol Clin Biol 2000;24(6–7):679.

354. Vander Els NJ, Gerdes H. Sarcoidosis and IFN-alpha treatment. Chest 2000;117(1):294.
355. Fiorani C, Sacchi S, Bonacorsi G, Cosenza M. Systemic sarcoidosis associated with interferon-alpha treatment for chronic myelogenous leukemia. Haematologica 2000;85(9):1006–7.
356. Eberlein-Konig B, Hein R, Abeck D, Engst R, Ring J. Cutaneous sarcoid foreign body granulomas developing in sites of previous skin injury after systemic interferon-alpha treatment for chronic hepatitis C. Br J Dermatol 1999;140(2):370–2.
357. Gitlin N. Manifestation of sarcoidosis during interferon and ribavirin therapy for chronic hepatitis C: a report of two cases. Eur J Gastroenterol Hepatol 2002;14(8):883–5.
358. Husa P, Klusakova J, Jancikova J, Husova L, Horalek F. Sarcoidosis associated with interferon-alpha therapy for chronic hepatitis B. Eur J Intern Med 2002;13(2):129–31.
359. Nawras A, Alsolaiman MM, Mehboob S, Bartholomew C, Maliakkal B. Systemic sarcoidosis presenting as a granulomatous tattoo reaction secondary to interferon-alpha treatment for chronic hepatitis C and review of the literature. Dig Dis Sci 2002;47(7):1627–31.
360. Noguchi K, Enjoji M, Nakamuta M, Sugimoto R, Kotoh K, Nawata H. Various sarcoid lesions in a patient induced by interferon therapy for chronic hepatitis C. J Clin Gastroenterol 2002;35(3):282–4.
361. Tahan V, Ozseker F, Guneylioglu D, Baran A, Ozaras R, Mert A, Ucisik AC, Cagatay T, Yilmazbayhan D, Senturk H. Sarcoidosis after use of interferon for chronic hepatitis C: report of a case and review of the literature. Dig Dis Sci 2003;48(1):169–73.
362. Li SD, Yong S, Srinivas D, Van Thiel DH. Reactivation of sarcoidosis during interferon therapy. J Gastroenterol 2002;37(1):50–4.
363. Boonen A, Stockbrugger RW, van der Linden S. Pericarditis after therapy with interferon-alpha for chronic hepatitis C. Clin Rheumatol 1999;18(2):177–9.
364. Johnson DM, Hayat SQ, Burton GV. Rheumatoid arthritis complicating adjuvant interferon-alpha therapy for malignant melanoma. J Rheumatol 1999; 26(4):1009–10.
365. Wandl UB, Nagel-Hiemke M, May D, Kreuzfelder E, Kloke O, Kranzhoff M, Seeber S, Niederle N. Lupus-like autoimmune disease induced by interferon therapy for myeloproliferative disorders. Clin Immunol Immunopathol 1992;65(1):70–4.
366. Conlon KC, Urba WJ, Smith JW 2nd, Steis RG, Longo DL, Clark JW. Exacerbation of symptoms of autoimmune disease in patients receiving alpha-interferon therapy. Cancer 1990;65(10):2237–42.
367. Nesher G, Ruchlemer R. Alpha-interferon-induced arthritis: clinical presentation treatment, and prevention. Semin Arthritis Rheum 1998;27(6):360–5.
368. Fukuyama S, Kajiwara E, Suzuki N, Miyazaki N, Sadoshima S, Onoyama K. Systemic lupus erythematosus after alpha-interferon therapy for chronic hepatitis C: a case report and review of the literature. Am J Gastroenterol 2000;95(1):310–12.
369. Beretta L, Caronni M, Vanoli M, Scorza R. Systemic sclerosis after interferon-alfa therapy for myeloproliferative disorders. Br J Dermatol 2002;147(2):385–6.
370. Friedman G, Mehta S, Sherker AH. Fatal exacerbation of hepatitis C-related cryoglobulinemia with interferon-alpha therapy. Dig Dis Sci 1999;44(7):1364–5.
371. Pateron D, Fain O, Sehonnou J, Trinchet JC, Beaugrand M. Severe necroziting vasculitis in a patient with hepatitis C virus infection treated by interferon. Clin Exp Rheumatol 1996;14(1):79–81.
372. Samson D, Volin L, Schanz U, Bosi A, Gahrtron G. Feasibility and toxicity of interferon maintenance therapy after allogeneic BMT for multiple myeloma: a pilot study of the EBMT. Bone Marrow Transplant 1996;17(5):759–62.
373. Morton AJ, Gooley T, Hansen JA, Appelbaum FR, Bruemmer B, Bjerke JW, Clift R, Martin PJ, Petersdorf EW, Sanders JE, Storb R, Sullivan KM, Woolfrey A, Anasetti C. Association between pretransplant interferon-alpha and outcome after unrelated donor marrow transplantation for chronic myelogenous leukemia in chronic phase. Blood 1998;92(2):394–401.
374. Rostaing L, Izopet J, Baron E, Duffaut M, Puel J, Durand D. Treatment of chronic hepatitis C with recombinant interferon alpha in kidney transplant recipients. Transplantation 1995;59(10):1426–31.
375. Dousset B, Conti F, Houssin D, Calmus Y. Acute vanishing bile duct syndrome after interferon therapy for recurrent HCV infection in liver-transplant recipients. N Engl J Med 1994;330(16):1160–1.
376. Féray C, Samuel D, Gigou M, Paradis V, David MF, Lemonnier C, Reynes M, Bismuth H. An open trial of interferon alfa recombinant for hepatitis C after liver transplantation: antiviral effects and risk of rejection. Hepatology 1995;22(4 Pt 1):1084–9.
377. Pohanka E, Kovarik J. Is treatment with interferon-alpha in renal transplant recipients still justified? Nephrol Dial Transplant 1996;11(6):1191–2.
378. Min AD, Bodenheimer HC Jr. Does interferon precipitate rejection of liver allografts? Hepatology 1995;22(4 Pt 1):1333–5.
379. Soriano V, Bravo R, Samaniego JG, Gonzalez J, Odriozola PM, Arroyo E, Vicario JL, Castro A, Colmenero M, Carballo E, et al. CD4+ T-lymphocytopenia in HIV-infected patients receiving interferon therapy for chronic hepatitis C. HIV-Hepatitis Spanish Study Group. AIDS 1994;8(11):1621–2.
380. Vento S, Di Perri G, Cruciani M, Garofano T, Concia E, Bassetti D. Rapid decline of CD4+ cells after IFN alpha treatment in HIV-1 infection. Lancet 1993;341(8850):958–9.
381. Marten D, Holtzmuller K, Julia F. Bacterial infections complicating hepatitis C infected hemodialysis dependent patients treated with interferon alfa. Am J Gastroenterol 2002;97(Suppl):163–4.
382. Parana R, Portugal M, Vitvitski L, Cotrim H, Lyra L, Trepo C. Severe strongyloidiasis during interferon plus ribavirin therapy for chronic HCV infection. Eur J Gastroenterol Hepatol 2000;12(2):245–6.
383. Serrano J, Prieto E, Mazarbeitia F, Roman A, Llamas P, Tomas JF. Atypical chronic graft-versus-host disease following interferon therapy for chronic myeloid leukaemia relapsing after allogeneic BMT. Bone Marrow Transplant 2001;27(1):85–7.
384. Beelen DW, Elmaagacli AH, Schaefer UW. The adverse influence of pretransplant interferon-alpha (IFN-alpha) on transplant outcome after marrow transplantation for chronic phrase chronic myelogenous leukemia increases with the duration of IFN-alpha exposure. Blood 1999;93(5):1779–10.
385. Hehlmann R, Hochhaus A, Kolb HJ, Hasford J, Gratwohl A, Heimpel H, Siegert W, Finke J, Ehninger G, Holler E, Berger U, Pfirrmann M, Muth A, Zander A, Fauser AA, Heyll A, Nerl C, Hossfeld DK, Loffler H, Pralle H, Queisser W, Tobler A. Interferon-alpha before allogeneic bone marrow transplantation in chronic myelogenous leukemia does not affect outcome adversely, provided it is discontinued at least 90 days before the procedure. Blood 1999;94(11):3668–77.
386. Johansson B, Fioretos T, Billstrom R, Mitelman F. Abberant cytogenetic evolution pattern of Philadelphia-positive chronic

myeloid leukemia treated with interferon-alpha. Leukemia 1996;10(7):1134–8.

387. Waysbort A, Giroux M, Mansat V, Teixeira M, Dumas JC, Puel J. Experimental study of transplacental passage of alpha interferon by two assay techniques. Antimicrob Agents Chemother 1993;37(6):1232–7.
388. Haggstrom J, Adriansson M, Hybbinette T, Harnby E, Thorbert G. Two cases of CML treated with alpha-interferon during second and third trimester of pregnancy with analysis of the drug in the new-born immediately post-partum. Eur J Haematol 1996;57(1):101–2.
389. Delage R, Demers C, Cantin G, Roy J. Treatment of essential thrombocythemia during pregnancy with interferon-alpha. Obstet Gynecol 1996;87(5 Pt 2):814–17.
390. Hiratsuka M, Minakami H, Koshizuka S, Sato I. Administration of interferon-alpha during pregnancy: effects on fetus. J Perinat Med 2000;28(5):372–6.
391. Mubarak AA, Kakil IR, Awidi A, Al-Homsi U, Fawzi Z, Kelta M, Al-Hassan A. Normal outcome of pregnancy in chronic myeloid leukemia treated with interferon-alpha in 1st trimester: report of 3 cases and review of the literature. Am J Hematol 2002;69(2):115–18.
392. Trotter JF, Zygmunt AJ. Conception and pregnancy during interferon-alpha therapy for chronic hepatitis C. J Clin Gastroenterol 2001;32(1):76–8.
393. Jacobson KR, Murray K, Zellos A, Schwarz KB. An analysis of published trials of interferon monotherapy in children with chronic hepatitis C. J Pediatr Gastroenterol Nutr 2002;34(1):52–8.
394. Barlow CF, Priebe CJ, Mulliken JB, Barnes PD, Mac Donald D, Folkman J, Ezekowitz RA. Spastic diplegia as a complication of interferon Alfa-2a treatment of hemangiomas of infancy. J Pediatr 1998;132(3 Pt 1):527–30.
395. Dubois J, Hershon L, Carmant L, Belanger S, Leclerc JM, David M. Toxicity profile of interferon alfa-2b in children: a prospective evaluation. J Pediatr 1999;135(6):782–5.
396. Worle H, Maass E, Kohler B, Treuner J. Interferon alpha-2a therapy in haemangiomas of infancy: spastic diplegia as a severe complication. Eur J Pediatr 1999;158(4):344.
397. Enjolras O. Neurotoxicity of interferon alfa in children treated for hemangiomas. J Am Acad Dermatol 1998;39(6):1037–8.
398. Grether JK, Nelson KB, Dambrosia JM, Phillips TM. Interferons and cerebral palsy. J Pediatr 1999;134(3):324–32.
399. Rostaing L, Chatelut E, Payen JL, Izopet J, Thalamas C, Ton-That H, Pascal JP, Durand D, Canal P. Pharmacokinetics of alphaIFN-2b in chronic hepatitis C virus patients undergoing chronic hemodialysis or with normal renal function: clinical implications. J Am Soc Nephrol 1998;9(12):2344–8.
400. Uchihara M, Izumi N, Sakai Y, Yauchi T, Miyake S, Sakai T, Akiba T, Marumo F, Sato C. Interferon therapy for chronic hepatitis C in hemodialysis patients: increased serum levels of interferon. Nephron 1998;80(1):51–6.
401. Anonymous. Interferon alfa-2b and ribavirin combination therapy—indications extended: previously untreated hepatitis C patients. WHO Newsletter 1999;1/2;9.
402. Chamberlain MC. A phase II trial of intra-cerebrospinal fluid alpha interferon in the treatment of neoplastic meningitis. Cancer 2002;94(10):2675–80.
403. Zylberberg H, Fontaine H, Thepot V, Nalpas B, Brechot C, Pol S. Triggering of acute alcoholic hepatitis by alpha-interferon therapy. J Hepatol 1999;30(4):722–5.
404. Casato M, Pucillo LP, Leoni M, di Lullo L, Gabrielli A, Sansonno D, Dammacco F, Danieli G, Bonomo L. Granulocytopenia after combined therapy with interferon and angiotensin-converting enzyme inhibitors: evidence for a synergistic hematologic toxicity. Am J Med 1995;99(4):386–91.
405. Bauckner JC, Schomberg PJ, McGinnis WL, Cascino TL, Scheithauer BW, O'Fallon JR, Morton RF, Kuross SA, Mailliard JA, Hatfield AK, Cole JT, Steen PD, Bernath AM. A phase III study of radiation therapy plus carmustine with or without recombinant interferon-alpha in the treatment of patients with newly diagnosed high-grade glioma. Cancer 2001;92(2):420–33.
406. Hassan M, Nilsson C, Olsson H, Lundin J, Osterborg A. The influence of interferon-alpha on the pharmacokinetics of cyclophosphamide and its 4-hydroxy metabolite in patients with multiple myeloma. Eur J Haematol 1999;63(3):163–70.
407. Chan TM, Wu PC, Lau JY, Lok AS, Lai CL, Cheng IK. Interferon treatment for hepatitis C virus infection in patients on haemodialysis. Nephrol Dial Transplant 1997;12(7):1414–19.
408. Desai RG. Drug interaction between alpha interferon and erythropoietin. J Clin Oncol 1991;9(5):893.
409. Nordio M, Guarda L, Lorenzi S, Lombini C, Marchini P, Mirandoli F. Interaction between alpha-interferon and erythropoietin in antiviral and antineoplastic therapy in uraemic patients on haemodialysis. Nephrol Dial Transplant 1993;8(11):1308.
410. Czejka MJ, Schuller J, Jager W, Fogl U, Weiss C. Influence of different doses of interferon-alpha-2b on the blood plasma levels of 5-fluorouracil. Eur J Drug Metab Pharmacokinet 1993;18(3):247–50.
411. Greco FA, Figlin R, York M, Einhorn L, Schilsky R, Marshall EM, Buys SS, Froimtchuk MJ, Schuller J, Schuchter L, Buyse M, Ritter L, Man A, Yap AK. Phase III randomized study to compare interferon alfa-2a in combination with fluorouracil versus fluorouracil alone in patients with advanced colorectal cancer. J Clin Oncol 1996;14(10):2674–81.
412. Ehrsson H, Eksborg S, Wallin I, Osterborg A, Mellstedt H. Oral melphalan pharmacokinetics: influence of interferon-induced fever. Clin Pharmacol Ther 1990;47(1):86–90.
413. Mannering GJ, Deloria LB. The pharmacology and toxicology of the interferons: an overview. Annu Rev Pharmacol Toxicol 1986;26:455–515.
414. Echizen H, Ohta Y, Shirataki H, Tsukamoto K, Umeda N, Oda T, Ishizaki T. Effects of subchronic treatment with natural human interferons on antipyrine clearance and liver function in patients with chronic hepatitis. J Clin Pharmacol 1990;30(6):562–7.
415. Tappero G, Ballare M, Farina M, Negro F. Severe anemia following combined alpha-interferon/ribavirin therapy of chronic hepatitis C. J Hepatol 1998;29(6):1033–4.
416. Sookoian S, Neglia V, Castano G, Frider B, Kien MC, Chohuela E. High prevalence of cutaneous reactions to interferon alfa plus ribavirin combination therapy in patients with chronic hepatitis C virus. Arch Dermatol 1999;135(8):1000–1.
417. Nathan PD, Gore ME, Eisen TG. Unexpected toxicity of combination thalidomide and interferon alpha-2a treatment in metastatic renal cell carcinoma. J Clin Oncol 2002;20(5):1429–30.
418. Israel BC, Blouin RA, McIntyre W, Shedlofsky SI. Effects of interferon-alpha monotherapy on hepatic drug metabolism in cancer patients. Br J Clin Pharmacol 1993;36(3):229–35.
419. Williams SJ, Baird-Lambert JA, Farrell GC. Inhibition of theophylline metabolism by interferon. Lancet 1987;2(8565):939–41.
420. Jonkman JH, Nicholson KG, Farrow PR, Eckert M, Grasmeijer G, Oosterhuis B, De Noord OE, Guentert TW. Effects of alpha-interferon on theophylline pharmacokinetics and metabolism. Br J Clin Pharmacol 1989;27(6):795–802.

421. Burger DM, Meenhorst PL, Koks CH, Beijnen JH. Drug interactions with zidovudine. AIDS 1993;7(4): 445–60.
422. Krown SE, Gold JW, Niedzwiecki D, Bundow D, Flomenberg N, Gansbacher B, Brew BJ. Interferon-alpha with zidovudine: safety, tolerance, and clinical and virologic effects in patients with Kaposi sarcoma associated with the acquired immunodeficiency syndrome (AIDS). Ann Intern Med 1990;112(11):812–21.

Interferon beta

See also Interferons

General Information

Interferon beta is used in the form of natural fibroblast or recombinant preparations (interferon beta-1a and interferon beta-1b) and exerts antiviral and antiproliferative properties similar to those of interferon alfa. Although its efficacy has been debated (1), interferon beta has been approved for the treatment of relapsing–remitting multiple sclerosis, and more recently for secondary progressive multiple sclerosis.

The general toxicity of interferon beta is very similar to that of interferon alfa (2), with no apparent differences between the two recombinant preparations with any route of injection (SEDA-20, 332) (3–6). In multiple sclerosis, fatigue and a transient flu-like syndrome responsive to paracetamol or the combination of paracetamol plus prednisone have been observed in about 60% of patients during the first weeks of treatment, and tachyphylaxis usually developed after several doses (7). Patients with chronic progressive disease are more likely to discontinue treatment because of adverse effects (8).

Clinically relevant adverse effects associated with interferon beta and their management have been lengthily reviewed (9). Interferon beta-1a and beta-1b, the two recombinant available forms of interferon beta, have not been directly compared. From the results of a randomized, crossover study in 12 healthy volunteers, a single injection of interferon beta-1a 6 MU (Rebif) was suggested to produce less frequent and less severe fever than interferon beta-1b 8 MU (Betaseron), but identical pharmacodynamic effects (10).

A flu-like illness is the most common adverse effect of interferon beta. In an open, randomized study of the effects of paracetamol 1 g or ibuprofen 400 mg before and 6 hours after interferon beta injection on interferon beta-induced flu-like symptoms in 104 patients, the two drugs were equally effective (11).

Organs and Systems

Cardiovascular

Cardiovascular adverse effects of interferon beta include isolated reports of severe Raynaud's phenomenon (SEDA-22, 374) and acute myocarditis (SEDA-21, 374).

Fatal capillary leak syndrome has been reported (12).

- A 27-year-old woman had an 8-month history of relapsing–remitting neurological symptoms and a monoclonal gammopathy. She started to take interferon beta-1b for multiple sclerosis, but had marked somnolence 30 hours after a single injection. She rapidly became unresponsiveness, and hemodynamic tests showed low central venous and pulmonary capillary wedge pressures with generalized peripheral edema, ascites, and bilateral pleural effusions. She died within 80 hours after injection from multiple organ failure. At postmortem she was found to have C1 esterase inhibitor deficiency.

In the light of the possible effects of interferon beta on cytokine release and complement activation, a cytokine-mediated reaction was discussed as the cause of the capillary leak syndrome in this case.

Respiratory

Bronchiolitis obliterans with organizing pneumonia has been reported in a patient taking interferon beta (13).

- A 49-year-old man had a progressive unproductive cough and right hemithoracic pain after 3 months of interferon beta-1a 30 micrograms/week for multiple sclerosis. A CT scan showed a right basal pulmonary infiltrate and transbronchial biopsies showed features consistent with bronchiolitis obliterans with organizing pneumonia. The lesions resolved fully on interferon beta-1a withdrawal and prednisone treatment.

Nervous system

Although direct toxic effects of natural interferon beta on the nervous system have been regarded as a possible risk of intraventricular and/or intratumoral injection (14), interferon beta is considered to be markedly less neurotoxic than interferon alfa (15).

Although headache was not specifically identified as an adverse effect of interferon beta in pivotal trials, the frequency, duration, and intensity of headache increased during the first 6 months of treatment in 65 patients (16). There was a 35% probability of aggravated headaches in patients with pre-existing headaches.

The possible deleterious effects of interferon beta-1b on increased spasticity have been examined in 19 patients with primary progressive multiple sclerosis, 19 untreated matched patients, and 10 patients treated with interferon beta-1b for relapsing–remitting multiple sclerosis (17). Patients with primary progressive multiple sclerosis had frequent (68%) and clinically relevant increased spasticity (seven required oral baclofen), usually after about 2 months of treatment, whereas only two (11%) of the untreated patients and none of the patients with relapsing–remitting multiple sclerosis had similar disabling spasticity. Seven patients had to discontinue treatment after 6 months because of spasticity, and symptoms improved over several months after withdrawal. The authors suggested that this possible adverse effect should be taken into account in clinical trials because it could mask the positive clinical effects of interferon beta-1b.

Neurosarcoidosis has been reported in a patient with chronic hepatitis C who was treated with interferon beta.

- A 56-year-old woman developed numbness and difficulty in swallowing and in closing her left eye several weeks after starting interferon beta for chronic hepatitis C (18). She had facial paresthesia, a left facial nerve palsy, dysphagia, and signs of radiculopathy on the left side. Serum angiotensin-converting enzyme activity was raised. She had bilateral hilar lymphadenopathy without interstitial changes and increased radiogallium uptake in hilar lymph nodes and the parotid glands. Although the cerebrospinal fluid was normal, a diagnosis of neurosarcoidosis was considered, and she recovered completely after interferon beta withdrawal and glucocorticoid therapy.

Moderate exacerbation of multiple sclerosis sometimes occurs in the first 3 months of interferon beta treatment.

- A 21-year-old man had an acute and very severe clinical relapse, with multiple disseminated demyelinating lesions and axonal injury on MRI and cerebral biopsy, after the third injection of interferon beta-1a (19).

Whether this case was due to interferon beta or resulted from spontaneous exacerbation was open to question.

Sensory systems

Retinal complications of interferon alfa in chronic viral hepatitis patients are well known, but few cases have been described with interferon beta.

- Bilateral retinopathy with similar features to those observed with interferon alfa has been reported in a 40-year-old woman treated with interferon beta-1b for multiple sclerosis (20).

In 49 patients, there was reversible otological impairment with tinnitus, mild-to-moderate hearing loss, or both in respectively 8, 16, and 20% of patients after administration of interferon alfa or interferon beta (SEDA-19, 336). These disorders tended to occur more frequently in patients on high cumulative doses, but led to withdrawal of treatment in only two patients.

Psychological, psychiatric

There have been reports of depression, suicidal ideation, and attempted suicide in patients receiving interferon beta (2,8,21). The lifetime risk of depression in patients with multiple sclerosis is high, and there has been a lively debate about whether interferon beta causes or exacerbates depression in such patients. Impressions of a possibly raised incidence of depression among patients treated with interferon beta for multiple sclerosis should be interpreted in the light of the spontaneous tendency to depressive disorders and suicidal ideation, which is encountered even in patients with untreated multiple sclerosis. Moreover, no raised incidence of these complications has been recorded in some studies (4,5). A critical review of the methodological limitations in studies that assessed mood disorders in patients on disease-modifying drugs for multiple sclerosis may help explain the widely divergent results from one study to another (22). Some results have argued against a specific role of interferon beta in the risk of depressive disorders.

A multicenter comparison of 44 and 22 micrograms of interferon beta-1a and placebo in 365 patients showed no significant differences in depression scores between the groups over a 3-year period of follow-up (23). In 106 patients with relapsing–remitting multiple sclerosis, depression status was evaluated before and after 12 months of interferon beta-1a treatment (24). According to the Beck Depression Inventory II scale, most of the patients had minimum (53%) or mild (32%) depression at baseline, and depression scores were not significantly increased after 1 year of treatment. There were no cases of suicidal ideation. In another study of 42 patients treated with interferon beta-1b, major depression at baseline was found in 21% of patients and was associated with a past history of psychiatric illness in most cases (25). Major depression was not considered as an exclusion criterion for interferon beta treatment when patients were on antidepressant therapy. There was a three-fold reduction in the prevalence of depression over the 1-year course of interferon treatment, suggesting a possible beneficial effect of treatment on mood. Finally, a single subcutaneous injection of interferon beta-1b did not alter cognitive performance and mood states in eight healthy volunteers (26).

The emotional state of 90 patients with relapsing–remitting multiple sclerosis has been carefully assessed with a battery of psychological tests at baseline and after 1 and 2 years of treatment with interferon beta-1b (27). In contrast to what was expected, and despite the lack of controls, there was significant improvement in emotional state, as shown by significant reductions in scores of anxiety and depression over time. In addition, there was no effect of low-dose oral glucocorticoids in a subgroup of 46 patients.

Depression has been quantified by telephone interview in 56 patients with relapsing multiple sclerosis 2 weeks before treatment, at the start of treatment, and after 8 weeks of treatment (28). Patients with a high depressive score 2 weeks before treatment significantly improved on starting treatment and returned to baseline within 8 weeks, whereas the depression score in non-depressed patients remained essentially unchanged. The investigators therefore suggested that patients' expectations had temporarily resulted in improvement of depression, and that increased depression during treatment is more likely to reflect pretreatment depression.

The clinical features, management, and prognosis of psychiatric symptoms in patients with chronic hepatitis C have been reviewed using data from 943 patients treated with interferon alfa (85%) or interferon beta (15%) for 24 weeks (29). Interferon-induced psychiatric symptoms were identified in 40 patients (4.2%) of those referred for psychiatric examination. They were classified in three groups according to the clinical profile: 13 cases of generalized anxiety disorder (group A), 21 cases of mood disorders with depressive features (group B), and six cases of other psychiatric disorders, including psychotic disorders with delusions/hallucinations ($n = 4$), mood disorders with manic features ($n = 1$), and delirium ($n = 1$) (group C). The time to onset of the symptoms differed significantly between the three groups: 2 weeks in group A, 5 weeks in group B, and 11 weeks in group C.

Women were more often affected than men. There was no difference in the incidence or nature of the disorder according to the type of interferon used. Whereas most patients who required psychotropic drugs were able to complete treatment, 10 had to discontinue interferon treatment because of severe psychiatric symptoms, five from group B and five from group C. Twelve patients still required psychiatric treatment for more than 6 months after interferon withdrawal. In addition, residual symptoms (anxiety, insomnia, and mild hypothymia) were still present at the end of the survey in seven patients. Delayed recovery was mostly observed in patients in group C and in patients treated with interferon beta.

One debatable case of visual pseudo-hallucinations occurred only, but not reproducibly, within 30–60 minutes after interferon beta-1a injection in a 37-year-old woman with disseminated encephalomyelitis (30).

Endocrine

While no evidence of thyroid dysfunction or antithyroid antibodies was found in 20 patients receiving interferon beta during 24 weeks for hematological malignancies (31), antithyroid antibodies were detected in 29% of patients with multiple sclerosis after a prospective follow-up performed at 6, 12, and 18 months of treatment (32). Biological thyroid abnormalities without antithyroid antibodies have also been found (SEDA-20, 332). Overall, thyroid disorders with antithyroid antibodies were reported in only three patients on long-term interferon beta treatment for multiple sclerosis (32,33).

Thyroid disorders before and during the first 9 months of interferon beta-1b treatment have been systematically investigated in eight patients with relapsing–remitting multiple sclerosis (34). Before treatment, one patient had positive thyroperoxidase antibodies and one was taking thyroxine for multinodular goiter. After 3 months three other patients developed sustained positive titers of thyroperoxidase antibodies, of whom one developed hypothyroidism after 9 months. These results are in accordance with a previous similar study and isolated case reports (SEDA-21, 374) (SEDA-22, 405), and suggest that interferon beta, like interferon alfa, can cause thyroid autoimmunity.

As suggested in a more comprehensive long-term follow-up study, interferon beta-induced thyroid dysfunction is often transient or has limited clinical consequences (35). Of 31 patients with multiple sclerosis regularly assessed for 30–42 months for thyroid function, 13 developed thyroid disorders during treatment with interferon beta-1b. None withdrew because of thyroid disorders. Of the eight patients with no previous thyroid disorders, one had a persistent but isolated increase in antithyroglobulin titer, six developed transient signs of hypothyroidism or hyperthyroidism during the first year of therapy, and only one had overt hypothyroidism after 12 months of treatment and required thyroxine replacement. Of the five patients with baseline signs of Hashimoto's thyroiditis, one had a transiently positive antithyroglobulin titer, one developed transient hyperthyroidism, and the three patients who had previously had or who newly developed subclinical hypothyroidism remained stable throughout the study. Overall, thyroid disorders occurred only during the first 12 months of treatment and no additional cases were detected after the first year of therapy. In the authors' opinion, pre-existing or new thyroiditis is not a contraindication to continuing interferon beta-1b treatment. Two patients took thyroxine replacement and continued to receive interferon beta-1b (36).

Metabolism

Severe hypertriglyceridemia, a well-known adverse effect of interferon beta, has been reported and fully investigated in a 39-year-old man receiving interferon beta for chronic hepatitis C (37).

Hematologic

Moderate reductions in white blood cell count (that is lymphopenia, leukopenia, and granulocytopenia) have been observed with recombinant interferon beta, and marked eosinophilia recorded in an atopic patient (SEDA-21, 374).

- A 42-year-old woman developed aplastic anemia after using interferon beta-1a for 1 year (38). There was hematological improvement after withdrawal and immunosuppressive therapy.

Reversible autoimmune hemolytic anemia (SEDA-20, 332) has also been reported.

Liver

Adverse hepatic effects of interferon beta were usually limited to a dose-dependent increase in transaminases, but transient autoimmune hepatitis has been described in one patient (39).

It has been suspected that interferon beta can accelerate hepatocellular carcinoma (40).

- A 62-year-old man with severe chronic hepatitis and positive serum anti-HCV, HBs, and HBc antibodies underwent unsuccessful treatment with interferon alfa for 3 months and then received interferon beta for 6 months with a partial response. During treatment, his alfa-fetoprotein (normal before treatment) progressively increased to seven-fold the upper limit of the reference range. There was also a slight increase in interleukin-6 serum concentration. A hepatocellular carcinoma was diagnosed 9 months later.

Liver carcinoma is an unexpected consequence of interferon beta in patients with chronic hepatitis C. However, the authors cited other published Japanese reports of hepatocellular carcinoma during or after interferon treatment. It is worth noting that interferon beta, but not interferon alfa, significantly increased serum interleukin-6 concentrations in patients with chronic hepatitis C (41), and that interleukin-6 has been suggested to promote the growth of hepatocellular carcinoma.

Fulminant liver failure has been attributed to interferon beta-1a (42), but it was subsequently confirmed that this case was confounded by concomitant exposure to nefazodone, which is hepatotoxic (43).

Urinary tract

Reversible hemolytic–uremic syndrome has been reported (SEDA-22, 405).

- Two women aged 24 and 44 years, whose primary diagnosis was relapsing multiple sclerosis, developed renal impairment and a thrombotic thrombocytopenic purpura-like syndrome within 2–4 weeks after starting interferon beta-1a (44). Thrombocytopenia and renal function normalized in the first patient, whereas the second patient had thrombotic angiopathy on renal biopsy and required dialysis while awaiting renal transplantation.

As interferon alfa has also been suggested to produce hemolytic–uremic syndrome with thrombotic thrombocytopenic purpura, it is tempting to speculate that either interferons or other cytokines may play a role in this syndrome.

Proteinuria, nephrotic syndrome, and various forms of renal lesions can be caused or exacerbated by interferon alfa (SED-14, 1252).

- Proteinuria with minimal–change nephrotic syndrome on renal biopsy has been attributed to interferon beta in a 64-year-old man with malignant melanoma (45). Although the proteinuria abated after withdrawal, the potential role of previous chemotherapy cannot be excluded.
- Nephrotic syndrome with segmental glomerulosclerosis has been reported in a 32-year-old woman with multiple sclerosis receiving interferon beta (46).

The clinicopathological features of proteinuria have been investigated in 23 patients with chronic hepatitis C who had new or worsened proteinuria during interferon treatment (interferon alfa 6–10 MU/day in three patients and interferon beta 6 MU/day in 20 patients (47)). Renal function and urinary findings were normal before treatment in 21 subjects. Proteinuria appeared after a mean of 12 (range 5–30) days after the start of treatment, and the mean value was 2.1 g/day. There was low selective proteinuria in 78% of the patients. Renal histopathology in 11 patients showed IgA glomerulonephritis in five, mesangial proliferative glomerulonephritis in four, membranoproliferative glomerulonephritis in one, and nephrosclerosis in one. There was only trace deposition of hepatitis C virus core antigen in three of nine patients, suggesting that hepatitis C was not the primary cause of these glomerulopathies.

Skin

Injection-site reactions are common after subcutaneous injection of interferon beta-1b, and are more frequent than with any other available interferons. In a multicenter placebo-controlled trial, 65% of patients receiving interferon beta-1b had reactions at the injection site compared with 6% in the placebo group (2). In contrast, only 5% of those who received interferon beta-1a had injection site reactions (3). The clinical features of injection site reactions to interferon beta-1b mostly consist of benign inflammatory reactions, but they can sometimes be more severe, with sclerotic dermal plaques, painful erythematous nodules, and deep cutaneous ulcers with skin necrosis (SEDA-21, 374) (48). Late severe reactions have included a case of squamous cell carcinoma at the injection site (SEDA-21, 375) and a case of panniculitis (49).

Since interferon beta-1b became available, 1443 instances of injection site reactions, 212 cases of injection site necrosis, and 10 cases of non-injection site necrosis were notified to the US Food and Drug Administration, and antibiotic therapy or surgery was required in 20–30% of patients (50). Severe necrotizing cutaneous lesions have also been attributed to subcutaneous interferon beta-1a (51).

In contrast to previous claims, even low-dose interferon beta-1b can produce severe local reactions and cutaneous necrosis, with no recurrence after interferon alfa injection and expected better tolerance to interferon beta-1a (52–55). The mechanisms of interferon beta-induced local skin reaction might involve a local vascular inflammatory process or platelet-dependent thrombosis, but positive intracutaneous tests to interferon beta have also been found (56).

There have been other isolated reports of skin lesions.

- Intravascular papillary endothelial hyperplasia with multiple lesions on both hands has been attributed to interferon beta-1b in a 50-year-old man with multiple sclerosis (57).
- Granulomatous dermatitis with disseminated pruritic papules and histological features resembling those of sarcoid granulomas has been described in a 57-year-old man who received interferon beta-1b (58). The first lesions were observed after 2 months of treatment, persisted for 2 years, and slowly improved after interferon beta withdrawal and treatment with hydroxychloroquine PUVA.
- Erythromelalgia has been attributed to interferon beta-1a in a 38-year-old woman (59). Complete recovery was obtained only after interferon withdrawal.
- In one patient, there was cutaneous mucinosis on skin biopsy, and skin lesions persisted for several months before healing spontaneously (60).

Other reports include exacerbation of quiescent psoriasis or induction of psoriatic lesions at the injection sites (SED-13, 1099) (SEDA-20, 332), and the development or exacerbation of lichen planus (SEDA-21, 375).

Musculoskeletal

Rhabdomyolysis associated with interferon beta has been reported (61).

- A 39-year-old man developed acute generalized myalgia and weakness in all four limbs 3 months after starting interferon beta-1a (22 micrograms three times a week) for relapsing–remitting multiple sclerosis. Serum creatine kinase activity peaked at about 95 times the upper limit of the reference range. Infectious and metabolic causes were ruled out and there was no argument in favor of an underlying metabolic muscle disorder. He recovered fully after interferon beta withdrawal and supportive treatment.

Although rhabdomyolysis has not been previously attributed to interferon beta, this case is in keeping with those described with interferon alfa.

- A 39-year-old man developed monoarthritis in his right elbow after receiving interferon beta for 16 days for chronic hepatitis C (62).

Although the arthritis resolved after withdrawal, this report casts doubt on the causal relation, as there was no recurrence on re-administration.

Reproductive system

Mild to moderate menstrual disorders were twice as frequent in patients receiving interferon beta compared with placebo (17 versus 8%). Severe persistent vaginal bleeding has been reported in a 19-year-old woman (SEDA-21, 375).

Immunologic

Hypersensitivity reactions

Hypersensitivity reactions to interferon beta are rare, with only two cases of immediate-type reactions (SEDA-20, 332) (63), and one case of urticaria associated with exacerbation of asthma (64).

- A 21-year-old woman had a severe anaphylactic-like reaction with laryngospasm and undetectable blood pressure within 10 minutes after interferon beta-1a injection (63). It is still uncertain that anaphylaxis was definitely attributable to interferon, because rechallenge and skin tests were not performed in this patient, who had tolerated the treatment for the 6 previous months.
- Urticaria developed after 9 months of treatment with interferon beta-1b in a 32-year-old woman with a previous history of penicillin allergy (64). She also had an exacerbation of asthma shortly after starting treatment. A positive intradermal test to interferon beta-1b, but not to interferon beta-1a or the diluents, suggested a specific IgE allergic reaction.

Another isolated case history has suggested that interferon beta-1b might have favored the development of a non-IgE-mediated anaphylactic reaction to previously well-tolerated injections of methylprednisolone (65).

Autoimmune disorders

In contrast to interferon alfa, the autoimmune consequences of interferon beta treatment have been poorly evaluated. Interferon beta does not appear to be associated with the appearance or increased titres of several auto-antibodies, and no clinical features of autoimmune disease were observed in patients receiving a 6-month course of interferon beta-1a or interferon beta-1b (66,67).

Subcutaneous lupus erythematosus reversible on withdrawal of treatment (SEDA-22, 405) and myasthenia gravis (SEDA-21, 375) have been described, but each only in a single patient receiving interferon beta.

The possible involvement of interferon beta in the occurrence of sarcoidosis has been noted in two patients (68,69).

Interferon beta antibodies

In multiple sclerosis, neutralizing antibodies to recombinant interferon beta occurred in 12–38% of patients treated for 2–3 years (3–5,70). There were no adverse consequences in patients who developed antibodies to interferon beta-1a (4), but there was reduced therapeutic efficacy in terms of clinical relapse rate or magnetic resonance imaging in several patients who had neutralizing antibodies to interferon beta-1b (SEDA-20, 332) (5,71).

The systemic availability of interferon beta-1b, measured by a myxovirus protein A assay, was completely inhibited in patients with neutralizing antibodies (72). The presence of increased titers of serum-binding antibodies increased the likelihood of neutralizing antibodies. From an in vitro study of nine patients who developed neutralizing antibodies against the available formulations of recombinant interferon beta (three on interferon beta-1a and six on interferon beta-1b), it appears that these antibodies systematically cross-react in both binding and biological assays (73). Although the sample size was small and lacked clinical confirmation, these results suggest that clinical benefit will not be obtained by switching to an alternative formulation when the absence of response or relapse during treatment is due to neutralizing antibodies.

The clinical significance of these antibodies is uncertain (74) and it has been proposed that decisions to discontinue treatment should be based on individual clinical responses and unequivocal demonstration of neutralizing antibodies with a reliable assay (70).

One study has shown that antibodies can spontaneously disappear in patients receiving long-term treatment. Of 24 of 51 patients who initially developed neutralizing antibodies, generally during the first year of treatment, only five still had antibodies after a mean treatment duration of 102 months (75). The mean time to antibody disappearance was 20 months.

A randomized study has been conducted in 161 patients to evaluate whether a monthly intravenous pulse of methylprednisolone reduces the frequency of neutralizing antibodies to interferon beta-1b (76). The patients who received both interferon beta and methylprednisolone had a 55% relative reduction in the development of neutralizing antibody and were significantly more likely to remain negative for neutralizing antibodies after 6 months of treatment compared with those who received interferon beta alone. The overall frequency of adverse effects and the number of withdrawals were similar between the groups, but headaches, fatigue, and myalgia were less frequent in the combination therapy group. A limitation of this study was that there was no difference in clinical outcome between the two groups.

Finally, possible differences in the immunogenic potential of recombinant and natural interferon beta preparations were found in a small study (77).

Second-Generation Effects

Teratogenicity

Data on outcomes in pregnancy after treatment with interferon beta-1a in patients with multiple sclerosis have been obtained from clinical trials (78). Of 29 pregnancies that occurred during or shortly after treatment withdrawal, 13 resulted in normal outcomes, two in premature births, one in fetal death, six in induced abortions, and seven in spontaneous abortions.

- A child whose mother had received interferon beta until 2.5 months before pregnancy had a right incomplete double renal pelvis and ureter (79). Although the authors discussed the possible role of interferon therapy, the timing of exposure was obviously not suggestive of a causal relation.

Although the data are still very limited, it is advisable to reassure exposed patients and to withdraw interferon beta up to the time of delivery.

Drug Administration

Drug dosage regimens

In 188 patients with relapsing–remitting multiple sclerosis assigned to receive interferon beta-1a 30 micrograms intramuscularly once a week or interferon beta-1b 44 micrograms subcutaneously three times a week, only injection site reactions and neutralizing antibodies to interferon beta were significantly more frequent in the interferon beta-1b group (80). These differences were probably related to the subcutaneous route of administration of interferon beta-1b. In contrast, there were significant differences in favor of interferon beta-1b for clinical outcomes after 2 years of treatment.

In a comparison of two regimens of interferon beta-1a (44 micrograms Rebif subcutaneously three times a week versus 30 micrograms Avonex intramuscularly once a week) in 677 patients with relapsing–remitting multiple sclerosis, Rebif was more effective on primary clinical outcomes (patients remaining relapse-free at 24 weeks), but produced significantly more frequent injection site reactions (88 versus 28%), asymptomatic and mild liver enzyme abnormalities (18 versus 9%), mild white cell abnormalities (11 versus 5%), and neutralizing antibodies to interferon beta (25 versus 2%) (81). However, the severity of adverse events and withdrawal due to an adverse event were similar in both groups.

Drug–Drug Interactions

Theophylline

Interferon beta reduced theophylline clearance by 29% in seven patients (SED-13, 1099).

References

1. Anonymous. Euromedicines evaluation: the striptease begins. Lancet 1996;347(9000):483 (see also Harvey P. Why interferon beta 1b was licensed is a mystery. BMJ 1996;313(7052):297–8 and Napier JC. Reputation of interferon beta-1b. Lancet 1996;347(9006):968).
2. The IFNB Multiple Sclerosis Study Group and The University of British Columbia MS/MRI Analysis Group. Interferon beta-1b in the treatment of multiple sclerosis: final outcome of the randomized controlled trial. Neurology 1995;45(7):1277–85.
3. Jacobs LD, Cookfair DL, Rudick RA, Herndon RM, Richert JR, Salazar AM, Fischer JS, Goodkin DE, Granger CV, Simon JH, Alam JJ, Bartoszak DM, Bourdette DN, Braiman J, Brownscheidle CM, Coats ME, Cohan SL, Dougherty DS, Kinkel RP, Mass MK, Munschauer FE 3rd, Priore RL, Pullicino PM, Scherokman BJ, Whitham RH, et al. Intramuscular interferon beta-1a for disease progression in relapsing multiple sclerosis. The Multiple Sclerosis Collaborative Research Group (MSCRG) Ann Neurol 1996;39(3):285–94
4. Ebers GC, Hommes O, Hughes RAC, et al.; PRISMS (Prevention of Relapses and Disability by Interferon beta-1a Subcutaneously in Multiple Sclerosis) Study Group. Randomised double-blind placebo-controlled study of interferon beta-1a in relapsing/remitting multiple sclerosis. Lancet 1998;352(9139):1498–504.
5. European Study Group on Interferon Beta-1b in Secondary Progressive MS. Placebo-controlled multicentre randomised trial of interferon beta-1b in treatment of secondary progressive multiple sclerosis. Lancet 1998;352(9139):1491–7.
6. Weinstock-Guttman B, Rudick RA. Prescribing recommendations for interferon-beta in multiple sclerosis. CNS Drugs 1997;8:102–12.
7. Rio J, Nos C, Marzo ME, Tintore M, Montalban X. Low-dose steroids reduce flu-like symptoms at the initiation of IFNbeta-1b in relapsing-remitting MS. Neurology 1998; 50(6):1910–12.
8. Neilley LK, Goodin DS, Goodkin DE, Hauser SL. Side effect profile of interferon beta-1b in MS: results of an open label trial. Neurology 1996;46(2):552–4.
9. Bayas A, Rieckmann P. Managing the adverse effects of interferon-beta therapy in multiple sclerosis. Drug Saf 2000;22(2):149–59.
10. Buraglio M, Trinchard-Lugan I, Munafo A, Macnamee M. Recombinant human interferon-beta-1a (Rebif) vs recombinant interferon-beta-1b (Betaseron) in healthy volunteers. A pharmacodynamic and tolerability study. Clin Drug Invest 1999;18:27–34.
11. Reess J, Haas J, Gabriel K, Fuhlrott A, Fiola M, Schicklmaier P. Both paracetamol and ibuprofen are equally effective in managing flu-like symptoms in relapsing-remitting multiple sclerosis patients during interferon beta-1a (AVONEX) therapy. Mult Scler 2002;8(1):15–18.
12. Schmidt S, Hertfelder HJ, von Spiegel T, Hering R, Harzheim M, Lassmann H, Deckert-Schluter M, Schlegel U. Lethal capillary leak syndrome after a single administration of interferon beta-1b. Neurology 1999; 53(1):220–2.
13. Ferriby D, Stojkovic T. Clinical picture: bronchiolitis obliterans with organising pneumonia during interferon beta-1a treatment. Lancet 2001;357(9258):751.
14. Matsumura S, Takamatsu H, Sato S, Ara S. [Central nervous system toxicity of local interferon-beta therapy. Report of three cases.] Neurol Med Chir (Tokyo) 1988;28 (3):265–70.
15. Liberati AM, Biagini S, Perticoni G, Ricci S, D'Alessandro P, Senatore M, Cinieri S. Electrophysiological and neuropsychological functions in patients treated with interferon-beta. J Interferon Res 1990;10(6):613–19.
16. Pollmann W, Erasmus LP, Feneberg W, Then Bergh F, Straube A. Interferon beta but not glatiramer acetate therapy aggravates headaches in MS. Neurology 2002;59(4):636–9.
17. Bramanti P, Sessa E, Rifici C, D'Aleo G, Floridia D, Di Bella P, Lublin F. Enhanced spasticity in primary progressive MS patients treated with interferon beta-1b. Neurology 1998;51(6):1720–3.
18. Miwa H, Furuya T, Tanaka S, Mizuno Y. Neurosarcoidosis associated with interferon therapy. Eur Neurol 2001;45(4):288–9.
19. Von Raison F, Abboud H, Saint Val C, Brugieres P, Cesaro P. Acute demyelinating disease after interferon beta-1a treatment for multiple sclerosis. Neurology 2000;55(9):1416–17.
20. Sommer S, Sablon JC, Zaoui M, Rozot P, Hosni A. Rétinopathie à l'interféron bêta au cours d'une sclérose en

plaques. [Interferon beta-1b retinopathy during a treatment for multiple sclerosis.] J Fr Ophtalmol 2001;24(5):509–12.
21. Lublin FD, Whitaker JN, Eidelman BH, Miller AE, Arnason BG, Burks JS. Management of patients receiving interferon beta-1b for multiple sclerosis: report of a consensus conference. Neurology 1996;46(1):12–18.
22. Feinstein A. Multiple sclerosis, disease modifying treatments and depression: a critical methodological review. Mult Scler 2000;6(5):343–8.
23. Patten SB, Metz LM; SPECTRIMS Study Group. Interferon beta1a and depression in secondary progressive MS: data from the SPECTRIMS Trial. Neurology 2002;59(5):744–6.
24. Zephir H, De Seze J, Stojkovic T, Delisse B, Ferriby D, Cabaret M, Vermersch P. Multiple sclerosis and depression: influence of interferon beta therapy. Mult Scler 2003;9(3):284–8.
25. Feinstein A, O'Connor P, Feinstein K. Multiple sclerosis, interferon beta-1b and depression. A prospective investigation. J Neurol 2002;249(7):815–20.
26. Exton MS, Baase J, Pithan V, Goebel MU, Limmroth V, Schedlowski M. Neuropsychological performance and mood states following acute interferon-beta-1b administration in healthy males. Neuropsychobiology 2002;45(4):199–204.
27. Borras C, Rio J, Porcel J, Barrios M, Tintore M, Montalban X. Emotional state of patients with relapsing-remitting MS treated with interferon beta-1b. Neurology 1999;52(8):1636–9.
28. Mohr DC, Likosky W, Dwyer P, Van Der Wende J, Boudewyn AC, Goodkin DE. Course of depression during the initiation of interferon beta-1a treatment for multiple sclerosis. Arch Neurol 1999;56(10):1263–5.
29. Hosoda S, Takimura H, Shibayama M, Kanamura H, Ikeda K, Kumada H. Psychiatric symptoms related to interferon therapy for chronic hepatitis C: clinical features and prognosis. Psychiatry Clin Neurosci 2000;54(5):565–72.
30. Moor CC, Berwanger C, Welter FL. Visual pseudo-hallucinations in interferon-beta 1a therapy. Akt Neurol 2002;29:355–7.
31. Pagliacci MC, Pelicci G, Schippa M, Liberati AM, Nicoletti I. Does interferon-beta therapy induce thyroid autoimmune phenomena? Horm Metab Res 1991;23(4):196–7.
32. Martinelli V, Gironi M, Rodegher M, Martino G, Comi G. Occurrence of thyroid autoimmunity in relapsing remitting multiple sclerosis patients undergoing interferon-beta treatment. Ital J Neurol Sci 1998;19(2):65–7.
33. Schwid SR, Goodman AD, Mattson DH. Autoimmune hyperthyroidism in patients with multiple sclerosis treated with interferon beta-1b. Arch Neurol 1997;54(9):1169–90.
34. Rotondi M, Oliviero A, Profice P, Mone CM, Biondi B, Del Buono A, Mazziotti G, Sinisi AM, Bellastella A, Carella C. Occurrence of thyroid autoimmunity and dysfunction throughout a nine-month follow-up in patients undergoing interferon-beta therapy for multiple sclerosis. J Endocrinol Invest 1998;21(11):748–52.
35. Monzani F, Caraccio N, Casolaro A, Lombardo F, Moscato G, Murri L, Ferrannini E, Meucci G. Long-term interferon beta-1b therapy for MS: is routine thyroid assessment always useful? Neurology 2000;55(4):549–52.
36. McDonald ND, Pender MP. Autoimmune hypothyroidism associated with interferon beta-1b treatment in two patients with multiple sclerosis. Aust NZ J Med 2000;30(2):278–9.
37. Homma Y, Kawazoe K, Ito T, Ide H, Takahashi H, Ueno F, Matsuzaki S. Chronic hepatitis C beta-interferon-induced severe hypertriglyceridaemia with apolipoprotein E phenotype E3/2. Int J Clin Pract 2000;54(4):212–16.
38. Aslam AK, Singh T. Aplastic anemia associated with interferon beta-1a. Am J Ther 2002;9(6):522–3.
39. Durelli L, Bongioanni MR, Ferrero B, Oggero A, Marzano A, Rizzetto M. Interferon treatment for multiple sclerosis: autoimmune complications may be lethal. Neurology 1998;50(2):570–1.
40. Malaguarnera M, Restuccia S, Di Fazio I, Di Marco R, Pistone G, Trovato BA. Rapid evolution of chronic viral hepatitis into hepatocellular carcinoma after beta-interferon treatment. Panminerva Med 1999;41(1):59–61.
41. Furusyo N, Hayashi J, Ohmiya M, Sawayama Y, Kawakami Y, Ariyama I, Kinukawa N, Kashiwagi S. Differences between interferon-alpha and -beta treatment for patients with chronic hepatitis C virus infection. Dig Dis Sci 1999;44(3):608–17.
42. Yoshida EM, Rasmussen SL, Steinbrecher UP, Erb SR, Scudamore CH, Chung SW, Oger JJ, Hashimoto SA. Fulminant liver failure during interferon beta treatment of multiple sclerosis. Neurology 2001;56(10):1416.
43. Francis GS, Grumser Y, Alteri E, Micaleff A, O'Brien F, Alsop J, Stam Moraga M, Kaplowitz N. Hepatic reactions during treatment of multiple sclerosis with interferon-beta-1a: incidence and clinical significance. Drug Saf 2003;26(11):815–27.
44. Herrera WG, Balizet LB, Harberts SW, Brown ST. Occurrence of a TTP-like syndrome in two women receiving beta interferon therapy for relapsing multiple sclerosis. Neurology 1999;52:135.
45. Nakao K, Sugiyama H, Makino E, Matsuura H, Ohmoto A, Sugimoto T, Ichikawa H, Wada J, Yamasaki Y, Makino H. Minimal change nephrotic syndrome developing during postoperative interferon-beta therapy for malignant melanoma. Nephron 2002;90(4):498–500.
46. Gotsman I, Elhallel-Darnitski M, Friedlander Z, Haviv YS. Beta-interferon-induced nephrotic syndrome in a patient with multiple sclerosis. Clin Nephrol 2000;54(5):425–6.
47. Ohta S, Yokoyama H, Wada T, Sakai N, Shimizu M, Kato T, Furuichi K, Segawa C, Hisada Y, Kobayashi K. Exacerbation of glomerulonephritis in subjects with chronic hepatitis C virus infection after interferon therapy. Am J Kidney Dis 1999;33(6):1040–8.
48. Elgart GW, Sheremata W, Ahn YS. Cutaneous reactions to recombinant human interferon beta-1b: the clinical and histologic spectrum. J Am Acad Dermatol 1997;37(4):553–8.
49. Heinzerling L, Dummer R, Burg G, Schmid-Grendelmeier P. Panniculitis after subcutaneous injection of interferon beta in a multiple sclerosis patient. Eur J Dermatol 2002;12(2):194–7.
50. Gaines AR, Varricchio F. Interferon beta-1b injection site reactions and necroses. Mult Scler 1998;4(2):70–3.
51. Radziwill AJ, Courvoisier S. Severe necrotising cutaneous lesions complicating treatment with interferon beta-1a. J Neurol Neurosurg Psychiatry 1999;67(1):115.
52. Berard F, Canillot S, Balme B, Perrot H. Nécrose cutanée locale après injections d'interféron béta. [Local cutaneous necrosis after injection of interferon beta.] Ann Dermatol Venereol 1995;122(3):105–7.
53. Sheremata WA, Taylor JR, Elgart GW. Severe necrotizing cutaneous lesions complicating treatment with interferon beta-1b. N Engl J Med 1995;332(23):1584.
54. Benincasa P, Bielory L. Necrotizing cutaneous lesions as a complication of subcutaneous interferon beta-1b. J Allergy Clin Immunol 1996;97:343.
55. Webster GF, Knobler RL, Lublin FD, Kramer EM, Hochman LR. Cutaneous ulcerations and pustular psoriasis flare caused by recombinant interferon beta injections in patients with multiple sclerosis. J Am Acad Dermatol 1996;34(2 Pt 2):365–7.
56. Feldmann R, Low-Weiser H, Duschet P, Gschnait F. Necrotizing cutaneous lesions caused by interferon beta

injections in a patient with multiple sclerosis. Dermatology 1997;195(1):52–3.
57. Durieu C, Bayle-Lebey P, Gadroy A, Loche F, Bazex J. Hyperplasie endothéliale papillaire intravasculaire: multiples lésions apparues au cours d'un traitement par interféron bêta. [Intravascular papillary endothelial hyperplasia: multiple lesions appearing in the course of treatment with interferon beta.] Ann Dermatol Venereol 2001;128(12):1336–8.
58. Mehta CL, Tyler RJ, Cripps DJ. Granulomatous dermatitis with focal sarcoidal features associated with recombinant interferon beta-1b injections. J Am Acad Dermatol 1998;39(6):1024–8.
59. Demirkaya S, Bulucu F, Odabasi Z, Vural O. An erythromelalgia case occurred during interferon beta treatment for multiple sclerosis. Eur J Neurol 2002;9(Suppl 2):220.
60. Benito-Leon J, Borbujo J, Cortes L. Cutaneous mucinoses complicating interferon beta-1b therapy. Eur Neurol 2002;47(2):123–4.
61. Lunemann JD, Schwarzenberger B, Kassim N, Zschenderlein R, Zipp F. Rhabdomyolysis during interferon-beta 1a treatment. J Neurol Neurosurg Psychiatry 2002;72(2):274.
62. Murata K, Shiraki K, Takase K, Nakano T, Tameda Y. Mono-arthritis following intensified interferon beta therapy for chronic hepatitis C. Hepatogastroenterology 2002; 49(47):1418–19.
63. Corona T, Leon C, Ostrosky-Zeichner L. Severe anaphylaxis with recombinant interferon beta. Neurology 1999;52(2):425.
64. Brown DL, Login IS, Borish L, Powers PL. An urticarial IgE-mediated reaction to interferon beta-1b. Neurology 2001;56(10):1416–17.
65. Clear D. Anaphylactoid reaction to methyl prednisolone developing after starting treatment with interferon beta-1b. J Neurol Neurosurg Psychiatry 1999;66(5):690.
66. Colosimo C, Pozzilli C, Frontoni M, Farina D, Koudriavtseva T, Gasperini C, Salvetti M, Valesini G. No increase of serum autoantibodies during therapy with recombinant human interferon-beta1a in relapsing-remitting multiple sclerosis. Acta Neurol Scand 1997;96(6):372–4.
67. Kivisakk P, Lundahl J, von Heigl Z, Fredrikson S. No evidence for increased frequency of autoantibodies during interferon-beta1b treatment of multiple sclerosis. Acta Neurol Scand 1998;97(5):320–3.
68. Abdi EA, Nguyen GK, Ludwig RN, Dickout WJ. Pulmonary sarcoidosis following interferon therapy for advanced renal cell carcinoma. Cancer 1987;59(5):896–900.
69. Bobbio-Pallavicini E, Valsecchi C, Tacconi F, Moroni M, Porta C. Sarcoidosis following beta-interferon therapy for multiple myeloma. Sarcoidosis 1995;12(2):140–2.
70. The IFNB Multiple Sclerosis Study Group and the University of British Columbia MS/MRI Analysis Group. Neutralizing antibodies during treatment of multiple sclerosis with interferon beta-1b: experience during the first three years. Neurology 1996;47(4):889–94.
71. Rudick RA, Simonian NA, Alam JA, Campion M, Scaramucci JO, Jones W, Coats ME, Goodkin DE, Weinstock-Guttman B, Herndon RM, Mass MK, Richert JR, Salazar AM, Munschauer FE 3rd, Cookfair DL, Simon JH, Jacobs LD. Incidence and significance of neutralizing antibodies to interferon beta-1a in multiple sclerosis. Multiple Sclerosis Collaborative Research Group (MSCRG) Neurology 1998;50(5):1266–72.
72. Deisenhammer F, Reindl M, Harvey J, Gasse T, Dilitz E, Berger T. Bioavailability of interferon beta 1b in MS patients with and without neutralizing antibodies. Neurology 1999;52(6):1239–43.
73. Khan OA, Dhib-Jalbut SS. Neutralizing antibodies to interferon beta-1a and interferon beta-1b in MS patients are cross-reactive. Neurology 1998;51(6):1698–702.
74. Cross AH, Antel JP. Antibodies to beta-interferons in multiple sclerosis: can we neutralize the controversy? Neurology 1998;50(5):1206–8.
75. Rice GP, Paszner B, Oger J, Lesaux J, Paty D, Ebers G. The evolution of neutralizing antibodies in multiple sclerosis patients treated with interferon beta-1b. Neurology 1999;52(6):1277–9.
76. Pozzilli C, Antonini G, Bagnato F, Mainero C, Tomassini V, Onesti E, Fantozzi R, Galgani S, Pasqualetti P, Millefiorini E, Spadaro M, Dahlke F, Gasperini C. Monthly corticosteroids decrease neutralizing antibodies to IFNbeta1 b: a randomized trial in multiple sclerosis. J Neurol 2002;249(1):50–6.
77. Fierlbeck G, Schreiner T. Incidence and clinical significance of therapy-induced neutralizing antibodies against interferon-beta. J Interferon Res 1994;14(4):205–6.
78. Sanberg-Wollheim M. Outcome of pregnancy during treatment with interferon-beta-1a (Rebif) in patients with multiple sclerosis. Neurology 2002;58(Suppl):A445–6.
79. Watanabe M, Kohge N, Akagi S, Uchida Y, Sato S, Kinoshita Y. Congenital anomalies in a child born from a mother with interferon-treated chronic hepatitis B. Am J Gastroenterol 2001;96(5):1668–9.
80. Durelli L, Verdun E, Barbero P, Bergui M, Versino E, Ghezzi A, Montanari E, Zaffaroni M; Independent Comparison of Interferon (INCOMIN) Trial Study Group. Every-other-day interferon beta-1b versus once-weekly interferon beta-1a for multiple sclerosis: results of a 2-year prospective randomised multicentre study (INCOMIN). Lancet 2002;359(9316):1453–60.
81. Panitch H, Goodin DS, Francis G, Chang P, Coyle PK, O'Connor P, Monaghan E, Li D, Weinshenker B; EVIDENCE Study Group. EVidence of Interferon Dose-response: Europian North American Compartative Efficacy; University of British Columbia MS/MRI Research Group. Randomized, comparative study of interferon beta-1a treatment regimens in MS: The EVIDENCE Trial. Neurology 2002;59(10):1496–506.

Interferon gamma

See also Interferons

General Information

Recombinant interferon gamma (interferon gamma-1b) is currently only approved as an adjunct to antibacterial therapy in chronic granulomatous disease (1), but its immunoregulatory potential has been investigated in other diseases. Clinical experience with interferon gamma is therefore limited and the most relevant information on long-term safety has been obtained from the ICGDSCG trial (2). In this study, adverse effects that were significantly more frequent with interferon gamma-1b (1.5 micrograms/kg or 50 micrograms/m^2) than with placebo included mild fever and flu-like symptoms, headache, and moderate injection site reactions. There were no adverse consequences on growth and development in children followed for a mean of 2.5 years (3,4). Several other adverse effects have been reported to the manufacturers, but causal evaluation is lacking (1).

Interferon gamma has been investigated in 27 patients with systemic sclerosis randomized to receive interferon gamma for 12 months. Most of them complained of symptoms consistent with a flu-like syndrome, namely headache (85%), fever (81%), and arthralgia and myalgia (70%) (5). There were adverse events (one or more per patient) leading to treatment withdrawal in four cases, including arthralgia, cardiac pain, atrioventricular block, reversible loss of hearing, and impotence; however, a causal relation with interferon gamma was not documented.

Organs and Systems

Cardiovascular

Heart rate, ventricular or supraventricular extra beats, and asymptomatic cardiac events were not significantly different during treatment compared with baseline in 20 patients receiving interferon gamma (6). Interferon gamma rarely produced cardiovascular adverse effects. Hypotension, dysrhythmias, and possible coronary spasm were sometimes observed, mostly in patients receiving high doses or with previous cardiovascular disorders (SEDA-20, 333) (SEDA-22, 405) (7,8).

Exacerbation of Raynaud's syndrome occurred in five of 20 patients with systemic sclerosis treated with interferon gamma (SEDA-20, 333).

Respiratory

Of 10 patients treated with interferon gamma-1b 200 micrograms three times a week for advanced idiopathic pulmonary fibrosis, four developed irreversible acute respiratory failure (9). All four patients had increasing dyspnea, fever, and rapidly progressive hypoxemia, and had new alveolar opacities on lung imaging. The symptoms occurred shortly after interferon gamma had been started in three patients, and after 35 injections in the fourth. Three patients died from refractory hypoxemia and the fourth underwent lung transplantation, but died a few weeks later. Pathological examination in two patients showed diffuse alveolar damage with pre-existing interstitial pneumonitis. Interferon gamma was suspected, as no other cause of abrupt pulmonary deterioration was found. Although the number of patients was small, the authors noted that before interferon beta pulmonary function tended to be worse in the four patients who developed acute respiratory failure than in the other six.

Psychological, psychiatric

Neuropsychiatric disturbances have not been consistently found in patients receiving interferon gamma, despite electroencephalographic monitoring and psychometric tests (10). However, careful examination led to the impression that interferon gamma can cause neurophysiological changes similar to those of interferon alfa (11), and data from the manufacturers also point to rare cases of nervous system adverse effects in patients treated with high-dose interferon gamma (1).

Endocrine

Interferon gamma can increase serum cortisol concentrations (12).

Metabolism

Reversible dose-dependent hypertriglyceridemia has been attributed to interferon gamma (13).

Hyperglycemia, reversible on interferon gamma withdrawal and a short course of insulin, has been reported in one patient (SEDA-22, 406).

Hematologic

Interferon gamma was supposedly the cause of asymptomatic non-immune hemolytic anemia in one patient receiving both interleukin-2 and interferon gamma (14).

Only minimal effects of interferon gamma on white blood cell counts have been observed (15).

Auto-immune thrombocytopenia occurred in a patient receiving interferon gamma (SEDA-22, 406).

Gastrointestinal

A convincing case of severe aphthous stomatitis has been reported in a patient receiving interferon gamma (SEDA-20, 333).

Urinary tract

Dose-related asymptomatic proteinuria was sometimes observed, and severe proteinuria with nephrotic syndrome has been reported once after low-dose interferon gamma (SED-13, 1100). Acute renal insufficiency is extremely rare (SEDA-20, 333) (16).

Skin

Induction of psoriatic lesions at the injection site has been observed in 10 of 42 patients treated with interferon gamma for psoriatic arthritis, while the joint symptoms were improved (17).

Single or multiple lesions of erythema nodosum leprosum occurred in 60% of patients given intradermal interferon gamma for lepromatous leprosy, and severe systemic symptoms required thalidomide treatment in two patients (18).

Severe erythroderma was observed in five of 10 patients after interferon gamma was added to ciclosporin for autologous bone marrow transplantation (19).

Immunologic

An anaphylactoid reaction and severe bronchospasm have been reported once after the first injection of interferon gamma (10).

Although interferon gamma is mainly used for its immunoregulatory properties, the possibility of clinical immune adverse consequences has been addressed in a limited number of prospective studies. In two studies involving patients with chronic hepatitis B treated for 4–6 months, most developed a new autoantibody (20,21), but none developed clinical evidence of autoimmune disease. However, other reports suggested that interferon gamma can either improve or aggravate immune or inflammatory conditions. Although no change in antinuclear antibodies was reported in a trial of 54 patients with rheumatoid arthritis (22), increased or new antinuclear antibodies were observed in three of six patients with rheumatoid arthritis who received interferon gamma for 2–8 months, and two patients had clinical exacerbations of the disease (23). Isolated cases of systemic lupus erythematosus have been reported in patients receiving interferon gamma for rheumatoid arthritis (24,25). Rheumatoid or lupus-like symptoms associated with raised antinuclear antibodies titers were also noted in 17% of patients receiving interferon alfa and interferon gamma for myeloproliferative disorders, and in only 8.3% of patients treated with interferon alfa alone (26). Interferon gamma was also involved in the induction or reactivation of seronegative arthritis in patients with cutaneous psoriasis (27) and the unexpected exacerbation of multiple sclerosis in 39% of patients (28). Finally, neutralizing antibodies have exceptionally been found (SEDA-20, 333).

References

1. Todd PA, Goa KL. Interferon gamma-1b. A review of its pharmacology and therapeutic potential in chronic granulomatous disease. Drugs 1992;43(1):111–22.
2. The International Chronic Granulomatous Disease Cooperative Study Group. A controlled trial of interferon gamma to prevent infection in chronic granulomatous disease. N Engl J Med 1991;324(8):509–16.
3. Bemiller LS, Roberts DH, Starko KM, Curnutte JT. Safety and effectiveness of long-term interferon gamma therapy in patients with chronic granulomatous disease. Blood Cells Mol Dis 1995;21(3):239–47.
4. Weening RS, Leitz GJ, Seger RA. Recombinant human interferon-gamma in patients with chronic granulomatous disease—European follow up study. Eur J Pediatr 1995; 154(4):295–8.
5. Grassegger A, Schuler G, Hessenberger G, Walder-Hantich B, Jabkowski J, MacHeiner W, Salmhofer W, Zahel B, Pinter G, Herold M, Klein G, Fritsch PO. Interferon-gamma in the treatment of systemic sclerosis: a randomized controlled multicentre trial. Br J Dermatol 1998;139(4):639–48.
6. Friess GG, Brown TD, Wrenn RC. Cardiovascular rhythm effects of gamma recombinant DNA interferon. Invest New Drugs 1989;7(2–3):275–80.
7. Sonnenblick M, Rosin A. Cardiotoxicity of interferon. A review of 44 cases. Chest 1991;99(3):557–61.
8. Yamamoto N, Nishigaki K, Ban Y, Kawada Y. Coronary vasospasm after interferon administration. Br J Urol 1998;81(6):916–17.
9. Honore I, Nunes H, Groussard O, Kambouchner M, Chambellan A, Aubier M, Valeyre D, Crestani B. Acute respiratory failure after interferon-gamma therapy of end-stage pulmonary fibrosis. Am J Respir Crit Care Med 2003;167(7):953–7.
10. Mattson K, Niiranen A, Pyrhonen S, Farkkila M, Cantell K. Recombinant interferon gamma treatment in non-small cell lung cancer. Antitumour effect and cardiotoxicity. Acta Oncol 1991;30(5):607–10.
11. Born J, Spath-Schwalbe E, Pietrowsky R, Porzsolt F, Fehm HL. Neurophysiological effects of recombinant interferon-gamma and -alpha in man. Clin Physiol Biochem 1989;7(3–4):119–27.
12. Krishnan R, Ellinwood EH Jr, Laszlo J, Hood L, Ritchie J. Effect of gamma interferon on the hypothalamic–pituitary–adrenal system. Biol Psychiatry 1987;22(9):1163–6.
13. Kurzrock R, Rohde MF, Quesada JR, Gianturco SH, Bradley WA, Sherwin SA, Gutterman JU. Recombinant gamma interferon induces hypertriglyceridemia and inhibits post-heparin lipase activity in cancer patients. J Exp Med 1986;164(4):1093–101.
14. Rabinowitz AP, Hu E, Watkins K, Mazumder A. Hemolytic anemia in a cancer patient treated with recombinant interferon-gamma. J Biol Response Mod 1990; 9(2):256–9.
15. Aulitzky WE, Tilg H, Vogel W, Aulitzky W, Berger M, Gastl G, Herold M, Huber C. Acute hematologic effects of interferon alpha, interferon gamma, tumor necrosis factor alpha and interleukin 2. Ann Hematol 1991;62(1):25–31.
16. Ault BH, Stapleton FB, Gaber L, Martin A, Roy S 3rd, Murphy SB. Acute renal failure during therapy with recombinant human gamma interferon. N Engl J Med 1988;319(21):1397–400.
17. Fierlbeck G, Rassner G, Muller C. Psoriasis induced at the injection site of recombinant interferon gamma. Results of immunohistologic investigations. Arch Dermatol 1990; 126(3):351–5.
18. Sampaio EP, Moreira AL, Sarno EN, Malta AM, Kaplan G. Prolonged treatment with recombinant interferon gamma induces erythema nodosum leprosum in lepromatous leprosy patients. J Exp Med 1992;175(6):1729–37.
19. Horn TD, Altomonte V, Vogelsang G, Kennedy MJ. Erythroderma after autologous bone marrow transplantation modified by administration of cyclosporine and interferon gamma for breast cancer. J Am Acad Dermatol 1996;34(3):413–17.
20. Weber P, Wiedmann KH, Klein R, Walter E, Blum HE, Berg PA. Induction of autoimmune phenomena in patients with chronic hepatitis B treated with gamma-interferon. J Hepatol 1994;20(3):321–8.
21. Kung AW, Jones BM, Lai CL. Effects of interferon-gamma therapy on thyroid function, T-lymphocyte subpopulations and induction of autoantibodies. J Clin Endocrinol Metab 1990;71(5):1230–4.
22. Cannon GW, Emkey RD, Denes A, Cohen SA, Saway PA, Wolfe F, Jaffer AM, Weaver AL, Manaster BJ, McCarthy KA. Prospective 5-year followup of recombinant interferon-gamma in rheumatoid arthritis. J Rheumatol 1993;20(11):1867–73.
23. Seitz M, Franke M, Kirchner H. Induction of antinuclear antibodies in patients with rheumatoid arthritis receiving treatment with human recombinant interferon gamma. Ann Rheum Dis 1988;47(8):642–4.
24. Graninger WB, Hassfeld W, Pesau BB, Machold KP, Zielinski CC, Smolen JS. Induction of systemic lupus erythematosus by interferon-gamma in a patient with rheumatoid arthritis. J Rheumatol 1991;18(10):1621–2.
25. Machold KP, Smolen JS. Interferon-gamma induced exacerbation of systemic lupus erythematosus. J Rheumatol 1990;17(6):831–2.
26. Wandl UB, Nagel-Hiemke M, May D, Kreuzfelder E, Kloke O, Kranzhoff M, Seeber S, Niederle N. Lupus-like autoimmune disease induced by interferon therapy for myeloproliferative disorders. Clin Immunol Immunopathol 1992;65(1):70–4.
27. O'Connell PG, Gerber LH, Digiovanna JJ, Peck GL. Arthritis in patients with psoriasis treated with gamma-interferon. J Rheumatol 1992;19(1):80–2.
28. Panitch HS, Hirsch RL, Schindler J, Johnson KP. Treatment of multiple sclerosis with gamma interferon: exacerbations associated with activation of the immune system. Neurology 1987;37(7):1097–102.

Interferons

See also Individual agents

General Information

The interferons, first described in 1957, include at least five natural human glycoproteins (alfa, beta, gamma, omega, and tau). Only the first three types are currently used, and they differ both structurally and antigenically. Interferon alfa is produced by macrophages, B cells, and null lymphocytes, interferon beta by fibroblasts, epithelial cells, and macrophages, and interferon gamma from T lymphocytes and macrophages after antigenic or mitogenic stimulation. The interferons share 30–40% of sequence homology and have antiviral and antiproliferative actions. Interferon gamma, produced by activated T cells and natural killer cells, is recognized by a different receptor and acts primarily as an immunoregulatory cytokine.

Uses

The uses of interferons are listed in Table 1.

Two authoritative reviews have outlined the therapeutic potential of interferons (1,2). A wide range of viral diseases or cancers are other candidates for interferon therapy (3–5).

Mechanisms of action

On binding to surface receptors, interferon alfa results in activation of cytoplasmic enzymes affecting messenger RNA translation and protein synthesis (6). The antiviral state takes hours to develop but can persist for days. Besides broad antiviral activity, interferons are of major importance in regulating immunological functions.

General adverse effects

The adverse effects of interferon are multifarious and the natural products seem to be less toxic than the pure synthetic compounds. Influenza-like symptoms with fever, chills, fatigue, myalgia, arthralgia, nausea, and lethargy, starting within 1 week after the start of treatment and lasting 1–7 days, seem to be very common (7,8). Adverse effects also include neurotoxicity (paresthesia, polyneuropathy), hepatic toxicity, renal toxicity, and an increase in eyelash growth (9–13). Neutralizing antibodies can lead to resistance in patients with hairy cell leukemia and chronic myeloid leukemia (14,15). The route of administration influences the provocation of an antibody response, and recombinant interferon beta is more likely to be immunogenic when given subcutaneously or intramuscularly than when given intravenously (16). Raynaud's phenomenon has been described after treatment with interferon alfa (17), and exacerbation of multiple sclerosis has been observed after treatment with interferon gamma.

The most common adverse effects reported in two large multicenter studies were fever (60%), leukopenia (43%), increased serum aspartate transaminase activity (30%), anorexia (30%), thrombocytopenia (25%), fatigue (21%), nausea, and vomiting (17%) (18,19). Compared with subcutaneous administration, intravenous interferon alfa is associated with similar adverse effects of greater severity and frequency (20,21).

Table 1 Names of different types of interferons and their indications

Generic name and trade name	Indications
Interferon alfa	Malignant diseases: hairy cell leukemia, chronic myelogenous leukemia, cutaneous T cell lymphoma, follicular lymphoma, multiple myeloma, Kaposi's sarcoma, diffuse melanoma, renal cell carcinoma, carcinoid tumors
Human natural leukocyte interferon alfa (IFN alfa-n3; Alferon)	Viral diseases: condylomata acuminata, chronic active hepatitis B and C
Lymphoblastoid interferon alfa (IFN alfa-n1; Welferon)	
Recombinant interferon alfa-2a (rIFN alfa-2a; Roferon)	
Recombinant interferon alfa-2b (rIFN alfa-2b; Intron A)	
Recombinant interferon alfa-2c (rIFN alfa,2c; Berofor)	
Interferon beta	Multiple sclerosis
Natural fibroblast (Fiblaferon)	
Recombinant interferon beta (rIFN beta; Avonex)	
Recombinant interferon beta-1b (rIFN beta-1b; Betaseron)	
Interferon gamma	Chronic granulomatous disease
Recombinant interferon gamma-1b (rIFN gamma-1b; Actimmune)	

References

1. Galvani D, Griffiths SD, Cawley JC. Interferon for treatment: the dust settles. BMJ (Clin Res Ed) 1988;296(6636): 1554–6.
2. Merigan TC. Human interferon as a therapeutic agent: a decade passes. N Engl J Med 1988;318(22):1458–60.
3. Agarwala SS, Kirkwood JM. Interferons in the therapy of solid tumors. Oncology 1994;51(2):129–36.
4. Urabe A. Interferons for the treatment of hematological malignancies. Oncology 1994;51(2):137–41.
5. Dorr RT. Interferon-alpha in malignant and viral diseases. A review. Drugs 1993;45(2):177–211.
6. Stiehm ER, Kronenberg LH, Rosenblatt HM, Bryson Y, Merigan TC. UCLA conference. Interferon: immunobiology and clinical significance. Ann Intern Med 1982; 96(1): 80–93.
7. Alexander GJ, Brahm J, Fagan EA, Smith HM, Daniels HM, Eddleston AL, Williams R. Loss of HBsAg with interferon therapy in chronic hepatitis B virus infection. Lancet 1987;2(8550):66–9.
8. Giles FJ, Singer CR, Gray AG, Yong KL, Brozovic M, Davies SC, Grant IR, Hoffbrand AV, Machin SJ, Mehta AB, et al. Alpha-interferon therapy for essential thrombocythaemia. Lancet 1988;2(8602):70–2.
9. Korenman J, Baker B, Waggoner J, Everhart JE, Di Bisceglie AM, Hoofnagle JH. Long-term remission of chronic hepatitis B after alpha-interferon therapy. Ann Intern Med 1991;114(8):629–34.
10. Scott GM, Ward RJ, Wright DJ, Robinson JA, Onwubalili JK, Gauci CL. Effects of cloned interferon alpha 2 in normal volunteers: febrile reactions and changes in circulating corticosteroids and trace metals. Antimicrob Agents Chemother 1983;23(4):589–92.
11. Ingimarsson S, Cantell K, Strander H. Side effects of long-term treatment with human leukocyte interferon. J Infect Dis 1979;140(4):560–3.
12. Cheeseman SH, Rubin RH, Stewart JA, Tolkoff-Rubin NE, Cosimi AB, Cantell K, Gilbert J, Winkle S, Herrin JT, Black PH, Russell PS, Hirsch MS. Controlled clinical trial of prophylactic human-leukocyte interferon in renal transplantation. Effects on cytomegalovirus and herpes simplex virus infections. N Engl J Med 1979;300(24):1345–9.
13. Smedley H, Katrak M, Sikora K, Wheeler T. Neurological effects of recombinant human interferon. BMJ (Clin Res Ed) 1983;286(6361):262–4.
14. Inglada L, Porres JC, La Banda F, Mora I, Carreno V. Anti-IFN-alpha titres during interferon therapy. Lancet 1987;2(8574):1521.
15. Steis RG, Smith JW 2nd, Urba WJ, Clark JW, Itri LM, Evans LM, Schoenberger C, Longo DL. Resistance to recombinant interferon alfa-2a in hairy-cell leukemia associated with neutralizing anti-interferon antibodies. N Engl J Med 1988;318(22):1409–13.
16. Konrad MW, Childs AL, Merigan TC, Borden EC. Assessment of the antigenic response in humans to a recombinant mutant interferon beta. J Clin Immunol 1987;7(5):365–75.
17. Roy V, Newland AC. Raynaud's phenomenon and cryoglobulinaemia associated with the use of recombinant human alpha-interferon. Lancet 1988;1(8591):944–5.
18. Taguchi T. Clinical studies of recombinant interferon alfa-2a (Roferon-A) in cancer patients. Cancer 1986;57(Suppl 8):1705–8.
19. Umeda T, Niijima T. Phase II study of alpha interferon on renal cell carcinoma. Summary of three collaborative trials. Cancer 1986;58(6):1231–5.
20. Mirro J, Dow LW, Kalwinsky DK, Dahl GV, Weck P, Whisnant J, Murphy SB. Phase I-II study of continuous-infusion high-dose human lymphoblastoid interferon and the in vitro sensitivity of leukemic progenitors in non-lymphocytic leukemia. Cancer Treat Rep 1986;70(3):363–7.
21. Muss HB, Costanzi JJ, Leavitt R, Williams RD, Kempf RA, Pollard R, Ozer H, Zekan PJ, Grunberg SM, Mitchell MS, et al. Recombinant alfa interferon in renal cell carcinoma: a randomized trial of two routes of administration. J Clin Oncol 1987;5(2):286–91.

Interleukin-1

General Information

Interleukin-1-alfa and interleukin-1-beta are produced by two distinct genes with only 25% homology, but they act through the same receptor and share similar in vitro biological properties. Interleukin-1 on its own has modest antitumor activity and limited hemopoietic effects. It also acts synergistically with other colony-stimulating factors (for example GM-CSF, G-CSF, interleukin-3, or interleukin-6) to promote colony formation and stimulate hemopoietic recovery in patients undergoing autologous bone marrow transplantation or receiving cytotoxic anticancer treatment (1).

General adverse effects

Both forms of interleukin-1 have been investigated in humans, and they produce a wide and very similar spectrum of adverse effects (SED-13, 1101) (2). Whatever the dose, fever and chills are universal but only occasionally treatment-limiting. Tachyphylaxis can develop during prolonged administration. Other frequent but moderate adverse effects include transient fatigue, myalgia, arthralgia, dose-dependent headache, nausea, vomiting, diarrhea, and abdominal pain. Injection site reactions included local phlebitis, while subcutaneous injection of interleukin-1-beta can cause local pain and erythema. Interleukin-1-alfa can cause transient and moderate increases in bilirubin, aspartate transaminase, and serum creatinine concentrations.

Organs and Systems

Cardiovascular

The most significant adverse effect of both forms of interleukin-1 is dose-limiting hypotension resulting from a capillary leak phenomenon with clinical features of septic shock (2). Although mild weight gain, dyspnea, and pulmonary infiltrates can occur, severe capillary leak syndrome is usually not observed. Shortness of breath requiring oxygen and benign supraventricular dysrhythmias were sometimes noted. The maximum tolerated dose of interleukin-1 with pressors is therefore 0.3 micrograms/kg/day. The most probable mechanism underlying these complications is an interleukin-1-induced increase in nitric oxide production by vascular smooth muscle.

Nervous system

A few patients given interleukin-1 complain of somnolence, agitation, delusional ideation, photophobia or subjective blurred vision, but at high doses some patients experienced a greater degree of central nervous system toxicity, with complaints of confusion, severe somnolence and seizures (3).

Endocrine

Various endocrinological effects have been observed, but without clinically apparent endocrinopathies (SEDA-20, 333).

Metabolism

Interleukin-1-beta has been associated with transient hypoglycemia (4).

Mouth and teeth

Interleukin-1-alfa can cause mucositis and xerostomia (3) and can increase the severity of chemotherapy-induced oral mucositis and erythema (5).

References

1. Curti BD, Smith JW 2nd. Interleukin-1 in the treatment of cancer. Pharmacol Ther 1995;65(3):291–302.
2. Vial T, Descotes J. Clinical toxicity of cytokines used as haemopoietic growth factors. Drug Saf 1995;13(6):371–406.
3. Smith JW 2nd, Urba WJ, Curti BD, Elwood LJ, Steis RG, Janik JE, Sharfman WH, Miller LL, Fenton RG, Conlon KC, et al. The toxic and hematologic effects of interleukin-1 alpha administered in a phase I trial to patients with advanced malignancies. J Clin Oncol 1992;10(7):1141–52.
4. Crown J, Jakubowski A, Kemeny N, Gordon M, Gasparetto C, Wong G, Sheridan C, Toner G, Meisenberg B, Botet J, et al. A phase I trial of recombinant human interleukin-1 beta alone and in combination with myelosuppressive doses of 5-fluorouracil in patients with gastrointestinal cancer. Blood 1991;78(6):1420–7.
5. Prussick R, Horn TD, Wilson WH, Turner MC. A characteristic eruption associated with ifosfamide, carboplatin, and etoposide chemotherapy after pretreatment with recombinant interleukin-1 alpha. J Am Acad Dermatol 1996;35 (5 Pt 1):705–9.

Interleukin-3

General Information

Interleukin-3 is produced by activated T lymphocytes and stimulates the proliferation and differentiation of the granulocyte, macrophage, eosinophil, basophil, erythroid, megakaryocyte, and mast cell lineages (1).

Observational studies

Subcutaneous recombinant interleukin-3 has been investigated in patients with chemotherapy-induced myelotoxicity, in the setting of autologous bone marrow transplantation or peripheral stem cell harvesting, or in patients with myelodysplastic syndrome, aplastic anemia, and Diamond–Blackfan anemia (1,2). Interleukin-3 given alone has limited clinical effects, but an enhanced hemopoietic response has been obtained with a genetically engineered GM-CSF/interleukin-3 fusion protein, PIXY321 (SEDA-21, 376) (3).

The specific toxicity of subcutaneous recombinant human interleukin-3 derived from *Escherichia coli* has been addressed in a 4-day study performed in healthy volunteers (4). All had mild-to-moderate dose-independent symptoms; flu-like symptoms, including fever, chills, headache, conjunctival congestion, myalgia, and diffuse aching, were the most frequent. Minor erythematous reactions at the injection site were also consistently described, and one patient had histological features of an allergic vasculitis resembling that reported with GM-CSF (SEDA-20, 335). Mild-to-severe skin rashes or urticaria were also sometimes observed, and there were bullae with hemorrhagic necrosis of the skin in one patient (5). In preliminary clinical trials, malaise, eye pain, nasal congestion, weakness or lethargy, tachycardia, and gastrointestinal disorders occurred in under 16% of patients (6). None of these effects was clearly related to dose, and withdrawal of treatment was not required. A similar safety profile was reported in patients who subsequently developed tachyphylaxis, and the adverse effect profile of yeast or interleukin-3 derived from *E. coli* did not appear to be different (6). Overall, the rate of withdrawal of treatment because of adverse effects was 17–50% in patients receiving 10 micrograms/kg/day. Constitutional symptoms, generalized skin reactions, and facial edema were the most frequent dose-limiting adverse events. In autologous bone marrow transplantation, the maximum tolerated dose was only 2 micrograms/kg/day. Interleukin-3-associated fever is supposedly the result of a dose-dependent increase in interleukin-6 and acute phase protein production.

Adverse effects related to interleukin-3 were observed in a comparison of G-CSF alone, GM-CSF alone, and sequential interleukin-3 and GM-CSF in 48 patients with cancer (16 in each group) receiving high-dose cyclophosphamide (7). In particular, fever above 38.5°C, skin rash, and headaches were more frequent during interleukin-3 administration. As a result, 90% of patients receiving interleukin-3 required pharmacological treatment for adverse effects.

Placebo-controlled studies

The potential hemopoietic benefits of postchemotherapy interleukin-3 are limited. In a phase III trial in 185 ovarian cancer patients treated with carboplatin and cyclophosphamide, premature withdrawal was significantly more frequent in patients randomized to received recombinant interleukin-3 (5 micrograms/kg from day 3 to day 12) than in the placebo group (8). The most frequent adverse effects were allergic reactions (50 versus 23%), which required interleukin-3 withdrawal in 21 patients compared with one in the placebo group, and headache (46 versus 19%). In this setting, interleukin-3 stimulated hemopoiesis, but did not reduce platelet transfusions or increase adherence to the chemotherapeutic regimen.

The benefit of interleukin-3 in promoting hemopoietic reconstitution after autologous bone marrow transplantation has been investigated in 198 patients with malignant lymphoma who received either interleukin-3 (10 micrograms/kg for 4 weeks, 130 patients) or placebo (68 patients) (9). There was no significant advantage of interleukin-3 over placebo in regard to the number of platelet transfusions before engraftment, the time to platelet engraftment, or the incidence of hemorrhagic complications. This confirms that interleukin-3 alone has limited clinical effects. In contrast, significantly more patients who received interleukin-3 had to discontinue treatment because of adverse events (26 versus 7%). Adverse events that were significantly more frequent with interleukin-3 than with placebo included mucositis (69 versus 44%), headache (38 versus 13%), and rash (25 versus 12%). It is not yet known whether the initial route of administration (continuous intravenous infusion for 7 days followed by subcutaneous administration for 21 days) might account for these findings.

General adverse effects

Constitutional symptoms, generalized skin reactions, and facial edema are the most frequent. Although they are not easily attributable to interleukin-3, other significant adverse events noted during treatment have included exacerbation of arthralgia in a seronegative patient (5) and transient thrombocytopenia in patients with myelodysplastic syndrome or aplastic anemia (10). Signs of meningism with neck rigidity were sometimes found (10).

As with G-CSF and GM-CSF, the presence of interleukin-3 receptors on leukemia cells suggests a theoretical risk of disease aggravation. However, accelerated tumor growth has not been noted in patients with non-hemopoietic tumors or newly diagnosed non-Hodgkin's lymphoma (6). Overall, some types of disease progression were observed in 11 of 86 patients with myelodysplastic syndrome, but no clear relation between interleukin-3 and disease acceleration can be assessed at the moment.

PIXY321

The clinical and hematological effects of PIXY321, a genetically engineered GM-CSF/interleukin-3 fusion protein, have been evaluated in 71 women with breast cancer (11). In addition to chemotherapy (four cycles of fluorouracil, doxorubicin, and cyclophosphamide), the patients received either PIXY321 or placebo from days 3–15. Although the incidence and/or duration of chemotherapy-induced severe neutropenia was significantly reduced by PIXY321, there were more frequent systemic adverse effects (fever, chills, abdominal pain, arthralgia, and injection-site reactions) and more severe thrombocytopenia during cycles 3 and 4. Based on these results and the lack of a demonstrable advantage of PIXY321 over GM-CSF (12), the development of PIXY321 as an adjuvant treatment in cancer was halted. In one study only insomnia and rash were more common in patients treated with subcutaneous PIXY321 compared with intravenous GM-CSF alone after autologous bone marrow transplantation (13).

Organs and Systems

Cardiovascular

Hypotension, exacerbation or new onset of atrial fibrillation, and dyspnea were infrequently observed in clinical trials (6). Although weight gain and peripheral edema can develop, only one fatal case, compatible with a capillary vascular leak syndrome, has been reported (SEDA-20, 335).

Thrombophlebitis was recorded in 45% of patients treated for advanced ovarian cancer who also received intravenous interleukin-3 (14), and deep venous thromboses were reported in children treated with maintenance interleukin-3 for Diamond–Blackfan anemia (15). In addition, one smoking breast-cancer patient developed severe hypotension and cerebellar and superior mesenteric thrombosis after subcutaneous interleukin-3 administration (SEDA-19, 340). Collectively, these case reports suggest that interleukin-3 may contribute to the development of thrombosis, but a possible increased risk of thrombosis with interleukin-3 remains to be demonstrated.

Hematologic

Interleukin-3 caused a transient rise in circulating atypical B lymphocytes, with enlargement of the spleen and lymph nodes in two patients with large-cell lymphoma and the development of a clonally-related transient plasmocytosis in one patient with relapsing follicular non-Hodgkin's lymphoma (SED-13, 1109) (10,16).

There has been one case of bone marrow histiocytosis in a patient treated with interleukin-3 for refractory aplastic anemia (SED-13, 1109).

Immunologic

An anaphylactoid reaction to recombinant human interleukin-3 (rHuinterleukin-3) has been described (17).

- A 66-year-old man with radiation-induced aplastic anemia and myelodysplastic features failed to respond to multiple therapeutic regimens. A trial of recombinant human interleukin-3 was begun, but he had transient shortness of breath and hypotension after the first subcutaneous injection. On the next day, 2 hours after the second dose, he had restlessness, dyspnea, spasticity, wheezing, cyanosis, hyperthermia, tachycardia, and hypotension (70/50 mmHg). Full recovery was obtained with fluids, adrenaline, promethazine, and glucocorticoids.

Histamine release from circulating basophils was the suggested mechanism.

Drug–Drug Interactions

Angiotensin-converting enzyme (ACE) inhibitors

Severe hypotension within hours after interleukin-3 injection has been observed in three of 26 patients treated with angiotensin-converting enzyme inhibitors (SEDA-19, 340). Indirect synergy between ACE and interleukin-3 on nitric oxide production was suggested to be involved.

Carboplatin

In patients with ovarian cancer, the combination of interleukin-3 with high-dose carboplatin was poorly tolerated; severe fever, malaise, protracted nausea, vomiting, severe hypotension, and nephrotoxicity required withdrawal of interleukin-3 in 60% of patients when interleukin-3 was given only 24 hours after high-dose carboplatin (18).

GM-CSF

Combined sequential administration of interleukin-3 plus GM-CSF in patients treated for myelodysplastic syndrome suggested unacceptable toxicity (19).

References

1. Gianella-Borradori A. Present and future clinical relevance of interleukin 3. Stem Cells 1994;12(Suppl 1):241–8.
2. de Vries EG, van Gameren MM, Willemse PH. Recombinant human interleukin 3 in clinical oncology. Stem Cells 1993;11(2):72–80.
3. Vadhan-Raj S. PIXY321 (GM-CSF/IL-3 fusion protein): biological and clinical effects of a novel cytokine. Forum Trends Exp Clin Med 1995;5:110–18.
4. Huhn RD, Yurkow EJ, Kuhn JG, Clarke L, Gunn H, Resta D, Shah R, Myers LA, Seibold JR. Pharmacodynamics of daily subcutaneous recombinant human interleukin-3 in normal volunteers. Clin Pharmacol Ther 1995;57(1):32–41.
5. Nimer SD, Paquette RL, Ireland P, Resta D, Young D, Golde DW. A phase I/II study of interleukin-3 in patients with aplastic anemia and myelodysplasia. Exp Hematol 1994;22(9):875–80.
6. Vial T, Descotes J. Clinical toxicity of cytokines used as haemopoietic growth factors. Drug Saf 1995;13(6):371–406.
7. Ballestrero A, Ferrando F, Garuti A, Basta P, Gonella R, Stura P, Mela GS, Sessarego M, Gobbi M, Patrone F. Comparative effects of three cytokine regimens after high-dose cyclophosphamide: granulocyte colony-stimulating factor, granulocyte–macrophage colony-stimulating factor (GM-CSF), and sequential interleukin-3 and GM-CSF. J Clin Oncol 1999;17(4):1296.
8. Hofstra LS, Kristensen GB, Willemse PH, Vindevoghel A, Meden H, Lahousen M, Oberling F, Sorbe B, Crump M, Sklenar I, Sluiter WJ, Kiese B, Trope CG, de Vries EG. Randomized trial of recombinant human interleukin-3 versus placebo in prevention of bone marrow depression during first-line chemotherapy for ovarian carcinoma. J Clin Oncol 1998;16(10):3335–44.
9. Brouwer RE, Vellenga E, Zwinderman KH, Bezwoda WR, Durrant ST, Herrmann RP, Kiese B, Maraninchi D, Milligan DW, Sklenar I, Tabilio A, Volonte JL, Winfield DA, Fibbe WE. Phase III efficacy study of interleukin-3 after autologous bone marrow transplantation in patients with malignant lymphoma. Br J Haematol 1999;106(3):730–6.
10. Ganser A, Seipelt G, Lindemann A, Ottmann OG, Falk S, Eder M, Herrmann F, Becher R, Hoffken K, Buchner T, et al. Effects of recombinant human interleukin-3 in patients with myelodysplastic syndromes. Blood 1990;76(3):455–62.
11. Jones SE, Khandelwal P, McIntyre K, Mennel R, Orr D, Kirby R, Agura E, Duncan L, Hyman W, Roque T, Regan D, Schuster M, Dimitrov N, Garrison L, Lange M. Randomized, double-blind, placebo-controlled trial to evaluate the hematopoietic growth factor PIXY321 after moderate-dose fluorouracil, doxorubicin, and cyclophosphamide in stage II and III breast cancer. J Clin Oncol 1999;17(10):3025–32.
12. Schuh JC, Morrissey PJ. Development of a recombinant growth factor and fusion protein: lessons from GM-CSF. Toxicol Pathol 1999;27(1):72–7.
13. Vose JM, Pandite AN, Beveridge RA, Geller RB, Schuster MW, Anderson JE, LeMaistre CF, Ahmed T, Granena A, Keating A, Fernandez Ranada JM, Stiff PJ, Tabbara I, Longo W, Copelan EA, Nichols C, Smith A, Topolsky DL, Bierman PJ, Lebsack ME, Lange M, Garrison L. Granulocyte–macrophage colony-stimulating factor/interleukin-3 fusion protein versus granulocyte–macrophage colony-stimulating factor after autologous bone marrow transplantation for non-Hodgkin's lymphoma: results of a randomized double-blind trial. J Clin Oncol 1997;15(4):1617–23.
14. Biesma B, Willemse PH, Mulder NH, Sleijfer DT, Gietema JA, Mull R, Limburg PC, Bouma J, Vellenga E, de Vries EG. Effects of interleukin-3 after chemotherapy for advanced ovarian cancer. Blood 1992;80(5):1141–8.
15. Gillio AP, Faulkner LB, Alter BP, Reilly L, Klafter R, Heller G, Young DC, Lipton JM, Moore MA, O'Reilly RJ. Treatment of Diamond–Blackfan anemia with recombinant human interleukin-3. Blood 1993;82(3):744–51.
16. Kramer MH, Kluin PM, Wijburg ER, Fibbe WE, Kluin-Nelemans HC. Differentiation of follicular lymphoma cells after autologous bone marrow transplantation and haematopoietic growth factor treatment. Lancet 1995;345(8948):488–90.
17. Mittelman M, Zeidman A, Fradin Z, Menachem Y. Anaphylactic shock due to recombinant human interleukin-3. Eur J Haematol 1999;62(3):199–200.
18. Dercksen MW, Hoekman K, ten Bokkel Huinink WW, Rankin EM, Dubbelman R, van Tinteren H, Wagstaff J, Pinedo HM. Effects of interleukin-3 on myelosuppression induced by chemotherapy for ovarian cancer and small cell undifferentiated tumours. Br J Cancer 1993;68(5):996–1003.
19. Nand S, Sosman J, Godwin JE, Fisher RI. A phase I/II study of sequential interleukin-3 and granulocyte–macrophage colony-stimulating factor in myelodysplastic syndromes. Blood 1994;83(2):357–60.

Interleukin-4

General Information

Interleukin-4 is a pleiotropic cytokine, mostly produced by activated T cells, which acts on the proliferation and differentiation of B and T lymphocytes and enhances the function of natural killer cells, eosinophils, and mast cells (1). It is being investigated for potential antitumoral and hemopoietic actions.

General adverse effects

Moderate fever with flu-like symptoms, arthralgias, fatigue, anorexia, nausea, vomiting, headache, and transient hypotension were frequent at all doses and by all routes of administration, but were more severe and prolonged at high doses (2). Periorbital, facial, and peripheral edema were also noted. Frequent discomfort caused by severe and resistant nasal congestion, supposedly due to edema and vascular engorgement from histamine stimulation, was sometimes dose-limiting. Mild asymptomatic increases in liver enzymes and minimal changes in serum creatinine concentrations can occur. No significant effects on serum hormone (ACTH, cortisol, thyrotropin, thyroxine, prolactin) or lipid concentrations have been noted (SEDA-20, 336). Other adverse events, as yet not clearly related to interleukin-4, included reversible Coomb's-positive hemolytic anemia, transient partial blindness, photophobia, and visual hallucinations. At the moment, only one report has suggested that long-term interleukin-4 may have stimulated the development of multiple myeloma (SEDA-21, 376).

Of 49 patients with advanced renal cell carcinoma treated with subcutaneous interleukin-4 (4 micrograms/kg/day for 28 days followed by a 7-day rest), nine had 13 episodes of grade 4 toxicity (3). Severe unexpected toxic effects included three cases of Bell's palsy and one episode of severe hypoglycemia in a previously well-controlled patient with diabetes mellitus.

Organs and Systems

Cardiovascular

The vascular leak syndrome was observed at a dose of 15 micrograms/kg by bolus or continuous intravenous administration, but a moderate capillary leak syndrome was also noted at lower subcutaneous doses (4).

Cardiac toxicity, consistent with myocardial infarction, was observed in three of seven patients with metastatic cancer receiving intravenous bolus interleukin-4 to a daily total of 800 micrograms/m^2 (5). A unique pattern of myocarditis with predominant polymorphonuclear, eosinophil, and mast cell infiltration was the possible cause of death in one case and suggested an allergic inflammatory myocardial process.

Endocrine

Permanent hypothyroidism associated with vitiligo was reported in a woman treated with interleukin-4 for metastatic malignant melanoma (SEDA-20, 336).

Hematologic

Unexpected severe neutropenia has been found in 33% of patients with AIDS-related Kaposi's sarcoma given interleukin-4 (SEDA-21, 376).

Isolated coagulation abnormalities with minor prolongation of prothrombin time were consistently observed, in patients given interleukin-4, particularly those with preexisting liver disease (2).

Gastrointestinal

Significant gastrointestinal toxicity was described in patients who received interleukin-4 alone or in combination with interleukin-2 for advanced malignancy (6).

Antral or prepyloric ulcers and erosive gastritis were identified after 12 of 84 courses of interleukin-4 in 72 patients, of whom three suffered from life-threatening bleeding. There were no treatment-related deaths and no clear correlation with the dose of interleukin-4. A possible protective effect of interleukin-2 on the gastrointestinal mucosa was suggested. Although all but one of these patients also took indometacin, there was no recurrence of symptoms in several patients who developed ulcers during interleukin-4 treatment and further received interleukin-2 and indometacin. The ability of interleukin-4 to affect prostaglandin E_2 synthesis strongly suggests that interleukin-4 alone can contribute to the development of digestive mucosal injury.

Skin

Rare dermatological adverse effects have been noticed and consisted of a papular eruption. One patient had a pruritic papulovesicular eruption, which recurred after interleukin-4 re-administration and was compatible with transient acantholytic dermatosis (7).

Vitiligo associated with permanent hypothyroidism was reported in a woman treated with interleukin-4 for metastatic malignant melanoma (SEDA-20, 336).

References

1. Peyron E, Banchereau J. Interleukin-4: structure, function and clinical aspects. Eur J Dermatol 1994;4:181–8.
2. Vial T, Descotes J. Clinical toxicity of cytokines used as haemopoietic growth factors. Drug Saf 1995;13(6):371–406.
3. Whitehead RP, Lew D, Flanigan RC, Weiss GR, Roy V, Glode ML, Dakhil SR, Crawford ED. Phase II trial of recombinant human interleukin-4 in patients with advanced renal cell carcinoma: a Southwest Oncology Group study. J Immunother 2002;25(4):352–8.
4. Prendiville J, Thatcher N, Lind M, McIntosh R, Ghosh A, Stern P, Crowther D. Recombinant human interleukin-4 (rhu IL-4) administered by the intravenous and subcutaneous routes in patients with advanced cancer—a phase I toxicity study and pharmacokinetic analysis. Eur J Cancer 1993;29A(12):1700–7.
5. Trehu EG, Isner JM, Mier JW, Karp DD, Atkins MB. Possible myocardial toxicity associated with interleukin-4 therapy. J Immunother 1993;14(4):348–51.
6. Rubin JT, Lotze MT. Acute gastric mucosal injury associated with the systemic administration of interleukin-4. Surgery 1992;111(3):274–80.
7. Mahler SJ, De Villez RL, Pulitzer DR. Transient acantholytic dermatosis induced by recombinant human interleukin 4. J Am Acad Dermatol 1993;29(2 Pt 1):206–9.

Interleukin-6

General Information

Interleukin-6 is produced by T cells, monocytes, fibroblasts, endothelial cells, and keratinocytes, and regulates pleiotropic biological functions. Recombinant interleukin-6 is being evaluated for thrombopoietic and antitumoral properties (1).

General adverse effects

During clinical trials, intravenous and subcutaneous interleukin-6 produced universal moderate fever and flu-like symptoms (2). Mild nausea, weight loss, and taste disorders sometimes occurred, and central nervous system symptoms (somnolence, restlessness, confusion, hallucinations) were dose-limiting in patients with advanced malignant cancer (SEDA-21, 376), but no clear dose-related effects have been demonstrated. Moderate injection site reactions usually followed subcutaneous interleukin-6 administration, and a diffuse maculopapular erythema occurred in one patient. In contrast to several other cytokines, interleukin-6 has not been associated with signs of vascular leak syndrome or hypotension. Neutralizing antibodies to interleukin-6 were rarely evidenced (SEDA-20, 336).

Whereas no major signs of toxicity appeared at doses up to 20 micrograms/kg/day in patients with malignant disease, the maximum tolerated dose of interleukin-6 was 5 micrograms/kg/day in patients with myelodysplasia or thrombocytopenia, and only 1 microgram/kg/day in autologous bone marrow transplant patients who developed hyperbilirubinemia and severe maculopapular rash with microvesicular steatosis as treatment-limiting adverse effects (2). Combination of interleukin-6 with G-CSF or GM-CSF was not associated with significant synergism or new forms of toxicity.

Biochemical effects of interleukin-6 included asymptomatic increases in liver function tests, transient proteinuria, and increased serum creatinine concentrations. Reductions in serum albumin and cholesterol concentrations, and increases in blood glucose concentrations were dose-related (SEDA-21, 376) (2).

Organs and Systems

Sensory systems

One isolated report documented reduced visual acuity and bilateral uveitis in a patient receiving a 2-week regimen of interleukin-3 and interleukin-6 for secondary myelodysplastic syndrome (SEDA-19, 341).

Endocrine

Interleukin-6 reduced serum thyrotropin and thyroid hormone concentrations and increased LH concentrations (SEDA-20, 336).

Hematologic

Dose-dependent and reversible normochromic normocytic anemia was consistently noted within several days after starting interleukin-6, and required blood transfusion at the highest dose (3). Hemodilution was considered as the primary mechanism.

Skin

Diffuse maculopapular erythema with histological features consisting of epidermal spongiosis and interstitial mixed inflammatory cell infiltrate was reported in one patient, and a causal role was suggested by the recurrence of symptoms after interleukin-6 re-administration (SEDA-19, 341).

Long-Term Effects

Tumorigenicity

The possibility of interleukin-6 might accelerate tumor growth was suggested by findings in two patients with solid tumors (SEDA-19, 341).

References

1. Veldhuis GJ, Willemse PH, Mulder NH, Limburg PC, De Vries EG. Potential use of recombinant human interleukin-6 in clinical oncology. Leuk Lymphoma 1996;20(5–6):373–9.
2. Vial T, Descotes J. Clinical toxicity of cytokines used as haemopoietic growth factors. Drug Saf 1995;13(6):371–406.
3. Nieken J, Mulder NH, Buter J, Vellenga E, Limburg PC, Piers DA, de Vries EG. Recombinant human interleukin-6 induces a rapid and reversible anemia in cancer patients. Blood 1995;86(3):900–5.

Interleukin-10

General Information

Interleukin-10 is a potent anti-inflammatory and immunosuppressive cytokine with beneficial effects expected in a wide range of diseases (1). In healthy volunteers, its adverse effect profile mostly consisted of flu-like symptoms at the highest dose (SEDA-20, 336). First-degree atrioventricular block was noted in a few patients. Due to immunomodulating properties, potential adverse immunological effects, namely an increased risk of infections, autoimmune disorders, or B cell lymphoproliferative disorders, can be anticipated.

Organs and Systems

Hematologic

The mechanisms of mild thrombocytopenia after multiple doses of interleukin-10 have been extensively explored in 12 healthy volunteers, of whom four received placebo and eight received subcutaneous interleukin-10 (8 micrograms/kg/day for 10 days) (2). Compared with placebo, there was a 40% fall in platelet count during interleukin-10 treatment and prompt normalization after interleukin-10 withdrawal. There were also moderate changes in hemoglobin concentration. Bone marrow function, platelet production, and serum thrombopoietin concentrations suggested that a reduction in bone marrow platelet production was the primary cause.

References

1. Goldman M, Velu T, Pretaloni M. Interleukin-10. Actions and therapeutic potential. Biodrugs 1997;7:6–14.
2. Sosman JA, Verma A, Moss S, Sorokin P, Blend M, Bradlow B, Chachlani N, Cutler D, Sabo R, Nelson M, Bruno E, Gustin D, Viana M, Hoffman R. Interleukin

10-induced thrombocytopenia in normal healthy adult volunteers: evidence for decreased platelet production. Br J Haematol 2000;111(1):104–11.

Interleukin-12

General Information

Interleukin-12, an immunomodulatory cytokine, has potential effects in several cancer and infectious diseases. Although interleukin-12 was considered to be reasonably safe in early clinical trials, severe and sometimes fatal multiple organ adverse effects have been described in subsequent studies (SEDA-20, 336). This unexpected profile of toxicity was later shown to result from schedule-dependent toxicity, which occurred only in patients with cancer who received multiple high doses without an initial single dose of interleukin-12 (1). This severe toxicity has since been avoided.

Organs and Systems

Hematologic

Single cases of agranulocytosis and Coombs' negative hemolytic anemia have been attributed to twice-weekly interleukin-12 in 28 patients with renal cell cancer or melanoma (2). The patients responded only to cyclophosphamide and/or glucocorticoids, and the causative role of interleukin-12 was therefore inconclusive.

Immunologic

Interleukin-12 has been involved in the pathogenesis of several autoimmune disorders.

- A 53-year-old woman with previously mild and stable rheumatoid disease had an exacerbation of severe rheumatoid arthritis after each course of interleukin-12 for cervical carcinoma (3).

References

1. Leonard JP, Sherman ML, Fisher GL, Buchanan LJ, Larsen G, Atkins MB, Sosman JA, Dutcher JP, Vogelzang NJ, Ryan JL. Effects of single-dose interleukin-12 exposure on interleukin-12-associated toxicity and interferon-gamma production. Blood 1997;90(7):2541–8.
2. Gollob JA, Veenstra KG, Mier JW, Atkins MB. Agranulocytosis and hemolytic anemia in patients with renal cell cancer treated with interleukin-12. J Immunother 2001;24(1):91–8.
3. Peeva E, Fishman AD, Goddard G, Wadler S, Barland P. Rheumatoid arthritis exacerbation caused by exogenous interleukin-12. Arthritis Rheum 2000;43(2):461–3.

Iodinated contrast media

General Information

The radio-opacity of X-ray contrast media depends on the fact that they contain substances that have high atomic numbers, which absorb X-rays. Bismuth, now largely obsolete, has an atomic number of 83, barium 56. Since the soluble salts of barium are poisonous, the insoluble salt, barium sulfate, is used as a suspension. Soluble contrast media are based on iodine, which has an atomic number of 53. This means that in principle they can have the various adverse effects of other iodine-containing compounds.

Iodinated water-soluble contrast agents are of four types:

- High-osmolar ionic monomers (for example amidotrizoate (diatrizoate) iodamide, iotalamate, ioxitalamate, metrizoate)
- Low-osmolar ionic dimers (for example ioxaglate)
- Low-osmolar non-ionic monomers (for example iobitridol, iohexol, iomeprol, iopamidol, iopromide, ioversol)
- Iso-osmolar non-ionic dimer (for example iodixonal, iotrolan).

These are mainly used intravascularly, but can also be injected into body cavities, including the bile ducts and pancreatic ducts, which can be outlined during endoscopic retrograde cholangiopancreatography (ERCP), particularly the low-osmolar contrast agents. The high-osmolar water-soluble contrast agent Gastrografin (sodium amidotrizoate and meglumine amidotrizoate in a ratio of 10:66) is suitable only for oral or rectal administration. Oil-based iodinated contrast agents, such as Lipiodol, are also available and can be used to outline the ducts of the salivary glands and the lacrimal ducts. Currently, the low-osmolar contrast agents are routinely used for these applications.

The high-osmolar ionic monomers, which are sodium and meglumine salts of tri-iodinated benzoic acid, have been available since the 1950s. They are very hyperosmolar, having 5–8 times the osmolality of the blood. The hyperosmolality greatly increases the hemodynamic and toxic effects of these agents. In the 1970s, low-osmolar contrast media became available. This was achieved through converting tri-iodinated benzoic acid into a non-ionic molecule by replacing the COOH radical with an amide ($CONH_2$). This molecule in solution will not dissociate, allowing the availability of three atoms of iodine with only one active particle (a ratio of 3:1). Another development was the introduction of the monoacid dimer, in which two tri-iodinated benzoic rings are linked with a bridge and the COOH of one ring is converted into an amide. This gives the same iodine:particle ratio of 3:1 in solution, since there are six iodine atoms and two active particles in one molecule. The osmolality of the ionic dimeric contrast media is almost the same as that of the non-ionic monomeric agents and is about twice that of blood at iodine concentration of 300 mg/ml. In the late 1980s the non-ionic dimeric contrast media were synthesized by attaching two non-ionic, tri-iodinated benzoic rings. These dimers give iodine:particle ratio of 6:1, since there are six iodine atoms and only one active particle in the molecule. The osmolality of the non-ionic dimers (iotrolan and iodixanol) at an iodine concentration of 300 mg/ml is equal to that of the blood. Iodixanol is the only non-ionic dimer currently in intravascular use (SEDA-21, 475) (SEDA-22, 502) (1–4).

Uses

For many types of investigation, contrast media have to be given intravascularly. Intravascular iodine-based contrast media are used for angiography and computed tomography, but since they are excreted mainly by the kidney, they are also used for excretory urography. Although the low-osmolar contrast media are safer than the high-osmolar contrast media, their use has not been universal because of high costs. However, the prices of low-osmolar contrast media are dropping, and in many countries high-osmolar ionic contrast media are no longer used intravascularly (SEDA-18, 441) (SEDA-22, 499). The media now used to outline cavities are mainly water-soluble and are preferred to water-insoluble or oily contrast agents.

- Cholecystography requires a contrast medium that is excreted primarily by the liver; iodipamide and ioglycamide have been long preferred, but the newer iodoxamate and iotroxate are more efficiently excreted by this route. However, cholecystography has become obsolete, with the availability of high quality real-time ultrasound scanning.
- In the gastrointestinal tract the insoluble barium sulfate is still most commonly used, but water-soluble iodinated media can be used in special circumstances.
- For retrograde urography, many different water-soluble iodinated media can be used, provided they are diluted sufficiently.
- For arthrography, ductography, and sinography, many different water-soluble iodinated media can be used, provided they are diluted sufficiently.
- For lymphography and ductography, iodinated oil is used. Iodinated water-soluble non-ionic dimeric media have also been used.
- Hysterosalpingography is now performed at most centers with low-osmolar water-soluble media.
- Bronchography was performed in the past with an aqueous or oily suspension, but these formulations have been withdrawn; the water-soluble non-ionic dimer iotrolan has been successfully used for fiberoptic bronchography.
- Myelography represents a special challenge, because of the sensitivity of nervous tissues to direct toxic effects; for this purpose the ionic media (which are neurotoxic) and the oily medium iophendylate have been superseded by non-ionic media, including the iso-osmolar non-ionic dimers (iotrolan and iodixanol), which are isotonic with cerebrospinal fluid and well tolerated by nervous tissues. However, myelography is rarely used in modern diagnostic imaging departments and has been widely replaced by magnetic resonance imaging (MRI).

Comparative studies

The authors of a large review of the comparative tolerability of contrast media used for coronary intervention recommended the use of ionic or non-ionic dimers over non-ionic low-osmolar monomeric agents, because of the antithrombotic advantage of the dimers (5). However, the recommendation to use ionic low-osmolar contrast media in preference to non-ionic contrast media is not widely endorsed, since the latter are less toxic than ionic media. In another study, there was no difference in the incidence of contrast media reactions between the non-ionic monomeric contrast agents iopamidol and iopromide, and both agents were well tolerated following left ventricle and coronary angiography (6). The authors concluded that both agents are perfectly acceptable for cardiac angiography.

Iodixanol 320 ($n = 307$) has been compared with the low-osmolar ionic dimer ioxaglate 320 ($n = 311$) in patients undergoing percutaneous coronary intervention (7). The two groups were well matched for basic demographic data and comparable in relation to cardiovascular state and other medical conditions. Fifteen patients (4.9%) in the iodixanol group and 27 patients (8.7%) in the ioxaglate group had reactions within 24 hours of the procedure; they were likely to have been due to the contrast medium, and included nausea, vomiting, flushing, facial edema, urticaria, and wheezing. There was no significant difference in the outcome of the procedure between the two groups. The authors suggested that in view of the higher incidence of adverse effects with ioxaglate, its automatic selection for percutaneous coronary intervention should be reviewed.

General adverse effects

The main types of collateral adverse effects of contrast media are listed in Table 1.

Low-osmolar contrast media are better tolerated than high-osmolar ionic media in cardiac and coronary angiography. However, it has been suggested that ionic contrast media may be advantageous during percutaneous transluminal coronary angioplasty, as they have some anticoagulant effect, which non-ionic media do not (SEDA-22, 501). The effects of the iso-osmolar non-ionic dimer iodixanol (iodine 320 mg/ml) and the low-osmolar ionic dimer ioxaglate (iodine 320 mg/ml) have been compared in 1411

Table 1 Adverse effects of soluble contrast media

Minor effects	Intermediate effects	Severe effects
Nausea, retching, and slight vomiting	Faintness	Collapse
Feeling of heat	Severe vomiting	Loss of consciousness
Limited urticaria	Extensive urticaria	Bronchospasm
Mild pallor or sweating	Edema of face or glottis	Edema of the glottis
Itchy rashes	Bronchospasm	Pulmonary edema
Arm pain	Dyspnea	Cardiac arrest
	Rigors	Myocardial infarction syndrome
	Chest pain	Cardiac dysrhythmias
	Abdominal pain	
	Headache	
	Tetany	

patients, mean age 62 years, undergoing percutaneous transluminal coronary angioplasty in a multicenter, randomized, double-blind study (8). The groups were comparable in relation to the prevalence of cardiac and other medical conditions, including diabetes, obesity, and smoking habits. All the patients received heparin and all but four received an antiplatelet agent (100 mg or more of aspirin and/or ticlopidine). There was no significant difference between the two groups—the incidence of major adverse cardiac events was 4.7% (192 patients) after iodixanol and 3.9% (197 patients) after ioxaglate. However, hypersensitivity reactions and adverse drug reactions were significantly less common with iodixanol ($n = 5$) than with ioxaglate ($n = 18$). The reactions to iodixanol were mainly rashes and urticaria-like reactions. The reactions to ioxaglate were anaphylaxis ($n = 1$), urticaria ($n = 12$), coughing and throat tightness ($n = 12$), and in one patient rigors, fever, vomiting, and flushing.

The diagnostic accuracy of bronchography with iotrolan is similar to that reported with Dionosil (9). No serious complications or significant change in spirometry measurements and oxygen saturation are observed with bronchography using iotrolan. The main adverse effects are nausea and vomiting. Pyrexia, pulmonary infection, and urticaria-like reactions are rare (9,10).

Serious delayed reactions have been reported from Germany and Japan in 26 cases; the features included shock, hypotension, angioedema, and dyspnea (11).

Time-course

Most reactions occur within 5–10 minutes of injection, but they can be delayed for up to 7 days; it is advisable for patients to be under close observation for about 20 minutes after injection. In 449 fatal reactions to ionic media, deaths occurred in all age groups, but the incidence peaked in the age group of 50–70 years; 80% of the reactions began in the first 5 minutes after injection, and the other 20% began at 5–15 minutes after injection (12). Late but mild reactions can also occur, notably those that are due to "iodism" (SEDA-11, 411).

Delayed reactions to both ionic and non-ionic media have an incidence of 0.4–18%. Most reactions are not serious or life threatening; they include a flu-like illness, parotitis, nausea and vomiting, abdominal pain, headache, and allergy-like reactions with skin manifestations. The incidence of delayed skin reactions to iso-osmolar non-ionic dimers is twice as high as the incidence of delayed skin reactions to low-osmolar non-ionic monomers, and twice as high in Japan and USA as in Europe. The pathophysiology of these delayed reactions is unknown. In response to reports of delayed skin reactions to the non-ionic dimer iotrolan, particularly in Japan, the manufacturer (Schering, Berlin) decided to withdraw it from the market as an intravascular agent (SEDA-21, 482).

The incidence of delayed adverse reactions has been investigated in 2001 patients who underwent cardiac angiography with either iopamidol 340 (a non-ionic monomer; $n = 738$, ages 22–88 years, mean dose 1.79 ml/kg), ioxaglate 320 (an ionic dimer; $n = 644$, ages 28–86 years, mean dose 1.8 ml/kg) or iodixanol 320 (a non-ionic dimer; $n = 619$, ages 26–85 years, mean dose 1.74 ml/kg) (13). The authors considered reactions that occurred within 24 hours as early reactions and those that occurred after 24 hours but within 1 week of the cardiac catheterization as late reactions. The incidences of early reactions were 22% with ioxaglate, 8.8% with iopamidol, and 7.6% with iodixanol. The commonest early reactions were urticaria and nausea and vomiting, the respective incidences being 6.8 and 4.0% with ioxaglate, 0.8 and 1.0% with iopamidol, and 0.5 and 1.1% with iodixanol. A few patients developed sudden hypotension, 0.5% with iopamidol, 1.4% with ioxaglate, and 0.3% with iodixanol. Cardiac arrest occurred in two patients with iopamidol, three with ioxaglate, and one with iodixanol. The frequencies of delayed skin reactions, which were generally benign, were 12% with iodixanol, 4.3% with ioxaglate, and 4.2% with iopamidol. The authors concluded that selection of a contrast agent for diagnostic cardiac catheterization should take account of adverse effects. Iodixanol was the best-tolerated agent in the early phase of the study, but it was associated with a higher incidence of delayed skin reactions. The authors did not consider that the skin reactions represented a contraindication to iodixanol, although patients should be advised of this particular adverse effect. Furthermore, no contrast agent was free from these effects. Ioxaglate was the least well-tolerated agent in the early phase, with a much greater chance of causing nausea/vomiting and allergic reactions.

Incidence

In various earlier surveys of conventional ionic contrast media, the incidence of minor reactions was one in 13–30 cases, the incidence of intermediate reactions one in 57–130 cases, and the incidence of severe reactions one in 1000–4000 cases. The figures for the non-ionic media are much more favorable. In 1990, the Japanese Committee on the Safety of Contrast Media surveyed 169 284 patients who had received ionic media and 168 363 who had received non-ionic contrast media (14). In patients with a previous history of reactions to contrast media, the incidence of severe reactions was 0.73% with ionic media and only 0.18% with non-ionic media. Among patients with asthma, severe and very severe reactions occurred in 1.88% with ionic media and 0.23% with non-ionic media. In a Canadian survey of 1992, the overall incidence of adverse effects to contrast media was 3.9% for ionic media and only 0.9% for non-ionic media, despite the fact that the proportion of patients with heart disease as a pre-existing susceptibility factor was much higher in the non-ionic group (SEDA-22, 500).

In a study from France the incidence of adverse drug reactions after 1480 injections of low-osmolar iodinated contrast media was 0.34%; the frequency was higher in patients with a history of allergy (1.5%) (15). In a similar study of the prevalence of adverse drug reactions amongst in-patients in a North Indian referral hospital over 3 years, 317 adverse reactions were reported (0.3%) (16). Skin reactions (123 cases, 39%) and gastrointestinal disturbances (90 cases, 28%) made up a large proportion of the reported adverse reactions. Of all the adverse reactions, 15% (48 cases) were due to iodinated contrast media (details of the types of contrast media used were not provided in the report) and the common reactions were nausea/vomiting (24 cases, 7.5%) and rashes

(16 cases, 5%); however, there was serious life-threatening anaphylaxis in three cases (0.9%).

The incidence of adverse reactions has been investigated in Taiwan in 28 364 patients after intravenous injection of contrast agents during intravenous urography and CT scanning (17). There were adverse reactions in 495 patients (1.75%), including 467 patients (2.03%) of 20 260 examined with ionic contrast agents and 28 (0.34%) of 8076 patients examined with non-ionic contrast agents. The authors concluded that the risk of adverse reactions to non-ionic contrast agents is significantly lower than with ionic agents. Skin rashes, such as urticaria, were the most common adverse effects, followed by nausea and vomiting. Shock requiring cardiopulmonary resuscitation was rare and occurred in only six patients (0.02%); there were no deaths in this series.

Adverse reactions to intravascular iodinated agents are usually classified as minor, intermediate, or severe life-threatening. All types of reactions to low-osmolar contrast media are five times less common than reactions to high-osmolar contrast agents (SEDA-22, 489) (SEDA-23, 494) (SEDA-24, 519), and very severe adverse reactions to contrast media are rare, with a frequency of about 0.04% with high-osmolar agents and 0.004% with low-osmolar agents. However, there are no important differences in the safety profiles of the different low-osmolar non-ionic monomers (18).

In one US study of cardiac angiography, the incidence of adverse events was 32% with diatrizoate and 10% with iohexol; it should be noted however that the diatrizoate used in that study (Renografin 76™) causes calcium binding, which may have increased the rate of cardiac complications (19). The non-ionic agent iodixanol 320, which is virtually iso-osmolar, has been tested in cardiac angiography against iohexol and seemed to be better tolerated (20).

The safety of the non-ionic contrast agents has also been emphasized in a review from Germany, in which the authors documented a reduced risk of adverse drug reactions with non-ionic contrast agents during interventional cardiology (21). According to reports to the FDA, the incidence of lethal complications was 3.9% with ionic monomers, 6.39% with the ionic dimer ioxaglate, and 2.07% with non-ionic monomers. The authors also stated that non-ionic contrast agents do not have thrombogenic potential, a previous concern; currently, most authors would support this view (SEDA-22, 501) (SEDA-23, 497).

There was no difference in the incidence of adverse effects between iotrolan 320 and iohexol 350 in cardiac angiography for ischemic heart disease in 120 patients (22). There were no serious adverse events. One patient developed mild urticaria after iotrolan. Five patients in each group had mild unspecified delayed reactions.

An analysis of adverse reactions associated with drugs in Poland (1997–98) has shown that 11.5% of these reactions were due to radiographic contrast media. People aged 36–65 were the largest group to have adverse drug reactions (23).

According to a survey conducted by the Royal Australian College of Radiologists in 1986, the incidence of severe reactions with high-osmolar ionic contrast media was 0.36% in high-risk patients (patients with a strong history of allergy or bronchial asthma or a history of reactions to contrast media) and 0.09% in low-risk patients (24). The incidence of these reactions with low-osmolar non-ionic media was 0.03% in high-risk patients, and 0% in low-risk patients.

In another survey, the incidence of contrast media reactions after intravenous administration was evaluated over 14 years (25). The incidence of all reactions to contrast media was 6–8% with high-osmolar contrast media and only 0.2% with low-osmolar non-ionic agents. Most of the reactions (over 90%) were allergic-like, and severe reactions were rare (0.05%). One death was reported after the use of a low-osmolar agent. These data are compatible with previous reports, which showed that low-osmolar contrast media have a much better safety profile than high-osmolar media and that there is no significant difference in the incidence of acute adverse reactions between non-ionic dimeric and monomeric contrast media.

In another study there was no significant difference in the incidence of adverse effects associated with the use of the non-ionic dimer iodixanol or the non-ionic monomer iopromide in femoral angiography (26).

Delayed reactions

There are conflicting data on the risk of delayed reactions, comparing non-ionic monomers and iso-osmolar non-ionic dimers (iotrolan, iodixanol). European studies (27) have shown no significant difference (0.62% iotrolan, 0.82% non-ionic monomers), but studies from Japan and the USA have suggested that delayed reactions are 2–5 times more common with iotrolan.

The incidence of delayed adverse reactions to various non-ionic monomers in Japanese patients undergoing contrast-enhanced CT has been compared with the incidence in control patients who did not receive contrast. Delayed reactions occurred in 12% of patients who received contrast compared with 10% in the control group. The authors concluded that the frequency of delayed reactions that can be attributed to contrast media is 2.1%. The most common reactions were itching and limited urticaria (28). This report highlights the difficulty of verifying that adverse events that occur many hours after contrast administration are directly caused by the contrast agent.

The incidence of delayed reactions has been assessed in 403 Italian patients who received intravenous iopamidol during CT or urographic examination (29). A total of 50 patients (12%) developed delayed reactions. Allergy, previous exposure to a contrast agent, and being female were associated with a significantly higher incidence of delayed reactions. The most frequently reported delayed reactions were nausea and vomiting, drowsiness, rash, itching, and headache. All reported reactions were mild and resolved spontaneously.

In a questionnaire study of 11 121 Japanese patients, 216 (1.4%) developed immediate adverse reactions and 1058 (9.5%) reported having had delayed reactions after intravenous contrast administration during various CT examinations (30). Delayed reactions were reported by 18 patients (13%) of the 136 patients with immediate reactions who answered the questionnaire. All the patients, with the exception of 360 who received the non-ionic dimer iotrolan, were given non-ionic monomeric contrast media. The dose was 60–200 ml. Delayed reactions were more frequent in patients with a history of allergy, past adverse reactions to contrast media or with a serum creatinine concentration over 180 μmol/l. Delayed reactions were also more frequent in women and in patients who had not previously received contrast media. There was no significant relation between the occurrence of immediate adverse reactions and the development of delayed reactions. The commonest delayed reactions were itching and skin reactions, which developed in 5.5% and 3.0% of the patients respectively. Skin reactions were observed twice as often in patients who were given iotrolan compared with those who were given monomeric agents. In the iotrolan group, 7.3% of the patients developed a skin reaction, 9.9% reported itching, and 60% of the reactions were severe or moderate. A quarter of the delayed reactions occurred within 6 hours after the examination and more than half occurred within 24 hours. Most of the reactions occurred within the first 3 days.

The incidence of delayed adverse reactions has been investigated in 2001 patients who underwent cardiac angiography with either iopamidol 340 ($n = 738$, aged 22–88 years, mean dose 1.79 ml/kg), ioxaglate 320 ($n = 644$, aged 28–86 years, mean dose 1.8 ml/kg) or iodixanol 320 ($n = 619$, aged 26–85 years, mean dose 1.74 ml/kg) (13). The authors considered reactions that occurred within 24 hours as early reactions and those that occurred after 24 hours but within 1 week as late reactions. The incidences of early reactions were 22% with ioxaglate, 8.8% with iopamidol, and 7.6% with iodixanol. The commonest early reactions were urticaria and nausea and vomiting, the respective incidences being 6.8 and 4.0% with ioxaglate, 0.8 and 1.0% with iopamidol, and 0.5 and 1.1% with iodixanol. A few patients developed sudden hypotension, 0.5% with iopamidol, 1.4% with ioxaglate, and 0.3% with iodixanol. Cardiac arrest occurred in two patients with iopamidol, three with ioxaglate, and one with iodixanol. The frequencies of delayed skin reactions, which were generally benign, were 12% with iodixanol, 4.3% with ioxaglate, and 4.2% with iopamidol. The authors concluded that selection of a contrast agent for diagnostic cardiac catheterization should take account of adverse effects. Iodixanol was the best-tolerated agent in the early phase of the study, but it was associated with a higher incidence of delayed skin reactions. The authors did not consider that the skin reactions represented a contraindication to iodixanol, although patients should be advised of this particular adverse effect. Furthermore, no contrast agent was free from these effects. Ioxaglate was the least well-tolerated agent in the early phase, with a much greater chance of causing nausea/vomiting and allergic reactions.

The Federal Institute of Drugs and Medical Devices in Germany has surveyed a total of 1135 adverse drug reactions (acute and late) associated with iotrolan 280 and 1354 reports associated with iodixanol at various iodine concentrations (31). There were late adverse reactions (observed later than 1 hour after injection) in 757 cases (67%) associated with iotrolan 280, and in 525 cases (39%) associated with iodixanol. Late reactions were observed mainly in the first 24 hours, with occasional reports at 24–72 hours after injection. Rarely, delayed contrast reactions have been reported more than 72 hours after injection, although they are difficult to substantiate. This study emphasizes the importance of extending the surveillance period for at least 72 hours after contrast administration. Most delayed reactions in this study were non-serious allergic-like reactions, with symptoms including itching, urticaria, erythema, edema, and bronchospasm. In a very few cases there were serious or life-threatening reactions, including Quincke's edema and hypotension.

The incidence of late adverse reactions to the iso-osmolar agent iodixanol has also been investigated in a retrospective comparison with the non-ionic monomer iohexol. Reactions after 3075 injections were reviewed. Patients were sent a written questionnaire to find out about the incidence of any acute or delayed reactions. Those who developed reactions were interviewed by telephone and specific second questionnaires were administered. The incidence of adverse reactions was low (2% for late adverse reactions and 2.3% for acute reactions). There was no significant difference in the incidence of acute or delayed adverse reactions to iohexol and iodixanol and there were no serious reactions (32).

Delayed reactions are generally benign, but not always. In a Japanese study, the incidence of delayed reactions was investigated in 6764 patients who received the low-osmolar non-ionic contrast medium iohexol intravenously (33). Delayed reactions (rash, pruritus, nausea, vomiting, fever, headache, and others) occurred in 192 patients (2.8%). There were no severe delayed reactions. A history of allergy and hay fever were risk factors for delayed adverse reactions.

Delayed adverse reactions to ioxaglate have been documented after coronary angiography with ioxaglate (34).

- A 63-year-old housewife had an acute myocardial infarction. Diagnostic coronary angiography was performed with ioxaglate and repeated 1 week later. On the morning after, she had intense shivering and generalized malaise, a temperature of 39.2°C, and hypotension. Several hours later she developed a non-pruritic maculopapular rash, starting on the face and extending within the next 48 hours to cover the entire body but sparing the mucous membranes. She had a mild eosinophilia (600×10^6/l) with a raised erythrocyte sedimentation rate (52 mm at 1 hour). Her IgE concentration was raised at 1593 kU/l. Blood cultures were negative. The initial clinical impression was that she had sepsis and she was therefore given vancomycin, netilmicin, and cefotaxime (dosages not stated). She improved rapidly and the fever and the rash resolved completely. She was discharged taking atenolol 100 mg/day and lysine acetylsalicylate 250 mg/day, but 3 days later she returned with a temperature of 39.8°C and recurrence of the skin rash. She had a marked eosinophilia (1.4×10^9/l) and raised liver enzymes, lactate dehydrogenase, and aldolase, but creatine kinase activity was in the reference range. She had a significantly raised concentration of circulating immune complexes. Atenolol and lysine acetylsalicylate were withdrawn and she was given acenocoumarol 2 mg/day and amlodipine 5 mg/day. The inflammatory syndrome rapidly disappeared and the enzymes and eosinophil count returned to normal. She had immunological investigations 2 months later. The total IgE was still raised. The leukocyte count and C-reactive protein concentration were within the reference ranges. The serum antinuclear antibody titer was 1/256 and the antimitochondrial antibody titer was 1/128. Tests for antinative DNA, antihistone, and anti-smooth muscle antibodies were negative. Skin prick tests, intradermal tests, and patch tests with lysine acetylsalicylate, atenolol, heparins, vancomycin, netilmicin, cefotaxime, and the contrast agents ioxaglate, sodium ioxitalamate, iopamidol, and iohexol were negative at 15 minutes, but at 48 hours indurated erythematous papules were observed with ioxaglate, ioxitalamate, and iopamidol. A biopsy from the ioxaglate skin reaction showed discrete spongiosis of the epidermis associated with slight lymphocytic exocytosis. The basal layer contained numerous apoptotic keratinocytes. The superficial dermis was edematous and there was a perivascular inflammatory infiltrate composed mainly of T lymphocytes. There were no mast cells or eosinophils. Immunohistological examination showed no staining with anti IgE, IgG, IgM, C1q, C3, or C4. During follow-up she was completely normal at up to 1 year, with a normal eosinophil count and an IgE concentration of 440 kU/l.

This report documents a rare clinical reaction to ioxaglate, with a combination of a maculopapular rash, fever, hepatic and muscle involvement, eosinophilia, and a very high serum IgE concentration. The intradermal tests confirmed a delayed hypersensitivity reaction to ioxaglate. Histological examination of a skin biopsy identified the predominantly T lymphocyte nature of the infiltrate. A contributing role of the beta-blocker atenolol to the seriousness of the clinical syndrome must also be considered.

Mechanisms and susceptibility factors

The mechanisms underlying idiosyncratic adverse reactions are far from clear. Although many resemble allergic or anaphylactic events, the evidence does not suggest that they are as a whole induced immunologically, though some certainly are, and there is no doubt that in some cases contrast media act as antigens. Lalli believes that all contrast media reactions are explicable on a neurological basis; this hypothesis is not generally accepted, but most would agree that anxiety can be an important predisposing factor, for example to cardiac dysrhythmias. It has been suggested that contrast media act as histamine liberators, and there is evidence from animal experiments that this is the case, the methylglucamine media being more potent in this respect than the corresponding sodium salts (though ioxaglate may apparently also elicit histaminoid reactions (35); the antihistamine diphenhydramine has been recommended both for preventing and treating reactions (see below) and may have some efficacy. A further theory is that bradykinin is an essential mediator in systemic contrast media reactions (36). There is also older experimental evidence that contrast media can activate serum complement by the "alternative pathway," and it is postulated that this may be one of the factors in systemic adverse reactions, possibly by liberation of anaphylatoxin and with a risk of disseminated intravascular coagulation.

Adverse reactions to contrast agents have been linked to an in vivo interaction with enzymes involved in cholinergic activity. However, experimental results on this topic are conflicting. In a study of the in vivo effects of the non-ionic monomer iohexol and the high-osmolar ionic monomer diatrizoate on human plasma acetylcholinesterase and butyrylcholinesterase, both contrast agents significantly inhibited the enzymes (37). The effect was more pronounced with iohexol, which has a lower incidence of adverse effects than diatrizoate. The significance of this observation is not certain, but activation of these enzymes is not likely to be important in mediating the adverse effects of contrast agents. Other enzymes that are inhibited by iodinated contrast agents include hexokinase, glucose-6-phosphate dehydrogenase, and alcohol dehydrogenase (38).

More minor adverse reactions to the second-generation non-ionic water-soluble contrast media, such as headache, nausea, and vomiting, are more frequent in women than in men, particularly in women aged 26–50 years. Early ambulation increases the incidence of headaches. In one study, there was a higher incidence of delayed headaches after iopamidol in comparison with iohexol. Long-distance travel also appeared to increase the incidence of headaches after myelography (SEDA-15, 503). Dizziness was more frequent in patients over the age of 50 years. In a meta-analysis of 25 published studies, the incidence of symptoms after myelography was significantly higher when needles larger than 22G were used.

The risks (expressed as risk ratios) of adverse effects of contrast media after intravenous injection related to some susceptibility factors are listed in Table 2.

Prevention and management

Intravenous pre-testing is unreliable in determining susceptibility; in one survey of 33 400 patients, most of the reactions were not predicted by pretesting, although a positive pre-test did indicate an increased risk of a reaction (39). The value of the lymphoblast transformation test is very limited, although it certainly provides interesting evidence that contrast media can sometimes act as antigens (SEDA-16, 531) (40).

The value of prophylactic use of glucocorticoids to reduce the risk of contrast reactions is contentious. The Contrast Media Safety Committee (CMSC) of the European Society of Urogenital Radiology (ESUR) considered this issue and produced guidelines on how to reduce the risk of generalized reactions to intravascular use of contrast media (Table 3) (41).

In high-risk patients, and more particularly those with a history of poor tolerance of contrast media, measures will

Table 2 Risk ratios for adverse effects of contrast media after intravenous injection related to susceptibility factors

History	Minor reactions	Intermediate reactions	Severe reactions	Death
Allergy (all types)	1.6	2.6	3.9	
Hay fever	1.7	1.8	2.3	
Urticaria	1.5	4.8	2.0	
Asthma	1.2	2.7	5.1	
Heart disease	1.1	0.9	4.5	8.5
Previous reaction to a contrast medium	6.9	8.7	11	
Previous reaction to other drugs	1.8	2.0	3.2	

Table 3 European Society of Urogenital Radiology (ESUR) Guidelines on prevention of generalized contrast medium reactions in adults

A. Susceptibility factors for reactions
Previous generalized reaction to a contrast medium, either moderate (for example urticaria, bronchospasm, moderate hypotension) or severe (for example convulsions, severe bronchospasm, pulmonary edema, cardiovascular collapse)
Asthma
Allergy requiring medical treatment

B. To reduce the risk of generalized contrast medium reactions
Use non-ionic agents

C. Premedication is recommended in high-risk patients (defined in A)
When ionic agents are used
When non-ionic agents are used, opinion is divided about the value of premedication

D. Recommended premedication
Glucocorticoids
Prednisolone 30 mg orally or methylprednisolone 32 mg orally 12 and 2 hours before contrast medium
Glucocorticoids are not effective if given less than 6 hours before contrast medium
Histamine H_1 and H_2 receptor antagonists may be used in addition to corticosteroids, but opinion is divided

E. Remember for all patients
Have a trolley with resuscitation drugs in the examination room
Observe patients for 20–30 minutes after contrast medium injection

F. Extravascular administration
When absorption or leakage into the circulation is possible, take the same precautions as for intravascular administration

be necessary to contain risks of hypersensitivity reactions. Apart from using non-ionic and low-osmolar media, and diluting media for certain purposes, one can consider prophylactic premedication. Glucocorticoid premedication alone has often been advocated, particularly in patients with asthma; although it has been condemned as unnecessary with the current generation of contrast media (SEDA-18, 442) (SEDA-19, 426) it seems to be well founded in experience, reducing both the frequency and severity of reactions, but it certainly does not eliminate risk (42). A double regimen based on prednisolone and the antihistamine diphenhydramine has been advocated in various centers (SEDA-16, 531) (SEDA-18, 442) (43,44). To be effective, glucocorticoids should be given sufficiently far in advance; in some cases, an intravenous injection of dexamethasone given immediately before an infusion of contrast media failed to prevent an anaphylactic reaction (45).

H_1 and H_2 receptor antagonists, aminocaproic acid, or hyposensitization have all been proposed as means of reducing risk prophylactically. Aminocaproic acid was formerly used prophylactically in France, but was associated with a risk of massive intravascular coagulation (46).

In severe reactions, intravenous glucocorticoids are usually given on an empirical basis, with oxygen as required. Non-cardiogenic hypotensive shock usually responds best to fluid replacement, but vasopressors are occasionally required. Adrenaline is primarily indicated for bronchospasm and other allergic-type reactions, but caution is required to avoid cardiac dysrhythmias. Intravenous antihistamines are useful in angioedema, but can aggravate hypotensive reactions. Chemotoxic convulsions require intravenous diazepam and oxygenation.

Systemic adverse effects of enteral contrast agents

Oral radiographic contrast media can intravasate during gastrointestinal examination. Septicemia has been reported (47).

- A 46-year-old patient developed ischemic necrosis of the small bowel complicating mesenteric volvulus. Small bowel resection was carried out and ileal and jejunal stomas were established. Six weeks after the operation Gastrografin was given through the jejunal stoma. A mesenteric vein filled with Gastrografin and this was followed by rapid washout of the intravascular contrast medium. The examination was stopped immediately and 60 minutes later the patient developed chills and a high fever. Hemodynamic instability required the use of vasoactive drugs and infusion of isotonic solutions. Blood cultures grew *Escherichia coli*, *Pseudomonas aeruginosa*, and *Enterobacter* species. Treatment included imipenem and after 48 hours the patient was stable and the vasoactive agents were stopped. Endoscopy through the jejunal stoma showed multiple stenoses, which required surgical treatment, and the jejunum in the area of intravasation was resected.

Gram-negative septicemia possibly related to oral Gastrografin has also been reported in a premature neonate with necrotizing enterocolitis (48).

- A baby born after 26 weeks of gestation received oral Gastrografin (0.5 ml 8 hourly) for gut stimulation. Three days after the last dose of Gastrografin there was sudden clinical deterioration leading to shock. Blood cultures grew *Enterobacter*. Progressive deterioration continued to occur, with multisystem failure, leading to death. Autopsy was not performed.

The authors suggested that the high osmolality of Gastrografin may have aggravated the pre-existing mucosal injury in the gastrointestinal tract, leading to complete loss of mucosal integrity and an increase in gut permeability to micro-organisms and toxins. Oral Gastrografin and other hyperosmolar contrast media should not be used in patients, particularly neonates, with compromised bowel integrity, since the high osmolarity may aggravate the bowel injury. Low-osmolar contrast media should always be used in such patients.

Disseminated intravascular coagulation and severe hypotension have been documented after intravenous administration of Gastrografin, which is suitable only for oral or rectal administration (47).

Cost to benefit ratio

At a time when reductions in the costs of medical care are critical, decisions about which classes of contrast media to use are not determined purely on clinical grounds, but by a consideration of the cost to benefit ratio. Concern about financial implications has been the major factor in preventing a universal conversion to non-ionic contrast agents, which are better tolerated but more expensive than high-osmolar ionic agents. In the USA, the Health Care Finance Administration (HCFA) has recommended that the use of the expensive non-ionic contrast media should be restricted only to patients with severe cardiac disease, a history of asthma, severe allergy, severe debility, sickle cell disease, or a previous severe adverse reaction to contrast media.

The results of a study in 1324 patients who underwent diagnostic arteriography have supported the selective use of non-ionic contrast agents following the HCFA guidelines. A cost saving of $41 per patient was possible without an increase in the incidence of complications (49).

Organs and Systems

Cardiovascular

Most severe reactions to contrast media are associated with cardiovascular manifestations, causing hypotensive shock and in some cases ventricular fibrillation and cardiac arrest; these events are reversible in most cases in which prompt treatment is given. In a case of hypotensive collapse reported in 1977, and followed by a small number of others, there was disseminated intravascular coagulation (50). In milder cases there is only hypotension, which can be transient and symptomless; in some cases there is bradycardia (due apparently to vagal overactivity) rather than tachycardia.

In more than 90 000 cardiac angiographies performed in US hospitals during 1991, the overall rate of complications with low-osmolar contrast media was 1.5%, including idiosyncratic reactions in 0.25%, vascular complications in 0.44%, neurological complications in 0.05%, dysrhythmias in 0.31%, and myocardial infarction in 0.06%; the death rate was 0.11%. In percutaneous coronary angioplasty major complications, generally of the same type, occurred in 5% of cases (51). In one large series of digital subtraction angiography examinations using iopamidol, the overall incidence of reactions was 2.5%; some occurred with a delay of 1 hour or more (52).

The safety of iodixanol 320 and iohexol 350 has been investigated in Swedish patients undergoing cardiac angiography for suspected coronary artery disease (53). Of 1020 patients, 502 aged 25–83 years received iohexol (median dose 105 ml, range 20–440) and 518 aged 18–85 years received iodixanol (median dose 115 ml, range 30–400). There were 134 patients with unstable angina in the iohexol group and 167 in the iodixanol group. Cardiac adverse events (angina pectoris, dysrhythmias, and dyspnea) within 24 hours of the examination were reported by 9% of the patients who received iohexol and 7% of patients who received iodixanol. There were two cases of ventricular fibrillation, both after iohexol. Cardiac adverse events in patients aged 65 years or more occurred in 11% with iohexol and 7% with iodixanol. The proportions of patients with unstable angina and cardiac adverse events were 18% with iohexol and 12% with iodixanol. The authors concluded that iodixanol could be advantageous in old patients and in those with unstable angina.

Iodixanol (a non-ionic dimer, 320 mg of iodine per ml) and ioxaglate 320 (a low-osmolar ionic dimer, 320 mg of iodine per ml) have been compared in a randomized study in 110 consecutive patients referred for coronary angiography and ventriculography (54). The incidence of adverse reactions was significantly higher with ioxaglate (28 versus 3%) but there was no difference in angiographic quality between the two agents. The increase in left ventricular end-diastolic pressure was significantly less with iodixanol than with ioxaglate. The QT interval was significantly prolonged by both agents, but the changes were less marked after iodixanol. The authors concluded that iodixanol and ioxaglate are of comparable diagnostic efficacy in coronary angiography and ventriculography but that iodixanol is better tolerated and has less marked hemodynamic and electrophysiological effects.

The hemodynamic effect of direct intra-arterial injection of contrast agents on capillary perfusion in man has been investigated (55). This was achieved through continuous recording of perfusion in the nail-fold capillaries of the right hand before and after a bolus injection of 20 ml of iodixanol 270 (a non-ionic dimer) or iopentol 150 (a non-ionic monomer) into the right axillary artery. The high-viscosity contrast agent iodixanol (5.8 mPa.s) caused a significant reduction in erythrocyte velocity, while iopentol, which has a much lower viscosity (1.7 mPa.s), had no effect. The authors concluded that high-viscosity contrast media can cause reduced organ perfusion. This effect could be significant in patients with atherosclerotic disease, as it might lead to reduced perfusion of the myocardium during coronary angiography.

Effects on blood pressure

Rapid peripheral intravenous injection of concentrated ionic contrast media produces a brief rise in systemic arterial pressure followed by a prolonged fall; the diastolic pressure decreases more than the systolic pressure and the heart slows; the pulse contour changes, and the venous pressure rises; the arterial hypotension is more marked if injection is rapid. The electrocardiogram can show flattening, splitting, or T-wave inversion; tachycardia is probably compensatory, as are the concomitant increases in venous pressure and pulmonary arterial pressure. Hypotension associated with a vasovagal reaction probably explained four deaths from acute coronary insufficiency (two each with iodoalphionic acid and iopanoic acid) in patients with ischemic heart disease.

- A 44-year-old man had a CT scan of the head with intravenous contrast enhancement (35 ml of ioversol 350) (56). He developed severe back pain 90 minutes later and then became acutely unwell, with nausea, vomiting, chills, tremor, and faintness. He rapidly became shocked (systolic blood pressure 80 mmHg, pulse 140/minute) and had a petechial rash over the trunk and upper limbs. He was given intravenous fluids (polygeline 2 liters and crystalloid 2 liters and adrenaline. Blood cultures were negative, and echocardiography, CT scan of the chest and abdomen, and abdominal ultrasound were normal. He continued to deteriorate, developed acute renal insufficiency with disseminated intravascular coagulation, and was given dopamine, aggressive fluid resuscitation, and antibiotics (gentamicin, ceftriaxone, and erythromycin). His general condition gradually improved and he recovered fully.

The authors attributed these events to a severe delayed reaction to the contrast medium, manifesting as prolonged hypotension.

Injection of contrast media into the right side of the heart or pulmonary artery can be followed by transient pulmonary hypertension but systemic hypotension. The pulmonary hypertension is partially due to an increase in the pulmonary vascular resistance from capillary blockage by the altered erythrocytes, which have a reduced elasticity due to the effect of a hypertonic contrast medium. Reduced cardiac output accompanied by cardiac slowing and diminished force of contraction seem to explain the initial systemic hypotension; persistence of hypotension thereafter is probably due to the vasodilator effect of the contrast medium on the systemic vessels. Pulmonary angiography is particularly dangerous when the right ventricular end-diastolic pressure exceeds 20 mmHg. Iohexol appears to be a safer medium for pulmonary angiography (SEDA-14, 423).

Injection into the left ventricle or the proximal aorta is likely to produce more marked effects. Cardiac rate, stroke volume, and cardiac output increase. There is a rise in right and left atrial pressures and left ventricular end-diastolic pressure. The pulmonary arterial pressure is also increased. The blood volume expands and peripheral blood flow increases and then decreases as systemic resistance falls. The hematocrit falls and venous pressure gradually rises. As the systemic arterial pressure falls, the heart rate increases. These responses are largely due to the injection of strongly hypertonic solutions, which promote a rapid expansion of the plasma volume; water shifts from the extravascular fluid spaces to the blood and moves out of the erythrocytes, which shrink and become crenated. Blood viscosity rises, but plasma viscosity does not increase significantly. The erythrocytes give up potassium to the plasma and this might contribute to the observed reduction in peripheral vascular resistance.

In two cases of severe hypotensive collapse with generalized itching after left ventricular angiography with 76% sodium methylglucamine diatrizoate, the hypotension failed to respond to vasoconstrictors, and measurements of right atrial and right ventricular pressures showed marked reduction in filling pressures. Rapid intravenous infusion of isotonic saline caused prompt improvement in the blood pressure. A similar case of hypotension with a beneficial response to plasma expanders occurred in a case of prolonged shock after intravenous urography. Severe and prolonged hypotensive collapse has also been seen after antegrade pyelography through a nephrostomy tube under general anesthesia, but the patient in question had a previous history of an acute reaction (SEDA-18, 445). In two cases, injection of diatrizoate during arteriography under general anesthesia caused severe hypotensive collapse (SEDA-7, 452).

Acetrizoate has a more marked effect in this respect than an equiosmolar solution of diatrizoate. Methylglucamine salts appear to be relatively less vasoactive in the peripheral vessels. All these changes are considerably less marked with low-osmolar media such as ioxaglate, iopamidol, or iohexol, but not necessarily absent. Abdominal aortography with iohexol has been found to produce both a decrease in the systemic blood pressure and an increase in the plasma concentration of atrial natriuretic peptide; this may be due to increased intravascular volume (SEDA-16, 533).

Intra-arterial injection of conventional ionic contrast media results in vasodilatation. This is due mainly to hypertonicity of the medium, but toxicity is also a factor. The vasodilatation may in addition be partly due to an anti-cholinesterase action, since it is partially blocked by atropine. In clinical practice, aortography and peripheral arteriography are usually associated with a slight fall in blood pressure, tachycardia and discomfort in the limbs, such as heat or pain.

During cerebral angiography with either ionic or non-ionic agents, hypotension, bradycardia, and even transient asystole can occur, though there can also be reflex tachycardia (57), which can result in hypertension. These changes are more marked during vertebral angiography when the posterior cerebral arteries have been filled, suggesting that they are due to involvement of centers in the hypothalamus or brain stem. Visual disturbances can also occur, due to involvement of the occipital cortex (58). The reflex cardiovascular changes may be more serious in patients with coronary artery disease and can give rise to left ventricular failure. Both electrocardiographic and electroencephalographic changes are less common when methylglucamine salts are used. Premedication with atropine reduces the incidence of the cardiovascular changes, but not that of focal electroencephalographic effects. Their incidence has also been reduced by use of very small doses of contrast agents and by premedication with hypertonic mannitol in patients with raised intracranial pressure. One patient with metrizamide encephalopathy developed severe hypertension (SEDA-11, 415) (SED-12, 1182).

Electrocardiographic effects

In a comparison of the effects of iodixanol and ioxaglate during coronary angiography, 22 patients received ioxaglate for the first injection into the left coronary artery and iodixanol for the next injections, and 20 patients received the media in the reverse order (59). Those who received ioxaglate first received a mean of 102 ml of contrast medium and the iodixanol group 104 ml. The first three injections into the left coronary artery were subjected to electrocardiographic analysis. Deviation from baseline was greater in those who received ioxaglate first. The most pronounced effects of ioxaglate were on the ST segment and T wave: the T wave change vector magnitude increased 11-fold from baseline after ioxaglate and 5-fold after iodixanol; the increase in ST change vector magnitude was 4-fold with ioxaglate and 3-fold with iodixanol. The authors concluded that iodixanol caused less pronounced electrocardiographic changes than ioxaglate. These findings are in accord with experimental evidence that iodixanol is well tolerated by the myocardium.

Certain contrast media, notably the high-osmolar products based on sodium methylglucamine, Renografin-76 and MD-76, have calcium-binding properties and cause more hemodynamic changes and a higher risk of ventricular fibrillation than the calcium-enriched media Angiovist and Hypaque-76 (60). In nine patients undergoing coronary arteriography, plasma measurements from the coronary sinus, there was a significant reduction in ionized calcium concentrations immediately after injection of Renografin 76 (sodium methylglucamine diatrizoate) into the coronary arteries. The effect was most marked and lasted longer in patients with vascular disease. The reduction in ionized calcium was attributed to the chelating agents (disodium EDTA and sodium citrate) present in some contrast media. This may have been a factor in causing electromechanical dissociation in cardiac muscle (SEDA-11, 412). The hypocalcemic effect of ionic contrast media can potentiate the effect of a calcium blocker such as verapamil (SEDA-8, 429) (SEDA-9, 410).

Non-ionic media cause fewer electrocardiographic changes than ionic media (SEDA-10, 424) (SEDA-11, 412). Non-ionic contrast media are almost sodium-free; they have little tendency to cause ventricular fibrillation or to depress cardiac contraction, and this small risk might (if in vitro animal studies are dependable) be further reduced by the addition of a very small amount of sodium (61). Following studies in dogs in which methylglucamine salts of diatrizoate or iotalamate produced only temporary T wave changes while sodium salts produced more marked changes with a fall in blood pressure and increase in coronary flow, the US manufacturers of a product containing sodium methylglucamine diatrizoate removed virtually all of its sodium content, but without announcing the change (62). Radiologists using the altered contrast medium noticed an unexpected increase in the incidence of ventricular fibrillation after coronary arteriography. Subsequent animal experiments confirmed that the new medium caused this effect, apparently by prolonging the time of depolarization. The addition of small quantities of sodium to the medium lessened this prolongation of the depolarization phase.

Prinzmetal angina with electrocardiographic changes has been seen 10 minutes after a dose of iodipamide (SEDA-2, 373). In another case an anaphylactoid reaction after left ventriculography was associated with electrocardiographic changes apparently due to coronary artery spasm (63).

In a comparison of the effects of ioxaglate (a low-osmolar ionic dimer) with iopamidol (a non-ionic monomer), iopamidol caused fewer electrocardiographic changes and a reduction in ventricular excitability compared with ioxaglate (64).

The electrocardiographic effects of different types of non-ionic low-osmolar contrast media have been investigated in 41 patients undergoing left ventricular angiography (65). There was transient prolongation of the QT interval in all of the patients. The effect did not cause important cardiac events and was less than 60 ms in most cases. The authors concluded that this effect was too brief to present any significant risk.

Left ventricular failure

Of 65 patients being investigated for intermittent claudication under general anesthesia, five developed pulmonary edema after retrograde aortic injection of sodium iotalamate (Conray 325 or 420). Three of the five had a history of myocardial disease and another had received 200 ml of Conray 420.

Although it is now widely acknowledged that low-osmolar non-ionic contrast media are better tolerated than high-osmolar ionic media, the choice of contrast agent does not affect the early results of percutaneous transluminal coronary angioplasty (66). However, the authors acknowledged that high-osmolar ionic agents carry higher risks of acute left ventricular failure. They retrospectively reviewed 401 patients who underwent percutaneous transluminal coronary angioplasty, 220 of whom received high-osmolar ionic media and 181 of whom received non-ionic contrast media. Acute left ventricular failure occurred more often in the high-osmolar group (1.4 versus 0%). There were no differences in the incidences of acute myocardial infarction (3.3% in each group) or urgent surgical intervention (0.5% with the high-osmolar agents and 0.6% with the low-osmolar non-ionic media). There were two cases of mild and transient central nervous system complications (loss of orientation and transient hemiparesis) with the high-osmolar contrast media. The authors concluded that in the majority of cases, the type of contrast medium used does not influence the early results of percutaneous transluminal coronary angioplasty in relation to its efficacy, the degree of revascularization, and residual narrowing. However, they acknowledged that the use of high-osmolar ionic media increases the risk of acute left ventricular failure after angioplasty. They attributed the finding that non-ionic contrast media increased the risk of abrupt vessel closure (4.5 versus 1.5%) to intravascular clotting. The suggestion that non-ionic agents are procoagulant is contentious, and there is no conclusive evidence to support this view (SEDA-22, 501).

Myocardial infarction

In spite of the safety of the non-ionic contrast media cardiac arrest can complicate the infusion of these agents.

- A 47-year-old man with chest pain and a myeloproliferative disorder had a CT scan of the abdomen with contrast enhancement (the type of contrast medium was not stated) (67). He had no significant past medical history or history of allergy. During a later CT scan of the abdomen infusion of 60 ml of the non-ionic monomer iohexol (iodine 300 mg/ml) caused a sudden cardiac arrest. Resuscitation was ineffective and post-mortem examination showed intramural acute and old organizing infarctions in the entire left ventricular wall.

Although the authors suggested that this event was an adverse effect of the contrast medium, it is possible that the cardiac arrest in this patient was secondary to an acute coronary event independent of the contrast agent.

Respiratory

Transitory changes in lung function can occur after bronchography due to retention of the contrast medium in the bronchi; normal diffusing capacity may not return for 3 days and it is better to avoid thoracic surgery during this period. When bronchography with propyliodone preparations is performed during fiberoptic bronchoscopy, there may be marked arterial oxygen desaturation (SEDA-15, 504).

Some contrast medium inevitably reaches the lungs after injection, and tracer studies in the early 1960s showed that some degree of pulmonary oil embolism occurred in every patient (68). Pulmonary function studies have shown abnormalities, in particular a reduction in pulmonary diffusing capacity and pulmonary capillary blood volume, even in the absence of clinical signs or symptoms (69). Most cases are symptomless, although there can be mild pyrexia, while X-rays show stippling or an arborization pattern. If hypotension, cyanosis, dyspnea, and pleuritic pain occur, infarction should be suspected. The risk that blockage of lung capillaries by oil will endanger the patient is naturally greater if pulmonary function is already compromised, for example by neoplastic or fibrotic disease, or by radiotherapy.

In some patients, this phase of mechanical obstruction is followed after some days or 3–4 weeks by a chemical reaction, presumably as the oil breaks down to irritant fatty acids, which cause exudation and hemorrhage. Interference with the production of lung surfactant can also occur and a marked intravascular cellular reaction has been described (70). The chemical irritative phase is marked by fever, cough with sputum (often blood) and a variable degree of respiratory distress; there may even be tachycardia and hypotension.

Non-cardiogenic pulmonary edema has been seen several times after contrast media in patients with a prior history of myocardial infarct (SEDA-16, 531); it can also be a component of anaphylactic shock. Non-cardiogenic pulmonary edema has been reported as a complication of intravenous injection of iomeprol (71).

- A 68-year-old man with chronic obstructive pulmonary disease underwent CT examination of the abdomen with intravenous infusion of iomeprol for suspected hepatocellular carcinoma and 2 hours later developed severe dyspnea. A chest X-ray showed bilateral diffuse shadowing of the lungs and the heart shadow was not enlarged. A diagnosis of non-cardiogenic pulmonary edema was made and he improved with glucocorticoids.

Contrast media can cause severe bronchospasm, particularly in patients with asthma (72). Subclinical bronchospasm can occur after bolus injections of ionic contrast medium; the incidence is lower with non-ionic media (SEDA-8, 427).

Life-threatening adult respiratory distress syndrome after intravascular radiographic contrast injection is rare. It has been successfully managed by extracorporeal membrane oxygenation (73).

- A 62-year-old man developed adult respiratory distress syndrome 5 minutes after receiving a low-osmolar ionic contrast medium (140 ml of ioxaglate 200) during coronary angiography. His respiratory rate was 35/minute, blood pressure 60/40 mmHg, pulse rate 125/minute, PaO_2 49 mmHg, main pulmonary artery pressure 21 mmHg, central venous pressure 9 mmHg, and pulmonary capillary pressure 10 mmHg. A chest X-ray showed pulmonary edema. Laboratory investigations, electrocardiography, echocardiography, and coronary angiography were normal. In view of life-threatening hypoxia, extracorporeal membrane oxygenation was given for 50 hours, and 2 weeks later he was discharged without pulmonary symptoms.

In one case adult respiratory distress syndrome was accompanied by disseminated intravascular coagulation (SEDA-16, 531).

- Respiratory arrest occurred after aspiration of water-soluble contrast material in a 12-year-old girl who had been injured in a traffic accident. Gastrografin diluted with tap water (540 ml) was given into the stomach via a nasogastric tube as part of CT-enhanced contrast examination of the abdomen. She also received 150 ml of non-ionic contrast media (iopamidol, iodine 300 mg/ml) intravenously, which was followed by vomiting attacks. She became irritable and had an acute fall in oxygen saturation and progressive respiratory distress, which required endotracheal intubation. The CT scan that was performed after she became stable showed contrast material in the lungs.

The authors concluded that aspiration of contrast material can be life-threatening and that administration of oral contrast media after trauma can increase the risk of aspiration of gastric contents (74).

Accidental inhalation of hypertonic contrast media during oral administration can cause fatal non-cardiogenic pulmonary edema (75).

In pediatric bronchography, segmental collapse occurs in half the cases, but is particularly common with the aqueous media. Collapse also seems to be more common when halothane and oxygen are used as the anesthetic agents (SEDA-15, 504); this has been attributed to the rapid absorption of the anesthetic gases combined with the partial bronchial block caused by the contrast medium.

Pulmonary fibrosis and microlithiasis has been reported as a late complication of lymphography with iodized oil, but a causative relation was uncertain (SEDA-12, 397).

Nervous system

Animal experiments with the ionic media have shown that these damage the blood–brain barrier, thereby creating a degree of risk to brain tissue when they are used in cerebral angiography, although they have often been used safely. Other evidence suggests that sodium increases the neurotoxicity of the contrast medium, possibly by increasing its diffusibility into the brain. Methylglucamine, on the other hand, reduces neurotoxicity. The addition of a small quantity of calcium also appears to reduce toxicity, at least when added to sodium. There are only marginal differences in neurotoxicity as measured in animal experiments between the diatrizoate, iotalamate, and metrizoate anions. Calcium methylglucamine metrizoate probably has the lowest neurotoxicity of the ionic media, followed closely by methylglucamine iotalamate. In clinical use, however, the calcium-containing formulations appear to cause a greater degree of discomfort because they cause a sensation of heat.

Although the non-ionic media produced less injury to the blood–brain barrier in animals, clinical studies have not generally shown them to be better tolerated when used for cerebral angiography, and it has been argued that these expensive media should now only be used where the blood–brain barrier is thought to be defective (76).

Transient neurological changes after myelography include asterixis, aphasia, and reversible visual defects. In one patient, asterixis and head bobbing were still present 3 months after myelography with metrizamide (SEDA-7, 453). An isolated case of persistent cervical myelopathy has also been reported after lumbar myelography with metrizamide.

A variety of other neurological complications have also been recorded. These include Guillain–Barré syndrome, auditory or visual disturbances, motor aphasia, sixth nerve palsy (SEDA-8, 431), mania, organic brain syndrome (SEDA-10, 425), confusional changes, and absence status. Absence status responds rapidly to intravenous diazepam (SEDA-14, 415).

Death has occurred following deterioration of neurological status. There has been a higher incidence of such complications in diabetics (SEDA-11, 415). Aspiration of 20–25 ml of cerebrospinal fluid after metrizamide myelography appears to reduce the incidence of neurological adverse effects (77).

All ionic contrast media are neurotoxic and they should not be injected into the subarachnoid space or intrathecally, and stern warnings against such use have been issued, for example by the American FDA (SEDA-18, 445). When they have accidentally been used, deaths have resulted (SEDA-18, 445) (78). Accidental misuse of diatrizoate for myelography, with fatal consequences, has been a serious problem (SEDA-22, 500). Lavage of the subarachnoid space with saline in such cases has been effective in reducing toxicity (SEDA-15, 504).

Accidental injection of diatrizoate into the subarachnoid space has occurred as a result of misplacement of the needle in arteriography, in discography, from inadvertent use in myelography, or during injection of a myelocele. Severe convulsions with extensor spasms occur and can result in death, particularly if the agent comes into contact with the brain; the onset of convulsions can be rapid, but they can also be delayed for several hours. Two patients developed renal insufficiency as an additional complication (SEDA-8, 1046).

The earliest water-soluble medium used for lumbar myelography or radiculography, sodium methiodal, had an irritant effect and required spinal anesthesia, which sometimes caused hypotension. Methylglucamine iotalamate was less irritant, while methylglucamine iocarmate had still lower neurotoxicity. However, even these two media could cause convulsions or muscle spasms if the contrast agent came into contact with the conus medullaris. For this reason the patient was postured with the head raised for several hours after the examination to prevent the contrast medium passing above the L-l vertebral level. Diazepam might also be given prophylactically. When convulsions did occur they could be severe, even resulting in fractures or dislocation of a hip. A convulsive pattern without actual convulsions has also been seen on the electroencephalogram in some patients.

Metrizamide was the first non-ionic contrast medium and became widely used for myelography and ventriculography. It was much less neurotoxic than iocarmate, although electroencephalographic changes lasting up to 3 days were found in some 16% of cases in early studies. Today, metrizamide is no longer used and has been succeeded by new generations of non-ionic monomers (iopamidol, iohexol) and dimers (iotrolan, iodixanol) which are well tolerated with low neurotoxicity (SEDA-22, 501). The need for intrathecal injection of contrast media in the developed world has dramatically fallen with the wide availability of MRI.

Visual evoked responses 20 hours after myelography can be delayed, with a correlation with the severity of headache after myelography; the delay in visual-evoked response is less marked with iopamidol than with metrizamide. It has been suggested that this technique may be useful in the assessment of myelographic contrast media toxicity (79).

In 439 myelographic procedures with metrizamide the most frequent adverse effect was headache, which could be differentiated into early-onset headache (related to hydrodynamic modifications in the spinal fluid following lumbar puncture) and late-onset headache (reflecting a specific metrizamide effect) (80). The frequency of late-onset headache was at least 27%, but altogether 46% of the patients had headache at one time or another. In this series, meningeal irritation was seen in 5%, sometimes in a severe form, mimicking a septic complication. There was spinal irritation in two cases and epileptic fits in one. An acute psychotic organic syndrome was common after cervical myelography with high doses of metrizamide. There was a severe anaphylactic reaction in one patient. The results of this study have generally been confirmed by others; seizures are clearly very rare with these non-ionic media, though they have occurred, even with iohexol (81), as have involuntary movements and facial twitching (82) and nystagmus (83). Meningeal irritation and paraplegia have both been seen with iohexol (SEDA-16, 536) and a case of aseptic meningitis with iotrolan (SEDA-16, 536).

In comparative trials, iopamidol and iohexol produced fewer adverse effects than metrizamide and they do not so far appear to have given rise to the psychosyndrome, but slight electroencephalographic changes can occur even with the newer media. Seizures and clonic jerks have been reported when relatively large doses of iopamidol have been used in myelography (SEDA-7, 455) (SEDA-13, 436).

Four cases of cauda equina syndrome have been described with methylglucamine iocarmate used for radiculography, although in two cases faulty technique was perhaps contributory.

Loss of consciousness can occur if there is hypotensive collapse; rarely there can be prolonged coma.

Convulsions, seen as part of an idiosyncratic reaction, tend to occur in patients with an existing tendency to epilepsy, or to occur as consequences of hypotensive collapse, cardiac arrest, or overdose.

Intraventricular metrizamide can cause perivascular mononuclear infiltration in the walls of the ventricles. This histological appearance may be mistaken for encephalitis if previous exposure to metrizamide is not considered (SEDA-7, 454).

A few cases of severe purulent meningeal reactions to iopamidol have been briefly described (84). In one exceptional report, a hemorrhagic meningeal reaction and thrombosis of the superior longitudinal sinus followed sacroradiculography with iopamidol (85). A case of transitory abducent nerve palsy has been reported after myelography with iopamidol (SED-12, 1183) (86).

Electroencephalographic changes

In 292 patients undergoing examinations with metrizamide, electroencephalography showed minor non-specific changes in 13% 24 hours after the injection. In 4% there were more marked abnormalities, such as spikes, spikes and waves, or paroxysms of bilateral synchronous high voltage rhythmic delta waves, apparently due to a direct toxic action of metrizamide on the cerebral cortex. They occurred shortly after the injection, and in the patients involved, a large amount of the contrast medium had flowed intracranially. Diazepam did not appear to have any significant effect on the electroencephalographic changes (SEDA-15, 504).

In a series of 308 cerebral angiograms in which metrizamide and meglumine metrizoate were compared on a randomized, double-blind basis, metrizamide caused a lower incidence of electroencephalographic changes, but the incidence of clinical complications showed no significant difference in the two groups, suggesting that the problems were mainly caused by other factors, such as thromboembolism; thromboembolism has indeed been suspected after cerebral angiography, even with iohexol (SEDA-13, 435).

Acute encephalopathy

Acute encephalopathy has been reported after intrathecal administration of non-ionic media (87).

- Six hours after 10 ml of iohexol (Omnipaque, iodine 240 mg/ml) had been injected into the left lateral ventricle during an operation on the thalamus of a 63-year-old man with Parkinson's disease, his level of alertness deteriorated and he became disorientated and confused. A CT scan of the head showed the surgical lesion and artefacts due to contrast medium, but no other abnormalities. After 24 hours, he became more alert, with coherent speech, but there was still mild disorientation. These symptoms resolved within the next 2 days.

According to the authors, this was the first case of encephalopathy after iohexol ventriculography, with the onset of symptoms several hours earlier than in myelography cases, probably owing to direct administration into the ventricular system. Awareness of this complication can be helpful in patient management after procedures in which iohexol is given intrathecally.

Transient contrast encephalopathy has been reported after carotid artery stenting (88).

- An 82-year-old right-handed man was given 50 ml of the ionic low-osmolar contrast agent ioxaglate 320 for carotid angiography. The next day his right internal carotid artery was stented and a total of 180 ml of ioxaglate was used. Aspirin, ticlopidine, and heparin 5000 units were given during the procedure. While he was still on the table he developed rapidly worsening confusion and a left hemiparesis. A CT scan without contrast 4 hours later showed marked cortical enhancement and cerebral edema in the distribution of the right anterior and middle cerebral arteries. He rapidly improved and had complete neurological recovery after 48 hours; 1 month later he was asymptomatic.

The cerebral contrast enhancement on the CT scan suggested disruption of the blood–brain barrier. This could have been due to the large volume of contrast medium used during the stenting procedure. This complication must be differentiated from massive cerebral infarction and hyperperfusion syndrome: the rapid radiological resolution and clinical recovery excluded cerebral infarction; hyperperfusion syndrome would have involved the carotid distribution exclusively, rather than both the ipsilateral carotid and posterior circulations. The authors recommended close follow-up of patients after such procedures. The safety of subsequent cerebral angiography in a patient with a history of such a reaction has not been studied extensively, and extreme caution must be exercised should the need for repeat angiography arise later.

Adhesive arachnoiditis

Methylglucamine iocarmate and methylglucamine iotalamate have both caused persistent arachnoiditis, leading to obliteration of nerve roots and constriction of the dural sac; operative treatment after myelography increases the risk of arachnoiditis, which is dose-dependent and varies with the contrast medium used (89,90).

Aseptic meningitis

Aseptic meningitis has been reported after iohexol myelography (91).

- A 74-year-old woman underwent lumbar myelography with iohexol (12 ml, iodine 240 mg/ml) for low back pain, having had iohexol myelography 2 years before with no complications, and 18 hours later developed headache, pyrexia (39°C), shivering, sweating, neck stiffness, nausea, and mild confusion. She had a leukocytosis (16.4×10^9/l) and a high C-reactive protein (145 micrograms/ml). There were leukocytes in the cerebral spinal fluid (11.5×10^9/l, 98% polymorphonuclear leukocytes), with protein 6.6 g/l and glucose 3 mmol/l, but a Gram stain was negative and no microorganisms were grown. She recovered spontaneously.

The authors suggested that this was a meningeal reaction to iohexol, since the interval between the injection of iohexol and the onset of symptoms was short, the symptoms resolved quickly, and there was no evidence of infection.

In the Netherlands, around 1979 there were several reports of aseptic meningitis after the use of metrizamide (SED-12, 1183) (92), and the complication has been reported since with iopamidol (93). Streptococcal meningitis has also been reported (94).

Convulsions

Up to 1979 it was estimated that some 360 000 cases of myelographies had been performed with metrizamide and that there had been 40 cases of epileptic attacks after its use (95); although they tended to relate to investigations in the upper part of the spine, three related to cases of lumbar myelography; a further case was later described. In some of these instances the use of other drugs may have played a role, including chlorpromazine, antihypertensive drugs, diphenhydramine, and pethidine (SED-12, 1182). The role of chlorpromazine in facilitating metrizamide-induced convulsions has been confirmed in animal studies; it was formerly recommended that phenothiazines should be withdrawn at least 48 hours before intrathecal use of metrizamide. Some, but by no means all, of the patients experiencing convulsions with metrizamide have a history of epilepsy.

- A 69-year-old man with idiopathic nasal bleeding underwent contrast-enhanced CT examination of the head with an intravenous non-ionic low-osmolar contrast medium (96). Convulsions and tremor developed 1 hour after the examination and lasted for 50 minutes.

There was an increased risk of seizures in patients with a previous history of seizures and in association with antineoplastic therapy (97). Patients with thrombotic thrombocytopenic purpura also appear to be at greater risk of seizures during contrast examination. Fatal status epilepticus can occur during CT (98). The non-ionic agent iopamidol appears to be less likely to cause seizures (76).

Cortical blindness

Cortical blindness after exposure to contrast agents has been reported to be as high as 1–4% in patients undergoing vertebral angiography, even with modern non-ionic low-osmolality contrast agents. It has been thought to be due to breakdown of the blood–brain barrier of the occipital cortex with subsequent direct neurotoxicity of the contrast medium. Repeated exposure to contrast agents did not cause recurrent episodes of cortical blindness. The outcome seems to be favorable, with return of vision within 24–48 hours and probably no increased risk on re-exposure. Occasionally cortical blindness can be caused by other procedures, for example coronary angiography (99).

- During coronary angiography, a 55-year-old man was given 280 ml of non-ionic contrast media iomeprol (iodine 350 mg/ml). Ten minutes later he became progressively confused and developed complete loss of vision. A CT scan of the head showed pronounced intracerebral enhancement of contrast media in the posterior third of the brain without evident relation to a vascular territory and a straight border towards normal brain tissue. Angiography of the right vertebral artery showed normal patency of the vertebrobasilar and venous systems, excluding thromboembolic events in the posterior cerebral circulation. Another CT scan of the head 1 day later showed clearing of the contrast medium. The neurological deficit resolved more slowly, but there was normal vision and minimal amnestic deficit after 5 days.

These findings were compatible with leakage of contrast medium through the blood–brain barrier, direct or indirect neurotoxicity of the contrast media being the most likely explanation for the neurological symptoms.

- A 64-year-old man developed transient cortical blindness after right subclavian, aortic, and femoral arteriography for ischemic pain in his left leg (100). Iopromide 250 ml (iodine 300 mg/ml) was used. The patient was hemodynamically stable throughout the procedure, at the end of which he had blurred vision and a slight headache. He could see shapes and colors but could not focus. There were no field defects. His pupillary reflexes and eye movements were normal. His vision improved 3 hours later and fully recovered after 48 hours.
- A 29-year-old man had a subarachnoid hemorrhage due to an arteriovenous malformation, which was embolized (101). During the procedure he suddenly lost consciousness, regained it 15 minutes later, but complained of total blindness. Cerebral angiography showed no arteriovenous malformation and no abnormality in the vertebrobasilar system. A CT scan of the head showed considerable contrast enhancement of the occipital lobes and 2 hours later the contrast had cleared. An MRI scan 12 hours later showed no evidence of infarction in the occipital lobes. Two days later his sight gradually returned and 7 days later he had completely recovered.

The authors of the second report thought that these adverse effects were probably due to the low-osmolar non-ionic contrast agent. Disruption of the blood–brain barrier is a factor in the pathophysiology of this complication.

- After difficult cardiac angiography in the supine position, an elderly man with arteriosclerosis developed transient cortical blindness (102). On CT scan there was contrast enhancement of the occipital lobes.

The best explanation of this observation is that a large amount of contrast medium entered the vertebral artery and passed upwards, passing a defective blood–brain barrier. Similar complications have been described in other patients, sometimes with amnesia, after cardiac catheterization and angiography (SEDA-18, 444).

- A 63-year-old woman with a left-sided spastic hemiparesis underwent cardiac and coronary angiography with a large volume (300 ml) of the non-ionic contrast medium iomeprole (iodine 350 mg/ml) (103). After the procedure her hemiparesis dramatically worsened, prompting emergency CT scanning of the head, which showed a marked hyperdensity in the right cerebral hemisphere. She recovered from this acute event, and follow-up CT of the brain showed complete resolution of the hyperdensity.

The right hemisphere was more affected in this case, because the contrast medium injected into the left ventricle or ascending aorta during angiography is likely to reach the right brachiocephalic artery first. The hyperdensity of the affected cerebral hemisphere seen on CT scanning was due to leakage of the iodinated contrast medium into the extracellular space, because of an increase in the permeability of the blood–brain barrier.

Paraplegia

Paraplegia can occur after angiography (104). In one series of five patients, four had tetraplegia (three being due to parathyroid arteriography and one after angiography of the posterior fossa), and in the fifth, paraplegia followed attempted renal angiography. When these neurological complications occur after angiography, the iodine content of the cerebrospinal fluid is raised.

There are various explanations, backed by animal studies, for this complication. When there is obstruction to the normal outflow of blood from the aorta, there is an increased risk that the contrast agent will be diverted into the spinal circulation. This effect can be aided by a gravitational factor if the examination is performed with the patient in the supine position.

The risk may not be the same for all contrast agents; the relation between the compound used and the neurotoxic effects is discussed below in connection with cerebral angiography.

Stroke

Cerebral effects can complicate thoracic aortography when excessive doses of concentrated agent are injected, particularly if the catheter is sited so that the major dose of contrast agent is directed into the cerebral circulation. In one case, 10 ml of sodium iotalamate 70% was injected into the carotid artery, being mistaken for methylglucamine iotalamate 60%; this was followed by an immediate convulsion, with loss of consciousness for 2 minutes. The patient at first appeared to have recovered completely, but hemiparesis followed and persisted for some 24 hours. Such changes are presumably due to cerebral edema after transient damage to the blood–brain barrier.

Cerebral oil embolism has been described in nine patients in one series of 3500 lymphograms (105) and in eight patients in another series of 16 501 investigations (106). All nine patients in the former series developed neurological signs, usually within 48 hours, reaching a peak in 4–7 days; the symptoms included motor dysfunction, paraplegia, and deep coma lasting for some weeks; three of the nine died. The electroencephalographic findings in these patients pointed to diffuse brain emboli. Evidence of retinal fat embolism can be useful in confirming the diagnosis and computed tomography can show collections of ethiodol in the brain. In the early phase after radiotherapy to the lungs, the vasculature is damaged, so that contrast agent is less effectively retained in the lungs. If lymphography is performed at this stage, there is an increased risk of cerebral embolism.

Sensory systems

Hearing impairment has been attributed to contrast agents.

- A 37-year-old man with recurrent attacks of low back pain underwent drip intravenous pyelography to exclude the possibility of stones of the urinary tract (8). Iohexol 300 was used, but the total volume was not documented. He had had drip intravenous pyelography for suspected urinary calculi 5 years before. A few hours after the procedure he suddenly had bilateral hearing loss and tinnitus in the right ear. He complained of dizziness and nausea but had no rotatory vertigo or skin rash. A pure-tone audiogram 2 days later showed complete right-sided and partial left-sided deafness. CT and MRI scans showed no abnormalities in the inner ear, internal auditory canal, or posterior fossa. He was given intravenous high-dose hydrocortisone sodium succinate, 10% dextran, and batroxobin, but there was no improvement in hearing. The dizziness and tinnitus in the right ear persisted, as did the deafness, for a further 2 months.

Hearing disturbances attributable to contrast agents are extremely rare. The hearing loss in this patient developed more than 1 hour after the injection of iohexol, without any evidence of other causes. The authors suggested that the hearing disturbance might have been attributable to cochlear impairment caused by a delayed allergic reaction or chemical toxicity of the contrast medium.

Psychological, psychiatric

To reduce the incidence of generalized reactions to contrast media in high-risk patients some authors have advocated the prophylactic administration of glucocorticoids (prednisolone 30 mg orally or methylprednisolone 32 mg orally, 12 and 2 hours before contrast injections). In one case an acute psychosis complicated glucocorticoid premedication to reduce the risk of contrast reactions (107).

- A 13-year-old girl with bipolar disorder and a history of adverse reactions to contrast media was given methylprednisolone (32 mg/day) and ranitidine (300 mg/day) before a CT scan of the head with intravenous contrast enhancement. One day after, she developed psychiatric symptoms, which were more severe than her initial symptoms, including extreme agitation and mental confusion. All medications were withdrawn and her symptoms resolved within 2 weeks.

The authors suggested that the recurrence of the manic symptoms could have been due to premedication with prednisolone. Exacerbation of manic symptoms after the use of glucocorticoids has been documented before, but never in a case of short-term premedication before contrast-enhanced radiographic examination. This report shows that even a short-term course of glucocorticoids can have significant adverse effects in patients with a history of mood disorders.

In 2500 cases of cervical myelography with metrizamide, there were transient mental reactions in 25, including 13 cases of confusion or disorientation, four of depression, two of hallucinations, two of psychosis, and one each of anxiety, drowsiness, dysphasia, and nightmares (108).

Of 18 German patients undergoing lumbar myelography with metrizamide, six had an organic psychosis, characterized by impaired memory and depression, but it was demonstrable only by psychometric tests and disappeared within 5 days (109). In four of the 18 patients there was hyporeflexia or areflexia and in three there were electroencephalographic changes; there was no correlation between these various types of effect.

Visual hallucinations are very rare adverse effects of contrast media, with isolated reports after vertebral angiography or myelography. The mechanism of this adverse reaction could be similar to that reported in transient cortical blindness after infusion of contrast agents. However, other possibilities include a toxic effect of contrast media on the optic nerve, transient impairment of cerebral blood flow, which could be mediated through the release of the potent vasoconstrictor endothelin, or the formation of microclots. Two cases of visual hallucinations after coronary angiography have been reported (110).

- A 70-year-old woman with a history of mastectomy developed syncope which lasted a few seconds. She had taken tamoxifen 10 mg bd for 10 years and had no history of allergic reactions. Doppler ultrasound showed aortic stenosis and coronary angiography was performed using 150 ml of iopromide (a non-ionic contrast medium, iodine 370 mg/ml). She had visual hallucinations (spiders on the wall, moving curtains) 30 minutes after the injection of iopromide. The symptoms resolved 72 hours later without any specific treatment. Neurological and psychiatric examinations were normal, as were brain MRI and Doppler ultrasound of the carotid and vertebral arteries.
- A 64-year-old man with a history of ischemic heart disease underwent coronary angiography with 150 ml of iopromide (iodine 370 mg/ml). One hour later he had visual hallucinations (moving objects, pictures of familiar persons), which resolved about 40 hours later without any treatment. He had taken the following drugs for a year: nifedipine 10 mg tds, metoprolol 50 mg bd, and aspirin 325 mg/day. His serum creatinine concentration was in the reference range and there was no history of allergies or previous exposure to contrast media.

Myelography with either iopamidol or metrizamide can cause transitory deterioration in memory as determined by psychological tests, but the effect is less with iopamidol (111).

Many of the psychiatric complications of cerebral angiography may be due to arterial trauma rather than to the toxic effect of the contrast agent. If the investigation is undertaken under general anesthesia, the use of a volatile anesthetic can in itself cause an increase in intracranial pressure and thereby constitute an aggravating factor (112). Focal electroencephalographic changes can occur on the side of the injection, and if these are prolonged they can be followed by evidence of neurological involvement. Transient global amnesia and confusional states have been reported after cerebral angiography, even with non-ionic media (SEDA-9, 410) (113).

Endocrine

Contrast agents contain very large amounts of iodine, though it is in a bound form. Liberation of iodine (114) from these agents can produce some inhibition of thyroid function in healthy subjects for up to 3 months, but can also increase hormonal synthesis in a thyroid adenoma, and cases of frank thyrotoxicosis have been attributed to these agents, the effect starting within a few days (115). Hypothyroidism has also been reported, particularly in neonates. Contrast medium-induced hyperthyroidism is rare and usually occurs in patients with autonomous thyroid function. Treatment is exclusively symptomatic. Prophylaxis with sodium perchlorate should be considered in cardiac patients with a goiter and a subnormal concentration of thyroid stimulating hormone (TSH) (SEDA-21, 478) (116). In premature babies and neonates thyroid complications can develop after intravascular administration of iodinated contrast media and great caution should be exercised during radiological examinations in infants (SEDA-20, 420).

Thyroid metabolism has been prospectively investigated in 102 patients undergoing diagnostic coronary angiography (117). Thyroid function tests (T3, rT3, T4, free T4, and TSH) and urinary iodine excretion were measured before and 3 weeks after diagnostic intra-arterial administration of iodinated contrast agents. Only euthyroid patients were included, in order to determine whether the administration of non-ionic iodine-containing contrast agents causes significant thyroid function changes in euthyroid patients and whether thyroid morphology is a prognostic factor for the risk of hyperthyroidism. Serum concentrations of thyroid autoantibodies (TPO-Ab, Tg-Ab, TSH-receptor-Ab) were measured. Thyroid ultrasound showed that 37 patients had normal thyroid glands. The gland was of normal size but nodular in 16 patients, there was a diffuse goiter in 15 patients, and a nodular goiter in 34 patients. In 25 patients Tg-Ab was positive and in 13 patients TPO-Ab was positive; TSH-receptor-Ab was not detected in any patient. T3 concentrations did not change significantly after the administration of iodine. T4 and free T4 concentrations underwent significantly different changes in the four groups. The amount of iodine given did not affect the changes in the serum concentrations of TSH, T3, T4, free T4, or rT3. Raised concentrations of urinary iodine correlated with the amount of contrast medium given. There were no cases of hyperthyroidism. The study showed that thyroid function was significantly altered after coronary angiography, independent of antibody status and the amount of contrast agent given, but dependent on thyroid morphology.

The effects of iopromide on thyroid function have been investigated in 20 pre-term infants with very low birth weights and 26 matched premature infants who did not receive contrast medium (118). The dose of iopromide (iodine 300 mg/ml) was 0.3–1.0 ml. Iopromide did not affect the concentrations of free thyroxine and thyroid stimulating hormone. This was attributed to the small amount of free iodide that iopromide contains (0.6 microgram/ml) compared with other contrast media, in which the free iodide concentration ranges from 1.8 micrograms/ml (iohexol) to 4 micrograms/ml (ioxaglate). Furthermore, hypothyroidism has previously been described after the injection of less than 1 ml of ioxaglate 320 in 13 premature infants of less than 34 weeks gestational age and in other children after the injection of iopamidol. The authors concluded that iopromide may be superior to other contrast media in protecting infants of very low birth weight from thyroid dysfunction. It is advisable to monitor thyroid function when contrast media are given to such infants.

- A 54-year-old man developed Graves' disease and hypoadrenalism secondary to adrenocorticotropin deficiency soon after a cranial CT scan with an iodine-containing contrast agent (119).

It was presumed that the iodine load (about 30 g) had precipitated thyrotoxicosis in this patient, who had antibodies to the thyrotropin receptor, which in turn precipitated collapse due to adrenal insufficiency.

In three women (aged 63, 72, and 75 years) with subclinical goiters, hyperthyroidism developed after the intravenous administration of iodinated contrast medium (120). There was a marked rise in the concentration of free T4. The hyperthyroidism improved spontaneously in all three.

In 51 sick neonates given two different non-ionic, iodine-containing contrast agents, metrizamide and iohexol, urinary iodine excretion was increased on day 5 after iodine exposure (121). In 17 term neonates given Amipaque, the median TSH concentration was normal after 5 days and 2 weeks, and there was only one case of transient hypothyrotropinemia; median concentrations of T3 and T4 were in the lower reference ranges. However, in 15 neonates given Omnipaque the median TSH was raised and T3 and T4 concentrations were very low. There was hypothyroidism in six of the eight preterm and one of the seven term neonates.

- Mild hypothyroidism with a goiter developed in a 15-year-old boy 6 weeks after lymphangiography with Lipiodol ultrafluid; the goiter disappeared after 3 months treatment with levothyroxine (SEDA-7, 454).

Metabolism

Iopanoic acid is as potent a uricosuric agent as probenecid and this effect might explain some renal complications; aspirin reduces the uricosuric effect but can also impair X-ray visualization because of competition at plasma protein-binding sites. Fluctuations of serum urate after oral cholecystography can interfere with diagnostic tests and even precipitate an attack of gout (122).

Electrolyte balance

Iodinated contrast media can cause increased release of potassium from blood cells and vascular endothelial cells, as has been investigated in vitro using blood, collected from 52 patients, mixed with iodinated contrast media for 30 minutes (123). The following contrast media were used: iopamidol (iodine 370 mg/ml), ioxaglate (iodine 320 mg/ml) and diatrizoate (iodine 370 mg/ml). Potassium release increased after exposure to the contrast media and the high-osmolar diatrizoate caused the greatest release, followed by iopamidol and then ioxaglate. The osmolality of contrast media may play an important role in the mechanism responsible for the release of potassium from blood cells. Chemotoxicity may also play a role. There are no data to suggest that the release of potassium is due to hemolysis, and it is most likely due to increased membrane permeability.

Mineral balance

Contrast agents can lower serum calcium and magnesium concentrations (124), which may be relevant to the occasional occurrence of tetany (SEDA-7, 452).

Hematologic

A single case of severe but reversible hypoplastic anemia has been attributed to sodium diatrizoate (125). Ionic contrast media have a disaggregating effect on erythrocytes, and hyperosmolar agents reduce their elasticity (SEDA-22, 501). When blood is diluted with 90% sodium diatrizoate in vitro, there is initially a reduction in erythrocyte diameter, due to the hypertonic environment, but as more contrast medium is added, the erythrocytes increase in diameter because of damage to the cell wall; this tallies with the fact that cases of hemolysis and hemoglobinuria have been reported with amidotrizoate (126).

Iodinated water-soluble contrast agents have traditionally been contraindicated in patients with sickle cell disease, because of possible shrinkage of erythrocytes secondary to the high osmolality of these agents, which can lead to impaired blood flow through the microcirculation and can precipitate or exacerbate a sickle cell crisis. The hematological and rheological effects in vitro of four contrast agents of different osmolalities (iodixanol 290 mmol/kg, ioxaglate 600 mmol/kg, iohexol 844 mmol/kg, and diatrizoate 1940 mmol/kg) have been compared (127). Blood was tested from 10 healthy and 10 sickle cell donors at drug concentrations of 0, 1, 10, and 30% w/v in an attempt to approximate the circulating concentrations of contrast medium that might occur during bolus injection. There were significant hematological effects in the blood of both the healthy and sickle cell donors: there was a concentration-related reduction in hematocrit and MCV and an increase in MCHC, all of which varied directly with the osmolality of the contrast medium (amidotrizoate > iohexol > ioxaglate > iodixanol). Only with amidotrizoate at concentrations of 10–30% was there marked echinocytosis. There was no significant increase in the number of irreversibly sickled cells in donors with hemoglobin S. The filterability of erythrocyte suspensions through capillary-sized pores was impaired in both healthy and sickle cell samples in direct proportion to the osmolality of the contrast medium. Filterability effects were greater with sickle cells than healthy erythrocytes. Iodixanol, which is iso-osmolar with blood, had little effect on erythrocyte volume and had no significant effect on the filterability of healthy or sickle cells. These results suggest that microcirculatory impairment after infusion of contrast agents can occur in sickle cell disease because of the unusual rheological sensitivity of HbSS erythrocytes and may be avoided by using low-osmolar or iso-osmolar contrast agents.

Acute thrombocytopenic purpura has been reported in three patients given contrast agents (SEDA-11, 413). Severe thrombocytopenia has rarely been reported after iopanoic acid (128), iocetamic acid (129), and sodium iopodate; in the last case there was evidence that the patient had developed platelet antibodies of the type associated with other drug-induced thrombocytopenias (130).

- Thrombocytopenia occurred 24 hours after 100 ml of iopamidol was given intravenously during cranial CT scanning to investigate a 9-month history of headache (131). The patient reported purpuric lesions on her legs, abdomen, and gingival bleeding within 24 hours of the scan, and examination of the peripheral blood at 48 hours confirmed severe thrombocytopenia. A bone marrow smear showed a prominent increase in megakaryocytes and dysmegakaryopoiesis. The bleeding time was longer than 15 minutes. Other laboratory values were within normal limits. Within 10 days, all the lesions disappeared spontaneously and the platelet count improved gradually and returned to normal within 2 months.

The pathogenesis of this complication is not understood but is most likely an immunological response to the contrast agent.

Clotting time is longer shortly after administration of ionic contrast agents (132). Non-ionic contrast agents do not have a similar anticoagulant action. In contrast, if blood is allowed to mix with a non-ionic medium in a syringe or catheter, thrombus formation can occur and this could be a cause of thromboembolism (SEDA-15, 502) (133). The non-ionic agents are not so much thrombogenic as less anticoagulant than their ionic predecessors (SEDA-19, 429). The risk of thromboembolism with ionic agents has been described in some contested studies as being 4–10 times higher (SEDA-17, 537) (SEDA-18, 444) (134). The non-ionic agents produce profound degranulation of platelets in vitro, but this is unrelated to thrombin generation (135). However, some prefer to heparinize when giving the non-ionic media. This issue is contentious, and although non-ionic agents are viewed as being less anticoagulant than ionic agents, they are not considered to be procoagulant (SEDA-22, 501). Adherence to a high standard of angiographic technique, with regular flushing of the catheter with isotonic saline is crucial to avoid thromboembolic complications during angiography.

The effects of contrast agents on leukocytes, platelets, and endothelium have been investigated in 19 subjects (mean age 63 years) undergoing angiography with the non-ionic contrast medium iohexol 350 (median volume 40–160 ml) for leg ischemia (136). Blood was obtained from the external iliac vein before and at several intervals after the injection of the contrast agent into the ipsilateral femoral artery. Markers of endothelial cell injury (von Willebrand factor), platelet activation (soluble P selectin), and leukocyte activation (neutrophil elastase and soluble L selectin) were measured in citrated plasma. Soluble intracellular adhesion molecule-1 and thromboxane B_2, which are non-specific markers of inflammation, were also measured. Compared with the sample before angiography, concentrations of soluble L selectin and soluble intracellular adhesion molecule-1 were reduced immediately after passage of the last bolus of contrast medium; 15 minutes later the concentrations returned to normal, but the concentration of von Willebrand factor had increased. After 30 minutes, only thromboxane B_2 concentrations were increased. On the next day both von Willebrand factor and soluble P selectin were increased. These data point to both early and late effects of contrast agents on markers of endothelial, platelet, and leukocyte function. The authors suggested that these adverse changes may increase the risk of coagulopathy and thrombosis after contrast examination and increase the risk of re-stenosis after angioplasty.

The hematological effects of ioxaglate (a low-osmolar ionic dimer) 105 (range 95–114) ml ($n = 15$) and iopromide (a low-osmolar non-ionic monomer) 102 (range 90–108) ml ($n = 16$) have been investigated in patients undergoing abdominal and femoral angiography (137). The aim was to investigate in vivo whether non-ionic contrast media are less anticoagulant or more prothrombotic than ionic agents. Activation of coagulation and platelets were found in almost 50% of patients before any contrast medium was given. Both iopromide and ioxaglate caused further increases in thrombin-antithrombin complex, prothrombin fragments 1 + 2, and beta-thromboglobulin; the degree of activation was similar with both agents. In contrast to the findings in in vitro studies, there were no significant differences between the effects of the non-ionic agent iopromide and the ionic agent ioxaglate. The results supported the notion that the catheterization procedure per se may represent a source of hemostatic activation and that ionic contrast agents have insufficient anticoagulant effect to prevent clotting activation being induced by the procedure. The study also yielded no support for the concept that non-ionic contrast media are less anticoagulant or more prothrombotic than ionic agents.

However, it has been suggested that anticoagulant effects are high with ionic media and low with non-ionic media (138). The authors also suggested that there is no direct activation of platelets with low-osmolar ionic and non-ionic dimeric contrast agents but a high degree of activation with non-ionic monomeric contrast media. They concluded that although the interaction between contrast media and coagulation has been widely studied in vitro and in vivo, this issue is contentious and further studies are required for better understanding.

Within a few hours after lymphography, the lymph nodes show dilatation of the marginal and intermediate sinuses and a giant-cell reaction, with diffuse reticulocytosis and sinus histiocytosis. Diffuse plasmacytosis and an increase in the eosinophil count can also occur. The response is maximal after 10–14 days, but the changes in the lymph nodes may not be eliminated for as long as 15 months (SED-12, 1184) (139).

The thrombotic complications after angioplasty have been investigated in patients with unstable angina (140). There was no significant difference in the incidence of thrombotic complications between patients who received the low-osmolar ionic dimer ioxaglate ($n = 103$) and those who received the non-ionic agent iopamidol ($n = 102$), although there was a non-significant trend towards more thrombus formation in the non-ionic group (21 of 129 patients) compared with the ionic group (15 of 141 patients). The two groups were well matched with respect to age, sex, class of unstable angina, and susceptibility factors. There was no significant difference between the two groups with respect to clinical outcome in the first 24 hours after percutaneous coronary angioplasty.

- Disseminated intravascular coagulation has been described in a 63-year-old man who received 50 ml of the non-ionic monomer iobitridol (iodine 300 mg/ml) for arteriography (141).

Mouth and teeth

Swelling of the parotid glands has been recognized as an occasional effect of contrast agents for very many years (142). It occurs particularly when there is renal insufficiency; the swelling usually occurs 2–4 days after the procedure and can last for several days, but evanescent salivary gland enlargement can also occur within a few minutes of injection and last for a number of hours. In one case the complication was associated with paralysis of the facial nerve, which largely subsided over the next 9 weeks.

Gastrointestinal

Nausea and vomiting can occur in reaction to contrast agents. Diarrhea is less common but has been repeatedly reported, sometimes with angioedema of the bowel (143).

Infarction of the bowel was formerly a very occasional complication of abdominal aortography and was due to injection of contrast medium into the mesenteric arteries. Most of these cases were due to the older media, such as acetrizoate; however, small bowel injury has occurred after injection of a concentrated bolus of sodium iotalamate (144). Ileus has been reported after mesenteric angiography in a patient with renal insufficiency (SED-12, 1177) (145).

Intra-arterial injection of lipiodol (iodized oil) has been used to enhance the accuracy of computed tomography in hepatic tumors. This can cause transient bowel ischemia with nausea, vomiting and diarrhea.

The use of Gastrografin for pre-operative mechanical bowel preparation has been investigated in 58 patients (aged 45–80 years) listed for elective colorectal operations (146). One group (30 patients, mean age 67 years) was given oral Gastrografin 200 ml and 3 liters of water for 2 days before the operation. The rest (28 patients, mean age 65 years) were given Ringer's solution 5–20 liters, warmed to body temperature, through a nasogastric tube; preparation was considered complete when the patient excreted clear fluid. All were given metronidazole and cefuroxime as antibiotic prophylaxis during the peri-operative period. There were no significant adverse effects in the Gastrografin group, apart from nausea in six patients. In the Ringer's solution group there was nausea in 15 patients and vomiting in eight. A clean colon was found at operation in 93% of patients in both groups. The authors concluded that Gastrografin is well tolerated and can be used successfully for mechanical bowel preparation before elective colorectal surgery.

The rectal administration of Gastrografin 400–1000 ml in patients with suspected diverticular disease before CT examination of the abdomen has been investigated in 308 patients (aged 19–97 years) (147). None of the CT scans showed extravasated contrast material in the peritoneal cavity as a sign of bowel perforation. No patient had sudden clinical deterioration after the examination. All tolerated the contrast medium well and there were no allergic reactions. High-quality diagnostic examinations were obtained in all patients.

Contrast agents caused release of vasoactive intestinal polypeptide in a patient with a vipoma of the pancreas and hepatic secondaries (SEDA-11, 411) (148).

The high-osmolar agents amidotrizoate and iotalamate were formerly recommended for oral use in preference to barium where there was a risk of perforation, but the osmotic effect of such material can lead to diarrhea and fluid loss, which can be dangerous in weak patients. Amidotrizoate, despite its cathartic action, can occasionally cause ileus when given postoperatively (149); it can also be precipitated as a solid mass in the stomach when gastric acidity is high, but also in an achlorhydric gastric stump following partial gastrectomy if there is stomal obstruction. On one occasion, when diatrizoate was used to fill the gastric balloon of a Sengstaken–Blakemore tube, hydrogen ions from the gastric content apparently penetrated the balloon, precipitated the contrast medium, and thus prevented the balloon's removal.

Low-osmolar media such as iohexol are now preferred for oral use; they can still cause some diarrhea, for example in 18 out of 40 cases in one series (SEDA-16, 529). Absorption can be increased if there is mucosal damage in the bowel, such as in Crohn's disease, resulting in delayed excretion but not apparently involving risk (SEDA-18, 441).

Amidotrizoate enemas are still sometimes used to treat meconium ileus or constipation, and it is important to give intravenous fluids so as to avoid dehydration. Hypomagnesemia can also occur (150). Osmotic effects lower in the gastrointestinal tract have even led to distention and cecal perforation (151). Stasis of amidotrizoate in dilated loops of bowel can cause inflammatory changes or necrosis (152,153).

Liver

Sulfobromphthalein retention is increased by sodium iopodate or iopanoic acid, probably by competition in the hepatic excretory pathway. The mechanism is not clear. Serum bilirubin concentration can rise, and there can be a slight increase in serum enzymes, persisting for a few days.

There have been several reports of hepatotoxicity of iodipamide, variously characterized by epigastric pain, nausea and vomiting, jaundice, pyrexia, and tenderness over the liver, with abnormal liver function tests. Biopsy has shown centrilobular necrosis (154). The incidence of abnormal liver function tests may be as high as 18% after a dose of 40 ml, and the quantity given should be as small as possible. Prior administration of glucocorticoids or sulfonylureas impairs hepatic excretion of ioglycamide. Both iodoxamate and iotroxate can affect liver function tests; in a small series of cases, the degree of intrahepatic cholestasis appeared to be relatively more marked after iodoxamate than after iotroxate (SED-12, 1168) (155).

- A 19-year-old woman without previous hepatic impairment developed abdominal pain and an acute rise in liver enzymes after an injection of iopromide (156). During intravenous infusion of iopromide she developed vomiting and hypotension, which resolved within a few hours. Repeat laboratory tests showed a rise in serum transaminases, which peaked on the second day and then rapidly fell. There was a slight prolongation of the prothrombin time and a moderate increase in total serum bilirubin. Serum gamma-glutamyl transpeptidase activity was normal. Ultrasonography of the liver and biliary tree was normal and serological markers for viral hepatitis were negative. Two weeks later, liver function tests were all in the normal range.

An acute rise in liver enzymes after intravascular iopromide is uncommon and has been previously reported only in some patients with concomitant hepatic impairment. In this case, the temporal association (rapid clinical onset and raised serum transaminases after the injection of iopromide) suggested that iopromide may have played a role in the occurrence of the hepatitis-like picture.

Biliary tract

Embolization of the cystic artery can cause acute acalculous cholecystitis (SEDA-15, 505).

Water-soluble contrast media are used to examine the pancreas and bile ducts during ERCP. Contrast media can affect the examination of bile for microlithiasis (157). Bile contaminated with contrast media during ERCP had pseudo-microlithiasis, mimicking calcium bilirubinate granules. This effect was observed with both the high-osmolar contrast medium sodium amidotrizoate and the low-osmolar medium iohexol. The authors concluded that bile collected during ERCP to be examined for microlithiasis should be collected without contamination by contrast agents. If this is not possible, pathologists should be aware that contrast media can cause pseudo-microlithiasis. Awareness of this effect may prevent unnecessary cholecystectomy.

Pancreas

Contrast agents can cause transitory enlargement of the pancreas (SEDA-11, 411). Oral and intravenous cholangiography have very rarely been reported to precipitate acute pancreatitis (158).

An experimental study has suggested that intravenous injection of contrast media can cause increased mortality associated with severe pancreatitis (SEDA-19, 425). There was little difference between ionic and non-ionic agents. The authors argue that contrast-enhanced CT should be avoided in patients with severe pancreatitis as it can exacerbate it.

Acute pancreatitis is a well-recognized complication of ERCP, and contrast media have been incriminated in its pathogenesis. It has been suggested that the use of low-osmolar non-ionic contrast media may minimize the risk. However, this has not been proven conclusively.

The iso-osmolar non-ionic dimer iotrolan and the low-osmolar ionic monomer iopromide (osmolarity about twice that of the blood) have been compared in 40 patients who underwent ERCP (159). They were randomized to receive either iopromide (iodine 300 mg/ml, 770 mosmol/kg, mean dose 15 ml) or iotrolan (iodine 300 mg/ml, 320 mosmol/kg, mean dose 12 ml). Pancreatitis after ERCP occurred in two patients given iopromide and in five given iotrolan. There were no significant differences between the groups in the time-course of changes in serum pancreatic enzyme activities, changes in acute-phase proteins, or the incidence of abdominal pain.

Experimental data suggest that high-osmolar ionic contrast media are more likely to cause chemical irritation of the pancreas, precipitating pancreatitis (159). However, clinical trials have not shown a clear advantage in using non-ionic media in ERCP. For example, in the above-mentioned study, iotrolan did not offer an advantage compared with iopromide (159). The authors suggested that overfilling of the pancreatic duct with contrast medium could be an important factor in the pathogenesis of ERCP-induced pancreatitis and that careful technique is important to avoid this complication.

Urinary tract

The kidney is the main route of elimination of water-soluble contrast agents. Ideally, the agents should be filtered without causing functional or structural changes in the kidney. Unfortunately, this is far from attainable and these agents cause altered renal function and structural changes in the renal tubules. These effects are usually of no clinical significance in patients with normal kidneys. However, in the presence of renal impairment, further significant deterioration in renal function can occur and can lead to significant morbidity and even mortality in some cases (4). Clinical experience has shown that non-ionic low-osmolar contrast media are less nephrotoxic than high-osmolar agents, particularly in patients with pre-existing renal impairment (SEDA-19, 428). However, renal tolerance of the different commercial formulations of non-ionic agents seems to be comparable.

Contrast medium-induced renal damage is associated with impaired renal function (an increase in serum creatinine by more than 25% or 44 μmol/l) within 3 days after the intravascular administration of a contrast medium in the absence of an alternative cause.

Presentation

A slight transitory increase in serum creatinine commonly occurs after the administration of contrast agents, and dysuria can occur. Acute renal insufficiency is uncommon with the agents currently in use, but some 100 fatalities were reported with bunamiodyl sodium. The mechanism is not clear; diffuse acute tubular necrosis, sometimes with crystals of calcium salts, has been found at biopsy or autopsy (160). A reduction in creatinine clearance within the reference range is common. The possibility that these agents might simply block the renal tubules has been advanced, but they are only present in the urine in small amounts in their non-conjugated, that is relatively insoluble, form. An effect on uric acid excretion might be involved. In any event, sufficient fluid should be given to ensure an adequate flow of urine.

The term "contrast nephrotoxicity" implies that impairment in renal function (an increase in serum creatinine by more than 25% or 44 μmol/l) has occurred within 3 days after the intravascular administration of contrast agents and the absence of an alternative cause (161). The increase in serum creatinine, which reflects a reduction in glomerular filtration rate, often peaks within 3–4 days after the administration of contrast agents. Mild proteinuria and oliguria can also occur. However, most patients with contrast nephrotoxicity tend to be non-oliguric, except those with pre-existing advanced chronic renal insufficiency. Heavy proteinuria is an unusual feature of contrast medium nephrotoxicity (162). Urinary enzymes are often increased after the administration of contrast agents. However, no relation has been established between a reduced glomerular filtration rate, a raised serum creatinine (the characteristic features of contrast nephrotoxicity), and the presence of enzymuria after the administration of contrast agents. It is therefore argued that the detection of urinary enzymes is of little importance to the clinical assessment and management of contrast medium nephrotoxicity (163). A persistent nephrogram on plain radiography or CT of the abdomen for 24–48 hours after the injection of a contrast agent has also been described as a feature of contrast nephrotoxicity

(162,164). This sign is now considered to be non-specific and can be observed in a number of cases without nephrotoxicity (165). However, the presence of this sign may discourage the administration of further doses of contrast agents (161). Fortunately, most episodes of contrast medium nephrotoxicity are self-limiting and resolve within 1–2 weeks. Permanent renal damage is rare and occurs only in a very few instances. However, contrast medium nephrotoxicity can increase the risk of severe non-renal complications and prolong hospital stay (4,161).

Contrast nephrotoxicity can be confused with the syndrome of atheroembolism that can occur after angiography. This condition is not caused by contrast agents, but results from trauma to atherosclerotic blood vessels, precipitating cholesterol microemboli. The clinical picture is characterized by acute renal insufficiency associated with distal digital infarction and skin mottling. Renal histology shows the pathognomonic microvascular cholesterol emboli (4).

Incidence

There are wide variations in the reported incidence of contrast nephrotoxicity because of differences in patient selection, the type of radiological procedure, and the definition of renal impairment. Contrast nephrotoxicity is relatively uncommon in people with normal renal function, in whom it is 0–10%. Pre-existing renal impairment increases the frequency, with a reported incidence of 12–27% in several prospective controlled studies. In some studies the incidence was as high as 50%, in spite of the use of low-osmolar contrast agents and adequate hydration. Dialysis may be required in some of these patients (SEDA-22, 502).

The causes of acute renal insufficiency have been surveyed in elderly patients (over 60 years) admitted to a hospital in India over 12 months (166). Of 4176 patients 59 (1.4%) developed acute renal insufficiency during hospitalization. Contrast medium injection was the culprit in 10 patients.

The incidence of contrast-induced renal damage has been investigated in 100 consecutive trauma patients (mean age 37 years) who underwent angiographic embolization (mean dose of contrast agent "non-ionic low osmolar" 248 ml) for bleeding in the abdomen or pelvis (167). None had diabetes or renal impairment before the injury (mean baseline serum creatinine 88 μmol/l). The serum creatinine increased by more than 25% of baseline in five patients, and returned to baseline within 5 days.

Comparative studies

The renal effects of iodixanol 40–100 ml and iohexol 42–102 ml have been compared in 116 patients undergoing renal and/or peripheral angiography (168). The two groups had the same baseline renal function and prevalence of diabetes. The serum creatinine rose by more than 10% in 15% of the patients given iodixanol and in 31% of the patients given iohexol and by more than 25% in 3.7% of the patients given iodixanol and in 10% of the patients given iohexol during the week after angiography. There was a correlation between the dose of contrast medium and the change in serum creatinine in both groups. These results suggest that iodixanol may be slightly less nephrotoxic than iohexol. However, previous reports have failed to show a significant difference between the non-ionic dimers and non-ionic monomers in relation to renal tolerance. The authors suggested that factors other than contrast media may have contributed to the rise in serum creatinine in some of their patients.

The renal effects of low-osmolar contrast agents (iopromide, ioversole, and ioxaglate) have been evaluated in 45 patients who underwent cardiac angiography (169). Iopromide (iodine 370 mg/ml, mean dose 1.9 g/kg) was used in 15 patients (mean age 62 years, mean serum creatinine 107 μmol/l, mean creatinine clearance 67 ml/minute), ioversole (iodine 320 mg/ml, mean dose 1.8 g/kg) in 15 patients (mean age 62 years, mean serum creatinine 103 μmol/l, mean creatinine clearance 71 ml/minute), and ioxaglate (iodine 320 mg/ml, mean dose 1.8 g/kg) in 15 patients (mean age 63 years, mean serum creatinine 100 μmol/l, mean creatinine clearance 71 ml/minute). All were normally hydrated and none had been examined with contrast agents in the months before the study or had been treated with nephrotoxic drugs. There were minor increases in serum creatinine 24 hours after ioversole (from 103 to 107 μmol/l) and ioxaglate (from 100 to 106 μmol/l) and at 48 hours after iopromide (from 107 to 115 μmol/l). Plasma concentrations of beta$_2$-microglobulin increased only with ioxaglate (from 1.9 to 2.0 micrograms/ml at 24 hours). There was a reduction in creatinine clearance from 71 to 55 ml/minute only with ioxaglate 6 hours after the administration, but it returned to baseline 24 hours later. There were no significant variations in creatinine clearance at 48 hours after angiography. There were increases in the activities of different tubular enzymes in the urine after angiography with all the contrast agents, but the changes were larger after ioxaglate. The tubular effects were maximum at 6–24 hours and returned to baseline within 72 hours after angiography. In summary, all three low-osmolar contrast agents caused reversible tubular damage, indicated by increased enzymuria, which was higher after ioxaglate. In addition, ioxaglate slightly impaired glomerular function. None of the observed changes in renal function were clinically relevant and they were not statistically significant. In summary, none of the three low-osmolar contrast agents caused significant changes in renal function. However, the authors suggested that ioxaglate is probably more nephrotoxic than non-ionic monomeric agents, and that other physicochemical properties beside osmolality play a role in nephrotoxicity due to contrast agents.

Placebo-controlled studies

The clinical and biological tolerance of iobitridol (Xenetix, a non-ionic medium, osmolality 915 mosmol/kg at an iodine concentration of 350 mg/ml) has been assessed in a placebo-controlled study in 21 patients with chronic renal insufficiency (glomerular filtration rate less than 60 ml/minute) (170). Serum creatinine and creatinine clearance remained stable 24 and 48 hours after the procedure. No patient had a nephrotoxic reaction or acute oliguria. Only one patient given iobitridol had an increase in serum creatinine of more than 15% from baseline; the serum creatinine normalized within 4 days of contrast administration. One patient given placebo had a similar increase in serum creatinine, which recovered within 48 hours. The author suggested that the use of non-ionic media such as iobitridol should result in a substantial reduction in the incidence of contrast nephropathy.

Susceptibility factors

There are several susceptibility factors for the development of contrast agent-induced renal damage, including pre-existing renal insufficiency, particularly if it is secondary to diabetes mellitus, dehydration, multiple repeat exposure to contrast media within a short period of time (72 hours), congestive heart failure, or concurrent administration of nephrotoxic drugs, such as non-steroidal anti-inflammatory drugs (171).

- A 45-year-old man with aggressive hypertension underwent abdominal aortography to assess the possibility of renal artery stenosis (172). His baseline renal function was reduced and the serum creatinine was 210 μmol/l. He received 1000 ml of saline solution intravenously as prophylaxis against contrast nephropathy. An unidentified high-osmolar contrast medium was injected into the abdominal aorta above the level of the renal arteries. There were atherosclerotic changes in the abdominal aorta and a discrete stenosis of left renal artery. Oliguria developed 24 hours later and the serum creatinine rose to 350 μmol/l. He was given isotonic saline (2 l/day) with 100 mg of furosemide. After 2 days the serum creatinine concentration fell to 190 μmol/l and his daily urine volume increased to 1.6 l/day.

The risk of contrast-induced acute renal insufficiency is particularly high in patients with diabetic nephropathy. Diabetes mellitus per se without renal impairment is not a susceptibility factor. The degree of renal insufficiency before the administration of contrast agents largely determines the severity of the nephrotoxicity. Old age (over 60 years), dehydration, and congestive cardiac failure are also risk factors. Multiple myeloma has been considered in the past as a risk factor for contrast nephrotoxicity. However, if dehydration is avoided, low-osmolar contrast agents rarely cause acute renal insufficiency in patients with myeloma. The concurrent use of nephrotoxic drugs, such as non-steroidal anti-inflammatory drugs (NSAIDs) and aminoglycosides, potentiates the nephrotoxic effects of contrast media. The importance of hypertension, hyperuricemia, or proteinuria per se as susceptibility factors for contrast nephrotoxicity is not clear (161,162). Large doses of contrast agents and multiple injections within 72 hours increase the risk of contrast nephrotoxicity. However, it has been reported that the intravenous administration of high doses of low-osmolality non-ionic iodinated contrast agent is safe in patients who have no pre-existing renal dysfunction or other underlying risk factors, even if doses as high as 800 ml are used (SEDA-21, 479). The route of administration is also important, and contrast agents are less nephrotoxic when administered intravenously than when given intra-arterially into the renal arteries or the aorta proximal to the origin of the renal blood vessels. The acute intrarenal concentration of contrast agent is much higher after intra-arterial injection than after intravenous administration. The type of contrast agent is also an important predisposing factor for contrast nephrotoxicity. High-osmolar contrast media are more nephrotoxic than low-osmolar contrast media, particularly in patients with pre-existing renal impairment. Whether the non-ionic dimers, which are iso-osmolar and highly hydrophilic, are less nephrotoxic is not yet clear. Clinical experience has so far shown no difference in the renal tolerance of non-ionic monomers and the iso-osmolar dimers (161).

The pharmacokinetics and safety of the low-osmolar non-ionic contrast agent iomeprole have been investigated in healthy volunteers and patients with various degrees of renal impairment (173). Six patients had normal renal function (glomerular filtration rate over 100 ml/minute, aged 22–58 years), six had mild renal impairment (glomerular filtration rate 51–75 ml/minute, aged 36–74 years), six had moderate renal insufficiency (glomerular filtration rate 26–50 ml/minute, aged 58–79 years), and four had severe renal impairment (glomerular filtration rate below 25 ml/minute; aged 34–73 years). Eight patients (aged 24–62 years) with end-stage renal disease who were receiving chronic hemodialysis were also studied. All received a single intravenous 50 ml bolus injection of iomeprole (iodine 400 mg/ml) and dialysis was performed about 2 hours later. The half-life of iomeprol increased progressively with increasing renal impairment. The half-life was 2 hours in patients with normal renal function, 4–6 hours in those with mild renal impairment, and 16–48 hours in those with severe renal impairment. Fecal excretion over 120 hours ranged from 1.6% of the total dose in healthy subjects to 7.2% in those with severe renal impairment. Thus, the pharmacokinetics of iomeprole are similar to those of other water-soluble contrast agents.

Hepatic cirrhosis is not a susceptibility factor, according to the results of a study in 72 patients with hepatic cirrhosis and 72 controls, who received 100–150 ml of low-osmolar contrast media intravenously for abdominal or chest CT scans (174). Serum creatinine was measured before and 48–72 hours after the administration of the contrast agent. The incidence of contrast nephrotoxicity was comparable in the two groups (two patients in the cirrhosis group and one control).

The type and dose of contrast media are important factors in the development of contrast nephrotoxicity. In patients with pre-existing renal impairment, low-osmolar non-ionic contrast agents are less nephrotoxic than high-osmolar agents and the iso-osmolar non-ionic dimers are less nephrotoxic than the low-osmolar non-ionic monomers. In 129 diabetic patients (mean age 71 years) with renal impairment (baseline serum creatinine 133–309 μmol/l) requiring angiographic examinations, the iso-osmolar dimer iodixanol ($n = 64$) was significantly less nephrotoxic than the low-osmolar non-ionic monomer iohexol ($n = 65$) (175). The incidence of contrast nephrotoxicity was 3% in the iodixanol group and 26% in the iohexol group. The authors concluded that iodixanol has low nephrotoxicity and should be the contrast agent of choice in patients at high risk of this complication.

Pathophysiology

The pathophysiology of contrast nephrotoxicity involves a reduction in renal perfusion caused by a direct effect of contrast agents on the kidney and toxic effects on the tubular cells. The mechanisms responsible for the reduction in renal perfusion involve tubular and vascular events. The endogenous vasoactive peptide endothelin seems to play an important role in mediating the nephrotoxic effects (SEDA-20, 421) (161).

Renal damage can occur in infants who receive large doses of ionic contrast agents during cardioangiography. Fatal cases after doses of more than 3 ml/kg had renal medullary necrosis or severe proximal tubular vacuolation. In other infants, such doses have produced microscopic hematuria. Renal necrosis has occurred in infants after intravenous administration of sodium diatrizoate 1–3 ml/kg, but these children were in very poor general condition. In high-risk adults, cardioangiography can similarly cause contrast nephropathy (SEDA-15, 501).

In abdominal aortography, the contrast agent reaching the renal parenchyma is relatively undiluted, so that factors of concentration and volume are more important, particularly if a bolus of high concentration is accidentally injected directly into the renal artery. In the early days of abdominal aortography, renal damage was a significant hazard, mainly because the agents then in use were relatively toxic, but at high doses or high concentrations the agents now used can also cause renal damage. In 400 patients undergoing angiography with high doses of an ionic contrast agent, the overall incidence of acute renal dysfunction was 11%, but in patients with pre-existing renal disease the incidence was 42%. Injections close to the renal arteries are more likely to cause renal damage than a similar dose of contrast agent injected intravenously for digital vascular imaging (SEDA-9, 408). In a patient with renal artery stenosis an intra-aortic injection of 30 ml of 50% methylglucamine diatrizoate at the level of the renal arteries resulted in oliguria with pyrexia within a few hours, and the urine output only gradually recovered over about 2 months (176). Diabetes was a predisposing factor in another case (SED-12, 1177) (177). In two other cases, renal insufficiency was followed by nephrogenic diabetes insipidus and nephrotic syndrome (SED-8, 1042) (178).

Contrast media, particularly high-osmolar agents, can cause a significant natriuresis and diuresis. In 42 patients who underwent cardiac angiography, the fractional excretion of sodium, the urinary excretion of the renal natriuretic peptide urodilatin, and the plasma concentration of atrial natriuretic peptide were measured before and after intravascular diatrizoate (an ionic high-osmolar contrast agent) 55 ml, or the non-ionic agent iopamidol 200 ml (179). None of the patients had diabetic nephropathy or multiple myeloma. Diuretics, angiotensin converting enzyme inhibitors, and non-steroidal anti-inflammatory drugs were withheld for at least 12 hours before the examination, and 11 patients received a mean of 600 ml of isotonic saline intravenously before and during angiography, because of mild chronic renal insufficiency. The other 31 received no volume expansion. Both groups received a similar volume of radiocontrast agent. After angiography the plasma concentration of atrial natriuretic peptide and the urinary excretion of urodilatin both increased. Urinary urodilatin excretion correlated with an increase in the fractional excretion of sodium. There was no correlation between the serum concentration of atrial natriuretic peptide and urinary sodium excretion. This study suggests that the intravascular administration of contrast agents causes a natriuresis associated with the urinary excretion of urodilatin. This is consistent with the hypothesis that urodilatin may contribute to sodium excretion after radiocontrast administration in a paracrine manner.

Transient proteinuria is common after aortography and selective nephroangiography, because of an increase in glomerular permeability. Ioxaglate, iopamidol, and iohexol cause only negligible proteinuria (SEDA-8, 428) (SEDA-11, 413).

Enzymuria has been reported after the intravascular administration of high-osmolar or low-osmolar contrast media (180). The study suggested that the brush-border enzyme gamma-glutamyl transpeptidase is a better marker for tubular toxicity due to contrast media than alanine aminopeptidase. However, no relation has been established between a reduction in glomerular filtration rate, a rise in serum creatinine (the characteristic features of contrast nephrotoxicity), and the presence of enzymuria. It has been argued that the detection of urinary enzymes is of little importance to the clinical assessment and management of contrast medium nephrotoxicity (161).

In patients who have received iodinated contrast media, urinary beta$_2$-microglobulin, albumin, epidermal growth factor, and gamma-glutamyl transpeptidase, *N*-acetyl-beta-D-glucosaminidase, and serum angiotensin-converting enzyme (ACE) activities are sensitive markers for the early detection of subclinical contrast medium-induced nephrotoxicity (181). At 24 hours after injection of contrast agents in 16 patients (aged 18–62 years, nine men), serum ACE and urinary beta$_2$-microglobulin, albumin, and enzymes were significantly raised. At 48 hours, serum creatinine concentrations increased significantly and urinary excretion of albumin remained significantly increased, but urinary enzyme excretion began to recover. Urinary excretion of epidermal growth factor was significantly reduced, due to tubular injury; healthy tubular cells release this factor into the urine and it is not filtered at the glomeruli. The observation that urinary albumin excretion continued to increase after the urinary enzymes started to recover suggests that the albuminuria induced by contrast media is probably due to glomerular and not tubular dysfunction. The mechanism of the rise in serum ACE activity is not known, but it may be due to damage to the vascular endothelial cells of glomeruli, ACE release from the brush borders of the epithelial cells of the proximal tubules, or an increase in vascular permeability and leakage of the enzyme into the blood.

Acute reduction in renal perfusion is considered important in the pathophysiology of contrast agent-induced nephrotoxicity. Color-coded duplex sonography has been used in assessing intrarenal vascular resistance in 10 patients (mean age 51 years) after intravenous injection of 100 ml of the low-osmolar contrast medium iopamidol (iodine 300 mg/ml) (182). The resistive index was measured at 1-minute intervals over 10 minutes after injection in each patient. There was a statistically significant rise in resistive index at 2, 3, 4, and 5 minutes after injection, mean values 0.74, 0.75, 0.72, and 0.75

respectively. The resistive index then fell progressively to baseline values (mean 0.70) within 10 minutes. The authors concluded that color-coded duplex sonography is a simple method for checking changes in renal flow resistance after intravascular contrast agents. They suggested that arterial Doppler flow measurement is ideal for investigating the pathophysiological mechanism of contrast agent-induced nephrotoxicity.

Prevention

Prevention of contrast nephropathy rests largely on the exclusion of high-risk cases, such as very ill patients with diabetic renal insufficiency, severe cardiovascular disease with reduced renal blood flow, jaundice, pre-existing uremia, and multiple myeloma. When the investigation is nevertheless needed in these conditions, the lowest possible dose of a low-osmolar non-ionic contrast medium should be used in patients at high risk of this complication. High-osmolar contrast media and large doses should be avoided. In addition, intravenous hydration with saline (1 ml/kg /hour for 4–6 hours before contrast injection to be continued for 12 hours afterwards) should be given. The concomitant use of other potentially nephrotoxic agents should be avoided. Finally, since the small amounts of contrast agent that remain in the body after a radiographic examination can potentiate renal damage resulting from subsequent events, there should be a delay of at least 12 hours after the examination before undertaking any surgery that could adversely effect the kidney, for example, procedures requiring temporary renal clamping or percutaneous balloon dilatation of the renal artery. A similar delay is advised between cerebral angiography and renal harvesting for transplantation. If renal glomerular filtration is reduced by 50% or more, a delay of 24 hours or more may be advisable after aortofemoral angiography (SEDA-15, 502).

Saline

Whether half-strength or isotonic saline should be used has been investigated in 809 patients who received half-strength saline and 811 patients who received isotonic saline (183). The two groups were matched in relation to baseline characteristics, and the mean serum creatinine before contrast injection was 80 μmol/l. All underwent coronary angioplasty using the low-osmolar non-ionic contrast medium iopromide (mean volume 234 ml). The incidence of contrast nephrotoxicity in those who received isotonic saline was 0.7% and in those who received half-isotonic saline it was 2%. The authors concluded that isotonic saline is superior to half-strength solution in reducing the incidence of contrast media nephrotoxicity.

Hemodialysis

Although hemodialysis is effective in removing contrast media from the body, its ability to prevent contrast nephrotoxicity has been disappointing. Hemodialysis after contrast administration in patients with pre-existing renal impairment does not prevent contrast nephropathy (SEDA-22, 502) because of the very rapid onset of renal damage (SEDA-21, 481) (SEDA-22, 501), since the effect of contrast media on the kidney after intravascular administration is almost instant and hemodialysis is usually offered at best 30–60 minutes after the procedure, which is too late to prevent the effects of contrast media on the kidney.

In patients with pre-existing renal impairment, hemodialysis did not influence the incidence or outcome of contrast-induced nephropathy, in spite of eliminating contrast agents effectively from the circulation. The same group has now confirmed their previous observation in a bigger study in 30 patients with pre-existing renal impairment (184). Hemodialysis did not influence the incidence or outcome of contrast-induced nephropathy, in spite of effective elimination of contrast medium from the circulation. The failure of hemodialysis to protect against the development of contrast nephropathy is due to the very rapid onset of renal injury after the administration of contrast medium.

The use of hemodialysis immediately after intravascular administration of contrast agents to prevent the development of nephrotoxicity in patients with renal impairment has been investigated in 15 patients with a mean serum creatinine of 234 μmol/l before contrast injection (185). The patients were randomized to receive either conservative treatment or hemodialysis for 2–3 hours, starting as early as possible (mean 106 minutes) after administration of the contrast agent. The increase in serum creatinine on days 2 and 3 after contrast injection was higher in the dialysed group. The incidence of nephrotoxicity, defined as an increase in serum creatinine by more than 44 μmol/l within 48 hours after administration of the contrast agent, was significantly higher in the dialysed group (43 versus 13%). The authors concluded that hemodialysis performed within 2 hours after contrast injection did not prevent the development of nephrotoxicity in patients with reduced renal function; indeed, it seems to have made things worse.

The use of prophylactic hemodialysis, in most cases starting more than 20 minutes after injection of a contrast agent, has been investigated in 113 patients with renal insufficiency (serum creatinine concentration over 200 μmol/l) (186). Hemodialysis did not reduce the incidence of contrast nephrotoxicity. This failure could have been related to the rapid onset of renal injury after the administration of the contrast agent.

The Contrast Media Safety Committee of the European Society of Urogenital Radiology (ESUR) has produced useful guidelines on dialysis and the intravascular use of contrast media (Table 4) and has reviewed the literature on this subject (187). In addition, they have produced guidelines on the prevention of contrast medium-induced renal damage (Table 5) following a consensus of experts in this field and of members and fellows of the society (188).

Acetylcysteine

The antioxidant *N*-acetylcysteine has also been recommended to reduce the risk of contrast nephrotoxicity. *N*-acetylcysteine 600 mg bd for 2 days, starting the day before the examination, in addition to hydration, reduced the incidence of contrast nephrotoxicity in 41 patients (189). The incidence of contrast nephrotoxicity was 2%

Table 4 European Society of Urogenital Radiology (ESUR) simple guidelines on dialysis and contrast media administration (188)

Patients on dialysis	Recommendations
Hemodialysis (all contrast media can be removed by hemodialysis)	Avoid osmotic and fluid overload Correlation of the time of contrast media injection with the hemodialysis session is unnecessary Extra hemodialysis session for removal of contrast media is unnecessary
Continuous ambulatory peritoneal dialysis (CAPD) (all contrast media can be removed by peritoneal dialysis)	X-ray examinations To protect residual renal function, refer to ESUR guidelines to avoid contrast medium-induced renal damage Hydration should be considered only after careful evaluation of fluid balance state of the patient Hemodialysis is unnecessary MRI scans To protect residual renal function, use doses under 0.3 mmol/kg of gadolinium-based contrast agents
Patients with severely reduced renal function	Refer to ESUR guidelines to avoid contrast medium-induced renal damage (hydration, use small doses of low-osmolar contrast media) Hemodialysis is unnecessary In MRI avoid doses over 0.3 mmol/kg of gadolinium-based contrast agents

Table 5 European Society of Urogenital Radiology (ESUR) simple guidelines to avoid Contrast Medium Nephrotoxicity (227)

Definition	Contrast medium nephrotoxicity is a condition in which an impairment in renal function (an increase in serum creatinine by more than 25% or 44 μmol/l) occurs within 3 days after the intravascular administration of a contrast medium in the absence of an alternative cause
Susceptibility factors	Raised serum creatinine concentration, particularly secondary to diabetic nephropathy Dehydration Congestive heart failure Age over 70 years Concurrent administration of nephrotoxic drugs, for example NSAIDs
In patients with susceptibility factors	*Do* Make sure that the patient is well-hydrated; give at least 100 ml/hour orally (for example soft drinks) or intravenously (isotonic saline) depending on the clinical situation, starting from 4 hours before to 24 hours after contrast administration; in hot climates increase the fluid volume Use low-osmolar or iso-osmolar contrast media Stop administration of nephrotoxic drugs for at least 24 hours Consider alternative imaging techniques that do not require the administration of iodinated contrast media *Do not* Give high-osmolar contrast media Administer large doses of contrast media Administer mannitol or diuretics, particularly loop-diuretics Perform multiple studies with contrast media within a short space of time

in patients who received acetylcysteine (baseline serum creatinine 220 μmol/l) following intravenous injection of 75 ml of low-osmolar non-ionic contrast media, and 21% in controls (baseline serum creatinine 211 μmol/l). However, the dose of contrast medium used was rather small and the patients did not have advanced renal impairment before contrast injection.

A study from Germany has shown that the antioxidant acetylcysteine plus intravenous saline 0.45% prevented the reduction in renal function induced by contrast agents (190). The authors prospectively studied 83 patients with chronic renal impairment (creatinine clearance under 50 ml/minute). The patients took oral acetylcysteine 600 mg bd for 1 day before and 1 day after the contrast medium. Saline 0.45% was given intravenously at a rate of 1 ml/kg/hour for 12 hours before and 12 hours after 75 ml of iopromide (iodine 300 mg/ml) intravenously. All the patients were encouraged to drink if they were thirsty. A matched control group received placebo and saline. The mean serum creatinine in the control group (42 patients, mean age 65 years) rose from a mean of 212–226 μmol/l 48 hours after contrast injection. In those given acetylcysteine (41 patients, mean age 66 years) the serum creatinine was 220 μmol/l before contrast injection and 186 μmol/l 48 hours after. One patient given acetylcysteine and nine controls developed contrast-induced nephrotoxicity. This suggests that the prophylactic oral administration of the antioxidant acetylcysteine in patients who are adequately hydrated with saline prevents contrast-induced nephrotoxicity in patients with chronic renal insufficiency. The main limitation of this study was the relatively small dose of intravenous contrast medium used (75 ml). It is important to determine whether acetylcysteine plus saline would still offer the same protection if higher doses of contrast media were used or if the agent was given intra-arterially.

Calcium channel blockers

In addition to using a small dose of low-osmolar non-ionic contrast medium and offering hydration, some authors have recommended the use of calcium channel blockers in patients at high risk of contrast nephrotoxicity. However, the effectiveness of this class of drugs in preventing contrast nephrotoxicity has not been consistently proven, particularly in patients with pre-existing advanced renal disease (191). Furthermore, some studies have suggested that the prophylactic administration of renal vasodilators, such as dopamine or calcium channel blockers, could have a deleterious effect, particularly in patients with diabetic nephropathy (SEDA-18, 444) (161). There is no conclusive evidence that these drugs are effective, particularly in patients with diabetic nephropathy who are at high risk of this complication (SEDA-19, 428).

Dopamine receptor agonists

In a study from the USA, dopamine was effective in preventing further deterioration in renal function in patients with a raised serum creatinine undergoing angiography for lower limb ischemia (192). Dopamine (2.5 mg/kg) was given to 28 patients beginning 1 hour before injection of contrast medium (Omnipaque 300, mean volume about 140 ml) and continuing for a total of 12 hours. Patients in the control group received an equal volume of isotonic saline. Serum creatinine was measured daily for 4 days after arteriography. Dopamine reduced the incidence of contrast nephrotoxicity (defined as an increase in the baseline serum creatinine concentration over 44 μmol/l) from 44 to 18%. Previous studies have not shown any protective effect of dopamine against contrast-induced nephropathy, in spite of marked increase in renal blood flow shown in a study of patients undergoing cardiac catheterization (161).

A report from Italy has suggested that intravenous saline 0.4% before and after administration of the contrast medium, an infusion of dopamine 3 micrograms/kg/minute for 24 hours after the contrast medium, intravenous furosemide 80 mg 30 minutes before the contrast medium, or intravenous mannitol (20%) 250 ml 1 hour before and 1 hour after the contrast medium each prevented the reduction in renal function caused by the non-ionic agents iobitridol, ioversol, or iodixanol (193). However, the protocol of the study was not described, and previous studies have shown that dopamine, furosemide, and mannitol do not offer good protection against contrast media-induced nephrotoxicity. On the other hand, volume expansion with intravenous saline has been found to offer some protection (190).

Fenoldopam, a selective dopamine D_1 receptor agonist, has also been advocated to reduce the risk of contrast nephrotoxicity. It is a renal vasodilator and increases glomerular infiltration rate. The authors of a review of studies that used fenoldopam to prevent contrast nephrotoxicity concluded that it offers good protection (194). In another study, the incidence of contrast nephrotoxicity was 4.7% in patients who received intravenous fenoldopam 0.1 micrograms/kg/minute starting 15–20 minutes before contrast injection and continued for 6 hours after and 19% in controls (195). However, fenoldopam has not been consistent in offering good protection against contrast nephrotoxicity, it has to be given by intravenous infusion, and it requires careful monitoring of blood pressure and dosage adjustment if hypotension develops.

Endothelin receptor antagonists

Although endothelin is considered to be an important mediator of the renal effects of contrast media, a report from the USA has shown that prophylactic administration of a non-selective endothelin receptor antagonist not only did not protect against contrast nephrotoxicity but exacerbated it (196). In this study, 158 patients with chronic renal insufficiency (mean serum creatinine 242 μmol/l) undergoing cardiac angiography were randomized to receive either the non-selective endothelin antagonist SB290670 (mean age 65 years, 51 men, 26 women) or placebo (mean age 67 years, 59 men, 22 women). The mean doses of contrast medium were 104 ml in the SB290670 group and 122 ml in the placebo group. Only low-osmolar radiographic contrast media were used. The dose of SB290670 was 100 micrograms/kg over 10 minutes followed by an infusion of 1 microgram/kg/minute starting 30–150 minutes before administration of contrast medium and continuing for 12 hours after. All the patients received intravenous hydration with saline 0.45% (1 ml/kg/hour) beginning 2–12 hours before contrast medium and continuing for at least 12 hours after. The mean increase in serum creatinine 48 hours after angiography was higher with SB290670 than placebo (64 versus 34 μmol/l). The incidence of radiocontrast nephrotoxicity was significantly higher with SB290670 than placebo (56 versus 29%). The authors concluded that a non-selective endothelin receptor antagonist may increase the incidence of contrast media nephrotoxicity and they questioned the role of endothelin in mediating the renal effects of contrast media. However, there were flaws in the design of this study. First, the endothelin receptor antagonist was administered only for a maximum of 12 hours after contrast examination—a longer period (2–3 days) should have been considered, since the reduction in renal function after contrast examination peaks at 48–78 hours, and in previous studies a single dose of nitrendipine 20 mg did not prevent contrast nephrotoxicity, whereas 20 mg/day for 3 days offered good protection. Secondly, a non-selective endothelin receptor antagonist is probably not suitable for the prevention of contrast nephrotoxicity. Blocking endothelin B receptors does not offer an advantage, since these receptors mediate renal vasodilatation and they also act as clearance receptors for endothelin. B receptor blockade could have caused the raised plasma endothelin concentrations that were observed in the treated group and may explain why the non-selective endothelin antagonist exacerbated contrast medium nephropathy. A selective endothelin A receptor antagonist should be studied before a role for this class of drugs in preventing contrast nephrotoxicity is excluded.

Theophylline

Theophylline, a non-selective adenosine receptor antagonist, has also been recommended, since adenosine has been suggested to be an important mediator of contrast-induced nephrotoxicity. Patients undergoing coronary angiography with the high-osmolar contrast medium diatrizoate (iodine 370 mg/ml) were randomized to receive either theophylline (200 mg bd orally 24 hours before and for 48 hours after coronary angiography, $n = 35$, mean age 54 years, mean dose of contrast medium 78 ml) or placebo ($n = 35$, mean age 52 years, mean dose of contrast medium 80 ml) (197). The glomerular filtration rate at 48 hours was reduced by 36% (from a mean of 85 ml/minute to a mean of 67 ml/minute) in the placebo group and by 9% in the theophylline group. Contrast nephrotoxicity, defined as a fall in glomerular filtration rate by 25% or more from baseline at 48 hours developed in 11 patients in the control group and only in one patient in the theophylline group. The authors concluded that nephrotoxicity induced by high-osmolar contrast media can be reduced by prophylactic administration of theophylline.

The protective effect of theophylline against contrast media nephrotoxicity has also been shown in another study (198). Intravenous theophylline 100 mg 30 minutes before intravascular administration of 100 ml of low-osmolar contrast medium offered good protection against contrast nephrotoxicity in patients with chronic renal insufficiency (mean serum creatinine 183 μmol/l). The incidence of contrast nephrotoxicity was 4% in the theophylline group and 16% in the placebo group (base line serum creatinine 110 μmol/l). The authors concluded that theophylline offers good protection against contrast nephrotoxicity in patients with pre-existing renal impairment. However, the dose of contrast medium was relatively small (100 ml) and the pre-existing renal impairment was not advanced. The consistency of theophylline in offering good protection against contrast nephrotoxicity has not been confirmed at higher doses of contrast media and in patients with more advanced renal disease.

Comparative studies

The protective effects of intravenous hydration alone (0.45% isotonic saline, 1 ml/kg/hour for 12 hours before and 12 hours after contrast administration), fenoldopam (0.1 microgram/kg/minute for 4 hours before and 4 hours after the procedure), and acetylcysteine (600 mg bd 24 for hours before and 24 hours after the procedure) have been compared in preventing contrast nephrotoxicity after intravascular administration of low-osmolar non-ionic contrast medium (199). The incidence of nephrotoxicity was 15% in the hydration group, 16% in the fenoldopam group, and 18% in the acetylcysteine group. All the groups were comparable and baseline creatinine clearance was about 60 ml/minute in all the patients who received a similar dose of the contrast medium (1.5 ml/kg). The authors concluded that fenoldopam and acetylcysteine do not offer extra protection against contrast nephrotoxicity over hydration alone.

Skin

The incidence of skin reactions to drugs has been analysed from spontaneous reports in Italy (200). Antibiotics most commonly caused skin reactions, followed by NSAIDs, analgesics, and radiocontrast agents, which were responsible for 2.7% of the reactions (71 cases); these included nine cases of exanthemas and 36 cases of urticaria.

Fixed drug eruption caused by non-ionic contrast media is rare (SEDA-22, 502), but has been attributed to the non-ionic contrast medium iomeprol (Iomerone, Bracco) (201).

- A 67-year-old Japanese woman developed multiple pea-sized erythematous plaques on the trunk and extremities 4 days after receiving 100 ml of iomeprol intravenously for a CT scan. She was treated with oral betamethasone 1.5 mg/day and glutathione 300 mg/day for 3 days. She then used topical betamethasone valerate ointment for a month until the erythematous plaques completely disappeared, leaving pigmentation. Six months later she was erroneously given 100 ml of iomeprol intravenously during a CT scan and the next morning developed erythematous plaques mixed with vesicles at the same sites as before. Biopsy showed histological changes compatible with a fixed drug eruption. In addition, both patch testing and intradermal testing were positive to iomeprol.

This report shows that non-ionic contrast media can cause multiple fixed eruptions and that repeated administration of the causative agent can be associated with a more severe eruption.

Rarely typical iododerma, sometimes with other skin and systemic complications, can occur (202) and causes a papulopustular eruption. Vegetating iododerma, in which pustules and vesicles coalesce to form large vegetating masses that later ulcerate, is very rare and its pathogenesis is unclear. A cell-mediated immune reaction, an inflammatory mechanism, and an idiosyncratic reaction in patients with other underlying diseases have been suggested. Iododerma occurs more often in patients with renal insufficiency, because of impaired clearance of contrast media. Oral or topical glucocorticoids have been of some benefit in treating this condition. Vegetating iododerma with a fatal outcome has been reported (203).

- A 65-year-old woman with a history of allergy to penicillin and abnormal renal function had cardiac angiography and a week later became breathless and slightly febrile and developed pustulovesicular lesions on the face, elbows, and legs. The lesions on the face coalesced into vegetating masses. Cultures from the skin lesions did not yield bacteria, fungi, or mycobacteria. Histological examination of the vegetating mass showed an inflammatory exophytic lesion with an ulcerated surface and an inflammatory infiltrate consisting mainly of neutrophils and eosinophils in the dermis. The lesions responded to 1:1000 copper sulfate solution. However, she continued to deteriorate despite hemodialysis and died 6 days later.

In this patient, renal insufficiency contributed to the development of iododerma and her death was due to poor cardiorespiratory function.

Delayed skin rashes have been noted in 5% of patients undergoing urography. Allergic-like skin reactions to intravascular contrast media can develop 24–96 hours after administration (204).

- A 73-year-old woman underwent CT scanning with contrast enhancement (250 ml of intravenous iopentol, a non-ionic contrast medium, iodine 300 mg/ml) for staging a malignant melanoma. Four days later she developed progressive pruritus beginning on the back and neck. On the sixth day she had a disseminated pruriginous papular partially confluent exanthema involving the trunk, neck, and proximal extremities. The eruption became generalized while she was receiving local corticosteroids and oral clemastine. Remission of the eruption was achieved with intravenous prednisolone 64 mg and dimethindene maleate 12 mg. Patch and intracutaneous tests to iopentol, but not to other contrast media, evoked a red indurated skin reaction after 48 and 72 hours. Histology and immunocytochemistry of the skin test site to iopentol showed an infiltrate consisting mainly of CD45RO+ and CD4+ lymphocytes together with eosinophils.

This reaction shared the features of a delayed hypersensitivity reaction (exanthematous rash, positive patch test) and of a late phase reaction (CD4+ lymphocytic infiltrate together with eosinophils). The authors emphasized the importance of skin testing in the diagnosis of delayed skin reactions to contrast media.

Other cases of delayed skin reactions have been reported.

- A 64-year-old woman with a history of an exanthematous skin eruption to an antibiotic and allopurinol had had a previous adverse reaction after angiography with radiographic contrast media. Her symptoms had included shivering and a generalized pruritic exanthema. Then, 30 minutes after intravenous angiography with iopromide (a non-ionic contrast medium), she developed shivering and dyspnea immediately followed by loss of consciousness; 3 hours later a generalized pruritic maculopapular rash developed.
- A 63-year-old woman with glomerulonephritis underwent angiography. She had a history of an immediate adverse reaction to lidocaine and of dyspnea, wheeze, and paresthesia of the fingers to repeated infusion of contrast media. Several hours after the last procedure she developed a generalized pruriginous maculopapular rash.
- A 60-year-old man underwent coronary angiography with iopamidol 200 ml. One day later he developed infiltrated erythema of the face with a generalized maculopapular rash. The skin symptoms receded within 1 week after treatment with a corticosteroid ointment. Coronary angiography with iopamidol was repeated 3 years later and again within 1 day a maculopapular rash developed and regressed within a few days with intravenous dimethindene and prednisolone-21-hydrogen succinate.
- A 54-year-old woman and a 68-year-old man developed rashes 24 hours after intravascular injection of iohexol (a non-ionic monomer) (205). The woman developed widespread pruritic erythema and eyelid edema. The man developed a maculopapular rash involving the trunk and legs. Both patients were treated with antihistamines, which resulted in complete recovery within 1 week. The man had slight desquamation of the affected area after his rash resolved. Patch tests were positive to iohexol in both patients. The man also had a positive patch test to iodixanol and the woman was positive to the non-ionic monomer ioversol.

Intracutaneous and patch tests were performed in the first two patients (206) with a series of ionic and non-ionic contrast media in concentrations of 1% according to international guidelines. In the first patient there were late positive intracutaneous and patch tests after 24–48 hours only to some of the tested contrast agents. In the second patient intracutaneous and patch tests showed late reactions to nearly the same contrast media. More than 20 patients with only immediate anaphylactoid reactions to contrast media gave negative results to these tests. The authors concluded that positive skin tests suggest an immunological basis for late reactions to contrast media. In the third case (207) patch and prick skin tests were performed using several iodinated contrast media. Intravenous provocation tests were also performed with several water-soluble contrast media using 5 ml in each case at strengths of 1:1000, 1:100, 1:10, and undiluted. Positive skin tests were observed with iopamidol, and the intravenous provocation test caused infiltrated erythema of the face and generalized maculopapular rashes. Skin biopsies showed heavy lymphohistiocytic infiltration at the site of positive skin tests. The authors concluded that the rashes represented delayed allergy to iopamidol.

Delayed skin reactions after contrast media have the features of true delayed hypersensitivity reactions, including positive skin tests (SEDA-24, 523). A generalized macular rash 24 hours after injection of ioversol with positive skin tests has been reported (208).

- A 61-year-old man received ioversol during a CT examination and 1 day later developed a generalized macular rash, which lasted for 2 weeks. Prick, intradermal, and patch tests with different types of non-ionic contrast media showed a delayed hypersensitivity reaction to ioversol, which lasted for 7 days.

Urticarial or erythematous rashes can occur and persist for a few days. Rarely acute vasculitis, Stevens–Johnson syndrome, and bullous lichen planus have been reported (SEDA-11, 411) (SEDA-14, 422).

- A 33-year-old man had three contrast-enhanced CT scans with iohexol over about 2 weeks, and developed a disseminated erythematous skin rash. Because drug allergy was suspected, all drugs were withdrawn (209). Because of a persistent fever a fourth CT scan was performed with iohexol, and 2 hours later he developed malaise, pruritic erythema, hypotension, and cutaneous bullae affecting 50% of his body surface and his oral mucosa. He was treated for toxic epidermal necrolysis and his skin healed without scarring or altered pigmentation. Skin patch tests, prick tests, intradermal tests, and intravenous and oral single-blind challenges with the antibiotics he had received were negative. However, a patch test with iohexol (iodine 300 mg/ml) was positive at 48 hours: erythema and multiple small flaking blisters appeared in the patch area. Identical patch tests in healthy controls were negative.

Other rarities reported sporadically (but all in more than one case) include the Koebner phenomenon (210), fixed drug eruptions (for example with iotalamate (211)), and delayed reactions of various types. Reports of severe drug eruptions have become more frequent since the introduction of the non-ionic contrast media, but this may simply be due to the fact that in recent years there has been greater awareness of such reactions (SEDA-16, 538) (SEDA-19, 427) (SEDA-22, 502).

Iocetamic acid seems more likely than other agents to cause skin reactions. Persistent urticaria has been seen in cases where iophendylate was used in myelography and the residue remained in situ (SED-12, 1180) (SEDA-16, 536).

Exacerbation of a lupus-like illness after injection of iodinated contrast agents has been reported (SEDA-9, 411) (SEDA-19, 427). All iodinated contrast agents should be used with caution in patients with systemic lupus erythematosus and perhaps in other types of vasculitis.

Reticulated purpura has been reported after the use of diatrizoate meglumine, a high-osmolar water-soluble contrast agent, for hysterosalpingography (212).

- Within 48 hours of a hysterosalpingogram using diatrizoate meglumine, a 34-year-old woman developed a burning sensation in her left leg, 4 days later developed tenderness and redness on the left posterior thigh and calf, and 4 days after that mottling of the skin of the thigh. Two weeks later she had marked tenderness and purpuric macules in a reticulated pattern on both legs. A skin biopsy showed changes suggestive of erythema multiforme. There was no evidence of vasculitis. The skin lesions persisted unchanged for about 1 week, after which they resolved without treatment.

This clinical picture of reticulated purpura with the formulation of a few bullae has not been previously reported after injection of contrast agents. The histological changes supported the diagnosis of a drug reaction. Although some of the histological findings are seen in erythema multiforme the patient's clinical presentation did not support that diagnosis.

The skin can be involved in allergic reactions after lymphography. Dermatitis has also been described some days after lymphography and apparently due to extravasation of the iodized oil into the tissues (SED-12, 1184) (213). Since lymphography requires an incision, wound infections can occur and rarely lymphangitis.

In 17 of 53 cases with obstructive lymphedema there was an increase in limb volume after lymphangiography with Lipiodol ultrafluid (iodinated poppy seed oil), and 10 cases had features resembling lymphangitis. In one patient there was an allergic reaction, with rapid development of edema and an increase in limb volume by 2 liters. Whereas contrast medium virtually disappears from normal lymphatics within 8 hours, in cases of obstructive lymphedema Lipiodol remains in the lymphatics for several days and it appears to cause a low grade chemical inflammation with obliteration of the lymphatics (SEDA-7, 454).

- A woman with an inoperable carcinoma of the cervix developed reticulohistiocytosis with arthritis and skin papules after lymphography with Lipiodol ultrafluid (214). Two later examinations with diatrizoate caused exacerbation of the disease within 24 hours. The condition receded spontaneously after 12 months, and subsequent examinations with metrizamide and iodamide were symptom-free.

Lymphatic obstruction is also an important factor in the etiology of oil embolism during lymphography causing shunting via distal lymphovenous communications.

Musculoskeletal

A transitory myopathy has been reported after iopamidol (215).

Immunologic

French workers investigating the causes of severe reactions to iodinated contrast agents suggested that any patient who has had a severe anaphylactoid or anaphylactic reaction after the injection of a contrast agent should undergo immunological assessment (216). The diagnosis of drug anaphylaxis is usually based on the history, proof of mediator release, and the presence of drug-specific IgE antibodies or positive skin tests. In five patients with severe anaphylactoid reactions after the intravascular injection of an iodinated contrast agent, the clinical symptoms, biology, and skin tests were consistent with anaphylaxis. The authors also reported that no premedication has proved effective in preventing subsequent allergic reactions to contrast agents.

In one study iodinated contrast agents were among the top 10 drugs responsible for anaphylaxis (161 cases due to contrast media out of 1338 reports of anaphylaxis) (217). Dextran was the most common cause of anaphylaxis (418 cases). The overall death rate was significantly higher in men than in women and increased with age. The report also suggested that since the introduction of low molecular weight dextran 1 the incidence of severe anaphylaxis to dextran has fallen markedly and that radiographic contrast agents may now be the most common agents causing anaphylaxis. Most of the anaphylactic reactions and all the fatal cases were due to ionic agents.

Patients allergic to additives, such as parabens in sodium iopodate, can react to them, for example with rash (218).

Hypersensitivity reactions seem to be less common after arteriography than after urography, perhaps because the agent does not pass directly through the lungs, although the data are limited. There were mild allergic reactions in six of 167 patients who underwent arteriography with iodamide (SED-12, 1175) (219). Two severe delayed generalized cutaneous reactions with blistering occurred after lumbar aortography with iopamidol and iohexol (SED-12, 1175) (220).

Three cases of mild allergic-like reactions to oral water-soluble iodinated contrast media during CT examinations of the abdomen have been documented (221). Two patients received Gastrografin and the third received the same agents under the brand name Gastroview. The main reaction was a skin rash that resolved within 2 days. The author advised that clinicians and radiologists should be aware of the potential for adverse reactions to oral iodinated contrast agents. In another case, a severe systemic allergic reaction occurred in a patient who was given oral iohexol (222). In a patient with known allergy to iodinated contrast media it would be prudent to consider barium suspension in preference to an iodinated agent to outline the bowel.

Allergic or even anaphylactic reactions can occur after lymphography, either to the contrast agent or to the dye; in hypersensitive patients, prior use of glucocorticoids and antihistamines may fail to prevent a severe reaction (223).

Non-IgE-mediated anaphylactic (anaphylactoid) reactions

A life-threatening anaphylactoid reaction occurred in a child after intravenous administration of a non-ionic contrast medium (ioversol) (224).

- A 3-year-old girl was investigated for hypertension and a renal arteriogram was performed. Her blood pressure before the study was 125/60 mmHg. She received 30 ml of ioversol (iodine 320 mg/ml). Within 30 seconds she developed tachycardia (200/minute) and hypotension (60/20 mmHg). She developed diffuse urticaria over her entire body and there was wheezing on auscultation. Cardiopulmonary resuscitation was begun and she received a saline infusion and adrenaline 1:1000 subcutaneously, 0.01 ml/kg, intravenous diphenhydramine 1 mg/kg, and intravenous hydrocortisone 5 mg/kg. She responded rapidly. Surprisingly, the authors thought that the contrast medium had not caused this response, and the patient was subsequently given a second injection of ioversol 320 in a dose of 1 ml/kg. Within 60 seconds she again became tachycardic and hypotensive and urticaria reappeared over the whole body with wheezing. Similar treatment was offered and she responded rapidly.

The authors claimed that this was the first case report of anaphylactoid shock after the administration of ioversol in a child.

A fatal anaphylactoid reaction to an intravenous non-ionic contrast medium occurred during a CT scan (225). The authors highlighted the value of measuring serum tryptase in the diagnosis of anaphylactoid reactions.

- An 81-year-old man underwent CT scanning of the head with intravenous contrast enhancement (100 ml of the non-ionic contrast medium iopamidol). After the injection he complained of sweating and nausea and had a cardiorespiratory arrest. Immediate resuscitation and intravenous dexamethasone and adrenaline were not successful. Mast cell tryptase activity in a sample taken 4 hours after death was high. At autopsy, the coronary and pulmonary arteries were patent. The right heart chambers were moderately enlarged. The lungs were hyperemic and edematous and there was obstructive edema of the larynx.

This patient had all the features of anaphylactoid reactions, which include pulmonary and laryngeal edema and a massive rise in serum tryptase. The half-life of tryptase is about 2 hours. Moderately raised post-mortem tryptase activity in the absence of anaphylaxis has been described. Therefore, only very high serum tryptase activity, as seen in this case, should be regarded as specific for fatal anaphylactoid reactions.

Graft-versus-host disease

Three cases of cutaneous graft-versus-host disease triggered by contrast agents have been reported (226).

- A 49-year-old man with acute myeloid leukemia underwent allogeneic bone marrow transplantation from his brother. Pre-existing pulmonary aspergillosis was treated with intravenous amphotericin. ACT scan of the chest and abdomen 120 ml of the non-ionic dimer iodixanol was performed and 6 hours after the injection he developed generalized erythema with a pruritic painful skin rash. Skin biopsies showed changes typical of chronic graft-versus-host disease. He received prednisolone 50 mg orally and the rash resolved within a few weeks.
- A 30-year-old woman with acute myeloid leukemia received an allogeneic bone marrow transplant from her brother. A CT scan of the abdomen was performed a few weeks after transplantation using 150 ml of iodixanol. Two days later she developed acute cutaneous graft-versus-host disease, which was treated with intravenous methylprednisolone 1 g/day for 4 days. Four months later, another CT was performed with 150 ml of iodixanol and 2 hours later she developed a generalized maculopapular rash over the whole body, which was diagnosed as grade-2 graft-versus-host disease. Intravenous methylprednisolone 1 g and clemastine 2 mg did not control the rash, which worsened. She was given daclizumab 50 mg/day for 2 days, prednisolone 100 mg/day, and mycophenolate mofetil 2 g/day. The rash resolved completely within 10 weeks.
- A 38-year-old man with acute myeloid leukemia underwent allogeneic bone marrow transplantation from his brother. He received iopromide 120 ml during CT scanning of the chest 15 months after the transplantation and 6 hours later developed generalized erythroderma, which was treated with oral prednisolone 50 mg. The lesion persisted and cholestatic jaundice developed. Graft-versus-host disease of the skin and liver was diagnosed. The patient still required immunosuppressive therapy and prednisolone 18 months after the event.

The authors suggested that the skin manifestations had been due to graft-versus-host disease triggered by the contrast medium and not a type-IV immunological reaction. Skin biopsy in one of the patients showed typical features of graft-versus-host disease. In addition, the reactions in these patients lasted for longer than one would expect in simple delayed reactions with skin manifestations, which usually resolve within 7–10 days.

Prevention

Prophylactic use of immunosuppression has been described to prevent delayed hypersensitivity reactions to contrast media (227).

- A 19-year-old man developed delayed hypersensitivity skin reactions to iopamidol (a low-osmolar contrast medium) after cerebral angiography for an arteriovenous malformation. Three months later he required embolization of the malformation. He was given prophylactic betamethasone (4 mg/day) for 2 days before the procedure in which iopamidol was used again. Three days after the embolization he developed a generalized maculopapular rash with severe itching. The rash resolved completely after intramuscular chlorphenamine 10 mg bd for 10 days and oral prednisone 25 mg bd. Skin tests confirmed a delayed hypersensitivity reaction to iopamidol and other types of contrast media. One month later he required further embolization and underwent immunosuppression with oral ciclosporin 100 mg bd and intramuscular methylprednisolone 40 mg/day for 1 week before and 2 weeks after the embolization. The contrast medium iobitridol, which gave negative results in skin tests, was used. The patient tolerated the procedure and did not develop further reactions.

Infection risk
Malarial relapse followed administration of iodipamide in two cases (228).

Body temperature

Several patients have developed hyperthermia after receiving metrizamide (SEDA-10, 425). A fatal case of malignant hyperthermia occurred after 100 ml of diatrizoate (229).

Death

There has been a review of 449 fatal reactions to ionic media (12). Deaths occurred in all age groups, but the incidence peaked in the 50–70 year age group; in this older group, cardiovascular collapse, cardiac arrest, and pulmonary edema were the most common features, but pulmonary edema appeared to be the commonest autopsy finding in all age groups (230). Of 53 deaths due to urography or computed tomography; 35 were of cardiac origin and eight were attributed to pulmonary edema. The presenting features in eight cases were nausea and vomiting, while seven patients developed shock or hypotension.

A fatal reaction has been reported in a case of Waldenström's IgM paraproteinemia (231). Ioglycamide produced fatal gel precipitation of the plasma in a case of Waldenström's IgM monoclonal paraproteinemia (232).

Long-Term Effects

Mutagenicity

An increased frequency of chromosomal aberrations and sister chromatid exchanges has been found in lymphocytes up to 1 week after intravenous urography; diatrizoate produced more changes than ioxaglate (SEDA-19, 430) (233). Earlier it was reported that the incidence of chromosomal aberrations in the lymphocytes of seven infants who underwent angiocardiography was higher than expected. Whether this means that contrast media produce significant cytogenetic damage is not at all clear.

Tumorigenicity

Some have suggested that the passage of contrast agents through malignant lymph nodes may facilitate metastases; one relevant case relates to Hodgkin's disease (234) and another to melanoma (235). There is also some animal evidence of this. However, it has generally been considered that lymphography is unlikely to be a significant factor in malignant dissemination and that its diagnostic value in planning treatment far outweighs any theoretical risk. Computed tomography and magnetic resonance imaging have now largely replaced lymphography for the demonstration of malignant lymph nodes.

Second-Generation Effects

Fetotoxicity

The main adverse effect of iodine-containing contrast agents after amniofetography is transient hypothyroidism, which has often been reported (236–246).

Iophenoxic acid, now obsolete, passes the placental barrier and can alter thyroid function in mothers and fetuses (247). In one case, a child was born with congenital hypothyroidism 5 years after the mother had undergone cholecystography (248); in a similar case the mother had been given iophenoxic acid 8 years before pregnancy (SED-12, 1167) (249).

Lactation

Contrast agents are excreted into breast milk, and they should not be used in breastfeeding women (SEDA-6, 404).

Susceptibility Factors

Genetic factors

Racial differences could be a factor in the high incidence of delayed skin reactions to contrast media in Japan, as 43% of Japanese are deficient in acetaldehyde dehydrogenase. This deficiency results in the accumulation of acetaldehyde, which potentiates the ability of contrast agents (especially dimers), to bridge proteins, which is a probable causative factor in many of their adverse effects (11).

In 1798 Indian patients the prevalence of adverse reactions to high-osmolar ionic iodinated contrast media was 21% (mild 19%, moderate 1.3%, and severe 0.3%) and there was only one death. The incidence of adverse effects was significantly higher in patients with risk factors, such as a history of previous contrast reactions (46%), bronchial asthma (69%), and diabetes mellitus (60%), compared with patients with no risk factors (21%). The authors tried to throw some light on the relation between race and incidence of contrast reactions. They showed that the incidence of mild reactions in the Indian patients (19%) was significantly higher than reported in white patients (5–15%) but that there was no difference in the incidence of moderate or severe reactions between the two populations (250).

The incidence of contrast reactions amongst patients of Indian origin in the UK was significantly higher than in the endogenous white population, with an eight-fold increase in severe reactions (251). There was also a significant increase in the incidence of reactions amongst patients of Mediterranean origin, but to a lesser degree.

There is no clear explanation for racial differences in the incidences of contrast agent reactions.

Age

Neonates are particularly sensitive to the effects of iodine, and transient hypothyroidism has often been reported, particularly in pre-term infants (237,252,253). The low glomerular filtration rate in infants can also result in delayed excretion of contrast agents.

The efficacy and safety of iodixanol has been documented in children. Iodixanol was well tolerated without any important adverse events in 25 children under 4-years-old undergoing excretory urography (254).

The use of low-osmolar contrast media in gastrointestinal imaging has been investigated in children under 16 years. One group received the iso-osmolar dimer iodixanol (74 patients, mean age 5.8 years, range 0–15, mean volume of contrast medium 87 ml) and the other group received the low-osmolar non-ionic monomer iohexol (78 patients, mean age 6.4 years, range 0–15, mean volume of contrast medium 93 ml) (255). There was a lower frequency of adverse events with iodixanol than with iohexol. Diarrhea developed in 16% of the patients given iodixanol and in 36% of those given iohexol.

The safety of the iso-osmolar dimer iotrolan in imaging the upper gastrointestinal tract has been investigated in neonates and young children (81 patients, age range 2 days to 14 years), 21 of whom were under 1 month old (256). The dose of contrast medium was 15–30 ml. There were no significant adverse effects and the authors concluded that iotrolan is a safe contrast agent for imaging the gastrointestinal tract in children.

Renal disease

In patients receiving hemodialysis, the mean plasma iomeprole concentration fell by 36% at 2 hours after administration when hemodialysis was started. The mean half-life on dialysis was 4.4 hours. The effective fall in plasma iomeprole concentration after a single dialysis was about 70%. The mean fraction of the dose recovered in the dialysate was 58%. The mean dialysis clearance was 81 ml/minute. The extraction efficiency of the dialyser was about 40%. The only adverse effect was infection of an arteriovenous fistula in a patient with end-stage renal disease, which was unrelated to the contrast agent. There were also mild to moderate adverse effects, but all resolved without sequelae. The most common adverse effects were headaches and sensations of warmth. Others were paresthesia, abdominal pain, taste disturbance, and nausea. None of the events was considered to be clinically important. There were no clinically important changes in vital signs, physical examination, electrocardiography, or clinical laboratory evaluations. The authors concluded that iomeprole is safe and well tolerated and can be almost completely eliminated both in patients with renal impairment and in patients receiving dialysis.

Hepatic disease

The risk of renal insufficiency after contrast agents is greater in the presence of hepatic insufficiency, apparently because in such cases both blood concentrations and renal excretion of the contrast medium are greater (SEDA-10, 422).

Other features of the patient

A high incidence of histamine release and anaphylactoid reactions to contrast media has been reported in patients with malignant tumors (257). Patients with malignant tumors were randomized into two groups. One group ($n = 66$) received non-ionic low-osmolar contrast media (iopamidol) and the other ($n = 64$) received high-osmolar ionic contrast media (ioxitalamate). An average of 100 ml of contrast medium (range 60–140 ml) was given before CT scanning in both groups. The incidence of reactions (tachycardia, bradycardia, hypertension and hypotension, a fall in oxygen saturation, nausea, vomiting, headache, and skin reactions) was similarly high in both groups (58% with iopamidol and 42% with ioxitalamate). The increases in plasma histamine concentrations were also similar: median 0.43 (range 0–13) ng/ml with iopamidol and 0.15 (0–12) ng/ml with ioxitalamate. The authors concluded that patients with malignancies are at risk of histamine-associated contrast reactions and suggested that antihistamine prophylaxis with histamine H_1 and H_2 receptor antagonists should be considered in these patients. However, there is no conclusive evidence that antihistamines offer effective prophylaxis against reactions to contrast media.

Routine electrocardiographic monitoring during intravenous urography shows that there are significant abnormalities in patients with heart disease and that the incidence of these abnormalities appears to be related to the dose of contrast agent and the speed of injection (258). Patients with a history of angina can develop ischemic electrocardiographic changes with or without chest pain after the injection of a contrast agent into the superior vena cava; one such patient developed ventricular fibrillation (259).

In patients with myasthenia gravis, crises may be precipitated by contrast agents (260). An acute myasthenic crisis with apnea was induced by contrast CT with diatrizoate in two patients with myasthenia gravis and this was followed by prolonged aggravation of the myasthenia (261). This has also occurred with iopamidol (SEDA-12, 396).

Patients with pre-existent thyrotoxicosis present a problem, since the condition may be aggravated by contrast agents, even to the point of precipitating a thyroid storm (262).

Patients with a history of previous reactions to contrast media have a 35–40% chance of reacting again if re-examined.

In patients with sickle-cell disease, a high local concentration of contrast medium in the blood during arteriography can cause sickling, with resulting thrombosis. One patient with sickle cell disease developed severe intravascular hemolysis, thrombocytopenia, leukocytosis, and pulmonary infiltrates after left ventriculography and coronary angiography with meglumine diatrizoate (263). In vitro studies suggest that the non-ionic agent iopamidol causes significantly less sickling than conventional ionic contrast agents, and iopamidol would therefore be preferable for arteriography in patients with this disorder (SEDA-7, 453).

There appears to be an increased risk of seizures due to vasospasm if cerebral angiography is performed during or shortly after an attack of migraine (SEDA-11, 412).

Drug Administration

Drug formulations

BR21 is a sterile pyrogen-free suspension containing iomeprol, both free in solution and entrapped in liposomal vesicles. The suspension ideally contains iodine 320 mg/ml with an osmolality of 560 mosmol/kg. The liposomes are 0.4 μm unilamellar vesicles in which the membrane is made of phospholipid. The total lipid concentration of the suspension is about 20 mg/ml. About

40 mg/ml of iodine are trapped within the liposomal vesicles and there is 280 mg/ml in the external phase. BR21 is taken up by the reticuloendothelial system and can enhance normal liver tissue, whereas neoplastic lesions, which lack reticuloendothelial cells, are not enhanced.

The safety and pharmacokinetics of intravenous BR21 have been evaluated in 30 healthy adult men in a phase I, single-blind, placebo-controlled, ascending-dose study (264). Four volunteers each received a single intravenous dose of BR21 (0.5, 1.0, 1.5, 2.0, or 2.5 ml/kg), and for each dose of BR21 two volunteers received saline 0.9%. All adverse events (headache, metallic taste, nausea, back pain, dizziness, tremors, sweating) were minor or mild and resolved rapidly without treatment. There was no difference in the incidence of adverse events from dose to dose of BR21 or between BR21 and saline. There were no significant changes in vital signs, electrocardiography, or laboratory findings.

A formulation of liposome-encapsulated iodixanol has been evaluated as part of a phase 1 assessment of diagnostic efficacy and safety (265). The formulation is a ready-to-use suspension of multilamellar liposomes with a mean size of 340 nm. The main constituents of the liposome wall are phosphatidylcholine and phosphatidylserine. The concentration of iodine in the formulation is 200 mg/ml (encapsulated iodine 80 mg/ml). The encapsulated iodine-to-lipid ratio is 1.5. This new formulation was injected in doses of 10, 30, 70, and 100 mg of encapsulated iodine per kg in 5, 8, 8, and 8 healthy volunteers (mean age 30 years). Saline was given to two volunteers in each dose group, in a volume matching that of iodixanol at the 70 mg dose. The intravenous injection was carried out using a power injector at a rate of 2 ml/second. There were dose-dependent changes in leukocyte count. During the first 2 hours the leukocyte count fell and then rose. At 10 and 30 mg doses the changes were small and in most of the volunteers did not exceed the reference range. At higher doses there was a prominent increase in neutrophils with rod-shaped nuclei, suggesting increased release from the bone marrow. C-reactive protein also rose dose-dependently, suggesting a cytokine-mediated reaction. Leukocyte count and C-reactive protein normalized spontaneously after 24 hours. The volunteers had subjective adverse events at doses of 70 and 100 mg; these included chills (88%), back pain (25%), flu-like symptoms (13%), and nausea and vomiting (38%); they started within 1 hour and recovered spontaneously within 3 hours. No adverse events were interpreted as severe, but they were judged to be too pronounced to be clinically acceptable. Research is needed to find a formulation that causes fewer adverse events without compromising diagnostic quality.

Another hepatocyte-specific contrast formulation, dysprosium ethoxybenzyltris(carboxylatomethyl)triazaundecanedioic acid diethylenetriaminepenta-acetic acid (Dy-EOB-DTPA), has been used for liver CT imaging (266). It contains calcium-EOB-DTPA (0.5 mg/ml), trometamol (1.2 mg/ml), and hydrochloric acid (final pH 7.4). It has been described as a stable metal chelate with high tolerability in vitro and in animal studies, in which a long-lasting increase in CT density of about 30 Hounsfield units has been reported. A total of 40 healthy male volunteers (mean age 33 years) received intravenous infusions of Dy-EOB-DTPA, 0.05, 0.1, 0.25, 0.375, or 0.5 mmol/kg over 10 minutes ($n = 6$ in each group), or placebo ($n = 2$ in each group). There were adverse effects in four of the 10 patients who were given placebo and 22 of the 30 who were given Dy-EOB-DTPA. The most common adverse events were nausea (25%), headache (18%), paresthesia (15%), loss of appetite, allergic reactions, back pain, and injection site hemorrhage (7.5%). The adverse effects were generally mild or moderate, but there was a slight increase in intensity at the higher doses. There were gastrointestinal adverse events in all six of the volunteers who received 0.5 mmol/kg. Nausea was the longest lasting and in one case it was severe. The results of laboratory tests did not exceed the reference ranges. Vital signs, hemodynamic parameters, and electrocardiography were not affected by the contrast agent. Over 50% of the adverse events were considered to be unrelated to the drug. The authors concluded that this liver-specific contrast formulation has a good safety profile.

Drug contamination

Contrast media used for arteriography contain a variety of microscopic particles. When glass ampoules are opened, they contain a larger number of particles than rubber-capped vials because of the vacuum effect on glass particles during the opening of the ampoule (267). This can theoretically cause microembolism. Angiographic catheters and guide wires also contain a very large number of particles derived from the manufacturing process, and the release of these particles is increased some sixfold after the insertion of the guide-wire into the catheter (SED-12, 1179) (268). Vials should be opened by removing the cap and not by puncture of the membrane, since the needle usually pushes large rubber particles into the solution. Ideally, contrast media should be filtered before injection, but this will often not be practicable.

In the case of glass ampoules, if the ampoule is allowed to stand for 30–60 seconds after opening, most of the larger particles will have sedimented to the bottom of the ampoule. These can then be avoided by leaving the lower 2–3 mm of contrast medium in the ampoule.

Drug administration route

Oral and rectal

The high-osmolar contrast agents diatrizoate and iotalamate were formerly recommended for oral use in preference to barium when there was a risk of perforation, but the osmotic effect of such material can lead to diarrhea and fluid loss, which may be dangerous in weak patients. Diatrizoate, which has a cathartic action, can occasionally cause ileus when given postoperatively (149); it can also be precipitated as a solid mass in the stomach when gastric acidity is high, but also in an achlorhydric gastric stump after partial gastrectomy if stomal obstruction is present. On one occasion when diatrizoate was used to fill the gastric balloon of a Sengstaken–Blakemore tube, hydrogen ions from the gastric content apparently penetrated into the balloon, precipitating the contrast medium and preventing the balloon's removal. Accidental inhalation of hypertonic contrast media during oral administration can cause fatal pulmonary edema (75).

Low-osmolar agents such as iohexol are preferred for oral use; however, they can still cause some diarrhea, for example in 18 out of 40 cases in one series (SEDA-16, 529). Absorption can be increased if there is mucosal damage in the bowel, such as in Crohn's disease, resulting in delayed excretion but not apparently involving risk (SEDA-18, 441).

Diatrizoate enemas are still sometimes used to treat meconium ileus or constipation and it is important to give intravenous fluids so as to avoid dehydration. Hypomagnesemia can also occur (150). Osmotic effects lower in the gastrointestinal tract have even led to distention and cecal perforation (151). Stasis of diatrizoate in dilated loops of bowel can cause inflammatory changes or necrosis (152,153).

Severe systemic reactions to enterally administered water-soluble contrast media are rare but they do occur, for example with oral iohexol (222).

Intra-arterial injection

Local vascular complications associated with angiography include intramural injection of contrast medium (leading to dissection of the arterial wall), arterial thrombosis, phlebitis, venous thrombosis, embolic phenomena, and damage to atheromatous plaques in the aorta leading to cholesterol embolism (SEDA-14, 423) (269). Injection of contrast material into an intervertebral disc during angiography can cause lumbar pain associated with disc necrosis. Acute pancreatitis has been reported after aortography with sodium acetrizoate 70% w/v accidentally injected into the celiac axis. A report from 1958 described a fatal case of bilateral adrenal necrosis following lumbar aortography (SED-12, 1178) (270). Aortography in patients with pheochromocytoma can produce hemorrhage into and around the adrenal tumor; in one case adrenal insufficiency followed bilateral adrenal venography (271).

Cerebral angiography

The risk of neurological complications after cerebral angiography is 0.55–3.2% but increases to 10% in patients with symptomatic carotid stenosis; the incidence of clinically silent cerebral embolism is unknown. Diffusion-weighted magnetic resonance imaging before and after cerebral angiography has been carried out to assess the prevalence of embolic events in 100 consecutive angiographies in 91 patients (272). The patients underwent neurological assessment before, immediately after, and 1 day after angiography. There were 42 bright lesions in 23 patients after 23 procedures in a pattern consistent with embolic events. There were no new neurological deficits after any angiographic procedure. The frequency of lesions correlated significantly with a history of atherosclerotic arterial disease, the complexity of the angiographic procedure, and the amount of contrast medium used. The authors concluded that after diagnostic and interventional cerebral angiography embolic events are more frequent than the neurological complication rate. The incidence of embolism is closely related to the vascular risk profile.

Intravenous injection

Subcutaneous extravasation of contrast media during rapid intravascular injection can cause local irritation and inflammatory responses. The severity of these effects depends on the volume and osmolality of the extravasated contrast medium. High-osmolality contrast media can cause skin ulceration and necrosis. Subcutaneous hyaluronidase, aspiration of fluid, elevation of the limb, and topical application of cold compresses are some of the measures used to treat this complication.

The frequency of extravasation of ionic and non-ionic contrast media during rapid bolus injection in 5106 CT contrast-enhanced scans was 0.9% (31 patients had extravasation of ionic media and 17 patients had extravasation of non-ionic media) (273). There was no correlation between the injection rate and the frequency of extravasation. None of the patients who had extravasation had permanent damage.

With highly concentrated sodium-containing media, such as sodium iotalamate 420, severe arm pain and late thrombosis can occur (274). In a comparison of the sodium and methylglucamine salts of diatrizoate, even with lower concentrations, the incidence of arm pain was higher with the sodium salt. Extravasation of ionic contrast medium in the soft tissues can cause a chemical cellulitis, leading to skin necrosis, particularly if the circulation is compromised (SEDA-10, 424); tissue damage is less severe with the non-ionic media. The risk of extravasation is greatest with the rapid injection of large doses needed in computed tomography. In rare cases, this has resulted in gangrene, particularly in venography. Arterial insufficiency probably results in slower removal of the agent and hence more prolonged exposure to it.

As in many other areas, the non-ionic media are less noxious in this respect; this has been shown in animal studies (SEDA-16, 530) and in a number of clinical cases in which extravasation of large volumes of iopamidol responded to palliative measures and had no lasting ill-effects (275). Among the ionic media, the methylglucamine media seem to have more local toxicity than their sodium equivalents.

Extravasation of ionic and non-ionic contrast media after rapid bolus infusion has been studied in 5106 CT studies in adults (276). The mean infusion rate was 2.8 ml/second and extravasation occurred in 48 patients (0.9%). Injection rate did not correlate with the frequency or amount of extravasation. Average age and use of ionic versus non-ionic contrast medium were identical in patients with and without extravasation. There was no sex difference. There was extravasation of ionic contrast medium in 31 patients, nine of whom had extravasation of at least 50 ml. There was extravasation of non-ionic contrast medium in 17 patients, of whom seven had extravasation of at least 50 ml. Hyaluronidase infiltration was often used to treat more extensive extravasation in 10 patients each with extravasation of ionic or non-ionic media. No patient required surgical intervention and none had severe or long-term effects.

The adverse effects of contrast agents during computed tomography (CT) are broadly similar to those during excretion urography, but the incidence of serious reactions and deaths may be higher, because reactions are harder to treat when the patient is in a scanner (SEDA-7, 451). Renal insufficiency can occur in patients with diabetes and pre-existing renal disease or as a result of multiple examinations. In *Herpes simplex* encephalitis, there can be prolonged retention of contrast medium in the brain. In patients with spinal tumors, stimulus-sensitive extensor spasms can occur in the trunk and limbs (SEDA-7, 453).

For computed tomography, large volumes of contrast medium have to be injected under pressure and this can lead to problems such as subclinical air embolism (SEDA-14, 422) and extravasation. In one series of 20 950 CT scans using non-ionic media, there was extravasation of 3–100 ml in 28 cases; the degree of extravasation depended on the pressure applied. When extravasation occurs, the extent of tissue damage depends primarily on the osmolarity of the contrast medium, but it is clear that of the ionic agents, the methylglucamine salts cause more damage than the sodium salts do (277).

Phlebography sometimes causes superficial thrombophlebitis in the injected vein. Of 61 previously healthy patients who had undergone phlebography, four had clear evidence of subsequent deep vein thrombosis and in two of these there were signs of non-fatal pulmonary embolism. The incidence of thrombosis may indeed have been higher, because there was abnormal fibrinogen uptake in 20 individuals, although the result could have been non-specific (278). The risk of thrombophlebitis is significantly less when low-osmolar media are used (SEDA-9, 410) (SEDA-11, 414).

Necrosis of the skin can follow peripheral venography (279); in these cases there had been some extravenous injection, and impaired circulation probably resulted in slower removal of the agent and hence more prolonged exposure to it. Gangrene of the toes has also occurred.

Polyarthropathy, in a severe and acute form, has been described as a rare complication of venography in patients with end-stage renal insufficiency (SEDA-18, 445).

Fat embolism is a rare complication of intra-osseous phlebography (280,281).

Orbital venography has been largely superseded by computed tomography and magnetic resonance imaging. This technique has usually been safe, but there have been reports of hemorrhage in a lymphangioma of the orbit and of transitory retinal artery spasm or retinal hemorrhage, the last two involving subjects with diabetes (SED-12, 1179) (282).

Priapism due to venous thrombosis has been reported after penile cavernosography with ioxaglate and diluted iotalamate (283). Contrast agents can cause endothelial damage in the corpus cavernosum. Prior injection of 1000–2000 units of heparin into the corpus cavernosum and the use of diluted non-ionic media have therefore been advocated for this procedure (284).

Subcutaneous or intramuscular injection

In the past, when intravascular injection proved difficult, contrast media were sometimes given by the subcutaneous or intramuscular routes. On occasion, severe sloughing of tissue resulted. Addition of hyaluronidase in order to alleviate this problem only aggravated it, and dilution with water, saline, or procaine solution also proved useless. If, in exceptional circumstances, these routes have to be used, the medium should be injected in small quantities at multiple sites.

Intra-articular injection

Minor reversible edematous changes have been noted in the synovial membrane after arthrography, and a chemical synovitis can occur (SEDA-10, 425).

Amniofetography

Ultrasound has superseded amniofetography, a procedure in which contrast media are injected into the amniotic sac during pregnancy to delineate fetal abnormalities. Diatrizoate, iotalamate, and, earlier, iodized oil were used. There is a theoretical risk of premature labor. Accidental injection of contrast medium into the fetal subcutaneous tissues could cause sloughing of the skin or subcutaneous necrosis. Cases of thyroid hyperplasia or hypothyroidism were also commonly described.

Arthrography

After injection of a contrast agent into a joint, the synovium becomes edematous and hemorrhagic within 2 hours. At 24 hours, there is tissue eosinophilia and vascular congestion. Eosinophilia of the synovial fluid can also occur. The complications reported in a survey of 126 000 examinations (285) are shown in Table 6.

Bronchography

Computed tomography of the lungs has reduced the requirement for bronchography, but it is still of value in selected cases. Iotrolan is most commonly used and is well tolerated. Adverse effects resulted from earlier products used in the field.

Hytrast (a mixture of iopydol and iopydone in aqueous suspension with carboxymethylcellulose) was generally withdrawn because it gave rise to a foreign body reaction. Iodized oil was formerly popular, but iodism was not uncommon and sometimes even fatal; sulfanilamide was added to one particular formulation of iodized oil to increase its viscosity and on occasion produced methemoglobinemia and cyanosis. Late granulomatous reactions in the lungs, followed by long-term fibrosis were also described with iodized oil, as were early allergic granulomatous reactions and other types of allergic reaction, such as pneumonitis and urticaria.

About one-third of patients undergoing bronchography have some type of reaction. The most common symptoms

Table 6 Complications of arthrography in 126 000 examinations

Complication	Number
Death	0
Severe reactions	
Hypotension	4
Vasomotor collapse and laryngeal edema	1
Air embolism	1
Vagal reactions	83
Subsequent seizures	6
Apnea	1
Urticaria	61
Cellulitis	1
Sepsis	3
Massive effusion	1
Severe pain	5
Sterile chemical synovitis	150

are headache, nausea and vomiting, fever, iodism, and dyspnea. Less frequent reactions include wheezing, diarrhea, dizziness, cyanosis, chest pain, and pneumonia. Aqueous propyliodone produces more reactions than the oily form, but as a rule the product that produces most reactions also produces the best visualization. Symptoms are also related to the volume of agent used and the degree of alveolarization.

In a survey of 100 000 bronchograms published in 1967, 18 deaths were attributed to the technique. However, half of the deaths were due to the local anesthetic, generally used in excessive amounts. Fatalities tended to occur in children, patients with limited respiratory reserves, or subjects with severe hypersensitivity reactions (SED-12, 1185) (286).

If the cricothyroid route is used for bronchography, contrast medium may be accidentally injected into the soft tissues of the neck; propyliodone has under these conditions produced an inflammatory reaction leading to dysphagia, pain on movement of the neck, and mediastinal spread, rarely with electrocardiographic changes suggesting pericarditis. Oral glucocorticoids with antibiotic cover usually produce dramatic relief of symptoms.

Heating lowers the viscosity of propyliodone and should be avoided. Death from progressive acute respiratory failure resulted from bilateral bronchography under general anesthesia using propyliodone which had been heated in an autoclave.

Cholecystography and cholangiography

Ultrasonography is now the primary imaging technique for the assessment of the gall bladder and bile ducts, and oral cholecystography is obsolete. Contrast agents that have been used for oral cholecystography are weak iodinated organic acids that are absorbed and then largely conjugated with glucuronic acid. The most widely used agents have been iopanoic acid and sodium or calcium iopodate; tyropanoate and iocetamic acid have also been used. Bunamiodyl sodium, which was nephrotoxic, has been withdrawn.

The use of intravenous cholangiography has fallen dramatically in recent years, largely because of the advent of new and safer techniques for imaging the biliary tree, including high-quality ultrasound. However, with the introduction of laparoscopic cholecystectomy, the technique is occasionally used to assess bile duct anatomy before surgery (SEDA-19, 426). Intravenous cholangiography with meglumine iotroxate was reported to be acceptably safe. Contrary to popular opinion, reactions are apparently no more frequent with modern agents for intravenous cholangiography than with angiographic agents (SEDA-20, 416).

In a national survey in Britain in 1970, when drugs were generally given for this purpose in a single injected dose, intermediate reactions to iodipamide occurred once in every 700 cases, severe reactions once in every 1600, and deaths once in every 5000 (SED-12, 1168) (72). The introduction of infusion cholangiography (in which the contrast medium is given over 15–30 minutes) reduced the incidence of minor reactions, allowing the liver to excrete the contrast medium more efficiently, so that doses as low as 3–5 ml of ioglycamide or 10 ml of 50% iodipamide can be used. According to a 1975 report from France, serious reactions nevertheless occurred once in every 310 infusion cholangiographies (SEDA-10, 422) (287).

Pyrexial reactions occurred in 5.3% of cases after postoperative cholangiography through a T-tube; in two patients there was endotoxic shock (SEDA-5, 420).

A fatal reaction occurred when diatrizoate was used for operative cholangiography and contrast medium entered the bloodstream (288).

Using a fine needle, with sodium diatrizoate as the contrast medium, percutaneous hepatic cholangiography is a relatively safe technique for use in cases of obstructive jaundice in which the high serum bilirubin precludes oral or intravenous techniques. The complications of bile peritonitis and internal hemorrhage are best avoided by decompression of dilated ducts. Bile blood fistula can lead to fatal endotoxic shock due to bacteria escaping from the obstructed biliary tract (289). The rapid appearance of a pyelographic shadow can be a useful diagnostic sign, calling for immediate antibiotic therapy. However, it is now usual to give a broad-spectrum antibiotic immediately before the examination. Acute renal insufficiency has been reported after transhepatic cholangiography (SEDA-10, 423).

Cholangiopancreatography

Although a severe contrast medium reaction with shock has been observed, this was the only contrast medium reaction in a series of 2000 cases of ERCP reported in 1977 (290). In some other reports, there were milder degrees of allergic reactions (291). In a series of 10 000 cases reported in the USA in 1976 (292), the most serious adverse effects were cholangitic sepsis (0.8%, fatal in 0.08%) and pancreatic sepsis (0.3%, fatal in 0.06%), but there was a 1% incidence of injection pancreatitis and other cases of drug interactions (diazepam, spasmolytic agents), instrumental injury, and aspiration pneumonia. Pancreatitis can result from over-filling of the pancreatic duct. To minimize the risk of pancreatitis after ERCP the examination should be performed with care. High-pressure injection of the contrast medium should be avoided to reduce the risk of overfilling and extraductile extravasation. In addition, low-osmolar non-ionic contrast agents should be used (SEDA-19, 425) (SEDA-20, 417). Significant quantities of contrast agent can be absorbed after ERCP. Transient asymptomatic hyperamylasemia can occur (SEDA-14, 422), and in one series there was a 15% incidence of mild renal dysfunction (293).

Discography

Subdural empyema with residual quadriparesis has been reported as a rare complication of discography (294).

Hysterosalpingography

Water-soluble agents are generally preferred for hysterosalpingography, agents such as diatrizoate or iotalamate being most commonly selected. It has sometimes been suggested that low-osmolar contrast media should be preferred; however, a double-blind comparison of the low-osmolar medium ioxaglate (Hexabrix 320) with methylglucamine diatrizoate (Conray 280) in 100 patients showed no difference in the incidence of early or late adverse effects between the two agents (295).

There is no justification for using specialized formulations based on the more toxic molecules acetrizoate or iodipamide; these cause more severe pain and can also cause hypotension and shock.

Iodized oil, at one time widely used, caused less pain but was suspected of causing adhesions and there was certainly some risk of oil embolism after intravasation, for example retinal embolism with visual impairment lasting for some months and several cases of pulmonary oil embolism (SEDA-16, 537). Skin testing with iodized oil on occasion resulted in both local and generalized reactions. Like later agents, lipiodol could also cause salpingitis.

The main remaining disadvantage of the currently used water-soluble media is their tendency to cause lower abdominal pain, which can be severe, during or shortly after the injection; it can last for 24 hours or longer. These adverse effects are likely to be less severe with low-osmolar non-ionic media. Vaginal bleeding can occur and the following menstrual period can be deranged. With all contrast media there is a possibility of hypersensitivity reactions, and dextran as an additive has on occasion produced anaphylactic symptoms (SEDA-15, 505). Salpingitis can occur with any contrast agent.

Lymphography

Lymphography is rarely required with the availability of modern CT and MRI scanners. However, intradermal injection of 2–4 ml (iodine 300 mg/ml) of iso-osmolar non-ionic dimers (iotrolan and iodixanol) at a rate of 0.1 ml/minute can be used to assess the lymphatics in limbs with lymphedema. The procedure is safe with no serious adverse effects, but idiosyncratic and allergic like reactions can occur.

Iodized oils are usually used as contrast media for lymphography and can cause iodism. Reactions can also occur to the dye "patent blue violet," which is injected subcutaneously before lymphography to enable the lymphatics to be visualized; it colors the skin and urine blue. The incidence of serious reactions to lymphography in 32 000 cases is shown in Table 7.

Myelography and ventriculography

Myelography and ventriculography are techniques that, irrespective of the agent used, have some unpleasant effects, including headache, nausea, and dizziness, which are frequent problems and are possibly more frequent in women, in people with multiple sclerosis, and in investigations at the higher levels of the central nervous system. Nevertheless, the nature and incidence of the adverse reactions depend on the contrast agent used, oily agents, the ionic water-soluble agents, and the non-ionic water-soluble agents. Today, MRI has substantially replaced these unpleasant invasive procedures (SEDA-19, 430).

The incidences of adverse effects in 4568 cases of lumbar myelography and 1232 cases of cervical myelography are shown in Table 8 and Table 9.

Oily media

Oily media are no longer used for myelography or other imaging techniques of the nervous system. Iofendylate was formerly widely used for myelography and to some extent for ventriculography. In the USA, where myelography was generally performed with large volumes of contrast agents, it was the custom to aspirate the iofendylate at the end of the investigation, whereas in some other countries smaller volumes were used under the assumption that these would be gradually absorbed. In patients with multiple sclerosis, myelography with iofendylate can cause particularly severe reactions.

Aseptic meningitis can occur 3–67 days after myelography, and in one case it was associated with evidence of cerebral vasospasm and infarction. An unusual ophthalmic complication in another patient followed the passage

Table 7 Frequency of serious complications in 32 000 episodes of lymphography

Event	Number	Frequency
Hypertensive crisis	6	0.0002
Pulmonary infarction	81	0.0025
Pulmonary edema	10	0.0003
Pneumonia	13	0.0004
Prolonged fever	24	0.0008
Hypersensitivity reactions		
Oily contrast medium	40	0.0012
Vital blue dye	57	0.0017
Cerebral disorders	9	0.0003
Death	18	0.0006

Table 8 Frequency of adverse effects after lumbar myelography (SEDA-4, 335)

Adverse effect	Frequency (%)
Headache	32
Nausea	11
Vomiting	7
Dizziness	7
Increased pain	7
Hypotension	<1
Micturition disturbance	1.1
Muscle fibrillation	0.35
Fever	0.26
Allergic reactions	0.13
Neck stiffness	0.11
Meningism	0.09
Numbness, paresthesia	0.07
Vasovagal attack	0.07

Table 9 Frequency of adverse effects after cervical myelography, other than tonic-clonic seizures (SEDA-4, 335)

Adverse effect	Frequency (%)
Headache	37
Nausea	20
Vomiting	14
Pain	7
Dizziness	5
Mental changes	2
Numbness, paresthesia	0.65
Micturition disturbance	0.65
Weakness in limbs	0.49
Myoclonus	0.32
Neck stiffness	0.16
Allergic reactions	0.16
Hematemesis	0.08
Eye flickering	0.08

of iofendylate into the region of the clivus and along the course of the optic nerve during cervical myelography; the patient had transient pain and flashes of light in the eye, followed by periorbital pain for 2 days. A month later, severe visual impairment with renewed pain occurred; the condition responded to systemic glucocorticoids (296).

Venous intravasation occurs rarely during lumbar myelography; pulmonary oil embolization has resulted and has also been described after ventriculography with iofendylate in a hydrocephalic child with a ventriculovenous shunt. In that case the symptoms were mild, but the agent can obstruct the valve and in any patient the medium should therefore be removed at the completion of the procedure.

Arachnoiditis is a recognized and much-discussed problem, which has given rise to group litigation. Extensive adhesions due to iofendylate have been described, leading to neurological complications and death; there are two cases on record with clinical changes resembling Sudeck's atrophy. Animal experiments have shown that the ability of iofendylate to cause arachnoiditis is especially pronounced if it is mixed with blood; it should therefore be avoided if there is the possibility that bleeding has occurred into the cerebrospinal fluid.

It is common to see evidence of iofendylate residues for many years after myelography. The residue problem extends to the skull and it is common to find symptomless deposits of iofendylate there after myelography; however, in several patients residues in the skull have apparently caused convulsions (SEDA-14, 424). They can also be associated with persistent headache (SEDA-8, 430) and perhaps with the development of vestibular disturbances many years later (SEDA-17, 538).

In two cases, ventriculography with iofendylate resulted in adhesions with obstruction to the outflow of cerebrospinal fluid (in one case at the level of the third ventricle, in the other at the level of the fourth) producing obstructive hydrocephalus (SED-12, 1180) (297).

An iofendylate cyst causing a thoracic radiculopathy has been reported (298).

- A 45-year-old woman had severe root pain at T10, which had gradually become more intense over the preceding 4 years. She had undergone spinal myelography about 30 years before. Clinical examination was normal. A plain X-ray of the thoracic spine showed a radio-opaque abnormality at the level of T10, which axial CT showed was in the vertebral canal, compressing the left posterolateral margin of the theca. At thoracic laminectomy, a well-circumscribed subarachnoid extramedullary cyst was identified, from which a small volume of oily material was removed. The cyst collapsed and its posterior wall was excised. Histology confirmed a benign arachnoid cyst. Within 24 hours the thoracic root pain had gone.

Recurrent febrile nodular non-suppurative panniculitis (Weber–Christian syndrome) has been described 1 month after myelography with iofendylate; the causal link was uncertain (299).

Persistent symptoms can be caused by residues of iofendylate after myelography; allergy with urticaria and anaphylactic episodes recurring for 17 years was described in one patient who was hypersensitive to iofendylate; after removal of most of the residue, the symptoms improved (300). In one unusual case of anaphylactic collapse, marked bilateral parotid enlargement was the presenting sign (SEDA-18, 442).

When metrizamide was used to outline the basal cisterns in association with computed tomography of the skull, headache occurred in about 50% of patients and vomiting in 26–56%, depending on the dose used; the symptoms occurred 2–6 hours after injection and cleared within 12 hours. Convulsions have occurred with this procedure (301).

Tolerance of non-ionic contrast media in myelography has been well documented (SEDA-22, 500). A report from India has documented the safety and diagnostic efficacy of the non-ionic monomer iohexol 7–10 ml (iodine 300 mg/ml) injected into the subarachnoid space in 25 patients (302). Only three patients developed minor adverse effects—headache and paresthesia in the legs.

Sialography

In randomized comparison of Lipiodol ultrafluid (ethiodized oil) with melumine diatrizoate 290 for sialography in 60 patients, pain and swelling of the parotid gland was more frequent after Lipiodol UF (303).

Extravasation of oil-based contrast agents used for sialography and dacryocystography can cause lipogranuloma formation (304).

- A four-year-old boy with epiphora had a left dacryocystogram with the iodinized oil-based contrast agent Lipiodol under general anesthesia. During injection, a false passage was inadvertently formed, with extravasation of the contrast agent from the lacrimal duct into the surrounding tissues. This was confirmed radiographically. He developed swelling and erythema, which gradually resolved over 6 months.

Iso-osmolar non-ionic dimers, such as iotrolan or iodixanol, are the safest contrast agents for such a procedure. Extravasation of these agents causes minimal tissue reaction.

Urography

The use of intravenous urography has been in decline for some years with the advent of high-quality real-time ultrasonography (SEDA-20, 417).

For retrograde and anterograde urography, only iodinated water-soluble contrast media should be used. The high-osmolar contrast agents, diatrizoate or iotalamate, are generally used in these procedures. Barium sulfate has been used for cystography in the past, but is inadvisable; if ureteric reflux occurs, the barium can become inspissated in the calyceal system of the kidney; in view of experimental findings, this might be expected to cause granulomatous reactions with fibrosis.

Retrograde urography is often followed by irritation and edema of the urethral and bladder mucosa. In animals this effect was maximal at 48 hours and persisted for at least 1 week. Factors that reduced the inflammatory response in the bladder were dilution of the medium and the use of smaller volumes instilled at lower pressure. In clinical use, diatrizoate has seemed to be less irritant than acetrizoate (305).

Retrograde pyelography can rarely cause deterioration of renal function, with acute renal insufficiency, particularly if there has been marked pyelorenal back flow; exceptionally, the complication can be fatal (306).

Retrograde pyelography with potassium bromide has caused renal insufficiency (SEDA-11, 413).

Small amounts of contrast agents can be absorbed after retrograde urography, mainly via the calyces. In one case, 12.5% of the contrast medium was absorbed (307). A severe generalized reaction has been reported after cystography with diatrizoate (SED-12, 1174) (308), and another in a patient with ureteric reflux given meglumine iotalamate; in the latter, there was circulatory collapse but it responded to simple change in posture and adrenaline was not required (SEDA-18, 445). Miliary dissemination of tubercle bacilli from an infected urinary system after retrograde pyelography with pyelovenous back flow is very rare. An anaphylactoid reaction to contrast medium injected into a ureter via a percutaneous nephrostomy has been reported (SEDA-19, 430).

Bladder rupture is a risk of cystourethrography. In two children with myelomeningoceles and ventriculoperitoneal shunts, bladder rupture had particularly serious consequences. The diatrizoate that was used passed into the peritoneal cavity and then via the shunt into the cerebral ventricles and subarachnoid space, causing tonic convulsions (SEDA-17, 538).

Autonomic dysreflexia (facial flushing, sweating, nasal congestion, headache and paroxysmal hypertension) can occur in quadriplegic patients in response to bladder distention during cystography (SEDA-19, 430).

Drug overdose

Fatal cases of accidental overdosage have been reported in infants; the complications leading to death were either pulmonary edema or convulsions. The latter can be due to hyperosmolarity (leading to hypertonic dehydration) or to the chemical toxicity of the contrast agent.

- In a fatal case, a massive overdose of 340 ml Renigrafin 76 was injected into a 7-year-old child with coarctation of the aorta, and computed tomography showed the presence of contrast agent in the brain (98).

A patient who was given 30 g of iopanoic acid, instead of 3 g, had severe nausea with vomiting and diarrhea but no more serious effects (SED-12, 1167) (309).

Drug–Drug Interactions

Antihistamines

Contrast media should not be mixed with antihistamines in a syringe, since precipitation can result (SED-8, 1034) (310).

Beta-blockers

Field experience, backed by a case-control study of 1991, strongly suggests that patients taking beta-blockers have a risk ratio of adverse reactions to contrast media of 2.7. Hypotension is the main effect, sometimes dangerously so, even with non-ionic media (SEDA-11, 411) (SEDA-17, 536) (311).

Cardiac glycosides

Diatrizoate and strophanthin K may have a synergistic toxic effect (312).

Heparin

Ionic contrast media cause temporary prolongation of clotting time in patients treated with heparin; this effect may last for 6 hours and may interfere with laboratory assays (132). Non-ionic media do not have this anticoagulant effect, and if blood is allowed to mix with a non-ionic medium in the syringe or catheter, thrombus formation can occur, which could be a potential cause of thromboembolism (SEDA-15, 502).

In contrast, in 664 patients undergoing percutaneous coronary intervention with insertion of a sirolimus-eluting stent, the addition of heparin was associated with significantly higher incidences of hematomas (8.5 versus 3.8%) and overall vascular complications (5.3 versus 0.01%), including pseudoaneurysm (2.6 versus 0.0%); more patients required surgical repair (1.8 versus 0.3%) and there was a trend toward a higher rate of blood transfusion (6.6 versus 2.6%) (313). The authors concluded that routine addition of low-dose heparin to contrast agents during percutaneous coronary intervention is associated with higher rates of bleeding and vascular complications.

Hydralazine

Hydralazine seems to increase the risk of acute cutaneous vasculitis in patients given iopamidol (314).

Interleukin-2

Prior interleukin-2 therapy can induce atypical contrast medium hypersensitivity in the form of toxic recall reactions of various types (SEDA-17, 537), and these cannot be prevented by glucocorticoid premedication (315).

Metformin

The use of contrast media in patients taking metformin should be carried out cautiously. Contrast-induced nephropathy can lead to retention of metformin and lactic acidosis. However, there is no conclusive evidence that intravascular contrast agents precipitate metformin-induced lactic acidosis in patients with normal serum creatinine concentrations (under 130 μmol/l). This complication was almost always observed in non-insulin dependent diabetic patients with abnormal renal function before injection of contrast media (4,316).

Lactic acidosis can occur after the use of intravascular iodinated contrast agents in patients taking metformin. Metformin is excreted by the kidneys, and renal insufficiency can lead to its retention, which can cause fatal lactic acidosis. The manufacturers have recommended that metformin should be withdrawn for 48 hours before and 48 hours after the administration of intravascular contrast media, which can cause renal damage, and treatment should not be restarted until normal renal function is confirmed. Reviews of reported cases of lactic acidosis after contrast administration have shown that there was pre-existing renal impairment in all cases. A retrospective evaluation of patients taking metformin who underwent contrast angiography has also confirmed this observation (317). Of 33 patients, 29 had a normal serum creatinine before the angiographic procedure and none had a rise after angiography. Four had an abnormal serum creatinine before angiography; all four had a significant deterioration in renal function and died, two from unrelated causes and two from acute renal insufficiency and acidosis. The authors concluded that administration of contrast media is hazardous in diabetic patients with pre-existing renal impairment and that patients with normal renal function taking metformin are not at risk of lactic acidosis. They recommended that serum creatinine should be measured in all patients before angiography. In patients taking metformin with a normal serum creatinine, intravascular contrast is not contraindicated.

NSAIDs

Non-steroidal anti-inflammatory drugs may increase the risk of contrast nephropathy (SEDA-15, 502).

Papaverine

Ioxaglate has been reported to be precipitated by papaverine, which has been used in penile cavernosography (SEDA-11, 413), but some cases may have been due to an interaction between heparin and papaverine, perhaps not involving the contrast medium (SEDA-18, 444); in one case, the use of iopamidol 370 immediately after an injection of papaverine was followed by extensive intra-arterial thrombosis (SEDA-17, 537).

Pethidine

When pethidine is given with iodipamide, a myocardial infarction-like syndrome can occur due to spasm of the sphincter of Oddi (SED-8, 1026) (318).

Protamine

Protamine sulfate has a pH of 3–4 and causes precipitation of diatrizoic acid; if injected into a catheter containing diatrizoate in heparinized patients, it could cause a precipitate which in theory might result in an embolus.

Uricosuric drugs

Drugs that increase uric acid excretion may precipitate contrast nephropathy (SEDA-7, 452).

Interference with Diagnostic Tests

Urinalysis

Urinalysis after intravenous urography can give misleading results. Increased specific gravity, false positive tests for protein (with the sulfosalicylic acid and nitric acid ring methods, but not the bromophenyl dye test), and the presence of needle-like crystals have been reported. Pseudo-albuminuria can occur with a false-positive sulfosalicylic acid test (319).

Black copper reduction test

A positive result in the black copper reduction test, suggesting alcaptonuria, can follow the use of diatrizoate, iotalamate or iodipamide (320).

Urinary catecholamines

Methylglucamine-based contrast media interfere with the estimation of urinary catecholamines in patients with pheochromocytoma (SEDA-10, 423).

Para-aminohippuric acid

Diatrizoate can interfere with *para*-aminohippuric acid extraction studies (SEDA-15, 502) (321).

References

1. Thomsen HS, Dorph S. High-osmolar and low-osmolar contrast media. An update on frequency of adverse drug reactions. Acta Radiol 1993;34(3):205–9.
2. Siegle RL. Rates of idiosyncratic reactions. Ionic versus nonionic contrast media. Invest Radiol 1993;28(Suppl 5):S95–8.
3. Cohen MD. A review of the toxicity of nonionic contrast agents in children. Invest Radiol 1993;28(Suppl 5):S87–93.
4. Thomsen HS, Morcos SK. Radiographic contrast media. BJU Int 2000;86(Suppl 1):1–10.
5. Esplugas E, Cequier A, Gomez-Hospital JA, Del Blanco BG, Jara F. Comparative tolerability of contrast media used for coronary interventions. Drug Saf 2002;25(15):1079–98.
6. Dyet JF, Carter EC, Hartley WC. Comparison of iopromide and iopamidol in left ventricular angiography and in coronary angiography. Appl Radiol 2002;31(Suppl):38–44.
7. Sutton AG, Ashton VJ, Campbell PG, Price DJ, Hall JA, de Belder MA. A randomized prospective trial of ioxaglate 320 (Hexabrix) vs. iodixanol 320 (Visipaque) in patients undergoing percutaneous coronary intervention. Catheter Cardiovasc Interv 2002;57(3):346–52.
8. Bertrand ME, Esplugas E, Piessens J, Rasch W; [Visipaque in Percutaneous Transluminal Coronary Angioplasty VIP.] Trial Investigators. Influence of a nonionic, iso-osmolar contrast medium (iodixanol) versus an ionic, low-osmolar contrast medium (ioxaglate) on major adverse cardiac events in patients undergoing percutaneous transluminal coronary angioplasty: a multicenter, randomized, double-blind study. Circulation 2000;101(2):131–6.
9. Morcos SK, Anderson PB, Ward P, Weber S, Wenzel-Hora BI. The efficacy of bronchography via the fibreoptic bronchoscope using water soluble non ionic dimer (iotrolan) in diagnosing airways disease. J Bronchol 1996;3:106–11.
10. Morcos SK, Anderson PB, Baudouin SV, Clout C, Fairlie N, Baudouin C, Warnock N. Suitability of and tolerance to iotrolan 300 in bronchography via the fibreoptic bronchoscope. Thorax 1990;45(8):628–9.
11. Stacul F. Currently available iodinated contrast media. In: Thomsen HS, Müller RN, Mattery RF, editors. Trends in Contrast Media. Berlin: Springer-Verlag, 1999:71–2.
12. Shehadi WH. Death following intravascular administration of contrast media. Acta Radiol Diagn (Stockh) 1985; 26(4):457–61.
13. Sutton AG, Finn P, Grech ED, Hall JA, Stewart MJ, Davies A, de Belder MA. Early and late reactions after the use of iopamidol 340, ioxaglate 320, and iodixanol 320 in cardiac catheterization. Am Heart J 2001;141(4):677–83.

14. Katayama H, Yamaguchi K, Kozuka T, Takashima T, Seez P, Matsuura K. Adverse reactions to ionic and nonionic contrast media. A report from the Japanese Committee on the Safety of Contrast Media. Radiology 1990;175(3):621–8.
15. Pelagatti V, Bagheri H, Fernandez P, Railhac N, Bregeon C, Railhac JJ, Montastruc JL. Effets indésirables des produits de contraste: bilan de 6 mois de suivi. [Adverse effects of contrast media: results of a 6 months study.] Therapie 2000;55(3):391–4.
16. Uppal R, Jhaj R, Malhotra S. Adverse drug reactions among inpatients in a north Indian referral hospital. Natl Med J India 2000;13(1):16–18.
17. Yang HC, Lee RC, Teng MMH, Chang CY. Adverse reactions to intravenous administration iodinated contrast media. Experience in a medical center. Chin J Radiol 2001;26:17–21.
18. Dooley M, Jarvis B. Iomeprol: a review of its use as a contrast medium. Drugs 2000;59(5):1169–86.
19. Hill JA, Winniford M, Cohen MB, Van Fossen DB, Murphy MJ, Halpern EF, Ludbrook PA, Wexler L, Rudnick MR, Goldfarb S. Multicenter trial of ionic versus nonionic contrast media for cardiac angiography. The Iohexol Cooperative Study. Am J Cardiol 1993;72(11):770–5.
20. Klow NE, Levorstad K, Berg KJ, Brodahl U, Endresen K, Kristoffersen DT, Laake B, Simonsen S, Tofte AJ, Lundby B. Iodixanol in cardioangiography in patients with coronary artery disease. Tolerability, cardiac and renal effects. Acta Radiol 1993;34(1):72–7.
21. Schraeder R. Contrast media selection in interventional cardiology. J Clin Basic Cardiol 2001;4:245–8.
22. Mezilis N, Salame MY, Dyet JF, Arafa SO, Oakley GD, Cumberland DC. Comparison of iotrolan 320 and iohexol 350 in cardiac angiography: a randomised double-blind clinical study. Eur J Radiol 1998;28(2):171–5.
23. Maciejczyk A, Arcab A, Czarnecki A. Analysis of adverse reactions associated with drugs in 1997/98. Acta Pol Pharm Drug Res 1999;56:303–6.
24. Palmer FJ. The RACR survey of intravenous contrast media reactions, final report. Appl Radiol 2002;31(Suppl):26–8.
25. Cochran ST, Bomyea K, Sayre JW. Trends in adverse events after IV administration of contrast media. Appl Radiol 2002;31(Suppl):55–9.
26. Pugh ND, Sissons GRJ, Ruttley MST, Berg KJ, Nossen JO, Eide H. Iodixanol in femoral arteriography (phase III): a comparative double-parallel trial between iodixanol and iopromide. Appl Radiol 2002;31(Suppl):81–6.
27. Niendorf HP. Delayed allergy like reactions to X-ray contrast media. Problem statement exemplified with iotrolan (Isovist) 280. Eur Radiol 1996;6(Suppl):S8–S10.
28. Yasuda R, Munechika H. Delayed adverse reactions to nonionic monomeric contrast-enhanced media. Invest Radiol 1998;33(1):1–5.
29. Bartolucci F, Cecarini M, Gabrielli G, Abbiati R, Barberio M, Busilacchi P. Reazioni tardive a un mezzo di contrasto radiologico (Iopamidolo-Bracco). Studio prospettico. [Late reactions to a radiologic contrast media (Iopamidol-Bracco). Prospective study.] Radiol Med (Torino) 2000;100(4):273–8.
30. Hosoya T, Yamaguchi K, Akutsu T, Mitsuhashi Y, Kondo S, Sugai Y, Adachi M. Delayed adverse reactions to iodinated contrast media and their risk factors. Radiat Med 2000;18(1):39–45.
31. Pohly JP. Onset of late adverse drug reactions to dimeric non-ionic contrast media: iotrolan, iodixanol. Pharmacoepidemiol Drug Saf 1998;7(Suppl 1):S18–22.
32. Rydberg J, Aspelin P, Charles J. Late adverse reactions observed retrospectively after use of monomeric and dimeric X-ray contrast media. Pharmacoepidemiol Drug Saf 1998;7(Suppl 1):S16–17.
33. Munechika H, Hiramatsu Y, Kudo S, Sugimura K, Hamada C, Yamaguchi K, Katayama H. Delayed adverse reactions to nonionic contrast medium (iohexol) in IV use: multicentric study. Acad Radiol 2002;9(Suppl 1):S69–71.
34. Kanny G, Marie B, Hoen B, Trechot P, Moneret-Vautrin DA. Delayed adverse reaction to sodium ioxaglic acid-meglumine. Eur J Dermatol 2001;11(2):134–7.
35. Spataro RF, Katzberg RW, Fischer HW, McMannis MJ. High-dose clinical urography with the low-osmolality contrast agent Hexabrix: comparison with a conventional contrast agent. Radiology 1987;162(1 Pt 1):9–14.
36. Lasser EC, Lyon SG. Inhibition of angiotensin-converting enzyme by contrast media. I. In vitro findings. Invest Radiol 1990;25(6):698–702.
37. Mironidou M, Katsimba D, Kokkas B, Kaitartzis C, Karamanos G, Christopoulos S. Effetti in vivo dello iohexolo e del diatrizoato sull'attivita plasmatica umana dell'acetil- e della butiril-colinesterasi. [Effects in vivo of iohexol and diatrizoate on human plasma acetyl- and butyryl-cholinesterase activity.] Radiol Med (Torino) 2001;101 (3):183–6.
38. Lasser EC. Metabolic basis of contrast material toxicity: status 1971. Am J Roentgenol 1971;113:415.
39. Katayama H, Tanaka T. Clinical survey of adverse reactions to contrast media. Invest Radiol 1988;23 (Suppl 1):S88–9.
40. Stejskal V, Nilsson R, Grepe A. Immunologic basis for adverse reactions to radiographic contrast media. Acta Radiol 1990;31(6):605–12.
41. Thomsen HS, Morcos SK, Almen T, Bellin MF, Clause W, Grenier N, Hietala SO, Jakobsen JA, Krestin GP, Lautrou J, Stacul F, Vik H, Webb JAW; Contrast Media Safety Committee of the European Society of Urogenital Radiology (ESUR). Prevention of generalized reactions to CM. Acad Radiol 2002;9(Suppl 2):S433–5.
42. Dunnick NR, Cohan RH. Cost, corticosteroids, and contrast media. Am J Roentgenol 1994;162(3):527–9.
43. Greenberger PA, Patterson R. The prevention of immediate generalized reactions to radiocontrast media in high-risk patients. J Allergy Clin Immunol 1991;87(4):867–72.
44. Bush WH, McClennan BL, Swanson DP. Contrast media reactions: prediction, prevention, and treatment. Postgrad Radiol 1993;13:137–47.
45. Melki P, Mugel T, Clero B, Helenon O, Belin X, Moreau JF. Parotidite aiguë bilatérale. Prodrome isolé d'un choc anaphylactoïde après injection de produit de contraste iodé. [Acute bilateral parotitis. Isolated prodrome to anaphylactoid shock following injection of iodinated contrast media.] J Radiol 1993;74(1):51–4.
46. Soyer PH, Levesque M, Rouleau P. Prevention of adverse reactions to intravascular contrast media. Int J Risk Saf Med 1991;2:21–8.
47. Glauser T, Savioz D, Grossholz M, Lopez-Liuchi J, Robert J, Huber O, Morel P. Venous intravasation of Gastrografin: a serious but underestimated complication. Eur J Surg 1999;165(3):274–7.
48. Tuladhar R, Daftary A, Patole SK, Whitehall JS. Oral gastrografin in neonates: a note of caution. Int J Clin Pract 1999;53(7):565.
49. Hartnell GG, Gates J, Underhill J. Implementing HCFA guidelines on appropriate use of nonionic contrast agents for diagnostic arteriography: effects on complication rates and management costs. Acad Radiol 1998;5(Suppl 2):S359–61.
50. Zeman RK. Disseminated intravascular coagulation following intravenous pyelography. Invest Radiol 1977;12(2):203–4.

51. Johnson LW, Krone R. Cardiac catheterization 1991: a report of the Registry of the Society for Cardiac Angiography and Interventions (SCA&I). Cathet Cardiovasc Diagn 1993;28(3):219–20.
52. Gross-Fengels W, Beyer D, Fischbach R, Lanfermann H. Akute Nebenwirkungen und Komplikationen der zentralvenösen DSA. Ergebnisse bei 2600 Untersuchungen. [Acute adverse effects and complications of central venous digital subtraction angiography (DSA). Results of 2,600 studies.] Med Klin (Munich) 1991;86(11):561–5.
53. Flinck A, Gottfridsson B. Experiences with iohexol and iodixanol during cardioangiography in an unselected patient population. Int J Cardiol 2001;80(2–3):143–51.
54. Roriz R, de Gevigney G, Finet G, Nantois-Collet C, Borch KW, Amiel M, Beaune J. Comparaison de l'iodixanol (Visipaque) et de l'ioxaglate (Hexabrix) en coronaro-ventriculographie: une étude randomisée en double aveugle. [Comparison of iodixanol (Visipaque) and ioxaglate (Hexabrix) in coronary angiography and ventriculography: a double-blind randomized study.] J Radiol 1999; 80(7):727–32.
55. Spitzer S, Munster W, Sternitzky R, Bach R, Jung F. Influence of iodixanol-270 and iopentol-150 on the microcirculation in man: influence of viscosity on capillary perfusion. Clin Hemorheol Microcirc 1999;20(1):49–55.
56. Burton PR, Jarmolowski E, Raineri F, Buist MD, Wriedt CH. A severe, late reaction to radiological contrast media mimicking a sepsis syndrome. Australas Radiol 1999;43(3):360–2.
57. Mitsumori M, Hayakawa K, Abe M. ECG changes during cerebral angiography; a comparison of low osmolality contrast media. Eur J Radiol 1991;13(1):55–8.
58. Wishart DL. Complications in vertebral angiography as compared to non-vertebral cerebral angiography in 447 studies. Am J Roentgenol Radium Ther Nucl Med 1971;113(3):527–37.
59. Flinck A, Selin K. Vectorcardiographic changes during cardioangiography with iodixanol and ioxaglate. Int J Cardiol 2000;76(2–3):173–80.
60. Matthai WH Jr, Hirshfeld JW Jr. Choice of contrast agents for cardiac angiography: review and recommendations based on clinically important distinctions. Cathet Cardiovasc Diagn 1991;22(4):278–89.
61. Baath L, Almen T, Oksendal A. Cardiac effects from addition of sodium ions to nonionic contrast media for coronary arteriography. An investigation of the isolated rabbit heart. Invest Radiol 1990;25(Suppl 1):S137–40.
62. Snyder CF, Formanek A, Frech RS, Amplatz K. The role of sodium in promoting ventricular arrhythmia during selective coronary arteriography. Am J Roentgenol Radium Ther Nucl Med 1971;113(3):567–71.
63. Druck MN, Johnstone DE, Staniloff H, McLaughlin PR. Coronary artery spasm as a manifestation of anaphylactoid reaction to iodinated contrast material. Can Med Assoc J 1981;125(10):1133–5.
64. Altun A, Ozbay G. Effects of ionic versus non-ionic contrast agents on dispersion of ventricular repolarization. Turk Kardiyol Dernegi Ars 1998;26:362–7.
65. Wiggins J, Beckmann R, Weinmann HJ, Lehr R. Electrocardiographic effects of diagnostic imaging agents. Acad Radiol 2002;9(Suppl 2):S444–6.
66. Lesiak M, Grajek S, Pyda M, Skorupski W, Mitowski P, Cieslinski A. Percutaneous transluminal coronary angioplasty: the influence of non-ionic and high osmolar ionic contrast media on the results and complication of the procedure. Kardiol Pol 1999;50:311–21.
67. Fukuda N, Shinohara K, Shimohakamada Y, Cochran ST, Bomyea K. Fatal cardiac arrest during infusion of nonionic contrast media in a patient with essential thrombocythemia. Am J Roentgenol 2002;178(3):765–6.
68. Richardson P, Crosby EH, Bean HA, Dexter D. Pulmonary oil deposition in patients subjected to lymphography: detection by thoracic photoscan and sputum examination. Can Med Assoc J 1966;94(21):1086–91.
69. Fraimow W, Wallace S, Greening RR, Cathcart RT. Pulmonary function studies. Cancer Chemother Rep 1968;52(1):99–105.
70. Hallgrimsson J, Clouse ME. Pulmonary oil emboli after lymphography. Arch Pathol 1965;80(4):426–30.
71. Ono K, Haraguchi M, Kimura M, Fujii K, Matsuzaki M. A case of survival from severe non-cardiac pulmonary edema caused by non-ionic contrast media. Respir Circ 2000;48:193–7.
72. Ansell G. Adverse reactions to contrast agents. Scope of problem. Invest Radiol 1970;5(6):374–91.
73. Machiels JP, Evrard P, Dive A, Bulpa P, Installe E. Venovenous ECMO in life-threatening radiocontrast mediated-ARDS. Intensive Care Med 1999;25(5):546.
74. Donnelly LF, Frush DP, Frush KS. Aspirated contrast material contributing to respiratory arrest in a pediatric trauma patient. Am J Roentgenol 1998;171(2):471–3.
75. Chiu CL, Gambach RR. Hypaque pulmonary edema. A case report. Radiology 1974;111(1):91–2.
76. Latchaw RE. The use of nonionic contrast agents in neuroangiography. A review of the literature and recommendations for clinical use. Invest Radiol 1993;28(Suppl 5):S55–9.
77. Numaguchi Y, Weems AM, Mizushima A, Keating J, Rege AB, Mather FJ, Rice JC. Myelography with metrizamide: effect of contrast removal on side effects. AJNR Am J Neuroradiol 1986;7(3):498–501.
78. Rosati G, Leto di Priolo S, Tirone P. Serious or fatal complications after inadvertent administration of ionic water-soluble contrast media in myelography. Eur J Radiol 1992;15(2):95–100.
79. Broadbridge AT, Bayliss SG, Firth R, Farrell G. Visual evoked response changes following intrathecal injection of water-soluble contrast media: a possible method of assessing neurotoxicity and a comparison of metrizamide and iopamidol. Clin Radiol 1984;35(5):371–3.
80. Gelmers HJ. Adverse side effects of metrizamide in myelography. Neuroradiology 1979;18(3):119–23.
81. Altschuler EM, Segal R. Generalized seizures following myelography with iohexol (Omnipaque). J Spinal Disord 1990;3(1):59–61.
82. Dalen K, Kerr HH, Wang AM, Olson RE, Wesolowski DP, Farah J. Seizure activity after iohexol myelography. Spine 1991;16(3):384.
83. Belanger JG, Blair IG, Elder AM, Fox AJ, Goldenberg MH, Mason JT, Nugent RA. Adult myelography with iohexol. Can Assoc Radiol J 1990;41(4):191–4.
84. Wallers K, Chaudhuri AKR, et al. Severe meningeal irritation after intrathecal injection of iopamidol. BMJ (Clin Res Ed) 1985;291:1688.
85. Glowinski J, Breuillard P, Delafolie A, Redondo A. Thrombose du sinus longitudinal supérieur après sacroradiculographie au iopamidol. [Thrombosis of the superior longitudinal sinus after sacculoradiculography with iopamidol.] Rev Rhum Mal Osteoartic 1986;53(3):183.
86. Bell JA, Dowd TC, McIlwaine GG, Brittain GP. Postmyelographic abducent nerve palsy in association with the contrast agent iopamidol. J Clin Neuroophthalmol 1990;10(2):115–17.
87. Schuurman PR, Speelman JD, Ongerboer de Visser BW, Bosch DA. Acute encephalopathy after iohexol ventriculography in functional stereotaxy. Acta Neurochir (Wien) 1998;140(1):98–9.

88. Dangas G, Monsein LH, Laureno R, Peterson MA, Laird JR Jr, Satler LF, Mehran R, Leon MB. Transient contrast encephalopathy after carotid artery stenting. J Endovasc Ther 2001;8(2):111–13.
89. Ahlgren P. Long term side effects after myelography with watersoluble contrast media: Conturex, Conray Meglumin 282 and Dimer-X. Neuroradiology 1973;6(4):206–11.
90. Hansen EB, Fahrenkrug A, Praestholm J. Late meningeal effects of myelographic contrast media with special reference to metrizamide. Br J Radiol 1978;51(605):321–7.
91. Cissoko H, Lemesle F, Jonville-Bera AP, Autret-Leca E. Aseptic meningitis after iohexol myelography. Ann Pharmacother 2000;34(6):812–13.
92. Circular from the Netherlands Public Health Service to hospitals and specialists. Amipaque, 1979.
93. Mallat Z, Vassal T, Naouri JF, Prier A, Laredo JD, Offenstadt G. Aseptic meningoencephalitis after iopamidol myelography. Lancet 1991;338(8761):252.
94. Schlesinger JJ, Salit IE, McCormack G. Streptococcal meningitis after myelography. Arch Neurol 1982;39(9):576–7.
95. Mejlhede A. Et tilfaelde med universelle krampeanfald efter lumbal myelografi med metrizamid (Amipaque). [A case with generalized seizures after lumbar myelography with metrizamide (Amipaque).] Ugeskr Laeger 1979;141(40):2761–2.
96. Shikaura S, Momodani A, Sawada S. Delayed adverse reaction of non-ionic low-osmolality media; a case report that showed convulsion and tremor. Jpn J Clin Radiol 2002;47:359–61.
97. Pagani JJ, Hayman LA, Bigelow RH, Libshitz HI, Lepke RA. Prophylactic diazepam in prevention of contrast media-associated seizures in glioma patients undergoing cerebral computed tomography. Cancer 1984;54(10):2200–4.
98. Junck L, Marshall WH. Fatal brain edema after contrast-agent overdose. AJNR Am J Neuroradiol 1986;7(3):522–5.
99. Sticherling C, Berkefeld J, Auch-Schwelk W, Lanfermann H. Transient bilateral cortical blindness after coronary angiography. Lancet 1998;351(9102):570.
100. Boyes LA, Tew K. Cortical blindness after subclavian arteriography. Australas Radiol 2000;44(3):315–17.
101. Nakai Y, Hyodo A, Okazaki M, Shibata Y, Matsumaru Y, Nose T. [Transient cortical blindness and convulsion mimicking a hemorrhagic complication during embolization of the cerebellar AVM.] No Shinkei Geka 1999;27(3):249–53.
102. Parry R, Rees JR, Wilde P. Transient cortical blindness after coronary angiography. Br Heart J 1993;70(6):563–4.
103. Heckmann JG, Bernhard N, Lang CJ, Werner D. Hyperdensity of cortex with a swollen hemisphere: what happened? Arch Neurol 2002;59(1):149–50.
104. Mishkin MM, Baum S, Di Chiro G. Emergency treatment of angiography-induced paraplegia and tetraplegia. N Engl J Med 1973;288(22):1184–5.
105. Koehler PR. Complications of lymphography. Lymphology 1968;1(4):116–20.
106. Rasmussen KE. Retinal and cerebral fat emboli following lymphography with oily contrast media. Acta Radiol Diagn (Stockh) 1970;10(3):199–202.
107. Mesurolle B, Ariche M, Cohen D. Premedication before i.v. contrast-enhanced CT resulting in steroid-induced psychosis. Am J Roentgenol 2002;178(3):766–7.
108. Nyegaard and Co. Summarising notes from the Amipaque Symposium 1977.
109. Richert S, Sartor K, Holl B. Subclinical organic psychosyndromes on intrathecal injection of metrizamide for lumbar myelography. Neuroradiology 1979;18(4):177–84.
110. Iliopoulou A, Giannakopoulos G, Goutou P, Pagou H, Stamatelopoulos S. Visual hallucinations due to radiocontrast media. Report of two cases and review of the literature. Br J Clin Pharmacol 1999;47(2):226–7.
111. Hammeke TA, Haughton VM, Grogan JP, et al. A preliminary study of cognitive and affective alterations following intrathecal administration of iopamidol or metrizamide Invest Radiol 1984;19(Suppl):S268.
112. Jennett WB, Barker J, Fitch W, McDowall DG. Effect of anaesthesia on intracranial pressure in patients with space-occupying lesions. Lancet 1969;1(7585):61–4.
113. Brady AP, Hough DM, Lo R, Gill G. Transient global amnesia after cerebral angiography with iohexol. Can Assoc Radiol J 1993;44(6):450–2.
114. Astwood EB. Occurrence in the sera of certain patients of large amounts of a newly isolated iodine compound. Trans Assoc Am Physicians 1957;70:183–91.
115. Fairhurst BJ, Naqvi N. Hyperthyroidism after cholecystography. BMJ 1975;3(5984):630.
116. Giroux JD, Sizun J, Rubio S, Metz C, Montaud N, Guillois B, Alix D. Hypothyroïdie transitoire après opacification iodées des cathéters epicutanéocaves au réanimation néonatale. [Transient hypothyroidism after iodine opacification of epicutaneo-caval catheters in neonatal intensive care.] Arch Fr Pediatr 1993;50(3):273.
117. Fassbender WJ, Schluter S, Stracke H, Bretzel RG, Waas W, Tillmanns H. Schilddrusenfunktion nach gabe jodhaltigen Röntgenkontrastmittels bei Koronarangiographie—eine prospektive Untersuchung euthyreoten Patienten. [Thyroid function after iodine-containing contrast agent administration in coronary angiography: a prospective study of euthyroid patients.] Z Kardiol 2001;90(10):751–9.
118. Dembinski J, Arpe V, Kroll M, Hieronimi G, Bartmann P. Thyroid function in very low birthweight infants after intravenous administration of the iodinated contrast medium iopromide. Arch Dis Child Fetal Neonatal Ed 2000;82(3):F215–17.
119. Beckers EA, Strack van Schijndel RJ, Weijmer MC. A contrast crisis. Lancet 2000;356(9233):908.
120. van Guldener C, Blom DM, Lips P, Strack van Schijndel RJ. Hyperthyreoidie door jodiumhoudende rontgencontrastmiddelen. [Hyperthyroidism induced by iodinated roentgen contrast media.] Ned Tijdschr Geneeskd 1998;142(29):1641–4.
121. l'Allemand D, Gruters A, Beyer P, Weber B. Iodine in contrast agents and skin disinfectants is the major cause for hypothyroidism in premature infants during intensive care. Horm Res 1987;28(1):42–9.
122. Kelley WN. Uricosuria and X-ray contrast agents. N Engl J Med 1971;284(17):975–6.
123. Hayakawa K, Nakamura T, Shimizu Y. Iodinated contrast medium-induced potassium release: the effect of mixing ratios. Radiat Med 2002;20(4):195–9.
124. Kutt H, Milhorat TH, McDowell F. The effect of iodinized contrast media upon blood proteins, electrolytes, and red cells. Neurology 1963;13:492–9.
125. Stemerman M, Goldstein ML, Schulman PL. Pancytopenia associated with diatrizoate. NY State J Med 1971;71(11):1220–2.
126. Cohen LS, Kokko JP, Williams WH. Hemolysis and hemoglobinuria following angiography. Radiology 1969;92(2):329–32.
127. Losco P, Nash G, Stone P, Ventre J. Comparison of the effects of radiographic contrast media on dehydration and filterability of red blood cells from donors homozygous for hemoglobin A or hemoglobin S. Am J Hematol 2001;68(3):149–58.

128. Hysell JK, Hysell JW, Gray JM. Thrombocytopenic purpura following iopanoic acid ingestion. JAMA 1977;237(4):361–2.
129. Insausti CL, Lechin F, van der Dijs B. Severe thrombocytopenia following oral cholecystography with iocetamic acid. Am J Hematol 1983;14(3):285–8.
130. Stacher A. Schwerste Thrombopenie durch ein perorales trijodiertes Gallenkontrastmittel. [Severe thrombopenia due to a peroral triiodized bile contrast media.] Wien Klin Wochenschr 1966;78(16):286–8.
131. Ural AU, Beyan C, Yalcin A. Thrombocytopenia following intravenous iopamidol. Eur J Clin Pharmacol 1998;54(7):575–6.
132. Parvez Z, Moncada R, Messmore HL, Fareed J. Ionic and non-ionic contrast media interaction with anticoagulant drugs. Acta Radiol Diagn (Stockh) 1982;23(4):401–4.
133. Robertson HJE. Blood clot formation in angiographic syringes containing non-ionic media. Radiology 1927;162:621.
134. Gasperetti CM, Feldman MD, Burwell LR, Angello DA, Haugh KH, Owen RM, Powers ER. Influence of contrast media on thrombus formation during coronary angioplasty. J Am Coll Cardiol 1991;18(2):443–50.
135. Chronos NA, Goodall AH, Wilson DJ, Sigwart U, Buller NP. Profound platelet degranulation is an important side effect of some types of contrast media used in interventional cardiology. Circulation 1993;88(5 Pt 1): 2035–44.
136. Blann AD, Adams R, Ashleigh R, Naser S, Kirkpatrick U, McCollum CN. Changes in endothelial, leucocyte and platelet markers following contrast medium injection during angiography in patients with peripheral artery disease. Br J Radiol 2001;74(885):811–17.
137. Hoffman JJML, Tielbeek AV, Krause W. Haemostatic effects of low osmolar non-ionic and ionic contrast media: a double blind comparative study. Appl Radiol 2002;31(Suppl):113–21.
138. Idee JM, Corot C. Thrombotic risk associated with the use of iodinated contrast media in interventional cardiology: pathophysiology and clinical aspects. Appl Radiol 2002;31(Suppl):102–12.
139. Kraus B, Klemencic J. The histologic picture of lymph node up to 15 months after lymphography with Lipiodol UF. In: Ruttmann E, editor. Proceedings, International Symposium on Lymphology, Zurich, 1966. Stuttgart: Georg Thieme Verlag, 1967:308.
140. Malekianpour M, Bonan R, Lesperance J, Gosselin G, Hudon G, Doucet S, Laurier J, Duval D. Comparison of ionic and nonionic low osmolar contrast media in relation to thrombotic complications of angioplasty in patients with unstable angina. Am Heart J 1998;135(6 Pt 1):1067–75.
141. De Meester A, Six C, Lismonde M, Lambot D, Vermonden J. Fatal disseminated intravascular coagulation during arteriography. Reanim Urgences 2000;9:141–4.
142. Navani S, Taylor CE, Kaufman SA, Parlee RH. Evanescent enlargement of salivary glands following triiodinated contrast media. Br J Radiol 1972;45(529):19–20.
143. Polger M, Kuhlman JE, Hansen FC 3rd, Fishman EK. Computed tomography of angioedema of small bowel due to reaction to radiographic contrast medium. J Comput Assist Tomogr 1988;12(6):1044–6.
144. Sewell RA, Killen DA, Foster JH. Small bowel injury by angiographic contrast medium. Surgery 1968;64(2):459–65.
145. Falchuk KR, Falchuk ZM. A complication of angiography in chronic renal failure; the acute abdomen. Am J Gastroenterol 1974;61(3):223–5.
146. Koussidis GA, Koussidis A. Preoperative bowel preparation with meglumine and sodium diatrizoate (Gastrografin): a prospective randomised comparison. Eur J Surg 2001;167(12):899–902.
147. Kircher MF, Kihiczak D, Rhea JT, Novelline RA, Maglinte DDT. Safety of colon contrast material in (helical) CT examination of patients with suspected diverticulitis. Emerg Radiol 2001;8:94–8.
148. Weinstein GS, O'Dorisio TM, Joehl RJ, Pokorney B, Koch KL. Exacerbation of diarrhea after iodinated contrast agents in a patient with VIPoma. Dig Dis Sci 1985;30(6):588–92.
149. Davies NP, Williams JA. Tubeless vagotomy and pyloroplasty and the "Gastrografin test". Am J Surg 1971;122(3):368–70.
150. Godson C, Ryan MP, Brady HR, Bourke S, FitzGerald MX. Acute hypomagnesaemia complicating the treatment of meconium ileus equivalent in cystic fibrosis. Scand J Gastroenterol Suppl 1988;143:148–50.
151. Seltzer SE, Jones B. Cecal perforation associated with Gastrografin enema. Am J Roentgenol 1978;130(5):997–8.
152. Creteur V, Douglas D, Galante M, Margulis AR. Inflammatory colonic changes produced by contrast material. Radiology 1983;147(1):77–8.
153. Leonidas JC, Burry VF, Fellows RA, Beatty EC. Possible adverse effect of methylglucamine diatrizoate compounds on the bowel of newborn infants with meconium ileus. Radiology 1976;121(3 Pt 1):693–6.
154. Sutherland LR, Edwards LA, Medline A, Wilkinson RW, Connon JJ. Meglumine iodipamide (Cholografin) hepatotoxicity. Ann Intern Med 1977;86(4):437–9.
155. Dohmen JP, Lemmens JA, Lamers JJ. A double-blind comparison of meglumine iotroxate (Biliscopin) and meglumine iodoxamate (Cholovue). Diagn Imaging 1981;50(6):305–8.
156. Re G, Lanzarini C, Melandri R. Liver injury after contrast-enhanced, computed tomography with iopromide. J Toxicol Clin Toxicol 1998;36(3):261–2.
157. Parasher VK, Romain K, Sukumar R, Jordan J. Can ERCP contrast agents cause pseudomicrolithiasis? Their effect on the final outcome of bile analysis in patients with suspected microlithiasis. Gastrointest Endosc 2000;51(4 Pt 1):401–4.
158. Muller K, Jorge A. Rezidive akuter Pankreatitis nach Cholezystographie. [Recurrent acute pancreatitis following cholecystography.] Med Klin 1965;60(42):1693–7.
159. Goebel C, Hardt P, Doppl W, Temme H, Hackstein N, Klor HU. Frequency of pancreatitis after endoscopic retrograde cholangiopancreatography with iopromid or iotrolan: a randomized trial. Eur Radiol 2000;10(4):677–80.
160. Schreiner GE. Nephrotoxicity and diagnostic agents. JAMA 1966;196(5):413–15.
161. Morcos SK. Contrast media-induced nephrotoxicity—questions and answers. Br J Radiol 1998;71(844):357–65.
162. Berns AS. Nephrotoxicity of contrast media. Kidney Int 1989;36(4):730–40.
163. Morcos SK, Epstein FH, Haylor J, Dobrota M. Aspects of contrast media nephrotoxicity. Eur J Radiol 1996;23(3):178–84.
164. Love L, Johnson MS, Bresler ME, Nelson JE, Olson MC, Flisak ME. The persistent computed tomography nephrogram: its significance in the diagnosis of contrast-associated nephrotoxicity. Br J Radiol 1994;67(802):951–7.
165. Jakobsen JA, Lundby B, Kristoffersen DT, Borch KW, Hald JK, Berg KJ. Evaluation of renal function with delayed CT after injection of nonionic monomeric and dimeric contrast media in healthy volunteers. Radiology 1992;182(2):419–24.
166. Kohli HS, Bhaskaran MC, Muthukumar T, Thennarasu K, Sud K, Jha V, Gupta KL, Sakhuja V.

Treatment-related acute renal failure in the elderly: a hospital-based prospective study. Nephrol Dial Transplant 2000;15(2):212–17.
167. Vassiliu P, Sava J, Toutouzas KG, Velmahos GC. Is contrast as bad as we think? Renal function after angiographic embolization of injured patients. J Am Coll Surg 2002;194(2):142–6.
168. Chalmers N, Jackson RW. Comparison of iodixanol and iohexol in renal impairment. Br J Radiol 1999;72(859):701–3.
169. Donadio C, Lucchesi A, Ardini M, Tramonti G, Chella P, Magagnini E, Bianchi C. Renal effects of cardiac angiography with different low-osmolar contrast media. Ren Fail 2001;23(3–4):385–96.
170. Deray G, Bellin MF, Zaim S, Raymond F, Grellet J, Jacobs C. Evaluation of the renal tolerance of Xenetix in patients with chronic renal failure. Nephron 1998;80(2):240.
171. Stouffer GA, Sheahan RG, Lenihan DJ, Agrawal M, Stouffer GA. Cardiology Grand Rounds from The University of North Carolina at Chapel Hill. Contrast induced nephropathy after angiography. Am J Med Sci 2002;323(5):252–8.
172. Kolonko A, Kokot F, Wiecek A. Contrast-associated nephropathy—old clinical problem and new therapeutic perspectives. Nephrol Dial Transplant 1998;13(3):803–6.
173. Lorusso V, Taroni P, Alvino S, Spinazzi A. Pharmacokinetics and safety of iomeprol in healthy volunteers and in patients with renal impairment or end-stage renal disease requiring hemodialysis. Invest Radiol 2001;36(6):309–16.
174. Najjar M, Hamad A, Salameh M, Agarwal A, Feinfeld DA. The risk of radiocontrast nephropathy in patients with cirrhosis. Ren Fail 2002;24(1):11–18.
175. Aspelin P, Aubry P, Fransson SG, Strasser R, Willenbrock R, Berg KJ; Nephrotoxicity in High-Risk Patients Study of Iso-Osmolar and Low-Osmolar Non-Ionic Contrast Media Study Investigators. Nephrotoxic effects in high-risk patients undergoing angiography. N Engl J Med 2003;348(6):491–9.
176. Stark FR, Coburn JW. Renal failure following methylglucamine diatrizoate (Renografin) aortography: report of a case with unilateral renal artery stenosis. J Urol 1966; 96(6):848–51.
177. Khan MA, Pillay VK, Wang F. Peripheral arteriography causing acute renal failure. S Afr Med J 1972;46(17):522.
178. Kovnat PJ, Lin KY, Popky G. Azotemia and nephrogenic diabetes insipidus after arteriography. Radiology 1973;108(3):541–2.
179. Haller C, Meyer M, Scheele T, Koch A, Forssmann WG, Kubler W. Radiocontrast-induced natriuresis associated with increased urinary urodilatin excretion. J Intern Med 1998;243(2):155–62.
180. Donadio C, Tramonti G, Lucchesi A, Giordani R, Lucchetti A, Bianchi C. Gamma-glutamyltransferase is a reliable marker for tubular effects of contrast media. Ren Fail 1998;20(2):319–24.
181. Duan SB, Wu HW, Luo JA, Liu FY. Assessment of renal function in the early stages of nephrotoxicity induced by iodinated contrast media. Nephron 1999;83(2):122–5.
182. Hetzel GR, May P, Hollenbeck M, Voiculescu A, Modder U, Grabensee B. Assessment of radiocontrast media induced renal vasoconstriction by color coded duplex sonography. Ren Fail 2001;23(1):77–83.
183. Mueller C, Buerkle G, Buettner HJ, Petersen J, Perruchoud AP, Eriksson U, Marsch S, Roskamm H. Prevention of contrast media-associated nephropathy: randomized comparison of 2 hydration regimens in 1620 patients undergoing coronary angioplasty. Arch Intern Med 2002;162(3):329–36.
184. Lehnert T, Keller E, Gondolf K, Schaffner T, Pavenstadt H, Schollmeyer P. Effect of haemodialysis after contrast medium administration in patients with renal insufficiency. Nephrol Dial Transplant 1998;13 (2):358–62.
185. Berger ED, Bader BD, Bosker J, Risler T, Erley CM. Kontrastmittelinduziertes Nierenversagen lasst sich durch Hämodialyse nicht verhindern. [Contrast media-induced kidney failure cannot be prevented by hemodialysis.] Dtsch Med Wochenschr 2001;126(7):162–6.
186. Vogt B, Ferrari P, Schonholzer C, Marti HP, Mohaupt M, Wiederkehr M, Cereghetti C, Serra A, Huynh-Do U, Uehlinger D, Frey FJ. Prophylactic hemodialysis after radiocontrast media in patients with renal insufficiency is potentially harmful. Am J Med 2001;111(9):692–8.
187. Morcos SK, Thomsen HS, Webb JA; Contrast Media Safety Committee of the European Society of Urogenital Radiology (ESUR). Dialysis and contrast media. Eur Radiol 2002;12(12):3026–30.
188. Morcos SK, Thomsen HS, Webb JAW. Contrast-media-induced nephrotoxicity: a consensus report. Appl Radiol 2002;31(Suppl):62–74.
189. Tepel M, Zidek W. Acetylcysteine and contrast media nephropathy. Curr Opin Nephrol Hypertens 2002;11(5):503–6.
190. Tepel M, van der Giet M, Schwarzfeld C, Laufer U, Liermann D, Zidek W. Prevention of radiographic-contrast-agent-induced reductions in renal function by acetylcysteine. N Engl J Med 2000;343(3):180–4.
191. Esnault VL. Radiocontrast media-induced nephrotoxicity in patients with renal failure: rationale for a new double-blind, prospective, randomized trial testing calcium channel antagonists. Nephrol Dial Transplant 2002;17(8):1362–4.
192. Hans SS, Hans BA, Dhillon R, Dmuchowski C, Glover J. Effect of dopamine on renal function after arteriography in patients with pre-existing renal insufficiency. Am Surg 1998;64(5):432–6.
193. Spoto S, Galluzzo S, De Galasso L, Zobel B, Navajas MF. Prevenzione della necrosi tubulare acuta da somministrazione di mezzi di contrasto radiologico non ionici. [Prevention of acute tubular necrosis caused by the administration of non-ionic radiologic contrast media.] Clin Ter 2000;151(5):323–7.
194. Generali J, Cada DJ. Fenoldopam: prevention of contrast media nephrotoxicity. Hosp Pharm 2002;37:75–80.
195. Kini AS, Mitre CA, Kim M, Kamran M, Reich D, Sharma SK. A protocol for prevention of radiographic contrast nephropathy during percutaneous coronary intervention: effect of selective dopamine receptor agonist fenoldopam. Catheter Cardiovasc Interv 2002;55(2):169–73.
196. Wang A, Holcslaw T, Bashore TM, Freed MI, Miller D, Rudnick MR, Szerlip H, Thames MD, Davidson CJ, Shusterman N, Schwab SJ. Exacerbation of radiocontrast nephrotoxicity by endothelin receptor antagonism. Kidney Int 2000;57(4):1675–80.
197. Kapoor A, Kumar S, Gulati S, Gambhir S, Sethi RS, Sinha N. The role of theophylline in contrast-induced nephropathy: a case-control study. Nephrol Dial Transplant 2002;17(11):1936–41.
198. Huber W, Ilgmann K, Page M, Hennig M, Schweigart U, Jeschke B, Lutilsky L, Weiss W, Salmhofer H, Classen M. Effect of theophylline on contrast material-nephropathy in patients with chronic renal insufficiency: controlled, randomized, double-blinded study. Radiology 2002;223 (3):772–9.
199. Allaqaband S, Tumuluri R, Malik AM, Gupta A, Volkert P, Shalev Y, Bajwa TK. Prospective randomized study of N-acetylcysteine, fenoldopam, and saline for

prevention of radiocontrast-induced nephropathy. Catheter Cardiovasc Interv 2002;57(3):279–83.

200. Naldi L, Conforti A, Venegoni M, Troncon MG, Caputi A, Ghiotto E, Cocci A, Moretti U, Velo G, Leone R. Cutaneous reactions to drugs. An analysis of spontaneous reports in four Italian regions. Br J Clin Pharmacol 1999;48(6):839–46.
201. Watanabe H, Sueki H, Nakada T, Akiyama M, Iijima M. Multiple fixed drug eruption caused by iomeprol (Iomeron), a nonionic contrast medium. Dermatology 1999;198(3):291–4.
202. Vaillant L, Pengloan J, Blanchier D, De Muret A, Lorette G. Iododerma and acute respiratory distress with leucocytoclastic vasculitis following the intravenous injection of contrast medium. Clin Exp Dermatol 1990;15(3):232–3.
203. Miranda-Romero A, Sanchez-Sambucety P, Esquivias Gomez JI, Martinez Fernandez M, Bajo del Pozo C, Aragoneses Fraile H, Garcia-Munoz M. Vegetating iododerma with fatal outcome. Dermatology 1999;198 (3):295–7.
204. Brockow K, Becker EW, Worret WI, Ring J. Late skin test reactions to radiocontrast medium. J Allergy Clin Immunol 1999;104(5):1107–8.
205. Anonymous. Cutaneous drug reaction case reports: from the world literature. Am J Clin Dermatol 2002;3(2):133–9.
206. Brockow K, Kiehn M, Kleinheinz A, Vieluf D, Ring J. Positive skin tests in late reactions to radiographic contrast media. Allerg Immunol (Paris) 1999;31(2):49–51.
207. Gall H, Pillekamp H, Peter RU. Late-type allergy to the X-ray contrast medium Solutrast (iopamidol). Contact Dermatitis 1999;40(5):248–50.
208. Erdmann S, Roos T, Merk HF, Grussendorf-Conen EII, Rubben A, Dahl T. Delayed hypersensitivity reaction to the non-ionic contrast medium ioversol. H G Z Hautkr 2000;75:169–71.
209. Rosado A, Canto G, Veleiro B, Rodriguez J. Toxic epidermal necrolysis after repeated injections of iohexol. Am J Roentgenol 2001;176(1):262–3.
210. Shah AM, Hutchison SJ. The Koebner phenomenon—an unusual localization of a contrast reaction. Clin Radiol 1990;42(2):136–7.
211. Benson PM, Giblin WJ, Douglas DM. Transient, nonpigmenting fixed drug eruption caused by radiopaque contrast media. J Am Acad Dermatol 1990;23(2 Pt 2):379–81.
212. Rinker MH, Sangueza OP, Davis LS. Reticulated purpura occurring with contrast medium after hysterosalpingography. Br J Dermatol 1998;138(5):919–20.
213. Redman HC. Dermatitis as a complication of lymphangiography. Radiology 1966;86(2):323–6.
214. Bork K, Hoede N. Paraneoplastische multizentrische Reticulohistiozytose: durch jodhaltige Röntgen-Kontrastmittel ausgelöst und provozierbar. [Paraneoplastic multicentric reticulohistiocytosis: induced and inductable by iodine containing x-ray contrast media.] Z Hautkr 1985;60(9):729–36.
215. Stinchcombe SJ, Davies P. Acute toxic myopathy: a delayed adverse effect of intravenous urography with iopamidol 370. Br J Radiol 1989;62(742):949–50.
216. Dewachter P, Mouton-Faivre C. Reactions sévères avec les produits de contraste iodes: l'anaphylaxie est-elle responsable? [Severe reactions to iodinated contrast agents: is anaphylaxis responsible?] J Radiol 2001;82(9 Pt 1):973–7.
217. Wang DY, Forslund C, Persson U, Wiholm BE. Drug-attributed anaphylaxis. Pharmacoepidemiol Drug Saf 1998;7(4):269–74.
218. Kuwano A, Sugai T, Mochida K. Systemic contact dermatitis induced by oral contrast media for the gallbladder. Skin Res 1993;35(Suppl 16):114–20.
219. Kaude J. Angiografi med jodamid—klinisk provning av ett trijoderat kontrastmedel. [Angiography with iodamide—clinical test of a triiodide contrast medium.] Lakartidningen 1971;68(Suppl 4):42–8.
220. Ansell G, Wilkins RA. Complications in Diagnostic Imaging. 2nd ed. Oxford: Blackwell, 1987.
221. Ridley LJ. Allergic reactions to oral iodinated contrast agents: reactions to oral contrast. Australas Radiol 1998;42(2):114–17.
222. Glover JR, Thomas BM. Case report: severe adverse reaction to oral iohexol. Clin Radiol 1991;44(2):137–8.
223. Lossef SV, Barth KH. Severe delayed hypotensive reaction after ethiodol lymphangiography despite premedication. Am J Roentgenol 1993;161(2):417–18.
224. Zuckerman GB, Riess PL, Patel L, Constantinescu AR, Rosenfeld DL. Development of a life-threatening anaphylactoid reaction following administration of ioversol in a child. Pediatr Radiol 1999;29(4):295–7.
225. Brockow K, Vieluf D, Puschel K, Grosch J, Ring J. Increased postmortem serum mast cell tryptase in a fatal anaphylactoid reaction to nonionic radiocontrast medium. J Allergy Clin Immunol 1999;104(1):237–8.
226. Vavricka SR, Halter J, Furrer K, Wolfensberger U, Schanz U. Contrast media triggering cutaneous graft-versus-host disease. Bone Marrow Transplant 2002;29(11):899–901.
227. Romano A, Artesani MC, Andriolo M, Viola M, Pettinato R, Vecchioli-Scaldazza A. Effective prophylactic protocol in delayed hypersensitivity to contrast media: report of a case involving lymphocyte transformation studies with different compounds. Radiology 2002;225(2):466–70.
228. Crosby DJ, Storm AH. Malarial relapse induced by intravenous cholangiography. Report of two cases. Arch Intern Med 1966;118(1):79–80.
229. Mozley PD. Malignant hyperthermia following intravenous iodinated contrast media. Report of a fatal case. Diagn Gynecol Obstet 1981;3(1):81–6.
230. Lalli AF. Contrast media deaths. Australas Radiol 1984;28(2):133–5.
231. Burchardt P, Flenker H, Schoop HJ. Todlicher Kontrastmittelzwischenfall bei unbehandeltem Morbus Waldenström. [Fatal contrast medium reaction in untreated Waldenstrom's disease.] Dtsch Med Wochenschr 1981;106(38):1223–5.
232. Bauer K, Tragl KH, Bauer G, Vycudilik W, Hocker P. Intravasale Denaturierung von Plasmaproteinen bei einer IgM-Paraproteinamie, ausgelost durch ein intravenos verabreichtes lebergangiges Rontgenkontrastmittel. [Intravascular denaturation of plasma proteins in a patient with IgM paraproteinaemia following the intravenous administration of a bile-excreted X-ray contrast medium.] Wien Klin Wochenschr 1974;86(24):766–9.
233. Nunez ME, Sinues B. Cytogenic effects of diatrizoate and ioxaglate on patients undergoing excretory urography. Invest Radiol 1990;25(6):692–7.
234. Engeset A. Dissemination of tumor cells by lymphangiography. In: Ruttmann E, editor. Proceedings, International Symposium on Lymphology, Zurich, 1966. Stuttgart: Georg Thieme Verlag, 1967:308.
235. Desmons M, Ramioul H. Essaimage néoplasique périlymphatique après lymphographie dans un cas de tumeur mélanique du pied. [Perilymphatic neoplastic spreading after lymphography in a case of melanotic tumor of the foot.] J Radiol Electrol Med Nucl 1964;45: 703–5.
236. Bona G, Zaffaroni M, Perona A. Neonatal transient hypothyroidism after excess iodide exposition by amniofetography. Panminerva Med 1988;30(3):192–3.
237. Storm W. Transitorische Hypothyreose des Neugeborenen nach Amniofetographie mit jodhaltigem

Kontrastmittel. [Transitory hypothyroidism of the newborn infant following amniofetography with an iodine-containing contrast medium.] Geburtshilfe Frauenheilkd 1986;46(3):185–6.
238. Miething R. Transitorische Hypothyreose bei Fruh- und Neugeborenen nach Amniofetografie wahrend der Schwangerschaft. [Transient hypothyroidism after amniofetography in preterm and newborn infants.] Klin Padiatr 1981;193(5):372–4.
239. Stubbe P, Heidemann P, Schurnbrand P, Ulbrich R. Transient congenital hypothyroidism after amniofetography. Eur J Pediatr 1980;135(1):97–9.
240. Lindinger A, Huhn W. Hypothyreote konnatale Struma nach Amniofetographie. [Hypothyreotic connatal struma after amniofetography.] Z Geburtshilfe Perinatol 1979;183(6):461–4.
241. Crepin G, Delahousse G, Decocq J, Delcroix M, Caquant F, Querleu D, Ahmed TL. Incidence de l'amniofoetographie sur la thyroide foetale. [The effect of amniofetography on the fetal thyroid.] J Gynecol Obstet Biol Reprod (Paris) 1978;7(8):1405–13.
242. Rodesch F, Camus M, Ermans AM, Dodion J, Delange F. Amniofoetographie et fonction thyroidienne foetale. [Adverse effect of amniofetography on fetal thyroid function.] Ann Endocrinol (Paris) 1978;39(2):145–6.
243. Maria B, Denavit MF, Leger A, Barrat J, Sureau C. Hypothyroidie foetale: une complication de l'amniofoetographie. A propos de 3 observations. [Fetal hypothyroidism: a complication of amniofetography. Apropos of 3 cases.] J Gynecol Obstet Biol Reprod (Paris) 1977;6 (7):951–62.
244. Denavit MF, Lecointre C, Mallet E, de Menibus C, Rossier A. Un accident de l'amniofoetographie: l'hypothyroidie. [A complication of amniofetography: hypothyroidism.] Arch Fr Pediatr 1977;34(6):543–51.
245. Leger FA, Denavit MF, Maria B, Savoie JC. Hypothyroidie neo-natale induite par l'iode apres amniofoetographie. [Neonatal hypothyroidism induced by iodine after amniofetography.] Nouv Presse Méd 1977;6(7):563–4.
246. Rodesch F, Camus M, Ermans AM, Dodion J, Delange F. Adverse effect of amniofetography on fetal thyroid function. Am J Obstet Gynecol 1976;126(6):723–6.
247. Shapiro R. The effect of maternal ingestion of iophenoxic acid with serum protein bound iodine of the progeny. N Engl J Med 1961;264:378.
248. De Jonge GA. Vruchtbeschadiging door farmaca. [Fetal damage caused by pharmaceutical agents.] Folia Med Neerl 1965;51:65–72.
249. Jankowski JJ, Feingold M, Gellis SS. Effect of maternal ingestion of iophenoxic acid (Teridax) on protein-bound iodine: report of a family. J Pediatr 1967;70(3):436–8.
250. Thomas M, Peedicayil J, Koshi T, Korah I. Adverse reactions to radiocontrast media in an Indian population. Br J Radiol 1999;72(859):648–52.
251. Ansell G, Tweedie MC, West CR, Evans P, Couch L. The current status of reactions to intravenous contrast media. Invest Radiol 1980;15(Suppl 6):S32–9.
252. Rohner G, Rautenburg HW, Hopfner B. Transiente Hypothyreose bei Sauglingen nach Röntgenkontrastmitteln. [Transient hypothyroidism in infants following administration of roentgen contrast media.] Rontgenpraxis 1983;36(9):301–4.
253. Oide S, Yamaguchi H, Niizu N, Takahashi S, Takashima K. [Transient neonatal hypothyroidism probably due to contrast media used in fetal radiography.] Horumon To Rinsho 1983;31(Suppl):76–9.
254. Dacher J, Sirinelli D, Boscq M, Hassan M, Garel C, Chateil JF, Amar C. Iodixanol in paediatric excretory urography: efficiency and safety compared to iohexol. Pediatr Radiol 1998;28(2):112–14.
255. Wright NB, Carty HM, Sprigg A, Kampenes VB, Friis M, Petersen KK, Stake G, Klaveness AJ. Iodixanol in paediatric gastrointestinal imaging: safety and efficacy comparison with iohexol. Br J Radiol 2002;75(890):127–35.
256. Kuwatsuru R, Katayama H. Evaluation of lotrolan after oral application to neonates, infants, and children: Japanese experience. Acad Radiol 2002;9(Suppl 1):S175–7.
257. Celik I, Hoppe M, Lorenz W, Sitter H, Ishaque N, Jungraithmayr W, Kapp B, Schmiedel E, Klose KJ. Randomised study comparing a non-ionic with an ionic contrast medium in patients with malignancies: first answer with a new diagnostic approach. Inflamm Res 1999;48 (Suppl 1):S47–8.
258. Pfister RC, Hutter AM Jr. Cardiovascular radiology. Cardiac alterations during intravenous urography. Invest Radiol 1980;15(Suppl 6):S239–42.
259. Hesselink JR, Hayman LA, Chung KJ, McGinnis BD, Davis KR, Taveras JM. Myocardial ischemia during intravenous DSA in patients with cardiac disease. Radiology 1984;153(3):577–82.
260. Eliashiv S, Wirguin I, Brenner T, Argov Z. Aggravation of human and experimental myasthenia gravis by contrast media. Neurology 1990;40(10):1623–5.
261. Chagnac Y, Hadani M, Goldhammer Y. Myasthenic crisis after intravenous administration of iodinated contrast agent. Neurology 1985;35(8):1219–20.
262. Shimura H, Takazawa K, Endo T, Tawata M, Onaya T. T4-thyroid storm after CT-scan with iodinated contrast medium. J Endocrinol Invest 1990;13(1):73–6.
263. Rao AK, Thompson R, Durlacher L, James F. Angiographic contrast agent-induced acute hemolysis in a patient with hemoglobin SC disease. Arch Intern Med 1985;145(4):759–60.
264. Spinazzi A, Ceriati S, Pianezzola P, Lorusso V, Luzzani F, Fouillet X, Alvino S, Rummeny EJ. Safety and pharmacokinetics of a new liposomal liver-specific contrast agent for CT: results of clinical testing in nonpatient volunteers. Invest Radiol 2000;35(1):1–7.
265. Leander P, Hoglund P, Borseth A, Kloster Y, Berg A. A new liposomal liver-specific contrast agent for CT: first human phase-I clinical trial assessing efficacy and safety. Eur Radiol 2001;11(4):698–704.
266. Krause W, Mahler M, Hanke B, Milius W, Kaufmann J, Rogalla P, Hamm B. Dy-EOB-DTPA: tolerance and pharmacokinetics in healthy volunteers and preliminary liver imaging in patients. Invest Radiol 2001;36(8):431–44.
267. Winding O. Intrinsic particles in angiographic contrast media. Radiology 1980;134(2):317–20.
268. Winding O. Particle release from angiographic utensils. Eur J Radiol 1981;1(2):114–16.
269. Harrington D, Amplatz K. Cholesterol embolization and spinal infarction following aortic catheterization. Am J Roentgenol Radium Ther Nucl Med 1972;115(1):171–4.
270. Ciccantelli MJ, Gallagher WB, Skemp FC, Dietz PC. Fatal nephropathy and adrenal necrosis after translumbar aortography. N Engl J Med 1958;258(9):433–5.
271. Goth M, Szilagyi G, Irsy G, Szabolcs I, Berentey E, Molnar F, Magyar E. Hypoadrenia following adrenal venography in Cushing's disease. Eur J Radiol 1984;4 (1):68–70.
272. Bendszus M, Koltzenburg M, Burger R, Warmuth-Metz M, Hofmann E, Solymosi L. Silent embolism in diagnostic cerebral angiography and neurointerventional procedures: a prospective study. Lancet 1999;354 (9190):1594–7.
273. Federle MP, Chang PJ, Confer S, Ozgun B. Frequency and effects of extravasation of ionic and nonionic CT contrast

media during rapid bolus injection. Radiology 1998;206 (3):637–40.

274. National Radiographic Survey (United Kingdom): unpublished reports up to 1990 made available by Dr G. Ansell.
275. Cohan RH, Dunnick NR, Leder RA, Baker ME. Extravasation of nonionic radiologic contrast media: efficacy of conservative treatment. Radiology 1990;176(1):65–7.
276. Fagan SC, Rahill AA, Balakrishnan G, Ewing JR, Branch CA, Brown GG. Neurobehavioral and physiologic effects of trifluoromethane in humans. J Toxicol Environ Health 1995;45(2):221–9.
277. Kim SH, Park JH, Kim YI, Kim CW, Han MC. Experimental tissue damage after subcutaneous injection of water soluble contrast media. Invest Radiol 1990;25(6):678–85.
278. Albrechtsson U, Olsson CG. Thrombotic side-effects of lower-limb phlebography. Lancet 1976;1(7962):723–4.
279. Gothlin J, Hallbook T. Skin necrosis following extravasal injection of contrast medium in phlebography. Radiologe 1971;11(4):161–5.
280. Thomas ML, Tighe JR. Death from fat embolism as a complication of intraosseous phlebography. Lancet 1973;2(7843):1415–6.
281. Young AE, Thomas ML, Browse NL. Intraosseous phlebography and fat embolism. BMJ 1976;2(6027):89–90.
282. Safer JN, Guibor P. Ocular complications of orbital venography. Radiology 1975;114(3):647–8.
283. Sellam R, Economou C, Amer M, Tobelem G, Arvis G. Priapisme après cavernographie. Raport d'un cas original. [Priapism after cavernography. Report of an original case.] Ann Urol (Paris) 1988;22(2):145–6.
284. Bookstein JS. Comment. Radiology 1990;174:286.
285. Newberg AH, Munn CS, Robbins AH. Complications of arthrography. Radiology 1985;155(3):605–6.
286. Olsen AM, O'Neil JJ. Bronchography. A report of the Committee on Bronchoesophagology. American College of Chest Physicians. Dis Chest 1967;51(6):663–8.
287. Nahum H, Desbleds MT, Marsault C. Les accidents de la cholangiographie intraveineuse: résultats de l'enquête de la Société Française de Radiologie. [Complications of intravenous cholangiography. Results of an inquiry launched by the French Radiological Society.] J Radiol Electrol Med Nucl 1975;56(8–9):595–7.
288. Sakahira K, Ebata T, Tsunoda Y, Amaha K, Meno K. Serum diatrizoate level during intraoperative cholangiography in patients without choledochal obstructions. Dig Dis Sci 1990;35(9):1085–8.
289. Keighley MR, Wilson G, Kelly JP. Fatal endotoxic shock of biliary tract origin complicating transhepatic cholangiography. BMJ 1973;3(5872):147–8.
290. Gmelin E, Kramann B, Weiss HD. Kontrastmittelzwischenfall bei einer endoskopischen retrograden Cholangiopancreatikographie. [Complication with contrast medium in endoscopic retrograde cholangiopancreaticography.] MMW Munch Med Wochenschr 1977;119(44):1439–40.
291. Lorenz R. Allergic reaction to contrast medium after endoscopic retrograde pancreatography. Endoscopy 1990;22(4):196.
292. Bilbao MK, Dotter CT, Lee TG, Katon RM. Complications of endoscopic retrograde cholangiopancreatography (ERCP). A study of 10,000 cases. Gastroenterology 1976;70(3):314–20.
293. Seibert DG, al-Kawas FH, Graves J, Gaskins RD. Prospective evaluation of renal function following ERCP. Endoscopy 1991;23(6):355–6.
294. Lownie SP, Ferguson GG. Spinal subdural empyema complicating cervical discography. Spine 1989;14(12):1415–17.
295. Davies AC, Keightley A, Borthwick-Clarke A, Walters HL. The use of a low-osmolality contrast medium in hysterosalpingography: comparison with a conventional contrast medium. Clin Radiol 1985;36(5):533–6.
296. Tabaddor K. Unusual complications of iophendylate injection myelography. Report of a case and review. Arch Neurol 1973;29(6):435–6.
297. Gupta SR, Naheedy MH, O'Hara RJ, Rubino FA. Hydrocephalus following iophendylate injection myelography with spontaneous resolution: case report and review. Comput Radiol 1985;9(6):359–64.
298. Fitzpatrick MO, Goyal K, Johnston RA. Thoracic radiculopathy caused by a Myodil cyst. Br J Neurosurg 2000;14(4):351–3.
299. Charles P, Ronne K, Kraft M. Weber–Christian's syndrom efter pantopaque-myelografi. [Weber–Christian's syndrome after Pantopaque myelography.] Ugeskr Laeger 1975;137(27):1540–1.
300. Lieberman P, Siegle RL, Kaplan RJ, Hashimoto K. Chronic urticaria and intermittent anaphylaxis. Reactions to iophendylate. JAMA 1976;236(13):1495–7.
301. Roberson GH, Taveras JM, Tadmor R, Kleefield J, Ellis G. Computed tomography in metrizamide cisternography—importance of coronal and axial views. J Comput Assist Tomogr 1977;1(2):241–5.
302. Yadav RK, Sharma A, Mishra DS, Airon RK, Kalra M, Dua S. An evaluation of myelography with non-ionic water soluble contrast medium—iohexol. J Indian Med Assoc 1999;97(1):16–19.
303. Nicholson DA. Contrast media in sialography: a comparison of Lipiodol Ultra Fluid and Urografin 290. Clin Radiol 1990;42(6):423–6.
304. Delaney Y, Khooshabeh R. Lipogranuloma following traumatic dacryocystography in a 4-year-old boy. Eye 2001;15(Pt 5):683–4.
305. Shopfner CE. Clinical evaluation of cystourethrographic contrast media. Radiology 1967;88(3):491–7.
306. Mihalecz K, Wolfer E, Czaszar J, Pinter J. Akute Niereninsuffizienz nach unilateraler retrograder Pyelographie. [Acute renal failure after unilateral retrograde pyelography.] Z Urol Nephrol 1967;60(11):783–8.
307. Lytton B, Brooks MB, Spencer RP. Absorption of contrast material from the urinary tract during retrograde pyelography. J Urol 1968;100(6):779–82.
308. Bettenay F, de Campo J. Allergic reaction following micturating cystourethrography. Urol Radiol 1989;11(3):167–8.
309. Hankins WD. Human tolerance of iopanoic acid (Telepaque). Radiology 1971;101(2):434.
310. Marshall TR, Ling JT, Follis G, Russell M. Pharmacological incompatibility of contrast media with various drugs and agents. Radiology 1965;84:536–9.
311. Pozzato C, Marozzi F, Brenna F, Gattoni F. Un caso di morte consequente all somministrazione endevenoza di mezzo di contrasto organiodato a basa osmolalita. [A case of death following the intravenous administration of an organo-iodinated contrast media of low osmolality.] Radiol Med (Torino) 1990;80(1–2):107–8.
312. Fischer HW, Morris TW, King AN, Harnish PP. Deleterious synergism of a cardiac glycoside and sodium diatrizoate. Invest Radiol 1978;13(4):340–6.
313. Rha SW, Kuchulakanti PK, Pakala R, Cheneau E, Pinnow E, Gebreeyesus A, Aggrey G, Pichard AD, Satler LF, Kent KM, Lindsay J, Waksman R. Addition of heparin to contrast media is associated with increased bleeding and peripheral vascular complications during percutaneous coronary intervention with bivalirudin and drug-eluting stents. Cardiovasc Radiat Med 2004;5(2):64–70.
314. Reynolds NJ, Wallington TB, Burton JL. Hydralazine predisposes to acute cutaneous vasculitis following urography with iopamidol. Br J Dermatol 1993;129(1):82–5.

315. Shulman KL, Thompson JA, Benyunes MC, Winter TC, Fefer A. Adverse reactions to intravenous contrast media in patients treated with interleukin-2. J Immunother 1993;13(3):208–12.
316. Jamet P, Lebas de Lacour JC, Christoforov B, Stern M. Acidose lactique mortelle après urographie intraveineuse chez une diabétique recevant de la metformine. [Fatal case of metformin-induced lactic acidosis after urography in a diabetic patient.] Sem Hop 1980;56(9–10):473–4.
317. Nawaz S, Cleveland T, Gaines PA, Chan P. Clinical risk associated with contrast angiography in metformin treated patients: a clinical review. Clin Radiol 1998;53(5):342–4.
318. Ansell G. A national survey of radiological complications: interim report. Clin Radiol 1968;19(2):175–91.
319. Sanen FJ. Considerations of cholecystographic contrast media. Am J Roentgenol Radium Ther Nucl Med 1962;88:797–802.
320. Lee S, Schoen I. Black-copper reduction reaction simulating alkaptonuria. Occurrence after intravenous urography. N Engl J Med 1966;275(5):266–7.
321. Tidgren B, Golman K. Effect of diatrizoate on renal extraction of PAH in man. Acta Radiol 1989;30(5):521–4.

Iodine-containing medicaments

General Information

Iodine is a non-metallic halogen element (symbol I; atomic no 53) which exists as a near-black solid but readily sublimates, giving a purple-colored vapor. It is found in nature both free (for example in large amounts in seaweeds such as kelp and in low concentrations in seawater) and in minerals such as iodyrite (silver iodide) and Chile saltpetre (sodium iodide).

Iodine-containing medicaments

Iodine must be present in the normal diet to prevent iodine-deficiency goiter or cretinism, and iodine deficiency-related disorders are still a worldwide (although preventable) group of diseases that affect about 150 million people in at least 40 countries. The WHO sponsored a program to control these disorders by the year 2000 (1,2), and since 1990 there has been a remarkable progress in prevention of iodine deficiency disorders. However, by the year 2000 one-third of the population affected by iodine deficiency disorders still did not have access to iodized salt (3).

Scepticism about the introduction of population-wide programs to prevent iodine-deficiency disorders is occasionally encountered in regions of mild iodine deficiency, especially in Europe (4). The main arguments against introduction of iodized salt are a temporary rise in the incidence of hyperthyroidism (5), a possible increase in the incidence of Graves' disease, and the fact that the remission rates with antithyroid drug therapy will fall (6). The value of preventing mild iodine deficiency has been supported by a longitudinal study from Switzerland, in which 109 000 people in a defined catchment area were studied before and for 9 years after correction of mild iodine deficiency (7). The incidence of toxic nodular goiter increased in the first year by 27%, but thereafter there was a steady fall in the incidence of both toxic nodular goiter (–73%) and Graves' disease (–33%). The range of optimal iodine intake is fairly narrow. Mild and moderate iodine excess are probably associated with higher frequency of hypothyroidism (8).

Some drugs contain iodine in amounts that considerably exceed the optimum daily intake of inorganic iodine. Such drugs include:

- most radiographic contrast media
- amiodarone and benziodarone
- iodoquinoline
- iodine-containing antiseptics (for example povidone-iodine).

Radioactive iodine

Different forms of radioiodine have been used at different times, including ^{123}I, ^{125}I, and ^{131}I. Radioactive iodine is used to scan the thyroid gland and in the treatment of thyrotoxicosis. See in the monograph on Radioactive iodine.

Potassium iodide and potassium iodate

Potassium iodide is the inorganic iodide most commonly used in high dosage for acute thyrotoxicosis. Indeed, large amounts of iodine cause reduced organification of iodine and a temporary block of thyroid hormone secretion (Wolff–Chaikoff effect) and therefore result in a more rapid thyrostatic effect than synthesis inhibitors. Potassium iodine is also used for preoperative treatment of goiter, especially to reduce preoperative bleeding. It can be used in combination with thyrostatic drugs but should never be prescribed in combination with potassium perchlorate, since each abolishes the other's effects. The thyrostatic effects of iodide are evident even at a dose of 6 mg/day, but doses between 50 and 100 mg/day are usually recommended. In some cases of intolerance to higher doses, perchlorate can be used, for example for preoperative treatment.

Potassium iodide has been widely used in asthma and chronic bronchitis as an expectorant. There is considerable controversy about its efficacy. It should not be used in adolescent patients because of its potential to aggravate and induce acne and its effect on the thyroid gland. In view of its doubtful efficacy and definite toxicity, it would be preferable if physicians stopped prescribing it as an expectorant.

Potassium iodide and potassium iodate are commonly added to table salt to prevent iodine deficiency and associated thyroid disease.

Iodine in protecting the thyroid against radioiodine

Accidents with nuclear reactors or nuclear bombs can expose large numbers of people to several decay products of uranium, and iodine isotopes are among the most abundant compounds released in such reactions. It is therefore logical to use salts of stable isotopes of iodine to prevent the accumulation of radioiodine in a person or population at risk of such exposure. The accidents in Windscale (UK), Three Mile Island (USA), and particularly Chernobyl (Ukraine) drew attention to such problems. The major question is therefore whether the potential adverse effects of stable iodine when given indiscriminately to large groups of people would outweigh the risk of radioiodine exposure. Stable iodine needs to be rapidly available when disasters occur, since, in order to be effective, it has to be given in sufficient amounts (100 mg) within a short time before or after (–12 to +3 hours) radioiodine exposure. Potassium iodate (KIO_3) is more stable than potassium iodide (KI), since the latter readily evaporates during prolonged storage. However, the dose recommended for radioprotection of 100 mg of iodine daily over several days (138 mg iodate per day) are close to retinotoxic doses of iodate reported in cases of accidental intoxication. In these doses iodate cannot be recommended. As an additive to salt for correcting iodine deficiency, much smaller doses of iodate are used (up to 1.7 mg/day), and in these doses iodate is probably safe (9).

The main adverse effects of stable iodine are shown in Table 1.

Iodine should be given to the general population if the risk of radioiodine exposure is sufficient (over 15–100 rem), but people with increased susceptibility to the adverse effects of iodine (previous thyroid disease or known serious allergies) should be excluded (10–15). In elderly people the benefit of stable iodine probably does not outweigh its potential adverse effects, while in pregnant women and infants the benefit to harm balance is not established; rapid evacuation of such people from fallout zones should be given the highest priority (SEDA-11, 358).

Tincture of iodine

Tincture of iodine (aqueous iodine oral solution, Lugol's solution) is a solution of iodine 5% plus potassium iodide 10% in water, which is used to reduce the vascularity of the thyroid gland in thyrotoxicosis before surgery.

Iodinated glycerol

Iodinated glycerol is used as a mucolytic agent in respiratory disorders, but its efficacy is controversial. Organically bound iodine is changed to unbound iodide after absorption.

Table 1 Adverse effects of iodine given for protection against radioiodine

Adverse effect	Susceptible individuals
Iodine-induced goiter	
Iodine-induced hypothyroidism	Fetus and neonate
Iodine-induced hyperthyroidism	People living in iodine-deficient areas; people with a history of hyperthyroidism
Sialadenitis and taste disturbances	
Nausea and abdominal pain	
Skin rashes	
Edema (including face and glottis)	
Allergic-like reactions (iodine fever, eosinophilia, serum sickness-like symptoms, vasculitis)	People with hypocomplementemic vasculitis

Iodoform

Iodoform is a lemon-yellow-colored crystalline organic salt of iodine (CHI_3), analogous to chloroform, with a saffron-like odor, used as an antiseptic.

Iodophors

Iodophors are labile complexes of elemental iodine with macromolecular carriers that both increase the solubility and provide sustained release of iodine. Povidone-iodine is a water-soluble iodophor that is used as an antiseptic and is said to be free of the undesirable effects of iodine tincture. However, iodine can be absorbed from it through burned areas (16), vaginal mucosa (17), oral mucosa (18), and in children even with normal skin (19). Povidone-iodine is discussed in a separate monograph under the title Polyvinylpyrrolidone.

Radiocontrast media

Many radiocontrast media contain iodine. These include iodixonal, iohexol, iomeprole, iopamidole, iopanoic acid, iopitridole, iopromide, iothalamate, iotrolan, ioversol, and ioxaglate. They are covered in a separate monograph.

General adverse effects

It has been estimated that in 1994 some 1.5 billion people in 118 countries were at risk of iodine deficiency, this being regarded as the world's most significant cause of preventable brain damage and mental retardation. Fortification of all salt for animal and human consumption has been chosen as the preferred method for the prevention of iodine deficiency disorders, and this approach is proving effective in reducing the incidence of such disorders. However, iodine supplementation is not without risks, which have been discussed (20) and which include allergic reactions and iodine-induced hyperthyroidism. It has been clearly shown that the benefits of iodine deficiency outweigh the risks on a population basis, but it is nevertheless evident that introduction of iodine supplementation is associated with clinical problems in individual subjects.

Because of its adverse effects, it is logical to omit iodine from all pharmaceutical formulations whenever possible, and at least clearly label its presence when it is necessary. The adverse effects of iodine include goiter and hypothyroidism (19,21), hyperthyroidism (SEDA-18, 176), neutropenia (22), metabolic acidosis (23), and generalized iododerma (16).

The term "iodism" covers a group of adverse effects that include irritation of the skin, the mucous membranes, and the conjunctiva. Allergic reactions are rare and mainly cause rashes, pruritus, fever, eosinophilia, and allergic vasculitis (24–27). Leukocytosis, swelling of the salivary glands, iodine coryza, and gastric upsets have also been reported. Headache can accompany the other reactions. In rare cases, jaundice, bleeding from the mucous membranes, and bronchospasm can occur. Inflammatory states may be aggravated by these adverse reactions.

Effects of iodine on thyroid function

Iodine excess can induce hyperthyroidism or hypothyroidism (SEDA-12, 355) (SEDA-13, 378). Pharmacological amounts of iodine induce only a temporary inhibition of thyroid hormone secretion, since even during continuous administration of iodine normal thyroid function reappears ("escape from inhibition"), at least in most healthy subjects. For some unknown reasons, thyroid function can remain suppressed, resulting in hypothyroidism, secondary hypersecretion of TSH, and development of goiter (28). Patients with autoimmune thyroiditis or partial thyroid resection and very young infants (or fetuses) are especially susceptible to iodine-induced hypothyroidism. That therapeutic doses of iodine could induce hyperthyroidism was already known in the nineteenth century shortly after its introduction for the prevention and treatment of iodine deficiency (5,29). Thereafter, similar observations were made in several other parts of the world when iodine supplementation was introduced in iodine-deficient areas. Such iodine-induced hyperthyroidism (the "Jod-Basedow" phenomenon) can also occur in patients with other thyroid diseases (especially multinodular goiter), even when the diet was sufficient in iodine before the excess intake of iodine. This can even be found in patients with apparently normal thyroid glands. The Jod-Basedow phenomenon is usually associated with a slight goiter, high concentrations of both free levothyroxine (T4) and triiodothyronine (T3) and a very low uptake of radioactive iodine. The disease disappears spontaneously weeks or months after interruption of the excess iodine (30–32). Such a disorder should be differentiated from the temporary increase in T4 and reciprocal fall in T3 that can occur 1–2 weeks after the administration of iodine or iodine-containing drugs and that is not associated with symptoms of thyroid dysfunction (33).

Organs and Systems

Cardiovascular

Cardiac dysrhythmias have been seen after accidental ingestion of a large amount of potassium iodide solution (34). In one case administration of iodide was associated with pulmonary edema and iododerma (SEDA-7, 190).

Endocrine

It has been estimated that in 1990 iodine deficiency affected almost one-third of the world's population and represented the greatest single cause of preventable brain damage and mental retardation. Fortification of all salt for animal and human consumption has been chosen as the preferred method for the prevention of iodine deficiency disorders, and this approach is effective in reducing the incidence of such disorders. However, iodine supplementation is not without risk, particularly iodine-induced hyperthyroidism and thyroiditis. The issue of benefit versus harm has been reviewed and the view, previously expressed, that the benefits of correcting iodine deficiency far outweigh risk of iodine supplementation has been reiterated (35). Complications of iodine administration are not confined to those taking dietary supplements to correct deficiency, but can also occur in those given iodine-containing contrast media and with the use of iodine-containing antiseptic solutions.

Shortly after the administration of iodine-containing drugs, there is a self-limited increase in serum thyroxine (T4), which sometimes exceeds the reference range, and a reciprocal fall in serum triiodothyronine (T3). This usually resolves spontaneously, but can persist during further treatment (so-called isolated hyperthyroxinemia). In some patients, true hyperthyroidism (increases in both T4 and T3 with clinical symptoms) occurs, for example in about 5% of patients taking long-term amiodarone, whereas evolution to iodine-induced hypothyroidism is less frequent (36–38). On the other hand, the frequency of iodine-induced hyperthyroidism can comprise about half of all cases of hyperthyroidism, at least in elderly patients taking several drugs (SEDA-7, 399).

The use of iodine has been held responsible for the increasing frequency of relapse of Graves' disease in the USA. Treatment of more severe cases of iodine-induced hyperthyroidism can be difficult, as thyroid synthesis inhibitors are not immediately active and ^{131}I cannot be used because of low thyroid uptake. The carefully supervised combination of perchlorate and methimazole is effective (39), but surgery has also occasionally been advocated.

A summary of the occurrence and epidemiology of iodine-induced hyperthyroidism has been published (40), based on the authors' experience in Tasmania, Zaire, Zimbabwe, and Brazil. Another review has more specifically examined the cardiac features of iodine-induced hyperthyroidism and has emphasized the importance of awareness, monitoring, and treatment of such hyperthyroidism in areas in which iodine supplementation has been recently introduced (41).

The complexity of the interaction between iodine intake and autoimmune thyroid disease has been highlighted by reports of evidence that iodide (compared with thyroxine) induces thyroid autoimmunity in patients with endemic (iodine deficient) goiter (42), while in those with pre-existing thyroid autoimmunity, evidenced by the presence of antithyroid (thyroid peroxidase) antibodies, administration of iodine in an area of mild iodine deficiency led to subclinical or overt hypothyroidism (43).

More importantly, in a study from Italy the use of iodine-containing disinfectants was responsible for transient neonatal hypothyroidism in more than 50% of cases identified (another common cause being transfer of maternal antibodies) (44). These findings led the authors to conclude that pregnant women should be advised of the adverse effects of using iodine-containing products and that their use should be generally discouraged.

Because of reports of severe hyperthyroidism after the introduction of iodized salt in two severely iodine-deficient African counties (Zimbabwe and the Democratic Republic of the Congo), a multicenter study has been conducted in seven countries in the region to evaluate whether the occurrence of iodine-induced hyperthyroidism after the introduction of iodized salt was a generalized phenomenon or corresponded to specific local circumstances in the two affected countries (45). Iodine deficiency had been successfully eliminated in all of the areas investigated and the prevalence of goiter had fallen markedly. However, it was clear that some areas were now exposed to iodine excess as a result of poor monitoring of the quality of iodized salt and of the iodine intake of the population. In these areas, iodine-induced hyperthyroidism occurred only when iodized salt had been recently introduced.

This complication of iodine administration is not confined to those receiving dietary supplements. Two of 788 unselected patients from a relatively iodine-deficient area of Germany who underwent coronary artery angiography with an iodine-containing radiographic contrast agent developed hyperthyroidism within 12 weeks (despite the absence of the typical risk factors of advanced age, preceding nodular goiter, or a low serum TSH) (46). While this represents a relatively low incidence, this series highlights the importance of recognizing the role of iodine-containing drugs in inducing hyperthyroidism, even in developed countries.

Iodinated glycerol

After the administration of iodinated glycerol organically bound iodine is changed to unbound iodide, causing thyrotoxicosis, hypothyroidism, or goiter in some patients (47). Reversible hypothyroidism has been reported in nursing-home residents, without a history of thyroid disease, who had been taking iodinated glycerol as an expectorant (48). Hypothyroidism has been reported after long-term treatment with iodinated glycerol (49).

Iodophors

Extensive iodine absorption from povidone-iodine can cause transient hypothyroidism or in patients with latent hypothyroidism the risk of destabilization and thyrotoxic crisis (SEDA-20, 226) (SEDA-22, 263). Especially at risk are patients with an autonomous adenoma, localized diffuse autonomy of the thyroid gland, nodular goiter, latent hyperthyroidism of autoimmune origin, or endemic iodine deficiency (50).

Hyperthyroidism from povidone-iodine is rarer than hypothyroidism (SEDA-20, 226), but a history of long-term use of iodine-containing medications should be considered when investigating the cause of hyperthyroidism.

- A 48-year-old woman developed palpitation and insomnia (51). The clinical history, physical examination, and laboratory tests supported hyperthyroidism. Since July 1994 she had been combating constipation by improper use of an iodine-containing antiseptic cream for external use only. She had inserted povidone-iodine into her rectum by means of a cannula. The iodine-containing cream was withdrawn and she was given a beta-blocker. The palpitation resolved within 2 weeks and her plasma thyroid hormone concentrations normalized within 1 month.

Hyperthyroidism in this patient was probably triggered by improper long-term use of an over-the-counter iodine-containing cream.

Potassium iodide

Iodine-induced hypothyroidism has been described as the result of prolonged intake of potassium iodide and iodinated glycerol as mucolytics (52).

Patients with an underlying disorder of the thyroid gland may be more predisposed to this complication.

The case of a severe iodine-induced thyrotoxicosis in a patient who had been using iodine-containing eye-drops for more than 10 years has been reported (53).

Mouth and teeth

Occasionally, after a high dose of iodine, sudden swelling of the parotid and submandibular glands develops (54).

- Acute sialadenitis ("iodide mumps") has been described in a 70-year-old man who underwent femoral artery angiography with an iodine-containing contrast agent; he gave a history of a similar episode 24 hours after a previous angiogram (55).

This effect is thought to be a hypersensitivity reaction due to formation of a complex between iodide and plasma proteins.

Urinary tract

Iodinated radiographic contrast media can cause acute renal insufficiency, perhaps as a result of reduced renal blood flow, an intrarenal osmotic effect, or direct tubular toxicity (56). Diuretics, calcium channel blockers, adenosine receptor antagonists, acetylcysteine, low-dose dopamine, the dopamine D_1 receptor agonist fenoldopam, endothelin receptor antagonists, and captopril have all been used to prevent contrast nephropathy.

Skin

A complication of the use of alcoholic iodine solution has been described in three women undergoing cesarean section, who developed painful, superficial, inflammatory reactions on their buttocks after skin preparation for surgery with 10% iodine in alcohol (57). These lesions were believed to have been caused by pooling of the solution underneath the patients, topical skin damage being exacerbated by heat and occlusive drapes.

Induction and aggravation of acne is a typical reaction to iodide (58).

Iododerma, which is thought to be an allergic reaction, starts with an acneiform lesion, localized in the area of the sebaceous glands, which spreads to form verrucous granulomatous lesions (59,60). After discontinuation of iodide, the skin clears over a few weeks. In addition to this typical picture of iodide sensitivity, iodide can cause urticaria and erythema and even hemorrhagic rashes. In order to verify the etiology of the skin conditions in certain cases, sensitivity testing may be required, but is not without risk.

Immunologic

Allergy to iodides can occur (61,62).

Of 126 participants in a study of the metabolism of radiolabelled proteins, four repeatedly developed urticaria and other symptoms after potassium iodide administration (63). Two of them were challenged with oral potassium iodide and developed urticaria, angioedema, polymyalgia, conjunctivitis, and coryza. Ten control patients were also challenged without adverse effects.

- Delayed hypersensitivity to potassium iodide occurred in a 66-year-old man who was given a cough syrup, Elixifilin, which contained potassium iodide (130 mg/15 ml), as well as theophylline and alcohol. Dyspnea, angioedema, itching, and erythema of the face and neck developed a few hours after the second dose. His symptoms disappeared 24 hours after treatment with parenteral glucocorticoids. Five hours after Elixifilin or iodide challenge, he developed edema of the face and neck, itching of the pharynx and eyes, and a sensation of heat (64).

Second-Generation Effects

Pregnancy

Iodine readily crosses the placenta, and the fetal concentration usually exceeds the maternal concentration. The placenta does not seem to have a regulating transfer mechanism, implying that excess maternal intake of iodine will also expose the fetus to iodine intoxication. This usually results in hypothyroidism and development of goiter. Such goiters may become very large and even create obstetrical problems during delivery or mechanical compression during early postnatal life (SEDA-4, 295) (SEDA-5, 328). In neonates iodine excess is a well-known cause of transient hypothyroidism. Iodine-containing antiseptics should therefore be avoided in both the delivery room and the neonatal ward. A similar warning against the use of iodine or iodine-containing drugs applies during lactation since iodine is actively secreted in milk.

Fetotoxicity

Large quantities of iodine reduce the organic binding of iodine (the Wolff–Chaikoff effect). Thus, the regular use of iodide during pregnancy can cause development of a goiter in the fetus. The size of the goiter in the child can be large enough to cause difficulty during delivery. Treatment of vaginitis with iodine-containing solutions in pregnant women can lead to goiter and hypothyroidism in the infant (17).

Neonatal goiter caused by the use of potassium iodine as an expectorant during pregnancy has been reported (65). The neonate, a girl, had acute hypothyroidism, with myxedema and respiratory distress. She was given levothyroxine for 6 months, with complete normalization of thyroid function.

Severe transient postnatal hypothyroidism has been reported in infants whose mothers have received high doses of iodine during pregnancy or multiple local applications of povidone-iodine during pregnancy and for delivery (SED-14, 472). Transient neonatal hypothyroidism during breastfeeding after postnatal maternal topical iodine treatment has also been reported (66).

- A baby girl was born prematurely at 29 weeks. Her weight, length, and head circumference were appropriate to her gestational age. Parenteral feeding was stopped at 20 days, and breastfeeding was gradually increased. TSH screening for congenital hypothyroidism on day 5 was negative (below 1 μU/ml; reference range 0.45–10.0), but a second screening on day 23 was high at 23 μU/ml. There were no signs of hypothyroidism and no palpable goiter. A confirmatory laboratory test on day 29 showed a high serum TSH concentration (288 μU/ml) and reduced concentrations of free thyroxine (2.8 ng/l; reference range 19–23) and free tri-iodothyronine (1.52 pg/ml; reference range 2.2–5.4). The mother had developed an abscess of the abdominal wall 1 week after cesarean section and had been treated with intravenous antibiotics and iodine tampons, 60 cm^2 daily to the abscess wound, containing about 10.5 mg of iodine. Maternal thyroid function was normal (TSH 1.59 μU/ml and free thyroxine 12 ng/l). Thyroid antibodies to thyroglobulin, TSH receptors, and thyroperoxidase were negative. Iodine concentrations in the maternal milk and infant urine were extremely high: 4410 (reference range 29–490) micrograms/l and 3932 (reference range below 185) micrograms/l respectively. Treatment with levothyroxine (25 micrograms/day) was started on day 32, breastfeeding was discontinued, and disinfection with iodine was stopped. Thyroid function normalized after 6 days, levothyroxine was withdrawn, and breastfeeding was restarted. Thyroid function remained normal over a follow-up period of 4 months.

Skin disinfection with iodine also caused goiter and hypothyroidism in five of 30 newborns under intensive care (67). Antiseptics containing iodine should be avoided not only during pregnancy and delivery but also after the delivery during breastfeeding.

Drug Administration

Drug overdose

- A patient who deliberately took potassium iodide solution 50 ml and a small dose of mefenamic acid (six capsules) as part of a suicide attempt developed acute renal insufficiency necessitating hemodialysis (68). Normal renal function returned after 10 days of hemodialysis.

The authors postulated that iodide toxicity had resulted in hemolysis and hemoglobinuria, which, together with acute interstitial nephritis secondary to inhibition of prostaglandin synthesis from mefenamic acid ingestion, had resulted in acute renal insufficiency. The mechanism of hemolysis resulting from toxic doses of iodine is not clear, although it may reflect inhibition of various red cell enzymes.

Interference with Diagnostic Tests

Thyroid function tests

Estimation of protein-bound iodine and tracer studies for the estimation of thyroid function are interfered with by the use of iodine-containing compounds (69).

References

1. Anonymous. Prevention and control of iodine deficiency disorders. Lancet 1986;2(8504):433–4.
2. HetzelBS. The Prevention and Control of Iodine Deficiency Disorders. Nutrition Policy Discussion Paper no. 3. Rome: United Nations ACC/SCN, 1988.
3. Delange F, Burgi H, Chen ZP, Dunn JT. World status of monitoring iodine deficiency disorders control programs. Thyroid 2002;12(10):915–24.
4. Laurberg P. Iodine intake—what are we aiming at? J Clin Endocrinol Metab 1994;79(1):17–19.
5. Kohn LA. A look at iodine-induced hyperthyroidism: Recognition. Bull NY Acad Med 1975;51(8):959–66.

6. Solomon BL, Evaul JE, Burman KD, Wartofsky L. Remission rates with antithyroid drug therapy: continuing influence of iodine intake? Ann Intern Med 1987;107(4):510–12.
7. Delange F. Correction of iodine deficiency: benefits and possible side effects. Eur J Endocrinol 1995;132(5):542–3.
8. Laurberg P, Bulow Pedersen I, Knudsen N, Ovesen L, Andersen S. Environmental iodine intake affects the type of nonmalignant thyroid disease. Thyroid 2001;11(5):457–69.
9. Burgi H, Schaffner TH, Seiler JP. The toxicology of iodate: a review of the literature. Thyroid 2001;11(5):449–56.
10. Yalow RS. Risks in mass distribution of potassium iodide. Bull NY Acad Med 1983;59(10):1020–7.
11. Robbins J. Indications for using potassium iodide to protect the thyroid from low level internal irradiation. Bull NY Acad Med 1983;59(10):1028–38.
12. Shleien B, Halperin JA, Bilstad JM, Botstein P, Dutra EV Jr. Recommendations on the use of potassium iodide as a thyroid-blocking agent in radiation accidents: an FDA update. Bull NY Acad Med 1983;59(10):1009–19.
13. Crocker DG. Nuclear reactor accidents—the use of KI as a blocking agent against radioiodine uptake in the thyroid—a review. Health Phys 1984;46(6):1265–79.
14. Helsing E, Dukes MNG. The Safety of Stable Iodine When Used to Provide Protection against Nuclear Fallout. Internal Advisory Report. Copenhagen: WHO Regional Office for Europe, 1986.
15. Wolff J. Risks for stable and radioactive iodine in radiation protection of the thyroid. In: Hall R, Kobberling J, editors. Thyroid Disorders Associated with Iodine Deficiency and Excess. Serono Symposia Publications. New York: Raven Press, 1985;22:111.
16. Bishop ME, Garcia RL. Iododerma from wound irrigation with povidone-iodine. JAMA 1978;240(3):249–50.
17. Vorherr H, Vorherr UF, Mehta P, Ulrich JA, Messer RH. Vaginal absorption of povidone-iodine. JAMA 1980; 244(23):2628–9.
18. Ferguson MM, Geddes DA, Wray D. The effect of a povidone-iodine mouthwash upon thyroid function and plaque accumulation. Br Dent J 1978;144(1):14–16.
19. Block SH. Thyroid function abnormalities from the use of topical betadine solution on intact skin of children. Cutis 1980;26(1):88–9.
20. Delange F. Risks and benefits of iodine supplementation. Lancet 1998;351(9107):923–4.
21. Safran M, Braverman LE. Effect of chronic douching with polyvinylpyrrolidone-iodine on iodine absorption and thyroid function. Obstet Gynecol 1982;60(1):35–40.
22. Alvarez E. Neutropenia in a burned patient being treated topically with povidone-iodine foam. Plast Reconstr Surg 1979;63(6):839–40.
23. Pietsch J, Meakins JL. Complications of povidone-iodine absorption in topically treated burn patients. Lancet 1976;1(7954):280–2.
24. Friend DG. Iodide therapy and the importance of quantitating the dose. N Engl J Med 1960;263:1358–60.
25. Utiger RD. The diverse effects of iodide on thyroid function. N Engl J Med 1972;287(11):562–3.
26. Horn B, Kabins SA. Iodide fever. Am J Med Sci 1972;264(6):467–71.
27. Eeckhout E, Willemsen M, Deconinck A, Somers G. Granulomatous vasculitis as a complication of potassium iodide treatment for Sweet's syndrome. Acta Dermatol Venereol 1987;67(4):362–4.
28. Vagenakis AG, Braverman LE. Drug induced hypothyroidism. Pharmacol Ther (C) 1976;1:149.
29. Coindet JF. Découverte d'une remàde contre le goitre. Bibl Univ Sci BL Arts 1820;14:90.
30. Ingbar SH. Autoregulation of the thyroid: the effects of thyroid iodine enrichment and depletion. In: Hall R, Kobberling J, editors. Thyroid Disorders Associated with Iodine Deficiency and Excess. Serono Symposia Publications. New York: Raven Press, 1985;22:153.
31. Savoie JC, Massin P, Thomopoulos P, et al. Hyperthyroïde induite par l'iode: une variété mal connue de pathologie iatrogène. Concours Med 1977;99–20:3227.
32. Evered D, Yeo PP. Drug-induced endocrine disorders. Drugs 1977;13(5):353–65.
33. Burger A, Dinichert D, Nicod P, Jenny M, Lemarchand-Beraud T, Vallotton MB. Effect of amiodarone on serum triiodothyronine, reverse triiodothyronine, thyroxin, and thyrotropin. A drug influencing peripheral metabolism of thyroid hormones. J Clin Invest 1976;58(2):255–9.
34. Tresch DD, Sweet DL, Keelan MH Jr, Lange RL. Acute iodide intoxication with cardiac irritability. Arch Intern Med 1974;134(4):760–2.
35. Delange F, Lecomte P. Iodine supplementation: benefits outweigh risks. Drug Saf 2000;22(2):89–95.
36. Jonckheer MH. Amiodarone and the thyroid gland. A review. Acta Cardiol 1981;36(3):199–205.
37. Andersen ED. Long-term antiarrhythmic therapy with amiodarone: high prevalence of thyrotoxicosis (11%). Eur Heart J 1981;2:199.
38. Karpman BA, Rapoport B, Filetti S, Fisher DA. Treatment of neonatal hyperthyroidism due to Graves' disease with sodium ipodate. J Clin Endocrinol Metab 1987;64(1):119–23.
39. Martino E, Aghini-Lombardi F, Mariotti S, Bartalena L, Braverman L, Pinchera A. Amiodarone: a common source of iodine-induced thyrotoxicosis. Horm Res 1987;26(1–4):158–71.
40. Stanbury JB, Ermans AE, Bourdoux P, Todd C, Oken E, Tonglet R, Vidor G, Braverman LE, Medeiros-Neto G. Iodine-induced hyperthyroidism: occurrence and epidemiology. Thyroid 1998;8(1):83–100.
41. Dunn JT, Semigran MJ, Delange F. The prevention and management of iodine-induced hyperthyroidism and its cardiac features. Thyroid 1998;8(1):101–6.
42. Kahaly GJ, Dienes HP, Beyer J, Hommel G. Iodine induces thyroid autoimmunity in patients with endemic goitre: a randomised, double-blind, placebo-controlled trial. Eur J Endocrinol 1998;139(3):290–7.
43. Reinhardt W, Luster M, Rudorff KH, Heckmann C, Petrasch S, Lederbogen S, Haase R, Saller B, Reiners C, Reinwein D, Mann K. Effect of small doses of iodine on thyroid function in patients with Hashimoto's thyroiditis residing in an area of mild iodine deficiency. Eur J Endocrinol 1998;139(1):23–8.
44. Weber G, Vigone MC, Rapa A, Bona G, Chiumello G. Neonatal transient hypothyroidism: aetiological study. Italian Collaborative Study on Transient Hypothyroidism. Arch Dis Child Fetal Neonatal Ed 1998;79(1):F70–2.
45. Delange F, de Benoist B, Alnwick D. Risks of iodine-induced hyperthyroidism after correction of iodine deficiency by iodized salt. Thyroid 1999;9(6):545–56.
46. Delange F, de Benoist B, Alnwick D. Risks of iodine-induced hyperthyroidism after correction of iodine deficiency by iodized salt. Thyroid 1999;9(6):545–56.
47. Kalant H, Roschlan W. Organically bound iodine. In: Principles of Medical Pharmacology. 5th ed. Washington DC: Decker, 1989:484–5.
48. Drinka PJ, Nolten WE. Effects of iodinated glycerol on thyroid function studies in elderly nursing home residents. J Am Geriatr Soc 1988;36(10):911–13.
49. Mather JL, Baycliff CD, Paterson NAM. Hypothyroidism secondary to iodinated glycerol. Can J Hosp Pharm 1993;46:177–8.
50. Gortz G, Haring R. Wirkung und Nebenwirkung von Polyvinylpyrrolidon-Jod (PVP-Jod). Therapiewoche 1981;31:4364.
51. Pagliaricci S, Lupattelli G, Mannarino E. Ipertiroidismo da uso impxoprio di iodio-povidone. [Hyperthyroidism due to

the improper use of povidone-iodine.] Ann Ital Med Int 1999;14(2):124–6.
52. Gomolin IH. Iodinated glycerol-induced hypothyroidism. Drug Intell Clin Pharm 1987;21(9):726–7.
53. Andre F, Bielefeld P, Besancenot JF, Belleville I, Sgro C, Martin F. Fausse inocuite des collyres: à propos d'une observation de thyrotoxicose induite par l'iode. [False innocuousness of eye drops. Apropos of 1 case of thyrotoxicosis induced by iodine.] Therapie 1988;43(5):431–2.
54. Bernecker C. Potassium iodide in bronchial asthma. BMJ 1969;4(677):236.
55. Chuen J, Roberts N, Lovelock M, King B, Beiles B, Frydman G. "Iodide mumps" after angioplasty. Eur J Vasc Endovasc Surg 2000;19(2):217–18.
56. Ide JM, Lancelot E, Pines E, Corot C. Prophylaxis of iodinated contrast media-induced nephropathy: a pharmacological point of view. Invest Radiol 2004;39(3):155–70.
57. Chilvers RJ, Weisz MT. Side-effects of alcoholic iodine solution (10%). Br J Anaesth 2000;85(1):178.
58. Papa CM. Acne and hidden iodides. Arch Dermatol 1976;112(4):555–6.
59. Baumgartner TG. Potassium iodide and iododerma. Am J Hosp Pharm 1976;33(6):601–3.
60. Wilkin JK, Strobel D. Iododerma occurring during thyroid protection treatment. Cutis 1985;36(4):335–7.
61. Toman Z. Alergicka reakcepo sukcinylcholinjodidu Spofa behem celkove anestezie. [Allergic reaction after succinylcholine iodide Spofa during general anesthesia.] Rozhl chir 1976;55(12):836–8.
62. Sicherer SH. Risk of severe allergic reactions from the use of potassium iodide for radiation emergencies. J Allergy Clin Immunol 2004;114(6):1395–7.
63. Curd JG, Milgrom H, Stevenson DD, Mathison DA, Vaughan JH. Potassium iodide sensitivity in four patients with hypocomplementemic vasculitis. Ann Intern Med 1979;91(6):853–7.
64. Munoz FJ, Bellido J, Moyano JC, Alvarez MJ, Juan JL. Adverse reaction to potassium iodide from a cough syrup. Allergy 1997;52(1):111–12.
65. Bostanci I, Sarioglu A, Ergin H, Aksit A, Cinbis M, Akalin N. Neonatal goiter caused by expectorant usage. J Pediatr Endocrinol Metab 2001;14(8):1161–2.
66. Casteels K, Punt S, Bramswig J. Transient neonatal hypothyroidism during breastfeeding after post-natal maternal topical iodine treatment. Eur J Pediatr 2000;159(9):716–17.
67. Chabrolle JP, Rossier A. Goitre and hypothyroidism in the newborn after cutaneous absorption of iodine. Arch Dis Child 1978;53(6):495–8.
68. Sinniah R, Lye WC. Acute renal failure from hemoglobinuric and interstitial nephritis secondary to iodine and mefenamic acid. Clin Nephrol 2001;55(3):254–8.
69. Davies PH, Franklyn JA. The effects of drugs on tests of thyroid function. Eur J Clin Pharmacol 1991;40(5):439–51.

Iodopropynylbutylcarbamate

General Information

Initially used as a preservative in wood paints and metalworking fluids, iodopropynylbutylcarbamate is being increasingly used in cosmetics (1).

Organs and Systems

Immunologic

Four contact allergic reactions were reported in a series of 3168 consecutively patch-tested patients (2). In another study there were 16 positive reactions (0.3%) in 4883 consecutive patients (3).

References

1. Badreshia S, Marks JG Jr. Iodopropynyl butylcarbamate. Am J Contact Dermat 2002;13(2):77–9.
2. Bryld LE, Agner T, Rastogi SC, Menne T. Iodopropynyl butylcarbamate: a new contact allergen. Contact Dermatitis 1997;36(3):156–8.
3. Schnuch A, Geier J, Brasch J, Uter W. The preservative iodopropynyl butylcarbamate: frequency of allergic reactions and diagnostic considerations. Contact Dermatitis 2002;46(3):153–6.

Ion exchange resins

General Information

The ion exchange resins colestyramine (rINN) and colestipol (rINN) are not absorbed, and their main adverse effects are therefore on the gastrointestinal tract. They can also interfere with the absorption of other drugs or fat-soluble vitamins.

Organs and Systems

Metabolism

The ion exchange resins tend to increase serum triglyceride concentrations, especially in patients with hypertriglyceridemia (1).

Nutrition

Serum total carotenoid and vitamin A concentrations fell by 30% in patients taking colestipol 30 g/day (2).

Acid–base balance

Colestyramine has been reported to have caused a hyperchloremic metabolic acidosis.

- A 70-year-old woman with a 2-year history of primary biliary cirrhosis confirmed by histological and immunological criteria took colestyramine sachets twice daily for 2 months and developed lethargy, confusion, and drowsiness (3). She had signs of chronic liver disease, portal hypertension, and hepatic encephalopathy. Laboratory investigations confirmed a metabolic acidosis (pH 7.15) and hyperchloremia. Multiple cultures failed to reveal sepsis, and a urinary pH of 4.85 together with tests of renal acidification excluded renal tubular acidosis. No other cause was found and she responded to 600 mmol of sodium bicarbonate intravenously over 36 hours.

Hematologic

Inhibition of vitamin K absorption can cause vitamin K deficiency, leading to hypoprothrombinemia and hence to bleeding (4).

Gastrointestinal

Patients taking colestyramine often have constipation, abdominal discomfort, and heartburn, but dietary fiber, such as psyllium, can reduce the symptoms (5,6). Other effects are flatulence, nausea, and fecal impaction; a mild laxative may be needed, particularly in the elderly. Many other patients complain of anorexia and occasionally there is diarrhea. Doses of colestyramine higher than the 10–16 g normally used can cause steatorrhea (7).

A small child died when impacted resin obstructed the colon (SEDA-8, 935) (8).

The most common adverse effect of colestipol is constipation (30%). In the first months of therapy nausea and bloating can also occur. There is disappointingly poor adherence to therapy in young patients (9). The encapsulated form of the drug is better tolerated (10).

Liver

- A 65-year-old man with type IIa dyslipidemia who took flavored colestipol granules 2 scoops/day for 3 months developed asymptomatic hepatotoxicity (11). Several of his liver enzymes were raised to 10 times the upper limit of the reference range. One week after withdrawal of colestipol, his serum transaminases fell dramatically and 3 weeks later all his liver function tests were normal.

Rechallenge was not attempted, but other potential causes of hepatocellular injury were ruled out.

Musculoskeletal

A degree of osteoporosis or osteomalacia can occur because of reduced vitamin D absorption (12).

Drug–Drug Interactions

General

Ion-exchange resins do not have systemic adverse effects, but they can affect the absorption of other drugs from the gut, particularly if they undergo enterohepatic or enteroenteric recirculation, since they will adsorb them in the gut and prevent their reabsorption.

There is reason to anticipate problems if the resin is given along with acidic drugs and some other drugs that have a narrow safety margin, such as oral anticoagulants (coumarins), cardiac glycosides, and thyroid hormones (thyroxine, triiodothyronine). Interference with the absorption of other acidic drugs, including the barbiturates, naproxen, phenylbutazone and its congeners, and the thiazide diuretics, can almost certainly occur, but is of little or no clinical importance, since the doses of these drugs can easily be adjusted as time goes by, to allow for any reduction in absorption, or alternative drugs can be used. Interference with anticoagulants and cardiac glycosides presents the most serious problems, because they have a low therapeutic index. It has often been said that problems can be avoided provided the drugs are not given simultaneously; however, this is not true when the drug in question undergoes enterohepatic circulation, as is the case with digitoxin and phenprocoumon, as a result of which these substances are present in the gastrointestinal tract for a long time and can be exposed to an ion exchange resin at any time. The interval principle for other drugs is useful, but the interval should be at least 1 hour and in the case of thyroxine 4–5 hours, in which case the drug should be given before the resin.

Cardiac glycosides

Colestyramine and colestipol bind digoxin and digitoxin and can affect their absorption. When the ion exchange resins and digoxin are co-administered the absorption of digoxin is reduced (13). However, even when they are not administered together, the resins can bind cardiac glycosides that have re-entered the gut after absorption by virtue of enterohepatic recycling and enteral secretion, increasing their rate of elimination. This action has been used to treat digoxin toxicity (14–16), digitoxin toxicity (17), and toxicity from derivatives of digoxin (18).

Coumarin anticoagulants

The interaction of colestyramine with coumarins is due to the enterohepatic recirculation of coumarins, which is interrupted by colestyramine.

Phenprocoumon undergoes enterohepatic recycling, and its elimination can be enhanced by ion exchange resins, sometimes with fatal consequences (19).

Warfarin also undergoes enterohepatic recycling, and its elimination can be enhanced by ion exchange resins (20); this has been used to treat warfarin toxicity (21).

Folic acid

Malabsorption of folic acid has been reported in patients taking colestyramine (SEDA-13, 1326) (22).

In children taking colestipol supplementary folic acid may need to be provided (23).

Valproic acid

The systemic availability of valproic acid is reduced by colestyramine unless they are given 3 hours apart (24).

References

1. Ryan JR, Jain A. The effect of colestipol or cholestyramine on serum cholesterol and triglycerides in a long-term controlled study. J Clin Pharmacol New Drugs 1972;12(7):268–73.
2. Probstfield JL, Lin TL, Peters J, Hunninghake DB. Carotenoids and vitamin A: the effect of hypocholesterolemic agents on serum levels. Metabolism 1985;34(1):88–91.
3. Eaves ER, Korman MG. Cholestyramine induced hyperchloremic metabolic acidosis. Aust NZ J Med 1984;14(5):670–2.

4. Vroonhof K, van Rijn HJ, van Hattum J. Vitamin K deficiency and bleeding after long-term use of cholestyramine. Neth J Med 2003;61(1):19–21.
5. Maciejko JJ, Brazg R, Shah A, Patil S, Rubenfire M. Psyllium for the reduction of cholestyramine-associated gastrointestinal symptoms in the treatment of primary hypercholesterolemia. Arch Fam Med 1994; 3(11):955–60.
6. Spence JD, Huff MW, Heidenheim P, Viswanatha A, Munoz C, Lindsay R, Wolfe B, Mills D. Combination therapy with colestipol and psyllium mucilloid in patients with hyperlipidemia. Ann Intern Med 1995;123(7):493–9.
7. Zurier RB, Hashim SA, Van Itallie TB. Effect of medium chain triglyceride on cholestyramine-induced steatorrhea in man. Gastroenterology 1965;49(5):490–5.
8. Cohen MI, Winslow PR, Boley SJ. Intestinal obstruction associated with cholestyramine therapy. N Engl J Med 1969;280(23):1285–6.
9. Kruse W, Kohlmeier M, Nikolaus T, Vogel G, Schlierf G. Langzeitbehandlung mit colestipol. Munch Med Wochenschr 1989;131:407–9.
10. Linet OI, Grzegorczyk CR, Demke DM. The effect of encapsulated, low-dose colestipol in patients with hyperlipidemia. J Clin Pharmacol 1988;28(9):804–6.
11. Sirmans SM, Beck JK, Banh HL, Freeman DA. Colestipol-induced hepatotoxicity. Pharmacotherapy 2001;21(4):513–16.
12. Heaton KW, Lever JV, Barnard D. Osteomalacia associated with cholestyramine therapy for postileectomy diarrhea. Gastroenterology 1972;62(4):642–6.
13. Brown DD, Schmid J, Long RA, Hull JH. A steady-state evaluation of the effects of propantheline bromide and cholestyramine on the bioavailability of digoxin when administered as tablets or capsules. J Clin Pharmacol 1985;25(5):360–4.
14. Roberge RJ, Sorensen T. Congestive heart failure and toxic digoxin levels: role of cholestyramine. Vet Hum Toxicol 2000;42(3):172–3.
15. Krivoy N, Eisenman A. [Cholestyramine for digoxin intoxication.] Harefuah 1995;128(3):145–7, 199.
16. Payne VW, Secter RA, Noback RK. Use of colestipol in a patient with digoxin intoxication. Drug Intell Clin Pharm 1981;15(11):902–3.
17. Hantson P, Vandenplas O, Mahieu P, Wallemacq P, Hassoun A. Repeated doses of activated charcoal and cholestyramine for digitoxin overdose: pharmacokinetic data and urinary elimination. J Toxicol Clin Exp 1991;11(7–8):401–5.
18. Kuhlmann J. Use of cholestyramine in three patients with beta-acetyldigoxin, beta-methyldigoxin and digitoxin intoxication. Int J Clin Pharmacol Ther Toxicol 1984;22(10):543–8.
19. Balmelli N, Domine F, Pfisterer M, Krahenbuhl S, Marsch S. Fatal drug interaction between cholestyramine and phenprocoumon. Eur J Intern Med 2002;13(3):210–11.
20. Jahnchen E, Meinertz T, Gilfrich HJ, Kersting F, Groth U. Enhanced elimination of warfarin during treatment with cholestyramine. Br J Clin Pharmacol 1978;5(5):437–40.
21. Roberge RJ, Rao P, Miske GR, Riley TJ. Diarrhea-associated over-anticoagulation in a patient taking warfarin: therapeutic role of cholestyramine. Vet Hum Toxicol 2000;42(6):351–3.
22. Kane JP, Malloy MJ. Treatment of hypercholesterolemia. Med Clin North Am 1982;66(2):537–50.
23. Glueck CJ. Colestipol and probucol: treatment of primary and familial hypercholesterolemia and amelioration of atherosclerosis. Ann Intern Med 1982;96(4):452–82.
24. Malloy MJ, Ravis WR, Pennell AT, Diskin CJ. Effect of cholestyramine resin on single dose valproate pharmacokinetics. Int J Clin Pharmacol Ther 1996;34(5):208–11.

Ipecacuanha, emetine, and dehydroemetine

General Information

Ipecacuanha is an extract of the root of *Psychotria ipecacuanha*, also known as *Cephaelis ipecacuanha*, a member of the Rubiaceae. It contains the emetic alkaloids cephaeline and emetine. It has often been used as a home remedy for various purposes, and not only as an emetic. It is a traditional ingredient of some expectorants, since expectoration often accompanies vomiting. Misuse of ipecacuanha by patients with anorexia nervosa and bulimia has resulted in severe myopathy, lethargy, erythema, dysphagia, cardiotoxicity, and even death. Use in infancy generally seems safe.

Emetine, once the drug of choice for the treatment of amebiasis, despite marked cardiotoxicity, has largely been replaced by metronidazole and related compounds for this indication. Large doses of emetine can damage the heart, liver, kidneys, intestinal tract, and skeletal muscle. Allergic reactions and tumor-inducing effects have not been described. Dehydroemetine is a little less toxic but also less effective than emetine; its adverse effects are similar (SED-11, 594).

Gastrointestinal decontamination in acute toxic ingestion has been reviewed (1).

- Although ipecac generally seems to have a good safety profile, it can be associated with protracted vomiting. Other reported adverse effects include drowsiness, agitation, abdominal cramps, diarrhea, aspiration pneumonia, cerebral hemorrhage, pneumoperitoneum, and pneumomediastinum. Its use is not currently recommended (2).

Gastric lavage can be useful in some patients who have taken life-threatening doses of highly toxic substances. However, toxin absorption can be enhanced by gastric lavage. Reported adverse effects mainly include laryngospasm, hypoxemia, aspiration pneumonia, bradycardia, electrocardiographic ST segment elevation, and rarely mechanical injury to the gastrointestinal tract.

- Activated charcoal has gained popularity as a first choice for gut decontamination, based on its efficacy and relative lack of adverse effects. Poor patient acceptance is a disadvantage. Frequent vomiting can rarely become a problem.
- Saline laxatives (magnesium citrate, magnesium sulfate, sodium sulfate, and disodium phosphate) or saccharide laxatives (sorbitol, mannitol, lactulose) are also used in poisoned patients. Common adverse effects are abdominal cramps, excessive diarrhea, and abdominal distension. Dehydration and electrolyte imbalance in children, and hypermagnesemia and magnesium toxicity (with magnesium-based cathartics) have also been reported.
- Whole bowel irrigation to wash the entire gastrointestinal tract rapidly and mechanically is similar to the methods used by gastroenterologists to prepare patients for colonic investigation or bowel surgery. It is safe, even in children, pregnant women, and patients with cardiac or respiratory failure. Polyethylene glycol isotonic electrolyte solution is commonly used. Complications are

usually minor and include nausea, vomiting, abdominal distension and cramps, and anal irritation.

Organs and Systems

Cardiovascular

Cardiotoxicity is the most serious and dangerous adverse effect of emetine. The clinical signs are tachycardia, dysrhythmias, and hypotension. Deaths have been described. Electrocardiographic abnormalities occur in 60–70% of cases; increased T wave amplitude, prolongation of the PR interval, ST segment depression, and T wave changes are all common. It seems possible that emetine influences the cell permeability of sodium and calcium ions, and this could be the basis of its effect on cardiac automaticity and contractility and on the electrocardiogram (SED-11, 594). The symptoms of emetine toxicity suggest that an effect on intracellular magnesium concentrations could be another possible explanation, but there are no data to support this hypothesis (SED-11, 594).

Respiratory

Asthma can occasionally be induced by ipecacuanha; when the compound was more widely used in medicine this was a familiar problem for those compounding medicines (3).

Gastrointestinal

Nausea and vomiting are frequent, perhaps in as many as one-third of all cases. In about half the cases, diarrhea is induced or existing diarrhea aggravated. Melena can occur, but this seems unlikely to be drug-induced (SED-11, 594).

Skin

Dermatitis has been attributed to emetine (4), as has cellulitis at the site of injection (5).

Musculoskeletal

Complaints of weakness, tenderness, and stiffness of skeletal muscles, especially in the neck and shoulder, are common. Following emetine aversion therapy for alcohol abuse, muscle weakness and pathological changes in muscle biopsy specimens have been described (SED-11, 594).

A reversible myopathy secondary to abuse of ipecacuanha by individuals with eating disorders has been noted (SED-12, 945) (SEDA-17, 421); the active alkaloid may have been responsible.

Long-Term Effects

Drug abuse

Munchausen's syndrome by proxy involving syrup of ipecacuanha has been reported in an 18-month-old child who was brought by his mother with persistent vomiting for 4 weeks with generalized myopathy and pneumonia (6). Its over-the-counter availability, low cost, and effective emetic properties give this drug a high appeal for such abuse.

Drug Administration

Drug overdose

There is some suggestion of cardiac impairment with overdosage, presumably also myopathic. Forced emesis can lead to esophageal damage or even complete rupture; pneumomediastinum and pneumoperitoneum have therefore sometimes complicated induced emesis (SEDA-10, 326). A bizarre case of neonatal vomiting, irritability, and hypothermia was attributed to the mother having added ipecacuanha surreptitiously to her baby's feed; at any age, however, emetine in excess can be very irritant to the gastrointestinal tract, resulting, for example, in bloody diarrhea.

Drug–Drug Interactions

Activated charcoal

Activated charcoal, sometimes used to treat self-poisoning, binds the active ingredients of ipecacuanha and inactivates them, at least partly (7). The administration of ipecacuanha also delays the administration of charcoal (8). They should not be co-administered.

References

1. Lheureux P, Askenasi R, Paciorkowski F. Gastrointestinal decontamination in acute toxic ingestions. Acta Gastroenterol Belg 1998;61(4):461–7.
2. Anonymous. Position paper: Ipecac syrup. J Toxicol Clin Toxicol 2004;42(2):133–43.
3. Persson CG. Ipecacuanha asthma: more lessons. Thorax 1991;46(6):467–8.
4. Schwank R, Jirasek L. Kožni přecitlivelost na emetin. [Skin sensitivity to emetine.] Cesk Dermatol 1952;27(1–2):50–6.
5. Anonymous. Drugs for parasitic infections. Med Lett Drugs Ther 1986;28(706):17.
6. Cooper C, Kilham H, Ryan M. Ipecac—a substance of abuse. Med J Aust 1998;168(2):94–5.
7. Krenzelok EP, Freedman GE, Pasternak S. Preserving the emetic effect of syrup of ipecac with concurrent activated charcoal administration: a preliminary study. J Toxicol Clin Toxicol 1986;24(2):159–66.
8. Kornberg AE, Dolgin J. Pediatric ingestions: charcoal alone versus ipecac and charcoal. Ann Emerg Med 1991;20(6):648–51.

Ipratropium bromide

See also Anticholinergic drugs

General Information

Ipratropium hydrobromide is a quaternary amine, the semisynthetic isopropyl derivative of atropine, which has low lipid solubility and is poorly absorbed. It has anticholinergic properties and is used to treat asthma.

The metered dose of ipratropium is some 20 micrograms. Its limited availability accounts for its relative bronchial selectivity when ipratropium is given in low doses by the aerosol route. In healthy volunteers, 120–280 micrograms given by intravenous injection reduced salivary secretion and increased heart rate. Inhaled doses, up to a total of 1.2 mg, had no significant effect on heart rate, although some patients reported dryness of the mouth (1). Only if substantial overdosage occurs (for example 1 mg by inhalation) do traces of generalized atropine-like effects begin to appear.

Ipratropium has established a place in the therapy of asthma as an alternative to $beta_2$-adrenoceptor agonist aerosols for patients who fail to respond adequately to these agents. Ipratropium may be more effective than $beta_2$-adrenoceptor agonists for patients with non-atopic asthma and chronic bronchitis. It has been reported to augment the effects of $beta_2$-adrenoceptor agonists when given by nebulized inhalation in acute asthma (2).

Therapeutic doses from an aerosol are free of systemic adverse effects because of the very low blood concentration after inhalation. Transient dryness of the mouth and scratching in the trachea can occur in up to 25% of patients receiving wet nebulizer treatment with the drug.

Therapeutic studies

There is continuing discussion about the role of inhaled antimuscarinic drugs combined with $beta_2$-adrenoceptor agonists in the treatment of acute asthma (3). Five trials involving 453 patients examined the efficacy of using a single dose (250 micrograms) of ipratropium bromide with a $beta_2$ agonist. There were no reductions in hospital admission rates when pooling the two trials that reported this outcome (RR = 0.93; CI = 0.65–1.32). In three trials in which pulmonary function was the major outcome measure, there was a significantly greater improvement in lung function at 60 minutes and 120 minutes after a single inhalation of a combination of an antimuscarinic drug and a $beta_2$ agonist. The addition of a single dose of an antimuscarinic drug was not associated with increased vomiting or tremor, but there was an apparent reduction in nausea (RR = 0.55; CI = 0.33–0.91). Five trials involving 366 children examined the effects of multiple treatments with combined ipratropium and a $beta_2$ agonist. Pooling of four trials using hospital admission as an outcome measure showed a 30% reduction (RR = 0.72; CI = 0.53–0.99). The authors cautioned that the total number and size of studies were small and that their conclusions could be modified by results of larger trials (3).

Comparative studies

Perennial rhinitis is common in both adults and children and is usually treated with intranasal corticosteroids, intranasal ipratropium bromide, antihistamines, intranasal cromones, and decongestants. Treatment-related adverse effects are common and monotherapy is often inadequate. There are few published studies of the comparative efficacy of rhinitis treatments.

Budesonide

Ipratropium bromide (42 micrograms per nostril bd) has been compared with budesonide (84 micrograms per nostril bd) for 6 months in a randomized, double-blind trial in 146 children with perennial rhinitis (4). Both treatments resulted in significant improvements in rhinorrhea, sneezing, and congestion (as rated by both patients and physicians) and improved quality of life. Budesonide achieved better control of sneezing than ipratropium throughout the study period and better control of congestion than ipratropium in the later part of the study. Of 36 patients who did not complete the study, largely for administrative reasons, six using ipratropium withdrew owing to lack of efficacy. There were no reports of systemic anticholinergic adverse effects. The commonest nasal adverse events in both groups were nasal congestion (23% with ipratropium and 18% with budesonide) and rhinitis (13% with ipratropium and 7% with budesonide). Of nasal adverse events considered to be related to treatment, epistaxis and nasal irritation were more common with budesonide (10 and 4% respectively) than with ipratropium (8 and 0%). Sneezing occurred in 5% of those using ipratropium and in none of those using budesonide, probably reflecting the better efficacy of budesonide for control of sneezing. Overall both drugs were well tolerated.

Ipratropium (42 micrograms per nostril tds), budesonide (84 micrograms per nostril bd), and ipratropium plus budesonide for 2 weeks have been studied in a randomized, double-blind, placebo-controlled trial in 533 patients with perennial rhinitis (5). As monotherapy, both ipratropium and budesonide produced significant reductions in rhinorrhea compared with placebo, and budesonide was more effective than ipratropium in reducing congestion and sneezing. Non-nasal adverse events occurred equally in all three groups. The incidences of epistaxis, nasal congestion, and nasal irritation were similar in all three groups (1–5%) but there was a greater incidence of nasal dryness (3 versus less than 1%) and blood-tinged mucus (4 versus 2%) with ipratropium. Combination therapy with ipratropium and budesonide reduced the severity and duration of rhinorrhea in 74 and 66% of patients compared with 57 and 50% for ipratropium, 64 and 54% for budesonide, and 47 and 38% for placebo. There were no other advantages for combination therapy over budesonide. Nasal adverse events occurred in all groups, including placebo, but patients who had two weeks of budesonide in the monotherapy arm of the study followed by combination therapy had more epistaxis (5%) and more nasal dryness (5%) than patients who had ipratropium before combination treatment. The authors concluded that combination therapy is superior to monotherapy, with no increase in adverse effects. However, the effect of combination therapy over monotherapy in this study is quite small and does not appear to have reached statistical significance. Nevertheless, most adverse effects seem to have been related to budesonide rather than to ipratropium. The addition of ipratropium in a patient already taking budesonide seems to be safe and may increase efficacy.

Salmeterol

A double-blind, double-dummy, parallel-group study in 144 patients with severe COPD (FEV_1 41% of predicted) has been conducted over 12 weeks to determine whether the combination of salmeterol 50 micrograms bd plus ipratropium 40 micrograms bd was better than salmeterol alone (6). At the beginning of treatment salmeterol increased FEV_1 (at peak 7% of predicted) for over 12 hours. Salmeterol plus ipratropium produced a greater bronchodilator response (at peak 11% of predicted) than salmeterol alone during the first 6 hours after inhalation. There were significant improvements in daytime symptom scores and peak flows with both salmeterol and salmeterol plus ipratropium compared with placebo. Adverse events were similar in the treatment groups; headache (six patients with salmeterol plus ipratropium, four with salmeterol, and 11 with placebo) and cough were the most common drug-related adverse events. Over the 12 weeks, 35 patients had an exacerbation of COPD, 36% with placebo, 23% with salmeterol, and 13% with salmeterol plus ipratropium.

Organs and Systems

Respiratory

In some patients with atopic asthma, bronchoconstriction can follow the use of ipratropium (SEDA-9, 127).

There has been concern that ipratropium and other antimuscarinics may cause drying and inspissation of sputum with resulting sputum retention. In vitro studies show no effect on ciliary activity. In healthy subjects and patients with chronic bronchitis, inhaled ipratropium did not affect the rate of tracheobronchial clearance of a previously inhaled radioactive carrier aerosol. In studies using therapeutic doses for 2–14 days sputum volume and viscosity did not change (1).

Sensory systems

Pupillary dilatation has several times been reported, possibly because the spray enters the eye; it is risky in cases of glaucoma (7).

Blurred vision can occur in patients given ipratropium by inhaler (8).

- A 68-year-old man's visual acuity dramatically improved (20/100 to 20/40) after he discontinued ipratropium bromide, which he had been taking in a dose of two puffs every 6 hours for chronic obstructive pulmonary disease.

Angle-closure glaucoma precipitated by ipratropium has been reported following both nebulizer and pressurized aerosol treatment (9,10); however, a specific study showed that in asthmatic children with no pre-existing ocular abnormalities, the risk of an ocular adverse effect from nebulized ipratropium is extremely small (11). A Turkish group studied the acute effects of inhaled ipratropium bromide, given both by metered dose inhaler and nebulizer, in 21 men (mean age 61 years) with a smoking history of 47 pack-years and FEV_1 values less than 50% of predicted at baseline (12). They did not have glaucoma. The doses of ipratropium bromide were 40 micrograms by inhaler and 250 micrograms by nebulizer. Intraocular pressure was measured at baseline and 120 minutes after drug administration. There was no increase in pressure with either dose, but this does not exclude the possibility that there may be a more pronounced effect in patients who have glaucoma, nor that chronic administration may have a greater effect.

A bad taste in the mouth has been reported by 20–30% of patients.

Psychological, psychiatric

Ipratropium produces no significant impairment of cognitive or psychomotor function in elderly patients with chronic airway obstruction (SEDA-21, 187).

Gastrointestinal

One case of paralytic ileus has been reported (SEDA-15, 137).

Urinary tract

In elderly men, who may have prostatic hyperplasia, ipratropium should be used with caution since it can cause urinary retention (SEDA-14, 122) (13).

Drug Administration

Drug administration route

The removal of chlorofluorocarbons from industrial and household products underlies the 1987 “Montreal Protocol on Substances that Deplete the Ozone Layer”. A reformulation of ipratropium bromide using an alternative, non-chlorofluorocarbon propellant, hydrofluoroalkane, 134a (1,1,1,2-tetrafluoroethane), has been compared with the marketed, chlorofluorocarbon-containing ipratropium bromide aerosol in a randomized, double-blind, placebo-controlled trial in 507 patients with moderate to severe obstructive airways disease (14). The patients were treated with hydrofluoroalkane/ipratropium bromide 42 micrograms, hydrofluoroalkane/ipratropium bromide 84 micrograms, hydrofluoroalkane/placebo, chlorofluorocarbon/ipratropium bromide 42 micrograms, or chlorofluorocarbon/placebo. The incidences of adverse clinical and laboratory events and significant cardiographic effects were not different across the groups.

A nasal spray (isotonic aqueous ipratropium pump) has been used in allergic and non-allergic rhinitis as well as the common cold. The spray caused no systemic adverse effects and only minor infrequent episodes of nasal dryness and epistaxis, which did not interfere with treatment (15,16).

References

1. Pakes GE, Brogden RN, Heel RC, Speight TM, Avery GS. Ipratropium bromide: a review of its pharmacological properties and therapeutic efficacy in asthma and chronic bronchitis. Drugs 1980;20(4):237–66.
2. Delacourt C, de Blic J, Lebourgeois M, Scheinmann P. Intérêt du bromure d'ipratropium dans la crise d'asthme de l'enfant. [Value of ipratropium bromide in asthma crisis in children.] Arch Pediatr 1994;1(1):87–92.
3. Plotnick LH, Ducharme FM. Should inhaled anticholinergics be added to beta2 agonists for treating acute childhood and adolescent asthma? A systematic review. BMJ 1998;317(7164):971–7.
4. Milgrom H, Biondi R, Georgitis JW, Meltzer EO, Munk ZM, Drda K, Wood CC. Comparison of ipratropium bromide 0.03% with beclomethasone dipropionate in the

treatment of perennial rhinitis in children. Ann Allergy Asthma Immunol 1999;83(2):105–11.
5. Dockhorn R, Aaronson D, Bronsky E, Chervinsky P, Cohen R, Ehtessabian R, Finn A, Grossman J, Howland W, Kaiser H, Pearlman D, Sublett J, Ratner P, Settipane G, Sim T, Storms W, Webb R, Drda K, Wood C. Ipratropium bromide nasal spray 0.03% and beclomethasone nasal spray alone and in combination for the treatment of rhinorrhea in perennial rhinitis. Ann Allergy Asthma Immunol 1999;82(4):349–59.
6. van Noord JA, de Munck DR, Bantje TA, Hop WC, Akveld ML, Bommer AM. Long-term treatment of chronic obstructive pulmonary disease with salmeterol and the additive effect of ipratropium. Eur Respir J 2000;15(5):878–85.
7. Mulpeter KM, Walsh JB, O'Connor M, O'Connell F, Burke C. Ocular hazards of nebulized bronchodilators. Postgrad Med J 1992;68(796):132–3.
8. Kizer KM, Bess DT, Bedford NK. Blurred vision from ipratropium bromide inhalation. Am J Health Syst Pharm 1999;56(9):914.
9. Malani JT, Robinson GM, Seneviratne EL. Ipratropium bromide induced angle closure glaucoma. NZ Med J 1982;95(718):749.
10. Hall SK. Acute angle-closure glaucoma as a complication of combined beta-agonist and ipratropium bromide therapy in the emergency department. Ann Emerg Med 1994;23(4):884–7.
11. Watson WT, Shuckett EP, Becker AB, Simons FE. Effect of nebulized ipratropium bromide on intraocular pressures in children. Chest 1994;105(5):1439–41.
12. Hvizdos KM, Goa KL. Tiotropium bromide. Drugs 2002;62(8):1195–203.
13. Pras E, Stienlauf S, Pinkhas J, Sidi Y. Urinary retention associated with ipratropium bromide. DICP 1991; 25(9):939–40.
14. Poli F, Longo G, Parmiani S. The safety and efficacy of immunotherapy with aluminum hydroxide-adsorbed venom extract of *Vespula* spp. An open, retrospective study. Allergol Immunopathol (Madr) 2001;29(5):191–6.
15. Bronsky EA, Druce H, Findlay SR, Hampel FC, Kaiser H, Ratner P, Valentine MD, Wood CC. A clinical trial of ipratropium bromide nasal spray in patients with perennial nonallergic rhinitis. J Allergy Clin Immunol 1995;95(5 Pt 2):1117–22.
16. Kaiser HB, Findlay SR, Georgitis JW, Grossman J, Ratner PH, Tinkelman DG, Roszko P, Zegarelli E, Wood CC. Long-term treatment of perennial allergic rhinitis with ipratropium bromide nasal spray 0.06%. J Allergy Clin Immunol 1995;95(5 Pt 2):1128–32.

Iprindole

See also Monoamine oxidase inhibitors

General Information

Iprindole is a 6,5,8 tricyclic compound, whose first two rings form an indole nucleus (SED-7, 27). It is of some theoretical interest, in that it is weak in its action on the amine pump mechanism. Adverse effects are reported as being similar to those of other tricyclic antidepressants (1,2).

Organs and Systems

Liver

The major adverse effect of serious concern has been jaundice. A review of 21 cases of liver damage during iprindole treatment showed that the onset was at 4–21 days after starting treatment (3). Recovery was rapid after withdrawal. Liver biopsy showed predominantly cholestasis. This complication seems to be similar to that seen after chlorpromazine. In one instance (4), jaundice was accompanied by a marked eosinophilia of 30% and laboratory signs suggesting some hepatocellular damage as well. Jaundice promptly recurred when the drug was re-administered. All the features of this case suggested an allergic reaction.

References

1. Martin ICA, Hossain M, Hart J. Treatment of marked, persistent mood depression: a double-blind comparison of iprindole (Prondol) with nortriptyline. Clin Trials J 1972;3:39.
2. Narayanan HS, Reddy GN, Rao BS. A comparative double-blind evaluation of iprindole and imipramine in the treatment of depressive states. Indian J Med Sci 1973;27(1):1–7.
3. Ajdukiewicz AB, Grainger J, Scheuer PJ, Sherlock S. Jaundice due to iprindole. Gut 1971;12(9):705–8.
4. Aylett MJ. Allergy to iprindol (Prondol) with hepatotoxicity. Br Med J 1971;1(740):112.

Irbesartan

See also Angiotensin II receptor antagonists

General Information

Irbesartan is a potent selective angiotensin II type 1 (AT_1) receptor antagonist. Its pharmacology is the same as that of other angiotensin II receptor antagonists (1). In the registration studies and other controlled trials adverse effects were not dose-related and not different from placebo.

An updated review of the pharmacology and therapeutic use of irbesartan in cardiovascular disorders has been published, including a brief section on drug tolerability, which referred to an unpublished postmarketing surveillance study in which 14% of the patients (1232 of 9009) had mostly mild adverse events (2). No further details were given on the nature of the adverse events.

Organs and Systems

Liver

Cholestasis with irbesartan has been reported (3).

- A 62-year-old woman developed deep icterus and hepatomegaly 1 month after starting to take irbesartan 300 mg/day. She had been hypertensive for 15 years and had no history of liver disease or risk factors for liver disease. Her bilirubin was 403 μmol/l, alkaline phosphatase 3193 IU/l, and aspartate transaminase 177 IU/l. Serology and autoimmune screens were negative, as were liver ultrasonography and computerized tomography. Cholangiopancreatography was normal. Irbesartan was replaced by amlodipine and metoprolol, and 2 months later she remained jaundiced (bilirubin 324 μmol/l). Liver biopsy showed portal tract expansion, minimal inflammation, ectatic ductules, and cholestatic rosettes. Within 16 weeks she fully recovered and continued to be anicteric more than 1 year later.

The temporal profile in this case and the lack of an alternative cause for liver dysfunction suggested a drug reaction.

Urinary tract

Renal insufficiency has been attributed to irbesartan.

- A 77-year-old woman took captopril 25 mg tds and furosemide 40 mg/day for decompensated heart failure (4). Irbesartan 75 mg/day then replaced captopril, and 3 days later she developed renal insufficiency. Irbesartan was withdrawn and her renal function normalized within 5 days. It was not stated whether her blood pressure also changed.
- A 78-year-old Caucasian man with insulin-treated type II diabetes, hypertension, and stable mild renal insufficiency took captopril 25 mg/day and torasemide 150 mg/day (5). His general physician substituted irbesartan 150 mg/day for the captopril. The basal average serum creatinine rose from 220 to 294 μmol/l 10 days after beginning irbesartan, and to 752 μmol/l 3 weeks later, at which stage he was admitted with acute renal insufficiency, oliguria, and edema with a 6 kg weight gain. Two days after withdrawal of irbesartan his creatinine reached a maximum of 907 μmol/l and then fell progressively to 570 μmol/l and never returned to basal values. The patient was started on chronic hemodialysis. Renal Doppler and MRI scans showed no renal artery stenosis, but there were signs of chronic renal ischemia, which may have contributed to the adverse drug reaction.

It is possible in the second case that irbesartan 150 mg/day produced abrupt and more pronounced inhibition of the renin–angiotensin system than the basal stable small dose of captopril 25 mg/day.

A further convincing case of ACE inhibitor-related renal insufficiency has been described with irbesartan and losartan (6).

- A 67-year-old woman with congestive heart failure developed oliguric renal insufficiency 2 days after the introduction of irbesartan. She rapidly recovered after withdrawal, and was then given losartan. The condition recurred shortly afterwards and subsided when losartan was stopped.

Drug–Drug Interactions

Simvastatin acid

A small well-designed study in 14 healthy subjects showed no significant effect of irbesartan on the single-dose pharmacokinetics of total simvastatin acid (7).

References

1. Johnston CI. Pharmacology of irbesartan. Expert Opin Investig Drugs 1999;8(5):655–70.
2. Markham A, Spencer CM, Jarvis B. Irbesartan: an updated review of its use in cardiovascular disorders. Drugs 2000;59(5):1187–206.
3. Hariraj R, Stoner E, Jader S, Preston DM. Drug points: prolonged cholestasis associated with irbesartan. BMJ 2000;321(7260):547.
4. Anglada Pintado JC, Gallego Puerto P, Zapata Lopez A, Cayon Blanco M. Fracaso renal agudo asociado con irbesartan. [Acute renal failure associated with irbesartan.] Med Clin (Barc) 1999;113(9):358–9.
5. Descombes E, Fellay G. End-stage renal failure after irbesartan prescription in a diabetic patient with previously stable chronic renal insufficiency. Ren Fail 2000;22(6):815–21.
6. Lee HY, Kim CH. Acute oliguric renal failure associated with angiotensin II receptor antagonists. Am J Med 2001;111(2):162–3.
7. Marino MR, Vachharajani NN, Hadjilambris OW. Irbesartan does not affect the pharmacokinetics of simvastatin in healthy subjects. J Clin Pharmacol 2000;40(8):875–9.

Iridaceae

See also Herbal medicines

General Information

The genera in the family of Iridaceae (Table 1) include *Crocus*, *Freesia*, and some types of lilies.

Table 1 The genera of Iridaceae

Acidanthera (acidanthera)
Alophia (alophia)
Aristea (aristea)
Belamcanda (belamcanda)
Calydorea (violet lily)
Chasmanthe (African cornflag)
Crocosmia (crocosmia)
Crocus (crocus)
Dietes (dietes)
Eleutherine (eleutherine)
Freesia (freesia)
Gladiolus (gladiolus)
Herbertia (herbertia)
Homeria (Cape tulip)
Iris (iris)
Ixia (African cornlily)
Libertia (libertia)
Nemastylis (pleatleaf)
Neomarica (neomarica)
Olsynium (grass widow)
Romulea (romulea)
Schizostylis (Kaffir lily)
Sisyrinchium (blue-eyed grass)
Sparaxis (wandflower)
Tigridia (peacock flower)
Trimezia (trimezia)
Watsonia (bugle-lily)

Crocus sativus

The stamens of *Crocus sativus* (Indian saffron) have been used primarily as a coloring and flavoring agent. Its potential use as an anticancer agent has been reviewed (1,2). No risks have been documented for daily doses up to 1.5 g, but 5 g is toxic, 10 g is abortive, and 20 g is lethal.

References

1. Abdullaev FI. Cancer chemopreventive and tumoricidal properties of saffron (Crocus sativus L). Exp Biol Med (Maywood) 2002;227(1):20–5.
2. Deng Y, Guo ZG, Zeng ZL, Wang Z. [Studies on the pharmacological effects of saffron (Crocus sativus L) — [T]a review.] Zhongguo Zhong Yao Za Zhi 2002;27(8):565–8.

Iron oxide

General Information

Ultrasmall superparamagnetic particles of iron oxide (USPIOs) of median diameter no less than 50 nm have been studied as blood-pool agents and are given intravenously to enhance liver imaging in patients with cirrhosis and to visualize lymph nodes. They consist of non-stoichiometric microcrystalline iron oxide cores, which are coated with dextrans (in ferumoxides) or siloxanes (in ferumoxsils). The most common form of iron oxide used is magnetite, which is a mixture of Fe_2O_3 and FeO; a mixture of Fe_2O_3 and Fe_3O_4 can be used instead.

After injection, the particles accumulate in the reticuloendothelial system. Liver tumors have few or no reticuloendothelial cells and so there is a contrast between normal liver and tumor.

These contrast agents are well tolerated, with no serious adverse effects. The reported adverse effects include low back pain, vomiting and diarrhea, urticaria, flushing, dizziness, and muscle spasm (SEDA-20, 419). The incidence of adverse effects is higher with these particulate iron oxide agents than with gadolinium chelates. However, that is not a great cause for concern, since few of the reactions are severe and all are self-limiting.

Ferristene

The USPIO contrast agent ferristene (Abdoscan, Amersham) is effective and safe in delineating the gastrointestinal tract after oral ingestion. Different rectal formulations of ferristene with different viscosities and iron concentrations have been evaluated in a phase II clinical study, in which ferristene enemas (200–500 ml) and intravenous gadodiamide (0.1 mmol/kg) were used in the evaluation and staging of rectal cancer in 113 patients (1). Five patients had 10 adverse events, including rectal pain, diarrhea, edema, a phobic reaction, nausea, and a skin rash; all recovered without further therapy. The high-viscosity formulation (70 g of granules/l) was better than the low-viscosity formulation in tumor staging, but the iron concentration (30 or 59 micrograms/ml) of the contrast agent was less important.

Ferucarbotran

Ferucarbotran (carboxydextran coated iron oxide nanoparticles, SHU 555 C, Resovist, Schering AG) is a contrast agent that consists of iron oxide microparticles coated with carboxydextran. After intravenous injection it is sequestered by the reticuloendothelial system, mostly in the liver and spleen. MRI iron oxide causes loss of signal intensity, especially on T1 and T2 weighted images, and the contrast between the lesions and the surrounding tissues is increased owing to loss of signal in the healthy tissues.

Feruglose

Feruglose (NC100150, Clariscan, Nycomed, Oslo, Norway) has been given to 18 healthy men in doses of 2, 3, and 4 mg/kg (2). There were no significant adverse effects during or after the scans. However, NC100150 interferes with iron metabolism, since iron is incorporated into the body after biodegradation. NC100150 shows promise for myocardial perfusion analysis. Studies in animals have also suggested a role for NC100150 in the detection and localization of intra-abdominal bleeding (3).

Ferumoxtran

Ferumoxtran-10 (Combidex, Advanced Magnetics, Cambridge, MA) is an ultrasmall superparamagnetic iron oxide agent. It targets the reticuloendothelial system but also functions as a blood-pool agent. In a phase 2 study in 104 patients with focal liver or spleen pathology who underwent MRI with ferumoxtran-10 (0.8, 1.1, and 1.7 mg of iron per kg), 15% reported a total of 33 adverse events, most commonly dyspnea (3.8%), chest pain (2.9%), and rashes (2.9%) (4). There were no serious adverse events during the 48-hour observation period and no changes in vital signs, physical examination, or laboratory parameters. The authors concluded that ferumoxtran-10 is safe and well tolerated.

SHU 555 A

The diagnostic efficacy and safety of SHU 555 A has been investigated in 19 patients aged 43–89 years who had been referred for investigation of hepatocellular carcinoma (eight patients), liver metastases (four patients), liver hemangioma (four patients), cholangiocarcinoma (two patients), and focal nodular hyperplasia (one patient) (5). The dose of iron was 6.0–11.7 μmol/kg. Patients under 60 kg received 0.9 ml as a bolus intravenous injection and patients over 60 kg received 1.4 ml. None of the 19 patients reported any pain or discomfort at the injection site. One had a diffuse erythematous rash associated with a feeling of pressure in the thorax, which lasted for 30 minutes. There was a significant increase in systolic blood pressure (from 137 to 141 mmHg) 5 minutes after injection; it returned to normal within 4 hours. There was a statistically significant fall in diastolic blood pressure from 75 to 70 mmHg at 4 hours after the injection. These changes were not considered to be of clinical importance. There were also minimal changes in the results of blood tests, which were not of clinical importance. High-quality diagnostic information was provided by the MRI examination.

References

1. Maier AG, Kersting-Sommerhoff B, Reeders JW, Judmaier W, Schima W, Annweiler AA, Meusel M, Wallengren NO. Staging of rectal cancer by double-contrast MR imaging using the rectally administered superparamagnetic iron oxide contrast agent ferristene and IV gadodiamide injection: results of a multicenter phase II trial. J Magn Reson Imaging 2000;12(5):651–60.
2. Panting JR, Taylor AM, Gatehouse PD, Keegan J, Yang GZ, McGill S, Francis JM, Burman ED, Firmin DN, Pennell DJ. First-pass myocardial perfusion imaging and equilibrium signal changes using the intravascular contrast agent NC100150 injection. J Magn Reson Imaging 1999;10(3):404–10.
3. Kroft LJ, de Roos A. Blood pool contrast agents for cardiovascular MR imaging. J Magn Reson Imaging 1999; 10(3):395–403.
4. Sharma R, Saini S, Ros PR, Hahn PF, Small WC, de Lange EE, Stillman AE, Edelman RR, Runge VM, Outwater EK, Morris M, Lucas M. Safety profile of ultrasmall superparamagnetic iron oxide ferumoxtran-10: phase II clinical trial data. J Magn Reson Imaging 1999;9(2):291–4.
5. Kehagias DT, Gouliamos AD, Smyrniotis V, Vlahos LJ. Diagnostic efficacy and safety of MRI of the liver with superparamagnetic iron oxide particles (SH U 555 A). J Magn Reson Imaging 2001;14(5):595–601.

Iron salts

General Information

Iron is a metallic element (symbol Fe; atomic no. 26). The symbol is derived from the Latin word for iron, ferrum.

Iron is found widespread in nature in ores such as almandine hercynite (iron aluminate); scorodite (iron arsenate); pyrites (iron disulfide); laterite (iron hydroxide); columbite (iron niobate); chromite, hematite, ilmenite, limonite, magnetite, mugearite, stilpnosiderite, and umber (iron oxides); lazulite (iron phosphate); babingtonite, crocidolite, cummingtonite, epidote, eudialyte, fayalite, gadolinite, glauconite, hornblende, hypersthene, olivine, pennine, piedmontite, and riebeckite (iron silicates); coquimbite, inkstone, and jarosite (iron sulfates); ankerite, arsenopyrites, bornite, chalcopyrite, pentlandite, and pyrrhotite (iron sulfides); marcasite (iron sulfite); and wolframite (iron tungstate).

The body has no physiological route for the excretion of excess iron, and iron overload is a constant risk of therapy. Long-term use of iron by any route in large amounts can lead to hemosiderosis, simulating hemochromatosis; the danger is greatest when the mucosal barrier is bypassed by parenteral injection. Even the safety of iron-fortified food is uncertain (SEDA-4, 171). As with other metals there is environmental exposure to iron in many forms. The use of iron cooking utensils is often considered a useful source of supplementary iron in the diet. Various iron oxides and hydroxides are used as pigments in cosmetics.

The molecular basis of iron overload and toxicity has been reviewed (1,2). Much attention has been paid to mechanisms of hemochromatosis (3,4). There have been reviews of the comparative tolerance and safety of iron salts (5) and their use in specific conditions, such as renal insufficiency (6).

In elderly people, iron deficiency is usually a sign of bleeding, and it is wiser to track down and correct the cause of the blood loss (for example gastric malignancy) than to prescribe iron, which can merely mask the problem and delay diagnosis.

In the following sections, adverse reactions are considered in connection with the types of iron therapy with which they have most commonly been associated, but any adverse effect of iron can in principle occur with any formulation or as a result of mixed medical and non-medical exposure.

Oral iron

New oral formulations with improved intestinal iron absorption are being marketed and their efficacy and toxicity are being studied (7).

Despite the use of recombinant erythropoietin, anemia remains a significant problem for patients with end-stage renal disease (8). Because oral iron formulations are relatively ineffective and poorly tolerated, intravenous iron dextran has been widely used, despite the risk of adverse effects.

Parenteral iron

Like oral iron, parenteral iron is used too widely. When iron is truly needed, oral administration is generally preferable (9). Intractable gastrointestinal intolerance to oral formulations, hyperemesis in pregnancy, very severe blood loss, and possibly ulcerative colitis are some of the few valid indications for parenteral iron. A low iron-binding capacity (for example due to prior saturating iron therapy or malnutrition), folic acid deficiency, and an allergic constitution predispose the patient to adverse reactions to parenteral iron. Iron injections have been reported to provoke hemolytic anemia in cases of paroxysmal nocturnal hemoglobinuria.

Most parenteral iron is administered intramuscularly, but intravenous injections have enjoyed a wave of popularity for no very good medical reason; it seems particularly likely to precipitate acute allergic or anaphylactic reactions in sensitive individuals, sometimes involving cardiac dysrhythmias, hypotension, circulatory collapse, and pulmonary edema.

The adverse effects of iron formulations have resulted in trials to optimize dose regimens. A large database of clinical variance reports from Fresenius Medical Care North America (FMCNA) has been analysed to determine the incidence of suspected adverse drug reactions of iron dextran and the associated patient characteristics, dialysis practice patterns, and outcomes (8). A case-cohort design was used, comparing individuals who had suspected adverse drug reactions with the overall population. Out of 841 252 intravenous iron dextran administrations over 6 months, there were 165 reported suspected adverse drug reactions, corresponding to an overall rate of about 20 per 100 000 doses. Hospital evaluation was required in 43 patients (26%), 18 (11%) required hospitalization, and one (0.6%) died. Dyspnea (43%), nausea (34%), vomiting (23%), flushing (27%), pruritus (25%), hypotension (23%), and neurological symptoms (23%) were the most common adverse reactions. Serious adverse reactions to intravenous iron dextran are rare and difficult to predict; the risk appears to depend on the specific formulation of intravenous iron dextran.

In a retrospective analysis of the incidence of adverse effects associated with 250 mg of ferric gluconate infused over 1–4 hours in 40 patients with severe chronic renal insufficiency, who received 79 treatments, four treatments in two patients were associated with adverse effects, including diarrhea, vomiting, low back pain, hypotension, and a burning sensation in the feet. The duration of the infusion did not influence the adverse effects profile.

Intramuscular iron

Iron compounds for intramuscular administration are iron sorbitol–citric acid complex (iron sorbitex), iron dextran, iron glycerin–citric acid complex, and iron polyisomaltose. The work on these formulations is largely old and has been reviewed in previous volumes in this series.

Intramuscular iron injections are often painful, can produce topical discoloration of the skin, and some local inflammation with lymphadenopathy. Rarely, more severe local reactions follow (SEDA-6, 224), such as transient lipomyodystrophy. An unpleasant metallic taste in the mouth is common and can persist for some hours or days. Some patients develop general symptoms, such as headache, flushing, sweating, nausea, vomiting, dizziness, generalized aches and pains, malaise, arthralgia, palpitation, and pericardial or abdominal pain. Although very rare, a severe anaphylactic reaction to intramuscular iron dextran can occur.

The safety and efficacy of iron dextran have been evaluated in patients on home renal replacement therapies, without any adverse effects (10).

Intravenous iron

Iron dextran is now the most commonly used iron compound for intravenous use, and most reported adverse reactions to intravenous iron relate to this formulation.

Local reactions to intravenous iron dextran include transient pain (in some 4% of cases) and phlebitis. The risk of the latter may be reduced by using saline instead of 5% dextrose as diluent. Nevertheless, deep vein thrombosis has been observed in a few patients infused with a dilution of iron dextran in normal saline (SED-8, 514).

Systemic reactions to iron dextran given intravenously are more common than those to intramuscular iron; they include non-immunological and immunological, immediate and delayed reactions. Flushing, a sensation of warmth, and a metallic taste are often associated with excessively rapid injection, but usually subside within less than a minute after slowing or stopping the injection. In about 1% of cases, including patients with no known prior exposure to dextran, life-threatening anaphylactoid reactions occur rapidly, with hypotension, cardiovascular shock, syncope, cyanosis, bronchospasm, respiratory arrest, urticaria, and angioedema; deaths have ensued. Milder allergic reactions comprise mild and transient hypotension, malaise, itching, and urticaria. Desensitization under an umbrella of glucocorticoids, antihistamines, and ephedrine has been carried out successfully (11).

Delayed systemic reactions to intravenous iron dextran appear to be more common, the reported incidence ranging from 5 to 15%. They start within 4–48 hours of injection and can last for 3–7 days. Characteristic symptoms are fever, arthralgia, myalgia, headache, and lymphadenopathy, singly or in combination, and a classic serum sickness has been seen (SEDA-16, 26). Chills may also occur and individual patients may experience dizziness, tinnitus, paresthesia, a feeling of stiffness in the arms and neck, pruritus, urticarial or other cutaneous eruptions, pallor, nausea, vomiting, and nasal irritation. There may be hepatosplenomegaly. These delayed reactions are more frequent in children and, for some reason, in patients of Chinese origin. They tend to be more severe in patients with low body weight given higher doses, and in patients with rheumatoid arthritis or other types of inflammatory disease.

Large doses of intravenous iron dextran and iron saccharate have been compared in a retrospective study of 379 patients who had attended peritoneal dialysis clinics in the past 5 years (12). Of these, 62 were selected to receive intravenous iron based on ferrokinetic markers of iron deficiency, non-adherence to oral iron, ineffectiveness of oral iron, or increased erythropoietin requirements. Intravenous iron was given as two injections of 500 mg each 1 week apart in 61 patients, 33 of whom received iron dextran, 23 iron saccharate, and five both iron dextran and iron saccharate. One patient developed anaphylaxis to a test dose of iron dextran and was excluded from further therapy. Blood samples were collected before and 3 and 6 months after iron infusions. Five of the 34 patients who received iron dextran developed minor adverse effects and one had an anaphylactic reaction to the test dose. Of the 23 patients who received iron saccharate, one had an anaphylactic reaction and two had transient chest pain, which subsided without therapy. There were more adverse effects with iron dextran (7.4% of injections) compared with iron saccharate (4.3% of injections), but this difference was not statistically significant. The number of episodes of peritonitis also increased during the 6 months after intravenous iron infusion, especially with iron dextran, compared with the number of episodes during the 6 months before iron infusions, although the difference was not statistically significant.

Other iron compounds for intravenous use

Saccharated iron oxide is strongly alkaline and hypertonic; if injected outside the vein it can cause marked local reactions. Significant serum hypophosphatemia has on occasion been observed during treatment, accompanied by reduced renal tubular reabsorption of phosphate. The mechanism of these changes, which were reversible after stopping the iron injections, has not been clarified (13).

Topical iron

Iron chloride is sometimes used topically as a hemostyptic after minor surgery. It can result in persistent brown staining at the site of application. Use of Monsel's solution (ferric subsulfate), another hemostyptic agent, can cause fibrovascular proliferation accompanied by strongly pigmented macrophages after an interval of up to 3–5 weeks; the condition may be mistaken for malignant melanoma.

Organs and Systems

Cardiovascular

Intramuscular iron

The major hazard of the intramuscular use of iron sorbitex consists of severe systemic reactions with cardiac involvement, which may be fatal; they occur in up to 1% of cases, they start 10–30 minutes after injection and a patient who has received an injection must be monitored for an hour. Nausea, chest pain, profuse sweating, cardiac dysrhythmias, and loss of consciousness can occur. Cardiac complications include complete atrioventricular block, ventricular tachycardia, and ventricular fibrillation.

Intravenous iron

Non-transferrin-bound iron, which increases after intravenous ferric saccharate, has been suggested to act as a catalytic agent in oxygen radical formation in vitro, and may therefore contribute to endothelial impairment in vivo (14). The effect of ferric saccharate infusion 10 mg has been investigated in 20 healthy volunteers. Ferric saccharate caused a greater than four-fold increase in non-transferrin-bound iron and transient significant reduction in flow-mediated dilatation 10 minutes after infusion of ferric saccharate. The generation of superoxide in whole blood increased significantly 10 and 240 minutes after infusion of ferric saccharate by 70 and 53% respectively. Thus, infusion of iron leads to increased oxygen radical stress and acute endothelial dysfunction.

Respiratory

Spontaneously regressing bronchial necrosis with granuloma formation has been associated with the aspiration of a tablet of ferrous sulfate in a single case (15).

Acute respiratory distress syndrome has been attributed to iron (16).

- A 3.5-year-old girl was admitted after accidental ingestion of 50–60 tablets of ferrous sulfate 200 mg. She was unresponsive and her serum iron concentration was 138 μmol/l. She required resuscitation and ventilation and an intravenous infusion of deferoxamine was started at a rate of 15 mg/kg/hour, reducing to 5 mg/kg/hour 20 hours later, when the iron concentration was 27 μmol/l. At that time, her liver function deteriorated, with raised alanine transaminase activity (57 IU/l), raised bilirubin (56 μmol/l), and a coagulopathy with an INR of 2.7. She was given an infusion of *N*-acetylcysteine 12.5 mg/kg/hour and her hepatic function stabilized. After about 40 hours she had acute respiratory deterioration with tachypnea and hypoxemia. A chest X-ray showed widespread bilateral infiltrates. A diagnosis of acute respiratory distress syndrome was made.

Aspiration of iron tablets can produce an acute reaction in the airways since they are highly irritative; immediate removal bronchoscopy is necessary to avoid permanent damage (SEDA-16, 236). Lung damage has been reported in a man who had inhaled an oral iron formulation containing 350 mg of elemental iron (17).

- A 75-year-old man developed chest discomfort and hemoptysis. A chest X-ray showed left lower lobe collapse and fiberoptic bronchoscopy showed that the left endobronchial mucosa was friable, edematous, and golden-yellow, with interspersed erythematous ulcerated areas with marked contact bleeding. There was heavy deposition of yellow–brown pigment on the basement membrane of the superficial bronchial epithelium, on the basement membrane of the bronchial glands, and on fibrillar material in the stroma. Pigment deposition was greatest in the necrotic fragments of mucosa, but was also seen in viable mucosa. This material stained strongly for ferric ion with Perls' stain. Iron was withdrawn and the left lower lobe collapse improved.

Metabolism

In erythropoietic protoporphyria, iron can cause a relapse of symptoms (18). An involvement of iron overload in the pathogenesis of some cases of porphyria cutanea tarda has been suggested (19).

Hematologic

Latent folic acid deficiency can become manifest during iron therapy due to additional demand for the vitamin secondary to increased erythropoietic activity (20).

Intramuscular iron

Thrombocytopenia has been attributed to intramuscular iron (21).

- A 30-year-old woman had a hemoglobin concentration of 3.1 g/dl, a mean cell volume of 77 fl, a reticulocyte count of 2.13%, a platelet count of 426 $\times$ 10^9/l, a serum iron concentration of 5 ng/ml, a transferrin saturation of 1%, and a ferritin concentration of 8 ng/ml. She was intolerant of oral iron and was given intramuscular iron dextran, 100 mg/day for 8 days, when she developed asymptomatic thrombocytopenia (platelet count 20 $\times$ 10^9/l). Iron dextran was withdrawn and she took oral ferrous fumarate 200 mg/day plus ascorbic acid 120 mg/day. Within 2 days her platelet count improved.

Mouth and teeth

Most liquid ferrous products stain dental enamel, but this is usually reversible (22).

Gastrointestinal

Severe gastrointestinal necrosis and strictures after iron overdose are well described. However, mucosal injury in patients taking therapeutic iron has received only scant recognition, despite its widespread use. In 36 upper gastrointestinal tract biopsies from 33 patients (24 gastric, nine esophageal, one gastro-esophageal junctional, and two duodenal) there was characteristic brown crystalline iron material (23). Most of the biopsies (32 of 36) contained luminal crystalline iron adjacent to the surface epithelium or admixed with luminal fibrinoinflammatory exudate. In 30 biopsies there was crystalline iron deposition in the lamina propria, either covered by an intact epithelium, subjacent to small superficial erosions, or admixed with granulation tissue. Three biopsies showed iron-containing thrombi in mucosal blood vessels. Erosive or ulcerative mucosal injury was present in 30 of 36 biopsies. The amount of iron accumulation in cases with mucosal injury was greater than in the cases without mucosal injury. About half of the patients (17 of 33) also had underlying infectious, mechanical, toxic, or systemic medical conditions that could have initiated or exacerbated tissue injury. Crystalline iron deposition was found in 0.9% of upper gastrointestinal endoscopic examinations (12 of 1300), and iron medication-associated erosive mucosal injury was present in 0.7% (nine of 1300). These results suggest that crystalline iron deposition in the upper gastrointestinal tract is not uncommon. It can cause or exacerbate a distinctive histological pattern of erosive mucosal injury, especially in patients with associated upper gastrointestinal disorders.

Oral iron

Though iron clearly does have the ability to irritate the mucous membranes, its widespread reputation for poor gastric tolerance is undeserved, generally reflecting its having been given in excess. Of patients taking up to 200 mg/day of elemental iron, only a few highly susceptible individuals will develop gastrointestinal adverse effects, and constipation is then the most usual feature. Higher doses can give rise to gastric discomfort, nausea, vomiting, or to either constipation or diarrhea. In sensitive individuals with complications in the upper gastrointestinal tract, histopathologically distinctive lesions are found in mucosal biopsies of the stomach and esophagus (24); there can be heavy iron accumulation within ulcer granulation tissue, in the connective tissue and blood vessels of the mucosal lamina propria, and within glandular and squamous epithelia. The appearance is similar to that seen after overdosage.

Oral iron can color the feces black, which can be mistaken for melena. Fewer gastrointestinal adverse effects occur if the iron dose is gradually increased to the desired level or if iron is taken with food, but since insoluble iron complexes may be formed with food it has been recommended that iron salts be taken between meals. Despite many claims for the better gastric tolerance of expensive iron formulations, it is still not entirely proven that they are any better tolerated than plain ferrous sulfate if the latter is properly dosed. Iron supplementation via a gastric delivery system did not produce any gastrointestinal adverse reactions while efficacy was similar to that of a ferrous sulfate elixir (25). Carbonyl iron has also been studied, although mainly as a means of reducing acute toxicity if such a product is accidentally taken by children (SEDA-16, 235). Iron protein succinylate is another iron derivative for oral use, providing protein-bound iron (26); it is more slowly absorbed than divalent iron, which probably explains the claimed improvement in gastrointestinal tolerability; again it is not at all clear that tolerance is truly improved as related to the amount of iron actually absorbed.

True gastrointestinal risks occur if a solid dosage form becomes lodged in the pharynx, esophagus, or intestinal diverticula; severe erosion can follow (SEDA-6, 224) (SEDA-20, 211). An accumulation of ferrous sulfate tablets with a non-soluble matrix has been the source of ileus in a case of Crohn's disease (SEDA-16, 236). This sort of risk is greatest with modified-release formulations and absent with liquid iron formulations; the latter should therefore be preferred in cases of delayed gastric emptying, pyloric stenosis, or diverticula of the alimentary tract.

Gut pigmentation has been attributed to an iron salt (27).

- An 80-year-old Japanese woman presented with epigastric discomfort and nausea. She had a history of hypertension, rheumatoid arthritis, iron deficiency anemia, chronic renal insufficiency, and had taken oral ferrous sulfite for 19 months. Endoscopic examination of the duodenum showed marked pigmentation of the duodenal mucosa. Histological examination showed that the pigment had histochemical features compatible with hemosiderin and was located mainly within macrophage lysosomes in the lamina propria. Ferrous sulfite was withdrawn and the pigmentation disappeared within 7 months.

Liver

There is much evidence that normal or even mildly increased amounts of iron in the liver can be damaging, particularly when combined with other hepatotoxic factors, such as alcohol, porphyrogenic drugs, or chronic viral hepatitis (28).

Oral iron

Chronic liver disease has been attributed to oral iron.

- A healthy 5-year-old girl, who had taken large doses of oral ferrous sulfate 300 mg five times a day (300 mg of elemental iron/day) for 5 years, developed severe hemosiderosis (29). Liver biopsy showed preserved lobular architecture, but the portal tracts were expanded by fibrosis and there was mild septal fibrosis. There was siderosis of the hepatic parenchymal cells and hemosiderin deposition in the Kupffer cells. She had no underlying hematological disease and her iron absorption was normal. HLA phenotypes and DNA analysis for the most common mutations associated with hemochromatosis excluded homozygous and heterozygous hereditary hemochromatosis. She was successfully treated by phlebotomy. Iron studies 10 years later were normal.
- A 22-year-old woman with adult-onset Still's disease and massive hyperferritinemia became progressively more anemic, with a fall in hemoglobin to 8.2 g/dl, and was given oral ferrous fumarate 300 g bd (30). She developed acute florid hepatitis with an intraparenchymatous histiocytic infiltration, which settled on withdrawal of the iron.

In the latter case iron may have exacerbated the macrophage hyperactivity that is presumed to be present in adult-onset Still's disease. Oral iron may be inadvisable in the acute phase of this disease.

Skin

Reversible skin eruptions have been described in occasional patients taking oral iron. One case presented with a generalized exanthematous pustular eruption following the use of ferrous fumarate (31), another with erythema and lichenification on sun-exposed areas after taking sodium ferrous citrate (32). Both these cases developed 2 weeks after starting treatment; it was suggested that in the latter case iron itself or the transferrin iron complex (diferric transferrin) might have acted as a photosensitizer.

Musculoskeletal

Parenteral iron

Intramuscular iron

The possible sarcoma-inducing potential of intramuscular iron was fully discussed 15 years ago (SED-9, 375) (33) and no new information on the topic has come to light. The conclusion at that time was that the evidance linking intramuscular iron to sarcomatous change was scanty.

Intravenous iron

Saccharated ferric oxide, an intravenous formulation of iron that is used when oral iron is not effective in anemia, can cause osteomalacia during long-term use. The underlying mechanism of nephropathy leading to bone toxicity has recently been reviewed (34).

Oral iron

Although total dose infusions of iron (see the section on Intravenous iron under Immunologic) can cause rheumatoid arthritis to flare up, this has not been demonstrated with oral iron. However, a patient who has reacted in this way to an infusion can subsequently relapse if given oral iron.

Immunologic

Iron enhances the pathogenicity of micro-organisms, adversely affects the function of macrophages and lymphocytes, and enhances fibrogenic pathways, all of which may enhance hepatic injury due to iron itself or to iron alongside other factors.

Oral iron

Skin reactions to oral iron are extremely rare.

- A 40-year-old woman with iron deficiency anemia due to menstrual blood loss took oral iron for 3 months without any adverse effects (35). Nine months later she became anemic again and 2 hours after an oral dose of ferrous sulfate 525 g (105 mg of elemental iron) she developed generalized pruritus and an erythematous maculopapular rash. This recurred 1 week later, when she took ferrous protein succinilate 800 g (40 g of iron). Desensitization with oral iron was carried out. Skin prick tests and patch tests with iron formulations were negative. Two single-blind, placebo-controlled oral challenges were performed and she began to have similar cutaneous symptoms. A slow desensitization protocol, using increasing doses, was tolerated without adverse effects. Chronic oral iron therapy once a day for 9 months sustained the desensitized state and the anemia disappeared.

Parenteral iron

Intravenous iron

Patients with a history of allergy may be at risk of developing undesired immunological reactions, for example attacks of asthma, after parenteral iron dextran; however, the incidence of such reactions seems to be low, and the risk probably also exists with other iron compounds as well. A test infusion is not recommended as it may or may not detect susceptibility to immediate reactions and can itself elicit violent reactions.

There was at one time impressive but limited case evidence that systemic reactions to iron dextran might be more frequent in patients with rheumatic or other inflammatory diseases; no further evidence has been published. There might be confusion with the ability of intravenous iron to induce a flare-up of an existing rheumatic condition (see the section on Oral iron under Musculoskeletal).

Single dose infusions of iron dextran appear to have increased the occurrence of malaria in endemic regions. There was an increased mortality after oral or parenteral iron therapy in children with severe malnutrition (kwashiorkor), perhaps due to overwhelming infections (36). Reactivation of quiescent infections of various other types has been observed in African nomads following ferrous sulfate therapy (SEDA-4, 171). Iron dextran has similarly been associated with a flaring up of latent tuberculosis in children.

Persistent hypogammaglobulinemia has been described in a patient receiving gold; a year after drug withdrawal the gamma-globulin concentrations were still unchanged (37).

An insulin autoimmune syndrome, marked by presence of insulin antibodies and small granulomas in the skin, has been documented in Japanese cases, many of whom had also received penicillamine (38,39).

Intramuscular iron

Iron dextran administration is associated with a high incidence of adverse reactions, including anaphylaxis and death (5). Although it is the dextran rather than the iron that is believed to be the cause of these reactions, which raises the question of whether patients who are sensitive to iron dextran can safely be given another form of parenteral iron, namely sodium ferric gluconate in sucrose. In a double-blind, controlled trial sodium ferric gluconate in sucrose or placebo was given to 144 iron dextran-sensitive patients for comparison with 2194 patients who had been tolerant to iron dextran. Serum tryptase concentrations were also measured. Of 144 patients who were sensitive to iron dextran and who were exposed to sodium ferric gluconate in sucrose, three were intolerant; all had suspected allergic reactions, including one with a serious reaction. One dextran-sensitive patient had a suspected allergic reaction after placebo. In contrast, among the 2194 iron dextran-tolerant patients, reactions to sodium ferric gluconate in sucrose were significantly less common, with intolerance in seven patients, including five who had suspected allergic events, but none who had serious events. Two iron-dextran tolerant patients had allergic-like reactions to placebo. Two of the three suspected allergic events in the iron dextran-sensitive group were confirmed as mast cell-dependent, by a 100% increase in serum tryptase, while there were no confirmed allergic events in the iron dextran-tolerant group. Long-term exposure to sodium ferric gluconate in sucrose in iron dextran-sensitive patients resulted in intolerance in only one additional patient and no serious adverse events.

Patients with a history of iron dextran sensitivity had about seven-fold higher rates of reaction to both placebo and sodium ferric gluconate in sucrose compared with iron dextran-tolerant patients. However, logistic regression analysis, performed to account for the higher reaction rate to placebo, suggested that this increased reactivity was neither drug-specific nor immunologically mediated, but represented host idiosyncrasy. These results support the conclusions that reactions to sodium ferric gluconate in sucrose can be attributed to pseudo-allergy, and that it is not a true allergen.

Iron dextran was particularly likely to cause hypersensitivity reactions when it was used in 537 dialysis patients (40), the most common adverse reactions were itching, dyspnea, wheezing, chest pain, nausea, hypotension, angioedema, dyspepsia, diarrhea, flushing, headache, cardiac arrest, and myalgia. Most of the reactions were mild, but of a subseries of 27 patients exhibiting adverse effects, three patients had to be hospitalized including the individual who had suffered cardiac arrest.

After intramuscular iron dextran, symmetrical allergic purpura of the lower limbs due to hypersensitivity vasculitis has been observed in a child (41).

Infection Risk

In a 10-year consecutive series of 263 allogeneic bone marrow transplant recipients, there were five cases of invasive mucormycosis (42). Only one infection occurred within the first 100 days after transplantation, while the rest complicated the late post-transplant course (median day of diagnosis, 343). Sites of infection were considered "non-classical" and included pulmonary, cutaneous, and gastric. There were no cases of fungal dissemination. Mucormycosis was the primary cause of death in three of the five patients. Corticosteroid-treated graft-versus-host disease, either acute or chronic, or severe neutropenia were present in all cases. However, compared with a matched control population, the most striking finding was severe iron overload in each patient. The mean serum ferritin concentration, transferrin saturation, and the number of transfused units of red cells in the study group were all significantly higher than in the control group. There was a striking association between the occurrence of mucormycosis in dialysis patients and the use of deferoxamine for the treatment of iron and/or aluminium overload. From experimental work and observational data, it appears that iron overload, either transfusional or due to dyserythropoiesis, may be an important risk factor in the development of mucormycosis in this transplantation patient population.

Long-Term Effects

Tumorigenicity

The risk of colorectal cancer due to iron has been specifically examined in a prospective investigation in more than 14 000 patients (43). Iron appears to confer an increased risk of colorectal cancer, and the localization of risk may be attributable to the mode of epithelial exposure. It seems that luminal exposure to oral iron increases the risk proximally, whereas an increased serum iron concentration increases the risk distally.

Genetic hemochromatosis constitutes a high risk factor for the development of hepatocellular carcinoma. It is widely accepted that venesection prevents the evolution of cirrhosis in hemochromatosis and indirectly protects against the development of hepatocellular carcinoma. However, three cases did not conform to the "siderosis-cirrhosis-carcinoma" sequence, and prompt and adequate iron depletion did not protect against the development of cancer (44).

- A 39-year-old army officer had bouts of palpitation and dizziness. There were no risk factors for chronic liver disease apart from a family history of hemochromatosis. His cardiovascular and nervous systems were normal but there was 5 cm hepatomegaly. Percutaneous liver biopsy showed grade 4 siderosis in parenchymal and non-parenchymal liver cells and a mild inflammatory infiltrate with minimal portal fibrosis. He had 45 liters of blood venesected over the next 18 months and a repeat biopsy 3 years later showed a non-cirrhotic liver with no stainable iron. He developed a non-resectable primary hepatocellular clear cell carcinoma 17 years after the initial diagnosis.
- The other two cases were male siblings. One presented with atypical chest pain and had 3 cm hepatomegaly. Liver biopsy showed parenchymal grade 4 siderosis with normal architecture. He had 170 liters of blood venesected over the next 27 years, but then his iron indices indicated reaccumulation. Ultrasound showed a hyperechoic lesion in the liver due to a moderately differentiated hepatocellular carcinoma. His elder sibling, who had grade 4 siderosis and normal hepatic architecture, also developed a well-differentiated hepatocellular carcinoma.

Second-Generation Effects

Pregnancy

The case once made against use of iron dextran in pregnancy because of a supposed risk of possible uterine cramps (SED-9, 377) or a greater risk of systemic reactions (SED-8, 513) has not been substantiated. However, in one case a pregnant woman had anaphylactic shock as a reaction to intravenous iron, and this resulted in fetal cerebral damage (SEDA-22, 246).

Susceptibility Factors

Age

Age is a possible risk factor regarding adverse reactions to total-dose infusions of iron dextran (45).

Renal disease

Iron deficiency is a common and important cause of poor response to erythropoietin in patients with severe chronic renal insufficiency, in whom oral iron supplements fail to correct iron deficiency (6). Ferric gluconate has a low adverse effects profile, but the recommended dose of 62.5–125 mg per treatment is not practical for patients who are not on hemodialysis. In a retrospective analysis of the incidence of adverse effects associated with 250 mg of ferric gluconate infused over 1–4 hours in 40 patients with severe chronic renal insufficiency, who received 79 treatments, four treatments in two patients were associated with adverse effects, including diarrhea, vomiting, low back pain, hypotension, and a burning sensation in the feet. The duration of the infusion did not influence the adverse effects profile.

Other features of the patient

Iron toxicity can be expected if the amount of free iron released into the plasma exceeds the plasma iron-binding capacity. This is more likely to occur when using iron sorbitol–citric acid complex (iron sorbitex), since the iron is less firmly bound than with iron dextran. Several conditions associated with low iron-binding capacity, such as malnutrition (kwashiorkor, malnutrition syndrome) and previous or simultaneous oral iron therapy appear to predispose to the development of these toxic reactions. In addition, folic acid deficiency has been reported to be a predisposing factor (SED-9, 516), the likely mechanism being altered iron utilization secondary to folic acid deficiency, which results in an increased saturation of iron-binding capacity.

Drug Administration

Drug administration route

Oral iron

Although modified-release formulations seem to be better tolerated, this is almost certainly a reflection of their less complete absorption. Iron is best absorbed in the duodenum, and most of the iron in modified-release tablets is released only when the tablets reach the lower parts of the gastrointestinal tract (46).

Parenteral iron

Total dose infusion of iron

With total dose infusion, the amount of iron that is required is delivered in a single infusion rather than by intermittent therapy. Although iron concentrations can rise to very high values, for example 100 000 micrograms/ml (45), there are unlikely to be signs of iron intoxication (SED-8, 513).

However, toxic reactions to intravenous iron occur when ionized iron exceeds plasma binding capacity. With iron dextran, the iron moiety is so firmly bound to dextran that ionized iron does not exceed plasma iron-binding capacity even when total plasma iron concentrations are extremely high. However, there are adverse effects, which were at first underestimated; whenever possible other routes or methods of iron dextran administration should be preferred.

Immediate reactions occurred in nine of 40 adults, variously in the form of anaphylaxis, chills, malaise, hypertension, gastrointestinal reactions, epistaxis, or chest pain. Monitoring for these early reactions is always necessary, but elderly patients require particular attention since they are more likely to react in this way.

Symmetric allergic purpura following the intravenous infusion of iron dextran has exceptionally been noted. In children, transient hepatosplenomegaly has been described as a common finding.

An adverse effect on rheumatic disorders of intravenous iron is well documented (SEDA-12, 190), with exacerbation of joint symptoms, perhaps by promoting lipid peroxidation (47). Of 11 patients with rheumatoid arthritis who received a total dose infusion of iron for anemia, nine experienced an exacerbation of the synovitis, and the two other patients had an anaphylactic reaction. The exacerbations occurred 24–48 hours after completion of the iron dextran infusion and settled in all patients within 11 days. One of these patients had synovial flares when challenged with oral ferrous sulfate. In a single reported case, total dose iron infusion was followed by prolonged polyarthritis, mainly of the large joints, in a patient with no previous evidence of rheumatoid arthritis or ankylosing spondylitis (48). Despite prolonged glucocorticoid therapy, clinical resolution of the problem took 6 months. It may also be relevant that when an iron infusion was given to 20 dialysis patients several of them developed muscular aches, an influenza-like condition or joint pain (SEDA-17, 278).

Organ calcification has very rarely been described after use of iron dextran in uremic patients (SED-8, 515).

Iron overload due to transfusions

Symptoms and signs of iron overload in transfusion-dependent anemias occur after a total transfusion burden of about 100–150 units of blood (49).

Drug overdose

The toxicokinetics and toxicodynamics of iron poisoning have been reviewed (50).

Oral iron

Acute poisoning of children who have taken iron tablets found in the medicine cabinet or elsewhere in the home has repeatedly been reported. The tablets, often attractively coloured and sugar-coated, are readily assumed to be confectionery.

The number of young children who have accidentally swallowed iron has more than doubled since 1986, since when more than 110 000 children under 6 years who accidentally swallowed iron tablets were reported to poison control centers. Many of the children were hospitalized and at least 33 died. The children who died had swallowed as few as five to as many as 98 tablets. In some cases, toddlers found tablets within their reach in uncapped or loosely capped containers. In other cases a young child managed to open a container. In 1995 the number of cases of unintended ingestion of iron by children was estimated at some 22 000 in the USA alone (51). Acute toxicity is associated with free radical formation. Emetics, gastric lavage, and even surgery may be called for to remove the excess.

Much more common is chronic poisoning due to excessive intake over a long period, with deposition of iron within cells. Iron has a toxic effect in almost all organs, especially the liver, heart, and endocrine glands. Histological evidence of iron-mediated tissue damage can be obtained before the clinical picture becomes evident. Combined management with ascorbic acid and deferoxamine can yield high rates of deferoxamine-induced urinary iron excretion without obvious adverse effects on the heart.

The FDA has proposed regulations requiring warning labels on iron formulations, such as tablets and capsules, and requiring unit dose packaging for products containing 30 mg or more of iron in each dosage unit (52). The proposed regulations apply to both dietary supplements and drugs containing iron, but not to iron-fortified foods, such as enriched flour. This proposal is based on findings that iron-containing drugs and supplements are the leading cause of accidental poisonings in children. In 1988–92, about 17% of childhood deaths reported to poison control centers in the USA were blamed on iron poisoning: in 1984–87 the incidence was only 5%.

The Consumer Product Safety Commission, which regulates child-resistant packaging for household substances, requires such packaging for any oral iron product that contains 250 mg or more iron per container. In addition, the FDA's proposed regulations would require manufacturers to wrap iron tablets and capsules containing more than 30 mg per dosage unit in individual units, such as in blister packs.

Drug–Drug Interactions

Antacids

Iron absorption is reduced by antacids (for example magnesium trisilicate and carbonate) (53).

Colestyramine

Iron absorption is reduced by colestyramine (54).

Penicillamine

Concomitant ingestion of iron reduces the copper-excretory effect of penicillamine (SED-12, 527) and penicillamine reduces iron absorption (55).

Tetracyclines

Concomitant oral administration of tetracyclines and iron grossly reduces the absorption of both, because complexes are formed (56,57); there should be an interval of 2–3 hours between the use of the two.

Interference with Diagnostic Tests

Urine

Urine can turn dark in color in the first 24 hours after parenteral iron injection. The reddish-brown color, which has been observed after the intramuscular injection of iron sorbitol–citric acid complex (SED-8, 515), is due to urinary excretion of part of the iron compound. It has to be distinguished from the black discoloration that may develop if urine of patients who have received iron-sorbitex is allowed to stand, assumed to be due to production of iron sulfide by bacterial growth. Phenomena of this kind are unlikely to occur after the use of iron dextran, which is not normally filtered by the renal glomerulus.

Blood grouping

If blood grouping is to be performed, samples should be taken before the intravenous iron dextran injection, since it interferes with the reaction.

Plasma discoloration

Single-dose infusion of iron dextran can cause plasma discoloration, which may be misinterpreted as a sign of severe hemolysis.

Calcium and phosphorus

In one case iron dextran administration falsely reduced total serum calcium concentration and increased the phosphorus concentration (58).

^{99}Tc-diphosphonate

The distribution of ^{99}Tc-diphosphonate in bone was reportedly altered by circulating iron dextran complex in an elderly woman patient undergoing scintigraphy (59).

References

1. Trinder D, Fox C, Vautier G, Olynyk JK. Molecular pathogenesis of iron overload. Gut 2002;51(2):290–5.
2. Eaton JW, Qian M. Molecular bases of cellular iron toxicity. Free Radic Biol Med 2002;32(9):833–40.
3. Whittington CA, Kowdley KV. Review article: haemochromatosis. Aliment Pharmacol Ther 2002;16(12):1963–75.
4. Bomford A. Genetics of haemochromatosis. Lancet 2002;360(9346):1673–81.
5. Coyne DW, Adkinson NF, Nissenson AR, Fishbane S, Agarwal R, Eschbach JW, Michael B, Folkert V, Batlle D, Trout JR, Dahl N, Myirski P, Strobos J, Warnock DG. Ferlecit Investigators. Sodium ferric gluconate complex in hemodialysis patients. II. Adverse reactions in iron dextran-sensitive and dextran-tolerant patients. Kidney Int 2003;63(1):217–24.
6. Jain AK, Bastani B. Safety profile of a high dose ferric gluconate in patients with severe chronic renal insufficiency. J Nephrol 2002;15(6):681–3.
7. Jeppsen RB. Toxicology and safety of Ferrochel and other iron amino acid chelates. Arch Latinoam Nutr 2001;51(Suppl 1):26–34.
8. Fletes R, Lazarus JM, Gage J, Chertow GM. Suspected iron dextran-related adverse drug events in hemodialysis patients. Am J Kidney Dis 2001;37(4):743–9.
9. Anonymous. Iron substitution therapy—parenteral use to be reserved for exceptional cases. WH Newslett 1996;5(6):3.
10. Sloand JA, Shelly MA, Erenstone AL, Schiff MJ, Talley TE, Dhakal MP. Safety and efficacy of total dose iron dextran administration in patients on home renal replacement therapies. Perit Dial Int 1998;18(5):522–7.
11. Altman LC, Petersen PE. Successful prevention of an anaphylactoid reaction to iron dextran. Ann Intern Med 1988;109(4):346–7.
12. Prakash S, Walele A, Dimkovic N, Bargman J, Vas S, Oreopoulos D. Experience with a large dose (500 mg) of intravenous iron dextran and iron saccharate in peritoneal dialysis patients. Perit Dial Int 2001;21(3):290–5.
13. Okada M, Imamura K, Iida M, Fuchigami T, Omae T. Hypophosphatemia induced by intravenous

administration of saccharated iron oxide. Klin Wochenschr 1983;61(2):99–102.
14. Rooyakkers TM, Stroes ES, Kooistra MP, van Faassen EE, Hider RC, Rabelink TJ, Marx JJ. Ferric saccharate induces oxygen radical stress and endothelial dysfunction in vivo. Eur J Clin Invest 2002;32(Suppl 1):9–16.
15. Lamaze R, Trechot P, Martinet Y. Bronchial necrosis and granuloma induced by the aspiration of a tablet of ferrous sulphate. Eur Respir J 1994;7(9):1710–11.
16. Ioannides AS, Panisello JM. Acute respiratory distress syndrome in children with acute iron poisoning: the role of intravenous desferrioxamine. Eur J Pediatr 2000;159 (3):158–9.
17. Clarke BE, Kim ST. Iron-induced bronchial injury. Histopathology 2002;41(5):472–3.
18. Milligan A, Graham-Brown RA, Sarkany I, Baker H. Erythropoietic protoporphyria exacerbated by oral iron therapy. Br J Dermatol 1988;119(1):63–6.
19. Ivanov E, Adjarov D, Kerimova M, Naidenova E. Rare cases of porphyria cutanea tarda associated with additional iron overload. Dermatologica 1982;164(2):127–32.
20. Scott JM. Iron-sorbitol-citrate in pregnancy anaemia. BMJ 1963;5353:354–7.
21. Go RS, Porrata LF, Call TG. Thrombocytopenia after iron dextran administration in a patient with severe iron deficiency anemia. Ann Intern Med 2000;132(11):925.
22. Editorial. Iron preparations for children. Drug Ther Bull 1966;4(3):9–11.
23. Abraham SC, Yardley JH, Wu TT. Erosive injury to the upper gastrointestinal tract in patients receiving iron medication: an underrecognized entity. Am J Surg Pathol 1999;23(10):1241–7.
24. Eckstein RP, Symons P. Iron tablets cause histopathologically distinctive lesions in mucosal biopsies of the stomach and esophagus. Pathology 1996;28(2):142–5.
25. Cook JD, Carriaga M, Kahn SG, Schalch W, Skikne BS. Gastric delivery system for iron supplementation. Lancet 1990;335(8698):1136–9.
26. Kopcke W, Sauerland MC. Meta-analysis of efficacy and tolerability data on iron proteinsuccinylate in patients with iron deficiency anemia of different severity. Arzneimittelforschung 1995;45(11):1211–16.
27. Hirasaki S, Koide N, Ogawa H, Ujike K, Okada H, Mizuno M, Ukida M, Tsuji T. A case of melanosis duodeni alleviated by the discontinuation of ferrous sulfite. Dig Endosc 1998;10:55–60.
28. Bonkovsky HL, Banner BE, Lambrecht RW, Rubin RB. Iron in liver diseases other than chemo chromatosis. Semin Liver Dis 1996;16(1):65–82.
29. Pearson HA, Ehrenkranz RA, Rinder HM, Riely CA. Hemosiderosis in a normal child secondary to oral iron medication. Pediatrics 2000;105(2):429–31.
30. Maclachlan D, Tyndall A. Acute hepatitis in adult Still's disease apparently resulting from oral iron substitution—a case report. Clin Rheumatol 2000;19(3):222–5.
31. Ito A, Nomura K, Hashimoto I. Pustular drug eruption induced by ferrous fumarate. Dermatology 1996;192(3):294–5.
32. Kawada A, Hiruma M, Noguchi H, Kimura M, Ishibashi A, Banba H, Marshall J. Photosensitivity due to sodium ferrous citrate. Contact Dermatitis 1996;34(1):77.
33. IARC Monographs on the Evaluation of Carcinogenic Risk of Chemicals to Man. Iron-Carbohydrate Complexes. Lyon: International Agency for Research on Cancer, 1973:161.
34. Sato K, Shiraki M. Saccharated ferric oxide-induced osteomalacia in Japan: iron-induced osteopathy due to nephropathy. Endocr J 1998;45(4):431–9.
35. Ortega N, Castillo R, Blanco C, Alvarez M, Carrillo T. Oral iron cutaneous adverse reaction and successful desensitization. Ann Allergy Asthma Immunol 2000;84(1):43–5.
36. Reddy S, Adcock KJ, Adeshina H, Cooke AR, Akene J, McFAarlane H. Immunity, transferrin, and survival in kwashiorkor. BMJ 1970;4(730):268–70.
37. Weber MH, Ammon A, Oppermann M, von Rothkirch T, Scheler F. Panhypogammaglobulinaemie: eine seltene Komplikation der parenteralen Gold-Therapie. [Panhypogammaglobulinemia: a rare complication of parenteral gold therapy.] Z Rheumatol 1991;50(4):207–10.
38. Yao K, Uchigata Y, Kyono H, Yokoyama H, Eguchi Y, Fukushima H, Yamauchi K, Hirata Y. Human insulin-specific immunoglobulin G antibody and hypoglycemic attacks after the injection of gold thioglucose. J Endocrinol Invest 1992;15(1):43–7.
39. Hirata Y. Autoimmune insulin syndrome "up to date". In: Andreani D, Marks V, Lefebvre PH, editors. Hypoglycemia. New York: Raven Press, 1987:105.
40. Fishbane S, Ungureanu VD, Maesaka JK, Kaupke CJ, Lim V, Wish J. The safety of intravenous iron dextran in hemodialysis patients. Am J Kidney Dis 1996;28(4):529–34.
41. Amitai A, Acker M. Adverse effects of intramuscular iron injection. Acta Haematol 1982;68(4):341–2.
42. Maertens J, Demuynck H, Verbeken EK, Zachee P, Verhoef GE, Vandenberghe P, Boogaerts MA. Mucormycosis in allogeneic bone marrow transplant recipients: report of five cases and review of the role of iron overload in the pathogenesis. Bone Marrow Transplant 1999;24(3):307–12.
43. Wurzelmann JI, Silver A, Schreinemachers DM, Sandler RS, Everson RB. Iron intake and the risk of colorectal cancer. Cancer Epidemiol Biomarkers Prev 1996;5(7):503–7.
44. Goh J, Callagy G, McEntee G, O'Keane JC, Bomford A, Crowe J. Hepatocellular carcinoma arising in the absence of cirrhosis in genetic haemochromatosis: three case reports and review of literature. Eur J Gastroenterol Hepatol 1999;11(8):915–19.
45. Shimada A. Adverse reactions to total-dose infusion of iron dextran. Clin Pharm 1982;1(3):248–9.
46. Begemann H. In: Praktische Haematologie. 8th ed. Stuttgart-New York: Thieme, 1982:355.
47. Blake DR, Lunec J, Ahern M, Ring EF, Bradfield J, Gutteridge JM. Effect of intravenous iron dextran on rheumatoid synovitis. Ann Rheum Dis 1985;44(3):183–8.
48. Brighton SW, de la Harpe AL. Development of an inflammatory synovitis following total-dose infusion of iron-dextran. A case report. S Afr Med J 1982;62(4):141–2.
49. Marcus RE, Huehns ER. Transfusional iron overload. Clin Lab Haematol 1985;7(3):195–212.
50. Tenenbein M. Toxicokinetics and toxicodynamics of iron poisoning. Toxicol Lett 1998;102-103:653–6.
51. Morse SB, Hardwick WE Jr, King WD. Fatal iron intoxication in an infant. South Med J 1997;90(10):1043–7.
52. Anonymous. Iron toxicity warnings. FDA Med Bull 1995;24:3.
53. Wallace KL, Curry SC, LoVecchio F, Raschke RA. Effect of magnesium hydroxide on iron absorption following simulated mild iron oversdose in human subjects. Acad Emerg Med 1998;5(10):961–5.
54. Thomas FB, Salsburey D, Greenberger NJ. Inhibition of iron absorption by cholestyramine. Demonstration of diminished iron stores following prolonged administration. Am J Dig Dis 1972;17(3):263–9.
55. Lyle WH. Penicillamine and iron. Lancet 1976;2(7982):420.
56. Neuvonen P, Mattila M, Gothoni G, Hackman R. Interference of iron and milk with absorption of tetracycline. Scand J Clin Lab Invest 1971;27(Suppl 116):76.
57. Campbell NR, Hasinoff BB. Iron supplements: a common cause of drug interactions. Br J Clin Pharmacol 1991;31 (3):251–5.

58. Newsom L, Erstad BL, Nakazato PZ, Daller JA. Falsely decreased total serum calcium concentration associated with iron dextran injection. Pharmacotherapy 1995; 15(6):789–92.
59. Forauer AR, Grossman SJ, Joyce JM. Altered biodistribution of Tc-99m HMDP on bone scintigraphy from recent intravenous iron therapy. Clin Nucl Med 1994;19(9):817–18.

Isepamycin

See also Aminoglycoside antibiotics

General Information

Isepamicin is similar to amikacin but has better activity against strains that produce type I 6′-acetyltransferase. It can cause nephrotoxicity, vestibular toxicity, and ototoxicity. However, it is one of the less toxic of the aminoglycosides (1). The antibacterial spectrum of isepamicin includes *Enterobacteriaceae* and staphylococci; anaerobes, *Neisseriae*, and streptococci are resistant (1). Isepamicin was as effective and safe as amikacin in the treatment of acute pyelonephritis in children and might prove an advantageous alternative in areas with a high incidence of resistance to other aminoglycosides (2).

Isepamicin is given intravenously or intramuscularly in a dosage of 15 mg/kg/day or 7.5 mg/kg bd. It is not bound to plasma proteins, it distributes in extracellular fluids, and it enters some cells (outer hair cells, kidney cortex) by an active transport mechanism (1); the transference of isepamicin to the bone marrow is excellent (3). Isepamicin is not metabolized and is renally excreted with a half-life of 2–3 hours in adults with normal renal function. Its clearance is reduced in neonates, and a dose of 7.5 mg/kg/day is recommended in children younger than 16 days. Its clearance is also reduced in elderly people, but no dosage adjustment is required. In patients with chronic renal impairment, isepamicin clearance is proportional to creatinine clearance.

The bone tissue penetration of isepamicin has been studied in an open, non-comparative study, and the results compared with microbiologic data to estimate the clinical efficacy of isepamicin in bone infections (4). In 12 subjects of similar age, body weight, height, and creatinine clearance, who were undergoing elective total hip replacement, a single parenteral dose of isepamicin 15 mg/kg achieved concentrations in both cancellous and cortical bone tissue greater than the minimum concentrations required to inhibit the growth of 90% of strains of most of the susceptible pathogens commonly involved in bone infections.

Organs and Systems

Sensory systems

Hereditary deafness is a heterogeneous group of disorders, with different patterns of inheritance and due to a multitude of different genes (5,6). The first molecular defect described was the A1555G sequence change in the mitochondrial 12S ribosomal RNA gene. Two cases of hearing loss after short-term exposure to isepamicin sulfate, an aminoglycoside with milder adverse effects than other aminoglycosides, have also been described in patients with the A1555G mutation (7).

Urinary tract

Fleroxacin had a protective effect on isepamicin-induced nephrotoxicity in rats (8).

Drug Administration

Drug dosage regimens

In a randomized, multicenter study 236 patients were randomly assigned to isepamicin in a calculated dose or a loading dose of 25 mg/kg (9). The calculated dose was estimated using a specific population model with a Bayesian method, including information about age, weight, height, sex, and serum creatinine. The Bayesian method was significantly more accurate and performed particularly well in ventilated patients and severely ill patients, compared with a loading dose of 25 mg/kg, in obtaining a first isepamicin peak concentration of 80 micrograms/ml in patients in an intensive care unit.

References

1. Tod M, Padoin C, Petitjean O. Clinical pharmacokinetics and pharmacodynamics of isepamicin. Clin Pharmacokinet 2000;38(3):205–23.
2. Kafetzis DA, Maltezou HC, Mavrikou M, Siafas C, Paraskakis I, Delis D, Bartsokas C. Isepamicin versus amikacin for the treatment of acute pyelonephritis in children. Int J Antimicrob Agents 2000;14(1):51–5.
3. Shibata Y, Midorikawa K, Naito M, Yatsunami M, Hamada K. [Concentration of isepamicin sulfate in bone marrow blood.]Jpn J Antibiot 2000;53(9):609–13.
4. Boselli E, Breilh D, Bel JC, Debon R, Saux MC, Chassard D, Allaouchiche B. Diffusion of isepamicin into cancellous and cortical bone tissue. J Chemother 2002;14(4):361–5.
5. Hardisty RE, Fleming J, Steel KP. The molecular genetics of inherited deafness—current knowledge and recent advances. J Laryngol Otol 1998;112(5):432–7.
6. Steel KP. Progress in progressive hearing loss. Science 1998;279(5358):1870–1.
7. Usami S, Abe S, Tono T, Komune S, Kimberling WJ, Shinkawa H. Isepamicin sulfate-induced sensorineural hearing loss in patients with the 1555 A→G mitochondrial mutation. ORL J Otorhinolaryngol Relat Spec 1998;60(3):164–9.
8. Yazaki T, Yoshiyama Y, Wong P, Beauchamp D, Kanke M. Protective effect of fleroxacin against the nephrotoxicity of isepamicin in rats. Biol Pharm Bull 2002;25(4):516–19.
9. Krishnan RS, Lewis AT, Kass JS, Hsu S. Ultraviolet recall-like phenomenon occurring after piperacillin, tobramycin, and ciprofloxacin therapy. J Am Acad Dermatol 2001;44(6):1045–7.

Isoetarine

General Information

Isoetarine is a beta-adrenoceptor agonist bronchodilator given orally in a modified-release formulation (SED-13, 363) (SEDA-21, 184). It is slightly more beta$_2$-selective than isoprenaline but has a beta-blocking metabolite.

When isoetarine was compared with salbutamol in the treatment of acute severe asthma in adults who received hourly nebulized isoetarine 5 mg or salbutamol 2.5 mg the two drugs were equally effective in relieving bronchoconstriction (SEDA-21, 184). However, adverse effects occurred in 36% of patients who used isoetarine and 4% of those who used salbutamol. The adverse effects included dizziness, nervousness, and bouts of palpitation, tremor, headache, and worsening shortness of breath.

Organs and Systems

Respiratory

In several patients, administration of isoetarine resulted in a pink coloration of the sputum, due to the presence of a reddish metabolite; in such cases, hemoptysis may be wrongly suspected (1).

Reference

1. Hooper PL, Harrelson LK, Johnson GE. Pseudohemoptysis from isoetharine. N Engl J Med 1983;308(26):1602.

Isoflurane

See also General anesthetics

General Information

Isoflurane is a potent inhalation anesthetic. An isomer of enflurane, it has many of the same adverse effects. It is hardly metabolized (about 0.2%), which has encouraged its prolonged use as a sedative agent or bronchodilator in patients with acute severe asthma. However, it may not be as inert in all patients.

Organs and Systems

Cardiovascular

Although atrial dysrhythmias have been reported in 3.9% of patients and ventricular dysrhythmias in 2.5% (1), the dysrhythmogenicity of isoflurane is less pronounced than that of halothane (2). Indeed, the incidence of dysrhythmias due to catecholamines in cardiovascular anesthesia and during oral surgery is reduced by using isoflurane rather than the other agents.

The most controversial adverse effect of isoflurane is its potential to cause coronary steal in patients with critical stenosis in the coronary circulation. Most recent work suggests that the risk of myocardial ischemia is not increased, as long as the hemodynamics, especially heart rate, are well controlled (3). However, there are still isolated reports, suggesting that the issue is not settled. In some cases isoflurane has caused a specific coronary steal even with good hemodynamic control (4).

Respiratory

Marked respiratory depression has been documented in children (5) and coughing associated with nausea and vomiting occurs in about 10% of subjects (1).

Like halothane, isoflurane is useful in cases of life-threatening acute severe asthma refractory to drug therapy.

- An 11-year-old girl with acute asthma, severe CO_2 narcosis, and ventricular fibrillation induced by hypoxemia was successfully treated with isoflurane in oxygen for 14 hours. Her recovery may have been due to bronchodilatation and the treatment that was possible because of the low dysrhythmogenic effect of isoflurane (6).

Nervous system

Seizures are uncommon with isoflurane, but reports continue to appear.

The neuromuscular blocking effects of vecuronium bromide can be enhanced by inhalation anesthetics.

- Symptoms suggestive of severe sensorimotor neuropathy developed in a 40-year-old woman 15 days after admission for a severe exacerbation of asthma (7). During this time she was given isoflurane 0.5–3% in oxygen, vecuronium bromide 4–6 mg/hour, and fentanyl 100 micrograms/hour. The neuropathy resolved spontaneously over the next 3 months.

In this case, isoflurane may have been the trigger.

- A fine tremor occurred when isoflurane was used in the management of a 3-year-old boy with pneumonia and underlying congenital myasthenia gravis (8).

Liver

Hepatic damage related to isoflurane anesthesia has very occasionally been described (9,10), including one report of hepatic necrosis and death (11). Hepatitis or hepatocellular injury has been described with all current volatile anesthetics. Among these, halothane-associated hepatitis has been best characterized and is probably caused by an immune reaction induced by hepatocyte proteins that have been covalently trifluoroacetylated by the trifluoroacetyl metabolite of halothane. The reactive acyl-halide metabolite of trifluoroacetic acid can trifluoroacetylate liver proteins, resulting in immune-mediated hepatic necrosis (12). However, isoflurane biotransformation to trifluoroacetate is less than 0.2%, compared with 15–20% for halothane.

In an interesting case report, clinical, histochemical, and immunohistochemical evidence supporting the role of trifluoroacetyl-modified proteins has been presented in a patient with hepatitis associated with isoflurane (13).

The role of CYP2E1 as the predominant route of metabolism of isoflurane to trifluoroacetic acid and inorganic fluoride ions has been confirmed using the enzyme inhibitor disulfiram as a metabolic probe in 22 adults randomized to either disulfiram 500 mg the evening before surgery or placebo. Anesthesia with 1.5% isoflurane lasted for an average of 8 hours. Postoperative plasma concentrations were increased and urinary excretion of trifluoroacetic acid was inhibited by 80–90% in the disulfiram group. Whether the use of disulfiram would reduce the incidence of hepatitis is unknown. Patients with increased activity of CYP2E1 or CYP2A6 appear to be at higher risk of isoflurane hepatotoxicity.

Acute hepatotoxicity has been reported with isoflurane (14). The authors hypothesized that induction of cytochrome P-450 by phenytoin had caused enhanced transformation of isoflurane to trifluoroacetic acid. They suggested that caution should be taken in the use of halogenated anesthetics in patients taking drugs that induce cytochrome P-450 isozymes.

- An obese 35-year-old diabetic woman developed isoflurane-induced hepatotoxicity (15). She had had four previous halothane anesthetics, the last two of which were associated with jaundice. She made a full recovery and during a subsequent anesthetic received an infusion of propofol. Unfortunately, trifluoroacetic acid antibody titers were not performed. Liver function does not appear to have been severely affected: peak alanine transaminase activity was 1410 IU/l.

Fatal hepatotoxicity associated with isoflurane has been reported (16).

- A 76-year-old woman with previous exposure to isoflurane 3 years earlier underwent an above-knee amputation for a liposarcoma using isoflurane anesthesia. On day 3 postoperatively she became febrile and confused. Bacterial cultures later showed *Staphylococcus aureus* in the sputum and *Escherichia coli* in the urine. Associated hypotension for 2 hours resolved with inotropic support and here renal function remained normal. On day 6 she became jaundiced and developed further hypotension. Despite intensive care treatment she died on day 7. An autopsy showed centrilobular necrosis consistent with drug-induced hepatitis. All liver serology was negative.

The clinical details in this case were similar to those seen in halothane hepatitis. The authors concluded that although there was no direct evidence that isoflurane was the causative agent, it was likely to have caused this type of hepatitis. Unfortunately, trifluoroacetic acid antibodies titers were not measured, because this test, if positive, would have confirmed the diagnosis.

Urinary tract

High concentrations of fluorine ions, potentially damaging to the kidney, can be found after prolonged use (17).

Four patients with renal dysfunction in an intensive care unit received isoflurane inhalation for sedation for 8–26 days. The concentrations of isoflurane used were 20–50% of the minimum alveolar concentration. Only small increases in fluoride ion concentration, the highest being 25 μmol/l, were recorded, well below the 50 μmol/l threshold associated with adverse effects on renal function (18).

Immunologic

Anaphylaxis has been reported in a patient who received isoflurane (19).

Body temperature

Malignant hyperthermia is a possible complication of isoflurane anesthesia (20).

Shivering after an anesthetic develops in as many as a half of patients recovering from isoflurane anesthesia. Most postoperative shivering appears to be thermoregulatory, although volatile anesthetics can themselves facilitate muscular activity. In 60 adult patients the incidence of postoperative shivering was 40% in a control group, 7% after physostigmine 0.04 mg/kg, zero after meperidine 0.5 mg/kg, and zero after clonidine 1.5 micrograms/kg (21). The centrally acting adrenoceptor agonist phenylpropylamine methylphenidate, the 5-hydroxytryptamine antagonist ketanserin, magnesium sulfate, doxapram, and hypercapnia also reduce the incidence of postoperative shivering.

Drug–Drug Interactions

Alfentanil and esmolol

The effects of alfentanil and esmolol on isoflurane requirements for anesthesia have been studied in a randomized trial in 100 patients (22). Alfentanil infusion to a targeted effect site concentration of 50 ng/ml, but not esmolol, reduced the minimum alveolar concentration of isoflurane required to suppress movement to surgical pain by 25%. The combination of esmolol and alfentanil caused a 74% reduction in isoflurane requirements. This study is interesting, because the beta-blocker esmolol had a profound effect on the isoflurane-sparing effects of alfentanil, while having little effect on its own.

Clonidine

In a randomized, double-blind, controlled trial in 61 patients, oral clonidine 5 micrograms/kg was given 90 minutes before surgery to reduce the concentration of isoflurane at which patients wake at the end of surgery by 8% (23). There was a 6–7 minute delay in waking in the clonidine group compared with the control group. Clonidine 2.5 micrograms/kg had no significant effect.

Rocuronium

The infusion requirements of rocuronium necessary to maintain twitch depression were reduced by 40% during anesthesia involving isoflurane (24). In another study in 60 patients undergoing maintenance anesthesia, isoflurane plus nitrous oxide anesthesia reduced the dosage requirement of rocuronium by 35–40% (25).

Suxamethonium

Isoflurane in nitrous oxide inhibited suxamethonium-induced muscle fasciculation in children (26).

References

1. Levy WJ. Clinical anaesthesia with isoflurane. A review of the multicentre study. Br J Anaesth 1984;56(Suppl 1):S101–12.
2. Rodrigo MR, Moles TM, Lee PK. Comparison of the incidence and nature of cardiac arrhythmias occurring during isoflurane or halothane anaesthesia. Studies during dental surgery. Br J Anaesth 1986;58(4):394–400.
3. Slogoff S, Keats AS. Randomized trial of primary anesthetic agents on outcome of coronary artery bypass operations. Anesthesiology 1989;70(2):179–88.
4. Inoue K, Reichelt W, el-Banayosy A, Minami K, Dallmann G, Hartmann N, Windeler J. Does isoflurane lead to a higher incidence of myocardial infarction and perioperative death than enflurane in coronary artery surgery? A clinical study of 1178 patients. Anesth Analg 1990;71(5):469–74.
5. Murat I, Beydon L, Chaussain M, Levy J, Saint-Maurice JP. Ventilatory changes during nitrous oxide isoflurane anaesthesia in children. Eur J Anaesthesiol 1986;3(5):403–11.
6. Shibata Y, Kukita I, Baba T, Goto T, Yoshinaga T. [A critical patient relieved from status asthmaticus with isoflurane inhalation therapy.] Masui 1993;42(1):116–19.
7. du Peloux Menage H, Duffy S, Yates DW, Hughes JA. Reversible sensorimotor impairment following prolonged ventilation with isoflurane and vecuronium for acute severe asthma. Thorax 1992;47(12):1078–9.
8. McBeth C, Watkins TG. Isoflurane for sedation in a case of congenital myasthenia gravis. Br J Anaesth 1996;77(5):672–4.
9. Gregoire S, Kennedy A, Smiley RK. Acute hepatitis in a patient with mild factor IX deficiency after anesthesia with isoflurane. CMAJ 1986;135(6):645–6.
10. Scheider DM, Klygis LM, Tsang TK, Caughron MC. Hepatic dysfunction after repeated isoflurane administration. J Clin Gastroenterol 1993;17(2):168–70.
11. Carrigan TW, Straughen WJ. A report of hepatic necrosis and death following isoflurane anesthesia. Anesthesiology 1987;67(4):581–3.
12. Kharasch ED, Hankins DC, Cox K. Clinical isoflurane metabolism by cytochrome P450 2E1. Anesthesiology 1999;90(3):766–71.
13. Njoku DB, Shrestha S, Soloway R, Duray PR, Tsokos M, Abu-Asab MS, Pohl LR, West AB. Subcellular localization of trifluoroacetylated liver proteins in association with hepatitis following isoflurane. Anesthesiology 2002;96(3):757–61.
14. Sinha A, Clatch RJ, Stuck G, Blumenthal SA, Patel SA. Isoflurane hepatotoxicity: a case report and review of the literature. Am J Gastroenterol 1996;91(11):2406–9.
15. Hasan F. Isoflurane hepatotoxicity in a patient with a previous history of halothane-induced hepatitis. Hepatogastroenterology 1998;45(20):518–22.
16. Turner GB, O'Rourke D, Scott GO, Beringer TR. Fatal hepatotoxicity after re-exposure to isoflurane: a case report and review of the literature. Eur J Gastroenterol Hepatol 2000;12(8):955–9.
17. Truog RD, Rice SA. Inorganic fluoride and prolonged isoflurane anesthesia in the intensive care unit. Anesth Analg 1989;69(6):843–5.
18. Fujino Y, Nishimura M, Nishimura S, Taenaka N, Yoshiya I. Prolonged administration of isoflurane to patients with severe renal dysfunction. Anesth Analg 1998;86(2):440–1.
19. Slegers-Karsmakers S, Stricker BH. Anaphylactic reaction to isoflurane. Anaesthesia 1988;43(6):506–7.
20. Boheler J, Hamrick JC Jr, McKnight RL, Eger EI 2nd. Isoflurane and malignant hyperthermia. Anesth Analg 1982;61(8):712–13.
21. Horn EP, Standl T, Sessler DI, von Knobelsdorff G, Buchs C, Schulte am Esch J. Physostigmine prevents postanesthetic shivering as does meperidine or clonidine. Anesthesiology 1998;88(1):108–13.
22. Johansen JW, Schneider G, Windsor AM, Sebel PS. Esmolol potentiates reduction of minimum alveolar isoflurane concentration by alfentanil. Anesth Analg 1998;87(3):671–6.
23. Goyagi T, Tanaka M, Nishikawa T. Oral clonidine premedication reduces the awakening concentration of isoflurane. Anesth Analg 1998;86(2):410–13.
24. Shanks CA, Fragen RJ, Ling D. Continuous intravenous infusion of rocuronium (ORG 9426) in patients receiving balanced, enflurane, or isoflurane anesthesia. Anesthesiology 1993;78(4):649–51.
25. Olkkola KT, Tammisto T. Quantifying the interaction of rocuronium (Org 9426) with etomidate, fentanyl, midazolam, propofol, thiopental, and isoflurane using closed-loop feedback control of rocuronium infusion. Anesth Analg 1994;78(4):691–6.
26. Randell T, Yli-Hankala A, Lindgren L. Isoflurane inhibits muscle fasciculations caused by succinylcholine in children. Acta Anaesthesiol Scand 1993;37(3):262–4.

Isometheptene

General Information

Isometheptene, used in the treatment of migraine, is an indirect sympathomimetic with a tyramine-like action and is also an agonist at alpha-adrenoceptors.

In one case an autonomic dysreflexic syndrome developed after the use of an isometheptene combination to treat migraine (1). In other respects its adverse reactions are similar to those of adrenaline and ephedrine.

Reference

1. Wineinger MA, Basford JR. Autonomic dysreflexia due to medication: misadventure in the use of an isometheptene combination to treat migraine. Arch Phys Med Rehabil 1985;66(9):645–6.

Isoniazid

See also Antituberculosis drugs

General Information

Isoniazid is the hydrazide of isonicotinic acid. It is a first-line drug for therapy and prophylaxis of tuberculosis. It is bactericidal for rapidly dividing mycobacteria, but bacteriostatic for "resting bacilli". Among non-tuberculous mycobacteria, only a few strains, such as *Mycobacterium kansasii*, are susceptible. As a rule, sensitivity should always be tested in vitro, since the minimum inhibitory concentration varies greatly.

Isoniazid diffuses rapidly into body fluids and cells, including cerebrospinal fluid. It is as effective against bacteria growing within cells as it is against bacteria in culture media. There is no cross-resistance between isoniazid and other antituberculosis drugs.

The daily dose of isoniazid is 5 mg/kg, with a maximum of 300 mg/day in adults with normal liver and kidney function. In children, 8–10 mg/kg/day is an appropriate dosage, with a maximum daily dose of 300 mg, since the metabolism of isoniazid in children is rapid. Untoward effects of isoniazid as a single antituberculosis drug can be evaluated in preventive tuberculosis therapy, since curative regimens usually consist of multiple drugs.

Pharmacokinetics

After oral administration, isoniazid reaches a peak plasma concentration of 3–5 micrograms/ml within 1–2 hours. It equilibrates into all body fluids and tissues and 75–95% is excreted in the urine within 24 hours. The most important urinary metabolites are products of acetylation (acetylisoniazid) and hydrolysis (isonicotinic acid). Isonicotinyl glycine, isonicotinyl hydrazones, and *N*-methylisoniazid appear in only small amounts. The rate of acetylation of isoniazid significantly alters its plasma concentrations and half-life. The mean half-life of isoniazid in rapid acetylators is about 70 minutes and in slow acetylators 3 hours.

General adverse reactions

In a survey of more than 2000 patients treated with isoniazid, the most frequent adverse effects were rash (2%), fever (1.2%), jaundice (0.6%), and peripheral neuropathy (0.2%). Seizures can also occur. Isoniazid prolongs the half-life of rifampicin and other drugs metabolized by the liver. Morbilliform, maculopapular, purpuric, and urticarial rashes, with or without fever, are considered to be of allergic origin. Hematological adverse effects consist of agranulocytosis, thrombocytopenia, pure red cell aplasia, and eosinophilia (SEDA-9, 268). Dyspnea, with thoracic pain, cough, fever, and eosinophilia, as well as micronodular densities in the chest X-ray, may also be due to an immunological process (1). Vasculitis associated with antinuclear antibodies has been observed, as well as arthritic symptoms (2). Liver injury (mainly hepatocellular) has been considered another form of hypersensitivity reaction, but usually occurs during combined antituberculosis treatment with rifampicin in combination with anticonvulsants or halothane, or in association with alcoholism. Some are of the opinion that the main factor that induces liver damage is the fast acetylator phenotype (3), while others have found no correlation (4). No increase in cancer deaths was observed in a series of 338 women treated with isoniazid for pulmonary tuberculosis (5). Isoniazid is a potent inhibitor of hepatic enzymes and interferes with the metabolism of many drugs (SEDA-8, 287) (SEDA-11, 271).

Organs and Systems

Respiratory

Symptoms suggestive of bronchial obstruction occur only very rarely during isoniazid treatment (1).

Nervous system

Untoward neurological effects (peripheral neuropathy and focal seizures) occur in 2% of patients if pyridoxine is not given and in 12–20% taking higher doses of isoniazid (10–15 mg/kg) (6).

Peripheral neuropathy due to isoniazid results from inhibition of the formation of the co-enzyme form of vitamin B6, pyridoxine. Numbness or tingling of the extremities in the "glove and stocking" distribution can occur early during treatment with isoniazid when pyridoxine is not given. Neuropathy was noted by several authors in up to 20% of malnourished patients and fast acetylators taking isoniazid in doses over 5–6 mg/kg. Only 2% of patients taking 5 mg/kg of isoniazid plus pyridoxine developed neuropathy. Symptoms generally consist of hyperesthesia, reduced vibration and position sense, and exaggerated or reduced tendon reflexes, but ataxia, muscle weakness, and even paralysis can develop (7). Shoulder–arm syndrome has also been described.

Neurohistology shows disappearance of synaptic vesicles, mitochondrial swelling or condensation, and fragmentation of axon endings. Alterations in the lumbar and sacral spinal ganglia and the spinal cord have also been reported (8).

The addition of pyridoxine to usual doses of isoniazid of 5 mg/kg/day in adults and 8–10 mg/kg/day in children markedly reduces neurotoxicity (9). Adherence to therapy is improved by prescribing combined tablets containing 20 mg of pyridoxine per 100 mg of isoniazid. In otherwise healthy people, prescription of pyridoxine is not mandatory. However, it should be routinely given to malnourished patients and those predisposed to neuropathy (for example pregnant women, elderly people, and people with diabetes, alcoholism, or uremia) (7).

Pellagra-associated encephalopathy has been suspected as an adverse effect of isoniazid administration in several patients with tuberculosis. Deficiency of niacin (nicotinic acid) is characterized by dermatitis, diarrhea, and dementia. Other symptoms can occur, such as seizures, hallucinations, spasticity, and glossitis. Pellagra induced by isoniazid is promoted by malnutrition or a vegetarian diet with low intake of the nicotinamide precursors tryptophan and nicotinic acid. Specific supplementation is essential (10).

Sensory systems

Optic neuritis and atrophy have occurred in patients taking isoniazid (11).

Psychological, psychiatric

Isoniazid can cause neuropsychiatric syndromes, including euphoria, transient impairment of memory, separation of ideas and reality, loss of self-control, psychoses (9), and obsessive-compulsive neurosis (12). Isoniazid should be used with caution in patients with pre-existing psychoses, as it can cause relapse of paranoid schizophrenia (13). Patients on chronic dialysis appear to be vulnerable to neurological adverse drug reactions, because of abnormal metabolism of uremic toxins. It is therefore recommended that a higher than usual dose of pyridoxine be given to patients on dialysis taking isoniazid (14,15).

Endocrine

Cushing's syndrome, gynecomastia, amenorrhea, and precocious puberty have been regarded as reflecting the enzyme-inhibitory activity of isoniazid, with resulting derangement of hormone metabolism in the liver.

Metabolism

Isoniazid can cause transient hyperglycemia in overdose (16).

In five volunteers taking isoniazid 15 mg/kg/day over a period of 6 weeks, serum cholesterol concentrations were reduced (SEDA-9, 268).

Hematologic

Agranulocytosis, thrombocytopenia, hemolytic anemia, sideroblastic anemia (17), pure red cell aplasia (18), methemoglobinemia, and eosinophilia can occur exceptionally during isoniazid treatment (SEDA-9, 268) (19). An acquired coagulation factor XIII inhibitor developed in a patient taking isoniazid and resulted in a bleeding disorder (20).

Gastrointestinal

No severe gastrointestinal adverse effects of isoniazid have been observed; symptoms are limited to such as epigastric distress, gastric burning, and dry mouth. Of 814 patients with pulmonary tuberculosis treated for 9 months with isoniazid and rifampicin, 18 had minor symptoms of gastrointestinal intolerance (21). Nausea can occur, particularly if the drug is taken before breakfast or in combination with other antituberculosis drugs; 5.5% of 912 patients taking a fixed tablet combination of isoniazid, protionamide, and diaphenyl sulfone plus rifampicin had sensations of fullness, nausea, or vomiting (22).

Liver

Abnormal liver function is the most commonly described adverse effect of isoniazid (23). It may be related to acetylator phenotype.

Hepatotoxicity caused considerable alarm after an episode in Washington DC, when 19 of 2231 government employees given isoniazid prophylaxis developed clinical signs of liver disease within 6 months; 13 were severely jaundiced and 2 died (23).

In a series of 13 838 individuals treated prophylactically, 114 developed overt hepatic disease (SED-9, 574) (24). There were 13 deaths, submassive necrosis in 9 cases, and massive necrosis in 4. The 20 other patients from whom hepatic tissue was available included 16 with moderately severe acute hepatocellular injury (four with a mixed hepatocellular-cholestatic pattern), and four with chronic hepatic damage (one with cirrhosis). The effects of liver disease before the onset of jaundice included vague digestive and "viral" disease-like complaints, some with and some without gastrointestinal symptoms. Jaundice was the presenting complaint in 10%, fever and rash were reported in under 4%, and there was a modest eosinophilia in about 10%. Liver damage was recognized during the first month of administration in 15% and during the second month in a further 31%. The other 54% had taken isoniazid for 2–11 months. Although liver damage in these patients may have been related to isoniazid, some probably had viral hepatitis.

In a study of isoniazid prophylactic therapy in Seattle, USA, only 11 patients of 11 141 had hepatotoxic reactions (25). The rate was 0.1% of those starting and 0.15% of those completing the course of therapy. The duration of therapy was not stated, but 10 of the 11 episodes occurred within 3 months of starting.

The mechanism responsible for hepatotoxicity is not known. A metabolite of isoniazid, acetylhydrazine, causes hepatic damage and may play a role. Alcoholic hepatitis is an aggravating factor. The sensitivity of chronic carriers of hepatitis B virus is controversial (26). In an investigation in which the urinary metabolic profile of isoniazid was assayed in patients who developed isoniazid-related liver damage, it was impossible to predict which patients would be susceptible. It was also impossible to show that rifampicin plays a significant role in inducing liver damage when added to isoniazid (27,28). Nevertheless, it is conceivable that enzyme induction by rifampicin alters the metabolism of isoniazid. Further risk factors are alcoholism, malnutrition, diabetes, previous liver damage, renal insufficiency, and drug abuse. Age is certainly another risk factor: hepatic damage seems to be rare in patients under the age of 20; the incidence of liver toxicity is 0.3% between the ages of 20 and 34, and increases with age to 1.2% between 34 and 49 and 2.3% over the age of 50 (9). Even in prophylaxis with isoniazid monotherapy, adverse effects are more frequent in patients aged over 35 years (29).

Liver damage usually appears 1–2 months after the start of therapy. In children, raised liver enzymes are common during the first few months of treatment, but withdrawal is seldom necessary. A careful watch should be kept for early symptoms of isoniazid-induced hepatitis, such as malaise, fatigue, nausea, and epigastric distress. The dangers of continuing isoniazid after the onset of symptoms of toxicity have been highlighted (30). The earliest symptoms of isoniazid toxicity should be clearly described to the patient, particularly to hepatitis B carriers, who may be more susceptible to hepatotoxicity (26).

It is advisable to measure the liver enzymes aspartate transaminase and alanine transaminase before treatment and monthly thereafter, for as long as isoniazid administration lasts. Isoniazid should be withdrawn if the transaminases increase to over five times normal (9).

Pancreas

Acute pancreatitis has been attributed to isoniazid (31,32).

- A 42-year-old Asian man developed clinical, biochemical, and imaging features of acute pancreatitis 11 days after starting to take rifampicin, isoniazid, and pyrazinamide for spinal tuberculosis (33). He had no history of excessive alcohol or other drug therapy. He improved after withdrawal of all drugs, but the pancreatitis recurred on reintroduction of isoniazid and resolved after withdrawal.

Causality here was difficult to establish. Pancreatitis has rarely been seen in patients who have taken an overdose of isoniazid. Rifampicin, also used in this case, is more likely to cause pancreatitis in usual doses.

Urinary tract

Isoniazid can rarely cause renal damage (34).

Urinary retention is a rare complication of isoniazid overdose (35).

Skin

Morbilliform, maculopapular, or urticarial rashes have been observed in up to 2% of patients (9). In one study, acneiform eruptions developed in only 11 cases (1.4%), including 0.5% of patients taking isoniazid, 1.5% of patients taking rifampicin, and 0.6% of patients taking ethambutol (36).

Acquired cutis laxa has been mentioned in a single child taking isoniazid, but it was probably coincidental (37).

Erythema nodosum and purpura have been described in patients taking isoniazid (38).

Pellagra has been reported in a patient taking isoniazid, despite concomitant pyridoxine prophylaxis (39).

- A 52-year-old man developed pellagra with a classical photosensitive distribution after taking isoniazid for 14 months; the first 6 months being treatment for possible tuberculous meningitis, the rest to provide antituberculosis protection while glucocorticoids were given for possible neurosarcoidosis. He was said to take alcohol only occasionally and took pyridoxine throughout the entire period of treatment. He improved rapidly on withdrawal of isoniazid and supplementation with nicotinamide.

The authors noted that isoniazid-induced pellagra was first described in 1956, shortly after the introduction of isoniazid for the treatment of tuberculosis, but that subsequent reports have been very uncommon.

Isoniazid has also been reported to cause subepidermal blistering (40).

- A 63-year-old man developed bullous lesions on the trunk and limbs and a six-fold rise in liver enzymes 15 days after treatment for tuberculosis. His skin recovered and his liver enzymes returned to normal within 2 weeks of withdrawal of all treatment, but the abnormalities recurred when treatment was resumed. At this point a skin biopsy showed subepidermal blistering. Once again withdrawal of treatment led to improvement, and when treatment was resumed without isoniazid the improvement continued.

Desensitization to isoniazid has been attempted in some patients with drug fever or rashes. A procedure of rush desensitization over a few days or a week can be used, starting with 1 mg orally and increasing the dosage every second day (41) or even every few hours.

Musculoskeletal

Arthritic symptoms, with back pain, bilateral proximal interphalangeal joint involvement, arthralgia of the knees, elbows, and wrists, and the so-called "shoulder–arm" syndrome with cervicobrachial neuralgia can occur (9).

Rhabdomyolysis occurred in subjects with isoniazid poisoning in a retrospective analysis of 270 patients seen over a 5-year period at the Phillipine General Hospital in Manilla (42). Skeletal muscle creatine kinase activity was raised in 31 of the 52 evaluable subjects who had taken more than 2.4 g/day of isoniazid. Creatine kinase activity peaked on days 5–6 and fell thereafter. Two patients developed acute renal insufficiency and required dialysis. Seizures occurred in all patients, and their duration, but not their frequency, correlated with raised creatine kinase activity. However, it is likely that factors other than seizures contribute to rhabdomyolysis in patients with isoniazid poisoning.

Immunologic

The expansion or new development of tuberculous lesions during ultimately successful therapy has been termed a "paradoxical response." It is most often reported in relation to intracranial tuberculomata, but is probably most common in tuberculous lymphadenopathy. It is also described in tuberculous pleurisy and in parenchymal lung disease. In most cases, the problem eventually settles, but sometimes glucocorticoid therapy is used empirically.

A lupus-like syndrome or vasculitis, with arthritis, rheumatic pain, fever, pleurisy, and leukopenia, has been reported in patients taking isoniazid (38,43). Tests for antinuclear antibodies are useful to distinguish idiopathic systemic lupus erythematosus and drug-induced lupus-like syndromes. However, many patients taking isoniazid have antinuclear antibodies, usually without signs or symptoms of systemic lupus erythematosus. Isoniazid can also exacerbate pre-existing systemic lupus erythematosus (38,43). Long-term glucocorticoid treatment may be necessary if symptoms persist after withdrawal of isoniazid.

- Two Japanese patients developed pleural effusions while taking antituberculosis therapy and were believed to have isoniazid-induced lupus-like syndrome (44). This diagnosis was based on the presence of antinuclear antibody in the effusate, and in one patient, a positive lymphocyte stimulation test using isoniazid; in the other patient it was negative. Both had moderately strongly positive serum antinuclear antibodies (1:160). In the first patient, the effusion disappeared 2 weeks after withdrawal of isoniazid; in the other treatment was continued but the effusion nevertheless resolved in 10 weeks.

It is worth checking for evidence of lupus-like syndrome in patients with paradoxical responses to antituberculosis therapy but it remains to be seen how many cases would be explained by it.

Long-Term Effects

Mutagenicity

Isoniazid is not mutagenic (SEDA-6, 276), but patients taking combined isoniazid and rifampicin therapy for 3–10 months developed an increased rate of chromosomal aberrations in peripheral blood lymphocytes (SEDA-9, 276). However, this effect is not known to have clinical consequences.

Second-Generation Effects

Fertility

Isoniazid has no effect on fertility (SEDA-6, 276).

Pregnancy

Isoniazid is the safest antituberculosis drug for use during pregnancy (45,46). During pregnancy, isoniazid with ethambutol is considered to be the preferred combination (45).

Teratogenicity

Isoniazid diffuses into blastocytes, but no teratogenic effects have been reported (46).

Lactation

Isoniazid is the safest antituberculosis drug for use during lactation (45,46). However, as isoniazid passes into breast milk, a watch must be kept for adverse effects in the infant when a nursing mother is taking isoniazid (47). However, the serum concentrations that occur in children have no therapeutic effect and cannot be considered as a form of preventive chemotherapy in infants of mothers with active tuberculosis.

Susceptibility Factors

Genetic factors

People are divided genetically into rapid and slow acetylators of isoniazid, depending on the amount of *N*-acetyltransferase they have. The rate of acetylation of isoniazid depends on race, but is not influenced by sex or by age after childhood. In Eskimos and Japanese, fast acetylators predominate. Slow acetylation is the predominant phenotype in most Scandinavians, Jews, and North African Caucasians (9). Slow acetylators are homozygous for an autosomal recessive gene, while fast acetylators are homozygous or heterozygous for a dominant gene. In the case of isoniazid (which has a low hepatic extraction ratio) the rate of acetylation significantly alters its plasma concentrations and half-life. The mean half-life of isoniazid in rapid acetylators is about 70 minutes and in slow acetylators 3 hours. Despite this, there is probably no difference in the effectiveness of isoniazid in the two phenotypes. The relation between isoniazid toxicity and acetylator status continues to be discussed (3,4,6).

Drug Administration

Drug overdose

Acute poisoning with isoniazid in children (48) and adults (13,26,35) causes recurrent seizures, profound metabolic acidosis, coma, and even death. In adults, toxicity can occur with the acute ingestion of as little as 1.5 g of isoniazid. Doses larger than 30 mg/kg often produce seizures and 80–150 mg/kg or more can be rapidly fatal. The first signs and symptoms of isoniazid toxicity usually appear 0.5–2.0 hours after ingestion, by which time peak absorption occurs (49), and include nausea, vomiting, slurred speech, dizziness, tachycardia, and urinary retention, followed by stupor, coma, and recurrent tonic-clonic seizures. The seizures are often refractory to antiepileptic therapy. However, pyridoxine, 20–1500 mg per gram of isoniazid ingested, usually eliminates seizure activity and helps to correct the metabolic acidosis (50).

Drug–Drug Interactions

Antacids

Absorption of isoniazid can be inhibited by aluminium-containing antacids (51).

Barbiturates

Barbiturates which induce liver drug-metabolizing enzymes increase the rate of metabolism of isoniazid, rifampicin, or combined antituberculosis treatment, since they may result in accelerated breakdown of these drugs (52).

Benzodiazepines

In healthy volunteers, the half-life of triazolam was prolonged from 2.5 to 3.3 hours when it was given with isoniazid (SEDA-9, 267). However, isoniazid did not affect the pharmacokinetics of oxazepam.

Beta-adrenoceptor antagonists

Lipophilic beta-adrenoceptor antagonists are metabolized to varying degrees by oxidation by liver microsomal cytochrome P450 (for example propranolol by CYP1A2 and CYP2D6 and metoprolol by CYP2D6). They can therefore reduce the clearance and increase the steady-state plasma concentrations of other drugs that undergo similar metabolism, potentiating their effects. Drugs that interact in this way include isoniazid (53).

Carbamazepine

Patients taking carbamazepine can develop signs of carbamazepine intoxication; serum concentrations of carbamazepine are increased by isoniazid, probably through enzyme inhibition (54).

Disulfiram

In seven patients taking isoniazid 0.6–1.0 g/day for at least 1 month, disulfiram 0.5 g/day caused dizziness, disorientation, staggering, insomnia, irritability, listlessness, lethargy, and in one case hypomania (55). This interaction may have been due to inhibition of isoniazid metabolism by disulfiram or to a complex interaction with dopamine metabolism.

Ethosuximide

In one case, isoniazid increased blood concentrations of the antiepileptic drug ethosuximide and caused hiccups, anorexia, nausea, vomiting, insomnia, and an acute psychosis (SEDA-9, 267) (56). This may have been due to inhibition of ethosuximide metabolism by isoniazid.

Monoamine oxidase inhibitors

Isoniazid inhibits monoamine oxidase, and hence reduces tyramine metabolism; this effect is enhanced by co-administration of other monoamine oxidase inhibitors (57).

Phenazone

Isoniazid significantly reduces the hepatic clearance of phenazone (antipyrine) by about 40% (SEDA-9, 267).

Phenytoin

Isoniazid inhibits the parahydroxylation of phenytoin. Symptoms of phenytoin intoxication, such as dizziness, incoordination, or excessive sedation, can occur, particularly in patients who are slow acetylators (SEDA-11, 271). Dosages of phenytoin should be adjusted according to plasma concentrations (58).

Stavudine

A five-fold increase in the risk of distal sensory neuropathy has been reported in patients taking stavudine plus isoniazid (55 versus 11%) compared with patients taking stavudine without isoniazid (59). In nine of 12 patients, the neuropathy resolved on changing antiretroviral drugs. Peripheral neuropathy is a distressing complication during treatment with stavudine and the risk is considerably increased with co-administration of isoniazid. This combination of drugs should be avoided, if possible, in patients with tuberculosis and AIDS.

Food–Drug Interactions

Tyramine-containing foods

Adverse reactions during treatment with isoniazid have been noted after ingestion of several kinds of cheese (60,61). Flushing, palpitation, tachycardia, and increased blood pressure have been observed 0.5–2 hours after cheese. The symptoms generally disappear within 2–4 hours. Interference by isoniazid with monoamine oxidase, and hence with tyramine metabolism, has been incriminated.

Histamine-containing foods

Headache, palpitation, erythema, redness of the eyes, itching, diarrhea, and wheezing can occur with isoniazid after skipjack fish (*Thunnidae*) (60,62), probably because of the high histamine content of this fish.

References

1. Schelling JL. Dyspnées médicamenteuses. [Medicamentous dyspnea.] Ther Umsch 1981;38(2):163–5.
2. Ueda Y, Fujita K, Kohno K, Ichinose K, Fukushima H, Nakatomi M. [A case of isoniazid-induced lupus.] Kekkaku 1989;64(10):613–19.
3. Mitchell JR, Thorgeirsson UP, Black M, Timbrell JA, Snodgrass WR, Potter WZ, Jollow DJ, Keiser HR. Increased incidence of isoniazid hepatitis in rapid acetylators: possible relation to hydrazine metabolites. Clin Pharmacol Ther 1975;18(1):70–9.
4. Gurumurthy P, Krishnamurthy MS, Nazareth O, Parthasarathy R, Sarma GR, Somasundaram PR, Tripathy SP, Ellard GA. Lack of relationship between hepatic toxicity and acetylator phenotype in three thousand South Indian patients during treatment with isoniazid for tuberculosis. Am Rev Respir Dis 1984;129(1):58–61.
5. Boice JD, Fraumeni JF Jr. Late effects following isoniazid therapy. Am J Public Health 1980;70(9):987–9.
6. Mitchell I, Wendon J, Fitt S, Williams R. Anti-tuberculous therapy and acute liver failure. Lancet 1995;345(8949):555–6.
7. Snider DE Jr. Pyridoxine supplementation during isoniazid therapy. Tubercle 1980;61(4):191–6.
8. Schroder JM. Zur Pathogenese der Isoniazid-Neuropathie. I. Eine feinstrukturelle Differenzierung gegenuber der Wallerschen Degeneration. [The pathogenesis of INH-neuropathy. I. Fine structural similarities and differences to Wallerian degeneration.] Acta Neuropathol (Berl) 1970;16(4):301–23.
9. Mandell GL, Sande MA. Antimicrobial agents: drugs used in the chemotherapy of tuberculosis and leprosy. In: Goodman Gilman A, Rall TW, Nies AS, Taylor P, editors. 8th ed. Chapter 49. Goodman and Gilman's The Pharmacological Basis of Therapeutics. New York: Pergamon Press, 1990:1146
10. Ishii N, Nishihara Y. Pellagra encephalopathy among tuberculous patients: its relation to isoniazid therapy. J Neurol Neurosurg Psychiatry 1985;48(7):628–34.
11. Leibold JE. Drugs having a toxic effect on the optic nerve. Int Ophthalmol Clin 1971;11(2):137–57.
12. Bhatia MS. Isoniazid-induced obsessive compulsive neurosis. J Clin Psychiatry 1990;51(9):387.
13. Bernardo M, Gatell JM, Parellada E. Acute exacerbation of chronic schizophrenia in a patient treated with antituberculosis drugs. Am J Psychiatry 1991;148(10):1402.
14. Siskind MS, Thienemann D, Kirlin L. Isoniazid-induced neurotoxicity in chronic dialysis patients: report of three cases and a review of the literature. Nephron 1993;64(2):303–6.
15. Cheung WC, Lo CY, Lo WK, Ip M, Cheng IK. Isoniazid induced encephalopathy in dialysis patients. Tuber Lung Dis 1993;74(2):136–9.
16. Ferner RE. Drug-induced diabetes. Baillière's Clin Endocrinol Metab 1992;6(4):849–66.
17. Sharp RA, Lowe JG, Johnston RN. Anti-tuberculous drugs and sideroblastic anaemia. Br J Clin Pract 1990;44(12):706–7.
18. Johnsson R, Lommi J. A case of isoniazid-induced red cell aplasia. Respir Med 1990;84(2):171–4.
19. Goldman AL, Braman SS. Isoniazid: a review with emphasis on adverse effects. Chest 1972;62(1):71–7.
20. Krumdieck R, Shaw DR, Huang ST, Poon MC, Rustagi PK. Hemorrhagic disorder due to an isoniazid-associated acquired factor XIII inhibitor in a patient with Waldenstrom's macroglobulinemia. Am J Med 1991;90(5):639–45.
21. Dutt AK, Moers D, Stead WW. Undesirable side effects of isoniazid and rifampin in largely twice-weekly short-course chemotherapy for tuberculosis. Am Rev Respir Dis 1983;128(3):419–24.
22. Hoose C, Eberhardt K, Hartmann W, Wosniok W. Kurz- und Langzeitergebnisse der Tuberkulosetherapie mit einer fixen Kombination aus Isoniazid, Prothionamid und Diaphenylsulfon (IPD) in Verbindung mit Rifampicin. [Short- and long-term results of tuberculosis therapy with a fixed combination of isoniazide, prothionamide and diaminodiphenylsulfone combined with rifampicin.] Pneumologie 1990;44(Suppl 1):458–9.
23. Snider DE Jr, Caras GJ. Isoniazid-associated hepatitis deaths: a review of available information. Am Rev Respir Dis 1992;145(2 Pt 1):494–7.
24. Black M, Mitchell JR, Zimmerman HJ, Ishak KG, Epler GR. Isoniazid-associated hepatitis in 114 patients. Gastroenterology 1975;69(2):289–302.
25. Nolan CM, Goldberg SV, Buskin SE. Hepatotoxicity associated with isoniazid preventive therapy: a 7-year survey from a public health tuberculosis clinic. JAMA 1999;281(11):1014–18.
26. Amarapurkar DN, Prabhudesai PP, Kalro RH, Desai HG. Antituberculosis drug-induced hepatitis and HBsAg carriers. Tuber Lung Dis 1993;74(3):215–16.

27. Gangadharam PR. Isoniazid, rifampin, and hepatotoxicity. Am Rev Respir Dis 1986;133(6):963–5.
28. Timbrell JA, Wright JM. Urinary metabolic profile of isoniazid in patients who develop isoniazid-related liver damage. Hum Toxicol 1984;3(6):485–95.
29. Mandell GL, Sande MA. Antimicrobial agents: drugs used in the chemotherapy of tuberculosis and leprosy. In: Goodman Gilman A, Goodman LS, Rall TW, et al., editors. The Pharmacological Basis of Therapeutics. 7th ed. New York: Macmillan Publishing, 1985:1201.
30. Halpern M, Meyers B, Miller C, Bodenheimer H, Thung SN, Adler J, Toth D, Cohen D, Baccardo L, Diferdinando G, Birkhead A; from the Centers for Disease Control and Prevention. Severe isoniazid-associated hepatitis—New York, 1991–1993. JAMA 1993;270(7):809.
31. Chan KL, Chan HS, Lui SF, Lai KN. Recurrent acute pancreatitis induced by isoniazid. Tuber Lung Dis 1994;75(5):383–5.
32. Rabassa AA, Trey G, Shukla U, Samo T, Anand BS. Isoniazid-induced acute pancreatitis. Ann Intern Med 1994;121(6):433–4.
33. Stephenson I, Wiselka MJ, Qualie MJ. Acute pancreatitis induced by isoniazid in the treatment of tuberculosis. Am J Gastroenterol 2001;96(7):2271–2.
34. Trainin EB, Turin RD, Gomez-Leon G. Acute renal insufficiency complicating isoniazid therapy. Int J Pediatr Nephrol 1981;2(1):53–4.
35. Romero JA, Kuczler FJ Jr. Isoniazid overdose: recognition and management. Am Fam Physician 1998;57(4):749–52.
36. Sharma RP, Kathari AK, Sharma NK. Acneiform eruptions and anti-tubercular drugs. Indian J Dermatol Venereol Leprol 1995;61:26.
37. Koch SE, Williams ML. Acquired cutis laxa: case report and review of disorders of elastolysis. Pediatr Dermatol 1985;2(4):282–8.
38. Rothfield NF, Bierer WF, Garfield JW. Isoniazid induction of antinuclear antibodies. A prospective study. Ann Intern Med 1978;88(5):650–2.
39. Darvay A, Basarab T, McGregor JM, Russell-Jones R. Isoniazid induced pellagra despite pyridoxine supplementation. Clin Exp Dermatol 1999;24(3):167–9.
40. Scheid P, Kanny G, Trechot P, Rosner V, Menard O, Vignaud JM, Anthoine D, Martinet Y. Isoniazid-induced bullous skin reaction. Allergy 1999;54(3):294–6.
41. De Weck AL. Approaches to prevention and treatment of drug allergy. In: Turk JL, Parker D, editors. Drugs and Immune Responsiveness, 13. Baltimore: University Park Press, 1979:211.
42. Panganiban LR, Makalinao IR, Corte-Maramba NP. Rhabdomyolysis in isoniazid poisoning. J Toxicol Clin Toxicol 2001;39(2):143–51.
43. Hoigne R, Biedermann HP, Naegeli HR. INH-induzierter systemischer Lupus Erythematodes: 2 Beobachtungen mit Reexposition. Schweiz Med Wochenschr 1975;105(50):1726.
44. Hiraoka K, Nagata N, Kawajiri T, Suzuki K, Kurokawa S, Kido M, Sakamoto N. Paradoxical pleural response to antituberculous chemotherapy and isoniazid-induced lupus. Review and report of two cases. Respiration 1998;65(2):152–5.
45. Des Prez RM, Heim CR. Mycobacterium tuberculosis. In: Mandell GL, Douglas RG Jr, Bennett JE, editors. Principles and Practice of Infectious Diseases. 3rd ed. New York: Churchill Livingstone, 1990:1877.
46. Kunz J, Schreiner WE. Pharmakotherapie während Schwangerschaft und Stillperiode. Stuttgart-New York: G Thieme, 1982.
47. Olive G. Interactions médicamenteuses chez le nouveau né. In: Comptes Rendus. 25e Congrès de l'Association des Pédiatres de Langue Française, Tunis, 1978. Paris: Expansion Scientifique Française, 1978:57.
48. Miller J, Robinson A, Percy AK. Acute isoniazid poisoning in childhood. Am J Dis Child 1980;134(3):290–2.
49. Shah BR, Santucci K, Sinert R, Steiner P. Acute isoniazid neurotoxicity in an urban hospital. Pediatrics 1995;95(5):700–4.
50. Gilhotra R, Malik SK, Singh S, Sharma BK. Acute isoniazid toxicity—report of 2 cases and review of literature. Int J Clin Pharmacol Ther Toxicol 1987;25(5):259–61.
51. Hurwitz A, Schlozman DL. Effects of antacids on gastrointestinal absorption of isoniazid in rat and man. Am Rev Respir Dis 1974;109(1):41–7.
52. Duroux P. Surveillance et accidents de la chimiothérapie antituberculeuse. [Surveillance and complications of antituberculosis chemotherapy.] Rev Prat 1979;29(33):2681–90.
53. Santoso B. Impairment of isoniazid clearance by propranolol. Int J Clin Pharmacol Ther Toxicol 1985;23(3):134–6.
54. Valsalan VC, Cooper GL. Carbamazepine intoxication caused by interaction with isoniazid. BMJ (Clin Res Ed) 1982;285(6337):261–2.
55. Whittington HG, Grey L. Possible interaction between disulfiram and isoniazid. Am J Psychiatry 1969;125(12):1725–9.
56. van Wieringen A, Vrijlandt CM. Ethosuximide intoxication caused by interaction with isoniazid. Neurology 1983;33(9):1227–8.
57. DiMartini A. Isoniazid, tricyclics and the "cheese reaction". Int Clin Psychopharmacol 1995;10(3):197–8.
58. Miller RR, Porter J, Greenblatt DJ. Clinical importance of the interaction of phenytoin and isoniazid: a report from the Boston Collaborative Drug Surveillance Program. Chest 1979;75(3):356–8.
59. Breen RA, Lipman MC, Johnson MA. Increased incidence of peripheral neuropathy with co-administration of stavudine and isoniazid in HIV-infected individuals. AIDS 2000;14(5):615.
60. Hauser MJ, Baier H. Interactions of isoniazid with foods. Drug Intell Clin Pharm 1982;16(7–8):617–18.
61. Lejonc JL, Schaeffer A, Brochard P, Portos JL. Hypertension artérielle paroxystique provoquée sous isoniazide par l'ingestion de Gruyère: deux cas. [Paroxystic hypertension after ingestion of Gruyère cheese during isoniazide treatment: a report on two cases.] Ann Med Interne (Paris) 1980;131(6):346–8.
62. Uragoda CG. Histamine poisoning in tuberculous patients after ingestion of tuna fish. Am Rev Respir Dis 1980;121(1):157–9.

Isoprenaline

See also Adrenoceptor agonists

General Information

As a non-selective beta-adrenergic receptor stimulant, isoprenaline produces a wide range of adrenergic effects. Those that involve the heart present the most marked problems in practice. Doses of up to 10 micrograms/minute are used to improve the peripheral circulation in shock. In respiratory disease, isoprenaline in sublingual tablets (up to 10 mg) and inhalers were used in the past, but have been supplanted by selective beta$_2$-adrenoceptor agonists. Isoprenaline inhalers sometimes provided more than the 20 micrograms needed for a maximum effect on the bronchi, resulting in adverse effects. Oral isoprenaline was also used to treat some forms of heart block, but is now obsolete.

Organs and Systems

Cardiovascular

Tachycardia, dysrhythmias, palpitation, flushing, and attacks of angina pectoris were disadvantages of isoprenaline when it was used in respiratory disease. Users tended to raise the dose (hence increasing the degree of cardiac toxicity), possibly because a metabolite (3-alpha-methylisoprenaline), which may act as a weak beta-blocker, accumulates and makes the original doses ineffective. Isoprenaline produces electrocardiographic changes compatible with myocardial infarction or can lead to ventricular fibrillation or even cardiac muscle necrosis if infusions are not given with the utmost caution (SED-12, 312) (1,2). Exceptionally, the tachycardia produced by an infusion of isoprenaline can be overshadowed by a reflex bradycardia, even while the drug is being given (SEDA-17, 163).

Respiratory

In relaxing bronchial smooth muscle, isoprenaline can impair the ventilation:perfusion ratio and aggravate hypoxemia even as it reduces airway resistance; thus, the patient may feel better but be worse off. In addition, paradoxical bronchospasm can occur, a response of this type having been found in 30% of patients in one series.

Nervous system

Headache, tremor, apprehension, dizziness, and faintness are common problems with isoprenaline.

Gastrointestinal

Quite apart from the fact that systemic adverse reactions appear to be more common when isoprenaline is given in the form of sublingual tablets, these commonly cause mouth ulcers. Their long-term use has also been reported on one occasion to have caused tooth destruction (SED-8, 305), but this was probably coincidental.

Second-Generation Effects

Teratogenicity

Isoprenaline has often been given in pregnancy, and animal studies do not suggest that it is teratogenic.

Susceptibility Factors

Isoprenaline is better avoided whenever stimulation of the heart or the central nervous system is undesirable, for example in patients with angina pectoris or thyroid disease. There is no reliable information on the risks in liver or renal disease.

Drug–Drug Interactions

Theophylline

The toxicity of isoprenaline in animals is increased if it is given with theophylline (3). There is no evidence of this in humans, although an interaction does occur at the cellular level (4).

References

1. Pentek L. Unsere Erfahrungen mit der Verwendung von Isoproterenol in der Behandlung des Schocks. [Use of isoproterenol in the treatment of shock.] Bruns Beitr Klin Chir 1969;217(4):355–62.
2. Jacobs RL, Koppes GM. Myocardial necrosis associated with isoproterenol abuse: a ten-year follow-up. Tex Med 1982;78(8):58–60.
3. Joseph X, Whitehurst VE, Bloom S, Balazs T. Enhancement of cardiotoxic effects of beta-adrenergic bronchodilators by aminophylline in experimental animals. Fundam Appl Toxicol 1981;1(6):443–7.
4. Trembath PW, Shaw J. Potentiation of isoprenaline-induced plasma cyclic AMP response by aminophylline in normal and asthmatic subjects. Br J Clin Pharmacol 1978;6(6):499–503.

Isopropamide iodide

General Information

A 5–10 mg oral dose of the anticholinergic drug isopropamide iodide produces typical anticholinergic adverse effects. In patients with Zollinger–Ellison syndrome the combination of cimetidine plus isopropamide 20–40 mg/day was generally more effective in suppressing acid secretion than cimetidine alone (1).

Organs and Systems

Urinary tract

The presence of isopropamide iodide in some over-the-counter cold remedies, for example alongside antihistamines, should be borne in mind as a hidden cause of urinary retention.

Immunologic

Isopropamide iodide can cause allergic reactions in patients who are sensitive to iodine.

Interference with Diagnostic Tests

Thyroid function

By virtue of its iodine content, isopropamide iodide can interfere with thyroid function tests.

Reference

1. McCarthy DM, Hyman PE. Effect of isopropamide on response to oral cimetidine in patients with Zollinger–Ellison syndrome. Dig Dis Sci 1982;27(4):353–9.

Isopropanolamine

General Information

Isopropanolamine is used in cosmetics, hair perms, hair sprays, and in tanning lotions as a buffering agent.

Organs and Systems

Immunologic

- Contact dermatitis to a gel containing biphenylacetic acid, a non-steroidal anti-inflammatory agent, carbomer, and isopropanolamine has been reported (1). Patch tests showed a positive reaction to isopropanolamine (1% aqueous) on day 4. Patch-testing of 22 patients as controls showed one case of slight irritation.

Reference

1. Cooper SM, Shaw S. Contact allergy to isopropanolamine in Traxam gel. Contact Dermatitis 1999;41(4):233–4.

Isoxepac

General Information

Evidence about the properties of the NSAID isoxepac is minimal; only increases in gastrointestinal blood loss over pretreatment levels have been described (1).

Reference

1. Mitchell H, Barraclough D, Muirden KD. Blood-loss studies for new non-steroidal anti-inflammatory drugs. Med J Aust 1982;1(8):328.

Isoxicam

See also Non-steroidal anti-inflammatory drugs

General Information

The oxicam NSAID isoxicam has a shorter half-life (30 hours) than piroxicam. However, there are large variations in half-life, clearance, and mean steady-state plasma concentrations. Except for edema, the incidence of adverse effects is unrelated to age (1).

Organs and Systems

Gastrointestinal

The main adverse effects of isoxicam are gastrointestinal (pain, dyspepsia, nausea, vomiting, stomatitis, constipation, and occasionally peptic ulcer), which occur in up to 80% of patients.

Skin

Serious skin reactions (Stevens–Johnson syndrome and Lyell's syndrome) caused temporary withdrawal of isoxicam in several countries, even though an analysis of 1800 patients with rheumatoid arthritis or degenerative joint disease failed to confirm an increased risk (2).

References

1. Haslock I. Tolerance of isoxicam with respect to age. In: Amor B, editor. Non-steroidal Anti-inflammatory Agents in the Elderly. Basel: Eular, 1984:114.
2. Burch FX. Evaluation of the safety of isoxicam. Am J Med 1985;79(4B):28–32.

Isoxsuprine

See also Adrenoceptor agonists

General Information

Isoxsuprine is a beta$_2$-adrenoceptor agonist that also has antagonist action at alpha-adrenoceptors. It has been variously presented as a beta-agonist, a specific vasorelaxant, a uterine relaxant, and an agent that reduces blood viscosity. In high dosages it also inhibits platelet aggregation. There is slim evidence that isoxsuprine improves cognitive function and mental performance in a limited number of patients, but the practical benefit is minor. There is no convincing proof of its efficacy in patients with claudication. It has been widely used in horses for treating navicular syndrome and laminitis, with little evidence of efficacy (1).

Since its efficacy has been doubted with respect to both its vascular and its obstetric use, one must suspect that underdosage of the drug is the best explanation for the low reported incidence of adverse reactions, which are generally of the type regarded as anecdotal (nausea, vomiting, palpitation, dizziness, weakness). Minor facial flushing and tremor are common. As patients tend to increase the dosage gradually, diarrhea, vomiting, headache, vertigo, and rash can occur (SEDA-3, 177) (SEDA-7, 228). The important adverse reactions of isoxsuprine are tachycardia and orthostatic hypotension, but they occur only at high dosages.

Second-Generation Effects

Fetotoxicity

The beta-adrenoceptor agonist effect is sufficient to cause fetal tachycardia when isoxsuprine is given intravenously in late pregnancy, although one large survey suggested that it may be better tolerated by the mother (as regards cardiac and stimulant effects) than salbutamol (SED-12, 313). The fact that maternal blood pressure can fall may reflect a direct relaxant effect on the blood vessels.

Reference

1. Erkert RS, Macallister CG. Isoxsuprine hydrochloride in the horse: a review. J Vet Pharmacol Ther 2002;25(2):81–7.

Isradipine

See also Calcium channel blockers

General Information

Isradipine is a dihydropyridine calcium channel blocker.

The MIDAS study (1) was a randomized trial of isradipine versus hydrochlorothiazide over 3 years in 883 patients, designed primarily to assess the effect on the rate of progression of medial intimal thickness in carotid arteries. The control of diastolic blood pressure was equivalent in both groups, but mean systolic blood pressure was 3.5 mmHg higher in isradipine group at 6 months, a significant difference that persisted throughout the study. This might explain the higher incidence of vascular events with isradipine, although there was no difference in the rate of progression of medial intimal thickness between the groups.

Drug–Drug Interactions

Ethanol

Studies in rodents and primates have suggested that calcium channel blockers, including darodipine, nifedipine, and verapamil, can attenuate the behavioral effects of ethanol. Isradipine seems to be the most effective. However, the results of published reports in man on the effects of calcium antagonists on the acute subject-rated, performance-impairing, and cardiovascular effects of ethanol have suggested that the behavioral effects of ethanol are not attenuated by verapamil, nifedipine, or nimodipine. The same conclusions have been reached from a study in nine healthy volunteers (2). Combined ethanol and isradipine produced increases in heart rate and reductions in blood pressure that were not observed with either drug alone. Isradipine significantly reduced peak breath alcohol concentrations, but it did not significantly alter the subject-rated performance-impairing effects of ethanol.

Phenytoin

An interaction of isradipine with phenytoin has been reported (3).

- A 21-year-old white man, who was taking phenytoin and carbamazepine for seizures, developed severe lethargy, ataxia, and weakness after isradipine was prescribed for blood pressure control. The interaction was verified 2 months later, when he was rechallenged with the same dose of isradipine, 2.5 mg bd, and developed the same symptoms. Phenytoin plasma concentrations were at the upper limit of the usual target range (maximum assayed 100 μmol/l) and did not fall when the dose of phenytoin was reduced while he was taking isradipine.

Both pharmacokinetic and pharmacodynamic mechanisms can explain these observations. Isradipine inhibits CYP450 isoforms that are responsible for the metabolism of phenytoin, and both isradipine and phenytoin can bind to calcium channels in the brain and thereby affect neurological function.

References

1. Borhani NO, Mercuri M, Borhani PA, Buckalew VM, Canossa-Terris M, Carr AA, Kappagoda T, Rocco MV, Schnaper HW, Sowers JR, Bond MG. Final outcome results of the Multicenter Isradipine Diuretic Atherosclerosis Study (MIDAS). A randomized controlled trial. JAMA 1996;276(10):785–91.
2. Rush CR, Pazzaglia PJ. Pretreatment with isradipine, a calcium-channel blocker, does not attenuate the acute behavioral effects of ethanol in humans. Alcohol Clin Exp Res 1998;22(2):539–47.
3. Cachat F, Tufro A, Dalmady-Israel C, Laplante S. Phenytoin/isradipine interaction causing severe neurologic toxicity. Ann Pharmacother 2002;36(9):1399–402.

Itraconazole

See also Antifungal azoles

General Information

Itraconazole is a triazole antifungal drug. It is used orally to treat oropharyngeal and vulvovaginal candidiasis, pityriasis versicolor, dermatophytoses unresponsive to topical treatment, and systemic infections, including aspergillosis, blastomycosis, chromoblastomycosis, coccidioidomycosis, cryptococcosis, histoplasmosis, paracoccidioidomycosis, and sporotrichosis. It is also used to prevent fungal infections in immunocompromised patients.

Pharmacokinetics

The systemic availability of itraconazole and the bioequivalence of single 200 mg doses of itraconazole solution and two capsule formulations have been evaluated in a crossover study in 30 male volunteers (1). Itraconazole and hydroxyitraconazole were 30–37% more available from the solution and were greater than from either capsule formulation. However, the values of C_{max}, t_{max}, and half-lives were comparable. There were no differences in safety and tolerance. The normal t_{max} of itraconazole is 1.5–4 hours and serum concentrations are dose-related. Steady-state concentrations are reached after about 10–14 days and are high in comparison with those attained after single doses. With single daily dose treatment the half-life is 20–30 hours. Itraconazole is highly protein bound. The tissue concentrations in lung, kidney, liver, bone, spleen, and muscle are 2–3 times higher than the corresponding serum concentrations. Concentrations in omentum and adipose tissue are particularly high, and higher concentrations are also found in various parts of the genital tract. Itraconazole is markedly keratinophilic; after withdrawal it will take 1–2 weeks before concentrations in the skin start to fall. Itraconazole concentrations in urine, saliva, eye fluids, and cerebrospinal fluid are low. Penetration of itraconazole into ocular tissues is low compared with those of ketoconazole and fluconazole (2,3). Itraconazole is degraded in the liver and excreted via the bile and to some extent in the urine. Its metabolism is not altered by renal dysfunction (4–6).

Observational studies

The pharmacokinetics, safety, and antifungal efficacy of intravenous itraconazole (400 mg for 2 days then 200 mg for 12 days), followed by 12 weeks of oral capsules (400 mg/day) have been investigated in 31 immunocompromised patients with invasive pulmonary aspergillosis (7). All received intravenous itraconazole and 26 then took oral itraconazole for a median of 79 days. Potentially therapeutic trough plasma itraconazole concentrations of 0.5 microgram/ml or more were achieved in 64% of the patients by day 2 and were generally maintained after switching to oral therapy. There was a complete or partial response in 15 patients. There were adverse events during intravenous therapy in 28 patients, and 13 had adverse events that were possibly related to the drug. The main events (at least 10% incidence) were fever, diarrhea, increased blood urea nitrogen, and nausea. Two of these 13 patients had intravenous therapy withdrawn. There were no consistent clinically relevant changes in laboratory parameters. During oral therapy, nine patients had similar adverse events that were possibly related to itraconazole. Treatment was withdrawn in seven patients because of adverse events during this phase. There were no deaths related to itraconazole.

The pharmacokinetics and safety of intravenous itraconazole for 7 days (200 mg bd for 2 days, then 200 mg od for 5 days), followed by itraconazole oral solution 200 mg od or bd for 14 days, have been assessed in 17 patients with hematological malignancies requiring antifungal prophylaxis (8). The mean trough plasma concentration at the end of the intravenous period was 0.54 microgram/ml. This concentration was not maintained during once-daily oral treatment but increased further during twice-daily treatment, with a trough itraconazole concentration of 1.12 micrograms/ml at the end of oral treatment. All patients had some adverse events, mainly gastrointestinal. The two patients who were withdrawn from the study during intravenous treatment both reported fever; one also had pneumonitis and died from pneumonia 2 weeks after withdrawal, but this was unrelated to the drug. Patients were withdrawn during oral treatment because of fever ($n = 3$), pneumonitis ($n = 2$), colitis ($n = 1$), and abdominal pain and diarrhea ($n = 1$). Biochemical and hematological abnormalities were frequent, but there were no consistent changes.

The efficacy and safety of intermittent itraconazole therapy have been investigated in 635 patients with onychomycosis (9). Intermittent itraconazole (400 mg/day for 1 week per month for 2 months) was effective and safe. Most adverse events were minor and occurred infrequently; there were no major changes in liver function tests.

Two dosages of itraconazole have been compared in the treatment of tinea corporis or tinea cruris in a multicenter, randomized, double-blind, parallel-group study, which showed that itraconazole 200 mg for 1 week (54 patients) is similarly effective, equally well tolerated, and at least as safe as the established regimen of itraconazole 100 mg for 2 weeks (60 patients) (10). In a similar study in tinea pedis or tinea manum, itraconazole 400 mg once a week (66 patients) and itraconazole 100 mg once every 4 weeks (69 patients) were both effective; the two schedules were equally well tolerated and safe (11).

Comparative studies

Amphotericin

Data on the safety of itraconazole have been collected in an open, randomized, multicenter study in 277 adults with cancer and neutropenia (12). Itraconazole oral solution (100 mg bd, $n = 144$) was compared with a combination of amphotericin capsules and nystatin oral suspension ($n = 133$). Adverse events were reported in about 45% of patients in each group. The most frequent were vomiting (14 versus 12 patients), diarrhea (12 versus 9), nausea (5 versus 12), and rash (2 versus 13 patients). There were no differences in liver function test abnormalities. Treatment had to be withdrawn because of adverse events (including death) in 34 patients who took itraconazole and 33 of those who took amphotericin plus nystatin; there were 17 deaths in each group and death was recorded as adverse event in 13 and 9 patients, respectively.

Itraconazole (400 mg intravenously for 2 days, 200 mg intravenously for up to 12 days, then 400 mg/day orally) and intravenous amphotericin deoxycholate (0.7–1.0 mg/kg) have been compared in 384 granulocytopenic patients with persistent fever in a randomized, multicenter trial (13). The median duration of therapy was 8.5 days. The incidence of drug-related adverse events (5 versus 54%) and the rate of withdrawal due to toxicity (19 versus 38%) were significantly lower with itraconazole. The most frequent reasons for withdrawal in patients taking itraconazole were nausea and vomiting (5%), rash (3%), and abnormal liver function tests (3%). Significantly fewer of the patients who received itraconazole had nephrotoxicity (5 versus 24%); however, more had hyperbilirubinemia (10 versus 5%). There was no difference in gastrointestinal adverse events between the two groups.

Itraconazole elixir 2.5 mg/kg bd ($n = 281$) has been compared with amphotericin capsules 500 mg qds ($n = 276$) for the prophylaxis of systemic and superficial fungal infections in a double-blind, randomized, placebo-controlled, multicenter trial for 1–59 days (14). While itraconazole significantly reduced the frequency of superficial fungal infections, it was not superior in reducing invasive fungal infections or in improving mortality. Adverse events were reported in 222 patients taking itraconazole (79%) and in 205 patients taking amphotericin (74%). The commonest adverse events were gastrointestinal, followed by rash and hypokalemia, with no differences between the two regimens. In both groups, 5% of the adverse events were considered to be definitely drug-related. Comparable numbers of patients in the two groups permanently stopped treatment because of adverse events (including death), 75 (27%) in the itraconazole group and 78 (28%) in the amphotericin group. Nausea (9 and 11%) and vomiting (8 and 7%) were the most frequently reported adverse events that led to withdrawal. Biochemical changes were comparable in the two groups.

Other antifungal azoles

The safety of continuous itraconazole (50–200 mg/day for up to 3 months) in the treatment of onychomycosis and dermatomycosis has been reviewed, using published and unpublished data from clinical trials (15). The overall incidence of adverse events in patients who took continuous itraconazole (21%) differed little from that in patients who took either topical miconazole or oral placebo (18%). The most frequently reported adverse events were gastrointestinal disorders (6.7%), headache (4.2%), and skin disorders (2.7%). No data were given on the incidence of serious adverse events attributed to itraconazole. Among laboratory abnormalities, clinically significant rises in liver function tests occurred in 3.4% of 527 patients treated with itraconazole (2.6% in patients treated with 50–200 mg/day for dermatomycosis versus 6.6% in patients treated with 200 mg/day for 3 months for onychomycosis).

Oral fluconazole 400 mg qds and oral itraconazole 200 mg bd have been compared in a randomized, double blind, placebo-controlled trial in 198 patients with progressive non-meningeal coccidioidomycosis (16). Overall, 57% and 72% of patients responded to 12 months of therapy with fluconazole and itraconazole, respectively. Relapse rates after withdrawal did not differ significantly. Both drugs were well tolerated. Serious adverse events occurred in eight of 97 fluconazole-treated patients and six of 101 itraconazole-treated patients. They included raised liver enzymes, gastrointestinal disturbances, hypokalemia, and skin rash. Alopecia was reported in 15 of 97 patients taking fluconazole and in only four of 101 patients taking itraconazole. Similarly, dry lips were reported in 11 of 97 patients taking fluconazole and in none of 101 patients taking itraconazole. Both adverse events have previously been reported with fluconazole.

In a double-blind comparison in oropharyngeal candidiasis in 244 patients with AIDS, itraconazole oral solution and fluconazole capsules (each 100 mg/day for 14 days) were equally efficacious; there were no significant differences in adverse effects (17).

Itraconazole oral solution and fluconazole tablets have been compared in oropharyngeal candidiasis in HIV/AIDS patients in a prospective randomized, blind, multicenter trial (18). Both regimens of itraconazole oral solution (100 mg bd for 7 days or 100 mg od for 14 days) were equivalent to fluconazole (100 mg od for 14 days). Itraconazole oral solution was well tolerated.

Oral itraconazole solution has been compared with intravenous/oral fluconazole for the prevention of fungal infections in a randomized, controlled trial in adult liver transplant recipients, who were randomized to receive either oral itraconazole solution (200 mg bd) or intravenous/oral fluconazole (400 mg/day) (19). Prophylaxis was started immediately before transplant surgery and continued for 10 weeks after transplantation. Proven fungal infection developed in nine of 97 patients given itraconazole and in four of 91 patients given fluconazole. Mortality from fungal infection was very low and occurred in only one of the 188 patients. Except for more frequent gastrointestinal adverse effects (nausea, vomiting, diarrhea) with itraconazole, both drugs were well tolerated and neither was associated with hepatotoxicity. Mean trough plasma concentrations of itraconazole were over 250 ng/ml throughout the study and were not affected by H_2 histamine receptor antagonists or antacids.

Terbinafine

Itraconazole (28 patients) and terbinafine (27 patients) have been compared in a double-blind, randomized study in tinea capitis (20). The cure rates at week 12 were 86% and 78% respectively. Adverse events were mild and did not warrant discontinuation of therapy.

Placebo-controlled studies

In a double blind, randomized, placebo-controlled, multicenter trial in plantar or moccasin-type tinea pedis in 72 patients, itraconazole 200 mg bd was significantly more effective than placebo; its safety and tolerability were comparable with placebo (21).

General adverse effects

Most of the reported adverse effects of itraconazole are transient. Gastrointestinal reactions, mild dyspepsia, pyrosis, nausea, vomiting, diarrhea, and epigastric pain are not uncommon. In many of the published reports mention is made of increases in serum liver enzyme activities and hypertriglyceridemia, and symptomatic liver toxicity has been reported. Itraconazole does not induce drug-metabolizing enzymes and is a weaker inhibitor of microsomal enzymes than ketoconazole (4,22). In rats given doses of up to 160 mg/kg, there was no induction or inhibition of the metabolism of xenobiotics (SEDA-16, 285). Hypokalemia has often been reported, without an explanation of the mechanism. The use of higher doses (400 or even 600 mg/day) causes an increased incidence of adverse effects; among those documented at these dosages are severe hypokalemia, reversible adrenal insufficiency, and (in one published case) arrhythmias, the latter being connected with an interaction with terfenadine (SEDA-16, 295) (SEDA-18, 198). Skin rashes and pruritus have been reported. Tumor-inducing effects have not been described.

In patients taking itraconazole capsules for prolonged periods the common adverse effects were nausea and vomiting (in under 10%), hypertriglyceridemia (9%), hypokalemia (6%), raised transaminases (5%), rashes and/or pruritus (2%), headache or dizziness (under 2%), and foot edema (1%) (23).

In a study using the UK General Practice Research Database to determine rates of rare, serious drug-induced, adverse effects on the liver, kidneys, skin, or blood, occurring within 45 days of completing a prescription or refill in 54 803 users of either fluconazole or itraconazole, one patient had an abnormal liver function test while taking itraconazole in whom a drug-induced etiology could not be ruled out, a rate of 3.2 per 100 000 prescriptions (95% CI = 0.6, 18) for serious adverse liver effects (24). Thus, itraconazole does not commonly have serious adverse effects on the liver, kidneys, skin, or blood.

Organs and Systems

Cardiovascular

Ventricular fibrillation has been attributed to itraconazole-induced hypokalemia (25).

- Pleural and subsequent pericardial effusion developed in a woman treated with itraconazole 200 mg bd for a localized pulmonary infection with *Aspergillus fumigatus* (SEDA-18, 282). After more than 9 weeks of treatment she developed a pericardial effusion, which necessitated drainage. Itraconazole was withdrawn. Six weeks later, and 2 weeks after the resumption of itraconazole, she developed signs of pulmonary edema and cardiac enlargement. These signs disappeared rapidly on discontinuation of itraconazole.

Studies in dogs and healthy human volunteers have suggested that itraconazole has a negative inotropic effect; the mechanism is unknown. A systematic analysis of data from the FDA's Adverse Event Reporting System (AERS) identified 58 cases suggestive of congestive heart failure in patients taking itraconazole (26). A simultaneous search did not identify any cases of congestive heart failure in patients taking fluconazole and ketoconazole, ruling out the possibility of a class effect. In consequence, the labeling of itraconazole has been revised. Itraconazole is now contraindicated for the treatment of onychomycosis in patients with evidence of ventricular dysfunction. For systemic fungal infections, the risks and benefits of itraconazole should be reassessed if signs or symptoms of congestive heart failure develop.

Nervous system

Headache due to itraconazole has been mentioned in some reports (27). Dizziness is an uncommon complaint, as are mood disturbances.

Psychological, psychiatric

Visual hallucinations with confusion have been reported in a 75-year-old woman, occurring on three separate occasions, each time about 2 hours after a 200 mg dose of itraconazole. Her symptoms abated spontaneously over about 8 hours (28).

Electrolyte balance

Hypokalemia, occurring either in isolation or with hypertension, has been reported regularly in a small fraction of patients (23). Marked ankle edema with weight gain was seen in a patient taking itraconazole 400 mg/day, in whom there was no explanation other than the use of the drug; after withdrawal of the itraconazole the symptoms disappeared. Hypokalemia and edema have also been observed in a number of patients taking high-dose therapy (600 mg/day) (SED-12, 680) (29) (SEDA-16, 295) (SEDA-17, 321) (4,25,29,30), associated with mildly depressed aldosterone concentrations (SED-12, 680) (SEDA-16, 295).

Gastrointestinal

Dyspepsia, pyrosis, nausea, vomiting, mild epigastric discomfort, and diarrhea can occur in patients taking itraconazole (31). These gastrointestinal complaints are generally mild, but they seem to be the most frequent adverse effects during treatment. The total incidence of adverse effects was 3–5% in patients treated for superficial mycosis and 8% in 99 patients treated for deep mycosis (SED-12, 680) (32). An incidence closer to 15% was reported in a multicenter trial (SEDA-17, 321).

In 50 women with acute vaginal candidiasis, adverse effects were reported in 17 (35%), nausea in seven, headache in six, dizziness in three, and bloating in three, while aspartate transaminase activity was raised in one (33).

Of 1108 patients with HIV treated for mucosal candidiasis, 239 reported gastrointestinal symptoms (34).

Pseudomembranous colitis has been reported in association with exposure to itraconazole (35).

- A 54-year-old man developed new abdominal pain and non-bloody diarrhea 1 month after exposure to a 7-day course of oral itraconazole 200 mg/day. He was taking stable chronic sertraline, valproic acid, and perphenazine, and had not taken antimicrobial drugs for 6 months. Flexible sigmoidoscopy after clinical progression showed pseudomembranes, and subsequent evaluation excluded other causes of diarrhea. Although *Clostridium difficile* culture and toxin assay were eventually negative, possibly because of delayed stool sampling, he responded to a 10-day course of anti-anaerobic drug therapy and was discharged with completely resolved symptoms.

The authors proposed that itraconazole had disrupted the resident fungal flora of the colon.

Liver

In most clinical reports, there were some cases of raised liver enzyme activities; the changes were transient or disappeared after withdrawal of itraconazole (36). More serious hepatotoxicity was not reported.

- Focal nodular hyperplasia of the liver has been reported in a 38-year-old woman who had taken itraconazole 200 mg/day for 4 months for a fungal infection of the fingernails (37). She had taken no other drugs in the year during which focal nodular hyperplasia developed.
- Of three patients, two women aged 62 and 57 and a man aged 75 years, who developed symptomatic hepatic injury 5–6 weeks after starting to take itraconazole, two had the biochemical pattern of cholestatic liver damage (38).

All itraconazole clinical trials sponsored by Janssen Research Foundation for the treatment of onychomycosis, in which there was an assessment of laboratory safety, have been analysed (39). There were no significant differences in the number of code 4 abnormalities (baseline value is in the reference range and at least two values, or the last testing in the observation period, exceed twice the upper limit of the reference range) in liver function tests (alanine transaminase, aspartate transaminase, alkaline phosphatase, and total bilirubin). The incidence of all the code 4 abnormalities was under 2%. Itraconazole pulse therapy for onychomycosis appears to be safe, especially from the perspective of potential liver damage. In the itraconazole package insert, liver function tests are recommended in patients receiving continuous itraconazole for over 1 month. There is no such monitoring requirement for the pulse regimen, unless the patient has a history of underlying hepatic disease, the liver function tests are abnormal at baseline, or signs or symptoms suggestive of liver dysfunction develop at any time.

Skin

Different types of rash, including a case of acneiform rash, have been reported in patients taking itraconazole. In one case there were bloody bullae (SED-12, 680) (40–43).

- A 29-year-old man developed an infiltrative maculopapular eruption after 1 week of itraconazole 100 mg bd for tinea corporis (44). Itraconazole was withdrawn, and the lesions disappeared within 7 days. Scratch tests, patch tests, scratch-patch tests, and drug induced lymphocyte stimulation tests for itraconazole were negative; however, rechallenge with systemic itraconazole induced a maculopapular eruption on the face, hands, and the dorsa of the feet. Empty itraconazole capsules had no cutaneous effects, suggesting an allergic reaction to a metabolite of the compound.

Photosensitivity has been attributed to itraconazole (200 mg qds for 5 days), with reduced minimal erythema dose for both UVB (0.12 J/cm^2) and UVA (20.1 J/cm^2), negative photopatch testing, and a positive photochallenge (45). The authors proposed a photoallergic mechanism because earlier exposure to itraconazole had been uneventful. However, details about sun exposure during the first exposure and about the intensity of sun exposure during the oral photochallenge procedure were not given. The eruption responded to oral steroids, which is more typical of photoallergic than phototoxic reactions.

The risk of serious skin disorders has been estimated in 61 858 users of oral antifungal drugs, aged 20–79 years, identified in the UK General Practice Research Database (46). They had received at least one prescription for oral fluconazole, griseofulvin, itraconazole, ketoconazole, or terbinafine. The background rate of serious cutaneous adverse reactions (corresponding to non-use of oral antifungal drugs) was 3.9 per 10 000 person-years (95% CI = 2.9, 5.2). Incidence rates for current use were 15 per 10 000 person-years (1.9, 56) for itraconazole, 11.1 (3.0, 29) for terbinafine, 10 (1.3, 38) for fluconazole, and 4.6 (0.1, 26) for griseofulvin. Cutaneous disorders associated with the use of oral antifungal drugs in this study were all mild.

Sexual function

There are inconsistent reports about the effects of itraconazole on sex steroids. Concentrations of testosterone, corticosterone, and progesterone were unchanged in rats and in six dogs in whom possible endocrine effects were studied (SED-12, 680). On the other hand, the administration of itraconazole to seven male volunteers for 2 weeks did not produce detectable changes in plasma testosterone or cortisol concentrations. There was a slightly reduced cortisol response to ACTH stimulation 2 weeks after the start of high-dose itraconazole therapy (600 mg/day) in one of eight patients with severe mycosis (29).

Erectile impotence, with normal steroid concentrations, has been reported, as has a reduction in libido (SEDA-17, 321) (47).

Immunologic

Itraconazole 200 mg bd for 2 weeks caused a serum sickness-like reaction in a 53-year-old woman with Menière's disease (48).

Second-Generation Effects

Teratogenicity

Since embryotoxicity and teratogenicity have been found in rats, albeit after the administration of high doses, itraconazole should be avoided during pregnancy (SED-12, 681) (49).

Susceptibility Factors

Age

The safety, tolerability, and pharmacokinetics of itraconazole and its active metabolite hydroxyitraconazole after administration of itraconazole solution in hydroxypropyl-β-cyclodextrin have been investigated in a multicenter study in 26 infants and children aged 6 months to 12 years with mucosal candidiasis or at risk of invasive fungal disease (50). There was a trend to lower minimum plasma concentrations in children aged 6 months to 2 years. The systemic absorption of the solubilizer hydroxypropyl-β-cyclodextrin was less than 1%. Given at 5 mg/kg/day, this formulation provided potentially therapeutic concentrations in plasma, somewhat lower than those attained in adults, and it was well tolerated and safe.

Itraconazole 100 mg/day has been studied in 24 children with *Trichophyton tonsurans* tinea capitis (51). Itraconazole was well tolerated, but 15 children required re-treatment due to persistent infection.

The safety, pharmacokinetics, and pharmacodynamics of an oral suspension of cyclodextrin itraconazole (2.5 mg /kg od or bd for 15 days) have been investigated in an open, sequential, dose-escalation study in 26 children and adolescents, 5–18 years old, infected with HIV (mean CD4 count 128 $\times$ 10^6/l) with oropharyngeal candidiasis (52). Apart from mild to moderate gastrointestinal disturbances in three patients, cyclodextrin itraconazole was well tolerated. Two patients withdrew prematurely because of adverse events. The oropharyngeal candidiasis score fell significantly from a mean of 7.46 at baseline to 2.8 at the end of therapy, demonstrating antifungal efficacy in this setting. Based on these results, a dosage of 2.5 mg/kg bd was recommended for the treatment of oropharyngeal candidiasis in children aged 5 years and over.

The safety and efficacy of oral cyclodextrin itraconazole (5 mg/kg/day) as antifungal prophylaxis has been assessed in an open trial in 103 neutropenic children (median age 5 years; range 0–15 years) (53). Prophylaxis was started at least 7 days before the onset of neutropenia and continued until neutrophil recovery. Of the 103 patients, only 47 completed the course of prophylaxis; 27 withdrew because of poor compliance, 19 because of adverse events, and 10 for other reasons. Serious adverse events (other than death) occurred in 21 patients, including convulsions ($n = 7$), suspected drug interactions ($n = 6$), abdominal pain ($n = 4$), and constipation ($n = 4$). The most common adverse events considered definitely or possibly related to itraconazole were vomiting ($n = 12$), abnormal liver function ($n = 5$), and abdominal pain ($n = 3$). Tolerability of the study medication at end-point was rated as good (55%), moderate (11%), poor (17%), or unacceptable (17%). There were no unexpected problems of safety or tolerability.

Other features of the patient

Adverse effects due to drug–drug interactions are not expected in diabetic patients using insulin and oral hypoglycemic drugs that are not metabolized by CYP3A4 (for example tolbutamide, gliclazide, glibenclamide, glipizide, and metformin). The pharmacokinetic and safety data from clinical trials and postmarketing surveillance have been reviewed to assess the safety of itraconazole in diabetic patients with onychomycosis or dermatomycosis (54). Postmarketing surveillance, including all adverse event reports in patients taking itraconazole concomitantly with insulin or an oral hypoglycemic drug, revealed 15 reports suggestive of hyperglycemia and nine reports suggestive of hypoglycemia. In most patients there was no change in antidiabetic effect. From clinical trials in 189 diabetic patients taking itraconazole for various infections, one itraconazole-related adverse event was recorded; this was a case of aggravated diabetes in a renal transplant patient who was also taking ciclosporin.

Drug Administration

Drug formulations

Itraconazole is poorly soluble in water and highly lipophilic. It is available as capsules, as oral and parenteral solutions that both contain hydroxypropyl-β-cyclodextrin as a solubilizer.

Absorption of itraconazole from capsules depends on a low gastric pH and is reduced by fasting and improved by the presence of food and acidic beverages; it is unpredictable in patients with hypochlorhydria. The t_{max} occurs at 1.5–2 hours. When polyethylene glycol is used as a solvent, the absorption is not as good. Inadequate plasma concentrations are often found in patients receiving cytotoxic drug therapy, which predisposes them to mucositis, poor food intake, and vomiting. The absorption of oral itraconazole seems to be reduced in patients with AIDS (2,3).

Systemic absorption of the cyclodextrin carrier after oral administration is negligible. After intravenous administration the cyclodextrin is not metabolized and is almost completely eliminated by glomerular filtration within 24 hours. Although the cyclodextrin enhances the systemic availability of itraconazole, it can have gastrointestinal adverse effects when used in escalating dosages exceeding 400 mg/day.

A dose-ranging study of itraconazole in antifungal prophylaxis in 123 neutropenic patients with hematological malignancies has been reported (55). The dosing regimens included itraconazole capsules 400, 600, or 800 mg/day and itraconazole cyclodextrin solution 400 and 800 mg/day (with an additional loading with 800 mg of the capsule formulation for 7 days). Ten of twenty-eight patients taking 800 mg/day as a solution withdrew after 1–6 days with severe nausea and vomiting in temporal relation to ingestion of the drug. All the patients who discontinued the solution continued medication with itraconazole capsules in the same dosage without gastrointestinal adverse effects.

Drug–Drug Interactions

Amphotericin

The in vitro effects of the combination of amphotericin with itraconazole was tested using six strains of *A. fumigatus*, and an antagonistic effect was found after pretreatment for all strains in vitro and for one strain in a mouse model of aspergillosis (56).

The effect of the combination of itraconazole with amphotericin on liver enzyme activities has been studied retrospectively in 20 patients with hematological malignancies or chronic lung disease complicated by fungal infection or colonization (57). They took itraconazole 200–600 mg/day for a median of 143 (range 44–455) days. Nine had no abnormal liver function tests, including periods of high concentrations of itraconazole (over 5000 ng/ml) and its active hydroxylated metabolite; only one had received concomitant amphotericin. All of the 11 patients with liver function abnormalities had received concomitant amphotericin. For each patient, liver function abnormalities were greatest during the time of concomitant therapy with both antifungal drugs. Although liver enzyme abnormalities are uncommon with amphotericin (58), and although this retrospective analysis was subject to several flaws and potential biases, it nevertheless suggests that hepatotoxicity should be carefully monitored if itraconazole and amphotericin are co-administered.

Antihistamines

It seems likely that combining itraconazole with astemizole (59) and terfenadine (60,61) will lead to increased effects of these antihistamines (62).

Barbiturates

Barbiturates lower itraconazole concentrations (SED-12, 681) (4,22).

Benzodiazepines

The effect of itraconazole on the single oral dose pharmacokinetics and pharmacodynamics of estazolam has been studied in a double-blind, randomized, crossover study in

10 healthy male volunteers, who took oral itraconazole 100 mg/day or placebo for 7 days and on day 4 a single oral dose of estazolam 4 mg (63). Blood samplings and evaluation of psychomotor function by the Digit Symbol Substitution Test, Visual Analogue Scale, and Stanford Sleepiness Scale were conducted up to 72 hours after estazolam. There was no significant difference between the placebo and itraconazole phases in peak plasma concentration, clearance, and half-life. Similarly, psychomotor function was unaffected. These findings suggest that CYP3A4 is not involved to a major extent in the metabolism of estazolam.

In a study of the effects of itraconazole 200 mg/day and rifampicin 600 mg/day on the pharmacokinetics and pharmacodynamics of oral midazolam 7.5–15 mg during and 4 days after the end of the treatment, switching from inhibition to induction of metabolism caused an up to 400-fold change in the AUC of oral midazolam (64).

Bupivacaine

The interaction of itraconazole 200 mg orally od for 4 days with a single intravenous dose of racemic bupivacaine (0.3 mg /kg given over 60 minutes) has been examined in a placebo-controlled crossover study in 10 healthy volunteers (65). Itraconazole reduced the clearance of *R*-bupivacaine by 21% and that of *S*-bupivacaine by 25%, but had no other significant effects on the pharmacokinetics of the enantiomers. Reduction of bupivacaine clearance by itraconazole is likely to increase steady-state concentrations of bupivacaine enantiomers by 20–25%, and this should be taken into account in the concomitant use of itraconazole and bupivacaine.

Buspirone

The interaction of itraconazole with the active 1-(2-pyrimidinyl)-piperazine metabolite of buspirone has been studied after a single oral dose of buspirone 10 mg (66). Itraconazole reduced the mean AUC of the metabolite by 50% and the C_{max} by 57%, whereas the mean AUC and C_{max} of the parent drug were increased 14.5-fold and 10.5-fold respectively. Thus, itraconazole caused relatively minor changes in the plasma concentrations of the active piperazine metabolite of buspirone, although it had major effects on the concentrations of buspirone after a single oral dose.

Busulfan

Reduced elimination and increased toxicity of busulfan co-administered with itraconazole has been postulated (67).

Carbamazepine

Low and sometimes very low serum concentrations of itraconazole have been seen during concurrent therapy of itraconazole with carbamazepine (68).

Ciclosporin

The combination of itraconazole with ciclosporin leads to a marked increase in blood ciclosporin concentrations, and this can result in a rise in serum creatinine, clearly pointing to renal damage as a result of the high ciclosporin concentrations (SED-12, 681) (69,70–72). However, an interaction has not been demonstrated in all cases (73).

Two cases of rhabdomyolysis caused by itraconazole in heart transplant recipients taking long-term ciclosporin and simvastatin have been reported (74,75). To avoid severe myopathy, ciclosporin concentrations should be monitored frequently and statins should be withdrawn or the dosage should be reduced, as long as azoles need to be prescribed in transplant recipients. Patients need to be educated about signs and symptoms that require immediate physician intervention.

Citrate-phosphate buffer

The citrate-phosphate buffer used to facilitate the absorption of dideoxyinosine (didanosine), prescribed for the treatment of AIDS, may interfere with the absorption of itraconazole (76).

Clarithromycin

A report of three HIV-negative patients has suggested that concomitant therapy with itraconazole and clarithromycin can lead to increased clarithromycin exposure, with an increased metabolic ratio, possibly related to itraconazole's effect on CYP3A4 (77). Nevertheless, in none of the three reported individuals were there adverse effects from this presumed interaction.

Clozapine

Itraconazole 200 mg had no significant effect on serum concentrations of clozapine 200–550 mg/day or desmethylclozapine in 7 schizophrenic patients (78).

Digoxin

Itraconazole inhibits the elimination of digoxin, eventually leading to toxicity (4,79–82) (SEDA-18, 198).

Itraconazole increases the digoxin AUC_{0-72} by about 50%, and reduces its renal clearance by about 20% (83). Apart from inhibition of the renal secretion of digoxin, which is probably mediated by inhibition of P glycoprotein, a study in guinea pigs also showed significantly reduced biliary excretion of digoxin by itraconazole, suggesting that the interaction between itraconazole and digoxin may not only be due to a reduction in renal clearance, but also to a reduction in the metabolic clearance of digoxin by itraconazole (84).

The importance of this interaction has been emphasized by a report of two renal transplant patients who had digoxin toxicity when they took itraconazole concurrently (85).

Famotidine

Famotidine 40 mg/kg/day reduced the peak and trough concentrations of itraconazole 200 mg/kg/day by about 35% in 18 patients undergoing chemotherapy for hematological malignancies (86).

Fentanyl

Fentanyl is a substrate of CYP3A4, CYP2C9, and CYP2C19. However, in one study, the pharmacokinetics and pharmacodynamics of fentanyl 3 micrograms/kg were similar after itraconazole 200 mg and placebo in 10 healthy volunteers (87).

- An interaction of itraconazole with fentanyl has been reported in a 67-year-old man with cancer on a stable dose of transdermal fentanyl 50 micrograms/hour (88). He took itraconazole 200 mg bd for oropharyngeal candidiasis, and 24 hours later developed signs of opioid toxicity, which was reversed by withdrawal of fentanyl and replacement with short-acting opioids.

This may be an interaction to which only some individuals are susceptible.

Flucytosine

The activity of itraconazole against black fungi can be augmented by combining it with flucytosine; the combination has prevented the development of flucytosine resistance (89).

Glucocorticoids

Itraconazole can inhibit the metabolic clearance of glucocorticoids by interfering with CYP3A4 and can directly inhibit steroidogenesis, thereby causing serious adverse effects. The effects on different glucocorticoids differ.

Budesonide

Two patients with cystic fibrosis developed profound adrenal failure and impairment of inhaled steroid clearance, resulting in paradoxical Cushing's syndrome, after long-term treatment with itraconazole and inhaled budenoside (90,91). Pituitary–adrenal axis and gonadal function was then assessed in 37 patients treated with itraconazole with or without budesonide (92). An adrenocorticotropic hormone (ACTH) test (tetracosactide 250 micrograms) was performed in 25 patients with cystic fibrosis taking itraconazole and budesonide and in 12 patients taking itraconazole alone (6 with cystic fibrosis and 6 with chronic granulomatous disease). Mineralocorticoid and gonadal steroid function were evaluated by measurements of plasma renin activity and follicle-stimulating hormone, luteinizing hormone, progesterone, estradiol, testosterone, and serum inhibin A and B concentrations. ACTH tests performed as part of a pretransplantation program in a further 30 patients with cystic fibrosis were used as controls. Eleven of the twenty-five patients who took both itraconazole and budesonide had adrenal insufficiency. None of the patients taking itraconazole alone and none of the control patients with cystic fibrosis had an abnormal ACTH test. Mineralocorticoid or gonadal insufficiency was not observed in any patient. Only one patient with an initial pathological ACTH test subsequently normalized; the other 10 patients improved but had not achieved normal adrenal function 2–10 months after itraconazole had been withdrawn.

The effects of itraconazole on the pharmacokinetics and cortisol-suppressing activity of budesonide by inhalation were further investigated in a randomized, double-blind, two-phase, crossover study in 10 healthy subjects who took oral itraconazole 200 mg/day or placebo for 5 days (93). On day 5, 1 hour after the last dose of itraconazole or placebo, they took budesonide 1000 micrograms by inhalation. Plasma budesonide and cortisol concentrations were measured up to 23 hours. Itraconazole increased the mean total AUC of inhaled budesonide 4.2-fold (range 1.7–9.8) and the peak plasma concentration 1.6-fold compared with placebo. The mean half-life of budesonide was prolonged from 1.6 to 6.2 hours. The suppression of cortisol production after inhalation of budesonide was significantly increased by itraconazole compared with placebo, with a 43% reduction in the AUC of plasma cortisol from 0.5 to 10 hours and a 12% reduction in the cortisol concentration measured 23 hours after budesonide, at 8 a.m. Thus, itraconazole markedly increased the systemic exposure to inhaled budesonide. This interaction resulted in enhanced systemic effects of budesonide, as shown by suppression of cortisol production.

Dexamethasone

Itraconazole markedly increases both systemic exposure to dexamethasone and its effects. This interaction has been investigated in a randomized, double-blind, placebo-controlled, crossover study (94). Eight healthy volunteers took either oral itraconazole 200 mg od or placebo for 4 days. On day 4, each subject was given oral dexamethasone 4.5 mg or intravenous dexamethasone sodium phosphate 5.0 mg. Itraconazole reduced the systemic clearance of intravenous dexamethasone by 68%, and increased its AUC and prolonged its half-life more than three-fold; the AUC of oral dexamethasone was increased nearly four-fold and its half-life nearly three-fold. Morning plasma cortisol concentrations at 47 and 71 hours after dexamethasone were significantly lower after itraconazole than placebo.

Methylprednisolone

The interaction of itraconazole with oral methylprednisolone has been examined in a randomized, double-blind, crossover study in 10 healthy volunteers taking either oral itraconazole 200 mg/day or placebo for 4 days (95). On day 4 each subject took methylprednisolone 16 mg. Itraconazole increased the total AUC of methylprednisolone 3.9-fold compared with placebo, the peak plasma methylprednisolone concentration 1.9-fold, and the half-life 2.4-fold. This effect was probably through inhibition of CYP3A4.

Similar effects were found in a study of the effects of itraconazole on the kinetics of intravenous methylprednisolone in a double-blind, randomized, crossover study in nine healthy volunteers (96). Itraconazole (200 mg for 4 days) increased the AUC of methylprednisolone (16 mg on day 4) 2.6-fold, and the AUC_{12-24} 12-fold. The systemic clearance of methylprednisolone was reduced to 40% by itraconazole and the half-life was increased from 2.1 to 4.8 hours. The mean morning plasma cortisol concentration was only 9% of that during the placebo phase. Thus, concomitant itraconazole greatly increased exposure to methylprednisolone during the night-time and led to enhanced adrenal suppression.

The effects of oral itraconazole (400 mg on the first day, then 200 mg/day for 3 days) on the pharmacokinetics of a single oral dose of methylprednisolone 48 mg have been studied in 14 healthy men in a two-period, crossover study (97). Plasma cortisol concentrations were determined as a pharmacodynamic index. Itraconazole significantly increased the mean AUC of methylprednisolone from 2773 to 7011 hours.ng/ml and the half-life from 3.2 to 5.5 hours. Cortisol concentrations at 24 hours were significantly lower after the administration of methylprednisolone with itraconazole than after methylprednisolone alone (24 versus 109 ng/ml).

Prednisolone

The effects of oral itraconazole (400 mg on the first day then 200 mg/day for 3 days) on the pharmacokinetics of a single oral dose of prednisolone 60 mg or methylprednisolone 48 mg have been studied in 14 healthy men in a two-period, crossover study (97). Plasma cortisol concentrations were determined as a pharmacodynamic index. The disposition of prednisolone was unchanged.

The effects of itraconazole on the pharmacokinetics and pharmacodynamics of oral prednisolone have been investigated in a double-blind, randomized, crossover study (98). Ten healthy subjects took either oral itraconazole 200 mg od or placebo for 4 days. On day 4 they took oral prednisolone 20 mg. Itraconazole increased the plasma AUC of prednisolone by 24% and its half-life by 29% compared with placebo. The peak plasma concentration and time to the peak of prednisolone were not affected. Itraconazole reduced the mean morning plasma cortisol concentration, measured 23 hours after prednisolone, by 27%.

The minor interaction of itraconazole with oral prednisolone is probably of limited clinical significance. The susceptibility of prednisolone to interact with CYP3A4 inhibitors is considerably smaller than that of methylprednisolone, and itraconazole and probably also other inhibitors of CYP3A4 can be used concomitantly with prednisolone without marked interaction.

Grapefruit juice

The effect of grapefruit juice on the systemic availability of itraconazole capsules has been investigated in a randomized, two-way, crossover design in 11 healthy volunteers (99). Grapefruit juice reduced the mean itraconazole AUC_{0-48} by 43% and the mean hydroxyitraconazole AUC_{0-72} by 47%. Grapefruit juice also significantly delayed the mean itraconazole t_{max} from 4 to 5.5 hours. The mechanisms for the impaired absorption of itraconazole in the presence of grapefruit juice remain to be elucidated; however, grapefruit juice is acidic and an inhibitor of CYP3A4.

Unexpectedly, in another study, grapefruit juice did not affect the pharmacokinetics of itraconazole in 22 healthy men while orange juice reduced the C_{max}, t_{max}, and AUC (100).

Haloperidol

The effects of itraconazole 200 mg/day for 7 days on the steady-state plasma concentrations of haloperidol and its reduced metabolite have been investigated in schizophrenic patients receiving haloperidol 12 or 24 mg/day (101). Itraconazole significantly increased trough plasma concentrations of both haloperidol and reduced haloperidol (17 versus 13 ng/ml and 6.1 versus 4.9 ng/ml respectively). There was no change in clinical symptoms, but neurological adverse effects of haloperidol were significantly increased during itraconazole co-administration. Similar findings in a similar study were reported for bromperidol and its reduced metabolite, although there were no differences in clinical symptoms or neurological adverse effects during concomitant itraconazole therapy (102).

Omeprazole

In 11 healthy volunteers, omeprazole 40 mg reduced the systemic availability of itraconazole 200 mg; these two drugs should therefore not be used together (103).

Oral contraceptives

Itraconazole can delay withdrawal bleeding in women using oral contraceptives (104). An analysis using data from a spontaneous adverse drug reaction reporting system in the Netherlands and logistic regression analysis showed an odds ratio of 85 (CI = 32, 230) for delayed withdrawal bleeding in women who used both drugs concomitantly compared with woman who used neither oral contraceptives nor itraconazole. Nine of the ten reports of delayed withdrawal bleeding concerned oral contraceptives containing desogestrel. In an open, crossover study in 10 young healthy subjects, fluconazole 150 mg increased the serum concentrations of ethinylestradiol at a close of 30–35 micrograms/day (105).

Phenytoin

Low and sometimes very low serum concentrations of itraconazole have been seen during concurrent therapy of itraconazole with phenytoin (68). At the same time, phenytoin concentrations may themselves be lowered when it is used with itraconazole (68).

Quinidine

In vitro studies have suggested that the oxidation of quinidine to 3-hydroxyquinidine is a specific marker reaction for CYP3A4 activity. In six healthy young men the pharmacokinetics of a single oral dose of quinidine 200 mg were studied before and during daily administration of itraconazole 100 mg (106). Itraconazole reduced quinidine total clearance, partial clearance by 3-hydroxylation, and partial clearance by *N*-oxidation by 61, 84, and 73% respectively.

Rifamycins

Rifampicin 600 mg/day for 14 days had a very strong inducing effect on the metabolism of a single dose of itraconazole 200 mg, indicating that these two drugs should not be used concomitantly (107).

Ropivacaine

The effects of clarithromycin (250 mg bd) and itraconazole (200 mg od) for 4 days on the pharmacokinetics of ropivacaine (given intravenously as a single dose of 0.6 mg/kg on day 4) have been studied in a double-blind, three-way, crossover study in eight healthy volunteers (108). There were no significant changes in the pharmacokinetics of ropivacaine after clarithromycin or itraconazole. Although clarithromycin and itraconazole inhibited formation of the (*S*)-2′,6′-pipelodoxylidide metabolite of ropivacaine, there were no significant changes in the pharmacokinetics of ropivacaine itself.

Saquinavir

The HIV protease inhibitor saquinavir has limited and variable oral systemic availability and ritonavir, an inhibitor of CYP450 and P glycoprotein, is widely used to increase its systemic exposure. A small pilot study in three HIV-infected patients has suggested that oral itraconazole can have similar effects on the oral availability of saquinavir (109). Concomitant use of itraconazole 200 mg/day with a combination of saquinavir and two nucleoside reverse transcriptase inhibitors led to a 2.5- to 6.9-fold increase in the AUC of saquinavir, a 2.0- to 5.4-fold increase in peak plasma concentrations, and a 1.6- to 17-fold increase in trough plasma concentrations. The effect of itraconazole on saquinavir was comparable to that of ritonavir.

Selegiline

The effects of itraconazole (200 mg/day for 4 days) on the pharmacokinetics of selegiline (10 mg on day 4) have been investigated in a randomized, placebo-controlled, crossover study (110). Itraconazole did not alter the pharmacokinetics of selegiline and its primary metabolites, desmethylselegiline and 1-metamfetamine. In human liver microsomes, itraconazole did not inhibit the formation of either metabolite. These findings suggest that selegiline is not susceptible to interactions with CYP3A4 inhibitors.

Statins

Itraconazole increases the risk of skeletal muscle toxicity of some statins by increasing their serum concentrations, but not all statins are equally affected. Concomitant use of atorvastatin, lovastatin, and simvastatin with itraconazole should be avoided or the doses should be reduced; fluvastatin and pravastatin have much less potential than other statins for clinically significant interactions with itraconazole and other CYP3A4 inhibitors; the effects of cerivastatin are intermediate.

In a randomized, open, three-way, crossover study, 18 healthy subjects took single doses of cerivastatin 0.8 mg, atorvastatin 20 mg, or pravastatin 40 mg without or with itraconazole 200 mg (111). Concomitant cerivastatin + itraconazole and pravastatin + itraconazole produced small increases in AUC, C_{max}, and half-life (up to 51%, 25%, and 23% respectively). However, itraconazole markedly increased atorvastatin AUC (150%), C_{max} (38%), and half-life (30%). Thus, itraconazole markedly increases systemic exposure to atorvastatin, but results in only modest increases in the plasma concentrations of cerivastatin and pravastatin.

Atorvastatin

Itraconazole increases serum concentrations of atorvastatin by inhibiting CYP3A4. In a randomized, double-blind, crossover study in 10 healthy volunteers, itraconazole 200 mg increased the AUC and half-life of atorvastatin 40 mg about three-fold, with a change in C_{max} (112). The AUC of atorvastatin lactone was increased about 4-fold, and the C_{max} and half-life were increased more than 2-fold. Itraconazole significantly reduced the C_{max} and AUC of 2-hydroxyatorvastatin acid and 2-hydroxyatorvastatin lactone and increased the half-life of 2-hydroxyatorvastatin lactone. The concomitant use of itraconazole and other potent inhibitors of CYP3A4 with atorvastatin should therefore be avoided, or the dose of atorvastatin should be reduced accordingly.

Cerivastatin

Cerivastatin uses a secondary CYP2C8-mediated metabolic pathway, which is unaffected by itraconazole (113). The effects of itraconazole on the pharmacokinetics of cerivastatin and its major metabolites have been investigated in a randomized, double-blind, crossover study (114). Inhibition of the CYP3A4-mediated M-1 pathway led to raised serum concentrations of cerivastatin, cerivastatin lactone, and metabolite M-23, resulting in increased concentrations of active HMG-CoA reductase inhibitors. However, the effect was modest.

Fluvastatin

The effects of itraconazole 100 mg on the pharmacokinetics of fluvastatin 40 mg have been studied in a randomized, placebo-controlled, crossover study in 10 healthy volunteers (115). Itraconazole had no significant effect on the C_{max} or total AUC of fluvastatin, but slightly prolonged its half-life.

Lovastatin

The effects of itraconazole 100 mg on the pharmacokinetics of lovastatin 40 mg have been studied in a randomized, placebo-controlled, crossover study in 10 healthy volunteers (115). Itraconazole, even in this low dosage, greatly increased plasma concentrations of lovastatin and its active metabolite, lovastatin acid, and increased the C_{max} of lovastatin about 15-fold and the total AUC by more than 15-fold; similarly, the C_{max} and total AUC of lovastatin acid were increased about 12-fold and 15-fold respectively.

Pravastatin

The effects of itraconazole 200 mg on the pharmacokinetics of pravastatin have been studied in a randomized, double-blind, crossover study in 10 healthy volunteers (116). Itraconazole slightly increased the AUC and C_{max} of pravastatin, but the changes were not statistically significant; the half-life was not altered.

Simvastatin

The effects of itraconazole 200 mg on the pharmacokinetics of simvastatin have been studied in a randomized, double-blind, crossover study in 10 healthy volunteers (116). Itraconazole increased the C_{max} and AUC of simvastatin and simvastatin acid at least 10-fold. The C_{max} and AUC of total simvastatin acid (naive simvastatin acid plus that derived by hydrolysis of the lactone) were increased 17-fold and 19-fold respectively, and the half-life was increased by 25%.

In two cases, rhabdomyolysis was caused by itraconazole in heart transplant recipients taking long-term ciclosporin and simvastatin (74,75). To avoid severe myopathy, ciclosporin concentrations should be monitored frequently and statins should be withdrawn or the dosage should be reduced, as long as azoles need to be prescribed in transplant recipients. Patients need to be educated about signs and symptoms that require immediate physician intervention.

Tacrolimus

Tacrolimus concentrations and toxicity are affected by itraconazole (117).

- In a 17-year-old man with cystic fibrosis who received a hepato-pulmonary transplant, there was an interaction of itraconazole 600 mg bd with tacrolimus (118). High trough concentrations of tacrolimus were noted, despite the relatively low dosage (0.1–0.3 mg/kg/day).
- Another patient experienced an interaction of tacrolimus 0.085 mg /kg bd with itraconazole 200–400 mg per day, with resulting ketoacidosis, neutropenia, and thrombocytopenia, requiring the withdrawal of both drugs (119).
- A 30-year-old man with a renal transplant had a more than two-fold increase in blood tacrolimus concentrations after starting to take itraconazole 200 mg/day, accompanied by a reduced glomerular filtration rate and biopsy-proven tacrolimus-associated tubulopathy (120).

Because of the narrow therapeutic index of tacrolimus, blood concentrations should be monitored particularly carefully when itraconazole is co-administered, and the dosage of tacrolimus may have to be altered (121).

The interaction of itraconazole (100 mg bd) with tacrolimus has been studied in 28 heart or lung transplant recipients (122). Tacrolimus blood concentrations were monitored on alternate days for up to 21 days after the start of itraconazole therapy ($n = 18$) or withdrawal ($n = 10$). The dose of tacrolimus was adjusted with the aim of keeping the 12-hour trough blood concentration at 7–12 micrograms/ml. The mean dose of tacrolimus during itraconazole therapy fell significantly from 8.4 to 2.9 mg/day. There was no significant change in serum creatinine or liver function tests. In patients in whom itraconazole was withdrawn, the mean dose of tacrolimus required increased significantly from 4.7 to 8.8 mg/day. Thus, substantial changes in the dose of tacrolimus were required both when itraconazole was begun and when it was withdrawn, and it was difficult to maintain tacrolimus blood concentrations within the target range during the first 2 weeks. However, major toxicity or rejection did not occur. Co-administration of itraconazole may reduce the cost of post-transplant immunosuppression. This interaction is probably due to inhibition of CYP3A4 by itraconazole.

Vinca alkaloids

Enhanced and potentially life-threatening neurotoxicity of vinca alkaloids through concomitant therapy with itraconazole has been the subject of several compelling reports (123–126). Enhancement of vincristine neurotoxicity results in polyneuropathy and paralytic ileus (80,127,128). The interaction is reversible, and readministration of vinca alkaloids may be safe after a prolonged washout (123). The mechanism has not been formally elucidated, but may be either competition for oxidative metabolism, leading to increased systemic exposure (129), or inhibition of the transmembrane P glycoprotein efflux pump (130), leading to increased intracellular concentrations of vinca alkaloids (130). The concomitant use of itraconazole and vinca alkaloids is therefore contraindicated.

Two adults with acute lymphoblastic leukemia developed unusually severe neurotoxicity caused by vincristine, which was probably the result of an interaction with itraconazole suspension (127).

Warfarin

Itraconazole can alter warfarin concentrations.

- Following the addition of itraconazole to a treatment regimen comprising warfarin, ranitidine, and terfenadine, cardiac dysrhythmias developed in a 62-year-old man. The signs and symptoms included prolongation of the QT interval and ventricular fibrillation (SEDA-18, 198).

This particular regimen apparently resulted in a second interaction, since unexpectedly very high concentrations of terfenadine were found (SEDA-18, 283). The phenomenon has been described by others, with a marked rise in terfenadine serum concentrations, and increased toxicity of the drug during concurrent ingestion of itraconazole. The mechanism is not known, but it is likely to be related to inhibition of CYP3A4 (62).

Zolpidem

Zolpidem is mainly transformed by CYP3A4. However, itraconazole 200 mg did not alter the pharmacokinetics and pharmacodynamics of zolpidem 10 mg in 10 healthy volunteers (131). Therefore, zolpidem may be used in normal or nearly normal doses together with itraconazole.

References

1. Barone JA, Moskovitz BL, Guarnieri J, Hassell AE, Colaizzi JL, Bierman RH, Jessen L. Enhanced bioavailability of itraconazole in hydroxypropyl-beta-cyclodextrin solution versus capsules in healthy volunteers. Antimicrob Agents Chemother 1998;42(7):1862–5.
2. Lyman CA, Walsh TJ. Systemically administered antifungal agents. A review of their clinical pharmacology and therapeutic applications. Drugs 1992;44(1):9–35.
3. Schafer-Korting M. Pharmacokinetic optimisation of oral antifungal therapy. Clin Pharmacokinet 1993;25(4):329–41.
4. Francis P, Walsh TJ. Evolving role of flucytosine in immunocompromised patients: new insights into safety, pharmacokinetics, and antifungal therapy. Clin Infect Dis 1992;15(6):1003–18.
5. Haria M, Bryson HM, Goa KL. Itraconazole. A reappraisal of its pharmacological properties and therapeutic use in the management of superficial fungal infections. Drugs 1996;51(4):585–620. Erratum in: Drugs 1996;52(2):253.

6. Dupont B, Drouhet E. Early experience with itraconazole in vitro and in patients: pharmacokinetic studies and clinical results. Rev Infect Dis 1987;9(Suppl 1):S71–6.
7. Caillot D, Bassaris H, McGeer A, Arthur C, Prentice HG, Seifert W, De Beule K. Intravenous itraconazole followed by oral itraconazole in the treatment of invasive pulmonary aspergillosis in patients with hematologic malignancies, chronic granulomatous disease, or AIDS. Clin Infect Dis 2001;33(8):e83–90.
8. Boogaerts MA, Maertens J, Van Der Geest R, Bosly A, Michaux JM, Van Hoof A, Cleeren M, Wostenborghs R, De Beule K. Pharmacokinetics and safety of a 7-day administration of intravenous itraconazole followed by a 14-day administration of itraconazole oral solution in patients with hematologic malignancy. Antimicrob Agents Chemother 2001;45(3):981–5.
9. Haneke E, Abeck D, Ring J. Safety and efficacy of intermittent therapy with itraconazole in finger- and toenail onychomycosis: a multicentre trial. Mycoses 1998;41(11–12):521–7.
10. Boonk W, de Geer D, de Kreek E, Remme J, van Huystee B. Itraconazole in the treatment of tinea corporis and tinea cruris: comparison of two treatment schedules. Mycoses 1998;41(11–12):509–14.
11. Schuller J, Remme JJ, Rampen FH, Van Neer FC. Itraconazole in the treatment of tinea pedis and tinea manuum: comparison of two treatment schedules. Mycoses 1998;41(11–12):515–20.
12. Boogaerts M, Maertens J, van Hoof A, de Bock R, Fillet G, Peetermans M, Selleslag D, Vandercam B, Vandewoude K, Zachee P, De Beule K. Itraconazole versus amphotericin B plus nystatin in the prophylaxis of fungal infections in neutropenic cancer patients. J Antimicrob Chemother 2001;48(1):97–103.
13. Boogaerts M, Winston DJ, Bow EJ, Garber G, Reboli AC, Schwarer AP, Novitzky N, Boehme A, Chwetzoff E, De Beule K. Itraconazole Neutropenia Study Group. Intravenous and oral itraconazole versus intravenous amphotericin B deoxycholate as empirical antifungal therapy for persistent fever in neutropenic patients with cancer who are receiving broad-spectrum antibacterial therapy. A randomized, controlled trial. Ann Intern Med 2001;135(6):412–22.
14. Harousseau JL, Dekker AW, Stamatoullas-Bastard A, Fassas A, Linkesch W, Gouveia J, De Bock R, Rovira M, Seifert WF, Joosen H, Peeters M, De Beule K. Itraconazole oral solution for primary prophylaxis of fungal infections in patients with hematological malignancy and profound neutropenia: a randomized, double-blind, double-placebo, multicenter trial comparing itraconazole and amphotericin B. Antimicrob Agents Chemother 2000;44(7):1887–93.
15. Nolting SK, Gupta A, Doncker PD, Jacko ML, Moskovitz BL. Continuous itraconazole treatment for onychomycosis and dermatomycosis: an overview of safety. Eur J Dermatol 1999;9(7):540–3.
16. Galgiani JN, Catanzaro A, Cloud GA, Johnson RH, Williams PL, Mirels LF, Nassar F, Lutz JE, Stevens DA, Sharkey PK, Singh VR, Larsen RA, Delgado KL, Flanigan C, Rinaldi MG. Comparison of oral fluconazole and itraconazole for progressive, non-meningeal coccidioidomycosis. A randomized, double-blind trial. Mycoses Study Group. Ann Intern Med 2000;133(9):676–86.
17. Phillips P, De Beule K, Frechette G, Tchamouroff S, Vandercam B, Weitner L, Hoepelman A, Stingl G, Clotet B. A double-blind comparison of itraconazole oral solution and fluconazole capsules for the treatment of oropharyngeal candidiasis in patients with AIDS. Clin Infect Dis 1998;26(6):1368–73.
18. Graybill JR, Vazquez J, Darouiche RO, Morhart R, Greenspan D, Tuazon C, Wheat LJ, Carey J, Leviton I, Hewitt RG, MacGregor RR, Valenti W, Restrepo M, Moskovitz BL. Randomized trial of itraconazole oral solution for oropharyngeal candidiasis in HIV/AIDS patients. Am J Med 1998;104(1):33–9.
19. Winston DJ, Busuttil RW. Randomized controlled trial of oral itraconazole solution versus intravenous/oral fluconazole for prevention of fungal infections in liver transplant recipients. Transplantation 2002;74(5):688–95.
20. Jahangir M, Hussain I, Ul Hasan M, Haroon TS. A double-blind, randomized, comparative trial of itraconazole versus terbinafine for 2 weeks in tinea capitis. Br J Dermatol 1998;139(4):672–4.
21. Svejgaard E, Avnstorp C, Wanscher B, Nilsson J, Heremans A. Efficacy and safety of short-term itraconazole in tinea pedis: a double-blind, randomized, placebo-controlled trial. Dermatology 1998;197(4):368–72.
22. Heykants J, Van Peer A, Van de Velde V, Van Rooy P, Meuldermans W, Lavrijsen K, Woestenborghs R, Van Cutsem J, Cauwenbergh G. The clinical pharmacokinetics of itraconazole: an overview. Mycoses 1989;32(Suppl 1):67–87.
23. Tucker RM, Haq Y, Denning DW, Stevens DA. Adverse events associated with itraconazole in 189 patients on chronic therapy. J Antimicrob Chemother 1990; 26(4):561–6.
24. Bradbury BD, Jick SS. Itraconazole and fluconazole and certain rare, serious adverse events. Pharmacotherapy 2002;22(6):697–700.
25. Nelson MR, Smith D, Erskine D, Gazzard BG. Ventricular fibrillation secondary to itraconazole induced hypokalaemia. J Infect 1993;26(3):348.
26. Ahmad SR, Singer SJ, Leissa BG. Congestive heart failure associated with itraconazole. Lancet 2001;357(9270):1766–7.
27. Odom RB, Aly R, Scher RK, Daniel CR 3rd, Elewski BE, Zaias N, DeVillez R, Jacko M, Oleka N, Moskovitz BL. A multicenter, placebo-controlled, double-blind study of intermittent therapy with itraconazole for the treatment of onychomycosis of the fingernail. J Am Acad Dermatol 1997;36(2 Pt 1):231–5.
28. Cleveland KO, Campbell JW. Hallucinations associated with itraconazole therapy. Clin Infect Dis 1995;21(2):456.
29. Sharkey PK, Rinaldi MG, Dunn JF, Hardin TC, Fetchick RJ, Graybill JR. High-dose itraconazole in the treatment of severe mycoses. Antimicrob Agents Chemother 1991;35(4):707–13.
30. Nelson MR, Smith D, Erskine D, Gazzara BG. Ventricular fibrillation secondary to itraconazole induced hypobalaemia. J Infect 1993;26(3):348.
31. Dismukes WE, Bradsher RW Jr, Cloud GC, Kauffman CA, Chapman SW, George RB, Stevens DA, Girard WM, Saag MS, Bowles-Patton C. Itraconazole therapy for blastomycosis and histoplasmosis. NIAID Mycoses Study Group. Am J Med 1992;93(5):489–97.
32. Cauwenbergh G, De Doncker P, Stoops K, De Dier AM, Goyvaerts H, Schuermans V. Itraconazole in the treatment of human mycoses: review of three years of clinical experience. Rev Infect Dis 1987;9(Suppl 1):S146–52.
33. Gryn J, Goldberg J, Johnson E, Siegel J, Inzerillo J. The toxicity of daily inhaled amphotericin B. Am J Clin Oncol 1993;16(1):43–6.
34. Barbaro G, Barbarini G, Calderon W, Grisorio B, Alcini P, Di Lorenzo G. Fluconazole versus itraconazole for *Candida* esophagitis in acquired immunodeficiency syndrome. *Candida* esophagitis. Gastroenterology 1996;111(5):1169–77.
35. Nguyen AJ, Nelson DB, Thurn JR. Pseudomembranous colitis after itraconazole therapy. Am J Gastroenterol 1999;94(7):1971–3.

36. Lavrijsen AP, Balmus KJ, Nugteren-Huying WM, Roldaan AC, van't Wout JW, Stricker BH. Hepatic injury associated with itraconazole. Lancet 1992;340(8813):251–2.
37. Wolf R, Wolf D, Kuperman S. Focal nodular hyperplasia of the liver after intraconazole treatment. J Clin Gastroenterol 2001;33(5):418–20.
38. Lavrijsen AP, Balmus KJ, Nugteren-Huying WM, Roldaan AC, van 't Wout JW, Stricker BH. Lever be schadiging tijdens gebruik van itraconazo (Trisporal). [Liver damage during administration of itraconazole (Trisporal).] Ned Tijdschr Geneeskd 1993;137(1):38–41.
39. Gupta AK, Chwetzoff E, Del Rosso J, Baran R. Hepatic safety of itraconazole. J Cutan Med Surg 2002;6(3):210–13.
40. Ganer A, Arathoon E, Stevens DA. Initial experience in therapy for progressive mycoses with itraconazole, the first clinically studied triazole. Rev Infect Dis 1987;9(Suppl 1):S77–86.
41. Marco F, Pfaller MA, Messer SA, Jones RN. Antifungal activity of a new triazole, voriconazole (UK-109,496), compared with three other antifungal agents tested against clinical isolates of filamentous fungi. Med Mycol 1998;36(6):433–6.
42. Kramer KE, Yaar M, Andersen W. Purpuric drug eruption secondary to itraconazole. J Am Acad Dermatol 1997;37(6):994–5.
43. Park YM, Kim JW, Kim CW. Acute generalized exanthematous pustulosis induced by itraconazole. J Am Acad Dermatol 1997;36(5 Pt 1):794–6.
44. Goto Y, Kono T, Teramae K, Ishii M. Itraconazole-induced drug eruption confirmed by challenge test. Acta Derm Venereol 2000;80(1):72.
45. Alvarez-Fernandez JG, Castano-Suarez E, Cornejo-Navarro P, de la Fuente EG, Ortiz de Frutos FJ, Iglesias-Diez L. Photosensitivity induced by oral itraconazole. J Eur Acad Dermatol Venereol 2000;14(6):501–3.
46. Castellsague J, Garcia-Rodriguez LA, Duque A, Perez S. Risk of serious skin disorders among users of oral antifungals: a population-based study. BMC Dermatol 2002;2(1):14.
47. Denning DW, Van Wye JE, Lewiston NJ, Stevens DA. Adjunctive therapy of allergic bronchopulmonary aspergillosis with itraconazole. Chest 1991;100(3):813–19.
48. Park H, Knowles S, Shear NH. Serum sickness-like reaction to itraconazole. Ann Pharmacother 1998;32(11):1249.
49. Van Cauteren H, Heykants J, De Coster R, Cauwenbergh G. Itraconazole: pharmacologic studies in animals and humans. Rev Infect Dis 1987;9(Suppl 1):S43–6.
50. de Repentigny L, Ratelle J, Leclerc JM, Cornu G, Sokal EM, Jacqmin P, De Beule K. Repeated-dose pharmacokinetics of an oral solution of itraconazole in infants and children. Antimicrob Agents Chemother 1998;42(2):404–8.
51. Abdel-Rahman SM, Powell DA, Nahata MC. Efficacy of itraconazole in children with *Trichophyton tonsurans* tinea capitis. J Am Acad Dermatol 1998;38(3):443–6.
52. Groll AH, Wood L, Roden M, Mickiene D, Chiou CC, Townley E, Dad L, Piscitelli SC, Walsh TJ. Safety, pharmacokinetics, and pharmacodynamics of cyclodextrin itraconazole in pediatric patients with oropharyngeal candidiasis. Antimicrob Agents Chemother 2002;46(8):2554–63.
53. Foot AB, Veys PA, Gibson BE. Itraconazole oral solution as antifungal prophylaxis in children undergoing stem cell transplantation or intensive chemotherapy for haematological disorders. Bone Marrow Transplant 1999;24(10):1089–93.
54. Verspeelt J, Marynissen G, Gupta AK, De Doncker P. Safety of itraconazole in diabetic patients. Dermatology 1999;198(4):382–4.
55. Glasmacher A, Hahn C, Molitor E, Marklein G, Sauerbruch T, Schmidt-Wolf IG. Itraconazole through concentrations in antifungal prophylaxis with six different dosing regimens using hydroxypropyl-beta-cyclodextrin oral solution or coated-pellet capsules. Mycoses 1999;42(11–12):591–600.
56. Schaffner A, Bohler A. Amphotericin B refractory aspergillosis after itraconazole: evidence for significant antagonism. Mycoses 1993;36(11–12):421–4.
57. Persat F, Schwartzbrod PE, Troncy J, Timour Q, Maul A, Piens MA, Picot S. Abnormalities in liver enzymes during simultaneous therapy with itraconazole and amphotericin B in leukaemic patients. J Antimicrob Chemother 2000;45(6):928–9.
58. Groll AH, Piscitelli SC, Walsh TJ. Clinical pharmacology of systemic antifungal agents: a comprehensive review of agents in clinical use, current investigational compounds, and putative targets for antifungal drug development. Adv Pharmacol 1998;44:343–500.
59. Lefebvre RA, Van Peer A, Woestenborghs R. Influence of itraconazole on the pharmacokinetics and electrocardiographic effects of astemizole. Br J Clin Pharmacol 1997;43(3):319–22.
60. Honig PK, Wortham DC, Hull R, Zamani K, Smith JE, Cantilena LR. Itraconazole affects single-dose terfenadine pharmacokinetics and cardiac repolarization pharmacodynamics. J Clin Pharmacol 1993;33(12):1201–6.
61. de Wildt SN, van den Anker JN. Wegrakingen tijdens simultaan gebruik van terfenadine en itraconazol. [Syncopes with simultaneous use of terfenadine and itraconazole.] Ned Tijdschr Geneeskd 1997;141(36):1752–3.
62. Bickers DR. Antifungal therapy: potential interactions with other classes of drugs. J Am Acad Dermatol 1994;31(3 Pt 2):S87–90.
63. Otsuji Y, Okuyama N, Aoshima T, Fukasawa T, Kato K, Gerstenberg G, Miura M, Ohkubo T, Sugawara K, Otani K. No effect of itraconazole on the single oral dose pharmacokinetics and pharmacodynamics of estazolam. Ther Drug Monit 2002;24(3):375–8.
64. Backman JT, Kivisto KT, Olkkola KT, Neuvonen PJ. The area under the plasma concentration-time curve for oral midazolam is 400-fold larger during treatment with itraconazole than with rifampicin. Eur J Clin Pharmacol 1998;54(1):53–8.
65. Palkama VJ, Neuvonen PJ, Olkkola KT. Effect of itraconazole on the pharmacokinetics of bupivacaine enantiomers in healthy volunteers. Br J Anaesth 1999;83(4):659–61.
66. Kivisto KT, Lamberg TS, Neuvonen PJ. Interactions of buspirone with itraconazole and rifampicin: effects on the pharmacokinetics of the active 1-(2-pyrimidinyl)-piperazine metabolite of buspirone. Pharmacol Toxicol 1999;84(2):94–7.
67. Buggia I, Zecca M, Alessandrino EP, Locatelli F, Rosti G, Bosi A, Pession A, Rotoli B, Majolino I, Dallorso A, Regazzi MB. Itraconazole can increase systemic exposure to busulfan in patients given bone marrow transplantation. GITMO (Gruppo Italiano Trapianto di Midollo Osseo). Anticancer Res 1996;16(4A):2083–8.
68. Tucker RM, Denning DW, Hanson LH, Rinaldi MG, Graybill JR, Sharkey PK, Pappagianis D, Stevens DA. Interaction of azoles with rifampin, phenytoin, and carbamazepine: in vitro and clinical observations. Clin Infect Dis 1992;14(1):165–74.
69. Kwan JT, Foxall PJ, Davidson DG, Bending MR, Eisinger AJ. Interaction of cyclosporin and itraconazole. Lancet 1987;2(8553):282.
70. Kramer MR, Marshall SE, Denning DW, Keogh AM, Tucker RM, Galgiani JN, Lewiston NJ, Stevens DA,

Theodore J. Cyclosporine and itraconazole interaction in heart and lung transplant recipients. Ann Intern Med 1990;113(4):327–9.
71. Kwan JT, Foxall PJ, Davidson DG, Bending MR, Eisinger AJ. Interaction of cyclosporin and itraconazole. Lancet 1987;2(8553):282.
72. Trenk D, Brett W, Jahnchen E, Bixnbaum D. Time course of cyclosporin/itraconazole interaction. Lancet 1987;2(8571):1335–6.
73. Navakova I, Donnelly P, de Witte T, de Pauw B, Boezeman J, Veltman G. Itraconazole and cyclosporin nephrotoxicity. Lancet 1987;2(8564):920–1.
74. Vlahakos DV, Manginas A, Chilidou D, Zamanika C, Alivizatos PA. Itraconazole-induced rhabdomyolysis and acute renal failure in a heart transplant recipient treated with simvastatin and cyclosporine. Transplantation 2002;73(12):1962–4.
75. Maxa JL, Melton LB, Ogu CC, Sills MN, Limanni A. Rhabdomyolysis after concomitant use of cyclosporine, simvastatin, gemfibrozil, and itraconazole. Ann Pharmacother 2002;36(5):820–3.
76. May DB, Drew RH, Yedinak KC, Bartlett JA. Effect of simultaneous didanosine administration on itraconazole absorption in healthy volunteers. Pharmacotherapy 1994;14(5):509–13.
77. Auclair B, Berning SE, Huitt GA, Peloquin CA. Potential interaction between itraconazole and clarithromycin. Pharmacotherapy 1999;19(12):1439–44.
78. Raaska K, Neuvonen PJ. Serum concentrations of clozapine and N-desmethylclozapine are unaffected by the potent CYP3A4 inhibitor itraconazole. Eur J Clin Pharmacol 1998;54(2):167–70.
79. Sachs MK, Blanchard LM, Green PJ. Interaction of itraconazole and digoxin. Clin Infect Dis 1993;16(3):400–3.
80. Woodland C, Ito S, Koren G. A model for the prediction of digoxin–drug interactions at the renal tubular cell level. Ther Drug Monit 1998;20(2):134–8.
81. Koren G, Woodland C, Ito S. Toxic digoxin–drug interactions: the major role of renal P-glycoprotein. Vet Hum Toxicol 1998;40(1):45–6.
82. Meyboom RH, de Jonge K, Veentjer H, Dekens-Konter JA, de Koning GH. Potentiering van digoxine door itraconazol. [Potentiation of digoxin by itraconazole.] Ned Tijdschr Geneeskd 1994;138(47):2353–6.
83. Jalava KM, Partanen J, Neuvonen PJ. Itraconazole decreases renal clearance of digoxin. Ther Drug Monit 1997;19(6):609–13.
84. Nishihara K, Hibino J, Kotaki H, Sawada Y, Iga T. Effect of itraconazole on the pharmacokinetics of digoxin in guinea pigs. Biopharm Drug Dispos 1999;20(3):145–9.
85. Mathis AS, Friedman GS. Coadministration of digoxin with itraconazole in renal transplant recipients. Am J Kidney Dis 2001;37(2):E18.
86. Kanda Y, Kami M, Matsuyama T, Mitani K, Chiba S, Yazaki Y, Hirai H. Plasma concentration of itraconazole in patients receiving chemotherapy for hematological malignancies: the effect of famotidine on the absorption of itraconazole. Hematol Oncol 1998;16(1):33–7.
87. Palkama VJ, Neuvonen PJ, Olkkola KT. The CYP 3A4 inhibitor itraconazole has no effect on the pharmacokinetics of i.v. fentanyl. Br J Anaesth 1998;81(4):598–600.
88. Mercadante S, Villari P, Ferrera P. Itraconazole–fentanyl interaction in a cancer patient. J Pain Symptom Manage 2002;24(3):284–6.
89. Viviani MA. Flucytosine—what is its future? J Antimicrob Chemother 1995;35(2):241–4.
90. Main KM, Skov M, Sillesen IB, Dige-Petersen H, Muller J, Koch C, Lanng S. Cushing's syndrome due to pharmacological interaction in a cystic fibrosis patient. Acta Paediatr 2002;91(9):1008–11.
91. Parmar JS, Howell T, Kelly J, Bilton D. Profound adrenal suppression secondary to treatment with low dose inhaled steroids and itraconazole in allergic bronchopulmonary aspergillosis in cystic fibrosis. Thorax 2002;57(8):749–50.
92. Skov M, Main KM, Sillesen IB, Muller J, Koch C, Lanng S. Iatrogenic adrenal insufficiency as a side-effect of combined treatment of itraconazole and budesonide. Eur Respir J 2002;20(1):127–33.
93. Raaska K, Niemi M, Neuvonen M, Neuvonen PJ, Kivisto KT. Plasma concentrations of inhaled budesonide and its effects on plasma cortisol are increased by the cytochrome P4503A4 inhibitor itraconazole. Clin Pharmacol Ther 2002;72(4):362–9.
94. Varis T, Kivisto KT, Backman JT, Neuvonen PJ. The cytochrome P450 3A4 inhibitor itraconazole markedly increases the plasma concentrations of dexamethasone and enhances its adrenal-suppressant effect. Clin Pharmacol Ther 2000;68(5):487–94.
95. Varis T, Kaukonen KM, Kivisto KT, Neuvonen PJ. Plasma concentrations and effects of oral methylprednisolone are considerably increased by itraconazole. Clin Pharmacol Ther 1998;64(4):363–8.
96. Varis T, Kivisto KT, Backman JT, Neuvonen PJ. Itraconazole decreases the clearance and enhances the effects of intravenously administered methylprednisolone in healthy volunteers. Pharmacol Toxicol 1999;85(1):29–32.
97. Lebrun-Vignes B, Archer VC, Diquet B, Levron JC, Chosidow O, Puech AJ, Warot D. Effect of itraconazole on the pharmacokinetics of prednisolone and methylprednisolone and cortisol secretion in healthy subjects. Br J Clin Pharmacol 2001;51(5):443–50.
98. Varis T, Kivisto KT, Neuvonen PJ. The effect of itraconazole on the pharmacokinetics and pharmacodynamics of oral prednisolone. Eur J Clin Pharmacol 2000;56(1):57–60.
99. Penzak SR, Gubbins PO, Gurley BJ, Wang PL, Saccente M. Grapefruit juice decreases the systemic availability of itraconazole capsules in healthy volunteers. Ther Drug Monit 1999;21(3):304–9.
100. Kawakami M, Suzuki K, Ishizuka T, Hidaka T, Matsuki Y, Nakamura H. Effect of grapefruit juice on pharmacokinetics of itraconazole in healthy subjects. Int J Clin Pharmacol Ther 1998;36(6):306–8.
101. Yasui N, Kondo T, Otani K, Furukori H, Mihara K, Suzuki A, Kaneko S, Inoue Y. Effects of itraconazole on the steady-state plasma concentrations of haloperidol and its reduced metabolite in schizophrenic patients: in vivo evidence of the involvement of CYP3A4 for haloperidol metabolism. J Clin Psychopharmacol 1999;19(2):149–54.
102. Furukori H, Kondo T, Yasui N, Otani K, Tokinaga N, Nagashima U, Kaneko S, Inoue Y. Effects of itraconazole on the steady-state plasma concentrations of bromperidol and reduced bromperidol in schizophrenic patients. Psychopharmacology (Berl) 1999;145(2):189–92.
103. Jaruratanasirikul S, Sriwiriyajan S. Effect of omeprazole on the pharmacokinetics of itraconazole. Eur J Clin Pharmacol 1998;54(2):159–61.
104. Van Puijenbroek EP, Egberts AC, Meyboom RH, Leufkens HG. Signalling possible drug–drug interactions in a spontaneous reporting system: delay of withdrawal bleeding during concomitant use of oral contraceptives and itraconazole. Br J Clin Pharmacol 1999;47(6):689–93.
105. Sinofsky FE, Pasquale SA. The effect of fluconazole on circulating ethinyl estradiol levels in women taking oral contraceptives. Am J Obstet Gynecol 1998;178(2):300–4.
106. Damkier P, Hansen LL, Brosen K. Effect of diclofenac, disulfiram, itraconazole, grapefruit juice and erythromycin

on the pharmacokinetics of quinidine. Br J Clin Pharmacol 1999;48(6):829–38.
107. Jaruratanasirikul S, Sriwiriyajan S. Effect of rifampicin on the pharmacokinetics of itraconazole in normal volunteers and AIDS patients. Eur J Clin Pharmacol 1998;54(2):155–8.
108. Jokinen MJ, Ahonen J, Neuvonen PJ, Olkkola KT. Effect of clarithromycin and itraconazole on the pharmacokinetics of ropivacaine. Pharmacol Toxicol 2001;88(4):187–91.
109. Koks CH, van Heeswijk RP, Veldkamp AI, Meenhorst PL, Mulder JW, van der Meer JT, Beijnen JH, Hoetelmans RM. Itraconazole as an alternative for ritonavir liquid formulation when combined with saquinavir. AIDS 2000;14(1):89–90.
110. Kivisto KT, Wang JS, Backman JT, Nyman L, Taavitsainen P, Anttila M, Neuvonen PJ. Selegiline pharmacokinetics are unaffected by the CYP3A4 inhibitor itraconazole. Eur J Clin Pharmacol 2001;57(1):37–42.
111. Mazzu AL, Lasseter KC, Shamblen EC, Agarwal V, Lettieri J, Sundaresen P. Itraconazole alters the pharmacokinetics of atorvastatin to a greater extent than either cerivastatin or pravastatin. Clin Pharmacol Ther 2000;68(4):391–400.
112. Kantola T, Kivisto KT, Neuvonen PJ. Effect of itraconazole on the pharmacokinetics of atorvastatin. Clin Pharmacol Ther 1998;64(1):58–65.
113. Gubbins PO, McConnell SA, Penzak SR. Antifungal Agents. In: Piscitelli SC, Rodvold KA, editors. Drug Interactions in Infectious Diseases. Totowa, NJ: Humana Press Inc, 2001:185–217.
114. Kantola T, Kivisto KT, Neuvonen PJ. Effect of itraconazole on cerivastatin pharmacokinetics. Eur J Clin Pharmacol 1999;54(11):851–5.
115. Kivisto KT, Kantola T, Neuvonen PJ. Different effects of itraconazole on the pharmacokinetics of fluvastatin and lovastatin. Br J Clin Pharmacol 1998;46(1):49–53.
116. Neuvonen PJ, Kantola T, Kivisto KT. Simvastatin but not pravastatin is very susceptible to interaction with the CYP3A4 inhibitor itraconazole. Clin Pharmacol Ther 1998;63(3):332–41.
117. Katari SR, Magnone M, Shapiro R, Jordan M, Scantlebury V, Vivas C, Gritsch A, McCauley J, Starzl T, Demetris AJ, Randhawa PS. Clinical features of acute reversible tacrolimus (FK 506) nephrotoxicity in kidney transplant recipients. Clin Transplant 1997;11(3):237–42.
118. Billaud EM, Guillemain R, Tacco F, Chevalier P. Evidence for a pharmacokinetic interaction between itraconazole and tacrolimus in organ transplant patients. Br J Clin Pharmacol 1998;46(3):271–2.
119. Furlan V, Parquin F, Penaud JF, Cerrina J, Ladurie FL, Dartevelle P, Taburet AM. Interaction between tacrolimus and itraconazole in a heart-lung transplant recipient. Transplant Proc 1998;30(1):187–8.
120. Ideura T, Muramatsu T, Higuchi M, Tachibana N, Hora K, Kiyosawa K. Tacrolimus/itraconazole interactions: a case report of ABO-incompatible living-related renal transplantation. Nephrol Dial Transplant 2000;15(10):1721–3.
121. Outeda Macias M, Salvador P, Hurtado JL, Martin I. Tacrolimus–itraconazole interaction in a kidney transplant patient. Ann Pharmacother 2000;34(4):536.
122. Banerjee R, Leaver N, Lyster H, Banner NR. Coadministration of itraconazole and tacrolimus after thoracic organ transplantation. Transplant Proc 2001;33(1–2):1600–2.
123. Jeng MR, Feusner J. Itraconazole-enhanced vincristine neurotoxicity in a child with acute lymphoblastic leukemia. Pediatr Hematol Oncol 2001;18(2):137–42.
124. Bosque E. Possible drug interaction between itraconazole and vinorelbine tartrate leading to death after one dose of chemotherapy. Ann Intern Med 2001;134(5):427.
125. Kamaluddin M, McNally P, Breatnach F, O'Marcaigh A, Webb D, O'Dell E, Scanlon P, Butler K, O'Meara A. Potentiation of vincristine toxicity by itraconazole in children with lymphoid malignancies. Acta Paediatr 2001;90(10):1204–7.
126. Sathiapalan RK, El-Solh H. Enhanced vincristine neurotoxicity from drug interactions: case report and review of literature. Pediatr Hematol Oncol 2001;18(8):543–6.
127. Gillies J, Hung KA, Fitzsimons E, Soutar R. Severe vincristine toxicity in combination with itraconazole. Clin Lab Haematol 1998;20(2):123–4.
128. Bohme A, Ganser A, Hoelzer D. Aggravation of vincristine-induced neurotoxicity by itraconazole in the treatment of adult ALL. Ann Hematol 1995;71(6):311–12.
129. Zhou-Pan XR, Seree E, Zhou XJ, Placidi M, Maurel P, Barra Y, Rahmani R. Involvement of human liver cytochrome P450 3A in vinblastine metabolism: drug interactions. Cancer Res 1993;53(21):5121–6.
130. Gupta S, Kim J, Gollapudi S. Reversal of daunorubicin resistance in P388/ADR cells by itraconazole. J Clin Invest 1991;87(4):1467–9.
131. Luurila H, Kivisto KT, Neuvonen PJ. Effect of itraconazole on the pharmacokinetics and pharmacodynamics of zolpidem. Eur J Clin Pharmacol 1998;54(2):163–6.

Ivermectin

General Information

Ivermectin, a dihydroavermectin B1, is an effective microfilaricide used in the treatment of strongyloides, scabies, and all types of filariasis except *Dipalonema (Mansonella) perstans* infections.

Over a number of years, ivermectin has shown excellent results in the treatment of onchocerciasis, both in controlled studies and in the field, including use in the WHO-sponsored program of treatment. This experience has provided a thorough picture of its adverse effects. The effective dosage is of the order of 50–200 micrograms/kg. After a single oral dose, skin microfilariae remain at low levels for up to 9 months.

As antihelminthic drugs go, ivermectin can be considered a reasonably safe drug, and it is generally better tolerated than diethylcarbamazine. Clinical experience has often shown relatively little toxicity, although mild adverse effects, presumably due to the killing of the microfilariae, involve at least one-third of patients; some work has suggested that neutrophil activation may play a role in the development of these reactions (1). It has also been well tolerated in combinations, for example when given with albendazole in order to kill adult worms (which cannot be achieved with ivermectin alone) or with diethylcarbamazine for bancroftian filariasis (SEDA-20, 281).

The principal reservation from the start was that ivermectin has a long half-life and that some late effects might occur in certain individuals. During the early phases it was recommended that in areas where the drug had been widely used the health workers involved should continue to observe patients for a time, in case problems did arise, but no late complications have in fact been documented.

Mode of action

The mode of action of ivermectin has been reviewed (2). It has tentatively been identified as agonism at GABA receptors, with inhibition of ion channels that control specific nerve cell connections. The functioning of chloride channels should thus be altered in most organisms, leading to paralysis and death of parasites. Several sites of action have been proposed:

- a postsynaptic agonist site either on the receptor or in its immediate neighborhood;
- a presynaptic site of activation of GABA release;
- potentiation of GABA binding to its receptor.

Another mechanism of action involves the binding of ivermectin to P glycoprotein.

Observational studies

Among the published studies some have specifically sought to define the pattern of adverse effects. In one such study (3), although a single dose of the drug was combined in some patients with diethylcarbamazine, the adverse effect pattern was similar to that when ivermectin was used alone (SEDA-18, 312). There now seem to be some circumstances in which a single low dose of ivermectin is sufficient to have a prolonged effect, for example in loaiasis a dose of 150 micrograms/kg resulted in a very much reduced level of microfilaria as much as a year later, and seemed to eliminate the infestation entirely in more than half the users (4,5). If further work confirms the validity of this approach, the adverse reactions problem may be lessened, since at these doses the few reactions experienced were limited to the skin and joints, although some calabar-like swellings were also noted.

Brugia malayi

In an open study from India 21 asymptomatic microfilaria carriers (with counts of 109–6934/ml of blood) were treated with a single oral dose of ivermectin 400 micrograms/kg and a single oral dose of diethylcarbamazine 6 mg/kg for infection with *Brugia malayi* (6). Twelve hours after treatment microfilaria counts fell by 96–100% in all patients and 12 patients had become afilaremic. All had an adverse reaction, lasting up to 48 hours after treatment: fever ($n = 20$), myalgia ($n = 19$), headache ($n = 17$), lethargy ($n = 15$), chills ($n = 13$), sweating ($n = 11$), anorexia ($n = 11$), sore throat and pharyngeal congestion ($n = 10$), arthralgia ($n = 6$), giddiness ($n = 4$), nausea and vomiting ($n = 3$), abdominal pain ($n = 2$), and cough ($n = 1$). Postural hypotension, lasting 1 day, was noted in two individuals. Transient dilated and painfully inflamed lymphatic channels, which stood out in cords, were seen in two individuals. Most adverse effects were mild and self-limiting.

Loa loa

The use of ivermectin and its adverse effects in patients infected with *Loa loa* have been reviewed (7). It was concluded that ivermectin in a single dose of 150–300 micrograms/kg is effective in reducing microfilaria counts by over 90% with suppressed counts to 25% of pretreatment values after 1 year. An even more sustained effect can be reached by more frequent dosing. There is also some evidence that ivermectin in higher doses (400 micrograms/kg twice yearly) can affect the adult *Loa loa*. Tolerance to ivermectin is generally excellent, but serious adverse effects, especially encephalopathy, can occur, principally in more heavily infected individuals.

Onchocerciasis

The impact of 5 years of annual community treatment with ivermectin on the prevalence of onchocerciasis and onchocerciasis-associated morbidity in the village of Gami (Central African Republic) has been assessed (8). Pruritus, onchocercal nodules, and impaired vision were all significantly reduced by annual treatment with ivermectin.

In a study of the effect of ivermectin on adult *Onchocerca* worms (9) the following regimens were compared:

- 150 micrograms/kg yearly (reference group; $n = 166$)
- 400 micrograms/kg then 800 micrograms/kg yearly ($n = 172$)
- 150 micrograms/kg 3-monthly ($n = 161$)
- 400 micrograms/kg then 800 micrograms/kg 3-monthly ($n = 158$)

After 3 years of treatment more female worms had died in those who were treated every 3 months than in the reference group; female worms were also less fertile. There was no difference between the two groups of patients who were treated yearly. There were no serious adverse events, even at high doses. However, subjective complaints of visual disturbances, such as blurred vision, ocular pain, or dyschromatopsia, were more frequent in those who were given 800 micrograms/kg than in those who were given 150 micrograms/kg; the effects lasted less than 1 week. Detailed ocular examination showed no differences between patients from the reference group and the three other groups.

Sarcoptes scabiei

In an uncontrolled open study 101 patients with scabies were treated with a single oral dose of ivermectin 200 micrograms/kg and then followed at 3 days and at 2 and 4 weeks (10). Two weeks after the start of treatment 89 patients were completely free of scabies, while another three had only mild lesions and pruritus with negative skin scrapings. The other nine patients had persistent pruritus and new lesions and were treated with a second dose, with a complete cure in all cases after 4 weeks. Twelve patients reported minor adverse effects, consisting of drowsiness ($n = 4$), arthralgia and bone aches ($n = 2$), dyspnea ($n = 3$), headache ($n = 1$), nausea ($n = 1$), and blurred vision ($n = 1$). The adverse effects were mostly reported at the first follow-up and were easily tolerated. Ivermectin appears to be a safe and effective treatment for scabies in a dose of 200 micrograms/kg, although a second dose is necessary for complete cure in a few patients.

- An 11-year-old girl developed severe crusted Norwegian scabies (11). Gamma-benzene hexachloride lotion and topical keratolytics had no significant effect. She was given a single oral dose of ivermectin 6 mg/kg with dramatic effect. The pruritus subsided in 4 hours and the lesions started to clear 2 days later. A second dose of 6 mg was given after 3 weeks when no skin lesions were found anymore. The only adverse effect was some edema of the skin after the first dose, which did not occur after the second dose, suggesting that the reaction was more related to the intensity of the infection then to the effect of the drug itself.

Outbreaks of scabies in elderly people require special management for disease control. Owing to the frequent failure of repeated non-synchronized therapeutic efforts with conventional external antiscabie treatments, special eradication programs are required. The management of outbreaks of scabies with allethrin, permethrin, and ivermectin has been evaluated (12). Healthy infested people ($n = 240$) were treated once simultaneously with an external scabicide, such as allethrin or permethrin; this was effective in 99%. Those with crusted scabies ($n = 12$) were hospitalized and treated with systemic ivermectin or ivermectin plus permethrin; seven patients received ivermectin twice after an interval of 8 days and one received permethrin three times. Unfortunately, no details of adverse effects were given.

Strongyloidiasis

The efficacy and adverse effects of ivermectin 200 micrograms/kg, repeated 2 weeks later, have been studied in 50 patients with chronic strongyloidiasis, aged 30–79 years (13). The eradication rate was 96% at 2 weeks after the first dose and 98% after the second dose. There was no recurrence after follow-up of 4 months. One patient had nausea and vomiting 3 hours after the first dose and again after the second dose, but they were transient and required no therapy. In four patients there were mild laboratory abnormalities (slight increases in liver function tests in two, microscopic hematuria in one, and mild leukopenia and lymphocytosis in one). Of the 50 patients 12 were positive for human T lymphotropic virus type-I.

Wuchereria bancrofti

Early-stage elephantiasis caused by bancroftian filariasis in a 27-year-old traveller was treated with a single-dose oral combination of ivermectin 24 mg plus albendazole 400 mg, followed by albendazole 800 mg for 21 days (14). To avoid a severe Mazzotti-like reaction, he was given oral glucocorticoids and antihistamines for 3 days. He had a transient rash, pruritus, and mild hypotension on the days after the initial treatment, but otherwise remained well and the swelling subsided. Within 1 month he was free of symptoms. At the last follow-up examination, 3 years after treatment, there was no clinical or laboratory evidence of relapse. The authors thought that this type of treatment should be evaluated on a wider scale, given the minimal adverse events and apparent therapeutic efficacy.

The efficacy of annual mass chemotherapy with a combination of diethylcarbamazine and ivermectin on bancroftian filariasis in rural southern India has been studied, as has the supplementary role of controlling the vector mosquito *Culex quinquefasciatus* (15). Nine villages, topographically and ecologically similar but reasonably isolated from each other, were selected and split into three comparable groups of three villages each. Group A received chemotherapy with diethylcarbamazine at about 6 mg/kg and ivermectin at 400 micrograms/kg. Group B received chemotherapy and vector control. The most important vector-breeding sites were soakage pits, which were treated with expanded polystyrene beads. Minor vector-breeding sources, such as domestic or irrigation wells, were treated by adding larvae-eating Talapia fish or a commercial insecticide based on *Bacillus sphaericus*. Group C received no intervention. After the first round of treatment, combination chemotherapy alone caused a 60% drop in the annual filarial transmission potential, whereas the combined strategy reduced the transmission potential by 96%. After two rounds of treatment, the reduction in transmission potential was similar with the two strategies (about 91–96% reduction), whereas the prevalence of microfilaremia was reduced by 88–92%. Adverse events after combination therapy were reported in 20% of those who had taken diethylcarbamazine and ivermectin for the first time. The patients with adverse events had increased microfilarial counts. The most common adverse effects were headache (72% of adverse events), giddiness (67%), fever, and weakness. The incidence of adverse events among those taking combination therapy for a second time was relatively low (5.5%). The adverse events were also less severe in the second round than in the first. When antifilarial treatment was withdrawn in the third and final year of the study, transmission was resumed in the absence of vector control, whereas no infective female mosquitoes were detected in villages with vector control. Vector control, although obviously not cost-effective in the short term, could therefore play an important supplementary role in an integrated program, by preventing re-establishment of transmission after chemotherapy has been completed.

Comparative studies

Sarcoptes scabiei

In a randomized trial a single oral dose of ivermectin (200 micrograms/kg) has been compared with 1% gamma-benzene hexachloride lotion for topical application overnight in 200 patients with scabies (16). The patients were assessed after 48 hours, 2 weeks, and 4 weeks. After 4 weeks, 83% showed marked improvement with ivermectin, compared with 44% of those treated with gamma-benzene hexachloride. There were no adverse events reported with gamma-benzene hexachloride. Headache was reported only once with ivermectin.

In 80 children aged 6 months to 14 years a single dose of ivermectin 200 micrograms/kg was compared with topical benzyl benzoate for the treatment of pediatric scabies in a randomized, controlled trial (17). Ivermectin cured 24 of 43 patients and topical benzyl benzoate cured 19 of 37 patients at 3 weeks after treatment. There were no serious adverse effects with either treatment, although benzyl benzoate was more likely to produce local skin reactions. These results are in line with those of another study, in which 18 children aged 14 months to 17 years with either scabies ($n = 11$) or cutaneous larva migrans ($n = 7$) were treated with a single dose of ivermectin 150–200 micrograms/kg (18). A single oral dose cured 15 patients, and three patients with crusted scabies required a second dose. None had significant adverse reactions.

Wuchereria bancrofti
In a study in which doses of 200 or 400 micrograms were used, with or without diethylcarbamazine, for *Wuchereria bancrofti* infection, there was a higher than average incidence of reactions (and a higher incidence with ivermectin than with diethylcarbamazine), but this perhaps reflected an unusually high success rate or the severity of the original infection (19). For similar reasons, repeated courses of treatment tend to show a falling incidence of adverse effects. Normally, such general symptoms as fever, weakness, anorexia, malaise, and chills occur in a substantial minority of patients on a first course, while at least one-third have muscle and/or joint pains. Vertigo, dyspnea, diarrhea and abdominal disturbances affect a few patients. The severity of adverse effects is not related to serum concentrations of the drug (20), which again reflects the fact that they are largely a consequence of the parasitic breakdown, rather than toxic effects of ivermectin.

Placebo-controlled studies

Emesis, ataxia, and mydriasis are cardinal signs of ivermectin toxicity. The safety, tolerability, and pharmacokinetics of escalating high-dose ivermectin have been studied in 68 healthy subjects in a randomized, double-blind, placebo-controlled study (21) in the following doses:

- 30 mg fasted ($n = 15$)
- 60 mg fasted ($n = 12$)
- 90 mg fasted ($n = 12$)
- 120 mg fasted ($n = 12$)
- 30 mg fed ($n = 11$)

Ivermectin was generally well tolerated. Quantitative pupillometry ruled out any mydriatic effect of ivermectin. There was no nervous system toxicity associated with oral ivermectin at any of the doses. There were no serious clinical or laboratory adverse events. Three of the fifty-one subjects who took ivermectin fasted reported minor adverse gastrointestinal events: fecal abnormality ($n = 1$), nausea ($n = 1$), and vomiting ($n = 1$); six reported minor neurological adverse events: headache ($n = 4$), anxiety ($n = 1$), and dizziness ($n = 1$). There were no adverse events in the subjects who took ivermectin 120 mg. The absorption of ivermectin was about 2.5 times higher when it was given after a high-fat meal.

Sarcoptes scabiei
In a randomized, double-blind comparison of the efficacy of oral ivermectin and topical gamma-benzene hexachloride 53 patients were randomly allocated to either a single oral dose of ivermectin 150–200 micrograms/kg and a placebo topical solution, or a single dose of gamma-benzene hexachloride topical solution 1% and placebo tablets (22). Patients who did not fulfil the criteria for clinical cure within 15 days, defined as the absence of both pruritus and clinical lesions or a reduction in signs and symptoms to a mild degree, repeated the initial treatment. Of the 53 patients 43 completed the study (19 of those treated with ivermectin and 24 of those treated with gamma-benzene hexachloride). After 15 days 74% of the patients treated with ivermectin and 54% of the patients treated with gamma-benzene hexachloride were considered to be cured. At 29 days both treatments were equally effective, with cure rates of 95% and 96% respectively. Adverse effects were mild and transient in both groups. One of the patients treated with ivermectin had hypotension, one had abdominal pain, one had vomiting, and one complained of headache. There were no abnormalities on routine laboratory testing.

Wuchereria bancrofti
In a double-blind, placebo-controlled study in Ghana single doses of ivermectin 150–200 micrograms/kg and albendazole 400 mg, either separately or in combination, were given to 1425 individuals for *Wuchereria bancrofti* infection (23). Of these, 340 were microfilariae-positive before treatment. Ivermectin and ivermectin plus albendazole both produced statistically significant reductions in mean microfilaria counts at follow-up; the effect of ivermectin was longer lasting. Albendazole produced a non-significant reduction. Adverse reactions were few and mostly mild, and there were no severe reactions.

General adverse effects

Acute symptoms, often flu-like or affecting the skin, are related almost entirely to the release of toxic products and allergens from the killed filariae, and can affect two-thirds of patients; in conditions in which this type of reaction does not occur one may suspect that the drug is ineffective. The mechanism of the effects also explains why they tend to occur early and sometimes briefly, that is immediately after the microfilariae die. For similar reasons, these effects are most severe in patients with a high microfilaria count (24).

Despite the sometimes transient and apparently tolerable nature of the skin effects, they can persist in patients requiring long-term treatment, for example for onchocerciasis, and under these conditions they are sufficient to impair compliance with treatment (SEDA-21, 317).

The effects of age, sex, dosing round, time of day, and distance from the nurse monitor on adverse event reporting during mass ivermectin administration in Achi in South-East Nigeria have been examined (25). There was a significant increase in adverse reporting with age, but not sex. Fewer adverse effects were reported after starting at night than after starting by day. There was no significant effect of distances up to 1 km on adverse events reporting. Both compliance and adverse reporting were less after the second dosing round than after the first. These variables should be included in the standardization of adverse events reporting.

Onchocerciasis

Although adverse reactions after ivermectin in onchocerciasis are usually less severe than after diethylcarbamazine, they still affect a significant number of patients with onchocerciasis after the first dose. With subsequent treatments, these reactions become less frequent and severe. The so-called Mazzotti reaction, which is often seen after treatment of *Onchocerca volvulus* with diethylcarbamazine or ivermectin, is characterized by fever, tachycardia, hypotension, adenitis, pruritus, arthralgia, a papular or urticarial rash, and lymphedema. It is ascribed to an inflammatory host response to microfilarial killing and tends to be more severe in those who have greater numbers of parasites. The roles of chemoattractants, such as eotaxin, RANTES, and MCP-3, in the recruitment of eosinophils to the site of parasite killing has been studied in 13 patients with onchocerciasis and two control subjects before and after ivermectin (26). There were adverse reactions in eight patients, but none were severe. The reactions were fever (54%), pruritus (62%), rash (46%), and lymphedema (46%). There was no significant postural hypotension. There was endothelial expression of both RANTES and eotaxin after ivermectin, suggesting that these chemoattractants have an important role in eosinophil recruitment into the skin during killing or degeneration of parasites after ivermectin.

A role for the release of *Wolbachia* bacterial endosymbionts has been suggested in the pathogenesis of the Mazzotti reaction (SEDA-26, 345). There was a good correlation between *Wolbachia* DNA, serum TNF-alfa, and the antibacterial peptides calprotectin and calgranulin after treatment with ivermectin or diethylcarbamazine, supporting a role for *Wolbachia* products in mediating these inflammatory responses (27).

There has been an epidemiological survey of the endemicity of human onchocerciasis and the effects of subsequent mass distribution of ivermectin in villages of the Nzerem-Ikpem community in Nigeria (28). Of 1126 people studied, 527 were positive for skin microfilariae, 329 had a leopard skin (characterized by focal skin depigmentation), 385 had nodules, and 167 had onchodermatitis. There were adverse effects in 362 patients (19%): pruritus in 13%, limb swelling in 8.5%, facial swelling in 2%, weakness in 4.8%, nausea and vomiting in 3.4%, headache in 5.8%, diarrhea in 3.4%, and rheumatism in 3.5%. There were no severe reactions.

Organs and Systems

Cardiovascular

Supine and postural tachycardia with postural hypotension can occur; in one large study, such effects were found in three of 40 patients (SEDA-14, 262) (SEDA-22, 327). In another there was hypotension in 13 of 69 cases (SEDA-20, 280), but in some series these effects have not been observed at all (SEDA-17, 356). A massive community study in Ghana noted hypotension in only 37 of nearly 15 000 patients treated (29). Transient electrocardiographic changes are sometimes seen.

Respiratory

In the treatment of *Wuchereria bancrofti* filariasis in 23 patients with single doses up to 200 micrograms/kg respiratory capacity was evaluated; there was a transient but significant fall in vital capacity some 24–30 hours after administration, apparently due to bronchodilatation (30). Frank dyspnea occurred in 2% of cases in the study cited above (3). In other studies, a few patients have developed a transient cough and in others pneumonitic patches have been seen in the chest X-ray (SEDA-18, 313).

Nervous system

Headache and vertigo are very common and even usual as part of the flu-like reaction to ivermectin.

A puzzling reaction was recorded in a small hospitalized Canadian population of elderly subjects treated for scabies with a single dose of ivermectin (150–200 micrograms/kg). Within 6 months, 15 of the 47 patients had died. All those who died had developed a sudden change in behavior, with lethargy, anorexia, and listlessness before death (31). The effect may have been an artefact with some extraneous cause, and it is notable that other groups using this treatment for scabies have not recorded similar reactions.

Loa loa encephalopathy

When treating *Loa loa* infections on a large scale with ivermectin, the encephalopathy that was a much-feared complication with diethylcarbamazine again seems to occur, especially with heavily infected or older individuals (32). For this reason, mass use of ivermectin in areas of endemic *Loa loa* infection is no longer recommended (33).

Ivermectin appears to promote the passage of *Loa loa* microfilaria into the cerebrospinal fluid, with a maximum after 3–5 days, followed by an intense allergic reaction to the dying microfilaria. The Mectizan Expert Committee defined a definite case of *Loa loa* encephalopathy related to ivermectin as having to satisfy two criteria:

1. encephalopathy in which there is microscopic evidence of vasculopathy in the brain associated with *Loa loa* microfilaria;
2. the onset of symptoms of disturbed nervous system function within 5 days after treatment with ivermectin, progressing to coma without remission.

A probable case of *Loa loa* encephalopathy was defined as having to satisfy four criteria:

1. coma in a previously healthy individual;
2. the onset of nervous system signs within 5 days of treatment with ivermectin progressing to coma;
3. an initial microfilaremia of over 10 000/ml, or 1000/ml in a blood sample taken within 2 months of treatment;
4. the presence of *Loa loa* microfilaria in the CSF.

Clinically common features of this condition are impaired consciousness appearing 3–4 days after treatment and lasting for 2–3 days.

There is no consensus on the proper management of ivermectin-associated *Loa loa* encephalopathy, and it is uncertain if co-administration of glucocorticoids is of any use. In several patients with more severe reactions, conjunctival hemorrhages were seen.

A systematic examination of the conjunctivae in 1682 patients complaining of any adverse reactions showed that these hemorrhages were closely correlated with the pretreatment microfilaria counts. This sign can be found 2 days after treatment and may thus single out patients susceptible to encephalopathy and needing closer follow-up. Although the incidence of such cases is very low (in the order of 1 in 10 000 treated patients), this serious adverse effect makes mass treatment of *Loa loa* infection problematic, and also mass treatment of onchocerciasis in areas in which *Loa loa* is endemic. To illustrate this point three probable cases of *Loa loa* encephalopathy after ivermectin treatment for onchocerciasis have been described (34). All three were young men treated with ivermectin 150 micrograms/kg in a mass-treatment campaign in onchocerciasis.

- A 26-year-old previously healthy man developed nervous system symptoms in the form of an inability to stand or eat and stiffness of the neck by the third day. On the fourth day he had difficulty swallowing and speaking. On the fifth day he could not speak and was incontinent of urine. He was given dexamethasone, diazepam, furosemide, and atropine. On the sixth day he became comatose. On the ninth day he developed a high fever, and was given penicillin and tube-feeding. His condition gradually worsened and he died on the 21st day. Serum microfilaria counts on day 13 after treatment were still high (3600/ml), and live *Loa loa* (10/ml) were found in the CSF.
- A 32-year-old man with alcoholism had a very high pretreatment serum microfilaria count (50 000/ml). After starting ivermectin he took to his bed and would not speak. On the third day he developed a fever, possibly attributed to malaria and treated with chloroquine. On the fourth day he was unable to stand, and alternately restless or somnolent; his CSF contained live *Loa loa* microfilaria. He became more incoherent and fidgety and had a marked grasp reflex. Later in the day he developed spastic hypertonia. On the fifth day he became incontinent and still would not speak. Over the following days he gradually improved and 4 months later had no neurological abnormalities, although his relatives found that his behavior had changed and that he was much calmer then in the past. An electroencephalogram on day 15 showed periodic diffuse discharges of large amplitude during hyperventilation and on day 146 an asymmetric tracing with focal activity in the right parieto-occipital area, which worsened during hyperventilation. On day 233 the electroencephalogram was normal.
- An 18-year-old previously healthy man was given ivermectin. On the second day he was unable to work and stayed at home. On the third day he was found unconscious in bed, incontinent of urine and feces. On the fourth day he did not move and had absent pain sensation. There was hypertonia in the arms with marked cogwheeling. On the fifth and sixth days there was a swinging horizontal movement of the eyeballs, but otherwise he appeared to improve. On the seventh day he could stay seated in bed with help and spoke several sentences. He could perform slow voluntary movements and his muscle strength and sensation returned to normal, although the cogwheel phenomenon still persisted. He gradually returned to normal over the following weeks. After 5 months the neurological examination was normal but he still complained of headaches and episodic amnesia. His pretreatment serum microfilaria counts were high (152 940/ml) and the CSF collected on the fourth day contained live *Loa loa* microfilaria. An electroencephalogram on the 19th day was slow with spontaneous, diffuse, paroxysmal, monomorphic theta activity, lasting 2–3 seconds. An electroencephalogram on the 105th day showed improvement, but focal abnormalities persisted in the left occipital region. On the 159th day all previously recorded abnormalities had disappeared.

Sensory systems

Careful ophthalmological examination shows a striking increase in the number of microfilariae in the anterior chamber of the eye in a significant minority of patients, and a new inflammatory infiltrate can appear during treatment in already damaged areas of the retina (SEDA-15, 334). However, no permanent ocular sequelae have been documented. Most of the other ophthalmic symptoms, including edema and local inflammation, are those of the primary infection.

Conjunctival hemorrhages have been recorded in patients living in areas in which loiasis is endemic. Although ivermectin is usually well tolerated, these patients had serious adverse reactions after taking ivermectin, including an encephalopathy similar to that seen after treatment with diethylcarbamazine. In retrospect, these cases all had high *Loa loa* microfilaremia and *Loa loa* microfilariae in the cerebrospinal fluid. The authors suggested that ivermectin might have provoked the passage of *Loa loa* microfilariae into the cerebrospinal fluid. In a subsequent study of 1682 patients with loiasis treated with ivermectin 150 micrograms/kg, conjunctival hemorrhages were found in 41, nine of whom had previously received a microfilaricidal drug (35). The initial mean *Loa loa* microfilaremia was 14 900 microfilariae/ml (range 0–182 400; median 37 500), compared with 14.5 microfilariae/ml (range 0–97 600; median 0) in those without conjunctival hemorrhage. In addition, male sex and *Dipalonema perstans* microfilaremia were associated with conjunctival hemorrhages. There was a close relation between conjunctival hemorrhages and retinal lesions. Based on observations in three patients who all developed coma after ivermectin the authors suggested that retinal lesions may reflect what occurs in the cerebral circulation in patients with high *Loa loa* microfilaremia and neurological problems after ivermectin.

Hematologic

When 28 Sudanese patients were treated with a single dose of ivermectin for onchocerciasis they developed a prolonged prothrombin time, which continued to lengthen significantly during the next 4 weeks; there were no changes in other clotting parameters (36). After a month, two of them developed hematomas, which continued to enlarge for the next 3–4 days. Both of these patients had received ivermectin 150 micrograms/kg. One was given a transfusion; the swellings in both cases resolved within a week. For a time it was considered that the prothrombin changes observed in some such cases were a potential problem; more recent work suggests that the prolongation of prothrombin ratio is in fact hardly more than with placebo, and that in fact ivermectin merely has a mild effect on vitamin K metabolism and little effect on coagulation (37). However, lymphadenitis has been noted in a few patients. In one Guatemalan study of biannual treatment of the population to eradicate *Onchocerca volvulus* infection, upper limb edema was noted in nearly 20% of cases receiving the treatment for the first time (38).

Gastrointestinal

In the late stages of *Strongyloides* hyperinfection, ileus can develop and hamper the absorption of oral medication (39).

- A 39-year-old Afro-Caribbean man with stage IVB T cell lymphoma due to HTLV-1 infection had invasive Strongyloides hyperinfection that did not respond to oral ivermectin plus albendazole because of concurrent ileus. He was treated with two 6 mg doses of a veterinary formulation of ivermectin subcutaneously. There were no adverse effects, apart from pain at the injection site.

Urinary tract

Proteinuria is unusual but has been described; it was detected 14 days after a single dose and disappeared during follow-up (SEDA-18, 313).

Observations that proteinuria and hematuria may occur in patients with filariasis bancrofti and loiasis, which may exacerbate after treatment with diethylcarbamazine or ivermectin, led to the study of kidney function in patients with onchocerciasis before and after treatment with ivermectin (40). The occurrence of renal abnormalities was studied in a population-based study in a meso-endemic village (40% microfilaria carriers), in a group of patients with a generalized or hyper-reactive form of onchocerciasis, and in 46 patients treated with ivermectin in a single oral dose of 150 micrograms/kg. All individuals in all three study groups were examined clinically and had skin snips, serological testing for onchocerciasis, and nodulectomy (when relevant). Tests for malaria, schistosomiasis, intestinal nematodes, and hepatitis B, and serum glucose, creatinine, IgE, and electrophoresis were also performed. The urine was tested for erythrocytes, leukocytes, protein, nitrites, pH, glucose, ketone bodies, urobilinogen, and creatinine. All the patients underwent renal ultrasound examination. There was no difference in renal function and renal ultrasound between patients with and without onchocerciasis. A raised urinary protein concentration (over 70 mg/g of creatinine) was common and occurred in 47% of the patients with onchocerciasis and 63% of the patients without onchocerciasis. In the 46 patients treated for onchocerciasis with a single dose of 150 micrograms/kg there was a slight but statistically significant increase in total urine protein after 2 and 5 days, especially in 16 patients with high pretreatment skin microfilaria counts. The abnormalities were minor and insignificant. Neither onchocerciasis itself nor treatment with ivermectin was associated with abnormalities of renal function.

Skin

A degree of pruritus, soreness, or burning sensation is common with ivermectin, and rashes or skin edema can occur, while pre-existing conditions of this type can be aggravated (SEDA-17, 355) (SEDA-22, 327). The skin over hematomas can be discolored. Swelling of the limbs and face, like the dermatological symptoms, is probably a reaction to breakdown products of the helminth (SEDA-20, 280).

Patients with severe skin involvement ("sowda") as a facet of their onchocerciasis can experience transient aggravation of the condition, but the course is favorable, and they are less likely to have the same problem if it is later necessary to repeat treatment (SEDA-20, 281).

Rashes and swelling of the lymph nodes seem to be more common in patients with AIDS who take ivermectin (41).

Musculoskeletal

Joint or bone pains are common but usually mild; in one study myalgia occurred in 33% of cases and arthralgia in 33% (3).

Reproductive system

Orchitis or epididymitis with scrotal tenderness occurs in a few patients as a manifestation of the acute reaction as the parasite succumbs (SEDA-17, 356) (SEDA-22, 327).

Second-Generation Effects

Teratogenicity

There is no evidence of second-generation injury from ivermectin, but it is prudent to avoid it in pregnant women.

Lactation

Only a small amount of ivermectin is excreted in the breast milk (42) and it has been suggested that it is unnecessary to exclude lactating mothers from mass chemotherapy with ivermectin.

References

1. Njoo FL, Hack CE, Oosting J, Stilma JS, Kijlstra A. Neutrophil activation in ivermectin-treated onchocerciasis patients. Clin Exp Immunol 1993;94(2):330–3.
2. Bounias M. Pragmatic efficacy against conceptual precaution in parasite control: the case of avermectins. J Environ Biol 2000;21:275–85.
3. Moulia-Pelat JP, Nguyen LN, Glaziou P, Chanteau S, Gay VM, Martin PM, Cartel JL. Safety trial of single-dose treatments with a combination of ivermectin and diethylcarbamazine in bancroftian filariasis. Trop Med Parasitol 1993;44(2):79–82.
4. Gardon J, Kamgno J, Folefack G, Gardon-Wendel N, Bouchite B, Boussinesq M. Marked decrease in Loa loa microfilaraemia six and twelve months after a single dose of ivermectin. Trans R Soc Trop Med Hyg 1997;91(5):593–4.
5. Duong TH, Kombila M, Ferrer A, Bureau P, Gaxotte P, Richard-Lenoble D. Reduced *Loa loa* microfilaria count ten to twelve months after a single dose of ivermectin. Trans R Soc Trop Med Hyg 1997;91(5):592–3.
6. Shenoy RK, George LM, John A, Suma TK, Kumaraswami V. Treatment of microfilaraemia in asymptomatic brugian filariasis: the efficacy and safety of the combination of single doses of ivermectin and diethylcarbamazine. Ann Trop Med Parasitol 1998;92(5):579–85.

7. Boussinesq M, Gardon J. Challenges for the future: loiasis. Ann Trop Med Parasitol 1998;92(Suppl 1):S147–51.
8. Kennedy MH, Bertocchi I, Hopkins AD, Meredith SE. The effect of 5 years of annual treatment with ivermectin (Mectizan) on the prevalence and morbidity of onchocerciasis in the village of Gami in the Central African Republic. Ann Trop Med Parasitol 2002;96(3):297–307.
9. Gardon J, Boussinesq M, Kamgno J, Gardon-Wendel N, Demanga-Ngangue, Duke BO. Effects of standard and high doses of ivermectin on adult worms of *Onchocerca volvulus*: a randomised controlled trial. Lancet 2002; 360(9328):203–10.
10. Molina JM, Chastang C, Goguel J, Michiels JF, Sarfati C, Desportes-Livage I, Horton J, Derouin F, Modai J. Albendazole for treatment and prophylaxis of microsporidiosis due to *Encephalitozoon intestinalis* in patients with AIDS: a randomized double-blind controlled trial. J Infect Dis 1998;177(5):1373–7.
11. Jaramillo-Ayerbe F, Berrio-Munoz J. Ivermectin for crusted Norwegian scabies induced by use of topical steroids. Arch Dermatol 1998;134(2):143–5.
12. Paasch U, Haustein UF. Management of endemic outbreaks of scabies with allethrin, permethrin, and ivermectin. Int J Dermatol 2000;39(6):463–70.
13. Zaha O, Hirata T, Kinjo F, Saito A, Fukuhara H. Efficacy of ivermectin for chronic strongyloidiasis: two single doses given 2 weeks apart. J Infect Chemother 2002;8(1):94–8.
14. Grobusch MP, Gobels K, Teichmann D, Bergmann F, Suttorp N. Early-stage elephantiasis in bancroftian filariasis. Eur J Clin Microbiol Infect Dis 2001;20(11):835–6.
15. Reuben R, Rajendran R, Sunish IP, Mani TR, Tewari SC, Hiriyan J, Gajanana A. Annual single-dose diethylcarbamazine plus ivermectin for control of bancroftian filariasis: comparative efficacy with and without vector control. Ann Trop Med Parasitol 2001;95(4):361–78.
16. Madan V, Jaskiran K, Gupta U, Gupta DK. Oral ivermectin in scabies patients: a comparison with 1% topical lindane lotion. J Dermatol 2001;28(9):481–4.
17. Brooks PA, Grace RF. Ivermectin is better than benzyl benzoate for childhood scabies in developing countries. J Paediatr Child Health 2002;38(4):401–4.
18. del Mar Saez-De-Ocariz M, McKinster CD, Orozco-Covarrubias L, Tamayo-Sanchez L, Ruiz-Maldonado R. Treatment of 18 children with scabies or cutaneous larva migrans using ivermectin. Clin Exp Dermatol 2002;27(4):264–7.
19. Addiss DG, Eberhard ML, Lammie PJ, McNeeley MB, Lee SH, McNeeley DF, Spencer HC. Comparative efficacy of clearing-dose and single high-dose ivermectin and diethylcarbamazine against *Wuchereria bancrofti* microfilaremia. Am J Trop Med Hyg 1993;48(2):178–85.
20. Njoo FL, Beek WM, Keukens HJ, van Wilgenburg H, Oosting J, Stilma JS, Kijlstra A. Ivermectin detection in serum of onchocerciasis patients: relationship to adverse reactions. Am J Trop Med Hyg 1995;52(1):94–7.
21. Guzzo CA, Furtek CI, Porras AG, Chen C, Tipping R, Clineschmidt CM, Sciberras DG, Hsieh JY, Lasseter KC. Safety, tolerability, and pharmacokinetics of escalating high doses of ivermectin in healthy adult subjects. J Clin Pharmacol 2002;42(10):1122–33.
22. Winstanley P. Albendazole for mass treatment of asymptomatic trichuris infections. Lancet 1998;352(9134):1080–1.
23. Dunyo SK, Nkrumah FK, Simonsen PE. A randomized double-blind placebo-controlled field trial of ivermectin and albendazole alone and in combination for the treatment of lymphatic filariasis in Ghana. Trans R Soc Trop Med Hyg 2000;94(2):205–11.
24. Chippaux JP, Boussinesq M, Gardon J, Gardon-Wendel N, Ernould JC. Severe adverse reaction risks during mass treatment with ivermectin in loiasis-endemic areas. Parasitol Today 1996;12(11):448–50.
25. Chijioke CP. Factors affecting adverse event reporting during mass ivermectin treatment for onchocerciasis. Acta Trop 2000;76(2):169–73.
26. Cooper PJ, Beck LA, Espinel I, Deyampert NM, Hartnell A, Jose PJ, Paredes W, Guderian RH, Nutman TB. Eotaxin and RANTES expression by the dermal endothelium is associated with eosinophil infiltration after ivermectin treatment of onchocerciasis. Clin Immunol 2000;95(1 Pt 1):51–61.
27. Keiser PB, Reynolds SM, Awadzi K, Ottesen EA, Taylor MJ, Nutman TB. Bacterial endosymbionts of *Onchocerca volvulus* in the pathogenesis of posttreatment reactions. J Infect Dis 2002;185(6):805–11.
28. Abanobi OC, Anosike JC. Control of onchocerciasis in Nzerem-Ikpem, Nigeria: baseline prevalence and mass distribution of ivermectin. Public Health 2000;114(5):402–6.
29. De Sole G, Awadzi K, Remme J, Dadzie KY, Ba O, Giese J, Karam M, Keita FM, Opoku NO. A community trial of ivermectin in the onchocerciasis focus of Asubende, Ghana. II. Adverse reactions. Trop Med Parasitol 1989;40(3):375–82.
30. Kumaraswami V, Ottesen EA, Vijayasekaran V, Devi U, Swaminathan M, Aziz MA, Sarma GR, Prabhakar R, Tripathy SP. Ivermectin for the treatment of *Wuchereria bancrofti* filariasis. Efficacy and adverse reactions. JAMA 1988;259(21):3150–3.
31. Barkwell R, Shields S. Deaths associated with ivermectin treatment of scabies. Lancet 1997;349(9059):1144–5.
32. The Mectizan Expert Committee. Central nervous complications of loiasis and adverse CNS events following treatment. Atlanta: Mectizan Donation Program, 1996.
33. Gardon J, Gardon-Wendel N, Demanga-Ngangue, Kamgno J, Chippaux JP, Boussinesq M. Serious reactions after mass treatment of onchocerciasis with ivermectin in an area endemic for Loa loa infection. Lancet 1997;350(9070):18–22.
34. Boussinesq M, Gardon J, Gardon-Wendel N, Kamgno J, Ngoumou P, Chippaux JP. Three probable cases of *Loa loa* encephalopathy following ivermectin treatment for onchocerciasis. Am J Trop Med Hyg 1998;58(4):461–9.
35. Fobi G, Gardon J, Santiago M, Ngangue D, Gardon-Wendel N, Boussinesq M. Ocular findings after ivermectin treatment of patients with high Loa loa microfilaremia. Ophthalmic Epidemiol 2000;7(1):27–39.
36. Homeida MM, Bagi IA, Ghalib HW, el Sheikh H, Ismail A, Yousif MA, Sulieman S, Ali HM, Bennett JL, Williams J. Prolongation of prothrombin time with ivermectin. Lancet 1988;1(8598):1346–7.
37. Whitworth JA, Hay CR, McNicholas AM, Morgan D, Maude GH, Taylor DW. Coagulation abnormalities and ivermectin. Ann Trop Med Parasitol 1992;86(3):301–5.
38. Collins RC, Gonzales-Peralta C, Castro J, Zea-Flores G, Cupp MS, Richards FO Jr, Cupp EW. Ivermectin: reduction in prevalence and infection intensity of *Onchocerca volvulus* following biannual treatments in five Guatemalan communities. Am J Trop Med Hyg 1992;47(2):156–69.
39. Chiodini PL, Reid AJ, Wiselka MJ, Firmin R, Foweraker J. Parenteral ivermectin in *Strongyloides* hyperinfection. Lancet 2000;355(9197):43–4.
40. Burchard GD, Kubica T, Tischendorf FW, Kruppa T, Brattig NW. Analysis of renal function in onchocerciasis patients before and after therapy. Am J Trop Med Hyg 1999;60(6):980–6.
41. Fischer P, Kipp W, Kabwa P, Buttner DW. Onchocerciasis and human immunodeficiency virus in western Uganda: prevalences and treatment with ivermectin. Am J Trop Med Hyg 1995;53(2):171–8.
42. Ogbuokiri JE, Ozumba BC, Okonkwo PO. Ivermectin levels in human breastmilk. Eur J Clin Pharmacol 1993;45(4):389–90.

IX 207-887

General Information

IX 207-887 (10-methoxy-4*H*-benzo-(4,5)-cyclohepta-(1,2–6)-thiophene-4 ylidene acetic acid) is a slow-acting drug for use in rheumatoid arthritis. Its mechanism of action involves inhibition of the release of interleukin-1. Adverse effects have occurred in 22% of cases, most commonly skin reactions, but also hepatitis and gastro-intestinal disorders (1).

Reference

1. Dougados M, Combe B, Beveridge I, Bourdeix I, Lallemand A, Amor B, Sany J. IX 207–887 in rheumatoid arthritis. A double-blind placebo-controlled study. Arthritis Rheum 1992;35(9):999–1006.

WITHDRAWN
FROM LIBRARY